CURRENT SURGICAL DIAGNOSIS & TREATMENT

current
SURGICAL
DIAGNOSIS
& TREATMENT

By

J. ENGLEBERT DUNPHY, MD

*Professor of Surgery and
Chairman, Department of Surgery
University of California School of Medicine
(San Francisco)*

LAWRENCE W. WAY, MD

*Associate Professor of Surgery
University of California School of Medicine
(San Francisco)*

And Associate Authors

Illustrated by **LAUREL V. SCHAUBERT**

Lange Medical Publications

LOS ALTOS, CALIFORNIA

1973

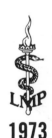

A Concise Medical Library for Practitioner and Student

Current Surgical Diagnosis & Treatment $14.00

Current Diagnosis & Treatment 1973 (12th annual revision). Edited by   1973
M.A. Krupp and M.J. Chatton. 996 pp.

Current Pediatric Diagnosis & Treatment, 2nd ed. Edited by C.H. Kempe,   1972
H.K. Silver, and D. O'Brien. 1008 pp, *illus.*

Review of Physiological Chemistry, 14th ed. H.A. Harper. 545 pp, *illus.*   1973

Review of Medical Physiology, 6th ed. W.F. Ganong. 578 pp, *illus.*   1973

Review of Medical Microbiology, 10th ed. E. Jawetz, J.L. Melnick, and   1972
E.A. Adelberg. 518 pp, *illus.*

Review of Medical Pharmacology, 3rd ed. F.H. Meyers, E. Jawetz, and   1972
A. Goldfien. 688 pp, *illus.*

General Urology, 7th ed. D.R. Smith. 436 pp, *illus.*   1972

General Ophthalmology, 6th ed. D. Vaughan, T. Asbury, and R. Cook.   1971
316 pp, *illus.*

Correlative Neuroanatomy & Functional Neurology, 15th ed. J.G. Chusid.   1973
429 pp, *illus.*

Principles of Clinical Electrocardiography, 8th ed. M.J. Goldman.   1973
400 pp, *illus.*

Handbook of Psychiatry, 2nd ed. Edited by P. Solomon and V.D. Patch.   1971
648 pp.

Handbook of Surgery, 5th ed. Edited by J.L. Wilson. About 780 pp, *illus.*   1973

Handbook of Obstetrics & Gynecology, 4th ed. R.C. Benson. 774 pp, *illus.*   1971

Physician's Handbook, 17th ed. M.A. Krupp, N.J. Sweet, E. Jawetz,   1973
E.G. Biglieri, and R.L. Roe. 728 pp, *illus.*

Handbook of Medical Treatment, 13th ed. Edited by M.J. Chatton. 648 pp. 1972

Handbook of Pediatrics, 10th ed. H.K. Silver, C.H. Kempe, and H.B. Bruyn. 1973
693 pp, *illus.*

Handbook of Poisoning: Diagnosis & Treatment, 7th ed. R.H. Dreisbach.   1971
515 pp.

Lithographed in USA

Table of Contents

Preface

This surgical text has been prepared with the needs of both medical students and practicing surgeons in mind. Each contributor has been asked to present, in as concise a manner as possible, the essential and most recent material in his field. It is hoped that the student will find in each chapter more than the core he needs to know and that the busy resident or practicing surgeon will appreciate the availability of up-to-date information on the less common conditions he may encounter and a practical recent review of everyday surgical problems for consultation, seminars, or rounds. The references are intended to serve as a guide to more complete discussions of basic or technical details.

The Editors are grateful to the contributors for their tolerant acquiescence to the alterations and deletions that were sometimes necessary in order to make the parts add up to a coherent whole.

In accordance with the policies of the publisher, the text will be translated into Spanish, and a Second Edition, with correction of the inevitable oversights, omissions, and errors, will appear within 2 years.

J. Englebert Dunphy, MD
Lawrence W. Way, MD

San Francisco, California
September, 1973

The Authors

John E. Adams, MD
Guggenheim Professor of Neurological Surgery, University of California School of Medicine (San Francisco).

Robert E. Allen, Jr., MD
Associate Clinical Professor of Surgery, University of California School of Medicine (San Francisco).

Delfin J. Beltran, MD
Clinical Assistant Professor of Anesthesia, Stanford University School of Medicine (Palo Alto).

Folkert O. Belzer, MD
Professor of Surgery, University of California School of Medicine (San Francisco).

Walter Birnbaum, MD
Clinical Professor of Surgery, University of California School of Medicine (San Francisco).

F. William Blaisdell, MD
Professor of Surgery, University of California School of Medicine (San Francisco).

Edwin B. Boldrey, MD
Professor of Neurological Surgery, University of California School of Medicine (San Francisco).

Barton A. Brown, MD
Assistant Clinical Professor of Neurological Surgery, University of California School of Medicine (San Francisco).

Jesse L. Carr, MD
Clinical Professor of Pathology & Legal Medicine Emeritus, University of California School of Medicine (San Francisco).

Norman L. Chater, MD
Associate Professor of Neurological Surgery, University of California School of Medicine (San Francisco).

Edward S. Connolly, MD
Chief, Section of Neurosurgery, Ochsner Clinic (New Orleans).

Herbert H. Dedo, MD
Associate Professor of Otolaryngology, University of California School of Medicine (San Francisco).

Alfred A. deLorimier, MD
Associate Professor of Surgery, University of California School of Medicine (San Francisco).

J. Englebert Dunphy, MD
Professor of Surgery and Chairman, Department of Surgery, University of California School of Medicine (San Francisco).

L. Henry Edmunds, Jr., MD
Associate Professor of Surgery, University of California School of Medicine (San Francisco).

William K. Ehrenfeld, MD
Assistant Professor of Surgery, University of California School of Medicine (San Francisco).

John M. Erskine, MD
Associate Clinical Professor of Surgery, University of California School of Medicine (San Francisco).

Peter H. Forsham, MD
Professor of Medicine & Pediatrics and Director of Metabolic Research Unit, University of California School of Medicine (San Francisco).

Maurice Galante, MD
Associate Professor of Surgery, University of California School of Medicine (San Francisco).

Leon Goldman, MD
Professor of Surgery Emeritus, University of California School of Medicine (San Francisco).

William P. Graham III, MD
Associate Professor of Surgery, The Milton S. Hershey Medical Center, The Pennsylvania State University College of Medicine, Hershey, Pennsylvania.

Orville F. Grimes, MD
Associate Professor of Surgery, University of California School of Medicine (San Francisco).

Neri P. Guadagni, MD
Associate Professor of Anesthesia, University of California School of Medicine (San Francisco).

Albert D. Hall, MD
Associate Clinical Professor of Surgery, University of California School of Medicine (San Francisco).

Harold A. Harper, PhD
Professor of Biochemistry, Departments of Biochemistry & Surgery, University of California School of Medicine (San Francisco).

Edward C. Hill, MD
Associate Professor of Obstetrics & Gynecology, University of California School of Medicine (San Francisco).

Yoshio Hosobuchi, MD
Assistant Professor of Neurological Surgery, University of California School of Medicine (San Francisco).

Thomas K. Hunt, MD
Associate Professor of Surgery, University of California School of Medicine (San Francisco).

Ernest Jawetz, PhD, MD
Professor of Microbiology and Chairman, Department of Microbiology, Professor of Medicine, and Lecturer in Pediatrics, University of California School of Medicine (San Francisco).

Floyd H. Jergesen, MD
Clinical Professor of Orthopedic Surgery, University of California School of Medicine (San Francisco).

Rayford Scott Jones, MD
Associate Professor of Surgery, Duke University Medical School (Durham, North Carolina).

Eugene S. Kilgore, MD
Associate Clinical Professor of Surgery, University of California School of Medicine (San Francisco).

Samuel L. Kountz, MD
Professor and Chairman, Department of Surgery, State University of New York, Downstate Medical Center (Brooklyn, New York).

Marcus A. Krupp, MD
Clinical Professor of Medicine, Stanford University School of Medicine (Palo Alto).

Robert C. Lim, Jr., MD
Associate Professor of Surgery, University of California School of Medicine (San Francisco).

Harold H. Lindner, MD
Clinical Professor of Topographical & Regional Anatomy & Surgery, University of California School of Medicine (San Francisco).

Carleton Mathewson, Jr., MD
Clinical Professor of Surgery Emeritus, University of California School of Medicine (San Francisco).

Wesley S. Moore, MD
Associate Professor of Surgery, University of California School of Medicine (San Francisco).

William J. Morris, MD
Associate Clinical Professor of Surgery, University of California School of Medicine (San Francisco).

Rowland K. Perkins, MD
Associate Clinical Professor of Neurological Surgery, University of California School of Medicine (San Francisco).

Byron C. Pevehouse, MD
Associate Professor of Neurological Surgery, University of California School of Medicine (San Francisco).

Theodore L. Phillips, MD
Professor of Radiology, University of California School of Medicine (San Francisco).

Malcolm R. Powell, MD
Assistant Professor of Radiology, University of California School of Medicine (San Francisco).

Victor Richards, MD
Clinical Professor of Surgery, University of California School of Medicine (San Francisco) and Stanford University School of Medicine (Palo Alto).

Benson B. Roe, MD
Professor of Surgery, University of California School of Medicine (San Francisco).

Theodore R. Schrock, MD
Assistant Professor of Surgery, University of California School of Medicine (San Francisco).

Robert J. Seymour, MD
Assistant Clinical Professor of Neurological Surgery, University of California School of Medicine (San Francisco).

George F. Sheldon, MD
Assistant Professor of Surgery, University of California School of Medicine (San Francisco).

Glenn E. Sheline, MD, PhD
Professor of Radiology, University of California School of Medicine (San Francisco).

Morley M. Singer, MD
Assistant Professor of Anesthesia & Medicine, University of California School of Medicine (San Francisco).

Donald R. Smith, MD
Professor of Urology and Chairman, Department of Urology, University of California School of Medicine (San Francisco).

Maurice Sokolow, MD
Professor of Medicine, University of California School of Medicine (San Francisco).

Francis A. Sooy, MD
Professor of Otolaryngology and Chairman, Department of Otolaryngology, University of California School of Medicine (San Francisco).

Samuel D. Spivack, MD
Assistant Clinical Professor of Medicine, University of California School of Medicine (San Francisco).

Emil A. Tanagho, MD
Professor of Urology, University of California School of Medicine (San Francisco).

Arthur N. Thomas, MD
Assistant Professor of Surgery, University of California School of Medicine (San Francisco).

Daniel G. Vaughan, MD
Associate Clinical Professor of Ophthalmology, University of California School of Medicine (San Francisco).

Ralph O. Wallerstein, MD
Clinical Professor of Medicine, University of California School of Medicine (San Francisco).

Lawrence W. Way, MD
Associate Professor of Surgery, University of California School of Medicine (San Francisco).

Charles B. Wilson, MD
Professor of Neurosurgery and Chairman, Department of Neurosurgery, University of California School of Medicine (San Francisco).

John L. Wilson, MD
Professor of Surgery, Stanford University School of Medicine (Palo Alto).

Edwin J. Wylie, MD
Professor of Surgery, University of California School of Medicine (San Francisco).

1...

Approach to the Surgical Patient

J. Englebert Dunphy, MD

All injuries, most congenital defects and cancers, many infections, and a substantial number of other lesions are best treated by surgery. The successful management of surgical disorders depends upon 2 equally important things: (1) the effective application of a broad knowledge of the basic sciences to the problems of diagnosis and total care before, during, and after the operation; and (2) a genuine sympathy for, understanding of, and indeed love for the patient. The surgeon must be a doctor in the old-fashioned sense, an applied scientist, an engineer, an artist, and a minister to his fellow man. Because life or death often depends upon the validity of his decisions, his judgment in reflection must be matched by courage in action and, of course, by a high degree of technical proficiency.

More mistakes are made in surgery because of failure to take an adequate history and perform a thorough physical examination than in the operative phase.

THE HISTORY

The surgeon's first contact with the patient is crucial. This is the time to gain the patient's confidence and to convince him that help is available and will be given and—above all—that the surgeon is concerned about the patient as a person who needs help and not just as a "case" to be processed through the surgical ward. This is not always easy to do, and there are no rules of conduct except to be gentle and considerate. What is most important is that the surgeon be a truly gentle and considerate man. Most patients are eager to like and trust their doctors and respond gratefully to sympathetic and affectionate words and gestures. Some surgeons are able to establish a confident therapeutic relationship with their patients with the first few words of greeting; others by means of a stylized and carefully acquired bedside manner. It does not matter how it is done so long as an atmosphere of sympathy, personal interest, and understanding is somehow created. Even in an emergency situation (unless the patient is unconscious), this subtle transmission of sympathetic concern can and does occur.

Eventually, all histories must be formally structured, but much can be learned about the patient by letting him ramble a little. Discrepancies and omissions in the history are often due as much to overstructuring and leading questions as to the unreliability of the patient. In the past, a common error the young physician made was to jump to a diagnostic conclusion early in the interview and then to make sure that what followed justified that conclusion. The enthusiastic novice asks leading questions; the cooperative patient gives the answer that seems to be wanted; and the interview concludes on a note of mutual satisfaction with the wrong answer thus derived.

BUILDING THE HISTORY

History-taking is detective work. Preconceived ideas, snap judgments, and hasty conclusions have no place in it. The diagnosis must be established by inductive reasoning. The interviewer must first determine the facts and then search for essential clues, realizing that the patient may conceal the most important symptom—eg, the passage of blood by rectum—in the hope (born of fear) that if it is not specifically inquired about or if nothing is found to account for it in the physical examination, it cannot be very serious.

Common symptoms of surgical conditions that require special emphasis in the history-taking are discussed in the following paragraphs.

Pain

A careful analysis of the nature of pain is one of the most important features of a surgical history. The examiner must first ascertain how the pain began. Was it explosive in onset, rapid, or gradual? What is the precise character of the pain? Is it so severe that it cannot be relieved by medication? Is it constant or intermittent? Are there classical associations, such as the rhythmic pattern of small bowel obstruction or the onset of pain preceding the limp of intermittent claudication?

The nature of abdominal pain is of particular importance and is dealt with in some detail in Chapter 31.

One of the most important aspects of pain is the patient's reaction to it. The overreactor's description of his pain is often obviously inappropriate. Smilingly he describes "excruciating" pain. If the patient shrieks and thrashes about, he is either grossly overreacting or suffering from renal or biliary colic. Very severe pain— due to infection, inflammation, or vascular disease— forces the patient to move as little as possible. He may writhe with pain, but he will not bounce around in the bed or climb the wall.

Moderate pain is made agonizing by fear and anxiety. Reassuring the patient and restoring his confidence are often a more effective analgesic than an injection of morphine.

Vomiting

What did the patient vomit? How much? How often? What did it look like? Was it projectile? It is especially helpful if the examiner can see the vomitus. There are many important clues which are described in detail in Chapter 31.

Change in Bowel Habits

A change in bowel habits is a common complaint that is often of no significance. However, when a person who has always had regular evacuations suddenly notices a distinct change, particularly toward intermittent constipation and diarrhea, he must be presumed to have a neoplasm of the colon. Too much emphasis is placed upon the size and shape of the stool—eg, many patients who normally have well-formed evacuations may complain of irregular small stools when their routine is disturbed by travel or a change in diet.

Passage of Blood

Bleeding from any orifice demands the most critical analysis and can never be dismissed as due to some immediately obvious cause. The most common error is to assume that bleeding from the rectum is attributable to hemorrhoids. The character of the blood can be of great significance. Does it clot? Is it bright red? Is it changed in any way, as in the coffee-ground vomitus of slow gastric bleeding or the dark, tarry stool of upper gastrointestinal hemorrhage? The full details and variations cannot be included here, but will be emphasized under separate headings elsewhere.

Trauma

Trauma occurs so commonly that it is often difficult to establish a relationship between the chief complaint and an episode of trauma. Children, in particular, are subject to all kinds of minor trauma, and the family may attribute the onset of an illness to a specific recent injury. On the other hand, children may be subjected to severe trauma and their parents be unaware of it. The possibility of trauma having been inflicted by the parent ("battered child syndrome") must not be overlooked.

When there is a history of trauma, the details must be established as precisely as possible. What was the position of the patient when the accident occurred? Did he lose consciousness? Retrograde amnesia (inability to remember events just preceding the accident) always indicates some degree of cerebral damage. If a patient can remember every detail of an accident, has not lost consciousness, and there is no evidence of external injury to the head, brain damage can be ruled out.

In the case of gunshot wounds and stab wounds, the nature of the weapon, its size and shape, the probable trajectory, and the position of the patient when hit may be very helpful in evaluating the probable nature of the resultant injury.

The possibility that an accident might have been caused by preexisting disease such as epilepsy, diabetes, coronary artery disease, or hypoglycemia must be carefully explored.

•   •   •

When all the facts and essential clues have been gathered, the examiner is in a position to complete his study of the present illness. By this time he may have been led inductively to consider only a few possible diagnoses. A third-year student, if asked the causes of shoulder pain, will include ruptured ectopic pregnancy in his thinking. The experienced physician will automatically consider the age and sex of the patient and not consider that possibility if the patient is an old man.

Family History

The family history is of great significance in a number of surgical conditions. Polyposis of the colon is a classic example, but diabetes, Peutz-Jeghers syndrome, chronic pancreatitis, multiglandular syndromes, and other endocrine abnormalities are often better understood and better evaluated in the light of a careful family history.

Past History

The details of the past history may illuminate obscure areas of the present illness. It has been said that patients who are well are almost never sick, and patients who are sick are almost never well. It is true that the patient who has a long and complicated history of diseases and injuries is likely to be a much poorer risk than even the aged patient experiencing his first major surgical illness.

In order to make certain that important details of the past history will not be overlooked, the "system review" must be formalized and thorough. By always reviewing the past history in the same way, the experienced examiner never omits a significant detail. Many skilled examiners find it easy to review the past history as they perform the physical examination, inquiring about each system as that part of the body is being examined.

In reviewing the past history, it is important to consider the nutritional background of the patient. There is an increasing awareness throughout the world that the underprivileged malnourished patient responds poorly to disease, injury, and surgery. Indeed, there is some evidence that various lesions such as carcinoma may be more fulminating in malnourished patients. Malnourishment may not be obvious on physical examination and must be elicited by questioning.

Acute nutritional deficiencies, particularly fluid and electrolyte losses, can be understood only in the light of the total (including nutritional) history. For example, a low serum sodium may be due to the use of diuretics or a sodium-restricted diet rather than to acute loss. In this connection, the use of any medications must be carefully recorded and interpreted.

A detailed history of acute losses by vomiting and diarrhea—and the nature of the losses—is helpful in estimating the probable trends in serum electrolytes. Thus, the patient who has been vomiting persistently but shows no evidence of bile in his vomitus is likely to have acute pyloric stenosis associated with benign ulcer, and hypochloremic alkalosis is to be anticipated. Chronic vomiting without bile—and particularly with evidence of changed and previously digested food—is suggestive of chronic obstruction, and the possibility of carcinoma should be considered.

It is essential for the surgeon to think in terms of nutritional balance. It is often possible to begin therapy before the results of laboratory tests have been obtained because the specific nature and probable extent of fluid and electrolyte losses can often be estimated on the basis of the history and the physician's clinical experience. Laboratory data should be obtained as soon as possible, but a knowledge of the probable level of the obstruction and of the concentration of the electrolytes in the gastrointestinal fluids will provide sufficient grounds for the institution of appropriate immediate therapy.

The management of electrolyte imbalances is discussed fully in Chapter 12.

The Patient's Emotional Background

Psychiatric consultation is seldom required in the management of surgical patients, but there are times when it is of immense help. Emotionally and mentally disturbed patients require surgical operations as often as others, and full cooperation between the psychiatrist and the surgeon is essential. On occasion, however, either before or after a surgical operation, patients develop major psychotic disturbances which are beyond the ability of the surgeon to appraise or manage. Prognosis, drug therapy, and overall management require the participation of a psychiatrist.

On the other hand, there are many situations in which the surgeon himself can and should deal with the emotional aspects of his patient's illness rather than resorting to psychiatric assistance. Most psychiatrists prefer not to be called upon to deal with minor anxiety states. As long as the surgeon accepts the responsibility for the care of the whole patient, such services are superfluous.

This is particularly true in the care of patients with malignant disease or those who must undergo mutilating operations such as amputation of an extremity, ileostomy, or colostomy. In these situations the patient can be supported far more effectively by the surgeon and the surgical team than by a consulting psychiatrist.

THE PHYSICAL EXAMINATION

The complete examination of the surgical patient includes the physical examination, certain special procedures such as gastroscopy and esophagoscopy, laboratory tests, x-ray examination, and follow-up examination. In some cases, all of these may be necessary; in others, special examinations and laboratory tests can be kept to a minimum. It is just as poor practice to insist on unnecessary "thoroughness" as it is to overlook those procedures that contribute to the diagnosis. Painful, inconvenient, and costly procedures should not be ordered unless there is a reasonable chance that the information gained will be useful in making clinical decisions.

THE ELECTIVE PHYSICAL EXAMINATION

The elective physical examination should be done in an orderly and detailed fashion. One should acquire the habit of doing the examination in exactly the same sequence with all patients, so that nothing of consequence will be overlooked. This routine must be modified, of course, in emergency situations, but the beginner should follow such a routine faithfully each time he performs a physical examination in other than emergency circumstances. This has the further advantage of familiarizing him with what is normal so that he can more readily recognize what is abnormal.

All patients are sensitive and somewhat embarrassed at being examined. It is both courteous and clinically useful to put the patient at his ease. The examining room and table should be comfortable, and drapes should be used if the patient is required to strip for the examination. Most patients will relax if they are allowed to talk a bit during the examination, and this is another reason why taking the past history while the examination is being done can be helpful.

A useful rule is to first observe the patient's general physique and habitus and then to carefully inspect his hands. Many systemic diseases show themselves in the hands (cirrhosis of the liver, hyperthyroidism, Raynaud's disease, pulmonary insufficiency, heart disease, and nutritional disorders).

The details of the examination cannot be included here, and the beginner is urged to consult special texts.

Inspection, palpation, and auscultation are the

time-honored essential steps in appraising both the normal and the abnormal. Comparison of the 2 sides of the body often suggests a specific abnormality. The slight droop of one eyelid that is characteristic of Horner's syndrome can only be recognized by careful comparison with the opposite side. Inspection of the female breasts, particularly as the patient raises and lowers her arms, will often reveal slight dimpling indicative of an infiltrating carcinoma which is barely detectable on palpation.

Successful palpation requires skill and gentleness. Spasm, tension, and anxiety caused by painful examination procedures may make an adequate examination almost impossible—particularly in children. Another important feature of palpation is the "laying on of hands" that has been called part of the "ministry of medicine." A disappointed and critical patient often will say of a doctor, "He hardly touched me—no wonder he made a mistake." Careful, precise, and gentle palpation not only gives the physician the information that he needs, but the manner in which he does it inspires confidence and trust.

When examining for areas of tenderness, it may be necessary to use only one finger in order to precisely localize the extent of the tenderness. This is of particular importance in examination of the acute abdomen. (See Chapter 31 for details.)

Auscultation, once thought to be the exclusive province of the physician, is now more important in surgery than it is in medicine. Radiologic examinations, including cardiac catheterization, have relegated auscultation of the heart and lungs to the status of preliminary scanning procedures in medicine. In surgery, however, auscultation of the abdomen and peripheral vessels has become absolutely essential. The nature of ileus and the presence of a variety of vascular lesions are revealed by auscultation. Bizarre abdominal pain in a young woman can easily be ascribed to hysteria or anxiety on the basis of "a negative physical examination and x-rays of the gastrointestinal tract." Auscultation of the epigastrium, however, may reveal a murmur due to severe obstruction of the celiac artery.

Examination of the Body Orifices

Complete examination of the ears, mouth, rectum, and pelvis is accepted as a part of a complete examination. Palpation of the mouth and tongue is as essential as inspection. Inspection of the rectum with a sigmoidoscope is now regarded as part of a complete physical examination. Every surgeon should acquire a familiarity with the use of the ophthalmoscope and sigmoidoscope and should use them regularly in doing complete physical examinations.

THE EMERGENCY PHYSICAL EXAMINATION

In an emergency, the routine of the physical examination must be altered to fit the circumstances.

The history may be limited to a single sentence, or there may be no history if the patient is unconscious and there are no other informants. Although the details of an accident or injury may be very useful in the total appraisal of the patient, they must be left for later consideration. The primary considerations are the following: Is the patient breathing? Is the airway open? Is there a palpable pulse? Is his heart beating? Is he bleeding massively?

If the patient is not breathing, airway obstruction must be ruled out by thrusting the fingers into the mouth and pulling the tongue forward. If the patient is unconscious, the respiratory tract should be intubated and mouth-to-mouth respiration started. If there is no pulse or heartbeat, cardiac resuscitation must be started.

The details of establishing and maintaining artificial respiration and external cardiac massage are described in Chapter 23.

The next consideration is to be sure that there is no serious external loss of blood which can be controlled by elevation of an extremity and local pressure over the wound. Tourniquets are rarely required.

Every victim of major blunt trauma should be suspected of having a vertebral injury capable of causing damage to the spinal cord if he is inappropriately manipulated.

Some types of emergencies are so threatening to life that action must be taken even before the surgeon can pause to verify patency of the airway and cardiac action or examine for massive external bleeding. Penetrating wounds of the heart, large open sucking wounds of the chest, and massive crush injuries with flail chest all require emergency treatment before any further examination can be done.

In most emergencies, however, after it has been established that the airway is open, the heart is beating, and there is no massive external hemorrhage—and after antishock measures have been instituted if necessary—a rapid survey examination must be done. Failure to perform such an examination can lead to serious mistakes in the care of the patient. It takes no more than 2 or 3 minutes to carefully examine the head, thorax, abdomen, extremities, genitalia (particularly in females), and back. If possible cervical cord damage has been ruled out, it is essential to turn the injured patient and carefully inspect his back, buttocks, and perineum.

Tension pneumothorax and cardiac tamponade may easily be overlooked if there are multiple injuries (eg, of the extremities).

Upon completion of the survey examination, control of pain, splinting of fractured limbs, suturing of lacerations, and other types of emergency treatment can be started.

LABORATORY & OTHER EXAMINATIONS

Laboratory Examination

Laboratory examinations in surgical patients have 3 main objectives: (1) screening for asymptomatic diseases that may affect the surgical result (eg, unsuspected anemia or diabetes); (2) appraisal of diseases that may contraindicate elective surgery or require treatment before surgery (eg, diabetes, heart failure); and (3) diagnosis of disorders that require surgery (eg, hyperparathyroidism).

Patients undergoing major surgery, even though they seem to be in excellent health except for their surgical disease, should have a complete blood and urine examination. A history of renal, hepatic, or heart disease requires detailed studies. Latent, asymptomatic renal insufficiency may be missed since many patients with chronic renal disease have varying degrees of nitrogen retention without proteinuria. A fixed urine specific gravity is easily overlooked, and preoperative determination of the BUN and creatinine is frequently required. Patients who have had hepatitis may have no jaundice but may have severe hepatic insufficiency that can be precipitated into acute failure by blood loss or shock.

Medical consultation is frequently required in the total preoperative appraisal of the surgical patient, and there is no more rewarding experience than the thorough evaluation of a patient with heart disease or gastrointestinal disease by a physician and a surgeon working together. It is essential, however, that the surgeon not become totally dependent upon his medical consultant for the preoperative evaluation and management of the patient. The total management must be his responsibility, and he cannot delegate it. Moreover, the surgeon is the only one with the experience and background to interpret the meaning of laboratory tests in the light of other features of the case—particularly the history and physical findings.

Radiologic Examination

Modern patient care calls for a variety of critical radiologic examinations. The closest cooperation between the radiologist and the surgeon is essential if serious mistakes are to be avoided. This means that the surgeon must not refer the patient to the radiologist, requesting a particular examination, without providing him with an adequate account of the history and physical findings. Particularly in emergency situations, review of the films and consultation are needed.

When the radiologic diagnosis is not definitive, the examinations must be repeated in the light of the history and physical examination. Despite the great accuracy of x-ray diagnosis, a negative gastrointestinal study still does not exclude either ulcer or a neoplasm; particularly in the right colon, small lesions are easily overlooked. At times the history and physical findings are so clearly diagnostic that an operation is justifiable despite negative x-ray findings.

Special Examinations

Special examinations such as cystoscopy, gastroscopy, esophagoscopy, colonoscopy, and bronchoscopy are often required in the diagnostic appraisal of surgical disorders. The surgeon must be familiar with the indications and limitations of these procedures and be prepared to consult with his colleagues in medicine and the surgical specialties as required.

• • •

THE PROBLEM-ORIENTED RECORD

The history and physical examination and the x-ray and laboratory studies provide the "data base" underlying the diagnosis and the surgeon's plan for the care of the patient.

The **problem-oriented record** is becoming the most accepted and reliable way in which to document and program management. It also lends itself to reliable peer review. According to this system, the word problem represents the most specific generalization available at any given time that will summarize the clinical data. It may be the name of a disease but often is less specific, indicating the diagnostic uncertainty that still exists. Management focuses on the problems, which should either be further defined by obtaining more data if necessary or resolved by appropriate therapy. Progress notes relate to each specific problem and are recorded as narrative notes and on flow sheets. The problem-oriented record is an improved logical and chronologic documentation of the care of the patient.

• • •

General References

Clain A (editor): *Bailey's Demonstrations of Physical Signs in Clinical Surgery*, 14th ed. Williams & Wilkins, 1967.

Dunphy JE, Botsford TW: *Physical Examination of the Surgical Patient*, 3rd ed. Saunders, 1964.

Morgan WL, Engel GL: *The Clinical Approach to the Patient*. Saunders, 1969.

Shackelford RT: *Diagnosis of Surgical Diseases*. 3 vols. Saunders, 1968.

Weed LL: *Medical Records, Medical Education, and Patient Care: The Problem Oriented Record as a Basic Tool*. Year Book, 1971.

2 . . .

Preoperative Care

John L. Wilson, MD, & Delfin J. Beltran, MD

The care of the patient with a major surgical problem commonly involves distinct phases of management which occur in the following sequence:

(1) Preoperative care
   Diagnostic work-up
   Preoperative evaluation
   Preoperative preparation
(2) Anesthesia and operation
(3) Postoperative care
   Postanesthetic observation
   Intensive care
   Intermediate care
   Convalescent care

Preoperative Care

The **diagnostic work-up** is concerned primarily with determining the cause and extent of the present illness. **Preoperative evaluation** consists of an overall assessment of the patient's general health in order to identify significant abnormalities which might increase operative risk or adversely influence recovery. **Preoperative preparation** includes treatments and procedures dictated by the findings on diagnostic work-up and preoperative evaluation and by the nature of the expected operation.

Postoperative Care

The **postanesthetic observation** phase of management comprises the few hours immediately after operation during which the acute reaction to surgery and the residual effects of anesthesia are subsiding. Patients who have had severe operations or whose general condition is precarious for other reasons should be transferred from the recovery room to an "intensive care unit." Duration of stay in an intensive care unit may vary from 1–2 days to many weeks depending upon the condition of the patient.

Large general hospitals now usually have a variety of specialized intensive care units adapted to the needs of medical, surgical, and pediatric patients. Intensive surgical care can of course be provided on a regular nursing unit by mobilizing the necessary personnel and equipment when needed by individual patients. If there is a constant census of 5–10 critically ill patients, it is more efficient and effective to establish an intensive care unit.

It should be noted that not all postoperative patients require intensive care. Uncomplicated operations for hernia, appendicitis, anal conditions, and other problems of similar magnitude ordinarily require only a few days of hospitalization and an intermediate level of care on a regular nursing unit.

Postoperative **intermediate care** can be described as that normally available on the regular nursing units of the hospital. This type of care, and the **convalescent care** provided to the ambulatory patient outside the hospital, will not be reviewed here because they pose no special problems not touched on in the following chapters on postanesthetic and intensive care or in Chapter 4.

The Continuum of Surgical Care

The continuum of surgical care has been represented above as progressing through a series of pre- and postoperative phases. In practice, these phases merge, overlap, and vary in relative importance from patient to patient. Morbidity, mortality, and therapeutic end result in the surgical patient depend upon the competence with which each succeeding phase is managed. The rapid progression and severe episodic stress of major surgical illness leave small margin for errors of management. The care immediately preceding and following operation, which includes preoperative evaluation and preparation and postanesthetic observation and intensive care, is especially critical. Improved surgical results in recent years are due chiefly to improvements in the management of these important phases of surgical care.

PREOPERATIVE EVALUATION

General Health Assessment

The initial diagnostic work-up of the surgical patient is concerned chiefly with determining the cause of the presenting complaints. Except in strictly minor surgical illness, this initial work-up should be supplemented by a complete assessment of the patient's general health. Such an evaluation, which should be completed prior to all major operations, seeks to identify abnormalities which may influence surgical risk or which may have a bearing on the patient's future well-being. Preoperative evaluation thus involves a comprehensive examination and should include at least a complete history and physical examination, urinalysis, complete blood count, serology, and chest x-ray. In patients over 40, it is advisable also to obtain an electrocardiogram, stool test for occult blood, and blood chemistry screening battery. Open wounds and infections usually require culture and determination of antibiotic sensitivity.

In addition to the foregoing studies, all significant specific complaints and physical findings should be adequately evaluated by appropriate special tests, examinations, and consultations. Bleeding tendencies, medications currently being taken, and allergies and reactions to antibiotics and other agents should be noted and prominently displayed on the chart. Psychiatric consultation is advisable in patients with a past history of significant mental disorder which may be exacerbated by surgery and in patients whose complaints may have a psychoneurotic basis.

Certain portions of the normal complete physical examination should always be included in examination of the surgical patient, eg, peripheral arterial pulses (carotid, radial, femoral, popliteal, posterior tibial, and dorsalis pedis). A rectal examination should always be done and a pelvic examination should be performed unless contraindicated by age, marital status, or other valid reason. Sigmoidoscopy is required for completeness of evaluation when there are rectal or colonic complaints. This can usually be accomplished at the time of the physical examination; if necessary, the rectum and lower sigmoid can be rapidly cleared by administration of a hypertonic sodium phosphate enema.

In summary, the preoperative evaluation should be sufficiently comprehensive to assess the patient's overall state of health, to determine the risk of the impending surgical treatment, and to guide the preoperative preparation.

Nonsurgical Diseases Affecting Operative Risk

Nonsurgical disorders frequently increase the risk of surgical procedures. An analysis of the causes of surgical mortality shows that fatal complications are often related to preexisting organic disease, particularly of the cardiovascular, respiratory, and genitourinary systems (see Chapter 5).

Other Factors Affecting Operative Risk

A. **The Pediatric Patient:** See Chapter 49.

B. **The Elderly Patient:** Operative risk should be judged on the basis of physiologic rather than chronologic age, and an elderly patient should not be denied a needed operation because of his age alone. The hazard of the average major operation for the patient over 60 is increased only slightly provided there is no cardiovascular, renal, or other serious systemic disease. Assume that every patient over 60—even in the absence of symptoms and physical signs—has generalized arteriosclerosis and potential limitation of myocardial and renal reserve. Accordingly, the preoperative evaluation should be comprehensive. Occult cancer is not infrequent in this age group; therefore, even minor gastro-

intestinal and other complaints should be thoroughly investigated.

Administer intravenous fluids with care not to overload the circulation in the elderly. Monitoring of intake, output, body weight, serum electrolytes, and central venous pressure is an important means of evaluating the cardiorenal response and tolerance in this age group.

Regarding medications, aged patients generally require smaller doses of strong narcotics and are frequently depressed by routine doses. Codeine is usually tolerated. Sedative and hypnotic drugs often cause restlessness, mental confusion, and uncooperative behavior in the elderly and should be used cautiously. Preanesthetic medications should be limited to atropine or scopolamine in the debilitated elderly patient, and anesthetic agents should be administered in minimal amounts.

C. **The Obese Patient:** Obese surgical patients have a greater than normal tendency to serious concomitant disease and a higher incidence of postoperative wound and thromboembolic complications. Obesity also usually increases the technical difficulty of surgery and anesthesia. For these reasons, it may at times be advisable to delay elective surgery until the patient loses weight by appropriate dietary measures.

D. **The Pregnant Patient:** See Chapter 5.

E. **The Compromised or Altered Host:** A patient may be considered a "compromised or altered host" if the capacity of his systems and tissues to respond normally to infection and trauma has been significantly impaired by some disease or agent. Preoperative recognition and special evaluation of these patients is obviously important.

1. **Increased susceptibility to infection**—Certain drugs may reduce the patient's resistance to infection by interfering with host defense mechanisms. Corticosteroids, immunosuppressive agents, cytotoxic drugs, and prolonged antibiotic therapy are associated with an increased incidence of invasion by fungi and other organisms not commonly encountered in infections. A combination of irradiation and corticosteroid therapy is found experimentally to produce lethal fungal infections. It is possible that the synergistic combination of irradiation, corticosteroids, and serious underlying disease may set the stage for clinical fungal infection. A high rate of wound, pulmonary, and other infections is seen in renal failure, presumably due to decreased host resistance. Granulocytopenia and diseases which may produce immunologic deficiency—eg, lymphomas, leukemias, and hypogammaglobulinemia—are frequently associated with septic complications. The uncontrolled diabetic is also observed clinically to be more susceptible to infection (see Chapter 5).

2. **Delayed wound healing**—This problem can be anticipated in certain categories of patients whose tissue repair process may be compromised. Many factors have been alleged to influence wound healing. However, only a few are of possible clinical significance. These include protein depletion, ascorbic acid

deficiency, marked dehydration or edema, and severe anemia. It has been shown experimentally that hypovolemia, vasoconstriction, increased blood viscosity, and increased intravascular aggregation and erythrostasis due to remote trauma will interfere with wound healing, probably by reducing oxygen tension and diffusion within the wound. Large doses of corticosteroids have been shown to depress wound healing in animals. This effect is apparently increased by mild starvation and protein depletion. Humans appear to react similarly to corticosteroid excess, and it is therefore reasonable to assume that wounds in patients who have received appreciable doses of corticosteroid preoperatively should be closed with special care to prevent disruption and managed postoperatively as though healing will be delayed.

Surgery may be required on a patient receiving cancer chemotherapy with cytotoxic drugs. These drugs usually interfere with cell proliferation and (theoretically at least) tend to decrease the tensile strength of the surgical wound. Although experimental evidence to support this assumption is equivocal, it is wise to manage wounds in patients receiving cytotoxic drugs as though healing will be slower than normal. Slow healing and decreased tensile strength during the healing stage are sometimes observed clinically in debilitated patients such as those with advanced cancer, renal failure, gastrointestinal fistulas, and chronic infection. Protein and other nutritional deficiencies are doubtless the chief cause of the sluggish wound repair. Preoperative assessment and correction of nutritional depletion may serve to minimize troublesome wound complications in such cases. On the whole, systemic factors are infrequently the cause of delayed wound healing because the healing wound receives high priority in the body economy of even the aged or depleted patient for the protein, catalysts, and other resources which are required for collagen synthesis and deposition. This knowledge serves to emphasize the paramount importance of adhering strictly to basic surgical principles in the creation, closure, and care of wounds.

Decreased vascularity and other local changes occur after a few weeks or months in tissues which have been heavily irradiated. These are potential deterrents to wound healing, a point which should be kept in mind in planning surgical incisions in patients who have been irradiated. Radiation therapy at levels of 3000 R and above are injurious to the skin and to connective and vascular tissues. Chronic changes include scarring, damage to fibroblasts and collagen, and degenerative changes with subsequent hyalinization in the walls of blood vessels. Capillary budding in granulation tissue and collagen formation are inhibited when these changes are well established, so that surgical wounds in heavily irradiated tissues may heal slowly or may break down in the presence of infection. When therapeutic doses of radiation are used as a surgical adjunct, it is generally agreed that there is an optimal delay period to minimize wound complications. This optimal period is 2–12 weeks after comple-

tion of the radiation therapy. In general, technical problems in correctly timed operations for cancer are not increased by low-dosage (2000–4000 R) adjunctive radiotherapy. With radiation dosage in the therapeutic range (5000–6000 R), increased wound complications can be expected although these can be minimized by careful surgical technic and proper timing.

F. Drug Effects: The surgical patient who is being evaluated and prepared for a major operation is about to face a formidable series of stresses in the course of which he will probably receive a variety of potent medications. Drug allergies, sensitivities, and incompatibilities and adverse drug effects which may be precipitated by surgery must be foreseen and, if possible, prevented. A history of skin or other untoward reaction or sickness after injection, oral administration, or other use of any of the following substances should be noted so that they may be avoided.

> Penicillin or other antibiotic
> Morphine, codeine, meperidine, or other narcotic
> Procaine or other anesthetic
> Aspirin or other analgesic
> Barbiturates
> Sulfonamides
> Tetanus antitoxin or other serums
> Iodine, thimerosal (Merthiolate), or other germicide
> Any other medication
> Any foods such as eggs, milk, or chocolate
> Adhesive tape

A personal or strong familial history of asthma, hay fever, or other allergic disorder should alert the surgeon to possible hypersensitivity to drugs.

Drugs currently or recently taken by the patient may require continuation, dosage adjustment, or discontinuance. Medications such as digitalis, insulin, and corticosteroids must usually be maintained and their dosage carefully regulated during the operative and postoperative periods. Prolonged use of corticosteroids such as cortisone (even though discontinued 1 month or more preoperatively) may be associated with hypofunction of the adrenal cortex, which impairs the physiologic responses to the stress of anesthesia and surgery. Such a patient should receive a corticosteroid immediately before, during, and after surgery. Anticoagulant drugs are an example of a medication to be strictly monitored or eliminated preoperatively.

The anesthesiologist is concerned with the long-term preoperative use of CNS depressants (eg, barbiturates, opiates, and alcohol), which may be associated with increased tolerance for anesthetic drugs; tranquilizers (eg, phenothiazine derivatives such as chlorpromazine); and antihypertensive agents (eg, rauwolfia derivatives such as reserpine), which may be associated with hypotension in response to anesthesia.

Consultations

The opinion of a qualified consultant should be

obtained when it may be of benefit to the patient, when requested by the patient or his family, or when it may be of medicolegal importance. The physician should take the initiative in arranging consultation when the treatment proposed is controversial or exceptionally risky, when dangerous complications occur, or when he senses that the patient or his family is unduly apprehensive regarding the plan of management or the course of events. Consultation with cardiac or other medical or surgical specialists preoperatively is important if the patient has abnormal findings in their fields of competence. It is also beneficial for the specialist consultant to become acquainted with the patient and his condition preoperatively when the possibility exists that the consultant will be called upon for advice later in connection with a postoperative complication or development.

Anesthesia consultation is always requested prior to major surgery if an anesthesiologist is available. In poor-risk patients, this consultation should be requested several days in advance of operation if possible. The patient's prospects for a smooth and uncomplicated anesthesia are greatly improved by the anesthesiologist's preoperative evaluation and advice. Respiratory, cardiovascular, and other complications related to anesthesia are forestalled or minimized when the anesthesiologist has an opportunity to adapt the anesthesia to the patient's special circumstances. When an anesthesiologist is available for preoperative consultation, he will usually write the orders for premedication, for the withholding of oral intake, and for other measures which relate directly to the anesthesia. When an anesthesiologist is not available, preanesthetic orders are written by the surgeon in accordance with the principles discussed in Chapter 14.

Preoperative Note

When the diagnostic work-up and preoperative evaluation have been completed, all details should be reviewed and a "preoperative note" written in the chart. This is usually done on the day before the operation. The note summarizes the pertinent findings and decisions and gives the indications for the operation proposed. This constitutes a final check on the adequacy of the analysis of the patient's problem and his need for treatment.

PREOPERATIVE PREPARATION

Major operations create surgical wounds and cause severe stress, subjecting the patient to the hazard of infection and metabolic and other derangements. Appropriate preoperative preparation facilitates wound healing and systemic recovery by making certain that the patient's condition at operation is optimal. Surgery also results in psychic trauma to the patient and his family and has significant medicolegal implications, all of which deserve special consideration preoperatively to avoid postoperative repercussions. In emergency conditions, time for preparation is limited but is usually sufficient to permit the principles of good surgical preparation to be followed. In elective surgery, meticulous preoperative preparation is both possible and mandatory and will normally include the following steps.

Informing the Patient

Surgery is a frightening prospect for the patient and his family. Their psychologic preparation and reassurance should begin at the initial contact with the surgeon. Appropriate explanation of the nature and purpose of preoperative studies and treatments establishes confidence. When all pertinent information has been gathered, it is the surgeon's responsibility to describe the planned surgical procedure and its risks and possible consequences in understandable terms to the patient and usually also to his next of kin. Similarly, prompt postoperative interpretation of pertinent findings and prospects to the patient and his family contributes to rapport and to intelligent cooperation during the recovery period.

Operative Permit

The patient or his legal guardian must sign (in advance) a permit authorizing a major or minor operation or a procedure such as thoracentesis, lumbar puncture, or sigmoidoscopy. The nature, risk, and probable result of the operation or procedure must be made clear to the patient or a legally responsible relative or guardian so that the signed permit will constitute "informed consent." A signed consent is not ordinarily valid except for the specific operation or procedure for which it was obtained.

Therapeutic abortions and operations which adversely affect the sexual or childbearing functions should usually be undertaken only with the concurrence in writing of the marital partner. It may not be required in a particular state or jurisdiction that the husband give his consent, but it is generally desirable that he be informed of the proposed procedure and its effects.

Emergency, lifesaving operations or procedures may have to be done without a permit. In such cases, every effort should be made to obtain adequate consultation, and the director of the hospital should be informed in advance if possible.

Legal and institutional requirements regarding permits vary. It is essential that the physician know and follow local specifications.

Preoperative Orders

On the day before surgery, orders are written which assure completion before operation of the final steps in the preparation of the patient. These orders will usually include the following:

A. Skin Preparation: See p 13.

B. Diet: Omit solid foods for 12 hours and fluids for 8 hours preoperatively. Special orders are written for diabetics and for infants and children.

C. Enema: Enemas need not be given routinely. Patients with well-regulated bowel habits do not require a preoperative enema except in the case of operations on the colon, rectum, and anal regions or operations (chiefly abdominal) likely to be followed by paralytic ileus and delayed bowel function.

Constipated patients and those scheduled for the above types of operations should be given a flushing enema 8–12 hours preoperatively with 500–1500 ml of warm tap water or, preferably, physiologic saline, or with 120–150 ml of hypertonic sodium phosphate solution conveniently available in a commercial kit (Travad Enema, Fleet Enema). Tap water enemas are contraindicated in congenital megacolon because of the danger of excessive water absorption. When thorough cleansing of the bowel is not essential, satisfactory evacuation on the evening before operation can usually be accomplished by use of a 10 mg bisacodyl (Dulcolax) rectal suppository. A hypertonic sodium phosphate enema or bisacodyl rectal suppository is also effective in the rapid preparation of the colon and rectum for sigmoidoscopy.

D. Bedtime and Preanesthetic Medication: If the anesthesia is to be given by a physician anesthesiologist, he will usually examine the patient and write the premedication order. If not, follow the guidelines laid down in Chapter 14.

E. Special Orders: In addition to the above more or less routine preoperative orders required for most major operative procedures, additional special orders related to the type and severity of the operation should be written. Antibiotic prophylaxis is discussed in Chapter 10. Other examples are given below.

1. Blood transfusion–If blood transfusions may be needed during or after operation, have the patient typed and arrange for a sufficient number of units to be cross-matched and available prior to operation.

2. Nasogastric tube–A nasogastric tube on suction is usually advisable after operations on the gastrointestinal tract to prevent distention due to paralytic ileus. If the patient has gastrointestinal obstruction with possible gastric residual, a nasogastric tube is passed preoperatively and the stomach aspirated or placed on continuous suction to reduce the possibility of regurgitation and aspiration during induction of anesthesia. If an emergency operation is to be undertaken on a patient who has eaten within the past 8–12 hours, lavage of the stomach with a large-bore Ewald tube followed by insertion of a nasogastric tube should be considered. When there is no indication for nasogastric intubation prior to surgery and the patient is to be under general anesthesia, the anesthesiologist can pass the tube into the stomach after the patient is unconscious.

3. Bladder catheter–If urinary retention or a need for hourly monitoring of urinary output postoperatively is anticipated, a Foley catheter is inserted for constant bladder drainage. If bladder distention will interfere with exposure in the pelvis (eg, during abdominoperineal resection), a catheter should be placed preoperatively. Catheterization can be done on the nursing unit just before the patient leaves for the operating room or after he has been anesthetized.

4. Venous or arterial catheter–Operations associated with marked blood loss call for preoperative placement of one or two 14 or 16 gauge intravenous plastic catheters for rapid administration of blood, fluids, or medication. Percutaneous insertion is usually possible; if not, a cutdown should be done to expose a vein, usually the antecubital. Central venous pressure monitoring may be required for assessment of the circulation during certain procedures such as complicated cardiovascular and pulmonary operations. For central venous pressure determination, a catheter should be passed into the superior vena cava via the subclavian or internal jugular vein (see Chapter 52). Arterial catheterization or cannulation, usually of the radial or brachial artery, is done primarily for monitoring blood pressure and obtaining blood gas measurements during and after operation in selected patients in whom repeated, accurate measurement of these parameters is essential. Central venous and arterial catheterization can usually be deferred until the patient is anesthetized.

5. Continuing medications–Certain patients will be receiving continuing medications whose dosage or route of administration must be altered as the result of operation. Insulin and corticosteroids are examples of hormone preparations requiring special preoperative orders. Digitalis, other cardiac drugs, antibiotics, etc may require shift to parenteral route of administration and altered dosage in the immediate preoperative period and during operation. Foresight in the adjustment of medication orders will minimize the possibility of under- or overdosage of potent and essential drugs.

6. Prophylactic antibiotics–See Chapter 10.

Asepsis & Antisepsis in the Prevention of Wound Infection

The protection of the surgical patient from infection is a primary consideration throughout the preoperative, operative, and postoperative phases of care. The factor of host resistance that influences the individual patient's susceptibility to infection has been discussed above. The incidence and severity of infection, particularly wound sepsis, are related also to the bacteriologic status of the hospital environment and to the care with which basic principles of asepsis, antisepsis, and surgical technic are implemented. The entire hospital environment must be protected from undue bacterial contamination in order to avoid colonization and cross-infection of surgical patients with virulent strains of bacteria which will invade surgical wounds in the operating room in spite of aseptic precautions taken during surgery. Prevention of wound infection therefore involves both application of general concepts and technics of antisepsis and asepsis in the hospital at large, and the use of specific procedures in preparation for operation.

A. Sterilization: The only completely reliable methods of sterilization in wide current use are by steam under pressure (autoclaving), by dry heat, and by ethylene oxide gas.

1. Autoclaving—Saturated steam at a pressure of 750 mm Hg (14.5 lb/sq inch above atmospheric pressure) at a temperature of 120 C (248 F) destroys all vegetative bacteria and most resistant dry spores in 13 minutes. Additional time (usually a total of 30 minutes) must be allowed for the penetration of heat and moisture into the centers of packages. Sterilization time is markedly shortened by the high-vacuum or high-pressure autoclaves now widely used.

2. Dry heat—Exposure to continuous dry heat at 170 C (338 F) for 1 hour will sterilize articles which would be spoiled by moist heat or which are more conveniently kept dry. If grease or oil is present on instruments, safe sterilization calls for 4 hours' exposure at 160 C (320 F).

3. Gas sterilization—Liquid and gaseous ethylene oxide as a sterilizing agent will destroy bacteria, viruses, molds, pathogenic fungi, and spores. It is also flammable and toxic, and will cause severe burns if it comes in contact with the skin. Gas sterilization with ethylene oxide is an excellent method for sterilization of most heat-sensitive materials, including telescopic instruments, plastic and rubber goods, sharp and delicate instruments, and miscellaneous items such as electric cords and sealed ampules. It has largely replaced soaking in antiseptics as a means of sterilizing materials that cannot withstand autoclaving. Care must be exercised in selecting items for gas sterilization because chemical interaction may occur with ethylene oxide or the agent with which it is mixed. For example, some acrylic plastic materials, polystyrene, certain lensed instruments, and pharmaceuticals may be damaged by ethylene oxide. Gas sterilization is normally carried out in a pressure vessel (gas autoclave) at slightly elevated pressure and temperature. It requires 1¾ hours for sterilization in a gas autoclave utilizing a mixture of 12% ethylene oxide and 88% dichlorodifluoromethane (Freon 12) at a temperature of 55 C (131 F) and a pressure of 410 mm Hg (8 lb/sq inch above atmospheric pressure). Following sterilization, a variable period of time is required for dissipation of the gas from the materials sterilized. Solid metal or glass items such as knives, drills, and thermometers may be used immediately following sterilization. Lensed instruments and packs including cloth, paper, rubber, and other porous items must usually be kept on the shelf exposed to air for 24—48 hours before use. Certain types of materials or complex instruments, such as a cardiac pacemaker, may require 7 days of exposure to air before use.

4. Boiling—Instruments should be boiled only if autoclaving, dry heat, or gas sterilization is not available. The minimum period for sterilization in boiling water is 30 minutes at altitudes less than 300 meters. At higher altitudes, the period of sterilization must be increased. The addition of alkali to the sterilizer increases bactericidal efficiency by raising pH so that sterilization time can safely be decreased to 15 minutes.

5. Soaking in antiseptics—Sterilization by soaking is rarely indicated and should never be relied upon if steam autoclaving, dry heat, or gas sterilization is suitable and available. Under some circumstances, it may be necessary or more convenient to sterilize lensed or delicate cutting instruments by soaking in a liquid germicide. A wide variety of such germicides are available. The liquid disinfectant of current choice for lensed instruments and certain other critical items which should be sterile when used is glutaraldehyde in 2% aqueous alkaline concentration (Cidex). This solution is bactericidal and virucidal in 10 minutes and sporicidal within 3 hours.

B. Antiseptics: Antiseptics are chemical agents which kill bacteria or arrest their growth; they may or may not be sporicidal. Antiseptics should not be used in wounds since their toxicity to host cells far outweighs the possible advantages of their antibacterial effect. Many new and more versatile antiseptics have been developed in recent years. The most promising of these are discussed below.

1. Antiseptics for general utility purposes—Soap solution is one of the best all-purpose cleansing agents, but it is a weak antiseptic. A number of basic chemicals, more bactericidal than soap, are now in general use in hospitals and offices for cleaning floors, furniture, and operating room equipment and for soaking contaminated utensils and materials. The most valuable of these germicidal chemicals are (1) synthetic phenolics, (2) polybrominated salicylanilides, (3) iodophors, (4) alcohols, and (5) quaternary ammonium compounds. An increasing number of institutions are using the synthetic phenolics and polybrominated salicylanilides (PBS) as general purpose disinfectants because of their effectiveness under actual working conditions. These agents retain high potency in the presence of organic matter and are notable for their excellent residual activities on surfaces. This is probably a reflection of their inherent stability, compatibility with ionic and alkaline agents, and their marked resistance to deactivation by organic matter. Synthetic phenolics and PBS compounds are compatible with soaps, detergents, and numerous other anionic and alkaline agents broadly used in hospitals. Iodophors and quaternary ammonium compounds tend to be rapidly diminished in activity by anionic or alkaline materials and are subject to a certain degree of volatilization. Glutaraldehyde preparations have the germicidal qualities of formaldehyde without the toxic and irritating properties.

a. Phenol compounds—Phenol (carbolic acid) is one of the most potent bactericidal chemicals available, but it is too caustic for safe use. The same is true to a lesser degree of cresol (Lysol). These have been superseded by synthetic phenolic germicides such as Lamar SP-63, Vestal Vasphene, and Western Polyphene. They kill gram-positive and gram-negative bacteria (including tubercle bacilli) and fungi. Surfaces properly treated with these compounds have demonstrated antibacterial properties for periods of 10—14 days. However, residual antibacterial activity should not be relied upon as a substitute for adequate routine cleaning and disinfection.

b. Polybrominated salicylanilide (PBS)—This is the newest class of antibacterial chemical. The antimicrobial spectrum and residual surface action are similar to those of the phenolics. When PBS preparations are used in laundries, textiles take on a self-sanitizing antibacterial finish. A disadvantage of PBS preparations is the white powdery film which remains on metal and other surfaces when the cleaning solution dries. PBS is the essential ingredient in Lamar L-300.

c. Iodophors—These are chemicals in which iodine is combined with a detergent (Wescodyne, Surgidine) or with polyvinylpyrrolidone (Betadine, Isodine). The toxicity of the iodine is practically eliminated, but surface and skin disinfection is efficient.

d. Alcohols—Seventy percent ethyl alcohol is a powerful germicide. Isopropyl alcohol should be used as 70–90%. Neither of these alcohols is effective against spores.

e. Quaternary ammonium compounds—These are less effective than phenol, iodine, and alcohol and are inactivated by soap and adsorbed by fibers. Benzalkonium chloride is the prototype.

f. Formaldehyde and glutaraldehyde—Aqueous solutions of formaldehyde are known as formalin, which, when purchased commercially, is approximately 40% formaldehyde in water. The high-level germicidal activity of formaldehyde is increased by adding alcohol; a combination of 8% formaldehyde (20% formalin) in 70% alcohol is rapidly bactericidal and is sporicidal within 3 hours. Irritating fumes and tissue toxicity limit the usefulness of formaldehyde preparations. Glutaraldehyde is chemically related to formaldehyde, but it has a low tissue toxicity and does not have an irritating odor. Glutaraldehyde in 2% aqueous alkaline concentration (Cidex) is approximately equivalent to 8% formaldehyde in alcohol. Glutaraldehyde is a good chemical sterilizing agent for soaking of instruments, cleaning of anesthesia equipment, and decontamination of operating room items such as basins, bottles, tubing, rubber goods, etc after exposure to septic fields.

g. Other chemicals—Hypochlorites, chloramine, mercury salts, and solutions of azo dyes have been largely replaced by more reliable compounds.

2. Skin antiseptics—The most important applications of skin antisepsis are the hand scrub of the operating team and the preparation of the operative field. Hexachlorophene is widely used in skin disinfection, usually in combination with a detergent (eg, pHisoHex) or with liquid or bar soap (eg, Septisol, Gamophen, Dial). Daily use of hexachlorophene produces a sustained lowering of the bacterial count on the skin. Sporadic or one-time use of hexachlorophene in soap or other preparation has no special value. Alcohol dissolves hexachlorophene and should not be applied if a prolonged surface effect is desired.

a. Hand scrub routine—Always scrub for 5 minutes if operating daily. If not operating daily, scrub for 10 minutes.

(1) Wash hands and forearms thoroughly with soap or a hexachlorophene preparation.

(2) Clean fingernails.

(3) Scrub for 5 minutes with a sterile brush or sponge, covering the entire surface of the hands and forearms repeatedly with soap, a hexachlorophene preparation, or an iodophor.

(4) Scrub for another 5 minutes with a second sterile brush or sponge (a total of 10 minutes by the clock) unless operating daily.

(5) Wash with 70% ethyl alcohol for 1 minute while rubbing the skin surface with a gauze sponge and allow to dry. This optional step in the scrub routine will improve its effectiveness. Omit alcohol rinse if hexachlorophene preparation is used regularly for prolonged effect.

b. Preparation of the operative field—

(1) On the day before operation—Initial preparation of the skin is usually done the afternoon or evening before operation. Designate the specific area to be prepared in the preoperative orders. The area should be washed with soap and water, making sure that it is grossly quite clean. A shower or tub bath is satisfactory. The type of soap used makes little difference. Soap is a weak antiseptic and it is useful because of its nonirritating detergent action, especially when washing is combined with mechanical friction.

Shaving is usually but not always required as part of the ward preparation. Shaving may be omitted where no hairs are present, as on the abdomen of a child. Where coarse hairs are present, shaving is necessary. Shaving must be skillfully done with a new blade and adequate soap lather. Slight nicks and scratches of the skin may be followed in a few hours by an abnormal increase in bacterial flora of the skin. For this reason, it is sometimes preferred—eg, by neurosurgeons—to have the patient shaved just prior to surgery. It is not necessary to apply antiseptics such as alcohol or other germicides to the skin or to cover the prepared area with a sterile dressing.

For elective operations involving areas with high levels of resident bacteria (eg, hands, feet) or likely to be irritated by strong antiseptics (eg, face, genitalia), preoperative degerming of the skin can be improved by repeated use of hexachlorophene soap or solution. Instruct the patient to wash the area several times daily for 3–5 days before operation exclusively with a soap or solution containing hexachlorophene.

(2) In the operating room—Use aseptic technic and prepare the operative field as follows:

(a) Wash for 10 minutes with gauze and detergent or with soap solution. Wipe off with 70% ethyl alcohol and dry with a sterile towel or gauze. (This step may be omitted without change in the wound sepsis rate if preoperative preparation has been meticulous.)

(b) Apply an antiseptic in one of the following ways:

(i) Apply 70% ethyl alcohol to the skin with a gauze swab for 3 minutes and allow to dry before draping. Several applications of tinted tincture of benzalkonium (1:1000) may be alternated with applications of 70% ethyl alcohol for the same effect.

(ii) Apply 1–2% iodine in 70% (by weight) ethyl alcohol. Repeat once. Iodine is one of the most efficient skin antiseptics available, but it occasionally causes skin reactions. Avoid streaming of iodine outside of operative field. Do not use iodine on the perineum, genitalia, or face; on irritated or delicate skin (eg, small children); or when the patient gives a history of iodine sensitivity. In practice, careful skin preparation with tincture of iodine is highly effective and safe. One percent iodine solution in 70% ethyl alcohol is an inexpensive all-purpose skin preparation. It has the same iodine concentration as the iodophors and is nonirritating unless there is a problem of sensitivity.

(iii) Apply an iodophor tincture to the skin.

(iv) For especially sensitive areas (perineum, around the eyes, etc), apply aqueous iodophor solution repeatedly; or apply 1:1000 aqueous benzalkonium solution (first swabbing the area with water to remove any residual soap).

C. Control of Hospital Environment: Hospital cross-infection with hemolytic, coagulase-positive *Staphylococcus aureus* and other organisms is always a potential problem. Strains endemic in hospitals are often resistant to many antimicrobial drugs as a consequence of the widespread use of these agents. Relaxation of aseptic precautions in the operating theater and wards and an unwarranted reliance on "prophylactic" antibiotics contribute to the development of resistant strains. The result may be a significant increase in the incidence of hospital-acquired wound infection, pneumonitis, and septicemia, the latter 2 complications especially affecting infants, the aged, and the debilitated.

Although the pyogenic cocci are the major offenders, the enteric gram-negative bacteria (particularly the coliform and proteus group and *Pseudomonas aeruginosa*) are increasingly prominent in hospital-acquired infections.

1. Hospital administration–

a. The surgical infection control program should be coordinated closely with that of other services through a Hospital Infection Committee set up to promulgate and enforce regulations.

b. All significant infections should be reported immediately. A clean wound infection rate of more than 1–2% is excessive and indicates a need for more effective control measures. The wound infection rate should be continuously observed on the surgical services.

2. Cultures–

a. Obtain culture and antibiotic sensitivity studies on wounds, ulcerations, and significant infections of all types.

b. Phage typing of staphylococci and detailed identification of other organisms may be useful in studying epidemics.

3. Isolation–

a. Isolate every patient with a significant source of communicable bacteria.

b. Isolate every case of suspected communicable infection until the diagnosis has been ruled out.

c. Isolate every patient in whom cross-infection will be serious.

4. Aseptic technic–

a. **Operating room**–The operating room should be considered an isolation zone which may be entered only by persons wearing clean operating attire (which may not be worn elsewhere).

b. **Ward procedures**–All open wounds should be aseptically dressed to protect them from cross-infection and to prevent heavy contamination of the environment. Eliminate dressing carts containing supplies and equipment for multiple bedside dressings.

c. **Hand washing**, preferably with hexachlorophene soap, before and after each contact with a patient is a simple but important routine measure in control of infection.

5. Housekeeping–

a. Bedding must be laundered, and mattresses, furniture, and cubicles cleaned with a general utility antiseptic after a patient is discharged.

b. Housekeeping procedures throughout the hospital must be thorough. Wet mopping and cleaning are required in order to prevent accumulation or raising of dust.

6. Antibiotics–

a. Prophylactic use of antibiotics should be minimized.

b. When possible, antibiotic therapy should be based on sensitivity studies.

c. Antibiotics should be given in adequate doses and discontinued as soon as possible.

7. Epidemiology–

a. Personnel with active staphylococcal infections should be excluded from patient contact until they have recovered. Personnel carrying staphylococci in their nasal passages or gastrointestinal tracts must observe personal hygiene, but need not be removed from duty unless they prove to be a focus of infection. The advisability of treatment of the carrier is uncertain since the carrier state is frequently transient; or recurrent in spite of treatment.

b. Every significant infection acquired in the hospital should be investigated to determine its origin and spread, possible contacts and carriers, and whether improper technics may have been responsible.

3...

Postoperative Care

John L. Wilson, MD

General Considerations

The postoperative care of patients who are seriously ill after a major surgical procedure usually progresses through several fairly well defined phases. The management of such patients is improved when appropriate facilities are available. The phases of progressive care and the optimum facilities are as follows:

Phases	Facilities
Postanesthetic observation	Recovery Room
Intensive care	Intensive Care Unit
Intermediate care	General Nursing Unit
Convalescent care	Home or Extended Care Unit

Postanesthetic observation and intensive care are discussed in some detail in this chapter because of their special features and because of their importance to the end results of major surgery. During these phases of postoperative care, attention is directed specifically to the prevention, early detection, and prompt treatment of the severe, life-threatening complications that are liable to occur in the hours and days immediately following operation. Such complications are chiefly responsible for prolonged morbidity and mortality in the postoperative period.

Patients who have received general anesthesia must be observed in the Recovery Room until out of danger. Upon recovery from anesthesia, patients without complications who are relatively self-sufficient can be well managed in the General Nursing Unit of a general hospital. Patients who are poor risks or who have been severely stressed by extensive surgery require close observation and meticulous management postoperatively. It is possible to achieve this level of care in the General Nursing Unit by arranging for special nursing and other supportive services. Experience has shown, however, that intensive care is most effectively provided in an Intensive Care Unit which is designed and staffed for the specific purpose of managing critically ill patients. The Recovery Room and the Intensive Care Unit are such important adjuncts to postoperative care that their functions will be reviewed.

Specialized Facilities for Postoperative Care; the Recovery Room & Intensive Care Unit

Intensive care concepts have gained increasingly wide acceptance since World War II. This trend has been encouraged by favorable experience in postanes-thesia recovery rooms, in centralized respiratory care of bulbar poliomyelitis during the 1950 epidemic, and, more recently, in coronary care units. Hospitals are rarely designed today without provision for special units in which seriously ill patients can receive close observation, intensive 24-hour nursing care, and emergency resuscitation and other complex treatment. In small hospitals, a single unit may serve for all types of intensive care. Large medical centers commonly have a variety of units such as Recovery Room, Intensive Care Unit, Coronary Care Unit, Respiratory Care Unit, Renal Dialysis Unit, Burn Unit, Pediatric Intensive Care Unit, Premature Nursery, etc.

The Recovery Room and surgical Intensive Care Unit provide environments in which qualified personnel and special equipment can be concentrated for the most effective surveillance and treatment of postoperative patients. The ready availability and frequent attendance of the anesthesiologist and surgeon are essential to the proper function of these units, which are more efficient when adjacent to each other. Also indispensable is the continuous presence of nurses experienced in identifying and interpreting the symptoms and signs of postoperative complications and in taking the necessary emergency action independently.

A. Recovery Room: The Recovery Room should be connected directly to the operating suite. Its dimensions are determined by the fact that one or 2 beds are generally required for each operating room. Most recovery rooms are open-style, with beds located so that all patients can be seen by the nurse. Patients who have had general anesthesia are kept in the Recovery Room until there is no longer a possibility of asphyxia, shock, or other complications requiring respiratory or circulatory resuscitation. The stay in the Recovery Room is usually a few hours at most; the patient is then transferred to either a general nursing unit of the hospital or, if continued close observation is needed, to an Intensive Care Unit.

B. Intensive Care Unit: The design and organization of an Intensive Care Unit (ICU) serving postoperative patients in a specific hospital will depend upon such factors as the number of acute medical and surgical beds and the characteristics of the patients being treated. As a general rule, a hospital with 300–500 acute beds will need an ICU of 10–15 beds, but requirements are quite variable. Ample space around each ICU bed is essential for treatment procedures and equipment. Ideally, each bed should be in a separate cubicle with a glass wall to assure quiet, isolation when necessary, and privacy while allowing continuous observation. Many ICUs have been created by remodeling existing space and present a distinct compromise in terms of location and layout. As new hospitals are built, joint planning by architects, physicians, nurses, and biomedical engineers is creating a new generation of facilities based on progressive care principles which emphasize the relationship of structure to function. Serious acute surgical and medical illnesses and severe trauma make up an increasing proportion of patients in general hospitals—hence the growing importance of intensive care services.

The staffing and equipment requirements of an ICU are dictated by the conditions and complications that must be treated. Almost all critically ill patients have severe involvement of one or more of the following systems: respiratory, cardiovascular, or renal. The major postoperative complications seen in an ICU are cardiac arrhythmias and failure, respiratory failure, shock; fluid, electrolyte, and acid-base imbalance; renal failure, invasive sepsis, and coagulation problems. The chief causes of death in postoperative patients in the ICU are cardiac, respiratory, septic, and hemorrhagic complications. Critically ill patients tend to deteriorate rapidly and may be impossible to evaluate without frequent or even continuous determination of physiologic variables not ordinarily crucial during the postoperative period. As a result, extensive effort is being made to develop monitoring technics that are sufficiently reliable and practicable for general use in the intensive care setting.

The purpose of the ICU is to care for patients who require the following types of life support services.

1. Continuous attendance by a registered nurse.

2. Continuous monitoring of vital signs, ECG, and fluid balance.

3. Continuous ventilatory support with maintenance and protection of the airway.

4. Management of shock, cardiovascular instability, and acute respiratory or renal failure.

5. Management of overwhelming infection or toxemia.

6. Management of severe metabolic, thermal, and other life-threatening disorders.

Monitoring

Continuous observation of the patient by an alert and competent team of nurses and physicians is the cornerstone of high-quality intensive care. However, future improvement in this care will be influenced significantly by technologic progress in monitoring. The term monitoring is used here in its broadest sense to mean close surveillance of the patient, using all available methods to obtain necessary data, either continuously or intermittently, regarding his changing condition. Monitoring of the critically ill patient is facilitated by a number of electronic devices now in general or experimental use and by repeated laboratory tests and bedside measurements. Assessment of data obtained in this manner informs the intensive care team of developments and trends that cannot be followed by the usual methods of examination. For example, continuous monitoring of the ECG can warn of dangerous arrhythmia or change in pulse rate which, if undetected, might lead to cardiac failure or arrest. Intermittent monitoring of the arterial pH, P_{O_2}, and P_{CO_2} provides invaluable and frequently unexpected evidence of respiratory insufficiency, permitting corrective measures before serious deterioration occurs.

A. Parameters Monitored: The following is a partial list of the observations and examinations which may be needed in the monitoring of difficult postoperative problems in the Recovery Room and ICU:

1. **Cardiovascular system—**
   Pulse rate
   Electrocardiogram
   Arterial blood pressure
   Central venous pressure
   Pulmonary arterial pressure
   Cardiac output (or index)
   Total peripheral resistance
2. **Respiratory system—**
   Respiratory rate
   Respiratory volume
   Respiratory flow rate
   Respiratory pressure
   Respiratory compliance
   Respiratory gases (P_{O_2}, P_{CO_2})
   Blood gases (pH, P_{O_2}, P_{CO_2})
   Chest tube drainage
   Chest roentgenography
3. **Central nervous system—**
   Electroencephalogram
   Ventricular pressure
4. **Gastrointestinal system—**
   Fluid intake by mouth
   Nasogastric or intestinal tube drainage and electrolyte analysis of recovered fluid
   Fistula drainage and electrolyte analysis of fluid
   Abdominal roentgenography
5. **Hematopoietic system—**
   Complete blood count
   Hematocrit
   Coagulation studies
   Platelet count
   Blood volume (red cell, plasma, total)
6. **Urinary system—**
   Urine output, hourly
   Urinalysis (routine and microscopic)
   Blood urea nitrogen (BUN)
   Serum creatinine
   Creatinine clearance
   Urine/plasma osmolality ratio
   Urine electrolytes (Na^+/K^+ ratio)
7. **Metabolism—**
   Temperature
   Body weight

Intravenous fluid volume (electrolyte,
colloid, blood)

B. Electronic Aids to Monitoring: Electronic
instruments make possible the continuous visual display—and permanent recording when required—of
physiologic variables such as pulse rate, ECG, and
blood pressure. An automatic feature can be incorporated so that variation in pulse rate or electrocardiographic complex beyond a predetermined range will
activate an alarm and start a permanent recording. The
commonest type of electronic monitoring equipment
now in use is the electrocardiographic monitor, which
is standard in operating theaters, recovery rooms, and
intensive care units.

Electronic devices are no substitute for direct
observation by trained personnel but do provide a convenient and accurate means of obtaining certain information. Biomedical engineering research will undoubtedly provide many new and improved electronic
instruments and systems for the continuous monitoring of patients and for the rapid performance of tests
and calculations that are too time-consuming and
costly by current methods. In view of the present frequent use of electronic instrumentation in postoperative care and the certainty that this will increase, some
of the principles involved will be discussed.

A basic electronic monitoring system has 3 parts:
transducer, signal conditioner, and readout device.

1. Transducer—The function of the transducer is
to interface with the patient, pick up the energy to be
measured, and transmit it as an electrical signal. A few
of the commoner types of transducers will be briefly
described:

If the energy is electrical, as in the case of the
ECG and EEG, the **bioelectric electrodes** applied to the
skin or elsewhere serve as transducers. **Pressure transducers** convert pressure change into electrical energy.
They are widely employed to measure blood pressure
via an indwelling needle or catheter. The device consists of a rigid chamber fitted at one end with a flexible
diaphragm. The chamber is filled with liquid or gas and
connected by tubing to the pressure source. Small
motions of the diaphragm due to pressure changes are
transmitted mechanically to electrical elements
attached to the diaphragm. Resistance in these elements is altered when they are deformed, with the
result that the output voltage of the transducer varies
proportionately to the pressure change. This produces
an electrical signal analogous to pressure. Since the
electrical signal is proportionate or analogous to the
mechanical variable, it is termed an analogue signal.
The transducer does not measure absolute pressure and
therefore requires calibration. **Temperature transducers**
or thermistors are simple, reliable, and very satisfactory for monitoring body temperature. They operate
on the principle that the electrical resistance of certain
materials varies widely with temperature change. Special probes are available for easy insertion into the rectum or esophagus or for application to the skin.
Electrochemical transducers are available to measure

pH, P_{O_2}, P_{CO_2}, Na^+, Cl^-, K^+, and certain other ions
and compounds. **Electromagnetic transducers** and
ultrasonic transducers can measure blood flow. **Photo-
sensitive transducers** react to changes in dilution of
exogenous dyes injected intravascularly in the determination of cardiac output.

The design of improved transducers for sensing
biologic signals is a promising field of research.

2. Signal conditioning—The signal-conditioning
section of the monitoring system receives the electrical
signal generated or transmitted by the transducer. It is
the function of this section to amplify, integrate, and
otherwise modify the signal so that it is of appropriate
energy level and quality for activation of the readout
device on which the signal will be displayed or
recorded. Intensive care personnel are often called
upon to manipulate the controls of the signal-conditioning equipment in order to calibrate the instrument
or to adjust the amplitude or other characteristics of
the displayed tracing.

3. Readout device—The standard readout instrument in operating theaters and intensive care areas is
the cathode ray oscilloscope. The commonest display
is the continuous electrocardiographic tracing. Pressure
pulse wave, arterial and venous blood pressure, EEG,
and other dynamic variables may be displayed when
required. Permanent records can be obtained by direct
writing methods employing hot styluses, ink pens, or
light beams. Information may also be stored on tapes
or disks for later replay. The analogue signal or tracing
of biologic variables can be converted to digital form
by a digital computer with the result that numerical
values for pulse rate, blood pressure, etc can be presented on a television screen. Because analogue to digital conversion is a continuous process and takes place
in a fraction of a second, the numerical values are
precise and current.

**C. Practical Application of Continuous Electronic
Monitoring:** Electronic monitoring systems which
record and analyze multiple physiologic variables are in
experimental use in many medical centers (Lewis FJ &
others: Surg Gynec Obst 130:333–341, 1970). Clinical application of the full range of currently available
monitoring technics is limited by a number of factors,
including cumbersome and invasive methods of inter-
facing with the patient and complexity and cost of
equipment. In an individual patient, it is important to
decide whether there is need to obtain a continuous
record of vital signs and other variables or whether
intermittent observations and tests will serve equally
well. In most patients, the latter will be the case.
Experience has shown that, except in the research setting, it is feasible and useful to monitor only a few
parameters on a continuous basis and that this is
required in only a selected group of critically ill
patients. In the majority of postoperative patients,
necessary information can be satisfactorily obtained by
clinical observation supplemented by repeated laboratory tests. The following are the physiologic variables
that can be monitored continuously in the usual well-
staffed and well-equipped ICU:

Physiologic Variable	Transduction
ECG and pulse rate	Chest wall electrodes.
Respiratory rate	Transthoracic electrical impedence from electrocardiographic electrodes.
Body temperature	Thermistor in the rectum, esophagus, or ear or on the skin.
Blood pressure	Pressure transducer connected to arterial catheter (an automatic blood pressure cuff device will provide intermittent blood pressure readings but is inaccurate when blood pressure drops significantly).

For practical purposes, the above is the scope of continuous monitoring available for routine clinical application in most hospitals. Monitoring of the other parameters listed on p 15 is on an intermittent basis.

Postoperative Orders

Postsurgical patients should be accompanied by a physician or other qualified attendant while en route to the Recovery Room, ICU, or General Nursing Unit. Detailed written orders should be sent with each postoperative patient, and the nurse receiving him should be given a verbal report of his condition. The postoperative orders should provide for appropriate observations and treatments which, in the case of the patient requiring intensive care, may include many of the procedures listed above under the parameters to be monitored. As a guide to the preparation of an inclusive set of postoperative orders, each of the following categories should be considered:

A. Special Observations:

1. Vital signs—Blood pressure, pulse, and respiration should be recorded at regular intervals after all major operations (eg, every 15–30 minutes until stable, and then hourly). A significant drop in blood pressure should be reported to the surgeon immediately. (Specify the level to be reported.)

2. Continuous monitoring of ECG—This is indicated in many critically ill patients. Other parameters to be monitored continuously will depend upon the patient's needs and the equipment available.

3. Central venous pressure—This requires percutaneous placement of an inlying catheter in the superior vena cava or right atrium via the internal jugular or subclavian vein (see Chapter 52). Record central venous pressure at stated intervals in patients in shock, those with a borderline cardiac or respiratory status, those who require large fluid volume replacement, or those with oliguria.

4. Miscellaneous—Orders should be given as indicated to observe closely for such developments as cardiac arrhythmias, respiratory distress, wound bleeding or drainage, impaired circulation in an extremity (eg, distal to a cast or vascular procedure), etc.

B. Position in Bed: Designate specifically, eg, flat or on side, sitting, or foot of bed elevated.

C. Mobilization: Prescribe bed rest, standing to void, up in chair, or ambulation. While recovering from general anesthesia, the patient should be turned from side to side every 30 minutes until conscious and then hourly for the first 8–12 hours. Require active position change and active motion of the feet and legs every 1–2 hours while awake until ambulated. Order elastic bandages or antiemboli stockings for the legs for elderly patients or when ambulation is delayed.

D. Respiratory Care: Hyperventilation, coughing, tracheal suction, and inhalation therapy should be ordered as required. Percutaneous placement of a small catheter in the trachea may be needed for injection of saline or water to stimulate cough.

E. Oxygen Therapy: See Chapter 14.

F. Intake and Output: Order either nothing by mouth or a specific diet. Record the fluid intake and output for as long after surgery as required for control of fluid balance. Prescribe the parenteral fluids to be administered during the first 24 hours. Continuous catheter drainage of the bladder may be required to follow urine output closely in suspected renal impairment due to shock or other cause. If the patient is on catheter drainage, specify intervals for measurement of urine volume (eg, hourly).

G. Voiding: Place an order for notification of the surgeon if the patient is unable to pass urine within a specified period (usually 6–8 hours) after operation.

H. Body Weight: Patients with fluid balance problems should be weighed daily.

I. Drainage Tubes: If a nasogastric or intestinal tube is in place, it should be connected to suction and irrigated every 1–2 hours with 15–30 ml of saline. Urethral, chest, biliary, and other drainage catheters call for specific orders.

J. Medications: A narcotic for pain relief is usually required. Other drugs frequently used include sedatives, antibiotics, and antiemetic drugs. Resume essential preoperative medications such as digitalis, insulin, and corticosteroids.

K. Special Laboratory Examinations: During the first 24 hours, it may be necessary to determine the hematocrit, complete blood count, blood pH, P_{O_2}, and P_{CO_2}; to order urinalyses and blood chemistries; and to obtain portable x-rays.

Special Postoperative Problems

Certain life-threatening complications occur with relative frequency in the early period after major surgery or trauma. The most important of these are the acute pulmonary, cardiovascular, and renal/electrolyte derangements which are chief causes of prolonged morbidity and increased mortality rates after severe operation or injury. Many of these patients have preexisting diseases or are elderly, and these factors compound the difficulty of their treatment.

An ICU environment is essential to the most effective management of these complications. Study of ICU activity in a major medical center will usually show that there has been a striking increase in the incidence of surgical patients with respiratory insufficiency and failure in recent years. There are many reasons for this. Blood gas and other respiratory tests are now widely used and have served to disclose marked deficits in function which were previously unrecognized. Older patients and those with multiple organ disease are being operated on more often. With improved management of cardiovascular, renal, and other complications, failure of the respiratory system is becoming a chief limiting element in recovery. Faster transportation and better resuscitation of trauma victims in military and civilian practice have resulted in survival of individuals whose lungs subsequently develop progressive posttraumatic changes.

Technical improvements in mechanical ventilatory support have accompanied significant advances in knowledge of the pathophysiology of pulmonary insufficiency. As a result, the ICU team is alert to the possibility of occult respiratory deficits and is more aggressive in the use of intubation and artificial ventilation in both prevention and treatment. Because management of respiratory failure has become one of the most demanding aspects of postoperative care, this condition has been selected for detailed discussion in this chapter. Various other serious postoperative complications such as cardiac arrhythmias and acute renal failure are discussed elsewhere in this text.

ACUTE RESPIRATORY FAILURE IN THE SURGICAL PATIENT

Essentials of Diagnosis

- Precipitating cause such as operation, trauma, or sepsis.
- Predisposing condition such as chronic obstructive pulmonary disease (frequently present).
- Dyspnea, tachycardia, and cyanosis are typical findings, but acute respiratory failure may be present without pathognomonic physical signs.
- Late signs include transient hypertension followed by hypotension, mental confusion or stupor progressing to coma, respiratory and cardiac irregularity, and cardiac arrest.
- Arterial blood gases show decreased oxygen tension or increased CO_2 tension (or both). A blood gas abnormality may be the only diagnostic sign of early respiratory failure.

General Considerations

Respiratory failure is the result of inability of the pulmonary system to maintain normal arterial oxygen or CO_2 tension. Acute respiratory failure is characterized by an arterial P_{O_2} of less than 60 mm Hg (normal, 85–110 mm Hg) or an arterial P_{CO_2} of more than 50 mm Hg (normal, 35–45 mm Hg) while the patient is breathing room air at rest—particularly if repeated arterial samples show the P_{O_2} to be falling and the

P_{CO_2} to be rising (and not due to respiratory compensation for metabolic alkalemia). In interpreting blood gas determinations, it is important to bear in mind that arterial P_{O_2} is normally decreased with age (Sorbin & others: Respiration 25:3–13, 1968) and that patients with long-standing lung disease may have chronic respiratory insufficiency with continuously abnormal blood gases.

From the standpoint of management, 2 groups of patients with acute respiratory failure may be identified. One group consists chiefly of medical patients whose acute respiratory failure is often due to an exacerbation of severe chronic obstructive pulmonary disease and in whom treatment usually involves carefully controlled oxygen therapy with delay in use of artificial ventilation. The other group consists chiefly of surgical patients in whom acute respiratory failure is precipitated by trauma, operation, or sepsis. Artificial ventilation is more frequently indicated in the latter group, who usually have slight or no preexisting lung disease. Patients who have severe chronic lung disease such as emphysema and chronic bronchitis are especially prone to develop acute respiratory failure after surgical stress.

Acute respiratory failure is commonly associated with certain major physiologic disturbances which occur singly or together. These include (1) increased physiologic shunting (most often due to atelectasis); (2) increased physiologic dead space (which may be caused by hypotension, pulmonary embolism, or atelectasis); (3) increased work of breathing (frequently due to decreased compliance associated with interstitial pulmonary edema); and (4) decreased oxygen transport (usually related to diminished cardiac output). The conditions predisposing to these physiologic disturbances will be discussed and their clinical manifestations described.

Predisposing Conditions

Numerous factors predispose to pulmonary insufficiency and contribute to the development of acute respiratory failure in surgical patients.

A. Pain: After operation or trauma, pain involving the chest or abdomen has a restrictive influence on respiratory function. Thoracic and abdominal incisions—particularly upper abdominal—are known to reduce vital capacity significantly in the immediate postoperative period with resulting decreased effectiveness of cough and increased incidence of retained secretions, atelectasis, and pulmonary infection. Statistics on the frequency of clinically important atelectasis and pneumonitis after major thoracic and abdominal operations are difficult to interpret because of variability among the reports in the literature, but it is reasonable to assume that the incidence is at least 15–20%.

B. Abdominal Distention: This is a frequent contributing cause of respiratory insufficiency and failure. Increased intra-abdominal pressure reduces lung volumes and capacities.

C. Restrictive Binders and Dressings: These inhibit pulmonary excursion and function.

D. Anesthetic Drugs and Narcotics: Ventilation is reduced and cough and other respiratory reflexes are suppressed by depressant drugs. Hypoxia and hypercapnia due to hypoventilation in the immediate postoperative period may become severe unless the patient's respiration is assisted until the effects of anesthetics and relaxants have subsided. Narcotics such as morphine must be used judiciously in the postoperative period in order to avoid ventilatory depression, hypercapnia, and atelectasis. Doses of narcotic which are normally well tolerated may have a marked depressant effect on pulmonary function in the very ill or debilitated patient.

E. Thoracic Conditions: Decreased lung volume and impaired ventilatory efficiency due to acute thoracic conditions have a direct effect on respiratory function. Flail chest, extensive pulmonary resection, large accumulations of pleural air or fluid, and other severe chest abnormalities create circumstances under which respiratory failure may develop rapidly.

F. Extrathoracic Trauma, Surgery, and Sepsis: When severe, these conditions often have an indirect but seriously adverse effect on the respiratory system. Pulmonary insufficiency, related in most cases to pulmonary vascular congestion and interstitial edema, is a leading cause of death in fatal cases of shock, trauma, and infection. Accordingly, patients suffering from these conditions should be observed with special care so that early evidence of failing lung function (eg, arterial blood gas derangement) will be discovered. Acute respiratory failure secondary to severe trauma or extensive operations has been variously termed post-traumatic pulmonary insufficiency, postoperative lung syndrome, shock lung, pump lung, and wet lung (see p 29).

G. Chronic Conditions: A variety of preexisting conditions have a significant influence on the incidence of respiratory problems after major surgery or trauma.

1. Chronic obstructive pulmonary disease is an increasingly common finding in surgical patients and is associated with an exceptionally high incidence of postoperative complications. Stein & others (JAMA 181:765–770, 1962) found that 70% of all patients with emphysema and chronic bronchitis developed atelectasis and pneumonia following operation, whereas the incidence was only 3% in patients with normal preoperative lung function. Chronic pulmonary disease, even though not severe, predisposes strongly to respiratory complications after trauma or operation.

2. Smoking is associated with an increased incidence of emphysema, chronic bronchitis, and postoperative respiratory difficulty. Morton (Lancet 1:368–370, 1944) found that the incidence of postoperative pulmonary complications was 3 times higher among heavy smokers than among nonsmokers.

3. Old age is related to a higher rate of postoperative complications in general, including respiratory.

4. Severe obesity decreases vital capacity and the efficiency of respiratory muscles and increases the work of breathing. Markedly obese patients have a higher than normal oxygen uptake and CO_2 produc-

tion. They are known to be especially susceptible to hypoventilation and to postoperative pulmonary complications.

5. Neurologic diseases and lesions such as poliomyelitis, multiple sclerosis, polyneuritis, and brain and spinal cord injuries may severely compromise the patient's pulmonary function and make him vulnerable to respiratory failure following trauma or surgery.

Clinical Findings

A. Symptoms and Signs: Pulmonary complications usually develop gradually over hours or days following surgery, trauma, or severe sepsis. Where predisposing conditions such as those described above are present, the patient must be evaluated with special care and arterial blood gas determinations performed if any suspicion of deteriorating pulmonary function arises even though definite evidence of acute respiratory failure is lacking. Mild to severe grades of respiratory failure may occur insidiously in the absence of pathognomonic symptoms or physical signs.

1. Hypoxia—The clinical findings in acute respiratory failure vary widely depending upon the cause and the patient's general condition. Dyspnea, tachycardia, and cyanosis form a classic triad of signs indicative of hypoxia of pulmonary or cardiac origin. A minimum of 5 g of reduced hemoglobin per 100 ml of blood must be present before cyanosis is clinically apparent. Although cyanosis is a manifestation of hypoxia, it ordinarily is not perceptible until the arterial oxygen saturation is below 80–85%, and severe tissue hypoxia can occur in the absence of detectable cyanosis. Stridor, wheezing, and retraction of supraclavicular and intercostal spaces are clear evidences of airway obstruction, respiratory insufficiency, and probable hypoxia. Decreased respiratory effort resulting in hypoventilation is also usually associated with hypoxia as well as CO_2 retention and is much more difficult to recognize and evaluate. Mild hypoxia usually causes an increase in heart rate, respiratory rate, cardiac output, peripheral resistance (vasoconstriction), and blood pressure. Tachycardia, tachypnea, and hypertension are thus common early signs of mild hypoxia. Late and severe hypoxia produces bradycardia, arrhythmias, and hypotension which may be followed by cardiac arrest. Old or debilitated patients often pass very rapidly into the late or terminal stage of hypoxia and circulatory failure.

2. Hypercapnia—Certain manifestations of acute respiratory failure may be due to CO_2 retention or hypercapnia. An early circulatory sign of CO_2 retention is vasodilatation with increased cutaneous blood flow and sweating. There is also stimulation of sympathetic activity with increased circulating catecholamines (epinephrine and norepinephrine), resulting in increased cardiac output, tachycardia, and hypertension. This reaction occurs only in those patients still able to respond to sympathetic activation. Increase of CO_2 content has a direct action on the respiratory center, leading to hyperventilation. However, the CNS depression and muscular weakness produced by hypercapnia may prevent hyperventilation. The degree of central depression caused by elevated blood levels of CO_2 is quite variable and ranges from mild sedation to deep coma. Respiratory arrest may occur. Other possible manifestations of hypercapnia are mental confusion, muscle twitching, visual defects, and cardiac arrhythmias. The combined depressant and stimulant effects of CO_2 retention, frequently accompanied by hypoxia, tend to produce a variable and unpredictable clinical picture.

3. Physical examination of the chest—Valuable clues to the presence of respiratory failure are usually found on chest examination. Increased tracheobronchial secretions and signs of atelectasis, pneumonitis, or pulmonary edema are common findings in respiratory failure. On the other hand, percussion and auscultation may occasionally disclose no significant changes. Physical examination of the chest must be integrated with other observations in order to develop a composite clinical impression of pulmonary status.

4. General evaluation—Certain categories of patients are known to be highly susceptible to respiratory failure and should be followed with special care. For example, the elderly patient with a long history of heavy smoking and of chronic obstructive lung disease is a likely candidate for respiratory failure after severe trauma or extensive surgery, particularly if conditions such as abdominal distention, obesity, and respiratory limitation by pain or narcotic are also present. Such patients require intensive preventive management and should be evaluated by appropriate laboratory studies before significant respiratory distress appears. In some patients, respiratory failure develops occultly in the absence of impressive symptoms and signs, and in such cases it is necessary to measure arterial blood gases to confirm or dispel the suspicion of respiratory failure. Usually, however, respiratory failure is associated with definite symptoms and signs, including at least dyspnea and tachycardia. Depending upon the severity of failure and other factors, there may also be cyanosis, stupor, or hypertension. Restlessness in the postoperative period is a common sign of hypoxia which should be ruled out before sedation is ordered. Marked hypoxia is also an important cause of hypotension and indicates a late stage of respiratory failure in which bradycardia, arrhythmia, and cardiac arrest are imminent.

B. X-Ray Findings: A baseline chest film should be taken prior to all major operations and as soon as possible after severe trauma. Chest x-ray is an important adjunct to physical examination in patients suspected of respiratory failure and will frequently disclose evidence of atelectasis, pulmonary congestion, chest fluid, and other abnormalities not otherwise detectable. Portable films are taken during the immediate postoperative or posttraumatic period if transport of the patient to the radiology department is impracticable. Patients with severe chronic lung disease usually require early and repeated chest films after major surgery or trauma. Chest x-ray during the first few hours following thoracotomy and periodically there-

after enables accurate assessment of lung expansion and of air and fluid accumulations.

There are no pathognomonic radiologic signs of acute respiratory failure, and there is frequently no correlation between x-ray findings and the blood gas values. However, chest x-ray is the only method of identifying many subtle parenchymal and other changes such as vascular congestion which accompany or contribute to respiratory failure. Furthermore, serial films are usually the only means available for following the course of these changes.

Pulmonary Function Tests

Pulmonary function tests are essential in patients with respiratory failure for purposes of diagnosis, for evaluating responses to treatment, and as an aid in deciding whether or not to start or to discontinue tracheal intubation and artificial ventilation. The most useful tests are listed in Table 3–1. Most of these tests can be performed at the bedside during both spontaneous and controlled respiration. Some of them are particularly helpful in determining when a patient in acute respiratory failure should receive ventilatory support by tracheal intubation and assisted respiration (Table 3–2). Predicted values for pulmonary function tests have been tabulated by Bates & others (*Respiratory Function in Disease,* 2nd ed. Saunders, 1971; pp 93–94). These tables of predicted norms provide useful baseline information with which to compare the findings in patients with respiratory problems.

Selected pulmonary function tests from Table 3–1 and the physiologic principles involved in their interpretation will be discussed in order to show how they may be used in the management of patients with acute respiratory failure. Preliminary to this discussion, it is advisable to review some of the standard symbols and abbreviations used in pulmonary physiology and testing to facilitate the recording of data and the calculation of results. The accompanying display (Table 3–3) of primary and secondary symbols can be arranged in various combinations to designate the blood and gas phases of physiologic variables. (See Federation Proceedings, Report Fed Proc 9:602–605, 1950.)

A. Tests of Oxygenation:

1. Measurement of inspired oxygen concentration (F_{IO_2})—In complex respiratory problems, particularly those requiring assisted or controlled ventilation, it is essential to be able to monitor and to adjust the concentration of inspired oxygen. The concentration of inspired oxygen can be measured by the Scholander technic or with the oxygen electrode. At the bedside, oxygen concentration being delivered to the patient can be determined by sampling the inspired gas line with the portable paramagnetic oxygen analyzer. In calculating the alveolar-arterial oxygen gradient ($A-a_{DO_2}$), it is necessary to be certain that all the nitrogen has been washed out during 100% oxygen breathing ($F_{IO_2} = 1.0$). Ten to 20 minutes of breathing 100% oxygen have been found to be sufficient for this purpose. This can be checked by attaching a nitrogen analyzer to the expired gas line if such an instru-

TABLE 3−1. Tests for assessing respiratory function in critically ill patients.*

Oxygenation
Inspired oxygen concentration (F_{IO_2})
Pa_{O_2} on controlled and spontaneous ventilation
$P_{(A-a_{DO_2})^{1.0}}$† or $P_{(A-a_{DO_2})^{0.5}}$†
Hematocrit or hemoglobin concentration
Arterial oxygen content (Ca_{O_2})‡
Right-to-left shunt ($\dot{Q}s/\dot{Q}_T$)‡

Ventilation
Tidal volume (V_T), frequency, minute ventilation ($\dot{V}_E$)
Pa_{CO_2}
Dead space to tidal volume ration (V_D/V_T)
Carbon dioxide production ($\dot{V}_{CO_2}$)
Ventilator dead space and compression volume

Ventilatory reserve and mechanics
Total vital capacity
First-second vital capacity (FEV_1)
Maximum expiratory flow rate (MEFR)
Inspiratory force
"Weaning time"
Effective compliance
Dynamic compliance‡
Check for ventilatory discoordination‡

Related diagnostic procedures
Chest x-ray and fluoroscopy‡
Sputum smear and culture; antibiotic sensitivity
Body weight
Water balance
Serum and urine electrolytes
Serum protein concentration
Central venous pressure‡
Mixed venous oxygen content‡
Cardiac output‡
Pulmonary artery and capillary wedge pressures‡

*Reproduced, with permission, from Pontoppidan H, Geffin B, Lowenstein E: New England J Med 287:743−752, 1972.
†Difference in alveolar-arterial oxygen tension measured during ventilation with 100% and 50% oxygen, respectively.
‡Tests performed under special circumstances in the critically ill, unstable patient with respiratory or circulatory failure or both; facilities and technics now available for doing these more complex tests at the bedside when indicated.

TABLE 3−2. Guidelines for ventilatory support in adults with acute respiratory failure.*†

	Normal Range	Tracheal Intubation & Ventilation Indicated
Mechanics		
Respiratory rate	12−20	> 35
Vital capacity (ml/kg body wt‡)	65−75	< 15
FEV_1 (ml/kg body wt‡)	50−60	< 10
Inspiratory force (cm water)	75−100	< 25
Oxygenation		
Pa_{O_2} (mm Hg)	100−75 (air)	< 70 (on mask O_2)
$P_{(A-a_{DO_2})^{1.0}}$§ (mm Hg)**	25−65	> 450
Ventilation		
Pa_{CO_2} (mm Hg)	35−45	> 55††
V_D/V_T	0.25−0.40	> 0.60

*Reproduced, with permission, from Pontoppidan H, Geffin B, Lowenstein E: New England J Med 287:743−752, 1972.
†The trend of values is of utmost importance. The numerical guidelines should obviously not be adopted to the exclusion of clinical judgment. For example, a vital capacity below 15 ml/kg may prove sufficient provided the patient can still cough "effectively," if hypoxemia is prevented, and if hypercapnia is not progressive. However, such a patient needs frequent blood gas analyses and must be closely observed in a well-equipped, adequately staffed recovery room or intensive care unit.
‡"Ideal" weight is used if weight appears grossly abnormal.
§See Table 3−1, note (†).
**After 10 minutes of 100% oxygen.
††Except in patients with chronic hypercapnia.

ment is available. When expired nitrogen levels fall below 1%, inspired oxygen has replaced all alveolar gas except CO_2 and water vapor. When nitrogen has been thoroughly washed out by breathing 100% oxygen, the Pa_{O_2} will reflect the alveolar-arterial gradient ($A-a_{DO_2}$) and the pulmonary shunt ($\dot{Q}s/\dot{Q}_T$).

2. Measurement of arterial oxygen tension (Pa_{O_2}) −Arterial blood samples may be obtained from a peripheral artery, preferably the radial, with a fine needle and heparinized syringe. For repeated samples, an indwelling plastic catheter may be inserted into the artery. Pa_{O_2} and other measurements listed below can be performed rapidly and accurately in the laboratory. All of the following examinations are usually done on each arterial blood sample obtained from the patient with a respiratory problem:

	Normal Range
Pa_{O_2}	On air: 85−110 mm Hg
	On 100% oxygen: 610−670 mm Hg
Percentage saturation	> 95%
Pa_{CO_2}	35−45 mm Hg
HCO_3^-	23−25 mEq/liter
pH	7.36−7.44

TABLE 3–3. Standard symbols in pulmonary physiology.

SYMBOLS FOR GAS PHASE

Primary symbols

V	Volume of gas
$\dot{V}$	Volume flow of gas per unit time
P	Pressure of gas
F	Fractional concentration of gas
R	Respiratory exchange ratio (volume CO_2/ volume O_2)
D	Diffusion capacity (volume per unit time per unit pressure difference)
f	Respiratory frequency (breaths per minute)

Secondary symbols (subscripts)

I	Inspired gas
E	Expired gas
A	Alveolar gas
T	Tidal gas
D	Deadspace gas
B	Barometric

SYMBOLS FOR BLOOD PHASE

Primary symbols

Q	Volume of blood
$\dot{Q}$	Volume flow of blood per unit time
C	Concentration of gas in blood
S	Percent saturation of hemoglobin with oxygen

Secondary symbols (subscripts)

b	Blood in general
a	Arterial blood
v	Venous blood
c	Capillary blood

GENERAL SYMBOLS

$\overline{X}$	Dash (−) over any symbol indicates a mean value
$\dot{X}$	Dot ($\cdot$) over any symbol indicates a time derivative
s	Subscript to denote steady state
STPD	Standard temperature, pressure, dry (0 C, 760 torr*)

*One torr = 1 atm/760, almost exactly equivalent to 1 mm Hg.

FREQUENTLY USED COMBINATIONS OF SYMBOLS
(See also Table 3–1.)

V_T	Tidal volume (ml)
V_D	Dead space volume (ml)
V_D/V_T	Dead space to tidal volume ratio
$\dot{V}_A$	Alveolar ventilation (liters/min)
$\dot{V}_{O_2}$	Oxygen consumption (ml/min, STPD)
$\dot{V}_{CO_2}$	Carbon dioxide production (ml/min, STPD)
$F_{I_{O_2}}$	Fractional concentration of oxygen in inspired gas
$\dot{Q}_T$	Cardiac output, total (liters/min)
$\dot{Q}_S$	Blood flow "shunted" through pulmonary capillaries exposed to nonventilated alveoli (liters/min)
$\dot{Q}_S/\dot{Q}_T \times 100$	Percentage of cardiac output perfusing nonventilated areas of the lung. The $\dot{Q}_S/\dot{Q}_T$ ratio in normal lungs measured while breathing 100% oxygen defines the anatomic intrapulmonary right-to-left shunt.
$P_{a_{O_2}}$	Partial pressure of arterial oxygen
$P_{a_{CO_2}}$	Partial pressure of arterial carbon dioxide
$P_{A_{O_2}}$	Partial pressure of alveolar oxygen
$P_{A_{CO_2}}$	Partial pressure of alveolar carbon dioxide
$P_{(A-a_{D_{O_2}})}$	Alveolar to arterial oxygen difference or gradient
P_B	Barometric pressure 760 mm Hg

ABBREVIATIONS

The following abbreviations are among many in common use:

VC	Vital capacity (total)
FEV	Forced expiratory volume
FEV_1	First-second vital capacity
MVV	Maximal voluntary ventilation; same as MBC, maximal breathing capacity
MEFR	Maximal expiratory flow rate
MMFR	Maximal midexpiratory flow rate
FRC	Functional residual capacity
CPPB	Continuous positive pressure breathing
IPPV	Intermittent positive pressure ventilation
PEEP	Positive end-expiratory pressure

Facilities for performing the above panel of tests should be available around the clock in close proximity to the operating theater, recovery room, and ICU. All blood gas determinations should be carried out as soon as possible after the sample is drawn, especially if the arterial oxygen tension is high. If delay is inevitable, the syringe containing the arterial sample should be kept in ice.

Measurement of $P_{a_{O_2}}$ serves as an index of the adequacy of arterial oxygenation when the hemoglobin content is known. Also, if inspired oxygen concentration ($F_{I_{O_2}}$) is known, alveolar-arterial oxygen difference ($A-a_{D_{O_2}}$) provides an estimate of the magnitude of the physiologic shunt (see below). $P_{a_{O_2}}$ must be high enough to maintain full oxygenation of the blood as measured by the arterial oxygen content ($C_{a_{O_2}}$). The arterial oxygen content depends upon the arterial oxygen tension, on the hemoglobin content, and, to a lesser extent, on arterial CO_2 tension and pH. The total content of oxygen in arterial blood is made up of 2 components: (1) oxygen combined with hemoglobin to form oxyhemoglobin, and (2) a very small amount of oxygen physically dissolved in plasma. The normal value for arterial oxygen content when breath-

"ASSISTED VENTILATION" & "CONTROLLED VENTILATION" DEFINED

Assisted ventilation is a form of respiratory support triggered by the patient's spontaneous respiratory effort in response to which a mechanical ventilator inflates the patient's lungs until a preset pressure has been reached, at which point the inspiratory phase stops and expiration begins. With the use of a pressure-limited ventilator, tidal volume is a function of airway resistance and pulmonary compliance. These parameters tend to change from time to time in acute respiratory failure, so that expired minute volume and tidal volume must be monitored frequently to assure adequate alveolar ventilation when a pressure-limited ventilator is used for ventilatory assistance.

Controlled ventilation is respiratory support provided by a mechanical ventilator which delivers a constant preset minute and tidal volume regardless of changes in airway resistance and pulmonary compliance. Respiratory rate is determined by the setting on the ventilator. In controlled ventilation, the patient's spontaneous respiratory effort must be completely overridden and not allowed to become asynchronous with the ventilator; otherwise, the patient will fight the respirator and respiratory insufficiency will be increased. If lung compliance is severely reduced, the volume-controlled or volume-limited ventilator may be the only means of providing adequate alveolar ventilation.

Assisted ventilation is indicated when impending or frank respiratory failure is associated with decreased tidal volume and an increased respiratory rate. **Controlled ventilation** is indicated when ventilation or oxygenation is inadequate on assisted ventilation at acceptable oxygen tensions. Flail chest and marked tachypnea are other indications. The energy cost of breathing is reduced by either assisted or controlled ventilation, but maximum reduction is achieved by controlled ventilation.

---

ing air and assuming a hemoglobin content of 15 g/100 ml is about 20 ml/100 ml. On 100% oxygen, the arterial oxygen content rises slightly in normal individuals to about 22 ml/100 ml due to an increase in O_2 dissolved in plasma at high Pa_{O_2}.

Transport to the tissues of an adequate supply of oxygen depends not only on arterial oxygen content but also on volume and distribution of cardiac output (normal cardiac output = 5–6 liters/min). Assuming an arterial-venous oxygen content difference of 6 ml/100 ml and a cardiac output of 5 liters, oxygen consumption is 300 ml/min at rest in a normal individual. When arterial oxygen content is decreased as a result either of low Pa_{O_2} or low hemoglobin content, there must be a compensatory increase in cardiac output to maintain adequate tissue oxygenation.

Maintenance of normal blood gases depends upon the relationship of effective alveolar ventilation ($\dot{V}_A$) to pulmonary blood flow or perfusion ($\dot{Q}$). The normal ventilation-perfusion ratio ($\dot{V}_A/\dot{Q}$) is about 0.80, based on normal values for $\dot{V}_A$ of 4 liters/min and for $\dot{Q}$ of 5 liters/min. *The most important cause of decreased Pa_{O_2} is abnormality of the ventilation-perfusion relationship ($\dot{V}_A/\dot{Q}$) in the lung.* Inspired oxygen concentration ($F_{I_{O_2}}$) is the other major factor related to pulmonary function which determines arterial oxygen tension (Pa_{O_2}). When there is a significant increase in physiologic shunt with resultant decrease in Pa_{O_2} due to abnormal $\dot{V}_A/\dot{Q}$, the use of 100% oxygen ($F_{I_{O_2}}$ = 1.0) increases Pa_{O_2} and decreases the effect of the shunt on arterial oxygen content.

3. **Estimation of physiologic shunt by measurement of alveolar-arterial oxygen tension difference ($P_{[A-aD_{O_2}]}$)**—The physiologic shunt is that portion of the cardiac output that does not participate in pulmonary blood gas exchange but returns to the left heart as unoxygenated venous admixture to arterial blood. The total physiologic shunt has 2 components: (1) the **anatomic shunt** through bronchial, pleural, and thebesian veins (approximately 2% of cardiac output); and (2) the **capillary shunt** via the pulmonary capillaries. The capillary shunt is normally minimal and unimportant, but it may be markedly increased by conditions that prevent ventilation of alveoli which continue to be perfused with blood. The following are the major causes of increased physiologic shunting in surgical patients:

a. Atelectasis (massive or patchy) is a common postoperative problem in which unventilated alveoli may be perfused by a significant portion of the cardiac output. The arterial P_{O_2} may be quite low. The arterial P_{CO_2} may remain normal or may even be decreased by hyperventilation.

b. Emphysema, pulmonary fibrosis, obesity, and mitral valvular disease may be associated with marked shunting as a result of *uneven distribution* of ventilation and perfusion. The shunt effect is caused by incomplete mixing of inspired air and its unequal distribution to alveoli.

c. A number of miscellaneous conditions associated with respiratory failure in the surgical patient are characterized by increased physiologic shunting. These conditions have been variously termed wet lung, respirator lung, postoperative lung, shock lung, pump lung, and posttraumatic pulmonary insufficiency. They are complex syndromes, and it is possible that some of them are separate entities. Precipitating circumstances vary as indicated by the descriptive titles. Pulmonary vascular congestion is a prominent component. Interstitial edema, alveolar exudate, and widening of alveolar-capillary septa are commonly present. Veno-arterial shunting occurs within the lung, which usually shows decreased compliance and either normal or increased respiratory resistance. Arterial blood gas studies when the patient is breathing room air frequently show low P_{CO_2} and low P_{O_2} accompanied by a base deficit secondary to hypoxia. Loss of normal alveolar surfactant, fat emboli, microembolism from intravascular coagulation, and oxygen toxicity are among the possible contributing factors.

d. Diffusion or alveolar-capillary block, presumably due to thickening of the alveolar-capillary membrane, is probably rarely responsible for significant physiologic shunting. Severe disturbance of the ventilation-perfusion ratio is usually the actual cause of what appears to be a diffusion block.

When cardiac output and arterial-venous oxygen content difference are relatively normal, the measurement of $P_{(A-aD_{O_2})}$ provides a convenient and reasonably accurate indication of ventilation-perfusion abnormalities in the lung and of the magnitude of physiologic shunting. The procedure consists of determining $P_{a_{O_2}}$ and $P_{a_{CO_2}}$ after the patient has been breathing 100% oxygen ($F_{I_{O_2}}$ = 1.0) for 15−20 minutes. Alveolar oxygen tension ($P_{A_{O_2}}$) is calculated by subtracting water vapor pressure (47 mm Hg at 37 C) and $P_{a_{CO_2}}$ (eg, 40 mm Hg) from the barometric pressure:

$$P_{A_{O_2}} = .760 - (47 + 40) = 673 \text{ mm Hg (normal)}$$

Actual values for $P_{a_{O_2}}$ in healthy subjects breathing 100% oxygen at sea level range from 610−670 mm Hg. Therefore, if $P_{a_{O_2}}$ after breathing 100% oxygen is normal (eg, 640 mm Hg), then

$$P_{(A-aD_{O_2})}{}^{1.0} = P_{A_{O_2}} - P_{a_{O_2}} = 673 - 640 = 33 \text{ mm Hg}$$

Under normal circumstances, the range for $P_{(A-aD_{O_2})}{}^{1.0}$ is 25−65 mm Hg. The alveolar-arterial oxygen difference rises when blood is shunted through unventilated alveoli. Values of $P_{(A-aD_{O_2})}$ greater than 450 mm Hg indicate severe ventilation-perfusion disturbance and are usually an indication for tracheal intubation and ventilatory support in patients with acute respiratory failure (see Table 3−2).

When $P_{(A-aD_{O_2})}$ is determined after breathing 100% oxygen, the shunt that is measured is caused chiefly by (1) the fixed anatomic shunt (2−3% of cardiac output) and (2) atelectasis. The shunt that occurs as a result of pulmonary congestion and interstitial edema in posttraumatic pulmonary insufficiency is also included in the measurement. In certain conditions such as obesity and chronic obstructive lung disease, significant shunting may occur as a result of uneven distribution of ventilation to perfusion when the patient is breathing room air. In such cases, it may be useful to determine $P_{(A-aD_{O_2})}$ when the patient is breathing room air (or 50% oxygen if ambient air is not tolerated).

When $F_{I_{O_2}}$ is substantially less than 100%, it is necessary for precise calculation of $P_{A_{O_2}}$ to use the alveolar gas equation (Nunn JF: *Applied Respiratory Physiology With Special Reference to Anesthesia.*

Appleton-Century-Crofts, 1969; p 108) and either to measure the respiratory exchange ratio or to assume it to be 0.8. For rough calculation of $P_{A_{O_2}}$, the following formula can be used:

$$P_{A_{O_2}} = F_{I_{O_2}} \times (P_B - P_{H_2O}) - P_{a_{CO_2}}$$

Although measurement of $P_{(A-aD_{O_2})}$ during temporary ventilation with 100% oxygen is a useful guide to the magnitude of right-to-left shunt under most circumstances, actual determination of the shunt ($\dot{Q}_S/\dot{Q}_T$) is necessary for accurate data. Oxygen content of arterial, mixed venous, and pulmonary end-capillary blood must be measured and substituted in the following "shunt equation":

$$\dot{Q}_S/\dot{Q}_T = \frac{C_{c_{O_2}} - C_{a_{O_2}}}{C_{c_{O_2}} - C_{v_{O_2}}}$$

where $\dot{Q}_S$ = portion of cardiac output perfusing nonventilated areas (ie, right-to-left shunt flow in liters/min),

$\dot{Q}_T$ = total cardiac output,

$C_{c_{O_2}}$, $C_{a_{O_2}}$, and $C_{v_{O_2}}$ = oxygen content (ml/100 ml STPD) of pulmonary end-capillary, arterial, and mixed venous blood, respectively, and

$\dot{Q}_S/\dot{Q}_T \times 100$ = % right-to-left shunt.

Precise calculation of the percentage of shunt by the above formula requires cardiac catheterization to obtain samples of pulmonary end-capillary blood and of mixed venous blood from the pulmonary artery. This may not be feasible in acutely ill patients—hence the frequent reliance on $P_{(A-aD_{O_2})}$ as a practical indicator of the magnitude of right-to-left shunting.

The relationship of $P_{(A-aD_{O_2})}$ to percentage of shunt ($\dot{Q}_S/\dot{Q}_T \times 100$) can be estimated by use of a set of curves calculated from the shunt equation and published by Pontoppidan & others (Advances Surg 4:163−254, 1970; p 173). It is also possible to calculate the percentage of shunt from a simplified version of the shunt equation which is reliable only when the $P_{a_{O_2}}$ is high enough to ensure full saturation of hemoglobin (ie, $P_{a_{O_2}}$ above 150 mm Hg):

$$\dot{Q}_S/\dot{Q}_T = \frac{P_{(A-aD_{O_2})} \times 0.0031}{P_{(A-aD_{O_2})} \times 0.0031 + C_{(a-vD_{O_2})}} \times 100$$

where 0.0031 is the factor for conversion of partial pressure into oxygen content at 37 C. By making the assumption that the arterial-venous oxygen content difference ($C_{[a-vD_{O_2}]}$) is normal (6 ml/100 ml) and thus avoiding the necessity for obtaining a mixed venous oxygen content on a pulmonary artery sample, the formula for determining the percentage of shunt can be further simplified as follows:

$$\dot{Q}_S/\dot{Q}_T = \frac{P_{(A-aD_{O_2})} \times 0.0031}{P_{(A-aD_{O_2})} \times 0.0031 + 6} \times 100$$

According to this formula, the percentage of shunt when $P_{(A-aD_{O_2})}$ is 450 mm Hg may be calculated as follows:

$$\dot{Q}_S/\dot{Q}_T = \frac{450 \times 0.0031}{450 \times 0.0031 + 6} \times 100 = 19\%$$

The limitations of $P_{(A-aD_{O_2})}$ as a measure of shunting must be kept in mind. Changes in cardiac output and arterial-venous oxygen difference may alter the values of both $P_{(A-aD_{O_2})}$ and $\dot{Q}_S/\dot{Q}_T$. On the other hand, the agreement of alveolar-arterial oxygen difference with percentage of shunt is good when the cardiac output and the arterial-venous oxygen difference are within fairly normal limits.

Physiologic shunting of 10–15% due to atelectasis and other factors occurs in almost all patients after major trauma and may even be present after uncomplicated upper abdominal surgery. Wilson & others (Current Topics in Surgical Research 1:361–374, 1969) found that patients with post-traumatic pulmonary failure with physiologic shunt fractions below 40% will generally survive when provided with intensive supportive care whereas few patients survive with shunts of greater than 50%. If the shunt fraction approaches 30–35% in any patient, some form of ventilatory assistance is usually indicated.

B. Tests of Ventilation:

1. Tidal volume (V_T)–Tidal volume (V_T) is the volume of gas inspired or expired during each respiratory cycle. It is easily measured at the bedside and is controlled at a prescribed level during ventilatory assistance. Tidal volume is usually 400–500 ml (7 ml/kg) in a healthy young adult. It varies with age and state of health. A nomogram is available from which the normal basal tidal volume can be predicted from the breathing frequency, body weight, and sex (Radford & others: New England J Med 251:877–884, 1954). This nomogram applies only to patients with normal lungs.

2. Minute expired volume ($\dot{V}_E$)–Minute expired volume ($\dot{V}_E$) is tidal volume multiplied by respiratory frequency ($\dot{V}_E = V_T \times f$). Normal ventilation is the minute expired volume required in a normal person to maintain normal arterial CO_2 tension (P_{aCO_2}). Because physiologic dead space (V_D) is frequently increased in patients with pulmonary disease and in acute respiratory failure, the "normal" minute ventilation as predicted from the above-mentioned nomogram is often grossly inadequate to prevent retention of CO_2 (hypercapnia). It is important to emphasize that adequacy of ventilation in the very sick patient cannot be determined simply by measuring the volume of ventilation. In a specific patient, adequate ventilation is defined as the minute expired volume which is in fact needed to maintain normal arterial CO_2 tension. Accordingly, when a patient is receiving respiratory assistance, the minute expired volume is adjusted upward or downward depending upon the arterial CO_2 values.

3. Measurement of arterial CO_2 tension (P_{aCO_2})–CO_2 tension in arterial blood is usually measured directly by means of a Severinghaus glass electrode. CO_2 tension can also be obtained from the Henderson-Hasselbalch equation when the CO_2 content and the pH of plasma are known. *Arterial CO_2 tension is the only valid measure of the adequacy of ventilation.* Normal ventilation is the minute volume of ventilation required to maintain normal arterial CO_2 tension in a normal person. In patients with respiratory disease and failure, there is frequently an increase in physiologic dead space (see below). Under these circumstances, the predicted volume of ventilation is grossly inadequate to eliminate CO_2, so that arterial CO_2 tension increases and hypercapnia results. Voluntary overbreathing and excessive ventilation–due, for example, to a brain lesion or to a poorly adjusted mechanical ventilator–are among the causes of hyperventilation and hypocapnia seen clinically.

In summary, the state of alveolar ventilation is defined by the CO_2 tension in arterial blood (P_{aCO_2}). The average normal value of P_{aCO_2} is 40 mm Hg, and the normal range is 35–45 mm Hg. A lower than normal value indicates alveolar hypoventilation or hypercapnia.

4. Dead space to tidal volume ratio (V_D/V_T)–Physiologic dead space (V_D) is that portion of each tidal volume which does not exchange gas and is a calculated quantity rather than an actual physical space. It consists of 2 components: anatomic and alveolar dead space. **Anatomic dead space** comprises the volume of the conducting airway (nose, mouth, pharynx, larynx, trachea, bronchi, and bronchioles down to the functional bronchiolar-alveolar junction). The anatomic dead space in an adult in milliliters is about equal to his ideal weight in pounds. Tracheostomy reduces the anatomic dead space by about 33%. At large tidal volumes, the anatomic dead space may be increased by as much as 50%, and at low tidal volumes it may fall below predicted values.

Alveolar dead space is the difference between the calculated physiologic dead space and the anatomic dead space. Alveolar dead space is small in normal humans at rest, so that under these conditions anatomic dead space is approximately equal to physiologic dead space, ie, about 30% of tidal volume.

The ratio of dead space to tidal volume (V_D/V_T) is a measure of the efficiency of CO_2 elimination and thus of ventilation. It represents that portion of the tidal volume that is not effective in the removal of CO_2 from the blood. The actual determination of the V_D/V_T ratio involves collection of expired gas in a balloon or chamber and simultaneous collection of an arterial blood sample. The pressure of CO_2 is measured in the expired air (P_{ECO_2}) and in the arterial blood (P_{aCO_2}), and the values are substituted in the following formula:

$$V_D/V_T = \frac{P_{aCO_2} - P_{ECO_2}}{P_{aCO_2}}$$

The test can be performed at the bedside on patients with artificial ventilation or spontaneous respiration. The normal range for V_D/V_T is 0.25–0.40 (see Table 3–2).

An increase in the V_D/V_T ratio results in alveolar hypoventilation and reduced elimination of CO_2. The arterial CO_2 level (Pa_{CO_2}) rises and remains high unless compensation is achieved by an increase in tidal volume and alveolar ventilation. In acute respiratory failure, the patient may be unable to compensate without artificial ventilation. Table 3–2 indicates that respiratory support should be considered when V_D/V_T exceeds 0.6. In most such patients, the ventilatory requirements are substantially greater than those predicted for normal individuals. The objective in the patient who is receiving respiratory support for respiratory failure is to adjust the minute volume of respiration to the level required to maintain normal arterial CO_2 tension. This requires measurement of Pa_{CO_2}, which is used as a guide to adjustment of tidal and breathing frequency. Ventilation requirements in such patients change from day to day or even from hour to hour, so that it may be necessary to determine Pa_{CO_2} and to adjust the minute volume several times a day. Each time the Pa_{CO_2} is measured in the patient on artificial ventilation, it is advisable also to measure minute ventilation and tidal volume (by attaching a ventilation meter to the exhalation part of the respirator) and to record the peak airway pressure (see p 27).

The following conditions are commonly associated with increased physiologic dead space (V_D) and increased dead space to tidal volume ratio (V_D/V_T): **(1) Pulmonary embolism** interrupts alveolar capillary blood flow, resulting in nonperfusion of ventilated alveoli and thus increasing V_D/V_T. **(2) Hypotension** due to hemorrhage and other causes lowers pulmonary arterial pressure so that blood flow is redistributed by gravity to the dependent portions of the lung. Perfusion of ventilated alveoli in the remainder of the lung is diminished, and V_D/V_T is increased. **(3) Atelectasis** is characterized by nonventilation of perfused atelectatic alveoli, which results in shunting (see p 23). When these atelectatic alveoli resist inflation during constant volume artificial ventilation, ventilation is redistributed to air spaces in other parts of the lung without a matching redistribution of perfusion. The net effect is an increase in V_D/V_T. It is also observed that increase in V_D/V_T may correlate with radiographic evidence of atelectasis, pneumonia, and pulmonary edema and that a substantial drop in abnormally elevated V_D/V_T may be accompanied by concomitant improvement in the chest x-ray. **(4) High mean airway pressure** during artificial ventilation, particularly in the hypotensive patient, may inhibit capillary perfusion of ventilated alveoli and thus raise the V_D/V_T.

C. **Tests of Ventilatory Reserve and Mechanics:** The following tests of ventilatory reserve and mechanics are useful (1) to disclose respiratory insufficiency which has not progressed to the point of decreased alveolar ventilation, and (2) to evaluate the progress of patients in whom spontaneous breathing is capable of providing adequate alveolar ventilation:

1. **Vital capacity (VC)**–Total vital capacity (VC) is the simplest and most frequently used lung volume measurement. It is the maximum volume which can be expelled after a maximum inspiration without limit of time. It is a gross index of the ventilatory reserve for inspiratory effort in the conscious and cooperative patient. For adequate reserve, the vital capacity should be at least 3 times the tidal volume. In other words, the patient's ventilatory reserve may be considered inadequate if his vital capacity is less than 3 times his average tidal volume. Adequate reserve is necessary for effective deep breathing and coughing and in order to permit an appropriate increase in minute ventilation when the ventilation requirement becomes greater as a result of enlarged dead space or increased metabolic demand. The normal range of vital capacity is 65–75 ml/kg body weight. For adequate sustained spontaneous ventilation, most patients require a total vital capacity of 20–25% of predicted normal or at least 15 ml/kg body weight. Vital capacity of less than 15 ml/kg suggests the need for ventilatory support (see Table 3–2).

2. **First-second vital capacity (FEV$_1$)**–The forced expiratory volume (FEV) is also known as the "timed vital capacity." It consists of the maximum volume which can be expelled in a timed interval by a maximally fast expiration starting from a full inspiration. The volume expelled may be measured at 0.50, 0.75, 1, and 3 seconds. The volume expelled in 1 second (FEV$_1$) is normally about 85% of actual vital capacity, and the volume expelled in 3 seconds (FEV$_3$) is normally about 95% of actual vital capacity. It has been demonstrated that FEV$_{0.75}$ multiplied by 40, or FEV$_1$ multiplied by 30, is usually approximately equal to the maximal voluntary ventilation (MVV) in liters per minute.

A reduced FEV usually but not always indicates increased airway resistance due to obstructive bronchopulmonary disease. Improvement in FEV after administration of a bronchodilator is consistent with some degree of reversibility. The FEV$_1$ is more informative than the VC in acute or chronic obstruction to air flow because decreased volume expelled per unit of time usually indicates not only resistance to air flow but also reduced capacity to cough and to generate the work of breathing. The normal range of FEV$_1$ is 50–60 ml/kg body weight, or 3–4 liters in the adult male. For sustained, adequate spontaneous ventilation, the FEV$_1$ should exceed 10 ml/kg. Values below 10 ml/kg suggest the need for ventilatory support (see Table 3–2).

3. **Maximal voluntary ventilation (MVV)**–The maximal voluntary ventilation is also termed the maximal breathing capacity (MBC). This test is performed by having the patient breathe in and out as rapidly and as deeply as possible, usually at a rate of 60–90 times per minute, for 15 seconds. The total volume breathed in or out during this period is expressed in liters per minute. Full cooperation by a well-coordinated patient

is necessary for the successful performance of this test, which may be too strenuous for a chronically or acutely ill patient. There is also considerable variation in the results of this test, so that a healthy person may deviate as much as 25–35% from the predicted normal value. The indirect MVV calculated from the $FEV_{0.75}$ or FEV_1 (as noted above) has been found useful in those patients who are too ill to undertake the MVV test. The MVV is another of the methods used to assess airway resistance and the presence of obstructive bronchopulmonary disease. The range of normal values for young and middle-aged adult males is 100–150 liters/min.

The "match test" is a simple bedside test which correlates grossly with the results of the FEV_1 and the MVV. The test consists of determining the ability of the patient to blow out a burning match held 4–6 inches from his mouth. Inability to do so constitutes a positive result. After inhaling as deeply as possible, the patient is instructed to exhale forcibly with his mouth kept widely open. To assure maximal patient effort, the test is repeated several times. If the match test is positive, it is advisable to obtain FEV_1 and, if possible, MVV. Snider & others (JAMA 170:1631–1632, 1959) found that 80% of patients with MVV greater than 60 liters/min could extinguish the match, whereas 80% of those with MVV of less than 60 liters/min could not. Eighty-five percent of those with FEV_1 greater than 1.6 liters/sec could extinguish the match, whereas 85% with FEV_1 less than 1.6 liters/sec could not.

The prognostic value of MVV was studied by Anderson & others (JAMA 186:763–766, 1963). They found a 2½ times greater incidence of postoperative pulmonary complications in patients with MVV less than 60% of predicted than in a comparable group of patients with MVV greater than 60% of predicted.

4. Maximal expiratory flow rate (MEFR)—This test is also a method of quantitating airway resistance and the severity of obstructive lung disease. The patient takes a maximal inspiration and, after a short pause, expires as fast and as forcefully as possible into a spirometer with a rapidly rotating drum. The MEFR is the flow between the first 200 ml and 1200 ml expressed in liters/min (normal for adult male: 350–550 liters/min). The maximal midexpiratory flow rate (MMFR) is the flow between the first 25% and 75% of the total forced expiratory volume (FEV) and is expressed in liters/sec. A reduced flow rate has the same significance as a reduced FEV_1 and is typical of increased airway resistance and obstructive lung disease. Normal MMFR is 2–4 liters/sec. Patients with significant chronic obstructive lung disease usually have an MMFR below 1 liter/sec and often below 0.5 liters/sec.

5. Inspiratory force—Inspiratory force is measured by simple equipment consisting of a face mask (or connector to an endotracheal tube) fitted with a manometer capable of registering below atmospheric pressure. Inspiratory force is the maximum inspiratory pressure below atmospheric which the patient can exert during a period of 10–20 seconds against a com-

pletely occluded airway. The method does not depend upon the patient's cooperation and is particularly useful in the comatose or anesthetized patient. The normal range of inspiratory force is 75–100 cm water below atmospheric. CNS depression or muscular weakness may cause low values. When lung compliance is decreased, greater inspiratory force is required to achieve adequate tidal ventilation. Experience has shown that artificial ventilation is usually required in patients with acute respiratory failure when inspiratory force is less than 25 cm water (see Table 3–2). It has also been found that successful weaning from intermittent positive pressure ventilation requires an inspiratory force exceeding 30–40 cm water.

6. Effective compliance—Lung compliance is defined as the volume change per unit pressure change:

$$\text{Compliance} = \frac{\text{Volume change}}{\text{Pressure change}} = \text{ml/cm water}$$

It is a measure of the elastic resistance (or distensibility) of the lungs and chest wall, either separately or together. Compliance of the lungs plus that of the chest wall can be measured in a spontaneously breathing patient by analyzing continuous recordings of airway pressure, gas flow, and tidal volume. In a patient with no spontaneous respiratory effort, total static compliance can be measured by using a large syringe to inject a predetermined volume of air (within the normal range of the patient's tidal volume) into the lungs while reading the airway pressure on a manometer.

In the patient on assisted ventilation, it is simple to determine the "effective compliance," which is defined as the ratio of tidal volume to peak airway pressure:

$$\text{Effective compliance} = \frac{\text{Tidal volume}}{\text{Peak airway pressure}} = \text{ml/cm water}$$

Average values for effective compliance are 40–50 ml/cm water for adult males and 35–45 ml/cm water for adult females with normal lungs. This measure may be misleading in the presence of high airway resistance.

A fall in effective compliance in the patient on assisted ventilation may be an early sign of atelectasis, pneumonia, or interstitial pulmonary edema (as in posttraumatic pulmonary insufficiency or "shock lung") before auscultative or radiographic evidence appears. These complications require prompt treatment. They are often associated with increased physiologic shunting. Decrease in effective compliance therefore indicates a need to determine arterial blood gases and possibly to readjust the pattern of ventilation and the concentration of inspired oxygen. Pontoppidan & others (New England J Med 273:401–409, 1965) found that decrease in effective compliance is significantly related to an increase in the dead space to tidal volume (V_D/V_T) ratio and indicates the need for reassessment of ventilation requirement. Finally, if an undetected fall in compliance occurs in a patient on a pressure-limited respirator, tidal volume will decrease, with possible rapid development of hypoxia and hyper-capnia, unless the respirator is properly readjusted. Relatively high airway pressures may be necessary to provide the required alveolar ventilation.

Differential Diagnosis

The etiologic differential diagnosis of acute respiratory failure after operation or trauma can usually be made by means of the history and physical examination and by taking special note of predisposing conditions (see p 18). However, it is again emphasized that laboratory studies—particularly blood gases—are essential to the identification of occult cases of respiratory failure when there are minimal or no physical findings and to the evaluation of patients with complex problems. Acute respiratory failure is usually due either to hypoventilation or to ventilation-perfusion disproportion—or, more frequently, to a combination of the two. Pulmonary function tests and blood gas analysis are especially helpful in following the patient's progress, in deciding when respiratory assistance should be started and discontinued, and in determining the pathogenesis (Tables 3–1 and 3–2). Tidal and minute volumes of ventilation are decreased in hypoventilation but are often increased in severe ventilation-perfusion defects. If the cause of respiratory failure is primarily hypoventilation, the usual finding is decreased arterial P_{O_2} and increased arterial P_{CO_2}. If the problem is due to ventilation-perfusion defect, the arterial P_{O_2} will be low whereas the arterial P_{CO_2} may be elevated but is frequently normal or low.

Hypoventilation and ventilation-perfusion disproportion will be discussed below in more detail. As an important example of ventilation-perfusion abnormality, posttraumatic pulmonary insufficiency will be specifically reviewed.

A. Hypoventilation: Simply stated, hypoventilation results from failure to move sufficient air in and out of the lungs with the result that respiratory exchange is inadequate to remove CO_2 and to oxygenate the blood. Hypoventilation is associated with low tidal and minute volumes, resulting in deficient alveolar ventilation. The patient's respirations are either too shallow or too slow to maintain a normal partial pressure of oxygen in the alveoli and to remove accumulating CO_2. On room air, arterial P_{O_2} tends to fall and arterial P_{CO_2} to rise. These blood gas changes are frequently the only indication of the seriousness of the ventilatory deficiency. When the $P_{a_{CO_2}}$ exceeds the normal range, there is respiratory acidosis. Severe and prolonged hypoxia (low $P_{a_{O_2}}$) produces metabolic acidosis characterized by a base deficit due to anaerobic glycolysis in the tissues with release of lactic acid. Such diverse signs as restlessness, depressed sensorium, hypertension, and hypotension may be manifestations of serious hypoventilation.

Hypoventilation is the commonest cause of respiratory failure in the immediate postanesthetic period. It is important to be alert to its insidious development caused by the residual effects of anesthetic agents and muscle relaxants, prolonged hyperventilation during anesthesia, narcotic administration, or ventilatory inhibition by wound pain. Hypoxemia secondary to hypoventilation in the postanesthesia recovery room may result in cardiac arrhythmias and death, and depressed ventilation may predispose to the development of atelectasis and other pulmonary complications later in the postoperative period. In a series of patients with abdominal operations, Thompson & Eason (Am J Surg 120:649–651, 1970) found $P_{a_{O_2}}$ levels as low as 60 mm Hg in the immediate postanesthetic period in some patients and observed that the longer the operation, the lower the $P_{a_{O_2}}$. From the clinical point of view, these patients all seemed to be ventilating adequately as indicated by absence of cyanosis and apparently good chest wall excursion. Marshall & Millar (Anesthesia 20:408–428, 1965) found that low arterial oxygen tensions in the immediate postanesthetic period persisted for up to 3 hours. Reduction in $P_{a_{O_2}}$ was greatest in older patients, after mechanical overventilation, and when there was preexisting lung disease.

During the early postoperative days and after complete recovery from anesthesia, the danger of hypoventilation and its sequelae persists. Such a problem is particularly common after thoracic and upper abdominal operations; less common after lower abdominal procedures; and still less likely to occur after surgery on the extremities. The duration of operation is again noted to be a significant factor. As an example of postoperative inhibition of ventilation, Anscombe (*Pulmonary Complications of Abdominal Surgery*, Year Book, 1957) observed a 50–60% reduction in vital capacity and in expiratory and inspiratory flow rates for several days after gastrectomy. The adverse effects of hypoventilation may be accentuated by higher tissue needs for gas exchange, which may increase to 120% of normal in the postoperative period and, in the presence of severe infection, may increase to 140%.

In summary, hypoventilation occurs frequently in the postanesthetic and early postoperative period and following severe trauma. It is characterized by decreased tidal and minute volumes, decreased $P_{a_{O_2}}$, and increased $P_{a_{CO_2}}$. Because it may exist to a marked degree even in the absence of physical signs, alertness to the possibility of hypoventilation is vital to its recognition. The causes of hypoventilation include the residual effects of anesthetic drugs, postoperative pain, narcotics given to relieve pain, mechanical restrictions such as abdominal and chest binders, pleural effusion, hemothorax, pneumothorax, abdominal distention, obesity, neuromuscular conditions causing paralysis or weakness of the muscles of respiration, and traumatic flail chest. Fortunately, hypoventilation can usually be corrected promptly if the diagnosis is suspected and, when necessary, confirmed by pulmonary function and blood gas measurements.

B. Ventilation-Perfusion ($\dot{V}_A/\dot{Q}$) Disproportion: Even though tidal volume and minute volume may be normal or increased, CO_2 elimination and oxygenation may be inadequate due to uneven distribution of ventilation and perfusion to the alveoli. This abnormality is common after major operations or severe trauma and may lead to acute respiratory failure. There are 2 main types of ventilation-perfusion defect, and they frequently occur simultaneously. In one type, some alveoli are well ventilated and poorly perfused. (*Examples:* hypotension, pulmonary embolism). The result is an increase in physiologic dead space, V_D/V_T ratio, and Pa_{CO_2}. Under these circumstances, high Pa_{CO_2} usually responds to increase in tidal volume and alveolar ventilation. Oxygen administration may also be necessary (see Chapter 14). Nonperfusion of ventilated lung may occur during mechanical ventilation if mean airway pressure is elevated sufficiently in some alveoli to cause redistribution of blood flow to the remainder of the lung (Werko L: Acta med scandinav, Suppl 193:1–125, 1947). If atelectasis is present and resists inflation by high mean airway pressure, the blood flow which is redistributed from the hyperinflated alveoli elsewhere in the lung will go to the atelectatic areas. Under these circumstances, there is both an increase in dead space to tidal volume ratio (V_D/V_T) and an increase in the physiologic shunt (Finley TN, Hill TR, Bonica JJ: Am J Physiol 205:1187–1192, 1963). High mean airway pressure is more likely to produce these redistribution effects on perfusion and ventilation when hypotension or hypovolemia is present.

In the other type of ventilation-perfusion defect, some alveoli are well perfused but poorly ventilated. (*Examples:* atelectasis, pulmonary fibrosis, and posttraumatic pulmonary insufficiency.) The result is a large veno-arterial shunt associated with low arterial P_{O_2} and increased alveolar-arterial oxygen difference ($A–a_{D_{O_2}}$). The arterial P_{CO_2} is usually relatively normal or below normal. If the shunt is extensive enough to require treatment, hypoxemia may be relieved by oxygen administration, and assisted or controlled respiration may also be necessary (see p 32). Identification and relief of the underlying cause of the ventilation-perfusion defect is, of course, a primary concern in every case.

C. Posttraumatic Pulmonary Insufficiency: Progressive pulmonary insufficiency culminating in acute respiratory failure may occur after severe trauma, extensive surgery, shock, cardiopulmonary bypass, and profound sepsis. There are thus a number of precipitating causes which result in similar pathophysiologic changes. The condition has a variety of synonyms such as posttraumatic pulmonary insufficiency, postoperative lung syndrome, shock lung, pump lung, and wet lung. Preexisting chronic lung disease is a predisposing factor.

Moore & others (*Post-Traumatic Pulmonary Insufficiency.* Saunders, 1969) have described 4 progressive phases of the posttraumatic pulmonary insufficiency syndrome: (1) an initial phase, occurring immediately after injury and resuscitation, usually characterized by high cardiac output, lowered peripheral resistance, hyperventilation, and mild hypoxemia and hypocapnia; followed by (2) a period of early respiratory difficulty with stable circulation; followed

by (3) continued progression of pulmonary failure; and, finally, (4) severe hypoxia, hypercapnia, lactic acidosis, and cardiac arrest. The pathophysiology of this syndrome is discussed on p 23. It is important to note that pulmonary vascular congestion and edema are characteristic features of the acute pulmonary insufficiency that follows a number of different types of nonthoracic trauma and certain other severe stresses. Most of the functional abnormalities observed have been attributed to disturbances in ventilation and perfusion. The role, if any, of diminished diffusion capacity or "alveolar-capillary block" in acute respiratory failure in general and posttraumatic pulmonary insufficiency in particular has not been established.

Posttraumatic pulmonary insufficiency has been recognized in recent years as a frequent and often fatal condition, especially in military and civilian hospitals that treat major trauma victims. It was reported to be the commonest cause of death following initial resuscitation of combat casualties in the Vietnam war. Early diagnosis depends upon anticipation of this type of pulmonary complication. Blood gas determinations and other respiratory tests are indicated on suspicion of developing respiratory failure. Factors which contribute to the pulmonary changes include fluid overload; pulmonary edema secondary to fluid retention associated with prolonged mechanical ventilation, head injury, and renal failure; aspiration of gastric contents; fat embolism; transfusion microembolism from debris in banked blood; and, very importantly, the low-flow states associated with hemorrhagic and septic shock.

Diagnostic & Monitoring Procedures

The onset of acute respiratory failure may be insidious. Early diagnosis requires not only alertness to premonitory physical signs but also the ready availability of test equipment in the postanesthetic and intensive care areas. Table 3–1 lists the examinations which are useful in diagnosis and in monitoring. The following basic pieces of apparatus will make it possible to perform the most frequently needed of the diagnostic and monitoring procedures: blood gas and pH analyzer, paramagnetic oxygen analyzer, low-resistance nonrebreathing and expired gas collection system, Wright respirometer for bedside determination of expired respiratory volumes, and a Collins spirometer for recording of measurements such as FEV_1 and MEFR. Improved results in recent years in the treatment of patients with respiratory failure are attributable to aggressive management based on physiologic principles and guided by objective data from respiratory function studies.

The indications for ventilatory support in patients with acute respiratory failure are summarized in Table 3–2. In Table 3–4, Pontoppidan & others (Advances Surg 4:163–254, 1970) have proposed a set of guidelines for the identification of patients who require preventive measures (see below) and close monitoring because of borderline respiratory compensation:

TABLE 3–4. Indications for preventive measures
and close monitoring.

	Acceptable Range	Preventive Measures and Monitoring Required
Mechanics		
Respiratory rate	12–25	25–35
Vital capacity (ml/kg)	70–30	30–15
Inspiratory force (cm water)	100–50	50–25
Oxygenation		
Pa_{O_2} (mm Hg)	100–75 (air)	200–70 (on mask O_2)
$P(A-a_{DO_2})^{1.0}$ (mm Hg)	50–200	200–350
Ventilation		
Pa_{CO_2} (mm Hg)	35–45	45–60
V_D/V_T	0.3–0.4	0.4–0.6

Prevention

Acute respiratory failure is largely preventable, and moderate pulmonary insufficiency can frequently be corrected promptly by relatively simple measures. A prime consideration in postoperative and traumatized patients is the prevention of atelectasis, which commonly sets the stage for a series of changes, including progressive collapse and pneumonitis, which may lead to respiratory failure. Avoidance of excess body fluid is another preventive measure which is of special importance in patients with borderline or failing pulmonary function—particularly those who are likely candidates for the development of posttraumatic pulmonary insufficiency. The prophylaxis of atelectasis and fluid overload can be briefly outlined as follows:

A. Atelectasis: The frequency with which atelectasis occurs in the postoperative period and its deleterious effects on pulmonary function have already been described. The aim of preventive measures is to minimize the occurrence of alveolar collapse, which may occur as a result of depressed respiratory excursions, small airway obstruction by secretions, or both.

1. Preoperative preparation—Chronic obstructive lung disease, chronic bronchitis, and acute respiratory infections should be brought under control by preoperative inhalation therapy, mist bronchodilator drugs, antibiotics, chest physical therapy, and other indicated methods of treatment so that secretions and respiratory obstruction will be minimized in the postoperative period. These measures should be continued postoperatively as required. Cooperation in deep breathing and coughing after operation is improved by preoperative instruction and practice.

2. Anesthesia and postanesthesia management—Endotracheal suction and frequent sighing and overexpansion of the lungs during and immediately after operation are indispensable procedures. Frequent turning of the patient and insistence on deep breathing and coughing in the recovery room (and throughout the

early postoperative period) are essential. The use of long rebreathing tubes postoperatively will stimulate ventilation by increasing the level of inspired CO_2. Laver & Bendixen (Progr Surg 5:1–37, 1966) noted that atelectasis is the commonest cause of hypoxia in the postoperative period and that the atelectasis is most frequently due to perpetuation of the periodic collapse of alveoli which is part of the normal pattern of ventilation. This is prevented by intermittent hyperventilation or deep breathing. Postanesthetic hypoventilation can usually be avoided by retaining the orotracheal or nasotracheal tube until spontaneous ventilation is well established. The tube not only facilitates tracheobronchial suction but also makes it possible to inflate the lungs several times every 15 minutes by hand compression of a self-inflating bag. When postoperative hypoventilation cannot be corrected by these simple means, continued intubation and prolonged ventilatory assistance become necessary.

3. Postoperative endotracheal intubation and artificial ventilation—The preventive value of prolonged controlled or assisted ventilation in selected patients after major surgery or severe trauma is firmly established. Some degree of respiratory failure can be predicted and often forestalled in patients with extensive injuries and operations, particularly if complicated by shock, sepsis, heart disease, obesity, muscular weakness, general debility, or chronic lung disease. The orotracheal tube can be left in place after operation, or a cuffed nasotracheal tube can be substituted for it. Mechanical ventilation, usually volume controlled, can then be continued for 48 hours—and several additional days if necessary—without undue hazard when proper equipment and experienced personnel are available. For example, mechanical ventilation for 24–48 hours after cardiac surgery is common practice and makes it possible to control the ventilatory pattern, lung expansion, and Pa_{CO_2}; to provide optimum oxygen intake (FI_{O_2}) and oxygenation (Pa_{O_2}); to remove secretions and prevent atelectasis by endotracheal suction; to reduce the work of breathing; and to facilitate accurate monitoring and control of the major parameters of pulmonary function. In controlled ventilation, the patient's respiratory effort must be eliminated so that the ventilator can completely take over the rhythm and depth of respiration. If sedation is necessary to depress the patient's respiratory drive or to prevent coughing or bucking on the endotracheal tube, small intravenous doses of morphine (2–3 mg) or meperidine (10–20 mg) should be given. It may occasionally be necessary to paralyze the patient, preferably with tubocurarine in repeated doses of 5–10 mg IV until the desired effect is obtained.

4. Oxygen therapy—Warm humidified oxygen prevents drying of the tracheobronchial mucosa and aids in mobilization of secretions, thus helping in the prevention of atelectasis. If hypoxia is suspected—or confirmed by a finding of Pa_{O_2} below 85 mm Hg—humidified oxygen may be delivered at a rate of 10 liters/min by a face tent which will provide about 40% inspired oxygen, which may be adequate; or by a snug mask which will raise inspired oxygen to 60–80%. A nasal catheter or cannula is simpler but provides less humidification; a flow of 100% oxygen at a rate of 5–10 liters/min results in inspired oxygen of 30–40%. A nasal cannula is more comfortable than a catheter and permits oxygen flow of up to 10 liters/min. Flow of oxygen through a nasal catheter should be limited to about 5 liters/min.

5. Nasotracheal suction—Introduction of a sterile 14F catheter into the tracheobronchial tree via the nose is an effective means of stimulating cough and aspirating sputum when the patient is unable or unwilling to cough up his secretions. This procedure should be performed early and as often as necessary in the postoperative period. Bronchoscopy may on rare occasion be required.

6. Transtracheal catheter—Some patients require cough stimulation and liquefaction of secretions but can then raise sputum without tracheal aspiration. Under these circumstances, transtracheal catheterization is a simple and useful procedure which should be done without undue delay. A standard No. 14 Intracath (Bard) is inserted percutaneously under local anesthesia into the trachea just below the cricoid cartilage. Alternatively, a plastic catheter can be passed through a No. 18 needle. Injection of 2–3 ml of sterile saline (or distilled water if necessary for stimulation) through the catheter will excite cough. The injection may be repeated as often as required to mobilize secretions and clear the airway. The catheter is too small to permit effective aspiration of secretions but may permit obtaining a specimen for culture.

7. Chest physical therapy—Encouragement of the patient to hyperventilate, cough vigorously, and raise secretions is a normal feature of good postoperative nursing care and, if done assiduously, will often obviate the need for mechanical aids. Blow bottles are a useful means of obtaining the cooperation of the patient in deep breathing. Inhalation of mist from an ultrasonic device or heated nebulizer is a useful adjunct to chest physical therapy. Intermittent positive pressure breathing has its advocates, but its value is uncertain and it is generally overrated as a postoperative measure.

8. Guides to prevention—Atelectasis should be anticipated and the above measures utilized appropriately in patients who are at risk by virtue of their circumstances. By the time physical signs and x-ray changes have occurred, atelectasis is an established and advanced process. Widespread patchy atelectasis due to alveolar collapse is a common early development that may be detected only by blood gas determination, which shows decreased P_{aO_2} and increased $P_{(A-aDO_2)}$.

B. Fluid Overload: Positive water balance should be avoided in postoperative and posttraumatic patients who are at risk of respiratory failure either because of the severity of their injury or the presence of chronic pulmonary disease. In shock or sepsis, water and protein may enter the interstitial space of the lung as a result of loss of integrity of the capillary endothelium. Under these circumstances, edema fluid accumulates primarily in the dependent portions of the lung even in the absence of increased capillary hydrostatic pressure (Cottrel & others: Circulation Res 21:783–797, 1967). For unknown reasons, patients on prolonged artificial ventilation also tend to retain water.

It is therefore important to maintain correct water and electrolyte balance in patients with impending or actual respiratory deficiency. This is usually accomplished through monitoring of intake and output, blood electrolytes, and body weight. Limitation of fluid intake and diuretic therapy may be necessary to maintain equilibrium. In the absence of damage to pulmonary capillaries, diuretic therapy and restriction of water lead to improvement of respiratory function. Colloid is administered only if there is circulatory evidence of hypovolemia or if hypoalbuminemia is present.

In patients with hemorrhagic or septic shock or drug intoxication, left-sided heart failure may exist in the presence of a low central venous pressure. If blood, albumin, or electrolyte solution is infused until arterial pressure and central venous pressure are normal, interstitial pulmonary edema and increased shunting (rising $A-aDO_2$) will almost invariably occur. In such patients, replacement should be considered adequate when urine output is satisfactory in spite of subnormal systemic arterial and venous pressure. If decreased urinary output is secondary to inadequate cardiac output and renal blood flow in the presence of adequate blood volume, it is frequently necessary to improve cardiac output by intravenous infusion of isoproterenol or epinephrine, or possibly transvenous cardiac pacing. Under these circumstances also, the best end point in terms of systemic blood pressure is the return of urinary flow (Pontoppidan & others: New England J Med 287:690–698, 1972).

Positive water balance in patients with impending or established respiratory failure should be recognized as a potentially serious problem and should be avoided. Prevention may involve limitation of fluid intake to 25–30 ml/kg/day. Body weight should decline by 350–500 g daily in patients with no caloric intake, and failure of such patients to lose weight means water retention. It should be remembered that the contribution of the nebulizer to body fluid may amount to 300–500 ml a day. Management by fluid restriction—and diuretics if necessary—are usually effective in reversing the trends toward fluid overload (Pontoppidan H: J Trauma 8:938–951, 1968).

Treatment

There are 2 major aspects to the treatment of respiratory failure. The first consists of measures for relief of conditions in the chest and elsewhere which are primarily responsible for the decrease in pulmonary function. These conditions include respiratory depression, thoracic disease or injury, atelectasis, and fluid overload, which have been discussed above. Measures to correct these conditions are essential in both prevention and treatment of respiratory failure.

The second aspect of treatment consists of procedures to maintain adequate ventilation and oxygenation while the patient recovers from the underlying causes of respiratory failure. These procedures will now be reviewed.

A. Indications for Mechanical Ventilation: Mild cases of hypoventilation and ventilation-perfusion disproportion usually respond to supplementary oxygen and other preventive measures (see above). When adequate ventilation and oxygenation cannot be maintained by these methods, respiratory support by mechanical ventilation is needed. The criteria for respiratory support are summarized in Table 3–2 and the criteria for monitoring in Table 3–4. The decision to provide an airway and begin mechanical ventilation should not be delayed until the patient's condition deteriorates. The preventive value of respiratory support in selected patients at high risk of respiratory failure has already been emphasized. Respiratory support is probably indicated if a patient who is receiving oxygen at 10 liters/min by face tent or mask has a Pa_{O_2} of 70–80 mm Hg or a Pa_{CO_2} of 50–55 mm Hg and the trend in these values is worsening, or if a poorly oxygenated patient has rapid, shallow respirations and is tiring. By the time the patient is gasping for breath and developing ventricular arrhythmias, there has been too much delay.

Once the diagnosis of acute respiratory failure and the need for respiratory support are established, treatment by mechanical ventilation is required to increase alveolar ventilation and to deliver greater amounts of oxygen to the arterial blood. The procedures involved are tracheal intubation and operation of a mechanical ventilator. Positive pressure ventilation by way of a tight-fitting face mask is useful in emergency resuscitation, but this technic is not efficient nor is it tolerated by the patient for very long. Therefore, tracheal intubation is necessary if mechanical support of respiration is required in respiratory failure.

B. Tracheal Intubation: A cuffed endotracheal tube is passed through the mouth if the situation is urgent. If feasible, intubation through the nose is more comfortable for the patient. However, tube size is limited by the nostrils and turbinates, and nasotracheal tubes are longer, narrower, offer greater resistance to gas flow, are harder to keep patent, and have a greater tendency to kink than orotracheal tubes. The tube can be left in place for 2–5 days if properly cared for. Once the tube is inserted and mechanical ventilation begun, it is possible to decide at greater leisure whether tracheostomy should be done. There is thus rarely a need for emergency tracheostomy.

1. Indications for tracheostomy—Elective tracheostomy is performed for the following reasons: (1) anatomic or traumatic abnormality precludes intubation from above; (2) obvious long-term need (ie, more than 4–5 days) for tracheal intubation; (3) failure to tolerate oral or nasal intubation; (4) inability to cope with excessive secretions or other problems without tracheostomy. Placement of an endotracheal tube prior to tracheostomy is of great advantage because it permits good ventilation and oxygenation during

tracheostomy and makes the procedure technically easier. Emergency tracheostomy is required when intubation from above is technically impossible or inadequate in such conditions as acute upper airway obstruction, massive aspiration, pulmonary hemorrhage, head and neck wounds, respiratory burns, and severe respiratory failure.

2. Management of the intubated patient—A competent attendant must *always* be present when an intubated patient is on mechanical ventilation. Disconnection or failure of the equipment can be rapidly lethal. Aseptic technic should be observed in handling the connections and during aspiration of the tube. The trachea should be suctioned as often as necessary to avoid accumulation of secretions and to prevent atelectasis. The patient should be well oxygenated prior to suctioning, and ventilation should be interrupted for no more than 15 seconds. In order to avoid drying of secretions in the airway, the respiratory gas mixture should be humidified by passage through heated water and delivered at 39 C. Mist should be visible but not densely so. Excessive volume of tracheal secretions suggests excessive humidification.

3. Complications of intubation—Laryngeal or tracheal ulceration and stenosis are common sequelae of intubation when extreme care is not taken to prevent these serious complications. Prolonged orotracheal or nasotracheal tubes may cause severe damage to the larynx, resulting in hoarseness, difficulty in swallowing, impaired laryngeal activity, and varying degrees of respiratory obstruction. By taking extreme care to reduce trauma due to the tube, the safe period of prolonged endotracheal intubation can in some cases be extended up to 8 days in adults and up to 3 weeks in children and infants. Maximal damage to the trachea from tracheostomy tubes typically develops at the level of the inflatable cuff. Tracheoesophageal fistula or erosion into a major artery may rarely occur, but the most frequent complication is fibrosis and stenosis of the trachea. By using low-pressure pliable cuffs on endotracheal and tracheostomy tubes, the incidence of these complications can be greatly reduced (Grillo & others: J Thoracic Cardiovas Surg 62:898–907, 1971). Inflation of the endotracheal or tracheal tube cuff should be just sufficient to prevent air leakage into the mouth during positive pressure ventilation. The cuff can be deflated when suctioning the patient and for about 5 minutes every hour if the patient can tolerate being off mechanical ventilation for that length of time. It may otherwise be necessary to deflate the cuff only briefly at hourly intervals. Suctioning of the oropharynx prior to letting the balloon down may prevent aspiration of material into the trachea.

C. Use of Mechanical Ventilators:

1. Type of ventilator—The best unit is a volume-limited ventilator with a variable inspiratory flow rate and a sighing device to produce periodic hyperinflations (eg, the Bennett MA–1). This type of ventilator will deliver a preset volume with each breath and is preferred to the pressure-cycled ventilator, which always requires the patient to perform some respiratory work.

2. Adjustment of the ventilator—

a. Assisted vs controlled ventilation—It must be decided whether ventilation should be assisted, with the patient initiating each breath, or controlled by the machine. If the patient's respiratory frequency is slow (12–15 breaths per minute), assisted ventilation can be tried. If not, controlled ventilation should be used at the most efficient frequency, which is 12–15 breaths per minute. It is advisable to use controlled ventilation initially in very ill patients. It may be necessary to depress the patient's respiratory drive and cough reflex by intravenous administration of morphine, meperidine, or tubocurarine (see p 30).

b. Ventilation—On controlled or assisted ventilation, the magnitude of the patient's ventilation is determined by adjustment of tidal volume and respiratory frequency. These are regulated to maintain a normal P_{aCO_2} of 35–40 mm Hg. P_{aCO_2} is thus the guide to the minute volume of ventilation required by the patient. Hyperventilation resulting in a P_{aCO_2} of 30–35 mm Hg is tolerable, but lower levels of P_{aCO_2} should be avoided.

c. Oxygenation—Oxygenation of the blood is maintained if possible at a minimum P_{aO_2} of 80–90 mm Hg. This is accomplished by increasing the fraction of oxygen in inspired air (F_{IO_2}) as required to raise the P_{aO_2}. It is usually appropriate to begin with 40% humidified oxygen. It is not useful to raise the P_{aO_2} above 130 mm Hg. Clinical experience suggests that oxygen concentrations of 50% or higher are likely to produce serious pulmonary damage due to "oxygen toxicity" when used for more than 2 days. The higher the F_{IO_2}, the more rapid the onset of damage (Clark & others: Pharmacol Rev 23:37–133, 1971). The morphologic changes presumably caused by oxygen toxicity include interstitial and intra-alveolar edema, hemorrhage, and hyaline membranes. These are nonspecific responses to a variety of injuries of which oxygen toxicity is only one. Except in chronically hypoxemic patients, it is generally advisable to select an F_{IO_2} that will result in a P_{aO_2} in the normal range. However, if the arteriovenous shunt is so large (marked elevation of $P_{[A-aDO_2]}$ and $\dot{Q}s/\dot{Q}T$) due to atelectasis or other cause that an F_{IO_2} above 50% is necessary to maintain a normal P_{aO_2}, it may be preferable to accept a P_{aO_2} in the hypoxemic range.

Certain alterations in the ventilatory pattern have been found to improve oxygenation. Patients on controlled ventilation at normal tidal volumes of 7 ml/kg complain of dyspnea and inadequate chest expansion even though P_{aO_2} and P_{aCO_2} are normal. Larger tidal volumes (10–15 ml/kg) are therefore advised and are well tolerated. Excessive hypocapnia can be corrected by introduction of mechanical dead space (Suwa & others: Anesthesiology 29:1206–1210, 1968). It has also been noted that the larger tidal volumes are associated with a reduction in $P_{(A-aDO_2)}$, whereas normal tidal volumes may be associated with a rise in $P_{(A-aDO_2)}$ indicative of progressive atelectasis. It is

possible that mechanical ventilators which automatically hyperinflate the lungs every 2–10 minutes may prevent progressive atelectasis and make it unnecessary to employ large tidal volumes and dead space.

Other variations in ventilatory pattern which may improve the efficiency of oxygenation are continuous positive pressure breathing (CPPB) and positive end-expiratory pressure (PEEP). On controlled ventilation with intermittent positive pressure ventilations (IPPV), airway pressure falls to zero during expiration, whereas normally the expiration is slowed by the continued action of the inspiratory muscles. In mechanically ventilated patients with stiff lungs due to decreased compliance, expiration is completed more quickly; with the ventilator pressure falling to zero during expiration, there is a greater tendency to alveolar collapse. It is possible that IPPV may in this way contribute to atelectasis. It has been observed clinically that CPPB with PEEP of 7–10 cm water is valuable in the treatment of hypoxemia and large $P_{(A-aDO_2)}$ in patients with severe respiratory failure not responding to other means of therapy (Ashbaugh & others: J Thoracic Cardiovas Surg 57:31–41, 1969). The chief mechanism by which PEEP (or CPPB) relieves hypoxemia is probably through prevention of alveolar collapse and shunting during the expiratory phase of respiration. Criteria for instituting PEEP include failure to maintain a P_{aO_2} of 70 mm Hg with an F_{IO_2} of 50% or more during IPPV; failure to reduce the shunt ($\dot{Q}s/\dot{Q}T$) by other measures such as treatment of cardiac failure, fluid overload, retained secretions, atelectasis, and pneumonitis; and inadequate blood volume as shown by circulatory response to PEEP (Kumar & others: New England J Med 283:1430–1436, 1970). The hazards of PEEP (as compared to IPPV) are an increased rate of complications such as subcutaneous and mediastinal emphysema and tension pneumothorax.

Pulmonary surfactant, a lipoprotein which lines the walls of the alveoli, has the unique property of reducing alveolar surface tension, thus offsetting the inherent instability of air spaces. It lowers the interfacial tension in the alveoli as they become smaller and tends to prevent alveolar collapse at low transpulmonary pressure. Impairment of surfactant function results in progressive closure of air spaces with shunting, particularly at end-expiration when lung volume and alveolar size are least. It has been suggested that high oxygen concentrations, mechanical ventilation, and excessively large tidal volumes may all cause surfactant depletion, but there is no convincing evidence in man that a primary defect in the surfactant system is an etiologic factor in pulmonary disease, including acute respiratory failure (Clements JA: Am Rev Resp Dis 101:984–990, 1970; Scarpelli EM: *The Surfactant System of the Lung*. Lea & Febiger, 1968). Morgan (New England J Med 284:1185–1193, 1971) has recently summarized experimental data that suggest that alveolar ventilation is sufficient to preserve surfactant synthesis in spite of loss of perfusion, whereas loss of both ventilation and perfusion results in rapid depletion of the surfactant system. In spite of continuing uncertainty regarding the role of surfactant deficiency in acute respiratory failure, it is appropriate to minimize the conditions which may possibly deplete surfactant, eg, high F_{IO_2} and continuous hyperinflation or collapse of alveoli.

Finally, it should be kept in mind that positive pressure breathing may decrease the venous return to the heart and the cardiac output. The central venous pressure will be elevated. The extent of these changes and the degree of circulatory support required to cope with them will be related to respiratory pressures and to the status of the lungs and circulation.

d. Weaning from the ventilator—The transition from mechanical to spontaneous ventilation should be attempted only when there is objective evidence that pulmonary function is adequate. Sustained spontaneous ventilation requires a minimal vital capacity of 10 ml/kg, or a volume essentially twice as large as the normal tidal volume. Ventilatory support can usually be permanently discontinued and the endotracheal or tracheostomy tube removed when the vital capacity exceeds 15–20 ml/kg. Although vital capacity has been found to be a more reliable guide to weaning than $P_{(A-aD_{O_2})}$ and V_D/V_T, it has been observed that weaning is rarely successful when $P_{(A-aD_{O_2})}$ is greater than 350 mm Hg and V_D/V_T is above 0.6 (see Table 3–2). Arterial P_{O_2} is also a valuable indicator of readiness for weaning. If P_{aO_2} is maintained at 200 mm Hg or above on the ventilator with F_{IO_2} of 40%, it is probable that the patient will tolerate a short trial period off the ventilator. On the other hand, if the patient can barely maintain a normal P_{aO_2} while on the ventilator and receiving a high F_{IO_2}, he cannot be expected to tolerate weaning.

Weaning is contraindicated when chest wall trauma has been the primary indication for controlled ventilation and paradoxic motion of the chest wall is still present. The average time for stabilization of the rib cage is usually at least 10 days for patients under 30 and 20 days for patients over 50. This will vary with the extent of injury.

The process of weaning must usually be gradual if the patient has had acute respiratory failure. The longer the period of mechanical ventilation, the more difficult will be the weaning. Weaning can begin with 5–15 minutes per hour or half-hour of spontaneous respiration off the ventilator but with a T connector to the tracheal tube delivering 60–80% humidified oxygen. The ECG, the depth and rate of respirations, and the patient's general reactions are observed for signs of distress. Periods of spontaneous respiration are lengthened and oxygen administration decreased as tolerated. If possible, the patient should be out of bed and ambulatory during this time. Blood gas determinations are often needed to evaluate the respiratory status at this stage. It may be advisable to return the patient to mechanical ventilation at night during the early weaning period so that he may sleep under good control. Weaning may take several days if mechanical ventilation has been used for a week or more.

Prognosis

Preventive measures and therapy based on physiologic principles have greatly improved the outlook for surgical patients with progressive pulmonary insufficiency or acute respiratory failure. Because many more patients are now receiving mechanical ventilatory support on a prophylactic basis than was formerly the case, it is difficult to quantitate the improvement in prognosis of acute respiratory failure which has taken place over the past 5–10 years. Reports from the Respiratory Unit at Massachusetts General Hospital are among the most specific in this regard. The majority of patients admitted to that unit are postoperative or posttraumatic, and most patients require tracheal intubation or tracheostomy and artificial ventilation for a large part of their stay. The average length of stay is 18 days. The mortality rate on the unit was 35–40% during the period 1961–1965 and fell to 11% in 1970 (Bendixen & others: *Respiratory Care.* Mosby, 1965; Pontoppidan & others: New England J Med 287:690–698, 1972). Other institutions have observed similar improvement in prognosis of patients with acute respiratory failure (O'Donahue & others: Chest 58:603–610, 1970). The decreased mortality rates can be ascribed to the fact that substantial progress has been made over the past decade in almost all aspects of management of pulmonary insufficiency.

• • •

General References

Ballinger WF, Drapanas T: Pages 157–174 in: *Practice of Surgery, Current Review.* Vol 1. Mosby, 1971.

Barnes RW, Merendino KA: Post-traumatic pulmonary insufficiency syndrome. S Clin North America 52:625–633, 1972.

Bates DV, Macklem PT, Christie RV: *Respiratory Function in Disease,* 2nd ed. Saunders, 1971.

Bendixen HH & others: *Respiratory Care.* Mosby, 1965.

Blaisdell FW, Lim RC Jr, Stallone RJ: The mechanism of pulmonary damage following traumatic shock. Surg Gynec Obst 130:15–22, 1970.

Boyd DR: Monitoring patients with posttraumatic pulmonary insufficiency. S Clin North America 52:31–46, 1972.

Kumar A & others: Continuous positive-pressure ventilation in acute respiratory failure: Effects on hemodynamics and lung function. New England J Med 283:1430–1436, 1970.

Lewis FJ & others: Automatic monitoring in the postoperative recovery room. Surg Gynec Obst 130:333–341, 1970.

Moore FD & others: *Post-Traumatic Pulmonary Insufficiency.* Saunders, 1969.

Pontoppidan H, Laver MB, Geffin B: Acute respiratory failure in the surgical patient. Advances Surg 4:163–254, 1970.

Pontoppidan H, Geffin B, Lowenstein E: Acute respiratory failure in the adult. New England J Med 287:690–698, 743–752, 799–806, 1972.

4 . . .

Postoperative Complications

F. William Blaisdell, MD

After successful surgery, the postoperative course should consist of rapid return to health. Anesthesia and surgery both have unavoidable temporary ill effects on normal physiology. A simple operation performed under local anesthesia causes minimal systemic effects. A major abdominal dissection such as that required for removal of a malignant retroperitoneal sarcoma can be expected to alter normal physiology markedly.

Incisional discomfort may be acute for 24–48 hours and should gradually subside over 3–4 days. During the period of acute discomfort, splinting of abdominal muscles may interfere with deep breathing and coughing. Intra-abdominal dissection and irritation of the peritoneum during the operation results in temporary paralysis of the peristaltic activity of the bowel (paralytic ileus). Some degree of ileus is normal following any intra-abdominal procedure. If the field of the operation is limited—eg, as in simple appendectomy—ileus may not persist longer than 12–24 hours. After major abdominal procedures associated with mechanical trauma to the bowel or peritoneum, paralysis of intestinal motility may continue for 3–4 days.

In addition to local changes which result from surgical trauma, a systemic ("stress") reaction is inevitable following major surgery. This reaction is proportionate to the magnitude of the surgical trauma and the extent of loss of blood, fluids, and electrolytes. The response to any injury is catabolic as the body mobilizes protein, fat, and carbohydrate to provide energy and repair damaged tissues. This mechanism is activated by certain metabolic and endocrine factors. After a few days to several weeks, an anabolic response follows. Caloric intake is increased, and nitrogen balance switches from negative to positive (see Chapter 13).

Increased metabolic activity is associated with the "stress response." Unless complications develop, body temperature rarely exceeds 37.8 C (100 F) even after major operations. The pulse and respiratory rates are only slightly above those recorded preoperatively. Cardiac output and oxygen utilization increase proportionately. A temperature elevation above 37.8 C or a marked elevation of the pulse or respiratory rate signifies a postoperative complication.

PREVENTION OF POSTOPERATIVE COMPLICATIONS

In order to avoid high morbidity and possible mortality from the operation, every effort must be made to prevent postoperative complications. It is far easier to prevent these complications than to treat specific problems once they develop. There is no substitute for good operative technic, and the principles of Halsted are just as applicable today as they were 50 years ago: meticulous hemostasis, gentle handling of tissues, careful approximation of wounds to avoid dead space, and rigid asepsis. Other important aspects of good operative technic are selection of the proper anesthetic, adequate preparation of the skin, good lighting, proper placement of incisions, adequate exposure, careful wound closure, care to avoid leaving foreign materials in the wound or body cavities, and team discipline and training.

The respiratory system should be evaluated at the completion of the operation.* Mucus plugs and accumulated secretions may obstruct bronchi, and respiration may remain depressed following major anesthesia. The conscious patient should be encouraged to breathe deeply and to cough; if he is not cooperative or has a depressed sensorium, nasotracheal aspiration should be instituted to remove retained secretions and stimulate the cough reflex. The patient's position should be changed frequently by encouraging him to sit up every 3 or 4 hours or by rolling him from side to side or changing the inclination of the bed.

The adequacy of peripheral perfusion should be assessed immediately after surgery by noting the skin color and warmth. Urine output and other fluid losses should be recorded. If the patient's condition is critical, hourly assessment of urinary output using an indwelling urethral catheter may be necessary. Blood volume deficits should be promptly replaced.

Overhydration may be manifested by rales in the dependent portions of the lung, excessive gain in weight, urine output over 100 ml/hour, dependent or sacral edema, or fullness of the neck veins. If overhydration is evident, fluids should be restricted and sodium withheld. If the fluid overload threatens cardiopulmonary function, diuretics may be required.

---

*Acute respiratory failure is discussed in the preceding chapter.

Antibiotic therapy should be given only as necessary to treat specific infections. Cultures should be taken at surgery whenever contamination is present; a smear should be made simultaneously, stained with Gram's stain, and examined microscopically so that antibiotics can be selected on the basis of the general nature of the organism while culture and sensitivity tests are being completed. Prophylactic antibiotics are rarely indicated in clean surgical operations, and the incidence of wound infections is not affected by their use. They have the disadvantage of encouraging the emergence of resistant strains, so organisms which do infect the patient are more virulent. If gross contamination has occurred during surgery or if the field is grossly infected, antibiotics may be advisable. When contamination is likely to be unavoidable, antibiotics should be started 2–3 hours before the operation so that high concentrations will be present in the blood and in the wound.

Overdistention of the bladder may develop in the anesthetized or sedated patient—particularly one who has been overhydrated during the operation—and the physician must be alert to this possibility. The lower abdomen should be percussed for bladder dullness in the immediate postoperative period; if a suprapubic mass is detected and the patient cannot void, immediate bladder catheter drainage is indicated. If the patient voids frequent small amounts (50 ml) postoperatively, overdistention should also be suspected. The patient is likely to be voiding small amounts from a grossly distended bladder.

As soon as possible in the postoperative course, the patient should be encouraged to sit up, cough and breathe deeply, and, if possible, to walk. The upright position permits expansion of basilar lung segments, which may be collapsed as a result of diaphragm elevation due to abdominal distention or splinting of the posterior aspects of the chest wall. Walking increases the circulation of the lower extremities and thus helps to prevent venous stasis and lessens the danger of venous thromboembolism.

Oral intake should be restricted postoperatively to prevent air swallowing and aggravation of abdominal distention. Return of function of the gastrointestinal tract after abdominal surgery is verified by the passing of flatus, spontaneous bowel movement, and normal peristalsis on auscultation. At this point, liquids can be instituted safely and the diet advanced as seems appropriate. Conversely, if abdominal distention develops postoperatively, nasogastric intubation may be necessary to decompress the upper gastrointestinal tract and prevent vomiting and undue distention, with its danger of compromise of ventilation.

Cutdowns utilized for intravenous fluids should be discontinued at 24–48 hours to minimize the risk of thrombophlebitis. It is preferable to switch the intravenous catheter every 1–2 days rather than to accept the risk of septic thrombophlebitis, which almost always occurs when prolonged intravenous catheterization is utilized. (See Chapter 52 for further details.)

COMMON POSTOPERATIVE COMPLICATIONS

A postoperative complication is arbitrarily defined as any untoward event that occurs within 30 days after the operation. It may seem that myocardial infarction 2 weeks following an uneventful operation should not be listed as a surgical complication. However, the incidence of myocardial infarction in the postoperative period is higher than in similar groups of patients who have not had an operation, and the surgeon must assume that this complication was related to the surgery.

Any interruption in the smooth postoperative course must raise the question of whether a complication has developed. Careful observation of the patient and his vital signs should make it possible to determine the nature of any given postoperative complication.

Postoperative complications can be manifested by temperature, pulse, or respiratory changes. The most common abnormality in the postoperative vital signs is fever. Any rectal temperature over 37.8 C (100 F) is abnormal, and a temperature over 38.3 C (101 F) indicates that a major problem is present. Tachypnea, tachycardia, hypertension, and hypotension are also frequent manifestations of surgical complications. Any change in one or more of these vital signs should be investigated and the cause determined.

Complications can occur in the wound, in any body cavity, or in organs adjacent to or far removed from the site of operation. Complications may be immediate or delayed and may be either a direct result of the surgery or of the disease being treated (eg, peritonitis following surgery for a ruptured appendix). Complications may occur as a result of immobilization (venous thrombosis) or exposure to an infectious agent in the hospital ("hospital acquired infections"). Complications can result from aggravation of some underlying condition such as an unsuspected bleeding disorder or from stress to a marginal psychiatric patient.

The most common complication seen in the postoperative period is **atelectasis**. This is usually considered to be a direct result of general anesthesia, but it also follows splinting of the abdominal wall following laparotomy or thoracotomy due to the patient's inability to take a deep breath or to cough up secretions. Its incidence varies from 5–10% to almost 100%, depending upon how carefully it is looked for and the extent and duration of the operation.

Wound infection is the second most common complication. It varies greatly in incidence and is related to specific procedures. It should occur in fewer than 2% of clean operations and probably occurs following 5–10% of "clean-contaminated" operations (those in which a hollow viscus is entered).

Postoperative ileus is a very common accompaniment of any operation involving the peritoneal cavity. If undue trauma or chemical or bacterial contamination occurs, it may be persistent and prolonged.

Urinary retention may occur following any operation, particularly if fluid overload has occurred during the period of anesthesia. It frequently complicates rectal operations and is particularly prone to occur in older males, many of whom have some degree of prostatic obstruction.

The use of catheters for the administration of intravenous fluids has resulted in a marked increase in **septic thrombophlebitis.** For this reason, the precautions outlined above should be rigidly adhered to.

Some complications are particularly common following catastrophic illness or secondary to other postoperative complications. These include hemorrhagic lung syndrome, stress ulcer, gastric dilatation, renal failure, and hepatic failure. Most of the cardiovascular complications (eg, cerebrovascular accidents, myocardial infarction, and pulmonary embolism) and almost all of the serious infections (eg, peritonitis) follow some grave complication such as anastomotic disruption, postoperative hemorrhage, or shock.

Specific postoperative complications are discussed in the following sections.

Altemeier WA & others: Infections: Prophylaxis and management: A symposium. Surgery 67:369, 1970.

Bolagny BL & others: The hazards of intravenous polyethylene catheters in surgical patients. Surg Gynec Obst 130:342, 1970.

Cole WH: Operability in the young and aged. Ann Surg 138:145, 1953.

Hamilton WK & others: Postoperative respiratory complications. Anesthesiology 25:607, 1964.

Johnstone FRC: Infection on a surgical service. Am J Surg 120:192, 1970.

Kinney JM: Ventilatory failure in the postoperative patient. S Clin North America 43:619, 1963.

Sheiner NM & others: Assessment of pulmonary function in postoperative patients. Am J Surg 120:714, 1970.

Subcommittee on Aseptic Methods: Aseptic methods in the operating room suite. Lancet 1:705, 763, 831, 1968.

PULMONARY COMPLICATIONS*

Most postoperative complications occur in the lungs. The incidence of these complications varies with the preoperative status of the patient, the quality of the anesthesia, the duration and type of operation, and the quality of the postoperative care. Patients with obstructive pulmonary airway disease—eg, chronic bronchitis with excessive tracheobronchial secretions—are particularly prone to develop respiratory difficulty postoperatively. Heavy smokers invariably have chronic bronchitis and fall into the high risk group. During anesthesia, failure to aspirate secretions, faulty placement of the endotracheal tube, or failure to deep-breathe or to sigh intermittently predisposes the patient to postoperative difficulty, as does extubation

in a still heavily sedated patient also. The longer the operation, the more vulnerable the patient becomes to minor omissions of these procedures.

Certain operations—particularly thoracic and upper abdominal operations—cause discomfort with respiration and impair the patient's ability to breathe deeply and to cough. As a result, pulmonary complications are much more frequent than in operative procedures carried out on the lower abdomen, perineum, neck, or extremities. Prolonged immobility in bed, abdominal pain, and abdominal distention all predispose to respiratory difficulty in postoperative patients; postoperative procedures such as encouraging deep breathing and coughing and, in selected patients, nasotracheal aspiration of the tracheobronchial tree are direct measures used to prevent respiratory complications. Appropriate use of analgesic agents, early mobilization of patients, and positional changes are of value in all patients and will lessen the incidence of postoperative pulmonary complications.

Atelectasis (Collapse of a Lung Segment or Lobe)

Atelectasis is the most common of all postoperative complications. It is thought to be due to inadequate ventilation during anesthesia, with collapse of lung segments or the accumulation of pulmonary secretions during or just after the operation. Accumulation of secretions results in obstruction of small bronchi, absorption of air, and collapse of the segment supplied by the occluded bronchus.

Atelectasis is the most common cause of postoperative fever. It usually develops in the first 24–48 hours following surgery. The first clinical sign of atelectasis may be present the evening after an operation. The patient may develop fever to 38.5–39 C (101.2–102.2 F), tachypnea (24–30/minute), and moderate tachycardia. Physical examination may reveal elevation or splinting of the diaphragm, scattered rales, and diminished breath sounds with bronchial breathing over the affected area—most commonly at the lung bases or at the posterior lung segments. There may be a shift of cardiac dullness to the affected side.

Studies in asymptomatic postoperative patients have demonstrated that arterial oxygen tensions are frequently much lower than expected. This is due to intrapulmonary shunting because it does not respond to the administration of 100% oxygen. This is presumably caused by miliary atelectasis because chest x-ray may be normal and physical signs absent.

The principal impact of atelectasis is its effect on oxygenation of the blood. The healthy patient usually has considerable reserve, and minor degrees of atelectasis are well tolerated. In patients with marginal reserve or cardiovascular disease, the consequences of atelectasis can be great, and hypoxia is the precipitating cause of many cases of cardiac arrhythmia and cardiac arrest.

Atelectasis is aggravated by a painful abdominal or thoracic incision with sufficient splinting of the chest wall or diaphragm to impair ventilation. Inability

*Acute respiratory failure is discussed in Chapter 3.

to breathe deeply and to cough results in progression of the process.

Treatment consists of stimulating the patient to cough and to breathe deeply. Frequent change in position of the bedridden patient facilitates ventilation of all portions of the lung. The patient should be moved from side to side and encouraged to sit up. If he cannot be moved easily or is uncooperative, endotracheal aspiration should be performed using a plastic catheter passed nasotracheally. This can be done easily by pulling the tongue forward with a sponge and asking the patient to inhale as the catheter is passed nasally. Analgesic drugs in small amounts may diminish incisional pain and improve the depth of spontaneous ventilation. Humidification of inspired air will assist in liquefying and mobilizing bronchial secretions. When the atelectasis involves an entire lung or lobe and is resistant to treatment, bronchoscopy may be indicated to remove secretions or mucus plugs.

Respiratory Distress Syndrome

Respiratory distress syndrome has been recognized only in the past few years. It has many names, eg, pump lung, shock lung, posttraumatic lung, fat embolism, and congestive atelectasis. This complication was at first thought to result only from cardiopulmonary bypass. Similar lesions are now being recognized in patients who have been in septic, hypovolemic, or cardiogenic shock or other types of catastrophic illness such as massive trauma or major burns.

Careful monitoring of postoperative patients with major illnesses has permitted definition of the clinical syndrome. Within 24 hours of clinical insult, the patient develops evidence of respiratory distress characterized by tachypnea and increased effort in breathing. Arterial blood gas measurements done at this time may show arterial desaturation. Chest x-ray shows diffuse, cloudy infiltrates in the lung, but—in contrast to pulmonary edema—there is no cardiac enlargement or increase in vascular markings. The compliance of the lungs is decreased, and increased pressures are often required to maintain adequate tidal volume. If the arterial P_{O_2} is below 60 mm Hg, an endotracheal tube should be inserted and positive pressure ventilation instituted with sufficient oxygen to maintain an arterial P_{O_2} of 70–100 mm Hg. With prompt institution of positive pressure ventilation, the lesion is usually reversible, and gradual recovery can be expected in 3–7 days. If the insult is severe and the patient's underlying disease is not fully reversible, a progressive downhill course may result until 100% oxygen arterial desaturation occurs and the patient dies. On gross examination, the lung is hemorrhagic and resembles liver. If autopsy is done within the first 24 hours, histopathologic examination reveals platelet and fibrin emboli filling the microcirculation of the lung. This is followed by congestion and then intra-alveolar hemorrhage at 24–72 hours. When death occurs between 3 and 5 days, intra-alveolar hemorrhage and hyaline membranes are the predominant lesions. If the patient is carried successfully through this insult, pneumonitis

develops, so that when death occurs more than 5–7 days following onset the principal changes are those of pneumonia.

Aspiration

Aspiration is a relatively common pulmonary complication. It usually occurs in the postanesthetic period when the patient's sensorium is depressed and vital reflexes such as swallowing and coughing are absent. Aspiration of oral secretions may precipitate pneumonia, usually mild, which can be managed by vigorous therapy similar to that described for atelectasis.

A far more lethal type of aspiration is that secondary to vomiting and inhalation of gastric contents. This can occur during induction of anesthesia in any patient who has recently eaten or one who has ileus and a stomach distended with intestinal contents. Aspiration of gastric contents produces a severe, often lethal pneumonitis. For this reason, access to the airway should be obtained immediately with an endotracheal tube or bronchoscope. This permits suctioning of aspirated material from the tracheobronchial tree and thorough cleansing with saline irrigations. Nonetheless, severe tracheobronchitis may result from breakdown of the mucosa and secondary infection.

Antibiotics and corticosteroids are advocated in the management of aspiration of gastric contents.

Pneumonia

Pneumonia may follow atelectasis or aspiration. Aspiration of nasopharyngeal secretions during or immediately following anesthesia or atelectasis may set the stage for the development of frank pneumonia. Abundant tracheobronchial secretions from preexisting bronchitis also predispose to this complication.

Atelectasis produces moderate fever in the first few postoperative days. If this is followed by higher temperatures, systemic toxicity, and respiratory difficulty, a presumptive diagnosis of pneumonia is justified.

As pneumonia develops, secretions become progressively more abundant and the cough becomes productive. Physical examination may reveal evidence of pulmonary consolidation, and numerous coarse rales are often present. Chest x-ray usually shows diffuse patchy infiltrates or lobar consolidation.

The treatment of pneumonia includes deep breathing and coughing. The patient should be encouraged to change position and move about as much as possible. Nasotracheal suction may be used to stimulate the cough reflex. Specific antibiotic therapy should be instituted on the basis of sputum smears and revised as dictated by subsequent cultures and sensitivity tests. In weak or debilitated patients with a poor cough reflex, emergency tracheostomy may be indicated to permit adequate ventilation and bronchoscopy. Positive pressure ventilation may improve the depth of respiration and eliminate the work of breathing in weak or extremely ill patients.

Pulmonary Embolism & Infarction*

Pulmonary embolism undoubtedly occurs far more commonly than is recognized. One prospective study demonstrated that 30% of patients with major illnesses have evidence of pulmonary embolism by the time of discharge.

It is probable that only about 10% of pulmonary emboli are recognized clinically. The remainder do not produce symptoms except for minor changes in respiratory rate. The patient may be assumed to have atelectasis or some other minor pulmonary condition. Fewer than 10% of emboli produce pulmonary infarction with the classical manifestations: hemoptysis, pleuritic pain, and a wedge-shaped density on chest x-ray. In most instances, the collateral circulation of the lung is adequate to prevent death of lung tissue and the classical changes of infarction.

Pulmonary embolism and infarction are most apt to occur late in the postoperative course—on the seventh to tenth postoperative days. The diagnosis of pulmonary embolism can only be made by maintaining a high index of clinical suspicion. The early manifestation is a rising respiratory and pulse rate out of proportion to the degree of fever. If pulmonary embolism is suspected and no contraindication exists, immediate anticoagulation with intravenously administered heparin is indicated. Anticoagulation should be continued until the patient has fully recovered and has resumed normal activity. For details of anticoagulant treatment of thrombophlebitis and pulmonary embolism, see Chapter 40. The infrarenal vena cava should be ligated if embolism recurs after anticoagulation or if anticoagulation is contraindicated.

Blaisdell FW, Lim RC Jr, Stallone RJ: The mechanism of pulmonary damage following traumatic shock. Surg Gynec Obst 130:15, 1970.

Blaisdell FW, Schlobohm RC: The respiratory distress syndrome. Surgery 74:(August), 1973.

Crane C & others: The management of major pulmonary embolism. Surg Gynec Obst 128:27, 1969.

Harbord RP, Bosworth PP: Therapy for atelectasis. Anesth Analg 45:684, 1966.

Jackson DR, Harrower HW: Pulmonary embolism following inferior vena caval interruption. Vasc Surg 3:129, 1969.

Sasahara AA: Clinical studies in pulmonary thromboembolism. Page 256 in: *Proceedings from the Symposium on Pulmonary Embolic Disease.* Sasahara AA, Stein M (editors). Grune & Stratton, 1965.

Wilson RF & others: Respiratory failure in clinical shock and trauma. Page 361 in: *Current Topics in Surgical Research.* Zuidema GD, Skinner DB (editors). Academic Press, 1969.

WOUND COMPLICATIONS

Wound complications include hematoma, seroma, infection, dehiscence, evisceration, and hernia.

*See Chapters 22 and 40 for detailed discussions of the causes, prevention, diagnosis, and treatment of pulmonary emboli.

Hematoma

Hematoma formation is the initial wound complication as it is manifested in the immediate postoperative period. Bleeding usually starts at the time of wound closure, and the hematoma presents within the first 24 hours. If the bleeding is in the deeper portions of a large wound, the presence of a hematoma may not be recognized until secondary infection occurs. The presence of blood in the wound increases local vascularity, and bleeding is potentiated by the presence of the hematoma. When the hematoma produces swelling and discomfort, the wound should be reexplored under sterile conditions, the hematoma evacuated, and the bleeding site controlled. When the hematoma is superficial, it may be possible to remove 1–2 sutures from the wound and express the blood. If bleeding continues despite local evacuation, wound reexploration is mandatory. Much morbidity can be averted by prompt definitive reoperation in such cases.

Seroma

Collection of serum in a wound is most apt to occur in incisions where it is difficult to avoid dead space, as in operations on the groin and breast where large flaps of skin are necessarily undermined. Meticulous closure of the wound in layers is the best way to avoid these collections. When a seroma is recognized, needle aspiration of the fluid and firm pressure may prevent recurrence. It is preferable not to open the wound because contamination of the tissue may lead to infection. When the seroma is large, it is appropriate to explore the wound in the operating room under sterile conditions. Operations on the groin, particularly along the course of the femoral artery and veins, are not only associated with a high incidence of seroma formation; because the lymphatics of the lower extremities are often divided, a frank leak of lymph with the formation of a lymphoma may occur. Careful ligation of divided lymphatics will reduce the incidence of this complication.

Some of the apparent accumulations of serum may be due to traumatized fat. Seromas in wounds which cross very few lymphatics such as longitudinal abdominal incisions are most apt to be due to traumatic fat necrosis.

Infection

Infection is the most common wound complication and may be due to poor surgical technic or gross contamination during the operation. The contribution of poor technic to the incidence of postoperative wound infection would be minimal if all surgeons mastered the fundamental surgical principles of gentle handling of tissue, careful hemostasis, approximation of tissues, and avoidance of dead space. Almost all wounds are contaminated to some degree; good aseptic technic ensures that wound contamination will be minimal. Given a fixed degree of contamination, the incidence of wound infection will vary from one surgeon to the next because wound infection is related to the presence or absence of dead space, which gives rise to collections of blood or serum—both ideal culture mediums for bacteria. Infection may be due to excessive trauma to the tissues or abuse of the electrocautery or ligatures. Another factor related to the incidence of wound infection is vascularity: the better the blood supply to a wound, the lower the incidence of infection. (See Chapter 9.)

A **clean wound** is an operative wound which has not become contaminated at any point in the operation. Herniorrhaphy and blood vessel surgery are examples of operations where the wound is clean. Infection is uncommon in these wounds; the incidence should not exceed 2%.

Contaminated operations are those in which gross contamination of the operative field has occurred. Appendectomy for rupture of the appendix and delayed laparotomy for perforated ulcer are typical examples. If the skin were closed, these wounds would be expected to become infected. Therefore, the skin and subcutaneous tissue should be left open whenever possible. Once wound defenses have been mobilized (4—5 days), delayed primary closure of the skin and subcutaneous tissue can be carried out or the wound can be left open to close secondarily.

Contamination of the wound is most likely at the time of surgery, yet wound infections usually appear about the fifth to the seventh postoperative day. The principal exception is streptococcal infection when erythema, fever, and systemic toxicity develop within 24—48 hours of contamination. Since streptococcal infections are nonnecrotizing, specific systemic antibiotic therapy is all that is needed and the wound does not require drainage. Wound infections which appear 5—7 days after surgery are invariably necrotizing and are due to staphyloccoci or gram-negative rods. These infections produce collections of pus in the wound, and treatment requires adequate drainage. This usually consists of opening the wound widely. These infections almost always occur in subcutaneous tissue and only rarely involve the fascial or muscle layers, so that opening the superficial layers of the wound establishes adequate drainage and permits the natural defense mechanisms of the body to become operative. This results in rapid control of the infection with or without specific antibiotics. The wound can sometimes be closed secondarily several days later.

When the wound is opened and infection seems to be coming from fascia or deep to the fascia, one should suspect an intraperitoneal source (see next section).

Dehiscence, Evisceration, & Hernia

Partial wound **dehiscence** implies disruption of several layers of the wound, such as peritoneum and fascia, without compromising the integrity of all layers. Without treatment, fascial dehiscence is usually followed by complete dehiscence of the skin closure and escape of viscera from the abdominal or thoracic cavity (**evisceration**).

Wound dehiscence and evisceration usually begins in the first 1—2 days following operation, when coughing or straining disrupts the peritoneum and fascial layers and a loop of bowel or omentum is pushed into the wound. However, it does not become evident until the fifth to tenth days, often just after the skin sutures are removed. A sudden discharge of serosanguineous fluid at this time heralds total dehiscence, and evisceration will follow unless the wound is opened and resutured.

Wound dehiscence or evisceration is usually precipitated by a sudden increase in intra-abdominal pressure caused by coughing or straining. The patient may describe a popping sensation during an episode of coughing. Once wound dehiscence starts, the wound usually opens like a zipper as additional strain is exerted on the remaining sutures. Prompt reoperation is imperative when dehiscence is recognized; evisceration requires reoperation to return abdominal contents to the peritoneal cavity. In rare cases in obese, poor-risk patients, dehiscence may be controlled by abdominal binders of the scultetus type, but this is inevitably followed by incisional hernia (see below).

Wound dehiscence or evisceration should not occur. Wound closure should be adapted to the requirements of the situation. For example, one would use a different closure for an emergency operation on an alcoholic who may have delirium tremens postoperatively than on a patient undergoing an elective cholecystectomy. Although retention sutures do not prevent the complications of dehiscence and evisceration, they can give considerable support to the wound and decrease the chances of a major disruption.

Incisional **herniation** occurs principally in abdominal incisions. It is the result of an unrecognized, unrepaired wound dehiscence, where the fascial layers have separated and the skin closure remains intact. Although the opening in the fascia may be small initially, progressive enlargement of a ventral hernia is inevitable. Therefore, unless some serious medical contraindication exists, all ventral incisional hernias should be repaired when recognized. Delaying repair always results in a larger, more complicated hernia. If major contraindications to surgery exist, it may be appropriate to control the ventral hernia with binders or girdles. (See Chapter 33.)

Alexander HC, Prudden JF: The causes of abdominal wound disruption. Surg Gynec Obst 122:1223, 1966.

Winegarner FG: Management of intraabdominal sepsis. Am J Surg 120:743, 1970.

PERITONEAL COMPLICATIONS

Following laparotomy—particularly one carried out for some type of septic condition such as a ruptured appendix, perforated ulcer, or perforated diverticulum—contamination may spread throughout the peritoneal cavity and cause generalized peritonitis or abscesses. Peritonitis and intraperitoneal abscess formation are rare complications after clean elective operations. The peritoneum is capable of withstanding large amounts of contamination, and infection usually occurs only when contamination is overwhelming. Overlooked collections of pus after rupture of a hollow viscus, contamination of the peritoneal cavity with intestinal contents or blood, and serum or lymph collections which provide culture media for bacteria are the usual sources of intraperitoneal infection. When laparotomy is done for a perforated viscus, careful cleaning of the abdominal cavity is mandatory; all foreign material and abscesses should be carefully aspirated. Undrained pockets of contamination set the stage for infection.

The complications which occur within the peritoneal cavity are peritonitis and localized infection or intraperitoneal abscess.

Whenever a patient develops unexplained fever or localized abdominal pain after laparotomy, the wound should be inspected. If no wound infection is present, digital examination of the rectum should be done to rule out the possibility of pelvic abscess. The presence of cul-de-sac fullness and tenderness is diagnostic. The abdomen and flanks should be carefully palpated. Absence of local tenderness suggests that the abscess is not within the portion of the peritoneal cavity below the costal margins. Because of the high incidence of subphrenic and subhepatic abscesses, these are the most likely possibilities if no other site is found.

Chest x-ray is often helpful because abscesses under the left diaphragm may be associated with fluid in the sulcus and atelectasis of the left lower lobe of the lung. The pulmonary changes may confuse the picture and suggest an intrapleural process, but primary pulmonary disease, for all practical purposes, rarely develops after the first few postoperative days unless some other complication supervenes. Inspiratory-expiratory films or fluoroscopy may reveal impaired motion of the diaphragm. Abnormal gas collections or air-fluid levels may also help localize the infection when gas-forming organisms are present. The manifestations of the subphrenic collection on the right are similar to those on the left, and there should be a reaction in the right pleural space on routine chest x-ray. Collections along the undersurface of the liver (the subhepatic space) are difficult to diagnose because there may be little evidence on the chest film to help localize the collection. Careful observation will usually reveal splinting on the appropriate side and a high diaphragm. The diagnosis and treatment of intraperitoneal abscess and peritonitis are discussed in Chapter 10.

CARDIAC COMPLICATIONS

Cardiac complications following major surgery are rare unless other major complications develop. Although any cardiac disability occurring during the postoperative period has been considered as being due to the "stress" of operation, most cardiac complications are secondary to some other major complication. If the patient's hydration is adequate and the operation is competently and cleanly done, the incidence of cardiac complications is low even in patients with advanced cardiac impairment. Patients with valvular heart disease and old myocardial infarctions tolerate surgery quite well. Myocardial infarction does present an increased risk if the operation is undertaken sooner than 3–6 months after the ischemic episode. Whenever possible, surgery should be delayed in patients who have had a recent infarction or who have ischemic changes on ECG.

Pulmonary Edema

In older patients with cardiac disease, excessive administration of fluids or blood during surgery or in the immediate postoperative period may precipitate pulmonary edema. This can be combated by administering digitalis and diuretics and by restricting fluids. Positive pressure ventilation may also be of great help if congestive failure does not respond promptly to conventional medical management.

Cardiac Arrhythmias

Cardiac arrhythmias may complicate the postoperative course. Many are secondary to anoxia caused by atelectasis or pneumonia. If the patient is on digitalis, hypokalemia may produce an arrhythmia. Other cases may be related to electrolyte imbalance, particularly hypokalemia, myocardial infarction, or pulmonary embolism.

Treatment consists of management of congestive failure. Paroxysmal atrial tachycardia may respond to carotid artery compression. Other arrhythmias may be reversed by cardioversion.

Myocardial Infarctions

Myocardial infarction is a serious complication of major surgery. If the patient is conscious, he may complain of chest pain. It is important to recognize myocardial infarction as such and not assume that the patient is complaining about incisional pain. If cardiovascular instability or an arrhythmia develops in any postoperative patient, an ECG should be obtained. Careful monitoring should be started once the signs of myocardial infarction are evident. Blood gas studies should be obtained, and oxygen and respiratory support administered as indicated. Careful fluid management is necessary. Anticoagulation should be considered in the postoperative patient with a massive myocardial infarct, particularly if low cardiac output and shock result, since there is a high incidence of thromboembolic complications in these patients.

Alexander S: Surgery in the cardiac patient. S Clin North America 50:567, 1970.

Dack S: Postoperative myocardial infarction. Am J Cardiol 12:423, 1963.

Merideth J: Cardiac arrhythmias in the postoperative patient. S Clin North America 49:1083, 1969.

GASTROINTESTINAL COMPLICATIONS

Gastrointestinal complications are most apt to occur after abdominal operations, but they may complicate other types of surgery also. In fact, any serious illness may cause malfunction of the gastrointestinal tract.

Gastric Distention

Gastric distention is one of the most common postoperative complications. It is caused by accumulation of air and, to a lesser extent, gastric juices in the stomach. Most patients with nausea or paralytic ileus will swallow air. If intestinal peristalsis is depressed, the swallowed gas accumulates in the stomach. As gastric distention increases, the movement of the diaphragm may be inhibited. When the patient develops hyperpnea and appears to be splinting his diaphragm, a nasogastric tube should be passed immediately and gastric aspiration continued as long as ileus persists.

Gastric Dilatation

Gastric dilatation, as opposed to gastric distention, is a grave postoperative complication that has been associated with a mortality rate as high as 50%. Gastric dilatation is defined as distention of the stomach with fluid to such a degree that secondary hemorrhage occurs. The gastric juice becomes brown or black from the contained hemoglobin. Gastric dilatation may follow untreated gastric distention, but it often is a complication of very serious illnesses of the type associated with low cardiac output. The cause may be extra-abdominal and may be associated with such procedures as open heart surgery.

Vomiting of brown or black material means gastric dilatation or intestinal obstruction. A nasogastric tube should be passed immediately. Decompression of the stomach reverses the gastric distention and secondary bleeding and prevents aspiration. Large quantities of fluid and electrolytes usually have been lost. Shock is often present, and correction of hypovolemia is an intrinsic part of therapy.

Postoperative Ileus (Paralytic Ileus)

Paralytic ileus consists of paralysis of intestinal peristalsis or lack of effective coordinated peristalsis. It usually follows an intraperitoneal irritative process such as laparotomy or intraperitoneal sepsis. It may result from low cardiac output and may occasionally be due to extra-abdominal causes such as pneumonia. The abdomen is distended and quiet. Faint or irregular bursts of peristalsis may be heard. An abdominal x-ray will demonstrate distended loops of bowel, but gas is typically distributed throughout both large and small bowel.

Air is often swallowed reflexly, and this accounts for many cases of gastric and bowel distention. When ileus is advanced, secretions may be "sequestered" in the bowel, adding to the distention.

Abdominal distention in the postoperative period is usually the result of ileus, and, if moderate or severe, should be treated by nasogastric decompression. Gastric aspiration usually reveals green to yellow fluid—as opposed to that seen with bowel obstruction or gastric dilatation, when the fluid is dark brown or black. The quantity aspirated is usually not more than 1–2 liters/24 hours; if larger quantities are obtained, bowel obstruction should be suspected. Once the nasogastric tube has been inserted, it should be kept on suction until intestinal peristalsis resumes and the patient begins to pass flatus.

Postoperative Intestinal Obstruction

Bowel obstruction may occur as a complication of any abdominal operation. It is most apt to occur as a consequence of peritonitis or generalized irritation of the peritoneal surface. These disorders produce varying degrees of adhesions between the loops of bowel. Obstruction results when these adhesions trap or kink a segment of intestine. Adhesions which form within the first few weeks after surgery are rubbery and seldom result in compromise of the circulation of the bowel. Dense, fibrous adhesions develop over 8–12 weeks or more, and these are more likely to entrap bowel and cause strangulation. For this reason, it is possible to treat postoperative bowel obstruction conservatively by nasogastric intubation or by the use of long intestinal tubes. Tube decompression will often result in realignment of the bowel and relief of the obstruction, or adhesions may give enough to allow spontaneous decompression. When conservative management is elected, an arbitrary period of tube decompression should be decided upon in advance; if the obstruction does not respond within that period (eg, 48–72 hours), reoperation is necessary. Intestinal obstruction is discussed in detail in Chapter 36.

Pancreatitis

Pancreatitis is an infrequent complication of surgery. It is seen just often enough to be considered in the differential diagnosis of postoperative fever or severe ileus, particularly when the surgery involved the biliary tract or when the dissection was carried out in the duodenal or pancreatic area. It can follow any type of surgery and has been described as a complication of appendectomy.

Postoperative pancreatitis causes symptoms in the first 24–48 hours following surgery. It can vary in severity from mild edematous to full-blown hemorrhagic pancreatitis. Pain may be negligible or, if present, may be thought to be incisional. The temperature may go as high as 39.5–40.5 C (103–105 F). Epigastric tenderness and ileus are consistent findings, although the epigastric tenderness may be confused with incisional tenderness.

Postoperative pancreatitis and its management are discussed further in Chapter 28.

Stress Ulcer

This complication is most apt to occur in the patient who has developed some other grave complication. For this reason, the mortality rate is high. The principal manifestation is gastrointestinal bleeding. A more detailed consideration of stress ulcer may be found in Chapter 25.

Pseudomembranous Enterocolitis

Pseudomembranous enterocolitis is diffuse ulceration with secondary fibrin membrane formation which may involve the small bowel, colon, or both. It was at one time believed to be due to overgrowth of staphylococci following administration of broad-spectrum antibiotics. Another possible explanation in some cases is that it results from mucosal damage following a decrease in circulation of the gut in unrecognized shock.

Mucosal ulceration combined with a change of bacterial flora with overgrowth of staphylococci is a toxic, depleting lesion which may rapidly overwhelm the patient. Specific antibiotic therapy is urgently required. Intravenous fluids should be administered as appropriate to correct fluid and electrolyte imbalance.

Fecal Impaction

Fecal impaction is a common cause of diarrhea in the postoperative patient. Whenever the patient develops diarrhea, digital rectal examination should be done immediately. If hard stool is encountered in the ampulla, the diagnosis of fecal impaction is verified. The condition is due to limitation of oral fluids and is especially prone to occur in elderly patients and others confined to bed. It may be aggravated by previous gastrointestinal series or barium enema with accumulation of barium in the colon.

The treatment of fecal impaction is digital disimpaction of the firm fecal masses after an oil retention enema.

Parotitis

Postoperative parotitis occurs mainly in elderly and debilitated patients. As is true of pancreatitis also, dehydration leading to parotid duct obstruction by viscous secretions may set the stage for parotitis. Poor oral hygiene with overgrowth of mouth organisms favors infection of the gland. In contrast to pancreatitis, parotitis usually develops late in the postoperative course and occurs in patients who have other debilitating complications. Fever may be moderate or high, with a septic swing. On inspection, the parotid gland is enlarged and diffusely swollen. The swelling extends anterior to the ear and downward and backward over the angle of the jaw. Inflammation of the orifice of Stensen's duct or purulent discharge from the duct is conclusive evidence of parotitis. The usual causative organism is *Staphylococcus aureus.*

Therapy consists of hydration, stimulation of parotid secretions by encouraging the patient to suck on hard candies, and specific antibiotics. Some have advocated x-ray therapy to decrease the function of the involved gland, but its effectiveness has not been verified. Refractory infection occasionally requires surgical drainage by means of incisions along the course of the facial nerve to avoid its injury. The capsule of the gland is exposed and punctured in multiple areas with the tip of a hemostat to release loculated pockets of pus.

Flowers RS, Kyle K, Hoerr SO: Postoperative hemorrhage from stress ulceration of the stomach and duodenum. Am J Surg 119:632, 1970.

Krippaehne WW, Hunt TK, Dunphy JE: Acute suppurative parotitis: A study of 161 cases. Ann Surg 156:251–257, 1962.

White TT, Morgan A, Hopton D: Postoperative pancreatitis: A study of 70 cases. Am J Surg 120:132, 1970.

HEPATIC COMPLICATIONS

Hepatic problems are rare but potentially lethal complications of surgery.

Liver Abscess

Intrahepatic abscess can occur as a complication of intra-abdominal sepsis and has the same causes as other intraperitoneal infections. Hepatic abscess may develop as a result of cholangitis secondary to biliary obstruction or septic thrombophlebitis of the portal vein (pylephlebitis) (see Chapter 33).

Hepatic abscess is difficult to recognize and is rarely diagnosed early. When it is suspected, hepatic radioisotope scanning should be done. Demonstration of an intrahepatic filling defect confirms the diagnosis, and drainage should be instituted.

Serum Hepatitis

Administration of blood or plasma carries the risk of serum hepatitis. This is usually a late postoperative complication; it rarely occurs earlier than 4 weeks and seldom later than 12 weeks following blood transfusion. This virulent infection is transmitted in the serum of donors, and the hepatitis which occurs following serum injection is far more lethal than infectious hepatitis. Its incidence varies with the quality of banked blood but is probably 0.1–0.5% of all patients who receive blood. It is fatal in about 10% of cases. Conservatism in the administration of blood or blood products and careful selection of blood donors can decrease the incidence of this complication.

Postoperative Jaundice

Postoperative jaundice may develop from various miscellaneous causes other than the above. Serum hepatitis can be ruled out if enzyme studies are normal. Halothane (Fluothane) anesthesia has been held responsible for postoperative liver necrosis, and this anesthetic agent may account for occasional jaundice, particularly if the patient has been anesthetized repeatedly with halothane.

Hemolysis due to transfusion reaction should

always be considered in the differential diagnosis of jaundice, and the Coombs test should be done to establish the presence or absence of transfusion antibodies.

Shock produces a characteristic lesion (centrilobular necrosis) that may simulate obstructive jaundice. The jaundice presumably results partially as a result of liver damage plus an increased bilirubin load, which follows blood transfusion. Most of the serum enzyme studies are normal, although the alkaline phosphatase is elevated.

Drug-induced cholestasis should always be considered and the drug history reviewed for drugs which can produce jaundice.

Allen JG: Post-transfusion hepatitis: a serious clinical problem. California Med 104:293, 1966.

Allen JG: Commercially obtained blood and serum hepatitis. Surg Gynec Obst 131:277, 1970.

Klion FM & others: Hepatitis after exposure to halothane. Ann Int Med 71:467, 1969.

Nunes G, Blaisdell FW, Margaretten W: Mechanism of hepatic dysfunction following shock and trauma. Arch Surg 100:546, 1970.

Strasberg SM, Silver MD: Postoperative hepatogenic jaundice. Surg Gynec Obst 132:81, 1971.

URINARY COMPLICATIONS

Urinary complications are common after surgery. Prompt diagnosis and treatment are essential to prevent serious residual disability.

Urinary Retention

Urinary retention is a frequent postoperative complication. It is most apt to occur after simple rectal operations such as hemorrhoidectomy, although it may occur after any type of surgery. It tends to occur in bedridden patients and in elderly males with prostatic disease. Excessive administration of fluids by the anesthesiologist during operation may result in distention of the bladder, causing bladder decompensation and urinary retention.

All sets of postoperative orders should include a request to record urine output. The patient should be examined immediately after operation and the suprapubic area percussed to determine bladder size. If the patient has not voided by the evening of the day of surgery and fluid therapy has been adequate, bladder distention should be suspected and confirmed by palpation or percussion.

The normal capacity of the urinary bladder is 500 ml. If this capacity is exceeded, permanent damage to the urinary tract may result. Therefore, if his condition permits, the patient should be encouraged to get out of bed to void on the evening after his operation. If the patient is unable to void, a catheter should be passed into the bladder using sterile precautions. If less than 300 ml of urine are found, the catheter should be

removed. If more than 500 ml are released from the bladder, the catheter should be left in place until acute abdominal pain has subsided or until the patient is able to move around or stand to void. Inadequate decompression of the bladder or unskilled catheterization may lead to urinary tract infection.

Urinary Tract Infection

Urinary tract infection may develop immediately in the postoperative period in a patient with preexisting contamination of the urinary tract. This is due to the urinary retention that follows surgery, anesthesia, or immobilization. The bladder is usually uncontaminated before surgery and remains so unless bacteria are introduced by instrumentation or catheterization. The systemic manifestations of urinary tract infection usually develop within 24–48 hours after removal of the urinary catheter. Fever due to urinary tract infections is usually high and may reach 39.5–40.5 C (103–105 F). Infection may be suspected when, despite high fever, the patient is not as toxic as would be expected with most other conditions that cause high fever. Flank tenderness may be present, suggesting pyelonephritis. Pus or bacteria are seen in the urine sediment. Residual urine, which is usually present, tends to perpetuate the infection and predisposes to ascending infection and pyelonephritis.

Treatment consists of forcing fluids and encouraging activity to facilitate complete emptying of the bladder. After urine specimens are obtained for culture, appropriate antibiotic therapy should be instituted based on the appearance of the organisms on a gram-stained smear. Reinstitution of catheter drainage may be necessary in patients with residual urine of 100 ml or more. Older patients with preexisting prostatic hypertrophy may require prostatic resection to permit complete emptying of the bladder. (See Chapter 44.)

Renal Failure

Renal failure is a relatively rare but serious complication of surgery. Oliguria is present when hourly urinary output drops below 30 ml/hour—the amount required to excrete metabolic wastes—and may reflect renal failure. It tends to occur in patients with other serious postoperative complications. With better fluid management and prompt treatment of shock, renal failure occurs much less frequently now than in the past. In patients with catastrophic illness, renal failure may occur as a terminal event.

Renal failure can be prevented by careful monitoring of the postoperative urinary output in all patients undergoing major surgery or patients with major surgical illnesses. If urinary output falls below 30 ml/hour, careful monitoring of cardiovascular function should be instituted. Using the central venous pressure as a guide to prevent fluid overload, plasma or blood should be added to restore vascular volume. With correction of hypovolemia, renal output usually returns promptly and renal tubular damage is avoided. Occasionally, drug reactions or prolonged shock may result in renal tubular necrosis, and the kidneys may not respond to the initial fluid load. If this is the case, fluid should be restricted to the amount required to replace insensible losses and fluid and electrolytes carefully monitored. A rising serum potassium which approaches 7 mEq/liter should be treated promptly.

Thornton GF, Andriole VT: Bacteriuria during indwelling catheter drainage. II. Effect of a closed sterile drainage system. JAMA 214:339–342, 1970.

CEREBRAL COMPLICATIONS

Cerebral changes occur relatively rarely in the postoperative period.

Cerebrovascular Accident

An older patient with underlying cerebrovascular disease may develop thrombosis of a cerebral vessel and suffer a cerebrovascular accident. This seems to occur more frequently after other serious complications, particularly those associated with shock.

Treatment is conservative and supportive. Hypertension should be treated to lessen the risk of secondary hemorrhage into the ischemic infarct, a lethal complication. The airway should be kept clear and oxygen administered as necessary to maintain normal arterial oxygenation.

Cerebral Fat Embolism

Cerebral fat embolism is a syndrome which has been thought to be a complication of long bone fracture in which there is release of medullary fat into the blood stream. However, fat embolism is far more complicated than this, for many of the fat droplets noted in the blood streams of patients following trauma are derived from the plasma. Fat embolism can occur in patients who have had a major episode of shock in which there has been no trauma. Fat embolism is most common in patients with the combination of extensive soft tissue injury and hypovolemic shock.

In many cases, fat droplets can be found simultaneously in urine and sputum. However, fat droplets can be seen in many patients who never develop the full-fledged syndrome. If these patients are monitored carefully, it is apparent that the primary lesion is not cerebral but pulmonary and that cerebral symptoms do not occur if anoxia is prevented. Fat embolism results when tissue damage has been extensive. The presence of gross fat and marrow droplets in the blood stream demonstrates that tissue thromboplastin release has been massive. Thromboplastin initiates intravascular clotting as the primary event which produces the organ damage in the fat embolism syndrome. The greatest impact is on the lung, and treatment is as described for respiratory distress syndrome.

POSTOPERATIVE PSYCHOSIS

Psychosis may occur in any postoperative patient, particularly if the patient is apprehensive about the operation or his ability to recover fully. It is most apt to occur in a previously marginally adjusted patient. Psychosis can also be toxic in origin or drug-induced.

Postoperative psychosis is usually self-limited. With support and sedation, the patient usually recovers without residual emotional disability.

VENOUS COMPLICATIONS*

The venous complications of surgery are due to clot formation, with local reaction and venous obstruction; thrombophlebitis; or minimal reaction and obstruction which leads to thromboembolism.

Thrombophlebitis may be caused by an intravenous foreign body such as an indwelling catheter or can be due to stasis of blood in the venous system.

At one time thrombophlebitis and phlebothrombosis were held to be 2 different clinical conditions. Phlebothrombosis was the term used to denote the clinical situation in which thrombi formed in veins with little local irritation (phlebitis); thrombophlebitis, the process in which inflammatory findings predominate. Actually, both conditions are due to venous clotting and may be regarded as variations or gradations of the same pathologic process.

A clot may form in a vein and lyse spontaneously or may embolize without presenting local signs in the vein of origin. In some instances, the clot irritates the vein wall and causes an inflammatory reaction adjacent to the thrombus. The thrombus gradually becomes adherent to the vein wall, and obstruction of venous return ultimately results. Impaired venous return in major deep veins produces limb edema and the clinical picture of acute thrombophlebitis.

If there has been no break in the skin in the vicinity of the vein involved with thrombophlebitis, the process can be assumed to be sterile despite the intense local reaction, tenderness, and even fever; no antibiotic therapy is indicated. Sterile thrombophlebitis tends to occur as a postoperative complication late in the postoperative course. It probably is iniated in the immediate postoperative period, but its manifestations tend to occur at the seventh to tenth days.

Superficial thrombophlebitis (involving only the subcutaneous veins) should be treated conservatively. Interruption of the vein is indicated when the process is extensive or involves the large superficial veins in the thigh. Otherwise, elastic support and ambulation are indicated. Superficial venous thrombophlebitis is not associated with swelling of the part, and this is the key to differentiation between superficial and deep thrombophlebitis.

*See also Chapter 39.

Deep venous thrombophlebitis causes limb edema. Homans' sign consists of pain on dorsiflexion of the foot and is present in most instances of lower limb involvement. Calf tenderness is also a common finding. Treatment consists of bed rest, elevation of the extremities, and anticoagulation.

Immobilization should be continued until swelling and tenderness have subsided, and anticoagulation must be continued until the patient is able to resume normal activity.

Septic thrombophlebitis is usually related to intravenous therapy. When plastic catheters are left in veins for longer than 24–48 hours or when the technic of introduction of the catheter is faulty, septic complications may develop which are manifested by redness and tenderness in the vein just above the point of entrance of the catheter. Systemic toxicity ranges from minimal to quite severe.

Treatment of septic thrombophlebitis involves immediate removal of the offending foreign body, application of warm moist compresses, and specific antibiotics based on the results of culture of the catheter. If the process does not respond within 24–48 hours, proximal ligation of the involved vein is indicated.

The consequences of thromboembolism are described in the section on pulmonary complications. In many patients, the emboli form silently, and, when the inflammatory reaction is minimal, the clot may not fix to the vein. Sudden physical exertion such as climbing out of bed or straining at stool may raise venous pressure, distend the lower extremity veins, and result in embolism of the clot. Thromboembolism is always a potentially lethal complication even though the symptoms are mild. Bed rest and anticoagulation are required. If anticoagulation is contraindicated or if recurrent embolism occurs on adequate anticoagulation, vena cava interruption is required.

Bergentz SE: studies on the genesis of post-traumatic fat embolism. Acta chir scandinav, Suppl 282, 1961.

Kakkar VV & others: Natural history of postoperative deep vein thrombosis. Lancet 2:230, 1969.

Tsapogas MJ & others: Detection of postoperative venous thrombosis and effectiveness of prophylactic measures. Arch Surg 101:149, 1970.

• • •

General References

Bartlett RH, Gazzinaga AB, Geraghty TR: Respiratory maneuvers to prevent postoperative pulmonary complications: A critical review. JAMA 224:1017–1021, 1973.

Byrne JJ & others: Symposium on postoperative complications. Am J Surg 116:325–406, 1968.

Doromal NM, Canter JW: Hyperosmolar hyperglycemic non-ketotic coma complicating intravenous hyperalimentation. Surg Gynec Obst 136:729–732, 1973.

Feller I, Richards KE, Pierson CL: Prevention of postoperative infections. S Clin North America 52:1361–1366, 1972.

La Mont JT, Isselbacher KJ: Postoperative jaundice. New England J Med 288:305–307, 1973.

Strode JE (editor): Symposium on unexpected complications of surgery. S Clin North America 50:289–533, 1970.

Walters MB, Stanger HAD, Rotem CE: Complications with percutaneous central venous catheters. JAMA 220:1455–1457, 1972.

Zarem HA: The management of complications in head and neck surgery. S Clin North America 53:191–201, 1973.

5...

Special Medical Problems in Surgical Patients

ENDOCRINE DISEASE & THE SURGICAL PATIENT
Peter H. Forsham, MD

Surgery on the endocrine glands is covered elsewhere in this text. General surgery performed on patients with endocrine diseases is the subject of this section. In any patient with endocrine disease, surgery carries the usual surgical hazards with some added risks. Endocrine abnormalities must be recognized and treated preoperatively if mishaps during and after surgery are to be prevented.

Blood Pressure & Circulatory Competence

These are endangered in patients with diminished blood volume as in adrenocortical insufficiency, pheochromocytoma, and diabetes insipidus.

In **adrenocortical insufficiency**, fluid depletion is due to sodium and water loss from the kidneys and from the intestinal tract. The preoperative management must include administration of saline and fludrocortisone, 0.2 mg orally, for 2 days preoperatively at least. Soluble hydrocortisone phosphate or hemisuccinate, 50 mg IM every 6 hours, may also be given on the day of surgery. When blood volume is adequately restored, one rarely has to use vasoconstrictors.

In a patient with **pheochromocytoma** whose plasma volume is decreased preoperatively, administration of human albumin and, on occasion, blood transfusions are indicated in order to prevent postoperative hypotension. This may prove lifesaving in view of the usual postoperative tendency to hypotension. Alphablocking agents such as phentolamine (Regitine) may also be used after restoration of blood volume.

In patients with **diabetes insipidus** and increased free water clearance, there is marked hemoconcentration and a low plasma volume. Administration of vasopressin (Pitressin), 10–20 units IM every 4 hours or an infusion of 5 units in 1000 ml of 5% dextrose in water, is indicated preoperatively until the elevated osmolality returns to normal.

Respiratory Exchange

Adequate respiratory exchange is severely reduced in patients with advanced **myxedema**. Surgery should be postponed until the patient has been made euthyroid with thyroid therapy. If surgery must be done within a week, give triiodothyronine (T_3), 50–100 μg/day orally. If it is possible to delay surgery for a month, sodium thyroxine (T_4), 0.2–0.4 mg/day orally, is used. In both instances, the dosage must be reduced if angina pectoris or cardiac irregularities appear.

Very **obese** subjects should be placed on assisted ventilation during and after surgery to guarantee adequate oxygenation.

Anesthesia

Anesthesia may be life-threatening in patients with untreated **adrenocortical** or **pituitary insufficiency** or a lack of **hypothalamic corticotropin releasing** factor. The cortisol response to stress is absent, and the anesthesia, with its accompanying vasodilatation, may lead to vascular collapse. There is little point in pretesting for such a possible collapse. Even if testing for an adrenocortical response with either metyrapone or insulin hypoglycemia shows an inadequate response, one may still find a good rise with the full stress of surgery. Most surgeons and anesthesiologists prefer to give hydrocortisone phosphate preoperatively whenever there is a possibility that hypotension due to adrenocortical insufficiency may occur during or after surgery. The dosage is 100 mg or more IV.

Hemostasis

Hemostasis may be particularly difficult in patients with excessive glucocorticoid activity, as in **Cushing's disease**, when their ability to constrict arterial and larger vessels is severely diminished. Severed blood vessels will thus produce increased bleeding in the surgical field unless one ties vessels with care.

Infections

Wound infection must be guarded against in **Cushing's disease**. The intrinsic protective mechanisms are markedly diminished in this condition because of excess glucocorticoid secretion. Phagocytosis and antibody formation are inadequate.

In uncontrolled **diabetes**, phagocytosis is markedly diminished and there is thus an increased danger of wound infection. In either case, the use of bactericidal rather than bacteriostatic antibiotics is preferable.

Wound Healing

Wound healing is definitely impaired in **Cushing's disease** because of impaired fibroplasia and enhanced tissue breakdown, in part as a result of increased lysosome membrane instability. Uncontrolled **diabetes mellitus** impairs wound healing, also reducing protein synthesis. Marked **hyperthyroidism** leads to a negative nitrogen balance. Hypogonadism definitely slows wound healing because of a lack of anabolic steroids.

Bowel & Bladder Functions

Abnormal bowel function may be related to endocrinopathies. Diarrhea is found in far-advanced **diabetic autonomic neuropathy** and at times in the presence of **hyperthyroidism**. Constipation is seen with excess calcium levels in hyperparathyroidism and with **hypothyroidism** or **myxedema**. Simple remedial treatment should precede surgery.

Bladder function may be inadequate in advanced long-standing diabetes because of impairment of the parasympathetic system.

Nutrition

Alimentation calls for specific management in several instances of endocrine disease before and after surgery. In patients with **hyperthyroidism**, a caloric intake as high as 4000 calories/day may be required during the acute stages of the disease, together with water-soluble vitamin supplementation since these vitamins are used up excessively in this condition. A high-protein diet with at least 120 g of protein and 2 g of calcium should be given to patients with **Cushing's disease** in order to affect the negative nitrogen balance and osteoporosis to some extent. A diet low in sodium and high in potassium must precede surgery in patients with **primary aldosteronism** in order to overcome the dangerously low serum potassium with its tendency to cause ascending paralysis of the extremities. In the presence of **hyperparathyroidism** with severe hypercalcemia, an attempt should be made to reduce the levels preoperatively. This involves overhydration with normal saline solution and the administration of hydrocortisone or one of its derivatives. Up to 200 mg daily of hydrocortisone or 60 mg of prednisone should be used for 3 days before surgery—but not longer, since these drugs have an adverse effect on wound healing. Preoperative **anemia** calls for iron supplementation and, more importantly, appropriate endocrine substitution therapy for many weeks preoperatively if the anemia is due to **myxedema, Addison's disease,** male **hypogonadism,** or **diabetes** associated with renal insufficiency.

Management of Surgery in the Diabetic Patient

Well-controlled diabetes mellitus probably does not increase operative risk. However, the uncontrolled diabetic must be properly treated and controlled before elective surgery. In emergency situations, constant vigilance is necessary to prevent complications. In all major surgical procedures, the patient must be under constant care to prevent ketosis or hypoglycemic reactions.

A clear distinction must be drawn between a diabetic controlled on **diet** and perhaps **oral medications** and one who is **insulin-dependent**. In the former group, an attempt should be made to minimize the period of overnight starvation so that it does not exceed 6–8 hours. After surgery, blood or urinary glucose levels should be determined. Catheterization should not be employed because the diabetic is prone to urinary tract infections. If possible, oral treatment should be maintained and, in addition, 10% glucose in water should be infused slowly intravenously up to 2000 ml/day at a slow rate. This will furnish the carbohydrate necessary to minimize ketoacidosis.

The diabetic who requires insulin should be given two-thirds of his usual insulin dosage on the morning of surgery, including both crystalline (rapid-acting) and intermediate-acting insulin. This should be followed at once by a slow intravenous infusion of 10% dextrose in water not to exceed 2000 ml/day. Additional crystalline insulin should be given every 6 hours. The amount needed should be determined by measuring blood glucose or testing free-flowing urine specimens for glucose. As soon as oral alimentation is resumed, insulin administration should revert to the preoperative regimen. At no time should either insulin or carbohydrate be withheld before, during, or after major surgery. Catheterization should not be resorted to unless it is surgically essential; antibiotic coverage is indicated.

Ambulation

Early ambulation after surgery is imperative in patients who undergo **total adrenalectomy** or removal of an **active adrenal adenoma** for Cushing's disease to minimize thromboembolic phenomena. Sudden reduction in cortisol apparently predisposes to thromboembolism, and adequate hydration and early ambulation are therefore necessary.

Sedation

Finally, depending on the endocrine abnormalities present, the question of sedation must be considered carefully. With **Cushing's disease**, where wakefulness and anxiety are extreme, one must use high doses of hypnotics. Unless **Addison's disease** is well treated, sedatives and cholinergics (eg, bethanechol [Urecholine]) have increased potency and must be used with care. In **hyperthyroidism**, because of the rapid metabolic rate, doses of hypnotics and analgesics must be markedly increased to be effective. This is true also in **hypoparathyroidism**, with its increased neuromuscular irritability. The reverse is true in **hypothyroidism** and in **hyperparathyroidism**.

CARDIAC DISEASE & THE SURGICAL PATIENT
Maurice Sokolow, MD

Anesthesia and general surgery are a hazard to any patient, but the risk in the cardiac patient is increased. Acidosis, arterial hypoxemia, hypercapnia, decreased systemic resistance, decreased cardiac contractility and conduction, and hypotension with decreased blood volume, which may result from bleeding—all are deleterious to cardiovascular function. Other important hazards are arrhythmias due to release of catecholamines, bradycardia due to the muscle-relaxing drugs, and impaired coronary perfusion as a result of decreased systemic flow. Postoperative problems that must be considered include thromboembolism, myocardial ischemia, and atelectasis. Because of these hazards, the physician is often asked to evaluate a surgical patient with heart disease preoperatively and judge whether the risk is warranted.

Key questions that must be answered are the following: (1) Is the operation urgent or elective? (2) If elective, does the patient have cardiac disease? (3) What is the risk of the underlying surgical disease if surgery is not performed? (4) What additional risk does the heart disease impose on the surgical procedure? (5) Is the surgical diagnosis correct, or could the symptoms, such as abdominal pain, be a manifestation of cardiac disease and not of surgical disease? The physician must distinguish between elective and emergency procedures and judge when the risk of surgery exceeds the risk of the underlying disease or vice versa.

Urgent operations must be done regardless of the underlying cardiac disease in such conditions as gross hemorrhage, strangulated hernia, perforation of the bowel or gallbladder, bowel obstruction, dissecting or ruptured aortic aneurysm, or removal of large arterial emboli which threaten life or limb.

The presence of heart disease does not mean that the patient will not tolerate the surgical procedure; one should not withhold a lifesaving procedure merely because of the presence of heart disease.

Cardiac Conditions Masquerading as Surgical Illnesses

Gastrointestinal symptoms, including acute abdominal pain, may so dominate the clinical picture that heart disease is not recognized or, if recognized, is thought not to be responsible for the symptoms. Early evidence of cardiac failure is often overlooked because it is overshadowed by the gastrointestinal symptoms. The most common causes of diagnostic confusion are the following:

(1) Angina pectoris or myocardial infarction presenting with epigastric pain.

(2) Fairly abrupt right heart failure presenting with right upper quadrant pain simulating gallbladder disease. This is particularly apt to occur in patients with tight mitral valve disease who develop atrial fibrillation or following exercise in patients with mild right heart failure.

(3) Slowly developing right heart failure, which may present with nonspecific gastrointestinal symptoms of anorexia, nausea, a sensation of heaviness and fullness after meals, and perhaps vomiting. These lead to weight loss and may seem to justify a diagnosis of carcinoma of the upper gastrointestinal tract. If there are no murmurs, the diagnosis of heart disease is often missed.

(4) Pulmonary infarction presenting as jaundice, leading to a diagnosis of biliary tract disease.

(5) Right heart failure or constrictive pericarditis presenting as ascites.

(6) Dysphagia, which may be the presenting symptom in a variety of heart diseases, eg, mitral stenosis with a large left atrium, pericarditis, aortic aneurysm, dissecting aneurysm, or anomalies of the aortic arch.

(7) Acute rheumatic fever, which may present with acute abdominal pain, especially in children.

(8) Acute abdominal pain, which may result from emboli to the splenic, renal, or mesenteric arteries in subacute bacterial endocarditis or atrial fibrillation.

(9) Nausea and vomiting, which may occur in cardiac failure, especially as a result of digitalis therapy.

Space does not permit a differential diagnosis of these conditions, but one should search for positive diagnostic evidence of heart disease: (1) A history of angina pectoris, dyspnea on effort, or orthopnea. (2) Cardiac enlargement with a left ventricular heave, with or without characteristic murmurs. (3) Evidence of right heart failure, with increased venous pressure, enlarged and tender liver, and edema or ascites. Orthopnea, decreased vital capacity, and rales and gallop rhythm may be present in left ventricular failure. (4) Signs of myocardial necrosis with fever, tachycardia, or enzyme changes. (5) Typical serial ECG changes of ischemia, infarction, hypertrophy, pericarditis, etc. (6) Radiologic evidence of cardiac enlargement or pulmonary venous congestion.

Considering the possibility of heart disease often leads to an adequate examination and appropriate therapy.

Preoperative Evaluation of the Surgical Patient With Cardiovascular Disease

The presence of heart disease is recognized on the basis of symptoms, significant murmurs, an enlarged heart or evidence of cardiac failure, hypertension, conduction defects, and ventricular arrhythmias. A history of angina pectoris or previous myocardial infarction, Stokes-Adams attacks, cardiac failure, intermittent claudication, or cerebral ischemic attacks may alert the physician to the possibility of cardiac disease. A history of antihypertensive treatment or treatment for cardiac failure may be obtained.

Preoperative ECGs are often valuable but may be difficult to interpret. A patient with known previous myocardial infarction may have a normal ECG; even more importantly, a patient with preinfarction angina may have a normal ECG. Conversely, grossly abnormal changes may be due to an old healed infarct and are therefore of less importance in deciding whether or not surgery should be performed. A baseline ECG is advisable to interpret postoperative changes. An ECG may also show evidence of digitalis therapy, electrolyte disturbances, conduction defects, or arrhythmias. In general, a stable abnormality in the ECG in the absence of cardiac failure or a change in the pattern of angina pectoris indicates that the patient will probably tolerate surgery almost as well as a normal individual. Such a patient with a healed previous myocardial infarction has an added mortality risk of about 3–5%.

The most important conditions which should contraindicate elective surgery are recent angina pectoris, a crescendo change in the pattern of angina pectoris in recent weeks or months, preinfarction angina, acute myocardial infarction, severe aortic stenosis, a high degree of atrioventricular block, untreated cardiac failure, or severe hypertension.

Specific Disease Problems

A. Coronary Heart Disease: The usual patient seen for preoperative evaluation is an older individual with possible coronary heart disease. One searches for a history of recent crescendo in the character of the anginal pain, pain at rest, preinfarction angina, or the possibility of recent myocardial infarction. If known coronary disease is stable, without change in the pattern of pain or in serial ECGs; if there are no symptoms or signs of cardiac failure; and if at least 6 months have elapsed since myocardial infarction, the surgeon can proceed if the indications for surgery are clear and definite.

Emergency surgery must often be done despite a recent myocardial infarction, but the mortality rate is high. Important but not lifesaving surgery is best delayed at least 3 weeks if possible. Purely elective surgery should be postponed for 3–6 months whenever possible.

B. Hypertension: Patients with uncomplicated chronic hypertension, even with left ventricular hypertrophy and an abnormal ECG, tolerate surgery without significantly increased mortality if there are no evidences of coronary heart disease or cardiac failure and if renal function is normal. Unless the diastolic pressure exceeds 110 mm Hg, it is best to decrease or even stop antihypertensive medication for a week prior to surgery and to be certain, if thiazides have been used, that the body potassium has been replenished. Anesthesiologists have found that the catechol depletion that follows reserpine, methyldopa, and guanethidine can be managed satisfactorily if they are forewarned and prepared to give vasopressors in the event of hypotension.

C. Arrhythmias: Chronic atrial fibrillation with a well-controlled ventricular rate does not increase the risk of surgery, nor does an asymptomatic isolated right or left bundle branch block. Second or third degree atrioventricular block is a warning sign, especially if associated with left ventricular conduction defects; a transvenous electrode catheter should be inserted into the right ventricle prior to the surgical procedure and the patient monitored with a pacemaker available in case ventricular standstill occurs. Infrequent atrial or ventricular premature beats usually do not require special treatment and can often be relieved with phenobarbital. If ventricular premature beats are frequent and from multiple foci, they are best depressed with drugs such as quinidine, 200–400 mg orally 2–4 times daily, or procainamide, 250–500 mg orally 3 or 4 times daily. They can be quickly abolished with lidocaine, 2% solution (20 mg/ml), 50 mg IV, followed by an intravenous infusion of 1–2 mg/minute.

D. Valvular Heart Disease: Severe aortic stenosis, tight mitral stenosis, and severe coronary ostial involvement due to syphilitic aortitis are the 3 major valvular conditions in which general surgery presents a considerably increased hazard. An aortic systolic murmur not associated with evidence of severe aortic valvular disease or significant left ventricular hypertrophy does not increase the mortality. Mitral insufficiency is usually tolerated well, but tight mitral stenosis, especially if the patient has sinus rhythm, may result in acute pulmonary edema if the patient abruptly fibrillates during surgery.

E. Congenital Heart Disease: In the absence of cardiac failure, ventricular septal defect and atrial septal defect usually pose no particular problems or extra hazard. Pulmonary hypertension with Eisenmenger's syndrome carries a significantly increased mortality risk, and surgery should be performed only upon urgent indications. Patients with coarctation of the aorta and patent ductus arteriosus should have their congenital lesions repaired before undergoing elective general surgical procedures. Mild pulmonic stenosis is not a contraindication to elective surgery, but severe pulmonic stenosis is a contraindication because of the hazard of acute right heart failure and a reversed shunt through the foramen ovale or a small atrial septal defect. Patients with tetralogy of Fallot are relatively poor surgical risks because of the polycythemia and because of the possibility of contraction of the infundibulum of the right ventricle with resulting poor cardiac output.

F. Cardiac Failure: Patients with mild cardiac failure whose symptoms and signs are controlled with digitalis and diuretics have only a slightly increased risk from general surgery provided ordinary activity does not cause symptoms. Patients with dyspnea on walking on level ground, orthopnea or nocturnal dyspnea, and signs of cardiac failure such as gallop rhythm, increased venous pressure, and rales are at a significantly increased risk, and surgery should be delayed if possible. Cardiac failure should be treated adequately before surgery. It is desirable to have the patient stabilized for at least a month before surgery, avoiding digitalis toxicity and potassium depletion by diuretics. Diuretics and digitalis can then be withheld for a few days before surgery. Digitalization of a patient with cardiac hypertrophy but no heart failure is probably unwise because of the hazard of digitalis toxicity, including arrhythmias. Although digitalis has a positive inotropic action even in normal hearts, clinical evidence of benefit from the drug has not been demonstrated when it has been given to patients with hypertrophy but no failure. If there is a question about whether or not heart failure is present preoperatively, a period of bed rest and restricted dietary sodium may be adequate treatment.

Special Precautions

With the emphasis on the surgical condition, one may overlook certain special precautions such as stopping anticoagulants, continuing corticosteroids, and inquiring about antihypertensive or insulin therapy and the patient's hypersensitivities to drugs, especially antibiotics or sedatives. Particular care should be taken to control the speed and volume of sodium-containing infusions used in preoperative preparation. Red cell mass rather than whole blood should be given to the cardiac patient if there is substantial blood loss or severe anemia preoperatively. The infusion should be given while the patient is supine so that he can be placed in the Fowler position if dyspnea or rales develop. The patient should be examined frequently during the infusion, being alert for dyspnea, orthopnea, rales, or elevation of venous pressure.

If urgent surgery is required in the patient with severe coronary disease, aortic stenosis, or atrioventricular block, the patient should be monitored with an arterial catheter, central venous pressure determinations, periodic blood gas measurements, and an electrode transvenous catheter in case ventricular standstill or arrhythmia occurs. Isoproterenol, pressor agents, lidocaine, and facilities for defibrillation should be readily available.

The choice and details of anesthesia are left to the anesthesiologist, but it is well to alert him to any possible problems he might expect.

Earley LE: Current concepts: Diuretics. New England J Med 276:966–968, 1023–1025, 1967.

Fisch C: Treatment of arrhythmias due to digitalis. J Indiana MA 60:146–152, 1967.

Fredrickson DS: On cultivating prognosis on cardiovascular research. Am J Cardiol 21:853–858, 1968.

Friedberg CK: *Diseases of the Heart*, 3rd ed. Saunders, 1966.

Friedberg CK: Prevention of heart failure. Am J Cardiol 22:190–194, 1968.

Harrison TR, Reeves TJ: *Principles and Problems of Ischemic Heart Disease.* Year Book, 1968.

Hurst JW, Logue RB: *The Heart, Arteries and Veins,* 2nd ed. McGraw-Hill, 1970.

Larragh JH: Ethacrynic acid and furosemide. Am Heart J 75:564–566, 1968.

Leonard JJ, deGroot WJ: The thyroid state and the cardiovascular system. Mod Concepts Cardiovas Dis 38:23–28, 1969.

Levine SA: *Clinical Heart Disease,* 5th ed. Saunders, 1958.

Lindsay J, Hurst JW: Drug therapy of dissecting aortic aneurysms. Circulation 37:216–219, 1968.

Marshall RJ, Shepherd JT: *Cardiac Function in Health and Disease.* Saunders, 1968.

Williams JF Jr, Morrow AG, Braunwald E: The incidence and management of "medical" complications following cardiac operations. Circulation 32:608–619, 1965.

RESPIRATORY DISEASE & THE SURGICAL PATIENT
John L. Wilson, MD

Operative morbidity and mortality are increased by acute or chronic respiratory tract diseases.

Specific Disease & Problems

A. Acute Conditions: Acute respiratory tract infections (colds, pharyngitis, tonsillitis, bronchitis, or pneumonitis) are contraindications to elective surgery because they are associated with an increased postoperative incidence of atelectasis and pneumonitis. The patient should be completely recovered from an acute respiratory tract infection for 1–2 weeks before operation. If emergency operation must be undertaken in the presence of acute respiratory tract infection, avoid inhalation anesthesia, if possible; employ prophylactic measures for atelectasis postoperatively, and administer an antibiotic (after obtaining throat or sputum culture) if the infection is marked or progressive. Penicillin G is usually given until the antibiotic sensitivity report on throat or sputum culture is obtained.

B. Chronic Bronchopulmonary Infection: Chronic bronchitis, bronchiectasis, emphysema, asthma, pulmonary fibrosis, and tuberculosis are among the disorders commonly associated with chronic bronchial or pulmonary infection in surgical patients. Many of these patients are elderly, and smoking is often an aggravating factor. Any patient who has smoked over 20 cigarettes a day for 10 years can be assumed to have chronic bronchopulmonary inflammation. Heavy smokers should abstain for at least 2 weeks before elective major surgery. The major hazard in the patient with chronic bronchopulmonary infection is excessive bronchial secretions during and after operation with a marked tendency to postoperative atelectasis and pneumonitis. Preoperative evaluation of these patients includes sputum culture and sensitivity with preoperative control of infection by administration of the appropriate antibiotic.

C. Chronic Pulmonary Insufficiency: Diminished pulmonary reserve is caused by a wide variety of disorders, particularly those mentioned above as associated with bronchopulmonary infection. When there is clinical evidence of chronically reduced lung function such as significant shortness of breath not due to extrapulmonary causes, pulmonary function tests are indicated in connection with preoperative evaluation. Reevaluation of lung function after treatment for infection and bronchospasm will frequently show improvement. During operation, the patient with chronic pulmonary insufficiency can usually be well oxygenated by the anesthesiologist. Problems begin to arise during the immediate postoperative period when atelectasis, hypoxia, and hypercapnia are the imminent dangers. These may be foreseen and minimized by careful preoperative evaluation and preparation and by intensive postoperative care. Consequently, with the exception of those thoracic resections which reduce pulmonary reserves to an intolerable level, pulmonary insufficiency is rarely severe enough to contraindicate necessary surgery.

Bates DV, Macklem PT, Christie RV: *Respiratory Function in Disease,* 2nd ed. Saunders, 1971.

Bendixen HH & others: *Respiratory Care.* Mosby, 1965.

RENAL DISEASE
& THE SURGICAL PATIENT
John L. Wilson, MD

The following types of renal disease are most frequently responsible for diminished reserve in surgical patients: chronic glomerulonephritis, chronic pyelonephritis, toxic nephritis, amyloid renal disease, obstructive uropathy, and acute renal failure. Before major operations, it is advisable to evaluate kidney function by one or more special examinations if any of the following is present: (1) a history of renal disease, (2) age over 60, (3) diabetes mellitus, (4) hypertension, or (5) abnormal urinalysis (proteinuria, casts, pyuria, hematuria, low or fixed specific gravity, and oliguria or polyuria not caused by variation in the fluid intake). The following special examinations are frequently of value in addition to the routine urinalysis: BUN, creatinine, PSP, a clearance test (urea or creatinine), blood and urine electrolyte determinations, urine culture, and an intravenous urogram.

Chronic impairment of renal function may be fully compensated and asymptomatic under normal conditions, but renal insufficiency may develop under the adverse conditions of surgical illness. About 700 ml/day of urine are normally required for the excretion of nitrogenous wastes in the adult. In patients with damaged kidneys, considerably larger volumes of urine (1500 ml or more) may be necessary as a result of the kidneys' inability to concentrate urine. Monitoring fluid intake and output and body weight will aid in evaluating such patients who tend to develop uremia if they become dehydrated or if the nitrogen load is increased, eg, in fever and as a catabolic response to trauma or infection. Metabolic acidosis is a common additional complication. Be alert for the dangerous accumulation of medications excreted by the kidneys in patients with diminished renal function, and be wary of the use of drugs having renal toxicity.

Extrarenal azotemia is the abnormal accumulation of nitrogenous waste products in the presence of normal or potentially normal renal function. The most common cause is inadequate glomerular filtration secondary to decreased effective circulating blood volume, as occurs in shock and dehydration. These conditions are not uncommon preoperatively in the acutely ill surgical patient. BUN, NPN, and blood creatinine are elevated. After massive gastrointestinal bleeding, extrarenal azotemia may occur as a result of protein digestion and absorption plus decreased circulating blood volume. Under these circumstances, the blood creatinine level is not elevated. Since no renal disease is present, treatment is aimed at improving circulating blood volume (transfusion), electrolyte balance, and urinary output (increased fluid intake).

Hollenberg NK, Epstein N: The use of drugs in the patient with uremia. Mod Treat 6:1011–1035, 1969.

Pitts RF: *Physiology of the Kidney and Body Fluids,* 2nd ed. Year Book, 1968.

Takacs FJ: Surgery with impaired renal function. S Clin North America 50:719–728, 1970.

Tucker RM: Management of renal insufficiency in surgical patients. S Clin North America 49:1095–1104, 1969.

HEMATOLOGIC DISEASE
& THE SURGICAL PATIENT
Ralph O. Wallerstein, MD

SURGERY IN PATIENTS WITH CHRONIC ANEMIA

In general, moderate anemia does not increase the hazard of surgery. If time permits, deficiencies of iron, folic acid, and vitamin B_{12} should be repaired before surgery. In an emergency, chronic anemia can be corrected by transfusion of red cells before surgery. If possible, surgery should be deferred for a day after transfusion to permit readjustment of blood volume and to give the transfused red cells a chance to accumulate a normal level of 2,3-diphosphoglycerate (2,3-DPG), which is necessary for efficient delivery of oxygen to tissues.

Patients with iron deficiency anemia and the various congenital and acquired hemolytic anemias do not ordinarily present any unusual risk at surgery provided their blood volumes and hemoglobin levels are adequate. In the case of megaloblastic anemias (pernicious anemia and folic acid deficiency), surgery should be deferred if possible until specific therapy (vitamin B_{12} or folic acid) has repaired the generalized tissue defect; this is because in these 2 conditions all the cells of the body are affected by the vitamin deficiency, and transfusions alone do not render surgery safe. It probably takes 1–2 weeks to reach adequate tissue levels.

Patients with sickle cell disease have an increased incidence of thrombosis, particularly pulmonary thromboses. Normally, only a few cells in the circulation are sickled; under the stressful conditions of surgery, excessive sickling, which leads to thrombosis, may be precipitated by anoxia and acidosis. The risk is greatest in a patient with sickle cell anemia, but it is appreciable also in hemoglobin S-C disease and in sickle cell thalassemia. If these patients must go to surgery, they should be transfused with whole blood to normal hemoglobin levels; this creates a relative dilution of their own sickled cells and prevents sickling of large columns of abnormal cells in the smaller blood vessels. A patient with sickle cell trait has an increased risk during surgery if the oxygen saturation falls to critically low levels.

A few hematologic disorders may simulate acute abdominal surgical conditions.

Sickle Cell Anemia

Painful abdominal crises in sickle cell anemia may suggest appendicitis, cholecystitis, a ruptured viscus, or other acute abdominal conditions. In a patient with this kind of pain, helpful diagnostic points are the following: (1) In sickle cell anemia, while the abdomen may be rigid and tender, peristalsis is usually normal. (2) The leukocytosis in sickle cell anemia has a relatively normal differential count—eg, with a white count of $20,000/\mu l$, only 65% granulocytes. (3) Leukocyte counts above $20,000/\mu l$ are seen in many patients with sickle cell anemia who are not acutely ill.

Henoch-Schönlein or Nonthrombocytopenic Purpura

These conditions are usually associated with obvious skin lesions or perhaps hematuria but may on occasion present with acute abdominal pain. The symptoms are apparently due to bleeding into the bowel wall. Intussusception may occur and may require surgical intervention. No reliably effective treatment is available to prevent or treat abnormal bleeding, although prednisone may be tried.

Lead Poisoning

Lead poisoning may cause acute abdominal pain. A history of possible exposure to lead may be of great importance. Laboratory clues are moderate anemia with striking stippling and a marked elevation of urinary coproporphyrin. The diagnosis is established by finding elevated lead levels in blood and urine.

Abdominal Wall Hemorrhage

Hemorrhage into the abdominal wall may simulate acute appendicitis in patients with thrombocytopenia, hemophilia, or other severe coagulation disorders.

SURGERY IN PATIENTS WITH HEMATOLOGIC MALIGNANCIES

Occasionally it is necessary to operate on patients who have leukemia, lymphoma, myeloma, or related disorders. Such patients can always undergo surgery without increased risk if they are in hematologic remission, and surgery may be relatively safe in partial remission. In acute leukemia, the risk of surgery is low if the white count is not excessive, the hemoglobin is over 10 g/100 ml, and the platelet count is near $100,000/\mu l$. Other coagulation factors are not usually disturbed in acute leukemia. If surgery must be done in spite of very abnormal blood counts and excessive bleeding develops, transfusions and platelet packs are used.

In patients with chronic myelocytic leukemia with platelet counts in excess of 1 million/μl or white counts above $100,000/\mu l$, bleeding may be a problem. In patients with chronic lymphatic leukemia and a normal platelet count, even white counts in excess of $100,000/\mu l$ are no contraindication to surgery.

Patients with polycythemia vera have a greatly increased incidence of bleeding and thromboses. A qualitative platelet defect can be detected when the red cell count and the platelet count are high. Occasionally, there is a fibrinogen deficiency. When blood counts have become normal (after phlebotomy, radiotherapy, or chemotherapy), surgery is safer, but the incidence of complications is still increased.

Patients with multiple myeloma or macroglobulinemia may bleed excessively in surgery because their elevated abnormal globulin may interfere with the coagulation process. Plasmapheresis before surgery should be considered.

Patients with all of the above have no increased difficulty with wound healing or postoperative infections as long as their total granulocyte count is at least $1500/\mu l$. The common anticancer chemotherapeutic agents—mercaptopurine (Purinethol), busulfan (Myleran), melphalan (Alkeran), methotrexate, and cyclophosphamide (Cytoxan)—do not interfere with wound healing.

SURGERY IN PATIENTS RECEIVING ANTICOAGULANTS

Heparin

Since the average dose of heparin (5000 units IV) maintains the whole blood clotting time at twice the control value for only 3–4 hours, a short wait will let the coagulation time return to normal. If a large dose has been administered, it may be necessary to neutralize its effect in a patient who suddenly becomes a candidate for emergency surgery.

Immediately after an intravenous dose of heparin,

the amount of protamine sulfate required (in milligrams) is equal to 1/100 the last dose of heparin (in units). The biologic half-life of heparin is less than 1 hour. The dose of protamine is reduced if some time has elapsed since the last dose of heparin: In 30 minutes, only about half the amount of protamine is required; in 4–6 hours, there is seldom need for neutralization. After the subcutaneous administration of heparin, the dose of protamine should be only 50–75% (in mg) × 1/100 of the last heparin dose (in units), but repeated doses of protamine may be required because of the continued absorption of heparin.

Protamine should always be given by slow intravenous injection. Rapid injection may cause thrombocytopenia. If given in excessive amounts, protamine may act as a weak anticoagulant.

During open heart surgery and extracorporeal circulation, large doses of heparin are required to prevent coagulation in the pump oxygenator and the patient's circulatory system; at the end of the procedure, the heparin must be neutralized. The dose of protamine should be based on the amount of heparin used. Neutralization is not required in some vascular operations if the dose is calculated and timed so as to lose its effect at the end of the operation.

Coumadin

Surgery in patients anticoagulated with coumadin derivatives is relatively safe when the prothrombin time is 25% or greater. In patients with lower values prophylactic measures are in order if surgery is necessary. Vitamin K, 5 mg IV, will return the prothrombin time to safe levels (40% or better) in approximately 4 hours and to normal levels in 24–48 hours. However, its administration may render the patient refractory to all coumadin therapy for a week or more. For immediate, transient (a few hours') restoration of normal prothrombin values, one may infuse 250–500 ml of plasma. Factors II, VII, IX, and X—the factors lowered by coumadin therapy—are quite stable in banked plasma. As an alternative, one may give the commercially available factor IX concentrate, Konyne. This material also contains factors II, VII, and X. The dosage is 20 ml (500 units), or 1 ampule. It carries a high risk of hepatitis.

SPECIAL PROBLEMS IN PATIENTS WITH LIVER DISEASE

Bleeding from the gastrointestinal tract in patients with cirrhosis of the liver is not usually due to abnormal coagulation but to vascular abnormalities, eg, esophageal varices, gastritis, or hemorrhoids. Factors II (prothrombin), V, VII, and X may be reduced and prolong the prothrombin time, but rarely to clinically important levels (below 20%). Factors IX and XI also may be reduced somewhat but do not constitute a bleeding hazard. Fibrinogen and factor VIII are not lowered by liver disease.

Platelets may be severely reduced, below 30,000/μl, with acute alcoholism and may be responsible for bleeding problems, but they rise spontaneously to normal levels in a few days when alcohol is withdrawn. Moderate thrombocytopenia (50–100,000/μl) that does not remit spontaneously may be a sign of hypersplenism secondary to cirrhosis; the spleen can either be felt, or its enlargement can be demonstrated by scanning it with ^{99m} technetium colloid.

Disseminated intravascular coagulation may occur in the course of very severe liver disease with the characteristic findings of that disorder: low factors V, VIII, fibrinogen, and platelets and increased levels of fibrin degradation products (FDP, "fibrin split products"). An elevated level of FDP alone is not enough to establish the diagnosis since these substances may be elevated when their clearance is impaired by severe liver disease.

A very rare hemorrhagic complication of hepatic necrosis is acute primary fibrinolysis, which may be difficult to differentiate from disseminated intravascular coagulation; in general, platelets and factors V and VIII are less strikingly decreased.

Clotting factor deficiency resulting from liver damage does not respond to vitamin K even when given parenterally in large doses. Vitamin K can only repair those deficiencies that result from impaired vitamin K absorption due to obstructive jaundice, as reflected in a prolonged prothrombin time.

Platelet deficiency may become a problem if more than 10 units of whole blood are given in rapid succession (see next section on transfusions). Factors V and VIII, the only factors that deteriorate significantly on storage, do not present an unusual problem in liver disease even with multiple transfusions. Factor V requires a minimum level of only 5–10% of normal for hemostasis, and factor VIII is usually elevated in liver disease.

TRANSFUSION OF BLOOD, BLOOD COMPONENTS, & PLASMA SUBSTITUTES

Transfusion of blood, blood components, and plasma substitutes for surgical patients may be required for one or more of the following reasons: (1) to restore and maintain normal blood volume, (2) to correct severe anemia, or (3) to correct bleeding and coagulation disorders. Certain other blood abnormalities such as granulocytopenia or hypoalbuminemia cannot be satisfactorily corrected by blood transfusion.

Decisions about the need for transfusion and selection of the proper type and amount of transfusion material must be based upon careful evaluation of the individual patient. Urgency of need and the availability of diagnostic and therapeutic resources are obviously the determining factors. Attention must be given to the total clinical picture:

(1) History of hemorrhage, bleeding tendencies, treatment with anticoagulant drugs or of systemic disease predisposing to blood loss.

(2) Determination of the presence and severity of anemia based on blood count.

(3) Estimation of effective circulating blood volume by monitoring blood pressure and central venous pressure or by direct measurement of blood volume (see below).

(4) Evaluation of bleeding time, clotting studies, prothrombin time (PT), partial thromboplastin time (PTT), or activated coagulation time (ACT).

Blood Volume

Determination of blood volume may be helpful in assessing the clinical status of the patient with anemia or shock, but these measurements are not infallible criteria of the requirements for blood transfusion for the following reasons:

(1) Values for normal blood volume vary widely, eg, the average volume in healthy persons 45–75 years of age is approximately 480 ml less than the average of those 19–36 years of age, even though their average hemoglobin concentrations are approximately the same. An obese patient has a relatively smaller blood volume per unit of weight than a lean one, because the blood flow in adipose tissue is only 20% of that in muscular tissue.

(2) It is difficult to measure and interpret blood volume variations in rapidly changing situations, as in a bleeding patient who is being transfused.

(3) Patients vary in their ability to accommodate to changes in blood volume. In a patient with chronic anemia, both total blood volume and red cell mass are often reduced, but a debilitated patient may have a greater than normal blood volume and may be bordering on cardiac failure even with low hematocrit values.

For these reasons, in the absence of acute blood loss, transfusions should not be given to correct assumed deficits in blood volume unless the deficits can be documented by accurate measurement. When such a deficit has been identified, transfusions should be calculated to increase red cell mass to not more than 70% of normal. *Caution:* For unknown reasons, the vascular system appears to need a greater volume of blood than was actually lost before stabilization can occur.

Choice of Transfusion Material

The routine use of whole blood to meet all transfusion requirements is not desirable since in most cases only one element of the blood is required for therapy and not whole blood.

Freshly drawn blood (ie, the same day's procurement) is seldom required, since most clinical situations can be treated optimally with blood components or relatively fresh stored blood (< 4–7 days old). Fresh blood is required only if functioning donor platelets are needed. The age of the blood (within the expira-

Abbreviations Used in This Section	
ACD	Acid-citrate-dextrose
ACT	Activated coagulation time
AHF	Antihemophilic factor
CPD	Citrate-phosphate-dextrose
HAA	Hepatitis-associated antigen (Australia antigen)
PC	Platelet concentrate
PRP	Platelet-rich plasma
PT	Prothrombin time
PTC	Plasma thromboplastin component (factor IX)
PTT	Partial thromboplastin time

tion period) is relatively unimportant if the need is only for correction of volume deficits or anemia.

Most urban centers have blood bank facilities for collection and fractionation of whole blood into components to meet specific clinical needs, and these components should be utilized whenever possible.

Plasma substitutes may be administered (1) on an emergency basis for the treatment of hypovolemic shock, or (2) to provide necessary fluid, electrolytes, and nutrients.

WHOLE BLOOD

Patients with presumably normal bone marrow activity who need blood transfusions because of acute blood loss may receive stored (bank) blood of any age up to the expiration date (usually 21 days). Hemolysis during storage is almost negligible, or less than 1% at 21 days. The increased content of lactic acid, inorganic phosphate, ammonia, and potassium in stored blood is usually clinically insignificant. Except for patients with severe hepatic or renal impairment or extreme debility, the use of acceptable aged blood imposes no significant metabolic burden on the recipient.

Most coagulation factors are stable in stored blood, but platelets, factor V (proaccelerin), and factor VIII (antihemophilic globulin) deteriorate. Bank blood which has been stored in the refrigerator for more than 2 days is essentially devoid of viable platelets. Massive replacement with this blood (eg, giving 10–15 units in rapid succession) may result in thrombocytopenia.

Loss of other clotting factors is usually less important. For factor V, only 5–10% of normal levels is adequate for hemostasis; reductions to this level rarely result from multiple transfusions, even of older blood. Factor VIII deficiency (hemophilia A) is better treated with cryoprecipitate (see below).

Serologic Considerations (Blood Typing)

The antigens for which routine testing should always be performed in donors and recipients are A, B, and D (Rh_O) for administration of group-specific blood. Pretransfusion compatibility tests use the serum of the recipient and the cells of the donor (major cross-match). To ensure a maximal margin of safety, each transfusion should be preceded (if possible) by a 3-part compatibility procedure: (1) at room temperature in saline; (2) at 37 C fortified by the addition of albumin; and (3) at 37 C followed by an antiglobulin test. It usually takes about 1½ hours to complete these procedures.

(1) ABO System Groups: Administration of low-titer type O ("universal donor") Rh-negative blood to A, B, or AB recipients is justified in emergency situations only after every effort has been made to secure type-specific blood. The administration of low-titer type O blood can lead to later complications which can be avoided by giving type-specific blood. Plasma of type O blood containing high titers of anti-A or anti-B isoagglutinins may cause hemolysis of the recipient's blood. If only 2 or 3 units of group O blood have been given successfully to a patient who is not group O, it is safe to return to group-specific blood, but the infusion set must be changed before specific blood is started.

After the uneventful transfusion of 4 or more units of group O to an adult who is not group O, the administration of group O blood is usually continued even though group-specific blood becomes available. The decision to change back to group-specific blood (if more transfusions are needed) is best based upon the presence or absence of anti-A or anti-B in subsequent samples of the recipient's blood as determined on the cross-match. If an AB recipient has received either group A or group B blood, his plasma will contain anti-A or anti-B. The decision to change to yet another blood group must be based upon consideration of the antibodies concerned.

(2) Rh System Groups: A few units of Rh-positive blood can be administered with relative safety to Rh-negative recipients if compatible on a Coombs cross-match. This substitution, however, must not be made in girls or in women of childbearing age.

Rh-negative blood may be administered to Rh-positive patients.

Amount of Blood for Transfusion

A. Adults: Two units (1000 ml) of whole blood will raise the hemoglobin by 2–3 g/100 ml in the average adult (70 kg). The red blood cell count will rise by 0.8–1 million/μl, and the hematocrit by 8–9%. Ten ml of whole blood per kg body weight will produce a 10% hemoglobin rise.

B. Children:
1. Over 25 kg–Give 500 ml of whole blood.
2. Under 25 kg–Give 20 ml/kg of whole blood.
3. Premature infants–Give 10 ml/kg of whole blood.

Rate of Transfusion

Blood is normally given at a rate of 80–100 drops per minute, or 500 ml in 1½–2 hours. In cardiac patients, one should allow 2–3 hours for the transfusion. For rapid transfusions in emergencies, it is best to use a 15-gauge plastic cannula and allow the blood to run freely. The use of added pressure to increase flow is dangerous unless it can be applied by gentle compression of collapsible plastic blood containers. Central venous pressure monitoring is a safeguard against overtransfusion; it is a measure of the heart's ability to handle venous return.

Massive Transfusions

An actively bleeding patient receiving over 10 units of bank blood in a few hours may have some difficulty with adequate oxygenation of his tissues because blood collected in acid-citrate-dextrose (ACD) gradually becomes more acid and loses some of its 2,3-diphosphoglycerate (DPG); the hemoglobin's affinity for oxygen increases ("hemoglobin dissociation curve shifts to left"), resulting in a fall of central venous oxygen tension. This process is reversible, and all values return spontaneously to normal after 1–2 days. In these clinical situations, blood only 1–3 days old—or blood collected with citrate-phosphate-dextrose (CPD) as an anticoagulant—is more desirable. Massive transfusions may also lead to thrombocytopenia and bleeding. (See Platelet Transfusion, below.) Whenever possible, fresh whole blood should be used for massive replacement, as in the patient with multiple severe injuries.

Complications of Blood Transfusion

Although some of the following complications of blood transfusion are not preventable, most of the fatal complications can be avoided by careful selection of donors, proper cross-matching of blood, and careful collection, storage, labeling, patient identification, and administration of blood:

(1) Hemolytic reactions are a serious complication of blood transfusion. The most severe reactions are due to ABO incompatibility, but serious hemolytic reactions may also be due to antibodies resulting from isoimmunization following previous transfusion or pregnancy. Symptoms may include apprehension, headache, fever, chills, pain at the injection site or in the back, chest, and abdomen, and shock; but in the anesthetized patient spontaneous bleeding from different areas and changes in vital signs may be the only clinical evidence of transfusion reactions. Posttransfusion blood counts fail to show the anticipated rise in hemoglobin. Free hemoglobin can be detected in the plasma within a few minutes. Hemoglobinuria and oliguria may occur. Exact identification of the offend-

ing antibody should be made, and this is usually possible when the Coombs test is positive.

(2) Other conditions where clots fail to form in vitro are circulating anticoagulant and heparin administration. In vitro clotting may be greatly prolonged to 1 hour or more in the hemophilias and in factor XII deficiency.

(3) Allergic reactions occur in about 1% of transfusions. They are usually mild and associated with itching, urticaria, and bronchospasm, but they may be severe or even fatal. (The reaction results from an antigen-antibody reaction between a protein in the donor plasma and a corresponding antibody in the patient. Some of these reactions are caused by an antibody to IgA.) If reactions are mild, the transfusion may be cautiously continued. Antihistamines, epinephrine, and corticosteroids may be required.

(4) Too rapid transfusions of large quantities of blood may result in circulatory complications (eg, cardiac or respiratory failure). This is particularly true of elderly or debilitated patients. Careful monitoring should help prevent this complication.

(5) Abnormal bleeding—ie, massive oozing of blood—may follow transfusion of large amounts of stored blood, which contain few platelets. Fresh blood is often needed, especially with massive transfusions. Here again, citrate-phosphate-dextrose is preferable to acid-citrate-dextrose as an anticoagulant.

(6) Transfer of viral, bacterial, spirochetal, or protozoal disease by blood from an infected donor can occur. Infectious hepatitis of the long incubation type (serum hepatitis) is the most common (0.5%) blood-transmitted infection in the USA. Testing of the prospective donor's blood for hepatitis-associated antigen (HAA or Australia antigen) reduces the incidence and the severity of this complication. Other transmitted diseases include rubella, syphilis, malaria, and brucellosis.

(7) Bacterial contamination of blood may occur through improper collection, storage, and administration. Reactions—noted early in the course of transfusions—are serious and may be fatal. Treat as for septic shock (see Chapter 16). Prevention is obviously the most important consideration.

(8) Unknown pyrogens may cause "nonspecific" febrile reactions which usually subside with symptomatic treatment within 24 hours. Other causes should be ruled out.

After antibody screening of the patient's serum, transfusions with compatible blood may be advisable. If no compatible blood can be found, plasma expanders (eg, dextran) and plasma may have to be used instead of whole blood. Pressor agents may be necessary.

Some studies suggest that osmotic diuretics such as mannitol can prevent renal failure following a hemolytic transfusion reaction. After an apparent reaction and in oliguric patients, a test dose of 12.5 g of mannitol (supplied as 25% solution in 50 ml ampules) is administered IV over a period of 3–5 minutes; this dose may be repeated if no signs of circulatory overload develop. A satisfactory urinary output following the use of mannitol is 60 ml/hour or more. Mannitol can be safely administered as a continuous intravenous infusion; each liter of 5–10% mannitol should be alternated with 1 liter of normal saline to which 40 mEq of KCl have been added to prevent serious salt depletion. If oliguria develops despite these efforts, treat as for acute renal failure.

PACKED RED BLOOD CELLS

Packed red cells also have a storage (shelf) life of 21 days. They are the treatment of choice for anemia without hypovolemia. Perhaps most blood transfusions can be given as packed red cells, even in patients with moderate degrees of blood loss.* The use of packed red cells instead of whole blood not only conserves a precious and limited resource of plasma but reduces the potential hazard of (1) circulatory overload; (2) excessive electrolyte and metabolic loads (eg, increased potassium and ammonium of stored blood); (3) exposure to certain antigens (eg, granulocytes and plasma proteins, and food or drug allergens in donor blood); and (4) transmission of infectious agents. It is possible to concurrently administer balanced salt solutions.

PLATELET TRANSFUSION

For the treatment of thrombocytopenia and thrombasthenia, freshly drawn whole blood, fresh platelet-rich plasma (PRP), or platelet concentrate (PC) may be needed. Enough must be given to raise the platelet count to 100,000/μl.

Platelets cannot be preserved for long periods, but survival may extend to several days if platelet-rich plasma is not refrigerated but stored at room temperature after collection. Compatibility tests are not mandatory for platelet concentrate or PRP if the recipient's blood has been screened for antibodies, but it should be type-specific because even platelet concentrate contains a few red cells. PC made from the blood of more than one donor carries a higher risk of transmitting hepatitis.

Administration of platelets is indicated for uncontrollable bleeding due to temporary thrombocytopenia following surgery; for purpura or bleeding in thrombocytopenic patients who require surgery; and for bleeding in patients who have developed thrombocytopenia after transfusion with 10 or more units of blood in a period of a few hours.

*Schorr JB, Marx GF: New trends in blood replacement. Anesth Analg 49:647–651, 1970.

Platelets should not be administered to patients with conditions associated with a very short life span of transfused platelets—eg, most cases of idiopathic thrombocytopenic purpura or disseminated intravascular coagulation. Platelets should not be transfused unless absolutely necessary lest isoantibody formation prevent their being effective at a time when they are critically needed.

Sources of platelets are as follows:

(1) Fresh whole blood: If transfused within 24 hours of collection, the number of viable platelets will be sufficient to maintain the platelet count at a safe level during massive transfusion. Correction of thrombocytopenia, however, cannot be accomplished with whole blood since it does not contain enough platelets per unit volume.

(2) Platelet-rich plasma: PRP has the advantage that it is easier to prepare than platelet concentrate and damages the platelets less. Its volume is only 50% of the original whole blood, yet it contains most of the platelets. Even so, its relatively large volume still limits the number of platelets that can be administered at one time.

(3) Platelet concentrate: PC is prepared by centrifugation of PRP at high gravitational force. The platelets are deposited in a small mass and plasma is then removed, leaving 25–30 ml in which the platelets are resuspended before transfusion. Platelet concentrate should be transfused within 4 hours of collection. Platelets may be administered in any quantity required. It usually takes 6–8 units of the concentrate to raise the platelet count to 100,000/μl. Platelet viability is approximately 50% of that in PRP. In general, one can expect only 30% of the platelets in the original unit to survive in the recipient. This form of replacement therapy is very expensive because of the many units required. The platelet mass must be resuspended in the remaining plasma by manual compression of the bag. Before transfusion, the suspension should be homogeneous (without visible clumps).

Platelets are usually transfused through a standard set containing a filter.

FIBRINOGEN

Hypofibrinogenemia, either congenital or acquired, is associated with faulty or absent clot formation. Prothrombin time, PTT, and thrombin time are prolonged. The administration of 4–5 g of fibrinogen should promptly raise the plasma fibrinogen level by 100–150 mg/ml. The fibrinogen deficiency must be demonstrated before administering this material. The commercial preparations are expensive and are associated with a high (5%) incidence of infectious hepatitis.

COAGULATION FACTOR CONCENTRATES

Stored blood or plasma provides all coagulation factors except factor V (proaccelerin) and factor VIII (AHF, antihemophilic factor). Frozen plasma preserves factors V and VIII. A concentrate prepared from fresh-frozen plasma (cryoprecipitate) contains 15–20 times the AHF concentration of fresh whole plasma and is very effective in the treatment of factor VIII deficiency (hemophilia A or "classic" hemophilia) and von Willebrand's disease (pseudohemophilia). One unit of the cryoprecipitate for each 6 kg body weight raises the AHF level to 50%—enough for most surgical procedures. For difficult cases, it may have to be followed by half that amount every 12 hours given as long as necessary.

Konyne is a concentrate in powder form which contains the vitamin K-dependent coagulation factors (II, VII, IX, and X) and is used for the treatment of bleeding due to the deficiency of these factors. The commonest deficiency of these 3 is that of factor IX (PTC) deficiency, which causes so-called Christmas disease (hemophilia B). It carries a high risk of hepatitis.

PLASMA

Any of the various plasma preparations such as fresh plasma, fresh-frozen plasma, or lyophilized or reconstituted plasma may be employed for the treatment of acute hypovolemia (shock), for the correction of plasma loss (eg, due to extensive burns), or for the correction of coagulation disorders. Pooled plasma is usually readily procurable, may be rapidly set up for administration, and does not require preliminary blood typing. However, pooled plasma carries a high risk of transmission of infectious hepatitis regardless of aging or processing with ultraviolet light. Although pooled plasma is still used on an emergency basis for the treatment of hypovolemic shock, its use has decreased in favor of more specific treatment with blood. Obviously, plasma cannot be substituted for whole blood if red cells are essential. Most centers now use lactated Ringer's injection until blood arrives.

Fresh plasma and fresh-frozen plasma are used to correct coagulation defects due to deficiency of certain of the blood coagulation factors (see above).

PLASMA SUBSTITUTES

Dextrans

Dextrans are fairly effective plasma "substitutes" for the emergency treatment of shock. These water-soluble biosynthetic polysaccharides have high molecular weights, high oncotic pressures, and the necessary viscosity, but they have not proved to be as useful as plasma, and their use is not without hazard because it is usually not safe to give more than 15 ml/kg/24 hours. They have the advantages of ready availability, of compatibility with other preparations used in intravenous solutions, and of not causing infectious hepatitis. They may also help prevent thrombosis by interfering with platelet aggregation.

Dextran 40 (Rheomacrodex, Gentran), a low molecular weight (40,000) dextran, is available as a 10% solution in either isotonic saline or 5% dextrose in water for intravenous use. It decreases blood viscosity and appears to assist the microcirculation. Rapid initial infusion of approximately 100–150 ml within the first hour is followed by slow maintenance for a total of 10–15 ml/kg/24 hours (preferably less than 1 liter/day). This preparation may also reduce the risk of intravascular coagulation in the severely injured or septic patient.

Dextrans must be used cautiously in patients with cardiac disease, renal insufficiency, or marked dehydration to avoid pulmonary edema, congestive heart failure, or renal shutdown, and patients must be observed for possible anaphylactoid reactions. Dextran 40 has considerably less antigenicity than high molecular weight dextran 75. Prolongations of bleeding time have been reported, and dextran should probably not be used in thrombocytopenic patients. Blood for typing and cross-matching must be obtained before dextran therapy since dextran may interfere with these tests.

Electrolyte & Dextrose Solutions

Experimental and clinical studies have shown that substantial blood losses can be effectively replaced or augmented with appropriate balanced salt solutions. With careful monitoring of central venous pressure, vital signs, urinary output, and serum electrolyte determinations, specific fluid and electrolyte abnormalities may be corrected and apparently normal blood volume maintained.

Balanced salt solutions may be augmented with specific electrolytes, vitamins, dextrose, and special protein nutriments to provide successful intravenous alimentation for prolonged periods. (See Chapters 12 and 13.)

PREGNANCY & THE SURGICAL PATIENT
Edward C. Hill, MD

The incidence of surgical illness is the same in pregnant women as in the nonpregnant women of the same age group. Pregnancy may alter or mask the signs and symptoms of the disease, so that recognition is more difficult. Furthermore, the fetus must be considered in planning a surgical procedure, and pregnancy

may modify the timing of a semi-elective operation or the surgical approach of an emergency abdominal procedure. Purely elective surgery should be deferred until the postpartum period. Any major operation represents a risk not only to the mother but to the fetus as well. During the first trimester, congenital anomalies may be induced in the developing fetus by hypoxia. It is preferable to avoid surgical intervention during this period; if surgery does become necessary, the greatest precautions must be taken to prevent hypoxia and hypotension. The second trimester is usually the optimum time for operative procedures.

Diagnostic radiologic examinations of the lower abdomen and pelvis should be avoided during pregnancy, if possible, especially during the first 6 weeks of gestation when the fetus is particularly susceptible to irradiation. There is statistical evidence that mothers of leukemic children had a higher incidence of abdominal radiologic studies during pregnancy.

The following surgical problems which may occur in pregnant women are discussed briefly in the following paragraphs: acute appendicitis, cholecystitis and cholelithiasis, intestinal obstruction, hernias, breast cancer, ovarian tumors, and congenital and rheumatic heart disease.

Appendicitis

Acute appendicitis occurs about once in every 2000 pregnancies. The signs and symptoms are the same as those that occur in nonpregnant women, but they may be considerably modified. Because of the nausea and vomiting and lower abdominal discomfort which are seen frequently in the first and second trimesters of normal pregnancy, as well as the moderate leukocytosis and elevated sedimentation rate, errors in diagnosis are more frequently made. Moreover, the enlarging uterus often carries the appendix higher in the abdomen, so that McBurney's point can no longer be used as a point of reference, and maximal tenderness is proportionately higher. For the same reason, the presence of the gravid uterus may effectively block off the omentum and loops of small intestine and thus hinder the walling-off process, particularly in the third trimester. Therefore, rupture of the appendix is more often associated with widespread dissemination of infection, generalized peritonitis, and a high mortality rate. If an abscess does form following perforation, the gravid uterus forms the medial wall of the abscess. The intense inflammatory process often initiates uterine contractions, with premature labor and the loss of the fetus. With evacuation, there is a sudden reduction in the size of the uterus; the abscess then ruptures into the free peritoneal cavity.

Because of the flaccidity of the anterior abdominal wall during the last trimester, there may be relatively little rigidity associated with inflammation of the appendix, and rebound tenderness may be difficult to define, so that one cannot rely upon these physical findings.

The treatment of acute appendicitis during pregnancy is immediate surgical intervention. Because of the extreme seriousness of perforation, it is better to remove a normal appendix than to wait for typical signs or symptoms and risk perforation.

Regional anesthesia is preferred, and the transverse or oblique muscle-splitting incision should be placed somewhat higher than in the nonpregnant individual. In fact, late in the third trimester the appendix may be in the right upper quadrant of the abdomen. Premature labor is not common following an uncomplicated appendectomy.

Cholecystitis & Cholelithiasis

Normal pregnancy may contribute to the formation of gallstones by encouraging bile stasis, increasing the concentration of cholesterol in the bile, and fostering changes in the solubility of the bile salts. Thus, cholelithiasis is more common in women who have borne children.

Acute cholecystitis in pregnancy occurs less often than acute appendicitis, the prevalence being about one in 3500–6500 pregnancies. It is associated with gallstones in the vast majority of instances.

The symptoms are the same as in the nonpregnant patient, with an abrupt onset of colicky right upper quadrant abdominal pain radiating to the right scapula, low-grade fever, and nausea and vomiting. Cholecystitis may be difficult to distinguish from acute appendicitis, with the high position of the appendix associated with the third trimester of pregnancy.

Unlike appendicitis, however, acute cholecystitis in pregnancy is best managed conservatively with hospitalization, parenteral fluids, nasogastric suction, antispasmodics, analgesics, and broad-spectrum antibiotics. In 3 out of 4 patients thus treated, there will be a definite improvement within 2 days, and a definitive surgical procedure can be deferred until the postpartum period. Surgery should be done whenever there is doubt regarding the differentiation from acute appendicitis or if there is no response to conservative therapy as manifested by an enlarging mass (empyema), jaundice (common duct obstruction), evidence of rupture, or associated pancreatitis. Cholecystectomy is the procedure of choice, but cholecystostomy may be performed if technical difficulties warrant it, the excision of the gallbladder being delayed until the puerperium.

Intestinal Obstruction

Intestinal obstruction occurs infrequently during pregnancy, but it should be considered in the differential diagnosis of any pregnant patient with an abdominal scar who develops abdominal pain and vomiting. Adhesive bands are the most common cause of intestinal obstruction, and displacement of the intestine is most likely to occur when uterine growth carries the pregnancy into the abdomen around the fourth or fifth month of gestation; near term, when lightening occurs; or postpartum, with sudden reduction in the size of the uterus. Other causes of intestinal obstruction during pregnancy are volvulus, intussusception, and large bowel malignancy.

The symptoms and signs of intestinal obstruction are the same as those that occur in the nonpregnant woman, although the clinical picture may be obscured by the nausea and vomiting of early pregnancy, round ligament pain, and the abdominal distention already produced by the pregnancy.

When surgical intervention is indicated, it should be performed without delay, ignoring the pregnancy. Near term, a cesarean section may be required in order to obtain necessary exposure.

Hernias

Hiatal hernias are common during pregnancy; perhaps 15–20% of pregnant women develop this condition as a result of pressure against the stomach by the enlarging uterus. The principal symptom is reflux esophagitis with severe heartburn, aggravated by recumbency or by the ingestion of a large meal and relieved by assuming an upright position or by taking antacids. Hematemesis may occur due to ulceration of the esophageal mucosa.

Elevation of the upper half of the body while reclining, frequent, small, bland meals, and antacids given liberally are usually effective treatment. Most hiatal hernias disappear following the pregnancy. Surgical correction is required only for those that persist and remain symptomatic.

Umbilical, inguinal, and ventral hernias usually are unaffected by pregnancy. Repair can be carried out electively after delivery. Surgery during pregnancy is indicated only in the rare event of an incarcerated or strangulated hernia.

Cancer of the Breast

Cancer of the breast occurs infrequently during pregnancy, but it is a significant complication when it does occur. The breast changes which occur during gestation make detection of early breast carcinoma much more difficult. The disease is more malignant during pregnancy, perhaps as a consequence of hormonal changes. Most cases are advanced by the time they are diagnosed. Biopsy and appropriate surgical treatment should be undertaken as soon as the cancer is suspected. If the malignancy is confined to the breast, the prognosis is good; if the axillary nodes are involved, the outlook is poor. Statistically, the overall cure rate for cancer of the breast developing during pregnancy is about half of that of nonpregnant women of comparable age.

Therapeutic abortion is not indicated in the patient with localized disease of a favorable microscopic type. Interruption of an early pregnancy may be of some palliative benefit to the woman with advanced disease, but if the pregnancy has progressed beyond the 20th week, the life of the fetus should take precedence.

Haagensen CD: Cancer of the breast in pregnancy and during lactation. Am J Obst Gynec 98:141–149, 1967.

Rosemond GD: Management of patients with carcinoma of the breast in pregnancy. Ann New York Acad Sc 114:851–856, 1964.

Ovarian Tumors

A cystic corpus luteum is the most frequent cause of ovarian enlargement during pregnancy. This structure rarely exceeds 6 cm in diameter and gradually diminishes in size as the pregnancy progresses. It is usually asymptomatic, and only careful observation is required to distinguish it from a proliferative type of cystic enlargement.

True ovarian neoplasms are encountered in 1:1000 pregnancies, the majority being detected during the first trimester. Some are not found until the immediate postpartum period, when the uterine size no longer masks its presence and the abdominal wall is flaccid. Most ovarian neoplasms are cystic; solid tumors are quite rare. Frequently they are silent, producing few symptoms unless there is hemorrhage into the tumor, rupture of the cyst, or torsion of the pedicle—complications which are definitely increased during pregnancy (see Chapter 45).

The cystic neoplasms most often seen during pregnancy are benign cystic teratomas (about 40% are of this variety), serous and mucinous cystadenomas, and endometrial cysts. Dysgerminoma is the most frequently encountered solid tumor. Malignant ovarian neoplasms rarely complicate pregnancy, constituting only 2–3% of ovarian neoplasms. Serous and mucinous cystadenocarcinomas and endometrioid carcinomas are the most common histologic types.

Because of the danger of inducing an abortion during the first trimester, surgical removal of a suspected true neoplasm should be deferred until the fourth month of gestation except in the event of an acute abdominal emergency caused by torsion, rupture, or hemorrhage. When discovered during the immediate postpartum period, removal should be done as soon as possible in order to avoid the complications of infection, hemorrhage, rupture, and torsion.

Heart Disease

In approximately 2% of women, pregnancy is complicated by heart disease. The vast majority of these (90%) are rheumatic in origin. Congenital heart disease is encountered rarely.

Most cardiac patients can be carried successfully through pregnancy by expert medical management. The indications for cardiac surgery during pregnancy are not well established, and there is still considerable difference of opinion about its merits. In general, it is advisable to postpone closed or open heart surgery until after delivery. However, operation during pregnancy should be considered in special circumstances. For example, a patient with pure mitral stenosis who is in heart failure despite good medical management may benefit from mitral commissurotomy done during pregnancy. There is little risk from this procedure, but the fetal mortality is about 9%. Procedures requiring open heart surgery are considered too hazardous to perform during pregnancy.

Rovinsky JJ, Guttmacher AF (editors): *Medical, Surgical and Gynecologic Complications of Pregnancy,* 2nd ed. Williams & Wilkins, 1965.

6 . . .

Legal Medicine for the Surgeon

Jesse L. Carr, MD

I apprehend it will be found that physicians and surgeons are often called upon to exercise appropriate duties which require not only a knowledge of the principles of jurisprudence, but of the forms and regulations adopted in our courts of judicature.
—Percival's *Medical Ethics*, 1803

Historically, the civil and criminal legal restraints on the practice of medicine have developed in parallel with the profession's own attempts at peer control by means of licensing procedures, accreditation of hospitals, and other means. The function of these forces has been to define and defend the rights and responsibilities of the 3 parties to every medical contract, written or otherwise: the patient, the physician or surgeon, and "society."

Thomas Percival was speaking particularly of the physician's social responsibilities in discussing advice to a dying patient about his last will and testament and the mental capacity requisite to making one; the difference between real and personal property; the time and under which circumstances to beat a lunatic; and a physician's responsibility in confining or ill-treating any of His Majesty's subjects. He also felt a growing concern with the success or failure of medical therapy, sudden death, abortions, bastardy, the physician's responsibility in treating injuries to duelists, and the chastity of the female sex and its violation by force, but in his time there was little or no concern about malpractice.

Since Percival's time, while medical responsibilities have multiplied, the social obligations have declined and the legal immunity which physicians once enjoyed has become so qualified that the physician must now also feel for himself the medicolegal concern which he once felt for his patients. Today the burden of the patient's safety and well-being rests jointly upon the patient, the physician, and the hospital, and intricate legal regulations and responsibilities involve everything and everyone engaged in or associated with the practice of medicine.

A vast and fluctuating mass of law affects the physician and his associates, the hospital and its staff, the private insurance company, the commonwealth as an insurer, and the patient. Since each statute and precedent has its individual importance, there is no way to succinctly present "the law." There is in fact no specific answer to the apparently simple question, "What is the law?"

Though Justice Oliver Wendell Holmes, Jr., came as close as anyone by saying that the law is "the prophecies of what the law will do in fact and nothing more pretentious." Within this concept, then, there is no law in the form of a static and reliable document upon which the physician may rely.

Common law, inherited largely from England and frequently augmented by statutory provisions, comprises most of our legal code. A steady progression of precedent-setting court decisions continually establishes new legal principles which in turn are either confirmed or overruled by subsequent judicial decisions. Legislatures passing new statutes will have them declared constitutional or unconstitutional by the courts, while the several State Supreme Courts and the United States Supreme Court continually add crucial new laws by edict, and these may be altered only by subsequent Supreme Court decisions or by constitutional amendment.

Medicine, then, is subject not only to regulation by the corpus of the existing law, which applies generally or to a specialty, but also to subtle—and, at times, sudden and frequently dramatic—changes in which the physician has had no part, over which he exercises little control, and of which unfortunately he may not even be aware. The legal principles presented here are currently in force, but they may be interpreted in various ways and in any case constitute only a small part of what the physician needs to know in order to avoid civil and criminal legal difficulties. Additional necessary legal information must be obtained from the physician's own legal counselor.

Essential protection comes in 3 forms: (1) current knowledge of legal hazards, (2) adequate insurance coverage, and (3) competent legal advice in organizational, administrative, and financial arrangements. Insurance coverage and legal advice do not imply litigation but represent the 2 most effective factors in avoiding dangerous complications and disastrous liabilities.

THE DOCTOR-PATIENT RELATIONSHIP

When a patient goes to a physician's office seeking wise counsel and suitable treatment, he knowingly offers to enter into an implied contract in which, for an appropriate consideration, the doctor will agree to exercise an ordinary degree of skill, care, and judgment in studying and treatment of his medical problem.

The physician, however, in legally obtaining a state license to practice medicine, does not agree to practice on this or any other patient, and, if he chooses to practice, he need do so only on limited terms of his choice as long as he meets acceptable medical standards. Therefore, he may accept the patient, establish a consent relationship, and enter into a contract; or reject an association with the patient for any reason or for no reason at all.

Outside of agreeing to use the "ordinary skill, care, and judgment" required by law, the physician who does accept responsibility for the patient's care does not guarantee a cure or even that the treatment will be beneficial or effective. He is required to make diagnoses and give treatment only according to the practice of the school to which he belongs, and his treatment may not be tested by the rules of other schools. He may err in diagnosis and still not be liable for injury to the patient unless his failure to make a correct diagnosis is due to lack of learning, skill, care, or perception. He is not liable for initial errors of judgment, but subsequent improper treatment is a proper basis for liability. A licensed physician either in general practice or any specialty is bound to keep abreast of the times but not to stride too far ahead of them, for a departure from an approved method in general use, however logical, will render him liable if he injures the patient.

Having once established contractual relations with the patient, the physician must assume the obligation of continued care unless he discharges the patient, is discharged by the patient, or gives the patient sufficient notice of his intent to terminate care so that he has ample time in which to obtain the services of another physician.

The surgeon must give postoperative care unless the patient knows and understands that his services will be limited to the performance of the operation or until, in the surgeon's judgment, postoperative care is no longer necessary. The physician who leaves the patient unattended during any specific illness without reason or without sufficient notice is negligent and guilty of abandonment. A physician must not accept more patients than he can care for, and he may not be excused if he neglects some of them because of an overload of work and harm to the patient results.

A physician's unexpected and severe illness may relieve him from rendering service or giving timely notice to his patients, but illness does not excuse him if his physical condition is such that he can either secure the patient's acceptance of a substitute or give him ample notice so that he may select another qualified physician. Vacations and attendance at symposia and professional meetings are permissible providing the physician makes proper provision for the attendance of another acceptable physician during his absence.

PRIVILEGED COMMUNICATIONS

The patient's chart, in addition to being a medical record, is a business record. These records are the property of either the physician or, if the patient is hospitalized, the medical institution, but the facts contained in the record are the private property of the patient or his designee at any time and under any circumstances, and the relationship between the 2 parties is privileged except in special circumstances.

The physician and his assistants cannot reveal information about a patient to others without the consent of the patient, nor can they be questioned in a civil action about any information acquired in attending the patient unless the patient gives his consent. This privilege is for the protection of the patient and not for the security of the doctor or the hospital. However, the patient under certain circumstances loses his privileged rights to nondisclosure.

An action to recover damages for personal injury, assault and battery, or malpractice implies the plaintiff's consent to testimony by any physician who has treated him. An action to recover for the death of any patient also implies consent to the testimony of any physician who attended the deceased. With some exceptions, being served a subpoena to appear in a trial court or at a pretrial action also relieves the physician from the restraints of the doctrine of privileged communication.

In any action involving the validity of a will transferring real or personal property, a physician may testify to the mental condition and competence of the testator either before or after probate. A physician may testify to the physical condition of the patient in any action brought to recover damages arising from the death of the patient.

A record made by a medical student or intern when he is not an attending, prescribing, or treating physician and when he is not being paid by the patient is not legally a part of the chart and is not privileged, though students and house officers are ethically obligated to respect a patient's right to privacy.

Under any circumstances, the original business record, whether it be a hospital or private office record, should never be released or relinquished to anyone, including the patient or the patient's designees or legal representatives. Only reasonable facsimiles certified by the institution's custodian of records should be provided.

Hospital records should, if possible, be kept indefinitely, but a minimum of 5 years for adults and 22 years for minors. Physicians' office records should be kept until retirement, the sale of a practice, or the death of the physician. If a practice is sold or otherwise transferred, the office records become available to the transferee after patients have been informed of the prospective transfer and have had the opportunity to approve or reject the transfer of their records from one physician to another. The retiring physician retains ownership of the records while the new physician assumes custody. In some instances it may be preferable to provide copies to the transferee.

If records are to be discarded, they should be destroyed past the point of legibility or reconstitution. Professional document disposal agencies are now available and represent the safest means of elimination. The identity of the record and the date of destruction should be recorded and retained.

CONFIDENTIAL INFORMATION

Confidential information about a patient differs from the privileged communication between physician and patient in that the latter is usually involved in some form of legal proceedings. A confidential communication, however, is one made by a physician about his patient in circumstances other than legal matters. Custom and medical ethics prohibit physicians from discussing their patients' affairs, but there are exceptions.

Such circumstances arise when the welfare of the patient or the public demands disclosure. Where a patient is reasonably believed to have a communicable disease, such as venereal infection, the physician is not liable if he advises those in close contact with the patient of the fact.

Reporting the medical condition of a patient to a spouse is not a breach of confidentiality even if the physician has reason to believe that the information may be used against his patient in an action to dissolve marriage, the principle being that during the existence of a marital relationship each spouse has a right to know of any disease affecting the other.

Medical reports written in good faith to agencies which have a legitimate interest in dealing with the patient are permissible, including reports involving both the physical and mental condition of the patient. If, however, a physician makes a mistake in a report and refuses to rectify it, malice may be proved. Whether or not the physician is justified in cooperating without the patient's consent with an insurance carrier who is investigating the patient's condition depends upon the problem. The point at issue is whether or not "the public interest" is involved. In cases where a physician's report has resulted in the carrier's refusing to pay, such as for a preexisting congenital defect, the courts have held that the public interest is involved.

When either the patient or members of the patient's family initiate insurance claims, they waive the right to nondisclosure. However, all patients have the right not to be the subjects of gossip, and the patient has the legal privilege to object to disclosure unless his interest or the public interest demands it.

INFORMED CONSENT

In placing his medical problem in the physician's hands, the patient gives implied consent to any medical proceedings the physician chooses to use, but the law maintains that the consent must be an informed one and that the patient is entitled not only to know what the physician is going to do but must be aware of the limits of the physician's therapeutics, his immediate objective, the real and potential hazards of possible alternative procedures, and the anticipated results. He must not only be informed—he must be informed in such a way that he will understand.

Any treatment requiring the "laying on of hands" which is done without the fully informed consent and understanding of the patient constitutes either negligence or assault and battery and represents the principal basis of malpractice actions. Implied consent does not fulfill all of the requirements, for it may not be truly "informed." Therefore, except in specific circumstances, consent for each medical act should be given by the patient himself or, in the case of a minor, by the parent or guardian. The consent for surgery may be either verbal or written, but consent in writing is preferable. If a patient is unconscious and no adult relatives are available at the time of a true emergency, consent is implied to the limits of emergency treatment of an existing condition, but no treatment other than that necessitated by the emergency is permissible.

Many patients expect greater benefit from medical and surgical treatment than is warranted by the facts. Publicity about "miracle drugs," mechanical life support systems, and organ transplants fosters this attitude, but the physician knows that not all drugs are curative and not all operations are successful. Some drugs, radical operative procedures, and artificial supports not only prove ineffective in some cases but may also cause deleterious side-effects. Deciding whether to risk the side-effects of drug therapy or surgery in order to achieve a desired result is the crux of the problem of consent, and this must be explained to the patient and understood by him. In this area of the law there are fine distinctions between assault and battery and negligence. Assault and battery are intentional unauthorized acts by the physician which constitute a trespass and which may include a breach of contract. Negligence is an unintentional act, not involving a breach of contract, resulting in personal injury to the patient which may be compensable.

The fundamental distinction is that civil assault and battery are intentional whereas medical malpractice may be either deliberate or unintentional. In an action for assault and battery, the plaintiff may rely entirely upon his own testimony and need not show actual physical injury, for an action in trespass is a violation of a fundamental right of freedom by an intentional touching of his person. Written proof of informed consent to an operation or to medical treatment is a specific defense that the physician may enter against an action alleging trespass upon the person of the patient or assault and battery upon him.

Obviously, operating on the wrong person, amputating the wrong limb, extracting the wrong tooth, or performing a herniorrhaphy on the wrong side are unintended negligence, but they are also assault and battery. Operating on paired organs or appendages when consent has been given for the treatment of only one is also assault and battery unless the condition can be proved to be one that endangers the life or the health of the patient. The law in effect assumes that the patient desires all treatment necessary in the judgment of his physician; however, the surgeon exceeds the limits of consent when an authorization for a minor operation is extended to a major operation which the patient may not have wanted.

In the case of an exploratory laparotomy when the diagnosis is in doubt or when a method of treatment cannot be chosen before the operation, the patient must be apprised of these circumstances. The patient may give the surgeon permission to do what he feels is best. By so doing he constitutes the surgeon as his agent, and this should be made clear in writing before the procedure.

The physician has some privileges in emergencies. If immediate care is required to preserve life and health, the physician is reasonably privileged to exercise his judgment. This is not the implied consent of a patient but consent derived from the duties and obligations assumed by the physician in such emergencies.

Intoxicated persons cannot authorize operations unless an emergency exists, and under no circumstances can consent be given by the mentally incompetent. Felonious acts by the physician are not made less criminal by the consent of the patient. The unlicensed or unqualified physician who perpetrates a fraud upon a patient by misrepresenting himself cannot legally obtain consent under any circumstances. In summing up the matter, the California District Court of Appeals has stated that, "The physician violates his duties to his patient and subjects himself to liabilities if he withholds any facts which are necessary to form the basis of an intelligent consent by the patient to the proposed treatment. Likewise, the physician may not minimize the known dangers of a procedure or operation in order to induce the patient's consent."

Conversely, the physician must not give an extravagantly dismal prognosis which predicts an early demise since no physician is capable of accurately estimating how soon a patient will die. The physician whose advice has caused a patient or his family to make legal, financial, and social rearrangements in expectation of impending death which did not occur may be held liable under the laws of negligence and malpractice.

A recent decision of the Appellate Division of the Supreme Court of New York reversing a jury verdict for the defendant and ordering a new trial on the issue of informed consent is not only significant but alarming. The court concluded: "As the trespass to the body arises from the unlawful touching itself, there need be no showing of negligence or malice and the plaintiff is entitled to any damages which flow from the unauthorized procedure regardless of the fact that the operation was performed with utmost care."

THE EMANCIPATED MINOR; STERILIZATION PROCEDURES

Under certain circumstances, minors have been emancipated by legislative action, and in California and other states a minor may give a physician authority to treat venereal disease, to perform obstetric deliveries, and to undertake certain emergency measures. A minor cannot consent to most other major medical procedures, including sterilization, and a parent or guardian cannot consent to the sterilization of a minor except by court order.

An adult can consent to personal sterilization, and in some states the court may order sterilization of an adult if procreation by the adult is deemed contrary to the public interest.

LIBEL & SLANDER

Libel and slander are malicious false reports issued with intent to injure the reputation of another. Slander is the spoken word, libel is written. Actions for libel and slander are most commonly suits between doctors or between doctors and patients in which one seeks damages from another for malicious and damaging writings and statements, but hospital staff committees—especially those with regulatory and disciplinary functions—have also become vulnerable. With the socialization and institutionalization of health care practices, public criticism of such practices and the restraint of this criticism by libel laws have become important.

For example, a physician who had examining cubicles side by side completed the examination and treatment of a contentious, ill-tempered, difficult woman and went to the adjacent cubicle to attend another woman. Assuming that the first patient had departed, he remarked to his nurse in the presence of the second patient that the first patient was a miserable, complaining, uncooperative old harridan and he hoped never to see her again. The first patient had not in fact left, and she heard what the doctor said. Although she was not identified to the second patient—to whom she was unknown—she felt that she had suffered irreparable harm and sued the doctor for slander.

Between doctors, a chance remark or written statement may be a basis for legal action.

A patient who had had a thyroidectomy for hyperplasia had a recurrence of the symptoms and went to another surgeon in a large clinic for an examination. The second surgeon, upon seeing a very prominent thyroidectomy scar, said, "What butcher did that?"—in the presence of a nurse, an intern, and several medical students. The patient reported the remark to the first surgeon, who brought action against the second for slander.

Since the function of tumor boards, tissue committees, and disciplinary review boards entails critical review and disciplinary action, members of these boards have been accused of making defamatory statements by both doctors and patients. However, physicians need not be reluctant to serve on such boards for fear of legal involvement.

Truth is a defense to a charge of libel or slander, but one who condemns a particular health care practice as being harmful or of no benefit to patients may find that the legal proof of such claims is difficult to establish even though many medical scientists may agree with the criticism. Proof that such a practice is not damaging may be equally difficult. Fortunately, recent decisions have modified the libel and slander laws to allow more freedom for criticism of health care practices, since the progress of medical science depends on the greatest possible freedom for scientific criticism of existing methods and procedures.

The important factors in actions for libel and slander are whether the charges are true and whether there is actual malice. The law attempts to distinguish between an intent to injure through falsehood and a statement motivated by a desire to protect a person or the public through disclosure of important matters affecting and possibly damaging the public interest. Physicians, hospital officers, and public officials may attack procedures or statements based on other than the truth as they see it, and public officials, institutional representatives, and committees have recently been held partially immune from libel laws provided they do not indulge in malicious statements and limit themselves strictly to the truth and provided that their comments bear solely on matters which affect public health.

Countercharges of malice and slander have arisen out of the charges of incompetence or unprofessional conduct made by disciplinary review boards, tissue committees, tumor boards, and peer review committees which have been authorized by statute or medical societies to investigate professional behavior and, if necessary, impose disciplinary actions. These boards have only the powers and jurisdiction conferred upon them by statutes, and they may not exceed this authority. Nevertheless, there is a broad range of discretion. The board is not bound by all the technical rules of evidence when accused by those under discipline of having issued a libelous or slanderous statement; it is not bound to find that the accusation is warranted beyond a reasonable doubt before it can act, nor is it necessary that the preponderance of evidence support the allegation. It is sufficient that the evidence be substantial. Hospital committees such as surgical, tissue, and utilization committees fall in the same legal category.

Finally, review boards may exercise discretion in determining the type and extent of discipline, if any, to be imposed. They may attempt to rehabilitate an erring physician who, if he is willing to actively seek self-improvement, can eventually regain his hospital staff privileges and return to active practice in the hospital or community.

In establishing that the evidence of improper conduct is substantial, hearsay must be excluded because of its unreliability, but a board may exercise discretion in determining whether or not evidence is proper and admissible. If, after a fair hearing, a review board finds that the evidence warrants imposing disciplinary action or suspension, this action has been supported by courts upon review as the proper exercise of administrative discretion.

In short, persons who serve upon hospital, medical society, and disciplinary review boards may act freely within the scope of their authority without fearing charges of libel or slander.

MALINGERING

"The forensic importance of malingering is attested to by an estimate that over one half the cases in civil litigation involve claims of psychic or physical disability."–(Michael Juviler, *Personal Injury Annual,* 1961, pp 352–404.)

A patient may charge that a diagnosis of malingering constitutes slander, yet the necessity for deciding upon a diagnosis of malingering versus physical illness or neurosis frequently arises, particularly in cases involving alleged injuries and compensation.

The essential point is whether malingering is a medical diagnosis or a social condemnation of the patient. If it is a medical diagnosis, a physician is entitled to express an opinion about the genuineness of the patient's complaints of pain without some objective evidence of injury. If it is not a medical diagnosis, it could be considered slanderous. The currently accepted legal attitude is that when one has complained of pain upon being examined by a competent medical expert who found no indication of injury, the expert's opinion about whether the complaint is real or feigned has a legitimate bearing on the issues. The Supreme Court of Missouri held in 1952 that such a conclusion may be best drawn by medical experts but that lay opinion may be relevant when the matter indicative of malingering is a matter of common knowledge, as in the case in observations made by friends, neighbors, and civil servants such as firemen, policemen, and hospital stewards.

Hospital records of malingering have been held inadmissible in court on the grounds of hearsay except when the record constitutes the expression of an expert opinion.

As the matter now stands, the expert may testify about malingering on the part of a plaintiff but may not testify to the lack of malingering by a plaintiff without external indications of injury. An evaluation of whether a pain is real or pretended may be made by the physician without liability, but its weight depends to some extent upon the physician's competence as a qualified expert.

DYING DECLARATIONS

Dying declarations have legal status as evidence; they are an exception to the hearsay rule and are free of the restrictions on privileged communications on the theory that a person who knows or thinks he is about to die will want to tell the truth. The physician may describe the serious nature of the declarant's injuries as part of his certification of death. He may relate the circumstances which indicate that the declarant was aware of his impending demise, and he may repeat the dying declaration the declarant made. The use of such testimony may be held as neither hearsay nor a violation of privileged communication laws in most states.

LIABILITY INSURANCE

The liability insurance field is now plagued by problems both for the insurer and the insured. The typical liability insurance policy undertakes to provide both legal defense and indemnification for certain liability claims which may arise in the future; however, because of unavoidable delays in judicial procedures, the insurance carrier must attempt to forecast the claims experience of its policyholders as long as 5 years in advance.

Premium rates are based on such forecasts, and both the carrier and the insured are in tenuous positions since forecasts of both rates and the necessary protection are difficult to estimate. In medicine, there is a great disparity between the group that pays the premiums and the group of potential claimants. About 310,000 physicians in the USA are engaged in the medical care of a population of more than 200 million, any one of which might become a claimant for liability compensation. Injured patients making claims against affluent physicians and insurance companies are apt to elicit sympathy from courts and juries, and exaggerated reports of medical advances in lay magazines without disclosures of their inherent risks sometimes lead the public to expect results that cannot always be achieved.

There is no specific answer to the question, "How much malpractice insurance should one buy?" There is no safe minimum, and the maximum should be set by the amount of coverage an insurance company is willing to provide rather than the size of the premium one believes he can afford. Onerous as paying continually increasing insurance premiums may seem, it is a lesser evil than the prospect that liability insurance protection might generally cease to be available. This is a real threat, for each year fewer companies are willing to write liability insurance for physicians, and those companies still in the field tend to be more selective in accepting applicants for insurance. Some companies will not write policies in certain localities or for certain specialties or types of practice.

The premium costs of liability insurance show a striking disparity in legal risks between physicians practicing in varied specialties and in different localities in the USA. Insurance companies take state laws and local influences into considerations, and their actuaries arrive at similar figures for similar areas, for they can only make insurance available to physicians if they can cover their underwriting costs and sell policies at a profit. Consequently, there is little possibility of shopping around for insurance on the basis of price alone. Immediate help from the government or the various medical associations appears unlikely.

Personal injury litigation as a method of providing compensation to patients injured in the course of medical care is unfair, inefficient, and unreasonably costly. Out of $75 million paid by physicians for liability insurance, only $18 million will ever reach the pockets of injured patients. Legal expenses may absorb 50%, and the insurers' costs reportedly may so exceed the income from premiums that the structure of malpractice insurance is in jeopardy. Obviously, a better system of compensation is needed, but the physician has no present alternative but to buy all the medical liability coverage he can get. He cannot afford less.

LIABILITY WITHOUT FAULT

Two current threatening decisions entail the granting of a plaintiff's claims for damages from a rare surgical accident even though no liability has been established and based solely on the designated defendant's capacity to assume financial responsibility. Since 2 significant cases in this field are still unresolved, no further comment is appropriate, but the results of litigation should be carefully followed since adverse decisions will substantially affect the insurance protection pattern of tomorrow.

INSURANCE COMPANY RELATIONS

An insurance policy covering the hospital's and the physician's professional liability usually includes a clause which requires that an insured physician or hospital "cooperate" with the insurance company.

Essential to this cooperation is the provision of prompt or "timely" notification to the insurance company (insurer) about any claim made against the doctor (insured) and notification about any accident or untoward event which might result in a claim.

Accurate and detailed information should accompany the notification. Further developments such as communications from the patient or an attorney should also be reported. Requests from the insurer for further information, for consultation, and for testimony at trials should be honored, and any inability to comply with such a request must be fully explained.

Failure to cooperate with an insurance company can result in serious consequences for the insured physician or hospital, even to the point of relieving the insurance company of all obligations under the policy to defend the claim and to pay any judgments rendered.

A physician's delay in giving notice after he becomes aware that he has caused injury to a patient has been held unreasonable by the courts. The same is true if a physician puts off notifying his insurance carrier of the receipt of letters from attorneys threatening suit or seeking settlement for alleged malpractice. Whether or not a physician believes that he is liable is immaterial. Regardless of the virtue of the action, the insured physician is required to assist in the defense, to attend trial, and to testify.

THE PHYSICIAN'S RESPONSIBILITY FOR OTHER PERSONNEL

A physician who employs another person assumes responsibility for any injuries to patients caused by the employee's negligence, whether the employee be another physician, a nurse, regular medical personnel, regular paramedical personnel, or, in certain instances, residents and interns—although the latter may be at times the employees of and directly responsible to the hospital in which they work.

In the case of employed physicians, the employing physician's responsibility for the negligence of physicians hired by him is well established. In such cases, the patient relies upon the skill and reputation of the employing physician and accepts the services of the employed physician on that basis. The fact that the employing physician is out of town or otherwise unavailable and is therefore unable to supervise directly the work of an employed physician does not relieve him of liability for the negligence of his employee.

The physician who employs a substitute to treat his patient not only authorizes the substitution but also ratifies the substitute's treatment by billing the patient for the substitute's services.

A physician who employs others not licensed in the state where they are employed may be held guilty of unprofessional conduct, and in many states, including California, a physician who employs unlicensed assistants can lose the benefits of his malpractice insurance insofar as the negligent acts of the assistant are concerned.

If two or more physicians are practicing as a partnership, each partner is liable for the negligence of any member of the partnership. However, if one of the physicians in the group is the employer of the other physicians, then only the employer and the physician allegedly guilty of negligence are liable. Employees are not liable for the malpractice of other employees.

THE HOSPITAL'S RESPONSIBILITY FOR MEDICAL CARE

A hospital is obliged to maintain the standards of good practice embodied in the regulations of the state licensing agency for accredited hospitals or in the standards of the Joint Commission on Accreditation of Hospitals. Under these terms, it is the responsibility of the hospital (through its medical staff) to evaluate the quality of medical care by the standard prevailing procedures and practices, not only in a specific locality but under similar conditions of practice elsewhere throughout the country.

Because the hospital has a responsibility for the quality of medical care given in the institution, appropriate mechanisms must exist for evaluation of the competency of candidates for staff appointments and privileges. The hospital governing board must make certain that the medical staff establishes guidelines for physicians practicing in the institution and must monitor their practice to identify offenses when they occur.

According to recent court decisions, hospitals can be held liable for injuries resulting from the imprudence or carelessness of members of the medical staff whether they be treating their private patients, providing care on an emergency service, or acting as employees of the hospital in intern or resident capacities.

The governing body of each hospital is responsible for the quality of care provided in the hospital. Consequently, the selection of staff members becomes one of the responsibilities of the hospital board. This control cannot be exercised unreasonably or capriciously, unjustly or with prejudice, but the responsibility is clear.

As matters now stand, both charitable and private hospitals are responsible for a physician's conduct and have a duty to determine his capabilities and to control the nature and extent of his practice in the institution. A license to practice medicine does not itself establish the right to membership on a hospital staff.

Hospitals operating emergency departments which provide proper physician coverage can incur liability for consequent injury to emergency patients. The governing board of the hospital has a legal duty to ensure competent physician coverage.

STATUTE OF LIMITATIONS IN MALPRACTICE

It is a general rule of law that a person who is injured by another should seek legal redress as soon as possible. Consequently, states have established time limits for filing suits by means of laws referred to as statutes of limitations. The statutes vary from state to state, but as originally conceived these time limits were intended to run from the time the cause of action occurred through a stipulated subsequent interval. Since a patient may not be aware of an injury until months or years later, in some states "the time the cause of action occurred" is now being interpreted as either the time of occurrence or the time that the injury was discovered. For example, a sponge left in the patient's abdominal cavity during a laparatomy may cause no symptoms and may not be discovered until months or years later.

The statute of limitations in California is now 4 years after treatment or upon the event of discovery. In the case of minors, the statute runs until the patient reaches majority.

Courts have further held that where negligence has been fraudulently concealed the statute does not begin to run until the fraudulent conduct is discovered. This doctrine applies to all forms of malpractice—not only to surgical mishaps but also to other forms of medical treatment such as untoward reactions to injections, failure to diagnose malignancy by timely biopsy, and negligence in the fields of roentgenology, immunology, and allergy. These changes in the statutes of limitations assume added importance when one considers the extended necessity for liability insurance protection. Within the present concept, the claim for liability may be made long after the negligent act occurred—at intervals so long, in fact, that it may extend into the previously regarded "safe" area in a physician's life when he has retired, has disposed of his practice, and is no longer engaged in the practice of medicine.

Any insurance policy should be examined to make certain that extended coverage is included.

FEES FOR THE MEDICAL WITNESS

The physician who performs services as a medical expert or a medical witness is entitled to compensation. Although requests for such services are made by an attorney, they are not performed for him even if he could not function as an attorney without them. The patient has the same obligation to pay for medicolegal services as for hospital services which are necessary to enable a surgeon to perform his duties. An attorney may advance the money as a matter of convenience, but the client must pay the fees of a medical witness as a proper cost of litigation.

Under the principles of medical ethics of the American Medical Association, it is unethical for a physician to enter into any arrangement in which the amount of his fee for medicolegal services is contingent upon the outcome of the litigation. However, there is no objection if a physician contributes his medicolegal services without charge, just as he may contribute other professional services.

Excessive charges for medicolegal services give the medical profession a bad image, but the physician should not suffer financial loss because of time spent in preparing or giving medical evaluations or testimony. He should be compensated on a roughly computed hourly basis depending upon his hourly income from medical practice. While most physicians consider medicolegal services burdensome and disagreeable, excessive compensation is not justified as an inducement to accept this burden. With the growing trend toward liability litigation, it is essential that all physicians cooperate in the solution of medicolegal problems on a reasonable fee basis.

Many medical societies have drawn up agreements with bar associations whereby they provide a panel of experts which may be consulted by all lawyers. Members of the panel may confer with attorneys on either side and give them an unbiased, impartial evaluation. This arrangement, together with a relative fee schedule worked out between the bar association and the medical society on an hourly rate, promises to make medicolegal evaluations available to the lawyer and be less stigmatizing to the physician.

THE GOOD SAMARITAN ACT*

Physicians and nurses are often reluctant to offer first aid or emergency care at the scene of an accident because they fear their involvement might lead to malpractice action if their intervention should prove ineffective or contribute to a bad result. Although it is every citizen's implied duty to offer aid and succor to the injured, the licensed physician has in the past been exposed to excessive risk because of his status.

California and many other states have Good Samaritan Acts which in general provide that people licensed under specific chapters of the Medical Practice Act "who in good faith render emergency care at the scene of an emergency which occurs outside both the place and the course of employment will not be liable for any civil damages as a result of acts or omissions by such persons in rendering emergency care." This provision does not guarantee immunity from civil damages if the person was grossly negligent. If the physician offers more than emergency care then or later, a

---

*Business and Professions Code, Annotated, of the State of California, Div 2, Ch 5, Art 3, #2144.

doctor-patient relationship is established and the Good Samaritan Act offers no subsequent protection.

According to a recent decision, providing an injured person or his companions with a ride to the hospital from the scene of an accident is not "emergency care" within the meaning of the Good Samaritan statute. Therefore, anyone who provides such transportation is liable for injuries sustained by any passenger in any accident subsequent to the emergency.

LOCALITY RULE

In the past, physicians in a given locality have been required by law to use only the skill, judgment, and care common to medical practice in their area—the reason being that a physician in a small or rural community may find it impossible to keep fully abreast of the advances of the profession and may not have the most modern facilities for treating patients.

Progress in medical education, the standardization of curricula, and the proliferation of opportunities for continuing education in the many medical centers—together with the effective dissemination of scientific knowledge through various journals—have, according to recent court decisions, broadened the scope of medical knowledge so that physicians may now be expected to use the skill and care common to their specialty generally and not limited to their locality.

In the case of general practice, a physician may be expected to exercise the skill and care of the average qualified practitioner, taking into account the advances in the profession. While the medical resources available locally are necessarily considered in determining the skill and care required, hospitals in turn may now be expected—not only by the Joint Boards of Accreditation but also by law—to provide current and modern facilities for the use of their medical staffs.

Liability may be incurred if the physician fails to apply the methods followed or approved by the school of medicine from which he graduated as well as those which are widely recognized as likely to produce the most favorable results.

Exotic and expensive practices such as using a laser or employing supervoltage irradiation may not be "standard practice" in a defined area, but the need for such procedures may be common knowledge, and liability may result from not recognizing the need and referring the patient to proper sources of diagnosis and treatment.

The ultimate criterion of whether or not a surgical operation or a medical procedure should have been performed is not whether errors in judgment and technic contributed to a bad result but whether or not the judgments were formed in accordance with generally recognized scientific principles and accepted procedures.

THE ANATOMY OF MALPRACTICE

Wherever there is practice, there is malpractice, and every physician commits malpractice at some time during his career—either socially (eg, carelessly driving an automobile) or professionally through negligence, assault and battery, or abandonment. "Malpractice" is just another way of saying that one failed to obey the established rules. Fortunately, most acts of malpractice go unnoticed, are forgiven, or are unlitigated.

If good rapport has been established between the physician and his patient, it is very difficult for anyone—even a skillful claimant's attorney—to convince the patient that his doctor is anything but a conscientious and deserving person who is not really to blame for a bad result. If there is bad feeling between the physician and patient, even a successful result may be regarded as unsatisfactory and cause a patient to think in terms of charges, litigation, and damages.

Physicians who are sued often do not realize that they have contributed to their difficulty because they lack tact, sensitivity, personality, or "bedside manner." They may be distracted by illness, overwork, or personal problems, or they may actually be negligent or unsympathetic.

A great scientist, an important professor, and a truly dedicated person may antagonize others because he fails to treat people with respect and courtesy. Every physician must at least seem to like his patients, and he will have to understand them—otherwise, he will be prone to damage suits. He must also extend this respect, courtesy, and cordiality to his peers since one of the major reasons for the increase of malpractice suits is the careless conversation and criticism by physicians of the work of their colleagues. Such practices breed and encourage an awareness of the benefits of malpractice suits, as do the various news media which are making the public malpractice conscious. All scripts and articles written by physicians for non-professional consumption should be carefully screened for statements or examples of malpractice action before they are included among the waiting room literature for patient consumption.

Any physician who feels recurring antagonism or who has recurring episodes of tension between himself and his patients is perhaps ill suited to his specialty, his profession, or his environs. Introspection and, if indicated, medical assistance in such instances may forestall disastrous litigation.

Second to bad rapport as a cause of malpractice action is the litigious patient. Some people are habitually alert for grievances—not only when they go to the doctor but always and everywhere in their lives. Such people are hard to recognize on an initial visit, but every physician should develop a habit of evaluating new patients for their suit-prone possibilities. If such an attitude is suspected, extra effort and caution are indicated in developing effective and cordial communication. If it becomes apparent at any time during the relationship that the physician and his patient are simply not getting along, the patient should be told in a polite and kindly manner that he would do better with another doctor. The patient who is suit-prone or antagonistic in his dealings with one physician may get along quite well with another. Good medicine requires a continuing close relationship characterized by strong mutual confidence on both sides.

The third major cause of malpractice is money. The physician must charge fairly and within the patient's circumstances, have a complete understanding of insurance coverage, handle insurance forms efficiently, and carefully evaluate extra charges. A preliminary or preoperative discussion of all medical and hospital costs is most important. Any unsettled dispute over fees may generate malpractice action.

Before a bill for medical services is turned over to a collection agency or a threat is made to sue the patient for an unpaid bill, the physician should check the medical records and think back over his conduct of the case. Could the patient think he has been negligent or careless? Routine business collection methods cannot always be used in medicine, and a threat of suit is often followed by a threat of countersuit. It may be better to forego a fee than to get involved in what may be an unwarranted but defensible malpractice action. Malpractice suits are always traumatic and embarrassing even though successfully defended.

A strong contributing factor to the decision to sue is family prodding. A patient may respect the physician and appreciate his care, but the spouse, relative, or even neighbor may provoke an attitude of discontent. Surgeons in particular must pay careful attention to the patient's family and associates both before and after surgery, since they will have a major impact on the physician's relationship with his patient.

If a malpractice action is instituted, the physician's position is always better if he has limited his practice to his competence, has called in consultants when indicated, has kept the patient and his family informed about the seriousness of the illness, and has kept meticulous records.

The physician who does not keep accurate, up-to-date records invites multiple hazards in court. It may be that he was sued in the first place because he relied on his memory and forgot something essential. He may not only have forgotten essential matters during the course of therapy, but without good records he is almost sure to forget significant facts when he appears in court. In the minds of a jury he is not primarily a medical witness but a doctor and an accused person, and jurors feel that when they themselves go to a doctor they are putting their lives in his hands. All juries react adversely when a physician's records are inadequate, sloppy, and incomplete. Records which have been altered after a claim has been made constitute irrefutable damaging evidence against the physician and the hospital.

The most infrequent but most costly of all occasions for malpractice claims is the major bad result, and bad results are usually worse than the patient's original problem. The toxicity of potent new drugs, the hazard of new anesthetic procedures, and the risks of radical surgical procedures have begun to contribute materially to morbidity and mortality statistics. New procedures are often less safe than time-tested ones and may bring the patient closer to the threshold of death. In the past, the patient usually died if the result was bad and a successful suit for wrongful death ended with the payment of a suitable death award. With current anesthetics, resuscitative methods, and artificial support mechanisms, the patient may not die but live on as a vegetative organism, incurring high costs for custodial care. He may be wheeled into the courtroom staring vacantly at the doctor and being stared at by a sympathetic jury. Awards in such cases are high, for the current verdicts include compensation for projected loss of companionship, services, and income to the family as well as provision for prolonged and expensive support and medical care.

Of paramount importance is honesty. Lawyers who advise a physician never to admit an error, an unintentional assault, or negligence may themselves be in error, for honest admissions of human error may either forestall a suit or contribute to a fair and amicable settlement.

Malpractice litigation is a problem area of medical practice in great need of medicolegal reform. The best hope for the future is that the disciplinary review boards of the state boards of medical examiners, the plaintiff's panels of county medical societies, peer control, and the development of arbitration agreements between doctor and patient established before treatment may lead to fewer actions for alleged malpractice and to the settlement of justifiable malpractice action without litigation.

●　●　●

General References

The Best of Law and Medicine. American Medical Association, 1968.

Curran WJ: *The Doctor as a Witness.* Saunders, 1965.

Hassard H: *Medical Malpractice: Risks, Protection, Prevention.* Medical Economics, 1966.

Lawyer's Medical Journal. Schwitzer SC (editor). Baker, Voorhis & Co. (New York). [Periodical.]

Shindell S: *The Law in Medical Practice.* Univ of Pittsburgh Press, 1966.

Slovenko R: *Psychotherapy, Confidentiality, and Privileged Communications.* Thomas, 1966.

Waltz JR, Inbau FE: *Medical Jurisprudence.* Macmillan, 1971.

Wasmuth CE: *Law for the Physician.* Lea & Febiger, 1966.

7...

Radiation Therapy: Basic Principles & Clinical Applications

Glenn E. Sheline, MD, PhD, & Theodore L. Phillips, MD

BASIC RADIATION THERAPY

Radiation therapy deals with the treatment of disease using ionizing radiations. Since most diseases treated by radiation therapy are malignant, radiation therapy is actually a branch of oncology. Radiation therapy is the treatment of choice for the control of cancer in many sites. In other situations it is used, with curative intent, in conjunction with surgery or chemotherapy. It is also used for the relief of symptoms resulting from cancer. In order to know when and how to apply radiation therapy, the radiotherapist must be familiar with the biologic behavior of various forms of cancer and with the results obtainable by all treatment methods available. The realization that cancer is the second most common cause of death and that over 60% of cancer patients will require radiation therapy during the course of their disease underscores the importance of this branch of medical science.

PHYSICAL PRINCIPLES & RADIATION SOURCES

The radiations commonly used in radiotherapy include x-rays, gamma (γ) rays, electrons, and beta (β) rays. X-rays and γ rays are identical in properties but are produced by different sources. Electrons and β rays also differ only in the source from which they are derived. The efficacy of other types of radiation—eg, neutrons, protons, alpha (a) particles, and pi mesons—is presently under investigation. All have the common property of producing ionization within tissue. Ionization and other effects, such as excitation and free radical formation, cause chemical changes in cellular components. The total amounts of energy absorbed are exceedingly small, and the biologic effects are caused by the sensitivity to ionization of certain portions of cells.

X-rays and γ rays are electromagnetic radiations with neither mass nor charge; electrons and β rays are charged particles. X-rays are derived from the interaction between moving electrons and matter, whereas γ

rays are emitted during the decay of radioactive isotopes (radium, cobalt 60, etc). In biologic material, these rays give up energy by ejecting electrons from atomic orbits; in turn, the ejected electrons deposit energy in creating charged ions (ionization) within the target material. Most of the total ionization is caused by these secondary electrons. The distribution of the absorbed energy is related both to the absorption pattern of the primary radiation and the distance the secondary electrons travel within the tissue. When a beam of x-rays enters tissue, the energy absorption at first increases because the secondary electrons are

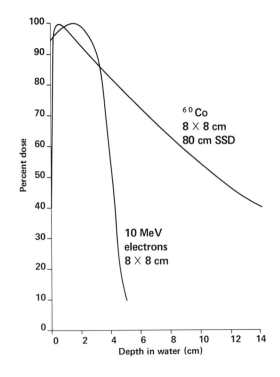

FIG 7—1. **Comparison of the depth dose distribution for an x-ray beam and an electron beam.** Dose is expressed as a percentage of the maximum and plotted against depth for an 8 × 8 cm ^{60}Co beam and an 8 × 8 cm 10 MeV electron beam. SSD = source-skin distance.

building to a maximum. The depth of this maximum point beneath the surface increases with the energy of the x-rays. After a maximum, the energy absorption decreases in an exponential fashion.

In the case of electron beams, the ionization within tissue is due in large part to the primary electrons. The energy is deposited fairly uniformly along the pathway of the electron. Such electrons travel a finite distance and then stop. With a monoenergetic electron beam, energy absorption in soft tissue is thus relatively constant from the surface to near the end of the electron's path, at which point the deposition of energy rises slightly and then falls abruptly to zero. The different absorption characteristics—exponential after an initial build-up interval for x-ray photons and approximately linear with rapid drop-off for electrons—can be adapted to fit various clinical situations (Fig 7–1).

In modern radiotherapy, 2 or more radiation beams are often combined to produce a more desirable distribution of absorbed energy than would result from a single beam. Furthermore, compensating or wedge-shaped filters are frequently used to compensate for body contour or to alter the shape of the absorption curve (Fig 7–2).

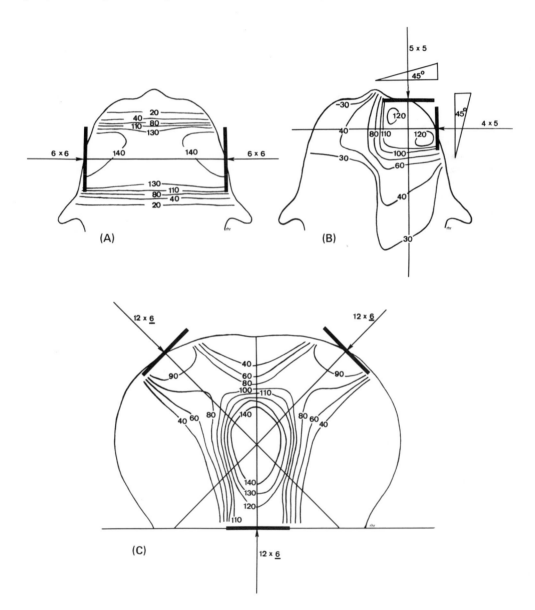

FIG 7–2. Isodose curves for several combinations of external radiation beams from ^{60}**Co.** *A:* Two 6 × 6 cm beams with opposed central axes. *B:* Two beams, 4 × 5 cm and 5 × 5 cm, with central axes at right angles utilizing 45 degree wedge filters. *C:* Three 12 × 6 cm beams with central axes at 120 degree angles to each other.

During the last 2 or 3 decades there has been an increasing trend to megavoltage (greater than 1 million volt) x-rays or γ rays for radiotherapy of deeply situated lesions. The advantages of the higher energy radiations are (1) "skin sparing," (2) less absorption in bone, (3) decreased energy absorption by healthy tissue, and (4) greater penetration. "Skin sparing" derives from the fact that the absorbed energy or dose at any depth depends largely on the secondary electrons. With x-rays generated by a 250 kilovolt peak (kVp) x-ray machine, the secondary electrons travel such short distances that the maximum energy absorption is essentially at the surface. With higher energies, the secondaries travel many millimeters or even centimeters; therefore, energy absorption builds up and does not reach its maximum until a considerable depth has been reached. In the case of ^{60}Co gamma rays, the maximum energy deposition is at 5 mm; for x-rays from a 25 million electron volt (MeV) betatron, the maximum is at 5 cm beneath the surface (Fig 7—3). Decreased absorption of megavoltage irradiation in bone compared to soft tissues is due to the difference in atomic number of the atoms within these 2 types of tissue. The fact that higher energy radiations undergo less side-scatter and hence have a more sharply defined beam contributes to a decrease in radiation dose to healthy tissue surrounding the target volume.

A detailed discussion of the sources of external beam therapy is beyond the scope of this book, but a few broad statements about presently available equipment may be useful.

Conventional x-ray machines produce x-rays with energies up to 300 kVp. This is known as "kilovoltage" or "orthovoltage." The radiocesium therapy machine gives radiation approximately equivalent to an 800 kVp x-ray generator. At present, the most common source for deep therapy is the artificial radioisotope ^{60}Co ("radiocobalt" therapy), which yields gamma rays of 1.17 and 1.33 MeV. Electron accelerators producing x-rays or electron beams with energies up to 10 MeV are also widely used. Less common but available in some centers are linear accelerators and betatrons capable of energies of 25, 35, or even 45 MeV. All photon or x-ray beams above 1 MeV are known as "megavoltage" beams.

Short distance radiotherapy (brachytherapy) takes advantage of the rapid decrease in dose with distance from a radiation source. For this purpose, the radiation source may be placed within a cavity (intracavitary) or inserted directly into tissue (interstitial). One or more sources may be used, with the geometric arrangement dictated by the clinical circumstances of the particular lesion. After a prescribed period of time, the sources are usually removed. They may be in the form of needles, narrow tubes, wires, or small seeds. While the most commonly used radioactive material is radium, interstitial and intracavitary sources may contain radon gas or artificially produced radioactive cessium, cobalt, gold, yttrium, or iridium. Beta ray applicators, such as the ^{90}Sr loaded eye applicator, are used for the treatment of thin superficial lesions.

Two units for describing radiation dosages are in

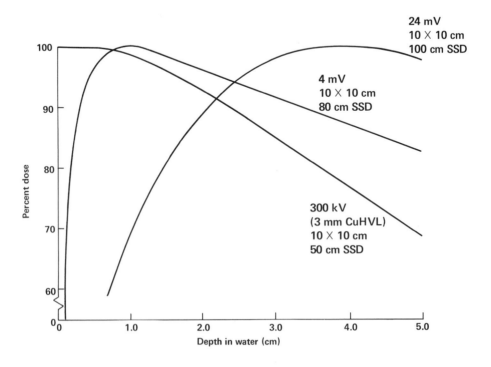

FIG 7—3. Comparison of the depth doses for x-ray beams of different energies. SSD = source-skin distance; CuHVL = copper half value layer.

common usage. One relates to the amount of radiation needed to produce a certain amount of ionization per unit volume of air; the other relates to the energy absorbed per unit mass. The roentgen (R), a unit of exposure, is defined only for x-ray and γ ray photons; it is the amount of radiation which will produce ionization equivalent to a charge of 1 electrostatic unit in 1 ml of air at standard temperature and pressure. Since different tissues will actually absorb different amounts of energy when exposed to the same beam of radiation, the concept of **absorbed dose** has been developed. The unit of absorbed dose is the rad, and represents the absorption of 100 ergs (energy units) per gram of matter. Ionizing radiation of all types can be measured in rads. For x-rays or gamma rays with energies of a few MeV, exposure of soft tissue to 1 R will result in the absorption of 0.96 rad. The ratio of rads to roentgens varies according to the energy of the x-ray and γ radiation and the composition of the substance irradiated. With low-energy x and γ rays and material of higher atomic number, such as bone, the ratio may be as high as 4:1.

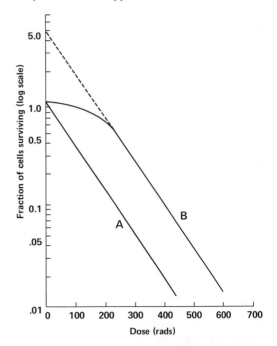

FIG 7–4. Examples of cell survival curves obtained following irradiation of cell cultures. *Curve A* shows the relationship between dose and the logarithm of the fraction of cells surviving in the situation where only one hit is required for killing. *Curve B* shows the response in cells requiring 5 hits before killing occurs. The slope of both lines is the same after the shoulder of curve B is passed.

BIOLOGIC BASIS OF RADIATION THERAPY

The amounts of energy involved in cell killing by radiation are far too small to account for death on the basis of temperature change. While a few cells may die immediately after irradiation because of direct effects, most of the injury caused by the doses used in clinical radiotherapy is to intranuclear structures such as the chromosomes and the mitotic apparatus. After irradiation, chromosomal abnormalities become evident only at the time of mitosis. Bridges occur between daughter cells, preventing completion of cell division. Genetic material in daughter cells may be altered or lost at mitosis. The use of microbeams to irradiate specific areas within cells has shown that, in terms of cell killing, the nucleus is 100–1000 times more sensitive than the cytoplasm. Other studies have shown that radiation can cause breaks in one or both DNA strands and that the number of double strand breaks, as well as the number of chromosomal aberrations, corresponds to the fraction of cells killed. These studies have also demonstrated that some breaks can be repaired.

In vitro studies of cell cultures have shown that when there is no threshold dose necessary for cell killing, the relationship between the dose given and the logarithm of the fraction of surviving cells (as measured by cellular ability to form clones or colonies) is a straight line (Fig 7–4). This indicates that cell killing is based on the probability of a vital area being hit. While in some cases the threshold dose is zero, for most mammalian cells a definite threshold or "shoulder" is seen on the dose response curve (Fig 7–4). This shoulder is thought to arise from the need for multiple hits within a cell before death is caused and the possibility of repair after one hit before a second hit occurs. Since

the dose-response curve, after the threshold dose has been reached, is logarithmic (as expressed in the following formula: surviving fraction = $1 - [1-e^{-D/D_o}]N$), the number of cells surviving any given dose is related to the number originally present. Experimentally, it has also been shown that all mammalian cells, with the exception of lymphocytes and germinal cells, have similar dose-survival curves and that, after the shoulder on the curve has been passed, it requires 100–160 rads to kill about 60% of the cells present. Thus, the dose required to kill a given number of tumor cells depends on the number of tumor cells initially present and is related to the tumor size.

In vivo, other factors affect the end result of irradiation, and the situation is far more complex than in a simple cell culture. Apparent growth or shrinkage of any normal tissue or tumor will depend upon the balance between new cell production and the natural cell death rate as well as upon cell killing by an outside agent. Two tumors with equal cellular sensitivity and equal numbers of cells but different cell growth and cell loss rates may show the effects of irradiation at different times; one may be misled if a judgment on sensitivity is made too soon.

Comparison of cell survival after doses given as a single exposure vs the same dose given in multiple exposures separated by various time intervals has shown that in most cell systems cellular repair and increased survival follow divided doses. With such fractionation, it may require a total dose 2−5 times greater than that given as a single dose to produce an equal effect (Fig 7−5). Ways of improving the therapeutic ratio* using various dose fractionation patterns are under study. Theoretical considerations suggest that the greatest advantage is obtained when the treatment is delivered in more than 10 fractions. Clinical experience over the last 50 years has rather consistently led to the conclusion that the optimal number of fractions is somewhere between 20 and 40. Most radiotherapists have adopted treatment plans in which the irradiation is given in about 30 fractions over 6 weeks' time.

One major factor influencing radiosensitivity remains to be considered (Fig 7−6). Mammalian cells in the presence of 1% or more oxygen (> 7 mm Hg partial partial pressure) are 2.5−3 times as sensitive as anoxic cells. Normal tissues, with a few exceptions, have an adequate oxygen supply. In animal tumors, 1−20% of cells are severely hypoxic, and the same presumably applies to human tumors. If it were not for a phenomenon known as reoxygenation, hypoxia

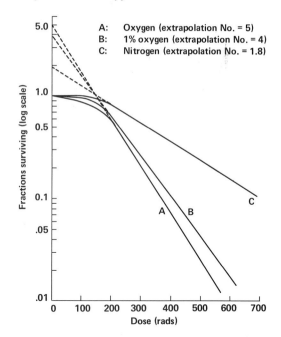

FIG 7−6. Cell survival curves following irradiation in various concentrations of oxygen. *Curve A* represents the response of a cell requiring 5 hits in the presence of 100% oxygen. *Curve B* represents the response to be observed in the presence of 1% oxygen, and *Curve C* the response observed in the presence of pure nitrogen. As the slope of the curve and the D_O increases, the extrapolation number decreases.

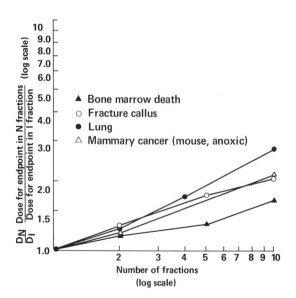

FIG 7−5. A demonstration of the effect of recovery between doses on radiation tolerance. The ratio of the dose for a given end point in N fractions to the dose for the same end point in one fraction is plotted against the number of fractions. Both are on logarithmic scales. The open circles represent bone marrow death in LAF_1 mice; the squares, 50% inhibition of fracture callus formation; the crosses, death from lung damage within 160 days; and the diamonds, the dose required for 50% cure of mouse mammary· cancer. The lung shows the greatest recovery and the bone marrow the least.

would tend to protect tumor cells. With fractionated radiation exposures, the death and subsequent absorption of oxygenated cells permits hypoxic ones to come into position nearer a capillary and thus regain sensitivity. The effectiveness of fractionated clinical radiation therapy is probably due in large part to reoxygenation. Failure of reoxygenation may account for the resistance of some tumors.

In summary, many interrelated factors play a role in the clinical application of radiation therapy: (1) The inherent sensitivity of the normal cells and tumor cells in the volume treated. (2) The total number of various types of cells present. (3) The ability of normal cells to migrate and tumor cells to metastasize. (4) The capability of repopulation of tumor vs normal tissue. (5) Rearrangement of cells in the cell cycle. (6) Repair of sublethal damage in tumor and normal cells. (7) Oxygen tension and reoxygenation. The extent to which these factors affect the sparing of normal tissue cells and the killing of tumor cells forms the basis of radiation therapy.

*Therapeutic ratio = $\dfrac{\text{Damage to tumor}}{\text{Damage to normal tissue}}$

NORMAL TISSUE REACTIONS & INJURY

Any cancer can be locally destroyed by radiation if the dose is sufficient. In clinical practice, the limiting factor is the damage unavoidably received by nearby normal tissues. When radiation therapy was done with medium-voltage radiation and by incompletely trained physicians, complication rates were understandably high; with fully trained radiotherapists and modern equipment, the incidence of clinically significant complications is very low.

The reactions in rapidly renewing cell systems which appear within days after exposure and heal early should be distinguished from the delayed late reactions that may be progressive and mean permanent damage. The extent of late radiation effects in all tissues is influenced by the degree of injury to the supporting structures, particularly the vascular system, where prevention of proliferation of endothelial cells, endarteritis, and obliteration of capillary lumens may occur. If the vascular injury is excessive, late damage appears in the form of atrophy, fibrosis, and even ulceration. Such changes due to the action of radiation on the vascular and connective tissue systems may appear many months or years after completion of treatment.

In tissues with rapid cell turnover—eg, the epithelium of gut and skin—injury reactions appear within a matter of days and, if the dose is not excessive, healing is equally rapid. In other tissues, such as brain, slow cell reproduction means that the damage will become evident only after many months or years. Permanent suppression of osteocyte production may contribute to the failure of a fracture to heal. Alteration in saliva may result in late severe changes in dental structures, even outside of irradiated areas, and this may in turn permit introduction of infection into devitalized bone. Since these late reactions appear only after long intervals of time, they are of no value in judging the conduct of a particular course of radiation therapy. Knowledge of them and of the frequency and severity with which they occur under various circumstances is essential in treatment planning.

Late reactions in the CNS may cause focal brain necrosis or radiation myelitis and spinal cord transection. Late changes in the thorax include pericarditis and radiation pneumonitis. Radiation nephritis can occur after abdominal irradiation. The total dose that leads to these late complications varies according to the organ included in the radiation beam. In general, the organs most sensitive to clinically significant late damage are the kidneys, liver, lungs, and lenses. Somewhat less sensitive are the bowel, spinal cord, brain, pericardium, cornea, and retina. Among structures least likely to show clinically significant late injury are skeletal muscle, subcutaneous connective tissue, and other supportive tissues in the body, including bone. The limiting doses when the weekly treatment is given as 5 fractions of 200 rads each (1000 rads per week) are 2000 rads for the kidneys, liver, and lungs and 4500 rads for structures of intermediate sensitivity

such as spinal cord. The resistant tissues usually withstand 6000 rads or more. These doses can be increased if the treated volume is small or the fractionation used involves smaller individual doses.

PRE- & POSTOPERATIVE RADIATION THERAPY

The rationale for combining radiation therapy and surgery in the treatment of cancer is that each method may compensate for deficiencies of the other. Irradiation may be used to sterilize the margins of a lesion; surgical resection may then be relied upon to remove the less radiosensitive central portion or extensions into bone and cartilage. Irradiation may, by killing the majority of cancer cells prior to resection, reduce the probability of seeding or dissemination of viable cancer cells during surgery. The use of such combined therapy is rational for highly invasive, poorly differentiated cancers with a high risk of spread and in situations where adequate surgical resection is impossible for anatomic reasons.

Pre- or postoperative radiation therapy may also be given to regional lymph nodes. This is not combination therapy in the sense that both methods are applied to the same area; rather, the radiation is used to extend the definitive therapy beyond the limits of the surgical excision. An example of such combination therapy is the irradiation of supraclavicular lymph nodes following radical mastectomy for breast cancer.

SELECTION & MANAGEMENT OF RADIATION THERAPY PATIENTS

Specific indications for the selection of patients for curative radiation therapy will be given below in the discussion of specific diseases. In general, the smaller, superficial, exophytic lesions are most amenable to radiation therapy; large, avascular, necrotic tumors and those with bone involvement are less likely to be controlled permanently by radiation therapy alone. Radiation should be used when it offers either a higher cure rate or the same cure rate as surgery with a lower morbidity or better functional result. Radiation therapy may occasionally be used instead of surgery if the patient's general condition contraindicates a radical operation.

Palliation involves the relief of symptoms by the use of a specific treatment method. Patients selected for palliative treatment with radiation should have a local problem, present or impending, that can be relieved or significantly delayed in onset by treatment. Palliative radiotherapy may be employed for pain due to local invasion or bone involvement, obstruction of hollow organs, involvement of functioning areas in the brain or spinal cord, irritation or ulceration of mucosal surfaces such as those of the bronchi or bladder, or local ulcerating, infected tumor masses. In certain cancers, such as those arising in the oral or pharyngeal mucosa, the dosage required for palliation is essentially the same as that used for cure. Palliation of obstructive or brain lesions also requires large doses. Lasting palliation of bone pain can often be achieved with substantially lower doses.

The proper selection of patients for radiation therapy requires close cooperation between the surgeon, radiotherapist, and chemotherapist. A combined plan, involving 2 or 3 methods of treatment, may offer the best chance of cure or palliation. It is usually best if the patient is seen jointly by all members of the oncology team and the treatment planned as a joint effort from the beginning.

A patient being considered for radiation therapy should have a thorough medical evaluation, including history, physical examination, and laboratory tests. Significant medical problems should be attended to and housing and transportation problems solved before treatment is undertaken. The most frequent problem arising during radiation therapy is the maintenance of adequate food and fluid intake. Patients irradiated around the head and neck often lose their appetite because of changes in saliva and impaired taste sensation. Specially prepared foods and suitable encouragement may be of value. Special diets may be needed for patients with bowel problems. Changes in diet or use of medication for the control of symptoms resulting from radiation should never be undertaken without first consulting the radiotherapist since he will be using the severity of the reaction as a guide to treatment.

Cancer patients are often ill and subject to numerous concomitant medical problems. Acute myocardial infarction, serum hepatitis, acute appendicitis, perforation of a peptic ulcer, and many other unrelated major medical or surgical problems may occur in patients undergoing radiation therapy. The tendency to ascribe such problems to the irradiation should be resisted so that definitive therapy will not be delayed.

RADIATION THERAPY
OF SPECIFIC DISEASES

This discussion of the radiation therapy of specific diseases is intended only to outline the place of radiation therapy, with enough comment to give the reader a general understanding of the levels of dose used, the areas or volumes treated, and the results obtainable. It is not intended for use as a manual of radiation therapy. In clinical practice, treatment planning is varied for each patient and each disease. Treatment plans, including the daily and total dose to be

delivered, are often altered during the course of treatment depending upon the response of the lesion and the effects on the patient. A discussion sufficiently detailed to permit conduct of treatment for a specific patient is beyond the scope of this book.

Before proceeding to the discussion of specific diseases, a final word of caution may be appropriate. The physician or physicians who are to be responsible for the management of a cancer patient should be consulted before any act, even biopsy, is performed. Seeing the intact, untouched lesion can be of immense help in planning the definitive treatment, whether it be surgery, radiation therapy, or a combination of the two. To excise the evidence and then refer the patient elsewhere for treatment imposes a severe handicap upon the therapist and the patient.

SKIN MALIGNANCIES

Basal Cell & Squamous Cell Carcinomas

Basal cell and squamous cell carcinomas are the most common malignancies of the skin. Basal cell carcinomas tend to invade slowly but they rarely metastasize. Metastases from squamous cell carcinomas, although more frequent than from basal cell lesions, are also rare. Both types are sufficiently radiosensitive to be controllable by radiation doses well within the limits of skin tolerance. While locally advanced carcinomas with infiltration into bone are more difficult to control, radiation therapy of the smaller lesions yields a cure rate of greater than 95%. Since surgical excision gives approximately equal control rates, the choice of treatment in a specific situation depends on the complexity of the surgical procedure and the resulting functional or cosmetic deficiency. In the absence of infection, radiation is the treatment of choice for lesions of the eyelids and over cartilage. Small carcinomas of the lip (eg, 1 cm) can be either excised or irradiated. Larger lip lesions which require a more complex surgical procedure are better treated by radiation, which provides a better functional result. Carcinomas of the trunk where there is adequate skin for closure are best treated surgically. Surgery is the preferred treatment for lesions on the backs of the hands. Surgical resection is preferred for the rare case of lymph node metastasis.

Carcinomas of the skin up to 2–3 cm in size may be treated with orthovoltage x-ray radiation delivering skin doses of about 4500 rads in 15 fractions over 3 weeks. The fields are shaped by lead sheeting to include a generous margin around the lesion. The details of treatment (kVp, filtration, etc) depend upon the particular situation. Larger lesions are treated more slowly and to higher doses. Deeply infiltrating ones are treated with higher kVp and more heavily filtered radiation. Protective lead shields are used under eyelids and behind the lips. Treatment over cartilage is not contraindicated but requires greater fractionation.

Malignant Melanomas

Malignant melanomas respond to radiation, but the doses required are high and the control less certain than for skin carcinomas. In most situations, surgical resection is the treatment of choice, with radiation therapy reserved for those patients who refuse surgery or in whom the disease is so extensive that surgery is not feasible. Radiation therapy of fixed nodes or of extensive local recurrence has resulted in local control for several years.

BREAST CANCER

Current opinions regarding the proper treatment for carcinoma of the breast vary widely. There are advocates for surgical procedures ranging from local excision of the breast mass to the supraradical mastectomy with or without pre- or postoperative irradiation. These matters are discussed and evaluated in Chapter 21.

The present opinion of the authors is outlined below. Since there is no evidence on which to base predictions of radiation response according to histologic type all varieties of breast cancer will be considered together. Most available data relate to the 95% that are adenocarcinomas. The large majority of these carcinomas respond well to radiation.

Carcinomas considered operable by the classic Halsted type of radical mastectomy or by modified radical mastectomy (see Chapter 21) should be treated in that way. If the primary lesion is in a medial quadrant or if the axillary lymph nodes contain metastases, there is a high likelihood that the ipsilateral internal mammary or supraclavicular-infraclavicular nodes are involved. These lymph node chains should be irradiated, starting when the surgical incision has healed. Megavoltage radiation is used, and the doses are carried to 5000–5500 rads to the nodes in 5–6 weeks. With operable lesions for which the surgeon has elected to do a simple mastectomy or wedge resection—or when he has not removed the pectoralis muscle—the chest wall is treated also via opposed tangential fields.

Unfortunately, convincing proof of the value of immediate postoperative irradiation versus irradiation if and when metastases appear has not been adduced. It appears that so many factors affect survival in breast cancer that even controlled clinical trials are hard to evaluate. In one such trial—the National Surgical Adjuvant Breast Project—no evidence of prolongation of survival after combined operation and postoperative irradiation could be shown. Local recurrence in the operative field was essentially eliminated by postoperative irradiation.

Inoperable carcinomas of the breast may be controlled for years or indefinitely by proper radiation therapy. In this event the breast, the chest wall, and the axillary, supraclavicular, and internal mammary lymphatics are treated. Dosage to the nodes is 5000–5500 rads and to the breast 6000 rads in 6 weeks. Residual disease in the breast or in the large fixed nodes may then receive additional treatment through smaller fields. Care must be taken to avoid lung tissue as much as possible and to prevent overlap of the rather complex set of treatment fields.

Radiation also plays an important and undisputed role in the treatment of local recurrence or metastases from breast carcinoma. Its use must be carefully coordinated with systemic therapy with hormones or anti-cancer drugs. With judicious use of radiation, soft tissue and bone metastases can often be controlled for years. Metastases in weight-bearing bones or the long bones of the upper extremities, especially if fracture appears imminent, are treated with doses of about 3000 rads in 3 weeks. If therapy is primarily for symptomatic relief, as in rib metastases, doses of 600–1000 rads may be sufficient. Radiation castration, while slower than surgical castration, is apparently as effective and may be accomplished by doses of 2000 rads in 2–3 weeks. Radiation castration is utilized when there is a contraindication to oophorectomy or other pelvic structures require radiation therapy.

Radiation therapy following biopsy or local excision for breast cancer has yielded 5-year survival rates of 20–75% depending upon the extent of the disease at the time of irradiation. Simple mastectomy plus radiation therapy for operable lesions has given 5-year salvage rates equivalent to those of radical mastectomy. The addition of radiation therapy to radical mastectomy results in a higher rate of control of regional lymph nodes and may, at least in cases with high axillary node involvement, produce increased survival. With proper technics and careful attention to treatment planning, the complications of curative radiation therapy are limited to mild atrophy, tanning and telangiectases of skin, mild fibrosis of the breast, and (usually asymptomatic) peripheral lung fibrosis. Severe changes of the skin, chest wall, or lungs, arm edema, or brachial plexus injury as a direct result of the irradiation should not occur.

BONE TUMORS

Reticulum Cell Sarcomas

Reticulum cell sarcomas primary in bone are moderately sensitive to radiation; a dose of 5000 rads given over a period of 5–6 weeks yields a local control rate of over 90%. Because of the tendency for these tumors to extend throughout the marrow cavity, the entire bone should be treated. The 5-year survival rate is about 50%. Metastases to other bones, lymph nodes, or organs may be treated similarly.

Ewing's Sarcoma

Ewing's sarcoma is also moderately radiosensitive; local control can be achieved in approximately 80% of cases by doses of 5000–6000 rads in 6–7 weeks. The entire bone is treated as in reticulum cell sarcoma. Chemotherapy with drugs such as cyclophosphamide (Cytoxan), vincristine (Oncovin), and dactinomycin (Cosmegen) is often given in conjunction with radiation and for 6 months to 2 years thereafter. Amputation is reserved for local radiation failure in the absence of distant metastases.

Because of the marked tendency to metastasize, actual cures in Ewing's sarcoma are rare. Occasional cures have been reported following irradiation of distant metastases, including those in the lungs. The maximum dose that can be delivered to the entire lungs is about 2500 rads in 20 fractions over 4 weeks. If given in conjunction with chemotherapy (eg, dactinomycin), the total dose to the lungs is reduced to 1500 rads. Small areas in the lung may be spot-treated to higher doses.

Osteogenic Sarcoma

Local control of osteogenic sarcoma by radiation alone is uncertain, and amputation is the treatment of choice. Radiation therapy is of value in the treatment of osteogenic sarcoma in nonresectable locations, in providing symptomatic relief for the patient who already has metastases, and as a preoperative measure. The purpose of preoperative radiation is to provide local control for 4–6 months while waiting to determine whether lung metastases have already occurred. In this way, needless amputation may be avoided. Large doses (7000–8000 rads) are given to the radiographically evident lesion plus a margin of at least 6–8 cm. The 5-year disease-free survival rate is 20–25% with or without preoperative radiation.

Chondrosarcoma & Fibrosarcoma

These tumors are preferentially treated by surgical means. They may respond to a large dose of radiation, which is used for inoperable tumors and for the occasional patient who refuses surgery. These sarcomas metastasize late, and there is little or no place for preoperative radiation.

Benign Bone Tumors

Certain benign bone tumors such as **benign giant cell tumors** and **aneurysmal bone cysts** are controllable with radiation therapy. With giant cell tumors it is exceedingly important to obtain an adequate biopsy to rule out malignancy. Doses of 4000 rads and 3000 rads, respectively, are used for giant cell tumors and aneurysmal bone cysts. Cure rates of 80% or more are reported.

SOFT TISSUE TUMORS

Soft tissue sarcomas such as **liposarcoma** and **fibrosarcoma** should be treated surgically if it can be done without excessive mutilation. Some of these sar-

comas do respond to radiation, and treatment by radiation is occasionally justified. Response is slow, and doses of about 7000 rads in 7–8 weeks are usually required.

When surgical excision is the primary treatment the local recurrence rate may be as high as 40%. Recent studies in which radiation was used postoperatively or for small local recurrences have shown a 90% local control rate.

Desmoid tumors inaccessible or too extensive for surgical extirpation may respond to moderately high doses of irradiation. Many months may be required before the response to therapy becomes evident.

CNS TUMORS

Radiation, after biopsy and decompression, is the treatment of choice for the radiosensitive medulloblastomas, ependymomas, and certain lesions of the pineal gland. Together with decompressive shunt, it is the accepted therapy for tumors in areas such as the pons, medulla, and brain stem, where attempts at biopsy carry prohibitively high mortality and morbidity rates. For most gliomas, postoperative radiation is thought to prolong useful survival and to increase survival rates. The notable exception is the cystic cerebellar astrocytoma, which has a high cure rate with surgery alone. Radiation of the highly malignant glioblastoma multiforme is of questionable value, but occasional cures have been claimed and survival may be prolonged. Meningiomas are primarily a surgical problem, but radiation may contribute to control in the incompletely resected lesion and, as a preoperative measure, may significantly reduce vascularity.

Ependymomas and **pinealomas** should be treated with large local fields, including the adjacent ventricular system. While intracranial ependymomas occasionally seed down the spinal canal, in our experience this has been evident clinically in less than 5% of patients. Treatment of the local area with doses of about 5000 rads has produced a 5-year survival rate of 85%; the failures usually have been at the primary site.

Unbiopsied tumors of the brain stem and most of the **differentiated gliomas** are treated with doses of 5000–5500 rads in 6–7 weeks. With these doses, complications from the radiation are few. In one well documented series, use of radiation yielded a 5-year survival rate of 25% for unbiopsied intrinsic brain stem tumors. For **glioblastoma multiforme,** most or all of the brain is treated to a dose fo 5000–6000 rads.

Radiation treatment of intracranial **metastases from carcinomas** and **lymphomas** is often rewarding. Lymphomas are usually controlled by relatively small doses, and many patients with metastatic carcinoma can be maintained in a functional state for long periods with 4500–5000 rads. Because of the frequency of multiple lesions, both of these entities require therapy to the entire intracranial volume. With lymphomas, it may be necessary to treat the spinal canal either at the same time or later.

NEUROBLASTOMA

Neuroblastomas are very radiosensitive tumors of childhood. They may arise in the adrenal gland or any sympathetic ganglion and commonly metastasize to bone. Local control is usually achieved by radiation in doses of 2500–3000 rads. If it is necessary to include the spine in the treatment field, symmetrical radiation of the vertebrae is thought to reduce the incidence of late scoliosis. With widespread metastases, radiation therapy is used for lesions which are symptomatic or threaten loss of function; in some patients (perhaps 10–20%), other metastases will undergo spontaneous maturation.

The cure rate for neuroblastoma is around 30–35%.

CARCINOMA OF THE THYROID

Papillary and follicular carcinomas are primarily surgical problems. Even in the presence of multiple bilateral cervical metastases cure is obtained in a substantial percentage of cases by thyroidectomy and neck dissection. Local invasion or inoperable recurrence and isolated distant metastases are treated with external irradiation, and control lasting many years may be achieved. In the case of widespread (especially pulmonary) metastases, radioactive iodine (^{131}I) may prove effective. Administration of thyroid hormone may control or at least retard the growth of metastases from some papillary and follicular carcinomas.

Undifferentiated adenocarcinomas with local invasion and **lymphosarcomas** of the thyroid are treated primarily with radiation. Radiation therapy should be offered for **spindle cell** and **giant cell carcinomas,** but these lesions have an exceedingly poor prognosis irrespective of the therapy applied.

OCULAR & INTRAORBITAL TUMORS

The tumors of importance to radiotherapy in this anatomic area include retinoblastoma, embryonal rhabdomyosarcoma of the eye muscles, adenocarcinoma of the lacrimal gland, and squamous cell carcinoma and melanoma of the conjunctiva. All are relatively rare. Retinoblastomas and embryonal rhabdomyosarcomas occur in childhood and are quite sensitive to radiation. These lesions spread along the optic nerve or metastasize via the blood stream, but regional lymph node metastases are rare. Because of the regional nature and radiosensitivity, both retinoblastoma and rhabdomyosarcoma are best treated by radiation therapy.

The control rate for **retinoblastoma** may be as high as 80% depending upon the size of the lesion. It is important to use a well-defined megavoltage radiation beam and a special shield to protect the lens. The optic nerve should be included. The dose to the retina is 5000 rads in 25 fractions over about 6 weeks. Enucleation is used for radiation failure.

Rhabdomyosarcomas are treated by irradiation of the entire orbit, with corneal shielding whenever possible. The dose is carried to 5000–6000 rads in 6–7 weeks. Data on control rates are scarce, but local control should be achieved in a high percentage of cases.

Superficial conjunctival lesions may be treated with ^{90}Sr applicators. **Lacrimal gland carcinomas** are irradiated postoperatively when surgical margins are not clear or surgical failure has occurred, or as primary treatment if the lesion is inoperable. Doses of at least 6000 rads to the entire orbit are required.

Possible complications of radiation include cataract, dry eye, and corneal ulceration. Depending upon the location and nature of the tumor, these can usually be prevented by careful beam placement and shielding, but surgical removal of a cataract or enucleation is an occasional unavoidable consequence of successful therapy.

MALIGNANT LESIONS OF THE HEAD & NECK

The great majority of malignant neoplasms of the mucosa of the head and neck are squamous cell carcinomas of various degrees of differentiation and moderate radiosensitivity. Primary lymphomas arising in the nasopharynx or tonsils and adenocarcinomas of salivary and mucous glands are relatively rare. The lymphomas are quite radiosensitive, but the response of adenocarcinomas is less predictable. Unless otherwise specified, the following comments apply to squamous cell carcinomas.

Radiation therapy is generally the treatment of choice for carcinomas arising in the nasopharynx, tonsils, the floor of the mouth, the soft palate, the hypopharynx, the epiglottis, the false vocal cords, the laryngeal ventricle, and the true vocal cords. Exceptions are those lesions which extend into the pre-epiglottic space, vocal cord lesions sufficiently advanced to cause fixation, and lesions involving bone. Carcinomas of the gingival ridge, the anterior tonsillar pillars, the piriform sinus, and the salivary glands (adenocarcinomas) should be treated surgically. Early carcinomas of the tongue are equally well controlled by radiation (radium implant or transoral cone) or surgery, but radiation usually offers the better functional result. A hard, deeply infiltrating carcinoma of the tongue is less likely to be controlled by radiation. Most carcinomas arising from the mucosa of the maxillary antra—especially those with extension into the posterior and superior bony walls—should be treated by radiation.

In many sites, radiation may be tried first and surgical excision performed subsequently if radiation is not successful. If the patient is observed closely and surgery is utilized as soon as radiation failure is evident and the early radiation reaction has subsided (usually after 4–6 weeks), the delay in excision rarely affects the outcome adversely. With an experienced surgeon and properly administered radiation, there is little difference in morbidity rates whether surgery is utilized for radiation failure or for primary treatment.

The 5-year disease-free control rates for radiation therapy vary according to the primary site, the size and extent of the primary lesions and the distribution and character of involved lymph nodes. The control rate for stage I carcinoma of the vocal cords is 90–95%. Smaller carcinomas of the borders of the tongue, the free portion of the epiglottis, the floor of the mouth without extension into the tongue or to the mandible, and early localized lesions of the soft palate can be controlled by radiation in about 80% of patients. Carcinomas of the piriform sinus, the subglottic area, and the gingival ridge are rarely controlled by radiation alone. Early lesions of the nasopharynx, antrum, tonsils, the base of the tongue, the hypopharynx, the false vocal cords, and the laryngeal ventricle have cure rates of 80–90%. More advanced lesions and those with lymph node metastases have lower cure rates.

CARCINOMA OF THE LUNG

Histologically, carcinoma of the lung may be classified as adenocarcinoma, squamous cell carcinoma, large cell undifferentiated carcinoma, and oat cell carcinoma. For the localized operable adenocarcinomas, squamous cell carcinomas, and oat cell carcinomas, surgery is the treatment of choice. Few cases of oat cell carcinoma are thought to be curable after clinical evaluation, and for this reason this tumor is treated mostly by radiation. This is because treatment can be directed to tissues beyond the lung and because these carcinomas are sensitive to radiation.

Unfortunately, most bronchogenic carcinomas are inoperable, and only about 5% are curable at the time of diagnosis. Factors that preclude surgical resection are involvement of the parietal pleura, extensively involved or fixed mediastinal lymph nodes, recurrent or vagus nerve paralysis, bronchial extension approaching the carina, invasion of major vessels or the trachea, and distant metastases. If the lesion is inoperable but still localized, an attempt at radiation cure is justified. Limited peripheral lesions involving the chest wall (as in some superior sulcus tumors) or lesions of the carina contribute a few radiation cures. Squamous cell carcinomas are treated with relatively small fields, usually

including the primary and hilum; in the case of undifferentiated and oat cell carcinomas, lymph node regions of the mediastinum and the supraclavicular area are included also. With conventional fractionation schemes, the differentiated and large cell carcinomas require doses of 5500–6000 rads, whereas 5000 rads is adequate for oat cell carcinomas. Survival rates up to 5% are reported.

THYMUS

Tumors arising in the thymus may be malignant in that they invade locally and seed over the pleural surfaces. Histologically, it is difficult to recognize malignancy in the epithelial tumors. The sites of local invasion include the pericardium, heart, great vessels, nerves, and other structures in the mediastinum. Distant metastases are rare in the early stages.

Encapsulated thymic tumors should be totally resected surgically, since rupture of the capsule may lead to seeding. It is questionable whether any surgery other than biopsy is indicated for tumors that invade important mediastinal structures. Many can be controlled by radiation. There is no place for surgery in the management of lymphosarcomas, Hodgkin's disease (including the so-called granulomatous thymomas), and seminomas that occur in the thymus. These lesions are treated with radiation therapy, utilizing large treatment fields and modest radiation doses.

About 40% of patients with thymomas have myasthenia gravis. On the other hand, approximately 15% of patients with myasthenia gravis have a thymoma. Thymic irradiation may be useful for symptomatic control of patients with myasthenia without a demonstrable thymoma. To lessen the possibility of myasthenic crisis, all patients scheduled for surgery for thymic tumors should receive preoperative irradiation; in these cases it is important to begin with small daily doses and limit the total dose to about 2500 rads.

GASTROINTESTINAL TRACT

Esophagus

With rare exceptions, malignant lesions of the esophagus are squamous cell carcinomas. Esophageal neoplasms give rise to symptoms only when deeply penetrating or when obstruction, which occurs late because of the inherent distensibility of the organ, is imminent. Because of the rich lymphatic supply and absence of serosal covering, these carcinomas tend to extend long distances up and down the esophagus and frequently infiltrate surrounding mediastinal structures by the time of diagnosis. For these reasons, radiation therapy must include long segments of the esophagus and adjacent soft tissues.

In the proximal third of the esophagus, surgical access and reconstruction are difficult and results with radiation therapy are at least as good as with excision. Therefore, radiation is the treatment of choice. Special tissue compensating filters are used, and a dose of 6000–6500 rads in 7 weeks is recommended. Care must be taken to avoid excessive radiation to the spinal cord.

In the middle third, the best results appear to be with a combination of preoperative radiation therapy followed, in resectable cases, by esophagectomy. The entire esophagus receives up to about 5000 rads in 6 weeks; 5–6 weeks later, esophagectomy is performed.

Primary surgery is probably preferable for lesions arising in the distal esophagus.

Even though cure rates of 25% or higher have been reported for well-selected series of patients, the overall cure rate for esophageal carcinoma is probably no better than 5%. Radiation therapy alone will reopen the esophagus and control local symptoms in 70–75% of patients. Thus, gastrostomy for feeding purposes is rarely indicated.

Stomach & Bowel

Most cancers of the stomach and bowel are adenocarcinomas. While these lesions are moderately radiosensitive, the radiation doses required are not well tolerated by the abdominal organs and surgery is usually the treatment of choice.

The lymphomas which occur in stomach or bowel should be treated by radiation. An effort is made to treat the entire abdomen to doses of 3000–4000 rads, with shielding of the kidneys after 2000 rads and of the liver after 3000 rads. Such large fields are not well tolerated, and the daily dose to the midplane of the abdomen is often limited to 150 rads or less.

Rectum & Anus

Preoperative irradiation with doses of about 4000–5000 rads may add to the cure rate of large, locally extensive rectal carcinomas. Radiation therapy is often of value in palliation of pain due to local recurrence and in temporary relief of a localized obstruction.

Evidence is accumulating that preoperative x-ray may improve survival following operation for carcinoma of the rectum and rectosigmoid. Controlled clinical trials are in progress.

Intracavitary irradiation may have a place in the treatment of small carcinomas of the rectum, especially in elderly or poor-risk patients and in those who refuse a colostomy.

Squamous cell carcinoma is the most common type of anal malignancy. Lesions originating in or extending above the pectinate line tend to spread upward along the rectal wall and into the rectal lymphatics and are primarily surgical problems. Those below the line behave like ordinary squamous cell carcinomas of skin and can be controlled by radiation with preservation of the anus and anal sphincter.

FEMALE GENITAL TRACT

Ovaries

Most **ovarian carcinomas** are of epithelial origin and are moderately sensitive to radiation. Because of their location and the poor tolerance of adjacent tissues to the necessary doses of radiation, surgery is the preferred method of treatment for localized tumors. For lesions which have been incompletely resected but are still localized to the pelvis, postoperative radiation therapy increases the local control rate. Preoperative radiation occasionally makes an inoperable lesion operable. In inoperable cases, palliative radiotherapy may provide long-term relief of symptoms and prevent bowel obstruction. The value of total abdominal irradiation for widely disseminated lesions and irradiation of the periaortic lymph nodes is uncertain.

Dysgerminoma of the ovary—the counterpart of the testicular seminoma—is highly radiosensitive. For this rare lesion, postoperative treatment of pelvic and abdominal lymph nodes should be done routinely. Pelvic radiation should include both sides of the pelvis with the dose carried to 3000–3500 rads. Irradiation of half of the pelvis in an attempt to spare the other ovary may leave that ovary functional, but scattered radiation may deliver a dose that causes genetic damage. If abdominal lymph nodes are involved, the treatment fields should be extended to include the mediastinum and supraclavicular areas. When peritoneal implants are present, the entire pelvis and abdomen are treated to 2500–3000 rads in 5–6 weeks with kidney shielding after 2000 rads. Control may still be achieved in the presence of distant metastases.

Uterus

Tumors of the uterine fundus that are subjected to radiotherapy are primarily the adenocarcinomas of endometrial origin. Radiation therapy may aid in local control of mixed mesodermal sarcomas and carcinosarcomas but adds little to the treatment of leiomyosarcomas, which are primarily surgical problems. **Endometrial adenocarcinomas** are potentially curable by radiation therapy alone, but hysterectomy is more reliable.

Cervix

Ninety-five percent of cervical malignancies are **squamous cell carcinomas**; most of the remainder are **adenocarcinomas**. Although adenocarcinomas tend to respond more slowly, both are about equally radiosensitive and their radiation-induced control rates are similar. Because of the great tolerance of the cervical and vaginal mucosa to radiation and the accessibility of the vagina and uterus for radium insertions, radiation therapy plays a major role in the treatment of cervical carcinoma. Recent studies have shown that metastases in pelvic lymph nodes may also be controlled by radiation.

For in situ carcinoma, total hysterectomy is an adequate procedure, has a low morbidity rate, and is generally the treatment of choice. Lesser surgical procedures may be done when the patient is desirous of retaining her uterus and can be kept under close observation (see Chapter 45).

With invasive carcinoma clinically limited to the cervix (stage I), there is a 15–20% chance that pelvic node metastases are present. Radical surgical procedures or radiation therapy for early lesions yield about equal 5-year survival rates (80–90%). Because of the lower rate of major complications (primarily ureteral obstruction or fistula formations in 8–10% following radical surgery; bowel damage or fistula formations in 1–2% following radiation therapy), radiation is the method of choice. Radical surgical procedures are reserved for radiation failures.

Radiation therapy typically includes 2 insertions of radium into the uterus and vaginal fornices supplemented with external irradiation to raise the dose to the lymph nodes in the lateral parts of the pelvis.

For advanced cervical carcinomas (stage II and beyond), radiotherapy is even more strongly preferred to surgery. Greater use is made of external radiation, with a corresponding reduction of the emphasis on radium. This is done by increasing the dose to the entire pelvis from external radiation and decreasing the dose from the radium applications.

Vagina

Vaginal carcinomas are chiefly squamous cell in type. Carcinoma of the proximal vagina tends to spread along the same lymphatic channels as carcinoma from the cervix; carcinoma of the distal vagina tends to metastasize to the inguinal lymph nodes.

In general, radiation therapy is the method of choice. It utilizes a combination of external radiation and intravaginal radium, with the relative emphasis determined by the extent and location of the lesion. External radiation is usually given first, with the entire vaginal axis and adjacent tissues carried to a dose of 4000–5000 rads. For lesions of the proximal vagina, treatment is extended to the whole pelvis. Radium is then inserted into the vagina in such fashion that the entire vaginal and cervical mucosa receives another 3000–4000 rads.

Accurate survival data are not available, but a high cure rate is obtainable for the early vaginal carcinomas.

Vulva

Because of the poor tolerance of the vulva to large doses of radiation, vulvar carcinomas are primarily surgical problems.

MALE GENITAL TRACT

Testis

Testicular tumors arising from the germinal epithelium are by far the most important for the radio-

therapist. These tumors include seminoma, embryonal carcinoma, teratocarcinoma, choriocarcinoma, and mixtures of these types. Seminomas are very sensitive to radiation, and the others exhibit variable degrees of sensitivity. Unless far advanced, testicular tumors are confined by the tunica vaginalis and lymphatic drainage is via the spermatic cord to the para-aortic and renal hilar lymph nodes.

When a tumor of the testis is suspected, orchiectomy should be done through an inguinal incision with ligation at the internal inguinal ring. **Seminomas** are then given radiation to the ipsilateral pelvic, renal hilar, and para-aortic lymphatics up to the diaphragm with doses of about 3000 rads. If abdominal lymph node metastases have been demonstrated at surgery or by intravenous urography or by lymphangiography, the mediastinum and supraclavicular areas should also be treated. Whether in the absence of demonstrable abdominal lymph node involvement the areas above the diaphragm should be treated prophylactically is currently under investigation.

In the case of **embryonal carcinomas** and **teratocarcinomas**, treatment of the abdominal lymph nodes is controversial. Various combinations of para-aortic node dissection and radiation are advocated. Some specialists prefer radiation alone for embryonal carcinoma and radiation plus dissection for teratocarcinomas. In either case, radiation of the mediastinal and supraclavicular lymphatics is advised.

Choriocarcinomas have a high tendency to disseminate via the blood stream, and prophylactic radiation therapy is of questionable value.

The 5-year survival rate for seminomas is about 90%. Even with distant spread, seminomas are curable by radiation therapy. The overall cure rate for other types of testicular cancer (except choriocarcinoma) treated by orchiectomy and radiation is about 50%, ranging from 10–75% depending upon the extent of disease at diagnosis.

Prostate

In the last few years it has been demonstrated that **adenocarcinoma of the prostate** may be locally controlled by radiation. These carcinomas respond slowly and require doses of about 7000 rads in 7–8 weeks. Such doses make megavoltage radiation, protection of adjacent tissues, and careful treatment planning absolutely essential.

The use of radiation for control of prostatic cancer is too recent to permit final conclusions regarding the indications for surgery vs irradiation.

TUMORS OF THE URINARY TRACT

Renal Parenchyma

Wilms's tumor (embryoma of the kidney) is a very radiosensitive tumor of childhood. It may invade locally and commonly metastasizes to the lungs and liver. Bilateral involvement occurs in about 5% of cases.

Surgical resection is indicated for primary Wilms's tumor. Since metastases do not rule out the possibility of cure, resection should be attempted even if metastases have already occurred. Preoperative irradiation may be used if the tumor is very large, highly vascular, or fixed. These tumors generally regress rapidly. Postoperative irradiation is given if there is capsular invasion or local lymph node involvement. Chemotherapy with dactinomycin is started at the time of surgery and continued intermittently for 2 years.

Bladder

The large majority of bladder carcinomas are transitional cell in type. These vary widely in characteristics from small, superficial grade I papillary tumors that may be cured by transurethral resection to the usually large, bulky, infiltrating grade IV carcinomas. Grade I papillary tumors have a tendency to recur and to become less well differentiated with time. Higher grade carcinomas spread through the lymphatics of the bladder wall as well as to adjacent pelvic lymphatics.

Early papillary tumors may be treated by local resection, but the more malignant ones require treatment of the entire bladder. Some of the intermediate lesions, especially in the bladder dome, may be controlled by segmental resection. Since cure rates with modern radiation therapy are as good as with total cystectomy and the functional result is better, most higher grade (III and IV) transitional cell carcinomas are treated with radiation. The usual dose is 6000–6500 rads in 6–7 weeks. Various combinations of multiple fixed fields and rotational therapy are used; selection is based on the anatomy of the lesion and the habitus of the patient.

The overall cure rate is about 30%, with better results in less extensive lesions. Significant complications with proper radiotherapy technics are rare.

Urethra

Carcinomas of the urethra are often treated with radiation. External irradiation, radium implants, or a combination of the 2 are used, depending upon the anatomic distribution of the involvement.

NONNEOPLASTIC DISEASES

In a few situations, radiation therapy is of value in the treatment of benign disease. **Local inflammatory lesions** such as acute parotitis and resistant staphylococcal infections often respond to a few hundred rads in fractionated doses. For acute parotitis in elderly debilitated patients, radiation may be lifesaving. **Subacute thyroiditis** usually responds favorably to similar treatment. The pain arising from **ankylosing spondylitis of the spine** is relieved in most patients by radiation, but the course of the disease is unaltered.

Overgrowth of fibrous tissue, as in **keloid** formation, may be prevented or subsequent symptoms relieved by a single dose of 600 rads of superficial radiation or by 5 doses of 200 rads at weekly intervals, depending upon the size and location of the scar. Cosmetic results are better with fractionated therapy.

After excision, 2000–3000 rads of very superficial β-ray irradiation may prevent recurrences of **pterygium**.

External radiation to the retrobulbar orbital tissues is helpful in reducing or preventing progression of the changes in severe progressing **infiltrative exophthalmos** associated with Graves' disease. Both orbits are treated with doses of about 200 rads daily for a total of 10 treatments. Care must be taken to avoid the lens. The treatment of **hyperthyroidism** with parenteral radioiodine has replaced thyroidectomy in selected patients, but a discussion of the advantages and disadvantages of such treatment is beyond the scope of this presentation.

Radiation is also used for prevention of a **threatened rejection of transplanted tissues**. It is thought to be of value in reversing the rejection process in transplanted kidneys. The usual dose is 150 rads given 3 times at daily intervals. If necessary, the course of therapy may be repeated twice.

Radiation therapy is often of considerable value in treating selected cases of gastrointestinal ulceration, especially of the duodenum, due to elevated gastric acidity. The treatment is 1800 rads in 2 weeks to the entire acid-secreting portion of the stomach.

●　●　●

General References

Ackerman LV, del Regato J: *Cancer: Diagnosis, Treatment, and Prognosis,* 4th ed. Mosby, 1970.

Alexander P: *Atomic Radiation and Life.* Penguin Books, 1957.

Andrews JR: *The Radiology of Human Cancer Radiotherapy.* Saunders, 1968.

Buschke F, Parker R: *Progress in Radiation Therapy,* vol 1. Grune & Stratton, 1958.

Casaret AP: *Radiation Biology.* Prentice-Hall, 1968.

Fabrikant J: *Radiobiology.* Year Book, 1972.

Fletcher GH: *Textbook of Radiotherapy,* 2nd ed. Lea & Febiger, 1973.

Hendee WR: *Medical Radiation Physics.* Year Book, 1970.

Johns HE, Cunningham JR: *Physics of Radiology,* 3rd ed. Thomas, 1969.

Moss WT, Brand WN: *Therapeutic Radiology,* 3rd ed. Mosby, 1969.

Pitzarillo DJ, Witkofski RL: *Basic Radiation Biology.* Saunders, 1968.

Rubin P, Casaret AP: *Clinical Radiation Pathology.* 2 vols. Saunders, 1968.

Selman J: *Basic Physics of Radiation Therapy.* Thomas, 1960.

8...

Nuclear Medicine in Surgical Diagnosis

Malcolm R. Powell, MD

Nuclear medicine is a medical specialty that uses radionuclides in medical diagnosis and treatment. Radionuclide tracers provide methods of studying the structure and function of internal organs. Tracer procedures differ from conventional x-ray studies in several fundamental respects. Radioactive tracers are physiologically insignificant and do not impose the chemical, osmolal, or volume stresses that occur when x-ray contrast materials are used. The emission images obtained with radiotracers are of lower resolution than roentgenograms, but many of the organs imaged are not as readily susceptible to x-ray examination. Radionuclide distribution is readily quantified, providing the basis for testing of physiologic function. Although nuclear medicine tests are sensitive in detecting pathologic conditions and defining their location, they do not usually provide a specific diagnosis. Nuclear medicine procedures are free of morbidity and can be readily performed on outpatients.

PRINCIPLES OF RADIOACTIVITY DETECTION & INFORMATION PRESENTATION IN NUCLEAR MEDICINE

Radioactivity

Radioisotopes are unstable forms of elements which have the same chemical properties (atomic number) as the stable isotope but a different atomic mass. They decay to other isotopes, emitting particles and electromagnetic radiation with each radioactive decay. Individual radioisotopes have characteristic half-lives (the time at which 50% of the original number of atoms of the radioisotope will have undergone decay to another isotope). Ideally, each isotope used in nuclear medicine would have a half-life similar to the time required for the test and would emit only useful types of radiation, thus limiting radiation exposure of the patient. If an isotope is given for a test that entails in vivo counting, the radiation should have a relatively low absorption in the patient, since it must escape to be counted. If a radioisotope is administered for therapy, it would be ideal if the emitted radiation were entirely absorbed within the target tissue.

Diagnostic tests such as thyroid uptake tests, radioisotope renograms, and organ imaging are generally performed by detecting gamma rays. The gamma ray is electromagnetic radiation with no charge and negligible mass, properties which allow it to pass through tissue without absorption. Gamma radiation is readily located and counted with external detectors.

The radioactive emissions used for therapy in nuclear medicine are beta particles. These have sufficient mass and charge that they penetrate only short distances through tissue and usually deliver their entire energy after traveling less than 1 mm.

Instrumentation

Knowledge of the instruments used in nuclear medicine is important to utilize these tests efficiently. Fig 8–1 shows the simplest form of detector for gamma rays. A sodium iodide crystal is used to absorb gamma rays and convert their energy to bursts of light (scintillations). The scintillations are detected by the photo-cathode of the multiplier photo tube. The photo-cathode converts each scintillation to a pulse of electrons which is multiplied in the tube. After amplification, the pulse is proportionate to the original gamma photon energy and may be identified as specific for the isotope. This allows detection of one isotope in the presence of others.

Radioisotope imaging devices provide planar projections of the radioactivity "seen" by the instrument. Radioisotope scanners do this by systematically moving a detector back and forth over the surface of the patient, detecting radioactive count rate and recording it as a pattern on paper or by exposing x-ray film proportionate to the radioactivity. Scanning devices detect radioactivity through a "focused" collimator which is most sensitive to radiation originating 3–5 inches from the surface of the collimator. Thus, as this type of detector moves across a patient, the image corresponds to a plane within the patient, and the rectilinear scan image is largely tomographic.

The scintillation camera employs a stationary detector containing a sodium iodide crystal 12 inches wide and ½ inch thick. An array of multiplier photo tubes is used to locate the position of scintillations within the crystal, and this information is displayed on an oscilloscope. The oscilloscope is photographed to collect the image information. Collimators for scintillation cameras are analogous to lenses in photographic cameras since they allow gamma photons to interact with the detector crystal in a pattern corresponding to radioactivity distribution in the subject. Gamma photons from meaningless orientations are absorbed in

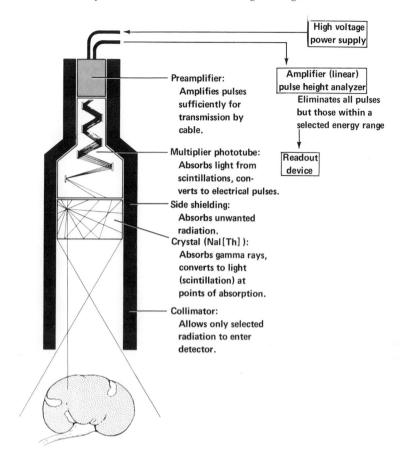

High voltage power supply

Preamplifier:
Amplifies pulses sufficiently for transmission by cable.

Amplifier (linear) pulse height analyzer
Eliminates all pulses but those within a selected energy range

Multiplier phototube:
Absorbs light from scintillations, converts to electrical pulses.

Readout device

Side shielding:
Absorbs unwanted radiation.

Crystal (NaI[Th]):
Absorbs gamma rays, converts to light (scintillation) at points of absorption.

Collimator:
Allows only selected radiation to enter detector.

FIG 8–1. Detector. NaI(Th) = thallium-activated sodium iodide crystal.

the lead collimator. Since the scintillation camera detector is stationary, rapidly changing radioisotope distributions may be recorded as "stop motion" photographs. Scintillation camera data may also be recorded by computer for numerical data analysis.

Table 8–1 compares rectilinear scans and scintiphotographs. The principal difference between scans and scintiphotos is that the scintiphotos are usually miniaturized. This is appropriate for the limited information density produced by nuclear medicine images. Fig 8–2 demonstrates the value of image minification: "life-size" or 1:1 scan is larger than desirable for the information density.

Scintiphotos are best used for primary acquisition of data on radioisotope distribution. In addition to obtaining images, scintillation cameras are increasingly used to obtain quantitative regional data for evaluation of physiologic processes such as pulmonary perfusion, ventilation, renal cortical function, and cardiac function.

Rectilinear scans are most useful for the following purposes: (1) Scans provide 1:1 images for exact correlation with topical or palpable anatomy such as a renal scan in the biopsy position for kidney localization or a thyroid scan for correlation with a palpable nodule (Fig 8–3). (2) Scans provide the best means of

TABLE 8–1. Comparison of scans and scintiphotos.

	Scans	Scintiphotos
Speed of image formation	Slow (static studies)	Fast (static or dynamic studies)
Data density; resolution	Lower	Higher
Image depth	Tomographic	Images as deeply as permitted by absorption of gamma photons in the subject
Image size	Usually 1:1	Usually one-tenth of life size
Image media	Paper print, x-ray film	Polaroid film, 35 mm film, videotape
Field of view	Larger (14 × 17 inches or more)	Smaller (10 inch circle)*

*With parallel hole collimator; larger with other collimators, but at expense of speed or image resolution.

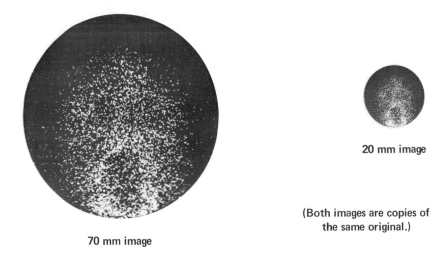

20 mm image

(Both images are copies of
the same original.)

70 mm image

FIG 8–2. Image size and pattern recognition. Despite the minified nature of scintiphotographs, the small images are somewhat larger than ideal for viewing at arm's length. For comparison, 2 copies of the same image are shown here, one more than twice the usual scintiphotograph size and the other reduced to approximately 40% of the usual size. Most interpreters will find it easier to recognize the pathology in the smaller image (or in the larger image at a distance of 5–10 feet). This is an illustration of the anterior view of a patient's head during the arterial phase of a brain blood flow study after the peripheral intravenous injection of ^{99m}Tc pertechnetate. Two curvilinear defects of arterial filling are seen laterally over each hemisphere with medial displacement of the middle cerebral artery arborizations. These defects are large subdural hematomas. This test is often a valuable aid in the diagnosis of acute neurosurgical problems.

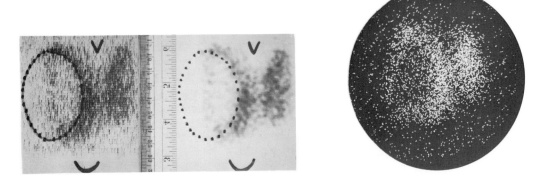

Scanning time, 15 minutes   **Scintiphotography time, 4 minutes**

FIG 8–3. Microfollicular adenoma of the thyroid. A large defect is easily recognized in the lateral right lobe of the thyroid. This large adenoma has displaced the right lobe of the thyroid gland to rotate it forward around the trachea. This illustration compares the presentation of information in scans and scintiphotographs after photographic copying at the same size. Scans show the linear pattern caused by detector motion and generally are obtained on x-ray film. Scintiphotographs are a continuous record for all areas of the field of view and are usually obtained on Polaroid film. Exact outlines of palpable findings can be drawn directly on scan images, a direct comparison of anatomic findings which is more difficult on scintiphotographs. Markers are conventionally shown on scans at the thyroid cartilage notch and at the suprasternal notch. The scintillation camera, in contrast, provides a more rapid image and often shows more effective resolution of abnormalities than the spatial resolution available in scans.

^{18}F fluoride localization in carcinoma metastatic to bone

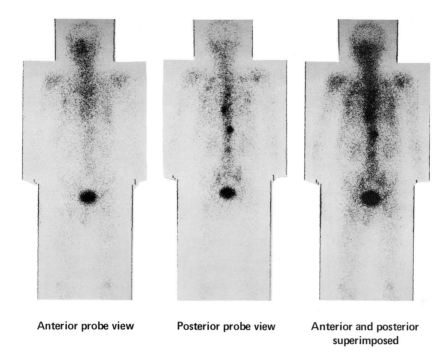

Anterior probe view   Posterior probe view   Anterior and posterior
                                                      superimposed

FIG 8–4. Whole body scan. This whole body scan was performed 1½ hours after intravenous administration of ^{18}F fluoride, which localizes in bone mineral much like phosphate. ^{18}F is not generally available and will soon be replaced by technetium polyphosphates. Either can be used to demonstrate localized or generalized increases in bone blood flow due to neoplastic disease, infection, inflammatory arthritis, Paget's disease, or other abnormalities. This illustration shows the laminographic nature of scans well. The lesions in the lower thoracic and upper lumbar spine are clearly recognized in the posterior probe view, which is a posterior laminograph. Anterior structures such as iliac crests, the sternum, the manubrium, and the facial bones are all more readily recognized in the anterior view. The lesions shown here were due to metastatic prostatic carcinoma and were not definitely recognizable on roentgenograms. Scanning has been shown to be a more sensitive way of localizing bone metastases than x-ray bone surveys.

scanning large areas such as the whole body scan, as needed for tumor scanning, bone scanning, or bone marrow scanning (Fig 8–4). (3) Because of the nature of the scanning apparatus, a scan provides a tomograph of the region examined and may be used to define deep lesions without interference from overlying structures.

Radiopharmaceuticals

Nuclear medicine procedures require preferential localization of a radiopharmaceutical in the organ or tissue which is to be studied. If a physiologic function is to be quantified, then the radiopharmaceutical must specifically label the process measured. When an imaging study is used to detect abnormal tissue within an organ, the abnormality may be detected either by (1) localization of the radiopharmaceutical in the lesion or (2) by less radiotracer in the lesion compared to the surrounding organ. Examples of increased uptake in abnormal tissue include the labeling of brain

lesions on a negative background of normal brain and increased bone uptake or labeling in abnormal bone. Examples of diminished localization in abnormal tissue include abnormal areas in the lung, liver, spleen, kidney, and pancreas.

Many radiopharmaceuticals are prepared in the nuclear medicine laboratories where they are used. This is particularly convenient for radioisotopes with short half-lives such as technetium-99m, which is obtained by separation from its longer-lived parent, molybdenum-99.

The common radiopharmaceuticals for static radionuclide imaging are listed in Table 8–2. Technetium-99m is especially useful because it will image so many organs or tissues, has a short half-life, and emits only a single gamma ray and, because of the absence of beta radiation, the radiation exposure to the patient is extremely low.

In addition to the static procedures tabulated in Table 8–2, a number of dynamic procedures are com-

TABLE 8–2. Radiopharmaceuticals for common static imaging procedures.

Organ or Tissue Imaged	Radionuclide	Chemical Form	Labeling Mechanism
Brain	6-hour ^{99m}Tc	Technetium pertechnetate	Increased capillary permeability in abnormal brain (normal brain unlabeled).
Thyroid	8-day ^{131}I 13-hour ^{123}I	Iodide Iodide	Incorporated in thyroid iodide metabolism.
Lung	6-hour ^{99m}Tc 8-day ^{131}I	Macroaggregates (various) Macroaggregated albumin	Particles (average diameter, 30 μm) lodge for 2–8 hours in one of every 10,000 pulmonary arterioles.
Liver, spleen marrow	6-hour ^{99m}Tc	Colloid	Phagocytosis by reticuloendothelial cells of liver (85%), spleen (10%), marrow (5%).
Pancreas	120-day ^{75}Se	Selenomethionine	Participates in pancreas (and liver) amino acid metabolism.
Kidney	2.7-day ^{197}Hg 47-day ^{203}Hg	Chlormerodrin Chlormerodrin	Uptake in renal tubular cells proportionate to renal blood flow. Long biologic half-life.
Bone	1.7-hour ^{18}F 6-hour ^{99m}Tc	Fluoride Technetium polyphosphate	Accumulate in regions of active bone deposition: increased labeling of most abnormal areas.
Placenta	6-hour ^{99m}Tc	Technetium pertechnetate, technetium albumin	Label vascular spaces in placenta
Tumor	3.2-day ^{67}Ga	Gallium citrate	Labels neoplasms (and some localized inflammations)—probably related to reticulum uptake.

monly performed using technetiated albumin for rapid imaging of vascular spaces and the heart, radioxenon gas and solution for pulmonary studies, radioiodinated rose bengal for hepatobiliary studies, radioiodinated hippurate for kidney function studies, and a variety of radioactive compounds to study CSF pathways.

PRINCIPLES OF RADIOISOTOPE IMAGING PROCEDURES

The size of the smallest lesion that can be detected in a scan or scintiphotograph varies depending upon whether it actively takes up the radiopharmaceutical or whether it appears as a "cold area" in a labeled organ. With sufficiently active uptake of the radiopharmaceutical, an infinitely small lesion can be seen. "Cold" lesions are more difficult to identify. They are seen most easily when on the surface or edge of a solid organ and least easily when located centrally. A central lesion in the liver 2.5 cm in diameter should be detectable, whereas a peripheral one half that size should be seen. Generally speaking, scintillation cameras provide better resolution of small detail than rectilinear scanners. The speed of the scintillation camera also allows more photographs and a faster rate of information accumulation, providing better opportunity to detect minimal abnormalities.

Brain

Brain imaging procedures are widely used as screening tests for CNS disease. Scintiphotography provides a cine study of arterial and venous distributions of the tracer immediately after intravenous injection. This permits determination of vascularity in any lesion that is later identified in the static scintiphotographs and also provides an angiographic evaluation which can identify displacement by subdural hematomas, lack of perfusion after a stroke, and prolonged transit time, such as occurs with ischemic brain disease. Abnormal capillary permeability reveals about 90% of primary brain tumors and approximately 75% of metastatic brain lesions, but also accompanies a variety of other diseases such as inflammation, ischemia, infection, and vasculitis. Brain imaging should precede elective craniotomy. The extent of a lesion or the multiplicity of lesions is often appreciated only in the scintiphotographs. Fig 8–5 shows the typical appearance of an abnormal focus of brain labeling; Fig 8–2 shows the appearance of a single frame in a vascular perfusion study which demonstrates bilateral subdural hematomas.

Thyroid

Thyroid scanning provides a regional evaluation of thyroid function. The functional status of a palpable nodule may be determined, and if the nodule is cold the scan provides supportive evidence for excisional biopsy. If a nodule is hot, with evidence of suppression of the remainder of the gland, an autonomous nodule is the likely diagnosis. This may be confirmed by administering thyroid hormone (25 μg of triiodothyronine 3 or 4 times daily for 7 days in adults) and repeating the neck ^{131}I uptake and scan to determine

Dynamic scintiphotos after intravenous injection of a bolus of ^{99m}Tc pertechnetate

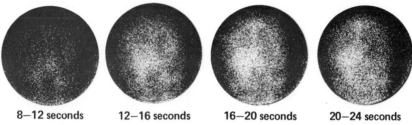

| 8–12 seconds | 12–16 seconds | 16–20 seconds | 20–24 seconds |

Static scintiphotos 90 minutes postinjection

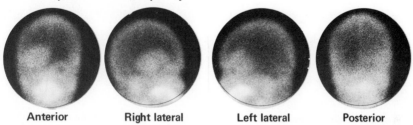

| Anterior | Right lateral | Left lateral | Posterior |

FIG 8–5. **Sphenoid ridge meningioma.** Scintiphotographic examinations allow both dynamic studies of brain blood flow patterns and static photographs of later localization of the radiopharmaceutical. A right sphenoid ridge meningioma is illustrated here which shows rapid filling during the arterial phase of brain vascular filling. There is actually some slight delay of filling of the right hemisphere—seen in the 8- to 12-second scintiphotograph, followed in the next scintiphotograph by a rapid "blooming" of the entire region of the meningioma which persists in its brightly labeled appearance through the 20- to 24-second picture. The static scintiphotographs show the bright frontotemporal abnormality in all projections, but the 2 projections that show it best are the anterior and the right lateral views, where the tumor is closest to the detector. This highly vascular appearance is typical of a meningioma.

whether the nodule has been suppressed. Autonomously functioning nodules are benign lesions and may be managed in a variety of ways, including long-term observation alone. Radioiodide ablation of autonomous nodules never leads to hypothyroidism since the normal tissue is suppressed and does not take up the ^{131}I. Nodules with limited function detected by scan are almost always benign since thyroid cancer does not take up radioiodide when thyrotropic hormone (TSH) levels are normal (euthyroid). Care must be exercised in interpretation of a thyroid scan so that a cold nodule superimposed over functioning tissue will not be misinterpreted as a "warm" nodule with limited function. Other uses of the thyroid scan include evaluation of goiters too large for accurate palpation, determination of the extent of a substernal goiter, and detection of carcinoma and ectopic thyroid tissue. Radioiodide labeling of thyroid cancer requires stimulation by elevated levels of TSH. The author prefers endogenous TSH in a state of temporary hypothyroidism and iodide depletion. Most follicular and papillary thyroid carcinomas show labeling with adequate patient preparation. Fig 8–6 shows examples of radio-iodide concentration in thyroid carcinoma and in ectopic areas.

Lung

The lung is most commonly imaged for diagnosis of suspected thromboemboli. Labeling of the lung with macroaggregates 30 μm in diameter shows the distribution of pulmonary arterial flow by lodging a tracer microembolus in one of every 10,000 (patent) pulmonary arterioles. Only partial and temporary arterial obstruction results from the particle localization The image, therefore, shows blood flow distribution in smaller vessels than those seen in angiograms. There are many other causes of defects of pulmonary perfusion, eg, bronchospasm, atelectasis, inflammation, and bronchogenic carcinoma. Comparison of regional ventilation using radioxenon gas with a perfusion study may help to differentiate the specific cause of decreased perfusion. Perfusion and ventilation studies often contribute unique information in the work-up of a patient before thoracotomy.

Liver

Liver scintiphotography may be performed using

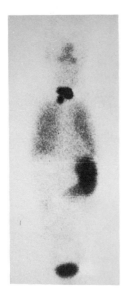 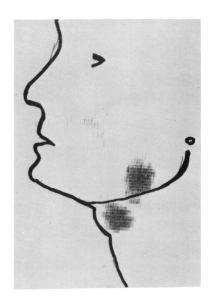

A   **Thyroid carcinoma metastatic**   B   **Ectopic thyroid, lingular**
     to cervical nodes and lungs   **and anterior cervical**

FIG 8–6. Scanning for detection of radioiodide uptake in abnormal locations. These 2 scans show different uses of the scanning technic. *A:* The whole body scan, which was discontinued below the bladder, shows thyroid carcinoma metastatic to cervical nodes. Recognizable normal structures are the paranasal mucosal areas, the salivary glands, the stomach, and the bladder. The labeling in cervical metastases is easily identified. There is a faint generalized labeling abnormality throughout each lung, indicating a general involvement of the lungs by metastatic thyroid carcinoma. This metastatic neoplasm is often amenable to treatment by combinations of neck dissection, radioiodide, and, in some cases, x-ray therapy. *B:* As an example of radioiodide scanning for identification of smaller abnormal localizations, a full-sized 1:1 scan can be performed, as in the illustration on the right. This patient has ectopic thyroid tissue in the superior anterior cervical region and on the tongue. There was no radioiodide uptake in the normal thyroid area, proving the ectopic nature of this patient's thyroid.

colloids which localize in the reticuloendothelial tissue or by using rose bengal dye, which is extracted from blood by hepatocytes and excreted into the bile. Technetium sulfur colloid delineates the liver and also the spleen and bone marrow. Irregularly decreased uptake of colloid is a sensitive indicator of parenchymal liver diseases. Space-occupying liver lesions produce "focal defects" with discrete margins. Other changes seen are distortion of normal liver anatomy, related changes in the size of the spleen and functioning bone marrow, and the degree to which these tissues accumulate the colloid. Fig 8–7 illustrates echinococcal cysts in the liver. Rose bengal I 131 dye provides information about hepatocyte function and the etiology of jaundice. Since the dye is secreted into bile and only small amounts are needed for identification of biliary structures, this test may be particularly useful in distinguishing between intrahepatic and extrahepatic causes of jaundice.

Kidney

Renal structure is best evaluated by an agent which labels the cortex and is retained long enough to obtain a high-resolution image. Chlormerodrin (labeled with radiomercury) and several newer technetium compounds are used for this purpose. Kidney function may be imaged during excretion of radioiodinated hippurate, and renal blood flow may be photographed after rapid peripheral intravenous injection of pertechnetate. Renal carcinoma causes a cold defect in a chlormerodrin image which shows both displacement of the normal cortex by the neoplasm and the influence of the carcinoma on perfusion of the remainder of the kidney. The degree of vascularity in perfusion studies may also be used to detect renal ischemia responsible for hypertension. In addition to diminished perfusion of the ischemic kidney or portion of the kidney, the rate of accumulation of hippurate will be diminished and transit time prolonged, causing late retention of the radiotracer in the ischemic tissue. Renal imaging may also be used for evaluation of kidney trauma, differentiation of cysts from neoplasms, study of transplants for competency of vascular and ureteral anastomoses, and for the evaluation of renal failure. Valuable

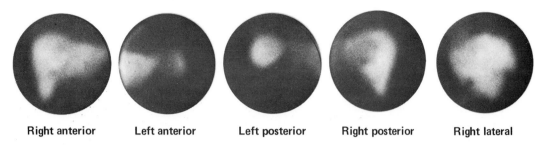

| Right anterior | Left anterior | Left posterior | Right posterior | Right lateral |

FIG 8–7. Echinococcal disease. Any mass lesion in the liver or spleen will show as a defect in the uniform uptake of colloid within these organs. In addition to demonstrating involvement by cancer, isotope scanning is useful in the diagnosis of many nonneoplastic lesions which are of interest to the surgeon, such as this grossly abnormal liver involved by echinococcal cysts. Small defects are appreciated at the inferior margin of the anterior segment of the right lobe in the right anterior view; in the posterior inferior margin of the posterior segment of the right lobe in the right lateral view; and in several other locations. There is a much larger defect approximately 6.5–7.5 cm in diameter occupying the medial and superior aspects of the posterior segment of the right lobe, as best visualized in the right posterior view. The spleen is normal in size, shape, and position in this illustration, and the vertebral bone marrow is not visible at these photographic settings, indicating that the amount of colloid uptake in the marrow is not increased. The presence of mass lesions within this liver does not appear to have greatly influenced either its normal functions or its size, since the amount of colloid uptake in unaffected areas of the liver is normal and liver size is not increased.

information may be obtained by hippurate imaging studies, even in the presence of severe degrees of renal failure.

Bone

Bone scanning is principally of value in the detection of asymptomatic foci of metastatic carcinoma before there is sufficient loss of mineral to show in roentgenograms. Carcinoma, infections, repair after trauma, and arthritis may cause focal abnormalities of bone labeling with any of several tracers. Abnormal bone labeling is recognized as an area of increased uptake of the tracer, as illustrated in Fig 8–4.

Miscellaneous

Many other organs, tissues, or spaces may be imaged: bone marrow, joints, parathyroid adenomas, pancreas, placenta, brain ventricles and cisterns, other CSF spaces (and leaks), salivary glands, urinary bladder, myocardium, and any abnormal space (such as pericardial effusion). Most of these tests have enjoyed limited use. We routinely obtain marrow views during liver and spleen examinations with technetium sulfur colloid and often identify sites of metastases and other bone marrow abnormalities. With attention to technical details, these less frequently utilized tests often provide valuable diagnostic information.

In Vivo Counting Procedures

In vivo counting refers to tests such as that for thyroid radioiodide uptake where the amount of isotope in an area is counted. In general, these tests require far less tracer than imaging tests since a more sensitive lead cylinder collimator is used that allows more exposure of the crystal than do imaging collimators.

The thyroid uptake test measures radioiodide uptake in the neck. The number of radioiodide counts detected in the thigh is subtracted from those detected simultaneously in the neck (assuming equal tissue volumes), and the difference is the content of radioiodide in the thyroid. Exposure to exogenous iodides will cause the radioiodide tracer to represent less of a fraction of the available iodide atoms and result in a decrease of measured percentage uptake in the thyroid. Conversely, a decreased iodide pool will cause elevation of measured percentage thyroid uptakes. Fortunately, iodide pool sizes are relatively constant in most populations. Common sources of increased plasma inorganic iodide are radiographic dyes, tincture of iodine, seafood, and various drugs. Decreased plasma inorganic iodide is most commonly due to diuretic therapy.

If thyroid uptake is in the upper normal range, euthyroid patients should respond to suppressive therapy by reduction of the neck uptake ("suppression test"). Similarly, patients with low radioiodide uptake may be restudied after administration of TSH. Response of a low uptake to TSH suggests secondary hypothyroidism due to pituitary disease; the thyroid does not respond to exogenous TSH stimulation in primary hypothyroidism. Table 8–3 summarizes in vivo thyroid counting tests in relation to the other common thyroid tests.

In vivo counting is also used for estimating radioiodide uptake by functioning metastases from thyroid carcinoma. The retention of radioiodide, as determined by measurement of 72-hour urinary excretion of a test dose, is sometimes equally helpful in deciding whether ^{131}I should be given as treatment for metastases.

Regional in vivo counting is also used to help decide whether to treat hemolytic anemia or thrombocytopenia by splenectomy. Red blood cells or platelets tagged with ^{51}Cr are used to study survival and

TABLE 8-3. Thyroid evaluation.

Condition	TT4	T3 Uptake (Resin)	Neck [131]I Uptake, 24 Hours	T3 Suppression	TSH Stimulation
Euthyroid	5.3–13.0 or 3.4–8.7 μg/100 ml I⁻*	90–110% or 25–35%	15–40%	Responds	Responds
Primary hypothyroidism	↓	↓	↓	Responds	No response
Reduced endogenous TSH	↓	↓	↓	Responds	Responds
Hyperthyroidism	↑	↑	↑	No response	Limited response†
Pregnancy, estrogen treatment	↑	↓	(N usually)	Responds	Responds†
Subacute thyroiditis	↑ early	↑ early	↓ or 0	Responds	Avoid†
Hashimoto's thyroiditis	N or ↓	N or ↓	N or ↓	Responds	Avoid†

*As iodide   ↓ = Reduced
† = No usual need to test or test undesirable   ↑ = Elevated
N = Normal

sequestration by the spleen. Splenectomy usually relieves hemolysis when spleen to liver count ratios are greater than 3:1. Since the counts obtained depend on spleen and liver size and position in addition to the extent of splenic sequestration, this test should be performed in laboratories with considerable hematologic experience.

The radioisotope renogram measures the rate (counts per minute) at which hippurate I 131 is excreted by the kidneys. No image of the kidney is obtained unless the test is performed during scintiphotography. The renogram is sensitive to renal abnormalities and is used for sequential studies of renal function in disease.

In Vitro Counting Procedures

Of the various in vitro counting tests, perhaps the most common are those that measure residual capacity for binding thyroid hormone by the serum proteins. Various resins are used to separate free ^{125}I-triiodothyronine (T3) from that bound to serum protein. T3 binding capacity is low in thyrotoxicosis and high in hypothyroidism. Extravenous factors that influence the serum proteins also affect T3 binding by resin. For example, estrogens increase binding capacity, causing low T3 uptakes.

The level of thyroid hormone in the serum may be measured by in vitro tracer tests. Both the total serum thyroxine and triiodothyronine may be measured, the former by displacement assays and the latter by radioimmunoassay. Displacement assays measure the displacement of a labeled molecule from binding sites in an equilibrium mixture by addition of an unknown amount of unlabeled molecules of the same type. In radioimmunoassays, a specific antibody to the unknown molecule is employed to react with it and allow its measurement. These tests rarely show artifacts in serum levels of the hormones except those related to changes in binding capacity. Free thyroxine remains constant despite differences in binding

capacity. The product of the binding capacity (measured by T3 uptake) and the total serum T4 is proportionate to the free thyroxine in the serum and is called the "free thyroxine index." This product remains normal in euthyroid patients, even when the binding capacity is abnormal.

Plasma volume can be determined by injecting radioiodinated human serum albumin (RISA) intravenously and then measuring its dilution after mixing but before protein loss. Extravascular loss of protein in edematous states, nephrosis, burns, and similar conditions will cause falsely high results.

Red cell mass is determined by tagging the patient's own red cells with chromium-51. The tagged cells are injected intravenously and whole blood, obtained after mixing, is counted to obtain the blood volume. The patient's hematocrit is used to determine the red cell mass and, indirectly, the plasma volume. Similarly, the red cell mass may be determined indirectly from the RISA plasma volume and hematocrit. The test is useful as a baseline before surgery where large changes in circulating volume are anticipated. Tagged red cells may also be used to quantitatively estimate gastrointestinal loss of blood since no reabsorption of the ^{51}Cr occurs from the gut.

The **Schilling test** estimates ileal absorption of vitamin B_{12}. Radioactive vitamin B_{12} tracer is given orally, and the amount excreted in the urine is measured after a "flushing" dose (1 mg) of unlabeled vitamin B_{12} given parenterally 1 hour later. Reduced excretion in the urine is interpreted to mean reduced intestinal absorption. If, in a repeat test, the addition of intrinsic factor to the vitamin B_{12} tracer raises urinary excretion to normal, the faulty absorption may be due to intrinsic factor deficiency. Strictures or blind loop syndrome due to diverticulosis of the small intestine may reduce vitamin B_{12} absorption, which is correctable with antibiotic therapy. Since vitamin B_{12} absorption is confined to the terminal ileum, ileal resection or disease (regional enteritis) may also lower its absorption. Occasionally, severe neurologic sequelae of vitamin B_{12} deficiency are seen in diseases other than classic pernicious anemia and could be avoided or treated after detection of the absorption defect. Displacement assays may also be used to estimate serum vitamin B_{12}, the intrinsic factor level in gastric juice, as well as anti-intrinsic factor antibodies. Direct in vitro assay of vitamin B_{12} does not require the administration of large "flushing doses" of vitamin B_{12} as in the Schilling test.

Other tests entailing stool counting include measurement of intestinal loss of serum protein in exudative enteropathy by ^{51}Cr albumin (already described above), rose bengal I 131 excretion in neonatal jaundice, and fat absorption using radioiodinated fats.

Endocrine surgery has benefited greatly from the development of radioimmunoassays (growth hormone, parathormone, ACTH, insulin, and gastrin) and by displacement assays (thyroxine and various steroid hormones). In the future, a greater variety of radioimmunoassays may be expected for proteins and displacement assays for smaller molecules.

Radioisotope Therapy

With the exception of limited use of agents such as ^{32}P colloid for therapy of effusions and of ^{32}P (as a soluble phosphate) for suppression of bone metastases and hematopoietic and reticuloendothelial malignancies, radioisotopes in nuclear medicine are limited to treatment of thyroid tissue with ^{131}I. This isotope limits several beta particles which deliver most of the therapeutic energy. Since beta particles penetrate tissue to a maximum of a few millimeters, over 90% of the dose of radiation from ^{131}I is restricted to the thyroid. Radioiodide therapy is used in the following circumstances: (1) Thyrotoxicosis in adults (diffuse or nodular goiters) and in juveniles when surgery is contraindicated. (2) Autonomous adenomas with toxicity symptoms from local pressure. (3) Goiters with local symptoms if surgery is contraindicated (uncommon). (4) Thyroid ablation. (5) Thyroid cancer.

Radioiodide is never used during pregnancy or in nursing mothers. The average course of therapy for Graves' disease delivers an ovarian radiation dose as high as a sacral roentgenographic examination. The radiation dose to the testicles is lower. Ophthalmopathy is not aggravated by radioiodide therapy, and there are no local effects (eg, hypoparathyroidism or recurrent laryngeal nerve injury). Large numbers of patients treated with radioiodide have been followed for many years without observation of an increase in leukemia or thyroid carcinomas. Most clinics have dropped the minimal age for therapy to the postadolescent age group.

Even skilled therapists find a 45—55% incidence of hypothyroidism 10 years after radioiodide therapy, but similar incidences of hypothyroidism were observed after surgery in the same studies. However, it is infrequent to have a complete loss of thyroid function after surgery as is sometimes seen after radioiodide therapy.

After proper patient preparation, radioiodide therapy is often curative for thyroid carcinoma metastatic to the lungs, frequently shows complete suppression of radioiodide uptake in metastatic lymph nodes, and is usually only palliative for metastatic bone lesions. Few follicular or papillary carcinomas show enough function for evaluation by ^{131}I iodide until normal thyroid tissue is removed and the patient becomes clinically hypothyroid. The thyroidectomized patient should be prepared by withdrawing long-acting thyroid hormone preparations. Exposure to exogenous iodide should be avoided for at least 3 months. Maintenance therapy with triiodothyronine for 2—3 weeks will allow metabolism of most previously administered tetraiodothyronine. All replacement therapy is then stopped for a further 2—3 weeks before evaluation with radioiodide. After discontinuing triiodothyronine, the hypothyroid patient will raise endogenous TSH production and stimulate ^{131}I uptake by the tumor. Sites of uptake may be evaluated by whole body scanning and regional in vivo counting, and can be quantitated by measurement of radioiodide excretion. Decisions about when to use ^{131}I therapy, its palliative or curative objectives in the individual case, the desirability of further surgical removal of metastatic deposits, and the possibility of radiation teletherapy should be made in conference between the surgeon, radioiodide therapist, and radiation therapist. If radioiodide therapy is elected, the best results are obtained when it is given in repeated courses to a hypothyroid and iodide-deprived patient until no further localization is detected.

• • •

General References

Belcher EH, Vetter H (editors): *Radioisotopes in Medical Diagnosis.* Appleton-Century-Crofts, 1971.

Blahd WH: *Nuclear Medicine,* 2nd ed. McGraw-Hill, 1971.

DeLand FH, Wagner HN: *Atlas of Nuclear Medicine.* Vol 3. *Reticuloendothelial System, Liver, Spleen and Thyroid.* Saunders, 1972.

Potchen EJ, McCready VR (editors): *Neuro Nuclear Medicine: Progress in Nuclear Medicine.* Vol 1. University Park, 1972.

Sodee B, Early PJ: *Technology and Interpretation of Nuclear Medicine Procedures.* Mosby, 1972.

9 . . .

Wound Healing

Thomas K. Hunt, MD

Without the capacity for repair and regeneration, no organism could survive the trauma of surgery. Only a century ago, complicated and incomplete healing after injury was the rule rather than the exception. Surgeons had little choice but to accept infected, draining wounds. Lister's first application of antisepsis changed surgery as dramatically as the discovery of anesthesia had 30 years before. Today, surgeons tend to ignore the healing process since it usually proceeds without obvious incident. Even so, poor healing and excessive healing continue to be leading causes of disability and death.

In the last 100 years, knowledge of the basic mechanisms of healing has grown rapidly. For the first time in history, surgeons who have a detailed knowledge of these mechanisms can influence healing and are able to anticipate and often prevent problems of incomplete and excessive repair.

THE NATURE OF THE WOUND

Healing is essentially a process in which injury and subsequent inflammation are followed by synthesis of new connective tissue and epithelium with its vascular and lymphatic supply. Inflammation and repair, however, are found in numerous places and conditions other than those usually considered injuries. The intravascular thrombus "organizes," ie, it heals. The hardness of the scirrhous carcinoma is due to intense "healing" and fibrosis in the tumor. Malformations of joints and heart valves in rheumatic conditions are the result of "healing." The word wound might even be defined as any event which is followed by healing. The common element of a "wound" in all of these illustrations is a tissue in which nutrition (or microcirculation) has become inadequate to the needs of living cells. For example, local hypoxia is a major feature of injured tissue. Cell death and inflammation then follow, with increased vascular permeability, appearance of fibroblasts, fibroplasia, and regrowth of local microcirculation.

The exact reason why cell death and loss of tissue nutrition trigger inflammation and subsequent healing is not known. Menkin, among others, postulated the existence of "wound hormones," but no proof of the existence of such substances has been found. The changing environmental conditions which exist after the disruption of normal tissue nutrition might stimulate enzyme induction and cell proliferation. On the other hand, it is equally possible that proteolysis, which follows injury, releases active polypeptides which may initiate the processes of repair. For example, bradykinin, a low molecular weight peptide which causes local vasodilatation, is found in large quantities in burned tissue.

FORMS OF HEALING

Surgeons customarily divide the types of wound healing into first, second, and third intention healing (Fig 9–1). **First intention** healing occurs when tissue is cleanly incised and reapproximated, and repair occurs without complication. **Second intention** healing is the healing of an open wound (or a closed [dead] space) through formation of granulation tissue* and eventual coverage of the defect by spontaneous migration of epithelial cells. Most infected wounds and burns heal in this manner. One can easily see that primary (first intention) healing is simpler and requires less time and material than secondary healing, in which the defect must be filled with new tissue before coverage can take place. It sometimes happens that primary healing is possible but insufficient reserve is present to allow secondary healing. For example, an ischemic limb may heal primarily, but if the wound opens or becomes infected, the wound might not heal. Amputation may then become necessary.

Healing by **third intention**, a little used term, occurs when a wound is left to accomplish the first phases of healing while open and is then closed to finish healing as if by first intention. Wound infection in contaminated wounds can often be avoided by leaving the wound open for 4 days and then closing it to heal by third intention (so-called secondary or

---

*Granulation tissue is the red, granular, moist tissue which appears during healing of open wounds. Microscopically, it contains new collagen, blood vessels, fibroblasts, and inflammatory cells, especially macrophages.

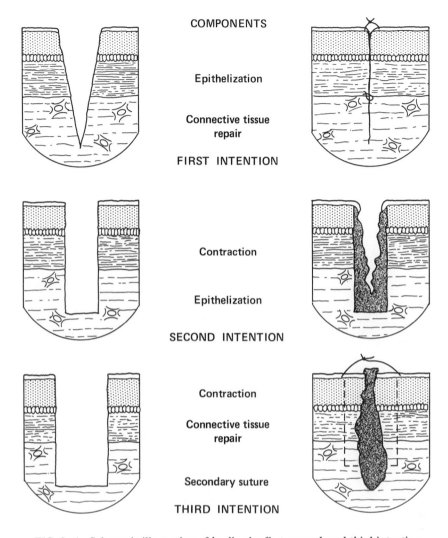

COMPONENTS

Epithelization

Connective tissue repair

FIRST INTENTION

Contraction

Epithelization

SECOND INTENTION

Contraction

Connective tissue repair

Secondary suture

THIRD INTENTION

FIG 9–1. Schematic illustration of healing by first, second, and third intention.

delayed primary closure). The wound is less likely to become infected while open than the wound closed primarily. The closed wound is most susceptible to infection in the first 4 days. Closure of a wound by skin graft is also an example of third intention healing.

THE PHASES OF HEALING

Normal primary healing is customarily divided into 3 phases: substrate phase (lag phase), proliferative phase, and resorptive phase. These are not really satisfactory divisions and cannot be defined precisely. They are useful only as descriptive terms in discussing the continuous process of healing.

Immediately after injury, damaged vascular structures thrombose, fluids exude into the damaged area from blood and lymph, and inflammation begins. Tis-

sue in the ischemic, injured area is lysed and removed. These events continue for 3–5 days. This is the **substrate phase**, in which the wound is prepared for subsequent healing.

The sequence of healing is essentially inviolable. If the events of the substrate phase are prevented—eg, by anti-inflammatory corticosteroids—subsequent healing will not occur.

The so-called **proliferative phase** begins as the first fibroblasts appear in the wound (as early as 2 or 3 days). Collagen synthesis begins shortly thereafter. The combination of preexisting and new collagen gives the wound its strength. By the fifth or sixth day, many fibroblasts have appeared, new collagen synthesis accelerates, and tensile strength increases rapidly—hence the name proliferative phase. This busy state continues for several weeks.

In the early proliferative phase, synthesis of new and lysis of old collagen take place simultaneously, and the bridging of the tissue discontinuity becomes a

struggle between the lysis and the synthesis of collagen. Any exaggeration of lysis of old collagen or
delay or diminution of synthesis may cause dehiscence
of the wound or leakage of an anastomosis. In the
section on factors affecting healing (see below), this
important concept is explained in more detail. A collagenolytic enzyme has been identified and characterized. One of the intriguing new aspects of collagenolytic phenomena is the recent discovery of a circulating collagenase inhibitor. For example, this system of
"collagenase and anticollagenase" may influence tensile strength, tissue synthesis, and wound remodeling
(Fig 9–2).

If all goes well, tensile strength increases rapidly
after a few days. Wounds in warm, highly vascular tissues such as the head and neck may be secure enough
so that skin sutures can be removed by the third day.
Wounds of the abdomen heal more slowly but are
usually secure enough so that skin sutures can be
removed by the seventh day, although they have now
gained only about 20% of the original strength of the
abdominal wall. Wounds of the extremities heal even
more slowly. Wounds in the gastrointestinal tract may
be even stronger than the normal tissue by 10 days.

The intense activity of the wound during this
phase causes a ridge of induration about 1 cm wide
around the wound. In a wound healing by first intention, this is called the healing ridge and can easily be
felt. If this ridge is complete along the length of the
wound, it implies good healing, and dehiscence will not
occur. If it is absent by 7–9 days, dehiscence becomes
a definite risk but is not inevitable.

In the last, or **resorptive phase**, the individuality
of the wound is slowly lost and it begins to resemble
normal tissue more and more closely. Fibroblasts and
macrophages disappear, and excessive collagen is
removed. Collagen is still synthesized more rapidly in
the wound than in normal tissue even after many
weeks, but a net resorption occurs during this phase. In
fact, the time at which the resorptive phase begins
might be defined as the time when net accumulation of

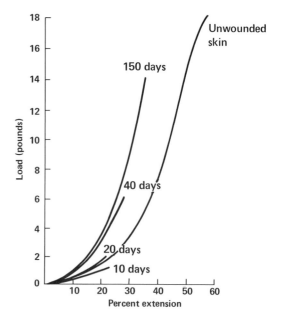

FIG 9–3. Tensile strength increases for at least 150
days after injury and suture. Extensibility also
increases. Obviously, collagen remodeling is
occurring. (See Fig 18–3.)

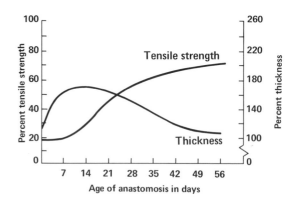

FIG 9–4. The strength of an anastomosis increases
while its thickness or mass decreases during the
resorptive phase.

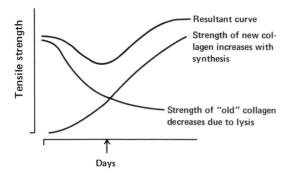

FIG 9–2. Tensile strength is the resultant between
the strength of old collagen as affected by lysis
and new collagen as affected by synthesis and
lysis.

collagen ceases and net collagen loss begins. As a consequence of the turnover of collagen in this phase, the
collagenous mass in the wound is remodeled. The
amorphous mass of collagen seen in the early wound
gradually becomes an interlocking network of large
collagen fibers joining the more normal-appearing collagen fibers at the edge of the wound. Presumably as a
consequence of remodeling, the breaking strength of
the skin or fascial wound increases for up to 6 months
even though the total amount of collagen in the area
decreases. Unfortunately, remodeling does not proceed
to the point of normality. Skin and fascia, for example, eventually achieve only about 80% of their normal

strength, and their other mechanical properties such as elasticity and capacity for energy absorption probably never return to normal. The end result is a serviceable but somewhat weak and brittle tissue (scar).

COMPONENTS OF REPAIR

The reparative process has 3 major components: epithelization, connective tissue regeneration, and contraction. Regeneration or hyperplasia of the parenchymatous remainder of an organ may also contribute, thus compensating for the loss of cellular function due to injury.

Epithelization

Within a few days following injury, epithelial cells at the edge of the wound become rounded and mitoses appear in the regenerative layers. Cells then migrate across the wound, remaining always in contact with (and partly controlled by) mesenchymal tissues. Squamous cells will advance deep to dead tissue, thus eventually covering a defect and debriding "eschar" at the same time. The new epithelium is usually thinner and less pigmented than normal.

Epithelial repair in special tissues such as the gastrointestinal tract has unique features which are beyond the scope of this chapter.

Connective Tissue Regeneration & Repair

Connective tissue regenerates to fill a tissue defect largely by the effect of inflammatory cells, vascular and lymphatic endothelial cells, and fibroblasts. Inflammatory cells are particularly prominent in the early phase of healing, and their presence is generally regarded as a response to injury. On the other hand, the macrophage is seldom far from the fibroblast when active tissue synthesis or remodeling is occurring. The exact relationship of the 2 cells is not known. The macrophage (among other functions) probably digests protein and supplies amino acids to the fibroblast.

Photomicrographs of "budding" and regenerating blood and lymph vessels are abundantly available, but very little is known about these cells. The re-formation of the nutritional transport system is absolutely essential to healing of all but the most minor wounds. The immense potential for lymph-vascular regeneration has been recognized only recently. The Vineberg myocardial revascularization procedure takes full advantage of it, as do operations employing omental implantation for relief of lymphedema.

The fibroblast is a large cell which is well endowed with protein-synthesizing endoplasmic reticulum. It synthesizes collagen and probably mucopolysaccharide as well. The fibroblast synthesizes the basic molecule—the "monomer"—of the polymeric collagen fiber, a long, thin, triple helix approximately 289 × 1.4 nm. These molecules are secreted into the extracellular space, where they slowly polymerize to form

large, strong, insoluble fibers (Fig 9–5). Recent evidence indicates that "vegetative" fibroblasts originate in the injured area.

The joining of the sides of a wound with collagen fibers is similar to building a bridge across a chasm. As each steel beam is locked into place, the bridge gains strength and span.

During collagen synthesis, proline is incorporated into the growing peptide chain. Proline molecules are subsequently converted to hydroxyproline by the action of protocollagen hydroxylase and molecular oxygen. Lysine is incorporated and hydroxylated similarly. This vital reaction requires iron, molecular (dissolved) oxygen, ascorbic acid, and α-ketoglutarate. If proline is not hydroxylated, collagen escape from the cell is hindered. Without hydroxylation of lysine, intramolecular and intermolecular bonding is diminished and a structurally poor collagen results. This suggests that healing would be impaired by severe iron and ascorbic acid deficiencies and states of local or systemic hypoxia. In practice, simple iron deficiency does not seem to impair healing. Ascorbic acid and oxygen deficiencies, however, are well known for their deleterious effects on healing.

Hydroxylysine molecules are oxidized to the aldehyde form and "condense" with other such lysine groups to form covalent cross-links within and between molecules. This step adds rigidity to the molecule and fiber. The reaction can be inhibited by β-aminopropionitrile (BAPN) and by penicillamine. A disease known as lathyrism that occurs naturally in animals

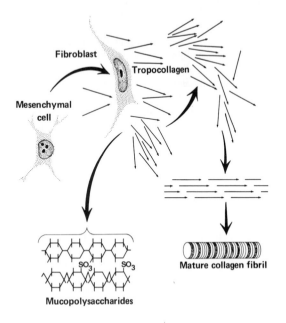

FIG 9–5. Schematic representation of collagen synthesis, deposition, and polymerization. The molecules polymerize with a "three-fourths stagger" overlap, which accounts for the cross-banding visible on electron microscopy.

fed peas containing BAPN is of great interest to surgeons because it may offer a clue to the control of the physical properties of scar tissue.

Several congenital defects of collagen bonding have been identified that lead to poor healing and easily broken collagen. They are extremely rare, but it seems reasonable to speculate that more subtle forms may contribute to hernia formation and occasional instances of poor fibrous repair.

In the differentiation phase of healing, a slow "tightening" of collagen fibers apparently occurs, which is why tensile strength increases despite a net loss of collagen. This "remodeling" may be due to a number of processes, including turnover of collagen, fiber shrinkage, and increasing intermolecular bonding. Remodeling is affected by mechanical stress, which partly determines the amount, form, and architecture of the final product.

The extracellular environment must be favorable for alignment and approximation of the collagen monomers. It is presumed that the ground substance, which is composed of sulfated and nonsulfated mucopolysaccharides of high molecular weight, provides this environment. These substances give the wound its characteristic metachromatic staining properties. A small amount of mucopolysaccharide is incorporated into the collagen fiber.

Nutritional substances necessary for collagen and mucopolysaccharide synthesis, cell replication, cellular nutrition, and energy metabolism must be delivered to the healing area, and waste products of metabolism must be removed. Unfortunately, as noted above, circulation to the area of injury has been partly disrupted. In connective tissue wounds (dermis, fascia, etc), the need for circulation is greater after injury but the perfusion capability is less.

Preexisting (and functioning) capillaries at the edge of the injured tissue send capillary buds toward the edge of the wound. The buds then bend and meet each other, thus forming new capillary arches capable of maintaining circulation. In primary healing, preexisting divided vessels "inosculate" and reacquire circulation, but in tissue defects this is not possible. The regenerating capillaries are fragile and easily injured. They must stay within the support of newly synthesized collagen to avoid bursting from transmitted blood pressure. At the same time, however, they must approach the advancing front of healing tissue in order to supply its needs. This tenuous situation of the microcirculation suggests that tissue nutrition at this point in the wound may be of borderline adequacy. In fact, oxygen tension at the advancing edge is quite low and hydrogen ion concentration and P_{CO_2} are quite high.

Contraction

Contraction is a mysterious process by which open skin wounds spontaneously shrink and close. The phenomenon in open wounds in man was recognized and described by John Hunter. It is perhaps better termed "intussusceptive" healing since normal tissue is pulled into the open area to achieve coverage. Huge defects on the back of the neck and other areas of loose skin will completely close by contraction. Contraction is not so rapid in other areas of the body.

Contraction should be distinguished from contracture, or loss of joint motion from shrinking scar tissue.

The contractile force has been measured and is roughly equivalent to forces exerted by known cellular systems. The currently popular view of contraction is that it depends on a contractile system in the fibroblast since contraction is independent of collagen content and other measurable biochemical components of the wound. The reparative fibroblast contains microfibrils indistinguishable from those of smooth muscle cells. Smooth muscle stimulators and inhibitors influence contraction. This similarity of function and appearance of fibroblasts and smooth muscle cells has also been noted in arterial injuries and atheromas. Cortisone and vinblastine stop contraction.

Experienced clinicians often remain patient and rely on contraction to close wounds in favorable areas. Skin grafts placed prematurely on rapidly contracting wounds will greatly inhibit contraction, and large skin graft scars remain where previously the wound was destined to be covered by normal skin.

HEALING OF SPECIALIZED TISSUES

Nerve

Brain heals largely through connective tissue scar formation in which glial and perivascular cells seem to differentiate to fibroblasts. When a peripheral nerve is severed, the distal nerve degenerates, leaving the axon sheaths to heal together by inosculation. The axon then regenerates from the nerve cell through the reconstituted sheaths, advancing as much as 1 mm/day. Unfortunately, because individual neural sheaths have no means of seeking out their original distal ends, the axon sheaths reconnect randomly, and motor nerve axons may regenerate in vain into a sensory distal sheath and end organ. The functional result of neural regeneration, therefore, is more satisfactory in the "purer" peripheral nerves.

Intestine

The intestine has received little attention from students of healing. The rate of healing apparently varies from one portion of the intestine to the other. Anastomoses of the colon and esophagus are quite precarious and likely to leak, whereas leakage of stomach or small intestinal anastomoses is rare. The intestinal anastomosis usually regains strength so rapidly that by 1 week it resists bursting more strongly than the more normal surrounding tissue. One reason for this is that the surrounding intestine participates in the reaction to injury, loses a large portion of its collagen by lysis, and consequently loses strength. For this reason, perforation is about as likely to occur a few millimeters from the anastomosis as it is in the anastomosis itself. The development of linear strength in intestine occurs at about the same rate as in skin, although the stomach and small bowel are somewhat quicker to "heal." Bursting strength is greatly enhanced early after injury because edema and induration in the wound limit distention of the segment and hence protect against bursting.

Any event which delays collagen synthesis or exaggerates collagen lysis is likely to increase the risk of perforation and leakage. The danger of leakage is greatest from the fourth to seventh days, when tensile strength is normally expected to rise rapidly. Local infection promotes lysis and delays synthesis; it often occurs near esophageal and colonic anastomoses, thus increasing the likelihood of perforation.

Bone

Healing in bone depends largely on connective tissue synthesis. Bone healing, however, also depends on a unique process, the condensation of hydroxyapatite crystals on specific points on the collagen fiber with an end result analogous to reinforced concrete. The long time required for attainment of full strength in healing fractures is well known, but it is not really much longer than that required for development of full strength in soft tissue wounds. Full calcification is so important clinically that the impression is given that bone healing is protracted. Bone healing also graphically illustrates the process of remodeling described above for soft tissue. The large callus seen after a month or so in a healing fracture often remodels until x-ray films must be examined quite carefully to see where the fracture was. The effect of mechanical stress on connective tissue healing is also well illustrated by the fact that, even though bone ends may be poorly aligned, the end result after months of remodeling shows that the bone has healed along the normal lines of stress.

The details of bone healing are thoroughly described in many texts and will not be discussed here.

Skin Grafts

The healing of skin grafts is unique in that their vascular supply has been completely interrupted. In the critical 3–4 days after a graft is placed, there is a remarkable inosculation of small vessels of the host to those of the graft. If enough vessels can be joined, the graft lives. We can now understand why immobilization of a skin graft is so important to its survival since very little collagen can be synthesized in these first few days and the graft is anchored only by the adhesiveness of fibrin. Immune mechanisms can attack a skin homograft only after circulation has been established. A second-set rejection usually occurs by 7 days, indicating that circulation is usually competent by that time.

SUTURE MATERIALS

The ideal suture material has not been designed. The ideal suture must be flexible and strong and must tie easily and securely. It should excite little tissue reaction, and should not be a nidus for infection. Monofilament suture is less likely to harbor bacteria, but it is also more likely to break and to tie poorly.

Stainless steel wire is inert and maintains strength for a long time. However, wire is difficult to tie, often causes the patient undue pain, and, being brittle, eventually fragments. It does not harbor bacteria, and it can be left in granulating wounds, when necessary, with the expectation that it will be covered by granulation tissue without causing abscesses.

Plastic sutures are generally inert and retain strength even longer than wire. However, they generally make insecure knots and must usually be knotted at least 4 times, resulting in large amounts of retained foreign body. Contrary to popular opinion, most multifilament plastic sutures are just as apt to become infected and migrate to the surface as silk sutures. Monofilament plastic, in common with wire, will not harbor bacteria. Nylon monofilament is extremely nonreactive and is a good suture material for skin and cornea, although it is difficult to tie. Polyethylene suture has a tendency to break. Monofilament polypropylene seems a satisfactory suture and ties well but is more reactive than nylon. Plastic sutures, because of their inertness, are best for cardiovascular work. Experiments are now being performed on synthetic polymers which can be resorbed. This is a promising new technic. The first such material, polyglycolic acid, is now widely used. Its absorption is more uniform and predictable than that of catgut.

Silk is an animal protein but is nearly inert in human tissue. It ties easily and is commonly used. Since it does lose its strength over a long period, it is unsuitable for suturing arteries to plastic implants or for insertion of prosthetic cardiac valves. Because fibrous tissue cannot securely anchor a plastic prosthesis to tissue, the sutures must maintain strength indefinitely. Silk sutures are multifilament and are a haven for bacteria, although even contaminated wounds sutured with silk will usually heal without infection. Occasionally, silk sutures form a focus for small abscesses which migrate and "spit" through the skin, forming small sinuses which will not heal until the offending silk is removed.

Catgut (made from the submucosa of sheep intestine) will eventually resorb, but the resorption time is highly variable. Catgut excites considerable inflammatory reaction, which is the means of resorption. Catgut suture is prepared in 2 ways: (1) plain catgut is simply twisted and dried before sterilization; (2) chromic catgut is "tanned" like leather in a strong solution of chromate ion. The chromic catgut causes less inflammation and absorbs slowly (20 days or more). Plain catgut causes more inflammation and is absorbed more rapidly. Unfortunately, the more reactive a suture, the more likely it is to be the site of infection. Contrary to popular opinion, catgut is used in contaminated wounds simply because it will resorb if it becomes the site of infection and will not "spit" to the surface. If a wound sutured with catgut becomes infected, the catgut is likely to resorb quickly and break before the wound is secure.

A new technic in the manufacture of absorbable sutures involves the ultrafine division of **bovine tendon** and its reconstitution into so-called **collagen suture**. This material, almost pure collagen, appears to cause less inflammation and has a somewhat more constant resorption time than collagen.

Skin tapes are the skin closure of choice for so-called clean contaminated wounds because they minimize the probability of subcutaneous infection. They are somewhat harder to use than skin sutures and cannot be used on actively bleeding wounds or wounds with complex surfaces, such as the perineum. They minimize infection by avoiding the presence of a foreign body in the form of a skin suture which connects the skin surface to the wound dead space.

Sutures are foreign bodies which strangulate tissue and cause inflammation. They are at best a necessary evil, and needless sutures should be avoided. Postlethwaite and his associates have published extensive investigations into the properties of suture materials.

IMPLANTS

New prosthetic materials are constantly being introduced. Among the metals, titanium, and among the alloys, Vitallium have shown the least tendency to corrode and wear. Solid implants such as joint replacements have worked well, but mesh implants have eventually fragmented.

Plastic implants are long-lasting and are well tolerated by tissue. Teflon, nylon, and Silastic are the most inert. Teflon has a nonwettable surface, and connective tissue will not penetrate fine Teflon mesh. As a result, the neo-intima in Teflon arterial prostheses tends to break off and embolize. High-density polyethylene has even been used for weight-bearing joint prostheses. Artificial joints made of a combination of plastic and metal are now being widely used to replace hips, knees, and even digital articular surfaces damaged by disease or injury.

Silastic seems to be the current material of choice for solid implants for plastic surgery since it can be easily molded and sutured in place.

Dacron has a wettable surface, and connective tissue will penetrate and envelop Dacron mesh. It is the current material of choice for vascular implants.

Even the best plastic is still a foreign body. Infection around plastic prostheses of all sorts remains a major problem. Autologous tissue is mandatory for grafting into a contaminated area.

CONTROLLABLE FACTORS AFFECTING HEALING

Nutrition

Mild to moderate nutritional deficiencies do not affect healing, which seems to have a high priority in the body economy. However, major acute nutritional depletion does retard healing.

Protein depletion (as opposed to protein starvation alone) inhibits healing if recent weight loss exceeds 20% of original body weight. Dehiscence occurs more often in patients who have quickly lost large amounts of weight and have a low serum albumin concentration. Some of the effects of protein depletion have been overcome in animals by feeding methionine, which is a particularly essential amino acid for wound healing. Methionine acts as a sulfur source and methylating agent.

The first nutritional substance discovered to be important to wound healing was ascorbic acid. In ascorbic acid deficiency (scurvy), wound healing is arrested in early fibroplasia. Many fibroblasts appear in the wound, but synthesis of collagen is grossly impaired. The scorbutic wound responds rapidly to treatment with ascorbic acid treatment. As noted above, ascorbic acid is essential in the formation of collagen, specifically because it is required for the hydroxylation of proline. It has other functions also.

Zinc deficiency also retards wound healing. An indolent open wound with "atrophic" granulations and a prominent yellow-gray exudate suggests zinc deficiency. Serum zinc levels below 100 $\mu g/100$ ml have been associated with poor healing. Zinc sulfate, 220 mg 3 times daily, is an effective and safe treatment. The actual mechanism of action is not known. There is no evidence that supplemental zinc will accelerate the healing of normal wounds.

Diabetes

Healing is often retarded in diabetics. Several mechanisms are probably operative. Diabetic vascular disease probably leads to oxygen deficiency, which retards healing. Poor circulation also lowers tissue temperature, and this too can retard healing. Intermediary carbohydrate metabolism is prominent in healing tissue and is necessary to fulfill energy requirements for protein synthesis. Any impairment due to insulin deficiency would be expected to impair healing. Certainly, the susceptibility to infection which occurs in diabetes presents a hazard to primary healing.

Temperature

The rate of healing in poikilothermic animals is directly dependent upon body temperature. It is assumed that this is why cutaneous wounds of the cooler extremities heal less rapidly than those in the normally warmer skin of the trunk.

Oxygen

Wounds in ischemic tissue heal poorly or not at

all. Recent research has shown that oxygen deficiency is a prominent feature common to most wounds. Any decrease in oxygen supply to the wound impairs healing, and increased oxygen supply can accelerate healing above the accepted normal rate. The place for supplemental oxygen in accelerating healing is not yet well defined, but it seems to be effective in open, poorly healing, nonnecrotic wounds where impaired blood supply is the major reason for inadequate healing. Extra oxygen appears to increase the "take" of skin grafts. On the other hand, oxygen supply can be impaired even when vascular disease is not present. Hypovolemia and vasoconstriction can rob a wound of its oxygen supply and virtually stop healing. Overly tight sutures can do the same.

One might expect that anemia would also produce hypoxia in wounds. In fact, this is not true. Studies on wound healing and anemia are of 2 types: (1) those in which anemia was produced by inducing hypovolemia and (2) those in which blood volume was kept normal. In the first group, all investigators have reported impaired healing. In the second group, healing is normal. The P_{O_2} of arterial blood rather than the oxygen content of blood reaching the wound seems to be the principal determinant of oxygen supply to the wound since oxygen tensions and collagen synthesis are essentially normal in wounds in anemic but normovolemic animals. Furthermore, increasing arterial P_{O_2} above the hemoglobin-oxygen dissociation curve enhances collagen synthesis far beyond the effect to be expected on the basis of increased oxygen volume delivered.

Corticosteroids

Exogenous corticosteroids impair healing. In the primarily closed wound, these drugs interfere with healing most profoundly when given in the first 3 days after injury. After 3 days, the effect is much reduced. They reduce the inflammatory reaction and impair subsequent collagen synthesis. On the other hand, corticosteroids impair contraction of open wounds no matter when they are given. Their effect on collagen synthesis and inflammation does not readily explain the effect on contraction.

Vitamin A & Cartilage Powder

Under certain circumstances, vitamin A can restore corticosteroid-retarded healing toward normal. The effect is clinically useful. It occurs both with systemic and local application of vitamin A. Systemic use of vitamin A for patients who are receiving corticosteroids for control of inflammatory disease must be undertaken cautiously since, if the vitamin can counteract the effects of the corticosteroid on the wound, it presumably may counteract other anti-inflammatory effects of the drug.

Vitamin A is probably important to repair since severely hypovitaminotic animals synthesize collagen poorly. Less extensive human studies indicate but do not prove a role for vitamin A in human repair.

Cartilage powder will accelerate normal healing

slightly in the first 7–10 days and will also antagonize the effect of corticosteroids. The mechanism is not known, but the active agent apparently is chitin.

INFECTION & RESISTANCE

The closed wound would seem an ideal site for bacterial growth. It is moist, dark, filled with serum, and the P_{CO_2} is high and the P_{O_2} low. However, although all wounds are contaminated, relatively few become infected. Resistance to infection is a property of the well-healing wound. Numerous studies have pointed out 3 major prerequisites for infection: (1) a receptive host, (2) contamination by microorganisms, and (3) some particular reason for susceptibility in the wound. All 3 are variable and act independently. The susceptible host is one who is debilitated, has a disease which is reducing the immune or inflammatory response, is taking corticosteroids, or is providing poor wound nutrition. The more bacteria contaminating the wound, the more likely is an infection. However, wound factors are extremely important. Clostridial infections will not occur unless dead tissue is present within the wound. Sutures obviously increase susceptibility. Trauma to the wound (producing a particular reason for susceptibility to infection) is as important a contributing factor in postoperative infection as is the introduction of bacteria.

Antibiotics reach the wound in effective concentrations. Antibiotics given in such a manner that effective concentrations exist at the time of wounding will prevent wound infection if the contaminating bacteria are sensitive to the antibiotic used. Antibiotic prophylaxis, to be effective, depends on the coincidence of the right antibiotic and the sensitive organism. Obviously, prophylaxis is unlikely to be effective in the vast majority of instances where the contaminants may be multiple and unpredictable. However, a few situations can be defined in which prophylaxis is useful. Penicillin should be given when streptococcal or clostridial infections are a definite risk (rheumatic heart disease, severe burns, severe tissue damage and contamination with dirt). It now appears that prophylaxis has some value in the high-risk situation of colon surgery. In prescribing prophylactic antibiotics, one must always balance the risks of side-effects and the emergence of resistant strains of bacteria against the probability of usefulness of the antibiotic. To be effective, antibiotics must be given long enough before operation to ensure high tissue concentrations when the wound is open and exposed. In most cases, less than one hour is required. For the clean surgical operation, antibiotic prophylaxis has little or no value.

There is increasing evidence that topical antibiotics reduce the incidence of infection in moderately contaminated wounds.

DECUBITUS ULCERS

Decubitus ulcers are disastrous complications of immobilization either in bed or in casts. They result primarily from prolonged pressure which robs an area of tissue of its blood supply. However, in practice, irritative or contaminated injections and prolonged contact with moisture, urine, and feces also play a prominent role. Most patients who contract decubitus ulcers are also poorly nourished. Pressure ulcers are becoming more common in drug addicts who take overdoses and lie immobile for many hours at a time. The ulcers vary in depth and often extend from skin to a pressure point such as the greater trochanter or the sacrum. Necrotic fascia is often eventually exposed.

Most decubitus ulcers are preventable. Hospital-acquired ulcers represent inadequate nursing care.

Treatment is difficult and usually prolonged. The first important step is to incise and drain any infected necrotic spaces. Dead tissue is then debrided until the exposed surfaces are all viable and granulating. Many will then heal spontaneously. However, deep ulcers may require closure, sometimes with removal of underlying protuberant bone. The defect is closed by judicious cutting of flaps and movement of thick tissue over the susceptible area.

SURGICAL TECHNIC

Good surgical technic remains the most important and the most immediately available means of achieving optimal healing. Most cases of healing failure are due to technical problems. In the conduct of every operation, the skin should be excluded from the operative field in order to avoid contamination. Tissue should be protected from drying and from internal or external contamination. Fine instruments, sharp dissection, minimal and skillful use of the electrocautery, and minimal and skillful use of ligatures and sutures with the avoidance of strangulation of tissues are essential. All of these contribute to one of the greatest assets of a surgeon—gentleness in handling tissue. Even the best ligature remains a foreign body which is tied tightly in order to strangulate tissue. Even the best suture has the same properties. The skillful operator who uses sutures minimally and gently will be rewarded with the best results. Perfect hemostasis is a laudable objective, but with patience, gentleness, and skill, it can be obtained by securing a minimal number of bleeding points. Too much sponging and electrocautery and tying of small vessels is traumatic and invites infection.

In common with many other points of surgical technic, the exact method of wound closure may be less important than how well it is performed. The tearing strength of sutures from fascia is no greater than 3—4 kg. There is little reason for use of sutures of greater strength than this. Tight closure strangulates tissue and leads to hernia formation and infection.

Wound Closure

If surgeons could foresee the future, dehiscence would not occur since technics to prevent dehiscence are well known. The surgeon can choose his technics to meet the needs and risks of the individual wound (Figs 9—6, 9—7, and 9—8).

The ideal closure for small wounds in healthy patients is done with fine, interrupted sutures placed loosely and conveniently close to the wound edge. In abdominal wounds, the peritoneum is usually closed with a running mattress of 0 or 00 catgut.

Unfortunately, the surgeon is often required to operate on patients who represent a major "wound healing risk." In these cases, closures must be more secure in order to avoid dehiscence. A more secure closure usually begins with a chromic catgut running mattress suture in the peritoneum (or joint capsule or submucosa). The closure is continued with vertical mattress buried retention sutures through fascia and peritoneum in which the farthest point of penetration is at least 1 cm from the wound edge. By placing the tension this far back, one avoids the fascial fibers which become weakened by postinjury collagen lysis. The lytic effect extends often for 5 mm to each side of the wound edge. The ideal suture is placed in far-far, near-near fashion, but simple, widely placed sutures alternating with single narrower sutures are also used. The subcutaneous layers can then be reasonably approximated by a few subcuticular sutures. The skin is preferably closed with adhesive strips unless bleeding from the wound or an uneven surface makes the adherence of the strips precarious. The advantages of this technic of closure are its security and the fact that with it the skin of severely contaminated wounds can easily be left open for delayed primary or secondary closure.

Another very secure closure is used in particularly difficult wounds. This consists of through-and-through mattress sutures of No. 22—26 steel wire placed through all layers, including skin and peritoneum. They are placed about 2.5 cm away from the wound and 2.5 cm apart. With these sutures held on tension to approximate the wound edges, the peritoneum can be closed with a running chromic catgut suture, and the fascia—if possible or desirable—can be closed with a few "catgut" sutures. The heavy retention sutures are twisted together at the side of the wound to produce coaptation of the wound edges. Wound edema will make these sutures too tight within the next few days, and the twisted wires can be partly untwisted to prevent strangulation of tissue and cutting through of sutures. For this reason, plastic sutures are not recommended for this closure since they cannot be twisted to tighten or loosen the closure as required. In the latter case, instead of the plastic sutures holding the wound together, they merely limit how far it can fall apart. Sutures strung across the open wound edge act as "bowstrings" and can cut through bowel, resulting in fistula formation. This "through-and-through retention" closure with very long wire is obviously rather painful to the patient and should be used only when

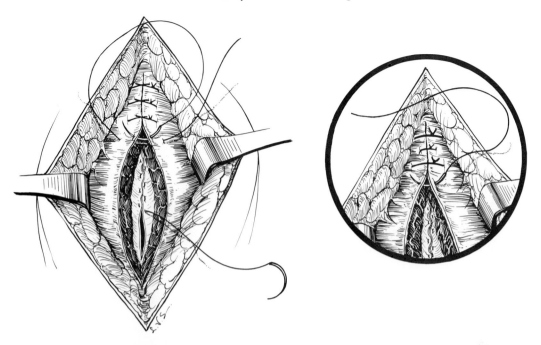

FIG 9–6. Closure of peritoneum with continuous suture. Fascia closure with figure-of-eight (*left*) and simple interrupted sutures (*right*) are illustrated.

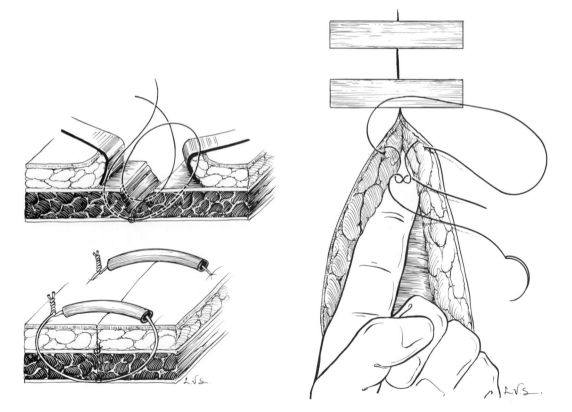

FIG 9–7. Types of retention sutures. Figure-of-eight suture is illustrated above and "through-and-through" retention sutures below.

FIG 9–8. Skin closure with interrupted subdermal sutures and Steri-Strips.

necessary. It is excellent for closing the abdomen rapidly, and it is the method of choice for closing the dehisced wound.

In all closures, sutures should be placed as far apart as possible consistent with approximation of tissue. Too close sutures obstruct blood supply to the wound. The 2 most common iatrogenic causes of dehiscence are infection and too tight sutures. In the vast majority of dehiscences, the suture material has cut through tissue and has not broken or become untied.

It is a useful exercise to assess the patient's "wound risk" in advance so that the proper choice of closure can be made easily at the end of the operation.

CARE OF THE WOUND

Postoperative care of the wound involves cleanliness, protection from trauma, and maximal support of the patient. Even closed wounds can be infected by surface contamination of bacteria, particularly within the first 4–6 days as the classical experiments of DuMortier show. The bacteria gain entrance through the suture tracts and the wound. If a wound is likely to be traumatized or contaminated, it should be protected during this time. Such protection may require special dressings such as occlusive sprays or repeated cleansings as well as dressings.

The ideal care of the wound begins in the preoperative period and ends only months later. One must prepare the patient so that optimal conditions exist when the wound is made. One must be clean, gentle, and skillful in surgical technic and thoughtful and ingenious in protecting the postoperative wound. Postoperatively, wound care includes maintenance of nutrition, blood volume, and oxygenation. Although wound healing is in many ways a local phenomenon, the ideal care of the wound is essentially the ideal care of the patient.

•   •   •

General References

Branemark PI: Capillary form and function: The microcirculation of granulation tissue. Bibl anat 7:9, 1965.

Brunius U: Wound healing impairment from sutures. Acta chir scandinav, Suppl 395, 1968.

Conolly WB & others: Clinical comparison of surgical wounds closed by suture and adhesive tapes. Am J Surg 117:318, 1969.

Converse JM, Rapaport FT: The vascularization of skin autografts and homografts: An experimental study in man. Ann Surg 143:306, 1956.

DuMortier JJ: The resistance of healing wounds to infection. Surg Gynec Obst 56:762, 1933.

Dunphy JE: The fibroblast: A ubiquitous ally for the surgeon. New England J Med 268:1367, 1963.

Edlich RD & others: Studies in the management of the contaminated wound (I and II). Am J Surg 117:323, 1969.

Ehrlich HP, Hunt TK: Effects of cortisone and vitamin A on wound healing. Ann Surg 167:324, 1968.

Forrester JC & others: Mechanical, biochemical, and architectural features of repair. In: *Repair and Regeneration.* Dunphy JE, Van Winkle W Jr (editors). McGraw-Hill, 1969.

Gillman T, Penn J: Studies on repair of cutaneous wounds. Med Proc 2:121, 1956.

Gross J, Lapierce CM, Tanzer ML: Organization and disorganization of extracellular substances: The collagen system. Page 175 in: *Cytodifferentiation and Macromolecular Synthesis.* Locke M (editor). Academic Press, 1963.

Hawley P, Hunt TK, Dunphy JE: Etiology of colonic anastomotic leaks. Proc Roy Soc Med 63 (Suppl): 28, 1970.

Hunt TK, Hawley P: Surgical judgment and colonic anastomoses. Dis Colon Rectum 12:167, 1969.

Jepsen OB, Larsen SO, Thomsen VF: Post-operative wound sepsis in general surgery. Acta chir scandinav Suppl 396:73, 1969.

Madden JW, Peacock EE Jr: Studies on the biology of collagen during wound healing. I. Role of collagen synthesis and deposition in cutaneous wounds in the rat. Surgery 64:288–294, 1968.

Majno G & others: Contraction of granulation tissue in vitro: Similarity to smooth muscle. Science 173:548, 1971.

McMinn RMH: *Tissue Repair.* Academic Press, 1969.

Menkin V: *Newer Concepts of Inflammation.* Thomas, 1950.

Niinikoski J, Hunt TK, Dunphy JE: Oxygen supply in healing tissue. Am J Surg 123:247, 1972.

Pareira MD, Serkes KD: Prediction of wound disruption by use of the healing ridge. Surg Gynec Obst 115:72, 1962.

Peacock EE Jr: Dynamic aspects of collagen biology. I. Synthesis and assembly. II. Degradation and metabolism. J Surg Res 7:433, 481, 1967.

Peacock EE Jr, Van Winkle W Jr: *Surgery and Biology of Wound Repair.* Saunders, 1970.

Polk HC Jr, Lopez-Mayor JF: Postoperative wound infection: A prospective study of determinant factors and prevention. Surgery 66:97, 1969.

Pories WJ & others: Zinc deficiency as a cause for delayed wound healing. Curr Top Surg Res 1:315, 1969.

Postlethwaite RW & others: Wound healing. II. An evaluation of surgical suture material. Surg Gynec Obst 108:555, 1959.

Schilling JA: Wound healing. Physiol Rev 48:374, 1968.

Trueblood HW, Nelson TS, Oberhelman HA: The effect of acute anemia and iron deficiency anemia on wound healing. Arch Surg 99:113, 1969.

Van Winkle W Jr: Wound contraction. Surg Gynec Obst 125:131, 1967.

10 . . .

Surgical Infections

Thomas K. Hunt, MD, & Ernest Jawetz, MD

A surgical infection consists of localized suppuration which is not likely to resolve with medical treatment and can be either surgically excised or incised and drained. Appendicitis, cholecystitis, diverticulitis, cutaneous or perianal abscesses, wound infections, and osteomyelitis are types of surgical infections. Empyema, peritonitis, ascending cholangitis, cavitating tuberculosis, hepatic, pulmonary, subphrenic, or pelvic abscesses, clostridial infections, and necrotizing fasciitis are other common examples.

PATHOGENESIS OF SURGICAL INFECTIONS

Three elements are common to surgical infections: (1) a closed space in the tissues, (2) an infectious agent, and (3) a susceptible host.

The Closed Space

Any wound—especially one that has been severely traumatized or poorly closed—contains at least a potential space which is separated from the circulation by hemostasis in small vessels surrounding the area of injury. Antibacterial defenses are to some extent excluded, and infectious organisms can multiply fairly rapidly in these protected conditions. Dead tissue left by trauma, such as chips of bone in a fracture, further exclude white cells, opsonins, antibodies, and antibiotics. Infarction, as in infected emboli, may cause lung and liver abscesses. Closely related to this is the easily infected collection of extravasated blood (hematoma).

Some natural spaces are particularly prone to become closed and infected. The appendix, the gallbladder, and intestinal diverticula often become obstructed, cannot drain, and may give rise to life-threatening infections.

The peritoneal and pleural cavities are not normally "closed spaces." Contaminants are usually spread over a wide area by movement of the viscera, so that natural defenses are more effective. Foreign bodies and dead tissue interfere with this spreading action and greatly potentiate peritoneal or pleural infections. When infection becomes established, inflammation may bind the moving surfaces, thus establishing a closed space which may then form an abscess.

Foreign bodies in tissue produce closed spaces and carry their own bacteria as well. Wood slivers are the most common example, but implanted vascular grafts or bullets may potentiate localized infections also. Foreign bodies of plant materials are particularly likely to become infected.

No matter what its origin, the space behaves essentially like a wound. (See Chapter 9.) Its internal environment is characterized by hypoxia, high P_{CO_2}, and low pH. These conditions favor the growth of bacteria. White cells, especially macrophages, require oxygen to kill injected bacteria. The P_{O_2} found in the dead spaces of most wounds is below the optimum for intracellular killing of bacteria.

The Infectious Agent

Almost any infectious agent can contaminate the closed space and cause infection. The more virulent organisms are the most likely to become established. Streptococci invade even minor breaks of the skin and spread through connective tissue planes and lymphatics. Staphylococci are common invaders. *Escherichia coli*, proteus, and klebsiella can cause primary infection when implanted in large numbers, or they can appear secondarily as opportunistic invaders in a susceptible host. Pseudomonas and serratia are seen most frequently as opportunistic invaders. Many fungi (histoplasma, coccidioides, actinomyces) and even parasites (amebas, echinococci) may cause abscesses or sinuses. Other rare diseases such as psittacosis, cat-scratch fever, and tularemia may become surgical infections when they cause abscesses in lymph nodes. The multiplicity of organisms found in surgical infections underscores the need for the surgeon to smear and culture the contents and the tissue wall of an abscess whenever he drains or excises one. The surgeon must inform the bacteriologist of the conditions under which he took the samples so that he can choose the optimal culture conditions to isolate and characterize the offending organisms.

The Susceptible Host

The dead space increases the susceptibility of tissue to infection, especially in patients with lowered systemic defenses.

Host resistance due to immune and inflammatory factors is dependent upon adequate tissue perfusion. Resistance is impaired in patients with multiple infections, severe malnutrition, low cardiac output, or poor tissue perfusion. It is not clear why malnutrition causes increased susceptibility, since even starved persons studied in World War II were able to adequately manufacture antibody in response to common pathogens. Patients with immature or depressed immune systems and those receiving anti-inflammatory steroids are also particularly susceptible. Alcoholism increases susceptibility by inhibiting leukocyte migration, ciliary motion, and the cough reflex. Streptococcal infections of the extremities are particularly common in alcoholics, and the organisms multiply rapidly because of poor hygiene, poor nutrition, dehydration, and exposure. Hypoxia may enhance susceptibility, perhaps because macrophages cannot inactivate ingested bacteria without adequate oxygen. Severe trauma, even remote from the infection, may increase susceptibility by causing hypoperfusion, hypoxia, and hypercapnia of the tissues. Extensive operations, hypovolemia, and multiple transfusions also impose a high risk of infection.

Recent research has shown disorders of white cell function in burned and severely injured patients. Such patients are highly susceptible to opportunistic infections. Rarely, patients may have genetic deficiencies of the enzyme systems that participate in bacterial killing. Granulomatous disease of childhood is the best known of many such examples.

COMPLICATIONS & SPREAD OF INFECTIONS

An established infection may spread locally or to distant sites or may exert secondary effects on the host.

Toxicity

"Toxicity" is one of the most obvious but least well understood effects of serious infection. In its clinical application, the word toxic denotes the appearance of a patient with severe infection and refers to lethargy or restlessness, weakness, or delirium in addition to fever, tachycardia, and leukocytosis. Toxemia is a broad term which refers to the spread via the blood stream of bacterial substances injurious to tissue. "Surgical scarlet fever" from streptococcal erythrogenic toxins is an example. The clostridia of gas gangrene produce a number of toxic enzymes, including a lecithinase which causes hemolytic anemia and jaundice. *Cl tetani* infection disseminates a potent neurotoxin. Septic shock may be associated with endotoxins released by gram-negative bacteria but can also follow gram-positive bacteremia. The basic mechanisms are not well understood. Complicated ulcerative colitis with toxic megacolon is another example of a surgical infection in which toxemia plays an important part.

Bacteremia

Bacteremia with chills and fever signifies dissemination beyond local defenses and intermittent presence of bacteria in the blood stream (ie, positive blood cultures). Systemic bacteremia may lead to bacterial endocarditis or other metastatic abscesses (brain, lungs, etc). Portal vein bacteremia may produce liver abscesses or suppurative portal phlebitis (pylephlebitis). Colonic infections such as amebic colitis may also spread to the liver through the portal vein.

Extension of Infection

Bacteria tend to spread along susceptible tissue planes. Streptococcal cellulitis which spreads in subcutaneous tissue and dermis is a common example. Invasive clostridial myositis spreads rapidly along muscle and in many cases requires amputation for control. Clostridial cellulitis, on the other hand, extends in the subcutaneous plane.

The lymphatics also serve as routes of spread of infection. Lymphangitis—the so-called blood poisoning of the preantibiotic era—is spectacular in the skin but may also occur where it is not seen, as in the pelvis or retroperitoneum.

Infections may spread along surfaces such as the peritoneum or pleura or even the skin to form satellite abscesses in the region of the original one.

In summary, the main dangers of surgical infection are (1) the spread to more and more seriously life-endangering sites and (2) "toxicity," which threatens the viability and functions of other tissues and organs.

GENERAL PRINCIPLES OF TREATMENT

Treatment is directed at control or containment of the infection.

Incision & Drainage

The simplest and often the most effective procedure for cure of an abscess is merely to open it and drain it to the outside. Bacteria, necrotic tissue, and toxins are thereby removed. The pressure in the infected space is lowered, thus decreasing the tendency of toxins and bacteria to spread and cause further damage to the local microcirculation.

An abscess with systemic manifestations is a surgical emergency. Fluctuation is a late sign of abscess. It may never appear, despite extensive abscess, in the parotid and perianal areas. If the surgeon waits for fluctuation to appear in these areas, serious complications or even death may result. Perianal "cellulitis" more than a few days old always harbors an abscess. Drainage creates an open wound, but the tissue will heal by second intention with remarkably little scarring.

Excision

A more definitive approach is to excise the infection, as is done in removing an infected appendix or gallbladder. In these cases, no further drainage may be necessary and the patient is cured on the operating table. On the other hand, excision of clostridial myositis may require amputation of the infected limb. The cure of cavitating pulmonary tuberculosis may require lobectomy. Surgical cure of bacterial endocarditis may require excision of an infected valve and replacement of the valve with a prosthesis. The success of such operations is greatly facilitated by intensive specific chemotherapy.

Ancillary Measures

On occasion, the cure of surgical infection may involve operation in another area. Stubborn infections in ischemic extremities may be best cured by restoring blood flow to the infected area. Surgery may be performed to diminish the bacterial contamination of an infected area, as in a colostomy for the treatment of diverticulitis. The most effective operation for complicated diverticulitis, however, is to excise the badly infected segment and place a colostomy proximal to the area of excision so that the surrounding inflammation can resolve and the tissues can heal before the colon is reconnected.

A well-drained abscess with no systemic effects needs no antibiotic therapy. The uncomplicated case of appendicitis without peritonitis needs only operation. An invasive infection, however, should be treated with antibiotics as well as surgery. One must obtain cultures at the earliest possible time and start specifically effective antibiotics as soon as possible. If it is necessary to start antibiotics chosen empirically, every attempt must be made to start cultures before antibiotics are given and obtain the results as soon as possible.

DIAGNOSTIC AIDS

Physical examination is the simplest effective means of detecting the site of surgical infection. When a surgical infection is suspected but cannot be found initially, repeated examination will finally reveal the subtle development of warmth, erythema, induration, tenderness, or splinting due to a developing abscess. Failure to repeat the physical examination is the most common reason for delayed diagnosis and therapy.

The most important diagnostic aids are smear and culture of pus or other infected material. The most common reason for inappropriate treatment of surgical infections is the failure to examine a gram-stained smear of the pus as an immediate guide to antibacterial and surgical therapy.

Radiologic examination is frequently helpful, particularly for the diagnosis of pulmonary infections. An elevated and immobile diaphragm is a clue to the presence of subphrenic abscess. Obliteration of the psoas shadow frequently indicates an appendiceal abscess. Whenever infection is close to bone, radiologic examination is indicated to detect early signs of osteomyelitis which might require aggressive surgical therapy. Scanning—particularly of the liver or brain—is useful for the detection of abscesses in these organs. On rare occasions, thermography can locate a hidden abscess.

Alexander JW, Meakins JL: Natural defense mechanisms in clinical sepsis. J Surg Res 11:148, 1971.
Cline MJ: Drug potentiation of macrophage function. Infection Immunity 2:601, 1970.
Hunt TK & others: Oxygen tension and wound infection. Surg Forum 23:47, 1972.
Lehrer RI: The role of phagocyte function in resistance to infection. California Med 114:17–25, June 1971.

SPECIFIC TYPES OF SURGICAL INFECTION

FURUNCLE, CARBUNCLE, & HIDRADENITIS

Furuncles and carbuncles are cutaneous abscesses. Furuncles are the most common surgical infections, but carbuncles are rare.

Furuncles can be serious when multiple and recurrent (furunculosis). Furunculosis usually occurs in young adults and is probably due to disease of the skin, altered glandular secretions, or impaired resistance to the common skin organisms, staphylococci and diphtheroids.

Hidradenitis suppurativa is a serious skin infection of the axillas or groins consisting of multiple abscesses of the apocrine sweat glands. The condition often becomes chronic and disabling.

Furuncles usually start in infected hair follicles, although some are caused by retained foreign bodies and other injuries. Hair follicles normally contain bacteria. If the pilosebaceous apparatus becomes occluded by skin disease or bacterial inflammation, the stage is set for development of a furuncle. Because the base of the hair follicle may lie in subcutaneous tissue, the infection can spread as a cellulitis or it can form a subcutaneous abscess. If a furuncle results from confluent infection of several hair follicles, a central core of skin may become necrotic and slough when the abscess is drained.

A furuncle which extends in the subcutaneous tissue, forming a long, flat abscess, is called a phlegmon. This name may be applied also to such abscesses in other organs.

Clinical Findings

Furuncles are usually readily apparent because of the pain and itching they produce. The skin first becomes red and then turns white and necrotic over the top of the abscess. There is usually some surrounding erythema and induration. Regional nodes may become enlarged. Systemic symptoms are rare.

A carbuncle usually starts as a furuncle, but the infection dissects through the dermis and subcutaneous tissue in a myriad of connecting tunnels. Many of these small extensions open to the surface, giving the appearance of a large furuncle with many pustular openings. As the carbuncle enlarges, the blood supply to its center is destroyed and the central tissue becomes necrotic. A carbuncle on the back of the neck is seen most often in diabetic patients. The patient is usually febrile and mildly toxic. This is a serious problem that demands immediate surgical attention.

The vast majority of furuncles and carbuncles are caused by staphylococci, but many other kinds of bacteria—especially diphtheroids—may participate.

Simple furuncles should not be treated with antibiotics. Invasive carbuncles must be treated with antibiotics as well as operation. Between these 2 extremes, there are many types of infection in which the use of antibiotics depends somewhat on the location of the abscess and the degree of sepsis. Large abscesses near the nose and face are best treated with antibiotics in addition to surgical drainage. However, surgical drainage is the mainstay of treatment.

In carbuncles, diabetes must be suspected and treated.

Differential Diagnosis

Identification of the specific cause of a furuncle is usually not important since all forms of abscesses require the same treatment.

On occasion, the surgeon may be confronted with a localized area of erythema and induration without obvious suppuration. The majority of such lesions will go on to central suppuration and become an obvious furuncle. On the other hand, when these lesions are located near joints or over the tibia or when they are widely distributed, one must consider such differential diagnoses as rheumatoid nodules, gout, bursitis, synovitis, erythema nodosum, fungal infections, some benign or malignant skin tumors, and, commonly, inflamed (not previously infected) sebaceous or epithelial inclusion cysts.

The differentiation of hidradenitis from furunculosis is best achieved by skin biopsy, which shows typical specific involvement of the apocrine sweat glands. One also suspects hidradenitis when abscesses are concentrated in the apocrine gland areas.

The experienced observer rarely confuses carbuncle with any other disease.

Complications

Any of these infections may cause suppurative phlebitis when located near major veins. This is particularly important when the infection is located near the nose or eyes. Central venous thrombosis in the brain is a serious complication, and abscesses on the face usually must be treated with antibiotics. Incision and drainage in this area should be done when there is fluctuation and an obvious abscess.

Hidradenitis may disable the patient but rarely has systemic manifestations. Carbuncles on the back of the neck may go on to epidural abscess and meningitis.

Treatment

The classic therapy for furuncle is incision and drainage; antibiotics can only reduce the infection around the abscess. All patients with recurrent furunculosis should be checked for diabetes or immune deficiencies. Frequent washing with soaps containing hexachlorophene or other disinfectants is advisable. It may also be necessary to advise extensive laundering of all personal clothing and disinfection of the patient's living quarters in order to reduce the reservoirs of bacteria. Furunculosis associated with severe acne may benefit from tetracycline, 250 mg orally daily.

Infection associated with primary immunologic deficiency requires specific therapy. Antibiotics and gamma globulin are of value for patients with isolated deficiencies of immunoglobulins.

A **collar-button abscess** is a small infected blister under the epidermis which is contiguous through a small opening with a deeper and larger subcutaneous abscess. In cross-section, it is shaped like a collar button with the narrow point at the dermis. Removal of the top of the infected blister is inadequate treatment. When an abscess fails to resolve after a superficial incision, the surgeon must look for collar-button abscess.

Hidradenitis is usually treated by drainage of the individual abscess followed by good hygiene. The patient must avoid astringent antiperspirants and deodorants. Painting with mild disinfectants is sometimes helpful. Fungal infections should be searched for if healing after drainage does not occur promptly. If none of these measures are successful, the apocrine sweat-bearing skin must be excised followed by skin grafting.

Carbuncles are often more extensive than the external appearance indicates. In the vast majority, incision alone is inadequate. Carbuncles are best treated by excision, usually done with the electrocautery. Excision is continued until the many sinus tracts are removed—usually far beyond the cutaneous evidence of suppuration. It is sometimes necessary to produce a large open wound. This may appear to be drastic treatment, but it achieves rapid cure and prevents further spread. Failure to excise usually leads to prolonged morbidity since incision is inadequate to drain the multiple sinuses of infection. The large wound usually contracts to a small scar and does not require skin grafting.

CELLULITIS

Cellulitis is a common invasive nonsuppurative infection of connective tissue. The term is loosely used and often misapplied. The microscopic picture is one of severe inflammation of the dermal and subcutaneous tissues. Although PMNs predominate, there is no gross suppuration except perhaps at the portal of entry.

Clinical Findings

Cellulitis usually appears on an extremity as a brawny red or reddish-brown area of edematous skin. It advances rapidly from its starting point, and the advancing edge may be vague or sharply defined (eg, in erysipelas). A surgical wound, puncture, skin ulcer, or patch of dermatitis is usually identifiable as a portal of entry. The disease often occurs in susceptible patients, eg, alcoholics with postphlebitic leg ulcers. Most cases are caused by streptococci, but other bacteria have been involved. A moderate or high fever is almost always present.

Lymphangitis arising from cellulitis produces red, warm, tender streaks 1 or 2 cm wide leading from the infection along lymphatic vessels to the regional lymph nodes. There is no suppuration. Bacteria are difficult to obtain for culture, but blood culture is often positive.

Differential Diagnosis

Since the visible features of cellulitis are all due to inflammation, the word cellulitis has come to be associated with visible signs of inflammation. This is unfortunate since cellulitis implies lack of suppuration and therefore is not an indication for incision and drainage. When the word is carelessly used it may lead to the inference that no suppuration is present when in fact incision and drainage are urgently required.

Thrombophlebitis is often difficult to differentiate from cellulitis, but swelling is usually greater with phlebitis, and tenderness may localize over a vein. Homans' sign does not always make the differentiation—nor does lymphadenopathy. Fever is usually greater with cellulitis, and pulmonary embolization does not occur in cellulitis.

Severe contact allergy, such as poison oak, may be indistinguishable from cellulitis in its early phase, but dense nonhemorrhagic vesiculation soon discloses the allergic cause.

Chemical inflammation due to drug injection may also mimic streptococcal cellulitis.

Treatment

Therapy should entail rest, elevation, massive hot wet packs, and penicillin, 2.4 million units per day IM (600,000 units every 6 hours). If a clear response has not occurred in 12–24 hours, one should suspect an abscess or consider the possibility that the causative agent is a staphylococcus or other resistant organism. The patient must be examined one or more times daily to detect a hidden abscess masquerading as cellulitis.

The appearance of hemorrhagic bullae and skin necrosis suggests necrotizing fasciitis as the correct diagnosis.

POSTOPERATIVE WOUND INFECTION

Postoperative wound infection results from bacterial contamination during or after a surgical procedure. The infection usually involves the subcutaneous tissues.

Despite every effort to maintain asepsis, most surgical wounds are contaminated with bacteria at the end of an operation. If contamination is minimal, the wound has been made without undue tissue injury, and there is no dead space, infection rarely develops. In clean surgical wounds—as in hernia or thyroid operations—the incidence of infection should be no more than 1 or 2%. In "clean-contaminated" wounds—eg, biliary or gastric surgery—infection rates as high as 5 or 6% are experienced. Rates higher than this for these types of operation indicate poor asepsis or poor operative technic. Severely contaminated wounds such as in operations on the unprepared colon or emergency operations for intestinal bleeding or perforation may have an infection risk of 15–30%. To confine these rates to an acceptable range, one must make liberal use of isolation technics and delayed primary closure.

Unnecessary trauma from retractors, inappropriate use of electrocoagulation, gross ligation of bleeding points, foreign bodies, and dead space contribute more to postoperative wound infection than the mere presence of excessive numbers of bacteria. Whenever gross contamination of the wound cannot be avoided, the skin subcutaneous tissues should be left open (see Prevention, below). Since even a minor postoperative wound infection prolongs hospitalization and occasions economic loss, every effort must be made to keep the infection rate low.

Clinical Findings

Wound infections usually manifest themselves between the fifth and tenth days after surgery, but they may appear as early as the first postoperative day or even years later. The first sign is usually fever, and every instance of postoperative fever requires inspection of the wound. The patient may complain of wound pain. The wound rarely appears severely inflamed, but edema may be obvious because the skin sutures appear tight.

Palpation of the wound is useful to detect abscess. A safe and rewarding method is to pour surgical soap on the wound and, using it as a lubricant, palpate gently with the gloved hand. Firm or fluctuant areas, crepitus, or tenderness can be detected in this way with minimal pain and contamination. The rare infection deep to the fascia may be difficult to recognize. In doubtful cases when a decision must be made, one can carefully open the wound in the suspicious area. If no pus is present, the wound can be closed immediately with skin tapes.

Infections are particularly common in contaminated wounds, ie, wounds used to expose and enter some portion of the intestinal tract, upper airway, or an area of infection such as the infected urinary tract.

Some patients are more susceptible than others.

The bacteriology of wound infection goes through cycles. Before the antibiotics became available, streptococcal and staphylococcal infections were the most feared. When antibiotics appeared, many surgeons felt the problem of surgical infection would disappear. Unfortunately, the problem of emerging resistance was not anticipated. Antibiotics were overused and were substituted for careful surgical technic. Severe problems with staphylococcal infections developed, requiring greater attention to housekeeping, preparation of the skin, surgical technic, and isolation. Soaps and antibiotics effective against resistant staphylococci were developed. Infections with gram-negative bacteria are now the major problem. Furthermore, the individual hospital or ward may have periodic outbreaks of infections due to one or another resistant organism.

Differential Diagnosis

Differential diagnosis includes all other causes of postoperative fever, wound dehiscence, and wound herniation (see Chapter 4).

Prevention

External bacterial contamination can be almost entirely eliminated by extraordinary precautions such as operating through ports in sterilized plastic chambers; but even then the patient contributes bacteria to his wound from deep in his skin and from his gastrointestinal, urinary, or respiratory tracts. As surgery is done today, one can assume that all wounds are contaminated to some slight extent. Nevertheless, prevention is still the most important aspect of wound infection.

There are 4 main aspects to prevention of infection: (1) careful, gentle, clean surgery; (2) reduction of contamination; (3) support of the patient's defenses; and (4) antibiotics. The first 2 are by far the most important.

The surgeon who traumatizes tissue, leaves foreign bodies or hematomas in wounds, uses too many ligatures, and exposes the wound to drying or pressure from retractors is exposing his patients to needless risks.

Many technics are directed at reducing contamination. They include housekeeping in the operating theater, hand scrubbing, skin preparation, wound protectors, dressings, isolation chambers, and special ventilating systems.

Closure technics also influence infection rates. The purpose of sutures is to approximate tissues and hold them securely, and the right number to use is as few as possible to accomplish this aim. Sutures should be tied as loosely as the requirements of approximation permit. Subcutaneous sutures should be used rarely and only when dead space is sure to result if they are omitted. Using skin tapes when possible instead of skin sutures lowers infection rates, especially in contaminated wounds.

Severely contaminated wounds in which infection is likely to develop are best left open initially and managed by delayed primary closure. In the abdomen, chest, or skull this means that the deep layers are closed while skin and subcutaneous tissues are left open, sterilely dressed, inspected on the fourth day, and then closed (preferably with skin tapes) if no sign of infection is seen. A clean granulating open wound is superior to a wound infection. Scarring from secondary healing is usually minimal.

Postoperative care is also important since wound infections can originate on the ward as well as in the operating room. The patient himself is the most common source of contamination. Most wounds can safely be left without dressings, but wounds are particularly susceptible to surface contamination for the first 24–48 hours. If contamination is likely, protective dressings should be used.

The patient has many defense mechanisms which the surgeon can support. Adequate blood volume, arterial oxygenation, nutrition, and antibody levels all help prevent infection.

The use of antibiotics as a means of preventing surgical wound infection is controversial. There is a tendency to use them just to make sure. For operations in which foreign substances are implanted, the inclination to use prophylactic antibiotics is even greater.

Well-controlled studies have shown that antibiotics are of no value in preventing infections after clean surgical procedures and that side-effects outweigh any benefit. The case may be different with heavily contaminated wounds. In controlled studies, if prophylactic antibiotics reached adequate concentrations by the time of wounding, infection rates after colon surgery were lowered. Prophylactic penicillin should be given for contaminated traumatic wounds with injured tissue. Most surgeons use antibiotics preoperatively for penetrating wounds of the abdomen. If an old wound which was once infected is to be re-entered, the patient should be given antibiotics effective against the old infection. Unless this is done, repeated wound infection due to the same organism is likely.

In the prophylaxis and treatment of wound infection, the amount of antibiotic which penetrates into the wound is obviously important. Most antibiotics can be made to penetrate the wound in therapeutic concentrations. If prophylaxis is desired, by far the highest concentrations will be found in the wound if a high blood level of antibiotic is present at the time the wound is made. If antibiotic administration is delayed until after the wound is made, there is a great diminution in the amount reaching the wound since the inevitable vascular injury of the wound causes a diffusion block to penetration of antibiotic.

After the wound is made, bolus doses of intravenous antibiotic will cause wound antibiotic concentration to rise rapidly to equal blood concentration about an hour after injection. The antibiotic is then trapped in the wound and remains there for a number of hours in higher concentrations than in serum until a new serum dose is given. The notable exceptions to this rule are the tetracyclines, whose wound levels (for unknown reasons) are always below blood levels; and gentamicin, whose wound levels are so extremely low that it is difficult to say whether trapping has occurred or not. Clindamycin and polymyxin appear to behave rather like tetracycline, but definitive data on these drugs are lacking.

Among those antibiotics having excellent access to the wound are the penicillins and the cephalosporins. Clindamycin reaches intermediate concentrations, and carbenicillin, nafcillin, oxacillin, gentamicin, erythromycin, and polymyxin seem to have the least potential efficacy in terms of concentration. In general, all of these antibitocis—except clindamycin and polymyxin—equilibrate with blood levels at about 90 minutes after bolus intravenous doses.

In general, antibiotics can be raised to slightly higher concentrations in early wounds than in older ones. This does not constitute an endorsement of prophylactic antibiotics. This knowledge should be of use in managing patients who are known to have contaminated wounds and therefore may benefit from prophylactic antibiotic administration.

During constant infusion of antibiotic, with a low blood level which has reached a plateau, wound concentration rises slowly to equal blood concentration at about 6 hours. Although the net amount of antibiotic reaching the wound is the same for equal doses regardless of manner of injection, the appearance rate and peak concentrations are far greater after bolus injection (Figs 10–1 and 10–2).

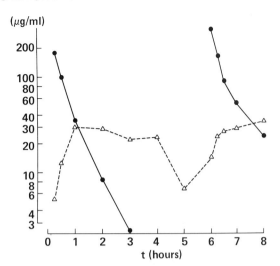

FIG 10–2. Antibiotic levels (cephaloridine in μg/ml wound interstitial fluid) after intravenous bolus dose of 8 mg/kg. Levels of 30 μg/ml are reached temporarily. Average level is 10–20 μg/ml. Solid line = blood; dotted line = wound.

There is a growing body of evidence that the local use of antibiotics for irrigating peritoneum and wounds may reduce the rate of infection in selected contaminated wounds (eg, after colon surgery and renal transplantation).

Treatment

The basic treatment for wound infection is to open the wound and allow it to drain. This is so effective that antibiotics are not necessary unless the infection is invasive. Culture is essential for several reasons: (1) to help locate the source and prevent further infection in other patients; (2) as a preview of the bacteriology in case other infections, such as pelvic abscess, develop deep to the wound; (3) for selection of preoperative antibiotics in case the wound must be entered again; and (4) in case the infection should become invasive.

As the wound granulates, a loose secondary closure with tapes can be used to shorten the time to complete closure.

Prognosis

Most wound infections increase morbidity. Wound infection correlates positively with mortality rates but is not often the cause of death. It is often the added factor that tips the scales against the success of an operation.

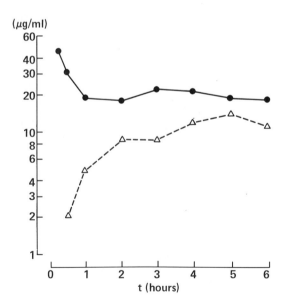

FIG 10–1. Antibiotic levels (cephaloridine in μg/ml wound interstitial fluid) after constant intravenous infusion with a small loading dose. Blood level is 10–20 μg/ml at 4–6 hours. Solid line = blood; dotted line = wound.

Alexander JW & others: Antibiotic concentration in wounds. J Trauma. [In press.]

Anderson B, Korner B, Östergaard AH: Topical ampicillin against wound infection after colorectal surgery. Ann Surg 176:129, 1972.

Burke JF: Wound infection and early inflammation. Monogr Surg Sc 1:301, 1964.

Conolly WB, Hunt TK, Dunphy JE: Management of contaminated surgical wounds. Surg Gynec Obst 129:593, 1969.

Edlich RF & others: Studies in the management of the contaminated wound. Am J Surg 117:323, 1969.

Ehrlich HP, Licko V, Hunt TK: Kinetics of cephaloridine in experimental wounds. Am J Med Sc. January 1974.

Jepsen OB, Larsen SO, Thomsen VF: Post-operative wound sepsis in general surgery. Acta chir scandinav Suppl 396:73, 1969.

CLOSTRIDIAL INFECTIONS

1. CLOSTRIDIAL INFECTIONS OTHER THAN TETANUS

Gas gangrene is generally associated with grossly contaminated injuries (eg, war wounds) since the organisms are found in soil and feces. However, it is an important problem in civilian surgical practice also. The rising civilian accident rate and the appreciable incidence of clostridial infection after elective surgery make the prevention and treatment of gas gangrene a matter of major concern to the surgeon.

The term gas gangrene should be restricted to spreading or diffuse clostridial myositis, although *Clostridium perfringens (Cl welchii)* is found in 90% of all anaerobic gas-forming bacterial infections. Clinically, there is a broad spectrum of disease caused by these organisms ranging from negligible surface contamination, through invasive "cellulitis" of connective tissue, to invasive anaerobic infection of muscle with massive tissue necrosis and profound toxemia.

Traditionally, anaerobic bacterial infections have been classified as diffuse clostridial myositis (gas gangrene), localized clostridial myositis, and clostridial cellulitis. Gas formation and crepitus may or may not be present in some forms of clostridial gangrene.

Pathophysiology & Bacteriology

Most clostridia are strict anaerobes, but some (eg, *Cl perfringens*) may multiply rapidly even in the presence of small amounts of oxygen as long as the oxidation-reduction potential is low.

There are several means by which tissue redox potentials are diminished: impaired blood supply, muscle injury, pressure from casts, severe local edema, foreign bodies, or the presence of oxygen-consuming organisms. Thus, clostridial infections frequently occur in the presence of other bacteria, eg, gram-negative rods.

Clostridia proliferate and produce toxins which diffuse into the surrounding tissue. The toxins devitalize cells and destroy the local microcirculation. This allows further invasion which can advance at an aston-

ishing rate. The alpha toxin, a necrotizing lecithinase, is thought to be particularly important in this sequence, but other so-called toxins, including collagenase, hyaluronidase, leukocidin, protease, lipase, and hemolysin, also contribute. When the disease has advanced sufficiently, toxins enter the systemic circulation, causing the systemic features of pallor, anxiety, restlessness, delirium, severe tachycardia, jaundice, and ultimately shock and death. The progress of the local lesion can often be judged fairly accurately by the general state of the patient as well as the local signs.

Clinical Findings

A. Diffuse Clostridial Myositis (Gas Gangrene): Diffuse clostridial myositis usually begins less than 3 days after the injury, with rapid increase of pain in the wound, edema, and a brown seropurulent exudate, often containing bubbles. There is marked tachycardia, but fever is variable. Crepitus may or may not be present. Profound toxemia often appears early and progresses to delirium and hemolytic jaundice. The surface edema, necrosis, and discoloration are usually less extensive than the underlying muscle necrosis. The disease characteristically progresses rapidly with loss of blood supply to the infected muscle. The swelling and edema may produce ischemia, especially under tight dressings or plaster casts. Following injury with vascular damage, delay in debridement or inadequate debridement furnishes the same critical factor—dead tissue. Since gas gangrene often develops under plaster casts, a sudden deterioration within 3 or 4 days of injury coupled with a muscle injury, an "autopsy room" odor, and a brown exudate require removal or windowing of the cast.

B. Localized Clostridial Myositis: Localized clostridial myositis occurs occasionally. The injury and infection involve muscle, but the infection is not invasive. The wound has the characteristic odor, edema, crepitation, and appearance, but the findings are localized and the limb appears well perfused, with intact pulses. The systemic reaction may include fever and tachycardia but not severe prostration, delirium, and other signs of toxemia.

C. Crepitant Clostridial Cellulitis: This type ("anaerobic cellulitis") is an invasive infection of subcutaneous tissue which has been made susceptible by injury or ischemia. The dissection occurs above the deep fascia and may spread at an exceptionally rapid rate, producing discoloration of the skin, edema, and crepitus.

D. Gas Abscess (Welch's Abscess): Gas abscess is a localized infection not usually thought of as invasive. In this case, muscle has not usually been injured and is not involved by the infection. This form is much less severe and requires less drastic treatment than clostridial myositis. The incubation period is usually a week or more. There is usually little pain; the edema is moderate; and the patient does not appear toxic, although he may have fever and tachycardia. The wound, however, has the characteristic brown seropurulent exudate and the characteristic autopsy room odor, and gas may be found diffused through the connective tissues. Except for the involved area, the limb appears well perfused.

E. Edematous Gangrene: Edematous gangrene is a variant caused by *Cl novyi (oedematiens)*. No gas is produced, but edema of muscle is prominent. This is a particularly aggressive and fatal infection requiring rapid and radical surgical debridement.

Many open wounds are superficially infected or contaminated with clostridia but there is no significant local or systemic disease. There is often a brown seropurulent exudate. The condition is not invasive because the surrounding tissue is basically healthy, and the clostridia are confined to necrotic surface tissue. Debridement of dead surface tissue is usually the only treatment necessary, but this condition can develop into invasive gangrene if a severe hemodynamic abnormality or further injury decreases the oxidation-reduction potential of the surrounding tissue.

Differential Diagnosis

Diffuse clostridial myositis ("gas gangrene") is most often confused with other gas-producing infections, which are usually due to mixtures of gram-negative bacilli and gram-positive cocci. These mixed infections are not usually as virulent as gas gangrene and respond well to incision and drainage. Crepitant cellulitis should not be confused with clostridial gangrene since it, too, is well treated by lesser means (see below). Gas in the tissues is not a good differentiating point since some species (eg, *Cl novyi*) do not produce gas, nonclostridial organisms (eg, *Escherichia coli*) often produce gas, and air can enter tissues through a penetrating wound or from the chest or joint areas.

Prevention

Almost all clostridial infections are preventable. The keystone of prevention is early debridement of dead tissue and support of the circulation.

Suspicion should be directed at any wound received out of doors and contaminated with a foreign body, soil, or feces and any wound in which tissue (particularly muscle) has been extensively injured. This type of wound should be carefully examined under sufficient anesthesia to permit full inspection and debridement. The minimum criteria for tissue viability are that the tissue bleeds freely when it is cut and that muscle contracts when gently pinched.

Antibiotic prophylaxis is valuable. Penicillin is most often used, although many antibiotics have prevented gas gangrene in laboratory animals. However, no antibiotic can prevent gas gangrene without adequate surgical debridement.

Polyvalent gas gangrene antitoxin has been advocated for both prevention and treatment, but there is little evidence of its effectiveness.

Treatment

The major emphasis in treatment is inevitably surgical. Antibiotics are essential but are ineffective without surgical control of the disease.

A. Surgical Treatment: The wound must be opened, and dead and severely damaged tissue must be excised. Tight fascial compartments must be decompressed. Immediate amputation is necessary when there is diffuse myositis with complete loss of blood supply or when debridement would have to be so extensive that a useless limb would result.

Surgical treatment for clostridial cellulitis must be aggressive, but amputation is not necessary. Extensive debridement, with excision of necrotic skin and wide-open drainage, is essential. One must be careful to determine whether muscle is involved, because myositis and cellulitis may coexist. This will usually determine whether amputation should be done or whether extensive debridement of skin is all that is necessary. Multiple debridements may be required. Localized gas gangrene requires only local debridement.

When clostridial infections follow penetrating injuries of the colon and rectum, diverting proximal colostomy is required with wide drainage of the flanks, buttocks, or perineum. On occasion, clostridial infections involve tissues which cannot be extensively debrided such as spinal cord, brain, or retroperitoneal tissues. Surgical drainage is required in such cases, but major reliance is placed on antibiotics and hyperbaric oxygenation.

B. Hyperbaric Oxygenation: Hyperbaric oxygenation is beneficial in treating clostridial infections, but it cannot replace surgical therapy since no amount of increased arterial P_{O_2} can force oxygen into dead tissue. Hyperbaric oxygen may contain the focus of bacteria but cannot eliminate it. It probably prevents production of alpha toxin by bacteria in environments where P_{O_2} is above 90 mm Hg. Treatment for 1 or 2 hours at 3 atmospheres repeated every 6–12 hours is recommended, and only 3–5 exposures are usually necessary. Where large hyperbaric chambers are available, surgery and hyperbaric oxygenation can be accomplished simultaneously. Early use of hyperbaric oxygen can reduce tissue losses.

Because even hyperbarically administered oxygen will fail to reach the tissues in hypovolemic patients, vigorous support of blood volume is necessary. Many patients with gas gangrene and extensive injuries require multiple blood transfusions. In this case, reduced 2,3-diphosphoglycerate stores in red cells diminish tissue oxygenation. Fresh blood must be given early, and serum phosphate must be measured and kept within the normal range. Depressed serum phosphate also leads to rigidity of the red cells, which probably diminishes tissue oxygenation.

C. Antibiotics: Penicillin (20–40 million units per day) should be given intravenously. If the patient is allergic to penicillin, tetracyclines or other antibiotics are given.

D. Gas Gangrene Antitoxin: Antitoxins are available against the toxins of *Cl perfringens, Cl novyi, Cl histolyticum,* and *Cl septicum,* usually in the form of concentrated immune globulins. Since the clinical picture is similar with all species of toxin-forming clostridia, polyvalent antitoxin (containing antibodies to several toxins) is usually relied on. While such antitoxin is often administered to individuals with contaminated wounds containing much devitalized tissue, the effectiveness of the antitoxin is uncertain. Surgical management and antibiotics are more effective.

Prognosis

Without treatment, clostridial cellulitis and myositis are fatal diseases. With adequate treatment, deaths are rare and should occur only when treatment is delayed, in patients who are already severely ill with other diseases, or in patients with advanced invasion of vital structures. The overall mortality rate is approximately 20%.

The prognosis for salvage of functioning limbs is not so favorable. When clostridial myonecrosis is added to injury, affected limbs often become useless and must be amputated to save life.

Altemeier WA: Diagnosis, classification, and general management of gas producing infections, particularly those produced by *Clostridium perfringens*. Page 481 in: *Proceedings of the Third International Conference of Hyperbaric Medicine.* Brown IW Jr (editor). National Academy of Sciences—National Research Council, Publication No. 1404, 1966.

Altemeier WA, Fullen WD: Prevention and treatment of gas gangrene. JAMA 217:806, 1971.

DeHaven KE, Evarts CM: The continuing problem of gas gangrene. J Trauma 11:983, 1971.

2. TETANUS

Essentials of Diagnosis

- Presence of puncture wounds which have not been debrided.
- Limitation of movements of the jaw, with painful muscle spasm and spasm of the facial muscles (risus sardonicus).
- Stiffness of the neck and laryngospasm.
- Tonic spasms and generalized convulsions.

General Considerations

Tetanus is a specific anaerobic infection caused by the neurotoxin of *Clostridium tetani* which leads to nervous irritability and tetanic muscular contractions. The causative organism enters and flourishes in hypoxic wounds contaminated with soil or feces. The tetanus-prone wound is usually a puncture wound or one containing devitalized tissue or foreign body.

The incubation period of tetanus varies from 1–54 days, with an average of 8 days. The greater the delay before debridement and antitoxin therapy, the shorter the incubation period is likely to be. The longer the delay from injury to the onset of symptoms, the better the prognosis.

Clinical Findings

A. Symptoms and Signs: The first symptom is usually pain or tingling in the area of injury and limitation of movements of the jaw (lockjaw) and spasms of the facial muscles (risus sardonicus). This is followed by stiffness of the neck, difficulty in swallowing, and laryngospasm. Hesitancy in micturition due to sphincter spasm is also seen. In the more acute cases, severe spasms of the muscles of the back produce opisthotonos. Spasms become increasingly frequent and involve more and more muscle groups. As chest and diaphragm spasms occur, longer and longer periods of apnea follow. The temperature is normal or slightly elevated. Sweating tends to be profuse. Marked elevation of the pulse rate is a grave sign. The severity of cases varies widely; some are very mild and easily handled.

B. Laboratory Findings: Polymorphonuclear leukocytosis may be present.

Prevention

Specific preventive measures for patients with wounds are outlined as follows by the Committee on Trauma of the American College of Surgeons (1972 Revision).

A. Previously Immunized Individuals:

1. Immunized within the past 10 years—

a. To the great majority, give 0.5 ml IM of adsorbed tetanus toxoid as a booster unless it is certain that the patient has received a booster within the previous 5 years.

b. To those with severe, neglected, or old (more than 24 hours) tetanus-prone wounds, give 0.5 ml IM of adsorbed tetanus toxoid unless it is certain that the patient has received a booster within the previous year.

2. Immunized more than 10 years previously—

a. To the great majority, give 0.5 ml IM of adsorbed tetanus toxoid.

b. To those with severe, neglected, or old (more than 24 hours) tetanus-prone wounds—Give 0.5 ml IM of adsorbed tetanus toxoid, 250 units of tetanus immune globulin (human), and consider the use of oxytetracycline or penicillin.

B. Individuals Not Previously Immunized:

1. Clean minor wounds (tetanus unlikely)—Give 0.5 ml of adsorbed tetanus toxoid as initial immunizing dose. Then give the patient a written record and tell him what to do to complete the immunization schedule. Basic immunization with precipitated toxoid requires 3 injections: one initially, one at 4–6 weeks, and one in 6 months to 1 year.

2. All other wounds—Give 0.5 ml IM of absorbed tetanus toxoid as initial immunizing dose, 250 units IM of tetanus immune globulin (human)—in a different syringe and at a different site—and consider the use of antibiotics.

C. Use of Tetanus Antitoxins: Equine antitoxin should never be used prophylactically unless tetanus immune globulin (human) is not available and cannot be obtained within 24 hours, and then only if the possibility of tetanus outweighs the considerable danger of immune reaction to the equine antitoxin. Question the patient and test for sensitivity to horse serum. If the patient is not sensitive to equine tetanus antitoxin, give 3000–6000 units IM. If the patient is sensitive, give large doses of penicillin or oxytetracycline and no antitoxin. In these patients, the danger of anaphylaxis probably outweighs the danger of tetanus.

Caution: Human tetanus antitoxin is gamma globulin. It should *never* be given intravenously.

Treatment

Intensive treatment should be started as soon as the diagnosis is made, since the respiratory paralysis may advance rapidly. Treatment often becomes extremely complicated and requires the combined efforts of a surgeon, an anesthesiologist, and an internist or clinical pharmacologist.

Treatment of tetanus is usually arranged in a sequence of priorities:

A. Fix toxin with human tetanus immune globulin. The usual dose of human immune globulin is 3000–6000 units IM, given preferably in the proximal portion of the wounded extremity or in the vicinity of the wound. Repeated doses may be necessary since the half-life of the antibody is about 3 weeks.

B. Excise and debride the suspected wound under anesthesia appropriate to a complete and unhurried excision. Ordinarily, surgery should be done approximately an hour after the systemic serotherapy has begun. The wound must be left open and may be treated with peroxide.

C. Medical control of the nervous system disorder should begin whenever necessary. The patient should be isolated from sudden stimuli and should be spared unnecessary movement and excitement. Barbiturates or other sedatives may be employed, but overdoses often cause cardiorespiratory failure. Diazepam (Valium) is also useful to help lower the amount of barbiturate necessary to control spasms. Curarization is preferable to cardiodepressant doses of barbiturates even though curarization necessitates the use of mechanical ventilation.

D. The patient with respiratory problems will usually require tracheostomy since mechanical ventilation, once it becomes necessary, must be continued for weeks. The patient should be intubated as soon as respiratory problems appear. All modern technics for proper control of respiration and prevention of pneumonia are required. Tracheal stenosis is common after prolonged intubation for tetanus.

E. Aqueous penicillin G, 10–40 million units a day by intermittent intravenous bolus injection. The penicillin is given to kill clostridial organisms and prevent the release of more neurotoxin. Penicillin has no effect on the already liberated toxin.

Prognosis

For the established case of tetanus with respiratory insufficiency, mortality rates are usually 30–60%. The mortality rate is inversely proportionate to the length of the incubation period and directly proportionate to the severity of symptoms. An attack of tetanus does not confer lasting immunity, and such patients after recovery require active immunization according to the usual recommended schedules.

Furste W, Wheeler WL: Tetanus, a team disease. Curr Probl Surg, October 1972.

Moore JH & others: Tetanus at Charity Hospital, New Orleans, La. (Collection of cases from 1962 to 1966.) Surgery 64:397, 1968.

NECROTIZING FASCIITIS

Necrotizing fasciitis is an invasive infection of fascia, usually due to multiple pathogens, characterized by thrombosis of vessels passing between the skin and deep circulation, producing skin necrosis superficially resembling ischemic vascular or clostridial gangrene.

Clinical Findings

Fasciitis usually begins in a localized area such as a puncture wound or leg ulcer. The infection spreads along the relatively hypoxic fascial planes, meanwhile causing the penetrating vessels to thrombose. The skin is thus devascularized, whereas the muscle and bone are usually unaffected. Externally, hemorrhagic bullae are usually the first sign of skin death. The fascial necrosis is usually wider than the skin appearance indicates. The bullae and skin necrosis are surrounded by edema and inflammation. Crepitus is occasionally present, and the skin may be anesthetic. The patient often seems alert and unconcerned, although he appears toxic and has fever and tachycardia.

Bacteriologic cultures and gram-stained smears are helpful for diagnosis and treatment. The infection is usually a mixed one with microaerophilic streptococci, staphylococci, or both, commonly in conjunction with gram-negative bacilli. This finding allows early choice of penicillin, but the sensitivities of the gram-negative bacilli are not predictable. Clostridia are sometimes seen, and the disease has many clinical features in common with clostridial cellulitis. Bacteroides may also be a part of the mixed flora. At surgery, the findings of edematous and dull-gray and necrotic fascia and subcutaneous tissue confirm the diagnosis. One can also see the thrombi in penetrating veins.

One may encounter related infections in which severe fascial or muscle gangrene may occur with relatively little evidence that such a severe process is occurring. Wide muscle necrosis may be encountered and should always be suspected.

Differential Diagnosis

Although it is essential to avoid underestimating the severity of the disease and confusing it with cellulitis, localized abscess, and phlebitis, it is also necessary not to confuse necrotizing fasciitis with clostridial cellulitis or myositis or vascular gangrene. Fasciitis advances rapidly; Meleney's ulcer (chronic progressive cutaneous gangrene) advances very slowly.

Treatment

No preventive measures are available. Treatment

consists of surgical debridement, antibiotics, and support of the local and general circulation.

A. Surgical Treatment: Debridement, under general or spinal anesthesia, must be thorough, with removal of all avascular skin and fascia. This may require extensive denudation of an extremity. Where necrotic fascia undermines viable skin, longitudinal skin incisions may be helpful in obtaining full debridement of fascia without sacrificing excessive skin. It is essential to avoid confusing fasciitis with deep gangrene. It is a tragic error to amputate an extremity when removal of dead skin and fascia will suffice. A functional extremity can usually be salvaged in fasciitis; if not, amputation can be safely performed later. If debridement is adequate, antibiotic irrigation of the wound should not be necessary.

It is often difficult to accurately distinguish necrotic from edematous tissue. Careful daily inspections of the wound will demonstrate whether repeated debridements will be necessary. If possible, all obviously necrotic tissue should be removed the first time. When viability of the remaining tissue is assured and the infection has been controlled, homografting is sometimes useful until autografting can be performed.

B. Antibiotics: Intravenous penicillin, 20–40 million units per day, is begun as soon as material has been taken for smear and culture. Because gram-negative bacteria are so often seen in this disease, another appropriate antibiotic (eg, kanamycin, 15 mg/kg/day, or gentamicin, 5 mg/kg/day) should be added and changed if indicated by reports of antibiotic sensitivity.

C. Circulatory Support: Blood volume must be maintained with blood or plasma. Debridement often leaves a large raw surface which may bleed extensively. Since tissue oxygenation is critical, it seems reasonable to transfuse early with fresh blood. Diabetes, if present, should be treated appropriately.

Prognosis

Reliable data on prognosis are not available since the proper diagnosis is so often missed. Death often results, especially in elderly patients.

Rea WJ, Wyrick WJ: Necrotizing fasciitis. Ann Surg 172:957, 1970.

Stone HH, Martin JD Jr: Synergistic necrotizing cellulitis. Ann Surg 175:702, 1972.

OTHER ANAEROBIC INFECTIONS

A number of bacteria can cause the typical features of anaerobic infection. Microaerophilic streptococci, gram-negative bacilli, and, more frequently, bacteroides (gastrointestinal strains) are being seen. Some of these are gas-producing and others are not. In general, they are less aggressive than clostridia, but they are also less easily treated. These bacteria may invade alone or in combination.

LUDWIG'S ANGINA

Ludwig's angina is an acute invasive infection, usually originating in the oropharynx, which causes severe edema in the upper neck that may cause airway obstruction. It is usually caused by streptococci or staphylococci, but other organisms, including anaerobes, may play a role. It is a cellulitis involving the deeper structures of the neck and usually remains localized to the upper neck and the floor of the mouth. Constitutional symptoms may be severe, however, and respiratory difficulty is common.

The disease usually begins in some form of oral lesion such as an alveolar abscess which spreads into the floor of the mouth and soft tissues of the neck. At times, the origin is obscure. Edema and swelling often increase rapidly, but there may be no fluctuation. Redness of the skin is a late sign. Edema of the glottis, respiratory obstruction, and bronchopneumonia with rapid demise of the patient occur unless treatment is instituted promptly.

The disease is now rare, but failure to recognize its lethal potential still results in fatalities.

The diagnosis is based largely on the clinical findings, with confirmation by smear and culture if pus can be found. Treatment should be started with penicillin, 10–20 million units daily IV if gram-positive cocci in chains are found on smear. If staphylococci are found, a penicillinase-resistant penicillin should be used.

The response to antibiotics is usually rapid, but because the infection produces tension in the deeper structures of the neck with respiratory insufficiency, radical incision and drainage are often indicated. Although a large amount of pus may not be released by drainage, improvement is usually prompt.

Tracheostomy may be lifesaving and should always be considered early if the response is not dramatically favorable to antibiotics and drainage.

VINCENT'S ANGINA & NOMA

Vincent's angina—also called trench mouth, ulceromembranous stomatitis, and necrotizing ulcerogingivostomatitis—usually presents as an acute inflammatory disease of the mouth or pharynx which starts as a red edematous area in which a grayish-white pseudomembrane develops over an ulcer. The ulcers are characteristically shallow and rarely larger than 0.5 cm in diameter. They are usually tender and painful. The disease usually lasts 8–16 days and rarely causes systemic symptoms.

Noma is a rapidly enlarging gangrenous infection of mucous membranes and skin usually occurring in the gingival and facial tissues of undernourished children. It has many names, including cancrum oris or gangrenous stomatitis. It can advance rapidly and is often extremely destructive.

The organisms found in the lesion of Vincent's angina or noma are usually fusiform bacilli and spirochetes. Penicillin is usually effective treatment. Surgery is rarely helpful.

RABIES

Rabies is a viral encephalitis transmitted through the saliva of an infected animal. Humans are usually inoculated by the bite of a rabid bat, skunk, raccoon, fox, wolf, dog, cat, or other animal. Since the established disease is almost invariably fatal, early preventive treatment is essential.

The incubation period varies in humans from 10 days to several months. Clinical symptoms begin with pain and numbness around the site of the wound followed by fever, irritability, malaise, and spasms of the muscles of swallowing. Paralysis and convulsions occur terminally.

Rabies and tetanus have many features in common. The history is the most useful differentiating point.

Prevention

Do not kill the animal, but confine it under veterinary observation for 10 days. If it becomes rabid, the animal should be sacrificed and its brain examined for rabies antigen by immunofluorescence. If the animal dies of any cause, or if it is inadvertently killed before 10 days have passed, the head should be sent to the nearest public health or other competent laboratory for examination. Consult local health authorities to determine if any cases of rabies have been reported recently.

The wound should be flushed immediately and cleaned repeatedly with soap and water. Tetanus prophylaxis should be given. For severe exposure, the area around the wound should be infiltrated with anti-rabies serum.

The indications for vaccine and serum are summarized in Table 10-1.

TABLE 10-1. Specific systemic treatment for rabies.*

Nature of Exposure	Status of Biting Animal (Vaccinated or Not)		Recommended Treatment
	At Time of Exposure	10-Day Observation Period	
No lesions (indirect contact)	Rabid	. . .	None
Licks			
Unabraded skin	Rabid	. . .	None
Abraded skin, scratches and unabraded or abraded mucosa	Healthy	Clinical signs of rabies or proved rabid (laboratory)	Start vaccine† at first signs of rabies in biting animal.
	Signs suggestive of rabies	Healthy	Start vaccine† immediately; stop treatment if animal is normal on fifth day after exposure.
	Rabid, escaped, killed, unknown	. . .	Start vaccine† immediately.
Bites			
Mild exposure	Healthy	Clinical signs of rabies or proved rabid (laboratory)	Start vaccine‡ at first sign of rabies in biting animal.
	Signs suggestive of rabies	Healthy	Start vaccine† immediately; stop treatment if animal is normal on fifth day after exposure.
	Rabid, escaped, killed, unknown	. . .	Start vaccine† ‡ immediately.
	Wild (wolf, jackal, fox, bat, etc)	. . .	Serum‡ immediately, followed by vaccine.†
Severe exposure (multiple, or face, head, finger, or neck bites)	Healthy	Clinical signs of rabies or proved rabid (laboratory)	Serum‡ immediately; start vaccine† at first sign of rabies in biting animal.
	Signs suggestive of rabies	Healthy	Serum‡ immediately, followed by vaccine.† Vaccine may be stopped if animal is normal on fifth day after exposure.
	Rabid, escaped, killed, unknown		
	Wild (wolf, jackal, pariah dog, fox, bat, etc)	. . .	Serum‡ immediately, followed by vaccine.†

*From WHO Expert Committee on Rabies, Fifth Report. World Health Organization Technical Report Series No. 321, 1966.

†Practice varies concerning the volume of vaccine per dose and the number of doses given. (See package insert for further details.)

‡In all severe exposures and in all cases of unprovoked wild animal bites, antirabies serum or its globulin fraction together with vaccine should be employed. Because both the serum and the vaccine can cause deleterious reactions, continued therapy in mild exposures is considered optional. As with vaccine alone, it is important to start combined serum and vaccine treatment as early as possible after exposure, but serum should still be used no matter what the time interval. Serum should be given in a single dose (40 IU/kg body weight) and the first dose of vaccine inoculated at the same time. Sensitivity to the serum must be determined before its administration. (See package inserts for further details.)

ANTHRAX

Anthrax (woolsorter's disease, malignant pustule) was once a common disease, particularly in Europe, but is now rare. The causative organism is *Bacillus anthracis,* a gram-positive spore-forming bacillus which is found in long chains on the smear. The infection is usually acquired by handling the wool or hides of infected animals. The reservoir includes sheep, cattle, horses, guinea pigs, hogs, and rabbits.

The disease is usually divided into 3 types: (1) The cutaneous type is most common and has a very low mortality rate. It usually begins as a furuncle which then develops a black, necrotic center. (2) The pulmonary form of the disease is presumably the result of inhalation of spores. The patient becomes rapidly ill, with chills, fever, tachycardia, cough, and pulmonary edema. This form is usually fatal because the diagnosis is made too late for effective treatment. (3) The intestinal infection causes chills, fever, diarrhea, and vomiting. This form also has a high mortality rate.

All forms of the disease respond to parenteral penicillin, 2–5 million units per day. Tetracycline is a somewhat less effective second choice.

TYPHOID FEVER

Typhoid fever is now much less common than formerly. Its initial manifestations are protean and are best described in textbooks of infectious diseases.

Typhoid fever is discussed here because of its surgical complications. It often causes necrosis of lymphoid tissue of the intestine. This develops into ulcers, usually of the ileum, which occasionally perforate. The signs of typhoid perforation may be occult but often are obvious, with abdominal pain and signs of spreading peritonitis. The diagnosis is confirmed by the discovery of free air on x-ray of the abdomen. Significant hemorrhage sometimes results from the mucosal ulcer and may require emergency operation. Small perforations can be simply closed if bacteriologic control has been achieved. Larger lesions may require resection.

Although cholecystitis due to typhoid is rarely diagnosed, it is a fairly common cause of the carrier state. When patients continue to excrete *Salmonella typhi* in the stool despite adequate treatment with chloramphenicol or ampicillin, cholecystectomy is indicated.

The other common surgical complications of typhoid are osteomyelitis and chondritis.

Either chloramphenciol (2–3 g/day orally) or ampicillin is effective.

ECHINOCOCCOSIS
(Hydatid Disease)

Echinococcosis is caused by a tapeworm, *Echinococcus granulosus,* which forms larval cysts in human tissue. Dogs and, in some areas, foxes are the definitive hosts which harbor adult worms in their intestines. Ova are passed in the feces and are ingested by intermediate hosts such as cattle, man, rodents, and particularly sheep. Dogs become infected by eating uncooked sheep carcasses which contain hydatid cysts.

Most human infection occurs in childhood following ingestion of materials contaminated with dog feces. The ova penetrate the intestine and pass via the portal vein to the liver and then to the lung or other tissues. In the tissue, the ovum develops into a cyst filled with clear fluid. Brood capsules containing scoleces bud into the cyst lumen. Such "endocysts" may cause secondary intraperitoneal cyst formation if spilled into the peritoneal cavity.

The disease may cause systemic allergic manifestations or local symptoms due to pressure by the cyst. The patient may complain of hives, or, if the cyst ruptures, he may go into anaphylactic shock. Eosinophilia is present in about 40% of infected patients. The liver and the lungs account for 90% of cases, but the cysts can occur in many other organs and tissues. Ordinarily, the cyst is solitary in man. In 25% of patients, the parasite dies, the cyst wall calcifies, and therapy is not required.

Diagnosis may be substantiated by immunologic tests. Intradermal reaction tests are inaccurate. Hemagglutination inhibition and complement fixation tests are accurate and useful since they become negative if treatment eradicates the parasite.

Hydatid Disease of the Liver

Hydatid disease of the liver usually presents with hepatomegaly and chronic right upper quadrant pain in a past resident of an endemic area. Liver scan will outline the cyst or cysts, usually in the right lobe. In about 15% of cases, there are 2 cysts. Selective hepatic arteriography should also be obtained.

The only effective treatment is surgical. Because of the dangers of anaphylaxis or implantation, great care must be taken to avoid rupturing the cyst and spilling its contents into the peritoneal cavity. The fluid in the cyst is aspirated and replaced by a scolicidal agent. Both formalin and phenol have been used, but hypertonic (20–30%) sodium chloride solution or sodium hypochlorite (0.5%) destroys the scoleces and causes no damage if spilled into the abdomen or accidentally injected into the bile ducts.

The cyst can usually be shelled out intact by developing a cleavage plane between the endocyst and ectocyst layers. The resulting cavity can be drained, but it is simpler to fill it with normal saline solution and close it with catgut sutures. Hepatic lobectomy may sometimes be required for especially large cysts.

If rupture occurs into the bile ducts, biliary colic

and jaundice develop. Treatment consists of common duct exploration and excision of the cyst.

Hydatid Disease of the Lungs

Hydatid cysts of the lung cause chest pain and dyspnea. They may secondarily communicate with bronchioles and become infected. Oral expulsion of the cyst fluid may follow rupture into a bronchus, after which an air-fluid level can be seen on chest x-ray.

Removal of pulmonary cysts presents fewer technical difficulties than those in the liver. The lung is incised over the cyst, and, while the anesthesiologist inflates the lung, the cyst can be slowly delivered intact. Large cysts may be managed by lobectomy, but pneumonectomy is rarely necessary. Secondary bacterial infection and abscess formation should be treated as for pulmonary abscess in general.

Heslop JH: An assessment of the efficacy of hydatid scolicidal agents used locally in surgery. Australian New Zealand J Surg 37:205–208, 1967.

Pissiotis CA & others: Surgical treatment of hydatid disease. Arch Surg 104:454–459, 1972.

Romero-Torres R, Cambell JR: An interpretive review of the surgical treatment of hydatid disease. Surg Gynec Obst 121:851–864, 1965.

Schiller CF: Complications of Echinococcus cyst rupture. JAMA 195:220–222, 1966.

Wolcott MW & others: Hydatid disease of the lung. J Thoracic Cardiovas Surg 62:465–469, 1971.

AMEBIASIS

Amebiasis is caused by the protozoal parasite *Entamoeba histolytica.* Ten percent of the world's population is infected. The active vegetative form—the trophozoites—often inhabit the colon where they subsist on bacteria, usually without causing symptoms. The trophozoites may develop into more resistant cystic forms which are passed in stools. The infection is transmitted by oral-fecal contact. Invasion by trophozoites produces disease principally in the colon and liver. Skin, brain, vagina, etc are involved rarely. Active disease is accompanied by elevated antibody titers, best detected by the hemagglutination test.

Clinical Findings

A. Intestinal Amebiasis: When the amebas invade the colon, they burrow through the colonic mucosa, producing ulcers by undermining the mucosa. The resulting colitis may vary in severity from chronic and indolent to acute and fulminating.

1. Amebic dysentery—The average case begins with intermittent cramps. After weeks to months, mild diarrhea with blood-stained mucus develops. Fever is usually less than 38.5 C (101.3 F), and the patient is rarely seriously ill. Tenderness is present to palpation in both lower quadrants, and the liver is often slightly enlarged.

Trophozoites can be demonstrated in stools examined in the fresh warm state. It may be necessary to examine 3 or 4 (or more) specimens obtained on different days without purgatives.

2. Severe amebic colitis—This uncommon variation of amebic dysentery may progress to colonic perforation and peritonitis. It may begin suddenly with severe diarrhea of blood and mucus. Abdominal pain, cramps, tenesmus, and dehydration are severe. The patient is toxic, with fever from 39–40 C (102.2–104 F) and leukocytosis in the range of 25,000/μl. The stools often contain sloughs of colonic mucosa produced by the undermining action of the ameba.

Sigmoidoscopy demonstrates the typical small, white-capped amebic ulcers, but the examination must be performed gently to avoid perforation of the fragile bowel. Stool or mucosa obtained by sigmoidoscopy may reveal the trophozoites. Colonic dilatation may closely resemble acute ulcerative colitis. The distinction is critical because administration of corticosteroid drugs severely aggravates amebic colitis and colectomy is usually fatal, whereas amebicides and tetracycline usually control the disease. Very rarely, operation may be necessary for perforation.

3. Localized intestinal disease—Occasionally the amebas invade only a short segment of colon—usually the cecum and sigmoid colon. A chronic inflammatory process may lead to stricture formation or a granulomatous mass called **ameboma.** The typical patient presents with pain in the right lower quadrant and an enlarged and tender cecum and ascending colon. A history of dysentery is usually obtained, and trophozoites can be demonstrated in stool specimens. Barium enema shows concentric narrowing of the affected bowel. Resection may be indicated for intestinal obstruction, but in most cases drug therapy is curative.

Rectal strictures are sometimes produced and may be confused with neoplasms or lymphogranuloma venereum.

B. Hepatic Amebiasis: Hepatic involvement results from seeding of the liver via the portal vein and is usually a single abscess. In less than 10% of cases, liver abscess develops, with right upper quadrant pain, fever, and tenderness. In 50%, the amebic abscess appears with no history of dysentery. The right lobe is involved 90% of the time. The abscess contains sterile pus ("anchovy paste") which varies from pink to chocolate-brown in color. Trophozoites are found only at the active periphery of the abscess. Even there, recovery is rare.

Fever usually ranges from 38–39 C (100.4–102.2 F), and the white count is elevated to 15,000–25,000/μl. There is tenderness in the right upper quadrant, maximal over the abscess. Motion makes the pain worse. Serum bilirubin is usually normal unless secondary pyogenic infection occurs. The serum alkaline phosphatase is often increased. X-rays show an elevated right diaphragm and pleural fluid in the right hemithorax. Radioactive hepatic scan shows the location of the abscess and helps in selecting the site for percutaneous aspiration.

The distinction from pyogenic abscess may be difficult. In fact, secondary pyogenic infection is common. The presence of infection elsewhere in the abdomen in a severely toxic patient suggests a bacterial abscess. The presence of trophozoites in the stool, sterile pus in the abscess, and serologic tests are the major differential features.

The abscess may burst into the peritoneal cavity or occasionally into the pleural space.

Treatment

Metronidazole (Flagyl), 400 mg orally 3 times daily for 5 days, is usually sufficient for hepatic abscess; 800 mg orally 3 times daily are needed for amebic dysentery.

Emetine is effective against the intestinal parasites, and chloroquine, 500 mg/day orally for 10 weeks, will cure most hepatic abscesses. Emetine has many serious side-effects.

The resolution of hepatic abscesses can be hastened by aspirating their contents through a needle inserted percutaneously through an intercostal space. This technic is especially beneficial for large abscesses or those thought to be close to rupturing. Laparotomy and surgical drainage should be reserved for abscesses which have become secondarily infected.

Barrett-Connor E: Amebiasis, today, in the United States. California Med 114:1–6, Mar 1971.

Juniper K Jr & others: Serologic diagnosis of amebiasis. Am J Trop Med 21:157–168, 1972.

Powell SJ: New developments in the therapy of amoebiasis. Gut 11:967–969, 1970.

Reynolds TB: Amoebic abscess of the liver. Gastroenterology 60:952–954, 1971.

Stamm WP: Amoebic aphorisms. Lancet 2:1355–1356, 1970.

Wilmot AJ: *Clinical Amoebiasis.* Blackwell, 1962.

TULAREMIA

Tularemia is caused by *Francisella (Pasteurella) tularensis,* which is endemic in many rodents and other animals. The organism can be transmitted by ticks or biting flies. Most human infections, however, result from handling or dressing infected animals. Cooking usually destroys the bacteria.

Clinical Findings

The patient usually gives a history of hunting or handling wild animals and minor injury of the hands. The incubation period varies from 4–30 days, and asymptomatic infections are common.

A. **Symptoms and Signs:**

1. **Ulceroglandular type (most common)**—The onset is sudden, with fever, chills, headache, muscle pains, and occasionally delirium. At the site of inoculation, a superficial ulcer forms. Occasionally, the primary lesion is not apparent. The lymph nodes draining the area of inoculation become enlarged, discrete, and slightly tender. The surgeon is called because the initial ulcer fails to heal and the lymph nodes suppurate.

2. **Other forms**—The primary lesion is inapparent or the adenopathy is not prominent. These forms are rarely seen by the surgeon. They occur when the organism primarily involves the gastrointestinal tract, the lungs, or the eyes.

B. **Laboratory Findings:** The diagnosis is usually made from smear and culture of the primary lesion or a suppurating lymph node. Blood cultures may be positive.

Treatment & Prognosis

The suppurative nodes may require incision and drainage or occasionally excision, but the mainstay of treatment is the use of tetracyclines or streptomycin. Sites of incision and drainage are characteristically slow to heal. With early treatment, the mortality rate is 1–2%.

ACTINOMYCOSIS & NOCARDIOSIS

Actinomycosis and nocardiosis are chronic, slowly advancing infections which invade multiple tissues and tend to form abscesses, sinuses, and fistulas. The organisms are filamentous bacteria which are part of the normal flora of the tonsils. They produce a granulomatous type of inflammatory response in man. Organisms may penetrate breaks in the mucous membranes of the mouth, pharynx, lungs, or lower gastrointestinal tract. The lesions are most commonly seen in the head and neck, and less commonly in the abdomen, where they usually involve the cecum or appendix. About 15% of clinical infections involve the thoracic cavity and chest wall. The surface manifestations of the disease usually begin as a hard nodule that slowly enlarges and softens over weeks or months, forms an abscess which may involve even bone, and penetrates to the outside, where it drains through a small nonhealing sinus. Multiple sinuses from the same center of infection are common. Pus may contain typical "sulfur granules." The surrounding inflammation is only mildly tender, causes little pain, and is characteristically woody hard. Systemic symptoms and fever may or may not be present. Once the sinus is formed, superinfection is the rule and destruction of the infecting organisms may make the diagnosis extremely difficult.

In the abdominal form, the first symptoms may simulate appendicitis and lead to appendectomy, which is curative if the appendix has not perforated. Following perforating appendicitis, sinuses of the abdominal wall develop insidiously.

Thoracic actinomycosis is usually secondary to an active lesion in the neck or abdomen. The disease is similar to tuberculosis and may produce cough, pleural pain, fever, sputum, night sweats, and weight loss. The sinuses eventually penetrate the pleural cavity and the chest wall.

Treatment

Cure can be expected if the diagnosis is made early and treatment with massive doses of penicillin or tetracycline is continued for several months.

When the disease is encountered in its advanced form with multiple sinuses and invasion of bone, cure can rarely be achieved by medical therapy alone but requires aggressive excision and drainage.

Medical Letter Handbook of Antimicrobial Therapy, Vol 14, No. 3, January 21, 1972.
Wangensteen OH: The role of surgery in the treatment of actinomycosis. Ann Surg 104:752, 1936.

INFECTIONS RESULTING FROM DRUG ABUSE

The recent increase of drug abuse has resulted in a number of atypical infections which demand unusual expertise on the part of the surgeon.

Clinical Findings

Infections associated with drug abuse commonly result from intravascular or extravascular injection of irritating or even necrotizing substances which may contain bacteria and foreign material. As a consequence, the local lesion is complicated in a high percentage of cases by large areas of necrosis, bacteremia, and septic emboli. The needle may penetrate the fascia, causing deep space infections in which fluctuation or other external signs of abscess may be absent. The patient is often debilitated and may be highly susceptible to infection.

Bacterial contamination occurs through commonly used unsterile syringes, needles, and drugs. Drugs are mixed with methamphetamine, talcum powder, lighter fluid, barbiturates, or milk, all of which kill tissue and provide an ideal medium for bacterial growth. The addict may give no history or signs of habituation, may give an inaccurate history, and may use drugs even while under treatment.

A typical problem is a grossly swollen, tense, immobile forearm which is acutely tender but shows no localizing signs of infection. Fever and tachycardia are usually not severe. Many such acute, possibly sterile reactions will subside with rest, elevation, and hot packs. On the other hand, if sepsis is suspected on the basis of the systemic effects, surgical drainage is mandatory even though localization may be difficult. Unfortunately, addicts have many reasons for fever, including other drug-related problems such as withdrawal, pneumonia, empyema, hepatitis, or endocarditis.

Complications

The infectious complications of drug abuse are multiple. The most important are injection abscess, pylephlebitis, pneumonia (with foreign body embolus), empyema, hepatitis, endocarditis, synovitis, meningitis, pelvic inflammatory disease, and tetanus.

Treatment

Drainage of abscesses is essential, but they are often difficult to find. When the abscess is not found in the subcutaneous tissue, the deep fascia and muscle compartments must be opened. Neurologic findings may help, eg, median nerve paresis is an indication for extensive deep exploration if the injection was in the antecubital fossa.

Infection may spread along the vein and necessitate its removal, often up to the next major tributary.

Necrotic skin indicates extensive deeper damage requiring extensive excision.

Fever that does not respond to drainage within 24 hours indicates additional sites of infection.

Bacteremia may arise from mycotic arterial aneurysms, especially in amphetamine addicts. Arteriograms followed by excision during specific antibiotic therapy may be required. Coexisting endocarditis (bacterial or candidal) must be considered. Drug-related valvulitis with destroyed valves may require emergency excision and replacement. Early diagnosis and aggressive therapy are extremely important.

Tetanus is also prevalent in addicts, and immunization is imperative.

Intra-arterial injection of barbiturates or methamphetamine may cause acute vascular obstruction which may at first mimic cellulitis or abscess. Heroin is often diluted with barbiturates, and inadvertent arterial injection of heroin may cause a serious reaction.

Prognosis

The prognosis for long-term survival is poor in heroin or methamphetamine addicts who have destroyed their veins to the point where extravasation occurs or they are reduced to "skin popping" (subcutaneous injection). Many limbs have been crippled or lost as a result of this pattern of abuse.

Butterfield WC: Surgical complications of narcotic addiction. Surg Gynec Obst 134:237, 1972.

VENEREAL DISEASES

Venereal diseases are now treated principally by medical means, but their complications may require surgery.

Syphilis

Syphilis is rarely a surgical disease, but the cutaneous lesions of syphilis may masquerade as skin tumors or as stubborn infectious lesions. The primary ulcer (chancre) occurs most often on the genitalia, face, or anus and is self-limited. Secondary lesions usually begin as indurated nodules which break down to form punched-out ulcers with sharp epidermal edges. They may occur anywhere but are particularly common on the legs and form part of the differential diagnosis of leg ulcer.

Syphilis is known as "the great imitator." It produces gummas (tumorous granulomas specific to syphilis) which may involve the gastrointestinal tract, skin, bones, joints, or nose and throat. They may invade tissues such as the nasal septum, where perforations occur, and may cause masses in liver or in bone.

The diagnosis is made by darkfield or immunofluorescent examination of smears or exudates and by serologic tests. Treatment is with penicillin.

Yaws

Yaws (frambesia) is not a venereal disease but is closely related to syphilis since it is caused by *Treponema pertenue*. It causes ulcerating papules resembling those of syphilis. The disease is endemic, particularly among children, in hot tropical countries.

Diagnosis and treatment are the same as for syphilis.

Gonorrhea

Although gonorrhea usually begins with urethritis, producing a creamy exudate, it may also cause a painful proctitis—now commonly seen both in women and in homosexual males. It may also cause epididymitis and prostatitis; may involve the joints or even the meninges; and can cause serious systemic symptoms. Surgery is rarely needed except for gonococcal strictures of the urinary tract or for excision of tubo-ovarian abscess.

The diagnosis is made by finding gram-negative intracellular diplococci on smear. Culture revealing *Neisseria gonorrhoeae* is also usually necessary. Treatment is with penicillin or tetracyclines.

Chancroid

Chancroid is not a surgical disease. In its primary phase, it can be differentiated from syphilis on the basis of its angular, very shallow genital ulceration, with purulent discharge and pain—as opposed to the usually painless chancre, with raised edges, of syphilis. Chancroid does not give a positive serologic test for syphilis, but patients with chancroid may have or have had syphilis. Darkfield examination is negative. Smear reveals a mixed flora including gram-negative rods in chains. The major organism is *Haemophilus ducreyi*.

Treatment usually consists of tetracyclines or sulfonamides.

Lymphogranuloma Venereum

Lymphogranuloma venereum (esthiomene, tropical bubo, lymphopathia venereum) can produce serious surgical lesions. It is caused by an organism (Chlamydia) similar to that which causes psittacosis. The disease may manifest itself in 2 major ways. In men, the most common feature is inguinal adenopathy progressing to suppuration and nonhealing sinuses. In women and homosexual males, the most common presentation is ulcerative proctitis. The proctitis, if improperly treated, frequently results in stricture of the anus and rectum and multiple perianal infections. The infections may form multiple anal fistulas which in turn cause the so-called "watering pot perineum." This complication may require colostomy and multiple plastic surgical procedures of the anus. Occasionally, condylomatous lesions about the anus occur. Elephantiasis of the genitalia may result from chronic lymphatic obstruction.

The diagnosis is confirmed by serologic tests. Treatment usually consists of tetracycline, chloramphenicol, or sulfonamides.

Granuloma Inguinale

Granuloma inguinale is a relatively uncommon infection caused by *Donovania (Calymmatobacterium) granulomatis*. The lesion usually begins as a pustule in or around the genitalia. It soon ulcerates, produces a milky secretion, and slowly invades the adjacent skin. Although it is an infectious disease, it can behave in almost a malignant fashion when not treated. It rarely causes pain or tenderness and usually advances radially from the genitalia or from the anus.

Diagnosis is best made by finding "Donovan bodies" in biopsy material. Treatment is usually with tetracyclines. Streptomycin and ampicillin are second-choice drugs.

Condylomata Acuminata (Venereal Warts)

Venereal warts are a common surgical problem. They are usually seen around the genitalia and anus as painful cauliflower-like papillomas with a rough papillated surface. The etiologic agent is a virus related to or identical with that of molluscum contagiosum. Rarely, these warts invade the urethra and bladder or rectum, where extensive operative procedures may be needed to eradicate them and their obstructive effects.

The differential diagnosis includes syphilitic or lymphogranulomatous condylomas, hemorrhoids, and skin cancer. All warts which fail to respond to podophyllin should be cultured and biopsied.

The vast majority of external venereal warts are best treated by painting with tincture of podophyllin. This is extremely effective, but the podophyllin can cause pain, and extensive cases should be treated in segments. Warts within the urethra, bladder, anal canal, or rectum usually require fulguration. In stubborn cases, other antiviral agents may be useful.

Brown WJ (editor): *Syphilis and Other Venereal Diseases.* Harvard Univ Press, 1970.

Medical Letter Handbook of Antimicrobial Therapy, Vol 14, No. 3, January 21, 1972.

ANTIMICROBIAL
CHEMOTHERAPY

Microbial infection has always been an accompaniment of surgical procedures, has either delayed or prevented successful results, and has often resulted in death of the patient. Conversely, localized infections of many types—ranging from simple pus collections to infected prosthetic heart valves—have required surgery for cure. The first major step in the control of infectious complications of surgery was the concept of antisepsis, sterilization of instruments, and asepsis. The second was the development of effective antimicrobial drugs which could be used for the control of systemic microbial infections.

Frequent reference is made to the use of antimicrobial drugs in surgery elsewhere in this book, and the cardinal principle often stated is that these drugs are effective adjuncts but not panaceas. Antimicrobial drugs never are a substitute for sound surgical technic, but they can be of help in the management of local infections and may be lifesaving in systemic disseminated infections. Improper application of antimicrobials not only fails to cure the patient but may contribute significantly to patient morbidity and mortality. Widespread improper administration of antimicrobials favors the emergence of drug-resistant organisms, enhances the risk of hospital infections, produces dangerous sensitization of the population, and carries the risk of serious direct toxic effects.

This section summarizes simple principles for the selection of antimicrobials and describes briefly the characteristics and clinical uses of the more important classes of drugs employed in the treatment of microbial infections.

PRINCIPLES OF SELECTION OF
ANTIMICROBIAL DRUGS

Selection of an Antimicrobial
Drug on Clinical Grounds

For optimal treatment of an infectious process, a suitable antimicrobial must be administered as early as possible. This involves a series of decisions: (1) The surgeon decides, on the basis of a clinical impression, that a microbial infection probably exists. (2) Analyzing the symptoms and signs, the surgeon makes a guess at the most likely microorganism causing the suspected infection; he attempts an etiologic diagnosis on clinical grounds. (3) The surgeon selects the drug most likely to be effective against the suspected organism, ie, he aims a specific drug at a specific organism. (4) Before ordering the drug, the surgeon must secure specimens which are likely to reveal the etiologic agent by laboratory examination. (5) He observes the clinical response to the prescribed antimicrobial. Upon receipt of laboratory identification of a possibly important microorganism, he weighs this new information against his original "best guess" of etiologic organism and drug. (6) The surgeon may choose to change his drug regimen then or upon receipt of further laboratory information on drug susceptibility of the isolated organism. However, laboratory data need not always overrule a decision based on clinical and empiric grounds, especially when the clinical response supports the initial etiologic diagnosis and drug selection.

Selection of an Antimicrobial by Laboratory Tests

When an etiologic pathogen has been isolated from a meaningful specimen, it is often possible to select the drug of choice on the basis of current clinical experience. Such a listing of drug choices is given in Table 10−2. At other times, laboratory tests for antimicrobial drug susceptibility are necessary, particularly if the isolated organism is of a type which varies greatly in response to different drugs. The most common laboratory test for antimicrobial susceptibility is the disk test. This test measures the ability of a drug that diffuses through agar to inhibit the growth of an isolated microorganism. The size of the zone of inhibition cannot be directly related to the in vivo activity of the drug. The zone of microbial growth inhibition by a given drug must be compared to a standard for this drug to estimate microbial susceptibility. Zone sizes are not comparable from one drug to another. The disk test determines only growth inhibition and therefore provides no direct guidance when bactericidal activity is required for cure, eg, in bacterial endocarditis, acute hematogenous osteomyelitis, or infection in severely debilitated individuals.

In general, disk tests give valuable results. At times, however, there is a marked discrepancy between the results of the test and the clinical response of the patient treated with the chosen drug. Some possible explanations for such discrepancies are listed below.

(1) The organism isolated from the specimen may not be the one responsible for the infectious process.

(2) Failure to drain a collection of pus, debride necrotic tissue, or remove a foreign body. Antimicrobials can never take the place of surgical drainage and removal.

(3) Superinfection occurs fairly often in the course of prolonged chemotherapy. New microorganisms may have replaced the original infectious agent. This is particularly common with open wounds or sinus tracts.

(4) The drug may not reach the site of active infection in adequate concentration. The pharmacologic properties of antimicrobials determine their absorption and distribution. Certain drugs penetrate poorly into phagocytic cells and thus may not reach intracellular organisms. Some drugs may diffuse poorly into such areas as joints, CNS, or pleural space unless injected directly into the area.

(5) Rarely, 2 or more microorganisms participate in an infectious process but only one may have been isolated from the specimen. The antimicrobial being

TABLE 10–2. Drug selections, 1972–1973.*

Suspected or Proved Etiologic Agent	Drug(s) of First Choice	Alternative Drug(s)
Gram-negative cocci		
Gonococcus	Penicillin[1], ampicillin	Tetracycline[2], erythromycin[3]
Meningococcus	Penicillin[1]	Chloramphenicol, tetracycline
Gram-positive cocci		
Pneumococcus	Penicillin[1]	Erythromycin, lincomycin
Streptococcus, hemolytic groups A,B,C	Penicillin[1]	Erythromycin, lincomycin
Streptococcus viridans	Penicillin[1]	Cephalosporin[4], vancomycin
Staphylococcus, non-penicillinase-producing	Penicillin[1]	Cephalosporin, vancomycin, lincomycin
Staphylococcus, penicillinase-producing	Penicillinase-resistant penicillin[5]	Cephalosporin, vancomycin, lincomycin
Streptococcus faecalis (enterococcus)	Ampicillin plus streptomycin or kanamycin	Penicillin plus kanamycin or gentamicin
Gram-negative rods		
Enterobacter (Aerobacter)	Kanamycin or gentamicin	Tetracycline, chloramphenicol, polymyxin
Bacteroides	Tetracycline	Clindamycin, chloramphenicol
Brucella	Tetracycline plus streptomycin	Streptomycin plus sulfonamide[7]
Escherichia coli sepsis	Kanamycin	Cephalothin, ampicillin
E coli urinary tract infection (first attack)	Sulfonamide[6]	Ampicillin, cephalexin
Haemophilus (meningitis, respiratory infections)	Ampicillin	Chloramphenicol
Klebsiella	Cephalosporin or kanamycin	Gentamicin, chloramphenicol
Mima-Herellea	Kanamycin	Tetracycline, gentamicin
Pasteurella (plague, tularemia)	Streptomycin plus tetracycline	Sulfonamide[7]
Proteus mirabilis	Penicillin or ampicillin	Kanamycin, gentamicin
P vulgaris and other species	Kanamycin or carbenicillin	Chloramphenicol, gentamicin
Pseudomonas aeruginosa	Polymyxin or gentamicin	Carbenicillin
Ps pseudomallei (melioidosis)	Tetracycline plus sulfonamide	Chloramphenicol
Ps mallei (glanders)	Streptomycin plus tetracycline	
Salmonella	Chloramphenicol	Ampicillin
Serratia	Gentamicin	Kanamycin
Shigella	Ampicillin	Tetracycline, kanamycin
Vibrio (cholera)	Tetracycline	Chloramphenicol
Gram-positive rods		
Actinomyces	Penicillin[1]	Tetracycline, sulfonamide
Bacillus (eg, anthrax)	Penicillin[1]	Erythromycin
Clostridium (eg, gas gangrene, tetanus)	Penicillin[1]	Tetracycline, erythromycin
Corynebacterium	Erythromycin	Penicillin, cephalosporin
Listeria	Ampicillin plus aminoglycoside	Tetracycline
Acid-fast rods		
Mycobacterium tuberculosis	INH plus rifampin/ethambutol[8]	Other antituberculosis drugs
Mycobacterium leprae	Dapsone or sulfoxone	Other sulfones
Nocardia	Sulfonamide[7]	Tetracycline, cycloserine
Spirochetes		
Borrelia (relapsing fever)	Tetracycline	Penicillin
Leptospira	Penicillin	Tetracycline
Treponema (syphilis, yaws)	Penicillin	Erythromycin, tetracycline
Mycoplasma	Tetracycline	Erythromycin
Psittacosis-LGV-trachoma agents (chlamydiae)	Tetracycline, sulfonamide[7]	Erythromycin, chloramphenicol
Rickettsiae	Tetracycline	Chloramphenicol

*Reproduced, with permission, from Krupp MA, Chatton MJ (editors): *Current Diagnosis & Treatment 1973.* Lange, 1973.

[1] Penicillin G is preferred for parenteral injection; penicillin G (buffered) or penicillin V for oral administration. Only highly sensitive microorganisms should be treated with oral penicillin.

[2] All tetracyclines have the same activity against microorganisms and all have comparable therapeutic activity and toxicity. Dosage is determined by the rates of absorption and excretion of different preparations.

[3] Erythromycin estolate and triacetyloleandomycin are the best-absorbed oral forms.

[4] Cephalothin and cephaloridine are the best-accepted cephalosporins at present.

[5] Parenteral methicillin, nafcillin, or oxacillin. Oral dicloxacillin or other isoxazolylpenicillin.

[6] For previously untreated urinary tract infection, a highly soluble sulfonamide such as sulfisoxazole or trisulfa-pyrimidines is the first choice.

[7] Trisulfapyrimidines have the advantage of greater solubility in urine over sulfadiazine for oral administration; sodium sulfadiazine is suitable for intravenous injection in severely ill persons.

[8] Either or both.

used may be effective only against the less virulent organism.

(6) In the course of drug administration, resistant mutants may have been selected from a mixed population of microorganisms, and these drug-resistant mutants continue to grow in the presence of the drug.

Assessment of Drug & Dosage

An adequate therapeutic response is an important but not always sufficient indication that the right drug is being given in the right dosage. Proof of drug activity in serum or urine against the original infecting organisms may provide important support for a selected drug regimen even if fever or other signs of infection are continuing. If drug therapy is adequate, the patient's serum will be markedly bactericidal in vitro against the organism isolated from that patient prior to therapy. In infections limited to the urinary tract, the patient's urine must exhibit marked activity against the organism originally isolated from the patient's urine.

Determining Duration of Therapy

The duration of drug therapy is determined in part by clinical response and past experience and in part by laboratory indications of suppression or elimination of infection. Ultimate recovery must be verified by careful follow-up. In evaluating the patient's clinical response, the possibility of adverse reactions to antimicrobial drugs must be kept in mind. Such reactions may mimic continuing activity of the infectious process by causing fever, skin rashes, CNS disturbances, and changes in blood and urine. In the case of many drugs, it is desirable to examine specimens of blood and urine and to assess liver and kidney function at intervals. Abnormal findings may force the surgeon to reduce the dose or even discontinue a given drug.

Oliguria, Impaired Renal Function, & Uremia

Oliguria, impaired renal function, and uremia have an important influence on antimicrobial drug dosage since most of these drugs are excreted—to a greater or lesser extent—by the kidneys. Only minor adjustment in dosage or frequency of administration is necessary with relatively nontoxic drugs (eg, penicillins) or with drugs that are detoxified or excreted mainly by the liver (eg, erythromycins or chloramphenicol). On the other hand, aminoglycosides (streptomycin, kanamycin, gentamicin), polymyxins, tetracyclines, and vancomycin must be drastically reduced in dosage or frequency of administration if toxicity is to be avoided in the presence of nitrogen retention. Some general guidelines for the administration of such drugs to patients with renal failure are given in Table 10–3. The administration of particularly nephrotoxic antimicrobials such as aminoglycosides to patients in renal failure may have to be guided by direct, frequent assay of drug concentration in serum.

In the newborn or premature infant, excretory mechanisms for some antimicrobials are poorly developed and special dosage schedules must be used in order to avoid toxic accumulation of drugs.

Intravenous Antibiotics

When an antibiotic must be administered intravenously (eg, for life-threatening infection or for maintenance of very high blood levels), the following cautions should be observed:

(1) Give in neutral solution (pH 7.0–7.2) of isotonic sodium chloride (0.9%) or dextrose (5%) in water.

(2) Give alone without admixture of any other drug in order to avoid chemical and physical incompatibilities (which can occur frequently).

(3) Administer by intermittent (every 2–6 hours) addition to the intravenous infusion to avoid inactivation (by temperature, changing pH, etc) and prolonged vein irritation from high drug concentration, which favors thrombophlebitis.

(4) The infusion site must be changed every 48 hours to reduce the chance of superinfection.

ANTIMICROBIAL DRUGS

PENICILLINS

The penicillins comprise a large group of antimicrobial substances some of which are natural products of molds and others semisynthetic compounds. They share a common chemical nucleus (6-aminopenicillanic acid) and a common mode of antibacterial action—the inhibition of cell wall mucopeptide (peptidoglycan) synthesis. The penicillins are in 1973 the most important and most widely applicable group of antibacterial drugs. They can be arranged according to several major criteria:

(1) Susceptibility to destruction by penicillinase (ie, hydrolysis by the β-lactamase of bacteria).

(2) Susceptibility to destruction by acid pH (ie, relative stability to gastric acid).

(3) Relative efficacy against gram-positive versus gram-negative bacteria.

Antimicrobial Activity

All penicillins have the same mechanism of antibacterial action. They specifically inhibit the synthesis of bacterial cell walls which contain a complex mucopeptide (peptidoglycan). This leads to lysis of the cell in an isotonic environment and to the formation of "cell wall deficient" forms (L forms, protoplasts) in a hypertonic environment. Penicillins are inactive against bacteria which are not multiplying and thus forming no new cell walls.

One million units of penicillin G equal 0.6 g. Other penicillins are prescribed in grams. A blood serum level of 0.01–1 μg/ml of penicillin G or ampicillin is lethal for a majority of susceptible microorganisms; methicillin and isoxazolylpenicillins are 1/5–1/50 as active.

TABLE 10–3. Use of antibiotics in patients with renal failure.*

	Principal Mode of Excretion or Detoxification	Approximate Half-Life in Serum		Proposed Dosage Regimen in Renal Failure		Significant Removal of Drug by Dialysis (H = Hemodialysis; P = Peritoneal Dialysis)
		Normal	Renal Failure†	Initial Dose‡	Give Half Initial Dose at Interval Of	
Penicillin G	Tubular secretion	0.5 hour	10 hours	6 g IV	8–12 hours	H no, P yes
Ampicillin, carbenicillin	Tubular secretion	1.5 hours	10 hours	6 g IV	8–12 hours	H, P yes
Methicillin	Tubular secretion	0.5 hour	10 hours	6 g IV	8–12 hours	H, P no
Cephalothin	Tubular secretion	0.8 hour	15 hours	4 g IV	18 hours	H, P yes
Cephalexin	Tubular secretion and glomerular filtration	1 hour	15 hours	2 g orally	8–12 hours	H, P yes
Streptomycin	Glomerular filtration	2.5 hours	3–4 days	1 g IM	3–4 days	H, P yes
Kanamycin	Glomerular filtration	3–4 hours	3–4 days	1 g IM	3–4 days	H, P yes
Gentamicin	Glomerular filtration	2.5 hours	2–4 days	2 mg/kg IM	2–3 days	H yes, P no
Vancomycin	Glomerular filtration	6 hours	8–9 days	0.5 g IV	8–10 days	H, P yes
Polymyxin B	Glomerular filtration	5 hours	2–3 days	2.5 mg/kg IV	3–4 days	H no, P yes
Colistimethate	Glomerular filtration	3 hours	2–3 days	5 mg/kg IM	3–4 days	H no, P yes
Tetracycline	Glomerular filtration	8 hours	3 days	1 g orally or 0.5 g IV	3 days	H, P no
Chloramphenicol	Mainly liver	3 hours	4 hours	1 g orally or IV	8 hours	H, P poorly
Erythromycin	Mainly liver	1.5 hours	5 hours	1 g orally or IV	8 hours	H, P poorly
Lincomycin	Glomerular filtration and liver	4.5 hours	10 hours	1 g orally or IV	12 hours	H, P no

*Reproduced, with permission, from Krupp MA, Chatton MJ (editors): *Current Diagnosis & Treatment 1973.* Lange, 1973.

†Considered here to be marked by creatinine clearance of 10 ml/minute or less.

‡For a 60 kg adult with a serious systemic infection. The "initial dose" listed is administered as an intravenous infusion over a period of 1–8 hours, or as 2 intramuscular injections during an 8-hour period, or as 2–3 oral doses during the same period.

Resistance

Resistance to penicillins falls into 3 different categories:

(1) Certain bacteria produce enzymes (penicillinases) which destroy penicillin G, ampicillin, and other penicillins. Clinical penicillin resistance of staphylococci falls largely into this category.

(2) Certain bacteria are resistant to some penicillins although they do not produce enzymes that destroy the drug. Resistance of staphylococci to methicillin and of gonococci to penicillin falls into this category.

(3) Metabolically inactive organisms that make no new cell wall mucopeptide are temporarily resistant to penicillins. They can act as "persisters" and perpetuate infection during and after penicillin treatment. Cell wall deficient (L) forms are in this category.

Absorption, Distribution, & Excretion

After parenteral administration, absorption of most penicillins is complete and rapid. After oral administration, only a portion of the dose is absorbed (from 1/3–1/20, depending upon acid stability, binding to foods, and the presence of buffers). In order to minimize binding to foods, oral penicillins should not be preceded or followed by food for at least 1 hour.

After absorption, penicillins are widely distributed in body fluids and tissues. With parenteral doses of 3–6 g (5–10 million units) per 24 hours of any penicillin injected by continuous infusion or divided intramuscular injections, average serum levels of the drug reach 1–10 units (0.6–6 μg) per ml.

In many tissues, penicillin concentrations are equal to those in serum. Lower levels are found in the eyes and CNS. However, with active inflammation of the meninges, as in bacterial meningitis, penicillin levels in the CSF exceed 0.2 μg/ml with a daily parenteral dose of 12 g. Thus, pneumococcal and meningococcal meningitis may be treated with systemic penicillin G and haemophilus meningitis with intravenous ampicillin, and there is no need for intrathecal injection. Penetration into inflamed joints is likewise sufficient for treatment of infective arthritis caused by susceptible organisms.

Most of the absorbed penicillin is rapidly excreted by the kidneys into the urine—90% by tubular secretion. Tubular secretion can be partially blocked by probenecid (Benemid) to achieve higher systemic levels.

Renal excretion of penicillin results in very high levels in the urine. Thus, systemic daily doses of 6 g of penicillin may yield urine levels of 500–3000 μg/ml—enough to suppress not only gram-positive but also many gram-negative bacteria in the urine (provided they produce no β-lactamase or amidase).

Indications, Dosages, & Routes of Administration

The penicillins are by far the most effective and the most widely used antimicrobial drugs. All oral penicillins must be given 1 hour away from mealtimes to reduce binding and acid inactivation. Blood levels of all penicillins can be raised by simultaneous administration of probenecid, 0.5 g every 6 hours orally (10 mg/kg every 6 hours).

A. Penicillin G: This is the drug of choice for infections caused by gonococci, pneumococci, streptococci, meningococci, non-β-lactamase-producing staphylococci, *Treponema pallidum* and many other spirochetes, *Bacillus anthracis* and other gram-positive rods, clostridia, listeria, and bacteroides.

1. Intramuscular or intravenous—Most of the above-mentioned infections respond to aqueous penicillin G in daily doses of 0.6–5 million units (0.36–3 g) administered by intermittent IM injection every 4–6 hours. Much larger amounts (6–120 g daily) can be given by continuous or intermittent intravenous infusion in serious or complicated infections due to these organisms. Sites for such intravenous administration are subject to thrombophlebitis and superinfection and must be rotated every 2 days and kept scrupulously aseptic. In enterococcal endocarditis, an aminoglycoside is given simultaneously with large doses of a penicillin.

2. Oral—Buffered penicillin G (or penicillin V) is indicated only in minor infections (eg, of the respiratory tract or its associated structures) in daily doses of 1–4 g (1.6–6.4 million units). Oral administration is subject to so many variables that it should not be relied upon in seriously ill patients.

3. Intrathecal—With high serum levels of penicillin, adequate concentrations reach the CNS and CSF for the treatment of CNS infection. Therefore, and because injection of more than 10,000 units of penicillin G into the subdural space may cause convulsions, intrathecal injection has been virtually abandoned.

4. Topical—Rarely, solutions of penicillin (eg, 100,000 units/ml) are instilled into joint or pleural spaces infected with susceptible organisms.

B. Benzathine Penicillin G: This penicillin is a salt of very low water solubility. It is injected intramuscularly to establish a depot which yields low but prolonged drug levels. A single injection of 2.4 million units IM is satisfactory for treatment of beta-hemolytic streptococcal pharyngitis and perhaps for early syphilis. An injection of 1.2–2.4 million units IM every 3–4 weeks provides satisfactory prophylaxis for rheumatics against reinfection with group A streptococci. There is no indication for using this drug by mouth. Procaine penicillin G is another repository form for maintaining drug levels for up to 24 hours. For highly susceptible infections, 300–600 thousand units IM are usually given once daily.

C. Ampicillin, Carbenicillin: These drugs differ from penicillin G in having greater activity against gram-negative bacteria, but, like penicillin G, they are destroyed by penicillinases.

Ampicillin is the drug of current choice for bacterial meningitis in small children, especially meningitis due to *Haemophilus influenzae;* 200 mg/kg/day are injected IV. Ampicillin can be given orally in divided doses, 3–6 g daily, to treat urinary tract infections with coliform bacteria, enterococci, or *Proteus mirabilis.* It is ineffective against enterobacter and pseudomonas. In salmonella infections, ampicillin, 6–12 g daily orally, can be effective in suppressing clinical disease (alternative to chloramphenicol in acute typhoid or paratyphoid) and may eliminate salmonellae from some chronic carriers. Ampicillin is more effective than penicillin G against enterococci and may be used in such infections in combination with streptomycin, kanamycin, or gentamicin.

Carbenicillin is more active against pseudomonas and proteus, but resistance emerges rapidly. A combination of carbenicillin, 12–30 g/day, with gentamicin is suggested in pseudomonas sepsis. Hetacillin is converted in vivo to ampicillin and should not be used.

D. Penicillinase-Resistant Penicillins: Methicillin, oxacillin, cloxacillin, dicloxacillin, nafcillin, and others are relatively resistant to destruction by β-lactamase. The only indication for the use of these drugs is infection by β-lactamase-producing staphylococci.

1. Oral—Oxacillin, cloxacillin, dicloxacillin, or nafcillin may be given in doses of 0.25–0.5 g every 4–6 hours in mild or localized staphylococcal infections (50–100 mg/kg/day for children). Food markedly interferes with absorption.

2. Intravenous—For serious systemic staphylococcal infections, methicillin, 8–16 g, or nafcillin, 6–12 g, is administered IV, usually by injecting 1–2 g during 20–30 minutes every 2 hours into a continuous infusion of 5% dextrose in water or physiologic salt solution. The dose for children is methicillin, 100–300 mg/kg/day, or nafcillin, 50–100 mg/kg/day.

Adverse Effects

The penicillins undoubtedly possess less direct toxicity than any other antibiotics. Most of the serious side-effects are due to hypersensitivity.

A. Allergy: All penicillins are cross-sensitizing and cross-reacting. Any preparation containing penicillin may induce sensitization, including foods or cosmetics. In general, sensitization occurs in direct proportion to the duration and total dose of penicillin received in the past. Skin tests with penicilloylpolylysine, with alkaline hydrolysis products (minor antigen determinants), and with undegraded penicillin can identify many hypersensitive individuals. Among positive reactors to skin tests, the incidence of subsequent penicillin reactions is high. Although many persons develop antibodies to antigenic determinants of penicillin, the presence of such antibodies is not correlated with allergic reactivity (except rare hemolytic anemia), and serologic tests have little predictive value. A history of a penicillin reaction in the past is not reliable; however, in such cases the drug should be administered with caution—ie, have available an artificial airway, 1% epinephrine in a syringe, running intravenous fluids, and competent personnel standing by.

Allergic reactions may occur as typical anaphylactic shock, typical serum sickness type reactions (urticaria, fever, joint swelling, angioneurotic edema, intense pruritus, and respiratory embarrassment occurring 7—12 days after exposure), and a variety of skin rashes, oral lesions, fever, nephritis, eosinophilia, hemolytic anemia, other hematologic disturbances, and vasculitis. The incidence of hypersensitivity to penicillin is estimated to be 3—5% among adults in the USA but is negligible in small children. Acute anaphylactic life-threatening reactions are fortunately very rare. Ampicillin produces skin rashes (mononucleosis-like) 3—5 times more frequently than other penicillins.

Individuals known to be hypersensitive to penicillin can at times tolerate the drug during corticosteroid administration.

B. Toxicity: Since the action of penicillin is directed against a unique bacterial structure, the cell wall, it is virtually without effect on animal cells. The toxic effects of penicillin G are due to the direct irritation caused by intramuscular or intravenous injection of exceedingly high concentrations (eg, 1 g/ml). Such concentrations may cause local pain, induration, thrombophlebitis, or degeneration of an accidentally injected nerve. All penicillins are irritating to the CNS. There is little indication for intrathecal administration at present. A rare patient receiving more than 50 g of penicillin G daily parenterally has exhibited signs of cerebrocortical irritation, presumably as a result of the passage of unusually large amounts of penicillin into the CNS. With doses of this magnitude, direct cation toxicity (Na^+, K^+) can also occur. Potassium penicillin G contains 1.7 mEq of K^+ per million units (2.7 mEq/g), and potassium may accumulate in the presence of renal failure. Carbenicillin contains 4.7 mEq of Na^+ per gram—a risk in heart failure.

Large doses of penicillins given orally may lead to gastrointestinal upset, particularly nausea and diarrhea. Oral therapy may also be accompanied by luxuriant overgrowth of staphylococci, pseudomonas, proteus, or yeasts, which may occasionally cause enteritis.

Superinfections in other organ systems may occur with penicillins as with any antibiotic therapy.

Barrett FF & others: Methicillin-resistant *Staphylococcus aureus* at Boston City Hospital. New England J Med 279:441—448, 1968.
Grieco MH: Cross-allergenicity of the penicillins and the cephalosporins. Arch Int Med 119:141—146, 1967.
Kunin CM: Clinical pharmacology of the new penicillins. Clin Pharmacol Therap 7:166—179, 1966.
Martin WJ: Newer penicillins. M Clin North America 51:1107—1126, 1967.
Pines A & others: Treatment of severe pseudomonas infections. Brit MJ 1:663—665, 1970.

CEPHALOSPORINS

Cephalosporins are a group of compounds closely related to the penicillins. In place of 6-aminopenicillanic acid, cephalosporins have a nucleus of 7-aminocephalosporanic acid. The mode of action is the same as that of penicillins, there is some (limited) cross-allergenicity, and they are resistant to destruction by β-lactamase.

Cephalosporins are bactericidal in vitro in concentrations of 1—20 μg/ml against most gram-positive microorganisms, except *Streptococcus faecalis,* and in concentrations of 5—30 μg/ml against many gram-negative bacteria, except pseudomonas, herellea, proteus, and enterobacter. There is partial cross-resistance between cephalosporins and β-lactamase-resistant penicillins, and methicillin-resistant staphylococci are also resistant to cephalosporins.

Indications, Dosages, & Routes of Administration

A. Oral: Cephaloglycin, 0.5 g 4 times daily orally, yields urine concentrations of 50—5000 μg/ml—sufficient for treatment of urinary tract infections due to coliform organisms. Cephalexin, 0.5 g orally 4 times daily (50 mg/kg/day), can be used in urinary or respiratory tract infections due to susceptible organisms.

B. Intravenous: Cephalothin, 8—16 g daily (for children, 50—100 mg/kg/day) by continuous drip, gives serum concentrations of 5—20 μg/ml. This is adequate for the treatment of gram-negative bacteremia or staphylococcal sepsis, or as a substitute for penicillin in serious infections caused by susceptible organisms in persons allergic to penicillin (although some cross-hypersensitivity exists). Cephaloridine, 4 g daily (for children, up to 100 mg/kg/day) IV, gives serum levels of 10—25 μg/ml. It is used for the same indications.

C. Intramuscular: Cephaloridine, 0.5—1 g IM every 6 hours, is used for the same indications as above in less severely ill patients. Cephalothin is too painful when injected intramuscularly.

Adverse Effects

A. Allergy: Cephalosporins are sensitizing and a

variety of hypersensitivity reactions occur, including anaphylaxis, fever, skin rashes, granulocytopenia, and hemolytic anemia. Cross-allergy also exists with penicillins and can produce the same hypersensitivity reactions. Perhaps 5–15% of penicillin-allergic persons are also hypersensitive to cephalosporins.

B. Toxicity: Local pain after intramuscular injection, thrombophlebitis after intravenous injection. Cephaloridine can cause renal damage with tubular necrosis and uremia.

Griffith RS, Black HR: Cephalexin. M Clin North America 54:1229–1244, 1970.
Meyers BR & others: Cephalexin. Clin Pharmacol Therap 10:810–816, 1969.
Steigbigel NH & others: Clinical evaluation of cephaloridine. Arch Int Med 121:24–38, 1968.
Thoburn R & others: The relationship of cephalothin and penicillin allergy. JAMA 198:345–348, 1966.

ERYTHROMYCIN GROUP
(Macrolides)

The erythromycins are a group of closely related compounds which inhibit protein synthesis and are bacteriostatic or bactericidal against gram-positive organisms—especially pneumococci, streptococci, staphylococci, and corynebacteria—in concentrations of 0.02–2 µg/ml. Neisseriae and mycoplasmas are also susceptible. Activity is enhanced at alkaline pH. Resistant mutants occur in microbial populations, including pneumococci and mycoplasmas, and tend to emerge during prolonged treatment. There is complete cross-resistance among all members of the erythromycin group.

Erythromycins are the drugs of choice in corynebacterial infections (diphtheroid sepsis, erythrasma) and in mycoplasmal pneumonia. They are most useful as substitutes for penicillin in persons with streptococcal and pneumococcal infections who are allergic to penicillin.

Dosages

A. Oral: Erythromycin base, stearate, succinate, or estolate, or troleandomycin, 0.5 g every 6 hours (for children, 40 mg/kg/day).

B. Intravenous: Erythromycin lactobionate or gluceptate, 0.5 g every 12 hours.

Adverse Effects

Nausea, vomiting, and diarrhea may occur after oral intake. Erythromycin estolate or troleandomycin can produce acute cholestatic hepatitis (fever, jaundice, impaired liver function). Most patients recover completely. Upon readministration, the hepatitis promptly recurs. It is probably a hypersensitivity reaction.

TETRACYCLINE GROUP

The tetracyclines are a large group of drugs with common basic chemical structures, antimicrobial activity, and pharmacologic properties. Microorganisms resistant to this group show complete cross-resistance to all tetracyclines. Tetracyclines are inhibitors of protein synthesis. Equal concentrations of all tetracyclines in blood or tissue have approximately equal antimicrobial activity. Because of the emergence of resistant strains, tetracyclines have lost some of their former usefulness. Proteus and pseudomonas are regularly resistant; among coliform bacteria, pneumococci, and streptococci, resistant strains are increasingly common.

Tetracyclines are absorbed somewhat irregularly from the gut. Absorption is limited by the low solubility of the drugs and by chelation with divalent cations, eg, Ca^{++} or Fe^{++}. The drugs are widely distributed in tissues and body fluids, but the levels in CNS, CSF, and joint fluids are only 3–10% of serum levels.

Demeclocycline, methacycline, minocycline, and doxycycline are well absorbed from the gut but are excreted more slowly than others, leading to accumulation and prolonged blood levels.

Indications, Dosages, & Routes of Administration

At present, tetracyclines are the drugs of choice in cholera, mycoplasmal pneumonia, infections with chlamydiae (psittacosis-LGV-trachoma), and infections with some rickettsiae. They may be used in various bacterial infections provided the organism is susceptible, and in amebiasis.

Tetracycline hydrochloride, oxytetracycline, and chlortetracycline are dispensed in 250 mg capsules. Give 0.25–0.5 g orally every 6 hours (for children, 20–40 mg/kg/day).

Demeclocycline and methacycline are long-acting tetracyclines available in capsules containing 50 or 150 mg. Give 0.15–0.3 g orally every 6 hours (for children, 12–20 mg/kg/day). Doxycycline and minocycline are available in capsules containing 50 or 100 mg or as powder for oral suspension. Give 100 mg every 12 hours on the first day and 100 mg/day in 1 or 2 doses for maintenance.

In renal failure, the dosage of tetracycline must be reduced or intervals between doses increased (Table 10–3).

Adverse Effects

Gastrointestinal side-effects, especially diarrhea, nausea, and anorexia, are common. These can be diminished by reducing the dose or by administering tetracyclines with food or carboxymethylcellulose, but sometimes they force discontinuance of the drug. After a few days of oral use, the gut flora is modified so that drug-resistant bacteria and yeasts become prominent. This may cause functional gastrointestinal disturbances, anal pruritus, and even enterocolitis which may result in shock and death.

Tetracyclines are bound to calcium deposited in growing bones and teeth, causing fluorescence, discoloration, enamel dysplasia, deformity, or growth inhibition. Therefore, tetracyclines should not be given to pregnant women or small children.

Tetracyclines can impair hepatic function or even cause liver necrosis in pregnant women, in the presence of preexisting liver damage, or with doses of more than 3 g IV. Outdated tetracycline preparations have been implicated in renal tubular acidosis and other forms of renal damage.

Tetracyclines, principally demeclocycline, may induce photosensitization, especially in blonds. Intravenous injection may cause thrombophlebitis, and intramuscular injection may induce local inflammation with pain.

Kunin CM: The tetracyclines. P Clin North America 15:43–56, 1968.

CHLORAMPHENICOL

Chloramphenicol is a potent inhibitor of bacterial protein synthesis which inhibits the growth of many bacteria and rickettsiae in concentrations of 0.5–10 μg/ml.

Because of its potential toxicity, chloramphenicol is at present a possible drug of choice only in the following cases: (1) symptomatic salmonella infection, eg, typhoid fever: (2) *Haemophilus influenzae* meningitis, laryngotracheitis, or pneumonia that does not respond to ampicillin; (3) occasional gram-negative bacteremia; (4) severe rickettsial infection; (5) meningococcal infection in patients hypersensitive to penicillin; and (6) rapidly progressing bacteroides infections. It is occasionally used topically in ophthalmology.

In serious systemic infection, the dose is 0.5 g orally every 4–6 hours (for children, 30–50 mg/kg/day) for 7–21 days. Similar amounts are given intravenously.

Adverse Effects

Nausea, vomiting, and diarrhea occur infrequently. The most serious adverse effects pertain to the hematopoietic system. Adults taking chloramphenicol in excess of 50 mg/kg/day regularly exhibit disturbances in red cell maturation after 1–2 weeks of blood levels above 25 μg/ml. There is anemia, rise in serum iron concentration, reticulocytopenia, and the appearance of vacuolated nucleated red cells in the bone marrow. These changes regress when the drug is stopped and are not related to the rare aplastic anemia.

Serious aplastic anemia is a rare consequence of chloramphenicol administration and represents a specific, probably genetically determined individual defect. It is not related to dose or time of intake but is seen more frequently with either prolonged or repeated use. It tends to be irreversible and fatal. It is estimated that fatal aplastic anemia occurs 13 times more frequently after the use of chloramphenicol than as a spontaneous occurrence. Hypoplastic anemia may be followed by the development of leukemia.

Chloramphenicol inhibits the metabolism of certain drugs. Thus, it may prolong the action and raise blood concentration of tolbutamide or diphenylhydantoin.

Chloramphenicol is specifically toxic for newborns. Because they lack the mechanism for detoxification of the drug in the liver, the drug may accumulate, producing the highly fatal "gray syndrome" with vomiting, flaccidity, hypothermia, and collapse. Chloramphenicol should only rarely be used in infants, and the dose must be limited to less than 50 mg/kg/day in full-term infants and less than 30 mg/kg/day in prematures.

Ingall D, Sherman JD: Chloramphenicol. P Clin North America 15:57–72, 1968.
Wallerstein RO & others: Statewide study of chloramphenicol therapy and fatal aplastic anemia. JAMA 208:2045–2050, 1969.

AMINOGLYCOSIDES

Aminoglycosides are a group of drugs with similar chemical, antimicrobial, pharmacologic, ototoxic, and nephrotoxic characteristics. Important members are streptomycin, neomycin, kanamycin, and gentamicin. All of the aminoglycosides inhibit microbial protein synthesis. All aminoglycosides are much more active at alkaline pH.

1. STREPTOMYCIN

Streptomycin can be bactericidal for gram-positive and gram-negative bacteria and for *Mycobacterium tuberculosis*. Its antituberculosis activity is described below.

In all bacterial strains there are mutants which are 10–1000 times more resistant to streptomycin than the remainder of the microbial population. These are selected out rapidly in the presence of streptomycin. Treatment with streptomycin for 4–5 days usually results either in eradication of the infecting agent or the emergence of resistant infection which is untreatable with the drug. For this reason, streptomycin is usually employed in combination with another drug to delay the emergence of resistance. Streptomycin may enhance the bactericidal action of penicillins, particularly against *Streptococcus faecalis*.

Activity is enhanced at alkaline pH.

Indications & Dosages

The principal indications for streptomycin at present are (1) serious active tuberculosis; (2) plague, tularemia, or occasional gram-negative sepsis; (3) acute brucellosis (used in conjunction with tetracycline); and (4) bacterial endocarditis caused by *Streptococcus faecalis* or *S viridans* (used in conjunction with penicillin).

The dose in the nontuberculous infections is 0.5–1 g IM every 6–12 hours (for children, 20–40 mg/kg/day), depending on the severity of the disease.

Adverse Effects

The principal side-effects are nephrotoxicity and ototoxicity. Renal damage with nitrogen retention occurs mainly after prolonged high doses or in persons with preexisting impairment of renal function. Damage to the eighth nerve manifests itself mainly by tinnitus, vertigo, ataxia, loss of balance, and occasionally loss of hearing. Chronic vestibular dysfunction is most common after prolonged use of streptomycin. Streptomycin, 2–3 g/day for 4 weeks, has been used to purposely damage semicircular canal function in the treatment of Ménière's disease.

Streptomycin should not be used concurrently with other aminoglycosides, and great caution is necessary in persons with impaired renal function.

2. KANAMYCIN

Kanamycin is an aminoglycoside for systemic use in gram-negative sepsis. Kanamycin is bactericidal for many gram-positive (except enterococci) and gram-negative bacteria in concentrations of 1–10 μg/ml. Activity is enhanced at alkaline pH. Some strains of proteus are susceptible, but pseudomonas and serratia are often resistant. In susceptible bacterial populations, resistant mutants are rare. Kanamycin exhibits complete cross-resistance with neomycin but not with gentamicin.

Kanamycin is not significantly absorbed from the gut. After intramuscular injection (0.5 g every 6–12 hours), serum levels may reach 5–10 μg/ml. The drug is distributed widely in tissues but does not reach significant concentrations in the CSF, joints, or pleural fluid unless injected locally. Excretion is mainly by glomerular filtration into the urine, where levels of 10–50 μg/ml are reached, and into the bile. In the presence of renal insufficiency, the drug may accumulate rapidly and reach toxic levels.

Indications & Dosages

The principal indication for systemic kanamycin is bacteremia caused by gram-negative enteric organisms or, occasionally, serious urinary tract infection with enterobacter, proteus, or other "difficult" organisms. The IM dose is 0.5 g every 6–12 hours (15 mg/kg/day). In renal failure, the dose is reduced and the interval between injections prolonged (Table 10–3).

Adverse Effects

Like all aminoglycosides, kanamycin is ototoxic and nephrotoxic. Kanamycin is believed to be less toxic than neomycin. Proteinuria and nitrogen retention occur commonly during treatment. This must be monitored and the dose or frequency of injection adjusted when creatinine clearance falls. Since kanamycin is often used in surgical patients who have had an episode of shock, monitoring is particularly important. In general, these nephrotoxic effects are reversible upon discontinuance of the drug. The development of deafness is proportionate to the level of drug and the time of its administration, but it can occur unpredictably even after a short course of treatment. Loss of perception of high frequencies in audiograms may be a warning sign. Ototoxicity is a particular risk in patients with impaired kidney function. The sudden absorption of large amounts of kanamycin (or any other aminoglycoside) can lead to respiratory arrest. This has occurred after of 3–5 g of kanamycin (or neomycin) have been left in the peritoneal cavity following bowel surgery. Neostigmine is a specific antidote.

3. NEOMYCIN

Neomycin is analogous in all pharmacologic and antibacterial characteristics to kanamycin. However, it is believed to be more toxic when given parenterally and is therefore used mainly for topical application or for oral use.

Indications, Dosages, & Routes of Administration

After oral intake, only a minute portion of neomycin is absorbed. Most of the drug remains in the gut lumen and alters intestinal flora. For preoperative reduction of the gut flora, give neomycin, 1 g orally every 4–6 hours for 2–3 days before surgery. In hepatic coma, ammonia intoxication can be reduced by suppressing the coliform flora of the gut with neomycin, 1 g orally every 6–8 hours, and limiting the protein intake. Oral neomycin, 50–100 mg/kg/day, is effective against enteropathic *Escherichia coli*. To control surface infections of the skin (pyoderma), ointments containing neomycin, 1–5 mg/g, are applied several times daily. Solutions containing 10 mg/ml of neomycin can be instilled (up to a total of 0.5 g/day) into infected joints, pleura, or tissue spaces.

Adverse Effects

All topically administered forms of neomycin may produce sensitization. Hypersensitivity reactions occur particularly in the eye and skin after repeated use of neomycin ointments. Topical or oral neomycin rarely produces systemic toxicity. However, oral neomycin alters the intestinal flora and thus predisposes to superinfection. Staphylococcal enterocolitis, occasionally fatal, has followed the use of neomycin for preoperative "bowel sterilization."

4. GENTAMICIN

Gentamicin is used in severe infections caused by gram-negative bacteria which are likely to be resistant to other, less toxic drugs. Included are sepsis, infected burns, pneumonia, and other serious infections due to coliform organisms, klebsiella-enterobacter, proteus, pseudomonas, and serratia. The dosage is 2–3 mg/kg/day IM in 3 equal doses for 7–10 days. In life-threatening infections, 5–7 mg/kg/day have been given. In urinary tract infections caused by these organisms, 0.8–1.2 mg/kg/day are given IM for 10 days or longer. It is necessary to monitor renal, auditory, and vestibular functions and to lengthen the interval between doses if renal function declines (Table 10–3).

For infected burns or skin lesions, creams containing 0.1% gentamicin are used. In meningitis due to gram-negative bacteria, 0.1–1 mg gentamicin has been injected daily intrathecally. For endophthalmitis, 10 mg can be injected subconjunctivally.

Renal function must be monitored by repeated creatinine clearance tests. About 2–3% of patients develop vestibular dysfunction (perhaps because of destruction of hair cells), and occasional cases of loss of hearing have been reported.

5. SPECTINOMYCIN

Spectinomycin is an aminocyclitol antibiotic (related to aminoglycosides) for intramuscular administration. It is proposed as an alternative to penicillin for the treatment of gonorrhea, and this is its sole indication. Injection of 2 g into each buttock just once results in blood levels of 100 μg/ml. About 5–10% of gonococci are probably resistant, but cure rates of 85% or more have been claimed. There is usually pain at the injection site, and nausea and fever may occur.

Cornelius SC, Domescik G: Spectinomycin hydrochloride in the treatment of uncomplicated gonorrhea. Brit J Ven Dis 46:212, 1970.

Finland M (editor): International symposium on gentamicin. J Infect Dis 119:335–540, 1969.

Mann CH (editor): Kanamycin: Appraisal after 8 years of clinical application. Ann New York Acad Sc 132:771–1090, 1966.

Weinstein L: Streptomycin. Chap 58, pp 1230–1240, in: *The Pharmacological Basis of Therapeutics,* 3rd ed. Goodman LS, Gilman A (editors). Macmillan, 1965.

POLYMYXINS & COLISTIMETHATE

The polymyxins are a group of basic polypeptides bactericidal for most gram-negative bacteria except proteus and especially useful against pseudomonas.

Indications, Dosages, & Routes of Administration

Polymyxins are indicated in serious infections due to pseudomonas and other gram-negative bacteria which are resistant to other antimicrobial drugs.

A. Intramuscular: The injection of polymyxin B is painful. Therefore, colistimethate (polymyxin E), which contains a local anesthetic and is more rapidly excreted in the urine, is given IM 2.5–5 mg/kg/day, for urinary tract infection.

B. Intravenous: In pseudomonas sepsis, polymyxin B sulfate, 2.5 mg/kg/day, is injected by continuous IV infusion.

C. Intrathecal: In pseudomonas meningitis, give polymyxin B sulfate, 2–10 mg once daily for 2–3 days, and then every other day for 2–3 weeks.

D. Topical: Solutions of polymyxin B sulfate, 1 mg/ml, can be applied to infected surfaces, injected into joint spaces, intrapleurally, or subconjunctivally, or inhaled as aerosols. Ointments containing 0.5 mg/g polymyxin B sulfate in a mixture with neomycin or bacitracin are often applied to infected skin lesions. Solutions containing polymyxin B, 20 mg/liter, and neomycin, 40 mg/liter, can be used for continuous irrigation of the bladder with an indwelling catheter and a closed drainage system.

Adverse Effects

The toxicities of polymyxin B and colistimethate are similar. With the usual blood levels there are paresthesias, dizziness, flushing, and incoordination. These disappear when the drug has been excreted. With unusually high levels, respiratory arrest and paralysis can occur. Depending upon the dose, all polymyxins are nephrotoxic, producing tubular injury. Proteinuria, hematuria, and cylindruria tend to be reversible, but nitrogen retention or severe electrolyte disturbances may force reduction in dose or discontinuance of the drug. In individuals with preexisting renal insufficiency, kidney function must be monitored (preferably by creatinine clearance) and the dose reduced or the interval between injections increased (Table 10–3).

Jawetz E: Polymyxins, colistin, bacitracin, ristocetin, and vancomycin. Pages 91–101 in: *Antimicrobial Therapy.* Kagan BM (editor). Saunders, 1970.

Ryan KJ & others: Colistimethate toxicity: Report of a fatal case. JAMA 207:2099–2101, 1969.

SULFONAMIDES & SULFONES

Since 1935, more than 150 different sulfonamides have been marketed. The increasing emergence of sulfonamide resistance (eg, among streptococci, meningococci, and shigellae) and the higher efficacy of other antimicrobial drugs have drastically curtailed the number of specific indications for sulfonamides as drugs of choice. The present indications for the use of these drugs can be summarized as follows:

(1) First (previously untreated) infection of the urinary tract: Many coliform organisms, which are the most common causes of urinary infections, are still susceptible to sulfonamides.

(2) Chlamydial infections of the trachoma-inclusion conjunctivitis-LGV group: Sulfonamides are often as effective as tetracyclines in suppressing clinical activity, and they may be curative in acute infections. However, they often fail to eradicate chronic infection and are ineffective in psittacosis.

(3) Parasitic and fungal diseases: In combination with pyrimethamine, sulfonamides are used in toxoplasmosis. In combination with trimethoprim, sulfonamides are sometimes effective in falciparum malaria. Alone or in combination with cycloserine, sulfonamides may be drugs of choice in nocardiosis.

(4) Bacterial infections: In underdeveloped parts of the world, sulfonamides, because of their availability and low cost, may still be useful for the treatment of pneumococcal or staphylococcal infections; bacterial sinusitis, bronchitis, or otitis media; bacillary (shigella) dysentery; and meningococcal infections. In most developed countries, however, sulfonamides are not the drugs of choice for any of these conditions, and sulfonamide resistance of the respective etiologic organisms is widespread.

(5) Leprosy: Certain sulfones are the drugs of choice in leprosy.

Dosages & Routes of Administration

A. Topical: The application of sulfonamides to skin, wounds, or mucous membranes is undesirable because of the high risk of allergic sensitization or reaction and the low antimicrobial activity. Exceptions are the application of sodium sulfacetamide solution (30%) or ointment (10%) to the conjunctivas, or mafenide acetate cream (Sulfamylon) to burned surfaces.

B. Oral: For systemic disease, the soluble, rapidly excreted sulfonamides (eg, sulfadiazine, sulfisoxazole) are given in an initial dose of 2–4 g (40 mg/kg) followed by 0.5–1 g (10 mg/kg) every 4–6 hours. Trisulfapyrimidines USP may be given in the same total doses. Urine must be kept alkaline.

For urinary tract infections (first attack, not previously treated), trisulfapyrimidines, sulfisoxazole, or another sulfonamide with equally high solubility in urine are given in the same (or somewhat lower) doses as shown above. Following one course of sulfonamides, resistant organisms usually prevail. Simultaneous administration of a sulfonamide, 2 g/day orally, and trimethoprim, 400 mg/day orally, may be more effective in urinary, respiratory, or enteric tract infections than sulfonamide alone.

Salicylazosulfapyridine, 6 g/day, has been given in ulcerative colitis, where it may be of value in maintaining a remission.

"Long-acting" and "intermediate-acting" sulfonamides (eg, sulfamethoxypyridazine, sulfadimethoxine, sulfamethoxazole) can be used in doses of 0.5–1 g/day (10 mg/kg) for prolonged maintenance therapy (eg, trachoma) or for the treatment of minor infections. These drugs have a significantly higher rate of toxic effects than the "short-acting" sulfonamides.

C. Intravenous: Sodium sulfadiazine and other sodium salts can be injected intravenously in 0.5% concentration in 5% dextrose in water, physiologic salt solution, or other diluent in a total dose of 6–8 g/day (120 mg/kg/day). This is reserved for comatose individuals or those unable to take oral medication.

Adverse Effects

Sulfonamides produce a wide variety of side-effects—due partly to hypersensitivity, partly to direct toxicity—which must be considered whenever unexplained symptoms or signs occur in a patient who may have received these drugs. Except in the mildest reactions, fluids should be forced, and—if symptoms and signs progressively increase—the drugs should be discontinued. Precautions to prevent complications (below) are important.

A. Systemic Side-Effects: Fever, skin rashes, urticaria; nausea, vomiting, or diarrhea; stomatitis, conjunctivitis, arthritis, exfoliative dermatitis; hematopoietic disturbances, including thrombocytopenia, hemolytic (in G6PD deficiency) or aplastic anemia, granulocytopenia, leukemoid reactions; hepatitis, polyarteritis nodosa, vasculitis, Stevens-Johnson syndrome; psychosis; and many others.

B. Urinary Tract Disturbances: Sulfonamides may precipitate in urine, especially at neutral or acid pH, producing hematuria, crystalluria, or even obstruction. They have also been implicated in various types of nephritis and nephrosis. Sulfonamides and methenamine salts should not be given together.

Precautions in the Use of Sulfonamides

(1) There is cross-allergenicity among all sulfonamides. Obtain a history of past administration or reaction. Observe for possible allergic responses.

(2) Keep the urine volume above 1500 ml/day by forcing fluids. Check urine pH—it should be 7.5 or higher. Give alkali by mouth (sodium bicarbonate or equivalent, 5–15 g/day). Examine fresh urine for crystals and red cells every 2–4 days.

(3) Check hemoglobin, white blood cell count, and differential count every 3–5 days to detect possible disturbances early.

SPECIALIZED DRUGS AGAINST GRAM-POSITIVE BACTERIA

1. BACITRACIN

This polypeptide antibiotic is selectively active against gram-positive bacteria, including penicillinase-producing staphylococci, in concentrations of 0.1—20 units/ml. Bacitracin is very little absorbed from gut, skin, wounds, or mucous membranes. Topical application results in local effects without significant toxicity. Bacitracin, 500 units/g in ointment base, is often combined with polymyxin or neomycin for the suppression of mixed bacterial flora in surface lesions. Systemic administration of bacitracin has been abandoned because of its severe nephrotoxicity.

2. LINCOMYCIN & CLINDAMYCIN

These drugs resemble erythromycin (although different in structure) and are active against gram-positive organisms (except enterococci). Lincomycin, 0.5 g orally every 6 hours (30—60 mg/kg/day for children), or clindamycin, 0.15—0.3 g orally every 6 hours are used. Lincomycin, 0.6 g, can also be injected IM or IV every 8—12 hours. The drugs are alternatives to erythromycin as a substitute for penicillin. Success has been reported in staphylococcal bone infections and some bacteroides infections.

Common side-effects are diarrhea and nausea. Impaired liver function and neutropenia have been noted. If 3—4 g are given rapidly intravenously, cardiorespiratory arrest may occur. Clindamycin may have a lower incidence· of gastrointestinal side-effects than lincomycin.

3. VANCOMYCIN

This drug is bactericidal for most gram-positive organisms, particularly staphylococci and enterococci. Resistant mutants are rare, and there is no cross-resistance with other antimicrobial drugs. Vancomycin is given orally (3—4 g/day) only for the treatment of staphylococcal enterocolitis. For systemic effect, the drug must be administered intravenously. In the presence of renal insufficiency, marked accumulation may occur and have toxic consequences.

The only indications for vancomycin are serious staphylococcal infection or enterococcal endocarditis untreatable with penicillins. Vancomycin, 0.5 g, is injected IV over a 20-minute period every 6—8 hours (for children, 20—40 mg/kg/day).

Vancomycin is intensely irritating to tissues. Intramuscular injection or extravasation from intravenous injection sites is very painful. Chills, fever, and thrombophlebitis commonly follow intravenous injection. The drug is both nephrotoxic and ototoxic, and renal function must be monitored.

URINARY ANTISEPTICS

These drugs exert antimicrobial activity in the urine but have little or no systemic antibacterial effect. Their usefulness is limited to urinary tract infections.

1. NITROFURANTOIN

Nitrofurantoin is bacteriostatic and bactericidal for both· gram-positive and gram-negative bacteria in urine. The activity of nitrofurantoin is greatly enhanced at pH 5.5 or lower. The drug has no systemic antibacterial activity.

The average daily dose in urinary tract infections is 100 mg orally 4 times daily (for children, 5—10 mg/kg/day), taken with food. If oral medication is not feasible, nitrofurantoin can be given by continuous IV infusion, 180—360 mg/day.

Oral nitrofurantoin often causes nausea and vomiting. Hemolytic anemia occurs in G6PD deficiency. Hypersensitivity may produce skin rashes and pulmonary infiltration.

2. NALIDIXIC ACID

Nalidixic acid inhibits many gram-negative bacteria in the urine, but has no effect on pseudomonas. In susceptible bacterial populations, resistant mutants emerge fairly rapidly. Nalidixic acid has no systemic antibacterial action.

The dose in urinary tract infections is 1 g orally 4 times daily (for children, 55 mg/kg/day). Adverse reactions include nausea, vomiting, skin rashes, drowsiness, visual disturbances, and, rarely, increased intracranial pressure with convulsions.

3. METHENAMINE MANDELATE
(Mandelamine)
& METHENAMINE HIPPURATE

These are salts of methenamine and mandelic acid or hippuric acid. The action of the drug depends on the liberation of formaldehyde and of acid in the urine. The urinary pH must be below 5.5, and sulfonamides must not be given at the same time. The drug inhibits a variety of different microorganisms except those (eg, proteus) which liberate ammonia from urea and produce strongly alkaline urine. The dosage is 2—6 g orally daily.

4. ACIDIFYING AGENTS

Urine with a pH below 5.5 tends to be antibacterial. Many substances can acidify urine and thus produce antibacterial activity. Ammonium chloride, ascorbic acid, methionine, and mandelic acid are sometimes used. The dose has to be established for each patient by testing the urine for acid pH with test paper at frequent intervals.

SYSTEMICALLY ACTIVE DRUGS IN URINARY TRACT INFECTIONS

Many antimicrobial drugs are excreted in the urine in very high concentration. For this reason, low and relatively nontoxic amounts of aminoglycosides, polymyxins, and cycloserine can produce effective urine levels. Many penicillins and cephalosporins can reach very high urine levels and can thus be effective in urinary tract infections.

ANTIFUNGAL DRUGS

Most antibacterial substances have no effect on pathogenic fungi. Only a few drugs are known to be therapeutically useful in mycotic infections. Penicillins and sulfonamides are used to treat actinomycosis; sulfonamides and cycloserine have been employed in nocardiosis.

1. AMPHOTERICIN B

Amphotericin B inhibits several organisms producing systemic mycotic disease in man, including histoplasma, cryptococcus, coccidioides, candida, blastomyces, sporotrichum, and others.

Amphotericin B solutions, 0.1 mg/ml in 5% dextrose in water, are given by slow intravenous infusion. The initial dose is 1—5 mg/day, increasing daily by 5 mg increments until a final dosage of 1—1.5 mg/kg/day

is reached. This is usually continued for many weeks. In fungal meningitis, amphotericin B, 0.5 mg, is injected intrathecally 3 times weekly; continuous treatment (many weeks) with an Ommaya reservoir is sometimes employed. Relapses of fungal meningitis occur commonly.

The intravenous administration of amphotericin B usually produces chills, fever, vomiting, and headache. Tolerance may be enhanced by temporary lowering of the dose or administration of corticosteroids. Therapeutically active amounts of amphotericin B commonly impair kidney and liver function and produce anemia. Electrolyte disturbances, shock, and a variety of neurologic symptoms also occur.

2. GRISEOFULVIN

Griseofulvin can inhibit the growth of some dermatophytes but has no effect on bacteria or on the fungi that cause deep mycoses. The absorbed drug has an affinity for skin and is deposited there, bound to keratin. Thus, it makes keratin resistant to fungal growth and the new growth of hair or nails is first freed of infection. As keratinized structures are shed, they are replaced by uninfected ones.

Oral doses of 0.5—1 g/day (for children, 15 mg/kg/day) must be given for 6 weeks if only the skin is involved and for 3—6 months or longer if the hair and nails are involved. Griseofulvin is most successful in severe dermatophytosis, particularly if caused by trichophyton or microsporum. Some strains of fungi are resistant.

Side-effects include headache, nausea, diarrhea, photosensitivity, fever, skin rashes, and disturbances of hepatic, nervous, and hematopoietic systems. Griseofulvin increases the metabolism of coumarin so that higher doses of the anticoagulant are needed.

3. NYSTATIN

Nystatin inhibits Candida species upon direct contact. Nystatin in ointments, suspensions, etc can be applied to buccal or vaginal mucous membranes to suppress a local candida infection. There is no good indication for the use of nystatin orally because increase in gut candida is rarely associated with disease unless the patient is immunosuppressed.

4. FLUOROCYTOSINE

5-Fluorocytosine inhibits some candida and cryptococcus strains. Dosages of 3—8 g daily orally have produced clinical remissions in cases of meningitis, sepsis, and chromoblastomycosis (Phialophora sp). Resistant organisms may appear, and toxic effects (bone marrow depression, loss of hair) are common.

·   ·   ·

ANTIMICROBIAL DRUGS USED IN COMBINATION

Indications

Possible reasons for employing 2 or more antimicrobials simultaneously instead of a single drug are as follows:

(1) Prompt treatment in desperately ill patients suspected of having a serious microbial infection. A good guess about the most probable 2 or 3 pathogens is made, and drugs are aimed at those organisms. Before such treatment is started, it is essential that adequate specimens be obtained for identifying the etiologic agent in the laboratory. Gram-negative sepsis is the most important disease in this category at present.

(2) To delay the emergence of microbial mutants resistant to one drug in chronic infections by the use of a second or third non-cross-reacting drug. The most prominent examples are miliary tuberculosis, tuberculous meningitis, and chronic active tuberculosis of any organ with large microbial populations.

(3) Mixed infections, particularly those following massive trauma. Each drug is aimed at an important pathogenic microorganism.

(4) To achieve bactericidal synergism (see below). In a few infections, eg, enterococcal sepsis, a combination of drugs is more likely to eradicate the infection than either drug used alone. Unfortunately, such synergism is unpredictable, and a given drug pair may be synergistic for only a single microbial strain.

Disadvantages

The following disadvantages of using antimicrobial drugs in combinations must always be considered:

(1) The surgeon may feel that since he is already giving several drugs he has done all he can for the patient. This attitude leads to relaxation of the effort to establish a specific diagnosis. It may also give the surgeon a false sense of security.

(2) The more drugs are administered, the greater the chance for drug reactions to occur or for the patient to become sensitized to drugs.

(3) Unnecessarily high cost.

(4) Antimicrobial combinations usually accomplish no more than an effective single drug.

(5) On very rare occasions, one drug may antagonize a second drug given simultaneously. Antagonism resulting in increased morbidity and mortality has been observed mainly in bacterial meningitis when a bacteriostatic drug (eg, tetracycline or chloramphenicol) was given with a bactericidal drug (eg, penicillin or ampicillin). However, antagonism is usually overcome by an excess dose of one of the drugs in the pair and is therefore a very infrequent problem in clinical therapy.

Synergism

Antimicrobial synergism can occur in at least 3 types of situations. Synergistic drug combinations must be selected by complex laboratory procedures.

(1) Sequential block of a microbial metabolic pathway by 2 drugs. Sulfonamides inhibit the use of extracellular para-aminobenzoic acid by some microbes for the synthesis of folic acid. Trimethoprim or pyrimethamine inhibits the next metabolic step, the reduction of dihydro- to tetrahydrofolic acid. The simultaneous use of a sulfonamide plus trimethoprim is effective in some bacterial infections (eg, urinary tract, enteric) and in malaria. Pyrimethamine plus a sulfonamide is used in toxoplasmosis.

(2) One drug may protect a second drug from destruction by a microbial enzyme. Penicillin G or ampicillin is rapidly destroyed by β-lactamase (penicillinase) of gram-negative bacteria. Methicillin, cloxacillin, or cephalosporins are resistant to that enzyme but bind it very effectively, thus protecting the enzyme-susceptible drugs. This can be used only on a limited scale in urinary tract infections due to the need for high concentrations of drug.

(3) One drug may greatly enhance the uptake of a second drug and thereby greatly increase the overall bactericidal effect. Penicillins enhance the uptake of aminoglycosides by enterococci. Thus, a penicillin plus an aminoglycoside may be essential for the eradication of enterococcal (Streptococcus faecalis) infections, particularly sepsis or endocarditis. Similarly, carbenicillin plus gentamicin may be synergistic against some strains of pseudomonas.

ANTIMICROBIAL CHEMOPROPHYLAXIS IN SURGERY

Several well-controlled studies have established that the overall incidence of postoperative infections is not diminished by the administration of antimicrobials during or after surgery in "clean" elective procedures. In compound fractures, penetrating wounds of body cavities, operations on a ruptured abdominal viscus, and other "contaminated" procedures, antimicrobial drugs are often aimed at the organisms most likely to produce serious infections. A penicillin (eg, ampicillin, 2 g orally daily) and an aminoglycoside (eg, kanamycin, 1.5 g IM daily) are often administered in such situations. This approach does not significantly alter the incidence of wound infections, but it may diminish the incidence of major bacteremia or life-threatening systemic infections. Claims for prophylactic use of a cephalosporin (eg, cephalothin, 4 g IV daily on the day of operation and for 2–4 days afterward) have been made (Ferguson, S Clin North America 51:49, 1971). It must be accepted, however, that universal antimicrobial prophylaxis to protect against any and all types of postoperative infection does not exist.

Before elective operations on the lower intestinal tract, some surgeons reduce the bowel flora by the preoperative oral administration of neomycin or kanamycin. It is assumed that the reduction in numbers of intestinal bacteria will reduce the hazard of peritoneal infection after accidental contamination with bowel contents. Oral insoluble drugs suppress the bowel flora only transiently and partially. The lowest number of bacteria are present within 2–3 days after starting neomycin, 1 g every 4–6 hours. Soon thereafter, bacterial numbers rise and the composition of the bowel flora changes. An empty bowel that is clean of feces and fluid and strict aseptic technic are far more important than antimicrobial drugs in preventing peritoneal infection. Preoperative oral neomycin may lead to implantation of neomycin-resistant staphylococci in the bowel and predisposes to the development of staphylococcal enterocolitis with high morbidity and mortality.

In cardiovascular surgery, endothelial damage predisposes to infection, particularly endocarditis due to viridans streptococci. When penicillin G (2–5 million units daily) is given for 5 days postoperatively, this complication is virtually unknown, although endocarditis and pericarditis due to staphylococci and gram-negative bacteria may develop. Specific drugs directed against staphylococci (methicillin, 6–12 g IV daily) or pseudomonas (gentamicin, 3 mg/kg/day) may prevent infection by these particular bacteria but favor the selection of other resistant microorganisms (eg, fungi).

Topical antimicrobials are sometimes used to prevent local infections. Application of bacitracin-neomycin-polymyxin creams to skin sites of intravenous needles, tubes, or catheters may delay infection of the site but should never be an alternative to the rotation of such puncture sites every 48 hours. For the prevention of urinary tract infection in the presence of an indwelling catheter, only sterile, closed drainage systems must be employed. Incorporation of neomycin-polymyxin solutions into such drainage systems may further delay the growth of contaminating bacteria. The topical application of ampicillin to surgical wounds (eg, after colorectal surgery) can diminish the incidence of wound infections.

●   ●   ●

General References

Andersen B, Korner B, Östergaard AH: Topical ampicillin against wound infections after colorectal surgery. Ann Surg 176:129–132, 1972.

Barnett JA, Sanford JP: Bacterial shock. JAMA 209:1514–1517, 1969.

Bauer AW & others: Antibiotic susceptibility testing by a standardized single disc method. Am J Clin Path 45:493–496, 1966.

Bennett WM: Practical guide to drug usage in patients with impaired renal function. JAMA 214:1468–1475, 1970.

Cameron R: Inflammation and repair. Pages 31–73 in: *Pathology,* 3rd ed. Robbins SL. Saunders, 1968.

Ericsson HM, Sherris JC: Antibiotic sensitivity testing. Acta path microbiol scandinav, Suppl No. 217, 1971.

Feller I (editor): Symposium on surgical infections. S Clin North America 52:1359–1538, 1972.

Finegold SM & others: Chemotherapy guide. California Med 111:362–387, 1969.

Garrod LP, O'Grady F: *Antibiotics and Chemotherapy,* 3rd ed. Livingstone, 1971.

Jackson GG & others: Prophylactic antimicrobial agents. Pages 306–312 in: *Proceedings of the International Conference on Nosocomial Infections.* Brachman PS, Eickhoff TC (editors). Waverly Press, 1971.

Jawetz E: Principles of antimicrobial therapy. Mod Treat 1:819–828, 1964.

Johnstone FRC: Infection on a surgical service. Am J Surg 120:192–197, 1970.

Kagan BM (editor): *Antimicrobial Therapy.* Saunders, 1970.

Levin HS, Kagan BM: Antimicrobial agents: Pediatric dosages, routes of administration, and preparation procedures for parenteral therapy. P Clin North America 15:275–290, 1968.

Meyers FH, Jawetz E, Goldfien A: *Review of Medical Pharmacology,* 3rd ed. Lange, 1972.

Miller ME: Enhanced susceptibility to infection. M Clin North America 54:713–722, 1970.

Perkins RL, Smith EJ, Saslaw S: Cephalothin and cephaloridine: Comparative pharmacodynamics in chronic uremia. Am J Med Sc 257:116–124, 1969.

Weinstein L: Common sense (clinical judgment) in the antibiotic therapy of etiologically undefined infections. P Clin North America 15:141–156, 1968.

Weinstein L, Dalton AC: Host determinants of response to antimicrobial agents. New England J Med 279:467–473, 524, 580–588, 1968.

11 . . .

The Metabolic Response to Injury

L. Henry Edmunds, Jr., MD

THE CONCEPT OF TOTAL INJURY

Injury, whether accidental or elective, initiates responses which act to restore homeostasis and normal organ function. In general, the responses of the body are proportionate to the **total injury**, which is defined as the sum of all of the factors which tend to derange homeostasis of the internal environment. Directly or indirectly, these factors threaten life. The concept of total injury includes not only the initial tissue damage and fluid losses but also the effects of partial or complete loss of organ function and any ensuing complications. Recovery occurs when wounds have healed and organ function has been restored. Thus, the ultimate outcome depends upon whether or not the total injury prevails over the body's response.

The magnitude of an injury is in part proportionate to the amount of traumatized tissue and blood lost. Massive tissue losses such as in burns and blast injuries demand much from the body if homeostasis is to be protected and the wound healed. Several attempts have been made to grade injuries primarily on the basis of tissue trauma and losses. For example, an inguinal hernial repair rates 1 on a scale of 10, whereas a pancreaticoduodenectomy rates 6 or 7. This simplified means of assessing the magnitude of injury fails to take into account other important aspects of the total injury and is difficult to apply to accidental wounds.

The effect of wounding on function of the injured organ is a major component of the total injury. The magnitude of the total injury depends upon which organs are injured and the degree to which function is impaired. Every organ and organ system has some degree of functional reserve and partial functional loss of a vital organ can be tolerated without derangement of homeostasis. Depending upon the organ, more severe functional impairment may unbalance the homeostatic mechanism and magnify the total injury. Absolutely vital organs and tissues whose functions cannot be suspended for more than very short intervals include the heart, lungs, blood, and probably the medulla oblongata and basal ganglia. Temporarily expendable organs whose function cannot be indefinitely suspended include the cerebral cortex, kidneys, liver, gastrointestinal tract, and skin. The limbs, spleen, bladder, eyes, and gonads are examples of expendable organs whose functions do not play a major role in maintaining homeostasis or in repairing wounds.

The complications of an original injury increase the magnitude and prolong the duration of the total injury. Shock resulting from blood loss or low cardiac output may cause ischemic damage of other organs and metabolic acidosis. Acute tubular necrosis with loss of renal function or damage to the lung from shock may complicate the original injury and add to the total injury. Infection, fever, malnutrition, coma, congestive heart failure, and wound dehiscence are other examples of complications which increase the total injury and prolong its duration.

Many factors influence the patient's ability to respond to a major injury. A young, previously healthy individual with a strong desire to recover is capable of the greatest response to acute injury. Extremes of age, preexisting disease, starvation, cachexia, marked obesity, heavy smoking, alcoholism, diabetes, and other factors adversely influence the patient's ability to respond. In general, the patient's response reflects the functional reserve of his organs and organ systems. An evaluation of the patient's ability to respond—in contrast to an assessment of the total injury—permits the experienced surgeon to estimate the patient's chances of recovery or "risk."

The patient's response to injury may be divided into 2 general categories: (1) the obligatory metabolic response of the whole body, and (2) the specific responses of the injured organs and tissues. The metabolic response occurs after every injury of sufficient magnitude to trigger this defense. The response varies quantitatively but not qualitatively from patient to patient. The metabolic response regulates the biochemical and physiologic environment in which the specific organ responses take place.

Specific organ responses are the changes which occur in various injured organs. Head injuries may cause loss of consciousness and lead to brain swelling, compression of the medulla, and death. Fractured ribs may reduce ventilation or cause tension pneumothorax. Severe burns call forth a tremendous wound edema which depletes the body of electrolytes, water, and protein. Depending upon the organ or tissue injured, these responses are specific and predictable, though they can vary in magnitude and in the degree of functional impairment that results. Most of the care given an injured patient is directed toward specific organ injuries in an attempt to support organ function and prevent complications while healing occurs. The metabolic response may go unrecognized because the clinical scene is dominated by the injuries and responses of specific organs.

The general metabolic response to injury is described below. No attempt will be made to describe the effects of trauma and the responses of individual organs and organ systems.

FOUR PHASES OF INJURY

Moore has divided convalescence from injury into 4 clinical phases: injury, turning point, anabolism or muscle rebuilding, and weight gain. These 4 phases are easily recognized clinically and correlate positively with the marked changes in hormone and energy production, water and electrolyte balance, and nutrition that occur after trauma or operation. The duration of each phase depends upon the magnitude of the total injury, the patient's ability to respond, and the complications, if any, that may occur. In a young, previously healthy person, the phase of injury after elective appendectomy may last 2 days or may be protracted over several weeks or months if peritonitis, pelvic abscesses, or other complications develop.

1. INJURY PHASE

A summary of the metabolic responses during the injury phase is presented in Table 11–1.

Initial Response & Pain

Surprise is the initial reaction of most people to accidental injury. After the initial moments of surprise, many become afraid, others remain calm, and some faint. Pain is perceived moments or minutes later and helps the patient to locate his injuries. Pain then becomes the dominant subjective symptom and crowds other matters from the patient's consciousness.

After elective operation or treatment of accidental injuries, pain remains the dominant symptom. Analgesics usually reduce pain and cause the patient to lie still and to limit his movements. If medication is inadequate, the patient may become restless, uncooperative, and disoriented. Generally, he protects his wounds and avoids anything which causes pain. The patient has no appetite, little or no interest in his environment, and usually sleeps. Temperature and pulse rate are usually elevated.

Endocrine Changes

A. Catecholamines: Injury stimulates the sympathetic system and causes an immediate increase in the circulating catecholamines: epinephrine and norepinephrine. Norepinephrine stimulates the alpha receptors of the sympathetic nervous system and causes vasoconstriction of some vessels and an overall increase in peripheral vascular resistance. In the

TABLE 11–1. Initial metabolic and endocrinologic responses to injury.

Clinical	
Pain, limited movement, anxiety	Present
Appetite	Absent
Temperature	Increased
Respirations	Increased
Pulse rate	Increased
Cardiac output	Increased
Wound	Sealed by clot
Endocrine	
Epinephrine, norepinephrine	Increased
Corticotropin (ACTH)	Increased
Cortisol	Increased
Aldosterone	Increased
Vasopressin	Increased
Glucagon	Increased
Growth, thyroid, parathormone, sex hormones	Unchanged
Water and electrolytes	
Water	Retained, dilutes blood and extracellular fluid
Sodium	Retained, serum concentration decreased
Chloride	Retained, serum concentration decreased
Potassium	Lost in urine, serum concentration varies
Calcium, magnesium	No significant change
Concentrations of blood constituents	
Glucose	Increased
White cells	Increased
Red cells	Decreased
Platelets	Transient decrease
Albumin	Decreased
Other serum proteins	Unchanged
Amino acids	Unchanged
Free fatty acids	Increased
Creatinine	Increased slightly
Ascorbic acid	Increased slightly
Thiamine and other B vitamins	Decreased slightly
Metabolism	
Oxygen consumption	Increased
CO_2 production	Increased
Gluconeogenesis	Increased
Glycogenolysis	Increased
Fat oxidation	Increased

absence of blood loss, systolic and diastolic pressures rise. Norepinephrine and epinephrine together redistribute blood flow within the body and preserve or increase blood flow to the heart, brain, and skeletal muscle at the expense of the kidneys, mesenteric vessels, and skin. Epinephrine increases the heart rate, and both catecholamines increase stroke volume, so that cardiac output increases. Epinephrine also increases the concentrations of glucose, glycerol, and free fatty acids in the blood. The marked increase in sympathetic activity may be accompanied by increased parasympathetic discharge and anorexia, nausea, vomiting, and loss of peristalsis. The serum catecholamines usually remain increased for 1–2 days after injury.

B. Adrenal Corticosteroids: Pain and other afferent stimuli reaching the CNS cause large neurons in the hypothalamus to release corticotropin-releasing factor (CRF), which in turn causes the anterior pituitary to release increased amounts of corticotropin (ACTH). Stimulation of afferent nerves from injured tissues, fright, anxiety, and other emotions cause a release of increased amounts of corticotropin and overcome the feedback inhibition of normal levels of serum corticosteroids. Increased corticotropin causes increased secretion of cortisol and aldosterone (see below) from the adrenal cortex.

The adrenal corticosteroids are essential for survival after accidental injury or operation. Patients with adrenal insufficiency are particularly vulnerable unless increased amounts of exogenous adrenal steroids are provided. The "glucocorticoids," which include cortisol and corticosterone, accelerate the breakdown of protein into amino acids and sugar (gluconeogenesis), increase the deposition of liver glycogen, and, in concert with catecholamines, participate in the mobilization and oxidation of fat. The net effect is to increase the production of glucose and carbohydrate intermediates. The glucocorticoids increase 3- to 7-fold immediately after wounding and remain increased during the injury phase.

ACTH also increases secretion of aldosterone, a "mineralocorticoid" produced in the zona glomerulosa of the adrenal cortex. After trauma, the most potent stimulus to aldosterone secretion is acute blood loss; shock may raise the secretion of aldosterone 30-fold. Reduced renal blood flow stimulates the release of renin, which eventually causes plasma angiotensinogen to be converted into angiotensin. Angiotensin causes vasoconstriction of the skin, renal, and mesenteric vessels and stimulates the adrenal cortex to produce aldosterone. Aldosterone causes renal tubular reabsorption of sodium and facilitates the excretion of hydrogen ion and potassium. Blood aldosterone levels usually return to normal 2–3 days after operation or injury if blood volume and cardiac output have returned to normal.

C. Antidiuretic Hormone: Trauma—particularly acute blood loss—stimulates the posterior pituitary to increase production of antidiuretic hormone (ADH, or vasopressin). Although the secretion of vasopressin usually responds to changes in serum osmolality, after injury afferent stimuli from atrial volume receptors travel to the CNS by sympathetic and parasympathetic pathways and stimulate the release of vasopressin. Vasopressin increases reabsorption of water by increasing renal tubular permeability to water. This effect reduces urine volume and increases urine osmolality.

D. Other Hormones: Other hormones are less important for survival after injury. Loss of red cells stimulates the production of erythropoietin, which increases the synthesis of red cells in bone marrow. Trauma reduces the secretion of sex hormones during the injury and turning point phases. Late in convalescence, during the period of anabolism, androgenic hormones facilitate rebuilding of muscle; however, normal serum levels of these hormones appear to be adequate. In females, menses may arrive prematurely during this phase of convalescence. Increased amounts of growth hormone are not needed for tissue repair, and the increase in body metabolism which occurs after injury is not related to thyroid function. Reduction of these hormones does not change systematically after injury. Furthermore, transient changes in serum calcium after injury do not correlate with changes in parathormone secretion.

Insulin and glucagon participate in energy production after wounding. Blood glucose rises initially (glycogenolysis and gluconeogenesis) but falls after several hours. Glucagon increases hepatic blood flow in shock. After injury, insulin, glucagon, catecholamines, and adrenal corticosteroids all play important roles in the mobilization, breakdown, conversion, and utilization of the body's carbohydrate, protein, and fat stores.

Water & Electrolytes

During the injury phase, vasopressin causes water retention and aldosterone causes retention of sodium and chloride and the excretion of potassium and hydrogen ions. Normally, 150–250 mEq of sodium are excreted in the urine daily; but after major trauma, less than 10 mEq of sodium may be lost in the urine. On the other hand, potassium is excreted in larger than normal amounts, and urinary potassium losses may exceed intake by amounts up to 100 mEq/day. The amount of potassium excreted exceeds the amount calculated to be produced by protein catabolism, but the source of the additional excreted potassium is not known.

Serum calcium may fall transiently after injury. Less calcium is absorbed from the gastrointestinal tract, and less calcium is deposited in bone. Magnesium absorption is likewise decreased after injury. Clinically, significant changes in serum calcium and magnesium after injury are unusual unless prolonged parenteral fluid administration is required.

Urine volume generally decreases, and urine osmolality increases. The principal solute in the urine is urea, produced by catabolism of muscle protein. This catabolism also increases urinary creatinine and, in males, urinary creatine. Breakdown of traumatized tissues may produce urinary hemoglobin and myoglobin.

Retention of water after injury usually dilutes blood so that the concentrations of sodium, chloride, proteins, and red cells fall slightly. Oxidation of fat (180 ml water/kg) and protein (150 ml water/kg) and release of cell water (approximately 750 ml/kg lean tissue) further increase total body water. However, after major trauma or hemorrhagic shock, water may be sequestered in traumatized tissue or in other ill-defined "third space" areas. Thus, although water is retained after trauma, the requirements of electrolyte-containing fluids may greatly exceed the sum of exogenous losses and daily maintenance requirements (urine, feces, sweat, and insensible losses). Sufficient fluid and electrolytes must be given to maintain normal serum electrolyte concentrations and to provide an adequate daily urine output. Since vasopressin secretion is increased, urine volume can only be augmented by increasing the solute load in the glomerular filtrate. Administration of electrolytes in excess of "third space" and balance requirements thus augments urine flow after injury, but fluids must be given carefully to avoid overloading and congestive heart failure.

Hematologic Changes

During the injury phase, the white cell count increases but, because of increased adrenocorticoids, lymphocytes and eosinophils are reduced in number. Platelet levels decrease immediately after injury, presumably because of consumption at the site of injury. Within 5 days, platelets increase slightly above normal levels. Concentrations of fibrinogen and other clotting factors may increase in response to trauma or decrease if intravascular coagulation occurs. Blood loss reduces red cell concentration, and if shock occurs additional red cells may be removed from the circulation by sludging or intravascular coagulation.

Energy Production

Injury enhances caloric requirements, but unless heat losses are excessive, as in burns or major infection, an additional 300–1000 Cal are required daily. This represents a 15–50% increase in metabolism. Oxygen consumption and CO_2 production increase proportionately. Since injury is usually associated with reduced intake of exogenous calories, energy requirements must be met from endogenous sources. The metabolism of body fat and protein to produce calories causes weight loss proportional to the severity of the total injury. Infusion of amino acids, fatty acids, and other energy substrates reduces the catabolism of fat and protein but cannot abolish it during the injury phase after wounding.

The body has limited carbohydrate stores. The main supply—approximately 400 g—is located in the liver as glycogen. Glycogenolysis, stimulated by epinephrine and glucagon, provides only 4 Cal/g. Production of carbohydrate intermediates by gluconeogenesis causes redeposition of liver glycogen, but, after a major injury, rapid glycogenolysis usually depletes liver stores within 18–24 hours.

Fat provides over 80% of endogenous calories after injury. Oxidation of 1 g of fat tissue produces 9 Cal and 1.08 ml of water. During starvation, 75–100 g of fat may be oxidized daily; after major injury such as a severe burn, up to 500 g of fat may be burned per day. Catecholamines and glucagon definitely increase lipolysis of stored triglycerides, and adrenocorticosteroids probably participate also. Blood lipase hydrolyzes triglycerides to free fatty acids and glycerol, and

serum concentrations of free fatty acids increase after injury. Free fatty acids can be metabolized by all tissues except the CNS, which preferentially utilizes glucose.

Injury initiates protein catabolism (gluconeogenesis) and loss of lean muscle tissue to provide calories and carbohydrate intermediates. As compared to starvation, trauma augments gluconeogenesis, but only 12–20% of daily caloric needs are provided by this process. Gluconeogenesis is particularly important after trauma since the carbohydrate products produced can be used by all tissues. In general, the role of gluconeogenesis and urinary nitrogen excretion reflect the need for calories and the severity of the total injury.

A normal adult daily ingests 60–90 g of protein which contains 10–15 g of nitrogen (6.25 g of protein contains 1 g of nitrogen). The need for additional calories causes catabolism of an additional 15–75 g of protein daily, and this protein is supplied by lean muscle tissue. Although muscles waste after trauma, cell structure and innervation remain to receive resynthesized protein during the phase of anabolism. Protein oxidation is less efficient than that of fat, and 1 g of protein produces only 4 Cal. Skeletal muscle is 1 part protein to 3 parts water, and oxidation of 1 kg of lean muscle produces 40 g of nitrogen and only 1000 Cal. Serum proteins and proteins in other organs are generally spared in the early period after injury. In the presence of renal insufficiency, protein catabolism may produce dangerously high serum concentrations of urea, creatinine, and potassium.

Wound healing proceeds normally in spite of massive protein catabolism. Serum proteins may be diluted by water retention but generally are not significantly reduced until other body protein stores are depleted. A severe total injury over a protracted period causes tremendous muscle wasting, weight loss, and eventually reduced concentrations of serum proteins, particularly albumin.

2. TURNING POINT

The end of the injury phase and the beginning of anabolism is marked by a transitory period which Moore calls the turning point. Although subjective improvement may be masked in some patients, clinically most patients feel better, show more interest in their surroundings and appearance, and may even feel hungry. Wound pain is less, and movements are less restricted. Temperature and pulse rate decrease toward normal. After elective abdominal operations that are free of postoperative complications, "the turning point" generally occurs 2–5 days after operation and coincides with restoration of peristalsis. Complications, particularly infection, postpone the arrival of "the turning point."

Metabolically, elevated levels of corticotropin, adrenocorticosteroids, and vasopressin return to normal. Reduced aldosterone and vasopressin levels permit diuresis of salt and water and conservation of potassium. Fluid sequestered in "third spaces" and other ill-defined areas is mobilized and excreted as dilute urine.

Caloric intake remains inadequate, and oxidation of endogenous protein and fat continues. Weight loss continues, but usually at a reduced rate. Urinary nitrogen excretion exceeds nitrogen intake. In general, potassium balance becomes positive before nitrogen balance, but the reasons for this phenomenon and for the disparate loss of potassium as compared to nitrogen during the injury phase are not known.

Fibroplasia begins in the wound, and the requirements for vitamin C increase. Thiamine and riboflavin requirements may be slightly increased also, but requirements of other vitamins are not usually elevated above normal daily needs.*

3. ANABOLISM

Positive nitrogen balance and the beginning of muscle rebuilding are evident clinically as the patient regains strength and appetite. Pain is gone, the temperature and pulse are normal, and the patient generally moves about freely. He resumes quiet activities, shows more interest in his environment, and asks to go home, though he usually tires easily and needs more sleep and rest than normally. Appetite is good, and for the first time caloric intake exceeds caloric requirements. Bowels function normally.

*See Chapter 13 for discussion of special nutritional and vitamin requirements.

Anabolism begins as nitrogen intake exceeds nitrogen loss. Endocrine secretions have returned to normal. Sutures are removed as the wound gains in tensile strength. As nitrogen intake reaches 7–12 g/day, urinary and fecal losses are reduced to leave a positive balance of 3–5 g of nitrogen per day. In males, creatine excretion stops. Anabolism proceeds one-third to one-sixth as rapidly as catabolism occurred in the injury phase and requires proportionately more time. Thus, the phase of muscle rebuilding may last several weeks or months depending upon the severity and duration of the phase of injury. After an elective abdominal operation, the phase of anabolism is generally 3–4 weeks. During this phase, weight is gained, but weight does not return to the preinjury level since fat stores are not replenished. Adequate exogenous calories, protein, vitamins, and minerals must be supplied to prevent deficiencies during this muscle rebuilding process.

4. WEIGHT GAIN

The last clinical phase of convalescence is the least well defined. The patient returns to normal activity and regains strength. Exercise tolerance is reduced initially, but may be restored by activity and conditioning. The wound is sound and at maximal strength. Weight is gained as fat stores are replenished by excess caloric intake. The end of convalescence shades imperceptibly into normal metabolism and activity as the patient adjusts, as best he can, to the physical and psychologic residua of his operation or injury.

●　　●　　●

General References

Moore FD: *Metabolic Care of the Surgical Patient*. Saunders, 1959.

Shires GT (editor): *Care of the Trauma Patient*. McGraw-Hill, 1966.

Kinney JM, Egdahl RH, Zuidema GD: *Manual of Preoperative and Postoperative Care*. Saunders, 1971.

Porter R, Knight J: *Energy Metabolism in Trauma*. Churchill, 1970.

12...
Fluid & Electrolyte Therapy

Marcus A. Krupp, MD

Normally, the body fluids have a specific chemical composition and are distributed in discrete anatomic compartments of relatively fixed volumes. Disease produces associated or independent abnormalities in the amounts, distribution, and solute concentrations of the body fluids. Correct diagnosis and treatment of fluid and electrolyte disorders depends upon an understanding of the chemical laws and physiologic processes which control volume, distribution, and composition. In addition, the pharmacologic or physiologic action of some components of body fluids must be considered.

TABLE 12–1. TBW (as percentage of body weight) in relation to age and sex.*

Age	Male	Female
10–18	59%	57%
18–40	61%	51%
40–60	55%	47%
Over 60	52%	46%

*Modified and reproduced, with permission, from Edelman & Liebman: Anatomy of body water and electrolytes. Am J Med 27:256, 1959.

BASIC CONSIDERATIONS

VOLUME & DISTRIBUTION OF BODY WATER

The volume of body water in an individual is quite constant, with intake (food, water consumed, and water produced by combustion) balanced by output (respiratory water vapor, perspiration, and urine). Body water content among individuals differs inversely with obesity. Since fat cells contain very little water and lean tissue is rich in water, it follows that bodies heavy with fat will contain a smaller ratio of water to body weight than lean bodies. After childhood, females usually have a higher ratio of fat to lean tissue. As humans age, they tend to lay down more fat. In the average well-nourished population of the USA, total body water varies as shown in Table 12–1.

The distribution of water among the body fluid compartments is dependent upon the distribution and content of solute. The ability of membranes and cells to restrict movement of solute into and from capillaries, interstitial fluid, and cells results in compartmentalization of solute with resultant distribution of water by osmosis to sustain (1) equal osmolal concentrations of solute in compartments and (2) equal concentrations of water in compartments. Differences in composition of solute in various compartments exist, but osmolality (concentration in compartment water) is equal on both sides of the membrane separating 2 compartments.

Solute concentration is expressed in terms of osmols. The term osmol refers to the relationship between molar concentration and osmotic activity of a substance in solution. The osmolarity of a substance in solution is calculated by multiplying the molar concentration by the number of particles per mol provided by ionization. Glucose in solution provides 1 particle per molecule; NaCl in solution—for all practical purposes—totally dissociates into Na^+ and Cl^-, yielding 2 particles per molecule. One mol of glucose in solution thus yields 1 osmol; 1 mol of NaCl, 2 osmols. As with electrolyte concentrations, the milliunit is more convenient. Osmols-per-kilogram-of-water is termed osmolal; osmols-per-liter-of-solution is termed osmolar. The normal osmolarity of body fluids is 285–293 mOsm/liter.

In all problems of altered osmolality, the alteration exists in all body compartments, and the excess or deficit of solute or of water must be calculated on the basis of total body water (TBW).

ELECTROLYTES

In clinical medicine, the measurement of concentrations of electrolyte in body fluids is expressed in milliequivalents per liter of the fluid. Salts in solution dissociate into ions with positive charges (cations) and negative charges (anions). The numbers of positive and negative charges are equal, ie, a divalent cation (++) will be balanced by 2 monovalent anions or 1 divalent anion (- -).

One mol (gram-molecule) of a substance is the molecular weight of the substance expressed in grams. One mol of a substance contains 6.023×10^{23} molecules of that substance. If the substance can exist in ionized form, its combining capacity with a substance of opposite charge will be determined by its valence, ie, the number of charges per atom or molecule. One mol of a monovalent ion is defined as an equivalent. Thus, 1 mol of a divalent ion will yield 2 equivalents, or, to put it otherwise, 1 equivalent of a divalent ion will be provided by one-half mol of the substance. The term equivalent, therefore, is an expression of concentration in terms of electrical charge. The concentrations of ions in body fluids are small and better expressed in terms of 0.001 equivalents or milliequivalents per liter. Dissociation of some complex ions such as phosphate and protein varies with pH, thus precluding the assignment of a specific valence. (At pH 7.4, the normal pH of plasma, phosphate exists as a buffer mixture of $H_2PO_4^-$ and $HPO_4^=$ to yield an effective valence of 1.8.)

BODY FLUID COMPARTMENTS

The principal fluid compartments include plasma and interstitial fluid, which comprise the extracellular fluid, and intracellular fluid. Body fluids also are distributed to dense connective tissue, bone, and "transcellular" spaces (gut lumen, CSF, intraocular fluid), but these are relatively inaccessible and usually do not enter into clinical situations involving body fluid abnormalities.

The clinical simplification of considering body water or fluid as intracellular (ICW) or extracellular (ECW) is justified by the fact that sodium salts constitute the bulk of osmotically active solute in ECW

TABLE 12–3. Body water distribution in an average normal young adult male.*

	ml/kg† Body Weight	% of Total Body Water
Total extracellular fluid	270	45
Plasma	45	7.5
Interstitial fluid	120	20
Connective tissue and bone	90	15
Transcellular fluid	15	2.5
Total intracellular fluid	330	55
Total body water	600	100

*Modified from Edelman & Liebman: Anatomy of body water and electrolytes. Am J Med 27:256, 1959.

†$\frac{ml/kg}{10} = \%$, eg, 45 ml/kg = 4.5% body weight.

whereas potassium salts constitute the bulk of osmotically active solute in ICW. Furthermore, almost all other solutes present in body water can be considered to be either freely diffusible between ICW and ECW (such as urea) or osmotically inactive (such as ICW magnesium, which is largely bound to protein) and consequently are not osmotically active in either compartment, ie, they do not produce an osmotic gradient because their osmolar concentration is equal in both compartments.

The composition of the body fluids differs among the compartments. Characteristics of the electrolyte concentrations within the compartments are shown in Table 12–4.

Interstitial fluids are not readily available for assay. Clinically, one relies on determinations on plasma or serum which will provide adequate information to assess water and electrolyte derangements in the light of the clinical situation.

PHYSIOLOGY OF WATER & ELECTROLYTE & TREATMENT OF ABNORMAL STATES

In keeping with the basic considerations reviewed above, it is useful to describe the role of body fluids in support of homeostasis in terms of 3 closely related factors: volume, concentration, and pharmacologic activity. The ensuing discussion will consider the following:

TABLE 12–2. Molar and milliequivalent weights.

	Valence	Molar Weights (g)	Milliequivalent Weights (mg)
Cations			
Na^+	1	23	23
K^+	1	39	39
Ca^{++}	2	40	20
Mg^{++}	2	24	12
Anions			
Cl^-	1	35.5	35.5
HCO_3^-	1	61	61
$H_2PO_4^-$	1	31 (as P)	
$HPO_4^=$	2		
$SO_4^=$	2	96	48

TABLE 12–4. Concentrations of cations and anions present in plasma, interstitial water (ISW), and intracellular water (ICW). (nd = not determined.)

| | Plasma, mEq/liter | | ISW, mEq/liter* | ICW, mEq/liter |
	Average	Range	Average	Average
Na^+	140	138–145	144	10
K^+	4	3.5–4.5	4	155
Ca^{++}	5	4.8–5.65	nd	3
Mg^{++}	2	1.8–2.3	nd	26
Total	151		*	194
Cl^-	103	97–105	114	3
HCO_3^-	27	26–30	30	10
$Protein^-$	16	14–18	nd	55
$HPO_4^=$	2	1.2–2.3		100
$SO_4^=$	1			20
Undetermined anions	2			
Total	151		*	183+

*Concentrations derived by converting plasma concentrations to mEq/liter of serum water and applying Donnan factors of 0.95 for cations and 1.05 for anions.

Water Volume

(1) Extracellular fluid: Plasma, interstitial fluid, transcellular fluid (CSF, intraluminal intestinal fluid, ocular fluid).

(2) Intracellular fluid.

Concentration

(1) Osmolality: Total solute concentration.

(2) Concentration of individual electrolytes.

Pharmacologic Activity

(1) Concentration of hydrogen ion (pH).

(2) Concentration of electrolytes which exert pharmacologic actions.

WATER VOLUME

"Volume" and "water" are substantially interchangeable in the context of this discussion. Volume of body water is maintained by a balance between intake and excretion. Water as such, in foods and as a product of combustion, is excreted by the kidneys, skin, and lungs. Electrolytes important in maintaining volume and distribution include the cations sodium for extracellular fluid and potassium and magnesium for intracellular fluid, and the anions chloride and bicarbonate for extracellular fluid and phosphate and protein for intracellular fluid.

Loss of water or excess of water results in corresponding change in volume in both extra- and intracellular compartments. Loss of sodium (with accompanying anion) or excess of sodium results in decrease or increase, respectively, of the volume of extracellular fluid, with water moving out of the extracellular compartment with sodium loss and into the extracellular compartment with sodium retention.

In response to changes in volume, appropriate servo or feedback mechanisms come into play. The principal elements in regulation are antidiuretic hormone for water, aldosterone and other corticosteroids for sodium (and potassium), vascular responses affecting glomerular filtration rate for water and sodium, and, perhaps, a natriuretic hormone ("third factor") originating in the kidney.

The average adult requires at least 800–1300 ml of water per day to cover obligatory water needs. A normal adult on an ordinary diet requires 500 ml of water for renal excretion of solute in a maximally concentrated urine plus an additional amount of water to replace that lost via the skin and respiratory tract.

Fluid losses most often include electrolyte as well as water. Sweat, gastrointestinal fluids, urine, and fluid escaping from wounds contain significant quantities of electrolyte. In order to ascertain deficits of water and electrolytes, one must consider the history, change in body weight, clinical state, and appropriate determinations in plasma of concentration of each of the electrolytes, osmolality, protein, and pH. Assessment of renal function is required before repair and maintenance requirements can be determined and prescribed. Fig 12–1 indicates the variation in water required to excrete different loads of solute. The capacity of the kidney to excrete a concentrated or a dilute urine sets the limits of water requirement.

1. WATER DEFICIT

Water deficit results in a decrease in volume of both extracellular and intracellular fluids with a corre-

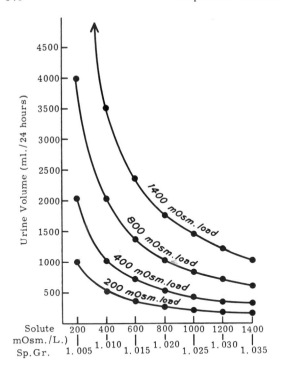

Solute mOsm./L.) / Sp.Gr.

FIG 12—1. Total solute excretion and urine volume per given sp gr. (Redrawn and reproduced, with permission, from Bland JH: *Clinical Recognition and Management of Disturbances of Body Fluids.* Saunders, 1956.)

sponding increase in concentration of both extracellular and intracellular solute in these fluids. In the blood, the loss of body water is reflected in an increased plasma osmolality as concentrations of plasma electrolyte and protein rise. With decreased blood volume, renal blood flow is reduced and excretion of urea falls, resulting in an elevation of urea in body fluids. Antidiuretic hormone secretion is stimulated, providing some protection from water loss by the kidney.

Water deficit results from reduced intake or unusual losses. Reduced intake is likely when the patient is unconscious, disabled, unable to ingest water because of esophageal or pyloric obstruction, or receives inadequate fluids to meet maintenance and replacement needs. Fever or a hot environment increases loss from the lungs and skin. The kidney fails to conserve water when there is inadequate ADH (diabetes insipidus) or insensitivity to ADH (nephrogenic diabetes insipidus), osmotic diuresis in diabetes mellitus, inadequate tubule function due to renal disease, and impaired capacity to reabsorb water secondary to potassium depletion, hypercalcemia, correction of obstructive uropathy, or from intensive diuretic therapy.

Water deficit is characterized by thirst, flushed skin, acute weight loss, "dehydrated" appearance, dry mucous membranes, tachycardia, and oliguria. As

dehydration increases, hallucinations and delirium, hyperpnea, and coma ensue.

Treatment

An essential guideline for treatment is acute change in weight, which is directly related to change in fluid volume. Water may be provided with or without electrolyte. If water alone is needed, 2.5—5% dextrose solution may be given intravenously; the dextrose is oxidized to yield water.

In the presence of normal renal function, 2000—3000 ml of water per day (1500 ml/sq meter of body surface) will provide a liberal maintenance ration. If dehydration is present with increased serum sodium concentration and osmolality, extra water replacement can be estimated on the basis of restoring normal osmolality for the total body fluid volume. The need for intracellular water is reflected in the extracellular fluid with which it is in osmotic equilibrium; therefore, any correction of deviation in osmolality must be considered on the basis of the total volume of body water.

The water requirement is increased in the presence of fever as a result of increased loss via the skin and lungs.

2. WATER EXCESS

Water excess (overhydration, dilution syndrome) results in expansion of the volume of body fluid and decreased concentration (dilution) of plasma electrolyte and protein, a reduced osmolality of plasma. Similar dilutions occur intracellularly. Normally, ADH secretion is inhibited, enabling the kidneys to excrete the excess water. Water excess results from intake in excess of capacity for excretion, usually from too large a water ration during parenteral administration; or from impaired excretory capacity resulting from acute or chronic renal insufficiency, renal functional changes (lowered glomerular filtration and increased water reabsorption) accompanying heart failure, liver disease with ascites, or administration of ADH or inappropriate secretion of "ADH-like" substance by neoplasms or in complex endocrine disturbances.

Water excess, particularly if severe or if it develops acutely, produces the syndrome of water intoxication, characterized by headache, nausea, vomiting, abdominal cramps, weakness, stupor, coma, and convulsions.

Treatment

The basic treatment consists of water restriction. If a real deficit of sodium exists as well, saline solutions should be employed. In the presence of severe water intoxication, administration of hypertonic saline solution may be useful to promote movement of excess intracellular water to the extracellular space, ie, to increase osmolality and diminish intracellular water volume.

CONCENTRATION

The total concentration of solute (osmolarity) is apparently the same in intracellular and extracellular water. In the intracellular compartment, protein concentration plays a more important osmolar role than in the plasma. The protein content of interstitial fluid is small, and osmolar effects are therefore negligible. The most accessible and best index of osmolarity is the measurement of the solute concentration in the plasma by ascertaining the depression of the freezing point. An indirect and useful measurement is that of plasma sodium concentration, provided due attention is paid to hyperglycemia and high urea concentrations, which cause a significant increase in osmolality; and lipemia and hyperproteinemia, which provide a nonaqueous addition to plasma volume. In the latter situations, sodium concentration determinations yield low values which must be interpreted with consideration of the concentration of the other constituents, ie, in terms of plasma or serum water rather than of the plasma specimen per se.

1. HYPERNATREMIA

Increased concentration of sodium in extracellular fluid and hyperosmolality may result from water loss without equivalent sodium loss (pure water volume deficit) or from excessive sodium administration with inadequate water replacement. Hypernatremia may be due to inappropriate regulation of osmolality, occasionally present with intracranial tumors.

Hypernatremia is not an index of total body content of sodium. Increased total body sodium is usually due to retention of sodium with heart failure, cirrhosis of the liver, and nephrosis. In these states, sodium concentration in extracellular fluid is usually normal or low as a result of expansion of the total volume of body fluid.

Treatment

Treatment must be based on accurate appraisal of the significance of the alteration of the plasma sodium concentration. The clinical history and examination and corroborating laboratory data provide a guide for therapy. Hypernatremia due to water deficit is treated by correcting the water deficit (see above). If treatment with excessive quantities of sodium salts produces hypernatremia, withholding sodium may suffice. Natriuretic drugs (diuretics) may be employed to hasten excretion of the excess sodium; attention must be paid to replacement of water when diuretics are so employed.

2. HYPONATREMIA

A decreased concentration of sodium in extracellular fluid may result from loss of sodium or from dilution by retention of water. Sodium loss occurs with adrenocortical insufficiency, vigorous diuretic therapy, unusual losses of gastrointestinal secretions, renal insufficiency, and unusual sweating. When the deficit of water is replaced with inadequate sodium replacement, hyponatremia ensues. Retention of water occurs with the therapeutic use of ADH or with the secretion of excess antidiuretic substances by some types of carcinoma of the lung, with chronic severe heart failure, cirrhosis of the liver with ascites, and nephrotic syndrome. These states produce dilution syndromes characterized by hyponatremia (dilutional hyponatremia) and usually normal or high total body sodium.

Treatment

If there is a deficit of sodium, sodium chloride with or without sodium bicarbonate may be used for replacement. For replacement of moderate deficits, 0.9% sodium chloride (155 mEq of Na^+ and Cl^- per liter), or Ringer's injection with or without lactate, may be employed. For severe sodium deficit, 3% sodium chloride (513 mEq/liter) or 5% sodium chloride (855 mEq/liter) may be used with caution. More comprehensive texts on water and electrolyte metabolism must be consulted for specific information on treatment.

Hyponatremia due to dilution of electrolyte because of water retention should be treated by restriction of intake of water. In states associated with dilutional hyponatremia, total body sodium is elevated or normal and, therefore, sodium should not be administered.

The concentrations of other electrolytes in extracellular fluids have insignificant osmolar effects.

PHARMACOLOGIC ACTIVITY OF FLUIDS & ELECTROLYTES

HYDROGEN ION CONCENTRATION

The hydrogen ion concentration (H^+) of body fluids is closely regulated with intracellular concentrations of 10^{-7} molar (pH 7.0) and extracellular fluid concentrations of 4×10^{-8} molar (pH 7.4). In spite of accumulation or loss of H^+, these concentrations are maintained at nearly normal by buffer substances which remove or release H^+. The capacity of buffers is limited, however, and regulation is accomplished principally by the lungs and kidneys. The principal buffer substances include proteins, the oxyhemo-globin-reduced hemoglobin system, primary and secondary phosphate ions, some intracellular phosphate esters, and the carbonic acid-sodium bicarbonate system.

Most of the food used for energy is completely utilized, with production of water, CO_2, and urea. Sulfate and, to a limited extent, phosphate end products are strong acid anions which must be "neutralized" by cation such as sodium. In the utilization of fat and carbohydrate, intermediate products include the strong acids acetoacetic acid and lactic acid. Buffers provide cation and remove H^+, which is ultimately excreted by the kidneys as acid or as ammonium ion and by the lung as CO_2 and H_2O, equivalent to carbonic acid. The anions of strong acids with cation such as sodium and ammonium are eliminated by the kidney.

The role of the lung and kidney in removal of H^+ and in regulation of H^+ concentration can be viewed as,

$$\frac{[H^+] \quad [HCO_3^-]}{[B^+] \quad [HCO_3^-]} \xrightleftharpoons{\qquad} P_{CO_2} \quad \begin{array}{l} \text{lung} \\ \\ \text{kidney} \end{array}$$

Respiratory control of the partial pressure of CO_2 (P_{CO_2}) in the pulmonary alveoli and therefore in the arterial plasma determines the H_2CO_3 concentration in body fluids:

$$CO_3 + H_2O \xrightleftharpoons{\qquad} H_2CO_3$$

The elimination of CO_2 via the lung in effect removes carbonic acid. The kidney is responsible for $BHCO_3$ concentration in body fluids, which, with H_2CO_3, constitutes one of the buffer systems for regulation of pH.

The kidney tubule cells produce carbonic acid from metabolic CO_2 and water by the following reaction:

$$CO_2 + H_2O \; \underset{\xrightarrow{\qquad}}{\xleftarrow{\boxed{\begin{array}{c}\text{Carbonic}\\\text{anhydrase}\end{array}}}} \; H_2CO_3$$

The carbonic acid serves as a source of H^+ which can be exchanged for Na^+ in the tubular urine so that H^+ is excreted and Na^+ reabsorbed. The exchange affects anions of weak acids: H^+ is excreted by the tubule cell into the tubular urine, and Na^+ is reabsorbed. The H^+ in the presence of HCO_3^- in the tubular urine forms H_2CO_3, which $\rightarrow H_2O$ and CO_2, which are reabsorbed. Similarly, H^+ is exchanged for 1 Na^+ of 2 $Na^+HPO_4^=$ to $\rightarrow Na^+H_2PO_4^-$. (See Fig 12–2.)

Although the pH of urine cannot be lowered below pH 4.5, additional H^+ can be excreted by combination with NH_3, generated principally from glutamine within the tubule cell. NH_3 diffuses from the tubule cell into the urine within the tubule, where it combines with $H^+ \rightarrow NH_4^+$, providing cation for excretion with anions of strong acids with no increase in H^+ concentration (no lowering of pH). These exchanges in the renal tubule involve active transport systems capable of maintaining a gradient in concentration of extracellular fluid H^+ of 4×10^{-8} molar (pH 7.4) against a tubular urine H^+ of 32×10^{-6} molar (pH 4.5), an 800-fold increase in H^+ concentration.

CLINICAL STATES OF ALTERED H^+ CONCENTRATION

The clinical term acidosis signifies a decrease in pH (increase in H^+) of extracellular fluid; the term alkalosis signifies an increase in pH (decrease in H^+) of extracellular fluid. The change in H^+ concentration may be the result of metabolic or respiratory abnormalities.

1. RESPIRATORY ACIDOSIS

Respiratory acidosis follows ventilatory abnormalities resulting in CO_2 retention and elevation of P_{CO_2} in alveoli and arterial blood (hypercapnia). Inadequate ventilation (1) during anesthesia, (2) following suppression of the respiratory center by CNS disease or drugs, or (3) resulting from respiratory muscle weakness or paralysis produces CO_2 retention. Anatomic changes in structure of the lung (emphysema) or pulmonary circulation and abnormal thoracic structure (kyphoscoliosis) may alter alveolar-capillary blood exchange or diminish effective ventilation to prevent CO_2 excretion. In association with impaired CO_2 excretion, there may be impaired O_2 exchange with low alveolar and arterial P_{O_2} (hypoxia). In the presence of CO_2 retention and the resultant increase in H_2CO_3 concentration, compensatory reabsorption of HCO_3^- by the kidney provides buffer to reduce H^+ concentration, but this protection cannot be accomplished rapidly and is effectively available only in chronic situations that develop slowly.

The hazard of acute hypercapnia cannot be overemphasized. Buffer protection is severely limited, and renal response is very slow. Thus, an increase in P_{CO_2} can quickly produce a sharp increase in H^+ concentration (decrease in pH) to levels incompatible with life. Respiratory inadequacy resulting in sudden increase in P_{CO_2} will usually result in a severe decrease in P_{O_2}, compounding the threat to life. It is apparent that periods of hypoventilation constitute a serious and often lethal complication in the immediate postoperative state, in thoracic surgery, in severe illness or shock accompanied by obtunded consciousness, in trauma to the CNS, and in the presence of heart failure, cardiac arrhythmias, and myocardial infarction.

Treatment

Treatment is directed toward improving ventilation with mechanical aids, bronchodilators, correction of heart failure, and antidotes for anesthetics or drugs suppressing the respiratory center. Tracheostomy or tracheal intubation is often required. Close monitoring of P_{CO_2}, P_{O_2}, and pH of arterial blood is essential. The respiratory center is readily rendered unresponsive by high P_{CO_2} (hypercapnia), and recovery may be very slow. In the presence of hypercapnia, relief of hypoxia with oxygen therapy may deprive the patient of the only remaining stimulus to the respiratory center and produce more severe hypoventilation with resultant CO_2 narcosis and death. Assistance with respiration is required until the respiratory center becomes normally responsive to normal CO_2 concentrations.

2. RESPIRATORY ALKALOSIS

Respiratory alkalosis is a result of hyperventilation which produces lowered P_{CO_2} and elevated pH of extracellular fluid. Anxiety is the usual cause. Hyperventilation during anesthesia or from incorrectly used mechanical respiratory aids occurs more commonly than is generally appreciated. Renal compensation by excretion of HCO_3^- (with Na^+ predominantly) is too slow a response to be effective, and elevation of pH may reach a point at which asterixis, tetany, and increased neuromuscular irritability appear.

Treatment

Treatment of spontaneous hyperventilation consists of reducing anxiety by drugs or psychotherapy. Tetany may be alleviated by rebreathing exhaled air, which will increase P_{CO_2} and lower blood pH. Regulation of devices used in assisting with respiration should be determined by measurement of the P_{CO_2} and pH of arterial blood.

3. METABOLIC ACIDOSIS

Metabolic acidosis occurs with starvation, uncontrolled diabetes mellitus with ketosis, electrolyte (including bicarbonate) and water loss with diarrhea or enteric fistulas, and renal insufficiency or tubular defect producing inadequate H^+ excretion. Cation loss (Na^+, K^+, Ca^{++}) and organic acid anion retention occur with starvation and uncontrolled diabetes mellitus. In the presence of renal insufficiency, phosphate and sulfate are retained and cation (especially Na^+) is lost because of limited H^+ secretion for exchange with cation in the renal tubule. A rare cause of metabolic acidosis is the ingestion of acid salts such as NH_4Cl or mandelic acid or acid precursors such as methyl alcohol; these are particularly likely to produce acidosis in the presence of renal insufficiency. Respira-

tory compensation for metabolic acidosis by hyperventilation provides reduction of P_{CO_2} and thereby reduction of H_2CO_3 in extracellular fluid.

Treatment

Treatment is directed toward correcting the metabolic defect (eg, insulin for control of diabetes) and replenishment of water and of deficits of Na^+, K^+, HCO_3^-, and other electrolytes. Anion replacement should include bicarbonate or lactate (bicarbonate equivalent), but large quantities of bicarbonate are needed only in unusual and threatening states. The "maintenance" solution described above is adequate for most needs; lactated Ringer's injection may be preferred if larger quantities of Na^+ are required. A mixture of half 0.9% saline and half 1/6 molar sodium lactate (or bicarbonate) provides an even greater fraction of HCO_3^-. Renal insufficiency requires careful replacement of water and electrolyte deficit and closely controlled rations of water, sodium, potassium, calcium, chloride, and bicarbonate to maintain normal extracellular fluid concentrations; the elevated serum phosphate may be lowered by interfering with phosphate absorption from the gut by oral administration of aluminum hydroxide preparations. In the presence of renal insufficiency, elevated extracellular K^+ concentrations may be reduced by either oral administration of ion exchange resins which bind K^+, either ingested or secreted, and prevent absorption in the intestine (see Hyperkalemia, below), or by hemodialysis or peritoneal dialysis.

Lactic Acidosis

A rare and serious form of acidosis is that due to large quantities of lactic acid. It is presumed that severe tissue anoxia (eg, in shock) leads to anaerobic glucose metabolism with production of lactic acid. Acidosis develops abruptly and is usually severe and highly resistant to therapy with HCO_3^-. Plasma lactate concentration may rise to 8 mM/liter.

Lactic acidosis must be considered in anoxic states, hypovolemic or endotoxin shock, severe pulmonary insufficiency or pulmonary edema, heart failure, severe hepatic failure, nonketotic diabetic acidosis, following phenformin therapy, and following poisoning with paraldehyde or salicylates. Diagnosis is confirmed in states of overt acidosis by actual lactate levels or by demonstrating that a large amount of unidentified anion is present in the serum (ie, not Cl^-, HCO_3^-, $HPO_4^=$, or ketone bodies).

Treatment is often ineffectual. The primary and contributing causes must be treated vigorously and sodium bicarbonate administered in large quantities despite the dangers of sodium overload.

4. METABOLIC ALKALOSIS

Metabolic alkalosis results from loss of gastric juice rich in HCl and occurs also in association with K^+

deficit (diuretics, adrenocortical excess, abrupt correction of hypercapnia), which is characteristically accompanied by increased urinary excretion of H^+. All of these result in renal retention of HCO_3^-, producing elevated extracellular fluid bicarbonate. Respiratory compensation by hypoventilation produces an elevation in P_{CO_2}, increasing the H_2CO_3 fraction of the bicarbonate buffer system.

Treatment

Alkalosis of metabolic origin requires adequate water, K^+, and Na^+. The anion should be exclusively Cl^- to replace the HCO_3^- excess and Cl^- deficit; no lactate or bicarbonate should be employed until normal blood pH and bicarbonate levels are obtained.

POTASSIUM

Potassium is one of the major intracellular cations, occupying a role that is parallel to that of sodium in extracellular fluid. Physiologic actions of potassium are related primarily to concentration of the cation in extracellular fluid, although the intracellular concentration may have some influence. Potassium plays an important part in muscular contraction, conduction of nerve impulses, enzyme action, and cell membrane function.

Cardiac muscle excitability, conduction, and rhythm are markedly affected by changes in concentration of K^+ in extracellular fluid. Both an increase and a decrease of extracellular K^+ concentration diminish excitability and conduction rate. Higher than normal concentrations produce a marked depression of conductivity with cardiac arrest in diastole; in the presence of very low concentrations, cardiac arrest occurs in systole. The effects of abnormal K^+ concentrations in extracellular fluid upon cell membrane potential of cardiac muscle and upon depolarization and repolarization are manifested in the ECG.

Membrane potential and excitability of skeletal and smooth muscle are profoundly affected by the concentrations of K^+, Ca^{++}, and Mg^{++}, with H^+ and Na^+ also involved. Conduction across the myoneural junction is under the influence of these cations as well. At both extremes of abnormal concentration of K^+ in extracellular fluid, muscle contractility is impaired and flaccid paralysis ensues.

Potassium concentration of extracellular fluid is closely regulated between 3.5–5 mEq/liter. Excretion of the 35–100 mEq of potassium contained in the daily diet of the average adult is predominantly via the kidney. There is good evidence that the potassium in glomerular filtrate is reabsorbed in the proximal tubule and that active secretion of potassium into the tubular fluid occurs in the distal portion of the tubule.

1. HYPERKALEMIA

Causes of increased extracellular K^+ concentration include failure of the kidney to excrete ingested potassium (acute and chronic renal failure, severe oliguria due to severe dehydration or trauma); unusual release of intracellular potassium in burns, crushing injuries, or severe infections; and overtreatment with potassium salts. In metabolic acidosis, extracellular K^+ concentration is increased as K^+ shifts from cells.

The elevated K^+ concentration interferes with normal neuromuscular function to produce weakness and paralysis; abdominal distention and diarrhea may occur. As extracellular concentration of K^+ increases, the ECG reflects impaired conduction by peaked T waves of increased amplitude, atrial arrest, spread in the QRS, biphasic QRS–T complexes, and finally ventricular fibrillation and cardiac arrest.

Treatment

Treatment consists of withholding potassium and employing cation exchange resins by mouth or enema. Kayexalate, a sodium cycle sulfonic polystyrene exchange resin, 40–80 g/day in divided doses, is usually effective. In an emergency, insulin may be employed to deposit K^+ with glycogen in the liver, and Ca^{++} may be given intravenously as an antagonist ion. Sodium bicarbonate can be given intravenously as an emergency measure in severe hyperkalemia; the increase in pH so induced results in a shift of K^+ into cells. Hemodialysis or peritoneal dialysis may be required to remove K^+ in the presence of protracted renal insufficiency.

2. HYPOKALEMIA

Potassium deficit may or may not be accompanied by lowered extracellular fluid K^+ concentration; however, when hypokalemia is present, total potassium deficit is usually profound. Exceptions to this common circumstance include the hypokalemia of alkalosis and that following administration of insulin. Causes of potassium deficit include reduced intake due to starvation or upper gastrointestinal obstruction; poor absorption in steatorrhea, short bowel syndrome, and regional enteritis; loss via the gastrointestinal tract due to emesis, diarrhea, and suction; loss via the kidney due to congenital tubule malfunction, diuresis resulting from diabetes or diuretics, accompanying metabolic alkalosis, and following excessive treatment with saline solutions containing little or no potassium; loss of interstitial fluid with burns or freezing; loss of K^+ due to adrenocortical hormone (cortisol or aldosterone) excess; and intracellular shifts in bouts of familial periodic paralysis. A low concentration of K^+ in extracellular fluid results in impaired neuromuscular function with profound weakness of skeletal muscle, leading to impaired ventilation, and of smooth muscle, producing ileus. The ECG shows decreased amplitude and broadening of T waves, prominent U waves, sagging S–T segments, atrioventricular block, and, finally, cardiac arrest. Metabolic alkalosis with elevated plasma pH and bicarbonate concentration develops as a result of potassium deficit which is accompanied by renal excretion of H^+ and reabsorption of bicarbonate and by movement of Na^+ and H^+ from extracellular fluid into cells as K^+ is lost. A defect of water reabsorption by the renal tubule also occurs, producing polyuria and hyposthenuria; this is only slowly ameliorated following treatment.

Treatment

Treatment requires replacement of potassium orally or parenterally. Because of the toxicity of potassium, it must be administered cautiously to prevent hyperkalemia. Furthermore, confirmation of adequate renal function is important when potassium is administered since the principal route of excretion is via the kidney. KCl in a total dose of 1–3 mEq/kg/24 hours may be given parenterally in glucose or saline solutions (or both) at a rate that will not produce hyperkalemia. Except in an emergency in which serum K^+ is extremely low and cardiac muscle and respiratory muscle activity seriously impaired, the administration of K^+ should be at a rate of 10–20 mEq/hour or less. Cl^- is always needed to relieve the hypochloremia that is associated with the accompanying metabolic alkalosis.

CALCIUM

Calcium constitutes about 2% of body weight, but only about 1% of the total body calcium is in solution in body fluid. In the plasma, calcium is present as a nondiffusible complex with protein (33%); as a diffusible but undissociated complex with anions such as citrate, bicarbonate, and phosphate (12%); and as Ca^{++} (55%). The normal total plasma (or serum) calcium concentration is 4.5–5.5 mEq/liter (9–11 mg/100 ml). The serum calcium level is responsive to 2 hormones: parathyroid hormone elevates and calcitonin lowers the concentration. Bone serves as a reservoir of calcium available to body fluids. Excretion of Ca^{++} is via the kidney.

Calcium functions as an essential ion for many enzymes. It is an important constituent of mucoproteins and mucopolysaccharides, and is essential in blood coagulation.

Along with other cations, calcium exerts an important effect on cell membrane potential and permeability manifested prominently in neuromuscular function. It plays a central role in muscle contraction as it is released from the sarcolemma to enter into the ATP-ADP reaction. During muscle relaxation, the calcium is actively transferred back to the sarcolemma and sarcoplasmic reticulum.

Neural function is sensitive to Ca^{++} concentration of interstitial fluid. Excitability is diminished by high Ca^{++} concentration and increased by low concentration. Signs of elevated Ca^{++} concentration include dulling of consciousness and stupor and muscular flaccidity and weakness. Low Ca^{++} concentration increases excitability to produce hyperirritability of muscle, tetany, and convulsions.

Cardiac muscle responds to elevated Ca^{++} concentration with increased contractility, ventricular extrasystoles, and idioventricular rhythm. These responses are accentuated in the presence of digitalis. With severe calcium toxicity, cardiac arrest in systole may occur. Low concentration of Ca^{++} produces diminished contractility of the heart and a lengthening of the Q–T interval of the ECG by prolonging the S–T segment.

1. HYPERCALCEMIA

Hypercalcemia results from hyperparathyroidism, invasion of bone by neoplasm (lung, breast, kidney, thyroid), production of a parathyroid-like hormone by isolated neoplasms (ovary, kidney, lung), sarcoidosis, multiple myeloma, and vitamin D intoxication.

Hypercalcemia affects neuromuscular function to produce weakness, and causes polyuria, dehydration, thirst, anorexia, vomiting, and constipation. Stupor, coma, and azotemia ensue.

Treatment

Treatment consists of control of the primary disease. Symptomatic hypercalcemia is associated with a high mortality rate; treatment must be promptly instituted. Until the primary disease can be brought under control, renal excretion of calcium with resultant decrease in serum Ca^{++} concentration can be promoted with a variety of agents. Excretion of Na^+ is accompanied by excretion of Ca^{++}; therefore, inducing natriuresis by giving Na^+ salts intravenously and by adjunctive use of diuretics is the emergency treatment of choice. Sodium chloride or sodium sulfate in large quantities (70–80 mEq/hour) with or without diuretics (furosemide) for 12–48 hours may be required. Replacement of water and of K^+ and Mg^{++} is usually necessary. The use of phosphate is hazardous and should be reserved for unusual cases refractory to saline therapy. When elevated Ca^{++} concentrations result from sarcoid or neoplasm, corticosteroids such as prednisone may be effective. Mithramycin is useful if elevated Ca^{++} is the result of neoplasm metastatic to bone.

2. HYPOCALCEMIA

Hypocalcemia results from hypoparathyroidism (idiopathic or postoperative), chronic renal insufficiency, rickets and osteomalacia, and malabsorption syndromes. Serum Ca^{++} concentration is reduced in association with decreased serum albumin concentrations, a physiologic relationship.

Hypocalcemia affects neuromuscular function to produce muscle cramps and tetany, convulsions, stridor and dyspnea, diplopia, abdominal cramps, and urinary frequency. Personality changes may occur. In chronic hypoparathyroidism and pseudohypoparathyroidism, cataracts may appear and calcification of basal ganglia of the brain may occur. Mental retardation and stunted growth are common in childhood.

Treatment

Treatment depends on the primary disease. Treatment of hypoparathyroidism with vitamin D and calcium is discussed in Chapter 20. For tetany due to hypocalcemia, calcium gluconate, $1-2$ g, may be given IV. A continuous infusion to sustain plasma calcium concentration may be required. Oral medication with the chloride, gluconate, levulinate, lactate, or carbonate salts of calcium will usually control milder symptoms or latent tetany. The low serum Ca^{++} associated with low serum albumin concentration does not require replacement therapy.

MAGNESIUM

About 50% of total body magnesium exists in the insoluble state in bone. Only 5% is present as extracellular cation; the remaining 45% is contained in cells as intracellular cation. The normal plasma concentration is $1.5-2.5$ mEq/liter, with about one-third bound to protein and two-thirds as free cation. Excretion of magnesium ion is via the kidney, with no evidence of active tubule secretion.

Magnesium is an important prosthetic or activator ion, participating in the function of many enzymes involved in phosphate transfer reactions, including those requiring ATP or other nucleotide triphosphate as coenzymes.

Magnesium exerts physiologic effects on the nervous system resembling those of calcium. Elevated Mg^{++} concentration of interstitial fluid produces sedation and central and peripheral nervous system depression. Low concentrations produce increased irritability, disorientation, and convulsions.

Magnesium acts directly upon the myoneural junction. Elevated levels produce blockage by decreasing acetylcholine release, reducing the effect of acetylcholine on depolarization, and diminishing excitability of the muscle cell. Calcium ion exerts an antagonistic action. Low levels of magnesium increase neuromuscular irritability and contractility, partly by increasing acetylcholine release. Tetany and convulsions may occur.

Cardiac muscle is affected by large increases in magnesium concentration in the range of $10-15$ mEq/liter. Conduction time is increased, with lengthened duration of P–R and QRS components of the ECG. As the concentration of Mg^{++} increases further, cardiac arrest in diastole occurs.

Elevated magnesium concentrations produce vasodilatation and a drop in blood pressure by blockade of sympathetic ganglia as well as a direct effect on smooth muscle.

1. HYPERMAGNESEMIA

Magnesium excess is almost always the result of renal insufficiency and inability to excrete what has been absorbed from food or infused. Occasionally, with the use of magnesium sulfate as a cathartic, enough magnesium is absorbed to produce toxicity, particularly in the presence of impaired renal function. Manifestations of hypermagnesemia include muscle weakness, fall in blood pressure, and sedation and confusion. The ECG shows increased P–R interval, broadened QRS complexes, and elevated T waves. Death usually results from respiratory muscle paralysis.

Treatment

Treatment is directed toward alleviating renal insufficiency. Calcium acts as an antagonist to Mg^{++} and may be employed parenterally for temporary benefit. Extracorporeal or peritoneal dialysis may be indicated.

2. HYPOMAGNESEMIA

Magnesium deficit may be encountered in chronic alcoholism in association with delirium tremens, starvation, diarrhea, malabsorption, prolonged gastrointestinal suction, vigorous diuresis, primary hyperaldosteronism, and hypoparathyroidism, particularly after parathyroidectomy for hyperparathyroidism and when large doses of vitamin D and calcium are consumed.

Magnesium deficit is characterized by neuromuscular and CNS hyperirritability with athetoid movements; jerking, coarse, and flapping tremors; positive Babinski response, nystagmus, tachycardia, hypertension, and vasomotor changes.

Treatment

Treatment consists of the use of parenteral fluids containing magnesium as chloride or sulfate, $10-40$ mEq/day during the period of severe deficit followed by 10 mEq/day for maintenance. Magnesium sulfate may also be given IM, $4-8$ g ($66-133$ mEq) daily in 4 divided doses.

THE APPROACH TO DIAGNOSIS & TREATMENT OF WATER, ELECTROLYTE, & ACID-BASE DISTURBANCES

In the diagnosis and treatment of water and electrolyte derangements, one must rely upon clinical appraisal of the patient, including details of the history, the presenting disease and its complications, recent and abrupt change in weight, the physical examination, and the laboratory data bearing upon altered volume, osmolarity, distribution, and physiologic manifestations. Although a thorough knowledge of the physiologic principles of water and electrolyte metabolism and of renal function is essential to sound management and direction of therapy, the science of therapy is far from exact, and the physician must always consider and be grateful for the homeostatic resources of the patient. If renal function is reasonably good, the range between acceptable lower and upper limits of amounts of water and electrolytes is broad and the achievement of "balance" not difficult. In the presence of renal insufficiency, some endocrinopathies influencing water and electrolyte metabolism, shock, heart failure, hepatic insufficiency, severe gastrointestinal fluid loss, pulmonary insufficiency, and some rarer diseases, the patient is deprived of his homeostatic resources and the physician is called upon to substitute as best he can with close observation and meticulous quantitative therapy.

Some general principles will be included here. For difficult and complicated problems, more specialized and more complete texts must be consulted.

MAINTENANCE

Most of those who require water and electrolyte are relatively normal people who cannot take orally what they require for maintenance.

It is apparent from Table 12–5 that the range of tolerance for water and electrolytes (homeostatic limits) permits reasonable latitude in therapy provided normal renal function exists to accomplish the final regulation of volume and concentration.

TABLE 12–5. Daily maintenance rations for patients requiring parenteral fluids.

	Per sq M Body Surface	Average Adult (60–100 kg)
Glucose	60–75 g	100–200 g
Na$^+$	50–70 mEq	80–120 mEq
K$^+$	50–70 mEq	80–120 mEq
Water	1500 ml	2500 ml

An average adult whose entire intake is parenteral would receive his maintenance ration in 2500–3000 ml of 5% or 10% dextrose in 0.2% saline solution (34 mEq Na$^+$ + Cl$^-$/liter). To each liter, 30 mEq KCl could be added. In 3 liters, the total chloride intake would be 192 mEq, which could be tolerated. An alternative would be to eliminate the KCl if parenteral fluids would be required for only 2–3 days. After 3 days of potassium-free parenteral fluids, total potassium loss may become significant and replacement is desirable. Other solutions available for maintenance therapy contain electrolyte mixtures designed to meet average adult requirements: in one example, each liter contains dextrose, 50 g; Na$^+$, 40 mEq; K$^+$, 35 mEq; Cl$^-$, 40 mEq; HCO$_3^-$ equivalent, 20 mEq; and PO$_4^\equiv$, 15 mEq. The daily administration of 2500–3000 ml satisfies the needs listed in Table 12–5.

In situations requiring maintenance or maintenance plus replacement of fluid and electrolyte by parenteral infusion, the total daily ration should be administered continuously over the 24-hour period in order to ensure the best utilization by the patient. Periodic large infusions result in responsive excretion by the kidney, reducing the opportunity for precise regulation by the kidney. Continuous infusion is desirable, particularly when losses are large and the total volume of the daily infusion is correspondingly large. With modern technics for continuous infusions, around-the-clock administration imposes little discomfort or hardship on the patient. The needle should be changed every 48 hours.

DEFICITS

To the maintenance ration one must add water and appropriate electrolyte for replacement of losses previously incurred and water and electrolytes to replace current losses. The amounts of water and electrolytes are dictated by clinical evaluation of deficits of each, and a further choice of anion would be dictated by the presence of metabolic acidosis or alkalosis and in some instances of respiratory acidosis.

The severity of dehydration (volume depletion) is assessed by means of the history, the magnitude of acute weight loss, and, on physical examination, the loss of elasticity of the skin and subcutaneous tissues, dry mucous membranes, tachycardia and hypotension, lethargy, and weakness. As dehydration becomes more severe, the decrease in plasma volume results in progression of hypotension and shock. Hemoconcentration progresses with loss of plasma water; electrolyte concentrations differ according to the losses incident to the primary disease; the increase in BUN reflects the decrease in glomerular filtration rate incident to circulatory changes associated with low blood volume.

A significant decrease of extracellular fluid volume and of circulating blood volume usually follows the redistribution of body fluids produced by burns, bowel obstruction, peritonitis, venous obstruction, and, rarely, lymphatic obstruction. The fluid sequestered in these conditions is derived from interstitial fluid and circulating plasma, producing volume deficits of physiologic importance.

Treatment consists of replacement of water deficit with appropriate electrolyte replacement according to serum osmolarity (Na^+ concentration), blood pH, and serum K^+ concentration. In the presence of hyperosmolarity (hypernatremia), electrolyte-free or hypotonic solutions should be employed; if serum Na^+ concentration is normal, repletion can be accomplished with isotonic solutions. If hypo-osmolarity (hyponatremia) exists due to sodium loss, hypertonic (3–5%) NaCl solutions or hypertonic $NaHCO_3$ solutions may be required. In addition to replacement needs, maintenance requirements must be met, requiring correlation of volume, electrolyte concentration, and rate of administration to effect a normal state.

One should aim for total replacement in 48–72 hours. Time is required for circulation, diffusion, equilibration, renal response, and restoration of normal homeostatic mechanisms; a general rule is to provide daily maintenance needs plus half the deficit in the first 24 hours and a quarter of the deficit daily for 2 days thereafter to complete restitution in 72 hours. To this must be added the equivalent of continuing losses.

Common situations in which deficits may be large are discussed below. Other less common derangements are beyond the scope of this chapter. For therapeutic guidance, consult more detailed texts and specific treatises.

1. DIABETIC KETOSIS

Characterized by significant losses of water, sodium, and potassium in addition to retention of ketone body acids and a decrease in bicarbonate and pH in the extracellular fluid. Therapy is complex, for it includes consideration of insulin requirement as well as the need for water and electrolyte. Refer to texts on management of diabetes for a full discussion.

2. GASTROINTESTINAL DISEASE

Often accompanied by large losses of water, sodium, and potassium. Loss of chloride or bicarbonate is related to the site of the disease or obstruction, eg, in pyloric obstruction with loss of HCl; small bowel fluid losses with loss of bicarbonate. (See Table 12–6.) Following intubation, the collected secretions should be assayed to determine the volume and losses of electrolyte that must be replaced.

3. BURNS

Edema accompanying the trauma to tissue results in sequestration of fluids in tissues beneath the burns with consequent decrease in circulating plasma volume and circulatory collapse. Therapy is described in Chapter 18.

4. PERITONITIS

Inflammation may produce a large collection of fluid in the peritoneal cavity. Prompt restoration of plasma volume and extracellular fluid is essential.

TABLE 12–6. Volume and electrolyte content of gastrointestinal fluid losses.*

	Na^+ (mEq/liter)	K^+ (mEq/liter)	Cl^- (mEq/liter)	HCO_3^- (mEq/liter)	Volume (ml)
Gastric juice, high in acid	20 (10–30)	10 (5–40)	120 (80–150)	0	1000–9000
Gastric juice, low in acid	80 (70–140)	15 (5–40)	90 (40–120)	5–25	1000–2500
Pancreatic juice	140 (115–180)	5 (3–8)	75 (55–95)	80 (60–110)	500–1000
Bile	148 (130–160)	5 (3–12)	100 (90–120)	35 (30–40)	300–1000
Small bowel drainage	110 (80–150)	5 (2–8)	105 (60–125)	30 (20–40)	1000–3000
Distal ileum and cecum drainage	80 (40–135)	8 (5–30)	45 (20–90)	30 (20–40)	1000–3000
Diarrheal stools	120 (20–160)	25 (10–40)	90 (30–120)	45 (30–50)	500–17,000

*Average values/24 hours with range in parentheses.

5. ASCITES

The association of liver disease with ascites and the consequences of therapy with diuretics may produce complex alterations of fluid distribution and electrolyte concentrations. (See Chapter 26.)

. . .

SUMMARY OF CLINICAL APPROACH

The following outline summarizes an approach to therapy with water and electrolytes. Listed are factors essential to an assessment of the state of the patient, of the urgency for treatment, and of the choice of the therapeutic agents and the quantities to be administered. This outline has been useful in planning the treatment and avoiding the ommission of essential elements of treatment.

Problems

(1) Simple maintenance.

(2) Repair of deficit plus maintenance.

(3) Repair plus replacement of continuing losses plus maintenance.

(4) Replacement of continuing losses plus maintenance.

Situations: Acute or Chronic

A. Acute:

1. Respiratory—Alteration of P_{CO_2} and pH. Often overlooked. H^+ concentration can change rapidly to life-threatening levels. *Caution:* Therapy must be immediate and adequate.

2. Organic ion acidosis (lactate, ketones), "anion gap." Normally, $Cl^- + CO_2 + 12 = Na^+$ in mEq/liter, or $Cl^- + 1/2\ CO_2 + 25 = Na^+$ in mEq/liter.

3. Plasma K^+ concentration deficit or excess.

4. Hyper- or hypo-osmolality, often iatrogenic.

5. Explosive gastrointestinal loss, Addison's disease in crisis.

6. Acute renal shutdown.

B. Chronic:

1. Renal insufficiency.

2. Pulmonary insufficiency.

3. Chronic gastrointestinal disease (gut, liver).

4. Endocrine abnormality, especially myxedema.

Determinants in Establishing Therapy

Sex: Females are usually fatter and, therefore, have lower total body water ratios (per kg) than males of equal weight.

Size: Fat or lean; more fat means lower ratios of total body water/kg. This must be considered in calculating replacement of osmolar deficit (ie, Na^+).

Renal and pulmonary function.

Cause of abnormal state, ie, shock, gastrointestinal obstruction, third space sequestration, diabetes or other endocrine abnormality, malnutrition, induced by drug effect or therapeutic error.

Observations

Weight.

Intake, output, and loss record.

Serum electrolytes, osmolality, urea or creatinine, protein, glucose.

Arterial blood P_{CO_2}, pH, P_{O_2} as indicated.

Urine specific gravity, osmolality, volume.

. . .

Tables 12–7, 12–8, 12–9, and 12–10 indicate the wide choices open to the physician in planning the restoration of water and electrolyte in the variety of clinical problems that may occur. A sound understanding of the physiologic mechanisms discussed above enables the physician to direct therapy rationally and with considerable skill. If renal and pulmonary function are comprised, the task becomes difficult and hazardous for even the best informed clinicians.

TABLE 12–7. Equivalents of salts used for therapy.*

Salt	g	mEq of Cation per Amount Stated
IV or oral		
NaCl	9	155
NaCl	5.8	100
NaCl	1	17
NaHCO$_3$	8.4	100
Na lactate	11.2	100
KCl	1.8	25
K acetate	2.5	25
K$_2$HPO$_4$	1.84	25
KH$_2$PO$_4$	0.4	
CaCl$_2$	0.5	10
Ca gluconate	2	10
MgCl$_2$	0.5	10
Oral		
K citrate	3	25
K tartrate	5	27

*Reproduced, with permission, from Krupp, Sweet, Jawetz, & Biglieri: *Physician's Handbook,* 16th ed. Lange, 1970.

TABLE 12–8. Examples of solutions for parenteral infusion.

	Na⁺	K⁺	Ca⁺⁺	Mg⁺⁺	NH₄⁺	Cl⁻	HCO₃⁻ Equiv*	PO₄⁼	Glucose (g/liter)
5% glucose in water									50
10% glucose in water									100
Isotonic saline (0.9%)	155					155			
Sodium chloride (5%)	855					855			
Ringer's solution	147	4	4			155			
Ringer's lactate (Hartmann's)	130	4	3			109	28		
Darrow's solution (KNL)	121	35				103	53		
Potassium chloride									
0.2% in dextrose 5%		27				27			50
0.3% in dextrose 5%		40				40			50
"Modified duodenal solution" with dextrose, 10%	80	36	5	3		64	60		100
"Gastric solution" with dextrose, 10%	63	17			70	150			100
Ammonium chloride, 0.9%					170	170			
Sodium lactate, 1/6 molar	167						167		
Sodium bicarbonate, 1/6 molar	167						167		
Examples of "maintenance solutions":									
Pediatric electrolyte "No. 48" with dextrose 5%	25	20		3		22	23	3	50
Maintenance electrolyte "No. 75" with dextrose 5%	40	35				40	20	15	50
Levulose and dextrose with electrolyte (Butler's II)	58	25		6		51	25	13	100
5% dextrose in 0.2% saline	34					34			50
10% dextrose in 0.45% saline	77					77			100

HCO₃⁻ equivalent may be lactate, acetate, gluconate, or citrate, or combinations of these.
A variety of modifications of multiple electrolyte solutions are commercially available.

TABLE 12–9. Examples of electrolyte concentrates.

	Ampule Volume	Na⁺	K⁺	Ca⁺⁺	Mg⁺⁺	NH₄⁺	Cl⁻	HCO₃⁻	Lactate	PO₄⁼
Potassium chloride*	10 ml		20				20			
KMC*	10 ml		25	10	10		45			
Potassium phosphate*	20 ml		40							40
Calcium gluconate, 10%	10 ml			4.5					4.5 (gluconate)	
Sodium bicarbonate, 7.5%†	59 ml	45						45		
Sodium lactate, molar†	40 ml	40							40	
Ammonium chloride*	30 ml					120	120			
Magnesium sulfate, 50%	. . .				8‡					

Note: The physician should always check the contents of the ampule as listed by the manufacturer.
*Dilute to 1 liter or more.
†Dilute as indicated by the manufacturer.
‡8 mEq/ml.

TABLE 12–10. Examples of oral electrolyte preparations.

Preparation	Supplied As	Electrolyte Content*					
		Na$^+$	K$^+$	NH$_4$$^+$	Ca^{++}	Cl$^-$	HCO$_3$$^-$
NaCl	Salt	17				17	
NaHCO$_3$	Salt	12					12
KCl	Salt		14			14	
K-triplex	Elixir		15 mEq/ 5 ml				
K gluconate (Kaon)	Elixir		7 mEq/ 5 ml				
Ca gluconate	Salt				4.5		
Ca lactate	Salt				10		
NH$_4$Cl (acidifying salt)	Salt			19†		19	
Kayexalate (ion-exchange resins)	Salt	1‡	‡				

*mEq/g unless otherwise specified.

†NH$_4$$^+$ is converted to H$^+$ in the body, mEq for mEq.

‡1 g resin removes 1 mEq K$^+$ and contributes 3 mEq Na$^+$ to patient.

• • •

General References

General

Black DAK: Symptoms and signs in disorders of body fluid. J Chronic Dis 11:340–347, 1960.

Bland JH: *Clinical Metabolism of Body Water and Electrolytes.* Saunders, 1963.

Gump FE & others: Caloric and fluid losses through the burn wound. S Clin North America 50:1235–1248, 1970.

Hutchin P: Metabolic response to surgery in relation to caloric, fluid, and electrolyte intake. Curr Probl Surg 1–51, April 1971.

Maxwell MH, Kleeman CR (editors): *Clinical Disorders of Fluid and Electrolyte Metabolism,* 2nd ed. McGraw-Hill, 1972.

Pitts RF: *Physiology of the Kidney and Body Fluids,* 2nd ed. Year Book, 1968.

Robinson JR: Metabolism of intracellular water. Physiol Rev 40:112–149, 1960.

Sunderman FW, Sunderman FW Jr (editors): *Clinical Pathology of the Serum Electrolytes.* Thomas, 1966.

Weiner M & others: Signs and symptoms of electrolyte disorders. Yale J Biol Med 43:76–109, 1970.

Windhazer EE: Kidney, water, and electrolytes. Ann Rev Physiol 31:117–172, 1969.

Fluid Volume

Bricker NS, Klahr S: The physiologic basis of sodium excretion and diuresis. Advances Int Med 16:17–41, 1970.

Clift GV & others: Syndrome of inappropriate vasopressin secretion. Arch Int Med 118:453–460, 1966.

Earley LE, Daugharty TM: Sodium metabolism. New England J Med 281:72–86, 1969.

Githers JH: Hypernatremic dehydration. Clin Pediat 2:453–462, 1963.

Kleeman CR, Fichman MP: The clinical physiology of water metabolism. New England J Med 277:1300–1307, 1967.

Kleeman CR: Hypo-osmolar syndromes secondary to impaired water excretion. Ann Rev Med 21:259–268, 1970.

Leaf A: The clinical and physiologic significance of the serum sodium concentration. New England J Med 267:24–30, 77–83, 1962.

Maffly RH, Edelman IS: The role of sodium, potassium, and water in the hypo-osmotic states of heart failure. Progr Cardiovas Dis 4:88–104, 1961.

Warhol RM, Eichenholz A, Mulhausen RO: Osmolality. Arch Int Med 116:743–749, 1965.

Welt LG: Hypo- and hypernatremia. Ann Int Med 56:161–164, 1962.

Hydrogen Ion

Albert MS, Dell RB, Winters RB: Quantitative displacement of acid-base equilibrium in metabolic acidosis. Ann Int Med 66:312–322, 1967.

Blumentals AS (editor): Symposium on acid-base balance. Arch Int Med 116:647–742, 1965.

Diarrhea and acid-base disturbances. Leading article. Lancet 1:1305–1306, 1966.

Elkinton JR: Hydrogen ion turnover in health and disease. Ann Int Med 57:660–684, 1962.

Kassirer JP, Schwartz WB: The response of normal man to selective depletion of hydrochloric acid. Correction of metabolic alkalosis in man without repair of potassium deficiency. Am J Med 40:10–26, 1966.

Manfredi F: Effects of hypocapnia and hypercapnia on intracellular acid-base equilibrium in man. J Lab Clin Med 69:304–312, 1967.

Schwartz WB, Waters WC: Lactate versus bicarbonate. Editorial. Am J Med 32:831–834, 1962.

Statement of acid-base terminology. Ann Int Med 63:885–890, 1965; Anesthesiology 27:7–12, 1966; Ann New York Acad Sc 133:251–258, 1966.

Steinmetz PR: Excretion of acid by the kidney-functional organization and cellular aspects of acidification. New England J Med 278:1102–1109, 1968.

Tranquada RE, Grant WJ, Peterson CR: Lactic acidosis. Arch Int Med 117:192–202, 1966.

Van Ypersele de Strihou C, Brasseur L, McConinck J: The "carbon-dioxide response curve" for chronic hypercapnia in man. New England J Med 275:117–122, 1966.

Potassium

Bellet S: The cardiotoxic effects of hyperpotassemia and its treatment. Postgrad Med 25:602–609, 1959.

Kassirer JP & others: The critical role of chloride in the correction of hypokalemic alkalosis in man. Am J Med 38:172–189, 1965.

Leaf A, Santos RF: Physiologic mechanisms in potassium deficiency. New England J Med 264:335–341, 1961.

Papper S, Whang R: *Hyperkalemia and Hypokalemia.* Disease-A-Month. Year Book, June 1964.

Surawicz B: Electrolytes and the electrocardiogram. Am J Cardiol 12:656–662, 1963.

Weatherall M: Ions and the actions of digitalis. Brit Heart J 28:497–504, 1966.

Calcium

Breuer RI, Bauer L: Caution in the use of phosphates in the treatment of severe hypercalcemia. J Clin Endocrinol 27:659–698, 1967.

Chakmakjian ZH, Bethune E: Sodium sulfate treatment of hypercalcemia. New England J Med 275:862–869, 1966.

Foster GV: Calcitonin (thyrocalcitonin). New England J Med 279:349–360, 1968.

Goldsmith RS, Ingbar SH: Inorganic phosphate treatment of hypercalcemia of diverse etiologies. New England J Med 274:1–7, 284, 1966.

Kleeman CR & others: The clinical physiology of calcium homeostasis, parathyroid hormone and calcitonin. California Med 114:16–43, March 1971; 114:19–30, April 1971.

Perlia CP & others: Mithramycin treatment of hypercalcemia. Cancer 25:389–394, 1970.

Rasmussen H: Ionic and hormonal control of calcium homeostasis. Am J Med 50:567–588, 1971.

Singer FR & others: Mithramycin treatment of intractable hypercalcemia due to parathyroid carcinoma. New England J Med 283:634–636, 1970.

Suki WN & others: Acute treatment of hypercalcemia with furosemide. New England J Med 283:836–840, 1970.

Magnesium

Gitelman HJ, Welt LG: Magnesium deficiency. Ann Rev Med 20:233–242, 1969.

MacIntyre I: Magnesium metabolism. Advances Int Med 13:143–154, 1967.

Wacker WEC, Parisi AF: Magnesium metabolism. New England J Med 278:772–776, 1968.

13 . . .

Nutrition in Surgery

Harold A. Harper, PhD

Metabolic Effects of Trauma

The rapid nutritional deterioration which so often follows severe injuries or acute infections is one of the most dramatic problems encountered clinically. Perhaps the first systematic investigation of this problem began early in the 20th century with measurements of nitrogen excretion in patients with typhoid fever. Later, Coleman and DuBois reported on their classic studies of the metabolic changes that occur in patients with acute and chronic medical illnesses, and Cuthbertson described the increased urinary nitrogen excretion that occurs following fractures. Since these pioneering studies, many investigators have described the metabolic changes that occur after injury.

The early metabolic response to injury of previously healthy adults includes the following: increased heat production; loss of weight; negative balances of nitrogen, potassium, sulfur, and phosphorus; impaired utilization of carbohydrate, possibly with ketosis; retention of water, sodium, and chloride; and changes in the metabolism of some of the water-soluble vitamins. The metabolic responses described may be accompanied by involution of lymphoid tissue and thymus, lymphopenia and eosinopenia, leukocytosis, hypertrophy of the adrenal cortex, and an increase in adrenocortical hormones in the blood and urine. Impairment of hepatic function is suggested by an increase in retention of sulfobromophthalein and a decrease in the rate of conjugation of adrenal corticosteroids. It thus appears that the metabolic reaction to injury is characterized by chemical and physiologic changes which involve protein, carbohydrate, fat, water, vitamins, and endocrine and electrolyte metabolism. Although the metabolic changes are qualitatively similar in patients with a wide variety of injuries or illnesses, their quantitative aspects tend to parallel the severity of the injury, with the most marked responses occurring in the previously healthy young adult male. The return to a normal metabolic state after injury or disease occurs after a variable length of time. Sodium metabolism, for example, becomes normal after a relatively brief period, whereas impaired metabolism of protein tends to be prolonged. Indeed, disturbances in protein utilization may constitute the most severe of the nutritional disturbances associated with altered metabolism in trauma or other disease states characterized by a significant catabolic response.

In the discussions that follow, references to metabolic changes will be made. For convenient reference,

TABLE 13–1. Some numerical constants useful in estimates of metabolic changes.

Protein catabolized = urinary nitrogen × 6.25
Wet lean tissue broken down = urinary nitrogen × 30 or protein × 4.75
Wet lean tissue is assumed to be 73% water and 27% protein

In muscle tissue:
Extracellular potassium = 3.8–4.3 mEq/liter
Intracellular potassium = 148–155 mEq/liter
Potassium content = 100 mEq/kg wet weight

Energy considerations:
Caloric equivalents of nutrients:

Carbohydrate	= 4 Cal/g
Fat (triglycerides)	= 9 Cal/g
Protein	= 4 Cal/g
Ethyl alcohol	= 7 Cal/g

Respiratory quotient (RQ) = CO_2/O_2 ratio
RQ for oxidation of carbohydrate = 1.00
RQ for oxidation of fat = 0.70
When carbohydrate is being converted to fat, RQ is > 1.00
On the usual mixed diet, RQ = 0.75–0.85
Basal Metabolic Rate (adults) = 36–41 Cal/sq m/hour (approximately 1600–1800 Cal/day)
For 1800 Cal energy expenditure, oxygen consumption = 250 ml/min

Carbohydrate consumption =	400 Cal (100 g)
Fat consumption	= 1160 Cal (130 g)
Protein consumption	= 240 Cal (60 g)
Total	= 1800 Cal/day

Table 13–1 lists some of the numerical data that may be useful in making estimates of these changes in various metabolic parameters of the surgical patient.

Protein Catabolic Response to Trauma

It has often been observed that the rate of excretion of nitrogen is increased after trauma or the stress of an operation. This is not due simply to starvation. Under normal circumstances, an individual on zero intake of nitrogen as protein maintains urinary nitrogen excretion at a normal or reduced rate (4–6 g/day) for a time, after which there occurs only a gradual reduction to low values. In contrast, after major trauma and with zero intake of protein, the urinary nitrogen may increase to as much as 7–15 g/day for 2–5 days. After extensive injury or trauma, nitrogen excretion may be increased to as much as 20 g/day. Fractures or major injury complicated by infection enhance the breakdown of lean tissue, which fosters very high urinary nitrogen excretion rates–to as much as 30 g/day, equivalent to the loss of 180 g of protein per day derived from about 1 kg (wet weight) of lean tissue, largely skeletal muscle.

Nitrogen Losses After Burns

Extensive losses of nitrogen constitute a very serious nutritional problem after extensive burns. The effect of trauma on nitrogen losses discussed above is certainly foremost in burns, as it is in other extensive injuries also. If there is simply soft tissue trauma progressing to uncomplicated convalescence and healing, the period of increased nitrogen excretion persists for only 2–5 days. However, this nitrogen catabolic period seems to be unduly prolonged after burns of even moderate severity. In a study of 5 patients, the excretion of nitrogen tended toward a maximum at the end of the first postburn week. During this period, 25–30 g of nitrogen per day were excreted. One patient excreted 36.9 g of nitrogen (equivalent to 230 g of protein) on the seventh day after the burn had occurred. While the degree of negative nitrogen balance lessened slowly, beginning about 7–10 days after the burn, positive nitrogen balance was not attained until 30–40 days after injury.

A second cause of nitrogen loss in the burned patient is the fact that the exudate from the burned surface is rich in protein derived directly from plasma and interstitial fluid. Furthermore, plasma protein leaves the circulation and passes directly into the injured tissues. Examples of the amounts of nitrogen lost in the exudate are reports of 7.8 g/day (equivalent to 49 g of protein) in an adult male with a 33% burn, to 0.7 g/day in a young girl with a 5% burn.

The nitrogen losses of the early postburn period undoubtedly result from extensive tissue catabolism. During the first 10 days after a severe burn, if a mean nitrogen loss of 18 g/day is assumed, a whole tissue loss of as much as 540 g/day would occur. In one study, burn patients lost a total of 8.2–11.7 kg of lean body tissue during the catabolic period following a burn.

Nitrogen Loss in Trauma

Even when large amounts of readily utilized calories and protein are provided during the nitrogen catabolic period, the amount of net nitrogen loss may only be decreased but not abolished. This suggests that the metabolic effects of trauma on protein nutrition are not attributable in any large degree to starvation. Because of the apparently obligatory nature of nitrogen catabolism during the early period after trauma, it seems undesirable–even if it were practicable–to attempt to supply the very large nutritional intake necessary to equal the losses. Certainly during the early

postburn period (7–10 days), excessive feeding may only result in nausea, vomiting, and diarrhea with consequent worsening of the nutritional status of the patient.

Because an increased rate of nitrogen excretion follows injection of corticotropin or certain of the adrenal corticosteroids such as cortisone or cortisol, and because adrenal hyperactivity is a component of the syndrome of stress, including infection and trauma, posttraumatic catabolism has been attributed to these endocrine effects. However, the nature of a wound, particularly its duration as an open wound, also affects nitrogen excretion, and later changes in nitrogen metabolism may occur as well, independently of demonstrable changes in corticosteroid production. The same may be said of the nature of posttraumatic nitrogen loss in the aged or previously debilitated patient, which does not correlate with corticosteroid production.

Reference was made above to the quantities of nitrogen lost in association with burns. In the first 5 days after other forms of major trauma, a patient may be expected to lose a total of about 50 g of nitrogen (equivalent to 312 g protein; 1500 g wet weight lean tissue).

Potassium Metabolism in Trauma

Potassium losses are excessive following any event associated with tissue breakdown and nitrogen loss. In the first day after moderately severe trauma, 2.7–3.5 g (38–50 mEq) of potassium may be excreted. A negative potassium balance of 2–5 g/day occurs immediately after burning. In contrast to nitrogen, potassium losses tend to decrease rapidly, so that if adequate amounts of potassium are provided, positive balance may be regained in 3–6 days.

Caloric Deficits in Trauma

It is virtually a certainty that an inadequate caloric intake will follow severe injury or extensive surgery, particularly if the surgery involves the peritoneal cavity. It follows that the patient should lose weight during the immediate posttraumatic or postoperative period. If he does not, overloading with water and salt should be suspected.

The exogenous deficit of calories will require that energy sources from within the body be mobilized to meet minimal energy needs. Carbohydrate–mostly as liver and muscle glycogen and glucose in the extracellular fluid–will be quickly utilized. The total available carbohydrate in these forms is no more than 300–500 g, equivalent to 1200–2000 Cal as energy. Within 8–16 hours after any significant surgical procedure, these readily available stores of carbohydrates will be exhausted.

Effects of Protein Catabolism on Muscle Tissue

The protein catabolic effects of trauma and stress, including that of surgery, have been discussed above. Most of the protein lost in this manner is derived from skeletal muscle. No other tissue could support such large losses of protein as have been observed in these catabolic states. After very severe trauma followed by a prolonged period of infection and illness, a decrease in skeletal muscle mass of as much as 30% or more has been observed.

The metabolic breakdown of the protein lost from muscle through the metabolic pathways for gluconeogenesis produces some carbohydrate which, of course, can be readily utilized for energy. As an example, when an amount of muscle tissue is sacrificed to account for a daily urinary excretion of 20 g of nitrogen, about 125 g of glucose (500 Cal of energy) are produced.

It should be apparent, however, that neither preformed carbohydrate nor that produced by gluconeogenesis from protein can supply a significant amount of calories. Consequently, as in starvation or any other metabolic circumstance characterized by an inadequate supply of energy, the fat stored in adipose tissue depots within the body serves as the main source of energy for bodily processes. After major trauma, endogenous fat may be mobilized and oxidized at rates of 250–500 g/day, accounting for the production of 2000–4500 Cal, a rate which exceeds that predicted from starvation alone. Most previously normal individuals carry a reserve of adipose tissue equivalent to 100–150 thousand Cal, an amount which is adequate to supply energy for 2–3 months at normal rates of consumption. Loss of half this amount or even more is not harmful.

The oxidation of 1 kg of fat in the body produces slightly more than 1000 ml of water of oxidation. One kg of lean tissue produces 730 ml of cellular water plus another 250 ml of water of oxidation from protein breakdown. All of this additional source of "endogenous" water must be taken into account in severe trauma, accompanied as it is by extensive breakdown of endogenous protein and fat, as a factor contributing to overhydration of patients in the immediate post-trauma period, particularly if excess fluid is given either by mouth or as parenteral fluid.

Surgery on the gastrointestinal tract may be expected to present special nutritional problems in addition to those associated with the metabolic responses discussed above. These special problems may include decreased efficiency of absorption of energy-yielding nutrients due either to changes in alimentation time or intrinsic changes within the gastrointestinal tissues themselves. Anemias may develop as a result of diminished absorption of iron or of vitamin B_{12}, in the latter instance particularly when the distal segments of the small intestine may be involved, since the ileum is the main absorptive area for vitamin B_{12}. Lack of an adequate amount of intrinsic factor—as might occur after extensive resection of the stomach—may also contribute to vitamin B_{12} deficiency.

Energy Considerations

A primary nutritional requirement is the provision of energy to support metabolic processes. Carbohydrate, fat, and protein of the diet are the calorific or energy-yielding components. The daily requirement for calories is the sum of that required merely to maintain life (so-called basal energy demand) plus that required for additional activity. Under normal circumstances, the caloric demand is increased during periods of growth or in pregnancy. In disease, the convalescent period requires extra energy to support the repair process. Metabolism requiring extra energy will be accelerated in hyperthyroidism or as a result of fever. In the latter instance, there is an increase of approximately 12% of the basal caloric requirement for each degree centigrade (7% per degree Fahrenheit) by which the temperature is above normal. The current recommended daily allowances for various nutrients in healthy individuals of varying ages and weights are given in Table 13–2. Twenty-five to 30 Cal/kg/day are required for maintenance purposes. In disease, however, these requirements are markedly altered. The daily requirements for calories in adult patients may increase to very high levels as indicated below:

Afebrile, minor injury or illness, at bed rest	2000 Cal
Severe injury or illness	2500–4000 Cal
Previously depleted	3500 Cal
Severe sepsis, fever	5000 Cal

When oral feeding is not possible in a surgical patient and nutrition is confined to the intravenous route, provision of adequate calories is extremely important, particularly in abnormal states characterized by heavy caloric demand. Inability to supply adequate exogenous energy from the diet often ranks as the primary problem in the nutrition of surgical patients.

Protein Requirements

Of almost equal nutritional importance to that of calories is the problem of supplying adequate protein to surgical patients. Protein is a unique constituent of the diet and cannot be replaced by any other food. The recommended daily intakes of protein for healthy individuals are shown in Table 13–1; however, as discussed above, the quantity of protein required by surgical patients may either be only slightly higher than that of normal individuals or very considerably increased up to 200 or 300 g/day or more, as in severe burns.

If possible, at least 100 g of protein per day should be given to all sick or injured persons. Patients with severe hepatic or renal disease and surgical patients who have had portacaval anastomoses are exceptions to this rule. The liver is the principal organ involved in the metabolism of protein. The action of intestinal bacteria on orally ingested protein produces ammonia, which normally is absorbed in the portal blood and carried directly to the liver, where the ammonia is promptly detoxified by conversion to urea. In advanced liver disease, the liver may perform this function inadequately; after portacaval anastomoses or the development of portal-systemic collateral vessels due to portal hypertension associated with long-standing chronic hepatic disease, the portal circulation bypasses the liver. In both instances, ammonia rises to toxic levels in the peripheral blood. It is under these circumstances that the oral intake of protein must be restricted even though a high-protein diet may otherwise be desirable. Caution should also be exercised, when giving high-protein diets, to provide adequate fluid to permit the renal excretion of the increased amounts of urea which will be produced from protein breakdown. It follows, of course, that adequate renal function to permit renal excretion of protein breakdown products must also be assured.

As was described above, the metabolism of protein is much affected by stress such as that after infections, injuries, major surgery, and burns. Prolonged bed rest will also induce increased protein breakdown with negative nitrogen balance. In all of these situations, there inevitably occurs some depletion of body protein stores, first from the very limited labile reserves but mainly from the breakdown of skeletal muscle. Depletion of the body protein leads to prolongation of convalescence, impaired wound healing, increased susceptibility to infection, skeletal muscle weakness, edema, anemia, impaired gastrointestinal motility, and a number of postoperative complications.

Reference was made above to the problem of providing adequate calories for surgical patients. Protein, although not intended primarily as a source of energy in the diet, will be utilized for this purpose unless adequate amounts of nonprotein calories are simultaneously supplied. In the immediate postoperative or post-traumatic period, the characteristic metabolic response appears to induce negative nitrogen balance which is difficult (if not impossible) to correct regardless of the amounts of protein and calories which may be supplied. During this so-called obligatory protein catabolic period, it does not appear desirable to attempt by nutritional means to reverse the metabolic process. However, after a variable period of time—usually only a few days after moderate stress—a protein anabolic period supervenes during which the body utilizes administered protein with much more efficiency if adequate calories are also provided. Nonetheless, during the postoperative period, an intake of as much as 0.5 g/kg of nitrogen (1 g of nitrogen equals 6.25 g of protein) and 45 Cal/kg may be necessary to restore positive nitrogen balance in a previously depleted patient.

Carbohydrate & Fat Requirements

Carbohydrates and fats serve as the main sources of energy in the normal balanced diet. In circumstances requiring significant increases in energy, a larger intake of fat is necessary. However, efficient utilization of fats requires at least small amounts of carbohydrate—said to be at least 5 g of carbohydrate/100 Cal in the total diet. Surgical patients who cannot take an adequate diet will compensate for the exogenous energy deficit by increased mobilization of their own endogenous fat. As little as 100 g of carbohydrate per day will provide for the efficient utilization of fat

derived from endogenous sources. This amount is easily provided even when only intravenous fluids are being administered since it is contained in 2000 ml of 5% dextrose, an amount well within the usual daily fluid prescription for adult patients.

Vitamins

Protein, carbohydrate, and fat provide nutritional sources for energy and repair of body tissues and special materials for other aspects of the metabolic machinery. However, the utilization of these nutrients requires other nutritional factors, such as vitamins and minerals, as well as water. When a normal individual is consuming an adequate balanced diet, all of the required vitamins, minerals, and water can be secured from dietary sources; supplementation must be considered in various abnormal states or when digestion or assimilation is impaired and the requirements for these nutrients must be increased. The recommended daily allowances for normal persons for various vitamins about which adequate information is available are given in Table 13–2. It is very likely, however, that increases in these recommended allowances will be necessary in abnormal states. In these situations, information is much less accurate with respect to appropriate vitamin requirements than is the case under normal circumstances of health.

A. Vitamin B Complex: The water-soluble vitamins of the B complex are directly involved as cofactors in important metabolic processes. Since these processes may be increased as a result of the abnormal metabolic state incident to disease, it is considered desirable to increase the intake of these vitamins. The recommended therapeutic daily doses of the most important of these vitamins are as follows:

Thiamine (B_1)	5–10 mg
Riboflavin (B_2)	5–10 mg
Niacinamide	100 mg
Pantothenic acid	20 mg
Pyridoxine (B_6)	2 mg
Folic acid (folacin)	1.5 mg
Vitamin B_{12}	4 µg

Because pantothenic acid is a constituent of a cofactor involved in the reactions leading to the production of acetylcholine, the suggestion has been made that increased amounts of this vitamin are of value in the therapy of paralytic ileus. There has been no demonstration of specific deficiency of pantothenic acid in surgical patients, nor has pantothenic acid or any of its derivatives proved to be of therapeutic benefit in ileus or any other definitive surgical complication.

B. Vitamin C: Vitamin C (ascorbic acid) appears to have particular value in connection with disease processes accompanied by accelerated metabolism and stress. One of the best-demonstrated functions of vitamin C is its role in maintaining the normal intercellular material of cartilage, dentine, and bone, as well as in collagen synthesis. This relates the vitamin specifically to wound healing. The observation that there are large amounts of vitamin C in the adrenal cortex and that

TABLE 13–2. Recommended daily dietary allowances, revised 1968.*[1]

	Age[2] (Years)	Weight (kg) (lb)	Height (cm) (in)	Kcal	Protein (g)	Fat-Soluble Vitamins			Water-Soluble Vitamins							Minerals				
						Vitamin A Activity (IU)	Vitamin D Activity (IU)	Vitamin E Activity (IU)	Ascorbic Acid (mg)	Folacin[3] (mg)	Niacin (mg eq[4])	Riboflavin (mg)	Thiamine (mg)	Vitamin B$_6$ (mg)	Vitamin B$_{12}$ (µg)	Calcium (g)	Phosphorus (g)	Iodine (µg)	Iron (mg)	Magnesium (mg)
Infants	0–1/6	4 9	55 22	kg × 120	kg × 2.2[5]	1500	400	5	35	0.05	5	0.4	0.2	0.2	1.0	0.4	0.2	25	6	40
	1/6–1/2	7 15	63 25	kg × 110	kg × 2.0[5]	1500	400	5	35	0.05	7	0.5	0.4	0.3	1.5	0.5	0.4	40	10	60
	1/2–1	9 20	72 28	kg × 100	kg × 1.8[5]	1500	400	5	35	0.1	8	0.6	0.5	0.4	2.0	0.6	0.5	45	15	70
Children	1–2	12 26	81 32	1100	25	2000	400	10	40	0.1	8	0.6	0.6	0.5	2.0	0.7	0.7	55	15	100
	2–3	14 31	91 36	1250	25	2000	400	10	40	0.2	8	0.7	0.6	0.6	2.5	0.8	0.8	60	15	150
	3–4	16 35	100 39	1400	30	2500	400	10	40	0.2	9	0.8	0.7	0.7	3	0.8	0.8	70	10	200
	4–6	19 42	110 43	1600	30	2500	400	10	40	0.2	11	0.9	0.8	0.9	4	0.8	0.8	80	10	200
	6–8	23 51	121 48	2000	35	3500	400	15	40	0.2	13	1.1	1.0	1.0	4	0.9	0.9	100	10	250
	8–10	28 62	131 52	2200	40	3500	400	15	40	0.3	15	1.2	1.1	1.2	5	1.0	1.0	110	10	250
Males	10–12	35 77	140 55	2500	45	4500	400	20	40	0.4	17	1.3	1.3	1.4	5	1.2	1.2	125	10	300
	12–14	43 95	151 59	2700	50	5000	400	20	45	0.4	18	1.4	1.4	1.6	5	1.4	1.4	135	18	350
	14–18	59 130	170 67	3000	60	5000	400	25	55	0.4	20	1.5	1.5	1.8	5	1.4	1.4	150	18	400
	18–22	67 147	175 69	2800	60	5000	400	30	60	0.4	18	1.6	1.4	2.0	5	0.8	0.8	140	10	400
	22–35	70 154	175 69	2800	65	5000	…	30	60	0.4	18	1.7	1.4	2.0	5	0.8	0.8	140	10	350
	35–55	70 154	173 68	2600	65	5000	…	30	60	0.4	17	1.7	1.3	2.0	5	0.8	0.8	125	10	350
	55–75+	70 154	171 67	2400	65	5000	…	30	60	0.4	14	1.7	1.2	2.0	6	0.8	0.8	110	10	350
Females	10–12	35 77	142 56	2250	50	4500	400	20	40	0.4	15	1.3	1.1	1.4	5	1.2	1.2	110	18	300
	12–14	44 97	154 61	2300	50	5000	400	20	45	0.4	15	1.4	1.2	1.6	5	1.3	1.3	115	18	350
	14–16	52 114	157 62	2400	55	5000	400	25	50	0.4	16	1.4	1.2	1.8	5	1.3	1.3	120	18	350
	16–18	54 119	160 63	2300	55	5000	400	25	50	0.4	15	1.5	1.2	2.0	5	1.3	1.3	115	18	350
	18–22	58 128	163 64	2000	55	5000	400	25	55	0.4	13	1.5	1.0	2.0	5	0.8	0.8	100	18	350
	22–35	58 128	163 64	2000	55	5000	…	25	55	0.4	13	1.5	1.0	2.0	5	0.8	0.8	100	18	300
	35–55	58 128	160 63	1850	55	5000	…	25	55	0.4	13	1.5	1.0	2.0	5	0.8	0.8	90	18	300
	55–75+	58 128	157 62	1700	55	5000	…	25	55	0.4	13	1.5	1.0	2.0	6	0.8	0.8	80	10	300
Pregnancy				+200	65	6000	400	30	60	0.8	15	1.8	+0.1	2.5	8	+0.4	+0.4	125	18	450
Lactation				+1000	75	8000	400	30	60	0.5	20	2.0	+0.5	2.5	6	+0.5	+0.5	150	18	450

*Reproduced from Publication 1694, Food and Nutrition Board, National Academy of Sciences, National Research Council, 1968.

[1] The allowance levels are intended to cover individual variations among most normal persons as they live in the USA under usual environmental stresses. The recommended allowances can be attained with a variety of common foods, providing other nutrients for which human requirements have been less well defined.

[2] Entries on lines for age range 22–35 years represent the reference man and woman at age 22. All other entries represent allowances for the midpoint of the specified age range.

[3] The folacin allowances refer to dietary sources as determined by *Lactobacillus casei* assay. Pure forms of folacin may be effective in doses less than ¼ of the recommended daily allowance.

[4] Niacin equivalents include dietary sources of the vitamin itself plus 1 mg equivalent for each 60 mg of dietary tryptophan.

[5] Assumes protein equivalent to human milk. For proteins not 100% utilized, factors should be increased proportionately.

the cortex is rapidly depleted of vitamin C when the adrenal gland is stimulated (as by stress) and the additional observation that increased losses of vitamin C accompany fever and infection favor the view that special attention should be given to the intake of this vitamin in disease states characterized by trauma and stress. For these reasons, at least 500 mg/day of vitamin C should be provided as a therapeutic dose.

If supplementation with vitamins is necessary for only a short period until a normal diet can be taken, only thiamine, riboflavin, niacinamide, and ascorbic acid need be given. It should also be noted that when these water-soluble vitamins are added to solutions to be given intravenously, large losses of the vitamins may occur into the urine. For this reason, intramuscular or subcutaneous injection is preferred if the oral route cannot be used.

C. Fat-Soluble Vitamins: Vitamins A, D, and K are the fat-soluble vitamins generally considered to be important in human nutrition, although a requirement in adult humans for vitamin D is questionable since it can be synthesized within the body. However, vitamins A and K do have generalized metabolic roles which are of continuing importance. A role of vitamin A in wound healing has recently been proposed, and vitamin K is essential to the production of prothrombin by the liver and therefore in coagulation of the blood. Under normal circumstances, vitamin A is present in adequate amounts in a balanced diet; the synthesis by intestinal bacteria of vitamin K assures production of adequate amounts of this vitamin. However, these fat-soluble vitamins are not adequately absorbed from the intestinal tract if fat digestion or absorption is impaired, as may occur in obstructive jaundice, biliary fistula, pancreatic disease, or any disease state which extensively involves the gastrointestinal tract. For surgical patients, a deficiency of vitamin K may be very significant because of its effects on prothrombin production. When circumstances as mentioned above are such as to induce a vitamin K deficiency, it is important to administer vitamin K preoperatively by injection until the prothrombin level is at least 60–70% of normal. The required dose of a water-soluble vitamin K preparation such as menadione sodium bisulfite (Hykinone) is only 2–5 mg IV or IM. If such a conservative dose does not produce a prompt response in the form of a rise in prothrombin, this suggests that the liver is severely damaged and unable to respond by production of prothrombin. This observation is of importance in assessing the danger of hemorrhage when operating on such patients.

Nutritional Importance of Potassium in Surgical Patients

Although the mineral elements are present in the tissues in relatively small amounts, they are essential to many body processes. The importance in surgical patients of certain of these elements such as sodium and potassium relates mainly to regulation of water metabolism and acid-base balance. There are, however, some considerations with respect to potassium that make it necessary to place nutritional emphasis on this element above all others in connection with surgical patients. Potassium deficiency is likely to develop in any illness, particularly in postoperative states, when patients are maintained for prolonged periods on intravenous fluids which do not contain potassium. Potassium deficiencies are likewise to be expected in chronic wasting diseases, malnutrition, prolonged negative nitrogen balance, gastrointestinal losses (including those incurred in all types of diarrhea, gastrointestinal fistulas, and continuous suction), and metabolic alkalosis.

In muscle, the proportion of potassium to nitrogen is 3 mM to each gram. Storage of nitrogen as muscle protein, such as must occur after muscle wasting incident to prolonged negative nitrogen balance, therefore demands that the diet contain not only protein but potassium as well. For example, it has been suggested that a loss of 5 kg of muscle protein requires 600 mEq of potassium together with the protein nitrogen necessary for its replacement.

Although potassium can easily be added to intravenous fluids, extensive deficiencies of potassium are most readily corrected when orally administered nutrients can be given. In the nutrition of surgical patients who may have incurred large deficits of potassium, it thus becomes important in prescribing a diet to consider the use of foods high in potassium. Those foods which have a high content of potassium (300–600 mg/serving) are meats, fish, and poultry, dried apricots, dried peaches, bananas, raisins, prunes, figs, and dates. Certain fruit juices such as prune, tomato, orange, and pineapple are also high in potassium. Among the vegetables, yams, squash, potatoes, brussels sprouts, cauliflower, lentils, and broccoli are high in potassium. Certain foods which are useful as sources of potassium may, however, also be high in sodium, which in some circumstances may not be desired. Examples are ham, bacon, milk, and tomato juice.

PARENTERAL NUTRITION

When the gastrointestinal tract cannot be used for nutritional purposes and only the intravenous route is available, certain nutrients can be added to the intravenous fluids. The principal problem under these circumstances is to provide sufficient calories. Normally, the dextrose contained within intravenously administered solutions can be expected only to provide calories to supplement the utilization of the patient's own reserves of fat, which may constitute a significant reserve of calories—in fact, as much as 100–150 thousand Cal in a normal man.

Administration of Glucose

One liter of 5% dextrose (glucose) provides only 200 Cal. On the assumption that a total fluid intake of 3 liters/day is the average maximum permitted an adult patient, such dextrose-containing solutions would provide only a total of 600 Cal/day. The minimum caloric requirement for a patient while confined to bed is 2000 Cal/day. Thus, even under relatively ideal circumstances, a substantial caloric deficit from exogenous sources always exists during ordinary parenteral nutrition. Even if only glucose is used as a source of calories, more concentrated solutions would of course yield more calories. The disadvantage to this approach is the fact that dextrose solutions exceeding isotonic concentrations ($> 5\%$) lead to phlebitis. There is also a limit to the rate at which dextrose can be given intravenously without causing excretion of excess glucose into the urine, which not only wastes the administered calories but may enhance dehydration because of the effect of glycosuria on increasing urine flow and a diuresis of electrolytes. To avoid glycosuria, dextrose should not be given at rates exceeding $0.5-0.75$ g (approximately $10-15$ ml of a 5% solution)/kg/hour. (Somewhat slower rates are preferred.) Thus, the higher the concentration of an intravenously administered solution of dextrose, the more slowly it must be given. Despite the disadvantages of using glucose solutions exceeding 5%, there may be circumstances where this will prove necessary for nutritional purposes. Examples are when parenteral nutrition must be maintained over a prolonged period or when maximal nonprotein calories are necessary to spare the breakdown of proteins, as may be the case in patients with acute renal insufficiency in whom the total fluid intake must be severely restricted. If hypertonic ($25-50\%$) solutions of dextrose are used in such special circumstances, phlebitis can be minimized by administering the hypertonic solutions very slowly through a small polyethylene catheter introduced directly into the subclavian vein.

Fructose Administration

Fructose, when administered intravenously, disappears from the blood faster than dextrose. It therefore can be administered more rapidly than dextrose and with less loss into the urine. For this reason, fructose has been studied for use as a possible substitute for dextrose in intravenous nutrition. The caloric value of fructose is the same as that of dextrose; however, it does not appear that the advantages attributed to fructose are significant enough to recommend its general use as a substitute for dextrose in parenteral fluids. Furthermore, there is evidence that considerable energy is required by the liver to convert fructose to glucose, which conversion is required for utilization of fructose by most tissues, including skeletal muscle.

Alcohol Administration

Ethyl alcohol may serve as a source of calories in intravenous solutions. It is metabolized when added to solutions of dextrose to provide 5.6 Cal/ml (7 Cal/g). However, alcohol should not be given intravenously in concentrations much exceeding 5% (50 ml 95% alcohol/liter). Because of this restriction, only an additional 280 Cal/liter would be obtained in this way.

This is not a significant addition to the caloric intake, and the fact that patients receiving alcohol-containing solutions intravenously must be carefully attended—as well as the possibility of undesirable reactions to other drugs that are being used—further limits the use of alcohol as a practical source of calories in intravenous regimens.

Fat Administration

As has already been pointed out, enrichment of the diet with calories is ordinarily accomplished by increasing the fat intake. Consequently, the addition of fat to an intravenous regimen would do much to ameliorate the caloric deficit which otherwise is inevitable under these circumstances. Emulsions of fat suitable for intravenous use have been prepared and found to serve effectively as a source of calories. Unfortunately, a fairly high incidence of untoward reactions has occurred in the course of the administration of some of these emulsions, and the total amount of fat that can be administered intravenously appears to be restricted. This is suggested by progressive development of lipemia in patients receiving fat intravenously for more than $7-10$ days. It is likely that the ability of the tissues to metabolize lipid administered by the intravenous route is limited. This is probably so because lipid is normally not presented to the tissues as "free" fat, as is true when triglycerides are administered intravenously. Fat taken orally is absorbed—after digestion—into the intestinal mucosal cells as fatty acids and glycerol, wherein these constituents of the dietary fat are recombined to form triglyceride (so-called "neutral fat"), which is then combined with a small (0.5%) but important quantity of protein to form a lipoprotein, the **chylomicron**, which appears first in the lymphatic vessels in the abdominal lymphatics and later in the systemic blood. The chylomicrons are responsible for the turbidity in the serum—the so-called alimentary lipemia—that is observed following a meal. Clearing of the lipemic serum is accomplished by the action of an enzyme, lipoprotein lipase (LPL) (so-called "clearing factor"), produced at the capillary border in adipose tissue. The action of LPL is similar to that of pancreatic lipase, ie, to hydrolyze triglycerides into fatty acid and glycerol, which enter adipose tissue cells to be resynthesized into triglyceride for storage in the adipose tissue cells. It might be expected that triglyceride injected intravenously would be treated similarly except that the substrate for the action of LPL is not free triglyceride but only that in the form of lipoprotein, mainly the chylomicron. Intravenously administered fat is thus, in a sense, unphysiologic. It is therefore not surprising that it is metabolized with difficulty. The occurrence of a so-called "overloading syndrome," wherein fat accumulates in tissues as if it were a foreign body, requires discontinuance of the use of intravenous fat in the affected patient if serious damage to vital organs because of thesaurosis of fat is to be avoided. At present, an emulsion of fat suitable for intravenous administration is not commercially available in the

USA, but a recently produced soybean emulsion (Intralipid, a 20% fat emulsion) used widely abroad appears to be safe and to produce a minimum of the undesirable side-effects observed with the previously available emulsions intended for intravenous administration.

Protein Administration

To administer a source of protein when only the parenteral route is available, amino acid mixtures prepared by enzymatic or acid digestion of protein (usually casein or fibrin) may be used. These solutions in 5% concentration in dextrose are generally well tolerated if given at rates not exceeding 300 ml/hour. Amino acids are not lost into the urine in any significant amount and are utilized for protein synthesis provided adequate amounts of calories from carbohydrates and fat are simultaneously available. As noted above, when only intravenously administered solutions are used for nutritional purposes, it is extremely difficult to provide adequate calories. As a result, there may be poor utilization of the administered amino acids. Despite the disadvantages attending their use, it seems appropriate to recommend that at least when parenteral nutrition must be prolonged beyond a few days, 2 liters of a 5% solution of amino acids in dextrose be added to the daily regimen. Plasma or purified fractions of the plasma such as albumin, when given intravenously, are used in part for nutritional purposes, but their utilization is such that they may be considered as nutritionally uneconomical as contrasted with other sources of protein nitrogen such as amino acids. Consequently, these proteins should not be administered solely for nutritional purposes.

Infusions of Carbohydrate & Amino Acids

In the above discussion, the problems associated with attempts to nourish adequately a patient who cannot be given nutrients except by the intravenous route were emphasized. Particularly difficult is the situation where there exists a massive catabolism of body protein as described above. In the severely traumatized individual during the immediate posttraumatic period, the extensive protein catabolic response to stress appears not to be substantially affected by large infusions of carbohydrate; as a result, administration of amino acids does not seem to reverse or even equal the protein nitrogen losses.

Despite these problems, it has been shown that the intravenous infusion of a fat-free amino acid and glucose solution could support normal growth and development. Dudrick & others (see 1968 reference, p 173) reported a study of 30 patients with chronic complicated gastrointestinal disease nourished exclusively by intravenous feeding for 10–200 days. Positive nitrogen balance was achieved in all, and this was associated with healing of wounds, closure of fistulas, and gain in weight as well as increased strength and activity. Caloric intakes up to 3300 Cal/day and nitrogen intakes of 16–25 g/day were achieved. The average positive nitrogen balance was 4 g/day.

Hypertonic Basal Solution

The method used for total parenteral (intravenous) nutrition is based on the infusion of glucose for calories and a protein hydrolysate as a source of nitrogen to provide for synthesis of protein. The hypertonic basal solution can be prepared in the hospital pharmacy by mixing routinely available solutions of glucose and 5% protein (fibrin) hydrolysates.

A. Method of Dudrick & Others: One liter of solution providing approximately 1000 Cal and 6 g of nitrogen (equivalent to approximately 35 g protein) is prepared by combining 860 ml of 5% fibrin hydrolysate (Aminosol) in 5% glucose with 165 g of anhydrous dextrose USP. Sterilization must be accomplished by the use of a 0.22 μm membrane since a glucose solution of such hypertonicity would undergo intense caramelization (browning [Maillard] reaction) if autoclaved. This is the stock solution to which additional nutrients can be added. There are approximately 8 mEq of Na^+, 14 mEq of K^+, and traces of other mineral elements such as chloride, phosphate, magnesium, and calcium in the protein hydrolysate added. These values may vary slightly depending on the type of protein hydrolysate used (eg, fibrin or casein digests).

B. Alternative Method: An alternative method for preparing the basic stock solution consists of discarding 250 ml from a 1 liter bottle of 5% protein hydrolysate in 5% glucose and then, using strict aseptic precautions, adding 350 ml of 50% glucose. The resultant 1100 ml of solution provides approximately 5.25 g of nitrogen (equivalent to 25 g as protein), 212 g of glucose, 7 mEq of Na^+, and 13 mEq of K^+ when fibrin hydrolysate is used. The caloric value is slightly less than 1 Cal/ml.

Unless contraindicated, 50 mEq of NaCl and 40 mEq of KCl, using concentrated solutions of the electrolyte, should be added per liter of solution prepared by either procedure.

Vitamins

Fortification with vitamins is most conveniently accomplished by the addition (to only one bottle of the daily infusate) of 10 ml of a commercially available multivitamin preparation* of fat- and water-soluble vitamins. Magnesium (4–8 mEq/day) may also be provided as magnesium sulfate. Vitamins B_{12}, K, and folic acid may be necessary during prolonged intravenous alimentation. These may be given intramuscularly. If plasma analyses so suggest, calcium gluconate and potassium acid phosphate (KH_2PO_4) may also be supplied as necessary. Unless there has been a preexisting iron deficiency or extensive hemorrhage, or both, iron is not required. Transfusions of whole blood will supply iron, as will intramuscular administration of iron dextran injection (Imferon). Trace mineral elements such as zinc, copper, manganese, cobalt, and iodine may be added if total nutrition by intravenous injection is prolonged beyond 1 month. Alternatively, 1 unit of plasma twice weekly will serve also as a source

---

*M.V.I. (multi-vitamin infusion).

TABLE 13–3. Average composition of adult nutrient solution.

Water	2500–3000 ml
Protein hydrolysate (amino acids)	100–130 g
Nitrogen	12–18 g
Carbohydrate (dextrose)	525–625 g
Calories	2500–3000
Sodium	125–150 mEq
Potassium	75–120 mEq
Magnesium	4–8 mEq
Vitamin A	5000–10,000 USP units
Vitamin D	500–1000 USP units
Vitamin E	2.5–5 IU
Vitamin C	250–500 mg
Thiamine	25–50 mg
Riboflavin	5–10 mg
Pyridoxine	7.5–15 mg
Niacin	50–100 mg
Pantothenic acid	12.5–25 mg

Calcium and phosphorus are added to the solution as indicated. ¶ Iron is added to the solution, or given intramuscularly in depot form as iron dextran injection, or given as blood transfusion as indicated. ¶ Vitamin B_{12}, vitamin K, and folic acid are given intramuscularly or added for intravenous administration as indicated. ¶ Trace elements such as zinc, copper, manganese, cobalt, and iodine are added only after total intravenous therapy exceeds 1 month. Alternatively, 1 unit of plasma twice a week will provide required amounts of trace elements.

of trace elements. Table 13–3 summarizes the average nutrient composition of 2500–3000 ml of the solution prepared as described above for hyperalimentation in adults. Solutions intended for use in children requiring long-term nutrition exclusively by the intravenous route are prepared as for adults with only minor modifications. This subject is discussed further in Chapter 52.

Technic of Administration*

Administration of the solution described above requires continuous infusion over the 24-hour day. The injection is made into a large-caliber vessel such as the superior vena cava, preferably using an indwelling catheter threaded carefully and with aseptic technic into the superior vena cava by way of the subclavian vein. For newborn infants or those less than 4.5 kg (10 lb) in weight, the superior vena cava may be reached via the jugular vein. Initially, only the normal amounts of fluid are given (2500 ml/day in adults; 125 ml/kg in infants); the volume infused is then slowly increased over a period of several days as tolerated, with careful attention to avoidance of overhydration. Measurement of plasma electrolytes and blood urea nitrogen every

*See Chapter 52 for illustrations of these procedures.

other day and serum glucose weekly should serve as monitors of the safety of the infusion. Testing for sugar in urine specimens collected at 6-hour intervals during the infusion is also recommended.

Rate of Glucose Administration

The rate of glucose utilization is between 0.5 g/kg/hour in adults and 1.2 g/kg/hour in infants, the average being 0.9 g/kg/hour in an adult. These are the rates for normal individuals, but infusion rates may have to be lower in seriously ill patients, and periodic adjustment in rate of administration of the nutrient solution may be required.

Giving glucose intravenously at a rate which permits less than 2% excretion of glucose in the urine avoids the danger of osmotic diuresis, with resulting dehydration and electrolyte imbalance. The normal pancreas will increase its output of insulin in response to the continuing infusion of glucose. If a diabetic patient is being treated, appropriate doses of insulin may be given subcutaneously every 6 hours, or the total dose may be added to the intravenous fluid. Indeed, 5–25 units of crystalline insulin per 1000 Cal may be added routinely to the nutrient solution to improve utilization of glucose and promote nitrogen retention in elderly patients with evidence of some degree of intolerance to glucose or in patients with severe nutritional depletion.

Potassium & Sodium

In patients receiving hyperalimentation, potassium is usually required in larger amounts than are used for maintenance. Forty mEq of KCl per liter of infusate is a minimum dose; more is required if there are substantial gastrointestinal fluid losses or extensive burns, with careful attention to the prevention of hyperkalemia. Although 50 mEq of sodium per 1000 Cal is a satisfactory intake in these patients, reduction of intake or even total elimination of sodium may be necessary in those clinical states which predispose to retention of sodium.

Hypoalbuminemia

Significant hypoalbuminemia or anemia may require initial administration of albumin or whole blood.

Complications of Hyperalimentation

A. Septicemia: The problem of septicemia developing during intravenous hyperalimentation must be kept in mind. Solutions to be used for parenteral alimentation are nutritionally very favorable to the growth of infectious organisms. Several reports (see Curry & Quie reference, p 173) emphasize infection as a dangerous complication of hyperalimentation. The infectious agents include not only bacteria but—even more commonly—fungi such as *Candida albicans*. The incidence of septicemia is related both to the duration of hyperalimentation and to the time elapsing between changes of an indwelling catheter. At present, there does not appear to be any absolutely safe method to prevent these infections, particularly when the pathogen is a fungus. Every effort must be made to maintain aseptic conditions when giving parenteral alimentation. The use of external arteriovenous shunts for injection of the nutritional solution may be preferred to direct catheterization of a vein.

Amphotericin B (Fungizone) (1 μg/ml) is fungicidal for candida. A transient "amphotericin flush" of the system every 3 days has been recommended.

B. Metabolic Hazards: In addition to the hazards of infection, there are reports of a peculiar metabolic disturbance associated with intravenous hyperalimentation. Silvas & Paragas (see p 173) observed 3 severely malnourished patients who were given the hyperalimentation solution described above intravenously. Although the patients appeared to be doing well for the first few days after the infusion was begun, between the fourth and seventh days each developed muscular weakness and paresthesias; 2 progressed to convulsions and coma, and one died in coma after 5 days. The most significant and characteristic finding was a profound decline in serum phosphate to mean levels of less than 0.3 mg/100 ml. None of the patients showed evidences of hyperosmolarity, uremia, or ketoacidosis.

In experimental studies with animal models (dogs or rats), effects similar to those observed with the patients were produced by intravenous hyperalimentation. The effects were particularly severe in previously starved animals as compared with those entering the experiment without a prior period of undernutrition. Attempts to correct the significantly low serum phosphate levels by including phosphate in the infusions did not prevent the syndrome. Balance studies on one dog indicated that the fall in phosphate was not attributable to negative phosphate balance since the amount of phosphate excreted fell far short of accounting for the fall in serum phosphate. It was concluded that an extravascular shift of phosphate had occurred.

In any case, it seems certain from these studies that a depression of CNS activity can occur in humans as a result of intravenous hyperalimentation and that the syndrome can be reproduced in experimental animals, although the causes of these occasionally fatal symptoms have not yet been elucidated. A possibly important clue is the observation in the rat experiments that the animals most susceptible to this fatal syndrome were those having a chronic and continuing weight loss at the time hyperalimentation was instituted. Both the animals totally fasted for a week and those allowed to stabilize at a constant albeit subnormal weight—ie, who have had an opportunity to adjust to the suboptimal intake of calories—were relatively resistant to the development of the full-blown fatal syndrome. Obviously, the metabolic circumstances in the patients who may be selected for intravenous hyperalimentation resemble those of the chronically malnourished rats. Further studies may better define all of the abnormal metabolic parameters that predispose to the development of this serious

complication of intravenous hyperalimentation.

Glycolysis in red blood cells differs somewhat from the classic Embden-Meyerhof (E-M) pathway as it occurs in other tissues, by the ability of the erythrocyte to form significant quantities of 2,3-diphosphoglycerate (2,3-DPG) from 1,3-diphosphoglycerate (1,3-DPG), which is the usual major product of the oxidation of glyceraldehyde-3-phosphate in the E-M glycolytic pathway. The formation of 2,3-DPG from 1,3-DPG is catalyzed by phosphoglycerate 2,3-mutase.

An important function of 2,3-DPG in red cells is its ability to enhance the dissociability of oxyhemoglobin by decreasing the tendency of oxygen to bind to hemoglobin, an effect similar to that of CO_2 (the so-called Bohr effect), or of a decline in intracellular pH. Thus, the P-50 for oxyhemoglobin (ie, the oxygen tension at which hemoglobin is 50% saturated with oxygen) is lowered. This is often referred to as a shift of the oxyhemoglobin dissociation curve "to the right." An important physiologic function of red cell 2,3-DPG, therefore, is to improve the delivery of oxygen to the tissues, particularly in circumstances where low oxygen tension prevails. Hypophosphatemia reduces the red cell 2,3-DPG content and thus may be considered as impairing oxygenation of the tissues. This is certainly a serious additional hazard in hypotension, ischemia, reduction of circulating red cell mass as in anemia, or after extensive hemorrhage uncorrected by adequate transfusions. While an increase in the amount of phosphate infused is said not to affect the CNS depression described above as being occasionally associated with severe hypophosphatemia, nonetheless it will prevent a fall in erythrocyte 2,3-DPG.

TUBE FEEDING

Feeding by nasogastric tube may occasionally be necessary to prevent serious malnutrition, eg, in severe anoxia, coma, obstructive lesions of the esophagus, fractures of the jaw, and after severe burns.

When liquid formulas are used, very small polyethylene nasogastric tubes (eg, K-30) which may be left in place for many days are suitable. These tubes may even be used for supplemental feedings in patients who can ingest some of their meals in the usual manner (eg, burned patients who may be unable to eat adequate quantities of protein).

Formulas for Tube Feeding

In preparing formulas for tube feeding, it is usually necessary to avoid the use of simple sugars, such as dextrose, and too much fat, such as cream, since both tend to cause diarrhea in tube-fed patients. The preferred source of carbohydrate is a dextrinized starch such as Dexin or Dextri-Maltose. A simple formula for feeding by gastric tube is as follows:

Homogenized milk	2200 ml
Half-and-half (cream and milk)	600 ml
Eggs	6
Dextri-Maltose	7 tbsp

(In a total volume of 3000 ml, this mixture contains 120 g protein and 3000 Cal.)

Homogenized milk alone is often the simplest substance to use at the beginning of a tube feeding regimen. It contains 3.5 g of protein and about 70 Cal/100 ml.

Rate of Feeding

During the first few days after an operation, the initial rate of feeding should not exceed 50 ml/hour. Thereafter, the rate may be increased gradually in accordance with the patient's tolerance until a maximum of 150–200 ml every 2 hours is reached, usually about 1 week later. If at this time the patient is tolerating the feedings well, the homogenized milk may be fortified with 50 g of a powdered protein hydrolysate and 30 g of Dextri-Maltose or Dexin per liter. If this is well tolerated, the carbohydrate may be gradually increased over a 3-day period to 60 g/liter. This final formula contributes 160 g of protein and about 2500 Cal in 2400 ml. Vitamins may be added to the formula, using a concentrated solution similar in composition to that given on p 164.

The formulas and rates of administration described above may also be used for jejunostomy feedings.

Use of Medium-Chain Triglycerides

Fat introduced into the formula, while valuable as a concentrated source of additional calories, is often difficult for patients to digest and absorb. This circumstance tends to favor fermentative activity within the bowel, leading to diarrhea, a complication that severely limits the usefulness of a tubal nutrient. However, triglycerides containing fatty acids of medium-chain length (C_6–C_{10}) have proved to be useful clinically since the fatty acids formed after digestion of a medium-chain triglyceride can be readily absorbed. Furthermore, they are transported as free fatty acids (rather than as chylomicrons) directly to the liver via the portal venous blood. Indeed, there is evidence that medium-chain triglycerides can be absorbed with no intestinal intraluminal hydrolysis whatsoever.

Using medium-chain triglycerides in a tubal nutrient formula, more extensive absorption of fat is possible in the presence of shortened lengths of small intestine or where there is an abnormally rapid transit time. It can also be expected that the use of medium-chain triglycerides will have the advantage of reducing the bulk of the stools as well as minimizing the foul quality of steatorrheic stools.

The dose of medium-chain triglycerides, like all tubal nutrients, must be adjusted to tolerance. These lipid materials occur as oily liquids, in which form they are usually given. Flavored preparations are available,

although their content of lactose may limit their tolerance in patients with a shortened small intestine.

A major use for formulas fortified with medium-chain triglycerides is in patients with short bowel syndrome or with internal or external fistulas. Illustrative of the benefit to be expected from the use of medium-chain triglycerides is the observation on a patient with total colectomy and ileostomy who after 70 g of ordinary triglyceride retained only 25% of the ingested fat, whereas 53.5% was retained using medium-chain triglyceride (see Morgan & others reference, p 173).

Concentrated Tube Feeding

A more concentrated tube feeding mixture can be used with the aid of a pump to maintain the flow of the mixture. A sample formula which utilizes commercially available puréed infant foods is as follows:

	Protein (g)	Calories
3½ oz strained beef	14.6	103
4½ oz beets	1.5	51
3 raw eggs	18.0	225
Homogenized milk (640 ml)	23.3	466
Totals	57.4	845

Other meats and vegetables can be used to vary the formula.

The commercial availability of amino acid preparations, usually as powdered hydrolysates of natural proteins but occasionally as mixtures of synthetic amino acids, has made it possible to construct "elemental diets" made up of amino acids as a source of protein, with the addition of sugars, minerals, and vitamins (see Stephens & Randall reference, p 173). Such an elemental mixture contains no fats, proteins, or higher peptides which require digestion before they can be absorbed. These dietary mixtures are of particular usefulness in nutritional balance studies. Stimulation of exogenous secretion by the pancreas is much reduced by the absence of lipid. There is also a diminution of enteric secretion. This reduces drainage from fistulas, and the absence of residue obviously reduces the volume of stools.

However, because a major disadvantage in using these elemental diets is their considerable hypertonicity, they should be given to patients very gradually and adequate water must be provided, particularly when normal thirst mechanisms are impaired. Although nitrogen is provided for protein synthesis from the constituent amino acids, the amounts may be inadequate when the metabolic demands are excessive, as after extensive trauma or stress or when there are large external losses of protein.

These elemental dietary mixtures are difficult to administer for prolonged periods unless given by tube because of their unpalatability. Nevertheless, they may be very useful adjuncts to the treatment of chronic pancreatic disease or of severe ulcerative colitis. While

TABLE 13–4. Types of surgical diets.

Diet	Indications
Regular or house	Normal maintenance.
High-protein, high-caloric, high-vitamin	Malnutrition; increased nutritional requirements.
Clear liquid Full liquid Surgical soft	Depressed or disturbed gastrointestinal function, eg, postoperatively.
Postgastrectomy	After gastric resection or gastroenterostomy.
Peptic ulcer regimens	Peptic ulcer.
Low-fat	Biliary tract disease.
Minimal residue	Colon preparation, rectal surgery, colitis.
Low-sodium	Cardiac disease, eg, congestive failure; edema.
Gastric tube feeding	Comatose, uncooperative, malnourished, or severely anorexic patients; markedly increased nutritional demands, eg, burns; gastrostomy.
Jejunostomy feeding	Jejunostomy.

the disadvantages of prolonged intravenous infusions are avoided, some gastrointestinal function is obviously required.

Precautions in Tube Feedings

(1) If given rapidly by gravity drip or by injection into the gastric tube, the formula should first be warmed to body temperature.

(2) Do not give over 200 ml at a time.

(3) Use special care to prevent aspiration in unconscious patients.

(4) Supply sufficient water in addition to the formula to permit excretion of nitrogenous end products. This is particularly important if the formula is high in protein.

(5) When stopping or starting a feeding, or whenever the question of gastric retention arises, aspirate the gastric tube and wash it out with water.

(6) Avoid constipation and fecal impaction in debilitated patients—if necessary, by introducing 30 ml of milk of magnesia into the tube.

THE NORMAL DIET

Parenteral and tube feedings should be discontinued as soon as possible in favor of a full normal diet taken by mouth. Foods should be palatable and attractively prepared as a stimulus to appetite. The physician should not overlook his responsibilities in this matter since a properly compounded nutritional prescription can be just as important to his patient's welfare as the drugs he may order.

TABLE 13–5. Daily allowance of certain foods according to requirements for sodium restriction.

Food Substance	2400–4500 mg Sodium	1000 mg Sodium	500 mg Sodium	250 mg Sodium
Milk	1 pint	1 pint	1 pint	Low-sodium ad lib.
Egg	One	One	One	One
Salt-free meat, fish, poultry	Ad lib.	6 oz	5 oz	5 oz
Bread	Ad lib.	Two slices plus low-sodium bread ad lib.	Low-sodium bread ad lib.	Low-sodium bread ad lib.
Butter, margarine, mayonnaise	Ad lib.	Two tsp regular; sweet ad lib.	Sweet ad lib.	Sweet ad lib.
Cream	Ad lib.	2 oz	2 oz	2 oz
Vegetables	Ad lib.	Low-sodium ad lib.	Low-sodium ad lib.	Low-sodium ad lib.
Fruits and juices	Ad lib.	Ad lib.	Ad lib.	Ad lib.
Desserts	One serving: cake, gelatin, ice cream, pie, pudding, sherbet	Special low-sodium only.	Special low-sodium only.	Special low-sodium only.
Cereals and starches	Ad lib.	Low-sodium only.	Low-sodium only.	Low-sodium only.

Daily Caloric Intake

The daily diet for the convalescent adult patient should contain 3000–5000 Cal and 100–150 g of protein. It is not sufficient merely to place these nutrients on a tray within the patient's reach; care must be taken to make certain that the entire nutritional prescription is actually consumed.

It is often difficult for surgical patients to eat large amounts of high-protein foods such as muscle meats. Intermittent feedings may have to be given, but must be carefully spaced so as not to spoil the patient's appetite for regular meals. Fruit juices and broths are of little value as supplementary nutrients because they contribute practically nothing toward remedying protein and caloric deficits, the major dietary faults in need of correction; in fact, these liquid supplements may actually dull the appetite and thus indirectly impair nutrition.

Supplementary Drink

A simple but useful supplementary drink may be prepared by stirring 50 g of skimmed milk powder into 200 ml of water. This supplies 17 g of protein and 26 g of carbohydrate—more than is available in 1 pint of milk but in only half the volume. Six glasses will supply over 100 g of protein of excellent nutritional quality. Other valuable protein supplements are ice cream, cottage cheese, and eggs.

The "Basic" Foods

As a guide to the formulation of an adequate diet, various foods have been arranged into 4 "basic" groups each of which makes a major contribution to the diet. To secure an adequate diet, some foods from each of the 4 groups should be taken each day as follows:

A. Milk Group: (Cheese, ice cream, and other foods derived from milk can supply part of the milk requirement.)

1. **Children**—3 or more 8 oz glasses of milk. (Smaller servings for some children under age 9.)

2. **Teen-agers**—4 or more glasses.

3. **Adults**—2 or more glasses.

B. Meat Group: Two or more servings of meats, fish, poultry, eggs, or cheese, with dry beans, peas, nuts as alternates.

C. Vegetables and Fruits Group: Four or more servings, including dark green or yellow vegetables; citrus fruits or tomatoes.

D. Bread and Cereal Group: Four or more servings. (One serving = 1 slice enriched or whole grain bread, ¾ cup enriched or whole grain dry cereal, ½ cup cooked enriched or whole grain cereal.)

The basic diet outlined above will provide approximately 1200 Cal. Additional calories may be derived from other foods as desired or by increasing the quantity of servings of the listed foods.

●　　●　　●

General References

Coleman W: Diet in typhoid fever. JAMA 53:1145, 1909.

Coleman W, Barr DP, DuBois EF: Clinical calorimetry, XXX. Metabolism in erysipelas. Arch Int Med 29:567, 1922.

Coleman W, DuBois EF: Clinical calorimetry, VII. Calorimetric observations on the metabolism of typhoid patients with and without food. Arch Int Med 15:887, 1915.

Cowan G Jr, Scheetz W (editors): *Intravenous Hyperalimentation.* Lea & Febiger, 1972.

Curry CR, Quie PG: Fungal septicemia in patients receiving parenteral hyperalimentation. New England J Med 285:1221, 1971.

Cuthbertson DP: *Minutes of the Fifth Conference on Metabolic Aspects of Bone and Wound Healing.* Page 43. Josiah Macy Foundation (New York), 1943.

Cuthbertson DP: Observations on the disturbance of metabolism produced by injury to the limbs. Quart J Med 1:233, 1932.

Dudrick SJ & others: Long term total parenteral nutrition with growth, development and positive nitrogen balance. Surgery 64:132, 1968.

Dudrick SJ & others: The use of carbohydrates and proteolysates for long-term parenteral feeding. Page 301 in:

Body Fluid Replacement in the Surgical Patient. Fox CL Jr, Nahas GG (editors). Grune & Stratton, 1970.

Moore FD: *Metabolic Care of the Surgical Patient.* Saunders, 1959.

Morgan A, Filler RM, Moore FD: Surgical nutrition. M Clin North America 54:1367, 1970.

National Academy of Sciences-National Research Council: *Recommended Daily Dietary Allowances,* rev ed. Publication No. 1694, NAS-NRC, 1968.

Pollack H, Halpern SL: *Therapeutic Nutrition.* Publication 234, National Research Council, 1952.

Reiss E, Pearson E, Artz CP: The metabolic response to burns. J Clin Invest 35:62, 1956.

Shaffer PA, Coleman W: Protein metabolism in typhoid fever. Arch Int Med 4:538, 1909.

Silvas SE, Paragas PV Jr: Fatal hyperalimentation syndrome: Animal studies. J Lab Clin Med 78:918, 1971.

Stephens RV, Randall HT: Use of a concentrated, balanced, liquid elemental diet for nutritional management of catabolic states. Ann Surg 170:642, 1969.

Williams SR: *Nutrition and Diet Therapy.* Mosby, 1969.

14 . . .

Anesthesiology

Neri P. Guadagni, MD

Every surgeon should have a thorough knowledge of the regional anesthetic procedures he performs himself but need not know the details and technicalities of general anesthesia conducted by a physician specialist in that field. The surgeon must understand the potentials, limitations, and hazards of all anesthetic technics and should be able to recognize good anesthesia or what is as good as a particular clinical situation permits. This chapter offers principles and guidelines for the conduct of anesthetic procedures performed by the surgeon and discusses basic concepts of the management of anesthetic procedures performed by others. The emphasis accorded to various aspects is not proportionate to their importance in anesthesiology as a branch of medical science.

PURPOSES OF ANESTHESIA

Most surgical procedures cause a degree of pain or discomfort that neither the patient nor modern society will accept. Advances in methods of relieving pain and sustaining life during surgery now embody an art and science which has broadened to a discipline concerned with more than relief of pain. It serves both patient and surgeon, offering the patient freedom from pain during surgery with or without awareness and with maximum safety and provides the surgeon with a "quiet field," often in otherwise inaccessible areas, for as long as required. The methods used to achieve these goals vary with the age, size, personality, and physical condition of the patient and with the location, duration, and technical intricacies of the operation. The same technics and skills essential to these goals also have application in the emergency room, recovery room, and the intensive care ward. In the form of "nerve blocks," they have both diagnostic and therapeutic uses.

ANESTHESIA BY THE SURGEON

Administration of anesthesia by the operating surgeon is a practical and safe expedient limited only by his knowledge and experience and by the magni-

tude of the surgical or anesthetic procedure. The limitations are obvious if either surgery or anesthesia requires the undivided attention of one person. General anesthesia, even when used for minor surgery, requires continuous attention and monitoring. No surgeon should attempt to give general anesthesia and also perform the surgery except in unavoidable emergency circumstances. He may have to assume the responsibility for anesthetic management when administered by a technician such as a nurse anesthetist who is not supervised by a qualified physician. In such a situation, the use of technicians of proved skill and reliability is of paramount importance, but the surgeon should have enough personal experience with general anesthesia to be able to help when necessary. The same holds true for regional anesthesia administered by the operating surgeon but monitored by a technician during the procedure.

Regional anesthesia performed by the surgeon is adequate for many procedures. It is particularly indicated for procedures performed on ambulatory patients, and is also useful for many operations done on hospitalized patients. A partial list of these operations includes surface surgery such as plastic procedures, biopsies, excision of moles and cysts, hernia repairs, many eye, ear, nose, and throat operations, and endoscopies of the respiratory, urinary, and gastrointestinal tracts.

Tissue infiltration of a small amount of local anesthetic for a minor procedure such as suturing a wound carries minimal risks. The risks increase with the amount of drug used and the extent of the procedure. The safety and practicality of regional anesthesia depend on the proper selection and preparation of the patient, the knowledge and skill of the surgeon, and his ability to diagnose and treat the complications of anesthesia as they arise.

SELECTION OF PATIENT

In general, young or emotionally unstable patients are poor candidates for regional anesthesia. However, hand lacerations can be sutured and wrist fractures can be manipulated following a brachial plexus block achieved with a fine needle by the axillary approach in a mildly sedated preschool child, whereas it is unreasonable to expect an older child to remain motionless under surgical drapes during a longer procedure done with regional anesthesia. Common sense and rapport with the child offer the best guidelines for the decision to use regional anesthesia. Emotionally unstable adults usually demand general anesthesia, and experienced surgeons seldom try to talk them out of it except for very minor operations.

The patient with severe cardiac or pulmonary disease presents a special problem that calls for sound clinical judgment. Such patients face a higher risk from general anesthesia than from regional anesthesia if the surgery is minor or limited to a small field or if it is of brief duration (eg, cataract extraction). If the procedure is extensive or prolonged, general anesthesia may be less hazardous. The systemic toxicity of local anesthetics used in large amounts becomes a factor, and the anxiety and discomfort of the patient during the administration of the local anesthetic and during surgery increase epinephrine release, oxygen consumption, and carbon dioxide production, imposing a greater burden on a decompensating cardiorespiratory system than a well-conducted general anesthetic procedure. Obvious exceptions include situations such as the amputation of a gangrenous leg using low spinal anesthesia which requires a simple injection of a small amount of drug and causes little discomfort.

PREPARATION OF THE PATIENT

The well-informed patient with whom the surgeon has established good rapport is a calmer, more cooperative subject for regional anesthesia. Anxiety can be reduced by sedatives such as barbiturates, which have the added advantage of reducing the incidence of convulsions caused by local anesthetics. However, if the barbiturate dose is excessive or if the patient is particularly susceptible, he may become confused or excited by painful stimuli and exhibit unpredictable and unmanageable behavior. Cautious dosage and the addition of a small amount of a narcotic usually prevent these problems and produce a mild euphoria which most patients find agreeable. Increments can be administered intravenously to achieve the desired effect before and during the procedure. Barbiturates are contraindicated if the patient is confused or experiencing pain. They increase the confusion and reduce pain tolerance. Tables 14–2 and 14–3 list some of the drugs and dosages used for premedication in adults and children. Table 14–4 offers a guide to which drugs should be used with various types of anesthetics.

The patient's stomach should be empty. During regional anesthetic procedures on a conscious patient in good physical condition, vomiting is not a serious matter; if the patient is debilitated or heavily sedated, vomitus may be aspirated into the lungs with disastrous results.

LOCAL ANESTHETIC AGENTS

Local anesthetic agents block the transmission of nerve impulses because the segment of a nerve axon exposed to the drug becomes incapable of generating the necessary action potential. The exact mechanism is not known, but it is proposed that these drugs act by altering the permeability of the cell membrane to the passage of ions, thus stabilizing the resting potential.

Susceptibility of individual nerve fibers is inversely proportionate to the cross-sectional diameter of the fibers: the smaller the fiber, the more susceptible it is to local anesthetics. Therefore, during regional anesthesia, perception of light touch, pain, and temperature and vasomotor control are abolished sooner and with a lesser concentration of the agent than are the perception of pressure or the function of motor nerves to striated muscles.

Many chemical substances are capable of interrupting nerve conduction, but only those that are completely reversible, nonirritating, and cause minimal systemic toxicity are used clinically. Rapidity of onset, predictability of duration, and ease of sterilization are other desirable properties.

Table 14–1 summarizes the uses and doses of the commonly used local anesthetics.

When absorbed into the systemic circulation, all local anesthetics have dose-related side-effects. All are capable of stimulating the CNS. At the medullary level, this may cause bradycardia, hypertension, and respiratory stimulation. At higher levels, it may produce anxiety, excitement, and convulsions. This stimulation resembles grand mal seizures in that it is followed by a period of depression that may include hypotension, loss of vasomotor control, respiratory depression, and coma. This indirect cardiovascular depression may be accentuated by a direct vasodilatory action and a direct myocardial depressant action. The latter is quinidine-like in its manifestations and is a property of local anesthetics which is used in the treatment of certain arrhythmias. Lidocaine (Xylocaine) is the recommended agent for this purpose.

The oldest local anesthetic, cocaine, has properties not shared by the others. The long-acting CNS stimulation that occurs produces a feeling of euphoria that can lead to addiction. Cocaine also possesses norepinephrine-like effects such as local vasoconstriction, pupillary dilatation, and potentiation of injected sympathomimetics. Its local vasoconstriction and excellent topical effectiveness make it ideal for "shrinking" and anesthetizing the mucosa of the nasal passages. Cocaine is not stable at the temperatures required for autoclaving, which is a minor disadvantage since it is only used as a topical agent.

TABLE 14−1. **Drugs used for local anesthesia.***

	Cocaine	Procaine (Novocain, Neocaine)	Tetracaine (Pontocaine)	Lidocaine (Xylocaine)	Dibucaine (Nupercaine)	Mepivicaine (Carbocaine)
Potency (compared to procaine)	3	1	10	2−3	15	1.5−2
Toxicity (compared to procaine)	4	1	10	1−1.5	10−15	1−1.5
Stability at sterilizing temperature	Unstable	Stable	Stable	Stable	Stable	Stable
Total maximum dose	100−200 mg	1 g	50−100 mg	500 mg	35 mg	500 mg
Topical						
Concentration	Eye, 1%; other, 4−10%	Not effective	Eye, 0.5%; other, 1−2%	Eye, 0.5%; other, 4%	Eye, 0.1%; other, 0.5−2%	Eye, 0.5%; other, 1−2%
Onset of action	Immediate	. . .	10−20 minutes	3−5 minutes	8−15 minutes	10−20 minutes
Duration	30−60 minutes	. . .	1−2 hours	30−60 minutes	2−3 hours	1−2 hours
Infiltration						
Concentration	. . .	0.25−1%	0.05−0.1%	0.5−1%	. . .	0.5%
Onset of action	. . .	5−15 minutes	10−20 minutes	3−5 minutes	. . .	5−10 minutes
Duration	. . .	45−60 minutes	1½−3 hours	30−60 minutes	. . .	1¼−2½ hours
Nerve block and epidural						
Concentration	. . .	1−2%	0.1−0.2%	1−2%	. . .	1−2%
Onset of action	. . . ·	5−15 minutes	10−20 minutes	5−10 minutes	. . .	5−10 minutes
Duration	. . .	45−60 minutes	1½−3 hours	1−1½ hours	. . .	1¼−2½ hours
Subarachnoid						
Concentration	. . .	3−5%	0.1−0.5%	5%	0.06−0.25%	. . .
Dose	. . .	50−200 mg	5−20 mg	40−100 mg	2.5−13 mg	. . .
Onset of action	. . .	3−5 minutes	5−10 minutes	1−3 minutes	7−15 minutes	. . .
Duration	. . .	45−60 minutes	1½−2 hours	1−1½ hours	2−3 hours	. . .

*Addition of vasopressor prolongs durations by 25−50% but not used topically.

REGIONAL ANESTHESIA TECHNICS

Pharmacologic interruption of nerve conduction is known as regional anesthesia, local anesthesia, or conduction anesthesia. The technics used to apply the drugs to the nerves include topical, infiltration, nerve and plexus blocks, and subarachnoid and epidural spinal anesthesia.

TOPICAL ANESTHESIA

Topical anesthesia is that achieved by absorption of the agent through the surface of an intact membrane. Skin is an effective barrier to such absorption, but the conjunctivas of the eye and the mucosa of the mouth, nose, throat, respiratory tract, urethra, and urinary bladder can be rendered insensitive by this method.

All local anesthetics are not equally effective when used topically. The agents, dosages, and concentrations are given in Table 14−1. Systemic absorption leading to toxic blood concentrations may be very rapid, particularly if the solution is swallowed. Application to the surface to be anesthetized can be done by spraying, gargling, application of soaked pledgets or packs, or direct instillation. When expertly

performed, topical anesthesia is ideal for bronchoscopy and laryngoscopy.

LOCAL INFILTRATION

Local infiltration, with a hypodermic needle, of tissues to be incised or of tissues surrounding an operative site (field block) requires little description or discussion. The need for sterility of solution and equipment is obvious. Dilute solutions yield satisfactory results because fine nerve fibers are the targets.

The hazards of systemic toxicity from overdosage must be kept in mind when large areas are anesthetized. This is best done by calculating in advance the number of milligrams of drug in the volume of solution that may be required and keeping to a limit below the toxic dose. Infiltration of tissues that are inflamed or are close to an inflamed area is contraindicated. Such injections lower local tissue resistance to infection, may result in rapid systemic absorption because of the increased vascularity of inflamed tissues, and may also be ineffective if the local tissue pH is low enough to reduce the anesthetic agent's ionic dissociation which is essential for anesthetic activity.

NERVE & PLEXUS BLOCKS

Most nerves of the body are accessible for blocking by the surgeon who is familiar with the anatomy of nerve distribution, the relation of nerves to surface or palpable landmarks, the tissue compartments and fascial planes that influence the spread of anesthetic solutions, and the surrounding structures that might be traumatized by the needle. The surgeon must also be aware of the possible complications. He must always aspirate before injecting to avoid intravascular injection. The need for sterility is again emphasized.

Figs 14–1 to 14–8 illustrate some common nerve blocks that are easily mastered.

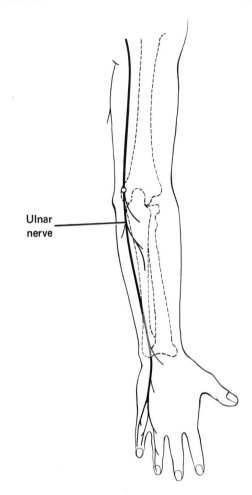

FIG 14–2. Ulnar nerve block at elbow.

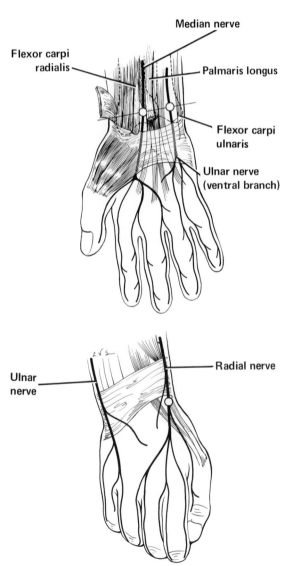

FIG 14–1. Nerve blocks at wrist. *Above:* Median and ulnar nerve block. *Below:* Radial nerve block.

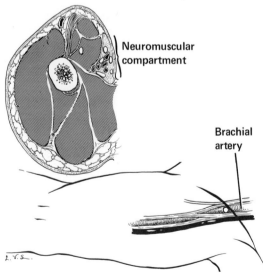

FIG 14–3. Brachial plexus block in axilla. *Above:* Cross-section of the arm at the axilla. *Below:* Surface landmarks for axillary block.

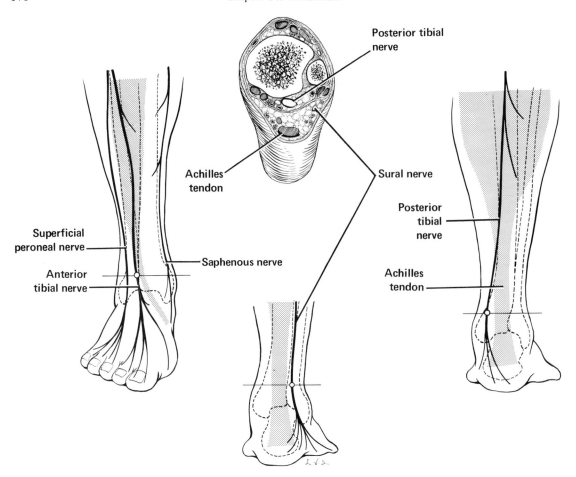

FIG 14—4. Nerve blocks at ankle. *Left:* Anterior tibial nerve block. *Right:* Posterior tibial nerve block. *Center, above:* Cross-section showing relationship of nerves to skin and bone. *Center, below:* Sural nerve block.

REGIONAL ANESTHESIA BY THE INTRAVENOUS METHOD

This technic has gained some popularity in recent years. It is accomplished by the intravenous injection of a dilute solution of a local anesthetic into the vein of an extremity kept ischemic by a tourniquet. It is particularly useful for the closed reduction of fractures.

A pneumatic tourniquet (eg, blood pressure cuff) is applied to the arm or thigh of the extremity to be anesthetized but left uninflated. A vein in the distal portion of the limb is cannulated, preferably with a pliable plastic needle. The limb is then elevated and drained of blood with the aid of an elastic bandage wrapped from distal to proximal. The tourniquet is then inflated rapidly to a pressure above systolic and kept inflated. Thirty to 50 ml of 0.5% lidocaine (Xylocaine) are then instilled into the vein. Excellent anesthesia below the tourniquet is achieved immediately and lasts 30–60 minutes.

After the procedure, the tourniquet is deflated momentarily and then reinflated. This is done 3 or 4 times at intervals of a few minutes so that the anesthetic is released intermittently and in small quantities into the systemic circulation. Sudden total release of the tourniquet may result in toxic manifestations and immediate disappearance of anesthesia. Anyone using this technic must be prepared to cope with these problems.

SPINAL ANESTHESIA ADMINISTERED BY THE SURGEON

In some communities and hospitals, spinal anesthesia by the subarachnoid or epidural method is administered by the surgeon, who then delegates the monitoring of the patient's condition to a technician while he operates. Where this is the accepted practice, the surgeon should have the same mastery of the entire management of spinal anesthesia as any physician who specializes in anesthesia. This subject is discussed more fully later in this chapter.

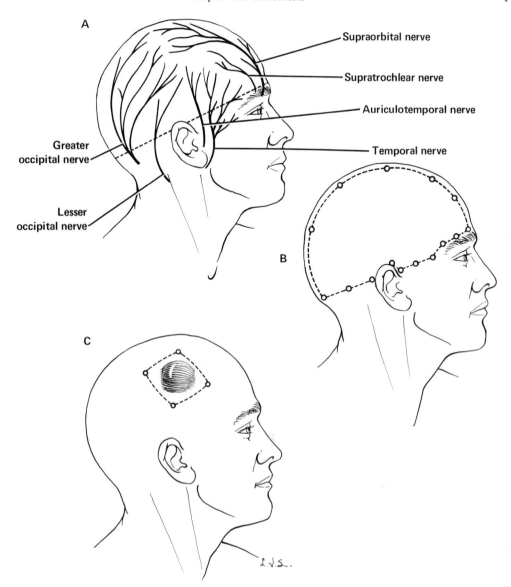

FIG 14–5. *A:* Sensory nerves of scalp. Dotted line shows sites of injection. *B:* Field block of scalp. *C:* Field block for excision of scalp lesion.

ADVERSE REACTIONS TO LOCAL ANESTHETICS

Clinical Manifestations

Allergic reactions to local anesthetics are rare. Vasovagal syncope may occur when the patient is very apprehensive or imaginative. Tachycardia and palpitations may be caused by the sympathomimetic vasoconstrictors added to the anesthetic solution.

Overdosage toxicity is the most serious and frequent adverse reaction to the local anesthetics. Table 14–1 gives the recommended maximum dosage for each of the commonly used agents when injected into tissues or used topically. Ten to 20% of this amount can produce overdosage symptoms if injected intravenously. The amount employed for dental anesthesia, suturing of minor lacerations, and most biopsies is usually less than the intravenously dangerous dose.

Overdosage toxicity is manifested by CNS stimulation followed by CNS and cardiovascular depression. The latter may appear without prior CNS stimulation. Excitement, apprehension, and nausea are the first symptoms, but they may be masked by sedative premedication. They may be accompanied by cardiovascular and respiratory changes. In most cases, the physician is first alerted by minor twitches of the muscles around the mouth and eyes. These spread and progress to full generalized convulsions whose duration varies with the amount of drug absorbed and the continuing

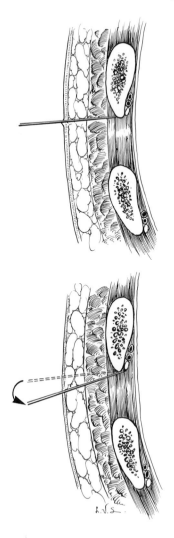

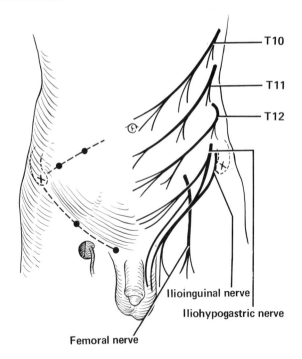

FIG 14—7. Nerves and sites for inguinal nerve block.

FIG 14—6. Intercostal nerve block. *Top:* Needle locating lower edge of rib. *Bottom:* Needle under edge of rib for injection of anesthetic agent.

absorption. A period of depression ensues which is characterized by a loss of consciousness, at times to the point of areflexia, coma, and a shock-like state. During the convulsive phase, the coordinated, rhythmic pattern of contraction and relaxation of the muscles of respiration is disrupted by random uncoordinated spasmodic contractions. If the abdominal muscles contract simultaneously with the diaphragm or with the adduction of the vocal cords, the increased intra-abdominal pressure causes evacuation of the bladder and rectum. Pulmonary ventilation ceases or is reduced, and oxygen consumption is increased. It is the resulting hypoxia and not the neuronal discharges nor the muscular movements that constitutes the threat to life. If the patient progresses to the stage of depression, this hypoxia predisposes to a more profound CNS and cardiovascular depression.

Prevention of Local Anesthetic Overdosage

Premedication with barbiturates or diazepam (Valium) offers some protection from convulsions (Table 14—2).

The ideal dosage of local anesthetics is the smallest amount of drug in the most dilute solution that will provide adequate anesthesia. The total maximum doses shown in Table 14—1 represent average safe limits. Obviously, the total safe dose for a big, young, healthy patient is not the same as for a small, elderly, and debilitated patient. The site of injection or application must also influence the calculation of a maximum single dose. Very rapid systemic absorption must be expected from highly vascularized tissues or from the stomach, which often receives much of the anesthetic used topically in the mouth, throat, and larynx unless the patient is encouraged to spit it out.

The addition of epinephrine to a resultant concentration of 1:200,000 in the anesthetic solution is indicated whenever near toxic amounts are injected. This will produce a local vasoconstriction that slows the rate of absorption, preventing systemic toxic levels of the agent and prolonging the anesthetic effect. However, the cardiac effects of epinephrine must be kept in mind if the patient has increased cardiac irritability due to other medications or to disease.

Treatment of Local Anesthetic Overdosage

A. Oxygen and Assisted Respiration: Treatment must be initiated with the first sign of overdosage reaction. Oxygen by mask may be all that is necessary since it supplies adequate alveolar oxygen in the presence of reduced ventilation. Assisted respiration by

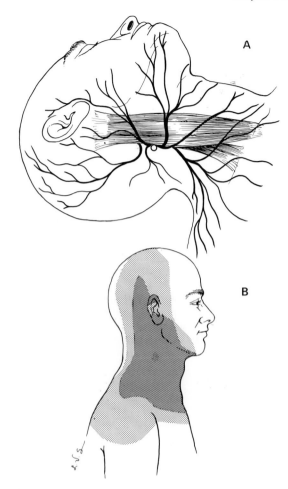

FIG 14—8. *A:* Site of injection for superficial cervical block. *B:* Total (dark area) and partial (light area) anesthesia after block due to overlapping innervation by other nerves.

positive pressure is seldom necessary if oxygen is given promptly, but it may be lifesaving if oxygen is not immediately available. If there is evidence of hypoxia (eg, cyanosis), it is better to perform artificial ventilation with a bag and mask or by means of mouth to mask or mouth-to-mouth breathing than to leave the patient to obtain oxygen equipment. Hypoxia can be prevented or treated by good pulmonary ventilation with air. The addition of oxygen is desirable but not essential.

B. Drugs: Intravenous barbiturates can control or terminate convulsions by a central action. Very small doses (eg, 25—50 mg of thiopental or pentobarbital) are sufficient. Criticism of their use is well deserved if oxygen therapy or artificial ventilation is delayed while the barbiturates are obtained, drawn into a syringe, and injected into a vein. Moreover, barbiturates, particularly in too large doses, add further depression to the postconvulsion depression. Other CNS depressants can be used to control convulsions, but all have the

same efficacy and hazards as the barbiturates.

Muscle relaxants such as succinylcholine can stop the gross muscular contractions, although their neurogenic cause persists. They do not add to the postconvulsion depression but should be used only by physicians who have the experience and equipment to perform artificial respiration.

Convulsions caused by local anesthetic overdosage can be managed with ease and safety by ensuring ventilation with or without drugs. Indecision, panic, and overtreatment are the real hazards.

C. Antishock Measures: The depression or shock stage requires symptomatic treatment. Hypoxia must be prevented. The Trendelenburg position or elevation of the legs seems beneficial. The value of vasopressors is not firmly established. (See Chapter 16 for a full discussion of shock and its treatment.)

ANESTHESIA BY THE ANESTHESIOLOGIST*

The remainder of this chapter will deal with the principles and practices of safe anesthesia conducted by anesthesiologists. It is not meant to instruct anyone in how to administer an anesthetic but only as background material for the surgeon's understanding of what transpires "on the other side of the ether screen."

The patient should be visited by the anesthesiologist before the date of surgery. In most instances, this is done the day preceding the day of operation. Whenever possible, the surgeon should consult with the anesthesiologist several days before the operation if he anticipates any problem related to anesthesia; better preparation of the patient and fewer last-minute cancellations can be achieved in this way. Any discussion of anesthesia between the surgeon and the patient should avoid committing the anesthesiologist to any particular agent or technic until he has been consulted or has seen the patient. This does not prevent the surgeon from listening to the patient's views concerning anesthesia and discussing with him "what anesthetic technics are usually used in similar cases" while at the same time stressing that every patient must be individually evaluated by whoever administers the anesthetic. The best rapport between the patient and his physicians occurs when the patient senses an agreement of opinion and mutual confidence between the surgeon, the anesthesiologist, and any other consultant. Faced by this united front, doubts and reluctance usually disappear.

---

*A person administering an anesthetic is an anesthetist. In the USA the physician anesthetist is called an anesthesiologist.

THE PREANESTHETIC VISIT

The preanesthetic visit by the anesthesiologist has several purposes. The patient gets to know the anesthesiologist, learns what to expect and how he can cooperate, can ask questions about anesthesia, and can have misconceptions corrected. The anesthesiologist gets to know the patient, evaluates his condition, institutes treatments, and plans the anesthetic management.

It is useful to review the patient's hospital record before the visit. This review may duplicate much of the information obtainable directly from the patient but may uncover details that the patient has forgotten or of which he is unaware. The anesthesiologist then obtains a history and does a physical examination (usually limiting himself to information relevant to anesthetic management), and discusses the anesthetic with the patient. The thoroughness of the chart review, the history, and the physical examination varies with the condition of the patient. It can be performed in a few minutes if the patient is a young healthy person facing a minor elective procedure. The most important inquiries concern previous anesthetic experiences, past or chronic illnesses, habits such as smoking or alcohol consumption, drugs used, allergies and sensitivities, and extent of physical activity. Previous anesthetics that posed technical difficulties and undesirable drug responses or complications should suggest using different agents and methods.

A history of myocardial infarction in the last 6 months is an indication for postponement of elective surgery. Asthma, hay fever, and other allergic conditions, neurologic disease, and a history of productive cough all influence the choice of anesthetic management. Heavy cigarette smoking should alert the anesthesiologist to expect a very active cough reflex. Barbiturate habituation or narcotic addiction suggests tolerance to these agents. Chronically used medications such as corticosteroids, insulin, reserpine, digitalis, quinidine, neostigmine, nitroglycerin, anticoagulants, and diuretics all have implications for anesthetic management. The underlying conditions for which they are used (eg, cardiac decompensation, myasthenia gravis), their continued need during surgery (eg, insulin, cortisone), their side-effects (eg, potassium depletion with certain diuretics), or their direct effects (eg, increased bleeding with anticoagulants) may influence the selection of agents and technics. Lastly, the patient's limit of physical activity is a remarkably good indication of the ability of his cardiorespiratory system to withstand the stresses of an anesthetic. The patient should be asked about his or her ability to do housework, climb stairs, play golf or tennis, etc to assess the general physical status.

The physical examination is directed toward and can be limited to finding variations and anomalies that have implications related to anesthetic management. Signs of diseases of the circulatory or respiratory system are most important, but certain minor findings have particular interest for the anesthesiologist. Bad teeth and delicate dental prostheses should be noted, and the patient should be warned that they may be damaged in spite of all precautions during general anesthesia. Conditions that might lead to technical problems of airway maintenance are looked for. The patient with inspiratory stridor should be told that he will undergo endotracheal intubation under local anesthesia before he can be put to sleep safely. The site of injection for regional anesthesia is examined for anatomic deformities or signs of infection.

A complete urinalysis and hemoglobin or hematocrit determination are the usual preanesthetic laboratory requirements. The preoperative examination by the anesthesiologist may turn up indications for chest x-rays, serum electrolyte determinations, blood volume determinations, ECGs, and other tests that were not necessary for the surgical diagnosis but whose findings influence anesthetic management, suggest pre- or postanesthetic therapy, or simply establish baselines. Simple bedside tests to determine the status of the cardiac or respiratory systems include pulse rate changes with minor exercise, analysis of arterial blood for P_{O_2}, P_{CO_2}, and pH, and measurements of respiratory rates, tidal volume, vital capacity, and forced expiratory volume during 1 second.

PREPARATION OF THE PATIENT FOR ANESTHESIA

The patient should be in the best physical condition possible within the limits of what medical treatment can accomplish and the urgency of the surgery. The preparation for anesthesia parallels the preparation for the operation, which is discussed in other chapters. Shock, hypovolemia, electrolyte imbalances, cardiac decompensation, diabetic acidosis, and fever are some of the conditions that require treatment before anesthesia if possible. The stomach should be emptied by suction or allowed to empty, remembering that pain and apprehension retard emptying time. Aspiration of vomitus is one of the most dangerous complications of general anesthesia for emergency surgery.

The pharmacologic preparation of the patient for anesthesia varies not only with the age and condition of the patient but also with the anesthetic technic planned. For this reason, it should be ordered by the physician who is to administer the anesthetic. Most patients prefer some sedation before surgery, and some demand to be made totally unaware of their surroundings before reaching the operating room. Since anesthetic management is easier if the patient is cooperative and oriented, a compromise must be reached. Respiratory depression must be avoided unless the anesthesiologist is in continuous attendance from the time the sedative drugs are administered. It may be desirable to reduce the secretions of the mouth and respiratory tract or to depress vagal reflexes with belladonna drugs. Tables 14–2, 14–3, and 14–4 list some of the drugs used for anesthetic premedication and

TABLE 14–2. Common drugs and average doses of drugs for premedication (adults).

Drug	Dosage	Route and Time
Barbiturates*		
Pentobarbital	50–200 mg	Give orally, 2–4 hours before induction; or IM, 30 minutes before induction; or IV, 15 minutes before induction.
Secobarbital	50–200 mg	
Amobarbital	50–200 mg	
Diazepam (Valium)	10 mg	Give orally or IM 1–2 hours before surgery.
Narcotics*		
Morphine	5–15 mg	Give subcutaneously, 1 hour before induction; or IM, 30–45 minutes before induction; or IV, 5–15 minutes before induction.
Meperidine (Demerol)	50–150 mg	
Alphaprodine (Nisentil)	30–60 mg	
Belladonna Alkaloids		
Atropine	0.2–0.6 mg	Give subcutaneously, 30–60 minutes before induction. (Can be combined with narcotic.)
Scopolamine†	0.2–0.6 mg	

*Dosages of barbiturates and narcotics should be reduced if premedication includes phenothiazines.
†Reduce or eliminate scopolamine dose in the elderly.

TABLE 14–4. Selection of premedication for various anesthetic agents.

Anesthetic Agent	Barbiturates	Narcotics	Atropine or Scopolamine
Ether	++	+	+++
Cyclopropane	++	+	++
Thiopental with N_2O	++	+++	++
Fluroxene	++	+	+++
Halothane	++	+	++
Methoxyflurane	++	+	++
Local anesthetic			
Less than 200 mg procaine or lidocaine or 20 mg tetracaine	++	++	+
More than 200 mg procaine or lidocaine or 20 mg tetracaine	+++	++	+

Legend:　+ None or reduced dosage
　　　　　++ Desirable
　　　　　+++ Indicated

TABLE 14–3. Anesthetic premedication for infants and children.*†

	Average Weight (lb)	Pentobarbital or Secobarbital	Atropine or Scopolamine	Morphine　or	Meperidine (Demerol)　or	Alphaprodine (Nisentil)
Newborn	7	. . .	0.1 mg	. . .	. . .	. . .
6 months	16	30 mg	0.2 mg	. . .	. . .	. . .
1 year	21	50 mg	0.2 mg	1 mg	10 mg	4 mg
2 years	27	60 mg	0.3 mg	1.5 mg	20 mg	8 mg
4 years	35	90 mg	0.3 mg	3 mg	30 mg	12 mg
6 years	45	100 mg	0.4 mg	4 mg	40 mg	15 mg
8 years	55	120 mg	0.4 mg	5 mg	50 mg	20 mg
10 years	65	150 mg	0.4 mg	6 mg	60 mg	25 mg
12 years	85	150 mg	0.6 mg	8 mg	80 mg	30 mg

*Modified and reproduced, with permission, from Smith: *Anesthesia for Infants and Children.* Mosby, 1959.
†Reductions must be made for underweight or poorly developed patients. Barbiturates are given rectally at least 90 minutes before induction, or IM (with two-thirds above dosage), 30 minutes before induction. Morphine and atropine or scopolamine are given subcutaneously 45 minutes before induction.

suggest which ones to use with different types of anesthesia. As a rule, infirmity and age diminish the need for and increase the hazards of premedication. These hazards include confusion, restlessness, respiratory depression, hypotension (with or without a postural component), nausea, vomiting, and delayed awakening.

SELECTION OF ANESTHETIC AGENTS & TECHNICS

Most surgical procedures can be performed with anesthesia provided by a variety of agents and technics. There are few absolute indications or contraindications, as shown by the comparable success of compe-

tent anesthesiologists who differ in their selection of methods. Each makes a decision based on the requirements of the surgery, the condition of the patient, and his skill and experience with the methods at his disposal. He is influenced by patient preference (eg, intravenous induction), the site of the surgery, the use of electrocautery, the need for muscular relaxation, etc. If ideal conditions for the surgery are not compatible with safe anesthesia, this should be discussed with the surgeon, who must realize that death during the operation is more often related to the anesthetic than to the operation itself. A cadaver-like operative field may produce a cadaver. Other physicians who consult on the case may render invaluable services but must not dictate the anesthetic management unless they are prepared to carry it out themselves.

GENERAL ANESTHESIA

General anesthesia is a drug-induced depression of the CNS that is reversible by the body's elimination or destruction of the drug. It is a state of analgesia, amnesia, and unconsciousness, with loss of reflexes and muscle tone. The drugs used must produce no permanent tissue damage and must not interfere with respiratory or vascular functions to the point of tissue hypoxia. The physical and chemical properties of the drugs should allow convenient, controllable, and predictable methods of introducing them into the circulation for transport to the CNS. Rapid onset of action is a desirable property not usually provided by absorption from tissues or from the gastrointestinal tract. Either the direct intravenous injection or the introduction into the respiratory tract for absorption from the lungs is the usual method.

INHALATION ANESTHESIA

Inhalation anesthetics diffuse from the lung alveoli to the blood, which transports them to the CNS. If the drug is a compressed gas provided in cylinders (nitrous oxide, cyclopropane, ethylene), it can be administered in any inhaled concentration up to 100% by an anesthetic machine (see below). If it is a liquid at room temperature (ethyl ether, halothane, fluroxene, etc), it requires vaporization before it can be inhaled by the patient. Vaporization may be achieved by dripping the liquid on a gauze mask held over the patient's mouth and nose. This open drop technic has been the method used in millions of ether administrations for over a century. It has been largely supplanted by methods of vaporization that flow other gases over the surface of the volatile liquid or that bubble other gases through the volatile liquid. If the system is efficient, the gas exposed to the volatile liquid by either method becomes saturated with the vapor of the liquid. The concentration of the agent so vaporized is a function of the agent's vapor pressure, which varies with its temperature as a liquid at the time of vaporization. At the usual operating room temperatures (20 C), halothane has a vapor pressure of 240 mm Hg. If 100 ml of oxygen are passed through an efficient halothane vaporizer, the oxygen becomes saturated with halothane vapor, which exerts a pressure of 240 mm Hg, or approximately one-third of an ambient atmospheric pressure of 760 mm Hg. Therefore, the mixture that emerges from the vaporizer will consist of 100 ml of oxygen and 50 ml of halothane, making the mixture two-thirds oxygen and one-third halothane (240 mm Hg). If a 150 ml/minute flow of halothane is desired, 300 ml of oxygen must be put through the vaporizer. Efficient vaporizers deliver approximately 33% halothane, 60% ethyl ether (vapor pressure 450 mm Hg), or 3% methoxyflurane (vapor

pressure 27 mm Hg). The desired inhaled concentration is achieved by dilution, but many anesthetic vaporizers (eg, Fluotec) are calibrated to deliver desired concentrations and relieve the anesthesiologist of having to calculate the dilutions necessary.

The transport of an inhalation anesthetic to the lung alveoli and from lung capillaries to the brain is passive. Its molecules are carried by the flow of gas in the airways and of blood in the vascular system. Passage of the agent from alveoli to blood and from blood to brain is accomplished by diffusion, which depends on active movement of molecules through liquid media. The direction and rate of this movement is wholly dependent on the diffusion of molecules from areas of higher tension, where they are more crowded, to areas of lower tension, where they are less crowded. This mechanism is the same for all gases in solution, including oxygen and CO_2. Each gas seeks equilibration of tension independent of other gases in solution in the same medium. Gas tensions must not be confused with number of molecules in solution, although for an individual gas the 2 are interdependent. The solubility of any gas in a particular liquid determines the number of molecules in solution at any chosen tension. For example, the solubility of ethyl ether in blood is so much greater than that of nitrous oxide that at equal tensions more than 30 molecules of the ether are held in solution for every molecule of nitrous oxide. For anesthetic purposes, solubility is best expressed as the blood-gas partition coefficient, which tells us the proportionate distribution of a sample of gas added to a volume of air exposed to an equal volume of blood at 37.5 C. This coefficient for ethyl ether is 12.5, which means that 12.5 as many molecules of ether will dissolve in blood for every molecule that remains in air when the volume of air and blood are equal.

Uptake, Distribution, & Elimination of Inhalation Anesthetics

The depth of anesthesia is dependent on the gaseous tension of the anesthetic in the brain. This is established by equilibration of tension with the arterial blood perfusing the brain. In turn, the tension of the agent in the arterial blood represents an equilibration with alveolar tension. It follows that controlling the alveolar tension of an inhalation agent will control the depth of anesthesia. Venous-arterial shunts that bypass the lungs or ventilation-perfusion anomalies that act as shunts interfere with alveolar-arterial equilibration of inhalation agents just as they do for oxygen.

Building and maintaining a desired alveolar tension of an inhalation agent depends on the inspired concentration, the pulmonary ventilation, the blood-gas partition coefficient (solubility), and the cardiac output. The first 2 require little explanation. A high inspired concentration and an active transport mechanism (pulmonary ventilation) obviously deliver more anesthetic agent to the alveoli than lesser inspired concentrations or lesser minute volumes of alveolar ventilation. If the gas is very soluble (eg, ethyl ether),

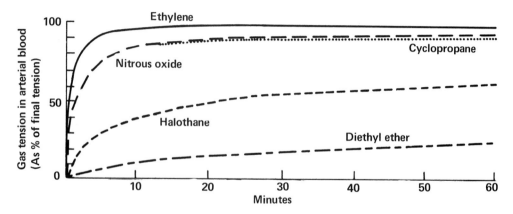

FIG 14–9. The rate of rise of tension of anesthetic in arterial blood with different agents administered at a constant inspired tension. (Reproduced, with permission, from Dripps, Eckenhoff, & Vandam: *Introduction to Anesthesia,* 3rd ed. Saunders, 1967.)

it will diffuse into the blood in such quantities that the alveolar tension and subsequent arterial blood tension rise slowly. Fig 14–9 plots the gas tension in arterial blood of several agents during induction under normal conditions.

During recovery, the soluble agents are "held" by the tissues and blood. Only a small portion of a highly soluble gas diffuses to the alveoli during the passage of any volume of blood through the lungs. The agents with low solubility are cleared from tissues and blood as rapidly as pulmonary ventilation clears them from the alveoli.

The distribution of cardiac output and its effect on anesthesia are worth noting here. About 70% of cardiac output goes to the brain, heart, kidneys, and liver. These organs are rapidly saturated with anesthetic so that the gas tension of the anesthetic is equal to the gas tension in the alveoli. During shock, the vasoconstriction of all organs except the brain and heart diverts an even greater share of cardiac output to the brain and heart and consequently their rapid and potentially dangerous saturation with anesthetic. Uptake continues for many hours at a reduced rate until all tissue gas tensions are equal. Failure to provide for this continuing uptake after the desired depth of anesthesia is reached results in diminishing depth as redistribution of the agent removes it from the brain.

When inhalation anesthesia is administered clinically, the depth is evaluated by observing the response of the patient and not by analysis of gas tensions. Progressive administration of an anesthetic agent depresses physiologic functions such as respiration, cardiac action, vasomotor tone, striated muscle tone, and reflexes. Changes in these functions are the signs of anesthesia. They are depressed by agents to different degrees and possibly in different sequences. For example, at the same level of respiratory depression, the muscle relaxant and circulatory effects of ether, cyclopropane, chloroform, and halothane are different. The clinical signs at various stages and planes of ether anesthesia (as classically described by Guedel)

are still useful signs for monitoring the patient's response to any agent, but their significance in determining the depth of anesthesia varies with the agent. By observing these signs, one strives to provide optimal surgical conditions commensurate with minimal depression of vital functions. Increases in the inspired concentration deepen the anesthetic level, and decreases in the inspired concentration lighten it.

The Anesthetic Machine

Most inhalation anesthetics are administered with an anesthetic machine, an apparatus that permits the administration of inhaled gases in known and controlled mixtures. The mixtures are prepared by accurately measuring flows of gases which may be available by piping from a central hospital source or from high-pressure tanks attached to the machine. In either instance, there must be foolproof safeguards against delivery of any but the desired gas or mixture, ie, it must be impossible to attach a nitrous oxide tank or hose to an oxygen inlet, or any other gas source to any but its own properly labeled flow system. Most anesthetic machines also have one or more vaporizers for the delivery of accurately measured concentrations of volatile liquid anesthetic agents such as ether, halothane, and fluroxene. If the anesthetic is administered by insufflation into the patient's mouth or throat, allowances must be made for dilution with room air. More commonly, the gases are administered by methods that exclude room air and contain the gas mixture in a system made continuous with the respiratory tract via a face mask or endotracheal tube. Such a system is a circle arrangement of a reservoir bag, a CO_2 absorber, a one-way overflow ("pop-off") valve, and 2 conducting tubes to the face mask with valves that allow circulation in one direction only. The reservoir bag allows the patient to breathe gases at flow rates which even during quiet respiration are greater (25–35 liters/minute) than the flow meters of most machines can deliver. The bag has additional functions when manually compressed. It then exerts a positive pressure on the contained gases, which is the usual method for applying positive airway pressure for controlled or assisted pulmonary ventilation during anesthesia. During spontaneous respiration, the bag gives visual evidence of rate and volume of respiration. The CO_2 absorber is essential whenever the flow of gas from the machine to the system is not sufficient to exhaust all of the patient's CO_2 exhalation out of the system through the overflow ("pop-off") valve. The absorber contains granules of the hydroxides of sodium, calcium, or barium, or mixtures of these substances. In the presence of moisture, CO_2 dissolves and forms carbonic acid (H_2CO_3), which reacts with the hydroxides to form carbonates and water. The freshness of the granules can be verified by indicators that change color when hydroxide is spent and the surface of the granules becomes acid. The conducting tubes ("elephant hoses") connect the mask or endotracheal tube to the reservoir bag. Unidirectional valves restrict one tube to inhalation only and the other to exhalation only. This arrangement prevents the rebreathing of

exhaled gas until it has gone "around the circle" to the other tube, has had its CO_2 content removed by the CO_2 absorber or by overflow, and fresh gas has been added. In other words, dead space is not increased by a circular absorber system.

Fig 14–10 illustrates the essentials of an anesthetic machine. All physicians, nurses, and technicians who work in operating rooms should know how to use an anesthetic machine for the administration of oxygen and artificial ventilation.

The Inhalation Anesthetics

The commonly used inhalation anesthetics are listed below. The brief description of each covers only those properties and clinical uses of interest to the surgeon.

A. Nitrous Oxide: Nitrous oxide (N_2O), one of the oldest inhalation anesthetics, is an inorganic gas that compresses to a liquid at about 50 atmospheres and is available in that state in cylinders. It is noncombustible (although it supports combustion by

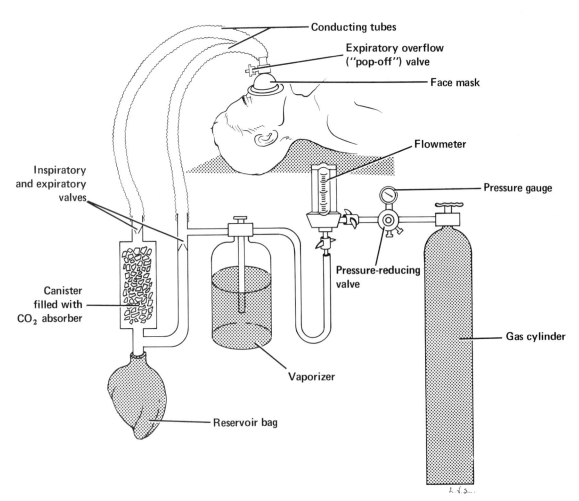

FIG 14–10. Diagram of the essential components of an anesthetic machine.

liberating oxygen) and has minimal side-effects outside the CNS. Its low solubility in blood permits rapid induction and recovery. The main drawback of nitrous oxide is its lack of potency. It can be administered in concentrations up to 80% if the remaining 20% of the mixture is oxygen. Even at these concentrations (which allow normal inspired oxygen), the addition of more potent inhalation agents or of narcotics or barbiturates is necessary to achieve surgical anesthesia. The patient in shock may be adequately anesthetized with a concentration of nitrous oxide as low as 50%. It is capable of reducing by approximately 50% the required concentration for surgery of other inhalation agents given with it. The potential for hypoxia is naturally greater with N_2O than with more potent agents that can be administered with higher oxygen concentrations.

B. Ethylene: Ethylene (CH_2CH_2) is available as a compressed gas in cylinders. It is more potent than nitrous oxide, with no greater toxicity. Its explosiveness and unpleasant odor have limited its popularity.

C. Cyclopropane: Cyclopropane (C_3H_6) is a highly explosive gas that liquefies at only 5 atmospheres at room temperature and consequently can be made available in light tanks. It offers smooth, rapid induction, minimal irritation of the respiratory passages, a wide margin of safety between anesthetic (5–25%) and toxic (40%) concentrations, and increased cardiac output with clinically useful concentrations. It is well tolerated by the patient in shock. The desirable circulatory responses to cyclopropane are not direct actions of the drug but responses to endogenous epinephrine release during anesthesia with this agent.

Cyclopropane is a potent respiratory depressant that leads to hypercapnia if the pulmonary ventilation is not augmented. If hypercapnia is allowed to occur, arrhythmias are frequent and hypotension ("cyclo shock") may occur in the postoperative period. The latter is probably caused by the sudden cessation of stimulation of epinephrine release by the cyclopropane and the hypercapnia. During anesthesia, ventricular fibrillation can result from catecholamine injections (epinephrine, levarterenol, etc). Noncatechol vasoconstrictors such as phenylephrine (Neo-Synephrine) are preferable during cyclopropane anesthesia.

D. Diethyl Ether: Diethyl ether ($CH_3CH_2OCH_2-CH_3$), usually referred to as ethyl ether or just ether, vies with nitrous oxide as the oldest anesthetic and is still one of the safest. It is the safest anesthetic in unskilled hands, with a wide margin between the concentration adequate for surgery and the concentration causing severe depression of the respiratory and cardiovascular systems. Ether is a liquid at room temperature and can be administered with a minimum of equipment, which, combined with low cost, is an attractive feature in many parts of the world. It provides excellent muscular relaxation.

The main disadvantages of ether are explosiveness; irritation of the respiratory passages, which can cause excessive secretions (blocked by belladonna drugs); induction laryngospasm and breathholding; slowness of induction and recovery (high solubility); and frequent postanesthesia nausea and vomiting.

E. Vinyl Ether (Vinethene): Vinyl ether ($CH_2CHOCHCH_2$) is a potent volatile liquid anesthetic whose principal advantage is rapidity of induction and recovery. It is as explosive as diethyl ether and more toxic, but it is useful for open drop inductions or for short procedures (less than 15 minutes) because it is rapid in action and less irritating to the respiratory passages.

F. Ethyl Chloride: Ethyl chloride (CH_3CH_2Cl) is a gas at room temperature but is provided as a liquid in well-stoppered bottles (boiling point, 12.3 C). Its low cost has encouraged its use as an induction agent in many countries, but its great potency, rapidity of action, and tendency to cause myocardial depression or irritability make it a hazardous agent except for induction by open drop administered by someone experienced in using it.

G. Trichloroethylene (Trilene): Trichloroethylene ($CHClCCl_2$) is a noncombustible volatile liquid anesthetic that has been used as an adjunct to nitrous oxide. It decomposes to toxic products when exposed to the heat and alkalies of CO_2 absorbers. It does not produce good muscular relaxation. It causes tachypnea which is believed to be due to sensitization of lung stretch receptors. In recent years it has been almost entirely supplanted by halothane.

H. Chloroform: Chloroform ($CHCl_3$) is the oldest of the halogenated liquid anesthetics. Its advantages are minimal irritation of the respiratory passages, rapidity of induction and recovery, low cost, ease of administration, and excellent muscular relaxation. A dose-related liver damage progressive to hepatic death limits the use of this otherwise excellent anesthetic.

I. Halothane (Fluothane): Halothane ($BrClHCCF_3$) is a nonexplosive volatile liquid. It provides smooth induction, almost no irritation of the respiratory tract, and moderate muscular relaxation which is adequate for surgery of infants and children. It causes minimal postanesthetic nausea.

Halothane depresses the circulation by both a direct action on the myocardium and by loss of vasomotor tone. It predisposes the myocardium to arrhythmias if epinephrine is injected or if the release of endogenous catecholamines is raised by hypercapnia. Cases of hepatitis severe enough to cause death have been traced to halothane, although the full explanation is not yet clear; case finding and proof of relationship to halothane are complicated by other causes of hepatitis such as viruses and other drugs. There is evidence that about one in 10,000 patients breaks down the halothane molecule to a product that causes liver damage, with increasing sensitization with each exposure. An otherwise unexplainable fever in the first 48 hours after halothane anesthesia suggests sensitivity and contraindicates future use. Other agents should be used when there is a possibility of jaundice due to other causes in order not to complicate the differential diagnosis in the postoperative period.

Many patients have had numerous uneventful halothane anesthesias. The many excellent characteristics of this drug have been amply demonstrated in millions of administrations; on balance, halothane has probably prevented more morbidity and mortality than have been caused by its potential for liver toxicity.

J. Fluroxene (Fluoromar): Fluroxene (CF_3CH_2-$OCHCH_2$) is a halogenated ether. It is a volatile liquid with properties between ethyl ether and halothane with respect to rate of induction, irritation of the respiratory tract, depression of the vascular system, and incidence of postanesthetic nausea. It has flammability hazards in concentrations above 4%.

K. Methoxyflurane (Penthrane): Methoxyflurane ($CHCl_2CF_2OCH_3$) is a halogenated ether that is a liquid with a very low vapor pressure at room temperature. It provides good analgesia that lasts into the postoperative period. It has been implicated as a cause of renal failure and is undergoing reevaluation.

Research continues in the field of new halogenated anesthetics. Several promising ones are undergoing clinical trials. All those mentioned above may be supplanted by better inhalation anesthetics in the near future.

Anesthetic Explosions

Several of the inhalation anesthetics discussed above are explosive in their effective concentrations. Explosions occur when a source of ignition (spark, flame, or heat) comes in contact with a highly combustible substance in the presence of oxygen. Anesthetic explosions may kill or injure not only the patient but others in the immediate vicinity. They can only be prevented by unremitting vigilance when explosive anesthetic mixtures are used. Spark-producing equipment such as electrocautery units and other electrical apparatus not declared spark-proof by the National Board of Fire Underwriters should not be used in the operating room when an explosive anesthetic is in use. To minimize sparks from static electricity, the relative humidity in operating rooms should be above 50% and all equipment and personnel should be grounded to a conductive floor. Drapes and external wearing apparel should not create static charges by friction. Floor conductivity, although sufficient to drain static charges, ought not be so great as to constitute an electrocution hazard for the personnel in the operating room.

INTRAVENOUS ANESTHESIA

Intravenous anesthesia has the advantage of ease of administration and great popularity with patients who desire general anesthesia but dislike the anesthetic mask and the slowness of induction of inhalation anesthesia. Intravenous anesthesia is also fatally easy to administer by the untrained or unskilled. Once injected

into a vein, the agent cannot be removed at will, whereas inhalation agents can be eliminated by ventilation of the lungs.

Intravenous Barbiturates

Thiopental (Pentothal) and thiamylal (Surital) are the most frequently used barbiturates for anesthesia. They are marketed as powders consisting of the sodium salts and are easily dissolved in water to make an alkaline solution. They are so similar in action that what is said here about thiopental applies also to thiamylal.

Thiopental is administered in a 0.2–2.5% solution. Accidental intra-arterial injections of higher concentrations can cause severe damage to peripheral tissues by arterial spasm, endothelial injury, and clotting. An intravenously injected dose of thiopental is distributed to all tissues, but the richly perfused organs such as the brain, heart, and kidneys receive a higher share of the dose. If the injected amount is sufficient (100–300 mg), loss of consciousness ensues. Awakening from a single dose is not due to destruction or excretion of the drug but is the result of a diminishing concentration of thiopental in the brain as distribution to other tissues takes place. Repeated or continued administration to maintain unconsciousness over a period of time will eventually saturate all body tissues to the same concentration as the brain. When that point is reached, awakening will be dependent on the metabolism of the barbiturate by the liver during the subsequent 24–48 hours. This is one of the reasons why thiopental is not a good choice as the sole agent for anesthesia of more than a few minutes' duration.

Thiopental is ideal for induction and as a basal anesthetic or adjunct to nitrous oxide anesthesia.

Thiopental induces a CNS depression that is characterized by better hypnosis than analgesia. Its failure to block afferent pathways except at great depth can lead to laryngospasm if the larynx is stimulated, overt movement following surgical stimulation, and retention of many other reflexes.

Hypotension frequently follows the administration of thiopental. The degree of hypotension depends on the amount and rate of injection and the physical condition of the patient. It is probably caused by a combination of central vasomotor depression, sympathetic ganglionic blockade, and direct myocardial depression. *Caution:* This hypotension can be disastrous in shock and hypovolemic states.

Intravenous Narcotics

Morphine, meperidine (Demerol), and other narcotics can be used intravenously for anesthesia, but, in contrast to the barbiturates, they provide excellent analgesia with little hypnosis. Increasing respiratory depression progresses in step with the analgesic effect. Narcotics are well tolerated in very large doses by poor-risk patients, causing minimal circulatory depression if the patient's pulmonary ventilation is maintained artificially during and after surgery.

Narcotic antagonists such as nalorphine (Nalline),

levallorphan (Lorfan), and naloxone hydrochloride (Narcan) can reverse the depressant actions of the narcotics.

Narcotics are not used as the sole agents for anesthesia but only in combination with nitrous oxide or barbiturates. A mixture of a narcotic (fentanyl) and a tranquilizer (droperidol), marketed as Innovar, has some popularity as an intravenous anesthetic. It provides good analgesia lasting into the postoperative period, causes no postoperative nausea and vomiting, and has the additional advantage of maintaining good cardiovascular stability. Its drawbacks are respiratory depression and poor muscular relaxation. Facilities for assisted or controlled respiration must be available when Innovar is used. Clinically, it is usually combined with nitrous oxide anesthesia.

Ketamine (Ketalar)

Ketamine is an intravenous agent that is almost as rapidly effective when administered intramuscularly. It causes an almost immediate trance-like analgesic state with no respiratory depression and no loss of muscle tone. Circulation is not depressed and blood pressure is raised, which contraindicates its administration to hypertensive patients. Pharyngeal and laryngeal muscle tone and reflexes are not lost, so that the airway remains patent even in awkward positions. Although the duration of anesthesia is only 5−10 minutes, repeated injections can be given to maintain analgesia for over an hour.

Ketamine analgesia is associated with unpleasant hallucinations during recovery in some patients (usually adults), which limits its usefulness.

Neuromuscular Blocking Agents

Neuromuscular blockers or muscle relaxants are a group of drugs that prevent striated muscles from contracting when their motor nerves are stimulated. They do not affect the sensorium. Their mode of action is by one of 2 mechanisms. Tubocurarine (curare) and gallamine triethiodide (Flaxedil) compete with acetylcholine at the neuromuscular junction but do not cause a depolarization of the end plate that initiates contraction. By outnumbering the acetylcholine molecules at these receptor sites, curare and gallamine effectively block neuromuscular transmission. A reversal of effect occurs if sufficient acetylcholine can accumulate at the neuromuscular junction for successful competition with the drugs. This is done clinically by the administration of neostigmine (Prostigmin), which inhibits cholinesterase, the enzyme responsible for the breakdown of acetylcholine. Neostigmine is therefore an effective antagonist to curare by this roundabout mechanism. Neostigmine has muscarinic effects (bradycardia, excessive salivation, etc) that must in turn be blocked by atropine administration before or simultaneously with the neostigmine used for curare reversal. Clinically, a mixture of 2.5 mg of neostigmine and 1 mg of atropine per 5 ml of solution is injected slowly over a period of minutes to reverse curare. Ten ml of the solution is the maximum useful

dose, but less than half of that is usually sufficient.

Succinylcholine chloride (Anectine) and decamethonium bromide (Syncurine) produce a neuromuscular block by acting like acetylcholine to depolarize the membrane of the motor end plate. However, unlike the action of acetylcholine, they do not permit the immediate repolarization necessary for another contraction. This type of neuromuscular block does not respond to neostigmine initially; however, when sustained by large doses over a period of time, it becomes curare-like and responds to neostigmine. This so-called phase II block is not fully understood. An occasional patient whose plasma is deficient in pseudocholinesterase will be unable to deactivate succinylcholine and may develop prolonged paralysis with a small dose. Mechanical ventilation and time are the antidotes.

The clinical use of the neuromuscular blocking agents has been one of the major advances in anesthesia of this century. Usually given intravenously, these drugs provide all degrees of muscular relaxation with minimal side-effects, thus diminishing the required dosage of general anesthetics with their many undesirable properties. Because they do not cross the placental barrier in effective concentrations, they are useful for cesarian sections. They should never be used by anyone without the means and experience to carry out mechanical ventilation.

Tubocurarine is the oldest and most commonly used muscle relaxant. It is partly excreted in the urine and partly metabolized. After a peak effect at about 10 minutes, its clinical action diminishes during the next hour, largely because of distribution away from the neuromuscular junctions. Therefore, prolongation of the neuromuscular block can be achieved with subsequent smaller doses. The degree of effectiveness of the block can be assessed objectively in clinical situations by observing the absence or fading strength of muscle twitches upon electrical stimulation of nerves. For example, the absence of contraction or the diminished strength of contraction of hand muscles in response to ulnar nerve stimulation can be observed.

A fall in blood pressure due to ganglionic blocking action and bronchospasm caused by histamine release are very rare adverse reactions to curare. A fall in blood pressure may also be due to the preservatives in some curare preparations. Ether anesthesia, quinidine, lidocaine, and a number of antibiotics (neomycin, kanamycin) intensify the effect of curare.

The paralyzing dose of curare is 15−30 mg IV.

Gallamine triethiodide (Flaxedil) has a curare-like action at the neuromuscular junction, a slightly shorter duration of action, does not liberate histamine, causes tachycardia by its vagolytic action, and is dependent on renal function for its elimination. The paralyzing dose is 100−200 mg IV.

Succinylcholine chloride (Anectine) has a duration of action of 3−5 minutes after a paralyzing dose of 20−50 mg. It is frequently administered by continuous intravenous drip of a solution containing 1−2 mg/ml.

BALANCED ANESTHESIA

Balanced anesthesia is a term applied to anesthesia produced by the combination of 2 or more drugs. Ideally, each agent contributes its most desirable property, and none is given in toxic amounts. The combined effect is tailored to suit the condition of the patient and the requirements of the surgery by variations in the dosages of the component agents. An example is the use of thiopental for a rapid, pleasant induction, nitrous oxide for its nontoxic, nonexplosive properties, a narcotic or potent inhalation agent to deepen the anesthetic level, and curare to provide muscular relaxation.

MANAGEMENT OF GENERAL ANESTHESIA

The desired depth of anesthesia for surgery is not difficult to achieve. Pushing the plunger of a syringe or turning the flow valve of an anesthetic machine to deepen anesthesia requires little knowledge. The experience and skill of the anesthesiologist is called into play in keeping the patient alive, safe, and relatively unharmed in spite of the necessary trauma of the operation and the anesthetic drugs used to facilitate it. During general anesthesia, the unconscious patient loses many protective reflexes, and vital respiratory and circulatory functions may be depressed. Corneal ulcers, pressure sores, nerve palsies caused by prolonged unphysiologic positioning, and injuries to joints and to intervertebral disks are examples of the damage the patient may sustain without complaint during anesthesia. Although protecting the patient from such trauma is important, the primary function of the anesthesiologist is the prevention of tissue hypoxia by maintaining adequate arterial blood oxygen tension and tissue perfusion. The signs of insufficient arterial blood oxygen tension progress from cyanosis (which is not reliable) and initial tachycardia to bradycardia, hypotension, dilated pupils, and cardiac arrest. The ventilatory causes of arterial oxygen desaturation are insufficient oxygen tension in the respired gases, insufficient pulmonary ventilation, or maldistribution of the ventilation in the lungs. A hypoxic inhaled mixture must be suspected immediately regardless of the contrary evidence of the flowmeters of the anesthetic machine whenever cyanosis develops in spite of good pulmonary ventilation and good circulation. Believing the machine instead of the clinical evidence has caused many fatalities.

Insufficient pulmonary ventilation may be due to central depression by the anesthetic drugs; to weakness or paralysis of the respiratory muscles caused by neuromuscular blockers or deep anesthesia; or, most commonly, to obstruction of the air passages. Although insidious, the first 2 are easily prevented or treated by assisted or controlled respiration. The signs of obstruction are absence of air movement (total obstruction) or noisy respiration (partial obstruction); noticeably increased muscular effort during inspiration; and indrawing of the soft tissues of the thoracic wall (suprasternal notch, supraclavicular fossas, and intercostal spaces) during inspiration. Deep anesthesia and muscle relaxants obscure the signs related to muscular efforts. Partial obstruction is diagnosed by auscultation of the air movement with ear or stethoscope over the trachea, the mouth, or the rebreathing tubes of the anesthetic machine. Total or partial obstruction of the paralyzed patient is diagnosed by noting the duration and degree of pressure required to inflate the lungs and also by listening for adventitious sounds. Obstruction of the airway may occur anywhere from the nose and lips down to the alveoli. The possible causes are numerous and include tongue obstruction, laryngospasm, inflammatory disorders, foreign bodies, and neoplasms. The anesthetic state itself causes some types of airway obstruction. During anesthesia, the tone of the lingual and mandibular muscles may be so diminished as to allow the tongue of the supine patient to sag back into the pharynx and obstruct air flow. This is the most frequent form of obstruction in anesthesia. It can be prevented or corrected by extending the patient's head and neck and drawing the mandible forward. Mechanical devices such as oropharyngeal and nasopharyngeal airways or endotracheal tubes may be required also.

Obstruction of the airway by laryngospasm occurs during light anesthesia. It can be corrected by deepening the anesthesia or by positive airway pressure. The expert anesthesiologist seldom resorts to paralysis with succinylcholine to relieve laryngospasm.

Airway obstruction may also be due to vomitus. Aspiration of vomitus may lead to severe postoperative pneumonitis. It is best avoided by withholding anesthesia until the stomach is empty or, if that is impossible, by intubating the trachea with the patient awake or following a rapid induction. General anesthesia should never be induced unless an efficient suction apparatus is available. The decision whether a tracheostomy should be done under local anesthesia before general anesthesia is administered to a patient with upper airway obstruction is a matter of clinical judgment.

One impediment to respiration that does not involve obstruction of the airway must be kept in mind during anesthesia. This is interference to lung expansion itself, the most common form of which is pneumothorax. It can occur during surgery of the neck or of the subdiaphragmatic area. It behaves like an airway obstruction except that adventitious sounds during respiration are absent. If it is caused by leakage of air from the lung, it can develop into a tension pneumothorax which embarrasses circulation. Treatment consists of removal of air from the pleural cavity. This is discussed in Chapter 22.

The circulatory deficiencies that interfere with tissue oxygenation are outlined in the chapter on shock. Anesthesia contributes to circulatory failure by causing myocardial and vasomotor depression. The anesthesiologist's role in its management is to maintain minimal anesthesia compatible with surgery, fluid and blood replacement, maintenance of a good arterial oxygen tension, and positioning the patient to assist venous return. Vasopressor drugs are useful in the treatment of hypotension during spinal anesthesia or of simple syncope, but are only stopgap measures in hypovolemic conditions.

.   .   .

ENDOTRACHEAL INTUBATION

Endotracheal intubation is done routinely as part of the management of general anesthesia for the majority of extensive surgical procedures. The technics of inserting the tube into the larynx are many and can only be mastered by practice. They are facilitated by deep anesthesia or muscle relaxants. Endotracheal intubation is frequently necessary for effective life-saving mechanical respiration in other areas as well as in the operating room. Skill in this technic should be part of the technical competency of any physician engaged in emergency medicine or the care of uncon-scious patients. During anesthesia, it provides better control of the upper airway, removes the anesthetic mask from the surgical field in oral and facial surgery, facilitates assisted or controlled ventilation, and pre-vents aspiration of foreign materials into the lungs.

SPINAL ANESTHESIA

Spinal anesthesia is a safe method of providing excellent operative conditions for many procedures. It is somewhat unpopular with patients who desire total unawareness or who are misinformed about the inci-dence of complications. The technics consist of block-ing the spinal nerves between their emergence from the spinal cord and their exit from the spinal canal through the intervertebral foramens. In the spinal canal, the spinal nerves course through the subarachnoid space where they are bathed in spinal fluid and then traverse the epidural space. They may be blocked in either location. Table 14–1 gives the dosages of drugs used in spinal anesthesia.

Subarachnoid spinal anesthesia is performed by doing a lumbar puncture with sterile technic and inject-ing the sterile anesthetic agent. Ampules of drugs used must be autoclaved and not stored in disinfectant solutions that might chemically contaminate the ampule contents through minute undetectable cracks. The lumbar puncture may be done in the sitting or lateral decubitus position at any level between L1 and S1. The anesthetic blocks all spinal nerves below the

site of injection as well as those reached by the ceph-alad spread of the anesthetic solution. This cephalad spread can be controlled by positioning the patient to allow the anesthetic solution to "sink" or "float" in the desired direction. For this purpose, the anesthetic solutions are either made heavier than the CSF (hyper-baric) by the addition of 10% dextrose or lighter than the CSF (hypobaric) by dissolving the anesthetic drug in distilled water to make a dilute solution (eg, 1 mg tetracaine per 1 ml distilled water). The effective spread is limited as dilution by the CSF occurs. After 20 minutes, the solution is "fixed" and further spread is unlikely.

Duration of anesthesia depends on the agent selected; larger doses than those given in Table 14–1 increase the duration of anesthesia only slightly. Addition of 0.2–0.4 ml of 1:1000 epinephrine or 3 mg phenylephrine (Neo-Synephrine) increases the duration 30–50%.

Epidural spinal anesthesia is administered by introducing a needle into the epidural space at any level of the spinal canal. It is easiest at the lumbar interspaces or through the sacral hiatus. In the lumbar area the space is recognized by advancing a blunt needle in the same manner as for a lumbar puncture but stopping when resistance to injection is no longer felt but no CSF can be aspirated. A test dose that would achieve subarachnoid spinal anesthesia but insufficient for epidural anesthesia is used for proof that the subarachnoid space has or has not been entered.

A catheter may be inserted through the needle for continuous epidural anesthesia with repeated injec-tions. The needle is withdrawn, leaving the catheter in position. Catheters should never be withdrawn through the needle for fear of cutting the catheter in the spinal canal.

The concentrations of local anesthetics used and the rate of onset of anesthesia are the same as for peripheral nerve blocks. The area anesthetized depends on the spread of the injected solution in the spinal canal and is therefore dependent on the volume, although considerable individual variations occur. The dangers of toxicity must be kept in mind because the total dose required may be large.

Subarachnoid and epidural anesthesia produce excellent analgesia and loss of motor function in the area of distribution of the spinal nerves affected. This can include the motor nerves to the diaphragm and cessation of respiration if the level reaches the fourth cervical vertebra. The minute volume of respiration is not diminished by loss of intercostal muscle activity.

Side-Effects of Spinal Anesthesia

Most of the side-effects of spinal anesthesia are related to block of the nerve fibers of the sympathetic nervous system as they accompany the anterior roots of the spinal nerves from the first thoracic to the second lumbar vertebrae (thoracolumbar outflow). This sympathetic block upsets many physiologic regulating mechanisms. Interruption of central vasomotor control to the affected areas leads to vasodilatation or at least to a loss of constriction of both resistance (arterioles) and capacitance (veins) vessels. The loss of resistance and the peripheral venous pooling (if not compensated by position) contribute to a fall in blood pressure. Moreover, cardiac rate and action are deprived of the stimulation of the cardiac sympathetic innervation and of the epinephrine normally released by sympathetic stimulation of the adrenal medulla. Meanwhile, the vagus has an unopposed parasympathetic effect of cardiac slowing. The hypovolemic or hypotensive patient reacts poorly to this situation. The arteriosclerotic hypertensive patient may have a precipitous blood pressure drop. The other effects of sympathetic loss such as increased intestinal peristalsis caused by unopposed vagal activity and the loss of sweating are of lesser consequence. Nausea and vomiting during spinal anesthesia may be related to the sympathetic blockade, but the mechanism is not entirely clear. They are frequently but not invariably associated with hypotension.

The general management of the patient under spinal anesthesia includes maintenance of good ventilation and oxygenation, positioning to favor good venous return, and the use of vasopressors if necessary. An intravenous infusion should be started before high spinal anesthetics are administered.

Subarachnoid Versus Epidural Blocks

The subarachnoid spinal is technically easier to accomplish, uses a much smaller amount of drug, and has a more rapid onset than the epidural. The epidural method avoids "spinal headaches" due to CSF leakage through the arachnoid puncture site and lends itself to a continuous technic for many hours by repeated injections through an epidurally placed catheter. It is generally felt that a continuous catheter technic for subarachnoid spinal anesthesia has an increased incidence of complications warranted only in selected cases.

Complications of Spinal Anesthesia

Headache occurring during the first week after a subarachnoid block, with onset usually in 24–48 hours and characterized by exacerbation in the erect position and amelioration in the recumbent, is reported in up to 15% of spinals. It is believed to be due to spinal fluid leak at the puncture site. Large caliber needles increase the incidence. Treatment consists of the recumbent position, hydration, sedation, and, in severe cases, epidural fluid injection to diminish the leak.

Nerve injuries and transverse myelitis have been caused by spinal anesthetics, resulting in transient or permanent disabilities ranging from minor paresthesias to complete paraplegia. These sequelae are rare, but their tragic impact gives them a notoriety out of proportion to their frequency. Their incidence is much lower than the incidence of cardiac arrest during general anesthesia. Contaminants, drug sensitivity, and excessive drug concentration have been held responsible. Cases have occurred following epidural as well as subarachnoid spinal anesthesia.

MONITORING DURING ANESTHESIA

Many methods are available for monitoring a patient's condition and responses to the drugs used for anesthesia and to the surgery. The experienced observer's senses and his ability to integrate the information obtained with them can be aided but not replaced by sophisticated electronic devices. Observations of the movements of the chest and of the reservoir bag together with continuous auscultation of breath sounds with a chest or esophageal stethoscope are the best monitors of pulmonary ventilation. Changes in volume and rhythm of breathing as well as the signs of airway obstruction are readily detected. Tissue color, bleeding (and the color of arterial blood at the surgical site), the quality of the pulse, the arterial blood pressure, the quality of the heart sounds (obtained with a precordial or esophageal stethoscope), the filling of neck veins and central venous pressure, the size and reactivity of the pupils, and urine outflow are all observable in most cases by the alert anesthesiologist with simple apparatus. The status of the heart, circulation, and tissue perfusion can thus be followed in a continuous manner. An earpiece molded to fit the observer's external ear canal is more comfortable than the binaural stethoscope during prolonged procedures. Continuous ECG and EEG tracings, arterial pressures obtained by intra-arterial catheters connected to pressure transducers, continuous analysis of expired CO_2 tension, and frequent sampling of arterial blood for determinations of P_{O_2}, P_{CO_2}, and pH provide critically important information in selected cases. However, artifacts and possible technical errors and failures must be kept in mind. The diagnosis of certain cardiac arrhythmias, the determination of the level of hypercapnia, and the determination of the degree of acidosis cannot be made without them.

POSTANESTHETIC MANAGEMENT

The anesthetic state cannot be terminated and the patient returned to his preanesthetic condition in an instant at the end of the surgical procedure. The central depressant drugs, the neuromuscular blockers, and the physiologic trespasses of regional anesthesia continue to act for variable periods of time. The trauma of the surgery, hemorrhage, and loss of circulating volume to the extravascular compartments are all additive to the residual anesthetic state. This situation may last many hours, during which time the patient requires the same monitoring of his condition and the same support of his vital functions as he did during the operation.

Complications that occur during the immediate postoperative period and related to the anesthetic drugs must be considered anesthetic rather than postanesthetic complications. The stage is still set for failure of any of the links of the oxygen transport mechanism. The cardinal sin in the management of the post-operative period is the administration of sedatives to control restlessness caused by hypoxia. Until proved otherwise, postoperative restlessness has a hypoxic basis that can be verified by a therapeutic test with higher inspired oxygen or assisted ventilation and analysis of arterial oxygen tension.

Atelectasis of patchy areas of lung or entire lobes is the most common postoperative complication. The causes include any impediments to good expansion of all parts of the lungs such as central sedation, neuro-muscular weakness, airway obstruction of any kind, secretions in the airways, pain caused by respiratory movements, and tight dressings. Treatment consists of the removal of the cause if possible and reexpansion of the lungs. The latter can be done by encouraging the patient to cough and to breathe deeply. Artificial means include tracheal suction, stimulation by admin-istration of 5% CO_2 or by increasing the dead space, and assisted ventilation with respirators. The broncho-scopic removal of bronchial obstruction is occasionally necessary. The use of a high inspired oxygen tension to compensate for shunting or inadequate ventilation neither prevents nor cures atelectasis.

OXYGEN THERAPY
Morley M. Singer, MD

Oxygen, like any other therapeutic agent, has specific indications, dosages, methods of administra-tion, hazards, and toxicity.

Indications

Any circumstance in which cellular oxygenation is impaired may be an indication for oxygen therapy. One cause of impaired cellular oxygenation is a decreased arterial oxygen tension (Pa_{O_2}). The Pa_{O_2} is normally 80–100 torr* when inspiring ambient air at sea level, and decreases gradually with age so that at age 70 a Pa_{O_2} of 70 torr may be regarded as normal. Hypoventilation or mismatching of ventilation and perfusion in the lung may result in a reduced Pa_{O_2}.

Tolerance to hypoxemia varies with the patient's age, hemoglobin concentration, the rate of onset, the presence of coronary or cerebrovascular disease, car-diac output, body temperature, and many other fac-tors. Since tolerance is not predictable, it is generally wise to administer oxygen to hospitalized patients with an acute decrease in Pa_{O_2} to less than 55–60 torr.

Cellular oxygenation may be impaired without significant decrease in Pa_{O_2}: low cardiac output, anemia, abnormal hemoglobin, shifts in the oxyhemo-globin dissociation curve, impaired cellular uptake of oxygen, and increased metabolic requirements of the

*One torr = 1 atm/760, almost exactly equivalent to 1 mm Hg.

cell are just a few examples. It may be appropriate or necessary to administer oxygen in these circumstances, but consideration of oxygen transport in the blood demonstrates the limitations. Each gram of normal hemoglibin can carry 1.34 ml of O_2 when fully satu-rated (Pa_{O_2} = 150 torr). Raising the Pa_{O_2} above this level adds very little oxygen to the blood—0.3 ml dis-solved O_2 for each 100 torr rise in Pa_{O_2}. It is evident that, whereas administering O_2 is appropriate, a greater effect on O_2 transport might be achieved by control-ling hemoglobin concentration and cardiac output or reducing tissue requirements when feasible.

The clinical signs of tissue hypoxemia are vari-able. The brain and the myocardium have relatively high O_2 consumptions, and the initial manifestations of inadequate oxygenation may be cerebral or myocar-dial dysfunction rather than signs of respiratory dis-tress. Arterial blood gas values should be checked in any patient with unexplained deterioration of CNS or cardiac function. Cyanosis is a late sign of severe hypoxemia, and absence of cyanosis does not exclude significant hypoxemia.

Dosages & Methods of Administration

In addition to the dose of oxygen required, patient comfort, economy, convenience of administra-tion, and reliability must all be considered.

Nasal cannulas or plastic face masks are adequate for the vast majority of patients. Other methods of oxygen administration are also described below.

It should be remembered that oxygen from a cylinder or wall supply is completely dry and must be passed through a humidifier to prevent drying of the airway mucosa.

A. Nasal Cannulas and Catheters: The nasal cannula is the best method of oxygen delivery for general use. Flow rates of 6–8 liters/min deliver 30–40% inspired oxygen. Higher rates are uncomfort-able and cause local irritation. Mouth breathing does not significantly affect the inspired concentration, but bilateral nasal obstruction obviously will.

Nasal catheters deliver similar concentrations but are less comfortable. These are inserted to the naso-pharynx (half the distance from nose to ear), and care must be taken to prevent accidental intubation of the esophagus.

B. Plastic Face Masks: Loose-fitting plastic face masks deliver 30–50% O_2 at a flow rate of 8–10 liters/min. A reservoir bag may slightly increase the O_2 concentration delivered, but a more important factor is the mask fit. It is important to keep in mind that, should the mask be removed for eating, coughing, suc-tioning, or other purposes, the patient is deprived of any supplemental oxygen.

C. Rubber Face Masks: The Boothby, Lovelace, Bulbulian (BLB) mask and the Barach and Eckman meter mask (OEM) are tighter-fitting masks which are capable of delivering high concentrations of oxygen (80%) but are too hot, heavy, and uncomfortable to use for more than 10–15 minutes.

D. Face Hood: The face hood is an unreliable

method of administering oxygen since it is difficult to keep in place. It is appropriate to use for the delivery of high humidity from mist generators.

E. Oxygen Tent: The oxygen tent is essentially obsolete for adults because of its bulk and inconvenience, the fire hazard involved, separation of the patient from nursing personnel and family, and inability to achieve high concentrations of oxygen. It is occasionally useful for small children. A minimum flow of 12 liters/min is required to achieve O_2 concentrations of 40%, and opening the tent lowers the concentration.

F. Venturi Masks: These are designed to deliver inspired oxygen, concentrations not exceeding 24%, 28%, 35%, or 40%. They are for specific use in patients with chronic hypercapnia when it is necessary to avoid raising the P_{aO_2} to greater than 60 torr (see below).

G. Plastic Head Box: A rigid clear plastic box with a cutout for the neck may be used for infants, usually up to 1 year of age. Oxygen flow of 5–10 liters/min can provide up to 100% inspired O_2 concentration; the inspired O_2 must therefore be monitored frequently.

H. T-Piece: A T-piece is commonly used for delivery of oxygen and humidity to patients with endotracheal tubes or tracheostomies. It provides a simple and safe system without valves. The inspired O_2 concentration will vary with the concentration and flow of oxygen delivered, the length of the T-piece connections, and the patient's inspiratory flow rate and respiratory frequency.

Hazards & Complications

A. Infection: The water in the humidifier can serve as a culture medium and source of infection. The humidifier should be changed every 24 hours to prevent this.

B. Retrolental Fibroplasia: Elevated *arterial* oxygen levels may produce blindness in premature infants. If it is necessary to administer O_2 to cyanotic premature infants, the P_{aO_2} must be monitored frequently, since a few hours of exposure may be harmful.

C. Ventilatory Depression: This is of concern **only** in patients with chronic hypercapnia. This does not mean that O_2 should not be administered when necessary but that it must be carefully titrated so that the P_{aO_2} does not exceed 60 torr. This can be done with a nasal cannula at flow rates of 1–2 liters/min or a Venturi mask. In either case, frequent monitoring of arterial blood gas values is essential.

D. Pulmonary Oxygen Toxicity: Pulmonary toxicity from O_2 does not occur with inspired concentrations of less than 50%. Since it is difficult or impossible to achieve higher concentrations for a significant length of time without an endotracheal tube or tracheostomy in place, pulmonary toxicity is not a concern with the standard methods of oxygen administration.

E. Fire: Flames and sparks must be kept away from high oxygen atmospheres.

VENTILATORS

In the past decade, the use of mechanical ventilators has played an increasingly important role in the management of surgical patients. Ventilators are used in 2 separate contexts: for the prevention and treatment of postoperative pulmonary complications, and for mechanical ventilation of patients with ventilatory insufficiency.

In the preoperative period, intermittent positive pressure breathing (IPPB) may be used by patients with chronic obstructive airway disease to deliver nebulized bronchodilators and to aid in expectoration of secretions. The forced expiratory volume at 1 second (FEV_1) can be measured before and after bronchodilator administration to observe the effects of therapy. It may be advantageous to familiarize patients predisposed to pulmonary complications with the use of IPPB preoperatively in anticipation of its use in the postoperative period. Routine use of IPPB for other than these purposes is to be discouraged. The patient with chronic lung disease characterized by increased pulmonary secretions will more likely benefit from cessation of smoking, chest physical therapy, and high inspired humidity, and these measures should be given priority over IPPB in preoperative preparation.

In the postoperative period, IPPB may be used to prevent or treat atelectasis. Some thought should be given to the rationale of this therapy. A number of factors (age, preexisting lung disease, immobilization, incisional pain, and abdominal distention) tend to produce decreased resting lung volumes and an increased tendency to atelectasis postoperatively. IPPB may be effective in preventing or treating atelectasis *only if it results in inflation to a larger lung volume than the patient can or will achieve with spontaneous respiration.* The vast majority of postoperative patients experience difficulty using IPPB with a mask or mouthpiece. Thus, if the patient has an inspiratory capacity of 1000 ml, one would not predict therapeutic benefit from inflation to an equal or lesser volume by IPPB. When used in this circumstance, IPPB probably functions as an indirect and expensive substitute for a "stir-up regimen," ie, encouragement of deep breathing, coughing, and early ambulation.

In selected patients, IPPB may be of value in the prevention and treatment of atelectasis. The inflation volume should be equal to or greater than the patient's postoperative respiratory capacity, and this volume should be written in the order chart and IPPB discontinued if this cannot be achieved. Treatment 3–4 times per day with the aid of an inhalation therapist is more likely to be effective than hourly use without assistance. Dramatic reinflation of atelectatic lung may be seen when IPPB is used *effectively.*

Once the patient becomes ambulatory, serious atelectasis is unlikely and IPPB may be discontinued. In the postoperative period, the patient who is alert, has no preexisting cardiopulmonary disease, and has an incision outside the thorax or abdomen would rarely if ever require or benefit from IPPB.

Hazards

IPPB should never be applied by mask to the obtunded or unconscious patient for fear of producing gastric distention, regurgitation, and aspiration.

It is prudent to avoid use of IPPB where surgical anastomoses are present in the upper gastrointestinal tract or after pulmonary surgery, but these are relative rather than absolute contraindications.

Treatment of Ventilatory Failure

Early recognition of impending ventilatory failure and preventive artificial ventilation via nasotracheal tube or tracheostomy is increasingly accepted in surgical practice. This has been practiced for several years in patients undergoing open heart surgery and is now being extended to other patients with a high probability of ventilatory failure. Factors predisposing to postoperative ventilatory failure include old age, obesity, preexisting cardiopulmonary disease, a smoking history, debility, thoracic and abdominal surgery, and peritonitis. A specific use of ventilators is the treatment of "flail" chest where the ventilator acts as a "pneumatic splint" preventing paradoxic movement of the chest wall. Use of a ventilator may be lifesaving in the management of intractable pulmonary edema which does not respond to customary conservative measures.

It is important to remember that almost any patient with terminal illness may have life prolonged temporarily by mechanical ventilation. Patients selected for ventilatory support should have a reasonable chance of functional recovery.

Types of Ventilators

A wide variety of ventilators are available, and there is frequent misunderstanding of their relative capabilities. Ventilators are commonly classified, by the mechanism producing cessation of inspiration, into pressure-cycled (Bird, Bennett) and time-volume cycled (Ohio 560, Bennett PR-4, Emerson, Engstrom). In the former, the operator determines a preset pressure, and the tidal volume delivered by the machine varies with the compliance of the lung-thorax and the airway resistance. If the compliance of the lung-thorax system decreases (from patient contraction of chest and abdominal muscles, airway secretions, atelectasis, pneumothorax, etc), the tidal volume delivered by the ventilator will decrease and the respiratory rate will increase. The time-volume cycled ventilator in this circumstance will generate higher pressures and deliver a more constant tidal volume with little or no change in respiratory rate. It seems obvious, therefore, that with use of pressure-cycled ventilators the tidal volume must be monitored and with time-volume cycled ventilators the inflation pressure must be monitored.

Another major difference between the 2 classes of ventilators is their response to leaks in the patient-ventilator system. The pressure-cycled machine will compensate for small leaks, taking a longer time to deliver the same volume, and will "stick" in the inspiratory phase if the leak is so large that the preset pressure cannot be achieved. The time-volume ventilator will not compensate for leaks, and the tidal volume will be decreased proportionate to the leak. (The tidal volume is *not* constant.) It is therefore essential to have an alarm system when the patient is dependent on the ventilator.

A third difference is that most of the presently available time-volume cycled ventilators are capable of generating higher inspiratory flow rates and inflation pressures than the pressure-cycled ventilators and are more effective in the presence of severely decreased compliance or increased airway resistance. Most models of pressure-cycled ventilators can generate peak pressures of approximately 50 cm water, whereas many time-volume cycled ventilators can double this value.

Thus, in the presence of severely decreased compliance, elevated airway resistance, or rapidly changing compliance or airway resistance, time-volume cycled ventilators may be more effective. Many other considerations enter into the selection of a ventilator: cost, size, power source, ease of sterilization, ability to control inspired O_2 concentration, ability to apply positive end-expiratory pressure, reliability, performance of the humidifier, etc. It should be borne in mind that the cost of time-volume cycled ventilators is approximately 10 times that of pressure-cycled machines. The success of ventilator care depends more on the quality and performance of the medical and nursing personnel involved than on the specific ventilator utilized.

Care of the Patient Requiring
Continuous Mechanical Ventilation

It is axiomatic that a patient dependent on a ventilator must be cared for in an environment where continuous observation is possible. Management of these patients consists of a multitude of measures aimed at preventing the complications of therapy, and the chances of success are improved if the patient is in an intensive care unit manned by highly skilled nursing and medical personnel.

Ventilatory Pattern

To prevent atelectasis, tidal volumes are set at 12–15 ml/kg. Periodic "sighs" are not necessary when these large tidal volumes are generated. If the patient has normal respiratory drive, it is generally safer to assist rather than control respiration, so that the patient's respiratory center "sets" the respiratory frequency and the arterial CO_2 tension (P_{aCO_2}). With assisted ventilation, the patient initiates each breath; the ventilator senses the negative pressure generated by the patient and completes inspiration to the preset pressure or volume. With controlled ventilation, the minute ventilation is entirely determined by the ventilator settings. Because of the frequent occurrence of increased wasted ventilation in patients on ventilators, nomograms predicting ventilatory requirements are of little value.

Endotracheal tubes can be left in for several days, after which tracheostomy is usually substituted. Both tubes should be flexible plastic and should have soft, low-pressure cuffs, inflated only to the volume required to prevent air leak.

Oxygen Toxicity

Inspired O_2 concentrations of 40–50% are tolerated for prolonged periods, and 24 hours' exposure to 100% O_2 does not produce clinically evident pulmonary changes. When the patient's clinical signs are stable, inspired O_2 concentrations should be decreased to the minimum required (determined by measurement of P_{aO_2} and clinical judgement). Pressure-cycled ventilators commonly used deliver 40–90% inspired oxygen when the Venturi is in effect. Air-oxygen "mixers" are available for more precise control of the inspired O_2 concentrations.

Circulatory Effects

Positive pressure ventilation may decrease venous return into the thorax and thereby decrease systemic blood pressure and cardiac output. This is most likely to occur in patients who are hypovolemic or lacking normal autonomic nervous system responses. This effect can be minimized by ensuring adequate intravascular blood volume and allowing the expiratory time to equal or exceed the inspiratory time.

Positive End-Expiratory Pressure (PEEP)

Preventing the airway pressure from returning to atmospheric at end-expiration will increase the resting lung volume. In selected patients, this may reduce the alveolar-arterial O_2 differences (presumably by reversing airway closure) and thus permit reduction of inspired O_2 concentrations to levels which decrease or eliminate the possibility of pulmonary oxygen toxicity. Possible adverse effects include depression of cardiac output and an increased incidence of pneumothorax.

General Care of the Patient Requiring Ventilatory Support

The patient fighting the ventilator should be regarded as having inadequate ventilation until proved otherwise and should not be sedated without careful assessment, including blood gas analysis. Small intravenous doses of morphine (2–3 mg), repeated as necessary, may be used when sedation is required. It is rarely (if ever) necessary to paralyze a patient in order to provide adequate ventilation, and doing so introduces unnecessary hazards. Adequate tidal volume, adequate oxygenation, and normal or slightly lower than normal P_{aCO_2} are of major importance in preventing patient distress.

Gastric distention is a common occurrence in patients on ventilators, and intubation of the stomach is frequently necessary.

The patient's body weight, hematocrit, serum electrolytes, and fluid intake and output must be monitored carefully to avoid inadvertent fluid overload and interstitial pulmonary edema.

Positive sputum cultures do not necessarily indicate pulmonary infection, and antibiotics should be administered only after careful assessment of clinical, radiologic, and laboratory findings.

Frequent (hourly) change of position and chest physiotherapy are useful in preventing atelectasis and promoting drainage of secretions.

Discontinuing Ventilatory Support

When the patient demonstrates some reserve of ventilatory function (vital capacity greater than 10 ml/kg) and adequate oxygenation of the arterial blood can be achieved with inspired oxygen concentration of 50% or less, increasing periods of spontaneous ventilation are allowed. Supplemental oxygen and close observation are mandatory during initial trials, as hypoxemia, cardiac arrhythmias, or deterioration of circulatory function may occur rapidly.

There is no evidence that any specific pulmonary lesions are induced by mechanical ventilators, and patients may recover from many months of ventilatory support without sequelae.

ELECTRICAL SAFETY

The increasing use of electronic instrumentation for diagnostic, therapeutic, and monitoring purposes creates some hazards for patients. In the operating suite, improper grounding of equipment has resulted in electrical burns from the electrosurgical cautery, ECG leads, and circulating water blankets. Patients with indwelling intravascular catheters in proximity to the heart or with cardiac pacemaker wires in place are "electrically sensitive" in that minor current leaks may produce serious arrhythmias. Such patients should be electrically isolated from direct contact with any AC-powered instrument. Contacts to be isolated include ECG leads and pressure transducers. Expert advice should be obtained concerning the safe use of biomedical devices and electrical installations.

15...

Emergency Management of the Injured Patient

Carleton Mathewson, Jr., MD

Each year the American public pays a frightful price in lives, pain, and money for accidents which appear to be part and parcel of the technologic sophistication of modern life. In the USA alone, the increase in the power and speed of vehicles and machinery, the mechanization of farm labor, and work at great heights and depths have brought with them an increase in the number and severity of injuries: 50 million injuries a year, 115,000 deaths, 400,000 permanent disabilities, and a financial cost of $13.6 billion.

Accident patients take up 22 million hospital beds a year—more beds than heart patients and 4 times more than cancer patients. During wartime, deaths from accidents always exceed battle deaths. In World War II, American battle deaths were 292,000. Accidental civilian deaths during the same period were 450,000. During the Korean conflict, the accidental death toll on the home front was 4 times the toll of the American dead on the Korean battlefields.

Accidental trauma has been rightfully called the neglected disease of modern society. Many studies have shown that death and disability are often attributable to lack of proper treatment at the scene of an accident, during transportation to a hospital, or in the hospital emergency room. Recent experience in the armed services has reemphasized the importance of the presence of trained personnel at the scene of an accident and the necessity for immediate institution of resuscitative measures. Rapid transportation, with the patient being given emergency care en route by trained personnel, has saved numerous lives under combat conditions. Similar facilities should be provided in civilian life, particularly in rural areas where quick transportation to and from the scene of an accident becomes a lifesaving factor. Furthermore, great efforts are being made by a number of agencies—including various medical societies (especially the American College of Surgeons), federal agencies, and lay organizations—to improve the care and transportation of the seriously injured.

Multiple injuries involving several body systems constitute a significant factor in mortality and prolonged or permanent disability. Yet our present knowledge of the management of multiple severe injuries is such that, if it were properly applied, many lives could be saved and residual disabilities avoided. The important steps in emergency care which should be familiar to every physician and surgeon are presented in the following pages.

IMMEDIATE MEASURES AT THE SCENE OF AN ACCIDENT

When first seen, the victim of an accident may not appear to be badly injured. There may be little or no gross external evidence of trauma. Therefore, when the mechanism of trauma has been such that severe injury might be expected, it is important that the victim be handled as if severe injury has occurred.

The injured person must be protected from further trauma. First aid at the scene of an accident should be administered by trained personnel whenever possible. Inexperienced persons should not move a victim of trauma. The simple act of moving an injured victim from one position to another, if done improperly, may compound a fracture, compress or lacerate the spinal cord, puncture a lung, or sever a major vessel—thereby converting a simple injury into a major surgical problem.

Wherever the patient is first seen—on the battlefield, beside a road, in the emergency ward, or in the hospital—the basic principles of initial management are the same:

(1) Is he breathing? If not, provide an airway and maintain respiratory exchange.

(2) Is there a pulse or heartbeat? If not, begin external cardiac massage.

(3) Is there gross external bleeding? If so, elevate the part if possible and apply external pressure over the major artery to the part. A tourniquet is rarely needed.

(4) Is there any question of injury to the spine? If so, protect before moving the patient.

(5) Splint obvious fractures.

As soon as these steps have been taken, the patient can be safely transported. In the emergency ward, shock is treated even as the emergency survey

---

*Eye injuries are discussed in Chapter 43. Penetrating and nonpenetrating wounds are discussed briefly here and in greater detail in Chapter 17.

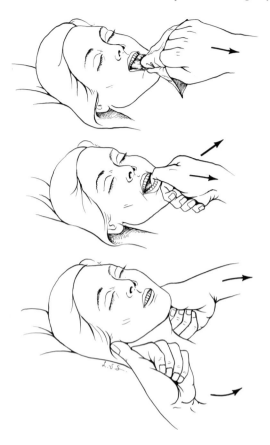

FIG 15−1. **Relief of airway obstruction.**

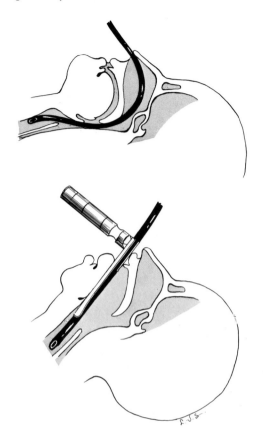

FIG 15−2. *Top:* Nasotracheal intubation. ***Bottom:*** Orotracheal intubation.

examination is performed, followed by definitive treatment.

The details of each step in management are as follows:

Asphyxia

A. Airway Obstruction: (Fig 15−1.) An open airway is essential to life and must be provided at once. This can often be done by simple manipulation of the mandible or traction on the tongue, particularly in unconscious or semiconscious patients. After the mouth is forced open, the tongue can be grasped between the thumb and forefinger covered with a handkerchief or gauze bandage. The tip of the tongue should be pulled forward beyond the front teeth. The mandible should be manipulated either by pulling forward the angles of the lower jaw or by inserting the thumb between the teeth, grasping the mandible in the midline, and drawing it forward until the lower teeth are leading. Often, however—particularly in the presence of severe facial injury—it may be necessary to introduce an artificial airway (Fig 15−2). This requires the immediate availability of trained attendants with the proper instruments. Tracheostomy should not be attempted at the scene of an accident. On rare occasions, the introduction of a large-bore needle (eg, 13

gauge) into the trachea may provide an adequate temporary airway (Fig 15−3).

Suctioning of the mouth and pharynx may clear them sufficiently of blood, mucus, or vomitus to permit normal respiration. Repeated suctioning may be required to maintain an adequate airway at the scene of the accident and during transit to a medical facility. Aspiration of vomitus is a frequent cause of sudden death and must be prevented at all costs. A lateral and slightly head-down position is best for patients who are liable to vomit. In respiratory arrest, a clear airway must be provided and mouth-to-mouth breathing instituted if other means of ventilation are not available (Fig 15−4).

B. Sucking Wound: An open or sucking wound of the chest must be closed as soon as it is recognized. This is best done at the scene of an accident by strapping or holding a sterile or clean dressing over the open wound. In desperate situations with marked respiratory distress, one should not hesitate to close the wound as nearly airtight as possible with any material available (towel, scarf, shirt, etc).

C. Tension Pneumothorax: Tension pneumothorax is a common cause of asphyxiation which is usually not recognized until a physician examines the patient. Increasing dyspnea and cyanosis are the prin-

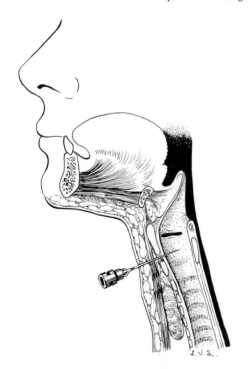

FIG 15–3. Needle in trachea to establish temporary airway.

cipal features. Absent breath sounds, hyperresonance, cardiac displacement, pallor, and a rapid, feeble pulse are other clinical signs. If untreated, tension pneumothorax can be fatal because the collapse of one lung is soon followed by a shift of the mediastinum to the opposite side and interference with cardiac filling and function of the opposite lung. Aspiration of air from the pleural cavity with a needle and syringe may be sufficient as a temporary measure to relieve the intrathoracic tension (Fig 15–5).

Cardiac Arrest (See also Chapter 23.)

Cardiac arrest, when encountered at the scene of an accident, is usually fatal because it is not recognized as such by lay personnel. Absence of heart sounds and pulse means cardiac arrest. Lives may be saved by immediate action. Blood flow to the brain must be reestablished within 4 minutes if permanent cerebral damage or death is to be avoided. Begin the following 2 procedures immediately: (1) Establish ventilation by mouth-to-mouth breathing. (2) Start closed chest cardiac massage (see Chapter 23).

Hemorrhage

Gross hemorrhage from accessible surface wounds is usually obvious and can be controlled in the great majority of cases by local pressure and elevation of the part. Firm pressure on the major artery in the axilla, antecubital space, wrist, groin, and popliteal space or at the ankle may suffice for temporary control of arterial hemorrhage distal to these points. When other measures have failed, a tourniquet may rarely be necessary to control major hemorrhage from extensive wounds or major vessels in an extremity. However, failure to release a tourniquet periodically may cause irreparable vascular or neurologic damage, and the tourniquet must therefore be kept exposed and loosened at least every 20 minutes for 1 or 2 minutes while the patient is in transit and permanently as soon as definitive care is given. It is wise to write the letters TK on the patient's forehead with skin-marking pencil or adhesive tape.

Restoration of blood volume at the scene of an accident and during transit to a hospital by the intravenous administration of lactated Ringer's injection or normal saline solution is at times a lifesaving measure and emphasizes the importance of the availability of proper equipment and personnel for immediate care.

Shock (See also Chapter 16.)

Some degree of shock accompanies most severe injuries and is manifested initially by pallor, cold sweat, weakness, lightheadedness, hypotension, tachycardia, thirst, air hunger, and eventual loss of consciousness.

A. Primary or Neurogenic Shock (Syncope or Fainting): Primary shock is due to the rapid pooling of blood in the splanchnic bed and voluntary muscles and is usually caused by psychic or nervous stimuli such as fright, sudden pain, or anxiety. It is self-limited and can be relieved by rest in the recumbent or Trendelenburg position. If the patient does not improve quickly, other types of shock must be considered.

B. Hypovolemic or Oligemic Shock: Hypovolemic shock is due to loss of whole blood or plasma. Blood pressure may be maintained initially by vasoconstriction. As hypotension ensues, tissue hypoxia increases; if prolonged, it may cause irreparable damage to the vital centers and shock becomes irreversible. Massive or prolonged hemorrhage, severe crushing injuries, major fractures, and extensive burns are the most common causes. The presence of any of these conditions is an indication for prompt institution of fluid replacement.

The patient must be kept recumbent and given reassurance and analgesics as necessary. Opiates, if necessary for relief of pain, are best administered intravenously in small doses. Subcutaneous injections are poorly absorbed in these circumstances and, if repeated, may accumulate and cause respiratory depression as circulating blood volume is restored.

Fractures

The recognition and splinting of major fractures and the immobilization of all injured parts before transportation are essential features of early management. Improper handling of the injured may increase or prolong shock and aggravate existing trauma beyond the possibility of definitive repair. "Splint 'em where they lie" is a time-honored rule of emergency care of fractures that has only a few exceptions—eg, when it is necessary to remove an injured patient from imminent danger of fire, explosion, escaping gas, etc. Improvised splints can be fashioned with boards, pillows, blankets,

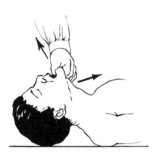
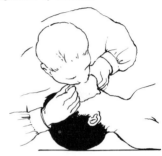

Method A: Clear mouth and throat. Place patient supine. Insert left thumb between patient's teeth, grasp mandible firmly in midline, and draw it forward (upward) so that the lower teeth are leading. Close patient's nose with right hand. Gauze (as shown) or airway may be used but is not necessary.

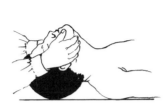
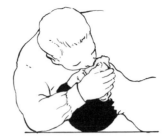

Method B: Clear mouth and throat. Place patient supine. Pull strongly forward at angle of mandible. Close patient's nose with your cheek. Gauze (as shown) or airway may be used but is not necessary.

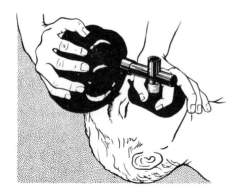

Instructions for Use of Manual Resuscitator
1. Lift the victim's neck with one hand.
2. Tilt head backward into maximum neck extension. Remove secretions and debris from mouth and throat, and pull the tongue and mandible forward as required to clear the airway.
3. Hold the mask snugly over the nose and mouth, holding the chin forward and the neck in extension as shown in diagram.
4. Squeeze the bag, noting inflation of the lungs by the rise of the chest wall.
5. Release the bag, which will expand spontaneously. The patient will exhale and the chest will fall.
6. Repeat steps 4 and 5 approximately 12 times per minute.

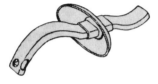

Airway for Use in Mouth-to-Mouth Insufflation. The larger airway is for adults. The guard is flexible and may be inverted from the position shown for use with infants and children.

FIG 15–4. Technic of mouth-to-mouth resuscitation and assisted ventilation with a bag and face mask.

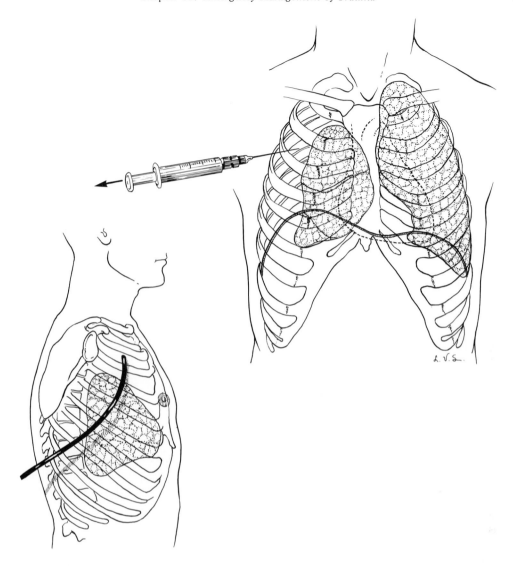

FIG 15–5. Relief of pneumothorax. Tension pneumothorax must be immediately decompressed by a needle
introduced through the second anterior intercostal space. A chest tube is usually inserted through the second
or third anterior intercostal space in the midclavicular line and directed toward the apex of the thorax. The
tube is attached to the suction device, and the rate of escape of air is indicated by the appearance of bubbles
in the second of the 3 bottles. When bubbling ceases, this suggests that the air leak has become sealed.

or other materials, but some sort of immobilization
must be provided even at the cost of a delay in transporting the patient to a hospital (Figs 15–6 to 15–9).

Transportation

Transportation by ground or air ambulance is
preferable when feasible. A station wagon or truck is
preferable to a passenger car. The manipulation necessary to load a seriously injured person into a passenger
car may be most harmful. Patients with internal
injuries, head injuries, spinal, pelvic, and lower extremity injuries, patients in shock, and patients with major
soft tissue wounds should be transported in the supine
position. The time lost in waiting for proper trans-

portation is rarely as harmful as the added trauma of
improper transportation. Resuscitation of the seriously
injured should be maintained during transportation,
and a constant effort must be made to avoid airway
obstruction and aspiration if the patient is vomiting.

EMERGENCY ROOM CARE

Temporary measures to control the immediate
effects of trauma have usually been taken before the
patient arrives in the emergency room. More definitive

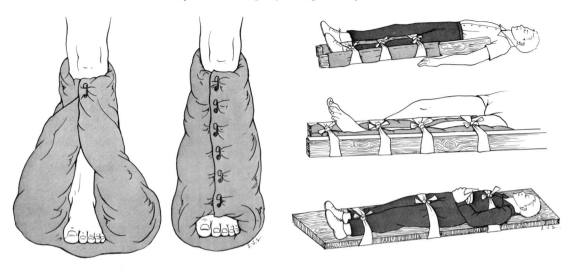

FIG 15–6. Pillow splint.

FIG 15–7. Fracture of femur. Emergency immobilization.

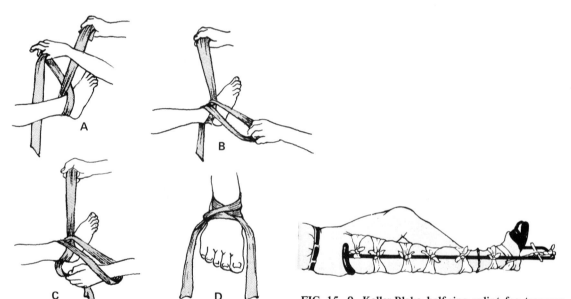

FIG 15–8. Method of tying Collins hitch.

FIG 15–9. Keller-Blake half-ring splint for transportation of patient with fracture of thigh or leg. Spanish windlass on a Collins hitch.

measures must be initiated as soon as he is delivered to a hospital. All clothing should be removed at once (cut off, if necessary) from the seriously injured patient, taking great care to avoid unnecessary movement. Immediate steps must be taken to correct life-endangering asphyxia, hemorrhage, and shock.

Asphyxia

Asphyxia due to any cause is the most urgent emergency situation, and its correction takes precedence over any other treatment or diagnostic measure. An adequate airway must be provided at once. If this cannot be accomplished by simple means, such as

extending the head and pulling the jaw forward (Fig 15–1) or by suctioning the trachea (Fig 15–10), the immediate introduction of an endotracheal tube with suction and the administration of oxygen are indicated (Fig 15–2). Massive hemorrhage and cardiac arrest should be controlled simultaneously.

Cardiac Arrest

Cardiac arrest is evidenced by the absence of peripheral pulses, blood pressure, and audible heart sounds, resulting from a sudden cessation of cardiac function in the form of (1) asystole, (2) ventricular fibrillation, or (3) ineffective myocardial contraction

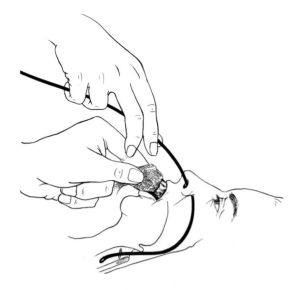

FIG 15–10. Tracheal aspiration.

with grossly inadequate cardiac output.

Treatment is described in detail in Chapter 23.

Tension Pneumothorax

Tension pneumothorax, if not already relieved, may require initial relief by aspiration with a large-bore needle. As soon as possible, however, in the emergency ward, this should be replaced by insertion of a thoracotomy tube in the second intercostal space anteriorly. Underwater suction should be applied. The technic of thoracotomy tube insertion is described in Chapter 52. If oxygen administered under positive pressure is required, there is danger of a sudden, severe tension pneumothorax which will lead to anoxia, cardiac arrest, and death if not relieved immediately. Whenever oxygen is administered under pressure, this complication must be anticipated. Tube drainage of one or both chests may be required as an emergency measure (Fig 15–5).

Flail Chest

Flail chest develops when several ribs or the sternum are fractured in more than one place. The unsupported chest wall segment behaves in paradoxic fashion, sucking in during inspiration (negative intrapleural pressure) and blowing out during expiration.

The major consequences of a flail chest are as follows: (1) Oxygen desaturation, caused by functional right to left shunt created by failure of the lung under the flail segment to ventilate. (2) Disturbed cardiac output, due to compromise of venous return because of swinging of the mediastinum. (3) Impaired coughing, resulting in retained secretions. (4) One of the major problems is the enormous increase in the work required to breathe. This is why the patient may arrive in the emergency room without oxygen desaturation and then suddenly develop severe cyanosis because sufficient energy is no longer available.

Relief of these consequences of flail chest is best accomplished by endotracheal intubation and controlled positive pressure ventilation (see Chapter 17).

Sucking Wounds

Sucking wounds of the chest also require immediate attention and should be sealed at least temporarily by the application of a clean dressing (sterile, if available). A petrolatum gauze dressing will prevent air leakage. Large wounds that cannot be controlled by dressings may require temporary closure of the skin by means of towel clips or large stitches in the skin. Definitive closure is accomplished best in the operating room. Control of respiration should be established with an endotracheal tube.

Mediastinal Emphysema

Mediastinal emphysema may cause sufficient tension to produce embarrassment to cardiac function and mediastinal vessels. Aspiration of air from the supraclavicular space or cervical mediastinotomy may be necessary to relieve compression.

Hemorrhage

A. External Hemorrhage: When the patient reaches the emergency room, definitive steps must be taken to control bleeding. Surface wounds should be inspected and major bleeding controlled with clamps and sutures. Subsequent debridement, followed by open or closed management of the wound, is best undertaken with anesthesia in the operating room under aseptic conditions. If bleeding is already controlled by pressure dressings, it may be best to leave these in place until shock is reversed and definitive care in the operating room can be undertaken.

B. Concealed Hemorrhage: Concealed hemorrhage must be suspected in all patients with signs of hypovolemic shock but no external blood loss. If signs of shock do not respond to resuscitative measures, open surgery in the operating room may be required for control. Delay in control of major bleeding into the thorax or abdomen may be fatal.

C. Hemothorax: Hemothorax is a common complication of open or closed injuries to the chest. The most serious forms are associated with injuries of large pulmonary vessels or intercostal arteries. Fairly large accumulations of blood in the pleural cavity may cause very little respiratory distress and, unless associated with pneumothorax, may not require immediate relief. The signs of respiratory impairment depend upon the amount of air and blood in the pleural cavity. Needle aspiration of the chest may be sufficient to afford temporary relief. However, blood and air are apt to reaccumulate, causing further respiratory distress. For this reason, tube drainage with an underwater seal (Fig 15–5) not only provides more efficient drainage but also demonstrates whether hemorrhage is still occurring. Continued bleeding may require open thoracotomy for control. Relief of hemothorax in the emergency room is required only when the accumulation of blood is sufficient to cause respiratory distress or hypovolemic shock.

Portable x-ray films of the chest are essential to determine the extent of hemothorax and the presence or absence of associated injury to the thoracic wall, the heart, and the mediastinum.

D. Cardiac Tamponade: Accumulation of blood in the pericardial space may occur when the heart is injured either by penetrating wounds or by compression injuries to the chest. The clinical features include pallor, sweating, cyanosis, dyspnea, hypotension, distant or inaudible heart sounds, and a weak and sometimes irregular or paradoxic pulse. The neck veins are usually distended. Aspiration of the pericardium (Fig 15—11) may be lifesaving and should be attempted as soon as cardiac tamponade is recognized; however, if aspiration fails, immediate steps should be taken to accomplish pericardial decompression by means of open chest resuscitation in the operating room.

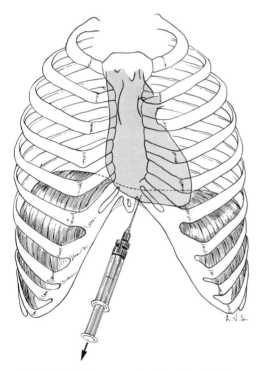

FIG 15—11. Removal of pericardial effusion.

E. Intra-abdominal and Retroperitoneal Hemorrhage: Intra-abdominal hemorrhage may be extremely difficult to detect in the absence of abdominal signs because the clinical manifestations are predominantly those associated with blood loss; therefore, intra-abdominal or retroperitoneal bleeding must be suspected and searched for in patients presenting with signs and symptoms of bleeding when the source is not evident.

Recognition and management are discussed in Chapter 17.

Shock (See also Chapter 16.)

Although initial steps may have been taken to relieve shock before admission to the emergency room, aggressive measures should be instituted at once. Impending shock should be suspected in all patients who have sustained severe trauma. Several intravenous routes should be established immediately. Large-bore needles are recommended. If the veins are collapsed, a cutdown should be performed immediately. When cutdowns are necessary, the superficial femoral or the antecubital veins (or both) should be used. In patients with major wounds of the abdomen and pelvis, only the veins of the upper extremities and neck should be utilized. This will prevent extravasation of transfused blood or fluids into the traumatized area. A catheter should be introduced via the right antecubital vein, right subclavian vein, or right external jugular vein into or near the right atrium so that central venous pressure monitoring can be started. Lactated Ringer's injection in large amounts may be required to provide volume replacement until blood becomes available. A urinary catheter should be kept in place to monitor urinary output. Fluid replacement should be rapid enough to obtain a blood pressure above 100 mm Hg, urinary flow of 30 ml/hour, and central venous pressure readings of 5—15 cm water. Absence of response to the administration of fluids and blood may mean massive internal hemorrhage requiring immediate surgery.

When massive transfusion is necessary, freshly drawn blood should be used exclusively if at all possible. If fresh blood is in short supply, use at least 1 unit to every 6—8 units of bank blood. The blood should be warmed during administration to avoid adverse effects in the cardiovascular system.

The nature of shock and its management are discussed more completely in Chapter 16.

TETANUS PROPHYLAXIS

Tetanus prophylaxis (see Chapter 10) should be given in all instances of open contaminated wounds, puncture wounds, and burns. No single prophylaxis plan can be applied to all patients.

EVALUATION OF THE INJURED PATIENT

A rapid and complete history and physical examination (with a written record of the findings) is imperative in patients with serious or multiple injuries. Progressive changes in signs and symptoms are often the key to correct diagnosis, and negative findings which change to positive may be of great importance in revising an initial clinical evaluation. This is particularly true in intra-abdominal, intrathoracic, and head injuries, which frequently do not become manifest until hours after the initial trauma.

Coma

Various stages of coma due to a variety of causes may accompany injury and will require treatment while initial steps are being taken to diagnose and treat the associated trauma.

Coma may be due to many causes. The most common are alcoholic intoxication, cerebrovascular accidents, diabetic acidosis, barbiturate poisoning, narcotic overdosage, and hypovolemic shock. Less common causes are epilepsy, eclampsia, and electrolyte imbalances associated with metabolic and systemic diseases. Other causes include anaphylaxis, heavy metal poisoning, electric shock, tumors, severe systemic infections, hypercalcemia, asphyxia, heat stroke, severe heart failure, and hysteria.

The differential diagnosis of unconsciousness depends upon (1) a careful history from available informants; (2) a careful and complete physical examination, with particular attention to the neurologic examination; and (3) laboratory tests such as urinalysis, blood counts, blood cultures, blood glucose, urea, ammonia, electrolytes, and alcohol, and CSF examination; and (4) skull x-rays. One should also search the patient for a medical card or medallion indicating known preexisting disease.

A. Immediate Care: If the injuries are extensive and there are signs of hypovolemic shock, coma is very likely due to cerebral ischemia. Resuscitation and blood volume replacement have first priority. If there are no signs of shock, head injury and other causes of coma are likely (see Chapter 41).

Early gastric lavage with activated charcoal may be helpful in preventing further absorption of alcohol or ingested drugs. Care must be taken to prevent aspiration. Deepening stupor in patients under observation should arouse suspicion of an expanding intracranial lesion requiring repeated thorough neurologic examinations. Too often one accepts obvious acute alcoholism as the cause of the unconscious state only to learn that increasing treatable intracranial hemorrhage has been overlooked.

B. Laboratory Studies in the Emergency Evaluation of Trauma: When coma is present, laboratory studies may be helpful in ruling out the following diseases: blood alcohol levels in acute alcoholism; blood and urine glucose levels in diabetic coma and hypoglycemic shock; and serum potassium, BUN, and creatinine in uremia.

DEFINITIVE CARE

Everyone who may have information about the circumstances of the injury should be questioned. Knowing the mechanism of the injury often gives a clue to concealed trauma. Unfortunately, obvious injuries may absorb the attention of the examiner and cause him to overlook less obvious but more serious head, spinal, abdominal, or thoracic lesions. Serious underlying medical problems may be overlooked in the absence of an accurate history. Distorted extremity fractures, bleeding lacerations, and head injuries are usually obvious and attract almost immediate attention. Too frequently, patients with these injuries are sent for prolonged x-ray studies while less apparent but more serious internal injuries go undetected.

Combined Injuries

Certain types of trauma are apt to cause more than one injury. Fractures of the calcaneus resulting from a fall from a great height are often associated with central dislocation of the hip and with fractures of the spine and the base of the skull. A crushed pelvis is often combined with rupture of the posterior urethra or bladder. Crush injuries of the chest are often associated with lacerations or rupture of the spleen, liver, or diaphragm. Penetrating wounds of the chest may involve not only the thoracic contents but also the abdominal viscera. These combinations of injuries occur frequently and should always be suspected.

Physical Examination

As soon as respiratory and circulatory function has been established and gross arterial bleeding controlled, a rapid survey examination as described in Chapter 1 should be performed. The initial appraisal of the extent of the injuries will then be completed, and plans for definitive care can be formulated.

Laboratory Studies

At the same time that intravenous needles or catheters are inserted for the treatment of shock, blood should be drawn for laboratory studies. If there is any indication that the injury is major or complex, the following should be obtained: hematocrit, P_{O_2}, P_{CO_2}, BUN, serum creatinine, serum electrolytes, and serum amylase. Arterial pH should be determined in critical cases. The urine should be examined for specific gravity, red and white cells, protein, and sugar. Catheterization may be necessary. If the patient is in critical condition, the catheter should be left in place for continuous recording of urinary output.

These determinations are a guide to the severity of the injuries and provide an essential baseline for continuing management.

X-Ray Examination

Films of the chest and abdomen are required in all cases of major injury. An intravenous urogram is of critical importance in abdominal injuries and pelvic fractures. It should not be done while the patient is in shock.

X-rays of the skull and long bones can usually be deferred until the more critical injuries of the thorax and abdomen have been cared for.

PRIORITIES FOR DEFINITIVE CARE

Certain injuries are so critical that operative treatment must be undertaken as soon as the diagnosis is made. In these cases, resuscitation is continued as the patient is being operated on. At times the situation is so urgent that anesthesia is induced after the operation has begun rather than beforehand. Profound shock may render the patient unconscious from cerebral ischemia. For example, with certain penetrating wounds of the heart, the chest should be opened in the emergency ward and the hole in the heart plugged with a finger. Resuscitation, induction of anesthesia, and a formal thoracotomy are then carried out simultaneously. Many abdominal wounds involving the aorta and vena cava cause such massive hemorrhage that shock cannot be corrected until the bleeding is controlled and surgical repair must become a part of resuscitation. Rarely, wounds near the hilum of the lung may produce the same type of exsanguinating hemorrhage. Usually, however, the life-threatening complications of chest injuries such as tension pneumothorax, open sucking wounds, or flail chest can be corrected immediately without operation as described above.

Cerebral injuries take precedence in care only when there is rapidly deepening coma. Extradural bleeding is a critical emergency requiring operation for its control and cerebral decompression. Subdural bleeding may produce a similar emergency. If the condition of the patient permits, arteriography should be performed for localization of the bleeding. In many cases of combined cerebral and abdominal injury with massive bleeding, laparotomy and craniotomy are carried out simultaneously.

On the other hand, fractures of the skull have a low priority and usually can be dealt with after the treatment of more critical abdominal or thoracic injuries.

Most urologic injuries are managed simultaneously with associated intra-abdominal injury. Pelvic fractures present special problems discussed in Chapters 44 and 46.

Unless there is associated vascular injury with threatened ischemia of the limb, fractures of the long bones can be splinted and treated on a semi-emergency basis. On the other hand, open contaminated wounds should be cleansed and debrided as soon as possible.

Injuries of the hand often present the critical problem of potential infection which, if not treated early, may result in lifelong handicap to the patient. Essential early treatment of the hand at the same time as the life-threatening injuries avoids infection and preserves the patient's means of livelihood as well as his life.

In all cases of multiple injury, there must be a "captain of the team" who directs the resuscitation, decides which x-rays or special diagnostic tests should be obtained, and establishes priority for care by continuous consultation with other surgical specialists and anesthesiologists. A general surgeon with extensive experience in the care of the injured patient usually has this role.

The details of definitive management of injuries are discussed in Chapter 17 and in the sections on trauma of the various organ system chapters.

MISCELLANEOUS SPECIFIC EMERGENCIES
George F. Sheldon, MD

ELECTRICAL INJURIES

The injury inflicted by electricity depends on amperage, voltage, resistance, type of current, current pathway through the body, duration of flow, and surface area of contact. The actual danger to life is mainly due to the amperage. (This can never be positively predicted, since body resistance at the moment of an accident is unknown.) Although high-voltage shocks are occasionally survived, voltages of over 40 V are considered dangerous. The risk of thermal injury is directly proportionate to the voltage. Extensive burns after high-tension accidents are caused partly by arcing of the current. The extremely high temperature in an arc can melt bone and volatilize metal.

Resistance

A person completing a circuit forms a resistance of which the skin is the most important part. Skin resistance will depend on its thickness, moisture, and cleanliness at the time of injury. A wet palm increases the conductivity by as much as 1000-fold. Because the resistance of the skin of the trunk is greater than that of the skin on other parts of the body, the amount of heat released is considerably less and thermal damage to internal organs is rare.

Type of Current

Alternating current is more dangerous than direct current because it has a tetanizing effect. A patient may be locked to the contact until the circuit is broken and may succumb to an injury which otherwise would not be lethal. The smaller the area of contact, the greater the density and the more energy transformed into heat. A child may bite through a live cord and sustain deep burns of the face but no systemic effects. An individual in a bathtub, however, may touch an electrical source and be killed immediately without local lesions.

Low-Tension Injuries

In low-tension injuries, a victim may become locked to his contact. The thermal injury is primarily at the contact point. The most characteristic injury is a small, deep burn which may involve vessels, tendons, and nerves. Current marks are often found near the contact point and may heal spontaneously with small injuries. Secondary hemorrhage may occur, particularly after a low-tension contact in the mouth.

High-Tension Injuries

Locking is uncommon in high-tension injuries; instead, the victim is usually thrown violently away from the contact point, often sustaining injuries from blunt trauma. In some instances, the circuit is completed by arcing and is not actually touched by the patient.

When the current passes through the head, injury is usually confined to the scalp and the skull. Resistance in the cranial bones is mainly in the outer and inner table, with the conductor being the vascular diploë, so that cerebral complications are rare. The rate of current flow through the trunk is generally insufficient to injure internal organs.

A frequent feature of contact with high tension is disturbance of the cardiac pacemaker with ventricular fibrillation and death.

In general, burns from high-tension contact are like those from low tension. Late lesions (eg, electrical cataract) occur in some victims.

Vascular injuries are common with both low-tension and high-tension contact. Inflammation of the vessels to an extremity produces ischemia and the need for delayed amputation. Extensive sloughing or false aneurysm may occur. Spastic narrowing of arteries involved in the electrical arc may persist for several months after the injury.

Nerve injuries and dysfunction can be transient or permanent depending on the intensity of heat produced by the current.

The hand is most commonly burned. Severely disabling spastic flexion contractures occur as a result of grasping a high-tension wire. Arcs may enter the wrist, causing acute flexion. Tendons may be involved, and necrosis may occur on the volar side of the hand. Simultaneous damage of nerves and arteries may render an extremity useless.

Treatment

Initial treatment of the victim begins at the site of the electrocution. If the victim is locked to a low-tension source, the current must be turned off. Cardiopulmonary resuscitation is instituted by conventional methods. If electrocution is due to high-tension contact, ventricular fibrillation or cardiac arrest may occur. Defibrillation must be accomplished using direct current countershock or by striking the chest. Cardiac arrest must be treated by cardiopulmonary resuscitation. Following a high-tension stimulus, the victim may fall or be thrown, producing fractures or other injuries of greater significance than the burn.

Patients with electrical burns usually require more fluids than their external injury would suggest since a large amount of deep tissue may be injured. Local treatment of the skin should be by the exposure method. The surgeon can visually observe the injury

and more accurately plan the timing of sequential debridement, which is usually necessary. The initial debridement is usually done within the first 2 weeks after injury. Damaged tendons, nerves, and vessels must be cared for with a view toward functional restoration during the staged debridements.

Artz CP: Electrical injury simulates crush injury. Surg Gynec Obst 125:1316, 1967.

Baxter CR: Present concepts in the management of major electrical injury. S Clin North America 50:1401–1418, 1970.

Mills W Jr, Switzer WE, Moncrief JA: Electrical injuries. JAMA 195:852–854, 1966.

Skoog T: Electrical injuries. J Trauma 10:816–830, 1970.

HEAT STROKE

Heat stroke is an uncommon but grave medical emergency. A crucial delay in therapy may be due to difficulty in differentiating the disorder from other causes of hyperpyrexia.

Heat stroke occurs when the temperature-humidity index is high (> 87). It commonly occurs in individuals who are not acclimatized to heat exposure. Older patients with cardiovascular disease are particularly vulnerable. Heat stroke frequently occurs in athletes, soldiers, and weekend sportsmen beginning conditioning. It may also be found in individuals with congenital absence of sweat glands, fibrocystic disease, or after sympathectomy of all 4 extremities.

Heat stroke results from a combination of increased environmental heat, increased humidity, and diminished ability to diffuse heat. When the external heat approaches 90% of body temperature, the ability to diffuse heat is markedly impaired.

Clinical Findings

The patient will usually present with CNS manifestations such as coma. Meningismus and convulsions may be present initially or develop later. The body temperature is usually above 40 C (104 F), although a somewhat lower body temperature does not exclude the diagnosis.

All patients with heat stroke do not have dry skin. In severe heat prostration, the patient will present in clinical shock. A coagulation disorder will be apparent from petechial hemorrhages or frothy sputum. Urinary output will be scant or absent, and proteinuria with casts and red blood cells is usually found.

Treatment

The heat stroke victim in coma is an extreme medical emergency. Central venous pressure monitoring should be instituted immediately, and, if the patient is dehydrated and volume-depleted, intravenous infusion of fluids must be started. A body temperature increase from 37 to 42 C will increase oxygen consumption by 40% and double the cardiac output.

When core temperature reaches about 41 C (106 F), cardiac muscle will begin to lose contractile force, and many of these patients are suffering from low-output syndrome when initially seen. Isoproterenol is the drug of choice to increase inotropic activity of the myocardium, and the concomitant peripheral vasodilatation will aid heat diffusion.

Endotracheal intubation should be instituted immediately to help support the failing cardiorespiratory system. When first examined, over half of these patients will have pulmonary consolidation, which may be due to bacterial pneumonia or to microemboli resulting from coagulation defects.

The severe metabolic acidosis which accompanies heat stroke requires correction with intravenous solutions containing bicarbonate. After the patient has been placed on a respirator, hypothermic therapy should be immediately instituted. Ice bags placed around his extremities will be effective treatment if chlorpromazine (Thorazine) is administered to obviate shivering. Diazepam (Valium) may be of use in controlling convulsions. Secondary rewarming may occur. If available, monitoring by temperature (thermistor) probes should be continued even if treatment is apparently successful.

The hematocrit is often elevated, reflecting dehydration. Serum electrolytes may show hypernatremia, although normal serum sodium values are common. Serum potassium levels will usually be low and should be monitored closely during cooling to prevent cardiac arrhythmias.

Hypofibrinogenemia and thrombocytopenia are commonly combined with other coagulation defects such as fibrinolysis. It is likely that consumption coagulopathy and disseminated intravascular coagulation are responsible. Appropriate therapy consists of heparin combined with transfusion of fresh blood.

Heat stroke can be averted by conditioning. Persons in sedentary occupations should not suddenly adopt a rigorous program of outdoor activity. Vulnerable individuals should be cautioned about the dangers of high heat-humidity exposure.

Eichler AC, McFee AS, Root HD: Heatstroke. Am J Surg 118:855–863, 1969.

Knochel JP & others: What are the important features of the optimal treatment of heat stroke? Mod Med 39:168–171, 1970.

Meikle AW, Graybill JR: Fibrinolysis and hemorrhage in a fatal case of heat stroke. New England J Med 276:911–912, 1967.

Schibolet S & others: Heatstroke: Its clinical picture and mechanism in 36 cases. Quart J Med 144:525–548, 1967.

Schrier RW & others: Renal, metabolic and circulatory responses to heat and exercise: Studies in military recruits during summer training, with implications for acute renal failure. Ann Int Med 73:213–223, 1970.

COLD INJURY

Cold injury is a significant military and civilian problem. First degree cold injury is manifested by simple erythema; second degree injury produces bullae, paresthesias, and hyperemia after rewarming; third degree injury causes edema and necrosis; and fourth degree injury consists of pallor and necrosis and implies an expected loss of a part. Such classifications, however, are of little prognostic value.

The risk of cold injury can be partly assessed from the patient's history. The duration of exposure and the extent of protective covering are most important; date, time, geographic location, and elevation are also significant. Predisposing patient factors include alcohol ingestion, drug intoxication, and vascular insufficiency.

Perhaps the most important secondary feature of hypothermic exposure is the contact of the part with metal (eg, rifle barrel) or water (eg, melted snow).

Cold injury is commonest when the temperature is less than 6.6 C (20 F). An occasional injury will be produced by exposure of moist skin surfaces to high wind velocities rather than extremes of cold. Significant cooling to 18–21 C (65–70 F) core body temperature can be achieved in moderate climates if exposure is pronounced. These patients often are alcoholics or drug addicts who are brought to the hospital in profound hypothermia and coma.

The treatment of the patient with generalized hypothermia consists of rapid rewarming in an environment with temperatures of 37.8–40 C (100–104 F). Sodium bicarbonate should not be administered unless arterial blood pH is below 7.1. With rewarming, metabolic functions will gradually return and the patient will improve.

Treatment of cold injury of an extremity should be by rapid rewarming in a warm water bath maintained at 37.8–40 C (100–104 F). In general, the slower the thawing, the greater the tissue damage that occurs. Anticoagulation with heparin or low molecular weight dextran has been recommended, but its effectiveness has not been established. Instability of the sympathetic nervous system has been observed in some patients, particularly following second degree immersion injury. Experimental evidence suggests that early sympathectomy may have some benefit.

Hardenbergh E, Miles JA: The effect of sympathectomy on tissue loss after experimental frost bite of the rabbit ear. J Surg Res 13:126–134, 1972.

Knize DM & others: Prognostic factors in the management of frost bite. J Trauma 9:749–759, 1969.

SNAKEBITE

Although venomous snakes are found in greatest numbers in tropical and subtropical countries, significant numbers may be found in temperate regions also. Only 4 poisonous snakes are indigenous to the USA. Three are pit vipers: the rattlesnake, the cottonmouth, and the copperhead. The coral snake is a member of the Elapid family (cobra-like) and has a venom unrelated to that of the pit vipers. Pit vipers can be distinguished from nonvenomous snakes by a rounded mouth with a pit between the eyes and the nares on each side.

Snake venom contains proteolytic enzymes and other substances which, when injected through the hollow teeth of the snake, can cause local tissue destruction and necrosis of blood vessels as well as profound neurotoxic or hemotoxic systemic reactions. Secondary edema spreads rapidly and may contribute to ischemia of an extremity. Bites on the fingers or toes may cause widespread destruction of digits, muscle compartments, and subcutaneous tissues. When intravascular injection occurs, bleeding secondary to low fibrinogen and platelet levels may ensue. Hemorrhage into tissue will exacerbate local pressure effects. Hemolysis of red cells may occur and produce acute tubular necrosis.

Treatment

A. First Aid Measures: There is much disagreement among authorities on the best way to treat snakebite. Physicians in snake-infested areas should be familiar with the types of snakes that may cause envenomation and be prepared to give advice or treatment based on their best understanding of the most responsible current practice.

1. Assess the extent of envenomation—A bite by a poisonous snake results in envenomation in only 50–70% of cases. Envenomation may be **mild** (scratch followed by a minimal swelling and not much pain); **moderate** (fang marks and local swelling and definite pain); or **severe** (fang marks, severe and progressive swelling, and severe pain).

2. Restrict activity—Provide reassurance and prevent exertion. The patient should be carried to a vehicle and transported to the nearest hospital.

3. Tourniquet—A flat tourniquet should be applied proximal to the bite, just tight enough to interrupt venous and lymphatic flow without affecting the arterial supply. It should be loosened every 30 minutes to avoid local tissue necrosis.

4. Local treatment of the wound—Incision and suction are recommended by some authorities and interdicted by others. After the tourniquet is in place, venom may be digitally expressed through the fang marks or after making a linear or cruciate incision through both fang marks and about 8 mm beyond. Mechanical suction may retrieve a significant amount of venom; mouth suction may be used but imposes a hazard of infection. Local treatment with ice has been said to increase the danger of necrosis, but some authorities feel that the risk of necrosis is outweighed by the advantages of holding the venom in situ until antivenin can be administered.

5. Antivenin—If envenomation has occurred and a commercial antivenin kit is available, administer the antivenin according to the instructions that accompany the kit after testing for horse serum sensitivity.

B. Hospital Treatment: Emergency hospital treatment consists of administering antivenin by intravenous drip as well as locally around the bite, plus fluids or blood as required. Antivenin should not be injected into a closed compartment such as a finger. Potential coagulation defects should be assessed and treated with appropriate component therapy or fresh blood.

The local injury should be assessed with a view toward further debridement. It may be necessary to debride the nearby fascia and subcutaneous tissue to prevent increasing edema and further tissue destruction.

Prognosis

The death rate following snake bite should be no more than 7% if adequate supportive care and specific antivenin are given. Significant morbidity may occur as a result of failure to perform early debridement and improper use of tourniquets.

Lockwood WE: Pitfalls in rattlesnake bite. Texas MJ 66:23, 1970.

Minton SA (editor): *Snake Venoms and Envenomation.* Dekker, 1971.

Reid HA: Snake bite. I: Clinical features. II: Treatment. Tropical Doctor 2:155–163, 1972.

ARTHROPOD BITES

Stings and bites of arthropods are most often merely a nuisance. Some arthropods, however, can produce death by direct toxicity or by hypersensitivity reactions. Because of their prevalence and widespread distribution, bees and wasps kill more people than any other venomous animal, including snakes.

Bees & Wasps

When a bee stings, it becomes anchored by the 2 barbed lancets so that withdrawal is impossible. In the struggle, a bee will usually avulse its stinging apparatus and die. After being stung by a bee, one should scrape the exuded poison sac with a sharp knife. Any attempt to pull the poison apparatus out will simply cause more venom to be squeezed into the tissue. The stinger, once imbedded, remains present. If this has occurred in an eyelid, it may irritate the globe of the eye months after the sting.

The stinging lancets of the wasp are not barbed and can easily be withdrawn by the insect to allow it to reinsert or to escape. It is unusual, therefore, to find a stinger left in place after a wasp sting. The females of the variety called yellow jackets are very aggressive. These insects sometimes bite prior to stinging.

The venom of bees and wasps contains histamine, basic protein components of high molecular weight, free amino acids, hyaluronidase, and acetylcholine. Antigenic proteins are species-specific and may lead to cross-reactivity between insects. Symptoms of arthropod stings may vary from minimal erythema to a marked local reaction or severe systemic toxicity (especially from multiple stings). Infection may occur, particularly from yellow jacket stings. A generalized allergic reaction may cause fatal anaphylaxis. A delayed reaction has been described which resembles serum sickness.

Early application of ice packs to reduce swelling is indicated. Elevation of the extremity is also useful. Oral antihistimines may be of some use in reducing urticaria. In exaggerated reactions, parenteral corticosteroids may be useful. If infection occurs, treatment consists of local debridement and antibiotics. Moderately severe reactions will present as generalized syncope or urticarial reactions. If an anaphylactic reaction or severe reaction is present, aqueous epinephrine, 0.5–1 ml of 1:1000 solution, should be given IM. A repeat dose may be given in 5–10 minutes, followed by 5–20 mg of diphenhydramine slowly IV. Administration of corticosteroids and general supportive measures such as oxygen administration, plasma expanders, and pressor agents may be required in case of shock. Previously sensitized patients should carry identifying tags and a kit for emergency intramuscular injection of epinephrine.

Spiders

The black widow spider (*Latrodectus mactans*) and the brown recluse spider (violin spider; *Loxosceles reclusa*) are most commonly incriminated as dangerous to man.

A. Black Widow Spider: The female black widow spider is characterized by a shiny black body with a red hourglass design on the under side of the abdomen. The male is smaller, less dark, and does not bite. The bite is usually followed by pain and muscular rigidity. Within 24 hours, the pain becomes severe, and a board-like abdomen is often present. A variety of symptoms such as convulsions, shock, and delirium may follow. Acute symptoms usually subside within 48 hours. Mortality may be as high as 5%.

Symptoms are usually self-limited. Initial treatment with debridement or tourniquet is to be condemned as the effect of black widow spider venom is instantaneous. Ice packs will reduce the pain. Intravenous injections of 10% calcium gluconate will relieve the muscle pain and spasm. A specific antivenin (horse serum) is available which is packaged with sterile water. Horse serum sensitivity testing and, if necessary, desensitization must precede use. The usual dose is 2.5 ml of restored serum given IM.

B. Brown Recluse Spider: The brown spider is dark tan in color and has 3 pairs of eyes on the ante-rior part of the cephalothorax. After biting, there is little local pain. At the puncture site, an erythematous bulla is present surrounded by a patch of ischemia. Within 8–10 hours after biting, this becomes dark, firm, and necrotic. An ulcer may form which may become indolent. A variety of severe systemic symptoms varying from hemoglobinuria to jaundice have been reported.

Corticosteroids should be given immediately to avert or alleviate systemic reactions. Treatment is with antibiotics, antihistamines, and often local debridement.

Denny WF & others: Hemotoxic effect of *Loxosceles reclusus* venom: In vivo and in vitro studies. J Lab Clin Med 64:291–298, 1964.

Frazier CA: Diagnosis and treatment of insect bites. Ciba 20:75–100, 1968.

Hershey FB, Aulenbacher CE: Surgical treatment of brown spider bites. Ann Surg 170:300–308, 1969.

Russell FE: Injuries by venomous animals. Am J Nursing 66:1322–1326, 1966.

BLAST INJURY

Blast injury is the result of the transmission of positive pressure waves during detonation of a high explosive. Injury is related to the nearness of the victim to the blast and the medium through which the pressure wave is transmitted. If the victim is in the water when exposed to a blast, great damage will occur since water is a high-density medium and much less compressible than air and will transmit the pressure waves with greater sustained intensity. Blast injuries may damage the contents of both the thoracic and abdominal cavities. If a victim is in water, he is more apt to sustain injury to intra-abdominal viscera. The viscera most commonly injured are the small and large bowel. Damage to the solid viscera (kidneys, spleen, and liver) is uncommon. The injuries to the bowel, primarily the colon, consist of subserosal hemorrhage and linear tears of the bowel wall.

Pulmonary injuries occur frequently when the positive wave medium is primarily the air. Rupture of alveoli and capillaries occurs, depending on the distance from the blast. Large bronchial and vascular structures may also be involved. The lung may be immediately transformed into a solidified structure.

Immediately following blast injury, the only symptom may be dyspnea. Rales are usually heard on auscultation of the chest, and hemoptysis may occur. As the process progresses, a frothy fluid and cyanosis develop. Chest x-ray may be normal initially and then progress to a picture of bilateral pulmonary infiltration. Pneumomediastinum from rupture of alveoli may occur. Progression to acute respiratory insufficiency may be rapid.

Treatment

If abdominal findings are present, the patient should have laparotomy and repair of injured intestine. Pulmonary care is supportive and requires endotracheal intubation, antibiotics, humidified oxygen, and careful monitoring of blood gases. Peak end-expiratory pressure should be employed from the outset to avoid alveolar edema.

Naclerio E: *Chest Injuries.* Grune & Stratton, 1971.

• • •

General References

American College of Surgeons Committee on Trauma: Essential equipment list for ambulances. Bull Am Coll Surg 55:7–13, 1970.

Borrie J: *Management of Emergencies in Thoracic Surgery.* Appleton-Century-Crofts, 1972.

Cole WH, Puestow CB: *Emergency Care: Surgical and Medical,* 7th ed. Appleton-Century-Crofts, 1972.

Committee on Trauma, American College of Surgeons: *Early Care of the Injured Patient.* Saunders, 1972.

Eckert C: *Emergency-Room Care.* Little, Brown, 1971.

Farrington JD, Hampton OP Jr: A curriculum for training emergency medical technicians. Bull Am Coll Surg 53:231–233, 1968.

Hampton OP Jr: The challenge of the trauma problem to organized medicine. J Trauma 10:926–931, 1970.

Levitt S: Fatal road accidents: Injuries, complications, and causes of death in 250 subjects. Brit J Surg 55:481–505, 1968.

Marshall SF, Nardi GL (editors): The management of surgical emergencies. S Clin North America 46:483–812, 1966.

Mathewson C: Early management of trauma patient. S Clin North America 52:531–537, 1972.

Mathewson C: Minor open wounds. Surg Gynec Obst 102: 369–371, 1956.

Mathewson C: Soft tissue injuries. Nebraska Med J 39:143, 1954.

Matthews DN (editor): Rehabilitation. Chap 24, pp 427–445, in: *Recent Advances in the Surgery of Trauma.* Little, Brown, 1963.

McNair TJ (editor): *Hamilton Bailey's Emergency Surgery,* 9th ed. Williams & Wilkins, 1972.

Moore FD: *Metabolic Care of the Surgical Patient.* Saunders, 1959.

Moore FD & others: *Post-Traumatic Pulmonary Insufficiency.* Saunders, 1969.

National Safety Council: *Accident Facts.* National Safety Council, 1969.

Shires T: Initial care of the injured patient. J Trauma 10:940–948, 1970.

Spencer JH: *The Hospital Emergency Department.* Thomas, 1972.

West IM & others: Natural death at the wheel. JAMA 205:266–271, 1968.

Wilson JL (editor): *Handbook of Surgery,* 4th ed. Lange, 1969.

Yarborough RW: Accidental injury: A major challenge to medicine. J Trauma 10:1010–1011, 1970.

16 . . .

Shock

F. William Blaisdell, MD

Shock is a breakdown of effective circulation at the cellular level. It occurs in association with many types of major illness such as trauma, hemorrhage, burns, infection, and cardiac disease and is the final event in most terminal illnesses.

Normal Physiology

The circulation is composed of the heart, the blood vessels (arteries, capillaries, and veins), and the blood. The arteries conduct blood to the tissues. Their terminal branches, the arterioles, provide effective resistance, control the blood pressure, and determine the perfusion of individual vascular beds. The veins act as the reservoir (capacitance) system, store at least half of the blood volume, and provide the priming pressure of the heart and thus help to determine cardiac output.

The normal blood volume averages about 8% of body weight and consists of 5−6 liters in the average adult. At any one moment, 10% of this volume will be in the arterial system, 20% in the capillaries, and 70% in the venous reservoir and heart. Since the venous system contains most of the blood, measuring the pressure in this system (central venous pressure, CVP) provides a rough estimate of the status of the blood volume.

The heart ejects 70−90 ml of blood with each beat at rest; this stroke volume correlates roughly with the blood volume and produces a systolic pressure of about 120 mm Hg. The arterioles provide the resistance in the circuit. The balance between cardiac output and peripheral resistance maintains pressure between cardiac contractions of roughly 80 mm Hg. This results in a mean pressure in the large arteries of about 95 mm Hg. Under normal circumstances, the blood vessels have the capacity for autoregulation−ie, through local reflexes which determine arteriolar tone, flow can be adjusted in accordance with tissue needs through a wide range of heart rates and blood pressures. The pressure in the arterioles is about 35 mm Hg.

The pressure in the capillaries averages about 25 mm Hg at the arterial end and 15 mm Hg at the venous end of the capillary bed. The higher pressure at the arterial end drives fluid out of the vessel into the interstitial space (filtration pressure). This is opposed by the oncotic pressure inside the capillary provided by the plasma proteins. Oncotic pressure exceeds filtration pressure at the venous end of the capillary and pulls fluid back into the vascular system. At any one

moment, an average of 20% of the capillaries may be open. This is all that is required to provide for normal cell nutrition and remove metabolic waste. Local accumulation of metabolites brings about dilatation of precapillary sphincters and increased perfusion of individual vascular beds.

Arteriovenous shunts are present in almost all vascular beds. These are capable of diverting blood directly from the arterial to the venous system. They open in response to certain stimuli such as heat and may open in those circumstances in which precapillary sphincters are closed.

The pressure in the venules is normally about 15 mm Hg. This pressure decreases progressively in the large veins and is normally about 4−5 mm Hg (5−6 cm water) in the great thoracic veins. Within normal physiologic limits, the higher the venous pressure, the greater the priming pressure of the heart, the greater the ventricular filling, and the greater the resulting stroke volume and cardiac output.

The vascular system acts to maintain tissue perfusion and fluctuations in volume elicit reflex mechanisms which tend to restore the circulation to normal. Any decrease in pressure or volume activates the sympathetic and renal defense mechanisms. Baroreceptors are located in the carotid sinus and the large thoracic arteries and sense changes in tension in the arterial wall. Decreased tension activates the sympathetic nervous system and the adrenal medulla. These stimulate the strength (inotropic) and the rate (chronotropic) of cardiac contraction and increase cardiac output. Vasoconstriction is produced successively in the skin and subcutaneous tissue, then in skeletal muscle and the splanchnic circulation. The splanchnic reservoir is emptied into systemic veins. The lowered filtration pressure in the peripheral capillaries favors oncotic attraction of fluid into the vessels, and this tends to restore vascular volume toward normal. The only vascular systems not constricted by the sympathetic nerves and catecholamines are the coronary and cerebral arteries, as the body's defense mechanism preserves flow to these organs at the expense of all others.

Control Mechanisms

A drop in renal artery pressure and flow produces renal artery vasoconstriction and results in decreased glomerular filtration and decreased urine output. The renin mechanism is simultaneously activated. This produces aldosterone secretion by the adrenal cortex

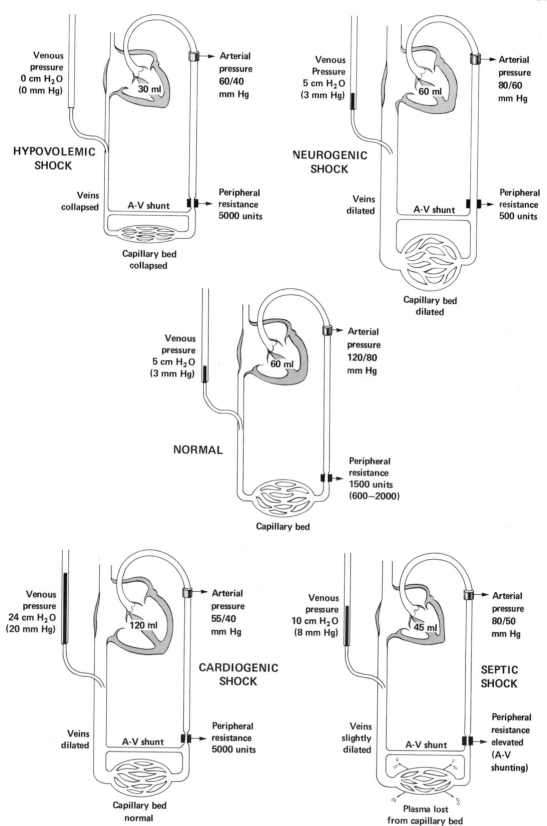

FIG 16–1. Hemodynamic changes in shock.

which promotes further salt and water retention. Renin release results in the production of angiotensin II, another potent vasoconstrictor which raises blood pressure.

Loss of blood volume also activates a generalized venous reflex; this produces venous constriction which increases the rate of venous return to the heart and increases the cardiac filling pressure which once again assists cardiac output.

In addition to these acute changes which result from loss of vascular volume, other long-term compensatory mechanisms are activated. The liver is stimulated, and increased protein synthesis results in a rapid rise in serum fibrinogen and other essential clotting factors. Albumin synthesis is increased; within 24 hours, serum proteins have returned to normal. Erythropoietin appears in the circulation, and the platelet count rises. Red cell volume returns to normal gradually over several weeks.

Shock Defined

Shock, then, can be defined as peripheral circulatory failure so that tissue perfusion is inadequate to provide the nutritional requirements of the cells and remove the waste products of metabolism. **In the simplest terms, shock can be defined as inadequate tissue perfusion.**

Aviado DM: Hypotension and the autonomic nervous system. Ann New York Acad Sc 66:998–1009, 1957.

Bassin R & others: Rapid and slow hemorrhage in man: I. Sequential hemodynamic responses. Ann Surg 173:325–330, 1971.

Moore FD: Effects of hemorrhage on body composition. New England J Med 273:567–577, 1965.

Types of Shock (Fig 16–1)

Various types of shock result from failure in one or more of the 3 major factors: pump, peripheral resistance, or blood volume. The major types are hypovolemic, cardiogenic, neurogenic, and septic shock.

A. Hypovolemic Shock: (Due to hemorrhage, burns, bowel obstruction, etc.) Hypovolemic shock results from decreased blood volume due to loss of blood, plasma, or acute and severe loss of body water and electrolytes. The characteristic changes noted in hypovolemic shock are a fall in venous pressure, a rise in peripheral resistance, and tachycardia.

B. Cardiogenic Shock: (Due to myocardial infarction, cardiac arrhythmias, congestive heart failure, etc.) The primary problem in cardiogenic shock is pump failure with a reduction in cardiac output. Blood backs up behind the heart, so that there is an increase in pressure in the venous bed. Peripheral resistance increases and directs remaining flow to critical vascular beds.

C. Neurogenic Shock: (Due to quadriplegia, spinal anesthesia, etc.) Neurogenic shock is due to a failure of arterial resistance. The result is a fall in blood pressure due to pooling of blood in dilated capacitance vessels. Cardiac activity increases and so maintains a normal stroke volume which serves to fill the dilated vascular system in an attempt to preserve perfusion pressure.

D. Septic Shock: (Due to infection, peritonitis, meningitis, etc.) Septic shock is most often due to gram-negative septicemia. Hypovolemia develops as a result of pooling of blood in the microcirculation and loss of fluid from the vascular space as a result of a generalized increase in capillary permeability. There may also be a direct toxic effect on the heart, with depressed cardiac function. Peripheral resistance is usually decreased as a result of the opening of arteriovenous shunts. Gram-positive sepsis occasionally produces hypovolemia, but in these instances loss of fluid is limited to the area of infection.

E. Miscellaneous Types of Shock: These include otherwise unclassified types of shock. Pulmonary embolism produces circulatory failure when the pulmonary vasculature is filled by thrombus, with obstruction to flow and right heart failure. Shock can occur secondary to inadequate cardiopulmonary bypass during heart surgery. Other types of shock include anaphylaxis (due to sensitivity to some allergenic agent) and insulin shock (shock due to severe hypoglycemia—a form of metabolic shock).

Table 16–1 summarizes the changes in the major parameters which occur in the principal types of shock.

TABLE 16–1. Major changes in the principal types of shock.

Type of Shock	Cardiac Function	Arteriolar Resistance	Venous Reservoir
Hypovolemic	↑	↑	↓↓
Cardiogenic	↓↓	↑	↑
Neurogenic	↑	↓↓	↑
Septic	↓	↓	↓

Carey LC: Hemorrhagic shock. Curr Probl Surg, Jan 1971.

Christy JH: Pathophysiology of gram-negative shock. Am Heart J 81:694–701, 1971.

Kwaan HM, Weil MH: Differences in the mechanism of shock caused by bacterial infections. Surg Gynec Obst 128:37–45, 1969.

Lillehei RC & others: Hemodynamic changes in endotoxin shock. Pages 442–462 in: *Shock and Hypotension*. Mills LJ, Moyer JH (editors). Grune & Stratton, 1965.

MacLean LD & others: The patient in shock. Canad MAJ 103:853–859, 1970.

Nickerson M: Vascular adjustments during the development of shock. Canad MAJ 103:853–859, 1970.

Scheidt S & others: Shock after myocardial infarction: A clinical and hemodynamic profile. Am J Cardiol 26:556–564, 1970.

Siegel JH & others: The surgical implications of physiologic patterns in myocardial infarction shock. Surgery 72:126–141, 1972.

Thal AP, Kinney JM: On the definition and classification of shock. Progr Cardiovas Dis 9:527, 1967.

MICROCIRCULATORY CHANGES IN SHOCK

The principal impact of all types of shock is on the microcirculation; unless there is insufficient microcirculatory flow, by definition there is no shock. The changes in the microcirculation progress in several phases (Fig 16–2).

Compensation Phase (Fig 16–2A)

This first phase occurs during the initial period of shock. When shock is mild, it may represent the only circulatory compromise. The first response of the circulation to hypovolemia is contraction of precapillary arterial sphincters. This causes the filtration pressure in the capillary to fall, and, since osmotic pressure remains the same, fluid moves into the vascular space with a corresponding increase in blood volume. If this compensatory mechanism is adequate to return blood volume to normal, the capillary sphincter relaxes and microcirculatory flow returns to normal. If shock is prolonged and profound, the next phase is entered.

Cell Distress Phase (Fig 16–2B)

If the precapillary sphincter contraction, with movement of interstitial fluid back into the vascular system, is not adequate to restore the volume and flow to normal, the precapillary sphincter remains closed. Arteriovenous shunts may open and divert arterial flow directly back into the venous system. The cells in the bypassed segment of the microcirculation must rely on anaerobic metabolism for energy. This decreases the amounts of glucose and oxygen available for the cell and results in the accumulation of metabolic waste products such as lactate. An inadequate supply of energy substrate results in a form of cell distress. Histamine is released, producing closure of the postcapillary sphincter. This serves to slow the remaining capillary flow and hold the red blood cells and nutrients in the capillaries longer. The empty capillary bed in this phase of shock totally constricts, and very few patent capillaries remain.

Decompensation Phase (Fig 16–2C)

In the agonal phase, just before cell death, local reflexes (perhaps due to accumulation of metabolites

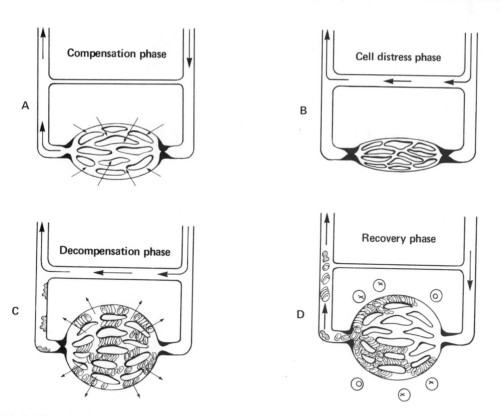

FIG 16–2. Microcirculatory changes in shock. *A:* Compensation phase. The precapillary sphincter closes, filtration pressure in the capillary drops, and fluid is drawn back into the vascular system by osmotic attraction. *B:* Cell distress phase. Arteriovenous shunts open, the postcapillary sphincter closes, and no fluid moves in or out of the capillary. *C:* Decompensation phase. The precapillary sphincter opens and the postcapillary sphincter remains closed. Fluid is lost from the damaged capillary bed with sludging of red blood cells in the capillary. *D:* Recovery phase. Normal volume has been restored. The precapillary and postcapillary sphincters are open. Sludged red cells and aggregates of platelets and white cells are washed into the systemic circulation.

and local acidosis) result in reopening of the precapillary sphincter while the postcapillary sphincter remains closed. Prolonged vasoconstriction of the capillary bed damages endothelial cells and results in increased capillary permeability. When the capillary finally reopens, fluid and protein are lost into the interstitial space and the capillary distends with red blood cells which pile up on one another and agglutinate ("sludge"). White cell and platelet aggregates accumulate in the venules, where acidosis is most profound. Many cells deprived of their circulation die. Arteriovenous communications which have opened during the cellular distress phase remain open during the decompensation phase, so that peripheral arteriolar flow is diverted directly back into the venous system for recirculation to vital areas such as the heart and brain.

Recovery Phase (Fig 16–2D)

If blood volume is restored at some point in the decompensation phase, while the effects on the microcirculation are still reversible, many of the badly damaged cells are capable of recovery. Capillary integrity may be regained as the "sludge" is washed into the venules, where red blood cell masses break up and return to the circulation. Some cell aggregates may be filtered out by the lungs or other microcirculatory beds. Platelet and white cell aggregates which form in the venules during the decompensation phase are also washed into the systemic circulation. If microcirculatory damage has been profound, large amounts of procoagulants from dead or dying cells, red cell sludge, and platelet aggregates may be released into the circulation and cause serious secondary morbidity (see Morbidity & Mortality, below). Other capillaries may be so badly damaged and filled with sludge that they remain permanently closed. Cells dependent upon these capillaries die.

Nickerson M: Vascular adjustments during the development of shock. Canad MAJ 103:853–859, 1970.

Shepro D, Fulton GP (editors): *Conferences on the Microcirculation as Related to Shock.* Academic Press, 1968.

METABOLIC FACTORS IN SHOCK

In shock there is depression of cell metabolism, and all metabolism ultimately reaches zero as death approaches. Before total collapse and death, individual metabolic factors are variably affected by shock.

(1) Protein metabolism is altered, for there is increased catabolism with cell breakdown and a rise in blood urea, serum creatinine, and serum uric acid.

(2) Changes in **fat metabolism** result as catecholamines initiate lipolysis. Tissue lipids and serum triglycerides are converted to free fatty acids. These changes are reflected in increased free fatty acids in the blood.

(3) Carbohydrate metabolism is profoundly

affected. Elevated catecholamine levels produce increased liver glycogenolysis with an increase in blood glucose. The metabolic pathway for glucose is compromised by the switch from aerobic to anaerobic metabolism in cells whose perfusion has been adversely affected. The ordinary metabolic pathway of glucose consists of breakdown into the 3-carbon pyruvate and then acetyl-coenzyme A. Further metabolism (the citric acid [Krebs] cycle) releases large quantities of high-energy ATP with CO_2 and water. When oxygen is not available, there is a block in metabolism so that the standard metabolic pathway cannot proceed further than pyruvate. During anaerobic metabolism, glucose is converted to pyruvate and then lactate with release of small quantities of high-energy ATP, a much less

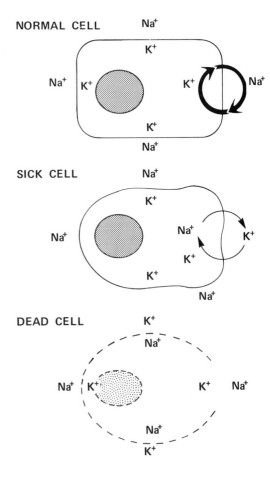

FIG 16–3. **Progressive cell damage and cell death in shock.** In the normal cell, energy is required to keep the membrane sodium-potassium pump functioning and to maintain the gradient between high intracellular potassium and high extracellular sodium concentrations. As shock progresses, adequate energy stores are no longer available to the cell and the pump breaks down. At the point of cell death, sodium and chloride move into the cell and water follows, leading to swelling.

efficient metabolic pathway but one that is capable of energy production in the absence of oxygen. As shock continues, there is a build-up of lactate in the blood stream. If liver perfusion is present, the lactate load can be further metabolized by the liver; otherwise there is progressive acidosis as lactate accumulates. This adds to the acidosis already produced by the changes in fat metabolism.

NORMAL CELL PHYSIOLOGY

Energy is required to maintain an osmotic differential between the cell and the surrounding interstitial fluid. This maintains the high intracellular potassium and extracellular sodium concentrations. Decreased nutrition of the cell results in decreased cell energy. Cell work diminishes, and cell membranes are thereby damaged by shock. Sodium moves into the cell and potassium moves out. Body water follows the sodium ion—so that, as sodium moves into the cell, obligatory cell edema occurs. At the same time, extracellular potassium rises. The serum sodium falls and the serum potassium rises progressively during the period of shock (Fig 16—3).

VICIOUS CYCLES IN SHOCK

Anoxia of cells in the CNS results in hyperventilation with respiratory alkalosis. Later, there is anaerobic metabolism and lactate accumulation. As the renal compensatory mechanism fails, there is progressive metabolic acidosis. Many vicious cycles are set in motion simultaneously. Examples are shown in Fig 16—4.

Baue AE & others: The dynamics of altered ATP-dependent and ATP-yielding cell processes in shock. Surgery 72:94–101, 1972.

Mela LM & others: Influence of cellular acidosis and altered cation concentrations on shock-induced mitochondrial damage. Surgery 72:102–110, 1972.

CLINICAL ASSESSMENT OF SHOCK

If the clinician fails to recognize the clinical signs of shock, proper treatment is delayed and the patient's chances of recovery may be severely compromised. In order to permit prompt recognition and effective treatment, shock may be classified as mild, moderate, or severe (Table 16—2).

Mild shock consists of decreased perfusion of nonvital organs and tissues such as skin, fat, skeletal muscle, and bone. These tissues can survive long

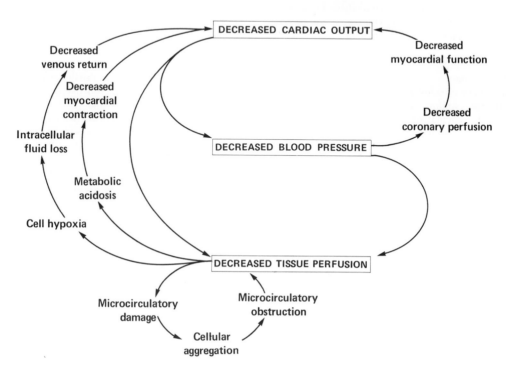

FIG 16—4. Vicious cycles in shock. The problem can be initiated at numerous points in any cycle: decreased tissue perfusion, decreased coronary perfusion, metabolic acidosis.

TABLE 16–2. Clinical classification of hemorrhagic shock.

Mild shock (up to 20% blood volume loss)
 Definition: Decreased perfusion of nonvital organs and tissues (skin, fat, skeletal muscle, and bone).
 Manifestations: Pale, cool skin. Patient complains of feeling cold.

Moderate shock (20–40% blood volume loss)
 Definition: Decreased perfusion of vital organs (liver, gut, kidneys).
 Manifestations: Oliguria to anuria and slight to significant drop in blood pressure.

Severe shock (40% or more blood volume loss)
 Definition: Decreased perfusion of heart and brain.
 Manifestations: Restlessness, agitation, coma, cardiac irregularities, ECG abnormalities, and cardiac arrest.

periods of decreased perfusion without undergoing irreversible changes.

Moderate shock encompasses all degrees of shock that involve decreased perfusion of vital organs other than heart and brain. The liver, gut, and kidneys are the principal examples.

Severe shock is defined as inadequate perfusion of the heart and brain. The compensatory mechanisms of shock act to preserve blood flow to these 2 vital organs at the expense of all others. Thus, in advanced shock there is constriction of all other vascular beds. The microcirculation of the coronary artery and CNS remains patent because vasoconstriction does not develop in these 2 vascular beds after sympathetic stimulation or catecholamine release.

In the young, healthy patient, a progressive decrease in circulating volume during hypovolemic shock produces predictable changes. The acute loss of up to 20% of blood volume is associated with mild shock; it is manifested by peripheral vasoconstriction. The patient is pale and has a cold skin. There may or may not be evidence of increased sympathetic activity, with sweating, tachycardia, and pupillary dilatation. The patient's chief complaint is that he feels cold.

Moderate shock in the young adult is generally found when there is a 20–40% blood volume loss. The manifestations of decreased vital organ perfusion are reflected in the kidneys. Careful evaluation of urinary output reveals that the hourly production of urine has fallen below the level required to excrete metabolic waste. In the adult, this is under 30 ml/hour. The principal sign of moderate shock is oliguria or anuria. There may be a slight to significant drop in blood pressure, but the young patient can, with vascular constriction, maintain an adequate blood pressure until 30% of blood volume is lost. The patient may complain of thirst.

In severe shock, the acute loss of blood volume usually exceeds 40%. Death generally occurs if about 50% of blood volume has been lost. Since the principal effect of severe shock is decreased perfusion of the heart and brain, the clinical manifestations are due to inadequate cerebral and coronary circulation. The first signs of decreased cerebral perfusion are restlessness, agitation, and excitability. The patient passes through this phase rapidly into semicoma and death. Unfortunately, if the patient has been drinking and has the odor of alcohol on his breath, the restlessness and agitation may be ascribed to the alcohol and the significance of the symptoms may not be recognized until coma or cardiac arrest occurs. The inexperienced clinician may attribute the cause to a head injury. Decreased perfusion of the heart may be manifested by cardiac irregularities or other ECG abnormalities which suggest myocardial ischemia and finally by cardiac arrest and death.

Monitoring the Shock Patient

Although treatment should be instituted as soon as shock is recognized, adequate treatment requires precise monitoring of the patient to avoid complications related to overenthusiastic therapy and to ensure optimal resuscitation of the vascular system.

A. Pulse and Blood Pressure: These are generally not reliable guides to the severity of shock. All patients with major illnesses, particularly at the time of initial presentation at the hospital, are apprehensive and have increased pulse rates whether or not actual shock is present. Decreased blood pressure is always significant; but the blood pressure may be normal, or relatively normal, until marked depletion of vascular volume occurs. This is particularly true of young patients, who by intense vascular constriction are able to maintain systolic pressure. In older, arteriosclerotic patients, a progressive drop in pressure usually parallels volume loss, but too much reliance on blood pressure in the past has resulted in gross undertreatment of shock. Arterial pressure results from the balance between the cardiac output and peripheral resistance. The diastolic pressure is a reflection of the status of the peripheral resistance; the pulse pressure, or the difference between the systolic and diastolic pressures, is related to the force and volume of cardiac systole and elasticity of the arterial vessels.

Warm skin with normal color indicates that peripheral perfusion is good. Since vasoconstriction is manifested first in the skin and subcutaneous tissues, good peripheral perfusion indicates normal peripheral resistance. A red, warmer than normal skin indicates a decrease in arteriolar resistance and is seen early in some cases of septic shock and in neurogenic shock. A cold, pale, moist skin signifies vasoconstriction with increased arteriolar resistance.

B. Urine Output: Urinary output is the most sensitive index of the adequacy of vital organ perfusion, and an indwelling urinary catheter is indicated for any patient in shock or in whom shock is likely to develop. Unless the patient has a history of renal disease, oliguria or anuria should be assumed to be due to inadequate perfusion resulting from myocardial failure or inadequate volume replacement. Vigorous treatment should be continued until the urine output exceeds 30 ml/hour.

C. Central Venous Pressure: Central venous pressure (CVP) has been a valuable guide to vascular volume replacement as a safeguard to prevent overloading the circulation. It is most reliable when colloids are used (blood, plasma, or plasma substitutes), as colloids remain in the vascular system and CVP accurately assesses the restoration of blood volume and can be relied upon to prevent overtreatment.

CVP can be most easily assessed by measuring the pressure in the venae cavae or intrathoracic veins. High CVP is reflected accurately in the extremities. However, when vasoconstriction occurs, measurement of the venous pressure in the extremities may give a falsely high value due to intense venous spasm. In order to accurately determine the status of the venous reservoir, a catheter should be threaded into a major vein (eg, the superior or inferior vena cava) and the CVP measured directly using a saline manometer.

Normal CVP is 5 cm water. Any venous pressure under 15 cm water with the patient supine is considered within the clinically optimal range. The zero point for venous pressure measurement in the supine patient is 5 cm below the sternal angle—roughly at the level of the anterior axillary line.

D. Blood Volume: Another means of evaluating the adequacy of the venous reservoir is to measure blood volume. Blood volume can be assessed by radioactive tagged serum albumin, which gives plasma volume, and by chromium labeling of the red blood cells, which determines red cell mass. Using the hematocrit of blood from the vena cava as a basis of calculation, the blood volume can be computed independently from a measurement of either plasma volume or red cell volume.

One practical disadvantage of the use of blood volume determinations as a guide to therapy is that red cells are trapped in the microcirculation and effective blood volume tends to be overestimated. In addition, increased permeability of the microcirculation results in transcapillary loss of albumin, leading to errors in the estimation of plasma volume. For these reasons, blood volume measurement is not a practical guide for monitoring or treating patients in shock.

E. Arterial Blood Gases: The partial pressures of oxygen (Pa_{O_2}) and CO_2 (Pa_{CO_2}) have become indispensable therapeutic guides. Using the Astrup nomogram, it is possible to calculate the base deficit and titrate it with appropriate amounts of bicarbonate solution. An arterial oxygen tension (Pa_{O_2}) of 80–100 mm Hg is normal; a tension below 60 mm Hg indicates a marginal respiratory reserve. If the Pa_{O_2} when breathing room air falls below 60 mm Hg, increased concentrations of oxygen are indicated.

The CO_2 blood gas tension (Pa_{CO_2}) should be monitored frequently and should be kept under 40 mm Hg. A Pa_{CO_2} over 45 mm Hg indicates that serious hypoventilation is present. In shock, unless there is underlying pulmonary disease, Pa_{CO_2} (as opposed to Pa_{O_2}) is usually within normal limits. A Pa_{CO_2} rising above 45 or 50 mm Hg with good ventilatory exchange is an ominous indication of severe pulmonary insufficiency.

F. Serum Lactate Levels: Serum lactate determination is often used as a prognostic guide. Prolonged, severe shock results in a switch to anaerobic metabolism. Initial lactate levels correlate well with subsequent mortality. (Normal = 0.44–1.8 mM/liter.) Levels of 2 mM/liter have been found to be associated with a mortality rate of 15%; 5 mM/liter or greater, a mortality rate of 75%; and 10 mM/liter or greater, a mortality rate of 95%. In shock, the initial lactate level may serve as a guide to the duration of preexisting shock and to the magnitude of the circulatory deficit. More effective therapy has improved the mortality, so that initial lactate levels are of less prognostic value.

G. Cardiac Output: Cardiac output has been used to monitor seriously ill patients in the hope that it might provide a better guide to the adequacy of the circulation. Unfortunately, this has not proved to be the case since, during shock resuscitation, preexisting ischemia opens a much greater circulatory bed. Moreover, the presence of arteriovenous shunting in areas of microcirculatory damage may result in deceptively high output measurements in the presence of inadequate perfusion at the microcirculatory level.

H. Packed Cell Volume (PCV, Hematocrit) and Hemoglobin: These clinical indices should be monitored serially. An abnormally high PCV indicates plasma loss in excess of red cell loss, as seen in septic shock and some types of cardiogenic shock. When the hematocrit is used to monitor hemorrhagic shock, there is a considerable lag before it reflects the true loss of red cell mass. Studies performed the first hour following massive hemorrhage may provide no clue whatever to the magnitude of the volume deficit; PCV may remain relatively normal, and only with appropriate hydration and support and 4–6 hours' observation will the hematocrit fall and correctly reflect the magnitude of blood loss. In the average adult, PCV falls 3–4% for every 500 ml of blood lost.

Cohn JN: Monitoring techniques in shock. Am J Cardiol 26:565–569, 1970.

Friedman E, Grable E, Fine J: Central venous pressure and direct serial measurements as guides in blood-volume replacement. Lancet 2:609–613, 1966.

MacLean LD: Blood volume versus central venous pressure in shock. Surg Gynec Obst 118:594–595, 1964.

MacLean LD & others: The patient in shock. Canad MAJ 105:78–83, 182–186, 1971.

Shoemaker WC: Indices of blood volume and measurements of hematocrit, plasma volume, and red cell volume. Chap 2 in: *Shock: Chemistry, Physiology and Therapy.* Thomas, 1967.

Weil MH, Afifi AA: Experimental and clinical studies on lactate and pyruvate as indicators of the severity of acute circulatory failure (shock). Circulation 41:989, 1970.

TREATMENT OF SHOCK

Ensure Airway

The first principle in resuscitation of the patient in shock is to ensure the adequacy of the airway. No resuscitation will be successful if the patient is not ventilating adequately. Blood gas (Pa_{O_2} and Pa_{CO_2}) and blood pH determinations should be done in any seriously ill patient, and oxygen should be administered by nasal catheter or by endotracheal tube depending upon the severity of any abnormality noted. Clinical evaluation alone is not adequate in the seriously ill patient, and direct arterial blood gas measurement is the fundamental means of assessment of the adequacy of pulmonary function.

Restore Blood Volume

Ordinarily, 20% of the blood volume is in the capillaries, 10% is in the arterial system, and the remainder is in the veins and heart. In the normal patient, only a fifth of the capillary bed is open at any one moment. Following shock and adequate resuscitation, there is dilatation of almost all of the capillary beds, which now can accommodate much of the blood volume. Sludging and anoxic damage result in increased permeability of the microcirculation and produce loss of red blood cells and plasma from the circulation. An obligatory cellular edema follows cell anoxia, and fluids in amounts several times the calculated loss may be required for resuscitation from shock. The longer shock persists, the greater the obligatory fluid deficit, so that there is no arbitrary rule which permits ready calculation of the volume required for adequate treatment. If a patient who is hemorrhaging has his blood volume replaced as rapidly as it is lost and is never permitted to go into shock, volume for volume replacement is sufficient. If, on the other hand, the patient has been allowed to remain in shock for several hours, optimal circulatory resuscitation may require fluid replacement which exceeds by several times the calculated loss.

Two types of fluids are used to resuscitate patients in shock: crystalloids and colloids.

A. Crystalloids: The crystalloids are electrolyte solutions such as 0.15 N sodium chloride solution or the so-called balanced salt solutions, eg, lactated Ringer's injection.* One liter of lactated Ringer's injection contains 130 mEq of sodium, 4 mEq of potassium, 3 mEq of calcium, 109 mEq of chloride, and 28 mEq of lactate. This is a buffering solution, for, as the lactate is metabolized, excess H^+ can be neutralized. It should be remembered that when crystalloid is used for resuscitation, 3 parts of crystalloid are lost to the

*Often called Ringer's solution in common hospital parlance. However, the NF XIII monograph on Ringer's solution (p 624) contains the following caution: "Do not use Ringer's Solution for parenteral administration or in preparations to be used parenterally. For such purposes use Ringer's Injection, USP XVIII."

extravascular space for every part that remains in the vascular system. Therefore, 2000 ml are required to increase the vascular volume by 500 ml. If the patient has been in shock for a matter of hours, the effective therapeutic ratio is even less and may approach 8:1 or 10:1.

In the treatment of hemorrhagic shock, initial resuscitation with crystalloids is favored because the solutions are readily available and effectively restore vascular volume for short periods. They lower blood viscosity and enhance resuscitation of the microcirculation. Time is thus gained for definitive typing and cross-matching of blood, and, if the patient continues to bleed during the period of resuscitation, the infused crystalloid solution is expendable—ie, blood reserves are not wasted and are available for restoration of blood volume after bleeding has been controlled. Provided the oxygen-carrying capacity of the blood is supplemented by increased oxygen in the airway, it is almost impossible to dilute the blood sufficiently to prevent adequate tissue oxygenation. However, as salt and water are lost from the circulation into the tissues, continued resuscitation with crystalloids promotes both pulmonary and tissue edema. Ideally, initial resuscitation with crystalloids should be promptly followed by colloid replacement.

B. Colloids: The colloids used to treat hypovolemic shock consist of blood, plasma, serum albumin, and plasma substitutes such as dextran. Although type O Rh-negative blood was at one time routinely used for resuscitation, major injury requires massive transfusion; the minor mismatches which often result from transfusion of type O Rh-negative blood may thus be magnified and result in serious morbidity or even fatal reactions. Type-specific blood should be used, even if it is not cross-matched. When possible, it is preferable to treat with crystalloid solutions and plasma or plasma substitutes while awaiting definitive cross-match.

The use of pooled plasma has recently come under criticism because of the risk of hepatitis. The quality of plasma varies greatly in different sections of the country, and the risk of hepatitis is difficult to assess. Plasma substitutes such as dextran or plasma fractions such as albumin are the principal colloids available.

Burn shock, which produces a greater deficit of plasma volume than of red cell volume, is the principal form of shock which still requires large quantities of colloid for treatment, although crystalloids can be used to replace much of the volume deficit.

Dextran is the most widely used plasma substitute at the present time. Two types are available in the USA: clinical dextran, with a molecular weight of 70,000; and low molecular weight dextran, with a molecular weight of 40,000. Clinical dextran is the most effective colloid since it stays in the vascular system for 24 hours. Its disadvantage in hemorrhagic shock is that it interferes with blood typing and may impair the coagulation mechanism. Low molecular weight dextran is a relatively short-acting colloid, staying in the vascular system approximately 8 hours. It is a low-viscosity solution which interferes much less with blood typing and does not depress the coagulation mechanism.

Improve Cardiac Function

Shock may result from primary pump failure due to cardiac damage or disease. In this instance, improving the efficacy of the pump and decreasing the load on the heart are the chief aims of therapy. Cardiogenic shock has been regarded as a condition in which there is a fluid overload. It is now recognized that cardiogenic shock may require blood volume replacement for adequate resuscitation. Blood pH should be carefully monitored and metabolic acidosis corrected, since acidosis has an adverse effect on myocardial contractility. Alkalosis may produce even more serious consequences than acidosis. Alkalosis interferes with the red blood cell's ability to give up oxygen to the tissues, and this can fatally aggravate the consequences of shock.

For chronic cardiac problems, digitalis is an appropriate drug; however, when myocardial failure is secondary to the shock state itself, more immediate forms of improving cardiac function should be considered such as correction of acidosis or administration of drugs such as isoproterenol. The CVP must be carefully monitored and fluids administered until the CVP reaches or exceeds 15 cm water. This improves cardiac function by stretching myocardial fibers and improving the strength of contraction (Starling's law). Once the priming pressure of 15 or 20 cm water is exceeded, the downward slope of Starling's curve may be reached, at which point cardiac function deteriorates and pulmonary edema develops.

Vasopressors & Vasodilators

There has been considerable controversy about the administration of vasopressors and vasodilators in shock. It is now recognized that vasopressors have almost no place in resuscitation if the patient is in shock. The only exception is cardiogenic shock, where a brief use of pressor drugs may increase aortic root pressure and coronary perfusion and thus improve cardiac function. Pressor drugs aggravate shock in most microcirculatory beds by intensifying preexisting vasoconstriction and may thus compromise ultimate recovery of the patient.

The vasodilator drugs are now in vogue in shock resuscitation. This is second-line therapy, for primary therapy is volume replacement. Unless volume replacement is adequate, the administration of vasodilators may result in prompt failure of the circulation due to the fall of blood pressure and circulatory collapse. Vasodilators are never indicated until vascular volume has been restored to normal and CVP is in the high normal range. At that point, use of peripheral vascular dilators may, by decreasing vascular resistance, decrease the work of the heart and improve cardiac output and tissue perfusion. If resuscitation has been adequate, it is rarely necessary to consider the use of vasodilating drugs.

The drug of choice for cardiac resuscitation has been isoproterenol (Isuprel). This drug has 2 methods of action in that it stimulates myocardial contractility and simultaneously lowers peripheral resistance. One 5 mg ampule of isoproterenol is added to 200–500 ml of fluid and administered IV at a rate which produces optimal circulatory benefit. Toxicity is manifested when the pulse rate exceeds 120/minute or cardiac arrhythmia develops.

Modify the Microcirculatory Lesion

Sludging of blood, platelet aggregation, and intravascular coagulation all follow microcirculatory damage and cell death. Increased attention is now being directed toward definitive treatment of microcirculatory perfusion. Low molecular weight dextran has been used to decrease blood viscosity and the tendency toward red cell sludging and platelet aggregation. It also decreases platelet adhesiveness. One to 2 units (500 ml each) are usually used in the initial resuscitation of shock. The maximal dose following initial priming by 2 units of dextran consists of 1 unit of dextran daily.

Heparin is being used to treat certain shock states, particularly shock due to gram-negative sepsis, where intravascular coagulation has been demonstrated to develop from gram-negative endotoxemia. Another type of shock which carries considerable morbidity as a result of intravascular coagulation has been traumatic shock or any form of shock which is associated with extensive tissue damage or necrosis. When heparin can be administered early in resuscitation of the patient in shock, it may well prevent or modify many of the secondary effects due to intravascular coagulation. The dose varies, but as a rule 1000–2000 units are given IV every 4–6 hours.

The secondary effects of blood cell aggregation and intravascular clotting are principally on the lung. Pulmonary function may be improved and pulmonary lesions may be modified by the early institution of mechanical ventilation. Therefore, endotracheal intubation and positive pressure ventilation are of value in profound shock.

Adrenal Corticosteroids

Adrenocorticosteroids have recently been advocated in the management of shock. There is some evidence that massive doses of these agents modify some of the adverse effects of gram-negative sepsis and lessen the morbidity following shock. This effect is presumably due to their ability to stabilize cell membranes. The doses used are 10–20 times the usual clinical doses. The dose advocated for dexamethasone is 1 gm IV every 6–8 hours.

There is no general agreement of the value of corticosteroids in treating septic shock. Those who are skeptical point out that all of the experimental evidence which establishes the effectiveness of corticosteroids in shock suggests that therapy must be initiated before shock occurs.

Carey JS & others: Comparison of hemodynamic responses to whole blood and plasma expanders in clinical traumatic shock. Surg Gynec Obst 121:1059–1065, 1965.

Christy JH: Treatment of gram-negative shock. Am J Med 50:77–88, 1971.

Hermreck AS, Thal AP: The adrenergic drugs and their use in shock therapy. Curr Probl Surg, July 1968.

Kinney JM: Problems of ventilation after injury and shock. J Trauma 2:370, 1962.

Kuhn LA: Shock in myocardial infarction: Medical treatment. Am J Cardiol 26:578–587, 1970.

MacLean LD & others: The patient in shock. Canad MAJ 105:78–83, 182–186, 1971.

Olcott C IV, Barber RE, Blaisdell FW: Diagnosis and treatment of respiratory insufficiency after civilian trauma. Am J Surg 122:260–268, 1971.

Schumer W, Nyhus LM: Role of corticoids in the management of shock. S Clin North America 49:147–162, 1969.

Sealy WC: The support of the lung during and after traumatic and hemorrhagic shock. Ann Thoracic Surg 3:578, 1967.

String T, Robinson AJ, Blaisdell FW: Massive trauma: Effect of intravascular coagulation on prognosis. Arch Surg 102:406–411, 1971.

Weil MH, Shubin H: Isoproterenol for the treatment of circulatory shock. Ann Int Med 70:638–641, 1969.

Yao ST, Shoemaker WC: Plasma and whole blood viscosity changes in shock and after dextran infusion. Ann Surg 164:973–984, 1966.

MORBIDITY & MORTALITY

As understanding of the pathogenesis of shock increases and therapy becomes more effective, "irreversible shock" is seen with decreasing frequency. Even so, patients still die of shock, principally as a result of irreversible damage to the brain or heart, because of respiratory failure from lung damage, or because of uncontrolled infection following profound shock. Such forms of shock as hemorrhagic shock should be reversible if the patient responds initially to resuscitation and cerebral damage has not occurred. Despite favorable response to initial resuscitation, patients still die days or weeks following an episode of shock, and more and more investigations are being conducted in an attempt to isolate the causes of irreversibility.

Organs that may at times be so badly damaged in shock as to cause death are discussed in the following paragraphs.

Brain

Four minutes of total circulatory arrest at normothermia are said to result in permanent cerebral damage. Death occurs when brain damage is irreversible. However, many patients who have apparently had circulatory arrest for more than 10 minutes have been successfully resuscitated. If the patient responds to resuscitation and awakens, irreversible brain damage has obviously not occurred.

Recent evidence suggests that injury to the microcirculation within the brain may itself be the major factor responsible for CNS damage. Brain cells in tissue culture can withstand 10–15 minutes of total ischemia, whereas clinical experience has documented that 4–5 minutes of circulatory arrest usually produces irreversible cerebral ischemia at normothermia.

Heart

The heart can be resuscitated 30–60 minutes after circulatory arrest. Cardiac transplantation has also demonstrated that, unless there is a myocardial lesion, cardiac resuscitation should be possible on most patients, and primary myocardial factors should rarely be a cause of irreversible shock except in the case of primary cardiogenic shock. Despite these observations, it is sometimes impossible to resuscitate the heart after relatively short periods of profound ischemia. Part of the problem may be brain stem damage with secondary depression of respiration and resulting anoxic compromise of myocardial function. Another factor may be related to microcirculatory damage. One investigator has demonstrated that ADP-induced platelet aggregation, although only transiently obstructive to the microcirculation, can produce myocardial infarction. This may explain the absence of vascular lesions in many of the patients who die.

Lungs

Respiratory failure is at present the most common cause of late death after an initially successful resuscitation of a patient in shock. In Vietnam and in general hospitals treating large numbers of trauma victims, most of the late deaths after initial successful resuscitation have been due to pulmonary damage and respiratory failure. All intensive care units nowadays are filled with patients on respirators, and anesthesiologists have taken an active interest in ICU care, principally because of the high incidence of pulmonary complications following any major illness.

Many different types of respiratory insufficiency are seen following shock. These are similar to those following any grave illness and include aspiration of gastric contents, airway obstruction due to plugs of mucus or blood, pulmonary edema due to overenthusiastic fluid therapy, atelectasis, oxygen toxicity, pulmonary contusion, pneumonia, and pulmonary embolism and infarction.

Respiratory distress syndrome (shock lung, hemorrhagic lung) is a distinct form of pulmonary failure which often follows shock but is also seen in various other circumstances. It usually becomes evident within the first 24 hours following an episode of shock. The early clinical signs are tachypnea and increased respiratory effort. Careful evaluation reveals a progressive decrease in pulmonary compliance, decreased Pa_{O_2}, and increased pulmonary arteriovenous shunting. In contrast with many of the other causes of respiratory insufficiency, the lungs sound dry to auscultation and pulmonary secretions are minimal. Chest x-ray shows diffuse alveolar infiltrates which may progress to complete consolidation. As the pulmonary lesion progresses, increasing inspiratory pressures are needed to maintain normal tidal volume. Greater inspiratory oxygen concentrations are required to provide adequate arterial oxygen tensions. With intensive support and meticulous respiratory care, the patient may recover gradually over 3–5 days. If he does not, respiratory insufficiency progresses so that inflation pressures of 50–60 cm of water are required and, despite the administration of 100% oxygen, oxygen tensions in the blood drop to critical levels and the patient dies. Autopsy reveals lungs which grossly resemble liver owing to intense hemorrhagic consolidation.

The primary lesion responsible for pulmonary insufficiency in shock is pulmonary microembolism. This is because dead cells release procoagulants and tissue thromboplastin, which results in intravascular coagulation in areas of circulatory stasis. Emboli also develop from sludging of red cells and from white cell and platelet aggregations which occur in the microcirculatory beds damaged by shock. Resuscitation washes the products of coagulation into the systemic circulation, where they are filtered out by the lung. The normal lung is capable of clearing a surprisingly large volume of such material. If the patient has underlying pulmonary insufficiency or the load is massive, the microcirculation of the lung may be overwhelmed. This produces secondary vascular damage with congestion, intra-alveolar hemorrhage, and bronchial constriction, resulting in arteriovenous shunting and decreased compliance. Ultimately, overgrowth of organisms in damaged stiff lungs results in death due to pulmonary infection.

Kidneys

The kidneys were at one time the organs most commonly affected by shock. This was undoubtedly because shock resulted in renal medullary shunting, with cortical ischemia and tubular necrosis. Since the concept of fluid resuscitation described above came into widespread application, renal failure has become a rare complication of shock. The use of artificial kidneys provides support until ultimate renal recovery in those few patients who do develop renal failure.

Liver

The liver is occasionally the organ which is most profoundly affected by shock. Because only 15% of its parenchyma is needed for survival, the liver can be markedly compromised before clinical catastrophe occurs. Jaundice occurs in 2–5% of patients with massive and prolonged shock. The derangement simulates obstructive jaundice because alkaline phosphatase and bilirubin rise in excess of the enzymes, indicating hepatocellular damage. Pathologic studies reveal centrilobular necrosis. Some degree of hemolysis occurs after massive transfusion, and an increased load of hemoglobin is presented to marginally damaged liver cells. Therefore, bilirubin rises and the increase is principally of the conjugated form. Conversion to bilirubin occurs, but excretion is more severely affected.

Despite the rather frequent appearance of jaundice, hepatic failure is rarely the primary factor in death due to shock.

Intestines

The bowel may be an important end organ in shock. The circulation of the gut is compromised early in the development of hypovolemia by intense splanchnic vasoconstriction. Since the mucosa is the most active tissue metabolically, the impact of decreased circulation is principally on the mucosa. If shock is prolonged, mucosal necrosis may occur. Ulceration of the gastrointestinal tract occurs with subsequent gastrointestinal hemorrhage ("stress ulcer"). The manifestations of stress ulcer secondary to mucosal ulceration usually occur approximately 5–7 days after the initial insult. It is of interest that the bowel may be responsible for much of the liver damage seen following shock; when the portal circulation has been diverted away from the liver, or when the bowel is isolated and perfused during the shock state experimentally in dogs, liver damage rarely occurs.

Adrenals

The adrenal glands have occasionally been the principal end organ affected by shock. Adrenal hemorrhage and insufficiency may result following profound shock, and in refractory cases small doses of corticosteroids should be administered to rule out the possibility of adrenocortical failure as the primary factor in irreversibility.

●　　●　　●

General References

Blaisdell FW, Lim RC Jr, Stallone RJ: The mechanism of pulmonary damage following traumatic shock. Surg Gynec Obst 130:15, 1970.

Byrne JJ (editor): The management of shock and unconsciousness. S Clin North America 48:245–459, 1968.

Glynn MF: Platelets and thrombosis: Mechanism and therapy. Ann Int Med 64:715, 1966.

Hershey SQ, Del Quercio LRM, McConn R (editors): *Septic Shock in Man.* Little, Brown, 1971.

Housman LB & others: Counterpulsation for intraoperative cardiogenic shock: Successful use of intra-aortic balloon. JAMA 224:1131–1133, 1973.

Mills LC, Mayer JH: *Shock and Hypotension.* Grune & Stratton, 1968.

Rocchio MA, DiCola V, Randall HT: Role of electrolyte solutions in treatment of hemorrhagic shock. Am J Surg 125:488–495, 1973.

Scheidt S & others: Intra-aortic balloon counterpulsation in cardiogenic shock. New England J Med 288:979–984, 1973.

Schloerb PR: Shock and metabolism. Surg Gynec Obst 128:315, 1969.

Schumer W: Evolution of the modern therapy of shock: Science vs empiricism. S Clin North America 51:3–14, 1971.

17 ...

Penetrating &
Nonpenetrating Injuries

Robert E. Allen, MD, & Albert D. Hall, MD

SURGERY OF THE NECK, CHEST,
& ABDOMEN AFTER TRAUMA
Robert E. Allen, Jr, MD

NECK INJURIES

All injuries to the neck are potentially life-threatening because of the many vital structures which course through from the head to the chest. Injuries to the neck may be classified as either blunt or penetrating, for each presents a different spectrum of management.

Penetrating injuries to the posterior neck generally endanger the vertebral column, the cervical spinal cord, the interosseous portion of the vertebral artery, and the neck musculature. Penetrating injuries to the anterior and lateral neck endanger the larynx, trachea, esophagus, thyroid, carotid arteries, subclavian arteries, jugular vein, and subclavian veins.

Blunt trauma can produce cervical fracture or dislocation with risk of spinal cord injury. Direct blows to the anterior neck can damage the larynx or trachea with hemorrhage and airway obstruction.

It is mandatory to examine patients closely for associated head and chest injuries. The initial level of consciousness is of paramount importance; progressive depression of the sensorium signifies intracranial bleeding and requires neurosurgical intervention. Injuries of the base of the neck may result in lacerations of major blood vessels. Hemorrhage into the pleural cavity may occur suddenly as contained hematomas suddenly decompress into a body cavity.

Clinical Findings

Injuries to the larynx and trachea may present without symptoms, or the patient may present with hoarseness, laryngeal stridor or dyspnea secondary to airway compression or aspiration of blood, or both. These symptoms may be accompanied by subcutaneous emphysema if disruption of the integrity of the larynx or trachea has occurred.

Esophageal injuries are rarely isolated ones and in themselves may not cause immediate symptoms. Hours later, as mediastinitis develops, progressive sepsis may become manifest. Mediastinitis results because the deep cervical space is in direct continuity with the mediastinum. Esophageal injuries are recognized promptly if the physician is alert to the possibility. Exploration of the neck or contrast examination of the esophagus confirms the diagnosis.

Cervical spine and cord injuries should always be suspected in deceleration injury or when there has been any violent trauma to the neck. If the patient complains of cervical pain or tenderness, the head and neck should be immobilized until cervical x-rays can be taken to rule out cervical fracture. The diagnosis is more difficult if the level of consciousness is depressed, and in this case the neck should be immobilized with sandbags until x-rays can be obtained.

Injuries to the great vessels (subclavian, common carotid, internal carotid, and external carotid arteries; subclavian, internal jugular, and external jugular veins) are possible whenever a penetrating injury is present. Blunt traumatic injuries of the clavicle or first rib may produce lacerations of the subclavian artery and vein. Typically, the patient presents with visible evidence of external blood loss, hematoma formation, and varying degrees of shock. In occasional cases, bleeding may be contained and the injury may temporarily go undetected. Auscultation of the head may reveal bruits which point to arterial injury.

Diagnosis

The differential diagnosis of penetrating injury to the neck is not difficult. The high density of major structures makes significant injury likely. The location of the trauma suggests which structures may be involved. Vascular injuries at the base of the neck require thoracotomy to obtain proximal and distal control of injured blood vessels before exposing the site of probable injury. Arteriography should be done, if possible, prior to exploration of any injury in which blood vessels may be damaged below the level of the cricoid cartilage or above a line connecting the mastoid process with the angle of the jaw. Arterial injuries above this line are inaccessible by ordinary surgical means. If injury to the carotid artery at the base of the skull is confirmed by arteriography, repair may not be possible and ligation may be required to control continuous hemorrhage. In addition, injured carotid arteries which have produced a neurologic deficit should be ligated.

Vertebral artery injuries should be suspected when there is bleeding from a posterior or lateral neck wound which cannot be controlled by pressure on the carotid artery, or when there is bleeding from a posterolateral wound associated with fracture of a cervical transverse process.

X-rays of the soft tissues and cervical spine should be taken routinely. Fractures of the cervical spine can be confirmed by x-ray. X-rays of the soft tissues can locate opaque foreign bodies if present and help determine the route of the missile.

The most important injuries resulting from blunt cervical trauma are (1) cervical fracture, (2) cervical spinal cord injury, (3) vascular injury, and (4) laryngeal and tracheal injury. X-rays of the cervical spine and soft tissues are of paramount importance in the differential diagnosis of blunt cervical trauma. Careful neurologic examination can differentiate between injuries to the cord, brachial plexus, and brain.

Complications

The complications of untreated neck injuries are related to the individual structures injured. Injuries to the larynx and trachea can result in acute airway obstruction, late tracheal stenosis, and sepsis. Cervicomediastinal sepsis can result from esophageal injuries. Carotid artery injuries can result in death from hemorrhage, brain damage, and arteriovenous fistula with cardiac decompensation. Major venous injury can result in exsanguination, air embolism, and arteriovenous fistula if there is concomitant arterial injury. Cervical fracture can result in paraplegia, quadriplegia, or death.

Prevention of these complications depends upon immediate resuscitation by intubation of the airway; prompt control of external hemorrhage and volume replacement; protection of the head and neck when cervical fracture is possible; accurate and rapid diagnosis; and prompt operative treatment when indicated.

Treatment

Any wound of the neck which penetrates the platysma requires prompt surgical exploration to rule out major vascular injury. If the patient presents with a neurologic deficit that is clearly not due to head injury, primary repair of the artery and reestablishment of blood flow to the brain will make the neurologic deficit worse since an ischemic area of infarction in the brain is thus converted into a more lethal hemorrhagic infarction; in such cases, the carotid artery should be ligated. Arteries damaged by high-velocity missiles require debridement. End-to-end anastomosis of the mobilized vessels is preferred, but if a significant segment is lost an autogenous vein graft can be used. Vertebral artery injury presents formidable technical problems because of the interosseous course of the artery shortly after it arises from the subclavian artery. It is best to ligate the vertebral artery rather than to attempt repair with restoration of blood flow. Unilateral vertebral artery ligation has been followed by fatal midbrain or cerebellar necrosis because of inadequate communication to the basilar artery. However, it is estimated that only about 3.1% of patients with left vertebral ligation and 1.8% of patients with right vertebral ligation develop these complications. In the face of massive hemorrhage resulting from a partially severed vertebral artery, immediate ligation becomes a surgical necessity with a reasonable prospect of "doing no harm."

Subclavian artery injuries are best approached through a combined cervicothoracic incision. Proper exposure is the key to success in the management of these difficult and too often fatal injuries. Ligation of the subclavian artery is relatively safe, but primary repair with restoration of pulsatile blood flow is preferable.

Venous injuries are best managed by ligation. The possibility of air embolism must be kept constantly in mind. A simple means of preventing this complication is to lower the patient's head until bleeding is controlled.

Esophageal injuries should be sutured and drained. Drainage is the cornerstone of treatment. Extensive injury to the esophagus is often immediately fatal because of associated injuries to the spinal cord. Systemic antibiotics should be administered routinely in such cases.

Minor laryngeal and tracheal injuries do not require treatment, but immediate tracheostomy should be performed when airway obstruction exists. If there has been significant injury to the thyroid cartilage, a temporary laryngeal stent (Silastic) should be employed to provide support. Mucosal lacerations should be approximated before insertion of the stent. Conveniently located small perforations of the trachea can be utilized for tracheostomy. Otherwise, the wounds can be closed after debridement and a distal tracheostomy performed. Extensive circumferential tracheal injuries may require resection and anastomosis or reconstruction using synthetic materials.

Primary neurorrhaphy should be attempted for nerve injury. Bilateral vagal nerve injury results in hoarseness and dysphagia. Cervical spinal cord injury should be managed in such a way as to prevent further damage. When there is cervical cord compression—from hematoma formation, vertebral fractures, or foreign bodies—decompression laminectomy should be performed.

Blunt trauma to the neck rarely requires surgical treatment. More commonly, the soft tissues are contused, and hematomas are formed which may cause tracheal compression and respiratory insufficiency. Tracheostomy is indicated in this instance. Cervical fractures are managed with skull tongs and traction. Surgical stabilization of cervical fractures is rarely indicated before 3 weeks after surgery unless there is progressive paraplegia. The common or internal carotid arteries can be torn or undergo disruption of the intima and require vascular reconstruction. Carotid arteriograms are essential to the diagnosis.

Prognosis

The prognosis after neck trauma varies with the extent of injury and the structures involved. Severance of the cervical spinal cord results in paralysis. Injuries to the soft tissues of the neck, trachea, and esophagus have a good to excellent prognosis if promptly treated. Major vascular injuries have a good prognosis if promptly treated before the onset of irreversible shock or neurologic deficit. The overall mortality for cervical injuries is about 10%.

Beall AC Jr, Roof WR, DeBakey ME: Successful surgical management of through and through stab wounds of aortic arch. Ann Surg 156:823, 1962.

Bricker DL & others: Vascular injuries of the thoracic outlet. J Trauma 10:1, 1970.

Fitchett V & others: Penetrating wounds of the neck. Arch Surg 99:307, 1969.

French AL, Haines GL: Unilateral vertebral artery ligation. J Neurosurg 7:156–158, 1950.

Harrington OB & others: Circumferential replacement of the trachea with Marlex mesh. Am Surgeon 28:217, 1962.

Hunt TK, Blaisdell FW, Okimoto J: Vascular injuries of the base of the neck. Arch Surg 98:586, 1969.

Monson DO, Saletta JD, Freeark RJ: Carotid vertebral trauma. J Trauma 9:987, 1969.

Shaw RR, Paulson DL, Lee JL: Traumatic tracheal rupture. J Thoracic Cardiovas Surg 42:281, 1961.

Shirkley AL, Beall AC Jr, DeBakey ME: Surgical management of penetrating wounds of the neck. Arch Surg 86:97, 1963.

Work WP, McCoy EG: Surgical repair of the cervical trachea following trauma. Ann Otol Rhin Laryng 65:573, 1956.

CHEST INJURIES

The chest is frequently injured by both penetrating and blunt trauma. About 60% of chest injuries are due to blunt trauma and 40% due to penetrating injury. Rib fractures are the most frequent injuries after blunt trauma to the chest. Parenchymal lung damage and vascular injuries are more common after penetrating wounds.

Twenty-five percent of deaths from automobile accidents are directly related to chest trauma. Blunt injuries of the thorax create different problems from those associated with penetrating injuries. In general, major nonpenetrating thoracic trauma produces more damage than penetrating trauma. The mortality is higher in the former group, and the hospital stay is longer. This is due in part to the high incidence of associated injuries to other organs with nonpenetrating trauma.

Pulmonary physiology is altered after chest trauma and, if not corrected, can cause severe complications and death. Injuries resulting in rib fractures may alter pulmonary physiology by decreasing ventilation. This results from "splinting" (spasm of the auxiliary muscles of respiration because of injury and pain) or paradoxic movement when the chest wall is flail due to unstable fractures; during respiration, the unstable segment moves in when the remainder of the chest wall is moving out and vice versa. These paradoxic respirations markedly decrease ventilation, and the patient must exert increased effort in order to breathe.

The physiologic changes that occur with flail chest are related to (1) inadequate ventilation of the lung and (2) blunt damage to the underlying pulmonary tissue caused by the initial trauma. Inadequate ventilation tends to cause atelectasis, congestion, and accumulation of secretions which, in turn, cause further atelectasis and stiffness of the lung. Direct damage to the underlying lung by the initial trauma can cause congestion, hemorrhage, edema, and atelectasis; it may also increase the rate of progression of atelectasis and other changes that follow inadequate ventilation. Shock and sepsis may further aggravate the above changes by causing (1) hypoxic damage to the lung; (2) embolization of platelet aggregates to the pulmonary capillaries; and (3) toxic or chemical changes from vasoactive substances, eg, histamine and bradykinin. Overloading of the circulation with fluids or the occurrence of congestive heart failure further reduces pulmonary function by increasing interstitial edema and transudation of fluid into the alveoli. Fat emboli from fractures or soft tissue injury may produce additional damage. Superimposed pneumonia causes local tissue necrosis and further accelerates the above pathophysiologic changes.

Penetrating wounds may release the negative pressure in the pleural space. This leads to collapse of the lung (pneumothorax) and the possibility of hypoxia. If the lung parenchyma is also damaged, tension pneumothorax can develop which causes collapse of the lung on the involved side and a decrease in venous return to the right heart. Pulmonary shunting caused by intraalveolar hemorrhage and atelectasis leads to hypoxia, hypocapnia, and respiratory alkalosis.

Injury to major blood vessels can occur, with resulting hemothorax. Injuries to the heart and great vascular structures in the mediastinum or lung hilum are usually immediately fatal. Most patients with penetrating cardiac wounds who survive to reach the hospital do so because of cardiac tamponade. Cardiac tamponade can cause death by restricting the pumping action and output of the heart.

Clinical Findings

Minimal trauma to the chest may produce few symptoms, or the patient may complain only of chest wall pain. After major trauma, the patient is more likely to be in respiratory distress; cyanosis may or may not be present.

Every patient with thoracic injury should have a careful physical examination and x-rays of the chest. Even though the initial x-ray examination shows no abnormalities, repeat x-rays in a few hours may reveal pneumothorax, hemothorax, or a widened mediastinum.

Penetrating wounds of the chest usually cause damage confined to the track of the wounding agent. High-velocity missiles are exceptions because they release enough kinetic energy to devitalize tissues for many centimeters surrounding the wound track. Lung parenchyma, however, is resistant to injury because of its low density. Shotgun wounds at close range can cause disruption of the chest wall and massive intra-thoracic injury. Considerations in penetrating wounds of the chest are (1) open pneumothorax (sucking wounds), (2) closed pneumothorax, (3) hemothorax, (4) pulmonary parenchymal damage, (5) esophageal injury, and (6) injury to the heart and great vessels of the thoracic cavity.

A. Chest Wall Injuries: Pain and hematoma formation over the ribs suggest rib fractures. A chest x-ray that shows rib detail will confirm the diagnosis. Dyspnea, multiple fractures of adjacent ribs, and paradoxic motion of a segment of the chest wall are diagnostic of flail chest (Fig 17–1). When the flail segment is the sternum, rib fractures may not be seen on x-ray. The diagnosis is a clinical one and is suggested by dyspnea and paradoxic motion of the sternum.

B. Pneumothorax: The diagnosis of open pneumothorax is self-evident (Fig 17–2). The patient is in respiratory distress, there is a penetrating wound, and there is a characteristic sucking sound with each inspiration. Hyperresonance to percussion and diminished breath sounds on one side suggest closed pneumothorax. Chest x-ray showing collapse of the lung is diagnostic (Fig 17–3).

Patients with tension pneumothorax generally have chest pain, air hunger, displacement of the trachea away from the involved side, and hyperresonance. The chest x-ray will show retraction of the lung from the parietal pleura and shift of the mediastinum to the opposite side (Fig 17–4).

C. Ruptured Bronchus: Rupture of a main stem bronchus (Fig 17–5) is associated with severe, persistent air leakage and mediastinal emphysema. Tension pneumothorax is present if the chest wall is intact. The diagnosis is confirmed by bronchoscopy and bronchography.

D. Hemothorax: Hemothorax should be suspected in every patient with rib fractures. Dullness to percussion, rib fractures, and fluid in the pleural space on x-ray indicate hemothorax (Figs 17–6, 17–7). Massive or prolonged bleeding almost always originates from the systemic vasculature of the chest wall, usually the intercostals or internal mammary arteries.

E. Pulmonary Contusion: A crushing injury to the chest, decrease in arterial oxygen tension, and saturation and the presence of fluffy infiltrates on the chest x-ray are sufficient for the diagnosis of pulmonary contusion.

F. Cardiac Injury: Extensive trauma to the sternum and left hemithorax should arouse suspicion of cardiac injury. Serial ECGs should be taken in all cases of chest trauma. Depressed or inverted T waves or arrhythmias following severe trauma to the anterior chest suggest cardiac injury. Muffled heart sounds, decreasing pulse pressure, paradoxic pulse, and increasing venous pressure point to cardiac tamponade.

G. Aortic Injury: Aortic rupture is suggested by a history of severe chest trauma and widening of the mediastinum on chest x-ray with or without hemothorax. Angiographic visualization of the brachiocephalic vessels can establish the diagnosis and pre-

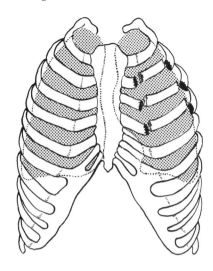

FIG 17–1. Flail chest.

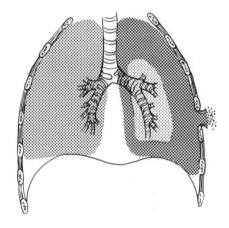

FIG 17–2. Open pneumothorax.

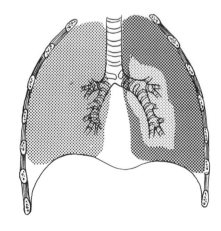

FIG 17–3. Closed pneumothorax.

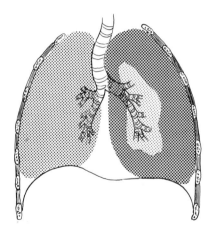

FIG 17−4. Tension pneumothorax.

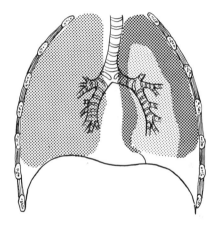

FIG 17−7. Hemopneumothorax.

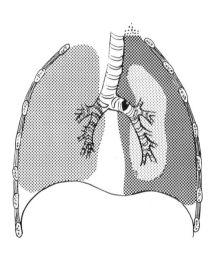

FIG 17−5. Ruptured bronchus.

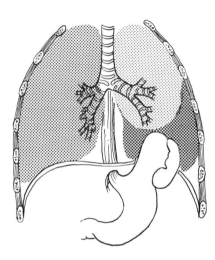

FIG 17−8. Ruptured diaphragm.

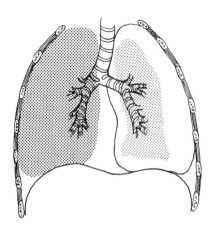

FIG 17−6. Hemothorax.

cisely locate active bleeding sites, accurately position foreign bodies, and define the nature of posttraumatic complications such as thrombosis or arteriovenous fistula formation.

H. Ruptured Diaphragm: (Fig 17−8.) Injury to the diaphragm should be suspected when there has been severe crushing injury or penetrating injury at or below the fifth rib anteriorly and the tip of the scapula posteriorly. A chest x-ray showing a "high diaphragm" may be the first evidence of diaphragmatic rupture. The appearance of abdominal viscera herniated into the chest on x-ray examination is diagnostic.

I. Esophageal Injury: The esophagus is usually injured by penetrating trauma. A chest x-ray showing mediastinal emphysema or hydropneumothorax suggests esophageal injury (Fig 17−9). Esophagoscopy and esophagography may confirm the diagnosis.

J. Respiratory Failure: Abnormalities in ventilation/perfusion relationships, including increased intrapulmonary shunting and physiologic dead space, are seen in most patients with significant thoracic trauma.

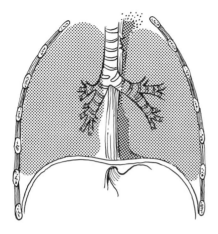

FIG 17-9. Esophageal injury.

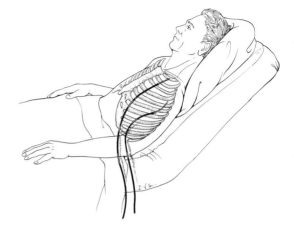

FIG 17-10. Intubation of patient with a chest injury.

Arterial oxygen tensions less than 60 mm Hg while breathing room air, increased CO_2 tension, decreased total lung compliance, or dependence on mechanical ventilatory assistance for more than 24 hours—all suggest the diagnosis of respiratory failure.

Complications

The sequelae of chest trauma are hypoxic brain damage, empyema, pulmonary abscess, constrictive pericarditis, and pulmonary fibrosis. Hypoxia can be minimized or entirely prevented by prompt and adequate ventilatory support. This can be accomplished with an endotracheal tube and controlled ventilation. Adequate surgical drainage of hemothorax, prompt reexpansion of collapsed lung, and aspiration of copious tracheobronchial secretions by bronchoscopy will minimize the complications of empyema and pulmonary abscess. Prompt use of ventilatory support for flail chest or rib fractures associated with progressive respiratory failure is a major advance in preventing serious complications and fatalities.

Treatment

Effective management of thoracic injury is based on precise understanding of the physiology and mechanics of respiration. The following principles must be observed in the treatment of these injuries: (1) preservation of airway and provision of adequate ventilation, (2) control of hemorrhage, (3) restoration of circulating blood volume, (4) aspiration of air and blood from the thoracic cavity, and (5) repair of major damage to intrathoracic viscera.

Acute respiratory distress requires immediate examination of the airway, removal of foreign body if present, and insertion of an endotracheal tube to give access to the airway and to permit aspiration of secretions and blood. An immediate airtight dressing should be applied to sucking wounds of the chest. Closed tube thoracostomy is the most effective method of treating most consequences of intrathoracic trauma (Fig 17-10). Tube thoracostomy is better than thoracen-

tesis for prompt, complete evacuation of intrapleural air or blood and provides an avenue of exit for continuing or recurrent air leaks or hemorrhage.

A. Chest Wall Injuries: Simple rib fractures not accompanied by vascular or lung injury may be completely innocuous and require only simple analgesics for relief of pain. Severe pain may interfere with pulmonary function, resulting in retained bronchial secretions, atelectasis, pneumonia, and pulmonary insufficiency. In such cases, intercostal nerve blockage is useful.

Flail chest should be treated by positive pressure ventilation administered through a cuffed endotracheal tube or tracheostomy and cuffed tracheostomy tube. Continuous positive pressure breathing provides better restoration of lung volume and stabilization of the chest wall. External stabilization of the chest wall usually is not indicated. Many patients find it difficult to adjust to the respirator. Deliberate hyperventilation to produce mild hypocapnia reduces the respiratory drive and permits a smoother adjustment to the respirator. If this is not sufficient, sedatives or muscle relaxants can be used as required.

The duration of treatment of flail chest is usually about 2 weeks, but this varies depending on the patient's response and the degree of pulmonary insufficiency. Ventilatory assistance should be continued until the patient can breathe spontaneously and maintain adequate arterial oxygenation according to the following criteria: (1) vital capacity of at least 10–15 ml/kg body weight; (2) A–a_{DO_2}* gradient less than 300 mm Hg; (3) maximum inspiratory force of at least 20 cm water (negative pressure); and (4) improvement in the clinical condition of the patient.

B. Pneumothorax: A small pneumothorax of 20% or less requires no treatment or may be aspirated by thoracentesis. Larger volumes of air should be removed

*A–a_{DO_2} = alveolar-arterial oxygen tension difference, which is used as an indirect measurement of the percentage of cardiac output that is shunted within the lung and is not oxygenated.

via closed tube thoracostomy. A chest tube is inserted in the second intercostal space in the midclavicular line. The chest tube is then connected to water-sealed (airtight) drainage under negative pressure. This procedure is done under local anesthesia and direct visualization. The index finger should be inserted through the opening into the pleural space and the chest tube guided into place. The incision is then closed by suture to prevent air leakage.

C. Ruptured Bronchus: Severe and persistent air leak suggests rupture of a main stem bronchus; bronchoscopy and bronchography are required to confirm the diagnosis. Bronchial rupture is treated by thoracotomy and suture. If the bronchus cannot be repaired satisfactorily by suture, pulmonary resection may be required.

D. Hemothorax: A large chest tube should be placed in the fifth or sixth intercostal space along the midaxillary line. The chest tube should be attached to water-sealed drainage under negative pressure. Small amounts of blood obtained initially are not a reliable indication of the magnitude of injury. If bleeding persists at the rate of 100 ml/hour or more, operative intervention is required. Clotted hemothorax is another indication for thoracotomy. Autotransfusion should be considered if there is a large amount of blood in the thoracic cavity. Only about 5% of patients with hemothorax will require thoracotomy.

E. Pulmonary Contusion: Small contusions usually require no treatment. Large contusions require vigorous respiratory support (positive pressure breathing and trachial toilet) to prevent hypoxia, atelectasis, and pulmonary sepsis. Contusions associated with marked intrabronchial hemorrhage and lung parenchymal destruction may be treated by thoracotomy and resection of the contused lung.

F. Cardiac Injury: The treatment of cardiac contusion is the same as that of myocardial infarction, with analgesia, bed rest, and control of arrhythmias and heart failure, if present. Pericardial tamponade is treated initially with pericardiocentesis, using a large needle and syringe. This is best accomplished via the substernal approach by inserting a needle upward and to the left from the angle between the costal arch and the xiphoid process. If tamponade is not relieved or if it recurs, open thoracotomy is required to control the bleeding.

G. Vascular Injury: Injuries to the subclavian artery require cervicothoracotomy. Thoracotomy and direct suture repair are required for injuries to the superior vena cava, innominate vein, pulmonary artery, and thoracic aorta. Extracorporeal circulation and the use of shunts are useful adjuncts in the treatment of thoracic aortic injuries.

H. Diaphragm: Diaphragmatic perforations or rupture can be repaired via a transthoracic or transabdominal approach. Diaphragmatic injuries are usually associated with injuries of the abdominal viscera. The transabdominal approach allows inspection of the abdominal viscera.

I. Esophageal Injury: Esophageal injuries are treated by thoracotomy and suture repair. Drainage of the area of repair is of paramount importance.

J. Respiratory Failure: Shock, fluid overload, aspiration pneumonitis, intravascular coagulation, infection, and pulmonary damage from high concentration of inspired oxygen and mechanical ventilation are factors that contribute to respiratory failure. Therapy is directed at (1) prevention or prompt treatment of circulatory failure; (2) limitation of fluid administration—particularly crystalloid solutions—so that only the minimum amount necessary to support good circulation is given; (3) use of mechanical ventilation when necessary to provide adequate arterial oxygenation and elimination of CO_2; (4) protection of the airway against aspiration by use of cuffed endotracheal and tracheostomy tubes; (5) prevention or treatment of associated intravascular coagulation; and (6) treatment of associated infection, particularly pneumonia.

Prognosis

The outlook for simple penetrating chest injuries and rib fractures is good. The overall mortality for penetrating wounds is about 4%, and the complication rate (empyema, pneumonia, atelectasis, and respiratory insufficiency) is about 15%. Severe nonpenetrating injuries have about a 10% mortality. The presence of associated injuries with nonpenetrating thoracic trauma greatly reduces the chances for survival.

Bassett JS, Gibson RD, Wilson RF: Blunt injuries to the chest. J Trauma 8:418, 1968.

Blair EM, Mills E: Rationale of stabilization of the flail chest with intermittent positive pressure breathing. Am Surgeon 34:860, 1968.

Breuner LA, Carter R: Wounds of the great vessels of the thorax. Am J Surg 114:340, 1967.

Burke JF: Early diagnosis of traumatic rupture of the bronchus. JAMA 181:682, 1962.

DeMuth WE Jr: Bullet velocity as applied to military rifle capacity. J Trauma 9:27–38, 1969.

DeMuth WE Jr: High velocity bullet wounds of muscle and bone: The basis of rational early treatment. J Trauma 6:744–755, 1966.

Fulton RL, Peter ET, Wilson JN: The pathophysiology and treatment of pulmonary contusions. J Trauma 10:719, 1970.

Garzon AA, Amer NL, Karlson KE: Treatment of penetrating wounds of the chest. Arch Surg 88:397, 1964.

Gerami S & others: The management of gunshot wounds of the chest. Ann Thoracic Surg 5:189, 1968.

Halter BL: Nonpenetrating trauma to the heart. Am J Surg 90:237–240, 1955.

Heberer G: Ruptures and aneurysms of the thoracic aorta after blunt chest trauma. J Cardiovas Surg 12:115, 1971.

Hopkins BR, Border JR, Schenk WG Jr: Experimental closed chest trauma. J Thoracic Cardiovas Surg 55:580–585, 1968.

Jones FL: Transmural myocardial necrosis after nonpenetrating cardiac trauma. Am J Cardiol 26:419, 1970.

Kirsh MM & others: Repair of acute traumatic ruptures of the aorta without extracorporeal circulation. Ann Thoracic Surg 10:227, 1970.

Lichtman M: The problem of contused lungs. J Trauma 10:731, 1970.

Lucido JL, Wall CA: Rupture of the diaphragm due to blunt trauma. Arch Surg 86:989–999, 1963.

McNamara J & others: Thoracic injuries in combat casualties in Vietnam. Ann Thoracic Surg 10:389, 1970.

Miller DR: Transection of the esophagus at the esophagastric junction by blunt trauma. J Trauma 8:1105, 1968.

Olcott C, Barker RE, Blaisdell FW: Diagnosis and treatment of respiratory failure following civilian trauma. Am J Surg 122:260–268, 1971.

Paton BC & others: Acute treatment of traumatic aortic rupture. J Trauma 11:1, 1971.

Sankaran S, Wilson RF: Factors affecting prognosis in patients with flail chest. J Thoracic Cardiovas Surg 60:402–410, 1970.

Schwindt W, Gale JW: Late recognition and treatment of traumatic diaphragmatic hernias. Arch Surg 94:330, 1967.

Sigelman SS, Rosenberg RF, Furman S: Angiographic evaluation of injury to the great vessels. Arch Surg 100:565, 1970.

Storey CF, Kuzman WJ: Traumatic coronary artery right atrial fistula: Successful repair of lesion caused by bullet wound of heart. Ann Thoracic Surg 4:352, 1967.

Wilson RF & others: Physiologic shunting in the lung in critically ill or injured patients. J Surg Res 10:571, 1970.

ABDOMINAL INJURIES

A major proportion of life-threatening traumatic injuries sustained in both civilian and military experience are abdominal. Most of the military injuries to the abdomen are penetrating wounds, whereas the vast majority of abdominal injuries in civilian life result from blunt trauma. The solid parenchymatous organs are wounded more frequently in civilian blunt casualties; injuries involving hollow viscera are seen more often in military practice, which deals primarily with penetrating wounds.

In trauma due to high-velocity missiles, susceptibility to injury is directly proportionate to the density of the tissues involved. Therefore, wounds caused by high-velocity missiles to the liver, spleen, and kidneys are most severe, whereas structures of lower specific gravity such as the lungs show greater resistance to injury.

Patients with abdominal injury may have major injuries involving many areas of the body and can present with shock, coma, or respiratory distress. The initial management is directed toward (1) maintenance of an adequate airway, (2) arrest of external hemorrhage, (3) restoration of circulating blood volume, (4) rapid and accurate diagnosis, and (5) definitive treatment.

Clinical Findings

Serious intra-abdominal injury is usually accompanied by abdominal pain, tenderness, and distention. Peristaltic sounds are diminished or absent. Nausea, vomiting, hematemesis, hematuria, melena, and shock may be associated with certain injuries. If the patient is unconscious, many of these signs and symptoms may not be present. Careful examination and consideration of the mechanism of injury will give some idea of the magnitude of intra-abdominal injury.

Blunt trauma to the abdomen may produce severe intra-abdominal injury with minimal physical findings. A patient with blunt abdominal injury may continue to have bowel sounds for several hours after injury.

The presence of abdominal tenderness and distention, with or without shock, should immediately suggest intra-abdominal injury. Fractures of the lower ribs, pelvis, and lumbar vertebrae can produce spasm of the abdominal wall which may be difficult to distinguish from intra-abdominal injury. In this clinical situation, exploratory laparotomy may be indicated.

In blunt trauma—characteristically, crushing injury—left shoulder pain, left lower rib fractures, and free blood in the peritoneal cavity on paracentesis suggest injury to the spleen. Left lower rib fractures are associated with splenic rupture in about 20% of cases. Right lower rib fractures and right shoulder pain should arouse a suspicion of hepatic injury.

X-ray examination is of assistance in arriving at an accurate diagnosis. Plain x-rays of the abdomen with upright and left lateral decubitus radiographic views will usually suffice for patients who can coherently relate their symptoms. Plain films of the abdomen may give evidence of skeletal injury, pneumoperitoneum, indirect evidence of rupture of a solid viscus, or alteration in the size, shape, or position of viscera. Intravenous urography should be added whenever major retroperitoneal injury is possible or hematuria is noted. The presence of hematuria may also be an indication for cystography whenever there is an associated pelvic fracture or suprapubic pain.

Abdominal paracentesis is a useful adjunct to diagnosis in blunt trauma. If the patient is intoxicated or unconscious or if abdominal symptoms are low-grade and persistent, abdominal paracentesis may provide objective evidence for operation. If blood is recovered, intra-abdominal injury is present in about 95% of cases. A negative paracentesis does not exclude significant visceral injury. In general, paracentesis is only contraindicated when there is already an obvious indication for surgery, tympanitic abdominal distention, or pulsatile abdominal mass.

In penetrating injuries caused by a bullet, assumptions concerning injury between the wounds of entrance and exit should not be made without knowledge of the wounding agent. Low-velocity missiles tend to cause local injury along the course of the wound. High-velocity missiles tend to cause damage far removed from the local area of injury. High-velocity missiles suck foreign material into the wound. In addition, in shotgun wounds, the wad and plastic caps which are used to separate the powder from the shot very often penetrate deeply into the wound, causing injury and infection.

Treatment

When the diagnosis of intra-abdominal injury is

seriously entertained, the patient should be given parenteral antibiotics immediately. In a few cases, intraperitoneal hemorrhage will be so severe that even rapid multiple transfusions will be ineffective until the abdomen has been opened and the hemorrhage controlled.

Operation should not be delayed in blunt abdominal trauma when there is good evidence that serious intraperitoneal hemorrhage or visceral rupture has occurred.

All gunshot wounds of the abdomen must be explored whether or not penetration is evident. Shock waves from nonpenetrating gunshot wounds of the abdominal wall may transect bowel or lacerate a viscus such as the liver or spleen.

Superficial stab wounds should be explored locally in the emergency room. If the extent of penetration cannot be determined or if the stab wound involves the posterior rectus sheath, the abdominal cavity must be explored.

In selected cases, stab wounds are followed expectantly by some authorities. If deep penetration is known to have occurred, exploration is the safer course.

At operation, a long incision should be made to ensure adequate exposure. The first objective is control of hemorrhage. This can be accomplished by gauze packing until adequate exposure is achieved. The second objective is to seal off all sites of bowel contamination. When the abdomen is opened, the organs of first priority are the liver, spleen, and pancreas. Laceration or rupture of hollow viscera can usually be managed by clamping and repair later.

A. Liver Injury: Minor injury to the liver requires ligation of the bleeding points (if actively bleeding) and drainage. Mass suturing of liver parenchyma to obtain hemostasis is contraindicated because the ischemic necrosis caused by the suturing often leads to subsequent infection. Extensive liver injury may require wide debridement of devitalized hepatic parenchyma and, in some instances, major liver resection (lobectomy). Liver injuries are covered in detail in Chapter 26.

B. Splenic Injury: Splenic injury is treated by splenectomy. When there has been extensive disruption of the spleen, it is important to remove all the accessible splenic tissue to prevent autotransplantation (splenosis). The pancreas and stomach must be carefully visualized and protected from injury. Injuries to the spleen are covered in detail in Chapter 29.

C. Gallbladder and Extrahepatic Bile Duct Injury: Injuries to the gallbladder and extrahepatic bile ducts are uncommon. Cholecystectomy will suffice for gallbladder injuries. Repair of injuries to the extrahepatic bile ducts is more complicated. When the duct is partially transected, simple primary repair with drainage is all that is indicated. If the duct has been completely transected, it can be repaired in an end-to-end fashion, with or without a stent.

D. Pancreatic Injury: The treatment of pancreatic injuries is determined by (1) the extent of injury,

(2) the extent of associated injury, and (3) the overall condition of the patient. The principles of treatment are control of hemorrhage, debridement of devitalized tissue, and drainage. In some cases, injuries of the pancreas to the left of the superior mesenteric artery are treated most expeditiously by distal pancreatectomy and splenectomy. Injuries of the head of the pancreas and duodenum are particularly difficult to treat, and the mortality rate is correspondingly high. These injuries may require pancreatoduodenectomy or a pancreatoenterostomy using a Roux-en-Y segment of jejunum, provided the posterior capsule is intact. The area of the pancreas must be drained externally.

E. Stomach and Duodenal Injury: The stomach and duodenum are frequently injured by penetrating wounds of the abdomen. Penetrating injury of the stomach and duodenum usually involves both the anterior and posterior surfaces. Extensive mobilization and inspection are required to make certain that a posterior injury has not been overlooked. Injuries to the stomach are debrided and closed.

Blunt trauma rarely involves the stomach, but the duodenum can be injured if it is trapped against the vertebral column. Duodenal injuries may be limited to contusions or intramural hematoma, or there may be intraperitoneal or extraperitoneal rupture. When possible, primary suture repair of the duodenum is preferable. An onlay serosal patch, using a segment of jejunum, is an alternative technic when primary suture repair is not feasible.

F. Injury to the Small and Large Intestines: Penetrating trauma to the small intestine and colon can result in multiple perforations through adjacent coils. Repair should consist of simple closure if surrounding tissue is not devitalized, or resection and end-to-end anastomosis if injury is complicated.

Rupture of the intestinal tract secondary to blunt trauma is relatively uncommon. The usual mechanism of disruption of the bowel is sudden compression of a segment of bowel filled with chyme, apparently leading to an increase in intraluminal pressure and rupture. Rupture characteristically occurs at points of fixation of the intestine. Fragments of bone from fractures of the pelvis occasionally cause penetrating injury to the cecum.

In general, wounds of the colon should be managed by exteriorization or resection if extensive injury has occurred. Primary anastomosis should be avoided in most cases. Injuries of the rectum should be managed with a proximal colostomy and presacral drainage.

G. Urogenital Tract Injury: (See Chapter 44 for additional comments on injuries to the urinary tract.) The kidney is frequently injured by blunt trauma and less frequently by penetrating trauma. Intravenous urography should be performed when injury to the upper urinary tract is suspected. Of paramount importance is the presence or absence of a kidney on the uninvolved side, an estimate of its functional capacity, and the gross integrity of the kidneys. If the contour of the kidney is grossly disrupted or there is extravasation of dye, operation is mandatory. Partial or complete nephrectomy may be indicated. However, every effort should be made to conserve renal tissue which is well vascularized and might be expected to return to good function. Ureteral injuries are managed by resection and end-to-end anastomosis, with or without a stent. External drainage is necessary.

With pelvic fractures and hematuria from blunt trauma, the most frequent urinary tract injury is to the bladder and bladder neck. A cystogram with right and left views will confirm the diagnosis. Bladder lacerations should always be approached transperitoneally so that other abdominal injuries will not be overlooked. Bladder lacerations should be sutured and drained suprapubically and through the urethra with a Foley catheter. Bladder neck injuries should be managed with a No. 22–24 Foley catheter with a 30 ml bag. Traction (0.5 kg) should be applied to the catheter for 5–7 days. The catheter is then left in place for 3 weeks.

H. Retroperitoneal Hematoma: Retroperitoneal hematomas secondary to blunt trauma should be managed conservatively if the hematoma is expanding and pulsatile and there is no injury to the urinary tract as shown by intravenous urography. Massive retroperitoneal hematomas are associated with pelvic fractures. Ligation of one or both hypogastric arteries is sometimes done to control massive hemorrhage associated with pelvic fractures.

Retroperitoneal hematomas resulting from penetrating injury should all be explored surgically.

I. Injury to the Diaphragm: Injury to the diaphragm is associated with penetrating trauma involving the upper abdomen. Thus, penetrating wounds of the upper abdomen are an indication for thorough exploration of the diaphragm.

Blunt abdominal injury can also result in diaphragmatic injury. Both immediate and late herniation of abdominal viscera are potential complications if the lacerations are not repaired.

Diaphragmatic injuries should be repaired with heavy mattress nonabsorbable sutures.

J. Vascular Injuries: Major vascular injury due to blunt trauma is not common. Rupture of the abdominal aorta and iliac arteries is occasionally seen when a pedestrian is struck by a rapidly moving vehicle. Venous injuries are more commonly seen after blunt trauma. Injuries of the inferior vena cava are frequently associated with extensive liver trauma.

Major vascular injury is more frequent after penetrating trauma than after blunt trauma. Patients with major intra-abdominal vascular injury often die soon after injury. Survival depends upon immediate recognition of the vascular injury and prompt control of the bleeding site.

Venous injuries are more difficult to treat than arterial injuries, particularly intrahepatic caval or hepatic venous injuries. Deliberate sacrifice of a portion of the liver, the use of an internal shunt, and occlusion of the portal triad constitute the accepted method of management. This technic maintains venous return to the heart, achieves hemostasis, and permits exposure of the site of venous injury for definitive repair. Ligation of the suprarenal vena cava is almost without exception fatal.

In uncomplicated lacerations of major vessels, simple lateral repair may be all that is necessary. In more extensive injuries, debridement with end-to-end anastomosis or autogenous vein grafting may be indicated.

Complications

The complications of abdominal injuries correspond to the organ injured. In general, they are wound infection, peritonitis, subphrenic abscess, pelvic abscess, delayed or secondary hemorrhage, wound dehiscence, intestinal obstruction, and enterocutaneous fistula formation.

Prognosis

The prognosis of abdominal trauma varies with the extent of injury and the magnitude of associated injuries. The mortality rate with penetrating abdominal trauma is 5%; with blunt abdominal trauma, 10%.

Allen RE & others: Retroperitoneal hemorrhage secondary to blunt trauma. Am J Surg 118:558–561, 1969.

Baker RJ, Boyd DR, Condon RE: Priority of management of patients with multiple injuries. S Clin North America 50:3–11, 1970.

Banowski LH, Wolfel DA, Lackner HL: Considerations in diagnosis and management of renal trauma. J Trauma 10:587, 1970.

Briggs FM & others: Surgical management of civilian colon injuries. J Trauma 3:484–491, 1963.

Bull JC Jr, Mathewson C Jr: Exploratory laparotomy in patients with penetrating wounds of the abdomen. Am J Surg 116:223, 1968.

Buscaglia L, Blaisdell FW, Lim RC Jr: Penetrating abdominal vascular injuries. Arch Surg 99:764, 1969.

Cerise E, Scully JH: Blunt trauma to small intestine. J Trauma 10:46, 1970.

Christensen N, Ignatius J, Mathewson C Jr: Treatment of injuries of the large bowel in civilian practice. Am J Surg 89:753–758, 1955.

Cooke RV, Southwood WFW: Closed abdominal injuries. Brit J Surg 51:767, 1964.

DeMuth WE Jr: Bullet velocity as applied to military life wounding capacity. J Trauma 9:27–38, 1969.

DeMuth WE Jr: The mechanism of shotgun wounds. J Trauma 11:219–229, 1971.

Duke JH, Jones RC, Shires GT: Management of injuries to the inferior vena cava. Am J Surg 110:759, 1965.

Freeark RJ, Love L, Baker RJ: An active diagnostic approach to blunt abdominal trauma. S Clin North America 48:97, 1968.

Gibbs BF, Crow JL, Rupnick EG: Pancreatoduodenectomy for pancreatoduodenal injuries. J Trauma 10:702, 1970.

Hawkins L, Pomerantz M, Eiseman B: Laparotomy at the time of pelvic fracture. J Trauma 10:619, 1970.

Jones RC, Shires GT: Management of pancreatic injuries. Arch Surg 90:502–508, 1965.

Kazarian KK & others: Stab wounds of the abdomen: An analysis of 500 patients. Arch Surg 102:465, 1971.

Macbeth RA: Blunt abdominal trauma. Canad J Surg 9:384, 1966.

Morton JR, Jordan GL: Traumatic accidental injuries. J Trauma 8:127–139, 1968.

Nelson JB & others: Diaphragmatic injuries and post-traumatic hernia. J Trauma 2:36–38, 1962.

Nelson JF: The roentgenologic evaluation of abdominal trauma. Radiol Clinic North America 4:415, 1966.

Ochsner JL, Crawford ES, DeBakey ME: Injuries of the vena cava caused by external trauma. Surgery 49:397–405, 1961.

Ramnath R, Walden EC, Caguin F: Ligation of the suprarenal vena cava and right nephrectomy with complete recovery. Am J Surg 112:88, 1966.

Rodkey GV: The management of abdominal injuries. S Clin North America 46:627, 1966.

Root HD & others: Diagnostic peritoneal lavage. Surgery 57:633–637, 1965.

Root HD, Keizer PJ, Perry JF: Peritoneal trauma: Experimental and clinical studies. Surgery 62:679, 1967.

Sheldon GF, Cohn LH, Blaisdell FW: Surgical treatment of pancreatic injuries. J Trauma 10:795, 1970.

Shires GT, Jones RC: Initial management of the severely injured patient. JAMA 213:1872–1878, 1970.

Starzl TE & others: Penetrating injuries of the inferior vena cava. S Clin North America 43:387, 1963.

Steicher FM & others: The management of retroperitoneal hematoma secondary to penetrating injuries. Surg Gynec Obst 123:581, 1966.

Thompson IM, Johnson EL, Ross G Jr: The acute abdomen of unrecognized bladder rupture. Arch Surg 90:371, 1965.

Thomsord NR, Curtiss PH, Marable SA: Injuries of the iliac and femoral arteries associated with blunt skeletal trauma. J Trauma 9:126, 1969.

Waltuck TL & others: Avulsion injuries of the vena cava following blunt abdominal trauma. Ann Surg 171:67, 1970.

Wanebo HJ, Hunt TK, Mathewson C Jr: Rectal injuries. J Trauma 9:700, 1969.

Weichert RF, Hewitt RL: Injuries to the inferior vena cava: Report of 35 cases. J Trauma 10:649, 1970.

ARTERIAL INJURIES
Albert D. Hall, MD

The repair of injured blood vessels to preserve normal circulation is an essential immediate extension of primary resuscitation. Until experience in the Korean conflict demonstrated the feasibility of repairing acute vascular injuries even under combat conditions, it was standard procedure to ligate disrupted arteries to control hemorrhage and accept the resulting 50% amputation rate recorded in World War II. This figure was reduced to 13% in the Korean experience largely because of more expeditious evacuation of casualties, the availability of blood for prompt resuscitation, a better understanding of blood vessel repair and bypass technics, the use of operative angiography, the appropriate use of heparin, and the more effective control of infections with the use of wound debridement, secondary closure, and antibiotics. Further improvement of survival and limb salvage rates has been achieved in recent years by more effective means of managing shock, the use of hemodialysis

units, and the introduction of the Fogarty balloon catheter for extraction of peripheral thrombi. When managed well, the casualty with major vascular injuries can have an uncomplicated course. Without proper assessment and optimum treatment, a reversible condition becomes irreversible.

Types of Injuries

A. Incisions and Lacerations: Incisions or lacerations, commonly caused by knives or glass, may or may not produce overt hemorrhage depending upon the extent of the injury and the location of the vessel. A completely divided artery can retract and constrict, so that bleeding is minimal; or an artery with a gaping lateral defect can bleed massively. If an adjacent vein has been incised simultaneously, an acute **arteriovenous fistula** is formed. Sharply lacerated arteries are readily treated by simple closure or anastomosis, and injured veins repaired or ligated.

B. Perforations: Perforations due to small, high-velocity missiles (bullets) or sharp instruments (ice picks, pointed knives) can produce life-threatening— even though initially occult—vascular injuries. External evidence of injury may be minimal and the significance of a wound not appreciated until hemorrhagic shock occurs or a pulsating hematoma, false aneurysm, or delayed arteriovenous fistula develops. Whenever a penetrating wound is located anywhere near the site of a major vessel, an important vascular injury may be present. Normal pulses do not rule out such injuries.

C. Puncture Wounds: Puncture wounds such as those produced by percutaneous catheterization of peripheral arteries during diagnostic procedures can cause defects in the arterial wall that bleed and form false aneurysms or pulsating hematomas. When a needle or catheter dislodges an arteriosclerotic plaque or elevates the intima, a vessel will thrombose, leading to acute ischemia of a limb. In either case, such an injury must be recognized promptly by careful observation of the patient after such a procedure. Restoration of blood flow is accomplished at emergency exploration.

D. Contusions or Crushing Injuries: These produce either transmural or partial disruption of arteries, resulting in elevation of the intima and formation of intramural hematomas which lead to occlusion of the lumen. Repair of these vessels may require replacement of the segment or a bypass graft. Contused arteries are seen with fractures, dislocations, or damage to muscles, nerves, and skin, leading to a less favorable prognosis for limb salvage. These complex problems—common in both military and some civilian casualties—may involve any vessel, including the extracranial cerebral arteries and the vasculature leading to any of the viscera. The brachial and popliteal arteries, coursing across joints and exposed to direct trauma, are particularly susceptible to injuries associated with fractures and dislocations.

E. Arterial Spasm: Segments of arteries, frequently within musculofascial compartments—and especially the muscular arteries (brachial, popliteal)—

may become narrowed by intense constriction of smooth muscle evoked by the injury. Such vessels may also be compressed by hematoma and edema. Although the involved artery may not be injured, it frequently supplies tissues that have been rendered ischemic by trauma, and a vicious cycle is created. Vasospasm alone is rarely sufficiently intense or persistent to produce numbness or paralysis of the distal extremity. When this occurs, objective evidence of patency of the system should be obtained since unnecessary delay in restoring perfusion may jeopardize the limb. An arteriogram can be performed when it is not clear whether an occlusion exists. A Doppler ultrasonic flow probe is a useful adjunct for detecting pulsatile flow.

F. Disruption of Thoracic Aorta or Brachiocephalic Vessels: Crushing blows to the chest or abrupt deceleration from high speed can disrupt the thoracic aorta, most often just distal to the ligamentum arteriosum. Forces are dissipated through points of fixation in a manner that disrupts the intima and media. This usually leads to fatal hemorrhage, but occasionally the adventitia and pleura contain the extravasated blood and a false aneurysm is formed. Such a lesion must be suspected when the upper ribs are fractured and the chest x-ray shows widening of the mediastinum. The diagnosis can be confirmed by arteriography and operative repair performed—usually with the aid of left heart bypass. The innominate, subclavian, and carotid arteries are subject to similar disruption by direct blows to the sternum.

G. Chemical Injury: Inadvertent intra-arterial injection of hypnotics (eg, thiopental) and other agents produces occlusion of small peripheral vessels which may be so severe that all or part of a limb may be lost. This can occur when the ulnar artery is superficial at the elbow in cases of high bifurcation of the brachial artery, and is a hazard that must be avoided by anesthesiologists in the operating room. Severe pain in the hand is associated with intense vasoconstriction, which may gradually subside after a few hours. When a high dose of the agent has been injected, thrombosis may progress to involve major vessels of the hand and forearm, ultimately requiring amputation. When such an injection is recognized, the needle should be left in place and 15,000 units of heparin injected through it. Reserpine (0.5 mg) has been recommended, although its only effect experimentally has been to protect against the release of catecholamines from the vessel walls when it is given before the injection of thiopental. Brachial plexus block or exploration of the vessel may be of some value in reducing the vasospasm.

Manifestations of Arterial Injury

A. Hemorrhage: Although the diagnosis of arterial injury is obvious when there is pulsatile external hemorrhage, a bleeding site may not be readily identified when blood is accumulating in deep tissues or draining freely into the thorax, abdomen, or retroperitoneum. In these cases, the primary presenting manifestation is hemorrhagic shock. The peripheral

vasoconstriction that accompanies such shock makes it difficult to evaluate peripheral pulses until the blood volume is restored. Recognition of arterial contusions and thromboses associated with multiple injuries is delayed by the difficulty in differentiating local from systemic factors. These effects of arterial injury are reciprocal, since ischemic tissue prolongs acidosis, venous stasis, and microembolization to the lungs, the latter compromising pulmonary function.

B. Ischemia: Until proved otherwise, ischemia of a part—whether of an extremity or a visceral organ—must be treated as though it were due to primary vascular injury. When an extremity is involved, paralysis or anesthesia rapidly develops, indicating anoxia of the peripheral nerves. It may not be possible to predict whether a given degree of ischemia will be tolerated by the part. For example, sudden occlusion of the carotid artery will result in brain damage within minutes unless collateral circulation provides a near physiologic perfusion pressure. Injury to a renal artery may produce a nonfunctioning kidney that can be restored by an arterial repair even several hours after the injury. An ischemic extremity may have sufficient perfusion to preserve some but not all muscle, the most susceptible to necrosis being those without major collateral arterial supply and located within nondistensible fascial compartments. Although 6 or 8 hours of ischemia may be tolerated by skeletal muscle, any delay in restoring perfusion risks the appearance of a vicious cycle consisting of subfascial edema, venous occlusion, propagation of thrombi within vascular spaces, and disruption of arterioles and capillaries which upon reperfusion will bleed and produce progressive swelling and necrosis. Time is a critical factor in the management of all vascular injuries to preserve life and organ function.

C. False Aneurysm: A false aneurysm may be formed by the outer layers of a partially disrupted artery or by the encapsulation of a **pulsating hematoma.** These may develop without interrupting distal blood flow, and in the acute phase are prone to rupture without warning. Although frequently tolerated for a time, they expand to produce symptoms either by compression of adjacent nerves or collateral circulation, and ultimately rupture.

D. Arteriovenous Fistula: Arteriovenous fistulas occur after simultaneous injury to adjacent arteries and veins, usually due to stab wounds or missiles. There may be little bleeding because the arterial pressure is decompressed into the vein. Fistulas are also produced by operative injuries—when a common ligature is applied to an artery and a vein (nephrectomy, thyroidectomy)—or by inadvertent injury of the vena cava or iliac veins and the aorta (removal of herniated intervertebral disks). Delayed arteriovenous fistulas are seen when infected hematomas erode into adjacent veins.

E. Venous Injury and Obstruction: When major venous drainage of a part is interrupted, tissue perfusion is compromised by the sequence of edema and compression of tissues in closed compartments. Propagation of thrombus from these veins can lead to pulmonary embolism. Venous injury should be suspected when peripheral veins in the extremity are abnormally prominent.

Principles of Diagnosis

(1) Vascular injury must be suspected in any wound in the vicinity of major blood vessels.

(2) Search for evidence of hemorrhage into body cavities.

(3) Suspect primary vascular injury whenever tissue perfusion or organ function is impaired (fractures, dislocations, penetrating wounds, direct trauma).

(4) Differentiate between the effects of hemorrhagic shock and vascular occlusion (monitor responses to blood volume restoration by observing urinary output and peripheral pulses).

(5) Search for physical signs of vascular injury (expanding or pulsating hematomas, to-and-fro murmurs of false aneurysms, continuous murmurs of arteriovenous fistulas, loss of pulses, progressive swelling of the part, unexplained ischemia or dysfunction).

(6) Differentiate between arterial injury and vasospasm (sympathetic block, topical or intra-arterial papaverine, ultrasonic Doppler flow probe, arteriogram).

(7) **Arteriography**, although of great value in elective cases, may unduly delay emergency operations (control of hemorrhage), and it is not always performed preoperatively unless definitive information concerning the injury is required to determine the operative approach (injuries at base of neck, thoracic aorta) or if confirmation of the clinical diagnosis of arterial injury is needed.

Treatment

A. Primary Care: The clinical assessment of the severity of acute injuries is accomplished without delay. The patient is immediately moved to the operating room if massive hemorrhage precludes resuscitation in the emergency room.

Restoration of blood volume and control of hemorrhage are carried out simultaneously. External bleeding is best controlled by continuous pressure or packing. Tourniquets—which may jeopardize the success of future arterial reconstruction—are avoided. Atraumatic vascular clamps are applied to bleeding vessels when they are accessible. Large-bore intravenous cannulas are inserted (superior or inferior vena cava), and blood is drawn for cross-matching. Blood volume is restored with lactated Ringer's injection, plasma, and type-specific blood. Cross-matched blood is given as soon as it is available. Resuscitation is not continued in the emergency room when the patient ought to be in the operating room, since surgical exposure of inaccessible bleeding vessels (thorax, abdomen, neck) must be accomplished without delay.

B. Associated Measures: Endotracheal intubation may be required to control ventilation or to prevent aspiration of blood from nasopharyngeal injuries. One or more thoracostomy tubes are inserted under local

anesthesia and attached to underwater suction when hemothorax or hemopneumothorax is diagnosed. Symptoms and signs of pericardial tamponade can be relieved by pericardiocentesis done from the perixiphoid approach using a long, thin-walled No. 17 needle.

If the clinical signs of intra-abdominal bleeding are not diagnostic (as in comatose patients), abdominal paracentesis may be used to detect free blood in the peritoneal cavity. An indwelling urinary catheter is used to assess the adequacy of renal perfusion and to detect possible urinary tract injuries.

Fractures are reduced and stabilized before arterial repair is accomplished in the extremities. Antibiotics are started, and tetanus prophylaxis (see Chapter 10) is administered preoperatively.

C. Operative Repair of Arterial Injuries: The feasibility of repairing injured vessels is determined by the magnitude of the wound. Extensive contamination and destruction of soft tissues, bones, blood vessels, and nerves—common in military casualties—preclude primary repair because thrombosis, gangrene, or delayed hemorrhage from infection will develop. Proximal arterial ligation and amputation are usually required as lifesaving procedures for these massive injuries.

Most vascular injuries seen in civilian practice and in certain military casualties are reparable because there is minimal contamination and tissue damage. When operated upon under optimal aseptic conditions with adequate anesthesia, qualified personnel, and proper instrumentation, such injured vessels are usually restored to normal function.

Adequate exposure of the involved vessel is required for control of bleeding and subsequent repair. In the extremities, incisions are placed parallel to the course of the vessel far enough above and below the lesion so that the damaged area is not disturbed. Control of the vessel is obtained proximal and distal to the injury by passing umbilical tapes around the vessel so that the lumen can be occluded with atraumatic clamps at these points. The injured area may then be dissected free without further bleeding in preparation for repair.

Proximal and distal thrombi are removed by flushing the proximal limb and backbleeding the distal limb. A Fogarty balloon catheter is then passed into the distal tributaries where thrombus is extracted. After completion of these maneuvers, a catheter the size of the artery lumen is inserted into the distal limb for injection of heparin solution (1000–2000 units). If there is concern about the adequacy of the distal thrombectomy and the status of a preexisting diseased arterial bed, an **operative arteriogram** is performed by injecting contrast media through the distal catheter.

Devitalized tissue is debrided from the wound and hematomas evacuated. Except in children or when a smaller vessel seems to be critical for limb survival, vessels under 5 mm in diameter are usually not repaired.

Simple lateral repair is permissible when a large

artery has a small incision and closure does not produce narrowing. To avoid narrowing the vessel, a lateral vein patch may be used if the vessel is not contused. When there are multiple defects in a segment or the vessel is contused, excision and end-to-end anastomosis gives the best results. If this produces tension, a replacement or bypass graft is used. The latter is less desirable because it requires that dissection be performed in normal tissues where collaterals may be interrupted.

When possible, autogenous tissue is used for grafting. The saphenous vein is used most commonly and the cephalic vein occasionally. Segments from the hypogastric or external iliac artery are sometimes used as autografts in visceral artery repairs. The iliac artery is then replaced by a prosthetic graft. Prosthetic grafts, although satisfactory when vein grafts are unavailable, are not favored in trauma cases because they are more prone to infection and thrombosis and disruption when used in a contaminated wound.

Cohen AC & others: Carotid artery injuries: An analysis of eighty-five cases. Am J Surg 120:210–214, 1970.

Connolly J: Management of fractures associated with arterial injuries. Am J Surg 120:33, 1970.

DeBakey ME, Simeone FA: Battle injuries of the arteries in World War II: An analysis of 2471 cases. Ann Surg 123:534–579, 1946.

Drapanas T & others: Civilian vascular injuries: A critical appraisal of three decades of management. Ann Surg 172:351–360, 1970.

Eastcott HHG: Arterial injuries. Pages 235–255 in: *Arterial Surgery*. Lippincott, 1969.

Hughes CW: Acute vascular trauma in Korean War casualties: An analysis of 180 cases. Surg Gynec Obst 99:91–100, 1954.

Hughes CW, Bowers WF: *Traumatic Lesions of Peripheral Vessels*. Thomas, 1961.

Hunt TK, Blaisdell FW, Okimoto J: Vascular injuries at the base of the neck. Arch Surg 98:586–590, 1969.

Mustard WF, Bull C: A reliable method for relief of traumatic vascular spasm. Ann Surg 155:339, 1962.

Rich NM & others: Acute arterial injuries in Viet Nam: 1000 cases. J Trauma 10:359–369, 1970.

18 . . .

Burns

Thomas K. Hunt, MD

The treatment of burn injuries is difficult and demanding, and an effective program of prevention is one of our most urgent public health needs. Because of vast technologic and social changes, the management of severe burns will become an increasing problem to the surgeon.

The diagnostic problems in burned patients are essentially evaluative: to determine the nature of the injuring agent (heat, cold, chemicals, electricity), the extent and depth of the burn, and whether the patient has associated illnesses (eg, stroke) or injuries which might have contributed to the accident or which might complicate its management.

The fundamental lesion in burns is loss of the protection afforded by the skin. Body fluids are exuded and evaporated, causing increasingly greater energy losses, and the victim becomes susceptible to overwhelming infection. Burns that involve extensive areas of the body are incompatible with life.

Thermal burns can be caused by heat or cold. Cell protein is easily denatured by great changes of temperature in either direction. Cold can be as injurious as heat, and the effects of both are similar. Obviously, it is the heat (caloric) exchange which determines the extent and depth of the damage. The depth of a burn is determined by the following formula:

$$\frac{\text{Specific heat} \times \Delta \text{ Temperature} \times \text{Time of contact}}{\text{Thermal conductivity of tissue}} \cong \text{Depth}$$

Δ Temperature = The difference between body surface temperature and the temperature of the burning agent.

This formula is useful for estimating the damage done by the burning agent. The specific heat of burning agents such as metals or steam is higher, and such burns tend to be deep. Warm or cool agents (Δ temperature not great) will not burn unless contact is prolonged. The inverse relationship of burn depth to thermal conductivity of tissue reflects the ability of the skin to conduct heat away from the burning agent (or to supply heat in the case of cold injury). Ischemic tissues have low conductivity and are particularly susceptible to deep thermal injury. Burns can be caused by constant exposure of skin to cold or by prolonged contact of a hypothermic patient with a warm heating pad at a normally tolerable temperature.

Burn depth is often difficult to determine (Fig 18–1). **First degree burns** cause only inflammation.

Second degree burns destroy epithelium, ranging from loss of superficial epithelial layers to loss of all but the deepest epithelium contained in hair follicles and in sweat and apocrine glands. In other words, in second degree burns the cleavage between necrotic and live tissue lies in a plane superficial to the deepest squamous elements seen in the skin. Second degree burns will epithelize spontaneously if given enough time. In **third degree burns**, all epithelium has been destroyed and the wound will not spontaneously epithelize. **Fourth degree burns** involve deeper structures such as fascia or tendon.

Unfortunately, the depth of a burn is determined not only by thermal exchange; secondary vascular changes tend to deepen the injury. In the thermal exchange, a vascular injury is produced. The extent of this injury is not immediately apparent: instead, vascular thrombosis increases through the first 48–72 hours. During this process, the burn depth tends to deepen at least partly by ischemic necrosis. Infection also deepens burns. Pseudomonas toxins, for example, thrombose even rather large blood vessels and can deepen the burn by causing ischemic necrosis. Inflammation or infection can destroy the remaining dermal elements of the deep second degree burn, converting it to a third degree burn. Obviously, the full extent of the burn is not always apparent immediately after the injury.

Burn wounds follow a predictable pattern of evolution. Injury (and necrosis) is followed by inflammation and increasing vascular damage as well as capillary permeability. These in turn are followed by loss of

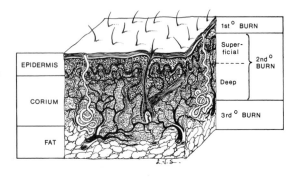

FIG 18–1. Layers of the skin showing depth of first, second, and third degree burns.

plasma into the burned area. In about 4 days, the depth of the burn is relatively fixed. Four to 7 days after injury, normal capillary permeability returns and retained fluid is reabsorbed and excreted (diuresis). Fluid loss into the burn is complicated, for reasons which are not well understood, by a tendency of other tissues to become edematous. These fluid losses add to the increased evaporative water loss from burned surfaces. Plasma is also lost in exudates from blisters and deeply burned tissue. These losses explain the great fluid requirements characteristic of patients with burns.

Pulmonary burns due to inhalation of heat or noxious fumes (such as plastic fumes) are becoming a major cause of death. For example, when polytetrafluoroethylene (Teflon) is heated above 427 C (800 F), it releases a vapor which can cause severe, often fatal pneumonitis. Any patient who is burned while in a closed space is particularly liable to pulmonary injury due to inhalation of hot gases. Pulmonary injury now causes 10–20% of deaths due to burns.

Many types of chemical agents can cause burns, including acids, alkalies, phosphorus, and tar. Electrical burns are becoming more common. Chemical burns are frequently extended by the use of solvents or mechanical forces necessary to remove the agent. For example, hot tar often cannot be removed without causing further injury.

Clinical Findings

A. First Degree Burns: These cause pain and erythema but are otherwise insignificant except when very extensive in very old or very young patients.

B. Second Degree Burns: Superficial second degree burns cause blistering. Deep second degree burns are often clinically indistinguishable from third degree burns. In general, superficial second degree burns retain sensitivity to touch or pinprick.

C. Third Degree Burns: Third degree burns result in pale or charred skin, thrombosed superficial vessels, and insensitivity to touch. They may be quite pink, but the color does not blanch under pressure.

D. Pulmonary Burns: Pulmonary burns are not always easy to diagnose immediately after burning. Acute respiratory failure at the time of injury is rare. The usual clinical signs of impending pulmonary damage are burned nasal hairs and dried or charred oral or nasal mucosa. As resuscitation continues and edema of the upper airway increases, hoarseness and "crowing" may herald pending upper airway obstruction. The mechanism of lower airway obstruction is not well understood. Pulmonary failure commonly occurs in the first 2 or 3 days after burning and then again approximately a week after burning, when pneumonitis from chemical burns, separation of burned bronchial mucosa, and pulmonary edema from excessive fluid administration are all likely to occur.

E. Electrical Burns: Electrical burns are deceptive. The damage is usually deeper than the surface appearance indicates. These burns often require extensive debridement of deep tissue and sometimes even amputation. The electrical currents tend to follow tissue interfaces such as vessels and periosteum, and quite deep damage may not be apparent on the surface. The surface burn is seen in 2 places: where the current enters and where it leaves the body.

Differential Diagnosis

Differential diagnosis is seldom a problem except in chemical burns, when the nature of the burning agent is important in initial treatment. For example, chemical burns may require specific chemical therapy. Unconscious burned patients may have been burned because of a stroke, alcoholism, or injury, and the examiner must always be alert to the possibility of major illnesses contributing to the injury. Such an illness is easy to overlook in the excitement of burn resuscitation.

Patients involved in explosions or automobile accidents may have internal injuries as well as burns.

Evolution of the Burn & Complications

The burned patient normally undergoes a series of "complications" over a period of weeks or months. This is the natural evolutionary process of the burn.

A. First 48 Hours: A typical sequence occurs during the first 48 hours. Shock is the major problem in the first 48 hours and results chiefly from loss of vascular fluid into tissue. During this time, resuscitation with intravenous fluids is the major treatment. Hemoglobin from burned red cells or myoglobin from muscle damage may appear in the urine and may threaten renal function. Fluid therapy has complications of its own, such as cardiac and respiratory failure, when excessive fluids are given.

Upper airway obstruction often occurs in the first 48 hours as increasing edema narrows the burned airway. Massive lower airway injuries cause early death, and little can be done about them. Fortunately, they are rare.

B. Evolution and Complications in the First Week: Once the patient is completely resuscitated, his fluid needs gradually decrease until the sequestered fluid is once again returned to the blood stream and diuresis results. Diuresis should be allowed to occur and should not be treated. At times diuresis must be encouraged or hastened, especially if fluid overloads threaten cardiac or pulmonary function.

Pericardial effusions and pancreatitis may develop in the first week. Pancreatitis is sometimes suspected only because the fluid needs are increased without obvious reason.

Infection becomes a problem toward the end of the first week. Streptococci are likely early invaders, and penicillin administration can control hemolytic streptococci but permits other organisms to supervene. Staphylococcal or gram-negative infections develop as time passes. Antibiotics can selectively control individual organisms, but no single antibiotic can control all organisms.

C. Later Complications:

1. Infection becomes an increasingly more serious

problem after injury. The burned patient possesses the anamnestic immunologic response but responds poorly to new antigenic stimuli. As the patient's general condition gradually deteriorates, infections may occur from less virulent gram-negative organisms such as pseudomonas or serratia. If these complications are successfully treated but the patient continues to deteriorate nutritionally, fungal infections develop next. Viruses have been implicated as serious infection risks in severely burned patients. The recent recognition that topical antibacterial substances can increase the survival from burns is an important step forward, but the problem is still far from solved.

2. Almost half of all seriously burned patients have blood in their stools, presumably from "stress" ulceration of the stomach. A few patients may develop peptic ulcer (Curling's ulcer) with all of its complications. The prognosis of a patient with severe bleeding or perforation from Curling's ulcer is very poor, and aggressive operative therapy may offer the only possibility for survival. The cause of this type of "stress" ulcer is obscure. Several investigators have shown that acid secretion does not increase in burned patients. Hypovitaminemia A has recently been implicated as one contributing cause of Curling's ulcer.

3. Malnutrition results from caloric losses from water evaporation, poor food intake, exudative losses, fever, and hypermetabolism secondary to toxicity and inflammation. Patients with major burns usually require hyperalimentation almost from the beginning. Hyperalimentation also has its dangers, particularly in the first week after burning, since the burn frequently causes a moderately severe ileus. Nasogastric suction is frequently indicated early, and attempts to feed large volumes of food must be instituted cautiously.

4. Adrenal failure occasionally occurs late in the burn course and is often due to sepsis.

5. Excessive healing is the major and most frequent serious complication in burned patients. Scarring and burn contracture cause long-term disability and require plastic surgery for correction. The spontaneous healing of burns and the mechanisms of healing of skin grafts are fundamental considerations of great importance in the care of burn wounds, and no physician who treats burns can understand the problems of long-term care unless he understands the problems of healing. (See Chapter 9.)

D. Other Complications: The physician treating the seriously burned patient must be ready for almost any complication. Such widely disparate complications as cerebral edema, mesenteric thrombosis, primary peritonitis, perforated ulcer, pyarthrosis, pleural effusion, pulmonary emboli, and septic thrombophlebitis will be seen.

Anesthetic complications from contractures of the neck and inability to place intravenous lines may also occur. Drug reactions are likely because of prolonged use during convalescence. Psychiatric complications (temporary organic psychoses) occur in almost all severely burned patients.

Prevention

The prevention of burns is a major public health problem, and any physician who has experience with burns in civilian practice realizes the importance of preventive measures. For example, flammable clothing is still being sold to unsuspecting buyers. Careless people still smoke in bed, and caustic chemicals are readily available in every household. Automobiles and other fire-prone enclosures are still manufactured with flammable and toxic plastics. Many feasible preventive measures have yet to be taken.

Treatment

A. First Aid Measures at the Scene: Minor burns can easily be treated at the scene of the injury. Cool water is usually sufficient to relieve pain. Chemical burns are often well treated with cool water. No other treatment should usually be given. If a physician is available, an intravenous infusion can be started. Certainly, no oily substances should be applied to the skin. The best emergency treatment for major thermal burns is usually to cover the burned area with a clean dry dressing and transport the patient to a hospital as soon as possible.

B. Care During the First 48 Hours: (See Table 18−1.)

1. Resuscitation−When the patient is first seen, the stage must be set for effective resuscitation. A complete physical examination is done to the finest detail, and the available history is recorded. As this is being done, resuscitation can proceed. The important physiologic functions are measured, including pulse, blood pressure (when unburned extremities are available for the measurement), respiratory rate, ECG, blood electrolytes, urinalysis, and body weight. The extent and the distribution of burns are carefully sketched on a drawing of the human figure (Fig 18−2). The diagram is used to determine the extent and distribution of burns so that fluid therapy can be calculated.

2. Intravenous fluids−An intravenous line is usually placed in patients with burns involving more than 20% of the body surface. In very old or very young patients, intravenous lines should be inserted even if the burn covers only 10% of the body surface. One of the intravenous lines should be usable for monitoring central venous pressure. The first solution given in the intravenous line is usually Ringer's injection. A urinary catheter is inserted if there is any danger of shock. The indications for urinary catheters are approximately the same as those for intravenous lines. If blood pressure cannot be measured because of extensive burns or if severe pulmonary injury is suspected, an arterial catheter is useful to measure blood pressure and for arterial gas measurement.

Fluid therapy for the first 24 hours may be planned according to the **Brooke formula** as follows: 1.5 ml electrolyte solution per kg body weight per degree of burn plus 0.5 ml colloid solution per kg body weight for each percent of body surface burned plus the normal daily water maintenance calculated for the age and size of the patient (eg, 2000 ml for the average

TABLE 18–1. Guide to initial therapy of burns, 1967.*
(Prepared by the Committee on Trauma, American College of Surgeons.)

Minor Burns

A. Put on cap and mask.
B. Consider cold packs for relief of pain.
C. Cleanse wound with bland soap and warm water.
D. Dress with sterile, nonadherent, fine-mesh gauze and secure bulky dressing firmly in place.
E. Have the patient return in 2 days.

Severe Burns

A. Assure an adequate airway. This may require tracheostomy (endotracheal tube), especially with respiratory tract injury following inhalation of noxious gases and with deep burns of the face and neck.
B. Perform venipuncture with a large-bore needle.
  1. Obtain blood for cross-match, hemoglobin, hematocrit, electrolyte determinations, and BUN tests.
  2. Start plasma, clinical dextran, or lactated Ringer's injection.
  3. Give morphine intravenously if needed.
C. Place an intravenous catheter for burns involving over 20% of the body surface.
  1. Choose the cephalic vein at the shoulder or wrist or the long saphenous vein at the medial malleolus.
  2. Use a long plastic catheter which accepts a 16- or 18-gauge needle.
  3. Infuse lactated Ringer's injection or colloid solution (plasma or dextran) if necessary.
D. Communicate with responsible attending physician.
E. Obtain adequate assistance. Put on cap and mask.
F. Remove patient's clothing, completely exposing all burned areas for evaluation.
G. Obtain history—ie, age; when, where, and how injury occurred; allergies; tetanus immunization status; prior state of health.
H. Insert a Foley catheter and send a urine specimen to the laboratory.
I. Cleanse the wound.
  1. Use bland soap and warm water.
  2. Gently remove dirt and loose devitalized shreds.

  3. Irrigate chemical burns with copious amounts of water.
J. Estimate percentage and depth of burn, making a chart for estimation of percentage of burn.
K. Early photographs are desirable.
L. Weigh patient or estimate weight.
M. Expose, dress, or excise wound, as indicated. *Caution:* Do not neglect to make decompression incisions on circumferential extremity burns if necessary.
N. Immunize against tetanus.
O. Write orders.
  1. Nothing by mouth initially.
  2. Record intake and output on chart.
  3. Record blood pressure, pulse, and urine output hourly.
  4. Cradle on bed.
  5. Mouth care.
  6. Procaine penicillin G, 600,000 units twice daily for 5 days.
  7. Vitamin B complex.
  8. Vitamin A, 50,000 units per day in adults.
  9. Vitamin C, 1000–1500 mg daily.
  10. Sedatives as necessary.
  11. Nasogastric tube if patient vomits.
  12. Humidified oxygen.
  13. Culture of burn wound.
  14. Watch for gastric dilatation.
  15. Critical list? Special nurses?
  16. Calculate fluids, number all intravenous fluid bottles—use any suitable formula, such as the Brooke, during first 24 hours.
  18. If blood pressure decreases and urine output falls below 30 ml/hour, increase colloid.
  19. If blood pressure is stable but urine output falls below 30 ml/hour, increase electrolyte solution.
  20. If hourly urine output exceeds 50 ml/hour, decrease fluid therapy unless a large volume is required to maintain urine free of hemoglobin.
P. Laboratory Work: Hemoglobin and hematocrit daily; BUN, CO_2 combining power, and serum potassium, sodium, and chloride every 2 days after second day.

*Copies of this table can be obtained from the American College of Surgeons.

adult male). About half of this is usually needed in the first 8 hours. Some experts have recently advocated that electrolyte solutions alone be used for the first 24 hours.

Formulas are simply estimates which have been averaged from patients successfully treated in burn centers. They are useful for planning the very broad outlines of fluid therapy, but they should be continued only as long as they keep the patient's pulse and blood pressure within relatively normal limits and the urine output within 35–50 ml/hour in adults. These formulas should be adhered to only as long as the patient's lungs are clear, his urinary specific gravity is within reasonable limits, and he is not developing intolerable edema. Formulas should be modified whenever the patient's response so indicates. Detailed records must

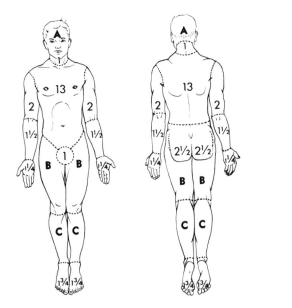

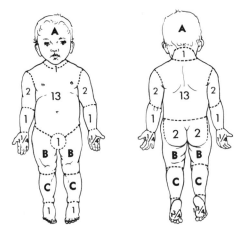

Relative Percentages of Areas Affected by Growth			
	Age		
Area	10	15	Adult
A = half of head	5½	4½	3½
B = half of one thigh	4¼	4½	4¾
C = half of one leg	3	3¼	3½

Relative Percentages of Areas Affected by Growth			
	Age		
Area	0	1	5
A = half of head	9½	8½	6½
B = half of one thigh	2¾	3¼	4
C = half of one leg	2½	2½	2¾

FIG 18–2. Table for estimating extent of burns. In adults, a reasonable approximation of these tables is the "rule of nines." In this "rule," each arm equals 9%, the head equals 9%, the anterior and posterior trunk each equal 18%, and each leg equals 18%. The sum of these percentages is 99%.

be kept of vital signs, input of each type of fluid, and output each hour. Falling urinary output and increasing specific gravity with normal vital signs usually indicate a need for more water and electrolytes. Falling blood pressure and rising pulse in the presence of a good urinary output usually requires some sort of blood volume expander. Crowing respirations and dyspnea usually indicate impending pulmonary edema. Some young patients can tolerate severe fluid overloads with only mechanical (compliance) problems in the lungs without developing the classic signs of pulmonary edema until gross overload exists.

Forcing fluids in the hope of lowering an elevated hematocrit is unwise and rarely effective. Blood transfusions in the first few days of burn therapy are rarely necessary unless the patient has blood losses from another injury. Special precautions in fluid therapy must be taken when either silver nitrate or mafenide (Sulfamylon) is used (see below). Urine volumes of more than 50 ml/hour in the first 48–72 hours generally indicate excessive use of fluids. It is false to assume that output greater than 50 ml/hour indicates good renal function and effective fluid therapy, since high urine output may also indicate dangerous overloads.

On occasion, salt-containing fluids can be given by mouth for resuscitation. Salt tablets and sodium bicarbonate can be used to make oral solutions. This is helpful in a mass disaster situation but is rarely used in ordinary practice.

Half the volume calculated by formula should be planned for the first 8 hours. The other half should be given in the succeeding hours. The patient will usually indicate his individual fluid needs (as opposed to calculated needs) within a few hours. It is rarely necessary to use the formulas after the first day. However, for those who prefer to depend on calculated amounts, the requirements of the second day are approximately half those of the first day. Overloading with resuscitation fluids is a common error. It occurs in the third to fifth days and may result in cardiac failure or electrolyte imbalance. It occurs when urine output does not increase after large amounts of fluid have been given. The way to avoid this problem is to arbitrarily halve fluid input for 1 hour every 12 hours if there is no shock or oliguria. Urine output will fall significantly if the fluid is necessary. If urine output does not change, fluid input can safely be diminished and overload avoided.

3. **Tetanus immunization**—Tetanus boosters should always be given with the initial therapy. This vital detail is easy to forget if postponed. Passive

immunization with tetanus-immune globulin (human) should be given simultaneously if it seems necessary.

4. Prophylactic antibiotics—Most authorities recommend small doses of penicillin (about 1 million units per day) for the first week or so after burning to prevent streptococcal and anaerobic infections. After the first week, antibiotics should be given on firm indications only. Fever or bacteria on the burn surface are not firm indications for antibiotic therapy.

5. Maintain airway—The airway must be watched carefully. In general, tracheostomy is inferior to endotracheal intubation unless it is abundantly clear that the tracheostomy can be done with reasonable leisure and that control of the airway will be necessary for more than 3 days. As soon as fluid therapy is begun, the danger of upper airway edema and obstruction in airway burns increases. The easiest way to determine the patency of the airway is to ask the patient to hyperventilate and to talk. If the airway is obstructed, hyperventilation produces stridor and hoarseness is apparent.

6. Nasogastric suction—In severe burns, a nasogastric tube should be passed to empty the stomach and prevent vomiting and aspiration. Antacid and nutritional therapy can be started in 24—48 hours.

7. Topical therapy—Topical burn therapy and debridement of major burns are of subordinate priority to the above emergency measures. Physicians have an unfortunate tendency to remove the burned patient to a cold operating room and wash him with cold fluids, thereby compounding his problems with hypothermia and fluid losses. The initial debridement should be a wash with antibacterial soap and debridement of loose skin only. In general, second degree burns heal slightly faster under an intact blister than if the blister is removed. This is particularly true of blisters on the hands, and most authorities now recognize that leaving blisters intact as long as they are not infected is a reasonable decision.

Special antidotes such as slightly alkaline solutions for treatment of acid burns are worth considering as emergency measures. Similarly, mild acid washes for known alkali burns should be considered. If the exact nature of the burning agent is not known, one can rarely go wrong by immediately flushing chemical burns with cool fresh water. This usually far outweighs the advantages of delayed but specific therapy. Copper sulfate, often held to be specific therapy for phosphorus burns, is only an adjunct intended to slow oxidation of the phosphorus and to identify retained particles of phosphorus since the interaction of copper with phosphorus causes the particles to turn black. Once again, even in phosphorus burns, flushing with copious amounts of cool water is the best treatment.

8. Dressings—Dressings may be applied after washing and debridement of loose skin and removal of burning chemicals. One must remember that chemicals in the dressing can be transported across the burn surface and subsequently be absorbed. Excessive washings with hexachlorophene, for example, can cause fever and convulsions. Topical antibiotics are absorbed.

Silver nitrate dressings transfer electrolytes and water across the burn, and mafenide (Sulfamylon) is absorbed and then acts as a diuretic and a carbonic anhydrase inhibitor.

Small and superficial burns can be treated in a number of ways. Cleansing with soap and water and application of loose, dry, protective gauze dressings are usually sufficient. The home remedies of butter and other greases have no particular value but neither are they harmful when used to treat first degree burns. Covering with oily substances tends to keep the burn area relatively soft and prevents the drawing feeling of the drying eschar. However, such dressings are prone to trap dirt and cause contamination. A clean, dry eschar in an ambulatory patient is the easiest and safest way to maintain the burn. For this, mafenide is often an ideal choice (see below).

9. Topical anti-infective agents—None of these topical applicants have been extensively tested for their effects on spontaneous healing of the burn. According to the reports that do exist, silver nitrate appears to allow better healing than mafenide. The ideal topical application for burns probably has not yet been developed.

a. Silver nitrate—Silver nitrate (0.5%) is often used for larger burns and is an improvement over older methods of simple dressing treatment. Silver nitrate dressing delays the onset of sepsis, but it must be started on the day of burning if it is to be maximally effective. Silver nitrate is comfortable, minimizes evaporative heat loss, and delays sepsis. Because silver nitrate leaches sodium, potassium, and chloride from the patient, electrolyte measurements may be necessary daily or sometimes even every 8 hours during the first few days. In fact, in poor-risk adults and in small children, a serum electrolyte measurement every 8 hours may be necessary to avoid convulsions or cardiac arrhythmias caused by hyponatremia and hypokalemia.

Large amounts of concentrated salt and potassium may be needed to maintain serum electrolyte concentrations. As much as 30 g of salt a day may be given in addition to the normal diet to maintain normal salt balance. The earliest chemical sign of excessive sodium loss is a fall in the urinary sodium concentration below 30 mEq/liter. This evidence can be used, however, only after 72 hours, since the hormonal response to stress usually results in sodium retention and low urinary sodium concentrations during the first 48 hours.

Silver nitrate gives its poorest results in elderly patients, who may have severe electrolyte and cardiac difficulties. It is generally agreed that silver nitrate therapy increases the survival rate of patients with burns up to about 50% of body surface.

The technic of applying silver nitrate dressings is to wrap the patient with a loose mesh gauze in which catheters with side holes are incorporated. Two or 3 layers of this gauze are covered with bias-cut stockinet, leaving the administration end of the catheter outside the dressings. The catheters are flushed with silver nitrate solution every 2–4 hours (cold or warm, depending on the patient's temperature). The dressings should be changed daily, or even oftener if local sepsis occurs.

b. Mafenide (Sulfamylon)–Mafenide cream is an excellent dressing for small to moderate-sized burns, particularly in young adults. It, too, is an effective agent for delaying sepsis. It is easy to apply, no dressings are necessary, and it is easily washed off. One disadvantage is that about 10% of patients become allergic to mafenide and develop a severe maculopapular skin rash. Some patients will insist that it be discontinued because of pain upon application. It is a mild diuretic, although rarely it may cause extreme diuresis even in the early burn phase. Since it is a carbonic anhydrase inhibitor, it causes the patient to hyperventilate to rid himself of CO_2. Mafenide rarely causes major electrolyte problems, but it may exaggerate pulmonary insufficiency. Caloric losses are usually increased because of evaporative heat loss from the lungs during hyperventilation and from the burned surfaces through the dry topical agent.

A typical clinical picture of a patient with a major burn treated with mafenide includes shivering and hyperpnea with a normal arterial pH and P_{CO_2}. Hypothermia and excessive caloric needs may occur, particularly in children and older patients. Radiation warmth from an infrared light placed over the patient helps prevent heat loss. If the patient is able to withstand the side-effects, mafenide is an excellent method of treatment for burns.

Potassium losses may occur because of the diuretic nature of mafenide. After the third day, supplemental potassium is usually necessary–especially during the diuresis.

c. Gentamicin (Garamycin)–Gentamicin cream and ointment are reasonably effective burn dressings. However, resistant bacteria exist and the problem of inducing resistant strains with topical therapy is a danger to other patients as well as to the burned patient. Furthermore, the resistant strains gradually contaminate the patient. Gentamicin has little or no effect on loss of fluid and electrolytes from the burn surface. However, it can impair renal function and hearing.

d. Silver-sulfadiazine–Silver-sulfadiazine, a combination of silver and sulfadiazine, has been extensively tested in the past few years. It causes less pain and less interference with electrolytes than mafenide or silver nitrate. Final evaluation is not complete, but it appears to be as effective as mafenide with fewer side-effects.

10. Burns of special areas–Special attention must be paid to certain critical areas in the initial evaluation and treatment of the burn.

a. Eye burns–Eye burns require specialized care, and the eyes should always be examined before lid edema covers them.

b. Hand burns–The hand should be splinted in the position of function (Fig 48–1) and should ordinarily be debrided and grafted early. The hand may need elevation to prevent chronic edema in the burned area. Since epithelization is slightly more rapid under intact blisters, blisters of the hand need not be debrided. Hand burns are discussed fully in Chapter 48.

c. Pulmonary burns–If respiratory distress continues even though the airway is open, the lower airway is probably burned. This demands immediate evaluation of blood gas tensions. If lower airway burns are either present or suspected, fluid loads should be avoided and digitalis should probably be given. Most authorities recommend giving one or 2 large doses of corticosteroids to patients with respiratory distress due to lower airway injury. Continuing high doses of corticosteroids for more than 1–2 days is harmful. Successfully treated airway burns predispose to bacterial pneumonia, which must be suspected and effectively treated.

11. Circumferential burns–Circumferential burns of the extremities may obstruct venous or arterial blood supply or both. Division of a constricting eschar (escharotomy) is easy and safe and requires no anesthesia. Done properly and at the right time, it may save a limb or a life. Escharotomy may be necessary within hours after fluid therapy is begun but is more likely to be needed toward the end of the first day. A constricting circumferential burn of the chest may cause pulmonary insufficiency. Occasionally, division of such a constricting eschar will remarkably improve the vital capacity and tidal volume.

C. Care During the Second to Fourth Days:

1. Fluid management–After the initial care, fluid administration should be decreased as far as the patient's tolerance will permit. It is often assumed that fluid therapy and urine output are interdependent; however, in many cases, by the second, third, or fourth day, all input can be stopped for an hour and the urinary output will continue. This is an excellent way of determining the patient's fluid needs and can help reduce fluid overloads.

Oral fluids should be given as soon as the patient can tolerate adequate volumes by mouth. If the patient can take oral fluids, antacids should be started.

2. Digitalis–In most elderly patients, digitalis should be given as soon as blood electrolytes show that the potassium is within normal limits and the electrolytes are stable. Digitalization should be relatively slow and should be aimed toward obtaining full effect by the fourth day when the need is greatest. The purpose is to avoid cardiac failure and pulmonary edema when the massive burn edema is resorbed.

3. Diet–Diet is an extremely important consideration in burn management. Energy expenditures are great in burned patients, and dietary requirements may be very high.

Patients who have burns of more than 30% of the body surface routinely require hyperalimentation. In most cases, this can be accomplished through oral intake. The objective of alimentation is weight gain or at least stabilization of weight. The physician must do whatever is needed to achieve this. Ordinarily, 4500 Cal/day, with at least 150 g of protein, will be neces-

TABLE 18–2. Suggested daily nutrition for adult patients with major burns.

Calories	4500–5500
Protein	150–200 g
Vitamins	
C	1500 mg
B_1	50 mg
B_2	50 mg
Niacin	500 mg
A	50,000 units
D	2000 units
Electrolytes	
Na^+	60–100 mEq*
K^+	80–200 mEq
Mg^{++}	10–20 mEq

*Greater in silver nitrate therapy.

sary for patients with massive burns and will require the help of a dietitian and much trial and error. Table 18–2 lists the components of a typical diet given a severely burned patient. Unfortunately, patients who take dietary supplements lose their appetite when they eat between meals. Dietary supplements are best given early after the evening meal and should be regarded as medicine. The patient then has time to become hungry again before breakfast.

The large dose of vitamin A shown in Table 18–2 is recommended because hypovitaminemia A is almost universal in seriously burned patients.

Oral feedings should be started gradually to avoid gastric distention, vomiting, and diarrhea. Intravenous hyperalimentation is effective for burn patients, but the complications from indwelling catheters are a formidable disadvantage. It is safer for any patient with a burn if he can take adequate food by mouth. If he cannot, intravenous alimentation may be unavoidable. If the patient simply refuses to take fluids by mouth, tube feedings can be given; however, they are dangerous because of the risk of gastric dilatation, vomiting, and aspiration. Tube feedings must be given carefully in small increments, with adequate attention to the amount of gastric residual. Although the small flexible feeding tube is well tolerated, it is not a good instrument for oral tube feeding. It is difficult to judge the residual, since aspirating through this small tube is not usually successful.

D. Psychiatric Care: The burned patient is under severe stress. He has pain with the slightest movement. He is often immobilized and totally dependent. Ordinary nursing care prevents sleep. He lives in the same room with the same people day after day.

He is also susceptible to other (treatable or preventable) causes of psychosis such as hypoxia, hyponatremia, sepsis, drug reactions, and hypomagnesemia. These causes must be routinely "ruled out" when psychosis occurs.

To prevent psychosis, the patient should be allowed to sleep in as normal a pattern as possible.

Distraction in the form of physical and occupational therapy, school teachers, and television should be provided, although this often requires imagination and ingenuity.

E. Prevention and Treatment of Infection: Recent improvements in therapy have diminished or somewhat delayed the problem of infection, but it remains a major problem in burned patients. Many methods of treating and preventing sepsis have been proposed. At present, most burn treatment centers use low doses of penicillin for prevention of streptococcal infections for the first week. Thereafter, antibiotics are used on specific indication only. Fever is not a specific indication. In fact, it is often difficult to diagnose sepsis early in its course. The burn, the urine, and the blood are cultured every few days. In this way, an "educated guess" can be made about the infecting organism and its antibiotic sensitivity.

Examination of the burn under ultraviolet light is an excellent means of detecting the fluorescent pseudomonas organism.

Infection is best prevented by early burn debridement and grafting. Good nutrition and blood volume support are initially important in prevention of infection.

Gamma globulin has been given for prevention and treatment of infection, but its present status is in some doubt. Polyvalent antipseudomonas immune globulins are now being tested with excellent success and may become an important facet of treatment.

F. Management of the Burn Surface: The burn surface is inspected daily, and loose tissue is debrided with forceps and scissors. This may be started as early as the second or third day. Frequently, the entire debridement can be done in small increments. and many patients managed in this way never require operative debridement under anesthesia.

G. Enzymatic Debridement: Enzymatic burn debridement is a promising recent development. When it is effective, operative debridement may be totally unnecessary.

Further Care of the Burn Wound

The remaining principles of burn care rest on an adequate knowledge of the healing process. A summary of this process follows.

Immediately following deep thermal injury, there is edema and exudation of plasma into the viable borderline area of injured but still perfused tissue. During the period of inflammation and fluid loss, the burn progressively deepens, and maximum vascular injury occurs in 48–72 hours. Tissues die to the depth at which the vascular supply is adequate for tissue survival. This level may be determined by any number of factors, but desiccation seems to be particularly important. A vascular supply which is merely adequate for survival is not adequate for healing. Healing is delayed until new vessels begin to appear and the wound neovasculature supplies the nutrition necessary for formation of granulation tissue. As damaged capillaries begin to "heal," they regain their normal permeability. Burn edema is reabsorbed (the diuretic phase). Shortly afterward, new vessels begin to proliferate in the live tissue and migrate toward the inflamed and necrotic areas, and more white cells, macrophages, and fibroblasts appear in the viable tissue.

At this point, the remainder of the healing process proceeds in 4 principal ways: (1) separation of dead tissue, (2) regeneration of connective tissues and vasculature, (3) epithelization, and (4) contraction.

Separation of dead tissue can occur through the natural mechanism by means of the enzymatic cleavage of collagen. A collagenolytic enzyme appears in the extracellular space in the area of inflammation and slowly cleaves the tough collagen bundles. The cleavage products are then susceptible to digestion by other extracellular and intracellular enzymes. Unfortunately, natural collagen lysis is too slow to be relied upon to do the entire job of separation except in small burns. In large burns, surgical or exogenous enzymatic debridement is also necessary. It is difficult, however, to determine the depth of a burn, and the surgeon must be careful not to deepen a second degree burn wound by overaggressive debridement. White cells and bacteria contain collagenolytic enzymes. Eschar separates more rapidly when it has become infected. Unfortunately, this speeding of one phase of healing is done at the expense of other phases in that infection also tends to deepen the burn. The regeneration of new connective tissue begins as the eschar is being separated. If the eschar separates, either spontaneously or by infection, granulation tissue is disclosed (see Chapter 9).

Granulation tissue can fill even rather large defects. However, the presence of epithelium over granulation tissue causes it to shrink, lose its vasculature, and essentially stop "healing." Therefore, most tissue defects are not totally filled since epithelization

by one means or another tends to occur before normal contours are reached. Deep in the granulation tissue layer is a dense layer of collagen. As is the case with all scar collagen, this collagen tends to shrink with time. Such shrinkage is probably the force behind contracture of burns which is responsible for the ugly scarring and loss of motion of joints so often seen after severe burns. The longer granulation tissue is allowed to exist, the longer it is exposed to drying and injury; the longer it remains inflamed, the thicker the layer of collagen is and the stronger the force of contracture will be.

Contracture tends to be balanced to some degree by remodeling of scar tissue. Scar collagen is a highly dynamic protein, and it is constantly being renewed for at least 6 months after its formation. Thus, early burn contractures can be easily stretched by constant light force.

If reinjury does not occur, scar collagen tends to decrease with time. This remodeling causes rather stiff collagen to become much softer, and on flat surfaces of the body, where reinjury and inflammation are not occurring, remodeling may even overbalance contracture. However, in areas which are likely to be injured, exposed, and inflamed, such as around joints or in the neck, contracture usually wins and plastic surgery is necessary to remove disabling scar tissue. The sooner granulation tissue can be covered with skin grafts, the less likely contracture is to occur. Fig 18–3 compares normal dermal collagen with scar collagen as seen with the scanning electron microscope.

Epithelial regeneration begins with mitoses near the injury and continues with migration of new epithelial cells toward and then over the defect. Each source of epithelium will cover a small area around it. Unfortunately, the farther the epithelium must migrate, the thinner the resulting layer of epithelium. Thickness does not increase much in time, and the

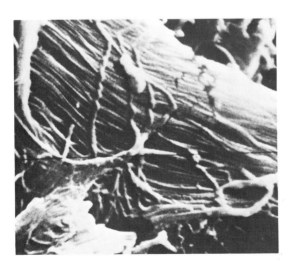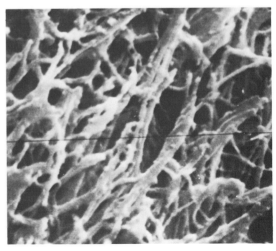

FIG 18–3. Normal dermal collagen appears on the left. Once it has been wounded, the typical wound collagen appears as on the right. Obviously, the mechanical properties of the natural and wound collagen differ markedly with the wound collagen being more brittle. (Magnification approximately × 12,000.)

poor quality of epithelium remains.

In second degree burns, many sources of epithelium persist in the depths of hair follicles, sweat glands, and apocrine glands. When proper local conditions permit, epithelial cells pour out of these hidden sources and small volcanoes of pearly gray epithelial cells are seen against the red granulation tissue. If the burn is superficial, only small distances remain between the volcanoes of epithelium and the burn heals quickly, with little scarring. In deeper burns, fewer sources of epithelium survive. Healing is slower, coverage is poorer, and the tendency to scar formation is greater. The recently epithelized burn remains red owing to the persistence of subdermal vessels. As time passes, these vessels disappear and the area becomes paler. Melanocytes regenerate but migrate less well than squamous cells. The end result of most burns is a scar which is lighter than the normal pigmented skin.

Contraction is the migration of normal tissue into an area previously occupied by injured and healing tissue. It is not to be confused with contracture. In open areas of the trunk or neck in particular, a small third degree burn wound will gradually shrink by contraction. These skin edges are drawn or pushed together by a somewhat mysterious force which is independent of the granulation tissue and collagen content of the wound. By this means, normal skin is brought into the defect and only a small scar is left. When contraction is occurring rapidly, it is often wise not to interfere since it leaves the most cosmetically acceptable scar one is likely to obtain. Unfortunately, placement of skin grafts slows contraction. Wounds of the extremities will not contract enough to justify reliance on this process.

The alternative to spontaneous healing is, of course, **skin grafting**. When a skin graft heals, its vessels inosculate with host tissue vessels and the blood supply to the graft is restored. This occurs in the first 3–5 days. The connective tissue of the host and graft then fuses as in primary healing. The advantages of immobilization to protect the delicate vascular anastomoses are obvious.

Allografts (homografts) go through the same process. First and second order rejections are usually delayed in patients with major burns—a reflection of the inability of burn patients to initiate immune responses to new antigens. The first set of allografts often survives for a month. The rejected allograft becomes hemorrhagic and gradually sloughs.

Thin skin grafts obviously will take better since fewer vascular connections are needed to support them. However, thin grafts (0.2–0.4 mm) give a thinner, less functional surface. They are used to obtain coverage of large areas. Thicker grafts are less likely to take but give a softer, more durable surface due to their thicker dermal component.

The management of the wound will vary according to the circumstances. The ultimate goal in burn therapy is to obtain epithelial coverage of the wound as quickly as possible with maximal return of both cosmetic and mechanical function. In major burns, coverage of the burn is necessary to save life. Function is of paramount but secondary importance. In less severe burns, the primary aim is to preserve function.

The first option in surgical management of the wound is dressing the fresh burn with skin. An extensive burn not suitably prepared for autografting can be dressed with allografts or xenografts which are changed every 2–4 days. These grafts do not take, but they do reduce surface bacteria and prevent water loss and subsequent desiccation of the burn surface. The end result is to minimize the depth of the burn, thus controlling sepsis and getting the area ready for permanent coverage with autografts.

The second option is to excise the burn and cover with autograft within the first few days. For small deep burns, this is an excellent alternative which minimizes the hospital stay and expense. However, one must be relatively sure one is not excising a second degree burn which would otherwise heal spontaneously and well. It is not always easy to tell the difference between second and third degree burns.

The next option is debridement or excision in the second or third week when the plane of cleavage is more apparent. Obviously, one could place either autografts, allografts, or heterografts on this surface. Autografts are preferable if enough skin is available. Grafts will take as well on the freshly debrided surface as on granulation tissue, and sometimes the take is even better.

Operative debridement is a stressful operation to the patient. Burned patients tend to become hypovolemic, and preoperative blood transfusions are often necessary. During the operation, the exposed patient loses heat, water, and blood with amazing speed. A warming blanket gives additional heat, and fluids and blood are forced as soon as the debridement is begun. Some surgeons limit debridements by stopping as soon as the patient's temperature drops below about 35 C (95 F) or when blood loss is more than 4 units of blood. Obviously, this is a serious and major procedure. The more debridement one can do during dressing changes, the better for the patient.

Lastly, the physician can wait for nonoperative debridement to occur and graft on granulation tissue. A portion at least of any major burn surface can be grafted this way, but there are several disadvantages. Time is lost during the wait for debridement, and during this interval the dense layer of connective tissue under the granulation thickens and contracts. Hence, scarring is greater.

Autografts and allografts give the best results. Heterografts also are being successfully used as burn dressings. Pigskin is commercially available. Skin can be stored up to about 2 weeks in ordinary refrigerators. If it is quick-frozen and kept in liquid nitrogen, it can be stored indefinitely.

During the entire grafting procedure, the burns and grafts can be dressed with the usual antibacterial dressings.

In general, it is best to graft broad areas first in major burns and areas of contracture formation first in minor burns. The usual areas of contracture formation are the face, anterior neck, axillas, elbows, hands, knees, and ankles. These are all areas of motion where the sensitive, fragile burn tissue is easily reinjured with subsequent inflammation, collagen deposition, and contracture.

The best way to prevent contracture is to graft early (before excessive collagen deposition) with flexible thick grafts. The contractured scars may be excised, and the grafts can be placed on the deeper soft tissues. On the other hand, it is surprisingly easy to stretch contractures by progressive splinting or by traction, usually skeletal. If splinting is maintained constantly for 4—6 months, when the biologic activity of the scar tissue recedes, contracture can often be avoided. Obviously, prevention is a better policy.

Constant pressure on biologically active scars will also cause hypertrophic scars to recede. Reddened, inflamed-looking tissue is biologically active, ie, it is vascular, inflamed, and is turning over collagen rapidly. It can be stretched and will lose collagen if pressure reduces its blood supply.

One of the most vigorous areas of investigation in burns is the manipulation of scar tissue. Physical means such as pressure and traction are used now. It is to be hoped that biochemical means of controlling scar overgrowth will be available in the future.

The principles of early debridement and grafting, prevention of edema, splinting, and often traction are particularly important in treatment of burns of the hand. Hand burns are particularly disabling and deserve special attention whenever they occur. (See Chapter 48.)

Prognosis

With modern methods of care, almost all patients except the elderly should survive third degree burns of up to 40% of the body surface if no pulmonary component is present. However, even small burns can be fatal to the elderly. Above 40%, mortality increases sharply until about half of even the young patients will succumb to 60% third degree burns. Only a few patients with over 70% third degree burns have survived.

● ● ●

General References

Artz CP, Moncrief JA: *The Treatment of Burns,* 2nd ed. Saunders, 1969.

Curreri PW, Asch MJ, Pruitt BA: The treatment of chemical burns: Specialized diagnostic, therapeutic and prognostic considerations. J Trauma 10:634—642, 1970.

Feller I: *International Bibliography on Burns.* American Burn Research Corp, 1969.

Fox CL: Silver sulfadiazine: A new topical therapy for pseudomonas in burns. Arch Surg 96:184—188, 1968.

Monafo WW Jr, Moyer CA: Effectiveness of silver nitrate in the treatment of major burns. Arch Surg 91:200—210, 1965.

Moncrief JA: Burns. (Medical progress article.) New England J Med 288:444—454, 1973.

Morton JJ: Radiation burns due to atomic explosions. Ann Surg 146:314—321, 1957.

Polk HC Jr, Stone HH (editors): *Contemporary Burn Management.* Little, Brown, 1971.

Polk HC Jr, Monafo WW Jr, Moyer CA: Human burn survival: Study of efficacy of 0.5% aqueous silver nitrate. Arch Surg 98:262—265, 1969.

Shuck JM, Moncrief JA: Safeguards in the use of topical mafenide (Sulfamylon) in burned patients. Am J Surg 118:864—870, 1969.

Skoog T: Electrical injuries. J Trauma 10:816—830, 1970.

19 . . .

Tumors of the Head & Neck

Maurice Galante, MD

Cancers of the lips, tongue, floor of the mouth, hard and soft palate, alveolar mucosa, and pharynx account for 5% of all malignant neoplasms recorded, or about 30,000 cases in the USA each year.

Death rates from cancer around the world suggest that the incidence of head and neck cancer is related to ethnic and environmental factors (Table 19–1). The cause of oral cancer is not known, but the disease is associated with exposure to various biologic, chemical,

TABLE 19–1. Incidence of oral cancer, 1964–1965. (Age-adjusted death rate per 100,000 population, 15 countries.)

	Males	Females
France	9.2	0.8
Puerto Rico	8.7	2.1
Hong Kong	18.0	6.3
Switzerland	7.0	0.8
South Africa	5.9	1.2
Italy	5.5	0.9
USA	4.6	1.3
Portugal	4.6	1.1
Ireland	4.3	2.1
Philippines	4.1	2.8
Canada	4.0	1.0
England, Wales	3.2	1.5
Denmark	1.9	1.0
Israel	1.5	0.8
Japan	1.4	0.7

and physical agents. An association between the use of tobacco and oral cancer was suspected as long ago as the early 18th century, when cancer of the lip was noted among smokers. A report to the Surgeon General (1964) based upon retrospective studies showed a significant association of oral cancer with smoking or chewing of tobacco or the use of snuff. The mortality rate from oral cancer is 4.2 times as high in cigarette smokers as in nonsmokers. For cigar and pipe smokers (compared with nonsmokers), oral cancer has the highest mortality ratio (3.3) of all causes of death, exceeding cancer of the esophagus, pharynx, and lungs.

No virus has been isolated that will induce oral cancer in humans, but an unusual type of oral cancer (Burkitt's lymphoma), perhaps caused by a virus, occurs in a narrow zone across Central Africa. This tumor affects children as well as adults of different racial backgrounds—European, Asian, and Indian— provided they live in an area with an elevation less than 5000 feet, an annual rainfall of more than 200 inches, and a temperature that does not fall below 15.5 C (60 F). These prerequisites suggest that the tumor may be transmitted by a vector such as a mosquito, and virus-like particles have been identified in cell cultures of Burkitt's tumor. Tumors similar to Burkitt's lymphoma have been identified in various countries.

Diagnosis

Even though tumors of the head and neck and of the oral cavity are readily accessible to inspection, one frequently encounters examples that are enormous and far-advanced when first seen by a physician. Most tumors of the head and neck are relatively asymptomatic early and are therefore ignored or overlooked by the patient even when readily accessible.

The diagnosis of head and neck tumors depends on 2 steps: (1) Careful inspection of all structures. The proper examination of the patient requires a thorough inspection of all the recesses of the oral and nasal cavities, nasopharynx, oropharynx, and hypopharynx. This requires proper lighting and a head lamp or a head mirror. Palpation should be utilized whenever possible. All triangles of the neck should be thoroughly inspected and palpated in the search for metastases or margins of direct spread. Direct or indirect endoscopy is necessary for areas that are not readily accessible to visual inspection. Diagnostic technics include indirect laryngoscopy, direct laryngoscopy, nasopharyngoscopy, roentgenography, arteriography, and laminography.

(2) **Histologic diagnosis by biopsy.** The biopsy should always be obtained from a representative area of the tumor. Regardless of the method utilized (incisional or excisional biopsy, punch biopsy, needle biopsy), it should always provide the pathologist with enough tissue so that he can adequately examine the lesion.

Cytologic examination is particularly helpful in detecting small lesions that are not readily seen by direct inspection and in follow-up care after treatment has been given. In general, definitive treatment should not be started on the basis of a cytologic diagnosis alone.

Fletcher GH: The place of roentgen diagnosis in treatment planning for cancers of the nasopharynx, paranasal sinus, and laryngopharynx. Radiol Clin North America 8:293–305, 1970.

Moore C: Cigarette smoking and cancer of the mouth, pharynx, and larynx. JAMA 218:553–558, 1971.

Rubin P: Cancer of the head and neck: General aspects. JAMA 215:450–462, 1971.

TUMORS OF THE SKIN

Both benign and malignant lesions of the skin are common on the head and neck. The incidence is much higher in sunny climates (5% of all cancers in England but 50% of all cancers in Australia) and in fair-skinned individuals (seldom seen in blacks).

Benign Tumors

Senile keratosis is the most common benign skin lesion. It appears grossly as an irregular gray area covered with fine scales. It is generally considered precancerous, and malignant change occurs in 1 out of 25 lesions. When excessive amounts of keratin are produced, a cutaneous horn results.

All premalignant lesions need definitive treatment. The skin of the face and neck should be carefully examined, and all suspicious areas excised and examined histologically.

Malignant Tumors

Malignant lesions occurring on the skin of the head and neck are as follows: basal cell carcinoma, squamous cell carcinoma, adenocarcinoma (arising in sweat or sebaceous glands), melanoma, mycosis fungoides, Kaposi's disease, lymphomas, and metastatic lesions.

Basal cell and squamous cell carcinomas—the most frequent skin malignancies—occur principally in elderly individuals (60s and 70s) and infrequently in patients under 40. They may present as small nodular or superficial plaques with or without ulceration and with or without deep infiltration into underlying soft tissues and cartilage.

It is occasionally difficult to distinguish clinically between basal cell and squamous cell carcinomas. Histologic diagnosis should be established before treatment is started. Both of these lesions may become large and invade vital structures.

Preventive measures for skin cancer consist of the following: (1) Avoidance of prolonged exposure to sunlight by susceptible individuals. (2) Careful observation of the skin to facilitate early diagnosis. (3) Use of protective skin creams. (4) Excision of precancerous lesions such as isolated keratoses. (5) Surgical planing of skin with multiple areas of involvement too numerous for individual excision.

Malignant lesions are curable if discovered early because they are accessible, grow slowly, and metas-tasize late. Some lesions may develop over a period of 10–20 years and present as an extensive, disfiguring, infected ulcerations. Metastases to lymph nodes from basal cell lesions are almost unknown. Particularly on the head and neck, squamous cell carcinoma of the skin metastasizes infrequently (5%).

Both radiation therapy and surgery are effective in the management of skin cancers. The selection of one method or the other depends upon the location and extent of the lesion, the feasibility of protection of vital structures (eye, middle ear, brain, cartilage, etc), previous treatment, the number of surgical procedures required for repair of the resulting defect, and patient factors such as availability for treatment and occupational hazards.

In most cases, surgical excision is preferred when it can be done simply. Primary closure of the surgical defect is preferable since it is more expeditious and results in a more satisfactory cosmetic effect. Larger surgical defects may require coverage with skin grafts or with flaps.

Although relatively advanced lesions can be successfully handled by radical surgery, radiation therapy, and plastic reconstructive procedures, some neglected lesions may be uncontrollable by the most radical surgery or radiation therapy.

CANCER OF THE ORAL CAVITY

The oral cavity extends from the vermilion border of the lips to and including the anterior faucial pillars which separate it from the oropharynx.

There are important biologic differences between tumors of the mucosa lining the oral cavity and that lining the oropharynx based on different degrees of cellular differentiation, tendency to infiltrate the adjacent tissues, and rate of spread to regional lymphatics.

Ninety percent of all tumors of the oral cavity are squamous cell carcinomas. They are usually better differentiated, more locally invasive, and less likely to metastasize to regional lymph nodes than malignant tumors of the oropharynx. One group of tumors—mucoepidermoid carcinomas—may be difficult to differentiate from epidermoid carcinoma because of epithelial metaplasia.

Salivary gland adenocarcinomas occur in 8% and constitute the next most frequent type of tumor. Along with mucoepidermoid carcinomas, they have a tendency to grow slowly, invade locally, and metastasize late to lymph nodes.

The remaining lesions are rare tumors originating in practically any tissue that is present in the oral cavity: muscle, blood vessels, nerves, connective tissue, etc.

Oral cancer usually occurs between the ages of 45

and 85 in individuals with associated vascular diseases, leukoplakia, heavy smoking and alcohol intake, and poor oral hygiene. Syphilis is not a significant contributing factor today.

Delay in diagnosis may be due to failure of the patient to seek medical help or to failure of the physician to appreciate the importance of early pathologic changes. The recent emphasis on oral cancer in the education of dentists has resulted in earlier detection of many lesions.

Although most lesions can be identified by their gross appearance, the diagnosis of intraoral cancer is established principally by biopsy. The physician who will provide definitive treatment should be the one who performs the biopsy so he can see the lesion before it is surgically altered. This is especially important for small lesions that could be totally removed by an excisional biopsy. Difficult problems of management may arise later if the physician responsible for definitive treatment cannot detect a residual lesion or even find the site of biopsy.

Biopsies should be obtained with a scalpel or biopsy forceps to avoid destruction or alteration of cellular detail and should be repeated if there is a suspicion of malignancy.

There is usually no need to biopsy palpable lymph nodes in the presence of a recognizable primary cancer. It may occasionally be necessary to do an aspiration biopsy of an involved cervical lymph node and, if negative, to do an excisional biopsy. Incisional biopsies should be avoided unless it is impossible to remove an intact lymph node because of its large size or infiltration into deeper structures.

Although cytology is never a substitute for an adequate biopsy, cytologic examination of exfoliated buccal cells is of great value in the early detection of cancer in the oral cavity.

Cady B: Carcinoma of the oral cavity. S Clin North America 51:537–551, 1971.

Clinical staging system for carcinoma of the oral cavity. Cancer 18:163–169, 1968.

Jesse RH & others: Cancer of the oral cavity: Is elective neck dissection beneficial? Am J Surg 120:505–508, 1970.

Jimenez JR: Roentgen examination of the oropharynx and oral cavity. Radiol Clin North America 8:413–424, 1970.

Millard J: Oral exfoliative cytology as an aid to diagnosis. J Am Dent A 69:547–550, 1964.

Rubin P: Head and neck cancer. Oral cavity: Primary lesion. JAMA 215:953–968, 1971.

Rubin P: Cancer of the head and neck. Oral cavity: Neck nodes. JAMA 217:451–465, 1971.

Trodahl JN, Sprague WG: Benign and malignant melanocytic lesions of the oral mucosa. Cancer 25:812–823, 1970.

CARCINOMA OF THE LIP

Carcinoma of the vermilion border of the lip is an entity distinct from cancer of the skin and is the most frequent of all intraoral malignant cancers (20–30%).

Most cancers of the lip are squamous cell carcinomas; fewer than 3% are basal cell lesions.

Cancer of the lip has the same relationship to exposure to actinic rays as cancer of the skin and is therefore more frequent in farmers, sailors, and individuals who are exposed to sunlight over long periods of time. Carcinoma of the lip is also more frequent in males than in females, and occurs primarily in the sixth and seventh decades of life; although it usually occurs on the lower lip, an occasional cancer may occur on the upper lip—more often in women than in men.

Carcinoma of the lip is usually a well-differentiated lesion presenting as an infiltrating or an ulcerating or exophytic tumor. It is small initially but may eventually become quite large, involve the entire lip from commissure to commissure, and destroy the soft tissues of the chin.

Metastases occur via the lymphatics in an orderly manner to the regional lymph nodes. First the submental, then the submaxillary, and eventually the cervical lymph nodes are involved. Distant metastases occur rarely. Carcinoma of the upper lip metastasizes to the facial and submaxillary lymph nodes—occasionally to the preauricular and parotid nodes. Metastases occur in 10–25% of cases depending on the size of the primary lesion and its histologic differentiation.

Treatment

Both surgery and radiation therapy are most effective in the control of carcinoma of the lip. The choice of treatment depends on the size of the lesion, the facilities available, occupational hazards of the patient, recurrence of the lesion following previous treatment, the presence of regional metastases, the presence of underlying bone involvement, and the condition of the skin (leukoplakia, atrophy, etc).

Small lesions are ordinarily best treated by localized surgical excision—a method which is simple, expeditious, and cosmetically satisfactory. Larger lesions can be managed most effectively with radiation therapy, avoiding unneccessary wide resections and multiple plastic procedures. Recurrence of disease in scar or in previously irradiated areas or involvement of bone ordinarily precludes the use of radiation therapy.

Cervical lymphadenectomy (radical neck dissection) is effective in the control of disease that involves the lymph nodes. The slow and orderly progression of metastases in the cervical chain of lymph nodes and their accessibility to frequent examination and evaluation make it possible to withhold surgery until the lymph nodes become clinically palpable (therapeutic neck dissection). Most patients who develop palpable nodes do so within 2 years after discovery of the primary tumor. Whereas 25% are found to have microscopically involved lymph nodes when the adenectomy is elective, tumor is found in 85% of patients undergoing therapeutic neck dissection.

Prognosis

The prognosis depends on the size of the tumor, the location of the lesion, the degree of differentiation, and the presence or absence of metastatic disease. Surgery and radiation therapy are about equally effective for comparable "curable" lesions.

The reported 5-year survival rates for cancer of the lip treated by surgery or by radiation therapy vary between 85 and 95% for lesions up to 2 cm in size. The cure rates are lower for larger lesions. The presence of metastases to the regional lymph nodes reduces the cure rate by 50% regardless of whether the neck dissection is elective or therapeutic.

Frazell EL: The care of patients with oral cavity and lip cancer: Surgical principles. JAMA 215:957–958, 1971.

CARCINOMA OF THE BUCCAL MUCOSA

The buccal mucosa lines the inner side of the cheek from the anterior commissure of the lip to the ascending ramus of the mandible and from the upper to the lower gingiva. This epithelium gives rise to carcinomas that are usually well differentiated and locally infiltrating. Larger lesions may extend from the superior to the inferior gingivobuccal sulci and gingivae, anteriorly to the commissure, and posteriorly to the "retromolar trigone"; they may infiltrate deeply through the buccinator muscle and be confused with tumors arising primarily in these regions.

Carcinoma of the buccal mucosa rarely metastasizes to the regional lymph nodes. When metastases do occur they do so in the form of isolated involvement of one or 2 lymph nodes (superficial facial, submaxillary, upper cervical nodes).

Treatment
Smaller lesions, particularly those surrounded by leukoplakia, can be excised surgically and closed primarily. Larger excisions require coverage of the resulting defect with skin grafts. Deeply infiltrating lesions may require excision of full thickness of cheek and repair of the resulting defect with mobilization of flaps previously prepared for that purpose.

Radiation therapy has been found to be as effective as surgery in the management of carcinoma of the buccal mucosa. It appears, however, that for highly differentiated tumors surgical extirpation is the treatment of choice.

Metastases to the cervical lymph nodes are best managed surgically.

The reported 5-year survival rates for both methods of treatment vary from 50–68%. Histologic involvement of the lymph nodes reduces the prospect of curability by about two-thirds.

Krishnamurthi S & others: Combined therapy in buccal mucosal cancers. Radiology 99:409–415, 1971.
Skolnik EM & others: Carcinoma of the buccal mucosa and retromolar area. Otolaryngol Clin North America 5:327–331, 1972.

CANCER OF THE ORAL TONGUE

For purposes of discussion the tongue should be considered as composed of an oral portion (mobile anterior two-thirds) and a pharyngeal portion (posterior third). The circumvallate papillae constitute the line of demarcation between the 2 segments.

Carcinoma of the oral tongue occurs from the fourth to the eighth decades of life, usually in males, in association with heavy smoking and alcohol intake and poor oral hygiene. The lesion is usually well differentiated and frequently arises along the lateral margin, although it may also occur on the tip, the dorsum, or the undersurface. Multiple primary carcinomas of the tongue are uncommon (3%). The lesion may progress in any direction and extend into the floor of the mouth to involve laterally the alveolus or posteriorly the anterior tonsillar pillar. Some lesions may be so large that it is impossible to determine the primary site of origin.

Metastases to the regional lymph nodes are frequent and may first appear on the contralateral side. At the time of initial diagnosis, 40–45% of patients have palpable lymph nodes. Another 20% will develop metastases to the cervical lymph nodes within a short time after control of the primary lesion.

Treatment
The location and size of the lesion, the condition of the adjacent tissues, the availability of treatment, and the general health of the patient determine the selection of treatment. In general, surgery and radiation therapy appear to be equally effective. However, radiation therapy has the advantage of permitting preservation of tissue which results in better function than after resection.

Surgical excision is the treatment of choice for small lesions, particularly those located at the tip of the tongue, because it is expeditious, effective, and produces negligible impairment of function.

Interstitial implantation of radium needles is indicated for lesions of moderate or larger size. This is a major surgical procedure requiring a general anesthetic, hospitalization, specialized training in the manipulation of radium needles, and expert nursing care for several days. The procedure may cause great discomfort, and its use in debilitated patients requires careful consideration.

If their location permits, smaller lesions can be treated by means of peroral irradiation.

In selecting the initial mode of treatment for the primary lesion, one should appreciate that surgery can still be utilized if radiation fails. Many experienced clinicians advocate prophylactic cervical lymphadenectomy because the lymph nodes are involved in 40–45% of cases before the disease is clinically apparent.

Prognosis
The rate of local control of the tumor depends on

its location and size. Whereas the 5-year survival rate for lesions of the tip of the tongue is 75–80%, it decreases to 55% for those at the lateral margins and to 40% for those on the dorsum. The 5-year survival rate is 78% for patients without metastases but drops to 14% for those with involved lymph nodes.

Horivchi J, Adachi T: Some considerations on radiation therapy of tongue cancer. Cancer 28:335–339, 1971.
Saxena VS: Cancer of the tongue: A study of the regional lymph node spread. Cancer 27:38–43, 1971.
Spiro RH, Strong E: Epidermoid carcinoma of the mobile tongue. Am J Surg 122:707–710, 1971.

CARCINOMA OF THE FLOOR OF THE MOUTH

The anterior and the 2 lateral gingivolingual sulci constitute the floor of the mouth. They are continuous posteriorly with the glossopharyngeal sulci and the piriform sinuses. The mucosa of the floor of the mouth has important anatomic relationships to the underlying musculature, the submaxillary gland, the lingual nerve, and the lingual artery.

Carcinoma of the floor of the mouth constitutes 15–20% of all intraoral malignant lesions. The tumor is usually a squamous cell carcinoma which is usually less well differentiated than tumors occurring on the oral tongue. It may extend medially to involve the undersurface of the tongue, laterally to involve the gingivae, the underlying periosteum, or the mandible itself to produce bone destruction. Inferior extension may involve the submaxillary duct, the lingual nerve, and the lingual artery, or the tumor may spread between muscle planes.

Most of these cancers arise in the anterior floor of the mouth. Invasion of lymphatics occurs early; 50–60% of patients have palpable lymph nodes at first examination. In some series, lymph node involvement has been reported in 90% of patients within 12 months after diagnosis. Metastases occur to the submaxillary, subdigastric, and upper deep cervical lymph nodes. Metastases to the contralateral side occur in 10–15% of cases.

Treatment

The propensity for carcinoma of the floor of the mouth to extend to the tongue and gingivae and to infiltrate deeply into the musculature of the submental and submaxillary regions makes most of these lesions unsuitable for local surgical or radiotherapeutic management as the primary treatment method.

The selection of treatment depends to a great extent on the size of the lesion and the presence or absence of involvement of the adjacent structures. Occasionally, a small lesion can be controlled by wide local excision or by peroral roentgen therapy or interstitial irradiation. Larger lesions may require either

(1) wide excision in continuity; or (2) external irradiation over the entire floor of the mouth and adjacent regional lymphatics, followed by a radical neck dissection. Extensive lesions of the floor of the mouth have been successfully treated with a combination of preoperative irradiation followed by radical surgery through tissues whose margins have been sterilized of tumor.

The treatment of choice of involved lymph nodes is therapeutic radical neck dissection.

Prognosis

Five-year survival rates between 40–75% have been reported, depending upon the size of the lesion and the presence or absence of cervical lymphadenopathy at the time of primary treatment.

Campos JL & others: Radiotherapy of carcinoma of the floor of the mouth. Radiology 99:677–682, 1971.
Fayos JV: Management of squamous cell carcinoma of the floor of the mouth. Am J Surg 123:706–711, 1972.
Harrold CC Jr: Management of cancer of the floor of the mouth. Am J Surg 122:487–493, 1971.

CANCER OF THE SOFT PALATE & ANTERIOR FAUCIAL PILLARS

The most frequent malignant tumors arising in these structures are squamous cell carcinomas. They are usually well-differentiated tumors with various degrees of local infiltration of the underlying musculature. They remain localized for a long time and metastasize late to regional lymph nodes. The presence of extensive adenopathy renders the prognosis grave.

The long period of localization of these tumors renders them amenable to wide surgical excision. Radiation therapy is frequently utilized as definitive treatment for superficial lesions or as preoperative treatment for those too extensive to be treated by surgery or radiation therapy alone. Planned preoperative irradiation of an extensive tumor may reduce its size significantly and permit its resection through margins sterilized of tumor cells.

Adenocarcinomas of salivary gland origin may occasionally arise in the soft palate. They are locally invasive and are best treated by surgical resection.

Lindberg RD & others: Evolution of the clinically negative neck in patients with squamous cell carcinoma of the faucial arch. Am J Roentgenol 111:60–65, 1971.

CARCINOMA OF THE "RETROMOLAR TRIGONE"

Lesions originating in the mucosa behind the last molar teeth constitute a special class of tumors presenting serious problems of management. Epidermoid carcinoma arising in this site is particularly radioresistant. It has a tendency to involve bone early, to infiltrate adjacent musculature, and to travel along nerve structures such as the mandibular and the lingual nerves. It may extend early along the pterygoid plate to the base of the skull. All of these features frequently make primary surgery of these tumors a futile effort. During the past 10 years, these tumors have been managed by intensive preoperative irradiation followed by radical surgical resection.

Skolnik EM & others: Carcinoma of the buccal mucosa and retromolar area. Otolaryngol Clin North America 5:327–331, 1972.

CARCINOMA OF THE LOWER GINGIVAE

It is important to distinguish between carcinoma of the gingivae and cancer of the jaw. The first is an epidermoid carcinoma arising in the epithelium covering the alveolus, whereas the latter signifies bone tumor arising in the mandible.

Epidermoid carcinoma of the mucosa of the lower gingivae is usually well differentiated and infiltrates underlying bone early and frequently (40–50%). It may first become apparent as a small ulceration adjacent to a tooth that was extracted after failure to recognize the true cause of local symptoms. The open socket then constitutes an avenue for invasion of bone by the cancer. The tumor may extend laterally to involve the buccal mucosa or medially to involve the floor of the mouth.

Metastases to the regional lymph nodes occur frequently (35–40% of cases). Extensive tumors involving the floor of the mouth to the midline may metastasize to the contralateral side.

Small superficial verrucous lesions of the gingivae can be controlled with radiation therapy.

Resection of the primary lesion (mandibulectomy) in continuity with radical lymphadenectomy is the treatment of choice for moderate-sized lesions of the alveolus with or without palpable lymph nodes.

For more extensive lesions, planned preoperative irradiation followed by combined resection yields the best results.

The overall 5-year survival rate is 35–45%.

CARCINOMA OF THE UPPER GINGIVAE & HARD PALATE

Cancers arising in the mucosa of the upper gingivae and the hard palate are usually well-differentiated epidermoid carcinomas which metastasize late. They frequently are confused with cancers that arise in the antrum and spread inferiorly. X-rays are necessary to distinguish between the 2 entities. Bone involvement may be extensive. The rare metastases are found in retropharyngeal, submaxillary, or subdigastric lymph nodes.

Wide surgical resection of the involved tissues is the treatment of choice. The resulting extensive surgical defects can be easily covered by prosthetic appliances. Five-year survival rates are about 60%.

CANCER OF THE OROPHARYNX

The oropharynx extends from the soft palate to the level of the hyoid bone and is delineated anteriorly by the lingual circumvallate papillae and the anterior faucial pillars. Epidermoid carcinomas, lymphoepitheliomas, and lymphosarcomas are the most common malignancies found in this region.

The epidermoid tumors are poorly differentiated, bulky lesions which metastasize early to both sides of the neck. They tend to be noninvasive but produce local symptoms by compression. Surgery is unsuccessful, but both primary and metastatic tumors usually respond to radiotherapy. Death often results from distant metastases.

Al-Saleem T & others: Malignant lymphomas of the pharynx. Cancer 26:1383–1387, 1970.

Banfi A & others: Malignant lymphomas of Waldeyer's ring. Brit MJ 3:140–143, 1972.

Fletcher GH, MacComb WS: *Radiation Therapy in the Management of Cancer of the Oral Cavity and Oropharynx.* Thomas, 1962.

Jesse RH Jr, Fletcher GH: Metastases in cervical lymph nodes from oropharyngeal carcinoma: Treatment and results. Am J Roentgenol 90:990, 1963.

Silva N: Pattern of lymphatic spread in pharyngeal cancer. J Surg Oncol 3:415–419, 1971.

Rubin P: Cancer of the head and neck: Oropharynx. JAMA 217:940–953, 1973.

CANCER OF THE BASE OF THE TONGUE
(Pharyngeal or Posterior Third)

The pharyngeal tongue originates from a different anlage than the anterior two-thirds and is covered by a squamous epithelium that is less well differentiated. The base of the tongue is infiltrated with lymphoid tissue and has abundant lymphatics that drain directly to the subdigastric lymph nodes. Because they are initially silent, tumors of the base of the tongue are usually detected late, after extensive infiltration has occurred into the deep musculature. The extent of infiltration is difficult to delineate clinically, and examination under general anesthesia is occasionally necessary to judge the size of the lesion and the extent of local spread. Pain, dysphagia, and voice changes may occur but are often preceded by unilateral or bilateral cervical lymphadenopathy. Lymph node involvement ranges from 40–90% depending on the stage of the lesion.

The treatment of choice for carcinoma of the pharyngeal tongue is external radiation to the primary lesion and to the cervical lymph nodes on both sides. Curative surgical excision would necessitate such an extensive resection that swallowing would be impossible without aspiration. The location of the primary tumor makes the use of interstitial radium needles very difficult.

The overall 5-year survival for treated carcinoma of the pharyngeal tongue is about 10%.

CARCINOMA OF THE VALLECULA

Lesions originating in the vallecula are often difficult to detect by inspection. Palpation and a lateral soft tissue x-ray film of the area may be necessary to establish the diagnosis. The characteristic roentgenographic finding is a pocket of air in the musculature of the tongue.

Lesions of this area are usually superficial rather than deeply infiltrating, and they spread in all directions to involve the pharyngeal wall and the tongue. They metastasize early to the cervical lymph nodes. The primary mode of treatment is external radiation therapy.

CARCINOMA OF THE TONSIL

Malignancies of the tonsil are often mistaken for inflammatory lesions until incontrovertible proof of tumor slowly appears. Both the anterior and posterior faucial pillars may be involved, and the tumor may spread into the soft palate and the uvula. Inferiorly, the tumor may extend into the glossopharyngeal sulcus and into the base of the tongue. Trismus may result from invasion of the pterygoid muscles. The tumor may spread to the base of the skull along nerve channels.

Histologically, malignant tumors of the tonsil are poorly differentiated epidermoid carcinomas (75%), lymphosarcomas (15%), and lymphoepitheliomas (10%).

It is most important to separate malignant lesions arising in the tonsil and tonsillar bed from those arising in the anterior tonsillar pillar since the 2 have entirely different biologic characteristics. This differentiation is not always possible because of the tendency of tonsillar carcinomas to spread widely into adjacent structures in all directions. In cancer of the tonsil, massive involvement of the ipsilateral lymph nodes is often the first clinical manifestation of the disease. Three-fourths of patients have palpable lymph nodes at the time of first examination. Distant metastases to bone, lungs, and liver occur frequently, particularly with lymphoepitheliomas.

Metastatic disease is occasionally found in a cervical lymph node even when the most meticulous examination has failed to detect a primary lesion. Histologic survey of a previously removed tonsil may reveal a small "occult" carcinoma.

Radiation therapy is the treatment of choice both for the primary lesions and the cervical metastases. Supervoltage external irradiation is given to large areas which include the primary and the neck to the level of the clavicle. Combined preoperative irradiation and surgery may be utilized in exceptional cases, but the exact place of this method of treatment is still under evaluation. Combined resection and radiation is better reserved for residual or recurrent disease.

Survival following treatment varies according to the extent of the primary lesion and the presence and extent of metastatic disease in the neck. Reported 5-year survival rates are 62% for patients without cervical adenopathy and 26% for patients with cervical adenopathy. The overall survival rate varies between 30–35%.

Fayos JV, Lampe I: Radiation therapy of carcinoma of the tonsillar region. Am J Roentgenol 111:85–94, 1971.

Perez CA & others: Malignant tumors of the tonsil. Am J Roentgenol 114:43–58, 1972.

CARCINOMA OF THE OROPHARYNGEAL WALLS

Lesions arising in the walls of the oropharynx are usually poorly differentiated carcinomas presenting a central ulceration surrounded by wide infiltration of the adjacent walls. They arise in the lateral or the posterior pharyngeal walls and have a tendency to metastasize early to the regional lymph nodes. They may extend to the nasopharynx superiorly or the hypopharynx inferiorly. Lesions arising in the lateral pharyngeal wall frequently extend to the epiglottis and piriform fossa and may exhibit an almost continuous induration with the involved midcervical lymph nodes. The deep prespinal fascia is rarely involved and is penetrated only late in the disease. Tumor may involve the ninth cranial nerve and extend to the base of the skull.

Exophytic lesions of the pharyngeal wall that are noninfiltrative and present discrete borders can be treated either by radiation therapy or by surgery if laryngectomy is not necessary for complete eradication of the tumor.

Infiltrating lesions are best treated by radiation therapy, which has the advantage of sparing the larynx. This is particularly true in patients with bilateral involvement of the cervical lymph nodes.

Larger lesions with wide involvement of the adjacent structures are treated surgically by means of laryngopharyngectomy and neck dissection, unilateral or bilateral as indicated.

No end results from large series have been reported. A 5-year survival rate of 32% has been reported in one series of 48 patients.

Wilkins SA: Carcinoma of the posterior pharyngeal wall. Am J Surg 122:477–481, 1971.

CANCER OF THE EPIGLOTTIS

Malignant lesions of the epiglottis are usually ulcerating or bulky tumors that may completely destroy the epiglottis. The lesions are usually well-differentiated epidermoid carcinomas and have a tendency to metastasize late.

Treatment of the primary lesion is usually by radiation therapy. Metastatic lymph nodes are treated by radical neck dissection.

· · ·

TUMORS OF THE NASOPHARYNX

The nasopharynx has been called a "blind spot" because tumors occurring in this area usually are diagnosed late and in an advanced stage. There is usually a delay of 8–10 months from the onset of signs to the time when the diagnosis is established. The initial signs and symptoms may vary depending on involvement by tumor of one or more of the following: cranial nerves III–VII and IX–XII, the mandibular and the auriculotemporal nerves, the levator muscle of the soft palate, the pterygoid muscles, the foramen lacerum and the carotid canal, and the eustachian tubes. No other tumor of the head and neck can present with such a variety of symptoms: nasal (obstruction), aural (hypoacusia, deafness, earache, tinnitus, pain, and headache), ocular (proptosis, diplopia, even blindness), neurologic (diplopia, facial paresthesias, Horner's syndrome), and olfactory.

Cervical adenopathy is the presenting symptom in over one-third of cases, and well over three-fourths may have lymphadenopathy at the time of the initial examination. The nasopharyngeal mucosa and submucosa are richly supplied by lymphatics which drain into the jugulodigastric chain (70%) and the upper deep cervical lymph nodes (65%). Lymph nodes in the spinal accessory and inferior cervical areas may also be involved. Lymphadenopathy—particularly if bilateral—in the absence of an obvious primary tumor should direct the search to the nasopharynx.

Epidermoid carcinoma, transitional cell carcinoma, and lymphoepithelioma are the most common nasopharyngeal tumors. Lymphosarcoma, adenocarcinoma, plasmacytoma, miscellaneous sarcomas, malignant melanomas, and other types also occur. Although the principal route of metastasis is via the lymphatics to the lymph nodes, regional or even distant hematogenous spread may occur with lymphomas and lymphoepitheliomas.

Treatment

The nasopharynx is surgically inaccessible except for biopsy, and the distribution of cervical metastases makes effective neck dissection impossible. Fortunately, these tumors are radiosensitive; treatment of the primary and its metastases consists of radiation. The entire nasopharynx is treated with fields that cover all possible areas of extension and the 2 sides of the neck down to the level of the clavicles.

Complications of treatment may include dry mouth, pharyngitis, epidermitis, and bone necrosis. A dread but infrequent complication is myelitis of the cervical spinal cord, which can occasionally result in death.

Curability depends on the stage of the lesion and the extent of tumor at the time of treatment. The overall 5-year survival in major centers in the USA is 30–35%. Lymphosarcomas have the best survival rate. Bilateral involvement of the cervical lymph nodes and of bone or nerves makes the prognosis poor. Local reappearance of the tumor may occur several years after the initial treatment and can sometimes be controlled with intracavitary radiation.

Chen KY, Fletcher GH: Malignant tumors of the nasopharynx. Radiology 99:165–171, 1971.

Jing B-S: Tumors of the nasopharynx. Radiol Clin North America 8:323–342, 1970.

Schnohr P: Survival rates of nasopharyngeal cancer in California. Cancer 25:1009–1106, 1970.

Wang CC, Meyer JE: Radiotherapeutic management of carcinoma of the nasopharynx. Cancer 28:566–570, 1971.

CANCER OF THE HYPOPHARYNX*

The hypopharynx is directly behind the larynx and is composed of the piriform sinuses, the aryepiglottic folds, the lateral and posterior pharyngeal walls, and the postcricoid mucosa.

Malignant lesions of the hypopharynx comprise approximately 4% of all malignant oropharyngeal tumors in man. Cancer of the hypopharynx is more frequent in men than in women but shows a peculiar geographic distribution in that it is more frequent in Scandinavian women in association with the Plummer-Vinson syndrome.

Unlike carcinomas occurring in the oral cavity, tumors of the hypopharynx have a tendency to be highly undifferentiated. Metastases occur to the regional lymph nodes along lymphatics that exit between the hyoid bone and the upper edge of the thyroid cartilage to the upper deep cervical lymph nodes.

Lesions arising in the hypopharynx are ordinarily silent in the early stages and may reach considerable size before they cause symptoms. Cervical adenopathy is occasionally the first clinical manifestation of the disease. Disturbances of the swallowing mechanism usually precede impairment of respiration or speech, the latter being symptoms of advanced lesions.

Malignant lesions of the hypopharynx can be divided into 2 groups: (1) carcinomas arising in the aryepiglottic folds and the upper lateral and posterior hypopharynx (prognostically more favorable); and (2) lesions which arise in the piriform sinus, the postcricoid and postarytenoid areas, and the lower reaches of the hypopharynx (prognosis is poor).

Attempts to control lesions arising in the hypopharynx by surgery or radiation therapy usually meet with little success. Survival rates have greatly improved since the advent of radical surgery, whereby laryngectomy, hypopharyngectomy, and radical neck dissection are performed in continuity at one stage. When these tumors are treated by radiation, surgery can be performed later in the event of radiation failure.

As for other lesions arising in the upper respiratory and digestive tracts, the combination of preoperative irradiation and surgery offers considerable promise for some of these lesions, but its exact value is yet to be established.

Futrell JW & others: Predicting survival in cancer of the larynx or hypopharynx. Am J Surg 122:451–457, 1971.
Jing B-S: Roentgen examination of the larynx and hypopharynx. Radiol Clin North America 8:361–386, 1970.
Leonard JR, Holt GP: Reconstruction of the hypopharynx and cervical esophagus. Otolaryngol Clin North America 5:435–446, 1972.
Macbeth R: Malignant disease of the hypopharynx. J Laryngol Otol 85:1215–1226, 1971.
Ogura JH & others: Elective neck dissection for pharyngeal and laryngeal cancers. Ann Otol Rhin Laryng 80:646–653, 1971.

*Carcinoma of the larynx is discussed in Chapter 42.

Rubin P: Cancer of the head and neck. Part 1: Hypopharynx and larynx. JAMA 221:68–85, 1972.

CANCER OF THE NASAL FOSSA

Although cancers of the nasal fossa represent only 1% or less of tumors of the head and neck, the mortality and morbidity they can produce is great. They present individual problems according to the areas in which they arise.

Primary tumors arising in the nasal fossa must be distinguished from those arising in adjacent sinuses, the nasopharynx, the oral cavity, and the skin and those extending into the nasal fossa because of uncontrolled growth.

According to the stage of the lesion, the symptoms vary from abnormal nasal discharge to bleeding, obstruction, and eventually pain.

Most are squamous cell tumors which are either bulky, obstructive, and exophytic tumors or deeply infiltrating and painful. Other types of tumors are lymphosarcomas, malignant melanomas, olfactory neuroblastomas (esthesioneuroepitheliomas) arising in the olfactory mucosa, plasmacytomas, sarcomas, and adenocarcinomas of salivary gland origin.

Malignant lesions of the nasal fossa chiefly present problems of local invasion, although they do sometimes metastasize to the regional lymph nodes and occasionally to distant sites via the blood stream.

Epidermoid carcinomas and lymphosarcomas of the nasal fossa are usually managed with radiation therapy, which is more successful here than for tumors arising in the paranasal sinuses or those invading the nasal fossa.

Radical surgery is the treatment of choice for mucous or salivary gland adenocarcinomas and malignant melanomas of the nasal cavity.

Considerable palliation can frequently be achieved with radiation therapy for nonresectable tumors.

Boone MLM & others: Malignant disease of the paranasal sinuses and nasal cavity: Importance of precise localization of extent of disease. Am J Roentgenol 102:627–636, 1968.
Jesse RH: Preoperative versus postoperative radiation in treatment of squamous carcinoma of the paranasal sinuses. Am J Surg 110:552–556, 1965.
Paulus DD Jr, Dodd GD: The roentgen diagnosis of tumors of the nasal cavity and accessory paranasal sinuses. Radiol Clin North America 8:343–360, 1970.

CANCER OF THE PARANASAL SINUSES

Tumors of the paranasal sinuses are more frequent in men than in women and constitute less than 1% of all head and neck tumors.

Histologically, most of these tumors are of the epidermoid squamous cell type. However, other types of tumors such as transitional cell carcinoma, lymphoepithelioma, adenocarcinoma, and lymphosarcoma may occur. These tumors spread by local invasion to adjacent areas and metastasize to the cervical lymph nodes and eventually to distant sites.

Most of these tumors arise in the maxillary sinus; an occasional tumor arises in the ethmoid sinus. Tumors arising in the frontal and sphenoid sinuses are extremely rare.

The symptoms of pain, nasal obstruction, and nasal discharge occur only when the tumor is relatively locally advanced and has destroyed surrounding structures. Radiologic findings usually are not conclusive until bone destruction has taken place. Early diagnosis is important since death is usually due to local growth. Often the patient has been treated for a long time with antibiotics for sinusitis while the underlying cause of symptoms is carcinoma.

Local spread causes the following symptoms: (1) Anterior extension: bone erosion and swelling. (2) Posterolateral extension into the infratemporal fossa: trismus and swelling. (3) Posterior extension into the pterygopalatine fossa: erosion of the base of the skull. (4) Medial extension into the ethmoid sinuses superiorly and into the nasal fossa medially: obstruction and bleeding. (5) Direct extension superiorly: erosion of the floor of the orbit, resulting in ocular signs. (6) Inferior extension: may involve the upper canines and molars, producing toothache, loosening of the teeth, and eventual protrusion into the gingivobuccal sulcus.

Treatment

Surgical excision is the major treatment for carcinoma of the maxillary sinuses, but it is utilized primarily for well-differentiated squamous cell carcinomas and adenocarcinomas. Radiation therapy rarely controls these tumors and is usually utilized only for palliation. The trend in recent years has been to treat patients with maxillary sinus carcinoma by radical surgery after preoperative irradiation.

Orbital exenteration is sometimes necessary when tumors arising in the superior portion of the maxillary sinus invade the floor of the orbit.

Because these tumors metastasize late, prophylactic neck dissection is not indicated. However, therapeutic neck dissections are indicated for clinically involved lymph nodes. Radiation therapy to the cervical region is used only for palliation.

The role of radiation therapy in palliation cannot be underestimated in a disease where a significant number of patients die of uncontrollable local tumor. It is most effective in controlling pain, discharge, proptosis, bleeding, etc. Preservation of the eye by protection of the cornea is feasible when management is by palliative radiation therapy.

Prognosis

Preoperative irradiation and radical surgery yields 5-year survivals of about 40–45%.

Boone MLM & others: Malignant disease of the paranasal sinuses and nasal cavity: Importance of precise localization of extent of disease. Am J Roentgenol 102:627–636, 1968.

Jesse RH: Preoperative versus postoperative radiation in treatment of squamous carcinoma of the paranasal sinuses. Am J Surg 110:552–556, 1965.

Kurohara SS & others: Role of radiation therapy and of surgery in the management of localized epidermoid carcinoma of the maxillary sinus. Am J Roentgenol 114:35–42, 1972.

Paulus DD Jr, Dodd GD: The roentgen diagnosis of tumors of the nasal cavity and accessory paranasal sinuses. Radiol Clin North America 8:343–360, 1970.

CANCER OF THE SALIVARY GLANDS

Salivary gland tissue is both ectodermal and entodermal in origin and is divided into 2 groups: (1) major salivary glands (parotid, submaxillary, sublingual) and (2) minor salivary glands (small deposits of salivary tissue scattered throughout the mucosa of the oral cavity, maxilla, and nasopharynx). About 80% of tumors occurring in major salivary glands are found in the parotid. Considering all salivary gland tumors, the parotid is the site of 50%.

The mixed tumor is a benign lesion that has the potentiality of malignant transformation even after many years.

Benign tumors may become large without invasion of the adjacent areas. Malignant tumors grow by local invasion of facial muscles, facial nerve, mandible, pterygoid muscles, or the base of the skull. They may enter the skull along the facial nerve or the mandibular branch of the trigeminal nerve.

Parotid carcinomas, especially epidermoid and mucoepidermoid lesions, tend to metastasize to the cervical lymph nodes. Hematogenous metastases may occur, particularly to lungs and bones. Peculiar cases have been reported where lung metastases progress slowly for 10–20 years.

MAJOR SALIVARY GLANDS

Classification

A. Parotid Gland: The parotid gland is the largest of the 3 major salivary glands. It is bounded by the masseter muscle, the ascending ramus of the mandible, and the pterygoid muscles. Inferiorly, the parotid may extend along the posterior belly of the digastric muscle. The gland is divided into 2 major portions, a superficial and a deep lobe joined by a bridge of tissue called the isthmus. The structure most closely related to the parotid gland is the facial nerve. In its course between the 2 lobes, it subdivides into 2 trunks, the zygomaticofacial and the cervicofacial. These in turn subdivide at the periphery of the gland into branches that supply the temporal, zygomatic, buccal, maxillary, and mandibular areas. The plane in which the main trunks of the facial nerve lie is not always easy to identify, and dissection of the nerve may be difficult.

The main lymphatics of the parotid gland drain first into the deep and superficial parotid lymph nodes and then into the superficial posterior cervical chain. The deep parotid lymph nodes drain to the subparotid node located below the angle of the mandible and ultimately into lymph nodes along the spinal accessory nerve or the deep jugular chain.

B. Submaxillary Gland: The submaxillary gland is located in the submaxillary triangle between the anterior and posterior bellies of the digastric muscle. The submaxillary duct lies close to the lingual and hypoglossal nerves, and tumor may spread along perineural spaces into the cranial cavity. The marginal mandibular nerve also lies close to the submaxillary gland and must be avoided during resection of the gland.

C. Sublingual Gland: This smallest of the 3 major salivary glands is located in the floor of the mouth beneath the deep buccal mucosa. It is rarely the site of a malignant process.

Types of Tumors

A. Mixed Tumors: "Mixed tumors" are the most frequent type arising in salivary glands. The epithelial cells may be spindle-shaped or stellate and arranged in sheets or in glandular patterns. The stroma may be myxoid, hyalinized, and even cartilagenous. Areas of necrosis can often be observed. Metaplasia of the epithelium into well-differentiated squamous cells occasionally occurs. The distinction between histologically benign and malignant tumors is often difficult, in which case the diagnosis can only be established by the clinical course.

B. Mucoepidermoid Carcinoma: The division of these tumors into low-grade and high-grade malignancy depends on the relative amounts of mucoid material secreted by the ductal cells and on the squamous cell component, which predominates in the more highly malignant lesions.

C. Squamous Cell or Epidermoid Carcinoma: These tumors evolve from squamous metaplasia of the ductal epithelium. Occasionally, the diagnostic dilemma arises of distinguishing a primary epidermoid carcinoma of the parotid gland from metastatic squamous cell carcinoma to an intraparotid lymph node.

D. Papillary Cystadenoma Lymphomatosum (Warthin's Tumor): This is the second most common benign tumor and is found only in the parotid. It is composed of proliferating salivary gland cells in lymphoid tissue and grossly appears as cysts with multiple papillary projections from the wall within the parotid gland. They are more common in males, and are bilateral in 10% of cases.

E. Adenocarcinoma:

1. Adenoid cystic carcinoma (cylindroma)—This tumor consists of small nests or strands of epithelial cells with relatively large nuclei and poorly defined cytoplasms. Mucicarmine stains are usually positive, and hyaline is often present.

2. Acinic cell carcinoma—This uncommon tumor resembles the acinic cells of the parotid gland. The cells are usually polygonal, with large eccentric nuclei, arranged in alveolar groups. They may metastasize to local lymph nodes and distant sites.

3. Miscellaneous adenocarcinomas varying according to the histologic pattern of the tumor—A small group of malignant lesions have been classified as trabecular, anaplastic, mucus carcinomas, etc. They are highly malignant tumors with great propensity for local and distant metastases.

F. Oxyphil Adenoma: These lesions are composed of eosinophilic cells showing considerable pleomorphism arranged in small groups separated by very thin fibrovascular septi.

G. Benign Lymphoepithelial Tumors (Godwin's Tumor): These tumors consist essentially of an enlargement of the parotid gland containing a mixture of inflammatory cells such as plasma cells and lymphocytes containing scattered reticulum cells. Islands of epithelial cells are found with zones of hyalinization.

Clinical Findings

The diagnosis of parotid tumors depends on the ability to differentiate inflammatory lesions from primary and metastatic neoplasms. Viral or bacterial parotitis and sialolithiasis are characterized by recurrent fever, pain, tenderness, and other symptoms which are not present with malignant lesions. Unless nerve structures are invaded, malignant lesions are asymptomatic.

The possibility of metastatic spread to the parotid lymph nodes from primary tumors located elsewhere in the head and neck should always be recognized.

The definitive diagnosis is established by histologic examination of the specimen. Needle or incisional biopsies must be performed with the utmost care to avoid seeding of malignant cells and eventual local recurrence. Biopsies should be planned so as not to interfere with the definitive cancer operation.

Treatment

Treatment of benign or malignant salivary gland tumors is surgical. Enucleation, particularly with mixed tumors, leads to a high rate of local recurrence.

A. Surgical Treatment: The entire parotid gland is exposed, the superficial lobe elevated, the facial nerve dissected, and the lobe excised en bloc with the intraglandular and paraglandular lymphatics and lymph nodes.

Occasionally, a tumor may be located deeply within the deep lobe and appear in the tonsillar fossa. In such cases it is always possible to preserve the facial nerve while removing the deeply located tumor. The facial nerve should never be sacrificed unless it is directly involved with malignant tissue.

Radical cervical lymphadenectomy is indicated whenever a malignant tumor of the parotid gland is accompanied by enlarged cervical lymph nodes. The yield of positive lymph nodes with prophylactic neck dissection is low, so that one may defer this operation until nodes become palpable.

B. Radiotherapy: Radiotherapy is indicated (1) when the primary tumor is not resectable, (2) for recurrent tumors not amenable to surgical extirpation, (3) when tumor is present at the surgical margins, and (4) for control of residual tumor in the surgical bed.

Complications of Surgery

The most frequent complications following surgery of the parotid gland are those resulting from temporary or permanent injury to the facial nerve and a peculiar set of symptoms grouped under the name of auriculotemporal nerve syndrome (Frey's syndrome).

Dysfunction of facial muscles may occur following extensive manipulation of the facial nerve even when the latter is not sectioned and may last from a few weeks to a few months. Function can be satisfactorily restored after accidental section of the facial nerve by immediate direct anastomosis. Function following the intentional sacrifice of the facial nerve can occasionally be reestablished by grafting from the greater auricular nerve.

Following parotidectomy, a few patients develop flushing and increased sweating in the parotid region at mealtime **(Frey's syndrome).** There is no satisfactory explanation for the symptoms, but it has been postulated that it is due to injury of the auriculotemporal nerve followed by abnormal regeneration of parasympathetic fibers which are carried in this nerve. It may appear from a few weeks to a year or more after operation.

A special feature of malignant tumors of the submaxillary gland is the 3–4 times higher incidence of metastases to the regional lymph nodes than for similar lesions occurring in the parotid. Radical neck dissection is therefore indicated whenever the submaxillary gland is removed for a malignant lesion.

Anderson R, Byars LT: *Surgery of the Parotid Gland.* Mosby, 1965.

Butler C: Salivary gland tumors. J Laryng 86:775–784, 1972.

Conley J & others: Analysis of 115 patients with tumors of the submandibular gland. Ann Otor Rhin Laryng 81:323–330, 1972.

Frazell EL: Clinical aspects of tumors of the major salivary glands. Cancer 7:637, 1954.

Frazell EL: Observations on the management of salivary gland tumors. Cancer 18:235–240, 1968.

Healey WV & others: Mucoepidermoid carcinoma of salivary gland origin. Cancer 26:368–388, 1970.

Leafstedt SW & others: Adenoid cystic carcinoma of major and minor salivary glands. Am J Surg 122:756–762, 1971.

Meine FJ, Woloshin HJ: Radiologic diagnosis of salivary gland tumors. Radiol Clin North America 8:475–485, 1970.

Thorvaldsson SE: Mucoepidermoid tumors of the major salivary glands. Am J Surg 120:433–438, 1970.

MINOR SALIVARY GLANDS

The 2 most frequent sites of origin of minor salivary gland carcinomas are the hard palate and the sinuses. These tumors may also occur at the base of the tongue, in the gums, the buccal mucosa, the larynx, the inner surface of the lip, the pharynx, the floor of the mouth, the nasopharynx, the soft palate, etc. Histologically, these tumors may be (in order of frequency) adenoid cystic carcinomas, mucoepidermoid carcinomas, benign mixed tumors, malignant mixed tumors, or various types of adenocarcinomas. Most tumors of minor salivary glands are malignant.

If left untreated, these tumors spread locally by invasion of muscle, bone, and nerves to areas inaccessible to surgical extirpation.

Contrary to common belief, a significant number of tumors arising in minor salivary glands metastasize to the cervical lymph nodes—an occurrence of very grave portent. Hematogenous spread to lung and bones is frequent.

The tumors consist usually of a bulky mass covered by an overlying intact mucosa of firm, rubbery consistency. They are diagnosed by direct or indirect visualization and occasionally—in the case of the paranasal sinuses—by x-ray examination. Radiologic examination may also be of help in detecting enlargement of the respective foramens when tumors extend to the cranial cavity along the mandibular or the maxillary nerves.

Treatment

The treatment of choice for minor salivary gland tumors, whether benign or malignant, is surgical excision. For malignant tumors, the excision should be radical and should include removal of adjacent nerves and tissues. Examination of the cut ends of nerves and the surgical margins is of paramount importance.

Radical cervical lymphadenectomy is indicated when there is lymphadenopathy.

Radiotherapy is reserved for postoperative management of lesions that are suspected to have been incompletely removed; recurrent tumors when surgery is no longer feasible; and for palliation of bulky tumors considered unresectable. The role of radiotherapy is thus limited to an adjuvant or palliative function.

Frable WJ, Elzay RP: Tumors of minor salivary glands. Cancer 25:932–941, 1970.

Kadish SP & others: Treatment of minor salivary gland malignancies of upper food and air passage epithelium. Cancer 29:1021–1026, 1972.

BENIGN TUMORS

Benign tumors of the head and neck are comparatively common. **Pigmented nevi, hemangiomas, der-**

moid cysts, inclusion cysts (nevi), and **keratoses** are particularly apt to be seen on the skin of the face, neck, and scalp. Surgical excision, often under local anesthesia, is usually appropriate (see Chapter 47).

Dermoid cysts occur frequently at the angle of the jaw, and particular care should be taken not to mistake an early parotid tumor for a dermoid cyst. In fact, a "dermoid cyst" at the angle of the jaw should be regarded as a parotid tumor until proved otherwise. Excisional biopsy should be done under circumstances permitting resection of the parotid gland if necessary.

A variety of **benign tumors and cysts** occur in the neck. Congenital cysts, branchial cleft cysts, and cystic hygromas are discussed in Chapter 49.

Benign peripheral nerve tumors are fairly common. Excision is usually required to establish the diagnosis and exclude other lesions, including lymph node metastasis from unknown sites.

Carotid body tumor is a painless neck mass attached to the carotid bifurcation. It is diagnosed by palpation and carotid arteriography (vascular "blush" and separation of internal and external carotid arteries by the mass). Its treatment is discussed in Chapter 39.

MALIGNANT NECK TUMORS WITH UNKNOWN PRIMARY

Because the cure rate is very low if metastatic carcinoma in the neck is treated without locating and controlling the primary lesion, patients with lumps in the neck must be examined very thoroughly. A thorough ear, nose, and throat examination must be done, including examination of the nasopharynx, nose, sinuses, pharynx, hypopharynx, larynx, and neck. If the primary tumor is not detected with diagnostic biopsies of the nasopharynx, the tonsillar fossa, the base of the tongue, and the area of the aryepiglottic fold, treatment is controversial. The best treatment is probably excisional biopsy of the mass to obtain a specimen for frozen section analysis, planning the incision appropriately for a radical neck dissection. If the lesion is a squamous cell carcinoma (metastatic to the lymph node), the incision should be extended and radical neck dissection done followed by full-course radiation therapy to the nasopharynx, the tonsillar fossa, the base of the tongue, and the piriform sinus.

Barrie JR & others: Cervical nodal metastases of unknown origin. Am J Surg 120:467–470, 1970.

Pico J & others: Cervical lymph node metastases from carcinoma of undetermined origin. Am J Roentgenol 111:95–102, 1971.

OPERATIONS ON THE HEAD & NECK

A multitude of operations are performed on the head and neck for the control of benign and malignant lesions. Although the description of the procedures are beyond the scope of this chapter, 2 operations deserve special mention: radical neck dissection and combined resection.

RADICAL NECK DISSECTION
(Radical Cervical Lymphadenectomy)

This operation was originally standardized by Crile in 1906 and was designed for the removal and control of metastatic deposits to the cervical lymph nodes from various primaries occurring in the head and neck. The deep cervical lymphatics and the cervical lymph nodes are removed from the level of the mandible superiorly to the level of the clavicle inferiorly, and from the midline anteriorly to the anterior border of the trapezius muscle posteriorly. The specimen usually includes the sternocleidomastoid muscle, the omohyoid muscle, the internal jugular vein, and frequently the spinal accessory nerve. The contents of the submental and submaxillary triangle are removed, along with the submaxillary gland and the tip of the parotid gland. The carotid vessels, the vagus and phrenic nerves, the sympathetic chain, the brachial plexus, the hypoglossal nerve, and the digastric muscle are preserved. Occasionally, the thoracic duct must be transected and ligated.

More limited, modified types of neck dissection done with the intention of preserving one or more structures listed above usually fail except when used for the control of papillary carcinoma of the thyroid gland.

When radical neck dissection is performed alone, control of the primary lesion by surgery or radiation therapy is a necessary prerequisite. The operation is not performed when there is extension of disease below the level of the clavicles or to more distant sites.

For midline lesions, bilateral neck dissection is occasionally indicated. The morbidity and mortality rates are higher for this operation, and the postoperative course is marked by profound facial edema. Sparing the jugular vein on one side or staging the operation by delaying the procedure on the second side for a period of several weeks reduces the morbidity and the mortality rate significantly.

COMBINED RESECTION

The removal of the primary tumor in continuity with a radical neck dissection constitutes a combined resection (also called "composite operation," "commando operation"). The principle underlying the combined resection is one of in-continuity removal of the primary lesion and the areas of lymphatic drainage. The mandible is frequently removed for lesions involving the floor of the mouth and the tonsillar fossa. For tumors involving the larynx, the latter is removed in continuity with the contents of the neck. The deformity resulting from mandibular resection depends on the extent and location of the resection: the more anteriorly the mandible is resected, the greater the resulting deformity. A temporary tracheostomy is usually indicated in combined operations.

For lesions that are too extensive to be safely removed with the combined operation, planned preoperative radiation therapy has been found to be most useful in reducing the size of the lesion and permitting resection through tumor-free margins. The advent of supervoltage and modern technics of irradiation permit major operative procedures with morbidity rates that are no greater than those following surgery through nonirradiated tissues.

• • •

General References

Ackerman LV, DelRegato JA: *Cancer*, 4th ed. Mosby, 1970.

Ansfield FJ & others: Treatment of advanced cancer of the head and neck. Cancer 25:78–82, 1970.

Buschke F, Parker RG: *Radiation Therapy in Cancer Management*. Grune & Stratton, 1972.

Buschke F, Galante M: Radical preoperative roentgen therapy in primarily inoperable cancers of the head and neck. Radiology 73:845–848, 1959.

Crews QE, Fletcher GH: Comparative evaluation of the sequential use of irradiation and surgery in primary tumors of the oral cavity, oropharynx, larynx and hypopharynx. Am J Roentgenol 111:73–77, 1971.

Dodd GD & others: The dissemination of tumors of the head and neck via the cranial nerves. Radiol Clin North America 8:445–461, 1970.

Farr HW, Arthur K: Epidermoid carcinoma of the mouth and pharynx 1960–1964. J Laryng 86:243–253, 1972.

Fayos JV, Lampe I: The therapeutic problem of metastatic neck adenopathy. Am J Roentgenol 114:65–75, 1972.

Fletcher GH: Elective irradiation of subclinical disease in cancers of the head and neck. Cancer 29:1450–1454, 1972.

Gaisford JC (editor): *Symposium on Cancer of the Head and Neck: Total Treatment and Reconstructive Rehabilitation*. Mosby, 1969.

Gollin FF & others: Combined therapy in advanced head and neck cancer: A randomized study. Am J Roentgenol 114:83–88, 1972.

Kerth JD, Sisson GA, Becker GD: Radical neck dissection in carcinoma of the head and neck. S Clin North America 53:179–190, 1973.

Lindberg R: Distribution of cervical lymph node metastases from squamous cell carcinoma of the upper respiratory and digestive tracts. Cancer 29:1446–1449, 1972.

McComb WS, Fletcher GH: *Cancer of the Head and Neck*. Williams & Wilkins, 1967.

Rubin P & others: Cancer of the head and neck: Nose, paranasal sinuses. JAMA 219:336–355, 1972.

Rush BF & others: Integrated radiation and operation in the treatment of carcinoma of the head and neck. J Surg Oncol 3:151–156, 1971.

Sanfilippo LJ & others: Treatment of advanced cancer of the head and neck with intensive preoperative irradiation and radical surgery. Am J Surg 118:701–707, 1969.

Wang CC: Primary malignant lymphoma of the oral cavity and paranasal sinuses. Radiology 100:151–153, 1971.

Wizenberg MJ & others: Treatment of lymph node metastases in head and neck cancer: A radiotherapeutic approach. Cancer 29:1455–1462, 1972.

Zarem HA: Current concepts in reconstructive surgery in patients with cancer of the head and neck. S Clin North America 51:149–173, 1971.

20 . . .

The Thyroid & Parathyroid

Leon Goldman, MD

THE THYROID GLAND

PHYSIOLOGY

The thyroid gland is concerned with iodine metabolism and with the synthesis, storage, and secretion of thyroxine (T_4) and triiodothyronine (T_3). The iodides absorbed from the gastrointestinal tract are trapped by the acinar cells of the thyroid gland and converted into thyroglobulin. Iodine combines with tyrosine to form monoiodotyrosine (MIT) and then diiodotyrosine (DIT). Two molecules of DIT form T_4. T_3 is probably formed by condensation of MIT with DIT. T_3 and T_4 are stored within the colloid of the gland. Thyroid-stimulating hormone (TSH) from the pituitary increases the secretion of T_3 and T_4 by the gland. Both of these are bound to plasma protein, although T_3 adheres to a lesser extent.

The function of the thyroid gland is regulated by a feedback mechanism which involves the hypothalamus, pituitary, and thyroid. Although the workings of the mechanism are not clear, an increase in circulating thyroid hormone inhibits the elaboration of TSH whereas a decrease stimulates it. It is thought that thyroid hyperfunction in Graves' disease is maintained by some abnormal thyroid-stimulating substance such as long-acting thyroid stimulator (LATS), although the exact role of LATS has not been definitely established.

EXAMINATION OF THE THYROID

In the patient with enlargement of the thyroid gland (goiter) the history and a careful examination of the gland are usually of more value than the many tests that are used to assist in the diagnosis. The surgeon must develop a systematic method of palpating the gland for size, contour, consistency, nodularity, and fixation or free mobility, as well as displacement of the trachea and examination of the rest of the neck for the presence of palpable lymph nodes.

Many laboratory tests of thyroid function are available, including protein-bound iodine (PBI), butanol-extractable iodine (BEI), T_4, T_4 by competitive protein binding (T_4-CPB, Murphy-Pattee), radio-

active T_3 uptake of red cells or resin, [131]I (radioiodine) uptake, T_3 suppression of radioiodine uptake, TSH stimulation of radioiodine uptake, radioimmunoassay of serum TSH, serum cholesterol, and the now infrequently performed basal metabolic rate (BMR). It is important to know not only the relative diagnostic value of these tests in thyroid disorders but also how these tests are influenced by many common drugs, pregnancy, cirrhosis, uremia, and certain other nonthyroid conditions (Table 20–1). Their use may wisely be restricted to unusual congenital or acquired types of thyroid dyshormogenesis.

Ackland JD: The interpretation of serum protein-bound iodine. J Clin Path 24:187–218, 1971.
Hershman JM, Pittman JA Jr: Utility of radioimmunoassay of serum thyrotropin in man. Ann Int Med 74:481–490, 1971.
Mayberry WE & others: Radioimmunoassay for human thyrotropin. Clinical values in patients with normal and abnormal thyroid function. Ann Int Med 74:471–480, 1971.

INFLAMMATORY THYROID DISEASE
(Thyroiditis)

Clinical Findings

A. Acute Thyroiditis: Acute bacterial thyroiditis is a rare condition which is due to bacterial infection,

TABLE 20–1. Effects of common drugs on thyroid tests.

Adrenal corticosteroids and ACTH	PBI and ^{131}I decreased
Antithyroid drugs	PBI, ^{131}I, and T_3 decreased
Antituberculosis drugs	[131]I decreased
Coumarin compounds	T_3 increased
Diphenylhydantoin sodium	PBI decreased, T_3 increased
Estrogens (and compounds)	PBI increased, T_3 decreased
Iodine compounds	PBI increased, [131]I ± decreased
Phenylbutazone	[131]I decreased, T_3 increased
Salicylates (excessive)	PBI decreased, T_3 increased
Testosterone	PBI decreased, T_3 increased
Thyroid hormones	PBI and T_3 increased, ^{131}I decreased
(except liothyronine)	PBI and ^{131}I decreased, T_3 increased

usually streptococcus or staphylococcus. It is characterized by painful swelling of all or part of the thyroid gland, causing signs of acute inflammation, fever, and leukocytosis. If fluctuation is present, aspiration may recover a purulent exudate. Another form of acute thyroiditis is thought to be viral in origin, although attempts to isolate a virus have not been successful. As the onset may be gradual, it is also sometimes referred to as "subacute thyroiditis."

B. Acute or Subacute Thyroiditis: Acute or subacute thyroiditis usually occurs in women with or without symmetric enlargement of the gland accompanied by a history of pain and tenderness over the gland. It may start following an upper respiratory infection as a localized process which quickly involves the entire gland. The gland usually becomes firm throughout. Its margins are easily outlined, it is symmetric and tender, and there may be symptoms of pressure on the trachea. Intermittent low-grade fever, malaise, and tachycardia may be present, and thyroid antibody tests are usually positive. Subacute thyroiditis may resolve spontaneously or may progress to chronic thyroiditis and hypothyroidism.

C. Chronic Thyroiditis: There are 3 types of chronic thyroiditis:

1. Hashimoto's thyroiditis—Hashimoto's thyroiditis usually occurs in women and children and may be followed by symptomatic tracheal compression. With thyroid administration, the process usually regresses in a few months, though it may last as long as 1 or 2 years. Finding thyroid antibodies in the blood supports the diagnosis and suggests that this may be an autoimmune disease.

2. Granulomatous thyroiditis—This type is usually limited to one lobe; it is asymmetric and may mimic carcinoma by its stony-hard consistency on examination or by radioisotope scan.

3. Riedel's (ligneous) thyroiditis—Riedel's struma is a rare form of thyroiditis that presents as a hard woody mass in the thyroid region with marked fibrosis and chronic inflammation in and around the gland. It infiltrates muscles and tends to encase the great vessels, and sooner or later usually causes symptoms of tracheal compression. Hypothyroidism is usually present.

Differential Diagnosis

Subacute thyroiditis is often confused with early acute cervical lymphadenitis or with infection or abscess formation in neighboring parts of the neck. The outstanding differential problem with chronic thyroiditis is carcinoma of the thyroid gland, which must be ruled out.

Treatment

A. Acute Bacterial Thyroiditis: Treatment consists of immobilization, local heat, and antibiotic therapy. If there is localization with abscess formation, drainage should be instituted.

B. Subacute Thyroiditis: Corticosteroids and x-ray therapy have been used, but there is no proof of their effectiveness. Antithyroid drugs may be of value

early if there is evidence of hyperthyroidism. After the condition has subsided, administration of thyroid may be indicated.

C. Chronic Thyroiditis: Operation is usually performed in chronic thyroiditis only to relieve pressure on the trachea by splitting and removing the isthmus. Subtotal thyroidectomy may be indicated for large goiters that do not respond to conservative treatment. Operation is occasionally necessary to rule out carcinoma. It is essential to make the diagnosis by frozen section examination during operation because total excision of the gland, as might be done for carcinoma, is nearly always impossible and is associated with a serious hazard of parathyroid injury. Tracheostomy may be necessary in some cases.

Thyroid administration is necessary to treat the hypothyroidism postoperatively.

Prognosis

Acute thyroiditis usually responds promptly to proper treatment. Spontaneous remissions and exacerbations may occur in the subacute type.

Hashimoto's thyroiditis may have a long, lingering course over a period of months, in which case hypothyroidism may develop because of destruction of parenchymatous tissue with replacement by fibrous tissue and lymphoid follicles. There is an association between this type of chronic thyroiditis and systemic collagen disease, and carcinoma is reported in 5–15% of cases.

Colcock BP, Penna O: Diagnosis and treatment of thyroiditis. Postgrad Med 44:83–92, 1968.

Doniach D: Thyroid autoimmune disease. J Clin Path 20: 385–390, 1967.

Greene JN: Subacute thyroiditis. Am J Med 51:97–108, 1971.

Hall R, Stanbury JB: Familial studies of autoimmune thyroiditis. Clin Exper Immunol 2:719–726, 1967.

Hirabayashi RN, Lindsay S: The relation of thyroid carcinoma and chronic thyroiditis. Surg Gynec Obst 121:243, 1965.

Thomas WC Jr & others: Clinical studies in thyroiditis. Ann Int Med 63:808–818, 1965.

NONTOXIC DIFFUSE GOITER
(Simple Goiter)

Simple goiter may be physiologic, occurring during puberty or the menses or during pregnancy; or it may occur in patients from endemic (iodine-poor) regions or as a result of prolonged exposure to goitrogenic foods or drugs. As the goiter persists, there may be a tendency to form lobulations. This type of goiter may occur early in life and may be due to a congenital defect in thyroid hormone production.

Symptoms are usually awareness of the neck mass and dyspnea or dysphagia. The thyroid is symmetric and has a smooth surface without areas of encapsulation. The PBI, BEI, T_3, and T_4 measurements may all be within normal limits, although the radioiodine uptake may be elevated.

Prevention & Treatment

A. Medical Measures: Endemic goiter may be prevented by the administration of iodine in the form of iodized salt, 1–2 g daily; or saturated solution of potassium iodide, 5 drops in water daily; or Lugol's solution, 5 drops daily. If signs of hypothyroidism are present, thyroid should be administered. Therapy may be necessary for a long time until the gland returns to normal size. Most patients respond more promptly to thyroid administration in the form of levothyroxine, starting with 0.1 mg orally daily and gradually increasing to 0.3 mg or to subtoxic levels.

B. Indications for Surgery:

1. To relieve the pressure symptoms of a large goiter, which may cause tracheal, esophageal, or vascular compression. The symptoms are dyspnea, dysphagia, or interference with venous return and development of collateral circulation.

2. To rule out malignancy. Localized areas of stony hardness, a "cold" area in the radioisotope scan, or rapid recent increased growth of the goiter should suggest possible malignancy.

Prognosis

Nontoxic diffuse goiter usually responds favorably to thyroid or iodine administration. This type of goiter, which may start in younger adult life, may develop into a multinodular goiter with or without toxicity in later years.

Astwood EB, Cassidy CE, Aurbach GD: Treatment of goiter and thyroid nodules with thyroid. JAMA 174:459–464, 1960.

Marchetta FC, Sako K: The enlarged thyroid in the elderly patient. Geriatrics 23:181–192, 1968.

HYPERTHYROIDISM
(Thyrotoxicosis)

Essentials of Diagnosis

- Nervousness, jitteriness, irritability, increased appetite, heat intolerance, sweating, weight loss, muscular weakness, and frequency of bowel movements.
- Warm, moist skin; tachycardia and hand tremors.
- Diffuse or nodular goiter with a thrill or bruit.
- Eye signs of staring, lid lag, exophthalmos.
- Elevated PBI, BEI, T_4, radio-T_3 uptake, and radioiodine uptake.

General Considerations

There are 3 forms of hyperthyroidism: toxic diffuse goiter (Graves' disease), toxic multinodular goiter, and the autonomous hyperfunctioning solitary ("hot") nodule. In all of these forms, the symptoms of hyperthyroidism are due to an increased secretion of thyroid hormone into the blood stream.

Clinical Findings

A. Symptoms: The onset of hyperthyroidism is usually gradual, although a full-blown picture may develop in 1–2 weeks. In the majority of instances, the diagnosis can be made without difficulty from the history and physical examination. The patient is restless, nervous, and irritable and displays increased muscular fatigability, weight loss in spite of increased appetite, unsteady fine and coarse tremors, impaired vision, diplopia, and palpitations or symptoms of cardiac failure.

B. Signs: The patient is flushed and has a staring appearance (exophthalmos) with or without lid lag and periorbital edema. A diffuse symmetric or a nodular goiter is almost always present. It is rubbery or elastic on palpation, and in the untreated patient a thrill and bruit are discovered over the gland. The skin is warm, thin, and moist, and the hair texture is fine. Other signs include tachycardia (which persists during sleep) and other arrhythmias, hypertension with increased pulse pressure, signs of heart failure, loud and forceful heart sounds, and pretibial edema. The patient may be on the verge of a thyroid "storm," which may represent an extreme accentuation of all the symptoms and signs of thyrotoxicosis with hyperpyrexia, thyrotoxic cardiac failure, neuromuscular excitation, delirium, and jaundice.

C. Laboratory Findings: Laboratory tests reveal elevation of the PBI, BEI, T_4, BMR, and the T_3 and radioiodine uptake. Question the patient regarding all medication received over the past several months. Organic iodinated compounds—eg, iodized oil (Lipiodol)—may produce abnormal values of PBI or radioiodine uptake for months or years. There is usually a lowering of the serum cholesterol, lymphocytosis, and occasionally glycosuria.

D. X-Ray Findings: If the goiter is large or if the lower poles are not palpable in the neck, barium swallow on x-ray (esophagograms) may show intrathoracic extension. In children or teen-agers demineralization of the skeleton may be found.

E. Electrocardiographic Findings: ECG may reveal tachycardia or paroxysmal or chronic atrial fibrillation.

Differential Diagnosis

Anxiety neurosis, heart disease without hyperthyroidism, primary gastrointestinal disease, hepatic cirrhosis, tuberculosis and other chronic respiratory disorders, myasthenia and other muscular disorders, menopausal syndrome, pheochromocytoma, and primary ophthalmopathy may be difficult to differentiate from hyperthyroidism. The clinical differentiation of these conditions from toxic goiter presents a special problem when thyroid enlargement is minimal or absent.

Anxiety neurosis is perhaps the condition most frequently confused with hyperthyroidism. It is characterized by persistent fatigue which is usually unrelieved by rest, cool and clammy palms, a normal sleeping pulse rate, and normal laboratory tests of thyroid function. The fatigue of hyperthyroidism is often relieved by rest, the palms are warm and moist, tachycardia persists during sleep, and thyroid function tests are abnormal.

Organic disease of nonthyroid origin which may be confused with hyperthyroidism must be differentiated largely on the basis of evidence of specific organ system involvement and normal laboratory tests of thyroid function.

Other causes of exophthalmos (eg, orbital tumors) or ophthalmoplegia (eg, myasthenia) must be ruled out by ophthalmologic and neurologic examination.

Complications

Without treatment, thyrotoxicosis usually causes progressive and profound catabolic disturbances and can ultimately cause severe cardiac, ocular, and psychiatric damage.

Thyrotoxic heart disease with myocardial failure is an avoidable complication which is difficult to treat without first correcting the hyperthyroidism. Asymptomatic coronary artery disease, latent myocardial disease, or valvular disease may become symptomatic in the presence of hyperthyroidism. Thyroid crisis and progressive exophthalmos may be complications of treatment as well as manifestations of the disease.

Treatment

Hyperthyroidism is treated by the administration of antithyroid drugs alone, radioactive iodine therapy, or thyroidectomy. Although the decision about what is the best method of treatment must be individualized, a widely accepted treatment method is subtotal thyroidectomy after adequate preparation with drugs which inhibit formation or release of thyroid hormone.

A. Antithyroid Drugs: Continuous propylthiouracil therapy alone (without surgery) has been advocated by some to avoid the risks and complications of surgery. This form of treatment may be indicated for patients who fear surgery and who can be relied upon to take the medication regularly. Frequent and prolonged observation over a period of 1–2 years is necessary. There is a 30–50% rate of recurrence and a slight but nonetheless significant possibility of propylthiouracil toxicity. The drug is given in dosages of 50–200 mg orally 3 times daily until the patient becomes euthyroid by clinical and laboratory criteria; the patient is then placed on a maintenance dosage of 50–150 mg daily and is observed periodically for evidence of hypothyroidism or drug toxicity.

B. Radioiodine: Recurrent hyperthyroidism and marked hyperthyroidism in poor-risk patients are best treated with radioiodine. The disadvantages of this form of treatment are that its use is still generally limited to medical centers; possible carcinoma may be missed; it cannot be used in pregnancy; its use should generally be limited to patients over 40 years of age (it has been used in patients in their 20s when other forms of treatment are inappropriate); its effects are slow to appear (often 2–3 months for maximum effect);

radiation thyroiditis may occur; retreatment may be necessary; and there is a relatively high incidence of hypothyroidism. Lifelong observation of all patients treated with radioactive iodine is an absolute necessity.

C. Surgery:

1. Preparation for surgery–Proper preparation of the patient and selection of the time for surgery, followed by a carefully performed subtotal thyroidectomy, should eliminate the risk of postoperative thyroid storm or other complications. Since the advent of the antithyroid drugs, the problem of adequate preparation of the patient has been greatly simplified. Prolonged bed rest and heavy sedation are not often required.

a. Diet–A high-caloric, high-protein, high-vitamin diet may be necessary to correct nutritional deficiencies.

b. Physical evaluation–Besides careful systemic appraisal, the vocal cords should be examined preoperatively for evidence of laryngeal nerve function.

c. Laboratory studies–Baseline studies of thyroid function should be obtained and followed carefully while the patient is receiving drug therapy until he is euthyroid from both a clinical and laboratory standpoint.

d. Thiourea drugs–Propylthiouracil, 100–200 mg orally 4 times daily, usually results in a euthyroid status in 4–6 weeks and is continued to the time of surgery. The appearance of leukopenia or granulocytopenia is an indication for cessation of the drug. Methimazole (Tapazole), 10–15 mg orally 4 times daily, may be used in its place.

e. Iodide–Saturated solution of potassium iodide (or Lugol's solution), 2–5 drops orally daily, is given for about 10–15 days before surgery in order to increase the firmness and reduce the vascularity of the gland.

f. Propranolol (Inderal)–Propranolol, a beta-adrenergic blocking agent, may be useful in alleviating severe or undesirable systemic manifestations of thyrotoxicosis until the antithyroid drugs take effect. Start with 10 mg orally 4 times daily and increase to as much as 120 mg 4 times daily if necessary. Simultaneous administration of the alpha-adrenergic blocker phenoxybenzamine (Dibenzyline), 10 mg orally 2–4 times daily, has also been recommended.

2. Indications for subtotal thyroidectomy–

a. The presence of diffuse toxic goiter (Graves' disease) with or without exophthalmos in patients 30 years of age or younger. The relationship between radiation to the neck in early life and the subsequent development of carcinoma of the thyroid gland contraindicates radioactive iodine treatment in young patients.

b. Failure to produce a remission by antithyroid drugs or radioactive iodine at any age.

c. Large goiter or severe cardiac manifestations. The patient with intrinsic heart disease is often seriously affected by hyperthyroidism. In such situations, surgery will bring about the most rapid corrective response.

d. **Toxic multinodular goiter.** These goiters are shown to contain malignancy in 0.5–2.5% of patients operated on. Surgical treatment removes the goiter with its nodules, whereas other methods of treatment affect only the hyperthyroidism.

e. Hyperthyroidism in a pregnant woman who does not respond to or is unable to tolerate antithyroid drugs.

3. Subtotal thyroidectomy—With careful technic in experienced hands, the risk of thyroidectomy is negligible. Injuries to the recurrent laryngeal nerve or parathyroid glands occurs in less than 2% of cases. Adequate exposure and precise identification of the vasculature, recurrent laryngeal nerves, and parathyroid glands is essential. Division of the prethyroidal muscles adds substantially to the exposure.

Complications of Thyroidectomy

Thyroidectomy patients require careful observation during the immediate postoperative period for acute complications such as wound hemorrhage, respiratory obstruction, recurrent laryngeal nerve palsy, acute hypoparathyroidism, and thyroid crisis. The patient must be followed for an indefinite period for evidence of progressive exophthalmos, chronic hypoparathyroidism, chronic hypothyroidism, and myxedema. Tests of thyroid function should be obtained from time to time.

A. Hemorrhage and Tracheal Obstruction: These complications rarely occur after a well-performed thyroidectomy. Marked swelling of the neck or signs of tracheal compression require that the patient be returned to the operating room so that the wound can be reopened. Respiratory obstruction is best handled by immediate tracheal intubation.

B. Recurrent Laryngeal Nerve Injury: Interference with the function of the recurrent laryngeal nerve may follow clamping, stretching, traumatic dissection, severance, edema, or hemorrhagic infiltration of the nerve. Recurrent laryngeal nerve injury produces an abductor paralysis of the ipsilateral vocal cord, which assumes a midline position and may be associated with some degree of respiratory obstruction. If a branch of the nerve has been injured, this paralysis may be partial. If both recurrent laryngeal nerves are injured and vocal cord paralysis is bilateral—as can be determined by indirect laryngoscopy—asphyxiation may result from obstruction of the glottis and tracheostomy should be performed immediately. Unilateral nerve palsy results in a whispering or hoarse voice. If the nerve has not been severed, vocal cord function will return between 3 and 12 months. This complication can be averted by purposely identifying the recurrent laryngeal nerve before the removal of the thyroid lobe as well as by staying within the capsule of the gland during the excision.

C. Hypoparathyroidism: (See p 272.)

D. Hypothyroidism: If the surgeon's estimate of how much thyroid tissue should be removed has been accurate, the patient will do better without thyroid administration. During the first 4–6 weeks after surgery, a mild state of hypothyroidism will correct itself by regeneration. If thyroid medication is given, TSH formation will be inhibited and regeneration will not take place and the patient will become permanently dependent on exogenous thyroid. If symptoms of hypothyroidism become overt and disconcerting during the postoperative period, small doses of thyroxine should be given.

Permanent total hypothyroidism with myxedema occurs about 10% of the time after subtotal thyroidectomies for diffuse toxic goiter (as compared with up to 50% treated with radioiodine). The incidence of hypothyroidism following ^{131}I therapy increases with each year and shows no inclination of reaching a plateau. The reports by surgeons and nuclear medical specialists differ widely within themselves, but in general it can be stated that hypothyroidism occurs less than half as frequently following surgical therapy. The incidence is less after thyroidectomy for toxic nodular goiter and most other forms of goiter.

Treatment consists of administration of thyroid or equivalent. Start cautiously with desiccated thyroid, 65 mg orally daily (or levothyroxine, 0.1 mg orally daily) for 1 week. Then increase by 65 mg (or 0.1 mg) daily to a total daily maintenance dose of 100–200 mg (0.15–0.3 mg), or just below the toxicity level. This dosage is continued until the symptoms of hypothyroidism are corrected and tests of thyroid function return to normal. Lifetime replacement therapy and observation are necessary.

If myxedema coma occurs, emergency treatment is necessary. Give sodium levothyroxine injection, 400–500 μg IV, plus hydrocortisone hemisuccinate, 100 mg IV, every 8 hours. Treat precipitating factors. The mortality rate from myxedema coma remains high despite current treatment methods.

F. Exophthalmos: Exophthalmos may occur as a complication of untreated hyperthyroidism, or it can begin immediately after treatment of hyperthyroidism by surgery or radiation. The pathogenesis of exophthalmos in hyperthyroidism is not clear, but one popular theory is that an exophthalmos-producing substance (EPS)—distinct from TSH or LATS—is formed by the pituitary. The fact that thyroid secretion exerts an inhibitory effect on the pituitary suggests that removal or destruction of the thyroid permits the pituitary to secrete some substance which aggravates the exophthalmos. Thyroid replacement, however, frequently fails to arrest progressive exophthalmos.

Mild exophthalmos is characterized by a staring expression, mild lid retraction, proptosis, and impaired ocular mobility. In progressive or severe exophthalmos, there may be marked proptosis, periorbital edema, chemosis, lid protrusion, conjunctivitis, keratitis, impaired vision, visual field changes, diplopia, papilledema, and ophthalmoplegia (malignant exophthalmos).

Mild cases usually present a minor cosmetic problem and require no treatment. Moderate to severe cases require ophthalmologic consultation. Protection of the eyes from light by dark glasses and from dust by eye shields is often indicated. Thyroid hormone, corticotropin (ACTH), corticosteroids, and estrogens have been beneficial for certain patients, but their effectiveness has been quite variable and unpredictable. Pituitary ablation is of no significant benefit. If exophthalmos progresses despite trials of medical treatment, surgical decompression of the orbit by the Ogura operation is currently considered to be the procedure of choice. Total ablation by radioiodine is used, but its beneficial effect has not been proved.

G. Thyroid Crisis (Thyrotoxic "Storm"): Thyroid crisis is an abrupt, dramatic, and life-threatening illness of hyperthyroid patients in whom thyrotoxicosis is apparently exacerbated by unusual stress such as surgery, severe infection, or drug reactions. The mechanism is not clear. It almost invariably occurs in patients who have not been treated—or who have been inadequately treated—for thyrotoxicosis. Patients taken to surgery who are not in a euthyroid state or who are otherwise not adequately prepared for surgery are most vulnerable.

The patient in thyroid crisis immediately after subtotal thyroidectomy displays both accentuation and distortion of the symptoms of hyperthyroidism: marked fever, profuse diaphoresis, tachycardia disproportionate to fever, tachypnea, hypertension, cardiac failure, nausea and vomiting, diarrhea, abdominal pain, hepatic abnormalities, tremor, restlessness, delirium, stupor, and coma. Laboratory tests of thyroid function, although abnormal, do not necessarily parallel the clinical severity.

Proper preoperative preparation of the patient should prevent this rare but unfortunate complication. If thyroid crisis does occur, the following steps must be taken immediately:

(1) Isolation in a cool, quiet area with moderate sedation as needed.

(2) Decrease hormone production by giving propylthiouracil, 400 mg every 8 hours, either orally or by nasogastric tube.

(3) Prevent release of preformed hormone by administration of Lugol's solution (strong iodine solution), 30 drops orally, or sodium iodide, 1—2 g by slow IV drip.

(4) Block peripheral adrenergic action of thyroid hormone by cautiously administering reserpine, 2.5 mg orally or IM 4—6 times daily, or guanethidine, 50—100 mg orally daily in divided doses. The action of reserpine is exceedingly slow. The beta-adrenergic blocking agent propranolol can be given in doses of 40—60 mg orally 4 times daily. The value of these drugs is perhaps subject to question.

(5) Support vital functions by giving oxygen, sedation, intravenous fluids (with glucose, electrolytes, and vitamins), and corticosteroids and by symptomatic reduction of fever.

(6) Treat specific precipitating causes (eg, infection, drug reactions).

Prognosis

The mortality rate following thyroidectomy is less than 0.25%. Postthyroidectomy deaths during the past 20 years have been rare. Complications are more apt to occur following operations for the removal of recurrent goiter, extensive malignancies, or intrathoracic goiter.

Das G, Krieger M: Treatment of thyrotoxic storm with intravenous administration of propranolol. Ann Int Med 70:985—988, 1969.

Harrison TS: The treatment of thyroid storm. Surg Gynec Obst 121:837, 1965.

Green M, Wilson GM: Thyrotoxicosis treated by surgery or iodine-131 with special reference to development of hypothyroidism. Brit MJ 1:1005, 1964.

Ingbar SH: Thyrotoxic storm. New England J Med 274: 1252—1254, 1966.

McDougall IR, Grieg WR, Gillespie FC: Radioactive iodine (^{125}I) therapy for thyrotoxicosis. New England J Med 285:1099—1104, 1971.

Nofal MM, Beierwaltes WH, Patno ME: Treatment of hyperthyroidism with sodium iodide 131. JAMA 197:605, 1966.

Ogura J, Wessler S, Aviola LV: Surgical approach to ophthalmopathy of Graves' disease. JAMA 216:1627—1631, 1971.

Roizen M, Becker CE: Thyroid storm: A review of cases at University of California, San Francisco. California Med 114:5—9, Jan 1971.

Senior RM & others: The recognition and management of myxedema coma. JAMA 217:61—65, 1971.

Thomas C: *The Thyroid.* Harper, 1972.

Wade JSH: Three major complications of the thyroidectomy. Brit J Surg 52:727, 1965.

NODULAR GOITER

Adenomatous goiter is usually associated with iodine deficiency, which causes generalized enlargement of the thyroid and, frequently, formation of gross nodules. Although goiters are worldwide in distribution, the incidence is significantly higher in certain areas where dietary iodine supplies are low—the Great Lakes region, the Pacific Northwest, the western slopes of the Rocky Mountains, the foothills of the Himalayas, the Swiss Alps, and the mountainous regions of Argentina. Certain foods and chemical compounds may interfere with the utilization of iodine. Women are much more commonly affected than men.

Goiters, although generally multinodular, are frequently asymmetric. In asymmetric glands—or when only a single enlarged nodule is palpable—it is clinically difficult or impossible to differentiate benign from cancerous lesions (see next section). The relationship of adenomas to the occurrence of malignancy is not known.

Unless the goiter is large enough to exert pressure on the trachea or esophagus, there are no symptoms. X-rays will sometimes reveal substernal extension. Hypothyroidism may occasionally occur, but hyperthyroidism is a much more frequent complication. Perhaps the most common complaint of patients with nontoxic diffuse or multinodular goiter relates to the cosmetic appearance.

Types of Nodular Goiter
  A. Adenoma:
    1. Involutionary.
    2. True—
      a. Follicular or colloid.
      b. Papillary.
      c. Atypical.
  B. Thyroiditis:
    1. Hashimoto's—
      a. Diffuse.
      b. Localized.
    2. Granulomatous.
    3. Riedel's.
  C. Malignancy.

Treatment

  A. Medical Treatment: Treatment must be individualized. If the goiter is of relatively recent development (eg, goiter associated with puberty or pregnancy) and malignancy is not seriously suspected, treatment with iodine and thyroid may cause satisfactory regression. Give potassium iodide or Lugol's solution, 5 drops in a glass of water daily, and desiccated thyroid (or equivalent), 60–120 mg orally daily, or levothyroxine, 0.1–0.2 mg orally daily, as long as the goiter continues to regress in size. Then advise the use of iodized table salt indefinitely.

  Suppressive therapy by the administration of thyroid produces variable results in the treatment of multinodular goiter. Astwood (see references) has noted a reduction in size in over 50% of cases; others report a good result in less than 25%. The decrease in size is often due to shrinkage of the gland proper while the encapsulated nodules remain unchanged. True adenomas, tumors, or large nodules are unlikely to be affected, whereas small involutionary hyperplastic nodules are apt to respond. Carcinoma may also shrink in size, and thyroid administration may in this way further delay surgical treatment.

  B. Surgical Treatment: The principal indications for surgical removal of nodular goiter are (1) hyperthyroidism, (2) suspicion of malignancy, (3) pressure symptoms, (4) substernal extension, and (5) cosmetic reasons. Other indications are the presence of a solitary nodule, a multinodular gland with a dominant hard nodule, or a cold nodule; nonregression of the gland after thyroid administration; and occurrence in a young age group.

  The most important aspect of the management of multinodular goiter is to determine whether carcinoma is present. The reported incidence of malignancy within a nodular goiter ranges between 4% and 30% in different series, depending upon how the patients are selected for operative treatment. At the University of California Medical Center in San Francisco, carcinoma was found in 18% of multinodular goiters and 27% of

TABLE 20–2. 100 thyroidectomies for nodular goiter, 100 cases, 1969–1971.

"Cold" nodules	75%
Proved carcinoma in "cold" nodules	27%
Carcinoma in the 100 cases	22%
Carcinoma in pathologically solitary nodules	27%

solitary nodular goiters among a recent series of 100 thyroidectomies for nodular goiter (Table 20–2). The possibility of malignancy is difficult to exclude in many patients short of microscopic examination of the gland itself. Recent onset, a history of rapid growth, a hard nodule on palpation, fixation of the tumor, enlarged cervical lymph nodes, and recurrent laryngeal nerve palsy arouse a suspicion of malignancy. In the series referred to, the "cold" nodule or nodules by scan proved to be carcinoma in 27% of patients. The rest are explained by cyst formation, hemorrhage, chronic thyroiditis, and inactive acini with large lakes of colloid, as in some colloid adenomas. There may be x-ray evidence of metastases to the bones, lungs, mediastinum, or abdominal viscera. The presence of metastasis may be detected in the scan if there is sufficient radioiodine uptake.

Astwood EB, Cassidy CE, Aurbach GD: Treatment of goiter and thyroid nodules with thyroid. JAMA 174:459–464, 1960.

Veith FJ & others: The nodular thyroid gland and cancer: A practical approach to the problem. New England J Med 270:431–435, 1964.

Welch CE: Therapy for multinodular goiter. JAMA 195:339–341, 1966.

Zacharewicz FA: Management of single and multinodular goiter. M Clin North America 52:409–416, 1968.

MALIGNANT TUMORS OF THE THYROID

Essentials of Diagnosis

- Painless nodule in thyroid region: more common in women; often of recent origin with recent rapid growth; usually asymmetric; often firm or hard and fixed; may be associated with vocal cord palsy and cervical lymphadenopathy; fails to respond to T_3 suppression.
- Past history of nodular goiter in childhood, thyroiditis, or radiation therapy to neck and mediastinum.
- Thyroid function tests are normal.

General Considerations

  An appreciation of the classification of malignant tumors of the thyroid is more pertinent than that of any other organ because the thyroid demonstrates the

TABLE 20–3. **Classification of malignant tumors of the thyroid.**

Carcinoma
Papillary adenocarcinoma
Pure papillary
Mixed papillary and follicular
Follicular adenocarcinoma
Pure follicular
Clear cell
Oxyphil cell
Medullary carcinoma
Undifferentiated carcinoma
Small cell
Large cell
Epidermoid
Lymphoma
Sarcoma
Metastatic tumors

widest discrepancy of tumor growth and behavior of any organ. At one end of the spectrum is the papillary adenocarcinoma, which usually makes its appearance early in life, grows very slowly, metastasizes late, and is compatible with long life even in the presence of metastasis (Table 20–3). At the other extreme is the undifferentiated carcinoma which appears late in life and is nonencapsulated and invasive, forming large infiltrating tumors composed of small or large anaplastic cells. The prognosis of this type is poor; the patient usually succumbs from local recurrence, pulmonary metastasis, or both. Between these 2 extremes there is a great variety of carcinomas whose prognosis depends upon the pathologic cell pattern as well as the biologic activity of the tumor.

The greatest problem in thyroid surgery today concerns the relationship of nodular goiter to carcinoma of the thyroid. One must be alert to the possibility of carcinoma in patients with nodular goiter. By careful attention to the salient features of the history and physical examination, patients with a reasonable likelihood of malignancy can be selected for thyroidectomy without resorting to surgery for every patient with nodular goiter.

Types of Thyroid Cancer

A. Papillary Adenocarcinoma: Papillary adenocarcinomas account for 60–70% of malignancies of the thyroid gland. The neoplasm starts to grow in childhood or early adult life, remains localized, and eventually metastasizes to the pericapsular and paratracheal lymph nodes, then along the internal jugular veins and into the lateral triangles of the neck, and later to the anterior superior mediastinum. Microscopically, the tumor is composed of papillary projections of columnar epithelium, and the sections may show a pure papillary pattern or may contain some follicular elements within the predominant papillary picture. Occasionally, the primary tumor may change

over to an anaplastic type, or the metastases may be follicular or anaplastic though the primary tumor is papillary. True benign papillary adenomas are rare and should be suspected of being malignant when first seen. According to Clarke, this tumor is unicentric and metastasizes by way of the lymphatics intraglandularly to other parts of the same lobe, the isthmus, or the opposite lobe and to the subcapsular and pericapsular lymph nodes. The rate of growth may be stimulated by TSH secretion.

Adequate surgical treatment of this type is followed by a 10-year survival rate of over 80% (Table 20–4).

B. Follicular Adenocarcinoma: Follicular adenocarcinoma accounts for approximately 20% of malignant thyroid tumors. It appears later in life than does the papillary form and may be elastic or rubbery or even soft on palpation. It may appear to be encapsulated and to contain colloid on gross examination. Areas may closely resemble normal thyroid tissue. Although it may metastasize to the regional lymph nodes, it has a greater predilection to spread by the hematogenous route to the lungs, skeleton, and liver. This type of neoplasm may demonstrate an avidity for radioactive iodine in metastases if total thyroidectomy has been performed. Skeletal metastases from follicular carcinomas may develop after 10 or 20 years and may follow a relatively benign course, although in general (as shown in Table 20–4) the prognosis is not as good as with the papillary type.

C. Medullary Carcinoma: Medullary carcinoma of the thyroid accounts for approximately 4–5% of malignant tumors of the thyroid. It contains amyloid and is a solid, hard nodular tumor which takes up radioiodine poorly. It is felt that cells of this type arise from the ultimobranchial bodies and are the same as those that secrete calcitonin. Familial occurrence of medullary carcinoma associated with pheochromocytoma and hyperparathyroidism is known as Sipple's syndrome.

D. Undifferentiated Carcinoma: This rapidly growing tumor occurs principally in women beyond middle life and accounts for 5% of all thyroid malignancies. It is a solid, quickly enlarging, hard irregular mass diffusely involving the gland and invading the trachea, muscles, and neurovascular structures early. The tumor may be painful and somewhat tender, may be fixed on swallowing, and may cause laryngeal or esophageal obstructive symptoms. Microscopically, the

TABLE 20–4. **Survival rates for papillary, follicular, and undifferentiated thyroid cancer in 390 patients (Hirabayashi and Lindsay) after surgical treatment.**

	10 years	20 years	30 years
Papillary	83.8%	62.6%	58.5%
Follicular	57.2%	36.6%	36.2%
Undifferentiated	14.3%	14.3%	. . .

cells are anaplastic, varying from a small to large or multinucleated cell type, all of which reveal frequent mitoses. Cervical lymphadenopathy is occasionally present, but pulmonary metastases are more common. Local recurrence after surgical treatment is the rule. External radiation therapy is helpful in controlling the local process. The prognosis is poor, and radioiodine therapy is ineffective. On occasion, this lesion is a transformation from a former papillary or follicular neoplasm.

Treatment

The treatment of thyroid carcinoma is operative removal. There is considerable controversy about the extent of excision necessary. Because of the high incidence of intraglandular metastasis, some authorities recommend total thyroidectomy for papillary, follicular, medullary, and undifferentiated carcinoma whenever possible. On the other hand, because long-term follow-up studies have not shown any increase in survival after total thyroidectomy compared with total lobectomy, a more conservative resection is sometimes advocated.

For papillary carcinoma grossly confined to one lobe, total thyroidectomy with excision of the isthmus and a subtotal excision on the opposite side is practiced by the majority of thyroid specialists. A conservative neck dissection preserving the sternocleidomastoid muscle is performed if grossly involved nodes are found.

In invasive follicular carcinoma, total thyroidectomy is preferred because of the multicentric spread and the frequency of distant metastases.

Medullary carcinoma has such a high incidence of nodal involvement that concomitant neck dissection is usually justified.

Undifferentiated invasive carcinoma is rarely controlled or ameliorated by surgical operation.

Frozen section study of all thyroid tumors is an essential adjunct to proper treatment, and in the hands of the experienced pathologist is remarkably reliable.

In all operations, particular attention must be directed to the identification and preservation of the parathyroid glands and the recurrent laryngeal nerve.

When malignant lymphoma or sarcoma occurs in the thyroid gland, it is excised as completely as possible and then treated by radiation and chemotherapy. Metastastic carcinoma is rare and develops by hematogenous spread from the kidneys, breast, lungs, or elsewhere; it is seldom a solitary metastasis.

External radiation therapy may be effective in controlling the undifferentiated, anaplastic type of carcinoma, which often cannot be completely removed because of its invasion of the vital structures of the neck. While chemotherapy has a somewhat limited role, some patients have developed regressions after 5-fluorouracil, vincristine, and chlorambucil therapy. The prognosis is poor.

Block GE: A modified neck dissection for carcinoma of the thyroid. S Clin North America 51:139–148, 1971.

Block MA & others: Familial medullary carcinoma of the thyroid. Ann Surg 166:403, 1967.

Clark RL, Ibanez ML, White EC: What constitutes an adequate operation for carcinoma of the thyroid? Arch Surg 92:23, 1966.

Crile G Jr: Late results of treatment for papillary cancer of the thyroid. Ann Surg 160:178, 1964.

Glassford GH, Fowler EF, Cole WH: The treatment of nontoxic nodular goiter with desiccated thyroid: Results and evaluation. Surgery 58:621, 1965.

Kaplan EL, Peskin GW: Physiologic implications of medullary carcinoma of the thyroid gland. S Clin North America 51:125–137, 1971.

Lindsay S: *Carcinoma of the Thyroid Gland: A Clinical and Pathologic Study of 293 Patients at the University of California Hospital.* Thomas, 1960.

Zacharewicz FA: Management of single and multinodular goiter. M Clin North America 52:409–416, 1968.

THE PARATHYROID GLANDS

EMBRYOLOGY & ANATOMY

The parathyroid glands arise from branchial pouches III and IV and may be arrested as high as the level of the hyoid bone during their descent to the posterior capsule of the thyroid gland. In 90% of people there are 4 parathyroid glands. One or more may be incorporated into the thyroid gland or thymus and hence may be intrathyroidal or mediastinal in location. Parathyroid III, which normally assumes the inferior position, may be found overlying the trachea in the suprasternal area, behind the clavicles, the upper sternum or esophagus, or in the anterior or posterior mediastinum. Parathyroid adenomas may lie in the anterior mediastinum in front of, within, or behind the thymus, along the arch of the aorta, or overlying the pericardium. The parathyroid glands may be separated from the thyroid gland lying anterior to or behind the internal jugular vein and common carotid artery.

The normal parathyroid gland has a distinct yellowish-brown color; is ovoid, tongue-shaped, polypoid, or spherical; and varies in size from 3–8 mm in length, 0.5–4 mm in width, and 2–5 mm in depth. Its capsule may be delineated, and a branch of the inferior or superior thyroid or thyroidima arteries can be seen entering a hilum-like structure, thus differentiating it from fat.

PATHOLOGY

When the normal gland becomes adenomatous, it loses some of its yellowish color because of the compactness of its cells and loss of fat and becomes reddish-brown, resembling the color of the normal liver as seen at the operating table. The size and shape of adenomas vary widely. Their delicate stroma and soft texture permit molding to the fascial planes of the neck, and vascular pedicles facilitate retrothyroidal descent down the neck. On cut section one may see a homogeneous gray or reddish-brown surface, occasionally surrounded by a thin rim of compressed cells, or cystic degeneration.

Adenomas may be single or multiple and are always accompanied by one or more normal parathyroids. In contrast, primary parathyroid hyperplasia involves all of the parathyroid glands; they are large and irregular. Glands found in hyperplasia secondary to renal insufficiency or intestinal malabsorption are one-third to one-half the size of the glands in primary hyperplasia and tend to have rounded borders, creating an oval, spherical, or kidney shape. The pathologist cannot differentiate adenoma from hyperplasia on the basis of the histology alone.

The surgeon must be able to distinguish a parathyroid tumor from lymph nodes, thyroid tissue, thyroid nodules, thymus, and fat. He should not depend on biopsy of the normal gland since this procedure may result in destruction and loss of function of the gland. The size of the tumor usually parallels the degree of hypercalcemia, but not always. Parathyroid adenomas may range from 35 mg to over 20 g. Pathologic examination by frozen section of all removed tissue should be done before the wound is closed.

HYPOPARATHYROIDISM

Essentials of Diagnosis

- Paresthesias of circumoral area, hands, and feet; carpopedal spasm, laryngeal stridor and wheezing, opisthotonos, muscle and abdominal cramps, tetany, urinary frequency, personality changes, and lethargy.
- Positive Chvostek and Trousseau signs, defective nails and teeth, cataracts.
- Hypocalcemia and hyperphosphatemia with normal alkaline phosphatase. Negative urine calcium (Sulkowitch).
- Calcification of basal ganglia, cartilage, and arteries.

General Considerations

Hypoparathyroidism occurs most commonly as an inadvertent loss of parathyroid function following thyroid surgery, especially that performed for carcinoma or recurrent goiter. Hypoparathyroidism occurs only rarely as a complication of the first operation for goiter and is even less common following surgery for hyperparathyroidism unless 3 or more normal, adenomatous, or hyperplastic parathyroids are

removed. An autoimmune cause is suspected in the idiopathic type because of the association of hypoparathyroidism with autoimmune adrenocortical insufficiency. Neonatal tetany may be associated with maternal hyperparathyroidism.

Clinical Findings

A. Symptoms and Signs: The manifestations of acute hypoparathyroidism are those due to hypocalcemia. Low serum calcium levels precipitate tetany. The state of latent tetany is indicated by mild or moderate paresthesias with a positive Chvostek and a positive Trousseau sign without evidence of cramps or muscle spasm. The early acute manifestations are paresthesias, muscle cramps, irritability, carpopedal spasm, convulsions, and opisthotonos. Personality change, dry skin, brittleness of the nails, and a high tubular resorption of phosphate are found objectively. A history of thyroidectomy is almost always present. Generally speaking, the sooner the symptoms and signs appear postoperatively, the more serious is the prognosis. After many years, patients may become adapted to a low serum calcium level so that tetany is no longer evident.

B. Laboratory Findings: Hypocalcemia and hyperphosphatemia associated with normal alkaline phosphatase may or may not be demonstrated. The urine phosphate is low or absent (due to the high tubular resorption of phosphate), and the urine calcium is low to nil (negative Sulkowitch test).

C. X-Ray Findings: X-rays may show calcifications of the basal ganglia, arteries, and the external ear.

D. Other Findings: ECG shows a prolonged Q–T interval and abnormal T waves. The EEG may show a generalized dysrhythmia. Ophthalmoscopic and slit lamp examination may reveal cataracts.

Differential Diagnosis

The differential diagnosis of hypoparathyroid tetany includes other causes of hypocalcemia, ie, intestinal malabsorption and renal insufficiency. Both are caused by failure of activation of vitamin D. Intestinal malabsorption can be substantiated by a history of steatorrhea, weight loss, and bone tenderness as well as megaloblastic or iron deficiency anemia and hypoproteinemia. The serum phosphate level is low. Other laboratory evidences of malabsorption may be present such as low serum cholesterol and carotene levels and an increase in the stool fat. The hypocalcemia of renal insufficiency is associated with high serum phosphate levels. With uremia, the acidosis usually prevents neuromuscular hyperirritability so that the Chvostek and Trousseau signs may be negative and muscle tone unaffected. Parathyroid hormone radioimmunoassay yields high values in patients with uremia due to secondary parathyroid hyperplasia and low or absent levels in hypoparathyroidism. Symptoms of tetany may be confused with those of alkalosis and hyperventilation. Sprue, rickets, osteomalacia, and early renal failure may be associated with hypocalcemia but can be differentiated by calcium and phosphorus blood studies, measurement of calcium and phosphorus in the urine, and by radioimmune parathyroid hormone assay.

Prevention

Technical operative care during thyroidectomy is necessary to avoid hypoparathyroidism. The operation most commonly responsible for hypoparathyroidism is total thyroidectomy. It is difficult to perform this operation and preserve the parathyroid glands, their blood supply, and their function. This relationship is so well established that total thyroidectomy should be reserved for operations for carcinoma of the thyroid gland.

Treatment

The aim of treatment is to raise the serum calcium level in order to bring the patient out of tetany and to lower the serum phosphate level to prevent metastatic calcifications. Most postoperative hypocalcemia is transient; if it persists longer than 2–3 weeks, it is apt to require long-standing treatment and periodic chemical determinations. When symptoms and signs of hypoparathyroidism appear postoperatively— usually between the second to fourth day after surgery—calcium is administered intravenously and by mouth.

Acute hypoparathyroid tetany. Acute hypoparathyroid tetany requires emergency treatment. Make certain that an adequate airway exists. Give calcium gluconate, 10–20 ml of 10% solution slowly IV, until tetany disappears. Ten to 50 ml of 10% calcium gluconate may then be added to 1 liter of saline or 5% dextrose solution and administered by slow IV drip. Adjust the rate of infusion so that hourly determinations of serum calcium are normal or the Sulkowitch test is positive for urine calcium. Avoid overtreatment. Switch to oral calcium (gluconate, lactate, or carbonate) 3 times daily as soon as the patient can take oral medication. Vitamin D, 100,000–150,000 units orally daily, is given together with the oral calcium. The maintenance dosage of vitamin D is about 50,000 units daily. Periodic estimation of serum calcium levels is necessary for regulation of proper vitamin dosage and to avoid vitamin D intoxication.

Prognosis

Vitamin D therapy alone usually reverses all the chemical changes found in hypoparathyroidism, but the response is slow.

Bronsky D, Kiamko RT, Waldstein SS: Familial idiopathic hypoparathyroidism. J Clin Endocrinol 28:61–65, 1968.

Fonseca OA, Calverley JR: Neurological manifestations of hypoparathyroidism. Arch Int Med 120:202, 1967.

Harrison HE & others: Comparison between crystalline dihydrotachysterol and calciferol in patients requiring pharmacologic vitamin D therapy. New England J Med 276:894, 1967.

Ireland AW & others: The calciferol requirements of patients with surgical hypoparathyroidism. Ann Int Med 69:81, 1968.

King LR & others: Serum calcium homeostasis following thyroid surgery as measured by EDTA infusion. J Clin Endocrinol 25:577–584, 1965.

Kleeman CR & others: The clinical physiology of calcium homeostasis, parathyroid hormone, and calcitonin. California Med 114:16–43, March 1971; 114:19–30, April 1971.

O'Malley BW, Kohler PO: Hypoparathyroidism. Postgrad Med 44:71–79, 182–190, 1968.

Schaaf M, Payne CA: Effect of diphenylhydantoin and phenobarbital on overt and latent tetany. New England J Med 274:1228, 1966.

Suh SM & others: Pseudohypoparathyroidism: No improvement following total thyroidectomy. J Clin Endocrinol 29:429–439, 1969.

PSEUDOHYPOPARATHYROIDISM

Pseudohypoparathyroidism is a genetically transmitted clinical syndrome characterized by the clinical and chemical features of hypoparathyroidism associated with a round face, short, thick body, stubby fingers, short metacarpal and metatarsal bones, and mental deficiency. Although the chemical features of hypoparathyroidism may be present, the physical appearance of the patient is usually diagnostic. The treatment is the same as for hypoparathyroidism.

Patients with pseudohypoparathyroidism do not respond to intravenous administration of 200 units of parathormone with phosphaturia (Ellsworth-Howard test).

PSEUDOPSEUDOHYPOPARATHYROIDISM

Pseudopseudohypoparathyroidism is a genetic disease with the same physical findings as pseudohypoparathyroidism but with normal serum calcium and phosphorus levels.

HYPERCALCITONINISM

Hypercalcitoninism is thought to occur with tumors involving cells of the thyroid gland that secrete calcitonin (thyrocalcitonin), found in certain adenomas or medullary carcinoma of the thyroid. While this is possible from a physiologic standpoint, there is some question that this exists as a distinct clinical entity.

PRIMARY HYPERPARATHYROIDISM

Essentials of Diagnosis

- History of renal colic or urinary stones, polyuria, polydipsia, nausea, vomiting, intractable peptic ulcer, constipation, bone and joint pains, pathologic fractures.
- Kyphosis, clubbing, "band keratopathy," hypertension.
- Serum calcium > 11 mg/100 ml, urinary calcium increased (positive Sulkowitch test), serum phosphate low or normal, and urine phosphate increased.
- X-rays show subperiosteal resorption of phalanges and other bones, loss of lamina dura of teeth, bone cysts, demineralization of the skull, and renal calcification or stones.

General Considerations

Primary hyperparathyroidism, a state of excess parathyroid function, occurs as a disease entity in patients with single (92%) or multiple parathyroid adenomas (4%), primary parathyroid hyperplasia (3%), or, rarely, carcinoma of the parathyroid glands (less than 1%). It may be one aspect of endocrine adenomatosis, often familial, involving other endocrine glands (see below). Hyperparathyroidism may also arise from ectopic malignancies of the lungs, kidneys, ovaries, uterus, colon, and thyroid. Parathyroid hormone hypersecretion mobilizes calcium from bone and inhibits tubular reabsorption of phosphate (TRP), so that hyperparathyroidism is characterized by elevated blood and urine calcium levels and hyperphosphaturia, resulting in hypophosphotemia in about half of cases. As a result of mild renal tubular acidosis, serum chloride levels usually exceed 106 mEq/liter. This process causes a wasting of both calcium and phosphate, so that osseous mineral loss becomes part of the process. If the disease is of sufficient severity and duration, overt osteitis fibrosa cystica may occur.

Endocrine adenomatosis. In order to rule out endocrine adenomatosis associated with hyperparathyroidism, the following diagnostic procedures are required: a lateral film of the sella turcica for possible pituitary tumor, a fasting blood glucose level for possible insulin-secreting tumor, and an evaluation of the gastrointestinal tract for possible gastrin-secreting islet cell tumor of the pancreas and adrenal adenoma.

Endocrine adenomatosis is more likely to be present when more than one adenoma is encountered or the hyperparathyroidism occurs later in life. A rare type of endocrine adenomatosis includes hyperparathyroidism, pheochromocytoma, and medullary carcinoma of the thyroid. The incidence of thyroid nodules and papillary adenocarcinoma of the thyroid gland in association with hyperparathyroidism is higher than the incidence of carcinoma of the thyroid in the general population.

The literature reports a high incidence of peptic ulcer in patients with endocrine adenomatosis; in the author's experience this occurs in only about 7% of cases. It is most commonly duodenal in location and often associated with Zollinger-Ellison syndrome.

Clinical Findings

A. Symptoms and Signs: Whereas in the past hyperparathyroidism was infrequently diagnosed by serendipity, routine laboratory screening now suggests the diagnosis in about half of cases. Even though the patient may deny the presence of symptoms of hypercalcemia preoperatively, after surgical correction he becomes retrospectively aware of preoperative muscle fatigability, bone pain, constipation, polydipsia, and polyuria. The disease should be suspected in all patients with hypercalcemia or symptoms and signs of nephrolithiasis, nephrocalcinosis, impairment of smooth muscle contractility and renal concentrating ability, muscle weakness, and bone and joint pain. Gastrointestinal complaints include anorexia, nausea, vomiting, abdominal pain, and constipation, which in extreme cases may go on to ileus with obstipation. Polydipsia, polyuria, nocturia, or diabetes insipidus (with severe dehydration) may occur. Hypertension is often present. There may be a history or findings of recurrent pancreatitis. In rare instances, mental aberrations and even psychosis may occur.

B. Laboratory Findings:

1. Serum calcium—While hyperparathyroidism is not the most common cause of hypercalcemia (Table 20–5), an elevated serum calcium on 3 successive examinations is still the keystone of the diagnosis. Hypercalcemia is usually relatively mild, being elevated by only 0.5–1.5 mg/100 ml; higher levels usually present fewer diagnostic problems. Hypercalcemia is usually persistent, although it can be reduced by increasing the dietary phosphate and fluid intake or by mobilizing the patient.

Hypercalcemia may be masked by a high phosphate intake. Three days of a low-phosphate diet plus aluminum hydroxide will serve to unmask the hypercalcemia.

Serum proteins and their electrophoretic pattern should always be measured in order to evaluate the ionized calcium level and to exclude myeloma and sar-

TABLE 20–5. Causes of hypercalcemia.

Condition	Approximate Frequency (%)
Malignancy	44
Hyperparathyroidism	38
Immobilization	7
Milk-alkali syndrome	5
Vitamin D overdose	5
Hyperthyroidism	4
Sarcoidosis	1
Adrenal insufficiency	1
Myxedema	1
Post renal transplant	1
Thiazide therapy	

coidosis by the globulin pattern. The hypercalcemia of hyperparathyroidism usually is resistant to cortisone, which abolishes the hypercalcemia of sarcoidosis, vitamin D intoxication, adrenal insufficiency, and in about half of cases, of ectopic malignancy. The hypercalcemia of breast cancer is associated with normal serum phosphate levels and is not accompanied by elevated parathyroid hormone levels.

2. **Serum phosphate**—The presence of both hypercalcemia and hypophosphatemia is practically diagnostic of hyperparathyroidism if one can rule out vitamin D overdosage, myeloma, sarcoidosis, and ectopic malignancies (Table 20–5). However, about half of patients with hyperparathyroidism have normal serum phosphate levels.

Hyperphosphaturia is demonstrated by subnormal tubular reabsorption of phosphate (TRP). In patients with normal renal function, the 12-hour night urine is collected and fasting blood is drawn in the morning for serum calcium, phosphorus, and creatinine determinations. The urinary creatinine and phosphorus is computed as milligrams excreted per minute, so that minor errors of collection do not affect the results.

$$\text{TRP (in \%)} = 100 \times 1 - \frac{\text{Urinary P} \times \text{Serum creatinine}}{\text{Urinary creatinine} \times \text{Serum P}}$$

This test is of no value when there is renal impairment. A high-phosphate diet (3 g daily for 3 days) will lower a normal TRP to below 70% in patients with hyperparathyroidism.

3. **Serum parathyroid hormone**—Determinations of parathyroid hormone in the serum by radioimmunoassay makes possible a direct laboratory diagnosis of hyperparathyroidism. The combination of hypercalcemia and a significant amount of parathyroid hormone in the serum is diagnostic of hyperparathyroidism whether from the parathyroid glands or from an ectopic source.

C. X-Ray Findings: Overt skeletal changes on x-ray are found in only 10% of patients. X-ray examination of the hands is the most valuable when it reveals subperiosteal resorption of the phalanges (Fig 20–1). Conventional roentgenograms of other bones demonstrate generalized decalcification and cysts. This may be associated with a high alkaline phosphatase level and increased urinary hydroxyproline excretion. Subperiosteal resorption is pathognomonic of hyperparathyroidism, either primary or secondary.

D. Electrocardiography: The Q–T interval is shortened, but ECG is of little diagnostic value in hypercalcemia.

Treatment

A. Preoperative Preparation: Special preoperative preparation of a patient with hyperparathyroidism is necessary if there is evidence of acute hypercalcemia, dehydration, electrolyte imbalance, or renal damage. Hydration and correction of hypokalemia and hyponatremia, if present, often result in lowering both serum calcium and creatinine levels. During the course

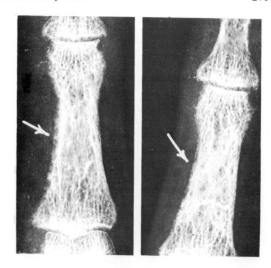

FIG 20–1. Subperiosteal resorption of radial side of second phalanges.

of hydration, fluids should not be withheld for blood chemistry or other purposes. Patients with dramatic symptoms of acute hypercalcemia should be operated on as soon as possible—even as an emergency—in order to utilize the most rapid and effective method of reducing the serum calcium level. Other patients require no special preoperative care except that serum calcium and phosphorus and TRP levels should be determined just before surgery.

B. Localization: (Figs 20–2 and 20–3.) Localization of a parathyroid adenoma is best done at operation by an experienced surgeon who is familiar with the normal and aberrant sites of the parathyroid glands. Although several preoperative and special operative diagnostic technics have been proposed—eg, arteriography, selenomethionine scans, esophagography, and injections of toluidine blue or radioiodinated toluidine blue—they have not proved dependable. It has also been proposed that localization can be determined preoperatively by massage of each side of the neck, which results in a higher parathyroid hormone level in the peripheral blood when the side containing the adenoma is manipulated, but this method is also not reliable. Measurement of parathyroid hormone in the regional venous drainage is of no value in localization of parathyroid adenomas except in the case of large tumors, and when the tumors are large the surgeon has little difficulty in recognizing them. Small tumors are difficult to find, particularly when they are in aberrant locations; they are not well localized by any of the above procedures.

C. Operative Treatment: The treatment of hyperparathyroidism consists of the operative removal of all excess functioning parathyroid tissue. The surgeon must be familiar with the clinical, chemical, and roentgen diagnosis of hyperparathyroidism and its applicability to the individual patient. If he is confident of the diagnosis, he can undertake to locate and remove all hyperfunctioning tissue at the first opera-

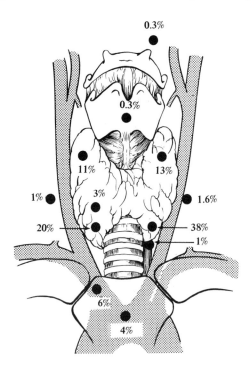

FIG 20–2. Locations of proved parathyroid
adenomas in 300 operated cases.

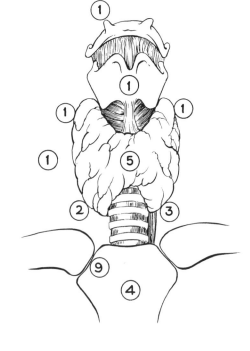

FIG 20–3. Locations of parathyroid adenomas in 28
patients who had had negative cervical
explorations before admission.

tion. He should be willing to spend whatever time is
necessary in exploration to avoid overlooking an
adenoma, for any subsequent search in a field of scar
tissue will be much more difficult (see ¶ F, below).

    D. Technic of Operation: The procedure is similar
to that for thyroidectomy. The exposure should be
greater, and dissection and hemostasis must be meticulously and painstakingly carried out in a dry field. If
tissues become blood-stained, the parathyroids may be
difficult or impossible to identify. The exploration is
conducted from the level of the bifurcation of the
common carotid artery downward into the posterior
and anterior mediastinum as well as behind the trachea
and esophagus. In over 80% of cases, the parathyroid
tumor is found attached to the posterior capsule of the
thyroid gland (Figs 20–2 and 20–3). In the remainder
it is truly aberrant, lying cephalad to the superior pole
of the thyroid gland, along the great vessels of the
neck, in thymic tissue, in the substance of the thyroid
gland itself (Fig 20–4), or in the posterior mediastinum behind the esophagus—where it is most often
overlooked. Exploration is conducted in a methodical
manner by first mobilizing the lateral lobes of the
thyroid gland so that they can be reflected medially
after division of the lateral veins. If necessary, the
superior and inferior thyroid artery and vein are
divided to obtain adequate exposure. Parathyroid
adenomas at this stage of the operation are usually
palpable before they are exposed. An adenoma of the
inferior gland often overlies the recurrent laryngeal

nerve, which should be intentionally identified before
excision of the tumor. Following the course of a
branch of the inferior thyroid artery may lead to the
adenoma.

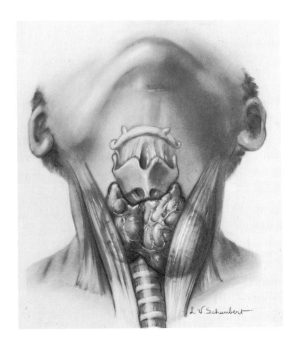

FIG 20–4. Intrathyroidal parathyroid adenoma.

An adenoma in the posterior mediastinum may be removed through the cervical incision because the blood supply arises in the neck. Before any tissue is removed, the exploration is completed on both sides of the neck. In many instances, the thin thyroid capsule covers the parathyroid gland so that one must dissect subcapsularly in order to expose the parathyroid; however, the tumor is usually attached and hangs from the capsule. One should attempt to identify 4 parathyroid glands, although there may be more or fewer than 4.

If a solitary adenoma is found, it is removed and the diagnosis confirmed by frozen section. If 2 adenomas are found, they are removed. The presence of normal parathyroid glands on frozen section indicates that the tumor removed is an adenoma rather than parathyroid hyperplasia, since in hyperplasia all the parathyroid glands are involved. When all parathyroid glands are hyperplastic, all but one should be removed and the remaining gland subtotally extirpated, leaving approximately 50 mg.

If exploration fails to reveal a parathyroid tumor, a conservative subtotal thyroidectomy is performed since these tumors are also found intrathyroidally. If thyroid nodules are present, they should be treated as nodular goiter and removed as well. The incidence of carcinoma of the thyroid in patients with hyperparathyroidism is high, and total thyroidectomy should be performed if thyroid cancer is found during exploration in a patient with hyperparathyroidism.

It is unwise to remove a normal parathyroid gland intentionally both because it has no beneficial effect and because it may be needed to maintain normal function when all the hyperfunctioning tissue is removed.

Occasionally, the cervical incision must be closed after painstaking exploration without a parathyroid tumor having been found.

Adenomas in the anterior mediastinum require mediastinotomy in only 2% of cases. If the cervical exploration is negative, the patient is allowed to leave the hospital and return in 2—4 weeks, when the diagnosis is again confirmed by laboratory studies. The mediastinum is then explored.

E. Postoperative Management: The postoperative management is quite similar to that following thyroidectomy, but the patient should be watched for signs of hypoparathyroidism.

Serum calcium and phosphorus levels are determined on the night of the operation and each morning thereafter, and a 12-hour urine collection is made each night for measurement of TRP. The TRP value usually rises above 95% on the first, second, or third day, indicating that there was parathyroid suppression by the tumor during the preoperative hypercalcemic period. It can be assumed that all of the excess functioning parathyroid tissue has been removed when the TRP rises, the serum calcium falls to below normal, and the phosphaturia drops markedly.

Patients with severe skeletal depletion ("hungry bones") or with long-standing hyperparathyroidism or high preoperative serum calcium levels are more apt to require temporary postoperative treatment with calcium.

F. Reoperation: The legacy of scar tissue in the neck following an unsuccessful exploration for hyperparathyroidism or following thyroidectomy compounds the difficulties encountered. If hyperparathyroidism persists after surgery, a parathyroid adenoma may still be found through the cervical incision in many patients. In most such patients, the important anatomic structures are found to be bound down by fibrous tissue, making it difficult to separate them to carry out adequate exploration. It is also difficult to dissect dense scar tissue from the usually soft and delicate parathyroid adenoma or recurrent laryngeal nerves, which could easily be torn or traumatized so that their recognition would be difficult. In such cases it is preferable to undermine the ribbon muscles en bloc, partially transect their cephalad insertion, mobilize the carotid sheath from the thyroid gland, and mobilize the gland after this is done rather than before.

Postoperative hypoparathyroidism requires prolonged treatment when normal parathyroid glands are removed at operations. In contrast, surgical removal of a hyperparathyroid gland rarely leads to long-standing hypoparathyroidism since normal glands are usually not removed.

Prognosis

Patients with hyperparathyroidism without renal damage are completely cured by parathyroidectomy. They should be carefully followed for many years, with special reference to blood pressure, serum calcium, and serum creatinine. Recurring hyperparathyroidism may be detected after many years in some patients, this time arising from an adenoma of a parathyroid gland previously observed to be normal at the operating table. In some of these cases, hyperparathyroidism may be familial.

After surgical cure, recalcification of eroded areas of the skeleton and of bone cysts—but not of brown tumors of bone—gradually takes place. Patients with very mild renal impairment often regain normal renal function during the postoperative period. Patients who already have some degree of uremia or severe renal impairment may or may not show renal improvement following parathyroidectomy. Although the bone lesions heal, the renal lesion may progress and eventually cause death from uremia or complications of hypertension. Early diagnosis and surgical cure are therefore essential.

Avioli LV: The diagnosis of primary hyperparathyroidism. M Clin North America 52:451—462, 1968.

Barnes BA, Cope O: Carcinoma of the parathyroid glands. JAMA 178:556—559, 1961.

Cope O & others: Primary chief-cell hyperplasia of the parathyroid glands: A new entity in the surgery of hyperparathyroidism. Ann Surg 148:375—388, 1958.

Cope O & others: Vicissitudes of parathyroid surgery: Trials of diagnosis and management in 51 patients with a variety of disorders. Ann Surg 154:491—500, 1961.

Dent CE: Some problems of hyperparathyroidism. Brit MJ 2:1419–1425, 1495–1500, 1962.

Egdahl RH, Canterbury JM, Reiss E: Measurement of circulating parathyroid hormone concentration before and after parathyroid surgery for adenoma or hyperplasia. Ann Surg 168:714–719, 1968.

Holmes EC & others: Parathyroid carcinoma: Collective review. Ann Surg 169:631–640, 1969.

Keating FR Jr: The clinical problem of primary hyperparathyroidism. M Clin North America 54:511, 1970.

Lafferty FW: Pseudohyperparathyroidism. Medicine 45:247, 1966.

Lloyd HM: Primary hyperparathyroidism: An analysis of the role of the parathyroid tumor. Medicine 47:53–72, 1968.

Owens MP, Sorock ML, Brown EM: The clinical application of in vivo parathyroid staining. Surgery 64:1049–1052, 1968.

Rienhoff WF & others: The surgical treatment of hyperparathyroidism. Ann Surg 168:1061–1074, 1968.

Steinbach HL & others: Primary hyperparathyroidism: A correlation of roentgen, clinical, and pathologic features. Am J Roentgenol 86:329–343, 1961.

Wilson RE & others: Hyperparathyroidism: The problems of acute parathyroid intoxication. Ann Surg 159:79–93, 1964.

PARATHYROID CARCINOMA

Parathyroid carcinoma is rare. Only 2 cases have been encountered in over 375 operations for parathyroid disease at the University of California Medical Center in San Francisco. The tumor is usually functional and may be indistinguishable from a parathyroid adenoma except for the finding of mitoses on pathologic examination. In some cases, the presence of extensive nodal metastases indicates malignancy. Excision of the ipsilateral thyroid lobe and neck excision are required if the diagnosis is made.

The prognosis must be guarded because recurrence with signs of hyperparathyroidism is common.

Secondary exploration may be helpful, but most patients succumb within 5–10 years after operation.

Holmes EC, Morton DL, Ketcham AS: Parathyroid carcinoma: A collective review. Ann Surg 169:631–640, 1969.

SECONDARY PARATHYROID HYPERPLASIA

The role of surgery in the treatment of secondary parathyroid hyperplasia and renal osteodystrophy during chronic hemodialysis or following renal homotransplantation remains to be clarified. Subtotal parathyroidectomy is warranted in rare instances when hypercalcemia and hyperparathyroid bone disease fail to respond to well-documented conservative measures, or in a patient in whom vascular calcification is progressing rapidly. The surgical risk for these patients is greater than the risk following operation for primary hyperparathyroidism because of the poor general condition of uremic patients and the possibility that permanent hypoparathyroidism can result from this ablative procedure.

The general principles of parathyroidectomy for this problem are controversial. Although total parathyroidectomy has been recommended, removal of 88% of the total parathyroid mass would appear to be more reasonable. When 3, 4, or more hyperplastic parathyroid glands are present, all but a portion of one hyperplastic gland should be removed, leaving an estimated 50 mg of parathyroid tissue.

After subtotal parathyroidectomy, the serum calcium level drops precipitously, and vigorous antitetanic treatment is necessary. For these reasons, parathyroid operations should be undertaken in patients with renal osteodystrophy only after the most careful consideration.

•   •   •

General References

Goldman L, Greenspan FS: Applied physiology of the thyroid and parathyroid glands. S Clin North America 45:317–326, 1965.

Goldman L & others: The parathyroids: Progress, problems and practice. Curr Probl Surg, Aug 1971.

Means JH, DeGroot LJ, Stanbury JB: *The Thyroid and Its Diseases,* 3rd ed. McGraw-Hill, 1963.

Pittman JA Jr (editor): Symposium on the treatment of thyroid disease. Mod Treat 6:441–549, 1969.

21 ...

The Breast

John L. Wilson, MD

CARCINOMA OF THE FEMALE BREAST

Essentials of Diagnosis

- Early findings: Single, nontender, firm to hard mass with ill-defined margins, usually in a middle-aged or older woman. The mass is discovered by the patient in 90% of cases.
- Nipple erosion (Paget's carcinoma) or discharge may be the only indication of early disease.
- Later findings: Skin or nipple retraction, skin edema or redness, axillary lymphadenopathy, fixation of mass to chest wall or to skin, ulceration of lesion, enlargement of breast, local pain.
- Late findings: Bone, liver, lung, brain, or other distant metastases.

General Considerations

A. Incidence: Carcinoma of the breast is the most common cancer in women in the USA and is the leading cause of death in women age 40–44. According to data from cancer registries in California, Connecticut, and New York, the peak incidence of the disease is in women 45–60 years of age. However, mammary cancer is frequent in women at all ages past 30, and the probability of developing the disease increases with age throughout life. There is evidence that the age-adjusted incidence rate for cancer of the female breast is gradually increasing in the USA. The reason for this trend, which is receiving careful study, is not apparent.

Large numbers of women are affected by breast cancer. It is estimated that in 1969 carcinoma of the breast was diagnosed for the first time in 66,000 women in the USA. The annual incidence of breast cancer is 70 per 100,000 females (Table 21–1). About 6% of newborn girls (1 out of 17) can be expected to develop breast cancer at some time during their lives.

Prevalence is distinct from incidence and is the number of cases that exist in a population at any given time. Based upon the estimated survival of all cases, the prevalence of breast cancer in the USA per 100,000 population is approximately 6 times the annual incidence.

Japanese women have a relatively low incidence of breast cancer (Table 21–1). Numerous studies have attempted without success to explain this observation in a definitive manner. High fertility, long periods of breast feeding, and dietary, endocrine, and genetic influences have all been considered as possible factors.

Breast cancer occurs 100 times more frequently in women than in men.

B. Bilateral Breast Cancer: It is not surprising that mammary cancer is often bilateral since both breasts are subject to the same genetic and hormonal influences. The literature shows an incidence of simultaneous bilateral breast cancer of about 1%, but there is an incidence of 5–8% of later occurrence of cancer in the second breast. Robbins & Berg (Cancer 17:1501, 1964), in a 20-year retrospective study, found that the risk increased about 10 times for the second breast; that bilaterality occurred more often in women under 50 years of age; and that it was more frequent when

TABLE 21–1. Age-adjusted average annual cancer incidence rates. Leading sites for Japanese and white females, Alameda County, California, 1960–1964. (Rates are per 100,000 population. Rates in parentheses are based on 5 or fewer cases. In situ cancers and basal and squamous cell carcinomas of the skin are excluded.)

Site	White	Japanese
Breast*	70	29
Stomach	9	39
Large intestine	26	(18)
Gallbladder and bile ducts	...	(26)
Cervix uteri	20	...
Corpus uteri	19	...
Ovary	14	...
Leukemia	...	(14)
Thyroid gland	...	(12)
Rectum	11	...

*The breast is the most common site of cancer among white females; the incidence rate for breast cancer is 70 per 100,000—almost 3 times the 26 per 100,000 rate for cancer of the large intestine, the second most common site. The incidence of breast cancer is considerably lower in women of other racial groups. The incidence rate of 29 per 100,000 for breast cancer in Japanese women is considerably lower than that of other races. (*Incidence of Cancer in Alameda County, California, 1960–1964.* State of California Department of Public Health [Berkeley], 1964.)

the tumor in the primary breast was multicentric or of comedo or lobular type.

Mammography and biopsy of the opposite breast are beginning to provide additional information on the simultaneous or later development of bilateral breast cancer. Mammography will occasionally show evidence of occult carcinoma preoperatively in the clinically uninvolved breast and is especially useful as a follow-up examination. Routine biopsy of the opposite breast has been debated for the past 2 decades and is of proved value in lobular carcinoma. According to reports in the literature, the incidence of bilateral involvement by lobular carcinoma ranges from 35–59% in the patients biopsied.

C. Occurrence During Pregnancy or Lactation: Only 1–2% of breast cancers occur during pregnancy or lactation. This overall low incidence in part reflects the fact that only 15% of mammary carcinomas occur during the reproductive years. When breast cancer occurs in women under age 35, it is concurrent with pregnancy in about 10–15% of cases. The diagnosis of breast cancer is frequently delayed in pregnancy because of a tendency of both patients and physicians to procrastinate in deciding on biopsy. When the lesion is confined to the breast, the 5-year survival after radical mastectomy is about 60%; therefore, the former extreme pessimism regarding outlook was not justified.

D. Etiology: The cause of breast cancer is not known, but certain conditions are associated with a higher incidence of the disease. A predisposition to breast cancer can be inherited, but the mechanism of inheritance is not clear. Numerous investigations have shown that female relatives of women with mammary carcinoma have a higher rate of disease than the general population. There is evidence that the average probability of breast cancer in mothers of patients with the disease is approximately double that of the general population; in sisters, the risk is about 2½ times that of the general population. Reports of symmetrical mammary cancer in monozygotic twins support the conclusion that inheritance plays a role in some cases.

Marital status and parity also influence the incidence of breast cancer. Single and nulliparous women have a slightly higher death rate from breast cancer than married and parous women. Women with 3 or more children have a lower risk than women with fewer children. Menarche after age 15 and artificial menopause are associated with a slightly lower incidence of breast cancer. These observations regarding fertility and ovarian function suggest that hormonal factors have some influence on the incidence of breast cancer. Lactation probably does not protect from breast cancer, as formerly thought. Breast cancer patients do not differ from unaffected women with respect to a history of lactation if account is taken of the fact that breast cancer patients tend to be of low parity.

Mammary dysplasia (cystic disease of the breast), particularly when accompanied by proliferative changes, papillomatosis, or solid hyperplasia, is prob-ably associated with an increased incidence of malignancy. This association is controversial because of the occurrence of varying degrees of mammary dysplasia in over 50% of breasts examined at autopsy in women dying of causes other than breast carcinoma. The apparent relationship between malignancy and mammary dysplasia again raises the question of hormonal factors in the etiology of breast cancer. Although the pathogenesis of cystic disease is not known, this disorder is believed to result either from a relative or absolute increase in estrogen or a relative or absolute decrease in progesterone. The inference is inescapable that the variations in hormonal environment which cause the pathologic changes of mammary dysplasia may under certain conditions also induce neoplasia.

Contraceptives containing estrogens and progestins may produce proliferation of epithelial elements within the breast and stimulation of the intralobular and interlobar connective tissues. The reaction in the ductal epithelium is particularly noticeable. Tenderness of the breasts, nodularity, galactorrhea, and fibroadenomas are among the gross breast changes which may rarely occur. While there is no definite evidence that oral contraceptives are related to human breast cancer, breast changes caused by these agents may be important to consider in differential diagnosis macroscopically and microscopically. Further information on the long-term effects of these hormonal preparations is needed. Administration of estrogens to postmenopausal women has not been found to increase the incidence of breast cancer, although fibrocystic and other benign changes in the breast are occasionally seen.

Many studies have been done in an attempt to determine whether women with breast cancer or with a predisposition to the disease show an abnormal pattern of excretion of estrogens, androgens, or hydroxycorticosteroids. These studies have proved very difficult to conduct, control, and interpret. As a result, evidence based on hormonal assays is conflicting, and it is not now possible to identify by these means those women with a high risk of developing malignancy of the breast. It does appear, however, that a significant percentage of women with carcinoma of the breast have an abnormal hormonal environment which may be of diagnostic importance when better understood.

There is no evidence that trauma to the breast causes cancer. Both breast trauma and cancer are common. When trauma precedes the discovery of cancer, it can be taken as coincidence rather than a cause and effect relationship.

E. Biologic Behavior: An understanding of the natural history of breast cancer is essential to the correct management of this highly variable disease. The growth rate and other behavior of the neoplasm is a result of biologic balance between growth potential of the tumor cell and host resistance. Both of these factors may vary initially over a wide range and may be altered in the course of the disease. For example, rates of tumor growth differ markedly from patient to patient as a result of the fact that the doubling time of malignant cells in breast cancer ranges from 23–209 days. Assuming that the rate of doubling is constant and that the neoplasm originates in one cell, a slowly growing carcinoma may remain localized to the breast and not reach a clinically detectable size (1 cm) for 8 years. On the other hand, rapidly growing lesions have a much shorter preclinical course and frequently metastasize to regional nodes or distant organs before a breast mass is discovered. Therapeutic plans and prognostications which do not take this diversity into account are unsatisfactory. For practical purposes, initial treatment is based chiefly on the clinical stage (gross extent) of the disease when the diagnosis is made with additional critical decisions dependent upon histologic study of the tumor and regional nodes.

Detection & Diagnosis

The primary complaint in about 80% of patients with breast cancer is a lump (usually painless) in the breast. Less frequent and later symptoms are breast pain; erosion, retraction, enlargement, discharge, or itching of the nipple; and redness, generalized hardness, enlargement, or shrinkage of the breast. Rarely, an axillary mass, swelling of the arm, or back pain (from metastases) may be the first symptom (Table 21–2).

Since about 90% of breast masses are discovered by the patient herself, continuing education of the public and the medical profession on the importance of prompt biopsy of suspect lesions is essential. A mean delay period of 6 or 7 months before consulting a physician has been reported in several large series of breast cancer. Delay in making the diagnosis also occurs when the physician minimizes the significance of a breast mass, failing to recognize that these lesions are extremely deceptive.

A. Early Detection:

1. Screening examinations–A number of mass cancer screening programs consisting of physical and mammographic examinations of the breasts of asymptomatic women have been conducted. These programs have demonstrated that breast cancer can be discovered at an earlier and more favorable stage by combined use of these procedures. About 70% of women discovered by screening methods to have breast cancer prove on operation to have negative axillary nodes, whereas only about 40% of patients with a self-discovered mass have negative nodes. Both physical examination and mammography are necessary for maximum yield of new cases in screening programs since about 40% of early breast cancers can be discovered only by mammography, whereas another 40% can be detected only by palpation.

The relatively low yield of new cases in proportion to the resources which must be committed to mass screening programs makes it unlikely that this method of breast cancer detection will be widely available in the near future. A practical alternative is for physicians to advise regular self-examination of the breast and annual physical examination for all their women patients, particularly those over 40. Women with a history of breast cancer in the immediate family or those who have already had cancer in one breast are in a high-risk group, and special effort should be made to ensure that they receive annual physical and mammographic examinations.

2. Self-examination–The high mortality rate of breast cancer can be most effectively reduced by earlier detection. All women over 30 should be encouraged to examine their breasts monthly–in premenopausal women, just after the menstrual period. The breasts should be inspected initially while standing before a mirror with the hands at the sides, overhead, and pressed firmly on the hips to contract the pectoralis muscles. Masses, asymmetry of breasts, and slight dimpling of the skin may become apparent as a result of these maneuvers. Next, in a supine position, each breast should be carefully palpated with the fingers of the opposite hand. Physicians should instruct their women patients in the technic of self-examination and advise them to report at once for medical evaluation if a mass or other abnormality is noted.

3. Mammography–A mammogram is a soft tissue radiologic examination of the breast. Mammography is the only reliable means of detecting breast cancer before signs and symptoms appear. Many breast cancers can be diagnosed by mammography as early as 2 years prior to their clinical recognition, and recent reports indicate that certain premalignant conditions of the breast may be identifiable in the future. These developments have led to increased interest in various experimental methods of earlier detection such as xeroradiography, thermography, ultrasonography, isotope scanning, and angiography. Wide practical application of certain of these new methods such as xeroradiography and thermography is imminent.

Indications for mammography include the following: (1) to survey the opposite breast at the time the diagnosis of breast cancer is made and annually thereafter; (2) to complement the annual physical examination of women, particularly those with a family history

TABLE 21–2. Initial symptoms of mammary carcinoma.*

Symptom	Percentage of All Cases
Painless breast mass	66
Painful breast mass	11
Nipple discharge	9
Local edema	4
Nipple retraction	3
Nipple crusting	2
Miscellaneous symptoms	5

*Adapted from report of initial symptoms in 774 patients treated for breast cancer at Ellis Fischel State Cancer Hospital, Columbia, Missouri. Reproduced, with permission, from Spratt JS Jr, Donegan WL: *Cancer of the Breast.* Saunders, 1967.

of breast cancer; (3) as an aid in the evaluation of ill-defined or questionable breast masses; multiple masses; nipple discharge, erosion, or retraction; skin changes; or breast pain; and (4) as an aid in the search for occult primary cancer in women with metastatic disease from an unknown primary.

Both false-positive and false-negative results are obtained with mammography, but, where mammography is employed proficiently and extensively, the yield of malignant lesions on biopsy remains around 35%–this in spite of the fact that more biopsies are done. The safest course is to biopsy all suspicious masses found on physical examination and, in the absence of a mass, all suspicious lesions demonstrated by mammography.

B. Symptoms and Signs: In addition to meticulous examination of the breasts, axillas, and supraclavicular regions, evaluation of the patient with a breast mass includes a careful history and a complete physical examination. In the history, special note should be made of menarche, pregnancies, parity, artificial or natural menopause, previous breast lesions, and a family history of breast cancer. Back or other bone pain may be the result of osseous metastases. Systemic complaints or weight loss should raise the

question of metastases, which may involve any organ but most frequently the bones, liver, and lungs. The more advanced the cancer in terms of size of primary and extent of regional node involvement, the higher the incidence of metastatic spread to distant sites.

Examination of the breast should be meticulous, methodical, and gentle. Inspection and palpation should be carried out with the patient sitting and supine. Axillary and supraclavicular areas should be carefully examined. These procedures should be followed on all physical examinations (Figs 21–1, 21–2, and 21–3). In some series, 5–10% of cases of breast carcinoma have been discovered during physical examinations performed for other purposes.

A lesion smaller than 1 cm in diameter may be difficult or impossible for the examiner to feel and yet may be discovered by the patient. She should always be asked to demonstrate the location of the mass; if the physician fails to confirm the patient's suspicions, he should repeat the examination in 1 month. During the premenstrual phase of the cycle, increased innocuous nodularity may suggest neoplasm or may obscure an underlying lesion. If there is any question regarding the nature of an abnormality under these circumstances, the patient should be asked to return after her

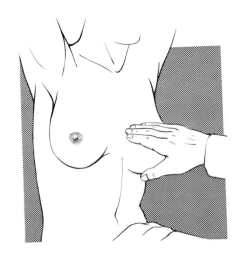

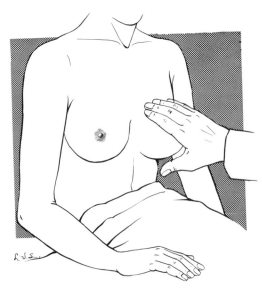

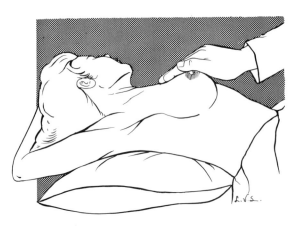

FIG 21–1. **Inspection and palpation of the breasts with patient sitting and supine.** Observe breasts for presence of mass, asymmetry, or nipple retraction. Skin retraction or dimpling may be accentuated by raising arms overhead.

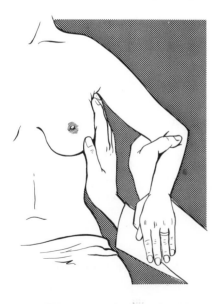

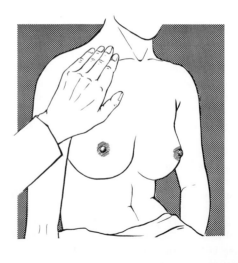

FIG 21–2. Palpation of axillary and supraclavicular regions for enlarged lymph nodes.

period. The location, size, consistency, and other physical features of all mammary lesions should be recorded on a drawing of the breast for future reference.

Breast cancer usually consists of a nontender, firm, or hard lump with poorly delimited margins (caused by local infiltration). Slight skin or nipple retraction is an important early sign. Minimal asymmetry of the breast may be noted. Very small (1–2 mm) erosions of the nipple epithelium may be the only manifestation of carcinoma of the Paget type. Watery, serous, or bloody discharge from the nipple is an infrequent early sign.

The following are characteristic of advanced carcinoma: edema, redness, nodularity, or ulceration of the skin; the presence of a large primary tumor; fixation to the chest wall; enlargement, shrinkage, or retraction of the breast; marked axillary lymphadenopathy; supraclavicular lymphadenopathy; and distant metastases.

C. Special Clinical Forms of Breast Carcinoma:

1. Paget's carcinoma–The basic lesion is intraductal carcinoma, usually well differentiated and multicentric in the nipple and breast ducts. The nipple epithelium is infiltrated, but gross nipple changes are often minimal and a tumor mass may not be palpable. The first symptom is often itching or burning of the nipple accompanied by a superficial erosion or ulceration. The diagnosis is readily established by biopsy of the erosion.

Paget's carcinoma is not common (about 3% of all breast cancers), but it is important because it appears innocuous. It is frequently diagnosed and treated as dermatitis or bacterial infection. This is disastrous, for the lesion metastasizes to regional nodes in up to 60% of cases and should be treated in the same manner as other forms of breast cancer. The prognosis of Paget's carcinoma is particularly poor when a mass is palpable

(about 25% 5-year survival after radical mastectomy).

2. Inflammatory carcinoma–This is the most malignant form of breast cancer and comprises about 3% of all cases. The clinical findings consist of a rapidly growing, sometimes painful mass which enlarges the breast. The overlying skin becomes red, warm, and edematous. The diagnosis should be made only when the redness involves more than one-third of the skin over the breast. The inflammatory changes, often mistaken for an infectious process, are caused by carcinomatous invasion of the subdermal lymphatics with resulting edema and hyperemia. These tumors

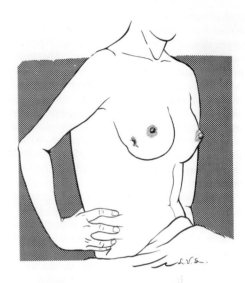

FIG 21–3. Skin retraction or dimpling may be accentuated by having the patient press her hand on her hip in order to contract the pectoralis muscles.

may be caused by a variety of histologic types. Metastases occur early and widely in all cases, and for this reason inflammatory carcinoma is rarely curable. Radical mastectomy is seldom indicated. Radiation and hormone therapy may have a transient palliative effect.

D. Laboratory Findings: Carcinoma localized to the breast and axillary nodes causes no abnormalities detectable by clinical laboratory examinations. Certain tests may be useful as clues to the presence of more widespread disease. A consistently elevated sedimentation rate may be the result of disseminated cancer. Liver metastases may be associated with elevation of alkaline phosphatase. Hypercalcemia is an occasional important finding in advanced malignancy of the breast. Fluorine-18 scanning of bone has demonstrated metastases in what appeared to be early cases with normal appearing x-rays of the skeleton by conventional technics. Such studies in the future may allow a better classification of cancer of the breast before operation.

E. Biopsy: The diagnosis of mammary carcinoma is established by histologic examination of a biopsy specimen of the primary lesion in the breast. The decision to obtain a biopsy is the critical one.

Every breast mass should be considered malignant until proved otherwise, usually by histologic section. About 30% of lesions thought to be definitely cancer prove to be benign, and about 15% of lesions believed benign are found to be malignant. These findings clearly demonstrate the fallibility of clinical judgment and the necessity for biopsy to settle the issue in most cases.

Biopsy specimens may be obtained by excision of small lesions, removal of a small portion of larger lesions, or by needle. A core of tissue is obtained with a special biopsy needle. There is no evidence that a properly done biopsy procedure causes metastatic spread of cancer. It has not been possible to show by retrospective studies that a delay of a week or so between diagnostic biopsy and definitive treatment of breast cancer has an adverse effect. The preferred approach is incisional or excisional biopsy of the breast mass in the operating room under general or local anesthesia with preparation to proceed immediately with mastectomy if frozen section is positive. However, incisional, excisional, or needle biopsy of the breast mass may be done under local anesthesia on an outpatient or inpatient basis with a view to scheduling definitive surgical or other treatment within a week (Fig 21—4).

Needle biopsy is diagnostic only if positive. A negative needle biopsy should be followed by an open biopsy of the lesion. Needle biopsy is especially useful in making a histologic diagnosis in advanced lesions for which no surgical treatment is planned.

Treatment of breast cancer should never be undertaken without an unequivocal histologic diagnosis. Fortunately, frozen section in this disease is highly reliable. On the rare occasion when diagnosis on frozen section or other type of histologic preparation is questionable, treatment should be deferred pending

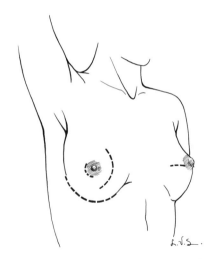

FIG 21—4. Incisions for biopsy and for removal of benign tumors.

further tissue examination.

Indications for biopsy of the breast include the following: persistent mass, (2) bloody nipple discharge, (3) eczematoid nipple, and (4) positive mammography. Thermography is an experimental procedure, apparently less reliable than mammography but potentially useful as a screening procedure. In the absence of physical or mammographic findings, positive thermography is a relative indication for biopsy of the suspicious area. Unexplained axillary adenopathy calls for biopsy of the enlarged node after mammography has been done. Random or mirror image biopsy of the contralateral breast is practiced in some centers when the diagnosis of operable breast cancer is established. In patients with a high risk of developing breast cancer, biopsy of the breast for minimal or equivocal change is justified.

In experienced hands, needle aspiration of discrete, spherical lesions of the breast is a useful means of distinguishing the benign cysts of mammary dysplasia from a solid tumor which may be cancer (Fig 21—5). Turbid greenish or amber fluid is characteristic of a benign cyst, which should disappear completely without residual mass when aspirated. Blood-tinged fluid or a persistent mass after aspiration is an indication for biopsy. In any case, patients who develop cysts have an increased risk of developing breast cancer and should be followed regularly. A baseline mammogram should be obtained. When in doubt regarding the diagnosis, biopsy should be performed.

Cytologic examination of nipple discharge is rarely helpful, and breast biopsy is preferred for bloody or questionable secretions.

In suspected bilateral involvement the preferred biopsy site, provided there are no physical or mammographic indications of a lesion elsewhere, is the upper outer quadrant of the breast since this is the commonest site of the initial lesion. Lobular carcinoma is frequently in situ, and its removal at this stage is generally

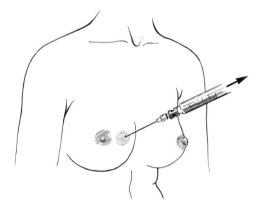

FIG 21–5. Needle aspiration of cyst.

curative. However, lobular carcinoma in situ may progress to infiltrating lobular carcinoma, the prognosis of which is no better than that of infiltrating ductal carcinoma and actually may be worse.

F. X-Ray Findings: Metastatic lesions occur most frequently in bones and lung and are identified by skeletal and chest films which should be obtained when symptoms or signs suggest the possibility of metastases. Mammography of the unaffected breast, either preoperatively or after the diagnosis has been established in a potentially curable lesion of the opposite breast, is advisable as an aid in identifying occult carcinoma. A baseline mammogram of the unaffected breast may also be of value for comparison with the results of future examinations.

Differential Diagnosis

A. Benign Lesions: The following benign lesions must be distinguished from breast cancer. The differentiation is made by biopsy in the great majority of cases.

1. Mammary dysplasia—This condition, also called chronic cystic disease of the breast, is common in premenopausal women age 30–50. It occurs as single or multiple masses or thickenings of one or both breasts, often associated with tenderness in the mass or in the breast. There is a tendency to premenstrual increase in discomfort or size of the mass. Lesions tend to fluctuate in size and may appear rapidly and subside spontaneously. Mammary dysplasia is the condition most frequently confused with carcinoma of the breast, and biopsy is often required to establish the diagnosis. Carcinoma and mammary dysplasia are both common and may coexist in the breast.

2. Mammary duct ectasia—This rare lesion (also called comedomastitis or plasma cell mastitis) is characterized by dilatation of the ducts, inspissation of breast secretions, intraductal inflammation, and periductal and interstitial chronic inflammation in which plasma cells are prominent. Inspissation of secretions within the duct is the probable cause. This view is supported by the fact that about half of patients have inverted or cracked nipples or difficulty in nursing.

The disorder tends to occur in the fifth decade and is of special clinical significance because it may produce a mass or induration, occasionally with skin or nipple retraction. Axillary node enlargement may further heighten the suspicion of cancer. Unlike cancer, however, the onset of mammary duct ectasia is usually associated with pain, tenderness, and redness, which suggest the inflammatory nature of the process. Biopsy may be required to establish the diagnosis.

3. Fibroadenoma—This benign neoplasm usually occurs in young women within 20 years after puberty. Fibroadenoma is characteristically a firm, round, discrete, nontender, fairly mobile lesion 1–5 cm in size. Occasionally it may be multiple. Excisional biopsy is advisable to confirm the diagnosis, which can be strongly suspected from the clinical appearance.

4. Intraductal papilloma—Papillomatosis is the most frequent cause of serous or bloody nipple discharge. The lesions are usually small and may not be palpable. The subareolar or para-areolar region is the usual tumor site; it is best localized by pressure directly over it so that a discharge from the nipple is expressed from the obstructed duct. Mammary dysplasia and carcinoma may also cause nipple discharge, which, if bloody, suggests malignancy. Biopsy or excision of the obstructed duct is usually required to settle the issue. Both ductal papilloma and cancer are capable of producing nipple discharge when too small to be palpable.

5. Fat necrosis—This is a rare condition which is usually indistinguishable from carcinoma without biopsy. The patient may or may not present with tenderness or with a history of trauma. Nipple or skin retraction may occur in fat necrosis, and this contributes further to its similarity in appearance to breast cancer.

B. Occult Carcinoma: Rarely, the first manifestation of breast cancer will be axillary node enlargement or distant metastases. No mass may be palpable in the breast. The mammary carcinoma in these circumstances is occult and only discovered by sectioning of excised breast tissue. Mammography may be useful in selecting the site for biopsy or may be used as a screening procedure to detect breast cancer in otherwise normal patients.

Prevention

Breast cancer cannot be "prevented," but a diagnosis can be made in an earlier stage provided certain procedures are followed. The most important of these are discussed under Detection & Diagnosis, above.

Clinicopathologic Correlations

A. Clinical Staging: Patients with breast cancer can be grouped into stages according to the characteristics of the primary tumor (T), regional lymph nodes (N), and distant metastases (M). Physical, radiologic, and other clinical examinations are used in determining the stage, which is based on all information available before therapy. Staging is useful in evaluating the prognosis and determining the type of treatment indicated. The International Union Against Cancer and the American Joint Committee on Cancer Staging and End Results Reporting have each formulated a standard TNM system to be used by physicians in breast cancer staging. The rules for staging of breast cancer as defined by the International and the American systems are given in Table 21–3. The TNM staging system is summarized in Table 21–4.

The 2 staging systems differ in several respects. The major differences are in the staging of patients with large tumors and those with involvement of the supraclavicular nodes. Under American rules, a patient with localized disease is stage I regardless of tumor size. Under the International System, the patient with localized disease is assigned to stage III if the primary tumor is larger than 5 cm. Patients with supraclavicular lymph node involvement but no other distant spread are assigned to stage III under the International System and to stage IV under the American System. Prognosis is significantly poorer when the primary tumor is greater than 5 cm in size; therefore, International rules on tumor size bear a closer relationship to prognosis than the American. In general, survival is inversely proportionate to tumor size. Available data on cases dependent for staging on supraclavicular lymph node involvement show a survival curve intermediate between that for patients who are in either stage III or IV according to both systems.

The records of 2038 patients subjected to radical mastectomy were examined by Zippen (J Natl Cancer Institute 36:53, 1966). These patients were staged according to both the International and the American classification. The percentage of cases falling into each

TABLE 21–3. Clinical staging of cancer of the breast.

Stage	International System*	American System†
I	0 No distant metastases.	0 No distant metastases.
	1 Tumor of 5 cm or less.	1 Tumor of any size.
	2 Skin fixation absent or incomplete.	2 Skin not involved or involved locally with Paget's disease.
	3 Nipple may be retracted, or Paget's disease may be present.	3 Skin attachment (dimpling) or nipple retraction.
	4 Pectoral muscle or chest wall fixation absent.	4 No pectoral muscle or chest wall attachment.
	5 No ipsilateral axillary nodes palpable.	5 No clinically palpable axillary lymph nodes (no metastases suspected).
II	0–4 As above.	0–4 As above.
	5 Ipsilateral axillary nodes palpable but movable.	5 Clinically palpable axillary lymph nodes that are not fixed (metastases suspected).
III	0 As above.	0 As above.
	1 Tumor more than 5 cm in diameter or	1 Tumor of any size.
	2 Skin fixation complete, or skin involvement wide of tumor or	2 Skin infiltration or ulceration or
	3 Peau d'orange present in tumor area or wide of tumor or	3 Peau d'orange or skin edema or
	4 Pectoral muscle fixation complete or incomplete, or chest wall fixation or	4 Pectoral muscle or chest wall attachment or
	5 Ipsilateral axillary nodes fixed or	5 Clinically palpable ipsilateral axillary nodes fixed to one another or to other structures (metastases suspected) or
	6 Ipsilateral supraclavicular or infraclavicular nodes movable or fixed or	6 Clinically palpable ipsilateral infraclavicular lymph nodes fixed to one another or to other structures (metastases suspected).
	7 Arm edema.	
IV	Distant metastases, regardless of the condition of the primary tumor and regional lymph nodes.	Clinical, radiographic evidence of metastases except those to ipsilateral axillary or infraclavicular nodes.

*Committee on Clinical Stage Classification and Applied Statistics, Malignant Tumors of the Breast, 1960–1964. International Union Against Cancer, Paris, 1960.

†American Joint Committee on Cancer Staging and End Results Reporting: *Clinical Staging System for Cancer of the Breast.* American College of Surgeons, 1962.

TABLE 21–4. TNM system of staging adopted by the American Joint Committee on Cancer Staging and End Results Reporting.

		Staging			
		I	II	III	IV
T: Primary tumor					
T1 Tumor of 2 cm or less in its greatest dimension; skin not involved, or involved locally with Paget's disease.	T1	X	X	X	
T2 Tumor over 2 cm in size or with skin attachment (dimpling of skin) or nipple retraction (in subareolar tumors); no pectoral muscle or chest wall attachment.	T2	or / X	or / X	or / X	Any
T3 Tumor of any size with any of the following: skin infiltration, ulceration, peau d'orange, skin edema, pectoral muscle or chest wall attachment.	T3			or / X	
N: Regional lymph nodes					
N0 No clinically palpable axillary lymph nodes (metastasis not suspected).	N0	X		X or	
N1 Clinically palpable axillary lymph nodes that are not fixed (metastasis suspected).	N1		X	X	Any
N2 Clinically palpable ipsilateral axillary or infraclavicular lymph nodes that are fixed to one another or to other structures (metastasis suspected).	N2			or / X	
M: Distant metastasis					
M0 No distant metastasis.	M0	X	X	X	
M1 Clinical and radiographic evidence of metastasis except those to ipsilateral axillary or infraclavicular lymph nodes.	M1				X

These designations are then combined to define 4 stages which are used for record purposes:

Stage I: T1/N0/M0; T2/N0/M0

Stage II: T1/N1/M0; T2/N1/M0

Stage III: T3/N0/M0; T3/N1/M0; T3/N2/M0; T1/N2/M0; T2/N2/M0; and includes any combination of T1, T2, or T3 with N2 and M0.

Stage IV: Any clinical stage of disease with distant metastasis (M1).

stage is shown in Table 21–5.

The 5-year survival data for Zippen's series (Table 21–6) show that there is little difference in prognosis between corresponding stages of the International and American staging systems (Cutler SJ, Myers MH: J Natl Cancer Institute 39:193, 1967).

The clinician must decide about treatment and estimate the prognosis in breast cancer patients whose extent of disease ranges from minimal to advanced. Judgment on management and outlook is improved if patients are systematically classified or "staged" in a manner which allows comparison with similar cases treated by others. Both the International and the American staging systems provide sound criteria for the clinical classification of patients with breast cancer. It will be advantageous if the International Union Against Cancer and the American Joint Committee on Cancer Staging and End Results Reporting can agree on a common staging system, which would doubtless rapidly gain world-wide acceptance. Meanwhile, the American TNM system of staging as described in Table 21–4 is widely used in the USA as the basis for comparing end results in the management of breast cancer.

From a practical point of view, it is useful to remember that the International and American systems of staging differ only in detail from the following brief

TABLE 21–5. Distribution of breast cancer according to International and American staging systems.

Stage	International System	American System
I	42%	48%
II	13%	17%
III	34%	22%
IV	11%	13%
Total	100%	100%

TABLE 21–6. Five-year survival rates according to stage of breast cancer.

Stage	International System	American System
I	80%	75%
II	70%	65%
III	50%	45%
IV	None	None

definition of stages:

Stage I: The tumor is confined to the breast. There may be early signs of skin involvement such as dimpling or nipple retraction, but there are no signs of axillary or distant metastases.

Stage II: The primary tumor is as in stage I, but there are movable, suspicious nodes in the ipsilateral axilla.

Stage III: The primary tumor is infiltrating the skin or chest wall, or the axillary nodes are matted or fixed.

Stage IV: Distant metastases are present.

1. Location and size of primary lesion—The relative frequency of carcinoma in various anatomic sites in the breast is approximately as shown in Fig 21–6.

Almost half of cancers of the breast begin in the upper outer quadrant, probably because this quadrant contains the largest volume of breast tissue. The high percentage in the central portion is due to the inclusion of cancers that spread to the subareolar region from neighboring quadrants.

Cancer occurs 5–10% more frequently in the left breast than in the right; there is no satisfactory explanation for this difference.

Tumor size at the time of surgery gives some indication of the alertness of both patients and physicians to the presence of breast cancer. In the series of 2578 patients treated surgically in the National Surgical Adjuvant Breast Project, about half of the tumors

were larger than 3 cm and about 5% were smaller than 1 cm (Fisher & others: ·Cancer 24:1071, 1969). Inasmuch as a 1 cm lesion should be readily identifiable by palpation if sought, it is clear that greater effort to discover small lesions is needed.

2. Metastases to regional lymph nodes—The axillary and the internal mammary lymph node chains are the major (but not the only) routes of primary lymphatic spread of breast cancer (Fig 21–7). Treatment and prognosis depend upon clinical and pathologic assessment of the status of the regional nodes with respect to metastases. The supraclavicular nodes are in direct continuity with the axillary chain and are usually involved secondarily only after the axillary nodes have been infiltrated. Involvement of the supraclavicular nodes almost invariably means that distant spread of the cancer has already occurred and that attempts at curative surgical treatment are futile. Involvement of the axillary or internal mammary nodes, although an extremely serious prognostic finding, calls for detailed discussion.

The axillary and internal mammary lymph node chains may be involved independently of each other, or both may be involved. Metastases occur more frequently in axillary than in internal mammary nodes in patients with operable breast cancer. Location in the breast of the primary lesion has relatively little effect on the incidence of axillary lymph node involvement as determined by pathologic examination of the nodes

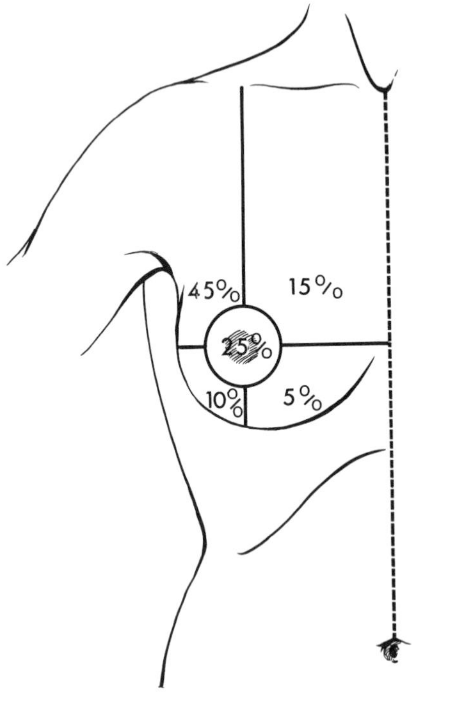

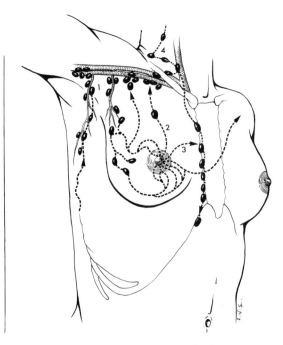

FIG 21–7. Lymphatic drainage of the breast to regional node groups. *1.* Main axillary group. *2.* Interpectoral node leading to apex of axilla. *3.* Internal mammary group. *4.* Supraclavicular group. (Modified from Ackerman LV, Del Regato JA: *Cancer,* 3rd ed. Mosby, 1962.)

FIG 21–6. Frequency of breast carcinoma at various anatomic sites.

after radical mastectomy. About half of the lesions located in any quadrant or centrally in the breast are associated with positive axillary lymph nodes on histologic examination. On the other hand, the incidence of spread to the internal mammary nodes is influenced by the location of the primary tumor. Cancers in the central and medial portions of the breast metastasize to internal mammary nodes more frequently than lateral lesions (Fig 21–8).

a. **Axillary lymph node metastases**—Evaluation of the axillary nodes is a significant feature of the physical examination in breast cancer. A clinical opinion based on palpation of the axilla should be formed regarding the presence or absence of metastases in the nodes. One or 2 movable, not particularly firm lymph nodes 5 mm or less in diameter can frequently be palpated in the normal axilla, but firm or hard nodes larger than 5 mm in diameter must be assumed to contain metastases until proved otherwise. As shown in Table 21–4, the presence of clinically positive axillary nodes places the patient at least in stage II. Unfortunately, evaluation of the axillary nodes by palpation is not always accurate. Histologic studies show that microscopic metastases are present in up to

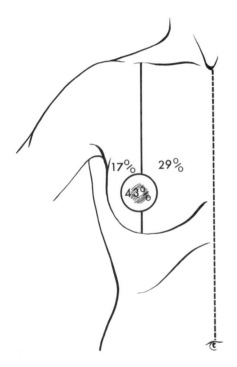

FIG 21–8. Percentage of internal mammary node metastases according to lateral, medial, or subareolar location of the primary tumor. The high percentage of metastases from central tumors is due to the fact that large tumors originating either laterally or medially and extending to the subareolar area are classified as central. (Haagensen CD & others: Ann Surg 169:174, 1969.)

30% of patients considered by the clinician to have "negative nodes." On the other hand, if the clinician thinks that the axillary nodes are involved, he will prove to be correct about 85% of the time. Thus, the examiner is frequently unable to detect early metastatic involvement of the axillary nodes and should recognize his limitations in this regard.

The relationship between primary tumor size and axillary node involvement is of interest. According to data obtained in the National Surgical Adjuvant Breast Project (Fisher & others: Cancer 24:1071, 1969), the incidence of axillary node metastases varied with tumor size as shown in Table 21–7.

It is of special importance that 22% of the patients with the smallest tumors (< 1 cm) had positive lymph nodes. When the extent of node involvement was studied for the entire series, patients with negative nodes were found to have significantly smaller tumors than those with 1–3 positive nodes. They in turn had smaller tumors than did patients with 4 or more positive lymph nodes. The proportion of patients with 4 or more positive nodes increased with increasing tumor size.

Stage of disease and initial therapy are decided on the basis of the clinical examination. Prognosis and subsequent therapy are influenced by histologic findings regarding the number and locations of involved axillary nodes when these are resected. Three anatomic levels of axillary nodes have been identified by Adair (Ann Roy Coll Surg Eng 4:36, 1949) as relevant to prognosis if involved by metastases in primarily operable cases treated by radical mastectomy (Table 21–8).

The surgeon who wishes to obtain the maximum amount of information from examination of the axillary contents should tag these 3 levels of nodes during operation as a guide to the pathologist.

b. **Internal mammary lymph node metastases**—As shown in Fig 21–3, medial or central lesions in the breast are associated with a higher incidence of internal mammary invasion than lateral tumors. The incidence of internal node metastases also increases in relation to the size of the primary tumor. Haagensen & others (Ann Surg 169:174, 1969) performed internal mammary node biopsies on 1007 patients with tumors of different sizes and obtained the results shown in Table 21–9.

When the axillary nodes are involved, the inci-

TABLE 21–7. Relationship of size of breast tumor to incidence of axillary node metastases.

Size of Primary Tumor	Percentage With Positive Axillary Lymph Nodes
< –1 cm	22%
1–1.9 cm	38%
2–2.9 cm	41%
3–3.9 cm	53%
6+ cm	63%

TABLE 21–8. Influence of anatomic location of involved axillary nodes on survival in breast cancer treated by radical mastectomy.

Level	Anatomic Location	Five-Year Survival if Nodes Positive
I	Nodes in low axilla up to the inferior border of the pectoralis minor muscle	65%
II	Nodes posterior to insertion of pectoralis minor muscle	45%
III	Nodes above superior border of pectoralis minor muscle	28%

dence of metastases to the internal mammary nodes is increased. Urban & Farrow (Acta Un Int Cancer 19:1551, 1963) reported on 258 cases of primary operable breast cancer treated by extended radical mastectomy which involved resection of both axillary and internal mammary nodes. When axillary nodes were negative histologically, the incidence of internal mammary node involvement ranged from zero to 22%, depending upon whether the cancer was in the lateral or medial portion of the breast. When axillary nodes were positive, the internal mammary nodes were positive in 33–67% of cases, with the higher incidence related to tumors in the medial portion of the breast.

The frequency of involvement of the internal mammary nodes in operable breast cancer (stages I and II) was first determined by Handley & Thackray (Lancet 2:276, 1949), who found that the internal mammary nodes were already invaded in about one-fourth of these cases and that radical mastectomy would consequently fail to remove all of the disease. As a result of this observation, Haagensen and his co-workers formerly performed internal mammary node biopsies in selected patients and refrained from radical mastectomy in those with positive internal mammary nodes. Haagensen now relies on clinical criteria in deciding on radical mastectomy and has abandoned internal mammary node biopsy on the grounds that it is helpful only in a few selected cases of borderline operability.

Other surgeons have advocated extended radical

TABLE 21–9. Relationship of size of breast tumor to incidence of metastases in internal mammary nodes.

Size of Primary Carcinoma	Percentage With Internal Mammary Metastases
3 cm	16%
3–5 cm	20%
5–8 cm	39%
7–8 cm	57%
All cases	33%

mastectomy which includes resection of the internal mammary chain of nodes. Kaae & Johansen (*Prognostic Factors in Breast Cancer.* Livingstone, 1968, pp 93–102) compared extended radical mastectomy with simple mastectomy plus radiotherapy in a controlled study of randomized patients and concluded that the results were virtually identical up to 10 years after treatment.

B. Pathologic Correlation: The behavior of breast cancer can be correlated with the histologic appearance of the lesion. Information on the microscopic characteristics of the neoplasm is therefore helpful in deciding on management and in estimating the prognosis. The pathologist can distinguish 4 types of mammary carcinoma on the basis of cellular differentiation and invasiveness, as shown in Table 21–10.

1. Relative frequency of pathologic types— Kouchoukos and his associates studied specimens from 432 radical mastectomies. It can be estimated from their data that the relative frequency of the various pathologic types in surgically treated patients is approximately as shown in Table 21–11.

2. Incidence of axillary metastases—Axillary metastases occur more frequently in patients with tumors of types III and IV, an indication of their greater metastasizing potential. Table 21–12 shows the approximate incidence of axillary spread by type in

TABLE 21–10. Classification of mammary carcinoma according to the cellular growth pattern. (Kouchoukas & others: Cancer 20:948, 1967.)

Type I: Rarely metastasizing (not invasive)
  1. Intraductal or comedocarcinoma without stromal invasion. Paget's disease of the breast may exist if the epithelium of the nipple is involved.
  2. Papillary carcinoma confined to the ducts.
  3. Lobular carcinoma in situ.

Type II: Rarely metastasizing (always invasive)
  1. Well differentiated adenocarcinoma.
  2. Medullary carcinoma with lymphocytic infiltration.
  3. Pure colloid or mucinous carcinoma.
  4. Papillary carcinoma.

Type III: Moderately metastasizing (always invasive)
  1. Infiltrating adenocarcinoma.
  2. Intraductal carcinoma with stromal invasion.
  3. Infiltrating lobular carcinoma.*
  4. All tumors not classified as types I, II or IV.

Type IV: Highly metastasizing (always invasive)
  1. Undifferentiated carcinoma having cells without ductal or tubular arrangement.
  2. All types of tumors indisputably invading blood vessels.

*Infiltrating lobular carcinoma has been moved from type II to type III because of growing experience with its metastasizing potential.

patients undergoing radical mastectomy (Kouchoukos & others).

3. Survival in relation to type—As expected, survival rates after radical mastectomy vary inversely with local invasiveness and a tendency to metastasize to regional nodes. The 5-year survival rate after radical mastectomy in patients with the 4 pathologic types of tumors is approximately as shown in Table 21–13.

4. Bilateral occurrence of type I tumors—Type I noninfiltrating neoplasms, particularly those of the intraductal and the lobular in situ variety, are of special interest because of their tendency to occur bilaterally. At the time of initial operation for breast cancer, Urban performed random biopsies of the opposite breast on 73% of 488 patients in his series. When an infiltrating type of carcinoma was present in the primarily involved breast, the overall rate of bilateral cancer was 12%—approximately 8% simultaneous and 4% asynchronous. However, when noninfiltrating cancer was found in the primary breast, the overall rate of bilateral involvement was 20–30% simultaneous and 10% asynchronous. Bilaterality is particularly likely to occur in patients with in situ lobular carcinoma, which should be recognized as a preinvasive form of breast cancer and treated accordingly. Lobular carcinoma may progress in time from an in situ to an infiltrating stage. It may be in situ in one breast and infiltrating in the other. Periods of 1–20 years may elapse between the diagnosis of in situ lobular carcinoma and the development of invasive cancer in the same or opposite breast.

TABLE 21–11. Relative frequency of pathologic types of breast cancer.

Type	Characteristics	Percentage of Total Cases
I	Rarely metastasizing (not invasive)	5%
II	Rarely metastasizing (always invasive)	15%
III	Moderately metastasizing (always invasive)	65%
IV	Highly metastasizing (always invasive)	15%
		100%

TABLE 21–12. Relationship of pathologic type of breast cancer to incidence of axillary node metastases.

Type	Percentage With Positive Nodes
I	13%
II	34%
III	58%
IV	57%

TABLE 21–13. Relationship of pathologic type of breast cancer to survival.

Type	Five-Year Survival Rate		All Cases
	Axillary Nodes		
	Negative	Positive	
I	95%	95%	95%
II	85%	70%	80%
III	80%	50%	60%
IV	80%	40%	55%

In addition to physical examination and mammography, there is a need to develop ways of diagnosing breast cancer during what may be, especially in type I tumors, a prolonged preclinical or "silent" stage. Biopsy of the opposite "negative" breast at the time of mastectomy for cancer is an approach to the problem of early diagnosis worthy of consideration in patients with lobular and intraductal carcinoma.

5. Implications of pathologic typing—In most statistical studies of survival after treatment for carcinoma of the breast, the various pathologic types are not separately identified. As a result, the influence of pathologic type on response to therapy is usually obscured. Those few studies which do correlate clinical stage and pathologic type reveal that stage I lesions less than 5 cm in size and of pathologic type I or II rarely metastasize beyond the nodes in the lower axilla. Such lesions, therefore, are in a particularly favorable category from the standpoint of such a surgical procedure as modified radical mastectomy.

Curative Treatment

Treatment may be curative or palliative. Curative treatment is advised for clinical stage I and II disease and for selected patients in stage III. Palliative treatment (discussed below) by irradiation, hormones, endocrine ablation, or chemotherapy is recommended for patients in stage IV (distant metastases), for stage III patients unsuitable for curative efforts, and for previously treated patients who develop distant metastases or ineradicable local recurrence.

A. Types of Curative Treatment:

1. Radical mastectomy—This operation involves en bloc removal of breast, pectoral muscles, and axillary nodes and has been the standard curative procedure for breast cancer since the turn of the century when W.S. Halsted and Willy Meyer independently described their versions of the technic. Experience with radical mastectomy is extensive, and, in properly selected patients, no other form of therapy has produced better results. Radical mastectomy removes the local lesion and the axillary nodes with a wide safety margin of surrounding tissue. Various breast incisions are used depending upon the location of the primary tumor and the preference of the surgeon (Fig 21–9). If the disease has already spread to the internal mammary or supraclavicular nodes or to more distant sites, radical mastectomy alone will not cure the patient.

2. Extended radical mastectomy—This procedure involves, in addition to standard radical mastectomy, removal of the internal mammary nodes. The extended operation has been recommended by a few surgeons for medially or centrally placed breast lesions and for tumors associated with positive axillary nodes because of the known frequency of internal mammary node metastases under these circumstances. Retrospective clinical comparisons suggest that the 5-year survival and incidence of chest wall recurrence may be slightly better after extended radical mastectomy than after standard radical mastectomy in selected patients, but a controlled prospective clinical trial is required to settle the issue. It does not appear that extended radical mastectomy is significantly more effective than irradiation in preventing recurrence from internal mammary metastases. For this reason, extended radical mastectomy has few advocates at this time.

3. Modified radical mastectomy—This procedure involves complete removal of all breast and subcutaneous tissue (as in standard radical mastectomy) and dissection in continuity of the axillary lymphatic bed up to the level of the coracoid process. The difference between the modified and the standard radical mastectomy is that the standard operation also removes the pectoralis major and minor muscles and the highest group of axillary nodes just inferior to the clavicle. There is now considerable evidence that morbidity, mortality, survival, and local recurrence rates for standard and modified radical mastectomy are essentially the same for stage I and II breast cancer. Prospective controlled clinical studies will be needed to settle the issue in a definitive manner, but there is already a notable shift in major centers to the use of modified radical mastectomy in patients who, a few years ago, would have been treated by standard radical mastectomy.

4. Simple mastectomy—If the malignancy is confined to the breast without spread to the adjacent muscles or to the regional nodes or beyond (true clinical stage I disease), simple mastectomy (or even wide local excision) should be effective in eradicating the cancer. Clinical experience bears this out in certain cases. The problem is the inability to determine with certainty, prior to their resection and pathologic examination, that the axillary nodes are uninvolved. Reference has already been made to the fact that physical examination is highly unreliable in detecting axillary metastases. Simple mastectomy must, therefore, be considered an inadequate operation for breast cancer until more is known of the risk associated with leaving axillary metastases until they become clinically evident. Nevertheless, Crile (JAMA 199:736, 1967) has advanced the controversial argument that simple mastectomy may be safely performed for stage I breast cancer, with axillary dissection undertaken only if axillary nodes are suspect when palpated through the wound or become clinically involved at a later date. The rationale for leaving the axillary nodes until they become clinically positive is that, theoretically, the regional lymph

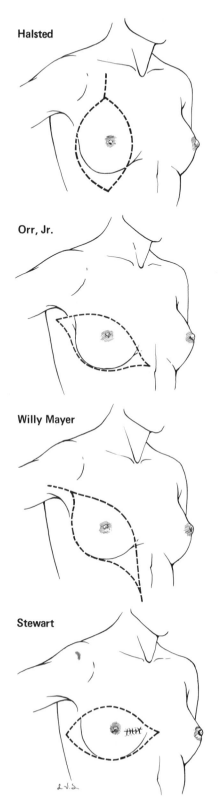

FIG 21–9. Types of incisions for radical mastectomy.

nodes are repositories of systemic immunity, which prevents the spread of early cancer.

Approximately 25% of patients judged clinically to be stage I develop axillary metastases after simple mastectomy alone. Crile has reported that after a second operation to remove the nodes, the prognosis in these patients is the same as in patients found to have microscopic metastases after radical mastectomy for clinical stage I cancer.

5. Supervoltage irradiation—In recent years, the proved efficacy of supervoltage irradiation in sterilizing the primary lesion and the axillary and internal mammary nodes (Guttman RJ: Am J Roetgenol 96:560, 1966; Cancer 20:1046, 1967) has made radiation therapy with or without simple mastectomy (or wedge resection) an important option for primary treatment of certain breast cancers, particularly those that are locally advanced or when the patient refuses mastectomy. The capability of radical irradiation to destroy or confine metastases in unresected regional nodes has largely eliminated the difference in survival between standard or modified radical mastectomy and simple mastectomy plus irradiation (Table 21–14). McWhirtir's policy (since 1941) of treating almost all stages of mammary cancer with simple mastectomy and radical irradiation has been much debated and contested, but the method appears to produce crude survivals at 10 and 15 years equal to those of radical mastectomy for comparable stages of disease (McWhirtir R: Am J Roentgenol 92:3, 1964).

B. Choice of Primary Treatment for Breast Cancer: There is evidence that control of mammary cancer confined to the breast and axillary nodes can be achieved by a number of different approaches including standard radical mastectomy, extended radical mastectomy, modified radical mastectomy, simple mastectomy with deferred therapeutic axillary node dissection, and radical irradiation with or without simple mastectomy. The variability in tumor-host relationship from patient to patient and the unpredictability of occult metastases make it difficult to determine with precision the relative merits of current competing forms of treatment without controlled prospective clinical trials.

Relying on evidence now at hand, modified radical mastectomy is recommended as the primary treatment of choice in stage I and II lesions. Results are apparently comparable to those obtained with standard radical mastectomy. Chest wall deformity and problems with shoulder mobility are less with modified radical mastectomy because the pectoral muscles are not removed. The best cosmetic result is achieved when a transverse incision can be used.

Stage III lesions are a borderline group and may or may not be suitable for surgical treatment by either a standard or modified radical mastectomy. Radical surgical treatment is usually contraindicated in stage III lesions with the following characteristics:

(1) Extensive edema involving more than one-third of the skin of the breast.
(2) Satellite nodules on the skin.
(3) Carcinoma of the inflammatory type.
(4) Parasternal tumor nodules.
(5) Edema of the ipsilateral arm.
(6) Palpable ipsilateral infraclavicular lymph nodes (metastases suspected or proved by biopsy).
(7) Two or more of the following grave signs of locally advanced carcinoma:
  (a) Ulceration of the skin.
  (b) Limited edema involving less than one-third of the skin of the breast.
  (c) Fixation of axillary lymph nodes to the skin or the deep structures of the axilla.
  (d) Axillary lymph nodes measuring 2.5 cm or more in transverse diameter.
  (e) Pectoral muscle or chest wall attachment.

The features listed above are signs of advanced disease and are almost invariably associated with spread to the internal mammary or supraclavicular nodes or other distant sites outside the scope of either standard or modified radical mastectomy. Under these circumstances, operation is not curative and may actually disseminate the disease locally or systemically. Radiotherapy with or without simple mastectomy (or wedge resection) is a more effective approach in these advanced stage III cases.

TABLE 21–14. Results of radical mastectomy versus simple mastectomy or wedge resection plus radical radiation therapy. (Powers WE: Cancer 24:1301, 1969.)

| | Five-Year Survival | | | |
| | Radical Surgery | | Local Surgery and Irradiation | |
	Number	% Survival	Number	% Survival
Brinkley & Haybittle* (Lancet 291, 1966)	91	54%	113	66%
Kaae & Johansen* (Acta radiol 80:155, 1959)	271	65%	288	62%
Peters (J Canad A Radiol 4:32, 1953)	308	76%	124	76%

*Only stage II patients studied. Patients selected for alternate mode of treatment by random allocation.

There remain those stage III lesions which do not exhibit the advanced signs listed above. A modified radical mastectomy may be performed if the primary tumor and the enlarged axillary nodes can clearly be excised with an adequate margin by this procedure. Attachment to the pectoral muscles, high axillary nodes, large primary tumor or nodes, or other technically unfavorable conditions would make standard radical mastectomy the preferred operation.

It is uncertain whether therapeutic abortion significantly improves the prognosis in pregnant patients with cancer which is apparently confined to the breast or to the breast and axillary nodes only. Practice varies widely. It seems reasonable to advise abortion when the child is nonviable. Obviously, the decision must be individualized.

Advice regarding pregnancy must sometimes be given to women who have undergone radical mastectomy or other treatment for cancer of the breast. The weight of the somewhat contradictory evidence is that pregnancy is hazardous and should be avoided or interrupted until the patient has been free of disease for at least 5 years. Thereafter, the presumed stimulating effect of pregnancy on residual cancer is less significant.

C. Radiotherapy as Adjunct to Radical Mastectomy: The purpose of preoperative or postoperative radiotherapy in association with modified or standard radical mastectomy is (1) to reduce the incidence of local recurrence from residual cancer in the operative field, and (2) to sterilize metastatic cancer in the internal mammary and supraclavicular lymph nodes. Patients are therefore selected for radiotherapy on the basis of the likelihood of local recurrence or of the existence of disease in unresected regional nodes. According to these criteria, completely resectable lesions confined to the breast (stage I) do not call for radiotherapy. On the other hand, stage II and stage III patients may be considered for radiotherapy before or after modified or standard radical mastectomy. Only supervoltage irradiation should be advised as adjunctive therapy. Orthovoltage irradiation for this purpose is outmoded.

1. Postoperative radiotherapy—The efficacy of postoperative irradiation in improving survival or recurrence rates has not been decisively demonstrated. However, in view of the proved ability of supervoltage radiotherapy to destroy cancer cells in the breast and regional nodes, postoperative radiotherapy is commonly recommended under the following conditions: (1) if the tumor has been cut through or there is a high likelihood that residual tumor has been left in the operative field; (2) if the tumor is larger than 5 cm or is located in the central or medial portion of the breast; or (3) if there are metastases to the axillary nodes. Some authorities advise postoperative radiotherapy if one or more axillary nodes are involved; others recommend radiotherapy only if 4 or more nodes are found to contain metastases.

Radiotherapy is begun as soon after operation as the patient's general condition and state of the wound

permit. A tumor dose in the range of 4000–6000 rads (usually 5000 or 5500 rads) is delivered over a period of 4–5 weeks to the internal mammary and supra- and infraclavicular nodal areas. The chest wall is also irradiated only if there is a high probability of chest wall recurrence such as would be the case if the breast lesion was large, cut through, or associated with extensive axillary node involvement. When irradiation is properly managed, delayed wound healing and pulmonary damage are infrequent problems. There is a slight increase in lymphedema of the arm following postoperative radiotherapy.

In a recent large cooperative study, Fisher found that although postoperative irradiation slightly reduced the incidence of local recurrence, it did not improve survival. There is an increasing trend to avoid postoperative irradiation except in selected cases with proved or high probability of internal mammary node involvement.

2. Preoperative radiotherapy—The beneficial results of preoperative radiotherapy are more definite than those of postoperative radiotherapy. Preoperative irradiation reduces the incidence of local recurrence. Fletcher (JAMA 200:140, 1967) demonstrated a 5% local recurrence rate after preoperative radiotherapy, compared to a 16% local recurrence rate following postoperative radiotherapy. Preoperative radiotherapy is possibly also of value in making inoperable patients curable by radical mastectomy, although in such patients the results may not be superior to those obtainable by radiotherapy alone. Indications for preoperative irradiation include the following: (1) primary tumor larger than 5 cm; (2) limited skin edema or direct skin involvement over tumor; (3) multiple low or midaxillary nodes; or (4) a previous surgical procedure which may have disseminated the tumor locally. A 4000–6000 rad tumor dose is delivered to the axillary, supraclavicular, and internal mammary nodes, and the chest wall and breast are treated tangentially. Radical mastectomy is performed 5–6 weeks after completion of radiotherapy. When cases are properly selected and managed and there is the necessary close cooperation between radiotherapist and surgeon, there is no significant increase in immediate postsurgical complications as a result of preoperative radiotherapy.

D. Preoperative Preparation for Radical Mastectomy: There are 2 objectives of the preoperative work-up: (1) to determine the patient's general condition, with special attention to operative risk; and (2) to search for possible distant metastases.

In patients with no evidence of systemic disease and only a small breast tumor, a complete work-up for metastatic disease is not usually necessary. Only about one in 5 or 6 of such patients is found on breast biopsy to have a malignant tumor. If the local lesion is highly suspicious or if enlarged axillary nodes or other suggestive signs of metastases are present, x-rays should be obtained of the chest (posteroanterior and lateral), skull (anteroposterior and lateral), and lumbar spine and pelvis (anteroposterior). Serum alkaline phosphatase determination and liver scan or needle biopsy are advisable if liver metastases are suspected because of hepatomegaly. Skeletal pain is an indication for films of the painful site, and, if these are negative, bone scans should be considered.

Preoperatively, full discussion with the patient and her next of kin regarding the possible necessity for mastectomy is essential. Because of the controversial nature of the relative benefits of simple, modified radical, or radical mastectomy, many patients wish to discuss the subject in detail and may insist that they wish one or another of the operations. It behooves the surgeon to be patient and understanding, stating his own position as he sees it.

E. Postoperative Management: Wound complications following modified or standard radical mastectomy such as marginal slough, fluid collection under the flaps, and infection are minimized by attention during operation to viability of skin flaps and to closure without tension. Suction drainage of the wound by means of catheters placed beneath the skin flaps reduce the collection of blood and serum. Bulky compression dressings are usually unnecessary. With careful, meticulous technic, closure without drainage may be done.

Active motion of the arm and shoulder on the operated side should be encouraged after the first few days, so that by 10–14 days postoperatively there is a full range of motion. Failure of the patient to cooperate or to make progress may necessitate physical therapy. The Service Committee of the American Cancer Society sponsors a rehabilitation program for postmastectomy patients called Reach for Recovery and will provide useful literature upon request. The patient's morale is improved by early provision of a breast prosthesis held in place by a comfortably fitted brassiere.

Radical mastectomy is well tolerated even by elderly patients. The operative mortality is 1% or less, and the immediate postoperative complications are not usually a serious problem.

F. Complications of Radical Mastectomy:

1. Local recurrence—Recurrence of cancer within the operative field following radical mastectomy is due to incomplete removal of tumor or involved nodes, to cutting across infiltrated lymphatics, or to spillage of tumor cells into the wound. The rate of local recurrence correlates with tumor size, the presence and number of involved axillary nodes, the histologic type of tumor, and the presence of skin edema or skin and fascia fixation with the primary. In one series of 704 patients treated with radical mastectomy without ancillary therapy and uniformly followed for at least 5 years, 17% developed local recurrence. When the axillary nodes were not involved at the time of mastectomy, the local recurrence rate was 7%, but the rate was 26% when they were involved. A similar difference in local recurrence rate was noted between small and large tumors. In general, local recurrence rate is a function of the stage of the patient's disease. (Spratt JS Jr, Donegan WL: *Cancer of the Breast.* Saunders, 1967.)

Chest wall recurrences usually appear within the first 2 years, with a peak incidence in the second year, but may occur as late as 15 or more years after radical mastectomy. Suspect nodules should be biopsied. If the biopsy is positive, disseminated disease must be suspected and a search for metastases made by chest and bone films. Local excision or localized radiotherapy may be feasible if an isolated nodule is present. If lesions are multiple or accompanied by evidence of regional involvement in the internal mammary or supraclavicular nodes, the disease is best managed by comprehensive radiation treatment of the whole chest wall including the parasternal, supraclavicular, and axillary areas. Although local recurrences usually signal the presence of widespread disease, when there is no evidence of metastases beyond the chest wall and regional nodes, radical irradiation for cure should be attempted.

2. Edema of the arm—Except for local recurrence, the only important late complication of standard radical mastectomy is edema of the arm. Significant edema occurs in 10–30% of cases. When it appears in the early postoperative period, it is usually caused by lymphatic obstruction due to infection in the axilla. Late or secondary edema of the arm may develop years after radical mastectomy as a result of axillary recurrence or of infection in the hand or arm with obliteration of lymphatic channels. After radical mastectomy, the lymphatic drainage of the arm is always compromised and the extremity becomes more than normally susceptible to infection following minor injuries. The patient should be warned of this and treatment instituted promptly if infection occurs. Specific instruction should be given to the patient who has had radical mastectomy to avoid breaks in the skin of the hand and arm on the operated side and to refrain from tasks likely to cause superficial wounds and infections. Injections for inoculation and immunization should not be given in that arm. Well-established chronic edema is managed by elevation and elastic support.

Palliative Treatment

A. Radiotherapy: Palliative radiotherapy may be advised for locally advanced cancers with distant metastases in order to control ulceration, pain, and other manifestations in the breast and regional nodes. Radical irradiation of the breast and chest wall and the axillary, internal mammary, and supraclavicular nodes should be undertaken in an attempt to cure locally advanced and inoperable lesions when there is no evidence of distant metastases. A certain number of patients in this group are cured in spite of extensive breast and regional node involvement.

Palliative irradiation is also of value in the treatment of certain bone or soft tissue metastases to control pain or avoid fracture, particularly when hormonal, endocrine ablation, and chemical therapy are inappropriate or ineffective.

B. Hormone Therapy: When distant metastases have occurred in breast cancer, the patient is incurable; however, disseminated disease may be kept under control or caused to regress for sustained periods by various forms of endocrine therapy, including administration of hormones or ablation of the ovaries, adrenals, or pituitary. About one-third of breast cancer patients will respond to one or more of these endocrine measures. The incidence of hormonal responsiveness is approximately the same in premenopausal women as in postmenopausal women, although the methods of treatment used may be quite different.

Ablation of ovarian secretion by oophorectomy or irradiation of the ovaries is, in the premenopausal patient, the simplest and most reliable method of obtaining tumor regression in advanced breast cancer. Administration of estrogen to premenopausal patients or to those whose tumor has responded favorably to castration may stimulate tumor growth. These observations have led to the hypothesis of estrogen dependence to explain the tumor regression seen in some breast cancers after castration, bilateral adrenalectomy, or hypophysectomy. According to this hypothesis, reactivation of tumor growth after control by castration is due to increasing estrogen secretion from the adrenal cortex. Bilateral adrenalectomy at this stage is known to cause further tumor regression in some cases. Subsequently, when the tumor reactivates after control by adrenalectomy, pituitary ablation may have an effect by eliminating secretion of both FSH and ACTH, which are capable of activating ectopic adrenal sources of estrogen. The assumption of estrogen dependence thus appears to explain the clinical remission of tumor growth seen after endocrine ablation therapy in some patients with late breast cancer. However, biochemical methods of estrogen determination have failed to show a correlation between clinical response and quantitative change in estrogen secretion. Furthermore, the estrogen dependence hypothesis cannot explain regression of some tumors after estrogen, androgen, or progestin therapy. Therefore, a combination of direct effect by metabolic products of the steroid on the tumor and of indirect effect via the pituitary (eg, alteration in prolactin or other pituitary secretion) is postulated as responsible for tumor regression in steroid therapy of breast cancer. Since different tumors probably vary in their response to hormonal therapy depending on the hormonal environment in which they have developed, the choice of a suitable steroid for therapy in each patient may be difficult. Nevertheless, certain general principles can be stated as guides to endocrine therapy.

Endocrine therapy is employed when surgery and irradiation have failed or when widespread metastases have rendered them useless. Many patients are candidates for a trial of hormone treatment because about half of all patients with breast cancer and 60% of those having positive axillary nodes at the time of mastectomy will develop metastatic lesions.

The major forms of hormone treatment are (1) estrogen, (2) androgen, and (3) corticosteroid therapy.

1. Estrogen therapy—Estrogens should be reserved for postmenopausal women. The best results of estrogen administration are obtained in women more than 5 years past the menopause. Estrogen is capable of causing exacerbation of tumor growth in 50% of premenopausal women and should not be given to them or to recently postmenopausal women until the vaginal smear ceases to show evidence of estrogenic activity. Tumor remission rates from estrogen (and androgen as well) tend to increase with increasing numbers of years past the menopause.

Estrogen administered as primary therapy will induce tumor regression in over 30% of postmenopausal patients with advanced breast cancer. Objective evidence of tumor regression is seen most commonly in soft tissue metastases in older patients, and over 40% of this group show remission of tumor growth. Both local soft tissue and visceral lesions show a higher remission rate from estrogen than from androgen therapy. The reverse is true for bone metastases.

Treatment usually consists of giving diethylstilbestrol (or equivalent), 5 mg 3 times daily orally, and continued as long as it is beneficial.

The first evidence of regression of metastatic cancer does not usually appear until about 4 weeks after beginning estrogen therapy, but the trial of estrogen should not be abandoned in less than 2 months except in case of obvious exacerbation or serious side-effects. The average duration of remission is about 16 months, but remissions of soft tissue lesions lasting more than 5 years are occasionally seen. The survival time of women who respond to estrogen therapy is about twice that of nonresponders.

The commonest side-effects are anorexia, nausea, and vomiting. These usually disappear within a few weeks, but when symptoms of toxicity are severe the dosage should be reduced temporarily until tolerance is acquired. Pigmentation of nipples, areolas, and axillary skin; enlargement of the breasts; and sodium and water retention are among the side-effects of estrogen therapy. Uterine bleeding occurs in the majority of postmenopausal patients when estrogen therapy is stopped, and patients should be warned of this possibility to avoid anxiety. Severe bleeding can usually be controlled by administration of testosterone propionate, 100 mg IM daily for 3 or 4 doses.

2. Androgen therapy—Androgen administration causes tumor regression in 10–20% of premenopausal women with advanced breast cancer. However, because of the more frequent and prolonged remission from castration, this procedure is preferred as initial treatment in the premenopausal group. Androgen therapy may sometimes be usefully added to castration in patients under 35 years of age, or in the presence of bone metastases, because of the frequently poor results from castration alone in such patients. Failure of response to castration may be considered an indication for a trial of androgen therapy because of the low likelihood of a favorable response by these patients to adrenalectomy or hypophysectomy. Androgen therapy causes temporary amenorrhea in premenopausal women.

Estrogen therapy is not advisable in recently postmenopausal women until the vaginal smear ceases to show evidence of estrogenic activity because of the danger of exacerbating the disease. A trial of androgen therapy is warranted in this group, but with the expectation of a favorable response in only about 15% of patients.

Since bone metastases are commonly more responsive to androgen than to estrogen therapy, a trial of androgen administration may be advantageous when osseous lesions are present, particularly before adrenalectomy or hypophysectomy is undertaken. About 25% of patients with bone metastases who are more than 5 years past the menopause will respond to androgen therapy. Patients failing to respond can still be subjected to operation if indicated, and surgery will usually have been delayed only about 6 weeks.

Postmenopausal patients who have shown a favorable response to castration or estrogen therapy and have then relapsed may be given a trial of androgen therapy with a 20–30% chance of responding favorably. In patients more than 5 years postmenopausal, bony metastases which have failed to respond to estrogens are more likely to regress on secondary androgen therapy than are soft tissue metastases. Occasionally, androgen administration will cause tumor regression in the completely hypophysectomized patient.

Androgen may be given continuously as long as tumor regression persists. It is probably preferable, however, to administer androgen until the tumor has regressed maximally and then to discontinue administration until reactivation occurs, at which time resumption of androgen therapy will often produce another regression. Intermittent therapy of this kind has the advantage of reducing the tendency to virilization while varying the hormonal environment of the tumor, thereby perhaps postponing the development of autonomy in the tumor.

The androgen preparation most frequently employed is testosterone propionate, 100 mg IM 3 times a week. However, it is simpler and equally effective to give fluoxymesterone, 20–40 mg daily by mouth. An orally administered nonvirilizing androgen, testolactone (Teslac), is reported to be as effective as testosterone propionate in causing tumor regression. The major reason for interest in this compound is that, since it appears to be relatively inert hormonally, it may have a direct effect on the breast cancer.

About 3 months of androgen therapy are usually required for maximal response. Pain relief may be achieved in up to 80% of patients with osseous metastases. In addition, androgen therapy usually results in a sense of well-being and an increase in energy and weight, particularly in postmenopausal patients. The principal adverse side reactions are increased libido and masculinizing effects—eg, hirsutism, hoarseness, loss of scalp hair, acne, and ruddy complexion. Virilization occurs in practically all women taking estosterone propionate for longer than 6 months but in only about one-third of patients receiving fluoxymesterone. Fluid retention, anorexia, vomiting, and liver damage are among the rarer side-effects of androgen therapy.

3. Corticosteroids—Corticosteroids are especially valuable in the management of the serious acute symptoms which may result from such conditions as hypercalcemia, brain and lung metastases, and hepatic metastases with jaundice. Corticosteroid therapy is also indicated for patients who are too ill for major endocrine ablation therapy and for those whose tumors do not respond to other endocrine therapy. The combination of systemic corticosteroid and the intracavitary injection of an alkylating agent (see below) may be very effective in controlling pleural effusion due to metastatic breast cancer.

The patient's age and previous response to sex hormone therapy are not correlated with response to corticosteroid therapy, which probably acts through a local effect upon the tumor or the tumor bed. A prior favorable response to adrenocorticosteroids does not guarantee a similar response to adrenalectomy. Objective evidence of tumor regression following corticosteroid administration is less than that following adrenalectomy. Remission on corticosteroid therapy averages about 6 months, whereas that following adrenalectomy is over 12 months.

The subjective response of the seriously ill patient to corticosteroid administration is often striking. Appetite, sense of well-being, and pain from bone or visceral metastases may be markedly improved. However, objective regression of soft tissue lesions occurs in only about 15% of patients. The relief of coma due to brain metastases and dyspnea due to lung metastases is often encouraging but transient. Hypercalcemia is probably improved by specific action on calcium metabolism.

Cortisone acetate, 150 mg daily orally, or prednisone or prednisolone, 30 mg daily orally, is an average dose. Twice or 3 times these amounts may be required temporarily for control of severe, acute symptoms. A variety of other corticosteroids have been employed in equivalent dosage with similar results. The dosage of corticosteroids must be reduced slowly if they have been used for prolonged periods because of the adrenocortical atrophy induced.

Adrenocortical hormones may cause numerous undesirable systemic effects and serious complications such as uncontrollable infection, bleeding peptic ulcer, muscle weakness, hypertension, diabetes, edema, and features of Cushing's syndrome.

The best overall tumor remission rate from hormonal therapy in postmenopausal patients can probably be obtained when treatment is individualized. In general, patients with soft tissue and intrathoracic metastases respond best to estrogen therapy. Androgen therapy is usually more effective in patients with bone metastases. Corticosteroid therapy should be considered especially for patients with brain and liver metastases.

C. Therapeutic Endocrine Ablation:

1. Castration—Oophorectomy in premenopausal women with advanced, metastatic, or recurrent breast cancer results in temporary regression in about 35% of cases, with objective improvement lasting an average of about 10 months. Life is definitely prolonged in patients who respond favorably. Patients not responding to castration usually but not always fail to respond favorably to adrenalectomy, hypophysectomy, or specific hormones. Authorities differ on whether castration should be given a trial in all premenopausal women before advising bilateral adrenalectomy or hypophysectomy. Of those patients responding favorably to castration, 40–50% will respond to bilateral adrenalectomy or hypophysectomy. Of those who do not respond to oophorectomy, only 10–15% show tumor regression after one of the major procedures. According to some authorities, simultaneous oophorectomy and adrenalectomy is the palliative treatment of choice in premenopausal women with disseminated breast cancer. Prophylactic castration of all premenopausal women with breast cancer is not of proved value and is not recommended.

Castration can be performed by bilateral oophorectomy or irradiation. Surgical removal of the ovaries is preferable because it rules out the possibility of residual ovarian function. Therapeutic castration is essentially confined to premenopausal women and is of no value in truly postmenopausal women. Ovarian function may persist for a few years after cessation of menses, and this can be determined by means of the vaginal smear; if evidence of persistent estrogenic activity is found, castration may be beneficial.

2. Adrenalectomy or hypophysectomy—Regression of advanced breast cancer occurs in about 30% of patients after either of these procedures. Patients who respond to castration or to hormone administration are most likely to benefit from removal of the adrenals or pituitary. This information is helpful in the selection of patients for one of these major ablation procedures.

Adrenalectomy is preferred over hypophysectomy because of its wider availability and greater ease of postoperative endocrine management. The mortality rate of both procedures is in the range of 5%. Transphenoidal implantation (under local anesthesia) of beta ray-emitting yttrium can now be performed with low morbidity and mortality in a few centers, and destruction of the pituitary with great precision by a proton beam is a possible future mode of therapy. Currently, however, adrenalectomy is the procedure of choice in most institutions. (See Chapter 38.)

The diet following adrenalectomy should include at least 3 g of NaCl daily, which may be achieved by liberal salting of food. Adrenal insufficiency will occur if the maintenance corticosteroid regimen is inadequate or is neglected. Resulting symptoms may include extreme weakness, nausea and vomiting, rapid weight loss, and hypotension. Increased stress calls for increased dosage. Acute crises of adrenal insufficiency require immediate hospitalization and intensive treatment.

In premenopausal women, when oophorectomy alone is followed by a remission and adrenalectomy withheld until progression of the tumor resumes, the overall palliation and length of survival are possibly somewhat better than when adrenals and ovaries are removed at the same operation. Postmenopausal women should be treated by simultaneous oophorectomy and adrenalectomy.

The response of metastatic breast carcinoma to administration of hormones or to ablation of endocrine glands is most likely to be favorable under the following circumstances: (1) slowly growing tumor (eg, free interval between diagnosis and development of metastases exceeds 24 months); (2) hormone therapy is begun promptly when metastases appear; (3) metastases localized to the soft tissues, bones, and pleuropulmonary region (as opposed to visceral areas such as liver and brain); (4) advanced age; and (5) previous response to hormone therapy or castration. However, favorable responses may occur occasionally when none of these favorable conditions exist.

D. Chemotherapy: (See also Chapter 50.) Chemotherapy should be considered for palliation in advanced breast cancer when hormone treatment is not successful or when the patient becomes unresponsive to it. Chemotherapy is most likely to be effective in patients who previously responded to hormonal therapy. The most useful chemotherapeutic agent to date is fluorouracil (5-FU), but thiotepa and methotrexate are also of value. These drugs are administered intravenously. Their side-effects include bone marrow depression and nausea and vomiting, which may be so severe as to limit or prevent their use.

Intrapleural injection of methotrexate will frequently control pleural effusion due to metastases. Control of pleural effusion due to metastatic breast cancer is best achieved by trocar thoracotomy to establish closed tube drainage. When the fluid has been practically completely removed, 20 mg of methotrexate freshly dissolved in 50–100 ml of diluent are injected through the tube, which is clamped for 2 hours and then reopened to water-seal drainage. The tube is removed in 1–2 days when all the fluid has been evacuated and the lung fully expanded.

E. Hypercalcemia in Advanced Breast Cancer: Hypercalcemia occurs transiently or terminally in about 10% of women with advanced breast cancer. The serum calcium level should be determined periodically in such patients or when suggestive symptoms occur. In the great majority of cases, the cause of the elevated serum calcium is not known, but there is a possible relation to (1) immobilization of the patient by progressive invalidism, (2) radiotherapy for osseous metastases, or (3) hormonal therapy. However, hypercalcemia develops in many women without these presumed causes and in the absence of bony metastases or changes in the parathyroid glands. This supports the theory that certain disseminated breast cancers elaborate an osteolytic substance. Some breast tumors have been found to produce parathormone; others elaborate a sterol with vitamin D-like activity.

The symptoms of hypercalcemia are protean, and its course is treacherous. Initial symptoms may include irritability, lethargy, anorexia, nausea, vomiting, nocturia, and dehydration. Many of these symptoms could be attributed to disseminated tumor and hypercalcemia overlooked. Rapid deterioration, anuria, coma, and death may occur unless the hypercalcemia is corrected.

Prevention is important and consists of (1) adequate hydration (at least 2 liters of fluid per day), (2) maintenance of as much physical activity as possible, and (3) a low-calcium diet (avoidance of milk, cheese, ice cream, and vitamin D).

Treatment of hypercalcemia is based on (1) immediate cessation of any hormone therapy, (2) increasing the rate of calcium excretion in the urine by maintaining a fluid intake of 5–6 liters per day, and (3) decreasing the mobilization of calcium from the bone by administration of corticosteroids in the form of 20–100 mg of prednisone (or equivalent) daily. Disodium edetate may, be given intravenously. For acute, severe, potentially fatal elevations of serum calcium, the intravenous injection of isotonic sodium sulfate may be lifesaving. Major endocrine ablation may be required after the hypercalcemia is controlled or may be necessary (though rarely) as a control measure.

After subsidence of an episode of hypercalcemia, many patients survive for months or years with essentially the same relationship to their disease.

Prognosis

In the USA, the annual mortality rate for breast cancer is about 26 per 100,000 females. Death rates are slightly higher among the nonwhite population (92% black) than among whites through ages 45–49, but lower thereafter. Age-adjusted death rates for female breast cancer differ throughout the world. In general, reported rates are high in developed countries (with the notable exception of Japan) and are low in underdeveloped countries. Reported differences may be due in part to underdiagnosis, under-reporting, and variable certification practices.

It has been difficult to substantiate by statistical studies the clinical deduction that delay in diagnosis of breast cancer reduces the prospects for survival or cure. However, evidence now available from screening programs and from studies which consider the many complex variables involved supports the common sense position that the incidence of metastatic spread to regional nodes and beyond increases with time and that the smaller the lesion and the earlier its discovery and treatment, the better the prognosis.

Prognosis is also correlated with the number of nodes involved by metastases. By careful dissection of the surgical specimen, the pathologist can recover 10–60 axillary lymph nodes. The more thoroughly the nodes are dissected and sectioned, the higher the yield of metastases on histologic study. When no axillary nodes are involved, the 5-year survival rate following radical mastectomy is 80% or more. If 1–3 nodes are involved, the survival rate is about 60%. In patients with 4 or more positive nodes, the 5-year survival rate falls to about 30%.

The internal mammary chain is frequently invaded by carcinoma of the breast and may occasionally be the only site of metastatic spread. With both axillary and internal mammary node involvement, prognosis is very poor. The overall 10-year survival is only 10–15% in such patients regardless of treatment.

Sixty to 70% of patients with breast cancer during pregnancy or lactation already have axillary metastases, and under these circumstances the 5-year survival rate following radical mastectomy falls to 5–20%. The course of patients who have disseminated disease is usually fulminating. Interruption of pregnancy and castration seem to have little beneficial effect. However, should castration produce a remission, adrenalectomy may be of value.

The prognosis of breast cancer in an individual patient depends upon many factors including genetic background, tumor-host relationship, age, parity, clinical stage, and pathologic type. The initial mode of treatment also influences the prognosis critically in potentially curable patients, but it is becoming increasingly apparent that various treatment programs are capable of achieving equivalent results when the disease is limited to the breast and regional nodes. Physicians and institutions adopt one or another therapeutic approach which in their hands seems optimal. Prospective, randomized clinical studies which compare different forms of treatment are just now beginning to determine their relative merits and to permit choice of therapy on more statistically valid grounds.

Table 21–14 shows the results of various surgical procedures and irradiation on the 5-year survival rate.

Radical mastectomy has dominated the field for over 50 years with unsurpassed results. The prognosis following other curative procedures of all kinds may thus be usefully compared to the results of radical mastectomy as a standard. The following statistics on survival following radical mastectomy are provided as an indication of the outlook for breast cancer patients when treatment is undertaken in a clinically curable stage of the disease.

Table 21–15 illustrates a fact which is well known to clinicians. Survival for 5 years after presumably curative treatment for breast carcinoma does not necessarily indicate that the cancer has been eradicated. Patients are still at risk of dying from the disease for at least 15 and occasionally more years after treatment. This must be kept in mind when evaluating treatment results.

Patients with breast cancer must be followed for life after curative treatment for at least 2 reasons: to detect recurrences and to observe the opposite breast for development of a second carcinoma. Most of the local and distant metastases occur during the first 3 years after radical mastectomy or other curative procedure. During this period, the patient should be examined every 3–4 months. Thereafter, a follow-up examination is done every 6 months for life. Special attention is given to the opposite breast on every visit because of the increased risk in such patients of developing a second primary. A mammogram is obtained annually or whenever there is suspicion of a mass in the remaining breast.

Vast efforts and resources are now committed to

TABLE 21–15. Probability of surviving 20 years and 5 years in 1458 breast cancer patients treated by radical mastectomy for cure.

1458 Patients	Probability of Surviving	
	5 Years	20 Years
Total group	61%	41%
Axillary nodes negative	82%	63%
Axillary nodes positive		
Level I (see Table 21–8)	61%	40%
Level II	43%	30%
Level III	31%	10%
Size of tumor		
Under 1 cm	84%	74%
1–1.9 cm	82%	60%
2–2.9 cm	70%	50%
3–3.9 cm	60%	31%
4–4.9 cm	52%	30%
5–5.9 cm	40%	29%
Over 6 cm	33%	20%

the treatment of breast cancer but with discouraging results. The breast is an accessible site, easy to examine by the patient herself, by the trained medical assistant, and by the physician. Mammography by roentgenograms and newer experimental technics are capable of detecting many lesions before they are palpable. Certain groups of women are known to be at increased risk. Knowledge and methods are thus at hand for a major reduction in the mortality from this disease through education of the public and the profession in the importance of regular examination of the adult female population for breast cancer. Screening programs have proved that the diagnosis can be made earlier and in a more favorable stage through appropriate organization of health care. The indications are that medical centers, health care programs, and practicing physicians are beginning to encourage fuller use of existing information and technology in order to reduce the attrition from breast cancer.

Auchincloss H: Significance of location and number of axillary metastases in carcinoma of the breast. A justification for a conservative operation. Ann Surg 158:37–46, 1963.

Barker WF & others: Management of nonpalpable breast carcinoma discovered by mammography. Ann Surg 170:385–395, 1969.

Breast Cancer—Early and Late: A collection of papers presented at the Thirteenth Annual Clinical Conference on Cancer, 1968, at The University of Texas M.D. Anderson Hospital and Tumor Institute at Houston, Houston, Texas. Year Book, 1970.

Crile GJ: Results of simple mastectomy without irradiation in the treatment of operative stage I cancer of the breast. Ann Surg 168:330, 1968.

Crowley LG: Current status of the management of patients with endocrine-sensitive tumors. Part I. Introduction and carcinoma of the breast. California Med 110:43–60, 1969.

Egan RL: Roles of mammography in the early detection of breast cancer. Cancer 24:1197–1200, 1969.

Egan RL: *Mammography.* Thomas, 1972.

Farrow JH: Current concepts in the detection and treatment of the earliest of the early breast cancers. Cancer 25:468–477, 1970.

Fisher B & others: Effect of radiotherapy following radical mastectomy. Ann Surg 172:711–732, 1970.

Fisher B: Prospects for the control of metastases. Cancer 24:1263–1269, 1969.

Fisher B: Present status of the management of regional lymph nodes and planned clinical trials. Am J Roentgenol 111:123–129, 1971.

Gershon-Cohen J, Hermel MB: Modalities in breast cancer detection: xeroradiography, mammography, thermography, and mammometry. Cancer 24:1226–1230, 1969.

Guttman R: Role of supervoltage irradiation of regional lymph node bearing areas in breast cancer. Am J Roentgenol 95:560–564, 1966.

Haagensen CD: A great leap backward in the treatment of carcinoma of the breast. JAMA 224:1181–1183, 1973.

Haagensen CD & others: Treatment of early mammary carcinoma. A cooperative international study. Ann Surg 170:875–899, 1969.

Handley RS: Observations and thoughts on cancer of the breast. Proc Roy Soc Med 65:437, 1972.

Hertz R: The problem of possible effects of oral contraceptives on cancer of the breast. Cancer 24:1140–1145, 1969.

Kennedy BJ: Hormone therapy in inoperable breast cancer. Cancer 24:1345–1349, 1969.

Moore FD & others: Carcinoma of the breast: A decade of new results with old concepts. New England J Med 277:293–296, 343–350, 411–416, 460–468, 1967.

Seideman H: Cancer of the breast: Statistical and epidemiological data. Cancer 24:1355–1378, 1969.

Shapiro S & others: Periodic breast cancer screening in reducing mortality from breast cancer. JAMA 215:1777–1785, 1971.

Surgical treatment of breast cancer. Med Lett Drugs Ther 15:19–20, 1973.

Watson TA: Cancer of the breast. The Janeway Lecture—1965. Am J Roentgenol 96:547–559, 1966.

CARCINOMA OF THE MALE BREAST

Essentials of Diagnosis

- A painless lump beneath the areola in a man, usually over 50 years of age.
- Nipple discharge, retraction, or ulceration may occur.

General Considerations

Breast cancer in men is a rare disease; the incidence is only about 1% of that in the female. The average age at occurrence is about 60—somewhat older than the commonest presenting age in the female. The prognosis, even in stage I cases, is worse in the male than in the female. Blood-borne metastases are commonly present when the male patient appears for initial treatment. These metastases may be latent and may not become manifest for many years.

As in the female, hormonal influences are probably related to the development of male breast cancer. A high estrogen level (as in liver disease), a shift in the androgen-estrogen ratio, or an abnormal susceptibility of breast tissue to normal estrogen concentrations may be of etiologic significance.

Clinical Findings

A painless lump, occasionally associated with nipple discharge, retraction, erosion, or ulceration, is the chief complaint. Examination usually shows a hard, ill-defined, nontender mass beneath the nipple or areola. Gynecomastia not uncommonly precedes or accompanies male breast cancer.

There is a high incidence of both breast cancer and gynecomastia in Bantu males, theoretically due to failure of estrogen inactivation by a damaged liver associated with vitamin B deficiency. Breast cancer is staged in the male as in the female patient. Gynecomastia and metastatic cancer from another site (eg, prostate) must be considered in the differential diagnosis of a breast lesion in the male patient. A biopsy should be performed to settle the issue when in doubt.

Treatment

Treatment consists of radical mastectomy in operable patients, who should be chosen by the same criteria as for female breast carcinoma. Radiation therapy is also advised as in female patients according to similar indications. Irradiation is the first step in the treatment of localized metastases in the skin, lymph nodes, or skeleton which are causing symptoms.

Since male breast cancer is so frequently a disseminated disease, endocrine therapy is of considerable importance in its management. Castration in advanced breast cancer is the most successful palliative measure and is more beneficial than the same procedure in the female. Objective evidence of regression may be seen in 60–70% of male patients who are castrated—approximately twice the proportion seen in the female. The average duration of tumor growth remission is about 30 months, and life is undoubtedly prolonged. Bone is the most frequent site of metastases from breast cancer in the male (as it is in the female also), and castration relieves bone pain in the vast majority of patients so treated. The longer the interval between mastectomy and recurrence, the longer the tumor growth remission following castration. As in the female, there is no correlation between the histologic type of the tumor and the likelihood of remission following castration. In view of the marked benefits of castration in advanced disease, prophylactic castration has been suggested in stage II male breast cancer, but there is no certainty that this approach is warranted.

Bilateral adrenalectomy (or hypophysectomy) has been proposed as the procedure of choice when tumor has reactivated after castration. Corticosteroid therapy is considered by some to be more efficacious than major endocrine ablation. Male breast cancer is too rare to enable this issue to be decided in a definitive manner at this time. Either approach may be temporarily beneficial. It is probably preferable to reserve corticosteroid therapy for those patients unfit for major endocrine ablation. The recommended dosage of prednisolone or prednisone is 30 mg daily orally, increased to 100 mg daily for urgent symptoms. The dosage is reduced to 20 mg daily when control is established, but it may be necessary to increase the dosage to maintain control over a long period. The side-effects of corticosteroid therapy must be kept in mind.

Estrogen therapy—5 mg of diethylstilbestrol 3 times daily orally—may rarely be effective. Androgen therapy may exacerbate bone pain. Castration, bilateral adrenalectomy, and corticosteroids are the main lines of therapy for advanced male breast cancer.

Prognosis

The absolute 5-year survival of men with breast cancer is about 30%. Following radical mastectomy, the 5-year survival is about 40%. Huggins & Taylor (Arch Surg 70:303, 1955) reported a 5-year survival in only 5 of 14 stage I cases of male breast cancer. Palliative therapy is frequently required in this disease because of the frequency of occult metastases and its tendency to present in an advanced stage.

Cortese AF, Cornell GN: Carcinoma of the male breast. Ann Surg 173:275–280, 1971.

Holleb AI & others: Cancer of male breast. Parts I and II. New York J Med 68:544–553, 656–663, 1968.

MAMMARY DYSPLASIA

This disorder, also known as chronic cystic disease of the breast, is the most frequent lesion of the breast. It is common in women 30–50 years of age but rare in postmenopausal women, which suggests that it is related to ovarian activity. Estrogenic hormone is considered to be an etiologic factor. The typical pathologic change in the breast is the formation of cysts in the terminal ducts and acini. Cysts may be gross or microscopic. Large cysts are clinically palpable and may be several centimeters or more in diameter.

Sclerosing adenosis is a rare form of mammary dysplasia which may produce a palpable lump and a microscopic picture suggestive of cancer. It also occurs in a diffusely disseminated form consisting of multiple small foci throughout a substantial part of the breast. The microscopic appearance of sclerosing adenosis is varied. Some examples of this lesion show changes quite suggestive of cancer such as marked hyperplasia of ducts. When sclerosing adenosis occurs clinically as a palpable lump in the breast with microscopy suspicious of cancer, the differential diagnosis can be quite difficult.

Clinical Findings

Mammary dysplasia may produce an asymptomatic lump in the breast which is discovered by accident, but pain or tenderness often calls attention to the mass. In many cases, discomfort occurs or is increased during the premenstrual phase of the cycle, at which time the cysts tend to enlarge rapidly. Fluctuation in size and rapid appearance or disappearance of a breast tumor are common. Multiple or bilateral masses are not unusual, and many patients will give a history of a transient lump in the breast or cyclic breast pain. Pain, fluctuation in size, and multiplicity of lesions are the features most helpful in differentiation from carcinoma.

Treatment

Because mammary dysplasia is frequently indistinguishable from carcinoma on the basis of clinical findings, it is advisable to prepare the patient for radical mastectomy and to explore the suspicious lesion in the operating room under general anesthesia with provisions for immediate diagnosis by frozen section. Discrete cysts or small localized areas of cystic disease should be excised when cancer has been ruled out by microscopic examination. Surgery in mammary dysplasia should be conservative, since the primary objective of surgery is to exclude malignancy. Simple mastectomy or extensive removal of breast tissue is rarely, if ever, indicated.

When the diagnosis of mammary dysplasia has been established by biopsy or is practically certain because the history is classic, aspiration of a discrete mass is justifiable. The skin and overlying tissues are anesthetized by infiltration with 1% procaine, and a 20 gauge needle is introduced. If a cyst is present, typical watery fluid (straw-colored, gray, greenish, brown, or black) is easily evacuated and the mass disappears. The patient is reexamined at intervals of 2–4 weeks for 3 months and every 6 months thereafter for life. If no fluid is obtained, if a mass persists after aspiration, or if at any time during follow-up an atypical, persistent lump is noted, biopsy should be performed without delay.

Breast pain associated with generalized mammary dysplasia is best treated by avoidance of trauma and by wearing (day and night) a brassiere which gives good support and protection. Hormone therapy is not advisable because it does not cure the condition and has undesirable side-effects.

Prognosis

Exacerbations of pain, tenderness, and cyst formation may occur at any time until the menopause, when the symptoms of mammary dysplasia subside. The patient should be taught to examine her own breasts each month just after menstruation and to inform her physician if a mass appears.

Davis HH, Simons M, Davis JB: Cystic disease of the breast: Relationship to carcinoma. Cancer 17:957–978, 1964.

Fechner RE: Fibrocystic disease in women receiving oral contraceptive hormones. Cancer 25:1332–1339, 1970.

Steinhoff NG, Black WC: Florid cystic disease preceding mammary cancer. Ann Surg 171:501–508, 1970.

MAMMARY DUCT ECTASIA

This rare disorder is also sometimes called plasma cell mastitis or comedomastitis. It is characterized by dilatation of ducts, inspissation of breast secretion, and inflammation within and around the ducts and in the interstitial tissues. Plasma cells are prominent in the inflammatory reaction, which produces a focal or diffuse area of pain, tenderness, induration, and tumor.

This condition tends to occur in the fifth decade of life. The most likely cause is inspissation of lipid debris within the duct. A sterile ductal inflammation is presumably followed by escape of lipid material into surrounding stroma with resultant more widespread inflammatory reaction. This view of etiology, as opposed to a viral or bacterial cause, is supported by the fact that about half of these patients have inverted or cracked nipples or have had difficulty nursing.

Although the lesion is benign and not precancerous, it is easily mistaken for breast carcinoma because of its tendency to cause skin or nipple retraction as a result of skin fixation. Inflammatory enlargement of axillary nodes may occur to heighten the resemblance to carcinoma with metastases. In mammary duct ectasia, however, there is usually a distinguishing history of pain, tenderness, and redness which suggests that the breast induration is due to inflammation. Nevertheless, biopsy will usually be necessary to differentiate mammary duct ectasia from cancer.

FIBROADENOMA OF THE BREAST

This common benign neoplasm occurs most frequently in young women, usually within 20 years after puberty. It is somewhat more frequent and tends to occur at an earlier age in black than in white women. Multiple tumors in one or both breasts are found in 10–15% of patients.

The typical fibroadenoma is a round, firm, discrete, relatively movable, nontender mass 1–5 cm in diameter. The tumor is usually discovered accidentally. Clinical diagnosis in young patients is usually not difficult. In women over 30, mammary dysplasia and carcinoma must be considered. Fibroadenoma does not normally occur after the menopause, but postmenopausal women may occasionally develop fibroadenoma after administration of estrogenic hormone.

Treatment in all cases is excision and frozen section to determine if the lesion is cancerous.

Cystosarcoma phyllodes is a type of fibroadenoma with cellular stroma which tends to grow rapidly. This tumor may become quite large, and if inadequately excised will recur locally. The lesion is rarely malignant. Treatment is by local excision of the mass with a margin of surrounding breast tissue.

INTRADUCTAL PAPILLOMA & NIPPLE DISCHARGE

Intraductal papilloma is a rare benign lesion arising from the ducts of the breast. The lesion is usually single and located in the region of the nipple, but multiple papillomas may occur throughout the breast. Papillomas are usually small, soft, and fragile, supported by filamentous fibrous trabeculae. They infrequently become large and may reach 4–5 cm in diameter. It may be difficult to distinguish intraductal papilloma from cancer on frozen section, and this difficulty increases with the size and complexity of the lesion. Malignant change in intraductal papilloma is very rare. Nipple discharge, which may or may not be bloody, is the commonest complaint associated with papilloma. A mass near the nipple is present in most patients, and pressure at this location usually causes a discharge from the nipple.

In order of decreasing frequency, the following lesions produce nipple discharge: intraductal papilloma, carcinoma, mammary dysplasia, and ectasia of the ducts. The discharge is usually serous or bloody. When papilloma or cancer is the cause, a tumor can frequently be palpated beneath or close to the areola.

The site of the duct orifice from which the fluid exudes is a guide to the location of the involved duct. Gentle pressure on the breast is made with the fingertip at successive points around the circumference of the areola (Fig 21–10). A point will be found at which pressure produces discharge. The dilated duct or a small tumor may be palpable here. The involved area should be excised by a meticulous technic that ensures removal of the affected duct and breast tissue immediately adjacent to it. If a tumor is present, it should be biopsied and a frozen section done to determine whether cancer is present. When localization is not possible and no mass is palpable, the patient should be reexamined at intervals of 1–3 months. When unilateral discharge persists, even without definite localization or tumor, exploration must be considered. The alternative is careful continued follow-up at intervals of 1–3 months. Mammography should be done. Cytologic examination of nipple discharge for exfoliated cancer cells is occasionally helpful in differential diagnosis.

Although none of the benign lesions causing nipple discharge are precancerous, they may coexist with cancer, and it is not possible to distinguish them definitely from malignancy on clinical grounds. Patients with carcinoma almost always have a palpable mass, but in rare instances a nipple discharge may be the only sign. For these reasons, chronic nipple discharge is usually an indication for exploration of the breast.

Atkins H, Wolff B: Discharges from the nipple. Brit J Surg 51:602–606, 1964.

Forrest H: Intraduct papilloma of the breast. Brit J Surg 53:1028–1032, 1966.

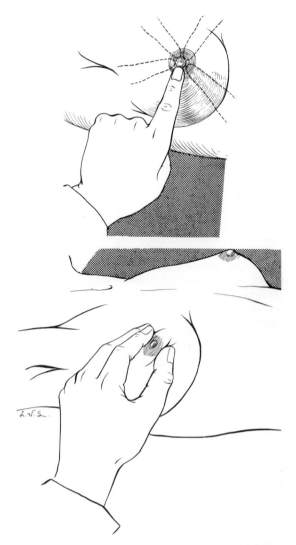

FIG 21–10. In patients with nipple discharge, the involved duct can usually be localized by fingertip pressure at successive points around the areola.

Funderburk WW, Syphax B: Evaluation of nipple discharge in benign and malignant disease. Cancer 24:1290–1296, 1969.

FAT NECROSIS

Fat necrosis is a rare lesion of the breast but is of clinical importance because it produces a mass, often accompanied by skin or nipple retraction, which is indistinguishable from carcinoma. Trauma is presumed to be the cause, although only about half of patients give a history of injury to the breast. Ecchymosis is occasionally seen near the tumor. Tenderness may be present. If untreated, the mass associated with fat necrosis gradually disappears. As a rule, the safest course is to obtain a biopsy. When carcinoma has been ruled out, the area of involvement should be excised.

BREAST ABSCESS

During nursing, an area of redness, tenderness, and induration not infrequently develops in the breast. In the early stages, the infection can often be reversed by discontinuing breast feeding and administering an antibiotic. If the lesion progresses to form a localized mass with increasing signs of infection, an abscess is present and should be drained.

A subareolar abscess may develop in a young or middle-aged woman who is not lactating. These infections tend to recur after incision and drainage unless the area is explored in a quiescent interval with excision of the involved collecting ducts at the base of the nipple.

Except for the subareolar types of abscess, infection in the breast is very rare unless the patient is lactating. Therefore, findings suggestive of abscess in the nonlactating breast require incision and biopsy of any indurated tissue. (See also Mammary Duct Ectasia, above.)

Benson EA, Goodman MA: An evaluation of the use of stilbesterol and antibiotics in the early management of acute puerperal breast abscess. Brit J Surg 57:255–258, 1970.

Benson EA, Goodman MA: Incision with primary suture in the treatment of acute puerperal breast abscess. Brit J Surg 57:55–58, 1970.

Habif DV & others: Subareolar abscess associated with squamous metaplasia of lactiferous ducts. Am J Surg 119:523–526, 1970.

GYNECOMASTIA

Hypertrophy of the male breast may result from a variety of causes. Pubertal hypertrophy is very common during adolescence and is characterized by a tender discoid enlargement 2–3 cm in diameter beneath the areola with hypertrophy of the breast. The changes are usually bilateral and subside spontaneously within a year in the majority of cases.

Men between 50 and 70 occasionally develop hypertrophy (often unilateral) similar to that occurring at puberty.

Certain organic diseases may be associated with gynecomastia: cirrhosis of the liver, hyperthyroidism, Addison's disease, testicular tumors (especially chorioepithelioma), and adrenocortical tumors.

If there is uncertainty about the diagnosis of the breast lesion, a biopsy should be done to rule out cancer. Otherwise, the treatment of gynecomastia is nonsurgical unless the patient insists on excision for cosmetic reasons. In this case, at least 2 years should be allowed before operation for possible subsidence.

Levy DM & others: Gynecomastia. Postgrad Med 36:234–241, 1964.

• • •

General References

Ackerman LV, Del Regato JA: *Cancer–Diagnosis, Treatment, and Prognosis,* 3rd ed. Mosby, 1963.

Benfield JR: National surgical breast project. California Med 118:5–9, March 1973.

Haagensen CD: *Diseases of the Breast.* Saunders, 1956.

Spratt JS Jr, Donegan WL: *Cancer of the Breast.* Saunders, 1967.

Stoll BA: *Hormonal Management in Breast Cancer.* Lippincott, 1969.

22 . . .

The Respiratory Tract, Pleura, & Mediastinum

Arthur N. Thomas, MD

ANATOMY OF THE CHEST & PLEURA

The chest wall is an air-tight, expandable, cone-shaped cage. Lung ventilation is accomplished by the generation of negative pressure within it by simultaneous expansion of the rib cage and downward diaphragmatic excursion.

The ventral wall of the bony thorax is the shortest dimension. It extends from the suprasternal notch to the xiphoid—a distance of approximately 18 cm. It is formed by the vertically aligned manubrium, sternum, and xiphoid and the costal cartilages of the first 10 ribs. The sides of the chest wall consist of the upper 10 ribs, which slope downward and forward from their posterior attachments. The posterior chest wall is formed by the 12 thoracic vertebrae, their transverse processes, and the 12 ribs (Fig 22–1). The upper ventral portion of the thoracic cage is covered by the clavicle and subclavian vessels. Laterally, it is covered by the shoulder and axillary nerves and vessels; dorsally, it is covered by the scapula.

The superior aperture of the thorax (also called either the thoracic inlet or the thoracic outlet), is a 5 X 10 cm kidney-shaped opening bounded by the first costal cartilages and ribs laterally, the manubrium anteriorly, and the body of the first thoracic vertebra posteriorly. The inferior aperture of the thorax is bounded by the twelfth vertebra and ribs posteriorly and the cartilages of the seventh to twelfth ribs and the xiphisternal joint anteriorly. It is much wider than the superior aperture and is occupied by the diaphragm.

The blood supply and innervation of the chest wall is via the intercostal vessels and nerves (Figs 22–2 and 22–3), but the upper thorax also receives vessels and nerves from the cervical and axillary regions.

The parietal pleura is the innermost lining of the chest wall and is divided into 4 parts: the cervical pleura (cupola), costal pleura, mediastinal pleura, and diaphragmatic pleura. The visceral pleura is the serous layer investing the lungs and joins the parietal pleura at the hilus of the lung. The pleural space is compressed to a capillary gap and normally contains only a few drops of serous fluid. This space may be enlarged when fluid (hydrothorax), blood (hemothorax), pus (pyothorax or empyema), or air (pneumothorax) is present.

PHYSIOLOGY OF THE CHEST WALL & PLEURA

Mechanics of Respiration*

Breathing entails expansion of thoracic volume by elevation of the rib cage and descent of the diaphragm. The former predominates in men and the latter in women. In infants, because the ribs have not yet assumed their oblique contour, diaphragmatic breathing is required to provide sufficient ventilation.

Expiration is mainly passive and depends upon elastic recoil of the lungs. With deep breathing, the abdominal musculature contracts and pulls the rib cage downward and simultaneously elevates the diaphragm by compressing the abdominal viscera against it.

Wade OL: Movements of the thoracic cage and diaphragm in respiration. J Physiol 124:193, 1954.

Physiology of the Pleural Space (See Fig 22–4.)

A. Pressure: The pleural cavity pressure is normally negative due to the elastic recoil of the lung and chest wall. During quiet respiration, it varies from −15 cm water with inspiration to 0–2 cm water during expiration. Deep breathing may cause large pressure changes (eg, −60 cm water during forced inspiration to +30 cm water during vigorous expiration). Because of gravity, pleural pressure at the apex is more negative when the body is erect and changes about 0.2 cm water per centimeter of vertical height.

B. Fluid Formation and Reabsorption: Transudation and absorption of fluid within the pleural space normally follow the Starling equation, which depends on hydrostatic, colloid, and tissue pressures. The net pressure is equal to approximately a 10 cm water drive of fluid into the pleural space, from the parietal pleura toward the visceral pleura and into the capillaries.

In health, pleural fluid is low in protein (100 mg/100 ml). When it increases in disease to about 1 g/100 ml, the net colloid osmotic pressure of the visceral pleural capillaries is equalled and pleural fluid reabsorption becomes dependent on lymphatic drainage. Thus, abnormal amounts of pleural fluid may accumulate (1) when hydrostatic pressure is increased, such as in heart failure; (2) when capillary permeability

---

*Pulmonary physiology and ventilation are described in Chapter 3.

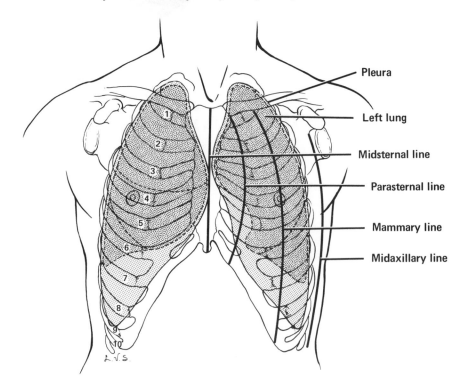

FIG 22–1. The thorax, showing rib cage, pleura, and lung fields.

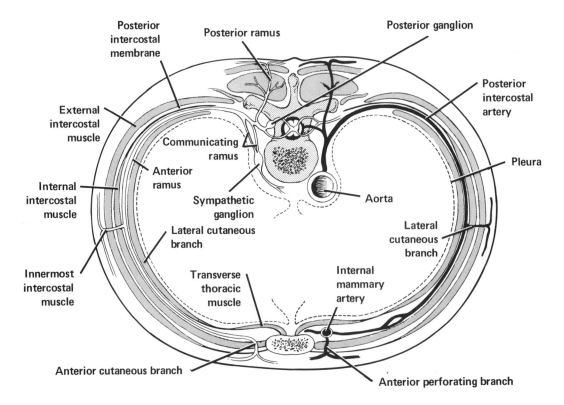

FIG 22–2. Transverse section of thorax.

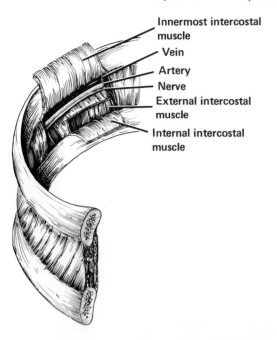

Innermost intercostal muscle

Vein

Artery

Nerve

External intercostal muscle

Internal intercostal muscle

FIG 22–3. Intercostal muscles, vessels, and nerves.

is increased, as in inflammatory or neoplastic disease; or (3) when colloid osmotic pressure is decreased.

Rutishauser WJ & others: Pleural pressures at dorsal and ventral sites in supine and prone body positions. J Appl Physiol 21:1500, 1966.

Stewart PB: The rate of formation and lymphatic removal of fluid in pleural effusions. J Clin Invest 42:258, 1963.

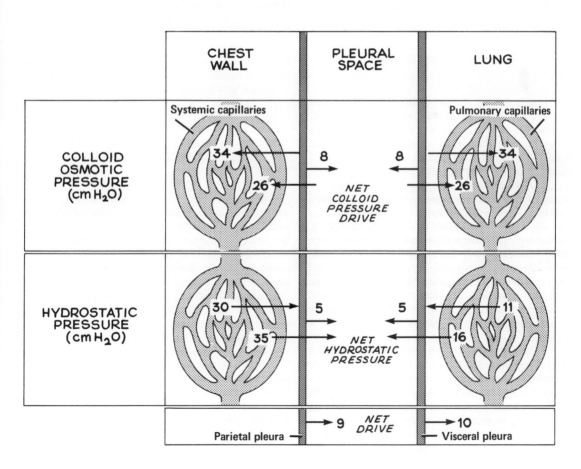

FIG 22–4. Movement of fluid across the pleural space, showing production and absorption of pleural fluid.

DISEASES OF THE CHEST WALL

Defects of development are described in Chapter 49. Neuromuscular syndromes of the inlet or shoulder are described in Chapter 39.

LUNG HERNIA (PNEUMATOCELE)

Pneumatocele or herniation of the lung can occur through defects in the chest wall caused by abnormal development, trauma, or surgery. Most lung hernias are thoracic in location, but cervical (defect of Sibson's fascia) or diaphragmatic herniation may occasionally occur. They are usually asymptomatic, but some patients experience local tenderness, pain, or mild dyspnea. Diagnosis is based on physical examination.

Although treatment has included various truss-like devices, operative repair is best if symptoms are present.

Shocket E, Hudseon TR: Lung hernia. Indust Med 26:556, 1957.

CHEST WALL INFECTIONS

Infections that appear to involve only the skin may actually represent outward extensions of deeper infection of the ribs, cartilage, sternum, or even the pleural space (empyema necessitatis). Inadequate drainage of superficial infection can lead to inward extension into the pleural space, causing empyema.

Subpectoral abscess is caused by suppurative adenitis of the axillary lymph nodes, rib or pleural infection, or posterior extension of a breast abscess, or may occur as a complication of chest wall surgery (eg, mastectomy, pacemaker placement). Hemolytic streptococci and *Staphylococcus aureus* are the usual organisms. The patient appears septic and the pectoral region is red and swollen, obliterating the normal infraclavicular depression. Shoulder movement is painful. Treatment consists of antibiotics and drainage by an incision along the lateral border of the pectoralis major muscle.

Subscapular abscess may arise from osteomyelitis of the scapula but most commonly follows thoracic operations such as thoracotomy or thoracoplasty. Winging of the scapula or paravertebral bulging of the trapezius muscle is usually present. The pus collection can be made more apparent by the bulge produced in adjacent soft tissues when the scapula is pressed against the chest wall. A pleural communication is suggested if a cough impulse is present or if the size of the mass varies with position or direct pressure. The diagnosis is

established by needle aspiration. Treatment consists of open drainage for pyogenic infections not involving the pleura. Tuberculosis should be treated by chemotherapy and drainage, which can sometimes be accomplished by needle aspiration.

INFECTIONS OF THE THORACIC CAGE

Sternal Osteomyelitis

Infection of the sternum now most commonly follows sternotomy incisions and presents as a postoperative wound infection or mediastinitis. Various gram-positive cocci and gram-negative bacilli have been isolated in individual cases. Treatment consists of antibiotics and either open drainage or closed drainage plus irrigation with antibiotic solution. In some cases, resection of involved sternum and a margin of adjacent normal bone is necessary.

Sanfelippo PM, Danielson GK: Complications associated with median sternotomy. J Thoracic Cardiovas Surg 63:419, 1972.

Osteomyelitis of the Ribs

In the past, osteomyelitis of the ribs was often caused by typhoid fever and tuberculosis. Except for a few cases in children, hematogenous osteomyelitis of the ribs is uncommon today. Most rib infections now occur as complications of thoracotomy incisions or occur in ribs adjacent to a draining empyema.

INFECTION OF THE COSTAL CARTILAGES & XIPHOID

Costal cartilage infections are relatively unresponsive to antibiotic therapy because once perichondral vascularity is interrupted the cartilage dies and remains as a foreign body to perpetuate the infection and sinus tract formation. The infection may be established during the course of septicemia, but the most common cause is direct extension of other surgical infections (eg, wound infection, subphrenic abscess). Surgical division of costal cartilages, as in a thoracoabdominal incision, may predispose to cartilage infection postoperatively if local sepsis develops. A wide variety of organisms have been implicated.

Pain, swelling, and erythema of overlying skin and subcutaneous tissue may be marked. This may be followed by fluctuance, spontaneous drainage, and sinuses which chronically discharge pus. The course may be fulminant or may be indolent over months or years with periodic exacerbations. There may be an associated osteomyelitis of the sternum, ribs, or clavicle.

The differential diagnosis includes local bone or cartilage tumors, Tietze's syndrome, chest wall metastasis, eroding aortic aneurysm, and bronchocutaneous fistula.

As a rule, the upper 5 costal cartilages (Fig 22–1) articulate separately with the sternum, but the sixth through the tenth cartilages are contiguous. Therefore, when one of the upper 5 costal cartilages is involved, local excision will usually suffice; but when cartilages 6 through 10 are involved, removal of the entire costal arch is usually required. If adjacent osteomyelitis is present, only grossly diseased bone need be excised.

Cure can be expected if surgery removes all the infected cartilage, but in many instances recurrence is prompt due to underestimation of the extent of the disease and inadequate resection.

Wilcox RE: Costal chondritis with associated osteomyelitis. J Thoracic Cardiovas Surg 49:210, 1965.

TIETZE'S SYNDROME

Tietze's syndrome is a painful nonsuppurative inflammation of costochondral cartilages of unknown cause. It affects adults of either sex. Local tenderness is the only symptom. The mass and tenderness eventually disappear without therapy. The syndrome may recur from time to time.

Treatment is symptomatic and may include analgesics and local or systemic corticosteroids. When symptoms persist longer than 3 weeks and tumefaction suggests neoplasm, excision of the involved cartilage may be indicated and is usually curative.

Wehrmacher WH: Significance of Tietze's syndrome in differential diagnosis of chest pain. JAMA 157:505, 1955.

MONDOR'S DISEASE
(Thrombophlebitis of the Thoracoepigastric Vein)

Mondor's disease consists of localized thrombophlebitis of the anterolateral chest wall. It is more common in women than in men and occasionally follows radical mastectomy. There are few symptoms other than the presence of a tender cord-like structure in the subcutaneous tissues of the abdomen, thorax, or axilla. The disease is self-limited and devoid of complications such as thromboembolism.

Abramson DJ: Mondor's disease and string phlebitis. JAMA 196:1087, 1966.

CHEST WALL TUMORS

Except for those of the breast, primary tumors of the chest wall are all sarcomas; carcinoma in this area not of breast origin is always metastatic. Only about 5–8% of skeletal and soft tissue tumors that occur in man involve the chest wall.

Most soft tissue tumors of the chest wall are benign, whereas half of skeletal tumors are malignant; most of the latter represent metastases from remote primaries. Benign tumors often occur in young adults; primary malignant tumors during middle age; and metastatic tumors in elderly people. Tumors in this area occur more often in males than females.

Classification

Tumors of the chest wall (excluding skin and breast) may be classified as follows:
  A. **Tumors of Soft Tissues:**
    1. **Benign**—Lipoma, neurolemmoma, neurofibroma, cavernous hemangioma, lymphangioma.
    2. **Malignant**—Fibrosarcoma, desmoid, neurofibrosarcoma, liposarcoma, leiomyosarcoma.
  B. **Primary Bony (Skeletal) Tumors:**
    1. **Benign**—Osteochondromas, fibrous dysplasia, eosinophilic granuloma, hemangioma, etc.
    2. **Malignant**—Chondrosarcoma, osteosarcoma, plasmacytoma (solitary), Ewing's sarcoma, reticulum cell sarcoma.
  C. **Metastatic Tumors (Usually Skeletal):** Lung, breast, prostate, kidney, stomach, uterus, colon.

Clinical Findings

A. Symptoms and Signs: Many tumors are asymptomatic and are first noted on a routine chest x-ray. When symptomatic, they present with local swelling or pain. In general, pain is more often associated with malignancy.

B. Laboratory Findings: There are no diagnostic findings on blood count, urinalysis, serum calcium, acid or alkaline phosphatase, or bone marrow biopsy. Radioactive ^{85}Sr or other bone scans may be useful to localize tumors not visible by ordinary roentgenographic studies.

C. X-Ray Findings: X-rays may be valuable for detection, diagnosis, or evaluation of tumors, but the diagnosis usually depends on complete histologic study.

D. Biopsy: Incisional biopsy or needle biopsy may not recover tissue representative of the most malignant portion of the tumor, and seeding of the adjacent soft tissue with malignant tumor cells sometimes occurs. Therefore, whenever possible, wide excisional biopsy is preferred.

Differential Diagnosis

Chest wall tumors may be simulated by enlarged

costal cartilages, chest wall infections, fractures, rickets, scurvy, hyperparathyroidism, and other conditions.

Specific Neoplasms

A. Benign Soft Tissue Tumors:

1. Lipomas–Lipomas are the most common benign tumors of the chest wall. Occasionally they are very large, lobulated, and may have dumbbell-shaped extensions that indent the endothoracic fascia beneath the sternum through a vertebral foramen. They may on occasion communicate with a large mediastinal or supraclavicular component.

2. Neurogenic tumors–These may arise from intercostal or superficial nerves. Solitary neurofibromas are most common, followed by neurolemmomas.

3. Cavernous hemangiomas–Hemangiomas of the thoracic wall are usually painful and occur in children. They may be isolated tumors or may involve other tissues (eg, lung), suggesting Rendu-Osler-Weber syndrome.

4. Lymphangiomas–This rare lesion is seen most often in children. It may have poorly defined borders that make complete excision difficult.

B. Malignant Soft Tissue Tumors:

1. Fibrosarcomas–Fibrosarcoma is the most common primary soft tissue malignancy of the chest wall. It is most common in young adults.

2. Liposarcomas–These tumors account for approximately one-third of all primary malignancies of the chest wall. They occur more often in men.

3. Neurofibrosarcomas–Neurofibrosarcomas involve the thoracic wall almost twice as often as other parts of the body. They often occur in patients with Recklinghausen's disease and usually originate from intercostal nerves.

C. Benign Skeletal Tumors:

1. Chondromas, osteochondromas, and myxochondromas–The combined frequency of these 3 cartilaginous tumors is nearly the same as that of fibrous dysplasia (ie, they comprise about 30–45% of all benign skeletal tumors). Cartilaginous tumors are usually single and occur with equal frequency in males and females between childhood and the fourth decade. The tumors are usually painless and tend to occur anteriorly along the costal margin or in the parasternal area. Wide local excision is curative.

2. Fibrous dysplasia–Fibrous dysplasia (bone cyst, osteofibroma, fibrous osteoma, fibrosis ossificans) accounts for a third or more of benign skeletal tumors of the chest wall. This cystic bone tumor can occur in any portion of the skeletal system, but approximately half involve the ribs. They must be clinically differentiated from cystic bone lesions associated with hyperparathyroidism. The tumor is usually single and may be related to trauma. Some patients complain of swelling, tenderness, or vague pain or discomfort, but the lesion is usually silent and is detected on routine chest x-ray. Treatment consists of local excision.

3. Eosinophilic granuloma–Eosinophilic granu-

loma may occur in the clavicle, scapula, or (rarely) in the sternum. It often represents a more benign form of Letterer-Siwe disease or Hand-Schüller-Christian syndrome. The patient may have fever, malaise, leukocytosis, eosinophilia, or bone pain. Rib involvement presents as an expansile lesion with cortical bone destruction and periosteal new growth. The clinical picture can resemble osteomyelitis or Ewing's sarcoma. When the disease is localized, excision will result in cure.

4. Hemangioma–Cavernous hemangioma of the ribs presents as a painful mass in infancy or childhood. The tumor appears on x-ray as either multiple radiolucent areas or a single trabeculated cyst.

5. Miscellaneous–Fibromas, lipomas, osteomas, and aneurysmal bone cysts are all relatively rare lesions of the skeletal chest wall. The diagnosis is established after excisional biopsy.

D. Malignant Skeletal Tumors:

1. Chondrosarcomas–Chondrosarcomas are the most common primary malignant tumors of the chest wall. About 15–20% of all skeletal chondrosarcomas occur in the ribs or sternum. Most appear in patients 20–40 years of age. They tend to occur anteriorly at the costochondral junction of the rib cage but may occur anywhere along the rib. Local involvement of pleura, adjacent ribs, muscle, diaphragm, or other soft tissue may develop. There may be pain, but most patients complain only of the mass. Chest x-ray shows destroyed cortical bone, usually with diffuse mottled calcification, and the border of the tumor is indistinct. Treatment consists of wide radical excision. Only occasionally are regional lymph nodes involved. The 5-year survival rate is 10–30%, depending largely upon the adequacy of the initial excision.

2. Osteosarcoma (osteogenic sarcoma)–Osteosarcoma occurs in the second and third decades, and 60% occur in males. It is more malignant than chondrosarcoma. X-ray findings consist of bone destruction and recalcification at right angles to the bony cortex which gives the characteristic "sunburst" appearance. Hematogenous metastasis with pulmonary involvement is common. Treatment is by radical local excision, but the prognosis is poor and 5-year survivals are rare.

3. Myeloma (solitary plasmacytomas)–These tumors are often found as a manifestation of systemic multiple myeloma, and patients with myeloma of the chest wall usually develop manifestations of systemic disease. The roentgenographic findings are punched-out, osteolytic lesions without evidence of new bone formation. The disease affects adults in the fifth to seventh decades and is seen nearly twice as often in males as in females. Solitary myeloma is quite rare, and systemic involvement eventually occurs in all cases. Treatment with antimetabolites relieves bone pain, although life is not prolonged. The 5-year survival rate is only about 5%.

4. Ewing's sarcoma (hemangioendothelioma, endothelioma)–Ewing's tumors are associated with systemic symptoms such as fever and malaise and, locally, a painful, warm chest wall mass. Roentgenographic

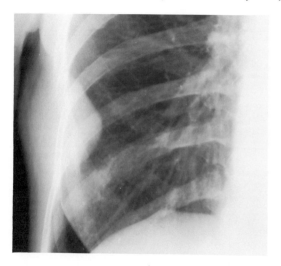

FIG 22–5. Rib metastasis and extrapleural mass from leiomyosarcoma of the uterus.

findings often show a characteristic "onion skin" calcification. These tumors are highly malignant, and evidence of other skeletal lesions is present in 30–75% when first seen. The diagnosis should be established by needle biopsy since surgical excision does not improve survival. X-ray irradiation is the only treatment available. Survival for as long as 5 years is rare.

5. Lymphoma–The diagnosis and treatment of chest wall lymphomas are essentially the same as for those lesions found elsewhere in the body.

E. Metastatic Chest Wall Tumors: Metastases to bones of the thorax are often multiple and are usually from tumors of the kidney, thyroid, lung, breast, prostate, stomach, uterus, or colon (Fig 22–5). Involvement by direct extension occurs in carcinoma of the breast and lung. Some cases of lung carcinoma involving the chest wall by direct extension have been cured by radical resection.

Groff DB III, Adkins PC: Chest wall tumors: A collective review. Ann Thoracic Surg 4:260, 1967.

Ochsner A Jr, Lucas GL, McFarland GB Jr: Tumors of the thoracic skeleton: Review of 134 cases. J Thoracic Cardiovas Surg 52:311, 1966.

Omell GH & others: Chest wall tumors. Radiol Clin North America 11:197–214, 1973.

Teitelbaum SL: Twenty years' experience with intrinsic tumors of the bony thorax at a large institution. J Thoracic Cardiovas Surg 63:776, 1972.

Teitelbaum SL: Twenty years' experience with soft tissue sarcomas of the chest wall in a large institution. J Thoracic Cardiovas Surg 63:585, 1972.

Vieta JO, Maier HC: Tumors of the sternum: Collective review. Internat Abstr Surg 114:513, 1962.

DISEASES OF THE PLEURA

The most common symptom of pleural disease is **pleuritic pain**–chest pain associated with respiratory excursion which sometimes reflexly inhibits respiration. Pleural pain is mediated through nerves to the parietal pleura or diaphragm since the visceral pleura does not contain pain fibers. When pulmonary processes become painful, it indicates involvement of both the visceral and parietal pleura. Pleuritic pain is felt in the shoulder over the distribution of the third through fifth cervical segments. Diseases involving the pleural surfaces can also produce an audible friction rub on auscultation. Both pleuritic pain and friction rubs may diminish if a pleural effusion forms.

Respiratory movement may lag on the affected side. Fullness or even bulging may appear with effusion. Long-standing pleural disease can even cause contraction and immobility of the involved hemithorax. The intercostal spaces are narrowed, and the ribs have a shingled relationship. Acute inflammation of the pleura may be associated with tenderness of the intercostal spaces or, in advanced cases, with swelling, redness, and local warmth. Tactile fremitus to the spoken voice is diminished with effusion, and there is dullness to percussion. Breath sounds may be exaggerated, bronchial, or amphoric in quality over a lung compressed by pleural effusion.

PLEURAL EFFUSIONS

The term pleural effusion denotes endogenous fluid in the pleural space. A more exact terminology is used when the character of the fluid is known. **Hydrothorax** denotes serous effusions, either transudates or exudates. **Pyothorax (empyema), hemothorax,** and **chylothorax** are other categories. These are discussed separately below.

Pleural effusions may occur with disease of the lungs, mediastinum, or chest wall. Identification of the specific type of effusion often depends on examination of fluid obtained by thoracentesis (Table 22–1). If this procedure is unsuccessful, either needle or open pleural biopsy must be considered.

Transudates have a specific gravity less than 1.016 and a protein content of less than 3 g/100 ml. Transudates contain only a few cells and are most often clear and yellow but occasionally are blood-tinged. Transudates occur in congestive heart failure, nephritis, and cirrhosis of the liver. Exudates may look clear, cloudy, or bloody. Examination of sediment after centrifugation may show such things as tumor cells, bacteria, fungi, tubercle bacilli, or parasites such as amebas.

Committee on Therapy, American Thoracic Society: Therapy of pleural effusion. Am Rev Resp Dis 97:479, 1968.

TABLE 22–1. Differential diagnosis of pleural effusions.*

	Tuberculosis	Malignancy	Congestive Failure	Pneumonia and Other Non-tuberculous Infections	Rheumatoid Arthritis and Collagen Disease	Pulmonary Embolism
Clinical context	Younger patient with history of exposure to tuberculosis.	Older patient in poor general health.	Presence of congestive failure.	Presence of respiratory infection.	History of joint involvement; subcutaneous nodules.	Postoperative, immobilized, or venous disease.
Gross appearance	Usually serous; often sanguineous.	Often sanguineous.	Serous.	Serous.	Turbid or yellow-green.	Often sanguineous.
Microscopic examination	May be positive for acid-fast bacilli; cholesterol crystals.	Cytology positive in 50%.	. . .	May be positive for bacilli.	. . .	. . .
Cell count	Few have > 10,000 erythrocytes; most have > 1000 leukocytes, mostly lymphocytes.	Two-thirds bloody; 40% > 1000 leukocytes, mostly lymphocytes.	Few have > 10,000 erythrocytes or > 1000 leukocytes.	Polymorphonuclears predominate.	Lymphocytes predominate.	Erythrocytes predominate.
Culture	Many have positive pleural effusion; few have positive sputum or gastric washings.	. . .	. . .	May be positive.	. . .	. . .
Specific gravity	Most > 1.016.	Most > 1.016.	Most < 1.016.	> 1.016.	> 1.016.	> 1.016.
Protein	90% 3 g/100 ml or more.	90% 3 g/100 ml or more.	75% < 3 g/100 ml.	3 g/100 ml or more.	3 g/100 ml or more.	3 g/100 ml or more.
Sugar	60% < 60 mg/100 ml.	Rarely < 60 mg/100 ml.	. . .	Occasionally 60 mg/100 ml.	5–17 mg/100 ml (rheumatoid arthritis).	. . .
Other	No mesothelial cells on cytology. Tuberculin test usually positive.	If hemorrhagic fluid, 65% will be due to tumor; tends to recur after removal.	Right-sided in 55–70%.	Associated with infiltrate on x-ray.	Rapid clotting time; LE cell or rheumatoid factor may be present.	Source of emboli may be noted.

Other transudates: (Sp gr > 1.016.)

    Fungal infection: Exposure in endemic area. Serous fluid. Microscopy and culture may be positive for fungi. Protein 3 g/100 ml or more. Skin and serologic tests may be helpful.

    Trauma: Serosanguineous fluid. Protein 3 g/100 ml or more.

    Chylothorax: History of injury or cancer. Chylous fluid with no protein but with fat droplets.

*Modified from Therapy of pleural effusion: A statement by the Committee on Therapy of the American Thoracic Society. Am Rev Resp Dis 97:479, 1968.

PLEURAL EFFUSION FROM NONPULMONARY DISEASES

Immunologic Diseases

Systemic lupus erythematosus is associated with pleural effusion in about half of cases. Only 10% represent isolated pleural involvement, and these are usually small (though they may be massive). In about 30–50% of cases, the heart is enlarged on x-ray.

Pleural effusion in patients with rheumatoid arthritis occurs almost exclusively in middle-aged men. The effusions are usually unilateral and involve the right side somewhat more often than the left. There appears to be no relationship between the pulmonary manifestations of rheumatoid disease and pleural effusion.

Cardiovascular Diseases

Pleural effusion is seen in constrictive pericarditis and congestive heart failure (Fig 22–6). The right side alone is most often affected, though the effusion may be bilateral. Fluid occasionally localizes in interlobar fissures, giving "phantom tumors" or "disappearing tumors." Interlobar effusions involve the right horizontal fissure in most cases but may be bilateral.

Pancreatitis

Pleural effusion secondary to pancreatitis usually affects only the left side but sometimes is on the right. The diagnosis rests on finding an amylase concentration in the fluid substantially above that in the serum.

Meigs' Syndrome

Meigs' syndrome (ascites and hydrothorax) was

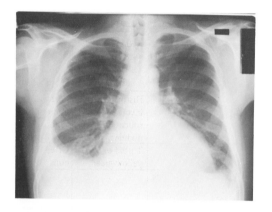

FIG 22–6. Pleural effusion secondary to heart failure (myocarditis).

first described in patients with fibroma of the ovary. Since then, a wide variety of pelvic tumors such as fibromas, thecomas, granulosa cell tumors, Brenner tumors, cystadenomas, adenocarcinomas, and fibromyomas of the uterus have also been implicated. Removal of the pelvic tumor is invariably followed by clearing of both effusions.

Cirrhosis of the Liver

Right-sided hydrothorax occurs in about 5% of patients with cirrhosis and ascites.

Renal Disease

Hydronephrosis, nephrotic syndrome, and acute glomerulonephritis are sometimes associated with hydrothorax.

Thromboembolic Disease

Pleural effusion following pulmonary embolism is usually serosanguineous and may be grossly bloody. These effusions are occasionally massive but usually are small and associated with characteristic x-ray findings in the lung. Treatment of the pleural effusion is usually not necessary, and the fluid is reabsorbed in a few days.

MALIGNANT PLEURAL EFFUSION

About half of all patients with carcinoma of the breast or lung develop pleural effusion during the course of their disease, and 25% of all effusions are the result of malignancy. Cytologic examination of pleural fluid is positive in 70% and pleural biopsy in 80% of malignant effusions. A definitive diagnosis is nearly always achieved by using both procedures if needed.

About 10% of malignant effusions are due to pleural mesotheliomas and the rest to metastatic tumors. About half of bilateral effusions associated with normal heart size are due to malignancy, and these are invariably associated with hepatic metastases.

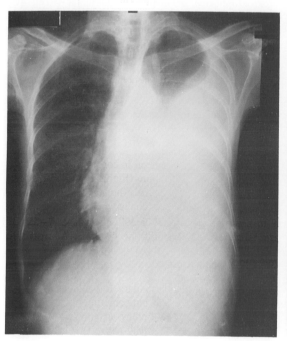
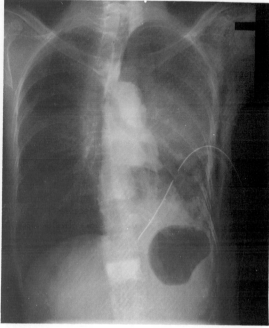

FIG 22–7. Malignant pleural effusion (carcinoma of lung). *Left:* Posteroanterior projection before treatment. *Right:* After chest tube drainage. Note left hilar mass and osteoblastic metastasis to the first lumbar vertebra.

The clinical findings are pleuritic pain, cough, fever, chest pain, and weakness.

Treatment

Multiple technics are used to treat malignant pleural effusions (Fig 22–7). The usual objective is to obtain full lung expansion and pleural synthesis so that the effusion does not recur. The most commonly used regimens are closed tube drainage for 4–7 days, with or without instillation of a sclerosing solution (eg, mechlorethamine) into the pleural space. Thoracentesis or tube drainage may be complicated by pneumothorax, fever, fluid loculation, and infection. Only rarely are thoracotomy, pleurectomy, and other aggressive surgical approaches indicated.

Prognosis

Recurrence of the effusion is inevitable after needle aspiration alone but drops to 15% in patients treated by tube drainage. However, the overall prognosis is very poor. The average duration of life in patients with malignant effusions due to solid tumors is about 6 months; with lymphomas, the average duration is 16 months.

Dollinger MR: Management of recurrent malignant effusions. CA 22:138–147, 1972.

Lambert CJ & others: The treatment of malignant pleural effusion by closed trochar tube drainage. Ann Thoracic Surg 3:1, 1967.

Mark JBD & others: Intrapleural mechlorethamine hydrochloride therapy for malignant pleural effusion. JAMA 187:858–860, 1964.

EMPYEMA

Essentials of Diagnosis

- Chest pain, hemoptysis, shortness of breath, weakness.
- Fever (may be very high).
- Patient may be toxic.
- Findings of pleural effusion.

General Considerations

The initial pleural response to infection may be an exudate, depending somewhat on the organism involved. Pleural exudates can form with nearby infection even before organisms have entered the pleural spaces; however, this is either transitory or bacterial invasion follows. **Empyema thoracis** is an acute or chronic suppurative pleural exudate which may be caused by many organisms, eg, pneumococci, streptococci, staphylococci, bacteroides, *Escherichia coli*, *Proteus vulgaris*, tubercle bacilli, fungi, and amebas.

Infections may involve the pleural spaces by (1) direct extension of pneumonia; (2) lymphatic spread from neighboring infections of the lungs, mediastinum, chest wall, or diaphragm; (3) hematogenous

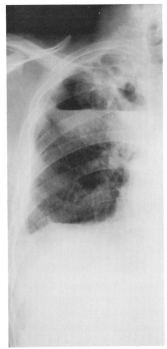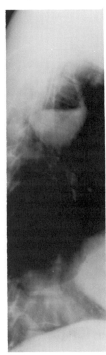

FIG 22–8. Postoperative loculated empyema with bronchopleural fistula. *Left:* Posteroanterior projection. *Right:* Lateral projection.

spread from a remote infection; (4) direct inoculation by penetrating trauma or surgical incision of a pulmonary abscess (Fig 22–8); (5) ruptured thoracic viscera (eg, esophagus) or displaced abdominal viscera (eg, strangulated traumatic diaphragmatic hernia); or (6) extension of subdiaphragmatic processes such as subdiaphragmatic abscesses, hepatic abscesses, or perinephric abscesses.

When empyema follows pneumonia it is known as **metapneumonic empyema.** In children, cystic fibrosis of the pancreas, congenital biliary atresia, agammaglobulinemia, Hodgkin's disease, and leukemia are predisposing factors. In adults, empyema usually develops in association with one of the following: alcoholism, chronic bronchitis, bronchiectasis, bronchial asthma, pulmonary emphysema with bullae, diabetes mellitus, inactive pulmonary tuberculosis, chronic corticosteroid therapy, congestive heart failure, carcinoma of the lung, heroin addiction, acute pelvic inflammatory disease, radiation therapy to the lung, Parkinson's disease, lymphomas, and cachexia.

Clinical Findings

A. Symptoms and Signs: Chest pain, shortness of breath, fever, weakness, and hemoptysis are usually present. Some patients are severely toxic or even comatose when first seen. They may be cyanotic, hypotensive, dehydrated, and oliguric. Temperature may reach 40.6 C (105 F) but is usually less. Respirations may be grunting. The physical findings of a pleural effusion are present (see above). In the absence of fever, empyema must be differentiated from pulmonary edema or pulmonary embolus with effusion.

B. Laboratory Findings: The hematocrit may be in the low 30s, particularly after rehydration. The white blood count is in the range of 14,000–18,000/µl, with a shift to the left. There may be azotemia.

The bacteriologic diagnosis is the most important part of the evaluation:

1. *Staphylococcus aureus*—S aureus is the most common organism involved in empyema in all age groups and accounts for over 90% of cases in infants and children. Staphylococcal pneumonia has a tendency to lead to empyema, abscesses, and pneumatoceles (Table 22–2). **Pneumatoceles** are thin-walled cystic spaces that form as a result of a check valve type of obstruction of small bronchi. They can produce localized overexpansion and rupture. The term pneumatocele is also used to refer to hernia of the chest wall, an unrelated condition.

2. *Streptococcus pyogenes*—Empyema is an especially frequent complication of streptococcal pneumonia. It is characterized by thick green pus which tends to become loculated within 2 or 3 days. Streptococcal organisms can often be diagnosed by sputum culture (60%), but throat culture is negative in about 80% of cases and blood cultures are rarely positive. The diagnosis is best made by culture of the pleural effusion. The antistreptolysin titer is greater than 250 Todd units in 97% of cases. The pneumonic component of streptococcal empyema may be minimal, and empyema may be the initial manifestation (Fig 22–9).

3. Bacteroides—Bacteroides empyema seems especially to affect young females with pelvic infections and elderly men with underlying respiratory disease, alcoholism, or malignancy. Identification of this organism is sometimes difficult because of its strict anaerobic requirement and slow growth. Its antibiotic sensi-

TABLE 22–2. Incidence of various complications of staphylococcal pneumonia in adults and children.

	Adults	Children
Abscess	25%	50%
Empyema	15%	15%
Pneumatocele	1%	35%
Effusion	30%	55%
Bronchopleural fistula	2%	5%

tivities are discussed in Chapter 10. Empyema with these bacteria develops more rapidly than with *Escherichia coli* or *Pseudomonas aeruginosa,* and loculation may be present almost from the beginning. The accumulation of pus is massive, thick, and foul-smelling, and it tends to return rapidly after evacuation. Mixed infection with anaerobic streptococci is common.

4. *Klebsiella pneumoniae*—Pneumonia and empyema from this organism principally affect debilitated, elderly, chronically ill, or alcoholic patients. One should suspect *K pneumoniae* when an effusion is associated with massive parenchymal consolidation. Abscess and cavitation occur in half of patients, and one-third of these develop empyema. Treatment must be aggressive but is often unsuccessful because of extensive parenchymal necrosis and the frequent development of a bronchopleural fistula.

5. Other bacteria—*Diplococcus pneumoniae* is now less often a cause of empyema than it was in the preantibiotic era. Pleural involvement following pneumococcal pneumonia usually occurred 7–10 days after onset, and most patients now have received effective antibiotic therapy by this time.

Escherichia coli, pseudomonas, and proteus may cause empyema in patients with underlying systemic disease.

C. X-Ray Findings: The roentgenographic appear-

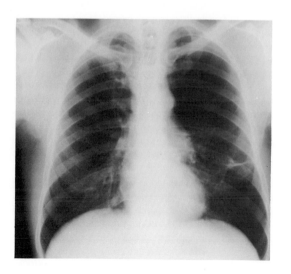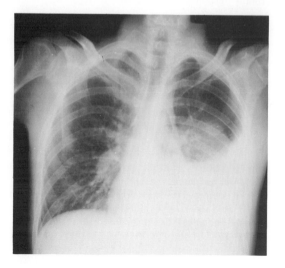

FIG 22–9. Streptococcal empyema. *Left:* Normal x-ray when admitted with high fever. *Right:* Chest x-ray 3 days after admission.

ance is characterized by opacification of a portion of the pleural space, sometimes with a fluid level. A pneumonic infiltrate is usually present but may be obscured by the effusion.

Complications

The complications of empyema are **empyema necessitatis** (invasion of the chest wall), bronchopleural fistula, pericardial extension, mediastinal abscess, osteomyelitis of ribs or cartilage, and chronicity. Formation of a bronchial fistula into an empyema requires emergency treatment to avoid flooding of the opposite lung with pus and subsequent fatal pneumonia.

Metastatic abscesses, particularly to the brain, are unusual when antibiotic coverage is adequate but can occur in neglected cases. Prolonged suppuration, such as may occur in postpneumonectomy empyema can result in amyloid deposition, particularly in the liver and kidneys.

Treatment

A. Antibiotic Treatment: Prompt diagnosis and treatment are essential. Cultures of throat, sputum, pleural fluid, and blood should be taken since no one of these is always positive. Initial antibiotic treatment should be chosen on the basis of the clinical findings and the results of smears. When not contraindicated by allergy, high doses of penicillin should be used since the organisms that most commonly cause empyema are sensitive to penicillin. When staphylococcal infection is suspected, penicillinase resistance must be considered and a drug such as methicillin included in the regimen. Drainage should be done promptly in all cases to prevent empyema necessitatis and to obviate general toxicity and other septic sequelae.

B. Drainage of Pleural Space: Evacuation of the pus by needle aspiration may be elected in cases where the pleural effusion is minimal and watery and a prompt response to antibiotic therapy can be expected. However, even in favorable cases such as streptococcal empyema in young men, hospitalization time is increased by almost 2 weeks when needle aspiration is used rather than closed tube drainage. In general, inadequate early drainage is the most frequent cause of subsequent therapeutic intractability from loculations, etc.

Prompt closed tube drainage of the pleural space to underwater seal is preferred in most cases (see Thoracentesis in Chapter 52). In cases failing to respond to simple drainage or where roentgenographic demonstration of multiple air-fluid levels indicate that loculation has already occurred, insertion of the tube may be combined with local rib resection (2.5–5 cm) and limited thoracic exploration to remove necrotic material and break down loculations. The chest tube can be brought through the chest wall by a separate incision or through the same incision, made airtight with layered absorbable sutures. Closed tube drainage with negative pressure minimizes residual pleural space.

When empyema is associated with parenchymal necrosis or lung trapping, the pleural space may not be

obliterated by the above measures and the residual space may require prolonged drainage to prevent sealing off and reactivation of the infection. By 5–7 days, the space communicating with the chest tube is usually isolated from the remaining pleural space and the underwater seal is no longer necessary to prevent lung collapse. At this point, the chest tube can be cut, leaving a portion protruding from the chest wall to maintain a chronic draining tract. Later, if the space does not seem to be shrinking or if debridement is required, it can be managed by a larger chest wall and rib resection, known as an **Eloesser flap.** This procedure consists of suturing a flap of skin to the pleura, creating a semipermanent epithelium-lined sinus into the empyema cavity for simpler long-term care.

C. Other Surgical Measures: More aggressive surgical approaches are reserved for unusual cases. Thoracoplasty, which involves collapsing the chest wall to obliterate pleural space, is rarely indicated. This procedure is discussed further in the section on tuberculosis. Empyemectomy involves resection of the empyema cavity en bloc and is usually reserved for empyemas localized to a lower lobe. This procedure may be especially appropriate when the associated lower lobe is destroyed and also requires resection. Decortication, or removal of the residual pleural peel, is indicated in the occasional case when ventilation of normal lung is prevented by a thick inelastic pleural scar or diaphragmatic fixation.

In occasional cases, bronchopleural fistula will not respond to therapy or may be so massive that pulmonary resection or reclosure of the postoperative bronchial stump is required. Bronchial stump closure may be buttressed by pedicle grafts of muscle or pleura, or other special procedures may be used. Postpneumonectomy empyema can occur with or without bronchopleural fistula. Initial treatment is by closed tube drainage, but once mediastinal stability is achieved an Eloesser flap can be performed to facilitate resolution of the infection. When pleural sepsis is controlled, the chest wall opening (Eloesser flap) may be closed without risk of recurrent empyema. This must be done by instillation of an appropriate antibiotic solution into the pleural space at the time of closure. This procedure is possible provided there is no bronchopleural fistula. In postpneumonectomy empyema without bronchopleural fistula, sterilization of the space is sometimes possible by antibiotic irrigation using chest tubes, thus eliminating the need for an Eloesser flap.

Chronic persistence of an empyema space is sometimes due to remediable causes of incomplete lung expansion. In cases with atelectasis due to aspiration of blood or mucus or when clearing of endobronchial secretions is inadequate, bronchoscopy should be performed early and should be repeated as necessary.

Prognosis

The average duration of hospitalization is 30–70 days. The mortality rate is higher in patients over age 40 and in those with predisposing conditions as outlined above. Those who arrive comatose, hypotensive, in pulmonary edema, or without leukocytosis have a poorer prognosis. Patients who succumb usually do so during the early part of the illness. The mortality rate is higher in infections with gram-negative organisms than with gram-positive ones.

The mortality rate in currently reported series ranges from 10–20% of patients developing empyema in association with pneumonia and from 25–55% in postoperative patients.

Rare Causes of Empyema

Almost any organism that infects the lungs can cause pleural effusion or empyema. *Mycobacterium tuberculosis* will be discussed with pulmonary tuberculosis. *Pasteurella tularensis* (causing tularemia) is associated with pleural involvement in 50% of cases of the typhoidal form. Organisms of the salmonella and clostridial groups have occasionally caused empyema.

Actinomyces israelii and Nocardia species may also cause pleural effusion and empyema. Pneumonitis is invariably present and usually is nonsegmentally distributed (homogeneous). The course of the disease may consist of lung abscesses followed by empyema and chest wall involvement with rib destruction (empyema necessitatis).

Entamoeba histolytica may cause secondary pleuropulmonary involvement by extension from a liver abscess. Lung cavitation and occasionally bronchobiliary fistula may occur. Sputum and pleural fluid may appear as "chocolate sauce." Amebic abscess often becomes secondarily infected with pyogenic organisms, in which case purulent empyema tends to mask the underlying amebiasis. *Paragonimus westermanii* and *Echinococcus granulosus* (see Chapter 10) are rare causes of pleural effusions or empyema.

CHYLOTHORAX

Accumulation of chyle in the pleural space may be (1) congenital, (2) traumatic postoperative, (3) traumatic nonsurgical, or (4) nontraumatic.

Congenital chylothorax is relatively rare. It is due primarily to congenital abnormalities of the lymphatic system such as absence of the thoracic duct or a fistula between the thoracic duct and the pleural space. Traumatic postoperative chylothorax follows operations or diagnostic procedures that injure the thoracic duct, most commonly cardiovascular and esophageal operations. Traumatic nonsurgical chylothorax follows either penetrating, blunt, or blast injuries. Fractures are not necessary for thoracic duct injury to occur. The usual mechanism is thought to be a shearing of the duct by the right crus of the diaphragm. This may occur with violent coughing or hyperextension of the spine. Nontraumatic chylothorax is generally regarded as ominous, since malignancy is the most frequent cause. However, there are many other causes such as

hepatic cirrhosis, thoracic aortic aneurysm and filariasis.

The treatment of nonmalignant chylothorax usually consists of removing sufficient fluid by needle or closed tube drainage to obtain full lung expansion. In many cases, the irritating nature of chyle will promote pleural synthesis and plug the leakage of chyle. During this time, the patient should be given a low-fat diet. In some cases, the patient may be fasted for several weeks and nutrition maintained by intravenous hyperalimentation. Surgical division and ligation of the duct should be considered early if drainage does not lead to prompt improvement.

Bessone LN, Ferguson TB, Burford TH: Chylothorax: A collective review. Ann Thoracic Surg 12:527, 1971.

Crosby IK, Crouch J, Reed WA: Chylopericardium and chylothorax. J Thoracic Cardiovas Surg 65:935, 1973.

HEMOTHORAX

Accumulation of blood in the pleural space is most commonly due to trauma, pulmonary infarction, neoplasms, or tuberculosis. It may also occur as a complication of surgery.

Treatment consists of closed tube drainage to evacuate the blood before clotting occurs. If no other specific treatment is required, relatively large amounts of blood or clot may be absorbed from the pleural space without significant sequelae if secondary infection does not occur. Occasionally, a persistent blood clot may result in fibrosis that impairs pulmonary function, in which case decortication should be considered.

PRIMARY PLEURAL TUMORS

There are 2 kinds of primary pleural tumors: localized mesothelioma and diffuse malignant mesothelioma. **Localized mesothelioma** most often arises from visceral pleura, is either pedunculated or sessile, and may either protrude into the pleural cavity or be embedded within the lung. It may achieve a gigantic size. Microscopically, this tumor is composed mainly of spindle cells and appears quite malignant, but usually the tumor is well encapsulated. Most do not recur after local excision, but about 30% of solitary mesotheliomas are malignant. Pleural effusion is present in only 10–15% of cases. The presence of blood in the effusion does not indicate incurability. The roentgenographic findings consist of a peripheral, well-demarcated mass, often forming an obtuse angle with the chest wall. Bone and joint pain, swelling, and arthritis have been described in as many as two-thirds of localized mesotheliomas.

Diffuse mesothelioma may arise anywhere within the pleura. It rapidly proliferates along the pleural surface to encase the lung. Pleural effusion is almost always present and is usually bloody. In cases without effusion, this lesion may present as diffuse pleural thickening. It is more common in areas where asbestos is mined.

All diffuse lesions are malignant. There is little evidence that they arise from originally benign localized mesothelioma. Diffuse mesotheliomas occur in all age groups but are often seen in relatively young patients, especially males, between 40–50 years. The patients complain of pleural pain, malaise, weight loss, weakness, anemia, fever, irritative cough, or dyspnea. The physical findings are those of pleural thickening or effusion.

Treatment of diffuse mesothelioma is rarely surgical but consists principally of relief of symptoms by controlling the pleural effusion, which may rapidly reaccumulate. Radiotherapy and intrapleural radioactive isotopes occasionally provide long-term remissions.

Hudspeth AS: Benign localized pleural mesotheliomas presenting as arthritis. Ann Thoracic Surg 2:691, 1966.

PNEUMOTHORAX

Essentials of Diagnosis

- Chest pain referred to the shoulder or arm on the involved side.
- Associated dyspnea.
- Hyperresonance, decreased chest motion, decreased breath and voice sounds on involved side.
- Mediastinal shift away from involved side.
- Chest x-ray revealing retraction of the lung from the parietal pleura is diagnostic.

General Considerations

Air or gas in the pleural space (pneumothorax) may originate from rupture of the respiratory system (eg, lung, bronchus, trachea), esophagus, or the chest wall or it may be generated by microorganisms in a pleural infection. Pneumothorax may be classified as spontaneous, traumatic, or iatrogenic, depending on the cause. It is referred to as "closed" when the chest wall is intact or "open" when a breach in the chest wall exists. The magnitude of pneumothorax is expressed as an estimate of the percentage of collapse of the lung. For example, a small rim of air around the lung would represent about a 5–10% pneumothorax; a total collapse, 90–100%. When the visceral and parietal pleuras are not adherent, pressure in the pneumothorax may be sufficient to displace the mediastinum to the opposite side (**tension pneumothorax**). Both open ("sucking") chest wounds and tension pneumothorax are surgical emergencies since they seriously compromise total ventilation.

In trauma patients, pneumothorax is often associated with blood in the pleural space (hemopneumothorax). (Traumatic pneumothorax is discussed in Chapter 15.) With esophageal rupture, the combination of pleural suppuration and air is known as pyopneumothorax. (Esophageal rupture is discussed in Chapter 24.)

Iatrogenic pneumothorax may occur as a result of inadvertent introduction of air into the pleural space, inadvertent puncture or rupture of the lung, or intentional introduction of air into the pleural space or mediastinum. Thoracentesis, placement of a subclavian vein catheter for central venous pressure monitoring, operations on the chest wall, neck, back, or upper abdomen, lung or pleural biopsy, thoracentesis, brachial block, arteriography, and intercostal nerve block are procedures that are often complicated by pneumothorax. Inadvertent rupture of the lung may occur with assisted ventilation for anesthesia or respiratory support. Pneumothorax may intentionally be induced for diagnosis or treatment.

Spontaneous pneumothorax may occur in any age group but is most common in males 15–35 years of age (Fig 22–10). In newborn infants, it may be asymptomatic and discovered as an incidental finding on a chest x-ray taken for other reasons, or it may cause acute respiratory distress. In young adults, spontaneous pneumothorax develops without known cause in association with localized emphysematous blebs near the apex of the upper lobe. In elderly patients, generalized emphysema, bullous emphysema, or some other predisposing cause is usually present. The left and right sides are involved with approximately equal frequency. Bilateral involvement and tension pneumothorax are both uncommon. Males predominate over females 10:1. An associated effusion which may contain blood is present in 10%.

About 30% of patients with spontaneous pneumothorax have chronic pulmonary disease, consisting largely of chronic bronchitis or emphysema. A history of smoking, pneumonia, recent upper respiratory infection, or asthma is often obtained. Secondary spontaneous pneumothorax (pneumothorax related to active disease) may occur in staphylococcal pneumonia, lung abscess, or a multitude of other less common pulmonary conditions ranging from sarcoidosis to thoracic endometriosis.

Clinical Findings

A. Symptoms and Signs: In one-third of cases, the pneumothorax occurs during mild to moderate exercise. Symptoms are chest pain, shortness of breath, cough, and shoulder pain, but in 5% of cases there are no symptoms at all. Severe cases may be associated with syncope, nausea, vomiting, or shock. Physical findings include evidence of diminished ventilation of the affected lung and hyperresonance, but the diagnosis may elude the examiner unless a chest x-ray is obtained. Tension pneumothorax may produce mediastinal shift and tracheal displacement away from the affected side with neck vein distention, cyanosis, and shock.

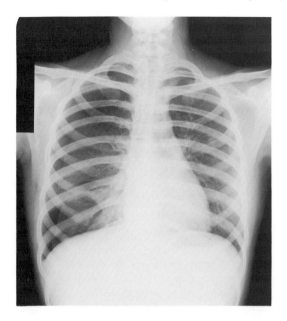

FIG 22–10. Spontaneous pneumothorax on right side.

B. X-Ray Findings: X-ray shows the extent of pneumothorax (Fig 22–10).

C. Differential Diagnosis: In cases where tension exists, the main disorders that must be differentiated are cardiac tamponade and acute congestive heart failure. The physical findings of tension pneumothorax are occasionally obscure, so that many clinicians have mistakenly thought tension pneumothorax to be excluded only to be proved wrong by the chest x-ray.

Complications

Pneumothorax may be complicated by tension pneumothorax, simultaneous bilateral pneumothorax, recurrent or persistent pneumothorax, pleural effusion or hemothorax, empyema, or pneumonitis.

Treatment

The objective of treatment is to relieve symptoms and promptly reexpand the lung by means of thoracentesis, closed tube drainage, or thoracotomy. General measures include bed rest, treatment of underlying diseases, relief of pain, and management of shock and hypoxia. Thoracentesis is used for diagnosis and as a definitive measure for reexpansion in mild cases when continuous observation is possible to detect recurrence. However, closed tube drainage is the most reliable treatment. The tube is usually placed anteriorly in the second anterior intercostal space, where air tends to accumulate. Air leaks that persist for 5–7 days and recurrent pneumothorax are usually treated by thoracotomy to excise apical blebs and to achieve pleural synthesis through pleural scarification, pleurectomy, or the use of pleural irritants.

Prognosis

The prognosis in properly managed patients with primary spontaneous pneumothorax is excellent for survival. In patients with secondary spontaneous pneumothorax, the prognosis is determined by the underlying disease but the overall mortality rate is 10–15%.

Recurrence is the most common indication for operative treatment, and the possibility of another recurrence increases with each attack. The average interval between attacks is 2–3 years, but pneumothorax can recur almost immediately or as long as 20 years afterward. Asynchronous bilateral involvement occurs in about 10%.

Gobbel WG & others: Spontaneous pneumothorax. J Thoracic Cardiovas Surg 46:331, 1963.

Seremetis JG: Management of spontaneous pneumothorax. Chest 57:65, 1970.

Timmis HH, Virgilo R, McClenathan JE: Spontaneous pneumothorax. Am J Surg 110:929, 1965.

PLEURAL CALCIFICATION OR PLAQUES

Pleural calcification occasionally occurs after long-term pleural infections, in organized collections of pleural blood, following empyema, in tuberculosis, and in asbestosis or silicosis. The costal and diaphragmatic pleura are involved more often than the visceral pleura.

Hyaline plaques may be seen at thoracotomy and may be confused with pleural metastatic implants. The cause of pleural plaques is not known, but the condition may follow tuberculosis or inhalation of asbestos fibers.

Rous V, Studeny J: Aetiology of pleural plaques. Thorax 25:270, 1970.

THE LUNGS

SURGICAL ANATOMY
(See Fig 22–11.)

The segment is the important functional unit of the lung. Clinical recognition of segmental anatomy has permitted thoracic surgeons to devise operative procedures that minimize unnecessary removal of normal lung parenchyma. Bronchopulmonary segments make up large lung units called the lobes. The right lung has 3 lobes: upper, middle, and lower. The left lung consists of 2 lobes: upper and lower. On the left, the lingular portion of the upper lobe is the homologue of the right middle lobe. Two fissures separate the

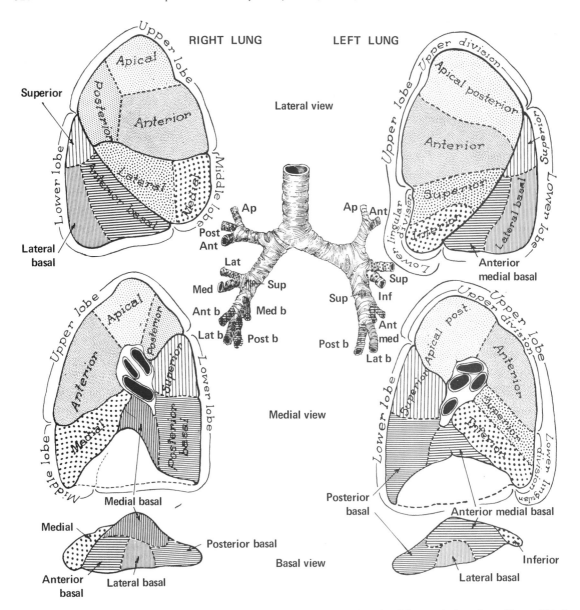

FIG 22–11. Segmental anatomy of the lungs. (Modified and reproduced, with permission, from Krupp MA & others: *Physician's Handbook,* 17th ed. Lange, 1973.)

lobes on the right side. The major or oblique fissure divides the upper and middle lobes from the lower lobe. The minor or horizontal fissure separates the middle from the upper lobe. On the left side, the single oblique fissure separates the upper and lower lobes.

The bronchopulmonary segmental anatomy is designated by numbers (Boyden) or by name (Jackson and Huber). The bronchial tree undergoes sequential division until the smallest unit of ventilation, the alveolus, is reached. The trachea and the main stem bronchi and their branches are prevented from collapse by horseshoe-shaped cartilages in their walls. Cartilaginous reinforcement of the airway gradually becomes less complete as the branches get smaller and ceases altogether with bronchi of 1–2 mm.

THE PULMONARY VASCULAR SYSTEM

The lungs have a dual blood supply: the pulmonary and the bronchial arterial systems. The pulmonary arteries transmit venous blood from the right ventricle for oxygenation. They divide in such a way as to closely accompany the bronchi. The bronchial arteries usually arise directly from the aorta or nearby intercostal arteries and are variable in number. They transmit oxygenated blood at systemic arterial pressure to the bronchial wall to the level of the terminal bronchioles.

The pulmonary veins travel in the interlobar septa and do not correspond to the distribution of the bronchi or the pulmonary arteries. The large bronchi may have bronchial veins that drain into the azygous system or—as occurs more distally in the bronchial tree—drain directly into the pulmonary venous system. Multiple rudimentary anastomoses exist between the pulmonary arteries and veins, the bronchial and pulmonary arteries, and the bronchial and pulmonary veins that may expand to transmit significant flow in disease.

THE LYMPHATICS

From the parenchyma, the lymphatics travel in intersegmental septa; those which reach the parenchymal surface form subpleural networks. Drainage continues toward the hilum in channels which follow the bronchi and pulmonary arteries. They eventually enter lymph nodes in the major fissures of the lungs, the hilum, and the paratracheal regions.

The direction of lymphatic drainage—irrespective of the primary site—is cephalad and usually ipsilateral, but contralateral flow may occur from any lobe. It appears from the spread of left lower lobe neoplasms that the lymphatics from this lobe may be almost equally distributed to the left and right. Otherwise, the usual sequence of lymphatic spread of pulmonary cancer is first to regional parabronchial nodes and then to the ipsilateral paratracheal, scalene, or inferior deep cervical nodes.

Baird JA: The pathways of lymphatic spread of carcinoma of the lung. Brit J Surg 52:868, 1965.
Baker NH & others: Pulmonary lymphatic drainage. J Thoracic Cardiovas Surg 54:695, 1967.

PHYSIOLOGY OF THE LUNG

The 7 major functions of the lung are as follows:
(1) Respiration and acid-base regulation, ie, to exchange oxygen and CO_2 between blood and the atmosphere.
(2) Blood reservoir.
(3) Excretion, eg, water vapor, ethanol, hydrocarbons.
(4) Temperature regulation.
(5) Detoxification and metabolic degradation.
(6) Secretion, eg, histamine, thromboplastin.
(7) Cleansing and filtering, eg, carbon, silica in air; blood clots, particulate matter in blood.

SYMPTOMS & SIGNS OF RESPIRATORY DISEASE

Occasionally, patients with advanced pulmonary disease have no symptoms. However, symptoms are usually present and help to establish a diagnosis.

Cough

Cough is a defensive mechanism mediated by the trigeminal, glossopharyngeal, superior laryngeal, and vagus nerves. It may be the first symptom of bronchial irritation by pulmonary disease. Cough is either dry or productive. Dry cough may be caused by any respiratory disease and often precedes a productive cough. Productive cough indicates irritation of the bronchial glands. Sputum should be described as to color, consistency, amount, time of occurrence, and special characteristics such as the presence of food particles or blood. Cough is sometimes described as hacking, loose, brassy, bovine, violent, spasmodic, irritative, persistent, or severe, but these features are rarely of diagnostic value.

Hoarseness or Voice Change

Voice change occurs when there is irritation or inflammation of the vocal cords or obstruction of nasal passages, or after interference with laryngeal innervation. Vocal cord paralysis may occur, especially on the left side, with carcinoma of the lung or esophagus, but also can be idiopathic or due to benign disease. Persistent voice change warrants examination of the vocal cords to rule out intrinsic lesions and abductor nerve paresis.

Shortness of Breath (Dyspnea)

Dyspnea must be distinguished from sighing, malaise, or anxiety. True dyspnea may connote important alteration of cardiopulmonary function. The character of the dyspnea, its duration, and its relationship to position, exertion, or other symptoms should be determined. Shortness of breath may be caused by chest pain (eg, angina pectoris, pleurisy, or peritonitis).

Chest Pain

Pleuritic pain is discussed on p 311.

The lung is relatively insensitive to pain, but in inflammatory diseases the tracheobronchial tree may be sensitive to contact or change in temperature.

Mediastinal pain is often felt retrosternally and may radiate to the back, neck, or arms. It may resemble myocardial ischemia and be described as squeezing, boring, pressing, or choking—much as in pulmonary embolism, pulmonary hypertension, pericarditis, or dissecting aneurysm. Esophageal pain is usually burning but may be spasmodic.

Chest wall pain, not pleuritic in origin, may be distinguished from pleuritic pain because it is not aggravated by cough and deep breathing and is usually poorly localized, constant, and dull or aching.

Hemoptysis

Hemoptysis must always be investigated since it is often the first sign of serious disease such as carcinoma, tuberculosis, or pulmonary infarction. It must be differentiated from nasal, upper airway, and gastrointestinal tract bleeding. Hemoptysis does not always indicate severe lung disease since it may be due to bronchitis or mitral stenosis or may be an idiopathic nonrecurrent event in a person without demonstrable disease. In general, about 90% of patients with hemoptysis have an identifiable underlying disease. Sometimes the amount of blood lost may be massive (ie, > 600 ml), as in tuberculosis, mitral stenosis, or broncholithiasis; or even exsanguinating, as when a thoracic aortic aneurysm ruptures into a bronchus.

Barrett RJ: A study of essential hemoptysis. J Thoracic Cardiovas Surg 40:468, 1960.

Wheezing

Diffuse wheezing occurs in patients with asthma, allergies, bronchitis, emphysema, or heart failure. A localized wheeze denotes isolated bronchial obstruction due to secretions, foreign bodies, strictures, or tumors.

Signs of Respiratory Disease

The physical findings in respiratory disease include local changes of the chest wall or diaphragm, evidence of mediastinal shift or widening, supraclavicular adenopathy, or percussive and auscultatory findings in the lungs themselves. Extrathoracic manifestations of pulmonary disease such as clubbing or hypertrophic pulmonary osteoarthropathy may be present. Cyanosis indicates at least 5 g/100 ml of reduced hemoglobin in the blood, often due to ventilatory insufficiency; right-to-left shunting, as in cardiac disease; excessive hemoglobin, as in polycythemia; abnormal hemoglobin, as in methemoglobinemia; or circulatory stasis due to cardiac disease or hypothermia.

SPECIAL DIAGNOSTIC STUDIES

Skin Tests

Skin tests are used in the diagnosis of tuberculosis, histoplasmosis, and coccidioidomycosis. Tuberculin testing is usually done with purified protein derivative (PPD) injected intradermally. Intermediate strength PPD should be used in patients who seem likely to have active disease. Induration of 10 mm or more at the injection site after 48–72 hours is called positive and indicates either active or arrested disease. Mumps antigen is usually placed on the opposite forearm to test for anergy. Because false-negative reactions are rare, a negative test fairly reliably rules out tuberculosis. Skin tests for histoplasmosis and coccidioidomycosis are carried out in a similar way, but tests for fungal infections are unreliable, and serologic tests should be done.

Freedman SO: Tuberculin testing and screening: A critical evaluation. Hospital Practice for May 1972, p 63.

Howard WL & others: The loss of tuberculin sensitivity in certain patients with active pulmonary tuberculosis. Dis Chest 57:530, 1970.

Endoscopy

A. Laryngoscopy: Indirect laryngoscopy is used to assess vocal cord mobility in patients suspected of having lung carcinoma, especially when there has been a voice change. It should also be performed to search for an otherwise occult source for malignant cells in sputum or metastases in cervical lymph nodes.

B. Bronchoscopy: Roentgenographic evidence of bronchial obstruction, unresolved pneumonia, foreign body, suspected carcinoma, undiagnosed hemoptysis, aspiration pneumonia, and lung abscess are only a few of the indications for bronchoscopy. The procedure can be done using either the standard hollow metal or the flexible fiberoptic bronchoscope and local or general anesthesia. Washings are usually obtained for bacterial or fungal culture and cytologic examination. Visible lesions are biopsied directly, and occasionally biopsies are taken of the carina even though it appears normal. Brush biopsies are obtained from specific bronchopulmonary segments. Occasionally, transcarinal needle biopsy of a subcarinal node is obtained. Thirty to 50% of lung tumors are visible bronchoscopically. Brushing, random biopsies, and sputum cytology may still yield a positive diagnosis of cancer or tuberculosis in the absence of a visible lesion.

C. Mediastinoscopy: Mediastinoscopy permits direct biopsy of paratracheal and carinal lymph nodes without thoracotomy. Tumor is found by this technic in about 40% of cases of lung cancer, and such a finding indicates surgical incurability. Persons with a negative biopsy have a relatively favorable prognosis with surgical treatment.

Mediastinoscopy is almost invariably accurate in the diagnosis of sarcoidosis. It is also useful to diagnose tuberculosis, histoplasmosis, silicosis, metastatic carcinoma, lymphoma, and carcinoma of the esophagus. It should not be used in primary mediastinal tumors, which should be approached by a surgical incision permitting definitive excision.

Mediastinoscopy is done through a suprasternal or parasternal incision. The mortality rate is 0.09% and the morbidity rate is 1.5%. The main complications are hemorrhage, pneumothorax, recurrent nerve injury, and infection.

Ashbaugh DG: Mediastinoscopy. Arch Surg 100:568, 1970.

Pearson FG & others: The role of mediastinoscopy in selection of treatment of bronchial carcinoma with involvement of superior mediastinal lymph nodes. J Thoracic Cardiovas Surg 64:382, 1972.

Scalene Lymph Node Biopsy

Scalene lymph node biopsy has been largely replaced by mediastinoscopy in the evaluation of pulmonary diseases since it attempts to obtain the same type of information but will do so less reliably. In the evaluation of lung cancer, about 15% of scalene node biopsies are positive when the cervical nodes are not palpable compared with 85% when the nodes are palpable. The risk of major complications with scalene lymph node biopsy is about 5%. Deaths are rare.

Boyd AD: Mediastinoscopy: Comparison with scalene fat pad biopsy. New York J Med 71:445, 1971.

Skinner DB: Scalene-lymph-node biopsy: Reappraisal of risks and indications. New England J Med 268:1334–1329, 1963.

Pleural Biopsy

A. Needle Biopsy: This procedure is indicated when the cause of a pleural effusion cannot be determined by analysis of the fluid or when tuberculosis is suspected. Any one of 3 needles can be used: the Vim-Silverman, Cope, or Abrams (Harefield) needle. A positive diagnosis can be obtained in 60–85% of cases of tuberculosis or malignancy. The principal complication is pneumothorax. Five to 10% of biopsy specimens are inadequate samples.

B. Open Biopsy: Open pleural biopsy is especially useful in those without pleural effusion, or when needle biopsy has failed. The quality of the specimen and the likelihood of its representing the pathology are better than with needle biopsy, but open biopsy is a more extensive procedure.

Hill HE, Hensler NM, Breckler IA: Pleural biopsy in diagnosis of effusion: Results in 50 cases of pleural disease observed consecutively. Am Rev Resp Dis 78:8, 1958.

Scerbo J, Keltz J, Stone DJ: A prospective study of closed pleural biopsies. JAMA 218:377, 1971.

Lung Biopsy

A. Needle Biopsy: The indications for percutaneous needle biopsy are not well established. It may be indicated in diffuse parenchymal disease and in some patients with localized lesions. The diagnosis of interstitial pneumonia, carcinoma, sarcoidosis, hypersensitivity lung disease, lymphoma, pulmonary alveolar proteinosis, and miliary tuberculosis has been established by this method.

In localized disease—particularly when carcinoma is suspected—there is controversy concerning the risks of spreading the tumor by needle biopsy. Until this is settled, needle biopsy of possible carcinoma should be reserved for patients with surgically incurable disease. Needle biopsies are done by any of 3 technics: aspiration with a cutting needle, by trephine, or by air drill. Needle biopsy of the lung is also possible by a transbronchial technic using a modified Vim-Silverman needle.

Complications following percutaneous needle biopsy include pneumothorax (20–40%), hemothorax, hemoptysis, and air embolism. Pulmonary hypertension or cysts and bullae are contraindications. Several deaths have been reported. There is about a 60% chance of success of obtaining useful information.

B. Open Lung Biopsy: A limited intercostal or anterior parasternal incision is used to remove a 3–4 cm wedge of lung tissue in diffuse parenchymal lung disease. The site of incision is selected for accessibility and the promise of giving information of diagnostic value. General or local anesthesia may be used. Open lung biopsy has a lower mortality rate, fewer complications, and greater diagnostic yield than needle biopsy. When a focal lesion is biopsied, a larger incision is used; peripheral lesions are totally excised by wedge or segmental resection; deeply placed lesions may be removed by lobectomy in suitable candidates.

Berger RL, Dargan EL, Huang BL: Dissemination of cancer cells by needle biopsy of the lung. J Thoracic Cardiovas Surg 63:430, 1972.

Gaensler EA, Moister VB, Hamm J: Open lung biopsy in diffuse pulmonary disease. New England J Med 270:1319– 133, 1964.

Krumholz RA & others: Needle biopsy of the lung: Report of its use in 112 patients and review of the literature. Ann Int Med 65:293, 1966.

Nordenstrom B: Transthoracic needle biopsy. New England J Med 276:1081, 1967.

Steel SJ, Winstanley DP: Trephine biopsy of the lung and pleura. Thorax 24:576, 1969.

Sputum Analysis

Exfoliative sputum cytology is most valuable for detection of lung cancer. Specimens are obtained by deep coughing, bronchial washings by either bronchoscopic or percutaneous transtracheal washing technics, or by abrasion with a brush. Specimens should be collected fresh in the morning and delivered to the laboratory promptly. Centrifugation or filtration can be used to concentrate the cellular elements.

In primary lung cancer, sputum cytology is positive in 30–60% of cases. Repeated sputum examination improves the diagnostic return. Examination of the first bronchoscopic washing material yields a diagnosis in 60% of cases.

Clark RE, Kyriakos M, Hendrix Y: The effect of anesthetic method upon the results of bronchial washing cytology. J Thoracic Cardiovas Surg 63:930, 1972.

Erozan YS, Frost JK: Cytopathologic diagnosis of cancer in pulmonary material: A critical histopathologic correlation. Acta cytol 14:560, 1970.

Ozgelen FN, Brodsky SL, DeGroat A: An examination of the merits and intrinsic limitations of explorative cytology in 465 cases of lung cancer. J Thoracic Cardiovas Surg 49:221, 1965.

DISEASES OF THE LUNGS

CYSTIC LESIONS OF THE LUNG

Broad usage of the term pulmonary cyst would include the following:

(1) Bronchogenic cysts: Congenital epithelium-lined developmental abnormalities.

(2) Pneumatoceles: Nonepithelized cavities in the parenchyma, often associated with staphylococcal pneumonia.

(3) Emphysematous bullae: Nonepithelized lung cavities resulting from degenerative changes in emphysema (Fig 22–12).

(4) Pulmonary blebs: Localized collections of air within lung interstitial tissue.

(5) Cystic bronchiectasis: Cyst-like bronchial dilatation which may be acquired or congenital.

(6) Lung cavities: Acquired lung spaces following destructive lung disease such as abscess, tuberculosis, fungal infection, malignancy.

(7) Parasitic cysts.

(8) Diffuse cystic disease: Seen in mucoviscidosis and Letterer-Siwe disease.

CONGENITAL CYSTIC LESIONS

Congenital cystic lesions of the lung are uncommon and usually not associated with cysts of other organs. The terminology of these lesions is confusing. Cysts that involve the lung can be derived from 3 sources: the air passages, pulmonary lymphatics, or pleural surfaces. Four distinct types of congenital cysts arising from the air passages are recognized: (1) Bronchogenic cysts, (2) sequestration of the lung, (3) congenital cystic adenomatoid malformation, and (4) infantile lobar emphysema. Except for the latter, all can present at any age but are more common in children and young adults. These lesions must sometimes be distinguished from pneumatoceles, blebs, bullae, or tumors.

The lungs and the trachea develop from the ventral bud of the primitive foregut. Abnormalities of ventral budding cause various types of bronchogenic cysts and pulmonary sequestrations. The ultimate location of the cyst or sequestration depends upon the extent of differentiation of the foregut. Early anomalies of budding lead to peripheral lung cysts or intralobar sequestration; later anomalies may cause cysts to remain extrapleural (bronchogenic) or sequestrations to be separate from the rest of the lung and to possess their own pleural coverings (extralobar sequestration). Abnormalities of development of the terminal bronchioles and alveolar ducts result in cystic adenomatoid formation. Alveoli develop by the 28th week of gestation, and abnormal alveolar development accounts for most cases of infantile lobar emphysema.

1. BRONCHOGENIC CYSTS

The term bronchogenic cyst includes both bronchial and lung cysts. They may be located in the mediastinum or hilum, but 50–70% are located in the lung. The more proximal cysts (bronchial) seldom have a bronchial communication and therefore are less likely to become secondarily infected. These cysts, usually considered mediastinal, are often in the right paratra-

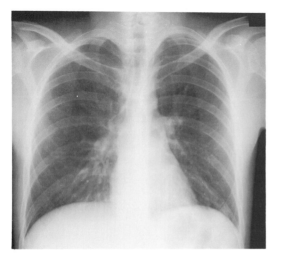
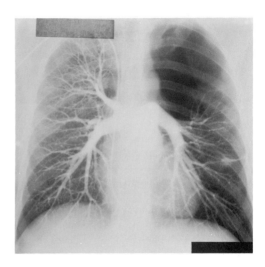

FIG 22–12. Emphysematous bullae of left lung. *Left:* Posteroanterior projection. *Right:* Pulmonary angiogram.

cheal, carinal, hilar, or paraesophageal locations. More peripheral bronchogenic cysts (congenital lung cysts) are thin-walled, often multiloculated or multiple, and usually have bronchial communications. They tend to become infected and to result in recurrent pneumonia, fever, sepsis, or other types of respiratory distress.

Clinical Findings

Congenital pulmonary cysts are manifested in infancy with respiratory embarrassment, pneumothorax, or compression atelectasis. If air trapping is the main feature, there will be dyspnea, cyanosis, and subcostal retraction. Less severe cases present as recurrent infection, hemoptysis, or an undiagnosed finding on chest roentgenogram.

Congenital lung cysts may occur anywhere in the lungs but involve the lower lobes twice as often as other sites. In adults, the lesion may be asymptomatic when detected by a chest roentgenogram. The mass may appear as a homogeneous density, a cavity with an air-fluid level, or an air cyst. It may be difficult to distinguish lung cysts from benign or malignant tumors, cavitary lesions due to fungi or tuberculosis, or pulmonary abscess.

Treatment

Treatment consists of local removal by enucleation, segmental resection, or in some cases lobectomy.

2. SEQUESTRATION OF THE LUNG

Masses of lung tissue that have no communication with the tracheobronchial tree are termed sequestrations. Two types are recognized. In intralobar sequestration, the abnormal lung is surrounded by normal lung and is supplied by anomalous systemic arteries; the venous drainage is into the pulmonary veins. Bronchial communication may be acquired through infection (about 15% of cases), but it is difficult to demonstrate radiologically. Repeated infections invariably occur because of poor drainage. Eighty-five percent of sequestrations are of the intralobar type. Extralobar sequestration consists of a separate or accessory mass of lung tissue invested by its own pleura. Anatomic and physiologic separation from adjacent lung tissue is complete, but vascular supply is the same as with intralobar sequestration.

The diagnosis is verified by arteriographic demonstration of a systemic arterial supply to the sequestered segment. Some cases are asymptomatic and are first discovered by chance on chest x-rays.

After infection is controlled, resection of the sequestration is indicated to prevent recurrent suppuration. Intralobar sequestration usually requires lobectomy; extralobar sequestrations can usually be locally excised. The main technical hazard is the aberrant blood supply.

3. CONGENITAL CYSTIC ADENOMATOID MALFORMATION

Congenital cystic adenomatoid malformation presents with manifestations of air trapping, progressive distention of the abnormal lung, and multiple cysts. It may be found in stillborns with anasarca, neonates with respiratory distress, or in older children and young adults as an asymptomatic chest x-ray finding, recurrent infection, or following pneumothorax.

4. INFANTILE LOBAR EMPHYSEMA

Infantile lobar emphysema with acute overinflation of the upper lobes or middle lobe is a cause of acute respiratory distress in infants. It is discussed in Chapter 49.

Carter R: Pulmonary sequestration: A collective review. Ann Thoracic Surg 7:68, 1969.

Hutchin P: Congenital cystic disease of the lung. Rev Surg, pp 79–87, March–April 1971.

Schmidt FE, Drapanas T: Congenital cystic lesions of the bronchi and lungs. Ann Thoracic Surg 14:650, 1971.

INFECTIONS OF THE LUNGS

BACTERIAL INFECTIONS

For many years, treatment of pleuropulmonary infections required a considerable portion of a thoracic surgeon's time, but drainage of pus from lung abscess, resection of bronchiectasis, and surgical treatment of tuberculosis have become relatively rare since the advent of effective antimicrobial therapy. Pulmonary infections are still common, but modern treatment is usually capable of preventing them from progressing to complications that require surgical treatment.

Among the infections, pneumonia is still the most lethal, and among all diseases it ranks fifth as a cause of death. At least half of all cases are bacterial, and 90% of these (40% of all cases) are due to pneumococci. Pneumococcal pneumonias are effectively treated with penicillin, but the other bacterial pneumonias are usually more resistant to therapy. *Staphylococcus aureus* (1–5%), *Klebsiella pneumoniae* (1–5%), *Haemophilus influenzae* (1%), *Neisseria meningitidis* (< 1%), *Streptococcus pyogenes* (< 1%), and the enterobacteriaceae (< 1%) are the pyogenic organisms most likely to lead to surgical complications. A major consideration in lung abscess and suppurative pneumonitis today is exclusion of bronchial carcinoma as an underlying cause.

LUNG ABSCESS

Essentials of Diagnosis

- Development of pulmonary symptoms about 2 weeks after possible aspiration, bronchial obstruction, or previous pneumonia.
- Septic fever and sweats.
- Periodic sudden expectoration of large amounts of purulent, foul-smelling or "musty" sputum.
- Hemoptysis may occur.
- X-ray density with central radiolucency and fluid level.

General Considerations

Lung abscess may result from aspiration (50%), bronchial obstruction (eg, from carcinoma), necrotizing pneumonia (20%), infection of cysts or bullae, or extension of infection from the subdiaphragmatic spaces or liver; or it may occur as a postembolic phenomenon or after trauma. In England, tuberculosis and carcinoma are the most common causes of lung abscess; the latter predominates in men over age 50.

To a large extent, the cause of lung abscess determines its location. In abscess secondary to aspiration, the patient's position at the time of aspiration is important. When the patient is supine, there is a tendency for aspirated material to enter the posterior segment of the right upper lobe or the superior segment of the right lower lobe. Carcinomatous abscess more frequently involves the anterior segments of the upper lobes. Embolic abscesses are often small and multiple and tend to involve the lower lobes. Basilar abscesses may suggest prior pneumonia. Abscesses often occur in alcoholics and other debilitated persons. Some follow aspiration during anesthesia and surgery. There may be other predisposing factors such as esophageal disease, hiatal hernia, carcinoma, achalasia, or tracheoesophageal fistula. Opportunistic pneumonia occurs in debilitated persons being given broad-spectrum antibiotics, those requiring tracheal tubes and ventilation therapy, those with systemic diseases, or those requiring treatment that affects host resistance. Diabetes, preexisting lung disease, dental caries, and epilepsy are also predisposing causes.

Although staphylococci, streptococci, and neisseriae are frequently found, the original causative organisms are often unknown because so many patients are treated with antibiotics without cultures and eventually a variety of gram-negative organisms emerge during antibiotic therapy. Pulmonary infarcts may become infected in patients with septic bacterial endocarditis or drug addicts who use the intravenous route of administration. Bland pulmonary infarcts also may become infected from adjacent bronchial disease. Lung abscesses following emboli are often near pleural surfaces; bronchopleural fistulas and emphysema can result.

Clinical Findings

A. Symptoms and Signs: The predisposing cause of lung abscess often contributes prominently to the clinical picture. During the development of an abscess, the clinical findings are indistinguishable from those of severe acute bronchopneumonia. The patient usually has fever, chills, pleuritic chest pain, and prostration. Sputum production may initially be minimal but can become putrid or fetid, which strongly suggests the diagnosis. Hemoptysis occasionally precedes the onset of productive cough. Physical findings may be indistinguishable from those of pneumonia.

B. Laboratory Findings: Leukocytosis is present.

C. X-Ray Findings: Chest x-ray initially shows only collapse or consolidation. If a solid or dense infiltrate is present, the diagnosis of carcinoma or tuberculosis may be suggested. Air-fluid levels develop once bronchial communication is established (Fig 22–13).

Differential Diagnosis

An abscess differs from bronchiectasis in that in abscess the infection is extrabronchial. The most common conditions causing abscess of the lung are tuberculosis, fungal infections, and carcinoma. Since carcinoma underlies 10–20% of lung abscesses, this should always be excluded. Bronchoscopy, sputum cytologic examination, and close follow-up are essential.

Complications

The complications of lung abscess are local spread, causing loss of additional parenchyma or even loss of an entire lobe; hemorrhage into the abscess, which can be massive; bronchopleural fistula; and emphysema, tension pneumothorax, pyopneumotho-

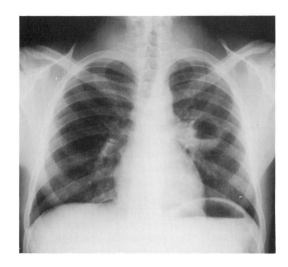

FIG 22–13. Lung abscess involving the superior segment of the left lower lobe.

rax, and pericarditis. Metastatic abscesses may occur, especially to the brain. Failure to heal, the most common complication, requires resection. Late complications are residual bronchiectasis, chronic abscess, chronic bronchopleural fistula, and recurrent pneumonitis.

Treatment

A. General Measures: Severely ill patients in shock, dehydration, or toxemia should receive immediate resuscitative measures. Sputum should be sent immediately for culture for aerobic and anaerobic organisms. Examination of stained smears of sputum or tracheal aspirates can suggest appropriate antibiotic therapy. Penicillin is given in most cases; when severe, 10 million units daily should be given by intravenous drip. General supportive measures are continued until the situation is stabilized. Within 2 or 3 days, it is usually safe to bronchoscope the patient to remove foreign material, obtain better cultures, promote drainage, or establish the diagnosis of an underlying disease. Bronchoscopy may be repeated at regular intervals to maintain drainage.

Postural drainage, assisted ventilation, and bronchodilators may be indicated. It is rare for a patient not to respond to such a regimen. The cavity will usually diminish in size within 2–3 weeks. If fever persists for 4 weeks, antibiotic therapy is often required for 6–8 weeks. However, failure to observe improvement on this regimen within 2–3 weeks should strongly suggest the presence of another aggravating factor, especially carcinoma.

B. Surgical Treatment: Occasionally, external closed drainage may be considered in severely ill patients with acute disease who are poor operative risks and have persistent sepsis because of inadequate bronchial drainage. Closed tube drainage is indicated only when it can be established that the drainage tract will traverse an area of synthesis of the parietal and visceral pleura so that empyema will not result.

Fewer than 5% of patients require surgical therapy unless an underlying carcinoma exists. Surgery is reserved for patients who show no signs of resolution radiologically or who have persistent evidence of inadequate resolution such as weight loss, anemia, and fever despite adequate antibiotic therapy or who cannot be withdrawn from antibiotic therapy. As long as improvement occurs on medical therapy, surgery is unnecessary. Large size of the abscess (> 6 cm), total lobe destruction, persistent bronchopleural fistula, persistent sepsis, or persistence of the abscess over several weeks are the surgical indications. Lobectomy is the usual procedure. Rarely, massive hemoptysis will make emergency lobectomy mandatory.

Prognosis

Medical therapy is successful in about 95% of cases; the remaining few require surgical treatment. There is a 10–15% mortality rate in those who need operation because of an inadequate response to antibiotics.

Bernhard WF, Malcolm JA, Wylie RH: Lung abscess: A study of 148 cases due to aspiration. Dis Chest 43:620–630, 1963.

Favell G: Lung abscess. Brit MJ 2:1032–1036, 1966.

May IA, Samson PC, Mittal A: Surgical management of the patient with complications of pulmonary infarction due to nonseptic pulmonary emboli. Am J Surg 124:223–228, 1972.

Schweppe HI & others: Lung abscess. New England J Med 265:1039, 1961.

BRONCHIECTASIS

The dilatation of the bronchial tree in bronchiectasis used to be considered irreversible, but this is now known to be false. Bronchiectasis often coexists with chronic bronchitis. Involvement is bilateral in 50% of cases, usually in the lower lobes, and in only 10% of cases is the lingular or middle lobe involved without ipsilateral lower lobe involvement.

Cases requiring surgical treatment have almost disappeared because antimicrobial therapy of pulmonary infections has largely prevented this disease. Bronchiectasis is mainly a pediatric disease, with 50% of cases having onset of symptoms before 3 years of age. Most cases begin with pneumonia complicating one of the childhood contagious diseases such as pertussis. Rarely, congenital defects such as mucoviscidosis and Kartagener's triad (situs inversus, sinusitis, and bronchiectasis) are involved in the pathogenesis. Patients with immunologic deficits and preexisting pulmonary disease such as lung abscess or bronchial obstruction by tuberculosis or foreign body sometimes develop bronchiectasis. The common feature in many of these is long-standing destructive bronchial infection.

The diagnosis of bronchiectasis depends on radiologic demonstration by bronchography of the typical irregular bronchial dilatations. Based on their shape, the disease is classified as (1) cylindric, (2) varicose, or (3) saccular or cystic bronchiectasis, but these distinctions are without prognostic significance. Patients with suspected bronchiectasis have cough, sputum production, and sometimes dyspnea; the symptoms are aggravated by frequent upper respiratory infections. Hemoptysis occurs in 50% of older patients. A few patients have little sputum ("dry bronchiectasis"). There may be associated pulmonary fibrosis or emphysema in advanced cases. Clubbing of the fingers is seen in about a third of cases.

There is no specific pattern of alteration of pulmonary function. Sputum cultures reveal multiple organisms, usually consisting of mouth flora.

Bronchiectasis secondary to bronchial obstruction (foreign body, tuberculosis, or tumor) should be ruled out.

Attacks of pneumonitis are often due to pneumococci or *Haemophilus influenzae*. Involvement of other segments of the bronchial tree, pulmonary fibrosis, and pulmonary insufficiency occur in advanced cases or when medical treatment has been inadequate.

Medical treatment consists of postural drainage, cessation of smoking, antibiotic therapy, and treatment of underlying conditions such as sinusitis. Humidification, bronchodilators, and expectorants may facilitate clearing of secretions. Upper respiratory infections may be treated with broad-spectrum antibiotics such as tetracyclines or ampicillin. Some patients are advised to seek warmer climates during the winter months.

Bronchoscopy may be indicated if secretions cannot be cleared or to search for aggravating causes. Surgical therapy is reserved for patients with localized disease (ie, involving one lobe) who have failed to respond to a strict medical regimen. The presence of diffuse pulmonary emphysema may limit the feasibility of surgery. In well-selected cases resection for bronchiectasis shows improvement in 95% with lobar disease. Bilateral involvement—particularly if the middle lobe or lingula are involved—has a poor prognosis following surgery, and most of these patients continue to produce large amounts of sputum. They may develop similar bronchial changes in previously uninvolved areas or in later years may develop increasing pulmonary insufficiency.

Ferguson TB, Burford TH: The changing pattern of pulmonary suppuration. Dis Chest 53:396, 1968.
Sealy WC & others: The treatment of multisegmental and localized bronchiectasis. Surg Gynec Obst 123:80–90, 1966.

MIDDLE LOBE SYNDROME

The middle lobe syndrome consists of repeated infections in this lobe which usually respond to antibiotics. It can be a manifestation of partial bronchial obstruction, to which the middle lobe is particularly susceptible. However, recurrent segmental infections can occur in other areas of the lung by a similar process. Secondary bronchiectasis is a frequent complication.

Broncholithiasis (see below) and middle lobe syndrome have been considered to be caused by compression or erosion of the bronchus by adjacent diseased lymph nodes. The middle lobe syndrome is seen less frequently now than formerly, and in some recently reported cases it was not associated with obstruction of the middle lobe bronchus. Other factors, such as poor natural drainage and lack of collateral ventilation, probably explain the frequency of middle lobe involvement and in some cases are sufficient to cause symptoms even though the bronchus is entirely patent. Bronchial obstruction may be demonstrable in as few as one-fourth of cases. It appears that in the middle lobe the presence of complete fissures limits collateral ventilation and favors the persistence of collapse, retained secretions, and infection.

Most patients who require surgical treatment are women over age 20 with symptoms of recurrent infectious bronchiectasis which include cough, hemoptysis, chest pain, and fever. Wheezing is occasionally reported. Chest roentgenography shows a midlung field density, middle lobe atelectasis, a small contracted middle lobe, or consolidated middle lobe. Bronchoscopy and bronchography show bronchiectasis in 40% of cases, incomplete filling in 20%, and occasionally a narrowed middle lobe orifice. Granulomatous disease, including tuberculosis and occasionally histoplasmosis, may be found.

Endobronchial tumors and foreign bodies must be ruled out by bronchoscopy or other means.

Most patients respond to intensive medical therapy (similar to that for bronchiectasis), and only a few require surgery. When surgery is required, lobectomy is performed. Indications for surgery include bronchiectasis, fibrosis (bronchostenosis), abscess, and unresolved or intractable recurrent pneumonia.

Bradham RR, Sealy WC, Young WG Jr: Chronic middle lobe infection: Factors responsible for its development. Ann Thoracic Surg 2:611–616, 1966.
Culiner MM: The right middle lobe syndrome: A non-obstructive complex. Dis Chest 50:57, 1966.
Johnson RM, Lindskog GE: Further studies on factors influencing collateral ventilation. J Thoracic Cardiovas Surg 62:321–329, 1971.

BRONCHOLITHIASIS

Broncholithiasis is an unusual condition in which a calcified parabronchial lymph node erodes into the bronchus and is either coughed up or lodges there. Rarely, inspissated and impacted mucoid material may undergo calcification and form a broncholith or "lung stone." In Europe, 10% of operated patients had documented tuberculosis. Histoplasmosis may be an equally important or even more important cause in the USA.

The criteria for diagnosis of broncholithiasis are (1) bronchoscopic evidence of peribronchial disease, (2) significant hilar calcifications, and (3) absence of associated pulmonary disease to explain the patient's symptoms.

Sudden unexpected hemoptysis in an otherwise healthy patient is the cardinal manifestation. The bleeding stops without specific measures and only rarely is massive.

Other frequent symptoms are cough, fever and chills, and purulent sputum. There may be localized pleuritic pain or localized wheezing. A history of expectoration of stones is present in one-third of cases. The chest roentgenogram invariably shows hilar calcification. One-third of cases have obstructive pneumonitis. Bronchoscopy demonstrates broncholiths in over 25%, and other endobronchial abnormalities in about 10% of cases.

The complications of broncholithiasis are suppurative lung disease, life-threatening hemoptysis, and bronchoesophageal fistula.

Medical treatment combined with bronchoscopic removal of the broncholith is usually indicated. In most patients symptoms are limited to a single attack of hemoptysis, since the invading lymph node becomes encased in scar tissue. Surgery is indicated to treat complications of broncholithiasis or when malignancy cannot be excluded. Of the 25% of patients that require surgery, most have lobectomy. Patients with bronchoesophageal fistula may require only fistula repair.

With adequate medical and surgical treatment, the prognosis has been greatly improved in recent years.

Arrigoni MG, Bernatz PE, Donoghue FE: Broncholithiasis. J Thoracic Cardiovas Surg 62:231–237, 1971.

MUCOVISCIDOSIS & MUCOID IMPACTION OF THE BRONCHI

Mucoviscidosis is a serious pulmonary disorder of children which may lead to bronchitis, bronchiectasis, pulmonary fibrosis, emphysema, or lung abscess.

Mucoid impaction occurs in adults and is associated with asthma and bronchitis. The mucoid plugs are rubbery, semisolid, gray to greenish-yellow in color, and round, oval, or elongated in shape. There is often a history of recurrent upper respiratory infection, fever, and chest pain. Expectoration of hard mucus plugs or hemoptysis may occur.

Most patients present with a history of respiratory infections, but nearly one-half have findings suggestive of bronchogenic carcinoma. The chest x-ray shows U-shaped lesions involving the second order bronchi. Bronchography helps to delineate the mass. Bronchoscopy is done to assess for malignancy and obtain cultures and for therapeutic purposes.

Bronchogenic carcinoma, fungal disease, tuberculosis, bronchiectasis, abscess, bacterial pneumonia, lipoid pneumonia, pulmonary eosinophilic granuloma, Löffler's syndrome, and cystic fibrosis must be ruled out.

Treatment is usually medical and includes expectorants, detergents, bronchodilators, antibiotics, and aerosol inhalation therapy. Acetylcysteine (Mucomyst) has largely converted this condition to a purely medical disease. Surgery is indicated when malignancy cannot be ruled out, for destroyed lung, or in the treatment of abscess. Long-term medical therapy gives good results, although occasional recurrences or indications for surgery occur.

Urschel HC Jr, Paulson DL, Shaw RR: Mucoid impaction of bronchi. Ann Thoracic Surg 2:1–16, 1966.

TUBERCULOSIS

Essentials of Diagnosis

- Presenting symptoms and signs may be minimal or absent.
- Minimal symptoms: malaise, lassitude, easy fatigability, anorexia, mild weight loss, afternoon fever, cough, apical rales, and hemoptysis.
- Positive tuberculin skin test; especially a recent change from negative to positive.
- Apical or subapical infiltrates, often with cavities.
- *Mycobacterium tuberculosis* in sputum or in gastric or tracheal washings.

General Considerations

Several species of the genus Mycobacterium may cause lung disease, but 95% are due to *M tuberculosis*. *M bovis* and *M avium* are seldom found in humans. Several less common species of Mycobacterium that are chiefly soil-dwellers have become clinically more important in recent years and have been less responsive to preventive and therapeutic measures.

Although tuberculosis is declining as a cause of death, an estimated 35 million persons are tuberculin-positive in the USA and form a reservoir from which about 5000–8000 relapses are expected. In addition, about 55,000 new cases occur annually (18 per 100,000 population). About one-third of cases are first reported at death. Although in the USA less than 20% of the population is tuberculin-positive, tuberculosis remains the most common infectious cause of death worldwide.

The initial infection involves pulmonary parenchyma in the midzone of the lung. When hypersensitivity develops after several weeks, the typical caseation appears. Regional hilar lymph nodes become enlarged. Most cases are apparently spontaneously controlled by the host at this stage. If the infection progresses, caseation necrosis develops and giant cells produce a typical tubercle. Although this has been called reinfection tuberculosis, postprimary tuberculosis, and secondary tuberculosis, it usually consists of continued activity or reactivation of a focus of latent disease. True reinfection or "superinfection" from repeated exposure seldom occurs. Destruction of additional tissue produces the varied clinical pattern. At this stage, the apical and posterior segments of the upper lobes and the superior segments of the lower lobes are the usual sites of infection.

Clinical Findings

A. Symptoms and Signs: In the vast majority of primary infections, there is no clinical evidence of disease. When present, symptoms are rarely impressive but may include fever, cough, anorexia, weight loss, excessive perspiration, chest pain, lethargy, or dyspnea. More severe symptoms may occur in extrapulmonary disease such as with involvement of the pericardium, bones, joints, urinary tract, meninges, lymph nodes, or pleural space. Erythema nodosum is seen occasionally in patients with active disease.

B. Laboratory Findings: The skin test with intermediate strength PPD is positive in more than 90% of patients with active tuberculosis. False-negatives are usually due to anergy or to improper testing or outdated tuberculin. Anergy is sometimes associated with disseminated tuberculosis, measles, sarcoidosis, lymphomas, or recent vaccination with live viruses (eg, poliomyelitis, measles, German measles, mumps, influenza, or yellow fever). Immunosuppressive drugs (eg, corticosteroids or azathioprine) may also cause false-negative responses.

Culture of sputum, gastric aspirate, and pleural fluid and pleural or lung biopsies are important to establish the diagnosis.

C. X-Ray Findings: Pulmonary tuberculosis often predominantly involves the apical and posterior segments of the upper lobes (85%) or the superior segments of the lower lobes (10%). Seldom is the anterior segment of the upper lobe solely involved, as in other granulomatous diseases such as histoplasmosis. Involvement of the basal segments of the lower lobes is uncommon except in women, blacks, and diabetics, but endobronchial disease usually involves the lower lobes, producing atelectasis or consolidation. Differing roentgenographic patterns are found which correspond to the pathologic variations of the disease: the local exudative lesion, the local productive lesion, cavitation, acute tuberculous pneumonia, miliary tuberculosis, bronchiectasis, bronchostenosis, and tuberculoma.

D. Bronchoscopy: Bronchoscopy may be required to rule out other diseases, improve the quality of specimens for culture, or assess endobronchial disease.

Differential Diagnosis

Localized tuberculosis is sometimes indistinguishable from bronchogenic carcinoma, particularly when it presents as a tuberculoma without calcification. When there is cavitation, carcinoma, coccidioidomycosis, and other granulomatous diseases must be considered as well as pyogenic abscess or cavitation of a pulmonary infarct. The manifestations of tuberculosis are so variable that in patients with a positive tuberculin test this disease is often difficult to totally exclude. One should suspect tuberculosis more strongly when there has been recent heavy exposure or when the tuberculin reaction has only recently converted, or is very strong.

Prevention

Ideally, prevention of tuberculosis would consist of elimination of contact with tubercle bacilli so that implantation is prevented. In the USA this is approaching reality, as shown by the fact that only 3.5% of young adults have positive reactions to intermediate strength PPD.

BCG vaccination is warranted to induce relative immunity in tuberculin-negative individuals subject to exposure. It is about 80% effective in preventing infection and almost 100% effective in preventing lethal infections.

Chemoprophylaxis is advocated in the following cases (1) Patients whose skin test recently converted from negative to positive. (2) Persons with known recent exposure, especially children and young adults. Chemoprophylaxis should be given for 6–12 weeks until retesting demonstrates a negative skin test. (3) Persons with positive skin tests and x-ray evidence for dormant tuberculosis. (4) Persons who are tuberculin-positive and especially predisposed to active tuberculosis, ie, patients with severe diabetes mellitus or nodular silicosis, those undergoing treatment with corticosteroids, postgastrectomy patients, patients with malignancies (especially lymphoma), strong tuberculin reactors, patients subject to continued heavy exposure, undernourished people, and alcoholics.

The regimen used for prophylaxis is isoniazid, 300 mg/day, given as a single dose.

Treatment

A. Medical Treatment: Prolonged bed rest, hospitalization, and isolation are no longer required in the average case. Chemotherapy is usually started in a hospital in order to establish the diagnosis, determine base-line laboratory values (white blood counts, hematocrit, BUN, and SGOT levels), and detect drug toxicity. Smears and cultures are best done and sensitivities of the organism determined where close medical supervision is possible. The impact of this changed approach can be appreciated by noting that in 1945, the average hospital stay was over 2 years; by 1970, it was reduced to 3 months or less.

Drug therapy (Table 22–3) usually consists of giving 2 or 3 drugs in combination to prevent the emergence of resistant strains and minimize toxicity. The duration of antituberculosis drug treatment is at least 18 months or until radiologic signs of activity are gone, whichever is longer.

The principal causes of failure of chemotherapy are as follows: (1) failure of the patient to take the medications; (2) single drug therapy interruptions, often caused by drug toxicity or hypersensitivity; (3) inadequate initial drug treatment; and (4) primary resistance (including atypical mycobacteria).

B. Surgical Treatment: The role of surgery in treatment of tuberculosis has diminished dramatically since chemotherapy became available. It is now confined to the following indications: (1) failure of chemotherapy, (2) diagnosis, (3) destroyed lung, (4) postsurgical complications, (5) persistent bronchopleural fistula, and (6) tuberculous bronchiectasis.

The surgical procedures available consist of (1) diagnostic procedures such as bronchoscopy, mediastinoscopy, scalene node biopsy, lung biopsy, lymph node biopsy, and pleural biopsy; (2) drainage operations such as closed tube drainage or open drainage (eg, Eloesser flap); (3) collapse therapy, including phrenic nerve crush, pneumoperitoneum, pneumothorax, thoracoplasty, or plombage; (4) decortication; and (5) pulmonary resection, which may be pleuropneumonec-

TABLE 22–3. Antituberculosis drugs and their side-effects.*

Drug	Dosage (Adult Daily)	Side-Effects (Usual)	Monitoring†	Remarks
Isoniazid (INH)	5–10 mg/kg; 300–600 mg	Peripheral neuritis, hepatitis, hypersensitivity, convulsions.	SGOT/SGPT (not as routine).	For neuritis, pyridoxine, 25–50 mg as prophylaxis; 50–100 mg as treatment.
Ethambutol (EMB)	25 mg/kg for 60 days, then 15 mg/kg‡	Optic neuritis (reversible with discontinuation of drug; very rare at 15 mg/kg); skin rash.	Visual acuity, red-green color discrimination (Snellen chart).	Ocular history and funduscopic examination before use; contraindicated with optic neuritis; use with caution if serious ocular problems.
Streptomycin (SM)	0.75–1 g (frequently given for initial 60 days with advanced disease)	Otic and vestibular toxicity, decreased hearing, vertigo, tinnitus (nephrotoxicity—rare).	Gross hearing (ticking of watch); if abnormal, audiograms; BUN and creatinine.	More common in older patients (> 60); decrease dose or avoid drug if renal function is not adequate.
Aminosalicylic acid (PAS)	12–15 g	Gastrointestinal, hypersensitivity (rash), hepatotoxicity, sodium load.	SGOT/SGPT.	For gastrointestinal irritation, temporarily reduce dose or use calcium, potassium, ascorbic acid, or resin combinations; avoid sodium salt in elderly patients or those with heart failure or renal disease.
Rifampin	600 mg once daily (children, 10–20 mg/kg to a maximum of 600)	Minimal; liver dysfunction rarely.	SGOT/SGPT.	Extremely effective.
Ethionamide §	750–1000 mg	Gastrointestinal, hepatotoxicity, hypersensitivity (rash).	SGOT/SGPT.	Temporarily stop or reduce dose with gastrointestinal irritation and hepatotoxicity.
Pyrazinamide § (PZA)	20–35 mg/kg; not over 3 g	Hyperuricemia, hepatotoxicity, arthralgia.	Uric acid, SGOT/SGPT.	Probenecid or allopurinol to reduce serum uric acid.
Cycloserine §	750 mg	Psychosis, personality changes, convulsions, rash.	Drug blood levels if poor renal function.	Pyridoxine, 50–300 mg/day, may help; mental problems more common with predisposition.
Capreomycin §	1 g daily for 60–120 days, followed by 1 g 2–3 times weekly	Nephrotoxicity, ototoxicity, hepatotoxicity, hypersensitivity.	Same as streptomycin with SGOT/SGPT in addition.	Effective, newly released drug; not for pediatric use.
Viomycin §	1 g every 12 hours twice a week	Similar to streptomycin but nephrotoxicity more common.	As for streptomycin, plus urinalysis.	As for streptomycin.
Kanamycin §	0.5–1 g			Rarely used.

*Reproduced, with permission, from Weg JG: Treatment and control of tuberculosis. National Tuberculosis and Respiratory Disease Association, 1972.

†The most important monitoring device is an informed patient having ready access to medical care supplemented by a careful history and appropriate physical examination.

‡FDA recommends 15 mg/kg for entire treatment period except for retreatment cases, when 25 mg/kg is recommended for the initial 60 days.

§These are the so-called second-line drugs which have more frequent and more severe side-effects; knowledge and experience in their use is a desirable prerequisite.

tomy, pneumonectomy, lobectomy, segmentectomy, or wedge resection. Resection is the preferred method of surgical treatment whenever feasible since the infection is actually removed.

Surgical resection for diagnosis may be necessary to rule out other diseases such as malignancy or to obtain material for cultures. Patients with destroyed lobes (Fig 22–14) or cavitary tuberculosis of the right upper lobe (Fig 22–15) containing large infected foci may sometimes be candidates for resection. Thin-walled cavities ("open negative") have a relapse rate of less than 2%, whereas infection relapses in about 10% of cases with thick-walled cavities, and selected patients in the latter category may occasionally be surgical candidates.

The disease becomes reactivated in some patients who have had thoracoplasty, plombage, or resection, and a few will require operation. The most common indications for surgery after plombage therapy are pleural infection (pyogenic or tuberculous) and migration of the plombage material, causing pain or compression of other organs. Following pulmonary resection, tuberculous empyema may develop in the post-pneumonectomy space, sometimes associated with a bronchopleural fistula or bony sequestration. Persistent bronchopleural fistula after chemotherapy and closed tube drainage may require direct operative closure. Tuberculosis-related bronchiectasis, particularly if localized to a lower lobe, may sometimes require surgery, particularly if there has been significant bronchial scarring or stricture.

Tuberculous empyema poses unique problems of management. Treatment depends upon whether the empyema is (1) with or without parenchymal disease, (2) mixed tuberculous and pyogenic or purely tuberculous, and (3) with or without bronchopleural fistula. In all cases, the ultimate objective is complete expansion of the lung and obliteration of the empyema space. Pulmonary decortication or resection may be used for tuberculosis, but open or closed drainage is necessary when the process is complicated by pyogenic infection or bronchopleural fistula. Extrapleural thoracoplasty may be used in rare cases to obliterate a cavity but should be avoided if possible.

Prognosis

In children with converted tuberculin tests by age 5, only 20% have roentgenographic changes in the chest; by the time they have passed age 30, 91% have no clinical disease, 5% have active disease, and 4% have died of tuberculosis.

The prognosis is excellent in most cases treated medically; the mortality rate decreased from 25% in 1945 to 10% in 1970. The operative mortality rate in pulmonary resections for tuberculosis is about 10% for pneumonectomy, 3% for lobectomy, and 1% for segmentectomy and subsegmental resections. The overall operative morbidity rate is low.

The relapse rate following modern chemotherapy is about 4%; following combined resectional therapy and chemotherapy, relapse occurs in about 2%.

Anderson RP, Leand PM, Kieffer RF Jr: Changing attitudes in the surgical management of pulmonary tuberculosis: Analysis of 425 consecutive patients. Ann Thoracic Surg 3:43–51, 1967.

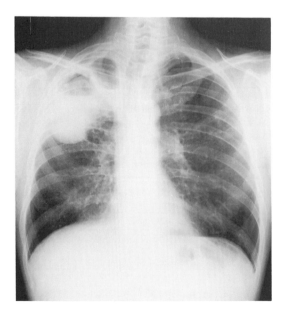

FIG 22–14. Cavitary tuberculosis of the right upper lobe.

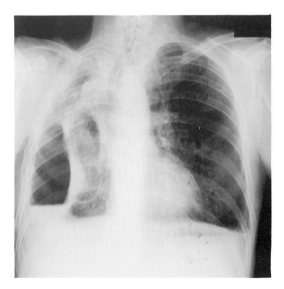

FIG 22–15. Tuberculosis of the right lung with empyema and bronchopleural fistula.

Barrett RN & others: Pulmonary resection in the treatment of tuberculosis: Experience with 1730 patients. J Thoracic Surg 38:803–817, 1958.

Fox RT & others: Surgical considerations in "atypical" mycobacterial pulmonary disease. J Thoracic Cardiovas Surg 59:1–6, 1970.

Freedman SO: Tuberculin testing and screening: A critical evaluation. Hosp Practice 7:63–70, 1972.

Howard WL & others: The loss of tuberculin sensitivity in certain patients with active pulmonary tuberculosis. Chest 57: 530–534, 1970.

Mitchell RS: Control of tuberculosis. New England J Med 276:842–848, 905–911, 1967.

Steele JD: The surgical treatment of pulmonary tuberculosis: Clinical review. Ann Thoracic Surg 6:484–502, 1968.

Steele JD (editor): U.S. Veterans' Administration Armed Forces Cooperative Studies of Tuberculosis. IV. Results of pulmonary resection, 1951–1955. Am Rev Tuberc 73:960–963, 1956.

Weg JG: The treatment and control of tuberculosis. National Tuberculosis and Respiratory Disease Association, 1972, pp 1–8.

Wiot JF: Spitz HB: Atypical pulmonary tuberculosis. Radiol Clin North America 11:191–196, 1973.

MYCOTIC INFECTION OF THE LUNGS

The increasing frequency of fungal disease is related to the widespread use of broad-spectrum antibiotics, corticosteroids, and immunosuppressive drugs. In the USA, each of the 3 most commonly encountered mycoses of surgical importance—histoplasmosis, coccidioidomycosis, blastomycosis—has a rather restricted endemic area. The surgeon becomes involved with fungal disease of the lung in 3 situations: (1) during diagnostic procedures, eg, bronchoscopy or biopsy; (2) in treatment of a lesion (eg, excisional biopsy) where the diagnosis is uncertain but neoplasm cannot be ruled out; and (3) in treatment of known fungal disease unresponsive to medical therapy. Special stains, special culture media, and special technics are essential for isolation and identification.

HISTOPLASMOSIS

Histoplasma capsulatum is found in soil contaminated by pigeon, chicken, or bat droppings. It is most prevalent in states bordering the Mississippi, Missouri, and Ohio River valleys. In the USA, 30 million persons are estimated to have been infected as shown by histoplasmin skin tests. Histoplasmosis has also been reported in South and Central America, India, Malaysia, and Cyprus. It is rare in Europe and Australia and almost nonexistent in England and Japan.

The symptoms and roentgenographic findings of histoplasmosis resemble those of tuberculosis, although the disease appears to progress more slowly. There may be cough, malaise, hemoptysis, low-grade fever, and weight loss. As many as 30% of cases coexist with tuberculosis. Pulmonary fibrosis, bulla formation, and pulmonary insufficiency occur in advanced cases. Mediastinal involvement is quite frequent and may take the form of granuloma formation, fibrosis with superior vena caval syndrome, or dysphagia. Erosion of inflammatory lymph nodes into bronchi may cause expectoration of broncholiths, hemoptysis, wheezing, or bronchiectasis. Traction diverticula of the esophagus may lead to development of tracheoesophageal fistula. Pericardial involvement may lead to constrictive pericarditis.

Histoplasmosis is a major diagnostic possibility in lesions that present as solitary pulmonary nodules, constituting about 15–20% of the total.

Radiologically, early infections appear as diffuse mottled parenchymal infiltrations surrounding the hila and enlargement of hilar lymph nodes. Cavitation indicates advanced infection and is the complication for which the surgeon is most often consulted. The diagnosis rests upon finding a positive skin test or complement fixation test and culturing the fungus from sputum or a bronchial aspirate.

Medical therapy with amphotericin B may be indicated.

Many cases appearing as solitary pulmonary nodules will require excisional biopsy to rule out neoplasm. Surgical therapy for unresolved cavitary disease or specific complications of mediastinal involvement must be planned to meet the criteria of feasibility of surgical correction.

Ahn C & others: The therapy of cavitary pulmonary histoplasmosis. J Thoracic Cardiovas Surg 57:42, 1969.

Forrest JV: Common fungal diseases of the lung. II. Histoplasmosis. Radiol Clin North America 11:163–168, 1973.

COCCIDIOIDOMYCOSIS

Coccidioides immitis is endemic to the southwestern part of the USA, especially the San Joaquin Valley of California. A few cases have been reported in Mexico and Central and South America. This soil-dweller produces arthrospores that are carried in the air and inhaled. Half of persons living in the endemic area have positive skin tests, and 25% of newly arrived individuals have a positive coccidioidin skin test after 1 year. Most conversions are asymptomatic, but about one-third develop flu-like symptoms. One percent of these go on to a prolonged illness lasting weeks or months. About 10 million people in the USA are estimated to have been infected.

Symptoms may be "flu-like," consisting of malaise, headache, and fever. There may be pleuritic pain

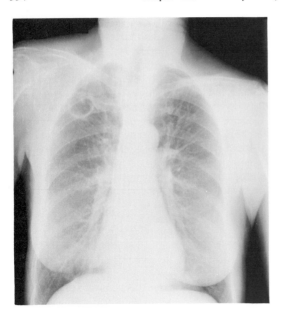

FIG 22–16. Thin-walled cavity of coccidioidomycosis.

and cough productive of mucoid bloody sputum. Physical signs are not helpful. The diagnosis is based on culture of sputum, fluids, or tissues obtained by biopsy. Roentgenographic findings are often indistinguishable from those of other granulomatous infections. Nodules may excavate to form thin- or thick-walled cavities (Fig 22–16), particularly in the upper lobes. Unlike tuberculosis, the anterior segments of the upper lobes are frequently involved. Cavitary disease is associated with pneumothorax and empyema in 2% of cases.

The only effective treatment is amphotericin B. Because of the drug's toxicity, it is given only on specific indications, ie, severe disease, disseminated disease, threat of dissemination, progressive pulmonary lesions, for surgical coverage, in patients with known disease who require corticosteroids, during pregnancy, or in diabetics.

Surgical treatment is reserved for patients with cavities that rupture into the pleural space, produce recurrent hemoptysis, or which are large or enlarging. Some bleeding occurs in 65% of coccidioidal cavities. Surgery may also be performed for undiagnosed solid lesions suspicious of carcinoma. Wide surgical excision of cavities or nodules—preferably lobectomy—is advised because of the frequent presence of satellite lesions which predisposes to postoperative complications. Ten to 15% of cases develop bronchopleural fistulas, coccidioidal empyema, or reactivation when wedge or localized excision is used.

Grant AR, Melick DW: The surgical treatment of cavitary pulmonary coccidioidomycosis. Arch Surg 94:559, 1967.

Sagel SS: Common fungal diseases of the lungs. I. Coccidioidomycosis. Radiol Clin North America 11:153–161, 1973.

NORTH AMERICAN BLASTOMYCOSIS

Blastomyces dermatitidis has a mycelial phase in soil and a yeast phase in humans and animals. Endemic areas are in the western hemisphere, particularly the central and southeastern USA and in Canada. It is considerably less common than histoplasmosis, but the exact incidence is not known. The disease has a cutaneous and a pulmonary form.

Pulmonary blastomycosis presents with symptoms of cough, chest pain, hemoptysis, and fever. Chest roentgenographic findings are nonspecific and may show cavitation, unresolved infiltrates, or consolidation. Calcification of parenchymal lesions is very rare. Skin lesions usually have a specific appearance, consisting of chronic indolent enlarging papulopustules with thick adherent crusts and elevated violaceous edges. The diagnosis is made by culture of the organism from sputum, skin lesions, abscesses, or biopsy material. The organism may also be demonstrated in urine, CSF, or blood. Pleural effusion occurs in 2% of cases, bony lesions in 25% of cases, and genitourinary tract lesions in 10% of males. When untreated, the clinical course is one of frequent remissions and exacerbations and a mortality rate of 30%. A positive blastomycin skin test should be considered significant only when stronger than that to histoplasmin and coccidioidin. Serologic tests may also be helpful.

Hydroxystilbamidine and amphotericin B should be considered for treatment.

Surgery is rarely indicated. It is more often employed for diagnosis to rule out bronchogenic carcinoma. Postoperative dissemination is minimized if drug therapy is used concomitantly with surgery; when not accompanied by adequate drug therapy, operative spread is common.

Busey JF & others: Blastomycosis. I. A review of 198 collected cases in Veterans' Administration hospitals. Am Rev Resp Dis 89:659, 1964.

Witorsch P, Utz JP: North American blastomycosis: A study of 40 patients. Medicine 47:169–200, 1968.

CRYPTOCOCCOSIS
(Torulosis)

Cryptococcus neoformans is a soil-dweller—particularly soil contaminated by pigeon droppings—that has a worldwide distribution. The organism enters the blood via the lungs and has a predilection for the CNS. It is a primary pathogen but also an opportunistic invader in debilitated patients, particularly those with lymphoma or collagen disease or those receiving antimetabolites, corticosteroids, or antibiotics.

Pulmonary symptoms are nonspecific or so insidious that they may not receive clinical recognition. When it affects patients ill from another disease, symptoms of the latter often overshadow those due to cryptococcosis. The disease is often discovered inadvertently on chest x-ray or by a pathologist examining tissue removed at thoracotomy. Cultures of sputum, bronchial washings, and spinal fluid may establish the diagnosis, but false-negatives are fairly common. Chest x-rays usually show a fairly well circumscribed mass, 2–8 cm in diameter, often single, in a lower lobe. Cavitation occurs in about 15% of cases. Pleural involvement is unusual and calcification is rare.

When extrapulmonary (especially CNS) disease is present, amphotericin B coverage is indicated. In the absence of CNS disease, amphotericin B may be withheld when cryptococcosis is found in a specimen of lung resected for diagnosis of a solitary nodule.

Campbell GD: Primary pulmonary cryptococcosis. Am Rev Resp Dis 94:236–243, 1966.
Hatcher CR Jr & others: Primary pulmonary cryptococcosis. J Thoracic Cardiovas Surg 61:39, 1971.

ACTINOMYCOSIS

Actinomyces israelii is a normal inhabitant of the oral cavity of man. The diagnosis is made from cultures of yellow-brown granules called "sulfur granules" from suppurative material or draining sinuses.

In man, cervicofacial, thoracic, and abdominal forms are recognized. The infections with this organism produce a marked fibroplastic response. Thoracic involvement, characteristically manifested by empyema or draining chest wall sinuses, is often associated with nonspecific pulmonary infiltrates, consolidation, or hilar manifestations.

Treatment

Penicillin is the drug of choice. Surgical treatment (with antibiotic coverage) may be required, ie, open drainage or wide excision. The diagnosis is sometimes made after thoracotomy for a lesion suspected to be bronchogenic carcinoma.

Villegas AH, Sala DA: Pulmonary actinomycosis of pseudotumoral form. J Thoracic Cardiovas Surg 49:677, 1965.

NOCARDIOSIS

Nocardia asteroides and less commonly, *N brasiliensis* or *N madurae* cause human infections. The organisms are found worldwide in soil, grasses, and in several species of animals. The lesions may resemble actinomycosis with sulfur granules and there is an acid-fast bacillus-like form resembling tuberculosis. They are often opportunistic.

Symptoms are often flu-like. Empyema develops in 25% of cases, often forming subcutaneous abscesses or fistulous tracts and sinuses. Nocardia has been isolated from broncholiths almost as often as histoplasma.

Sulfadiazine is the drug of choice. Pulmonary resection is rarely indicated. As a rule, surgical treatment is restricted to drainage of empyema or abscesses.

Freese JW & others: Pulmonary infection with *Nocardia asteroides:* Findings in eleven clinical cases. J Thoracic Cardiovas Surg 46:537, 1963.

ASPERGILLOSIS

Aspergillus fumigatus is the most commonly found species, but *A flavus, A niger,* and *A nidulans* also cause clinical disease. Three clinical forms occur: (1) bronchitis secondary to aspergillus sensitivity; (2) aspergillomas or fungus balls, which present as saprophytes in long-standing cavitary lung disease (Fig 23–17); and (3) opportunistic invasive infections causing a necrotizing pneumonia, infarction, and hematogenous dissemination.

Medical treatment has been unsatisfactory but iodides, nystatin, hydroxystilbamidine, and amphotericin B have all been reported to produce cures. Surgical therapy is indicated in suitably selected patients with aspergilloma, particularly if recurrent hemoptysis has occurred.

Davies D & others: Aspergillus in persistent lung cavities after tuberculosis. Tubercle (London) 49:1–11, 1968.

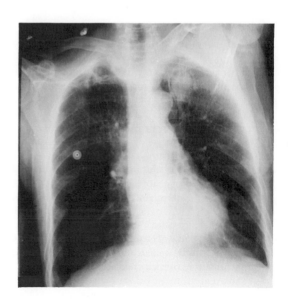

FIG 22–17. Aspergilloma (fungus ball) in tuberculous cavity of the left upper lobe.

Kennedy WPV: Necrotizing pulmonary aspergillosis. Thorax 25:691–701, 1970.

Solit RW & others: The surgical implications of intracavitary mycetomas (fungus balls). J Thoracic Cardiovas Surg 62:411–422, 1971.

OTHER MYCOTIC INFECTIONS

Candida albicans and other species of Candida usually cause opportunistic infections involving the lungs of patients treated by endotracheal tube, assisted ventilation, and broad-spectrum antibiotics. Localized bronchopulmonary candidiasis is extremely rare. Other relatively rare mycotic infections of thoracic surgical interest are sporotrichosis, which produces a localized cavity, phycomycosis or mucormycosis, South American blastomycosis, and geotrichosis.

Penta AQ: The mycotic infections of the broncho-pulmonary tract. Am J Surg 90:77–91, 1955.

Razzuk MA, Urschel HC Jr, Paulson DL: Systemic mycosis: Primary pathogenic fungi. Ann Thoracic Surg 15:644–660, 1973.

Takaro T: Mycotic infections of interest to thoracic surgeons. Ann Thoracic Surg 3:71–93, 1967.

PARASITIC INFESTATIONS*

PULMONARY & PLEURAL AMEBIASIS

Entamoeba histolytica is a protozoan infection that may have pleuropulmonary involvement in 10–20% of cases. About 75% of cases of thoracic involvement are secondary to transdiaphragmatic rupture of hepatic abscesses and only about 15% of cases of thoracic involvement occur without hepatic abscesses.

Clinical and roentgenographic manifestations are those of pleurisy, pleural effusion, empyema (25% have secondary pyogenic infection), bronchopleural fistula, or pulmonary abscess. There may be right upper quadrant pain, pleuritic pain, dry cough, or a cough productive of material resembling "chocolate sauce" or "anchovy sauce."

Medical treatment consists of metronidazole, emetine, chloroquine, and antibiotics for secondary bacterial infections (see Chapter 10).

Thoracentesis is used if no secondary infection is present. Surgical treatment in secondarily infected cases usually consists of closed tube drainage (occasionally followed by open drainage), decortication, or pulmonary resection.

The survival rate with pulmonary involvement is 90%. About 25% need only medical treatment, 35% chemotherapy and thoracentesis, 15% closed drainage, and 12% require more extensive procedures. Deaths are most common in patients with secondary bacterial infection.

Herrera-Lierandi R: Thoracic repercussions of amebiasis. J Thoracic Cardiovas Surg 52:361, 1966.

McIver WJ, Love JW, Ziperman HH: Profuse hemoptysis as an infrequent manifestation of hepatopulmonary amebiasis. Ann Thoracic Surg 4:454–457, 1967.

SARCOIDOSIS
(Boeck's Sarcoid, Benign Lymphogranulomatosis)

Sarcoidosis is a noncaseating granulomatous disease of unknown cause involving the lungs, liver, spleen, lymph nodes, skin, and bones. The distribution is worldwide, but the largest series are reported from Scandinavia, England, and the USA. Sarcoidosis is more prevalent in rural areas, particularly in the southeastern USA. The incidence in blacks (especially females) is 10–17 times that in whites. Half of patients are between the ages of 20 and 40.

Clinical Findings

A. Symptoms and Signs: Sarcoidosis may present with symptoms of pulmonary infection, but usually these are insidious and nonspecific. Erythema nodosum may herald the onset, and weight loss, fatigue, weakness, and malaise may appear later. Fever occurs in 15% of cases. Pulmonary symptoms occur in 20–30% and include dry cough and dyspnea. Hemoptysis is rare. One-fifth of cases have myocardial involvement, and heart block or failure may occur. Peripheral lymph nodes are enlarged in 75%; scalene lymph nodes are microscopically involved in 80%; mediastinal nodes in 90%; and cutaneous involvement is present in 30%. Hepatic and splenic involvement can be shown by biopsy in 70% of cases. There may be migratory or persistent polyarthritis, and CNS involvement occurs in a few patients.

B. Laboratory Findings: Laboratory findings are hypercalciuria (30%), hypercalcemia (15%), abnormal serum proteins, elevated alkaline phosphatase, leukopenia, and eosinophilia. The Kveim test is positive in 75% of cases.

C. X-Ray Findings: Chest roentgenographic findings are bilateral, symmetric hilar and paratracheal lymph node involvement (75–90%), diffuse pulmonary disease without enlargement of hilar nodes (25%), combined diffuse pulmonary disease and hilar lymph node involvement, or pulmonary fibrosis (20%). Pleural effusion is rare unless due to heart failure.

*Echinococcosis and amebiasis are discussed in Chapter 10.

D. Biopsy: If peripheral adenopathy or skin lesions are present, histologic diagnosis should be sought by biopsy of these lesions. Otherwise, biopsy via mediastinoscopy or of scalene lymph nodes will provide the answer in over 90% of cases.

Differential Diagnosis

Tuberculosis, coccidioidomycosis, histoplasmosis, cryptococcosis, and brucellosis may present a picture identical to that of sarcoidosis. Metastatic cancer, foreign body granulomas (especially in heroin addicts), or multiple hamartomatosis may be difficult to exclude.

Treatment

Medical treatment consists of observation, general supportive measures, and, in severe cases, corticosteroids. Preventive antituberculosis therapy should be used when corticosteroids are given or when a positive tuberculin reaction is present. Surgical management, in addition to procedures to establish the diagnosis and rule out other diseases (eg, biopsies of lymph nodes, lung, or liver), involves treatment of heart block by pacemaker implantation or, rarely, treatment of the complications of bullous emphysema in advanced cases.

Prognosis

The prognosis is poorer in blacks and when relapses have occurred. The mortality rate is about 5–10% in patients followed for 20 years. Cardiac failure is the leading cause of death. Superimposed tuberculosis is common and should be anticipated. About 65% of patients recover fully; 20–25% have some degree of permanent disability.

Bower G: Intrathoracic sarcoidosis: A review of 69 cases. Dis Chest 44:457–469, 1967.

Kent DC & others: The definitive evaluation of sarcoidosis. Ann Rev Resp Dis 101:721–727, 1970.

Lam CR: The surgical aspects of sarcoidosis. Arch Surg 97: 459–468, 1968.

Sones M, Israel HC: Course and prognosis of sarcoidosis. Am J Med 29:84–93, 1960.

PULMONARY THROMBOEMBOLIC DISEASE

Essentials of Diagnosis

- Large pulmonary embolus: Sudden onset of dyspnea and anxiety, with or without substernal pain. Signs of acute right heart failure and circulatory collapse may follow shortly.
- Pulmonary infarction: Less severe dyspnea, pleuritic pain, cough, hemoptysis, and an x-ray density in the lung are characteristic of pulmonary infarction.
- Recurrent minor emboli: Gradually developing, unexplained, with or without pulmonary x-ray densities.
- A history or clinical findings of thrombophlebitis is common in patients with pulmonary embolism.

General Considerations

Pulmonary embolism is the most frequent cause of death, established at autopsy. Half of cases are not suspected clinically, and in 20% no physical findings preceded the embolism. Pulmonary thromboembolism does not necessarily result in pulmonary infarction, which occurs in only 10–15% of cases. The site of origin of the clot is usually the lower extremity or pelvic veins; rarely, the upper extremities or cervical veins. The right atrium is the source in some cases.

Clotted blood is by far the most common embolus to the pulmonary vasculature, but fat, air, bits of tumor, amniotic fluid, bone marrow, parasites, and, in addicts, foreign materials such as starch, cotton, glass, rubber, etc may be found. Bacterial vegetations may embolize in bacterial endocarditis. Clot may even originate within the lungs by intravascular coagulation in mitral stenosis, or in diseases involving the arterial wall.

Clinical Findings

A. Symptoms and Signs: Pulmonary thromboembolism is manifested in 4 main ways: (1) acute massive embolism, (2) segmental emboli with or without infarction, (3) multiple small emboli that present as pulmonary insufficiency, and (4) silent or asymptomatic emboli. The clinical findings of pulmonary embolism or infarction are usually either cardiac or respiratory; hypoxia may lead to restlessness or anxiety. When 65–70% of the pulmonary vasculature is occluded, acute pulmonary hypertension occurs, cardiac output decreases, and hypotension, cardiac arrhythmias, shock, and death may ensue. This may occur within a few minutes or a few days. When embolism results in infarction, dyspnea, tachycardia, fever, pleuritic chest pain, cough, and sometimes hemoptysis develop. Dyspnea and chest pain are the most common symptoms, and dyspnea is always present in severe cases. When emboli are recurrent and small, the onset of dyspnea may be insidious. Chest pain is of 2 types. Retrosternal pain may be identical to that of myocardial infarction and is due to acute pulmonary hypertension or coronary insufficiency caused by diminished cardiac output. The second type of pain is pleuritic. Hemoptysis occurs in 20–35% of cases, and cough is present primarily as a result of hemoptysis.

Physical signs include decreased breath sounds, rales, rhonchi, rubs, or signs of pleural effusion. Evidence of right heart failure and pulmonary hypertension may be present, eg, a loud second pulmonic sound, venous distention, and acute liver enlargement. Cyanosis is often present.

B. Laboratory Findings: Laboratory tests are usually not diagnostic. Arterial blood gases may reveal a low oxygen tension, and there may be a gradient in P_{CO_2} between arterial blood and the end tidal gas. Electrocardiographic changes are helpful only in one-third of cases, but classically show an S wave in lead I, an inverted Q wave or T wave (or both) in lead III, and T wave inversion over the right side of the heart.

Roentgenographic findings may show either nothing abnormal, evidence of diminished vascularity, or, later, typical wedge-shaped peripheral infiltrates with or without effusion. The lower lobes are most often involved, especially the right. Ten to 15% of cases involve primarily the upper lobes. Evidence of acute enlargement of the pulmonary artery or a sudden termination of the pulmonary artery may be present. There may be signs of cor pulmonale in severe cases.

Pulmonary angiography is the only means of definitive diagnosis and should precede surgery in all patients being considered for thoracotomy (Fig 22–18). It may be necessary to institute cardiopulmonary bypass to accomplish this procedure. The angiogram shows the clot or an occlusion in the pulmonary arteries.

Radioisotope scanning using macroaggregated albumin tagged with ^{131}I isotopes is useful in less severe or doubtful cases. A normal scan rules out a massive embolism, but the presence of a defect does not prove the diagnosis. Diminished perfusion may occur for many reasons, including bullae (Fig 22–12), diminished cardiac output, etc. Serial scans may be more valuable.

Differential Diagnosis

The most common mistaken diagnosis in massive embolism is myocardial infarction. Thoracotomy in these patients carries a high mortality rate and must be avoided. In less severe cases, congestive heart failure, pneumonia, and asthma must be considered.

Treatment

The patient is immediately anticoagulated with heparin (see p 718) to prevent further thrombosis and for the pharmacologic effect of heparin that reduces pulmonary vascular resistance. Acid-base abnormalities are corrected. The patient is constantly monitored. Treatment should include cardiopulmonary resuscitative measures to support circulation and improve oxygenation. Hypotension is treated by pressor agents and hypoxia by intubation, assisted ventilation, or oxygen mask.

Surgical treatment is used to prevent recurrent episodes of embolism in patients who have emboli while adequately anticoagulated. The procedures available include caval ligation or caval filters.

Embolectomy requiring thoracotomy and cardiopulmonary bypass is reserved for patients receiving adequate medical therapy whose deterioration is indicated by hypotension, severe hypoxemia, or cardiac arrest and arteriographic evidence of occlusion of 50% or more of the pulmonary vasculature.

Prognosis

The overall prognosis is poor. About 47,000 people die every year of pulmonary embolism in the USA, and most of these are not clinically detected or

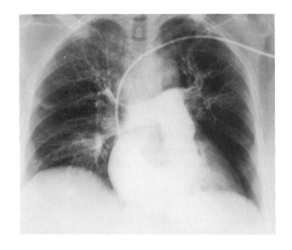

FIG 22–18. Pulmonary angiogram in a patient with massive thromboembolism.

treated. It is estimated that 75% of patients die within 1 hour. In recognized cases of massive embolism, the extent of embolism is most critical. In patients who withstand the initial episode, resolution and recanalization of the pulmonary vasculature can occur promptly, and most patients do not have lasting disability.

Accumulated statistics since 1967 for embolectomy with cardiopulmonary bypass show that survival was 70% using cardiopulmonary bypass and 60% with medical therapy.

Bergan JJ & others: Prevention of pulmonary embolism: Comparison of vena caval ligation, plication, and filter operations. Arch Surg 92:605–610, 1966.

Fred HL & others: Arteriographic assessment of lung scanning in the diagnosis of pulmonary thromboembolism. New England J Med 275:1026–1032, 1966.

Fred HL & others: Rapid resolution of pulmonary thromboemboli in man. New England J Med 280:1194–1199, 1969.

Houk VN & others: Chronic thrombotic obstruction of major pulmonary arteries. Am J Med 35:269–282, 1963.

Murray JF: The pathogenesis, diagnosis and treatment of pulmonary embolus. California Med 114:36–44, June 1971.

Paraskos JA & others: Late prognosis of acute pulmonary embolism. New England J Med 289:55–58, 1973.

Turnier E & others: Massive pulmonary embolism. Am J Surg 125:611–622, 1973.

THE SOLITARY PULMONARY NODULE
("Coin Lesions")

Solitary pulmonary nodules or "coin lesions" are peripheral circumscribed pulmonary lesions that encompass a wide variety of conditions, especially granu-lomatous diseases and neoplasms. The latter includes benign or malignant primary or secondary tumors. Many characteristics denote probable benignity or malignancy, but often the diagnosis is not certain. Since 5-year survival following resection of a solitary nodule that turns out to be bronchogenic carcinoma may be as high as 90%, prompt surgical therapy is warranted when malignancy cannot be excluded. In the average patient, the risk of thoracotomy is less than 1%, and if the chance of malignancy is 5% the probability of cure will outweigh the risk of thora-cotomy.

The overall incidence of malignancy in solitary nodular lesions seen on x-ray is about 5–10%. How-ever, in patients ultimately selected for resection of the nodules, the probability of malignancy is considerably higher. The breakdown is as follows: 35% primary carcinomas, 35% nonspecific granulomas, 20% tubercu-lous granulomas, about 5% mixed tumors (hamar-tomas), and 5% metastatic carcinomas. A small miscel-laneous category includes adenomas, cysts, and other lesions. The overall incidence of solitary nodules is 3–9 times higher in males than females. Malignancy is almost twice as frequent in males as in females.

Clinical Findings

A. Symptoms: Symptoms are usually not present, but cough, weight loss, chest pain, or hemoptysis favors a diagnosis of malignancy.

B. Past History: There may be a history of living in an endemic granuloma area. Previous tuberculosis favors granuloma, whereas smoking favors malignancy. Ninety percent of patients with solitary metastatic lesions have a history of extrapulmonary malignancy.

C. Signs: Clubbing is uncommon in benign lesions and is seen occasionally in malignant ones. Hypertro-phic osteoarthropathy signifies an 80% or greater probability of malignancy.

D. Laboratory Findings: Positive skin tests do not rule out malignancy, but granulomatous disease is less likely when skin tests are negative. In granuloma of known cause, the skin test is positive in 90% of cases of tuberculosis, 80% of cases of histoplasmosis, and 70% of cases of coccidioidomycosis.

Sputum cultures are usually negative. Cytologic examination of sputum yields a diagnosis in only 5–20% of cases.

E. X-Ray Findings: Coin lesions can rarely be diagnosed with certainty—whether benign or malig-nant—by radiologic findings (Fig 22–19). Some useful x-ray features are as follows:*

1. Size—Lesions 1 cm or less in diameter are prob-ably granulomas; those greater than 1 cm have a signifi-cant probability of cancer, and a lesion 4 cm or more in diameter is very likely malignant (Fig 22–20A and B).

---

*The most persuasive radiologic evidences of benignity are (1) calcification, especially if concentric or laminated; and (2) documented absence of growth for 1 year.

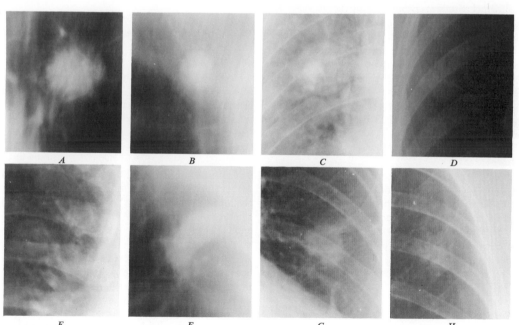

FIG 22–19. Coin lesions. *A:* Large cell undifferentiated carcinoma in RUL (tomogram). *B:* Histoplasmosis (tomogram). *C:* Hamartoma. *D:* Solitary metastasis from epidermoid carcinoma of the cervix. *E:* Tubercu-loma (tomogram). *F:* Foreign body granuloma in heroin addict (tomogram). *G:* Adenocarcinoma of LUL (present 6 years). *H:* Alveolar cell carcinoma of LUL (present 3 years). (RUL = right upper lobe; LUL = left upper lobe.)

2. Cavitation and radiolucent areas—These are seen in both benign and malignant lesions (Figs 22—19 and 22—20).

3. Calcification—The presence of calcification tends to favor benignity but does not exclude carcinoma unless it appears as concentric laminations. Calcification may be misinterpreted on plain films, and tomograms should be obtained when considered important. Calcifications of the "target" or "popcorn" variety are very unlikely to be malignant (Fig 22—19B and C). Lesions that are completely or heavily calcified are most likely benign. Malignant lesions with calcifications are most often squamous cell carcinomas. Adenocarcinomas are next most common. Calcification in malignancies generally consists of small flecks located eccentrically or at the periphery of the nodule.

4. Density—Dense lesions less than 3 cm in diameter favor a diagnosis of malignancy (Fig 22—19D and E).

5. Margins—Irregular shape is often seen in inflammatory lesions and benign lung tumors (Fig 22—19F). A rounded lesion with umbilication suggests malignancy (Fig 22—19G). Indistinct margins favor malignancy (Fig 22—20H), whereas discrete margins favor benignity (Fig 22—19B), although circumscribed margins are seen in about 30% of malignant lesions.

6. Growth—Documented absence of growth for more than 1 year means that malignancy is highly unlikely, but slow growth has been seen in malignant lesions followed for 6 years or more.

7. Satellites—The presence of satellite densities favors a diagnosis of granuloma.

F. Other Studies: Bronchoscopy is of value in about 10% of solitary cases, and mediastinoscopy may be diagnostic of malignancy in 6—15% of cases. In the absence of a pertinent history, a search should not be made for a primary lesion by roentgenographic studies of the upper gastrointestinal tract, urinary tract, or skeletal system. Percutaneous needle biopsy should not be done in potentially curable surgical candidates because of possible intrathoracic dissemination of the tumor.

Treatment

A decision must often be made about whether or not to give therapy for tuberculosis. The risks of the patient's being lost to follow-up, indecisive results even after 3—6 months, and the possibility of spread of tumor are factors favoring early resolution of the diagnostic dilemma by excisional biopsy. The overall risk of thoracotomy is less than 1%. Patients with a higher operative risk are in the age group of 50 years or older, but these patients also have a 50—60% chance of having carcinoma.

Surgical diagnosis may be made by excisional wedge biopsy in peripheral lesions and may constitute definitive therapy for benign lesions, for solitary metastasis, and for primary malignancy in poor-risk patients. Centrally placed lesions or those suspected of being coccidioidomycosis should be treated by lobectomy. Primary malignancies are treated by lobectomy

in good-risk patients with regional node dissection. Pneumonectomy should not be done until a tissue diagnosis of malignancy has been established.

Prognosis

The prognosis for malignant coin lesions is 3—6 times more favorable than that for lung cancer in general. The 5-year survival rate in those less than 2 cm in diameter is about 70%.

Bateson EM: An analysis of 155 solitary lung lesions illustrating the differential diagnosis of mixed tumours of the lung. Clin Radiol 16:51—65, 1965.

Burdette WJ, Evans C: Management of coin lesions and carcinoma of the lung. Ann Surg 161:649—673, 1965.

Davis EW, Peabody JW Jr, Katz S: The solitary pulmonary nodule. J Thoracic Surg 32:728—771, 1956.

Jackman RJ & others: Survival rates in peripheral bronchogenic carcinomas up to four centimeters in diameter presenting as solitary pulmonary nodules. J Thoracic Cardiovas Surg 57:1—8, 1969.

Mitchell RS, Taylor RR: The solitary circumscribed nodule. Arch Surg 100:780—792, 1957.

O'Connor TM & others: The malignant solitary nodule: Follow-up study. Arch Surg 86:985—988, 1963.

Steele JD: The solitary pulmonary nodule. J Thoracic Cardiovas Surg 46:21—39, 1963.

LUNG NEOPLASMS

BENIGN NEOPLASMS

Benign tumors of the lung are very uncommon and account for only 1—2% of all pulmonary neoplasms. Over half of the cases that are included in this category are bronchial adenomas, which are in fact low-grade malignant tumors since about 15% metastasize. Considering only coin lesions of the lungs, 5—10% are benign neoplasms.

Most truly benign lesions of the lung are hamartomas (mixed tumors). Other types are fibrous mesotheliomas, xanthomatous and inflammatory pseudotumors, and miscellaneous rare lesions such as lipomas and benign granular cell myoblastomas.

Benign lung tumors may occur at almost any age. Hamartomas occur in males twice as often as females. Symptoms are absent in 60% and nonspecific in many other cases. Bronchial obstruction by the lesion, pneumonitis, and hemoptysis may occur. Clubbing or hypertrophic osteoarthropathy does not occur in benign tumors except in fibrous mesotheliomas. X-ray may show calcification.

The differential diagnosis is discussed in the context of solitary pulmonary nodules in the preceding section.

Surgical excision should be conservative, and

enucleation or wedge excision done when possible. The prognosis is excellent.

Arrigoni MG & others: Benign tumors of the lung: A ten-year surgical experience. J Thoracic Cardiovas Surg 60:589–599, 1970.

Bateson EM: An analysis of 155 solitary lung lesions illustrating the differential diagnosis of mixed tumours of the lung. Clin Radiol 16:51–65, 1965.

Steele JD: The solitary nodule. J Thoracic Cardiovas Surg 56:21–39, 1963.

MALIGNANT LUNG NEOPLASMS

Essentials of Diagnosis

- Insidious onset with cough, localized wheeze, or hemoptysis; often asymptomatic.
- May present as an unresolved pneumonia, atelectasis, or pleurisy with bloody effusion, or as a pulmonary nodule seen on x-ray.
- Metastases to other organs may produce initial symptoms.
- Endocrine, biochemical, and neuromuscular disorders (see below) may be the presenting features of bronchogenic carcinoma.

General Considerations

The incidence of lung cancer is increasing, and lung cancer has become the most common fatal malignancy in males. In England during 1966, 39% of all male cancer deaths and 8% of all deaths were caused by lung cancer. The United Kingdom mortality rates are the highest of all, and Finland, Austria, several western European countries, and the Union of South Africa all have higher mortality rates from lung cancer than the USA.

It is believed that the rate of increase has reached a peak and that the twentieth century increase was due to cigarette smoking, air pollution, and specific industrial hazards. By far the most important etiologic factor in lung cancer is cigarette smoking. Cigarette smoking is related causally to bronchogenic carcinoma of the squamous cell and oat cell types but not to adenocarcinoma or alveolar cell carcinomas. Various materials in mining and industrial exposure that have been associated with bronchogenic carcinoma include asbestos, radioactive materials, arsenic, chromates, and nickel.

Classification

The most widely accepted classification of malignant lung tumors today is that proposed in 1958 by the World Health Organization (Table 22–4).

Pathologic Features

A. Squamous Cell Carcinomas: These tumors may be well differentiated or not depending upon the presence of keratin and epithelial pearls; intracellular

TABLE 22–4. Classification of malignant tumors of the lung.

Epidermoid carcinoma (squamous cell).
Keratinizing squamous carcinoma.
Oat cell carcinoma.
Adenocarcinoma.
Bronchiolar or bronchoalveolar carcinoma.
Undifferentiated large cell carcinoma.
Bronchial carcinoid.
Tumors of tracheobronchial mucous glands.
Adenoid cystic carcinoma (cylindroma).
Mucoepidermoid carcinoma.
Bronchial mucous gland adenocarcinoma.
Papilloma and papillary carcinoma.
Sarcoma.
Malignant lymphoma.
Leiomyosarcoma.
Others.
Teratomas, embryonal tumors, and mixed tumors.
Pleural mesothelioma.
Epithelial or diffuse.
Fibrosarcomas.
Other pleural sarcomas.

bridges; cell size and uniformity; or mitosis. About 45% of all lung tumors are squamous cell. Two-thirds are located centrally near the hilum and one-third peripherally. Growth rate and rate of metastases tend to be slower than those of other lung tumors.

B. Oat Cell Carcinomas: These are highly malignant tumors composed of small round or oval cells that often resemble lymphocytes. The origin of these cells is unknown, but they resemble carcinoid tumors and also have a similar distribution and propensity to cause endocrine disturbances. Anaplastic tumors of this type represent about 3.5% of all bronchial carcinomas. About 80% are centrally located and 20% peripheral.

C. Adenocarcinomas: Adenocarcinomas containing glandular elements comprise about 15% of malignant lung tumors. Histologically, they are acinar, papillary, or large giant cell in type. Tumors arising in the periphery and in scars are often adenocarcinomas. Adenocarcinomas are peripheral in 75% of cases and central in 25%. They are intermediate in malignant potential between squamous cell and oat cell types. They often spread along vascular channels. Bronchiolar or alveolar cell carcinomas are well-differentiated papillary adenocarcinomas and represent perhaps 2.5% of all malignant tumors. Giant cell tumors are highly malignant. They have pleomorphic or multinucleated cells and represent about 1% of all lung carcinomas.

D. Large Cell Undifferentiated Tumors: This is a poorly defined group of tumors. Some resemble anaplastic or squamous cell tumors with cells characterized by abundant cytoplasm—unlike the oat cell undifferentiated tumors. These tumors are seen more often peripherally; comprise 3–5% of all lung tumors; and are less malignant than small cell undifferentiated tumors.

E. Bronchial Adenomas: These comprise about 1% of lung tumors. They are slow-growing and have a low propensity to metastasize. They are sometimes erroneously classified as benign tumors. Bronchial carcinoid is the most common (85%); adenoid cystic carcinomas (cylindromas) are next in frequency (10–15%); and mucoepidermoid tumors are rare. Carcinoid tumors are usually centrally located in the main stem or lobar bronchi, but 5–10% may be located peripherally. The clinical course is often indolent, extending over years. Adenoid cystic tumors or cylindromas resemble analogous neoplasms in the salivary gland and are either pseudoacinar or medullary in type. These tumors are more malignant than carcinoid tumors but also tend to grow slowly. They have a distribution similar to that of the carcinoids. Mucoepidermoid tumors are most often centrally located and are usually of low-grade malignancy, resembling their salivary gland counterpart. Three cell types may be identified: squamous cells with keratin, mucin-producing cells, and intermediate cells arranged in nests or cords. Bronchial adenomas—especially carcinoid tumors—are twice as common in women as in men.

F. Isolated Bronchial Papilloma and Papillary Carcinomas: These rare tumors are usually part of generalized papillomatosis of the larynx or trachea.

G. Sarcomas: Sarcomas of the lung constitute less than 1% of all lung cancers. Involvement of the lung is not uncommon (7–40%) in disseminated lymphoma but rarely is seen confined to the lung. Most are lymphosarcomas or reticulum cell sarcomas. Other sarcomas arising from soft tissues or primitive mesenchymal cells may be (1) spindle cell sarcomas of the fibro-, lipo-, or myxosarcomatous type; (2) myosarcomas of either smooth or skeletal muscle type; (3) neurosarcomas; (4) chondrosarcomas or osteosarcomas; (5) vascular tumors of hemangiosarcomatous or lymphangiosarcomatous types; or (6) malignant histiocytomas.

Clinical Findings

A. Symptoms and Signs: In 10–20% of patients, no symptoms are present when lung cancer is first diagnosed. The malignancy is usually detected by chest roentgenogram or, very occasionally, by positive cytology. The first symptom may be cough (29%), chest pain (13%), dyspnea (12%), or hemoptysis (6%). A few cases present with pneumonia and malaise, symptoms of brain metastases, bronchitis, epigastric pain or anorexia, weight loss, pain from bone metastases, swelling of the upper body, shoulder pain, flu, hoarseness, or pleurisy.

When symptoms become established, the principal complaints are cough (usually productive) and hemoptysis.

The symptoms can be divided into thoracic and extrathoracic categories. Thoracic symptoms include cough, hemoptysis, wheezing, and pneumonia. Bronchial occlusion may cause dyspnea or tightness of the chest. Extension to the pleura may cause pleuritic pain and symptoms of pleural effusion. Pleural effusion is seen in bronchial obstruction or lymphatic obstruction and is more likely to be serous than bloody. Bloody effusion is usually caused by direct pleural involvement. Oat cell carcinoma most frequently invades the lymphatics and has the highest incidence of pleural effusion. Mediastinal involvement may give symptoms of retrosternal pain, hoarseness from recurrent laryngeal involvement (usually the left), or vena caval obstruction (often oat cell).

Tumors involving the thoracic or superior pulmonary sulcus at the root of the neck may cause **Pancoast's syndrome,** which consists of an apical lung tumor that involves the brachial plexus, the sympathetic ganglia at the base of the neck, and sometimes destruction of ribs and vertebrae. Symptoms are pain, loss of strength in the arm, and **Horner's syndrome** (ptosis, miosis, enophthalmos, and ipsilateral decreased sweating on the involved side). There may be swelling of the involved arm.

Extrathoracic manifestations of lung cancer may be due either to metastatic or to nonmetastatic causes. Extrathoracic metastases occur from either hematogenous or lymphatic dissemination. Lung cancer commonly metastasizes to the cervical and abdominal lymph nodes, liver, adrenals, kidneys, brain, or bone. The exact sequence of metastases differs somewhat with different pathologic types, but the patterns are the same. Lymph node involvement at autopsy is 75% hilar, 60% mediastinal, 15% mesenteric, 5% pancreatic, 3% axillary, and 1% inguinal. Blood-borne metastases at autopsy are to the brain (85%), adrenals (45%), liver (45%), and bone (35%). The bones most frequently involved are the vertebrae (20%), ribs (10%), pelvis (5%), and skull (less than 1%). Metastases are commonly widespread; the pancreas, heart, pericardium, thyroid, spleen, and bowel are often involved.

Nonmetastatic extrathoracic manifestations related to lung cancer include the following: (1) Connective tissue syndromes: dermatomyositis, scleroderma, hypertrophic pulmonary osteoarthropathy. (2) Neuromyopathies: cerebellar degeneration, encephalomyelopathy, polyneuropathy, and myopathy. (3) Endocrine effects and associated metabolic disorders: hyperadrenocorticism (oat cell), inappropriate antidiuretic hormone secretion (oat cell), hypercalcemia (with or without skeletal metastases), gynecomastia, hypoglycemia, excessive gonadotropin secretion, and carcinoid syndrome (weight loss, anorexia, explosive diarrhea, cutaneous flushing, and tachycardia) secondary to excessive secretion of 5-hydroxytryptamine. (4) Vascular and hematologic manifestations: migratory thrombophlebitis, thrombocytopenia, anemias, and chronic consumptive coagulopathies. The prognostic importance of these must be individually determined since some, eg, clubbing or hypertrophic osteoarthropathy, have no adverse prognostic implications whereas others—particularly hormone-secreting tumors—are often associated with oat cell carcinoma and for that reason have a poor prognosis.

B. X-Ray Findings: The roentgenographic manifestations of lung cancer are quite variable (Fig

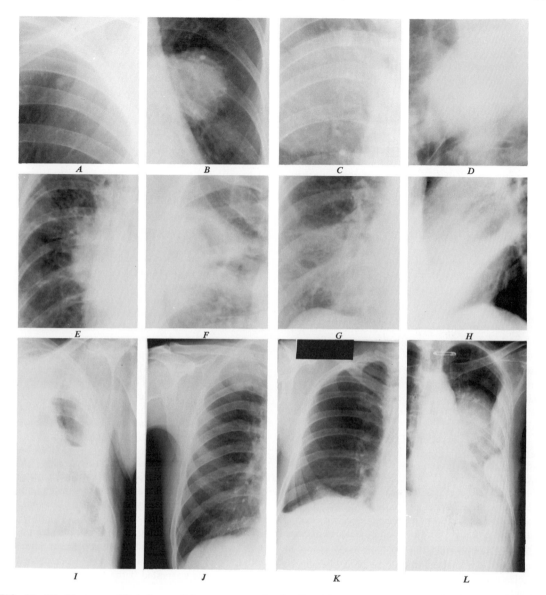

FIG 22–20. X-ray manifestations of lung cancer. *A:* Small epidermoid carcinoma in LUL (posteroanterior projection). *B:* Large coin lesion; adenocarcinoma in superior segment of LLL (lateral projection). *C and D:* Epidermoid carcinoma in RUL. *E:* Right hilar mass; oat cell carcinoma. *F:* Large cavitary epidermoid carcinoma in RUL. *G* (posteroanterior projection) and *H* (lateral projection): Middle lobe atelectasis from bronchial carcinoid (not visible). *I:* Opacification of left hemithorax; large cavitary epidermoid carcinoma. *J:* Pancoast's tumor; poorly differentiated epidermoid carcinoma with erosion of third rib and pathologic fracture of fourth rib. *K:* Right phrenic nerve paralysis caused by epidermoid carcinoma. *L:* Pleural metastasis caused by adenocarcinoma of LLL. (LUL = left upper lobe; LLL = left lower lobe, etc.)

22–20). They have been classified as hilar, parenchymal, and intrathoracic and extrapulmonary. A hilar abnormality with or without a mass is present in about 40% of cases; a parenchymal mass greater than 4 cm in diameter in 20% and smaller than 4 cm in 20%; and an apical mass in 2.5%. Extrapulmonary intrathoracic manifestations are present in 10%.

Treatment

Evaluation for treatment must be individualized. The objectives are to establish the diagnosis of lung cancer and to assess the curability of the tumor and the general health and suitability of the patient as a surgical candidate. This assessment must be done without undue delay since the best chance for cure is with surgery. It is very important to determine if the extent of tumor will permit possible cure so that unnecessary thoracotomy is avoided.

Unfortunately, two-thirds of patients with lung cancer are incurable when first seen. Evidence of incurability is as follows: (1) Regional lymph node involvement (enlarged supraclavicular, axillary, or abdominal lymph nodes). (2) Malignant pleural effusion diagnosed by cytologic examination. (3) Recurrent laryngeal nerve paralysis. (4) Phrenic nerve paralysis. (5) High paratracheal, contralateral hilar extension, or lymph node involvement. (6) Any distant metastasis synchronous with the appearance of the primary (most commonly the brain, adrenals, liver, and skeleton). (7) Superior vena cava syndrome. (8) Involvement of the main pulmonary artery.

The prognosis is less favorable if the lesion is bronchoscopically visible; if the chest wall is involved by direct extension; if Pancoast's tumor (superior sulcus tumor) is present; if cytologic examination of the sputum has established the presence of oat cell tumor; or if a biopsy diagnosis has been made. Some consider oat cell carcinoma to be incurable, and it is true that 90% of patients will be incurable by the above criteria when properly evaluated. However, in those patients who undergo resection for cure, the overall 5-year survival rate is 10%. Patients with peritracheal node involvement, carinal involvement in adenocarcinoma, or undifferentiated tumor are very unlikely to be curable.

The medical condition of the patient may impose a relative contraindication to surgery, but the assessment must be based on general health status, not on chronologic age.

Despite careful preoperative assessment, 5–10% of patients who undergo thoracotomy are found to be incurable. It is essential that low-risk diagnostic procedures such as bronchoscopy, laryngoscopy, scalene or mediastinal lymph node biopsy, and examination of pleural fluid for malignant cells be used liberally to minimize unnecessary thoracotomy since the operative mortality rate in such patients is 2–3 times higher than in patients who undergo curative resection.

Indications of incurability found at the time of operation include nonresectability (ie, unable to proceed safely or with a chance for cure) because of parietal pleural seeding, vena caval involvement, vertebral body extension, contralateral or high peritracheal lymph node involvement, aortic arch involvement, hepatic metastases palpable through the diaphragm, and the necessity for pneumonectomy in a patient who will tolerate only a lobectomy.

A. General Measures: There is no curative medical therapy for lung cancer. Medical treatment should be limited to preoperative preparation of the patient for surgery and must include assessment and measures to improve pulmonary function, heart failure, nutrition, and metabolic or acid-base disturbances.

B. Radiotherapy: Radiotherapy in lung cancer is used for palliation, as adjuvant therapy in combination with surgery, or occasionally for cure. Palliation of symptoms is the most frequent use of radiotherapy and may be for pain, for symptoms due to metastases to bone or brain, or for relief of obstruction of the airway or of the superior vena cava. Radiotherapy when used as an adjuvant to surgery may be given either pre- or postoperatively. Preoperative radiotherapy has not been proved to be of value except possibly preceding resection of Pancoast tumors. Preoperative therapy (exceeding 3000 rads) has been implicated in bronchial stump complications when the operative area is treated directly. Postoperative radiotherapy may be of benefit for patients who have mediastinal involvement or Pancoast tumors. Radiotherapy is curative of lung cancer in only 1–2% of cases, and these occur most often in undifferentiated tumors. Oat cell carcinoma has a grim outlook with any form of therapy, but surgery is preferable if patients are selected for operation by the criteria outlined above.

C. Surgical Treatment: If there is no evidence of incurability, the surgical treatment of lung cancer consists of thoracotomy and resection of the involved lung with regional lymph nodes or contiguous structures. Lobectomy is the procedure of choice in good-risk patients with localized disease. Pneumonectomy or bilobectomy (eg, right upper and middle lobes or right lower and middle lobes) is used when the tumor is situated at a fissure or in such a way as to require wide excision. Wedge resection or segmentectomy is used for localized disease in poor-risk patients, for low-grade malignancy, and when conservative surgery is indicated because the tumor is probably metastatic.

Bronchoplastic procedures such as sleeve resection are used to conserve lung tissue, eg, in the resection of a tumor involving the take-off of the upper lobe bronchus when pulmonary function is limited or the tumor is of low-grade malignancy (eg, carcinoid).

Extended resections are sometimes indicated in special situations. In-continuity resection of a lobe or lung with the chest wall, intrapericardial resection, extrapleural dissection, and, rarely, other procedures are sometimes warranted if the tumor is well differentiated.

Prognosis

Improvements in patient evaluation, anesthesia, and postoperative care in the past decade have made most reported operative morbidity and mortality statistics obsolete. Intensive care facilities with trained personnel, monitoring equipment, ventilatory support, blood gas analysis, and around-the-clock laboratory and radiologic facilities have greatly improved results. These advances, together with better selection of curable patients, permit many centers to report 5% or less operative mortality rates following major pulmonary resections in patients 40–60 years of age. In young good-risk patients or when thoracotomy is done for diagnostic purposes or for benign disease, the mortality rate should approach zero.

Five-year survival is about 35% following lobectomy and 20% after pneumonectomy. These rates are determined largely by the histologic type of tumor and operative or pathologic evidence of extension or invasiveness. The age of the patient, the anatomic location of the tumor, tumor doubling time, and the presence or absence of symptoms also have a bearing on the outcome. The prognosis is poor in children, young adults, and women, but adenocarcinoma and undifferentiated tumors predominate in these patients. Histologic evidence of lymph node involvement and blood vessel invasion adversely affect the prognosis.

It must be emphasized that overall curability of lung cancer is less than postoperative 5-year survival since two-thirds of all patients with lung cancer are not candidates for surgical treatment. Overall survival is only about one-fourth to one-third of the cure rate of surgically treated patients.

The natural history of lung cancer varies with the histologic type, the age of the patient, the location of the tumor, and other factors. Without surgery, 95% of patients with primary lung cancer are dead in 2 years. The average reported delay between the first visit to a physician and the operation is 4–6 months. In view of the short natural history of lung cancer and the known progression of disease in patients with favorable disease–ie, coin lesions, carcinoma in situ, occult primaries, or normal chest x-ray but positive cytology–prolonged observation to observe the rate of growth or the response to antituberculosis therapy can only be condemned.

Arrigoni MG & others: Benign tumors of the lung: A ten-year experience. J Thoracic Cardiovas Surg 60:589–599, 1970.

Arrigoni MG, Woolner LB, Bernatz PE: Atypical carcinoid tumors of the lung. J Thoracic Cardiovas Surg 64:413–421, 1972.

Burford TH & others: Results of treatment of bronchogenic carcinoma. J Thoracic Surg 36:316–324, 1958.

Claggett OT & others: The surgical treatment of pulmonary neoplasms: A 10-year experience. J Thoracic Cardiovas Surg 48:391–400, 1964.

Geha AS, Bernatz PE, Woolner LB: Bronchogenic carcinoma involving the thoracic wall. J Thoracic Cardiovas Surg 54:394–401, 1967.

Gibbon JH Jr, Templeton JY III, Nealon TF Jr: Factors which influence the long term survival of patients with cancer of the lung. Ann Surg 145:637–643, 1957.

Higgins GA, Beebe GW: Bronchogenic carcinoma: Factors in survival. Arch Surg 94:539–549, 1967.

Jackman RJ & others: Survival rate in peripheral bronchogenic carcinomas up to 4 centimeters in diameter presenting as solitary pulmonary nodules. J Thoracic Cardiovas Surg 57:1–8, 1969.

Jensik RJ & others: Sleeve lobectomy for carcinoma. J Thoracic Cardiovas Surg 64:400–412, 1972.

Kennedy JH: Extrapulmonary effects of cancer of the lung and pleura: Endocrine, muscular, cutaneous, hematologic and cardiovascular manifestations not due to metastases. J Thoracic Cardiovas Surg 61:514–529, 1971.

Kern WH, Jones JC, Chapman ND: Pathology of bronchogenic carcinoma in long-term survivors of cancer. Cancer 21:772–780, 1968.

Kirsh MM & others: Treatment of bronchogenic carcinoma with mediastinal metastases. Ann Thoracic Surg 12:11–21, 1971.

Kreyberg L: Histological lung cancer types. Acta path microbiol scandinav, Suppl 157, 1962.

Lennox SC & others: Results of resection for oat-cell carcinoma of the lung. Lancet 2:925, 1968.

Meyer JA: The concept and significance of growth rates in human pulmonary tumors. Ann Thoracic Surg 14:309–322, 1972.

Paulson DL, Urschel HC Jr: Selectivity in the surgical treatment of bronchogenic carcinoma. J Thoracic Cardiovas Surg 62:554–562, 1971.

Paulson DL & others: Bronchoplastic procedures for bronchogenic carcinoma. J Thoracic Cardiovas Surg 59:38–48, 1970.

Sensing DH, Rossi NP, Ehrenhoft JL: Pulmonary resection for bronchogenic carcinoma in geriatric patients. Ann Thoracic Surg 2: 508–513, 1966.

Shaw RR, Paulson DL, Klee JL Jr: Treatment of the superior sulcus tumor by irradiation followed by resection. Ann Surg 154:29–40, 1961.

Shields TW & others: Preoperative x-ray therapy as an adjuvant in the treatment of bronchogenic carcinoma. J Thoracic Cardiovas Surg 59:49–61, 1970.

Steele JD: *The Solitary Pulmonary Nodule.* Thomas, 1964.

Vincent TN, Satterfield JV, Ackerman LV: Carcinoma of the lungs in women. Cancer 18:559–570, 1965.

Watson WL (editor): *Lung Cancer.* Mosby, 1968.

Wellons HA Jr & others: Prognostic factors in malignant tumors of the lung: An analysis of 582 cases. Ann Thoracic Surg 5:228–235, 1968.

Woolner LB & others: In situ and early invasive bronchogenic carcinoma. J Thoracic Cardiovas Surg 60:275–290, 1970.

SECONDARY MALIGNANT NEOPLASMS OF THE LUNG

The lungs harbor metastases in about 30% of all patients with malignancy. Depending upon the primary lesion, the number of metastases may be limited, and a few of these may be surgically curable. The most frequent sources of solitary metastatic lesions are the colon, kidneys, uterus and ovaries, breasts, testes, malignant melanoma, pharynx, and bone. In coin lesions, solitary metastasis is the ultimate diagnosis in about 5%. Five to 15% of malignant coin lesions are solitary metastases, and in 90% of these cases a history of the primary is available.

Certain criteria for selection of patients suitable for resection have been developed: (1) The initial primary must be controlled, and no other metastases can be present. (2) When the initial primary was a squamous cell tumor, the lung lesion should be evaluated as a new primary. (3) When the initial lesion was an adenocarcinoma, other common sites of metastasis must be sought. (4) A waiting period of 3–6 months is advisable before thoracotomy if the primary lesion was treated within 2 years. (5) Total lung tomograms or stereoscopic views of the lung must be obtained to rule out additional metastases. (6) Synchronous appearance of a pulmonary metastasis and the primary lesion must be evaluated individually, but in general the prognosis improves as the interval between control of the primary and the appearance of the lung metastasis increases. (7) Multiple lesions, particularly when bilateral or involving different lobes, usually mean that the prognosis is poor. Recently, however, multiple resections for metastases from osteogenic sarcoma have been shown to be worthwhile.

About 80% of coin metastases meeting the above criteria are found to be susceptible to complete removal. Eighty percent are carcinomas and 20% sarcomas. The 5-year survival rate following removal of the carcinomas is 35%; for the sarcomas, 25%. Only a few 5-year survivals following removal of lung cancers metastatic from malignant melanoma or the breasts have been reported.

Claggett OT & others: The surgical treatment of pulmonary neoplasms: A 10-year experience. J Thoracic Cardiovas Surg 48:391–397, 1964.

Martini N & others: Multiple pulmonary resections in the treatment of osteogenic sarcoma. Ann Thoracic Surg 12:271–280, 1971.

Mitchell RS, Taylor RR: The circumscribed solitary nodule. Arch Surg 100:780–792, 1957.

Steele JD: The solitary pulmonary nodule. J Thoracic Cardiovas Surg 46:21–39, 1963.

Turney SZ, Haight C: Pulmonary resection for metastatic neoplasms. J Thoracic Cardiovas Surg 61:784–794, 1971.

THE MEDIASTINUM
Orville F. Grimes, MD

The mediastinum is the central portion of the thorax between the 2 pleural cavities. It extends posteriorly from the sternum to the vertebral column and from the base of the neck to the diaphragm. The lateral borders are formed by the mediastinal pleura, which is a continuation of the parietal pleura that lines the chest cavity on each side. The heart and great vessels occupy a large part of the mediastinum. The esophagus, the trachea, the origins of both main stem bronchi, the thoracic duct, lymph nodes, adipose tissue, and a network of lymphatic channels also lie within the mediastinum. The trunks of the vagus and phrenic nerves as well as the sympathetic ganglia pass through the area.

The anatomic area is divided into the superior and the inferior mediastinum. The superior mediastinum lies anteriorly above the level of the sternomanubrial angle and posteriorly above the upper portion of the fifth thoracic vertebra. The distance between the anterior and posterior borders is so short that the entire compartment is designated as the superior mediastinum without further division.

The inferior mediastinum is divided into anterior, middle, and posterior portions. This compartmentation is of clinical value since tumors of the mediastinum have a predilection for a specific division (Fig 22–21).

Important structures in the superior mediastinum include the trachea, esophagus, and thymus gland in the midline. To each side are the great vessels: the innominate artery on the right, the subclavian and common carotid arteries on the left. The left innominate vein crosses obliquely behind the manubrium and joins the right innominate vein to form the superior vena cava. The thoracic duct lies near the posterior surface of the esophagus, passes obliquely behind it, and eventually empties into the left subclavian vein. The trachea bifurcates at the level of the junction of the manubrium and the body of the sternum. The transverse portion of the aortic arch rises as high as the midportion of the manubrium. The phrenic and vagus nerves pass downward through the superior mediastinum; sympathetic ganglia lie on each side of the vertebral column.

In the inferior mediastinum, the anterior portion extends from the lower border of the superior mediastinum to the diaphragm and from the posterior border of the sternum to the pericardium. The compartment contains the triangularis sterni muscle, the internal mammary vessels, and a series of lymph nodes that lie in close proximity to the internal mammary and the medialmost portion of the intercostal vessels.

The middle mediastinum extends from the anterior surface of the pericardium backward to the posterior pericardium and roots of the lungs. It contains the heart, the lower half of the superior vena cava, the azygos vein, and the ascending aorta. The right and left main stem bronchi, the lymph nodes which surround the roots of the lung, and the origins of the pulmonary arteries and veins also lie in this compartment. The phrenic nerves pass directly downward beneath the mediastinal pleura and are closely applied to the pericardium.

The posterior mediastinum extends from the posterior pericardial surface and the roots of the lungs to the anterior surface of the vertebrae. The esophagus lies behind the heart and aorta. Between the aorta and the vertebral bodies the thoracic duct passes up from its origin in the cisterna chyli. Immediately to its right is the azygos venous system.

MEDIASTINAL EMPHYSEMA

The significance of air in the mediastinum depends on its cause. Mediastinal emphysema following external blunt or penetrating trauma or after diagnostic endoscopy almost always indicates injury to the trachea, the main stem bronchi, or the esophagus. Immediate operation is mandatory.

Intrapulmonary terminal alveoli may rupture spontaneously, and air released in the periphery of the lungs may dissect proximally along the bronchovascular structures and enter the mediastinum. If air enters the vascular system, air embolism, primarily to the brain, may result. Air may also enter the pleural

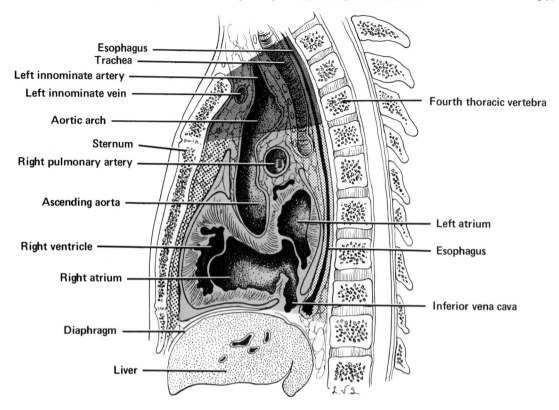

FIG 22–21. Divisions of the mediastinum.

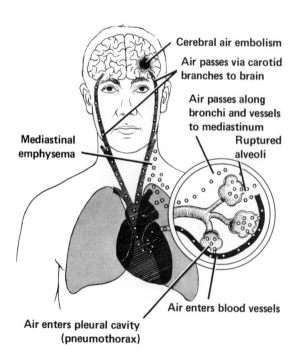

FIG 22–22. Mediastinal emphysema. (After Netter.)

space to form a pneumothorax (Fig 22–22). It can be recognized radiologically by mediastinal air shadows and clinically by the presence of crepitus in the base of the neck. Crepitus is almost always minimal and self-limiting. If progressive, the pressure thus produced in the mediastinum can be relieved by an incision in the suprasternal space to release the air contained in the fascial compartments.

When pneumomediastinum is suspected or recognized, immediate radiologic studies, including esophagrams, should be undertaken to locate the site of injury and the source of the air. Without immediate treatment, fatal mediastinitis may result. Cerebral emboli may cause severe distress.

Gray JM, Hanson GC: Mediastinal emphysema: Aetiology, diagnosis and treatment. Thorax 21:325, 1966.

INFECTIONS OF THE MEDIASTINUM

The fascial planes of the neck communicate directly with the superior mediastinum; the inferior mediastinal compartments are in fascial continuity with the retroperitoneal space. Infections may thus spread from one anatomic area to another. Infections in the neck frequently drain by gravity into the mediastinum, aided by the negative intrapleural pressure.

Infections of the mediastinum are classified as acute or chronic. Mediastinitis often develops from direct contamination, commonly as a consequence of rupture of the esophagus during endoscopy or dilatation or as a result of erosion of the esophageal wall by a foreign body. Postoperative anastomotic disruption of the esophagus is a common cause of fatal mediastinitis. After operations in the cervical region, infections that spread downward are usually contained within the superior mediastinum. Osteomyelitis in ribs or vertebrae that involves the adjacent soft tissues accounts for only a small number of mediastinal infections. The mediastinum may become secondarily infected through lymphatic channels that connect with those of the head and neck, neighboring intrathoracic structures, portions of the stomach and liver, and the subdiaphragmatic spaces. Pleural empyema occasionally ruptures into the mediastinal pleura. Abscesses that develop in the medial segments of the lungs may spread directly into the mediastinum.

1. ACUTE MEDIASTINITIS

Essentials of Diagnosis

- Rapidly rising temperature, chest pain, prostration, chills, and shock, especially after esophageal instrumentation or direct wounding.
- Substernal pain, dyspnea, tachycardia, and leukocytosis may be severe.
- Distention of superficial neck veins and crepitus if bronchial or esophageal perforation has occurred.
- Most cases occur after esophageal surgery, injury, instrumentation, or following spontaneous rupture.
- Chest films often show widening of the superior mediastinum, air in the mediastinum and subcutaneous tissues, and, occasionally, air-fluid levels.

General Considerations

The fascial planes of the neck are in direct continuity with the anatomic planes and spaces of the upper mediastinum. The lower mediastinal compartments and planes are similarly in fascial communication with the upper retroperitoneal region. Infections arising in one area may dissect progressively from one anatomic space into another. This is especially true of infections originating in the neck, since downward drainage into the mediastinum not only is affected by gravity but also is accentuated by the negative intrapleural pressure.

Acute suppurative mediastinitis most often develops as a result of direct contamination following injuries of the cervical or thoracic esophagus during instrumentation or as a result of erosion of the esophageal wall by a foreign body. Disruption of the suture line following operations upon the esophagus may cause severe and often fatal mediastinitis. Mediastinitis from external penetrating trauma usually results from complications of injuries to the esophagus, trachea, or main stem bronchi.

Acute infections of the mediastinum require immediate and vigorous management if prolonged and complicated convalescence or death is to be avoided. Sepsis is often severe since it is usually caused by instrumental or perforating wounds of the esophagus, resulting in contamination by the highly virulent mixed flora of the oropharynx, including bacteroides, streptococci, and neisseriae. Absorption of bacteria and toxic products through the generous lymphatic network of the mediastinum may cause almost immediate bacteremia and rapidly developing septicemia. Massive broad-spectrum antimicrobial therapy is mandatory and should be initiated immediately. After the organisms have been identified by cultures and sensitivity tests on the mediastinal fluid and blood have been performed, the antibiotic regimen can be appropriately altered if necessary.

Clinical Findings

A. Symptoms and Signs: Prostration, shock, high fever, and signs of sepsis develop rapidly, and substernal pain is often severe. As the infection spreads, pleuritic pain often occurs. Respiratory obstruction and dysphagia may result from compression of the trachea, bronchi, or esophagus due to the expanding inflammatory process. Tachypnea, tachycardia, and cardiac arrhythmias frequently develop. The soft tissues at the base of the neck anteriorly are swollen and edematous. Crepitus may be palpated if the cause of the acute mediastinitis is related to esophageal or tracheal perforation. Auscultation over the heart and the adjacent mediastinum may reveal a loud crunching, clicking sound due to the movements of the heart against air-containing tissues (Hamman's sign). The auscultative noises are synchronous with the heartbeat.

Acute infections involving the inferior mediastinum produce less definite symptoms and signs. Upper abdominal pain, tenderness, and muscular rigidity resulting from downward extension of the infection suggest an acute abdominal catastrophe.

B. Laboratory Findings: Leukocytosis invariably develops and may exceed $30,000/\mu l$ with a marked shift to the left.

C. X-Ray Findings: Radiologic studies show widening of the superior mediastinum and obliteration of the aortic knob. The increased distance between the vertebral column and the barium-filled esophagus indicates accumulation of fluid in this area. Interstitial emphysema is often present, both in the mediastinum and in the soft tissues of the neck. In acute infections involving the inferior mediastinum, x-ray studies, including water-soluble contrast examination of the esophagus, stomach, and duodenum, are often necessary to rule out acute upper abdominal disease.

Complications

Acute mediastinal infections may be fatal unless recognized and treated immediately. Rapid development of sepsis from absorption of bacteria and toxic products into the extensive lymphatic channels may produce overwhelming septic shock. Extension of sepsis into one or both pleural cavities may result in empyema. If massive hemorrhage from erosion into one of the great vessels occurs, it is usually fatal.

Treatment

Most acute infections of the mediastinum result from esophageal tears or wounds during diagnostic esophagoscopy or therapeutic dilatations. Immediate surgical repair and drainage is the preferred treatment of esophageal injuries, along with antibiotic therapy.

Prognosis

Early recognition of acute mediastinitis and its cause is essential. With prompt treatment, the results are excellent.

Leigh TF, Weens HS: *The Mediastinum.* Thomas, 1959.
Payne WS, Larson RH: Acute mediastinitis. S Clin North America 49:999–1009, 1969.

2. CHRONIC MEDIASTINITIS

Acute mediastinitis, by partial resolution, may localize as a chronic mediastinal phlegmon or abscess. Most cases of chronic mediastinitis, however, are granulomatous, with either tuberculous or fungal infections predominating. Cases are occasionally reported in which a nonspecific diffuse fibrotic inflammatory process involves part or all of the mediastinum.

Clinical Findings

A. Symptoms and Signs: Pain, fever, dysphagia, and cough may accompany the usual signs of chronic sepsis depending on the location, extent, and virulence of the infection. Obstruction of the superior vena cava may develop from the induration and inflammatory reaction in the superior mediastinum. Pneumonitis in the adjacent lung, localized empyema, and pericarditis may be produced by local extension of the chronic inflammatory process.

B. X-Ray Findings: Radiologic studies may show a localized mediastinal mass, often containing an air-fluid level. Varying degrees of widening of the mediastinal shadow may be seen. The mediastinum may show little or no widening in chronic diffuse granulomatous or nonspecific fibrous mediastinitis since these processes, though densely indurated, often do not project outward to any appreciable extent.

Differential Diagnosis

Chronic mediastinitis (with or without abscess formation) must be differentiated from mediastinal tumors and various lesions of the esophagus, trachea, and bronchi. Lymphadenopathy, either benign or malignant, may mimic chronic mediastinitis. Carcinoma of the upper lobe of the right lung adjacent to the superior vena cava may cause an obstruction identical to that caused by chronic infections of the superior mediastinum. Plain films of the chest are often diagnostic, especially if an air-fluid level is present which indicates the presence of a chronic abscess. Tomography, angiography, and endoscopy are often helpful. Surgical exploration is often necessary to establish a proper histologic diagnosis.

Complications

Abscesses may erode the trachea, bronchi, or esophagus to produce various types of fistulas. Erosions into major vascular trunks may result in massive, often fatal hemorrhage. In chronic granulomatous or fibrous mediastinitis, the most common complication is obstruction of the superior vena cava.

Treatment

Chronic mediastinal abscesses, especially those in the inferior mediastinum, often must be drained by a posterior paravertebral approach. Adequate biopsies of the fibrotic or granulomatous encasement must be obtained since malignant processes may grossly resemble benign lesions. Chronic fibrosing or granulomatous mediastinitis causing superior vena cava obstruction often does not require surgery, as the collateral venous circulation that develops adequately drains the upper portions of the body.

Prognosis

Most chronic infections of the mediastinum can be managed successfully either by an appropriate operative procedure, specific antibiotic therapy, or both.

Ferguson B, Burford TH: Mediastinal granuloma: A 15-year experience. Ann Thoracic Surg 1:125–141, 1965.
Goodwin RA & others: Mediastinal fibrosis complicating healed primary histoplasmosis and tuberculosis. Medicine 51: 227–246, 1972.
Nelson WP, Lundberg GD, Dickerson RB: Pulmonary artery obstruction and cor pulmonale due to chronic fibrous mediastinitis. Am J Med 38:279, 1965.
Sakulsky SB & others: Mediastinal granuloma. J Thoracic Cardiovas Surg 54:279, 1967.
Schowengerdt CG, Suyemoto R, Main FB: Granulomatous and fibrous mediastinitis: A review and analysis of 180 cases. J Thoracic Cardiovas Surg 57:365–379, 1969.

TUMORS OF THE MEDIASTINUM

Essentials of Diagnosis

- Benign tumors are often asymptomatic.
- Malignant tumors frequently produce pain,

erosion of adjacent structures, and distant metastases.

- Tumor often seen on plain chest films. Tomography and angiography are helpful.
- The exact diagnosis can be made only by biopsy.

General Considerations

Identification by radiologic studies of the mediastinal compartment in which the mass is located provides a fairly good clue to its exact type. In the superior mediastinum, the most common tumor is an intrathoracic goiter. Parathyroid enlargements and occasionally bronchogenic cysts are also found in this compartment.

The anterior portion of the superior mediastinum characteristically contains teratomas, thymomas, and tumors of dermoid origin. Pericardial and bronchogenic cysts are frequently seen in the middle mediastinum along with lesions involving the hilar lymph nodes. Neurogenic tumors are usually restricted to the posterior mediastinum. Bronchogenic, esophageal, and gastroenteric cysts occur less frequently in the posterior than in the middle mediastinum.

Clinical Findings

Tumors may reach a large size and remain almost asymptomatic if important mediastinal structures are not involved. Tumors of any size may cause symptoms if there is compression of the tracheobronchial tree, esophagus, superior vena cava, or chambers of the heart. Dyspnea, wheezing, and cough suggest encroachment upon the trachea or bronchi. Hemoptysis is uncommon but can occur with both benign and malignant lesions. Vascular compression is uncommon in benign tumors; when present, it suggests that the lesion is an invasive neoplasm.

Metabolic disturbances may accompany a mediastinal mass. Thymomas are occasionally associated with myasthenia gravis. Intrathoracic goiter is only rarely associated with hyperthyroidism. Malignancies such as Hodgkin's disease or anaplastic carcinomas may produce a generalized hypermetabolic state.

Differential Diagnosis

The intrathoracic goiter in the superior mediastinum often is an extension of a palpable neck mass. The substernal goiter appears radiologically on the lateral projection as a rounded mass projecting downward into the middle mediastinum. Displacement of the trachea is almost universal. Histologically, the lesions are usually composed of involutionary nodules. The lesions move upward and downward with swallowing, which is an important observation in ruling out other lesions of the superior mediastinum. Although bronchogenic cysts may occur in the superior compartment, they are more common in the middle mediastinum near the bifurcation of the trachea. Radiologically, bronchogenic cysts have a smooth, rounded contour. An opaque density is characteristic unless secondary infection has developed, in which case an

air-fluid level may be present. Esophageal cysts or gastroenteric duplications can be differentiated from bronchogenic cysts only by histologic examination following excision. Esophageal cysts or duplications often do not have a communication with the foregut. Biopsy or total excision is necessary for diagnosis of mediastinal lesions as the radiologic features are not sufficiently constant to be unequivocally diagnostic.

Complications

Both benign and malignant masses in the mediastinum may cause respiratory stridor from compression of the trachea or bronchi. Dysphagia may result from extrinsic pressure on the esophagus. Bronchogenic cysts occasionally rupture into the tracheobronchial tree and become secondarily infected. Cysts or reduplications of the esophagus may also become infected, resulting in hemorrhage and rupture. Invasive tumors of the mediastinum may produce hemorrhage and infection. They may involve the pleural spaces, causing esophagobronchial fistulas to develop, and, by venous compression, may produce the superior vena cava syndrome. Dermoid cysts occasionally rupture, usually into the lung; hemoptysis, purulent sputum, and dermoid elements such as hair and sebaceous material are then found in the sputum. Malignant thymomas in the anterior mediastinum often cause severe vascular, tracheal, or esophageal compression, with invasion into the mediastinal pleura, pericardium, and adjacent lung.

Myasthenia gravis is often accompanied by benign or, more commonly, malignant thymomas. Lymphosarcoma invades adjacent tissues extensively, and, since mediastinal lymph nodes are only a small part of the overall lymphatic disease, the intrathoracic lesions are ordinarily nonresectable. The trachea, major bronchi, esophagus, and great vessels are often involved. Pleuropericardial cysts rarely cause complications. Sufficiently large posterior mediastinal neurogenic tumors may produce compression of the trachea or esophagus. They may also produce rib erosion from posterior pressure; growth into the intervertebral foramina occasionally causes partial spinal cord paralysis.

Treatment

Masses arising in the mediastinum cannot be diagnosed with certainty except by histologic examination following biopsy, either simple or excisional. It follows that the treatment of most lesions of the mediastinum is surgical. Intrathoracic goiter in the superior mediastinum can usually be excised through a cervical approach. A sternal splitting incision or a standard posterolateral thoracotomy provides excellent exposure for tumors arising in the other mediastinal compartments. Nonresectable lesions often are treated with high-voltage cobalt therapy following biopsy.

Prognosis

The outlook depends entirely upon the benign or malignant nature of the lesion. In the case of malignant tumors, the prognosis is influenced by whether the lesion is completely removed, its response to radiation or chemotherapy, and the degree of local involvement of important mediastinal structures.

Boyd DP, Midell AI: Mediastinal cysts and tumors: An analysis of 96 cases. S Clin North America 48:493–506, 1968.

Cohn LH, Grimes OF: Surgical management of thymic neoplasms. Surg Gynec Obst 131:206–215, 1970.

Grosfeld JL & others: Primary mediastinal neoplasms in infants and children. Ann Thoracic Surg 12:179–190, 1971.

Kent HP, Nanson EM: Mass lesions of the mediastinum. Curr Probl Surg, June 1969.

Oldham HN Jr, Sabiston DC Jr: Primary tumors and cysts of the mediastinum, presenting as cardiovascular abnormalities. Arch Surg 96:71–75, 1968.

Rubush JL & others: Mediastinal tumors. J Thoracic Cardiovas Surg 65:216–222, 1973.

Sawyers JL, Foster JH: Surgical treatment of thymomas. Arch Surg 96:814–817, 1968.

VanHeerden JA & others: Mediastinal malignant lymphoma. Chest 57:518–529, 1970.

Wychulis AR & others: Surgical treatment of mediastinal tumors. J Thoracic Cardiovas Surg 62:379–392, 1971.

SUPERIOR VENA CAVA SYNDROME

The principal cause of the syndrome produced by superior vena caval obstruction is malignancy, usually invasive carcinomas of adjacent lung tissue. Edema of the face, neck, and arms develops along with varying degrees of venous stasis. The amount of venous distention and edema depends upon the degree of caval obstruction and the rapidity with which it develops. Edema of the conjunctivas and tearing are early signs. As the caval obstruction progresses, blood from the upper portions of the body drains through progressively enlarging and dilated collateral trunks. Huge venous channels may develop, especially in the lower neck and upper thorax. Benign lesions of the superior mediastinum rarely produce caval obstruction. A large substernal goiter may cause sufficient obstruction of the superior thoracic strait to provide some element of venous obstruction.

Aneurysms of the aortic arch are the second most frequent cause of obstruction of the superior vena cava. In addition to caval obstruction, tracheal compression from the aneurysm may cause dyspnea. Blunt or penetrating trauma with direct injury to the cava or compression of the cava by a mediastinal hematoma produces obstruction in a small percentage of cases. Phlebitis with scar contracture may produce a slowly progressive obstruction from which diffuse collateral channels develop.

In about 20% of cases, the superior cava syndrome is caused by inflammation. Primary phlebitis of the vena cava or secondary inflammation from mediastinal inflammatory processes (eg, histoplasmosis, tuberculosis) may produce idiopathic fibrous mediastinitis which often results in benign caval obstruction.

The superior vena cava syndrome can usually be recognized clinically. Radiologic study of the chest often reveals the cause of the obstruction, which frequently is an invasive carcinoma of the upper lobe of the right lung. The roentgenogram is not always specific and may show only slight superior mediastinal widening or irregularity. In these cases, angiography aids in localizing the site as well as identifying the type of obstruction.

Malignant lesions causing superior vena cava obstruction are seldom resectable. Radiation therapy is the treatment of choice and occasionally is administered as an emergency measure. Because of the generous development of collateral circulation in benign obstructions of the superior vena cava, the patient seldom experiences significant distress.

Effler DB, Groves LK: Superior vena cava obstruction. J Thoracic Cardiovas Surg 43:574, 1962.

Failor HJ, Edwards JE, Hodgson CH: Etiologic factors in obstruction of the superior vena cava. Proc Staff Meet Mayo Clin 33:671, 1958.

Hanlon CR, Danis RK: Superior vena caval obstruction: Indications for diagnostic thoracotomy. Ann Surg 161:771, 1965.

Levitt SH & others: Treatment of malignant superior vena cava obstruction: A randomized study. Cancer 24:447–451, 1969.

Pate JW, Hammon J: Superior vena cava syndrome due to histoplasmosis in children. Ann Surg 161:778, 1965.

●　●　●

General References

Blades B: *Surgical Diseases of the Chest*, 3rd ed. Mosby, 1973.

Borrie J: *Management of Emergencies in Thoracic Surgery*, 2nd ed. Appleton-Century-Crofts, 1972.

D'Abreu AL, Collis JL, Clarke DB: *A Practice of Thoracic Surgery*, 3rd ed. Arnold, 1971.

Felson B: *Chest Roentgenology*. Saunders, 1973.

Fraser RG, Paré JAP: *Diagnosis of Diseases of the Chest*. Saunders, 1970.

Fraser RG, Paré JAP: *Structure and Function of the Lung*. Saunders, 1971.

Gibbon JH Jr & others (editors): *Surgery of the Chest*, 2nd ed. Saunders, 1969.

Johnson J & others: *Surgery of the Chest*, 4th ed. Year Book, 1970.

Kubik S: *Surgical Anatomy of the Thorax*. Saunders, 1970.

Leigh TF, Weens HS: *The Mediastinum*. Thomas, 1959.

Lindskog GE, Liebow AE, Glenn WWL: *Thoracic and Cardiovascular Surgery With Related Pathology*, 2nd ed. Appleton-Century-Crofts, 1962.

Shields TW: *General Thoracic Surgery*. Lea & Febiger, 1972.

Spencer H: *Pathology of the Lung*, 2nd ed. Pergamon Press, 1968.

Watson WL: *Lung Cancer*. Mosby, 1968.

23 . . .

The Heart:
I. Acquired Diseases

Benson B. Roe, MD

GENERAL CONSIDERATIONS

During the past decade, the surgeon's role in the management of acquired heart disease has progressed from crude attempts at palliation by removing mechanical obstructions to his present ability to offer definitive therapy of all but the rarest forms of cardiac disease. We can now reasonably expect that even the patient with diffuse coronary artery disease or advanced myocardiopathy will be treated satisfactorily by replacement pumps or improved methods of managing cardiac transplantation. Not only must the cardiac surgeon be able to recognize the subtle nuances of cardiac symptoms and physical signs; he must also be able to detect ECG and radiographic abnormalities which characterize the primary disease and its postoperative complications.

Information obtained under operative conditions is not reliably diagnostic, and surgical success is predicated upon accurate anatomic and physiologic identification of disease before operation. The essential information provided by cardiac catheterization and cineradiography is as crucial to the cardiac surgeon as are the guidance and navigational instruments to the aircraft pilot. The rash surgeon who makes action decisions "by the seat of his pants" is destined to failure.

The selection of patients, choice of operative procedure, reduction of surgical risk, and prognosis for functional improvement are significantly aided by quantitative assessment of obstructive processes, regurgitant flow, ventricular ejection, pulmonary hypertension, and coronary artery patency in addition to the usual pressure and shunt measurements.

These methods of evaluation and long-term postoperative assessment have made it possible to identify operable heart disease before it causes irreversible secondary complications and is beyond surgical treatment. Surgical benefits have been greatly extended while becoming more sharply defined, and the lower operative mortality has lessened the tendency to defer operation.

EXTRACORPOREAL CIRCULATION

There are obvious temporal and technical limitations to operating within the heart while it remains beating or during brief periods of inflow occlusion. Satisfactory substitution technics to support circulation and oxygenation were long sought but slowly achieved. The functions provided by the enormous surface area of the human lung were not easy to reproduce mechanically, and unpredictable pathologic damage often followed the early use of extracorporeal oxygenation.

Several types of pumping mechanisms have been used, but all have now given way to the simple roller pump which damages blood only slightly.

Extracorporeal oxygenation by cross-circulation between parent (donor) and child (patient) was used clinically by Lillehei in a small series of operations in 1953. Experimental attempts were made to utilize an animal lung as an oxygenator, but these technics were abandoned when mechanical oxygenators became available. An important step in this achievement was the recognition by DeWall that tubing and containers made of plastic material were far less damaging to blood elements than were those made of glass.

Three basic methods of oxygenation have been employed clinically, and each has important advantages and disadvantages. Blood-gas exchange can occur (1) on the surface of a film of blood, (2) on the surface of gas bubbles in a column of blood, or (3) across a thin plastic membrane separating alternating thin layers of blood and oxygen. The filming technic is further subdivided into (a) gravity flow down a stainless steel screen with a cascade effect which supposedly keeps the surface layer mixed and changed, and (b) repeated reexposure on a series of rotating disks which dip into a trough of moving blood. Because the diffusion rate of oxygen through blood is less than 10 μm/second and the thinnest film is about 100 μm thick, the method is inefficient and requires multiple reexposures of the poorly mixed blood. Priming volumes are large and oxygenation is slow, but many consider this method less destructive to blood elements than the bubble technic.

Bubble oxygenation has the advantage of a large cumulative surface area and more efficient gas exchange; thus, priming volumes are smaller and recirculation is not required. However, embolization of residual microbubbles or of the antifoaming agent is a potential hazard. Furthermore, some surgeons contend that blood is damaged by this method, which renders it dangerous for perfusions of more than 1 hour. (Our own satisfactory experience with patients who have

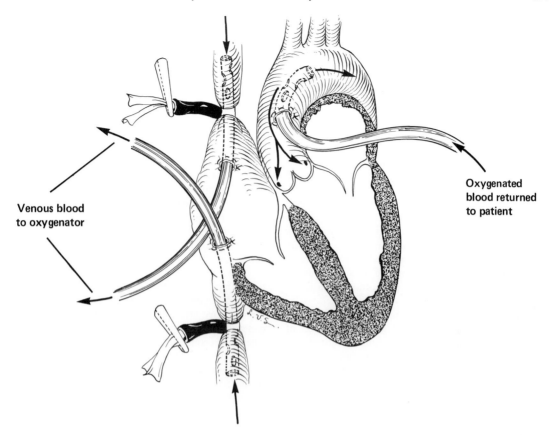

**Venous blood
to oxygenator**

**Oxygenated
blood returned
to patient**

FIG 23–1. Cannulation sites commonly used in connecting the extracorporeal circuit. Venous blood is drained through tubes introduced into both vena cavas. Oxygenated blood is returned to the arterial system through a tube in the aorta.

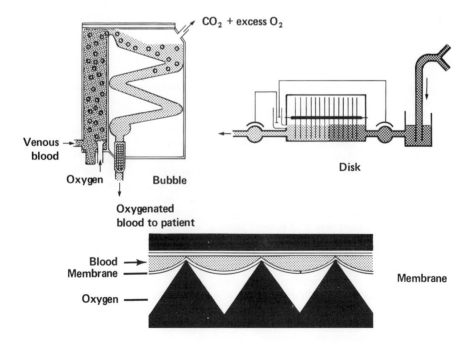

CO_2 + excess O_2

**Venous
blood**

Oxygen   **Bubble**

Disk

**Oxygenated
blood to patient**

Blood
Membrane

Oxygen

Membrane

FIG 23–2. Heart-lung bypass circuit.

sustained few or no complications after 4 or 5 hours of bubble oxygenation does not support this belief.) The availability of relatively inexpensive disposable bubble oxygenators has added to the popularity of this method. Generous heparinization (3.5 mg/kg plus another half dose every hour of bypass), high flow rates (2 liters/sq m of body surface per minute), and hemodilution (priming the oxygenator with acellular physiologic solutions) have contributed to the reduction of complications. The persistence of wide variations in technics of extracorporeal circulation used by cardiac surgeons attests to the continued unsettled and developmental state of the art.

Membrane oxygenators have the theoretical advantage of minimizing damage to blood elements and are expected to be the eventual method of choice. At present, however, they are cumbersome to assemble, need a large priming volume, and have a high resistance to flow. They are seldom used for surgical perfusion but may prove effective for long-term perfusion in treating pulmonary insufficiency.

No method of extracorporeal circulation is without its complications. Hemorrhagic consolidation of the lung and other tissues is the ultimate result of prolonged (12 hours or more) perfusion by currently available technics. However, recognition and avoidance of the many pitfalls in technical application have reduced what was once a formidable undertaking to a safe routine method which has few detrimental effects even after 6 hours or more of total body perfusion. Air embolization, intravascular coagulation, inadequate perfusion, ventricular distention, hypokalemia, and myocardial damage are usually caused by faulty application of the method rather than by the method itself. In the last few years, very few cardiac surgical deaths have been attributed to the extracorporeal system per se.

Postoperative Complications & Management Following Extracorporeal Circulation

During the early use of extracorporeal circulation, serious and fatal pulmonary, renal, and neurologic complications were common. Improved technics and better knowledge have materially reduced both the incidence and severity of these problems, many of which were related to unrecognized microembolism, inadequate heparinization, poor flow rates, and neglected intracardiac decompression.

Some degree of pulmonary shunting and congestion is almost invariable after open heart procedures but is effectively managed with a brief period of positive pressure respiration in the postoperative period and now only rarely causes severe respiratory insufficiency. The histopathology of this phenomenon consists of alveolar wall thickening with deposition of leukocytes and cellular debris with red cells in the alveolar spaces.

Neurologic sequelae are now seen only rarely and usually can be correlated with systemic air embolization. Meticulous and extensive procedures are routinely employed to evacuate air from its multiple areas

of potential entrapment within the heart and pulmonary veins before restoring cardiac output. Despite these efforts, however, we have identified the passage of air bubbles through the ascending aorta (with a Doppler flow probe) for 10 or 15 minutes after discontinuing bypass. This finding, in conjunction with a low incidence of neurologic complications, suggests that the body tolerates micro air embolism quite well.

Low cardiac output syndrome (cardiogenic shock) is the most common cause of postoperative death, particularly after manipulation or replacement of the mitral valve. The complication is recognized by delayed responsiveness, oliguria, peripheral constriction, and hypotension. For this reason, it is customary to monitor central arterial pressure, venous pressure, and urinary output with close observation of the patient's general appearance and peripheral color changes.

The many explanations advanced for this development have had little to substantiate them. Undoubtedly, coronary air emboli, iatrogenic damage to the coronary arteries, prolonged cardiac ischemia, and underlying myocardial disease all play a role. Hypovolemia certainly accounts for most cases with this difficulty. The postperfusion state is associated with "third space" sequestration of blood, and large volumes of additional fluid are necessary to maintain adequate circulating blood. The left atrial pressure should be monitored and fluid replacement continued until this value is elevated above 20 mm Hg to push the output "up the Starling curve."

Excessive postoperative bleeding is a common complication which in many cases requires reopening the incision for evacuation of clot and further hemostatic control. Although it is not uncommon to discover a surgical source, such as bleeding from a suture line, a transected coronary vessel, or a cannulation site, in most cases only diffuse oozing is found, and the probability of inadequate neutralization of heparin must be considered. Before reoperation, the clotting time and prothrombin time should be determined to reveal any correctable deficiency in protamine or vitamin K. It is interesting, however, that persistent and unremitting bleeding usually subsides after reexposure of the operative field and evacuation of clot, even when no significant bleeding point is identified.

Varying degrees of cardiac arrhythmia are exceedingly common and require constant monitoring for recognition. Their occurrence is related to the operative procedure, the underlying disease, and the medications in use. Repairs in the region of the conduction system (aortic valve replacement) may produce transient or permanent third degree heart block. Mitral valve disease is likely to be associated with atrial fibrillation, which, if not present preoperatively, may develop postoperatively; postperfusion hypokalemia can lead to digitalis toxicity and ventricular fibrillation; and tachycardia can result from inadequate digitalization.

Disseminated intravascular coagulation with secondary pulmonary consolidation and diffuse bleeding into the gastrointestinal tract is a devastating complication which is sometimes difficult to recognize. Its cause is not well established but may be related to a homologous blood reaction, infection, low output with sludging, inadequate heparinization during perfusion, or hypoxia.

Gibbon JH Jr: Application of a mechanical heart and lung apparatus to cardiac surgery. Minnesota Med 37:171, 1954.

Roe BB: Whole body perfusion with heart-lung machines: Present status and future trends. Chap 1, vol 1, in: *Cardiovascular Surgery, Current Practice.* Burford TH, Ferguson TB (editors). Mosby, 1969.

VALVULAR HEART DISEASE

Valvular heart disease manifesting itself for the first time in adult life has usually been attributed to rheumatic fever in childhood. It is now evident, however, that in a significant proportion of cases the disorder is congenital or due to degenerative disease. Some congenital anatomic variations produce no hemodynamic abnormalities or even murmurs in early life, when the leaflet structure is relatively flexible. Later, deposition of fibrin and calcium, presumably a consequence of turbulent flow around the tethered leaflets, results in loss of flexibility and narrowing of the orifice. However, no information is available to explain how or why fibrocalcific deposits develop in and around valves. The resulting clinical lesions are described as valvular stenosis or insufficiency depending on the mechanics of the pathologic process. Pure stenosis can occur in a totally competent valve, and a regurgitant valve may be unrestrictive, but the latter is seldom rheumatic in origin. In many instances, the anatomic abnormality consists of a fixed orifice which may both restrict forward flow and fail to prevent backward flow. The size, shape, flexibility, and position of the opening determine the relative degrees of stenosis and regurgitation.

From a prognostic standpoint, valvular stenosis is less well tolerated than valve incompetence because the impairment to flow raises intraventricular pressure. More cardiac work is required to overcome increased pressure than is required to handle the increased volume load resulting from regurgitation.

AORTIC STENOSIS

Essentials of Diagnosis

- Loud, harsh basal systolic murmur, often radiating to the neck.
- Evidence of left ventricular strain or overactivity by ECG or physical examination.
- Diminished or dampened peripheral pulse wave.

General Considerations

Aortic stenosis may appear at any stage of adulthood, and there is no clear distinction between the congenital and acquired forms of the disease. It is more common in men than in women. Symptoms are characteristically absent or minimal until myocardial failure heralds the terminal stages of the disease. Transient bouts of syncope or angina during exertion may occur when limited cardiac output cannot meet the requirements of muscular activity or other demands along with the basic perfusion needs of the brain or heart. Sudden unheralded cardiac arrest (presumably due to ventricular fibrillation) is a common complication of aortic stenosis and adds to the urgency for elective correction.

Clinical Findings

A. Symptoms and Signs: A systolic ejection type of murmur is heard in the right second interspace and frequently is transmitted to the neck vessels. Peripheral pulses may be dampened, with a delayed upstroke, and left ventricular hypertrophy is manifested by cardiac enlargement with a left ventricular lift. The shock-like symptoms and moist palms in patients with peripheral vasoconstriction occur when obstruction has critically reduced cardiac output. The effects of gradually impaired cardiac output are not as clinically dramatic or distressing as those of congestive failure and may lead to dangerous complacency about the severity of the disease.

B. X-Ray Findings: The chest film shows left ventricular enlargement after long-standing stenosis, but (remarkably) there may be little or no visible hypertrophy in far-advanced disease of recent onset. Calcific deposits are frequently seen in the aortic valve area on fluoroscopy or in overpenetrated films, but neither

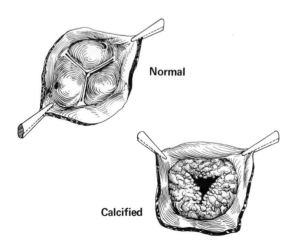

Normal

Calcified

FIG 23–3. Aortic valve (normal and calcified).

hypertrophy nor calcium is essential to making the diagnosis.

C. Cardiac Catheterization: Left ventricular systolic pressure is significantly higher than in the aorta. It is sometimes difficult or impossible to pass a catheter retrograde through a stenotic valve, so that this determination may have to be made by a transseptal or percutaneous approach. In advanced disease, the early evidence of left ventricular failure will be reflected by an elevated left ventricular end-diastolic pressure to levels as high as 40 mm Hg or more. Pulmonary wedge pressures without ventricular tracings might, therefore, misleadingly suggest mitral disease. When severe myocardial failure is thus manifested, the prognosis is grave and the operative risk is high. Interpretation of the systolic gradient across the aortic valve must be based on a knowledge of cardiac output. In advanced disease, a low output (below 2 liters/sq m/minute) may reduce this gradient. Aortic pressure curves have a slow upstroke and a characteristic anacrotic notch (Fig 23–4).

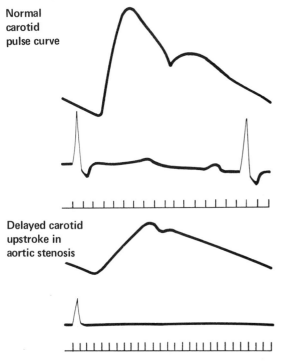

Normal carotid pulse curve

Delayed carotid upstroke in aortic stenosis

FIG 23–4. Abnormal aortic pressure curve in aortic stenosis with delayed upstroke.

Treatment

Surgical replacement of the diseased valve is urgently recommended when the disease first becomes symptomatic. Evidence of decompensation should be interpreted as end stage disease, and prompt response to supportive treatment does not obviate the need for surgery. When a characteristic systolic murmur is associated with left ventricular hypertrophy or signs of

failure, cardiac catheterization should be performed to identify a stenosis which can be treated before it reaches the dangerous symptomatic stage. A resting systolic gradient above 50 mm Hg warrants surgical consideration, but this criterion should not be used alone because its magnitude is influenced by the flow rate; such a gradient at basal resting cardiac output may double or treble during exercise. In advanced disease, the murmur may be deceptively diminished since the output and gradient are depressed by the impaired performance of the failing ventricle.

Attempts to reconstruct the diseased valve by opening commissures and excising calcific deposits have been virtually abandoned because of unsatisfactory long-term results and rapid recurrence. The pathologic process usually obliterates any semblance of valve structure, and it is futile to expect that function can be restored.

Prognosis

Early experience with this high-risk group of patients was associated with a significant operative mortality, but recently the risk has been reduced to less than 5% and patients over 70 have tolerated the procedure remarkably well. Associated coronary artery disease or secondary cor bovinum militates against a good long-term functional result, but (surprisingly) these disorders have not been a major surgical hazard.

Long-term results are difficult to assess in a disease process in the older age groups with a wide spectrum of severity. Replacement devices (or homografts) are undergoing constant change, and the risk factors of thromboembolism versus anticoagulation are not yet established. Embolization or thrombus formation on the prosthesis, hemorrhagic complications of anticoagulation, disruption or mechanical failure of the prosthesis, and arrhythmias account for late deaths at a rate of 1–3% per year. There seems little doubt, however, that life expectancy has been extended by surgical replacement of the calcified, stenotic aortic valve. The value of caged ball valve prostheses and homograft and heterograft transplants is now well documented, although there is still disagreement about which is the most effective replacement.

Perloff JK: Clinical recognition of aortic stenosis: The physical signs and differential diagnosis of the various forms of obstruction to left ventricular outflow. Progr Cardiovas Dis 10:323, 1968.

Ross J Jr, Braunwald E: Aortic stenosis. Circulation 38 (Suppl 5):61–67, 1968.

AORTIC INSUFFICIENCY

Essentials of Diagnosis

- Visible overactivity of the left ventricle.
- Left ventricular heave with an apical impulse displaced to the axilla.

- Peripheral pulses collapse in diastole, and a diminuendo blowing diastolic murmur is heard in the aortic area of the precordium.

General Considerations

When aortic incompetence develops gradually, even severe hemodynamic derangement may be tolerated for long periods without disability. The muscle development and energy requirements for increased volume work are significantly less than those needed for the greater pressure load imposed by aortic stenosis.

Acute aortic insufficiency, on the other hand, is very poorly tolerated, and a much less severe degree of valve leakage may be fatal unless it is corrected promptly. Impaired coronary perfusion secondary to the lowered diastolic (coronary-filling) pressure and the normally small ventricular chamber whose volume is inadequate to accommodate increased output requirements are major factors complicating the acute illness. One must not apply the traditional criterion of compensatory cardiac enlargement as an index of severity in the acute state. Congestive failure and aortic diastolic murmur are alone sufficient to justify semiemergency valve replacement if salvage is to be expected. In the presence of bacterial endocarditis, the hazards of embolization from bacterial vegetation or sudden further loss of valve integrity by erosion may offset the theoretical desirability of deferring operation until the infection is controlled.

Clinical Findings

In the chronic state of aortic insufficiency, the chest film shows gross cardiac enlargement with a prominent left ventricular shadow. In advanced disease, evidence of pulmonary congestion may be present, and wedge pressure (ventricular end-diastolic pressure) is elevated (as high as 45 mm Hg) on cardiac catheterization. Arterial pressure curves are sharply peaked, and the dicrotic notch is delayed or absent. It is a deceptive paradox that the arterial diastolic pressure, which may have been nearly zero, rises as the patient becomes symptomatically worse. This rise is a manifestation of failure with elevated ventricular end-diastolic pressure below which the arterial pressure cannot fall, even with wide-open incompetence. Whenever a patient with aortic insufficiency begins to have symptoms or shows radiographic progression of his heart size, he should be studied by cardiac catheterization. If the left ventricular end-diastolic pressure is elevated significantly above 15 mm Hg, valve replacement should be recommended.

Treatment

Surgery is strongly recommended when the first evidence of decompensation is recognized and certainly should not be delayed after the first episode of frank failure. Although most patients will respond promptly to digitalization, this does not justify postponing valve replacement because left ventricular function will deteriorate progressively and the functional

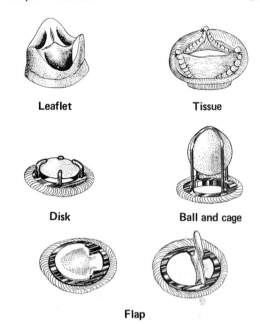

Leaflet   **Tissue**

Disk   **Ball and cage**

Flap

FIG 23–5. Examples of commercially available artificial heart valves.

benefit of valve replacement will be significantly impaired. The hospital mortality rate for valve replacement in aortic insufficiency is well below the 5% estimate for aortic stenosis, but long-term survival has been disappointing when the process has been allowed to progress to the "cor bovinum" stage; a successful operative result merely delays the inexorable progress of myocardial fibrosis and intractable muscular failure. For this reason, replacement is now recommended as soon as progressive and significant ventricular enlargement is recognized.

Procedures directed at preserving and reconstituting the patient's own valve have now been abandoned because of poor long-term results. Plications, suspensions, and other reconstruction devices have all broken down and have required later replacement. Except in small children, diseased aortic valves are best removed. Replacement may employ prostheses, homografts, heterografts, or autogenous fascia lata.

Prognosis

The immediate surgical risk is low. Long-term rehabilitation after correcting valve dysfunction is impaired by the degree of preoperative myocardial degeneration and thus tends to respond inversely to the degree of preoperative chronic cardiomegaly.

Late complications and death can occur from malfunction of the replacement valve, paravalvular leakage, thrombotic occlusion, congestive failure, arrhythmia, embolism, or hemorrhage secondary to prophylactic anticoagulation. Surgical experience, improved valve construction, earlier operation, better management practices, and the use of tissue valve replacements are helping to reduce these hazards. This author has never experienced significant paravalvular leakage in his patients, and no valve dysfunctions have occurred with the Smeloff-Cutter ball valve during the past 7 years.

Busse EFG: Acute aortic insufficiency. Ann Thoracic Surg 4:242–248, 1967.

Hegglin R, Scheu H, Rothlin M: Aortic insufficiency. Circulation 38 (Suppl 5):77–92, 1968.

Rees JR & others: Haemodynamic effects of severe aortic regurgitation. Brit Heart J 26:412–421, 1964.

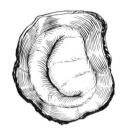 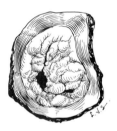

Normal   **Calcified**

FIG 23–6. Mitral valve (normal and calcified) as viewed from the left atrium.

MITRAL STENOSIS

Essentials of Diagnosis

- Dyspnea, orthopnea, and paroxysmal nocturnal dyspnea.
- Radiographic evidence of prominent superior pulmonary vessels.
- Enlarged left atrium.
- Prominent mitral first sound, opening snap (usually), and apical crescendo diastolic rumble.

General Considerations

The most common lesion caused by rheumatic fever is stenotic scarring of the mitral valve which is involved in the inflammatory process of rheumatic disease. It is usually years or decades after the bout of active carditis before progressive scarring and contracture produce a significant functional abnormality. Why the frequency and severity of late rheumatic pathologic change is greatest in the mitral valve, less in the aortic valve, uncommon in the tricuspid valve, and virtually absent in the pulmonic valve is not known. Because the incidence parallels the relative stress sustained by the 4 valves, this factor has been invoked as a possible basis but without valid explanation. Symptoms are often well controlled by unconscious or deliberate restriction of activity; thus, advanced stenosis can develop insidiously without apparent disability until late in the disease.

Clinical Findings

A. Symptoms and Signs: The characteristic murmur of mitral stenosis is sometimes difficult to localize at the cardiac apex, but the diagnosis should be suspected in the presence of an accentuated mitral first sound, a loud opening snap at the beginning of diastole, and an increased intensity of the pulmonic second sound. The diastolic murmur is a low-pitched rumble with presystolic accentuation. Development of atrial fibrillation with consequent loss of atrial systole to overcome the obstruction characteristically precipitates symptoms. Dyspnea, wheezing, orthopnea, and paroxysmal nocturnal dyspnea are characteristic complaints; hemoptysis, chest pain (not anginal), and peripheral edema are manifestations of chronic congestion.

B. X-Ray Findings: The cardiac silhouette is enlarged in the region of the left atrial appendage and pulmonary artery. Left atrial and right ventricular enlargement are sometimes seen in the lateral view. Penetrated films may show calcific deposits in the region of the mitral valve. In advanced stages, pulmonary congestion is evident and the pulmonary venous shadows become prominent in the upper lobes. Kerley "B" lines may be present in the lung periphery, manifesting lymphatic engorgement.

C. Cardiac Catheterization: Cardiac catheterization shows elevation of pulmonary artery and pulmonary capillary wedge pressures from normal values of 25/10 mm Hg and 7–10 mm Hg (respectively) to resting values of more than double those figures, which characteristically rise with mild exercise to values as high as systemic pressure in the pulmonary artery and 45 mm Hg in the capillary wedge.

Differential Diagnosis

Because auscultatory findings are often subtle, the symptoms of congestive heart failure are often attributed to myocardial or pericardial disease. The characteristic murmurs of mitral stenosis are similar to those heard with atrial tumors or tricuspid stenosis.

Complications

Chronic mitral stenosis commonly causes atrial fibrillation, and the latter may contribute to the development of atrial thrombi which can produce arterial embolization. Pulmonary hypertension with vascular changes and impaired ventilation ("cardiac asthma") can occur in the late stages of the disease.

Treatment

Symptoms precipitated by arrhythmia can be temporarily controlled with digitalis or quinidine. Diuretics and salt restriction will reduce pulmonary congestion. However, since the disease is one of mechanical obstruction, definitive therapy is necessarily surgical.

Mitral commissurotomy (reopening of the fused valve leaflet) has been accomplished with significant success by closed technics consisting of blind fracture of the valve structures with a finger or instrument in the heart. Because symptoms develop at a critical degree of valve stenosis, significant functional improvement can be derived from a slight increase in the effective valve area from slightly more than 1 sq cm to perhaps 2 sq cm, even though considerable obstruction remains. Before the days of safe, effective extracorporeal circulation, closed commissurotomy was usually preferable. However, the complex and extensive nature of the valvular pathologic process, the embolic hazard from unsuspected atrial thrombi, and the danger of producing mitral insufficiency are all reasons to recommend the open approach to every diseased valve. This method provides for meticulous mobilization of the valve leaflets, removal of thrombi before they become dislodged, and repair of any secondary commissural leakage. Direct visualization has focused attention on the intricate and extensive nature of subvalvular fusion. Short chordae tendineae to both leaflets from a single papillary muscle may tether valve mobility and require meticulous sharp separation. Thickened chordal and papillary structures frequently show no evidence of cleavage and must be divided deeply into the ventricle before an effective orifice can be developed.

Many surgeons will undertake commissurotomy for primary isolated mitral stenosis even with the expectation that eventual valve replacement will be necessary. However, growing satisfaction with replacement devices and the predictability of their performance have led to valve replacement in a higher proportion of patients with mitral stenosis. It is now considered desirable to replace almost all recurrently stenotic valves, almost all stenotic valves in patients over 55 or 60 years of age, and most heavily calcified valves or stenotic valves associated with significant aortic valve disease requiring replacement.

Prognosis

Mitral stenosis characteristically recurs after valvotomy in 3–10 years, presumably because of the behavior of scar tissue which is an integral part of the lesions. The incidence of systemic embolization is reduced but not obliterated by valvotomy. Some degree of mitral insufficiency is a frequent consequence of valvotomy, and its severity may be incorrectly assessed; subsequent replacement may be necessitated by this complication.

Atrial fibrillation is reversible in less than one-third of patients who had this condition before operation, and medical management is necessary indefinitely.

See references at end of next section.

MITRAL INSUFFICIENCY

Essentials of Diagnosis

- Loud systolic murmur at the apex, radiating into the axilla.
- Pulmonary congestion from elevated left atrial pressure.

- Cardiac enlargement consisting of left ventricular distention with hypertrophy and giant left atrium.

General Considerations

In mitral insufficiency, the valve fails to close because of (1) rheumatic inflammation, secondary scarring, and leaflet retraction (usually associated with mitral stenosis); (2) myxomatous degeneration with prolapse of leaflets; (3) attenuation and elongation of subvalvular structures with prolapse; (4) rupture of chordae tendineae or papillary muscles; (5) myocardiopathy with annular distention and secondary leaflet insufficiency; and (6) bacterial endocarditis.

Clinical Findings

A. Symptoms and Signs: Symptoms characteristically occur late in the disease and consist of dyspnea, orthopnea, wheezing, and paroxysmal nocturnal dyspnea. Insidious fatigability may precede any of these. Cardiac enlargement, left ventricular heave, and apical systolic murmurs are easily identified. Atrial fibrillation is common.

B. X-Ray Findings: The enlarged left atrium and left ventricular hypertrophy are identifiable on the chest film. Vascular congestion in the lungs is accompanied by prominent superior pulmonary veins and Kerley "B" lines in advanced disease.

C. Cardiac Catheterization and Cineangiocardiography: Cardiac catheterization shows an elevated mean left atrial pressure of 20–30 mm Hg with a high V wave up to 60 mm Hg, but the magnitude and distensibility of the enlarged atrial chamber have a significant damping effect on this regurgitant jet. Thus, the volume of regurgitation does not correlate well with the height of the V wave, particularly in the acute lesions of sudden onset where an undistended atrium may reflect a high pressure wave with a relatively small backflow.

Cineangiocardiography will demonstrate a regurgitant jet of contrast medium through the mitral valve when it is injected into the left ventricle. It is sometimes possible to identify the location of the jet.

Differential Diagnosis

Characteristic findings are not often mistaken for other diseases, but the systolic murmur can easily be confused with that of aortic or pulmonic stenosis. In the postinfarction state, it is often difficult to distinguish the systolic murmur of a ruptured ventricular septum from that of a ruptured papillary muscle (see p 365) and mitral regurgitation. When the anterior leaflet of the mitral valve is incompetent, the regurgitant jet is directed anteriorly and may easily be mistaken for the murmur of aortic stenosis. Since definitive identification of the lesion by angiographic and cardiac catheterization technics has become a standard procedure, the surgeon is seldom concerned with problems in differential diagnosis.

Treatment

Medical supportive measures such as digitalization, diuretics, and salt restriction can control symptoms satisfactorily for many years. If disability progresses or if cardiomegaly increases, surgical correction is indicated.

A wide variety of reconstructive surgical procedures have been attempted and advocated for the regurgitant mitral valve, but nearly all have been abandoned in favor of replacement. The thick muscular cone that constitutes the left ventricle does not lend itself to the distortion of true "annuloplasty." There are, however, tethered leaflets that can be mobilized by dividing subvalvular structures and by inserting a gusset of autogenous tissue to correct incompetence. However, the only circumstance in which nearly total success can be expected with nonreplacement technics is a ruptured chorda tendinea on the mural leaflet; the long concave curve of this valve edge lends itself admirably to wedge resection, shortening the curve and providing apposition to the septal leaflet in systole without impairing diastolic flow. Most operations for mitral insufficiency now result in replacement because of its more predictable outcome and generally acceptable long-term results. It remains to be determined which mechanical device or tissue valve will have the best long-term performance. Several alternatives can provide a 5-year life expectancy in at least 70% of patients, and the choice of method remains a matter of surgical judgment.

Prognosis

The secondary effects of elevated left atrial pressure and left atrial distention are progressive, and the patient will eventually die in congestive heart failure if the defect is not corrected. Operative mortality from valve replacement in this disease is less than that in stenosis (5–10%), but long-term complications are similar and the functional result, although almost invariably one of improvement, is variable; the size and performance of the replacement device and the degree of underlying myocardial disease are undoubtedly factors. For reasons not clearly understood, the left ventricular performance after mitral valve replacement is characteristically impaired for some weeks or months, in sharp contrast to the performance after replacement of the aortic valve. It has been thought by some that the cage of the ball valve extending into the ventricle interferes with ventricular function; this stimulated the development of so-called "low-profile" disk valves, but recent studies have indicated that there is no functional difference between the 2 mechanisms. However, the inability of the valve annulus to contract against a rigid ring could cause functional impairment.

Aldridge HE, Goldman BS, Bigelow WG: Progress in cardiovascular surgery: The course of patients following replacement of the mitral valve by a Starr-Edwards prosthesis. Dis Chest 50:186–193, 1966.

Belcher JR: What are the indications for mitral valve replacement? Brit MJ 2:1486–1489, 1966.

Dekker A, Black H, von Lichtenberg F: Mitral valve restenosis: A pathologic study. J Thoracic Cardiovas Surg 55:434–446, 1968.

Glenn WWL & others: Mitral valvulotomy. II. Operative results after closed valvulotomy: A report of 500 cases. Am J Surg 117:493, 1969.

Harken DE, Collins JJ Jr: Mitral valve replacement. Progr Cardiovas Dis 11:263, 1969.

Hubka M & others: Replacement of the mitral valve with an aortic valve homograft implanted into the left atrium. J Thoracic Cardiovas Surg 53:260–267, 1967.

Joassin A, Edwards JE: Late causes of death after mitral valve replacement: Analysis of 36 cases. J Thoracic Cardiovas Surg 65:255–263, 1973.

Kirklin JW, Pacifico AD: Surgery for acquired valvular heart disease. New England J Med 288:133–140, 194–199, 1973.

Morgan JJ: Hemodynamics one year following mitral valve replacement. Am J Cardiol 19:189–195, 1967.

Roy SB, Gopinath N: Mitral stenosis. Circulation 38 (Suppl 5):68, 1968.

Sanders CA & others: Mitral regurgitation secondary to ruptured chordae tendineae. New England J Med 276:943–949, 1967.

Wood P: An appreciation of mitral stenosis. Brit MJ 1:1051–1063, 1113–1124, 1954.

TRICUSPID STENOSIS & INSUFFICIENCY

Malfunction of the tricuspid valve is much less common than aortic and mitral valve malfunction, but the principles of recognition and management are similar to those in mitral disease, with less emphasis on replacement.

Clinical Findings

Right-sided heart failure is manifested by elevated venous pressure, hepatic enlargement, edema, and ascites. Murmurs of tricuspid valve disease are heard on the right side of the sternum and are similar to those of the mitral valve. Tricuspid insufficiency results in a venous pulse wave which produces a pulsating liver. X-rays show an enlarged right atrium. Cardiac catheterization demonstrates elevation of right atrial pressure with a high V wave of 10–20 mm Hg in the presence of valve incompetence (with variable factors similar to those of mitral insufficiency according to chamber size).

The functional significance of tricuspid insufficiency is influenced by the degree of concomitant pulmonary vascular resistance (either primary or secondary to mitral valve disease). In the presence of normal pulmonary arterial pressure, pulmonary perfusion can be maintained by modest elevation of systemic venous pressure without requiring effective pumping action of the right ventricle; thus, the need for definitive treatment is limited to patients with additional hemodynamic abnormalities.

Treatment

Tricuspid valve disease is seldom seen without associated mitral or aortic disease (or both). The exceptions are bacterial endocarditis (frequently associated with narcotic addiction) and associated tumor. Symptoms may respond to medical management as readily as in mitral disease. Surgical correction is sometimes indicated in conjunction with operations on the mitral valve.

Tricuspid stenosis usually appears as a conical structure with a central fibrous ring which presents no evident commissural lines for simple incisional relief, and some cardiac surgeons tend to replace the diseased tricuspid valve with the same alacrity as in mitral disease. It is evident, however, that the systemic effects of tricuspid insufficiency (or even total tricuspid excision) are well tolerated in the absence of high pulmonary vascular resistance and that the right ventricle is less suitable for the usual prosthetic devices. For these reasons, most surgeons are conservative about tricuspid replacement except in the presence of advanced organic disease.

Functional tricuspid insufficiency with flexible, intact leaflets lends itself well to improvement with true annuloplasty because of the crescentic shape of the valve annulus which (unlike the mitral annulus) provides for effective plication.

Prognosis

Tricuspid valve disease alone may be well tolerated. Congestive symptoms which do not involve the lung are less likely to be fatal, and the necessity for replacement is less pressing. Because of disputed indications for replacement, greater adaptability to annuloplasty, lower incidence of disease, and the almost invariable association with mitral valve disease, it is difficult to assess the surgical experience. Tricuspid valve replacement in combination with mitral or aortic valve replacement (or both) has an immediate surgical mortality rate of 15–25%, which reflects the risk of multivalve disease. Even so, it is apparent that the right ventricular cavity is less suited to a round (and particularly a caged) replacement device than is the left ventricle, and that late thrombosis in this area is more common. It is also notable that all fascia lata valves in the tricuspid position deteriorate. Successful total excision of the tricuspid valve for acute bacterial endocarditis has been reported.

. . .

THORACIC AORTIC ANEURYSM

Essentials of Diagnosis

- Enlarged mediastinal silhouette.
- Chest pain radiating to the back (not invariable).
- Angiographic demonstration of abnormal aorta.

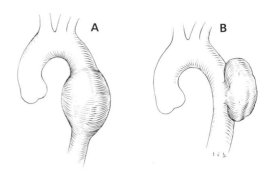

FIG 23–7. Types of thoracic aortic aneurysms. *A:* Fusiform. *B:* Saccular.

General Considerations

Pathologic distention of the aorta tends to be progressive because, at a given pressure, tension on the diseased aortic wall increases in direct proportion with its diameter; thus, the pathologic process is almost invariably progressive.

Thoracic aortic aneurysm may be due to (1) syphilis, (2) arteriosclerosis, (3) a degenerative process (cystic medial necrosis, Marfan's syndrome), or (4) trauma.

Aneurysms may be saccular outpouchings of an otherwise normally contoured aorta (usually syphilitic) but more commonly are a fusiform enlargement of the entire lumen. The latter are sometimes localized, but diffuse enlargement and tortuosity of the aorta also occur.

Clinical Findings

A. Symptoms and Signs: The manifestations of thoracic aortic aneurysm are related to its size and location. Bony erosion of the sternum or vertebral bodies can cause pain. Stretching of the recurrent laryngeal nerve may result in hoarseness. Coughing may occur because of compression of bronchi, and erosion into a lung may cause hemoptysis.

B. X-Ray Findings: Aortography is the only definitive study which can verify and delineate the aneurysm. Multiple views may be necessary to identify the nature and relationship of the arch vessels as well as the nature of the aorta at the limits of the aneurysm.

Differential Diagnosis

A space-occupying lesion in the mediastinum can be any of several mediastinal tumors or cysts as well as an aortic aneurysm. The signs, symptoms, and appearance on plain roentgenograms are often indistinguishable, so that aortography is always mandatory when the slightest doubt exists.

Treatment

Supportive measures to treat the secondary effects of an expanding mass are obviously of no avail since response is based on removal of the offending process. Systemic hypertension must be controlled because it compounds the hazard and accelerates the expansion of an aneurysm; however, surgical relief provides the only opportunity for definitive management. Replacement with a polyester tube graft is necessary for fusiform aneurysm. Saccular aneurysms can frequently be obliterated by closure of the neck at its connection to the aorta without total excision. Because of the related structures, the surgical hazards and results vary according to the location and pathologic nature of the disease process. Localized aneurysms of the ascending and descending aorta are more easily and safely treated than those of the arch, which require establishment of new connections to the head vessels. Aneurysms involving the sinuses of Valsalva are frequently associated with malfunction of the aortic valve and invariably result in displacement of the coronary ostia. It is, therefore, frequently necessary to replace the aortic valve and to transpose the coronary ostia into the cloth graft.

Operations for thoracic aortic aneurysm pose many technical and logistical challenges. A large aneurysmal mass may displace the heart and mediastinal structures so as to preclude the usual cannulation routes or to prevent access for clamping the aorta beyond the aneurysm. Under these circumstances, it is essential to initiate perfusion through the groin in order to induce profound total body hypothermia, which permits extended circulatory arrest; thus, the hazardous dissection can be carried out under "cadaveric" conditions.

Aneurysms of the distal aortic arch and descending aorta which must be approached from the left side require either left heart bypass (left atrium to femoral artery) or lower body cardiopulmonary perfusion (femoral vein to femoral artery through an oxygenator). Both of these technics require far greater skill than total body perfusion because of the distributional problem between the 2 pumping systems (the normal heart and lungs for the upper extremities and the extracorporeal perfusion system for the lower body).

Prognosis

Without surgical correction, progressive distention and eventual rupture are inevitable, but the course is unpredictable. Evidence of progressive enlargement should make operation compelling.

Cooley DA & others: Surgical management of aneurysms of the ascending aorta, including those associated with aortic valvular incompetence. S Clin North America 46:1033, 1966.

DeBakey ME & others: Resection and graft replacement of aneurysms involving the transverse arch of the aorta. S Clin North America 46:1057, 1966.

AORTIC DISSECTION
("Dissecting Aneurysm")

Essentials of Diagnosis

- Sudden severe chest pain with radiation to the back, abdomen, and extremities.
- Shock may be present, though often not until the later stages.
- CNS changes may occur.
- A history of hypertension is common.
- Dissection occurs most frequently in males.

General Considerations

Intramural splitting or dissection of the aorta usually arises from an intimal tear either just distal to the aortic valve or adjacent to the take-off of the left subclavian artery. Over 60% of dissections arise in the ascending aorta, roughly 20% in the transverse or distal arch, and the remainder in the descending thoracic or abdominal aorta. The process is commonly called dissecting aneurysm, but the term is inappropriate because aortic dissection does not always result in significant dilatation. The disease process consists of a degenerative weakness of the muscularis layer of the aorta (cystic medial necrosis). Hypertension is usually the triggering mechanism, but the patient may present in a state of shock with deceptively "normal" blood pressure.

Clinical Findings

A. Symptoms and Signs: Silent "dissections" have been encountered, but characteristically the onset is accompanied by chest pain (sometimes described as "tearing") which may extend into the back and abdomen. Discrepancies in character, timing, and magnitude of pulse waves may be present among the extremities, depending upon the location and consequences of the dissection. When the dissecting process selectively obliterates the central lumen, obstructing pulsatile flow to major vessels of the extremities, the brain, or abdominal organs, there will be varying degrees of impaired perfusion to these areas depending upon the circulatory mechanics. If the dissection process provides effective flow into the peripheral false lumen and if the false lumen communicates with the involved pathways, there may be little or no evidence of impaired organ function. If, however, the dissection effectively obliterates the flow to the involved organ system, evidence of ischemia or infarction will be seen, prompting immediate operation.

B. X-Ray Findings: Chest films do not always show mediastinal widening. Aortography may opacify the true lumen, false lumen (external pathway), or both. Multiple injections at different sites may be necessary to locate the intimal tear and to establish patency of essential vascular pathways. Several views may also be required to identify these landmarks.

Differential Diagnosis

The presenting signs and symptoms of acute myocardial infarction are similar to those of aortic dissection, so that the latter diagnosis may be missed. A normal ECG and abnormal pulse pattern suggest dissection.

Treatment

In simple dissection, both immediate salvage and long-term survival are greater after nonsurgical treatment and vigorous antihypertensive management than after surgical replacement. Because of its diffuse nature and the poor aortic tissue which characterizes the disease, the technical problems of surgical reconstruction are significant and the operative risk is high (15–20%). However, surgery is necessary if the patient develops secondary aortic insufficiency, obstruction of a major vascular pathway, or evidence of impending rupture suggested by intrapleural bleeding—or if, in spite of therapy, further extension is suggested by continued pain or expanding mediastinal shadow. It is desirable—though not always feasible—to resect the origin of the dissection and to obliterate the false lumen which may extend in both directions from this point. Occasionally the 2 ends can be reconnected, but the space usually must be filled with a synthetic graft. If the dissection is chronic or of long standing, it is important to map and identify the outflow to each of the major aortic branches because of the possibility that the false lumen has become the only pathway to one or more of these vessels. Obliteration of the false lumen in the procedure will then result in necrosis of the involved organ.

Prognosis

After prompt and vigorous antihypertensive therapy in uncomplicated cases, the immediate survival rate is 85% and the long-term survival rate 58%. Operative intervention, where indicated, results in a salvage rate of approximately 80%, depending on the origin and extent of dissection. The prognosis is necessarily guarded because of the diffuse and degenerative nature of the underlying disease process. Uncontrolled hypertension in the presence of a diseased arterial tree has a predictable outcome, and yet clinically unrecognized dissections are not infrequently discovered at autopsy, either with reentry pathways and patency of both lumens or with thrombosis and scarring of the false lumen.

DeBakey ME & others: Dissecting aneurysms of the aorta. S Clin North America 46:1045–1056, 1966.

Lindsay J Jr, Hurst JW: Clinical features and prognosis in dissecting aneurysm of the aorta: A reappraisal. Circulation 35:880–888, 1967.

Symbas PM & others: Rupture of aorta. Ann Thoracic Surg 15:405–410, 1973.

Wheat MW Jr, Palmer RF: Drug therapy for dissecting aneurysms. Dis Chest 54:372–377, 1968.

Wheat MW Jr & others: Acute dissecting aneurysms of the aorta: Treatment and results in 64 patients. J Thoracic Cardiovas Surg 58:344, 1969.

CORONARY INSUFFICIENCY; ANGINA PECTORIS

Essentials of Diagnosis

- Oppressive anterior chest pain associated with exercise or stress and relieved by rest or nitroglycerin.
- Seventy percent have diagnostic ECG abnormalities after mild exercise; the remaining 30% have normal tracings or nondiagnostic abnormalities.

General Considerations

Only a small percentage of the millions of people afflicted with coronary artery disease have persistent symptoms of classic angina. Limitation of physical capacity and the ultimate poor prognosis in these patients warrant definitive therapy. In a desperate endeavor to help in the management of a devastating disease, a multitude of ill-conceived surgical procedures such as pericardial poudrage (talc operation) or excoriation, internal mammary artery ligation, coronary sinus occlusion, acupuncture, and sympathectomy have been tried with no effort to obtain controlled evaluations. All of these measures have been abandoned for lack of demonstrable benefit.

Clinical Findings

Symptoms of pain related to exertion are usually reproducible, but the pattern of pain is sometimes bizarre and inconsistent. Signs are absent. ECG abnormalities may be absent, but transient evidence of ischemia can sometimes be demonstrated with exercise. Identification of the location, severity, and extent of coronary artery occlusion must be made by selective coronary angiocardiography. Complete mapping of the coronary artery branches, collateral pathways, and distal filling is essential before definitive surgery can be considered, planned, or ultimately assessed.

Differential Diagnosis

Since angina pectoris is a symptomatic disease with few objective findings, it may be difficult to distinguish it from a variety of conditions producing anterior chest pain, such as peptic esophagitis, duodenal ulcer, gallbladder disease, pericardial inflammation, and pleurisy. These lesions must be excluded by appropriate tests, particularly if the anginal pain is not typical in character or related to effort.

Treatment

Factors influencing the development of collateral circulation are not well understood. Collateral flow can be produced with implantation of internal mammary arteries into the myocardium: these arteries develop collateral pathways to ischemic areas of the myocardium in 80% of patients after 6–10 weeks, but the volume of flow through these collaterals appears to be variable and small. This operation has been all but abandoned but may still have limited application in patients with diffuse small vessel coronary disease which is not amenable to anastomotic grafting.

Bypass grafting of autogenous vein from the ascending aorta to the coronary arteries distal to a major occlusion is the first surgical procedure that offers an excellent expectation of helping patients with ischemic disease. Its opportunities are limited only by the distal runoff, and evidence is rapidly accumulating to document its efficacy in the relief of anginal symptoms. Significant flows are provided immediately to underperfused areas of the coronary vascular bed. Long-term evaluation is currently limited to 4 years, and graft patency rates of 80–90% after 1 year have been documented. The influence of bypass grafting on life expectancy is still not known, but there is reason to expect that it is favorable.

Endarterectomy, either as a definitive procedure or in conjunction with appropriate grafting, has been used with some success; however, the risk of injuring branch vessels increases the potential hazard and may limit the effectiveness of this procedure. Onlay patch grafts over stenotic areas of coronary artery have met with temporary success, but the frequency of late thrombosis suggests that this approach is undesirable.

Prognosis

The ultimate effect of the currently employed surgical procedures for coronary artery disease in terms of life expectancy is still to be demonstrated. A very large experience with surgical bypass grafting of obstructed coronary arteries (either with autogenous saphenous vein jump grafts, internal mammary artery grafts, or splenic artery grafts) has not been accompanied by control studies to ascertain the prognosis of unoperated patients with similar disease. Relief of anginal pain can be expected for 70–80% of patients. The surgical mortality rate is about 4%, and 80% of the grafts appear to be open after 1 year.

Recent emphasis has been directed to "preinfarction angina" or "crescendo angina" and the urgency of surgery before impending total occlusion occurs in a major coronary artery. The validity of this phenomenon has been documented in a few cases by the appearance of progressive ischemic changes on the ECG, but the incidence of eventual infarction in this group without surgery and the potential to develop adequate collateral pathways has not been documented. It is logical, however, that major vascular obstructions to a vital organ are dangerous and should be relieved.

Coronary bypass grafting has been tried in the treatment of impaired ventricular function secondary to occlusive coronary disease. Dysfunction is occasionally reversible after improved perfusion, but the results are usually poor under these conditions, presumably because of irreversible pathologic changes, and the new blood supply has little or no effective myocardium to perfuse.

Before the advent of direct anastomoses to the coronary arteries, Vineberg had popularized the intramyocardial implantation of mammary arteries. He reported that 86% of these implants were patent after 10 years and that effective symptomatic relief of angina occurred in 60–70% of patients. This procedure has now been virtually abandoned but is occasionally used when no suitable vessel for grafting can be found.

Alderman EL & others: Results of direct coronary-artery surgery for angina pectoris. New England J Med 288:535–539, 1973.

Messer JV & others: Effect of exercise on cardiac performance in human subjects with coronary artery disease. Circulation 28:404–414, 1963.

MYOCARDIAL INFARCTS; MECHANICAL COMPLICATIONS

Functional disability appearing late in convalescence after myocardial infarction should suggest the loss of ventricular wall function. Intractable decompensation may seem to rule out surgery, but immediate operation to correct a mechanical dysfunction is potentially lifesaving. The efficacy of acute infarctectomy remains in doubt, but where true dyskinesia (aneurysm) is demonstrated angiographically, functional improvement is to be expected after resection. Coronary angiography should be performed about 2 months postinfarction even if they do not have persistent angina. Most of these patients have had major occlusion of more than one coronary artery, and when collateral flow to the infarcted area is through a significantly (if not yet critically) occluded vessel, this vessel should have a saphenous vein bypass graft on a preventive basis.

Ellis FH Jr: Surgery for chronic asynergy of the left ventricle: A current appraisal. Surgery 70:801, 1971.

Enright LP & others: Human coronary artery bypass grafts and left ventricular function. Surgery 72:404, 1972.

Johnson WD & others: Extended treatment of severe coronary artery disease: A total surgical approach. Ann Surg 170:460, 1969.

Mundth ED & others: Myocardial revascularization for treatment of cardiogenic shock complicating acute myocardial infarction. Surgery 70:78, 1971.

Najafi H & others: Surgical management of complications of myocardial infarction. M Clin North America 57:205–218, 1973.

Rossi NP, Flege JB Jr, Ehrenhaft JL: Surgically treatable complications of myocardial infarction. Surgery 65:118–126, 1969.

Spencer FC & others: Coronary artery bypass for congestive heart failure: A report of experiences with 40 patients. J Thoracic Cardiovas Surg 62:529, 1971.

VENTRICULAR ANEURYSM

Essentials of Diagnosis

- Discrete bulge in the ventricular aspect of the cardiac silhouette on x-ray.
- Characteristic ECG pattern.

General Considerations

A large myocardial infarction which does not rupture causes fibrosis and contraction, or distention of the necrotic myocardium when the scarring process yields to ventricular pressure and produces aneurysm.

Any patient who has persistent cardiac failure after myocardial infarction and an enlarged cardiac silhouette should be studied by (1) cardiac catheterization, to determine ventricular competence (reflected by end-diastolic pressure) and to rule out a shunt through ventricular septal rupture; (2) ventricular angiography, to rule out ventricular aneurysm, mitral incompetence, and ventricular septal defect; and (3) selective coronary angiography, to determine the patency of the coronary vessels.

Clinical Findings

Since aneurysms arise in the area of damaged or infarcted myocardium, the ECG pattern of healed infarct is essential to the diagnosis. Occasional paradoxic systolic thrust over the precordium can be recognized in the thin-chested patient. Paradoxic motion of the cardiac border by fluoroscopy is a classic finding, although its absence does not rule out the disease. Cardiac catheterization combined with cineangiocardiography will document left ventricular failure with an elevated left ventricular end-diastolic pressure. This study will distinguish the characteristic localized paradoxic bulge of ventricular aneurysm from the generally impaired contractility of advanced myocardial failure. Although the aneurysm is characteristically filled with laminated clot, peripheral embolization from this material occurs only rarely (5–10% of cases). Intractable congestive heart failure is the most common indication for surgery in ventricular aneurysm.

Complications

Rupture of ventricular aneurysms, in contrast to the fate of aortic aneurysms, is exceedingly rare. The pericardium almost always becomes fused to the infarcted area and provides a sturdy viable support. This should be remembered when approaching the lesion surgically because, if the pericardium is dissected off the aneurysm before cardiopulmonary bypass is instituted, fatal hemorrhage may occur.

When the aneurysm (usually posterior) involves the attachment of papillary muscles, a secondary mitral insufficiency can develop.

Treatment

Excision of ventricular aneurysm (with extracorporeal circulation) has a mortality rate of about 5% and usually results in significant improvement. Concomitant mitral valve replacement may be necessary when papillary muscle is involved. The size of the aneurysm is no contraindication to surgical resection; if the patient can survive with a large nonfunctioning area of myocardium, his condition will be improved with a smaller chamber. However, when a small aneurysm is resected in the presence of diffuse ventricular dysfunction, failure is to be expected.

Prognosis

Small ventricular aneurysms may remain asymptomatic indefinitely without enlargement, and the patient's prognosis is dependent upon the progress of his underlying coronary artery disease.

Cooley DA, Hallman GL, Henly WS: Left ventricular aneurysm due to myocardial infarction: Experience with 37 patients undergoing aneurysmectomy. Arch Surg 88:114–121, 1964.

Dunaway MC, Dillon ML Jr, Greenfield JC Jr: Repair of postinfarction interventricular septal rupture. Arch Int Med 122:147–149, 1968.

Groden BM, James WB, McDicken I: Cardiac aneurysm after myocardial infarction. Postgrad MJ 44:775–784, 1968.

Loop FD & others: Posterior ventricular aneurysms: Etiologic factors and surgical treatment. New England J Med 288:237–239, 1973.

MITRAL INSUFFICIENCY
(Ruptured Papillary Muscle)

The development of a murmur after myocardial infarction, particularly when coincident with a late onset of decompensation, suggests mitral valve regurgitation secondary to avulsion of an infarcted papillary muscle.

As with ventricular aneurysm, the opportunities for surgical correction of a mechanical complication should be appreciated and cardiac catheterization should be undertaken immediately.

The lesion is identified by the same criteria listed above for organic mitral valve disease leading to incompetence. Mitral insufficiency can sometimes be distinguished from postinfarction ventricular septal defect (see below) only by cardiac catheterization with angiocardiography. In either instance, prompt identification is essential to appropriate planning and management. Any patient who develops a murmur secondary to myocardial infarction is in danger of significant hemodynamic embarrassment.

Treatment

Surgery to plicate or replace the mitral valve is indicated when functional disability is significant. Surgery should be undertaken on an urgent basis when supportive medical therapy is not successful in managing congestive failure. When possible, however, it is desirable to defer operation for approximately 2 months in order to permit healing of the underlying myocardial infarction and maximal development of collateral circulation.

The infarction process is only rarely limited to the papillary muscle itself and usually involves a significant area of myocardial wall surrounding the base of the muscle. This area should be carefully inspected for evidence of significantly impaired function and paradoxic motion. It may be desirable to excise this area of ventricular wall; if so, the valve replacement can be carried out from the ventricular side.

Prognosis

The relative rarity of this complication and its relationship to the degree of associated coronary artery disease make it impossible to generalize about surgical risks. In relatively young patients with well-healed small infarcts, the risk is that of routine mitral valve replacement ($< 10\%$). In the older patient with diffuse coronary artery disease and extensively destroyed myocardium, the chance of salvage is low. In either case, the prognosis with surgery is at least an improvement over the available alternatives.

Austen WG & others: Surgical treatment of papillary-muscle rupture complicating myocardial infarction. New England J Med 278:1137–1141, 1968.

Morrow AG & others: Severe mitral regurgitation following acute myocardial infarction and ruptured papillary muscle: Hemodynamic findings and results of operative treatment in four patients. Circulation 37 (Suppl 2):124–132, 1968.

VENTRICULAR SEPTAL DEFECT
(Rupture of Infarcted Septum)

A myocardial infarction involving the ventricular septum can undergo central necrosis and breakdown, creating a sudden communication between the ventricles. The resulting left-to-right shunt may precipitate a hemodynamic crisis.

As with mitral insufficiency—for which it is easily mistaken—the onset of ventricular septal defect is typically heralded by a new apical murmur and sudden signs of decompensation. The right-sided aspects of the failure (hepatomegaly and venous distention) may be more prominent than in mitral insufficiency, but all of these clinical findings may be present in either lesion.

Diagnostic confirmation requires prompt cardiac catheterization and angiocardiography in order to plan management intelligently. If this information is delayed and the patient's condition deteriorates rapidly, his chances for successful surgery may be jeopardized.

Treatment

The indications for closure of ventricular septal defect are obviously related to the degree of hemodynamic abnormality it produces. If congestive failure can be successfully managed, it is desirable to postpone surgery for 2 months or more to allow scar tissue to develop which will adequately support surgical repair. The development of collateral circulation and resolution of the infarct will also reduce the operative risk.

Although successful cases of early closure have been reported, the integrity of such a surgical closure is tenuous because sutures must be placed in soft, edematous, and ischemic myocardium. Under the latter circumstances the surgical technic of choice is similar to that used for multiple congenital muscular defects, ie, through-and-through heavy sutures across external buttresses.

Lewis AJ, Burchell HB, Titus JL: Clinical and pathologic features of postinfarction cardiac rupture. Am J Cardiol 23:43–53, 1969.

Oldham HN Jr & others: Surgical correction of ventricular septal defect following acute myocardial infarction. Ann Thoracic Surg 7:193–201, 1969.

•   •   •

CARDIAC TUMORS

As with tumors elsewhere in the body, tumors of the heart are manifested primarily by their space-occupying effects and may remain asymptomatic until they become large. If pedunculated, a tumor can produce transient symptoms of obstruction to blood flow; if friable, it can deliver emboli into the blood stream; and if rapidly invasive on the epicardial surface, it can produce hemopericardium and pericardial tamponade.

Tumors can occur at any age. They have been reported in children as young as 6 and in adults over 70.

TABLE 23–1. Types of heart tumors.

I. **Primary**
  A. Benign—75%
    1. Myxoma
    2. Rhabdomyoma (Purkinje hamartoma)
    3. Papillary tumor of heart valve (Lambl excrescence)
    4. Fibroma
    5. Lipoma
    6. Teratoma
  B. Malignant—25%
    1. Sarcoma: angiosarcoma, rhabdomyosarcoma, fibrosarcoma, liposarcoma, neurosarcoma, leiomyosarcoma
    2. Teratoma
II. **Metastatic**
  A. Carcinoma—67%
  B. Sarcoma—20%
  C. Melanoma—12%

Benign **myxoma** is by far the most common lesion and accounts for nearly 75% of primary benign cardiac tumors (Table 23–1). Its physical characteristics range from a smooth, firm, spherical, encapsulated mass to a loose conglomeration of gelatinous material with the cohesiveness of jellied consommé. Eighty percent are pedunculated. Over 75% are attached to the septum in the left atrium, but they do also occur in the right atrium and rarely in the ventricles.

Malignant tumors are predominantly sarcomas, most commonly rhabdomyosarcoma and angiosarcoma. Malignant teratomas of the heart occur rarely.

A full spectrum of metastatic tumors to the heart has been reported. Hepatomas will extend directly into the heart through the hepatic veins.

Clinical Findings

Systemic symptoms reported with some myxomas include fever, weight loss, and anemia. Laboratory studies may show an increased sedimentation rate, increased gamma globulin, and variable elevations of SGOT and LDH.

The onset and clinical findings of cardiac tumors are variable, and the latter are frequently bizarre. Classically, a pedunculated left atrial myxoma has a ball valve action in the mitral orifice which obstructs flow and mimics mitral stenosis or distorts a leaflet to produce mitral insufficiency. Subtle differences in the murmurs produced may identify a tumor, particularly when the position of the patient alters the murmur.

Sudden onset of vascular obstruction, particularly in a young person with no history of cardiovascular disease, should raise a suspicion of fragmenting left atrial myxoma. If the diagnosis is verified histologically from the embolus, immediate intervention is indicated without further study.

Bizarre cardiac symptoms, distortions of the cardiac silhouette, or unexplained tamponade or signs of obstruction should lead to angiographic study, which usually makes the diagnosis.

Differential Diagnosis

A cardiac tumor may be mistaken for a variety of valvular lesions, and even angiocardiography cannot distinguish it from an atrial thrombus.

Treatment

Surgical removal of the tumor is indicated because of its obvious hemodynamic hazards. The malignant potential of a myxoma is uncertain, but recurrences have been reported. For this reason, excision of the pedicle with its base should be done whenever possible. The urgency of the necessity for removal depends upon how the tumor manifests itself. Embolization represents an imminent hazard of being repeated and should be considered an emergency. Severe hemodynamic symptoms, even if intermittent, should also be considered pressing; but mild intermittent symptoms can be dealt with electively. An asymptomatic calcified mass discovered incidentally can probably be observed without risk.

In contrast to intraluminal myxomas, sarcomas are seldom favorably localized by the time they are identified, and complete resection is almost never possible. Surgery is indicated to provide palliative relief of tumor compression and to obtain a tissue diagnosis. Radiation therapy may provide effective palliation in some instances.

Casteneda AR, Varco RL: Tumors of the heart: Surgical considerations. Am J Cardiol 21:357–362, 1968.

Comer TP, Arbegast NR, Schinalhorst WR: Left atrial myxoma: Diagnostic and surgical aspects. California Med 118:18–20, April, 1973.

Goodwin JF: The spectrum of cardiac tumors. Am J Cardiol 21:307, 1968.

Laws JW, Annes GP, Bogren HG: Primary malignant tumors of the heart. California Med 118:11–17, April 1973.

Mundth ED & others: Clinical aspects of left atrial myxoma. Ann Thoracic Surg 5:255–261, 1968.

CARDIOPULMONARY RESUSCITATION

Cardiac arrest is either a precipitous event which may lead to immediate death or the terminal result of a gradual dying process. Experience derived largely from the management of patients undergoing chest surgery has demonstrated that circulatory arrest is both preventable and reversible in a substantial number of patients, particularly when it is not the consequence of progressive and irreversible disease. It is now feasible to deal effectively with this disaster when it occurs elsewhere in the hospital. Every physician must, therefore, be familiar with the measures which may salvage the patient who "dies" unexpectedly. This responsibility includes being able to use a laryngoscope and pass an endotracheal tube, to administer effective external cardiac compression, and to apply electrical defibrillation, as well as familiarity with the drugs and fluids that should be given.

"Cardiac arrest" is manifested by asystole, ventricular fibrillation, or profound cardiovascular collapse with continued but ineffective cardiac function. Many of these terminal events may be precipitated by or associated with severe pulmonary dysfunction, and it is obviously essential to consider the heart and lungs as a single unit in providing the body's oxygen needs. Thus, attention must be directed to both organs in considering the cause and administering resuscitation.

Etiology of Cardiac Arrest

Although unrecognized or unpreventable hypoxia probably accounts for the substantial majority (perhaps 75%) of cardiac arrests, much remains to be learned about the neurohumoral and electrical mechanisms which precipitate the event. It is almost impossible to reconstruct a complete picture of the patient's cardiac status immediately prior to cardiopulmonary arrest. Nevertheless, a number of causative factors have been recognized and are worthy of attention. Conduction abnormalities are produced by hyperkalemia and hypermagnesemia. Myocardial irritability and digitalis toxicity are augmented by hypokalemia, and vasodilatation and impaired perfusion can result from sedatives, narcotics, and anesthetic agents. Respiratory acidosis and hypoxia result from the ventilatory depression produced by narcotics.

Diagnosis of Cardiac Arrest

Any patient who fails to respond to commands or painful stimulus, who becomes pale without palpable pulse or blood pressure, whose respiratory activity ceases, or whose ECG shows ventricular fibrillation or cardiac arrest should be considered to be in cardiac arrest, and resuscitation should be started. Prompt treatment produces the best results. Confirmation of the arrest or fibrillation is made by palpating for the carotid or femoral pulses.

Treatment of Cardiac Arrest

Suspected cardiopulmonary arrest requires that a series of effective measures be instituted immediately without moving the patient but while simultaneously calling for assistance. Results will be closely related to prompt recognition of the problem and to the performance of a well-trained resuscitation team which should be on 24-hour call in every hospital. Persistence of resuscitative efforts should be encouraged. Patients have been saved after more than 80 depolarizing shocks or after efforts lasting over 1 hour.

Resuscitation consists of the following steps:

A. Airway: (See Fig 15–4.) The essential first step in the treatment of cardiac arrest is to establish an open airway. This can often be done by simply tilting the head backward and pulling the lower jaw forward. If the airway is still blocked, it may be necessary to manually extract vomitus or a foreign body (eg, false teeth) from the pharynx with a finger, at the same time displacing the tongue to secure an open airway. Insertion of an endotracheal tube is preferable since it gives better control of ventilation.

B. Breathing: Oxygen should be administered through the endotracheal tube or with a tight-fitting mask. If oxygen is not immediately available, ventilation can be maintained by mouth-to-mouth breathing either directly or via a Resuscitube.

C. Cardiac Resuscitation:· (Fig 23–8.) Closed chest massage should be started at once. This is accomplished by placing the patient on a hard surface, being certain that adequate ventilation has been established. A sharp blow with the fist to the sternum may stimulate the heart to beat. If this is not effective, place the base of the hand on the lower end of the sternum (not the xiphoid process) and press directly downward 4–5 cm toward the spine about once per second. The pressure exerted should be enough to depress the sternum but not enough to fracture a rib. Positive action requires more than arm motion, especially in robust

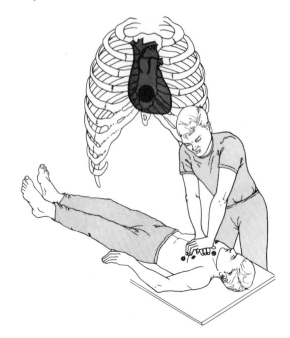

FIG 23–8. Technic of closed chest cardiac massage. Heavy circle in heart drawing shows area of application of force. Circles on supine figure show points of application of electrodes for defibrillation. (Reproduced, with permission, from Krupp MA, Chatton MJ: *Current Diagnosis & Treatment 1973.* Lange, 1973.)

adult patients; it is recommended that the physician kneel on the bed astride the patient so he can exert the weight of his shoulders against the patient's chest.

An attempt should be made to coordinate the massage with respiratory assistance so that one respiratory cycle is interposed between every 5 cardiac compressions. The carotid or femoral pulse should be palpated between each compression to determine the pressure necessary to produce a palpable pulse. Observe the pupils; persistent dilatation is a sign that adequate ventilation and perfusion have not been achieved.

Excessively vigorous compression can fracture ribs or costal cartilage and may even rupture the liver or spleen. Damage to other organs such as the lung and stomach has also been reported.

If flail chest, bilateral pneumothorax, or lacerations of the heart make external massage impossible, immediate thoracotomy and direct cardiac massage may be required.

D. Drug Therapy: Medications and electrolytes must all be administered intravenously, since absorption from the tissues in this state is limited and delayed. Persistent ventricular irritability should be treated with injections of 50–100 mg of lidocaine followed, if necessary, by an intravenous drip of this drug. If there is reason to suspect hypokalemia, potassium chloride can be administered in doses of 10–20 mEq. Impaired perfusion will result in metabolic acidosis, which should be treated by injection of 1 ampule of sodium bicarbonate intravenously. (Ampules usually contain 44 mEq.) Except in severe degrees (pH < 7.2), acidosis itself is not particularly harmful, and it is recommended that more attention be directed toward treating its cause (poor perfusion).

Inotropic drugs may be essential to stimulate adequate cardiac contraction or may be necessary to initiate systolic activity. Isoproterenol is the drug of choice because of its ancillary vasodilatory action, but epinephrine is an excellent substitute. The dosage of isoproterenol is 2 mg IV in 500 ml of 0.5 N saline or 5% dextrose and water at a rate of 10–20 drops per minute. It may be necessary to double or quadruple this dose–or, conversely, the drug may induce ventricular fibrillation and have to be discontinued.

E. Defibrillation: If the patient is in ventricular fibrillation, restoration of normal cardiac rhythm is essential but should not be attempted until effective circulation has been provided to the heart and brain (manifested by the patient's responsiveness). An ischemic heart will neither defibrillate nor respond to inotropic drugs. During the initial resuscitation efforts, while circulation and ventilation are being supported, ECG leads can be connected, effective intravenous pathways established, and arterial pressure monitoring provided.

Defibrillation should be attempted only after it is determined that the heart is fibrillating and after sufficient circulatory support has been provided to perfuse the heart and reverse hypoxia. Defibrillator electrodes must be applied with conductive jelly or over wet saline sponges. The electrodes should be placed in the midaxillary line of the left lower rib cage and over the upper sternum. The defibrillator (usually a condenser discharge system) should be set between 200 and 400 watt-seconds. Respiratory support is temporarily suspended during the shock but instantly resumed thereafter while the result is being assessed. Only one or 2 attempts at defibrillation should be made without an interval to attempt further improvement of circulation, volume loss, acidosis, or electrolyte imbalance.

Skin burns from the electrodes can be minimized by making certain that their entire surfaces are covered with conductive paste and are completely in contact with the body surface, leaving no gap for a spark to cross. On the other hand, the paste must not be smeared so as to form a conductive bridge between the 2 electrodes and thus cause a short circuit.

F. Pacemaker: Electrical pacing may be necessary when an asystole total heart block or sinus bradycardia persists. Conventional electrodes may be introduced intravenously, and percutaneous electrodes can be introduced through the apex.

Grossman JI, Rubin IL: Cardiopulmonary resuscitation. 2 parts. Am Heart J 78:569, 709, 1969.

Jude JR, Nagel EL: Cardiopulmonary resuscitation, 1970. Mod Concepts Cardiovas Dis 39:133, 1970.

● ● ●

General References

Beall AC Jr & others: Prosthetic replacement of cardiac valves: Five and one-half years' experience. Am J Cardiol 23:250, 1969.

Behrendt DM, Austen WG: *Patient Care in Cardiac Surgery.* Little, Brown, 1972.

Braunwald E: Mitral regurgitation: Physiologic, clinical, and surgical considerations. New England J Med 281:425, 1969.

Diethrich EB & others: An analysis of operated and nonoperated patients with documented coronary arterial disease. J Thoracic Cardiovas Surg 57:115, 1969.

Duvoisin GE & others: The advantages and disadvantages of prosthetic valves for aortic valve replacement. Progr Cardiovas Dis 11:294, 1969.

Effler DB, Groves LK: Coronary artery surgery utilizing saphenous vein graft techniques: Clinical experience with 224 operations. J Thoracic Cardiovas Surg 59:147, 1970.

Johnson WD & others: Extended treatment of severe coronary artery disease: A total surgical approach. Ann Surg 170:460, 1969.

Kaplan S (editor): Symposium on pediatric cardiology. P Clin North America 18:1009–1310, 1971.

Nelson CL, Esselstyn CB Jr (editors): Symposium on cardiac and renal surgery. S Clin North America 51:1007–1242, 1971.

Oldham HN Jr & others: Surgical correction of ventricular septal defect following acute myocardial infarction. Ann Thoracic Surg 7:193, 1969.

Selzer A & others: Clinical, hemodynamic, and surgical considerations of rupture of the ventricular septum after myocardial infarction. Am Heart J 78:598, 1969.

Symbas PN: *Traumatic Injuries of the Heart and Great Vessels.* Thomas, 1972.

Terzaki AK & others: Combined mitral and aortic valve disease. Am J Cardiol 25:588, 1970.

Vineberg A: The rationale of revascularization surgery. Dis Chest 55:245, 1969.

23...

The Heart:
II. Congenital Diseases

L. Henry Edmunds, Jr., MD

GENERAL CONSIDERATIONS

Developmental defects of the heart and great vessels encompass a wide spectrum of anatomic malformations that produce varying degrees of circulatory dysfunction. The different malformations are classified by anatomic characteristics, but the severity of individual lesions within each classification varies widely. Most importantly, the severity of the anatomic malformation often does not correlate with the degree of circulatory dysfunction. The same type of anatomic malformation may cause disabling symptoms in one patient and no symptoms in another. For proper management of patients with congenital heart disease, both the anatomic diagnosis and the pathologic physiology of the abnormal circulatory system must be understood.

The cardiac surgeon must clearly understand the pathologic anatomy of a given lesion in order to correct the structural deformity. However, the pathologic physiology of the abnormal circulation is far more important for understanding the symptoms, signs, laboratory findings, and complications of a particular anatomic lesion and the basis of medical or surgical management. To facilitate this understanding, congenital heart defects have been classified as (1) obstructive lesions, (2) lesions which increase pulmonary blood flow, (3) lesions which reduce pulmonary blood flow, and (4) complex malformations. A few rare anomalies that are not easily included in the above classification are grouped as miscellaneous lesions.

Incidence

Approximately 8–10 newborns out of every 1000 have some type of congenital heart disease. Some lesions are more common in one sex than the other; however, no racial predilection is recognized. High mortality in the first weeks and months after birth and occasional spontaneous cures reduce the incidence of congenital heart disease in school-age children to approximately 4.5 per 1000. The most reliable figures for the incidence of different lesions at birth and at school age are presented in Table 23–2.

Etiology

Most congenital heart lesions occur sporadically and are not associated with other disease. With few exceptions, the cause is not known. Maternal rubella causes 1–2% of all congenital heart lesions. Characteristically, these babies have patent ductus arteriosus and peripheral pulmonary stenosis (with or without ventricular septal defect), deafness, and cataracts. Other lesions occur in association with chromosomal anomalies; the most common is the association of persistent atrioventricular canal with 21 trisomy (Down's syndrome). Some diseases such as Marfan's syndrome, gargoylism, and certain cases of supravalvular aortic stenosis are inherited diseases.

In families without known genetic defects, 14% of persons with congenital heart lesions have a relative with a congenital heart defect. This incidence is much higher than that of the general population but much lower than can be explained by genetic laws.

Clinical Diagnosis

A congenital heart lesion may produce different degrees of circulatory dysfunction and different clinical features at different ages. The clinical manifestations of different types of anatomic malformations

TABLE 23–2. Incidence of various types of congenital heart disease.*

	Percentage at Birth	Percentage at School Age
Ventricular septal defect	30.8	12.5–28.1
Patent ductus arteriosus	8.0	11.2–14.1
Atrial septal defect†	10.9	15.1–20.0
Pulmonary stenosis and atresia	8.9	17.5–20.0
Aortic stenosis and atresia	6.5	11.7–17.5
Coarctation of aorta	6.0	2.5–7.5
Tetralogy of Fallot	6.1	3.8
Transposition of great arteries	4.6	
Truncus arteriosus	0.9	
Tricuspid atresia	1.2	
Miscellaneous	7.0	7.2–7.5
Undiagnosed	9.1	

*From Hoffman JIE: Natural history of congenital heart disease: Problems of its assessment with special reference to ventricular septal defects. Circulation 37:97–125, 1968.

†Includes ostium secundum, ostium primum, and total anomalous pulmonary venous connection.

vary widely, and few lesions produce pathognomonic symptoms or signs. Although anatomic changes in some lesions occur during infancy and early childhood, most of the variance in symptoms and signs is due to changes in circulatory dynamics. The circulatory physiology of a newborn differs from that of an older infant or child. At birth, pulmonary vascular resistance is nearly equal to systemic resistance, and both the foramen ovale and the ductus arteriosus are patent. As the ductus closes and pulmonary vascular resistance decreases, profound changes in circulatory dynamics may occur in patients with congenital heart defects. Similarly, activity affects circulatory physiology and the clinical manifestations of most congenital heart lesions.

Some newborns have obvious heart disease; others—even those with complex lesions—may appear normal at birth and show no evidence of abnormal circulation for days or weeks. In some cases, the possibility of congenital heart disease is not suspected until a murmur or abnormal finding is discovered at well baby, routine, or school examinations weeks or years after birth. Respiratory and feeding problems, cyanosis, absent or weak femoral pulses, enlargement of the liver and heart, murmurs, and failure to gain weight suggest the presence of heart disease in newborns. Frequent respiratory infections, irritability, fatigue, and poor growth and weight gain are common manifestations of congenital heart disease in older infants.

The diagnostic process should start with a thorough history and physical examination, ECG, posteroanterior and lateral chest x-rays, and hematocrit. Arterial blood P_{O_2}, P_{CO_2}, and pH determinations are often helpful. Clinical information frequently leads to an accurate diagnosis in children, but in newborns and infants these data usually only narrow the differential diagnosis. "Classic" findings of specific anatomic lesions often are absent or masked in newborns and young infants, and the differential diagnosis must include complex and potentially lethal malformations which are seldom observed in older children. Cardiac catheterization and cineangiocardiography add the necessary information to define the anatomic and physiologic pathology. Definition of both the structural and functional pathology is essential for proper management of congenital heart lesions in patients of all ages.

Cardiac Catheterization & Cineangiocardiography

These special studies can be performed at any time after birth in all infants, including small prematures. Local anesthesia with or without sedation is used routinely. There are virtually no contraindications to the procedure in patients with suspected heart disease regardless of the severity of circulatory dysfunction. Catheters are introduced through the saphenous, femoral, or brachial vein for study of the right heart chambers. The aorta and left heart are usually catheterized from the femoral or umbilical artery (occasionally the axillary or brachial artery). In this approach, the catheter is passed retrograde across the aortic valve into the left ventricle and occasionally into the left

atrium. The left atrium can also be entered by passing a catheter from the right atrium across a patent foramen ovale or by perforating the interatrial septum with a special needle (older children only). Catheters are maneuvered into specific chambers and vessels under fluoroscopic vision to obtain phasic and mean pressures and blood samples and to inject contrast material for biplane (usually anteroposterior and lateral) cineangiocardiograms. During the catheterization procedure, accumulated data may prompt additional measurements, cineangiocardiograms, or special studies to make certain that the anatomic and functional abnormalities of the lesion are clearly defined.

Mean and phasic pressures in various cardiac chambers provide quantitative information that is diagnostic of many lesions. In normal individuals, mean and phasic pressures in the different cardiac chambers differ with age (Table 23–3).

Cardiac output is generally measured by either the Fick or Stewart-Hamilton method. Both measurements are subject to considerable error (15–100%). Cardiac output is corrected for differences in body size by dividing the measured cardiac output (liters/min) by body surface area (sq m) to produce the cardiac index (liters/min/sq m). Normal cardiac indices range from 3–5 liters/min/sq m.

Pulmonary vascular resistance (PVR) in Wood units is calculated by dividing the difference between mean pulmonary arterial (PA) and left atrial (LA) pressures by the cardiac index. Normal pulmonary vascular resistances are 1–3 Wood units. Systemic vascular resistance is calculated by dividing the difference between mean aortic and right atrial pressures by the cardiac index. Normal systemic vascular resistances are 12–20 Wood units. The arbitrary Wood unit can be converted into dyne-sec/cm^{-5} by multiplying by 80.

Abnormal communications or shunts between the left and right heart chambers and great vessels can be detected by indicator dyes. More commonly, shunts are calculated by measurements of blood oxygen saturations (the percentage of hemoglobin that is saturated with oxygen). Normally, blood oxygen saturations are 70–75% in the right heart chambers and above 96% in the left heart chambers and systemic arteries. An increase in the blood oxygen saturation in the right heart chambers indicates a left-to-right shunt; similarly,

TABLE 23–3. Normal phasic and mean pressures.*

Location	Newborn (mm Hg)	One Month After Birth (mm Hg)	Children (mm Hg)
Right atrium	(2)	(2)	(1–5)
Right ventricle	50/3	30/3	15–28/0–5
Pulmonary artery	50/30 (38)	30/12 (18)	15–28/5–15
Left atrium	(4)	(4)	(5–8)
Left ventricle	70/5	80/5	80–120/0–8
Aorta	70/45 (55)	80/50 (60)	80–120/60–75

*Numbers in parentheses are mean pressures. Other numbers are systolic/diastolic pressures.

a decrease in oxygen saturation in the left heart chambers indicates a right-to-left shunt. The increase in blood oxygen saturation required to diagnose a left-to-right shunt varies between 5 and 15% depending upon the cardiac chamber sampled and the number of measurements.

Using the Fick principle, both pulmonary blood flow (Qp) and systemic blood flow (Qs) can be calculated from measurements of blood oxygen saturation. Blood oxygen content is calculated by multiplying the saturation percentage by 1.34 and by the hemoglobin concentration (g/liter).

$$\frac{Qp}{\text{(liters/min)}} = \frac{\text{Oxygen consumption (ml/min)}}{\text{Pulmonary venous } O_2 \text{ content (ml/liter)} - \text{Pulmonary arterial } O_2 \text{ content (ml/liter)}}$$

$$\frac{Qs}{\text{(liters/min)}} = \frac{\text{Oxygen consumption (ml/min)}}{\text{Systemic arterial } O_2 \text{ content (ml/liter)} - \text{Mixed venous } O_2 \text{ content (ml/liter)}}$$

Effective pulmonary blood flow is defined as the amount of mixed systemic venous blood (upstream to any shunt) that passes through the lungs. Effective pulmonary blood flow (Qep) is calculated as follows:

$$\frac{Qep}{\text{(liters/min)}} = \frac{\text{Oxygen consumption (ml/min)}}{\text{Pulmonary venous } O_2 \text{ content (ml/liter)} - \text{Mixed venous } O_2 \text{ content (ml/liter)}}$$

The magnitude of a left-to-right shunt equals Qp minus Qep, and the amount of a right-to-left shunt equals Qs minus Qep.

Since oxygen uptake by the lungs always equals oxygen consumption by the tissues, the relative magnitudes or ratio of pulmonary and systemic blood flows can be calculated without measuring oxygen consumption. The flow ratio is inversely proportionate to the arteriovenous differences in oxygen saturation:

$$\frac{Qp}{Qs} = \frac{\text{Systemic arterial } O_2 \text{ saturation} - \text{Systemic venous } O_2 \text{ saturation}}{\text{Pulmonary venous } O_2 \text{ saturation} - \text{Pulmonary arterial } O_2 \text{ saturation}}$$

Flow ratios can be calculated directly from oxygen saturations because the constants (1.34 and the hemoglobin concentration) used to convert blood oxygen saturation to blood oxygen content cancel out.

Cardiac catheterization is associated with an overall mortality rate of 0.06–0.44%. Infrequent complications include cardiac arrhythmias and arrest, perforation of the heart, adverse reactions to contrast material, injection of contrast material into the myocardial wall, embolism, thrombosis or injury of a peripheral vessel, local hematoma formation, false aneurysm, arteriovenous fistula formation, and sepsis.

Medical Management

Drugs, diet, and activity are regulated to achieve optimal performance of the abnormal circulation and maximal growth and development of the child. Special care is required for emergencies such as congestive heart failure, arrhythmias, hypoxic spells, syncopal episodes, and infections. Careful observation may prevent development of irreversible complications such as pulmonary vascular disease, cerebral thrombosis, and bacterial endocarditis. The timing of special diagnostic and surgical procedures, recommendations to parents and school authorities, and care during unrelated illnesses are important factors in good medical management.

Operative Management

The surgical treatment of congenital heart disease is conveniently divided into 2 categories: palliative operations and corrective operations.

A. Palliative Operations: Palliative operations are designed to improve circulatory function without correcting the anatomic malformation in patients with severe malformations that cannot be corrected or in patients in whom the risk of a totally corrective operation is high. With few exceptions, palliative operations create further anatomic abnormalities to help compensate for poorly tolerated circulatory dysfunction. In general, palliative operations are designed to reduce or increase pulmonary blood flow, improve mixing of oxygenated and poorly oxygenated blood within the heart, or relieve obstructions.

B. Corrective Operations: Corrective operations which do not use temporary cardiopulmonary bypass are applicable to extracardiac lesions such as patent ductus arteriosus, coarctation of the aorta, and vascular ring anomalies.

Correction of intracardiac congenital defects generally requires temporary cardiopulmonary bypass. Venous blood is shunted from both vena cavas or the right atrium into a mechanical oxygenator and then is pumped to the patient via a cannula in the aorta or femoral artery. Cardiopulmonary bypass provides satisfactory conditions for intracardiac surgery and can be performed with little risk in infants over approximately 6 months.

Because of the small size and reduced reserve of some organs and organ systems, newborns and small infants generally cannot tolerate prolonged periods of cardiopulmonary bypass. Three different methods that were designed to eliminate or reduce the period of bypass have been used for intracardiac procedures in these patients. Although the circulation cannot be interrupted safely at 37 C (98.6 F) for more than 3 or 4 minutes, very rapid operations such as incision of a stenotic pulmonary valve or creation of an atrial septal defect can be performed during temporary occlusion of both vena cavas. The period of circulatory arrest can be extended by surface cooling (hypothermia), but at around 30 C (86 F) the heart is electrically unstable and often develops ventricular fibrillation. If a special anesthetic and cooling technic is used, some patients can be safely cooled by surface means to 18–20 C (64.4–68 F) (deep hypothermia); at that temperature, the circulation can be safely suspended for 60 minutes.

A more rapid, safer, and preferred method is to combine surface cooling with core cooling during a short period of cardiopulmonary bypass. The circulation is interrupted during the intracardiac repair at 18–20 C, but only 30–40 minutes of bypass are required to cool and rewarm the patient.

If the anatomic lesion can be totally or substantially corrected, this operation is preferred to a palliative procedure in nearly all cases. The risk of a corrective operation is usually greater in newborns and young infants than in older infants and children, and a palliative operation is sometimes available at lower risk. Even so, a corrective operation may be preferred because the additive risks of a palliative operation and later corrective procedure equal or exceed the risk of an initial corrective operation. Furthermore, a definitive operation performed when the patient develops unmanageable symptoms has important psychologic, sociologic, and economic benefits for the parents and family and spares the patient the risks of serious complications during the interval between the palliative and corrective procedures. Palliative operations are therefore recommended principally for patients for whom no corrective operation exists.

C. Intraoperative Care: At present, halothane, ketamine, and intravenous morphine are most commonly used for anesthesia during cardiac operations in newborns, older infants, and children. ECG, arterial blood pressure, pulse, and rectal and nasopharyngeal temperatures are monitored continuously. In premature infants and newborns, the radial artery is catheterized; in older infants, a catheter is inserted into the femoral or brachial artery by the Seldinger technic which does not obstruct the vessel after the catheter is withdrawn. A venous catheter and one additional intravenous line are inserted for administration of blood, fluids, and drugs. During open heart surgery, central venous pressure is monitored constantly and arterial pH, PO_2, and PCO_2 are measured intermittently. Serum potassium and hematocrit are measured during and after cardiopulmonary bypass. A defibrillator, blood, sodium bicarbonate, isoproterenol, epinephrine, calcium, lidocaine, heparin, and protamine sulfate should be available in the operating room. Blood replacement and administration of fluids must be carefully controlled, particularly in very small patients. A sterile needle connected to a pressure transducer and recorder is useful for measuring particular vessel or chamber pressures during operation. Before closing the wound, the surgeon may elect to leave small polyvinyl catheters in the right or left atria (or both) and the pulmonary artery for use during the early postoperative period.

D. Postoperative Care: Operation for congenital heart disease requires careful postoperative nursing care and observation. This is best carried out in an intensive care unit where specially trained nurses and doctors and monitoring and resuscitative equipment are constantly available. In the early postoperative period, cardiac output, ventilation, and fluid and electrolyte balances require particular attention. The management program is designed to detect abnormalities early, before irreversible damage occurs, and to support organs and organ systems that have reduced or marginal function.

Upon arrival of the patient in the intensive care unit, several monitors are connected to the patient and blood is sent for laboratory examination. The ECG and the arterial blood pressure are continuously displayed on an oscilloscope. Central venous pressure and, usually, left atrial pressure are measured frequently. Temperature, pulse rate, arterial blood pressure, central venous pressure, left atrial pressure, and the respiratory rate are charted every 15–60 minutes. A portable chest x-ray and a 12-lead ECG are taken. Arterial blood is analyzed for pH, PO_2 and PCO_2. The hematocrit and serum electrolytes (including calcium and magnesium) are measured.

1. Blood and fluid balance—Blood losses are carefully measured and replaced with filtered, fresh heparinized blood. If blood loss has been excessive, a protamine titration test is done and blood is sent to the laboratory for platelet count, partial thromboplastin time, prothrombin time, fibrinogen concentration, and detection of fibrin split products.

In infants and children, bladder catheters are not used. Urine is collected in adhesive plastic bags and diapers are weighed. Intravenous fluids and flush solutions are carefully measured and recorded.

In infants, intravenous and intra-arterial fluids are best administered by a precision pump. Drug dosages are calculated and measured carefully and are usually given intravenously early after operation. The stomach is aspirated periodically of air and fluid. Oral feedings are started as soon as peristalsis returns.

2. Cardiac output—Special attention is required to evaluate and maintain an adequate cardiac output early after operation. Cardiac output is a function of heart rate and ventricular stroke volume. Arrhythmias reduce ventricular filling, and bradycardia (less than 60) or rapid tachycardia (over 180) reduce cardiac output. Arrhythmias require prompt treatment with appropriate drugs, electrical pacing wires, and, occasionally, electrical defibrillation. The amount of blood ejected with each beat is affected by the volume of blood within the heart during diastole (end-diastolic volume), the force of the myocardial contraction, and the resistance to the forward progress of blood (afterload). Within limits, expansion of the blood volume and elevation of atrial pressures increase ventricular end-diastolic volume. A variety of drugs (including digoxin, catecholamines, and calcium) and pathologic states (hypoxia, acidosis, hypercapnia) alter the contractility of myocardial sarcomeres. Postoperatively, ventricular afterloads are usually not manipulated, but occasionally a peripheral vasodilator is used temporarily to reduce systemic blood pressure. The ECG, atrial pressures, arterial pressure, peripheral pulses, urine output, arterial pH (and PCO_2), and a subjective impression of the adequacy of the circulation in the distal extremities form the basis of the clinical evaluation of cardiac output.

3. Respiratory care—The objectives of postoperative respiratory care are to maintain pulmonary gas transfer and to prevent pulmonary complications. After operation, the soft polyvinyl endotracheal tube is not removed but is connected to a system of continuous positive airway pressure (CPAP). This system provides positive airway pressure throughout the respiratory cycle and reduces the likelihood that individual alveoli will collapse at end-expiration. Arterial P_{O_2}, P_{CO_2}, and pH are measured frequently, and these values determine stepwise changes in the inspired oxygen concentration and the amount of positive airway pressure. The patient is constantly observed for clinical signs of excessive respiratory work or obstruction of the endotracheal tube or major airway: flaring nares, subcostal retraction, restlessness, asymmetric chest expansion, bradycardia, cyanosis, or inability to pass the tip of the aspirating catheter beyond the tip of the endotracheal tube. Occasionally, a patient will not breathe spontaneously and will require mechanical ventilation with positive end-expiratory pressure temporarily.

Outward transport of mucus is extremely important in the prevention of airway obstruction and pulmonary infection. Inspired gases are warmed and humidified, and the patient's position is changed each hour. Chest physical therapy, hyperinflation of the lungs, and instillation of small amounts of 0.9% saline solution into the endotracheal tube aid mucus transport. Aspiration of the endotracheal tube is performed frequently with sterile catheters and gloves. Suspicious mucus is examined by stained smear and culture, and appropriate antibiotics are given if organisms are found.

Extubation is not performed until the patient's cardiac output is adequate and circulatory dynamics are stable. Arterial blood gases must be in the normal range when the inspired oxygen concentration is 0.4 or less. After extubation, the patient is carefully observed for evidence of respiratory insufficiency or hypoventilation. Arterial blood gases are measured every 2–4 hours, and the patient is reintubated if P_{O_2} falls below 50 mm Hg or if severe respiratory acidosis develops. Chest physical therapy, encouragement of cough, and gentle oropharyngeal aspiration are continued until respiratory function is clearly adequate.

4. Prevention of complications—Careful observation and monitoring are necessary to prevent postsurgical complications. The most frequently observed respiratory complications are hypoventilation, hypoxia due to airway obstruction, pulmonary edema, pneumothorax (in infants), aspiration of stomach contents, and pneumonia.

Arrhythmias, hypovolemia, hypervolemia, and low cardiac output, pericardial tamponade, and continuing blood losses are the most common postoperative circulatory problems.

Relatively infrequent complications include oliguria, anuria, severe electrolyte imbalance, jaundice, wound infection, seizures, coma, and CNS deficits.

Campbell M: The causes of malformations of the heart. Chap 6, pp 84–88 in: *Paediatric Cardiology*. Watson H (editor). Mosby, 1968.

Gregory GA: Respiratory care of newborn infants. P Clin North America 19:311–324, 1972.

Hoffman JIE: Natural history of congenital heart disease: Problems of its assessment with special reference to ventricular septal defects. Circulation 37:97–125, 1968.

Kidd BSL, Keith JD (editors): *The Natural History and Progress in Treatment of Congenital Heart Defects*. Thomas, 1971.

Rudolph AM: The changes in the circulation after birth: Their importance in congenital heart disease. Circulation 41: 343–359, 1970.

I. OBSTRUCTIVE CONGENITAL HEART LESIONS

Obstructive lesions impede the forward flow of blood, increase ventricular afterloads, and cause turbulence within the vascular system. The impedance of the obstructive lesion is inversely proportionate to the cross-sectional area or squared diameter of the lumen. A 60% reduction in cross-sectional area causes a small pressure difference across the lesion during peak systole. Further obstruction causes progressively higher pressure differences which vary in proportion to changes in blood flow velocity during the cardiac cycle. Turbulence and cavitation develop when the degree of obstruction and velocity of flow exceed critical values.

In the absence of a ventricular septal defect, an obstructive lesion at the aortic or pulmonary valve initially causes the proximal ventricle to hypertrophy. Progressive hypertrophy compensates for the increased systolic pressure and ventricular work required to maintain forward flow but eventually may cause the heart to become "muscle-bound." Severe ventricular hypertrophy reduces diastolic filling volume, ventricular wall compliance, and the contractile force of myocardial sarcomeres. Under certain physiologic conditions, subendocardial areas of the hypertrophied muscle may become ischemic. Eventually, the ventricle fails when the systolic pressure required to maintain adequate forward flow exceeds that which the ventricle can produce. Ventricular end-diastolic volume and pressure increase, ventricular stroke volume decreases, and blood accumulates in the atrium and veins upstream to the decompensated ventricle.

The most common congenital obstructive lesions of the heart and great vessels are aortic and pulmonary valvular stenosis and coarctation of the aorta. Tricuspid atresia and pulmonary atresia are discussed below in the section on lesions that decrease pulmonary blood flow. Congenital mitral stenosis and cor triatriatum are rare lesions which produce pulmonary venous hypertension; these lesions are included in this section.

PULMONARY STENOSIS

Essentials of Diagnosis

- No symptoms in patients with mild or moderately severe lesions.
- Cyanosis and right-sided heart failure in patients (usually infants) with severe lesions.
- High-pitched systolic ejection murmur that is maximal in the second left interspace. S_2 delayed and soft. Ejection click often present. Increased right ventricular impulse.
- No ejection click and inaudible S_2 in severe cases.

General Considerations

Pulmonary stenosis with intact ventricular septum is a relatively common congenital heart lesion (Table 23–2) that affects boys and girls with equal frequency. There are 2 main types: valvular and infundibular (Fig 23–9).

Valvular pulmonary stenosis occurs in approximately 95% of patients. In most patients, the commissures of a flexible tricuspid semilunar valve fuse to produce a dome-like structure with a central opening of varying size (Fig 23–9A). Rarely, the valve is bicuspid, severely malformed, or associated with a hypoplastic pulmonary annulus. Infundibular stenosis associated with a normal pulmonary valve occurs infrequently and is most often caused by a distinct fibrous or muscular band in the outflow tract of the right ventricle below the pulmonary valve (Fig 23–9B). More often, hypertrophy of the right ventricular musculature narrows the infundibulum upstream to valvular pulmonary stenosis.

Most patients with pulmonary stenosis have a patent foramen ovale; a few have a true atrial septal defect. Turbulence produced by blood passing through the narrowed valvular orifice at high velocity causes poststenotic dilatation of the main pulmonary artery. As the child grows, the stenotic orifice sometimes fails to enlarge proportionately, and right ventricular pressure increases disproportionately to the increase in resting cardiac output.

In infants, severe valvular pulmonary stenosis may be associated with underdevelopment of the right ventricle.

Clinical Findings

A. Symptoms and Signs: Most children with pulmonary stenosis and an intact ventricular septum have no symptoms and grow and develop normally. A few complain of fatigue and dyspnea on exertion. Patients with very severe pulmonary stenosis may have anterior chest pain (angina), dizziness, and episodic dyspnea. These patients occasionally die suddenly. Patients with less severe obstruction who develop right ventricular failure often develop slight cyanosis. Infants with severe pulmonary stenosis feed poorly, are often lethargic, and occasionally have hypoxic spells.

Pulmonary stenosis causes a high-pitched systolic

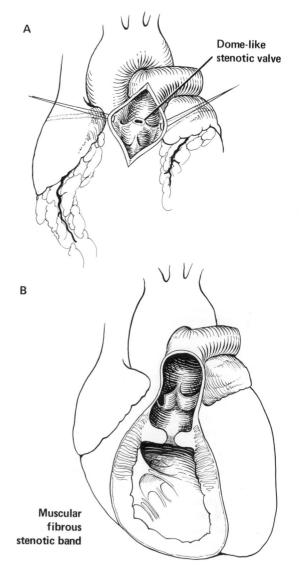

FIG 23–9. Pulmonary stenosis. *A:* Valvular pulmonary stenosis. *B:* Infundibular pulmonary stenosis.

ejection murmur which is maximal in the second left anterior interspace and widely transmitted. An ejection click is frequently present but may not be audible in patients with severe stenosis. The pulmonary second sound is delayed and is usually soft. The right ventricular impulse is usually increased.

In early infancy, severe pulmonary stenosis may cause right ventricular failure and cyanosis from right-to-left shunting of blood through a patent foramen ovale. These infants have a systolic ejection murmur (which may be less intense than that found in older children), hepatomegaly, cardiomegaly, cyanosis, and poor peripheral perfusion.

B. X-Ray Findings: Most children have abnormal chest roentgenograms. Dilatation of the main pulmonary artery and enlargement of the right ventricle, atrium, or entire heart are the most common findings. The degree of cardiac enlargement is not always proportionate to the severity of the right ventricular hypertension. The aortic arch is on the left. In infants with right-to-left shunting, pulmonary vascular markings may be reduced.

C. Electrocardiography: ECGs indicate right atrial and ventricular hypertrophy, and with few exceptions the changes are proportionate to the severity of the obstructive lesion and the pressure in the right ventricle. In neonates, the ECG may show left ventricular or biventricular hypertrophy.

D. Cardiac Catheterization and Cineangiocardiography: Cardiac catheterization reveals the magnitude of the right ventricular pressure, which may exceed left ventricular pressure, and the site of the obstruction. Cineangiocardiograms demonstrate severe malformations, hypoplastic annuli, secondary infundibular muscular hypertrophy, and other lesions.

Differential Diagnosis

In children, pulmonary stenosis must be differentiated from aortic stenosis, small ventricular septal defect, and tetralogy of Fallot. In neonates, severe pulmonary stenosis must be distinguished from aortic stenosis, pulmonary atresia, tricuspid atresia, tetralogy of Fallot, and hypoplastic right ventricle.

Natural History

Approximately half of deaths due to pulmonary stenosis occur in infants under 1 year of age. The remainder occur in asymptomatic children or adults who develop severe right ventricular hypertension and reduced cardiac output. The frequency with which moderate pulmonary stenosis progresses to severe pulmonary stenosis is not known. Available evidence suggests that progressive stenosis, severe right ventricular hypertension, and failure rarely develop in patients with differential pressures below 50–60 mm Hg.

Treatment

Infants who have severe right ventricular failure or hypoxic spells require urgent operation. Cardiac catheterization and angiographic studies are necessary to exclude other lesions such as pulmonary atresia or hypoplastic right ventricle. Valvotomy may be performed by either of 2 methods. The preferred method permits incision of the fused leaflets under direct vision while the venous return (both vena cavas) to the heart is interrupted for 2 or 3 minutes at 37 C (inflow occlusion). Less frequently, a valvulotome (a spear-like instrument) is introduced through the right ventricle of the beating heart and guided through the stenotic pulmonary valve (Brock procedure). After blind incision of the fused leaflets, a dilator is used to open the orifice further. Infants with associated underdevelopment of the right ventricle require a systemic-pulmonary arterial anastomosis in addition to the pulmonary valvotomy.

Operation is generally recommended for children or adults who have a pressure difference of 60 mm Hg or more across the pulmonary valve. Temporary cardiopulmonary bypass is used. The stenotic valve is exposed through a pulmonary arteriotomy. Every effort is made to completely relieve the obstruction without causing pulmonary regurgitation, but a small amount of regurgitation is preferable to incomplete relief of the stenosis. The infundibulum is palpated through the opened pulmonary valve to detect the presence of a localized muscular or fibrotic obstruction. Most surgeons do not perform right ventriculotomy and infundibular resection to remove secondarily hypertrophied infundibular muscle. With rare exceptions, hypertrophied infundibular muscle regresses after valvular or localized infundibular obstruction is adequately removed. Occasional patients who have a hypoplastic pulmonary annulus require a pericardial patch across the annulus. At operation, the atrial septum should be explored to close possible atrial septal defects or a patent foramen ovale.

Prognosis After Surgery

The hospital mortality rate following operations for relief of pulmonary stenosis in children and adults is 2–3%. Patients with severe stenosis who do not have resection of secondarily hypertrophied infundibular muscle often have right ventricular hypertension at the operating table and for weeks or months postoperatively; this regresses, but it may cause some degree of right ventricular failure postoperatively. Serious operative complications include neurologic injuries, hemorrhage, wound infection, postpericardiotomy syndrome, transient arrhythmias, and respiratory problems.

In over 90% of patients, operation relieves symptoms and results in regression of ECG and x-ray abnormalities. Most patients have postoperative systolic murmurs and often diastolic murmurs which were not present preoperatively. Only 10% of patients have significant residual abnormalities.

Gilbert JW, Morrow AG, Talbert JL: The surgical significance of hypertrophic infundibular obstruction accompanying valvular pulmonic stenosis. J Thoracic Cardiovas Surg 46:457–467, 1963.

Mustard WT, Jain SC, Trusler GA: Pulmonic stenosis in the first year of life. Brit Heart J 30:255–257, 1968.

Nadas AS: Pulmonic stenosis: Indications for surgery in children and adults. New England J Med 287:1196–1197, 1972.

Tandon R, Nadas AS, Gross RE: Results of open-heart surgery in patients with pulmonic stenosis and intact ventricular septum. Circulation 31:190–201, 1965.

AORTIC STENOSIS

Four types of congenital aortic stenosis are generally recognized (Fig 23–10). Valvular aortic stenosis is the most common; subaortic and supravalvular aortic stenosis and idiopathic hypertrophic subaortic stenosis occur infrequently.

1. VALVULAR AORTIC STENOSIS

Essentials of Diagnosis

- Usually asymptomatic in children; angina and syncope indicate severe stenosis.
- May cause severe heart failure in infants.
- Prominent left ventricular impulse, narrow pulse pressure.
- Harsh systolic murmur and thrill along left sternal border.
- Systolic ejection click.

General Considerations

Valvular aortic stenosis occurs predominantly in males. In about 20% of patients, the lesion is associated with other congenital heart defects (endocardial fibroelastosis, patent ductus arteriosus, coarctation of the aorta, ventricular septal defect, and pulmonary stenosis). The aortic leaflets are thickened, fibrotic, and malformed. All 3 commissures may be fused, but more often one commissure is absent or poorly formed, so that the aortic valve is bicuspid. Stenosis results if the remaining commissures are fused or if the leaflet tissue becomes stiff and calcified in adult life. Calcification of the valve does not occur in childhood, but post-stenotic dilatation of the ascending aorta may occur. Occasionally, hypoplasia of the aortic annulus, absence of 2 commissures, or aortic regurgitation may be associated with valvular aortic stenosis.

Clinical Findings

A. Symptoms and Signs: Many individuals have bicuspid aortic valves which are not stenotic during childhood and early adult life. Most children with congenital valvular aortic stenosis are asymptomatic and

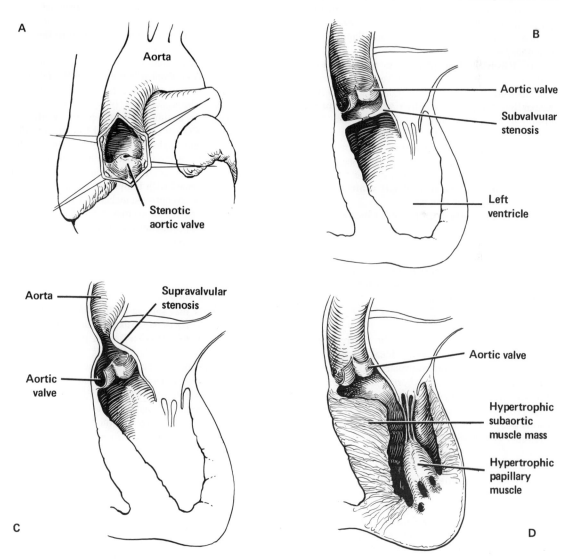

FIG 23–10. Types of congenital aortic stenosis. *A:* Valvular aortic stenosis. *B:* Subaortic stenosis (discrete fibrous band). *C:* Supravalvular aortic stenosis. *D:* Idiopathic hypertrophic subaortic stenosis.

have normal growth. A few patients with relatively severe stenosis develop dyspnea, angina, or syncope with effort. Neonates with severe aortic stenosis develop severe heart failure and cyanosis with associated feeding difficulties and respiratory distress.

A harsh, basal systolic murmur with a palpable thrill, a prominent left ventricular impulse, and a narrow pulse pressure are characteristic physical findings. The heart may not be enlarged. The murmur is usually transmitted into the neck, but in infants the murmur may not be audible because of heart failure and low cardiac output. Infants have tachypnea, hepatomegaly, cardiomegaly, cyanosis, poor peripheral perfusion, and often an increased right ventricular impulse.

B. X-Ray Findings: In children, chest x-rays are normal or show some degree of left ventricular hypertrophy. In some patients, the elevated left ventricular end-diastolic and atrial pressures cause pulmonary venous congestion. The ascending aorta may be dilated (poststenotic dilatation). Infants with severe aortic stenosis usually have dilated cardiac silhouettes and pulmonary venous congestion.

C. Electrocardiography: The vectorcardiogram correlates better with peak left ventricular pressure than does the ECG. The ECG usually shows left ventricular hypertrophy in children who have a pressure difference across the aortic valve of more than 50 mm Hg, but occasionally the ECG is normal in these patients. In infants, the ECG does not show left ventricular hypertrophy with aortic stenosis and may show right ventricular hypertrophy. The presence of symptoms or ECG evidence of left ventricular strain indicates severe aortic stenosis.

D. Cardiac Catheterization and Cineangiocardiography: With patience, a catheter can usually be passed retrograde through the stenotic aortic valve into the left ventricle. These studies are necessary to confirm the diagnosis, to differentiate valvular stenosis from other types, to measure pressure differences, and to identify associated lesions.

Differential Diagnosis

Valvular aortic stenosis must be differentiated by cardiac catheterization and cineangiocardiography from subvalvular and supravalvular aortic stenosis and pulmonary stenosis. In newborns, the absence of a murmur and the difficulty in detecting cyanosis may cause confusion between aortic stenosis and other lesions such as total anomalous pulmonary venous connection or double outlet right ventricle.

Natural History

Six to 10% of infants born with congenital aortic stenosis develop heart failure within the first year of life, and most of these will die without operation. Many of these infants have associated fibroelastosis. Few of the remaining patients develop heart failure until adulthood. All patients are susceptible to bacterial endocarditis of the deformed valve.

Sudden death occurs in 1–7% of children who have congenital aortic stenosis. Most of these children

develop symptoms before death. About 20% of patients with congenital aortic stenosis develop some degree of aortic valvular regurgitation. Patients with bicuspid aortic valves and minimal aortic stenosis may develop symptomatic aortic stenosis after their fifth decade from fibrosis and calcification of the abnormal valve.

Treatment

Infants who develop severe heart failure which cannot be controlled with digoxin and diuretics require urgent operation. Although excellent results have been obtained with inflow occlusion for approximately 10 minutes at 2 atmospheres of oxygen, most surgeons utilize temporary cardiopulmonary bypass. Commissures of the stenotic valve are incised to relieve the obstruction caused by the thickened abnormal valve. Undeveloped commissures cannot be cut because unsupported leaflets will prolapse to produce aortic regurgitation, which is poorly tolerated. Successful relief of the obstruction is directly related to the structural pathology of the valve.

Asymptomatic children with congenital aortic stenosis should refrain from severe exercise. Most of these children do not require operation until after 8–10 years of age. The appearance of symptoms (particularly syncope or angina) or signs of left ventricular strain on the ECG indicates the need for cardiac catheterization and cineangiocardiography. Patients with a systolic pressure difference of over 50 mm Hg at rest are candidates for aortic valvotomy. Operation is uniformly performed with temporary cardiopulmonary bypass. With few exceptions, incision of fused commissures results in partial or complete relief of the aortic stenosis without producing severe aortic regurgitation. Rarely, a prosthesis must be inserted for a badly deformed or torn valve or for associated hypoplasia of the aortic annulus.

Prognosis After Surgery

Valvotomy may salvage up to 80% of infants with isolated valvular aortic stenosis who develop failure in the first year of life. However, most infants have associated lesions such as fibroelastosis, mitral valve disease, or aortic coarctation, and in these the mortality rate is much higher. During childhood, the mortality rate of aortic valvotomy is less than 5%. Since the valve leaflets are deformed, many, if not all, will require reoperation and probably prosthetic replacement of the aortic valve in adult life.

Braunwald E & others: Congenital aortic stenosis: Clinical and hemodynamic findings in 100 patients. Circulation 27:426–462, 1963.

Coran AG, Bernhard WF: The surgical management of valvular aortic stenosis during infancy. J Thoracic Cardiovas Surg 58:401–408, 1969.

Fisher RD, Mason DT, Morrow AG: Results of operative treatment in congenital aortic stenosis. J Thoracic Cardiovas Surg 59:218–224, 1970.

2. SUBAORTIC STENOSIS

A discrete muscular or fibrous membrane or a diffusely narrowed segment of the left ventricular outflow tract (Fig 23–10B) causes a pressure difference between the body of the left ventricle and the aortic valve. The lesion seldom causes symptoms in infants, but in children the symptoms and findings are similar to those in patients with valvular aortic stenosis. The majority of patients with subvalvular aortic stenosis have both systolic and diastolic basal murmurs and frequently have additional cardiac defects. Turbulence in the left ventricular outflow tract often causes thickening of the normal aortic leaflets and poststenotic dilatation of the ascending aorta. Occasionally, valvular and subvalvular aortic stenosis may occur simultaneously. The diffuse or tunnel type of subvalvular aortic stenosis is sometimes associated with anomalous insertion of the anterior leaflet of the mitral valve. At cardiac catheterization, a pressure difference is found as the catheter is withdrawn from the body of the left ventricle to the ascending aorta. Cineangiocardiograms and the absence of pressure changes after administration of isoproterenol differentiate subaortic stenosis from valvular aortic stenosis and idiopathic hypertrophic subaortic stenosis.

Approximately two-thirds of patients have a discrete subvalvular fibrous or muscular membrane which is attached to the lateral edges of the anterior leaflet of the mitral valve and ventricular septum. This membrane is excised during temporary cardiopulmonary bypass after the aorta has been opened and the normal aortic leaflets have been retracted. Excision of the tunnel type of subvalvular aortic stenosis is more difficult. Occasionally, the left ventricle must be opened to excise obstructive tissue deep within the ventricular cavity, and sometimes the mitral valve must be excised and replaced. In patients with discrete subvalvular aortic stenosis, the operative mortality rate is less than 5%, the pressure difference is relieved, and the lesion does not recur. The operative mortality rate is considerably higher in patients with the tunnel type of subaortic stenosis, and some of the survivors do not get satisfactory relief of the obstruction.

Reis RL & others: Congenital fixed subvalvular aortic stenosis. Circulation 43 (Suppl 1):11–18, 1971.

3. SUPRAVALVULAR AORTIC STENOSIS

In most patients, supravalvular aortic stenosis is an isolated lesion and is not associated with mental retardation or genetic factors. The sexes are affected with equal frequency. Occasional patients have familial supravalvular aortic stenosis which occurs as an isolated lesion or in association with peripheral pulmonary arterial stenoses. Mental retardation, "elfin facies," strabismus, dental anomalies, inguinal hernia, and narrowing of peripheral systemic and pulmonary arteries occur in approximately 20% of patients with supravalvular aortic stenosis. Hypercalcemia in early infancy has been found in many of these patients.

The aorta usually has an hourglass deformity just above the aortic valve (Fig 23–10C); less commonly, the lesion is caused by a localized fibrotic membrane or hypoplasia of the ascending aorta. Symptoms and physical findings are similar to those of valvular aortic stenosis with the exception that the aortic second sound may be accentuated. The diagnosis is confirmed by cardiac catheterization and cineangiocardiography.

Localized fibrotic membranes and discrete hourglass deformities can be alleviated by insertion of a prosthetic patch in the ascending aorta. Hypoplasia of the ascending aorta cannot be corrected by operation. Asymptomatic patients who have pressure gradients less than 70 mm Hg at rest are not candidates for operation.

Rastelli GC & others: Surgical treatment of supravalvular aortic stenosis. J Thoracic Cardiovas Surg 51:873–882, 1966.

4. IDIOPATHIC HYPERTROPHIC SUBAORTIC STENOSIS (IHSS)

Muscular hypertrophy of the ventricular septum in the left ventricular outflow tract (Fig 23–10D) causes obstruction during systole. The severity of the obstruction increases throughout systole and is proportionate to the volume of the left ventricular cavity, the force of ventricular contraction, and the cross-sectional area of the left ventricular outflow tract during systole. Exercise, digitalis, isoproterenol, epinephrine, and nitroglycerin alter these dynamic relationships and generally increase the pressure difference across the obstructive area. During the normal systole which follows the premature ventricular beat, arterial pulse pressure decreases in patients with IHSS and increases in patients with valvular aortic stenosis. The hypertrophied muscle occasionally obstructs the right ventricular outflow tract as well as the left and may interfere with the function of the mitral valve. The cause of the progressive muscular hypertrophy is not known, and the histologic structure of the muscle fibers is not distinctive. The disease may be congenital or acquired and, in a few families, has been transmitted as an autosomal dominant trait.

A basal systolic murmur which was not previously present may be the first clinical sign of IHSS. The most common symptoms are fatigue, syncope, angina, and dyspnea on exertion. Variable physical findings include prominent left ventricular impulse, a basal systolic murmur with thrill, and a bifid carotid arterial pulse. Many patients have no physical signs or symptoms in childhood, but others develop the murmur in the first decade of life.

The left ventricle is usually enlarged on chest roentgenograms. The ECG is always abnormal; conduction disturbances, left axis deviation, and left ventricular hypertrophy are the most common findings. During cardiac catheterization, the diagnosis can be established by finding characteristic pressure changes in response to premature ventricular contraction and infusion of isoproterenol. Lateral cineangiocardiograms demonstrate systolic narrowing of the left ventricular outflow tract opposite the mitral valve.

The natural history of the disease is variable, but the disease tends to be progressive. Sudden death occurs, and most patients do not reach their fifth decade. Propranolol, a beta-adrenergic blocking agent, has alleviated symptoms in some patients but does not reverse the progressive hypertrophy. Symptomatic patients must not be given digitalis, isoproterenol, or nitroglycerin.

Operation requires temporary cardiopulmonary bypass. The abnormal hypertrophied muscle is widely excised. The operation is preferably done through an aortotomy, but a left ventriculotomy is sometimes necessary. Occasionally, the subvalvular mechanism of the mitral valve contributes to the left ventricular obstruction, and the mitral valve must be replaced.

The operative mortality rate is less than 10%. Complications include residual stenosis and iatrogenic heart block, ventricular septal defect, or mitral regurgitation. The duration of symptomatic benefit is uncertain, and in some cases is disappointingly short.

Braunwald E & others: Idiopathic hypertrophic subaortic stenosis. I. A description of the disease based upon an analysis of 64 patients. Circulation 30 (Suppl 4):3–119, 1964.
Kelly DT, Barratt-Boyes BG, Lowe JB: Results of surgery and hemodynamic observations in muscular subaortic stenosis. J Thoracic Cardiovas Surg 51:353–365, 1966.

COARCTATION OF THE AORTA

Essentials of Diagnosis

- Infants may have severe heart failure; children are usually asymptomatic.
- Absent or weak femoral pulses.
- Systolic pressure higher in upper extremities than in lower extremities; diastolic pressures are similar.
- Harsh systolic murmur heard in the back.

General Considerations

Coarctation or stenosis of the aorta is a relatively common congenital heart lesion (Table 23–2) that occurs twice as frequently in males as in females. Ninety-eight percent of all aortic coarctations are located at or near the aortic isthmus (the segment of aorta adjacent to the ligamentum arteriosum or ductus arteriosus). Rarely, coarctation may occur in other aortic locations or in multiple sites. In over 50% of patients, the aortic valve is bicuspid.

Patients with coarctation of the aorta are divided into 2 relatively distinct groups by the clinical course of the disease during the first year after birth. Associated lesions are present in about 90% of infants that develop heart failure during the first year. About two-thirds of these infants have patent ductus arteriosus, and in the majority the aortic constriction is upstream to the ductus or ligamentum arteriosum. Tubular hypoplasia of the aortic arch, anomalous origin of the right subclavian artery, ventricular and atrial septal defects, left ventricular outflow obstructions, fibroelastosis, transposition of the great arteries, and double outlet right ventricle (Taussig-Bing type) are the most frequently encountered associated lesions.

The majority of patients with coarctation of the aorta do not develop life-threatening symptoms during infancy. With the exception of bicuspid aortic valves and patent ductus arteriosus, associated lesions are not common. The aortic constriction is usually well localized and produced by both external narrowing and an intraluminal diaphragm. In nearly half of patients with coarctation, the internal diameter of the constricted segment is between 0.5 mm and 5 mm. About one-fourth are larger, and another fourth are atretic. In older children, the aortic wall upstream to the fibrous diaphragm develops intimal thickening and atheroma formation. Downstream, the aorta usually dilates and may have a plaque of intimal thickening where the jet of blood passing through the coarctation hits the aortic wall. In older children and adults, the aorta downstream to the coarctation becomes thin, friable, and eventually calcified. In these patients, intercostal arteries frequently become aneurysmal.

Coarctation causes systolic and diastolic hypertension in the proximal aorta and upper extremities and stimulates the enlargement of collateral vessels that connect branches of the subclavian arteries to arteries that originate from the aorta downstream to the coarctation. In most patients, blood flow to the lower body is not reduced, but pulse pressure downstream to the aortic coarctation is decreased and peak systolic pressure is delayed after peak pressure in the upstream aorta. Left ventricular work is increased.

The pathophysiology of the proximal hypertension is not understood. In some infants that have poorly developed collateral vessels, blood flow to the lower body is reduced, but even in these patients the presence of the coarcted segment does not explain the magnitude of the proximal hypertension. Most patients with aortic coarctation have normal plasma angiotensin concentrations and normal renal blood flow and function. The role of aortic and carotid baroreceptors in the autonomic nervous system in the development and maintenance of proximal hypertension is not known.

Clinical Findings

A. **Symptoms and Signs**: Most children with aortic coarctation are asymptomatic and well developed. Occasionally, children complain of headaches, fatigue, pains in the calves when running, or frequent nosebleeds. The disease is usually detected during routine physical examination by detecting weak or absent femoral pulses, measuring elevated arm blood pressures, or auscultating a harsh systolic murmur along the left sternal border and in the back. The femoral pulse, if palpable, is delayed as compared to the radial pulse. In the upper extremities, systolic blood pressure is 20 mm Hg or more higher than that in the lower extremities, but diastolic pressures are similar. A systolic murmur with thrill in the suprasternal notch is usually present; occasionally, the murmur is continuous. If collateral vessels are well developed, flow murmurs may be heard in the axillas, medial to the scapulas, and over the lateral ribs. A few patients have apical systolic murmurs from mitral regurgitation or precordial systolic murmurs from aortic stenosis.

Most symptomatic infants with coarctation develop severe heart failure within the first 6 weeks after birth. Signs include tachypnea, dyspnea, respiratory distress, pulmonary rales, hepatomegaly, poor feeding, poor weight gain, and poor peripheral perfusion. The heart is enlarged and usually has a gallop rhythm. Murmurs are generally not diagnostic because of associated lesions. Femoral pulses are generally weak or absent, but the amplitude may vary at different observations. Infrequently, right-to-left shunting through a patent ductus arteriosus that is downstream to the coarctation causes cyanosis of the lower body.

B. X-Ray Findings: Chest x-rays usually show left ventricular enlargement with or without notching of ribs between T3 and T8 in children with coarctation. Occasionally, the aorta bulges proximal and distal to the coarcted segment to produce a 3 sign in the plain chest film. The reverse, or E sign, is seen in the barium-filled esophagus.

The heart is greatly enlarged in symptomatic infants, and the peripheral lung fields appear congested. Rib notching is not present, and the contour of the descending thoracic aorta is usually obscured by the thymus gland.

C. Electrocardiography: The ECG shows left ventricular hypertrophy which is proportionate to the severity of the coarctation and proximal hypertension in children. In infants, particularly those less than 6 months of age, the ECG shows an abnormal increase in right ventricular hypertrophy with or without left ventricular hypertrophy. Isolated left ventricular hypertrophy is rare in infants with aortic coarctation.

D. Cardiac Catheterization and Cineangiocardiography: In children, cardiac catheterization is often not performed if clinical findings are diagnostic of coarctation. However, in atypical cases, cardiac catheterization and cineangiocardiography document the pressure difference across the coarctation, illustrate the local anatomy and the adequacy of collateral vessels, and often are diagnostic of an associated bicuspid aortic valve. In symptomatic infants, cardiac catheterization and cineangiocardiography are necessary to demonstrate the length of the coarcted segment and to define associated intracardiac and extracardiac lesions. Left ventricular end-diastolic pressures are always

greatly elevated in these patients. Pulmonary venous blood is often partially unsaturated because of associated respiratory problems.

Differential Diagnosis

Clinical signs, particularly proximal hypertension and reduced, delayed femoral pulses, establish the diagnosis of coarctation in children. In symptomatic infants, the differential diagnosis must include other diseases which cause severe heart failure, particularly aortic stenosis, interrupted aortic arch, hypoplastic left heart, and fibroelastosis.

Natural History

Children that survive infancy rarely die before their second decade; however, the mean age at death in these patients is about 40 years. Patients die of congestive heart failure, cerebral hemorrhage or thrombosis, ruptured intercostal arterial aneurysms, or dissecting aneurysms of the ascending aorta. Pregnant women with coarctation are more susceptible to complications. Since the advent of antibiotics, bacterial infections of the coarcted segment or bicuspid aortic valve are rare causes of death.

In symptomatic infants, congestive heart failure is the most common cause of death. Cerebral hemorrhage and hypertensive encephalopathy are rare causes.

Treatment

Resection of the stenotic segment of the aorta is recommended for nearly every patient with coarctation of the aorta. The optimal age for elective operation is between 4 and 8 years. In children, the elastic aorta can be brought together for a primary anastomosis in nearly all cases. Very rarely, a prosthetic graft is required to bridge the distance between the 2 ends of the aorta. If collateral vessels are poorly developed or if operation is required for restenosis of the aorta, hypothermia to 31 C, partial cardiopulmonary bypass, or a temporary shunt is recommended to protect the spinal cord from ischemic injury during cross-clamping of the aorta.

An intensive trial of medical measures (digoxin, diuretics, morphine, and oxygen) is recommended for all infants with severe heart failure associated with coarctation of the aorta. The infant often improves dramatically within a few hours, and operation can be postponed until childhood. Infants who do not respond to medical therapy within 12–24 hours require immediate operation. Although some of these infants may improve temporarily with intravenous isoproterenol, the mortality rate approaches 100%. Operation consists of resection of the aortic coarctation and division of a patent ductus arteriosus if this lesion is also present. Additional palliative procedures (eg, pulmonary arterial banding) are added depending upon specific associated intracardiac lesions.

Prognosis After Surgery

In children, operative mortality for elective resection of aortic coarctation is 1–2%. The operative mortality rate increases in adult patients who have friable, atheromatous aortas. All patients obtain some relief of the proximal hypertension, and over 80% of children eventually have normal systolic blood pressures. However, blood pressures may remain elevated immediately after operation and gradually decrease over a 6-month period.

Hemorrhage is the most frequent postoperative complication. Paraplegia or paraparesis is a rare (0.4%) but catastrophic complication and is related to the adequacy of the collateral circulation and the duration of aortic clamping during construction of the anastomosis. Necrotizing arteritis of mesenteric vessels occurs rarely, although up to one-fourth of patients develop abdominal pain 2–7 days postoperatively. Patients who have unexplained (paradoxic) hypertension after operation are more likely to have abdominal pain. These patients nearly always respond to sympatholytic drugs which reduce blood pressure and reduce the likelihood of severe necrotizing arteritis with gangrenous bowel. Injury to the left recurrent laryngeal nerve and chylothorax are infrequent complications.

The operative mortality rate is 25–50% in symptomatic infants who require resection of aortic coarctation for heart failure that is unresponsive to medical therapy. The mortality rate is lowest in the occasional infant who develops severe heart failure and does not have associated intracardiac lesions. The mortality rate increases in proportion to the severity of the associated lesions, and occasional patients with hypoplastic left hearts or severe fibroelastosis are inoperable.

Restenosis develops at the suture line in a few patients–particularly infants who require emergency operation. In children, restenosis is usually due to technical factors, the use of continuous sutures, or progressive fibrosis and scarring. Rarely, infants may develop rapid restenosis and recurrence of the symptoms of heart failure within a few weeks or months after operation. More commonly, progressive stenosis occurs, and most infants who survive resection of aortic coarctation have small systolic pressure differences across the anastomosis at follow-up cardiac catheterization during childhood. The pathogenesis of rapid or progressive restenosis is not known.

Brewer LA III & others: Spinal cord complications following surgery for coarctation of the aorta. J Thoracic Cardiovas Surg 64:368–381, 1972.

Hartmann AF Jr & others: Recurrent coarctation of the aorta after successful repair in infancy. Am J Cardiol 25:405–410, 1970.

Schuster SR, Gross RE: Surgery for coarctation of the aorta: A review of 500 cases. J Thoracic Cardiovas Surg 43:54–70, 1962.

Sinha SN & others: Coarctation of the aorta in infancy. Circulation 40:385–398, 1969.

AORTIC ATRESIA

Atresia of the aortic valve is associated with hypoplasia of the ascending aorta, hypoplasia or atresia of the left ventricle, and atresia or severe stenosis of the mitral valve. Coronary arteries arise from the base of the hypoplastic ascending aorta. A large patent ductus and an atrial septal defect are required for life, and most patients die within a few days. Systemic and pulmonary venous blood are mixed in the atria and then pumped by the right ventricle to the pulmonary arteries and systemic arteries via a patent ductus arteriosus. Aortic atresia and other variants of hypoplastic left heart are the most common causes of death from congenital heart disease in the first week of life. Infants may appear normal at birth but soon develop congestive heart failure with poor peripheral pulses and variable cyanosis. Physical, radiographic, and electrocardiographic findings are not diagnostic; cardiac catheterization and cineangiocardiography are required to establish the diagnosis and to rule out other lesions for which effective therapy exists. At present, medical management is ineffective, and operations are not usually recommended.

Cayler GG, Smeloff EA, Miller GE Jr: Surgical palliation of hypoplastic left side of the heart. New England J Med 282:780–783, 1970.

MITRAL ATRESIA & STENOSIS

In approximately 50% of patients with congenital mitral stenosis, the lesion is associated with hypoplasia of the left heart and aortic atresia. Patients who have mitral atresia with a normal aortic valve often have a hypoplastic left ventricle that communicates with the large right ventricle through a ventricular septal defect. Other anomalies–particularly of the systemic and pulmonary veins–are often present. Patients with mitral atresia with normal aortic valves seldom survive early infancy.

In congenital mitral stenosis not associated with aortic atresia, the funnel-shaped valve is thickened, with short, fused chordae tendineae and poorly defined commissures. Patients frequently have associated lesions (patent ductus arteriosus, aortic stenosis, coarctation of the aorta). The principal symptoms are dyspnea and frequent respiratory infections due to pulmonary hypertension and pulmonary congestion. An apical diastolic rumble with associated thrill is invariably present; an opening snap, loud first sound, and mitral systolic murmurs are also usually present. Chest x-rays show a dilated left atrium and increased pulmonary venous markings. In time, pulmonary vascular disease can occur if the stenosis is not relieved.

Over half of these infants die in their first year, and few survive childhood. A few mitral valves can be improved by valvuloplasty; more often, the deformed valve must be excised and replaced with a prosthesis. A few infants and young children have survived mitral valve replacement.

Tsuji HK & others: Congenital mitral stenosis. J Thoracic Cardiovas Surg 53:850–857, 1967.

COR TRIATRIATUM

In this rare anomaly, pulmonary veins enter a small accessory left atrial chamber which communicates with the normal-sized true left atrium through a small opening. Pulmonary venous hypertension causes pulmonary congestion and, eventually, increased pulmonary arterial and right ventricular pressures. Patients have severe dyspnea and frequent respiratory infections but do not have an apical diastolic rumble. An elevated pulmonary arterial or pulmonary capillary (wedge) pressure and a normal left atrial pressure at cardiac catheterization strongly suggest the diagnosis, which is proved by cineangiocardiography. Operation requires cardiopulmonary bypass and consists of excision of the obstructing membrane between the accessory chamber and the normal left atrium. Without operation, over half of patients die in infancy.

Brickman RD & others: Cor triatriatum. J Thoracic Cardiovas Surg 60:523–530, 1970.

II. CONGENITAL HEART LESIONS WHICH INCREASE PULMONARY ARTERIAL BLOOD FLOW

Approximately 50% of all congenital heart lesions shunt blood from the systemic arterial circulation into the pulmonary circulation (left-to-right shunt). The most common lesions in this group are patent ductus arteriosus and defects of the atrial septum, atrioventricular canal, and ventricular septum. Rare lesions include ruptured sinus of Valsalva, aortic-pulmonary window, truncus arteriosus, and some types of transposition of the great vessels, double outlet right ventricle, and other complex lesions.

Because compliance of the thick-walled left ventricle is less than that of the right ventricle and because systemic vascular resistance is normally about 10 times higher than pulmonary vascular resistance, pressures in the left heart chambers and systemic arteries are higher than corresponding pressures in the right heart and pulmonary arteries. These higher pressures cause some of the oxygenated blood in the left heart and systemic arteries to shunt through abnormal anatomic communications and to recirculate through the lungs without passing through systemic capillaries. The excessive pulmonary circulation causes pulmonary vascular congestion, resulting in frequent respiratory infections, and places an additional burden on the involved ventricle (the right ventricle in atrial septal defects; the left ventricle in patent ductus arteriosus; and both ventricles in atrioventricular canal and ventricular septal defects). The increased "volume load" or "preload" increases the diastolic volume of the involved ventricle. As the ventricle dilates, end-diastolic pressure increases; eventually, the ventricle may fail (ie, at the point at which an increase in ventricular volume at end-diastole no longer causes an increase in ventricular stroke volume).

In the circulation, resistance, flow, and pressure are related by the formula $R = P/F$, where R is resistance of a specified segment of the circulatory system (impedance when flow is pulsatile), P is the pressure difference across the resistance (in mm Hg), and F is the flow in liters/min/sq m. Conventionally, resistance is calculated in "Wood units" (mm Hg/liter/min/sq m). Resistances vary in different segments of the circulatory system. When no abnormal communications or shunts are present, blood passes through these resistances serially. When an abnormal communication is present, the relative downstream resistances of the normal and abnormal pathways largely determine relative blood flows in each pathway. This simplistic but useful concept is clearly illustrated in patients who have large ventricular septal defects in which the pressures in the right and left ventricles are nearly equal throughout the cardiac cycle. If we assume equal atrial pressures, the mean pressure difference across the pulmonary vascular bed is the same as that across the systemic vascular bed. Under these conditions, the ratio of pulmonary to systemic blood flow (10:1) is inversely proportionate to the ratio of the pulmonary to systemic resistance (1:10). In actual practice, the pulmonary-systemic flow ratio is less because of blood streaming within the ventricles, unequal atrial pressures, compliance of the pulmonary vasculature and ventricles, and other dynamic factors.

Because blood flow is pulsatile, pressures, flow, velocity, and impedance within the circulatory system change throughout the cardiac cycle. As indicated above, if dynamic factors are ignored by using mean pressures, flows, and resistances, the ratio of downstream resistances largely determines the ratio of net flows through normal and abnormal (shunt) pathways. Because the mean left atrial pressure is 2–3 mm Hg higher than the mean right atrial pressure, the net flow across an atrial septal defect is from left to right. However, during the cardiac cycle, phasic tracings of right and left atrial pressures show moments when right atrial pressure exceeds the simultaneous left atrial pressure. At these times, blood flows from right to left across the defect. Thus, although the net shunt is from left to right, atrial septal defects and many other shunts within the vascular system are actually bidirectional because of dynamic factors.

Increased pulmonary blood flow increases pulmo-. nary arterial blood pressure. Although pulmonary vessels are very distensible (and therefore compliant), pulmonary arterial pressure in the normal lung approximately doubles when pulmonary blood flow triples. Elevation of left atrial pressures from excessive flow—or increased left ventricular end-diastolic pressure—also increases pulmonary arterial blood pressure. These 2 mechanisms do not increase pulmonary vascular resistance. However, if pulmonary arterioles constrict in response to the increased blood flow, pulmonary vascular resistance increases (hyperkinetic pulmonary hypertension) and pulmonary arterial pressure may increase further unless flow decreases. Pulmonary vasoconstriction can be reversed by inhalation of oxygen or intravenous tolazoline, and this test is used to differentiate hyperkinetic pulmonary hypertension from pulmonary vascular disease. The elevation in pulmonary arterial pressure increases the afterload of the right ventricle, which already may have an increased "volume" or "preload" if the septal defect is in the atrium or ventricle.

In some patients, increased pulmonary blood flow and increased pulmonary arterial pressure eventually cause muscular hypertrophy of the media of pulmonary arterioles (stage 1), proliferation of intima (stage 2), and, eventually, hyalinization and fibrosis of the media and adventitia (stage 3). These morphologic changes, termed "pulmonary vascular disease," are acquired, but they are more likely to occur in congenital lesions which produce both high pulmonary arterial pressure and large flows (ventricular septal defect, complete persistent atrioventricular canal, truncus arteriosus) than in those that produce increased pulmonary blood flow only (atrial septal defect, total anomalous pulmonary venous connection). Pulmonary venous hypertension and chronic hypoxemia from residence at high altitudes also favor the development of pulmonary vascular disease. As the cross-sectional area of the pulmonary vascular bed decreases as a result of the morphologic changes, pulmonary vascular resistance increases and the ratio of pulmonary vascular resistance to systemic vascular resistance increases. The amount of blood shunted from left to right decreases. When pulmonary vascular resistance equals or exceeds systemic vascular resistance, left-to-right blood flow across the lesion ceases or reverses. Patients who have advanced pulmonary vascular disease (stage 3) and balanced or reversed shunts (Eisenmenger's syndrome) cannot be helped by operation and frequently do not survive the attempt. Often these patients live many years as they develop progressive cyanosis and polycythemia from their lesion which now shunts blood from right to left.

Pulmonary arterial banding is a palliative operation which is designed to reduce pulmonary arterial blood flow by increasing the total resistance to blood flow across the lungs (Fig 23–11). The band constricts the main pulmonary artery downstream to the valve and adds a resistance in series to the vascular resistance of the lung. Ideally, total resistance of the band and

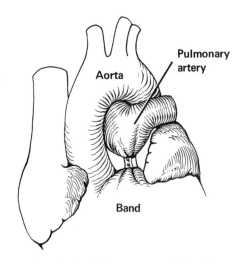

FIG 23–11. Pulmonary arterial banding.

the lungs should equal systemic vascular resistance. If vascular resistance in the lungs is already high, only a small resistance can be added by the band. Because of dynamic changes in cardiac output pressures and resistances within the circulation, addition of a fixed resistance (the band) cannot produce balanced pulmonary and systemic flows under all physiologic conditions. However, a good band can reduce pulmonary arterial blood flow sufficiently to alleviate ventricular failure and prevent rapid progression of pulmonary vascular disease. Unfortunately, preexisting pulmonary vascular disease may not regress after banding.

Congenital heart lesions which thoroughly mix systemic and pulmonary venous blood (eg, total anomalous pulmonary venous connection, single ventricle, truncus arteriosus) cause cyanosis. In these lesions, the oxygen saturation of aortic and pulmonary arterial blood may be similar, and the severity of the cyanosis is directly proportionate to the relative amounts of fully saturated pulmonary venous blood and unsaturated systemic venous blood that are mixed. If the amount of blood which flows through the lungs is 3 or more times the amount of systemic blood flow, the resulting oxygen saturation of the mixed blood will be high and cyanosis will be minimal. (For example, 3 parts oxygenated blood [20 ml O_2/100 ml] added to 1 part systemic venous blood [14 ml O_2/100 ml] saturates 92% of the hemoglobin in the mixed blood [18.5 ml O_2/100 ml].) Conversely, if an associated obstructive lesion or pulmonary vascular disease reduces the amount of pulmonary arterial blood flow in relation to systemic arterial blood flow, the mixed systemic and pulmonary venous blood will be much less saturated and cyanosis will be severe. (For example, 1 part oxygenated blood [20 ml O_2/100 ml] added to 3 parts systemic venous blood [14 ml O_2/100 ml] saturates only 77% of the hemoglobin in the mixed blood [15.5 ml O_2/100 ml].)

ATRIAL SEPTAL DEFECT, OSTIUM SECUNDUM TYPE

Essentials of Diagnosis

- Acyanotic, asymptomatic.
- Right ventricular lift.
- S_2 widely split and fixed.
- Grade 1–3/6 ejection pulmonary systolic murmur.
- Diastolic flow murmur at the lower left sternal border.

General Considerations

These defects occur in the region of the fossa ovalis. They may be single or multiple and vary in size from a few millimeters to 5 cm in diameter. Secundum defects are distinguished from (1) sinus venosus defects, which occur cephalad at the inlet of the superior vena cava into the right atrium; (2) patent foramen ovale, which is present in approximately 20% of the population; and (3) ostium primum defects, which are discussed below (Fig 23–12). In approximately 10% of patients, atrial septal defects are associated with either right hemianomalous pulmonary veins or persistent left superior vena cava.

Clinical Findings

A. Symptoms and Signs: Uncomplicated atrial septal defects seldom cause symptoms. Rarely, infants will develop heart failure, and children will become fatigued and dyspneic upon exertion more easily than normal children. Characteristic physical signs include a midsystolic ejection murmur over the upper left heart border with a loud and widely split second heart sound

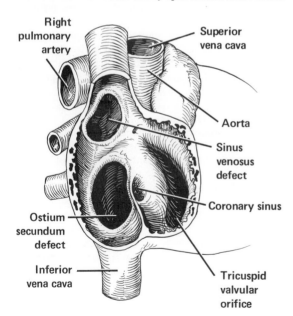

Right pulmonary artery

Superior vena cava

Aorta

Sinus venosus defect

Coronary sinus

Ostium secundum defect

Inferior vena cava

Tricuspid valvular orifice

FIG 23–12. Sinus venosus and ostium secundum defects in the atrial septum as viewed from the opened right atrium.

which does not change with respiration. The systolic murmur is due to turbulence at the pulmonary valve caused by the high-velocity ejection from the right ventricle. Fixed splitting of the second sound is an important diagnostic sign and is due to the fact that inspiration delays the sound of aortic valve closure (A_2) in patients with atrial septal defect. Thus, inspiration delays both A_2 and P_2; consequently, the interval between the 2 sounds does not change during the respiratory cycle. In patients with large left-to-right shunts (> 2:1), a soft diastolic murmur caused by blood passing through the tricuspid valve is also heard.

B. X-Ray Findings: Plain chest films reveal increased pulmonary vascularity and often an enlarged right atrium and ventricle.

C. Electrocardiography: The ECG is either normal or shows right axis deviation and right ventricular hypertrophy without conduction abnormalities.

D. Cardiac Catheterization and Cineangiocardiography: At cardiac catheterization, the catheter usually passes easily into both atria across the atrial septum. Blood samples from the right atrium and ventricle show an increase in oxygen saturation of at least 10% as compared to samples from the superior vena cava. Cineangiocardiograms after left atrial injection show simultaneous opacification of both atria.

Differential Diagnosis

Ostium secundum defects must be distinguished from common atrioventricular canal, total anomalous pulmonary venous connection, small ventricular septal defects, and left ventricular to right atrial shunts. Ostium primum defects, sinus venosus defects, and hemianomalous pulmonary veins are easily recognized and corrected at operation; preoperative recognition is not essential. In total anomalous pulmonary venous connection, blood oxygen saturation is the same in the right atrium, both ventricles, the pulmonary artery, and the aorta. Cineangiocardiograms after left ventricular injections are particularly useful for detecting small ventricular septal defects or left ventricular-right atrial shunts.

Natural History

Heart failure from uncomplicated ostium secundum defects is rare in childhood but occurs in approximately 40% of adults over 30 years of age. Pulmonary vascular disease does not occur in children but does occur in 5–10% of adults with untreated lesions. Patients who have small left-to-right shunts (< 2:1) do not require operation. Bacterial endocarditis is rare, but atrial arrhythmias may occur in adults.

Treatment

Ostium secundum defects are closed during temporary cardiopulmonary bypass. The heart is approached through a midline sternotomy or a right thoracotomy. The margins of the defect usually can be approximated by direct suture; occasionally, a patch of pericardium is necessary. Hemianomalous veins are redirected into the left atrium by shifting the atrial septum to the right of the orifices of the pulmonary veins. Sinus venosus defects are usually patched, and occasionally the entrance of the superior vena cava must be enlarged as well.

Prognosis After Operation

The mortality rate following open repair of ostium secundum defects should not be higher than 1–2%. Complications include air embolism with subsequent CNS damage, postoperative atrial arrhythmias, wound infection, and hemorrhage.

Sellers RD & others: Secundum type atrial septal defects: Results with 275 patients. Surgery 59:155–164, 1966.

Zaver AG, Nadas AS: Atrial septal defect–secundum type. Circulation 31 (Suppl 3):24–32, 1965.

ATRIAL SEPTAL DEFECT, OSTIUM PRIMUM TYPE

Essentials of Diagnosis

- Acyanotic; asymptomatic, or dyspnea on exertion.
- Fixed, widely split second sound.
- Apical systolic murmur (often).
- ECG shows left axis deviation; QRS frontal vector is counterclockwise.

General Considerations

Ostium primum defects are part of a group of lesions which occur during development of the atrioventricular canal. Ostium primum defects (occasionally called incomplete persistent atrioventricular canal) are less severe than complete atrioventricular canal defects, which involve the interventricular septum as well as the atrial septum. Ostium primum defects are located low in the atrial septum, caudad to the fossa ovalis and adjacent to the coronary sinus and the orifice of the tricuspid valve. The aortic leaflet of the mitral valve is usually cleft; occasionally, the septal leaflet of the tricuspid valve is cleft also. The septal defect is usually 2–4 cm in diameter. The incidence of ostium primum defects is approximately one-third that of ostium secundum defects.

Clinical Findings

A. Symptoms and Signs: Most children are asymptomatic or complain of dyspnea on exertion and easy fatigability. Occasional infants develop severe congestive heart failure from mitral regurgitation and a large left-to-right shunt across the ostium primum defect. Physical signs include a systolic ejection murmur which is maximal in the second left intercostal space, fixed wide splitting of the second sound, and often a systolic murmur at the apex of the heart which is transmitted to the left axilla.

B. X-Ray Findings: Plain chest films usually show cardiomegaly with increased pulmonary vasculature. Both atria and both ventricles may be enlarged.

C. Electrocardiography: The ECG is characteristically abnormal: the mean QRS axis is shifted to the left (usually 0 to −60 degrees); the P–R interval is often prolonged; and P waves are often tall. The frontal QRS loop of the vectorcardiogram is oriented superiorly and is inscribed in a counterclockwise direction. These findings are suggestive (but not pathognomonic) of an ostium primum defect or persistent atrioventricular canal.

D. Cardiac Catheterization and Cineangiocardiography: During cardiac catheterization, an increase in oxygen saturation nearly always occurs in the right atrium. Left atrial pressures may be elevated, and the v wave may be prominent. Cineangiocardiograms taken after left ventricular injection often demonstrate mitral incompetence and opacification of the atria before the right ventricle is seen. The mitral valve often appears deformed.

Differential Diagnosis

Ostium primum defects must be distinguished from more severe defects of the atrioventricular canal, ventricular septal defects, ostium secundum defects, and congenital mitral valvular regurgitation. The ECG, vectorcardiogram, and cineangiocardiographic findings are particularly important in the differential diagnosis.

Natural History

Ostium primum defects with associated severe mitral regurgitation or tricuspid regurgitation may cause heart failure in infancy and childhood. Bacterial endocarditis is rare, and pulmonary vascular disease generally does not develop until adult life.

Treatment

Ostium primum defects in children are repaired through a median sternotomy using cardiopulmonary bypass. When mitral regurgitation is present, the cleft in the mitral valve is approximated with interrupted sutures in such a way as to correct regurgitation without narrowing the mitral valvular annulus. The primum defect is closed with a pericardial patch.

Prognosis After Operation

The mortality rate of repair of ostium primum defects in children is approximately 3%. Aside from air embolism, the most important operative complication is complete heart block due to ligature of the conduction bundle during repair of the primum defect.

Many patients have a residual apical systolic murmur after operation, but mitral regurgitation is usually trivial.

Braunwald NS, Morrow AG: Incomplete persistent atrioventricular canal. J Thoracic Cardiovas Surg 51:71–80, 1966.

Gerbode F & others: Endocardial cushion defects. Ann Surg 166:486–495, 1967.

COMPLETE PERSISTENT ATRIOVENTRICULAR CANAL

Essentials of Diagnosis

- Heart failure common in infancy.
- Cardiomegaly, blowing pansystolic murmur, other variable murmurs.
- Loud S_2 with fixed splitting.
- ECG shows left axis deviation and counterclockwise frontal QRS vector loop.

General Considerations

Maldevelopment of the atrioventricular canal may result in a common defect of both the ventricular and atrial septa and a common atrioventricular valve or severely deformed mitral and tricuspid valves (Fig 23–13). Many gradations of the deformity (also called complete endocardial cushion defect) exist. About a third of these patients have additional cardiovascular anomalies. The atrioventricular valve or valves are incompetent, and blood is shunted from left to right at both the atrial and ventricular levels. Right ventricular pressure equals left ventricular pressure and pulmonary arterial pressure is elevated, often to systemic levels.

Clinical Findings

A. Symptoms and Signs: Most infants with complete persistent atrioventricular canal develop heart failure during the first few weeks or months of life. Symptoms include poor feeding, failure to grow, and frequent respiratory problems. These babies have tachypnea, hepatomegaly, an active, enlarged heart, and a blowing pansystolic murmur which is often associated with a thrill at the left sternal border. Slight cyanosis may be apparent during crying or feeding. If pulmonary arterial flow is greatly increased, the second sound is loud and split through all phases of respiration. An apical systolic murmur, a fourth left interspace soft systolic murmur, and a diastolic murmur are present.

B. X-Ray Findings: Plain chest films show moderate to severe cardiomegaly, increased pulmonary vasculature, and pulmonary congestion. Heart size may be normal at birth.

C. Electrocardiography: The ECG nearly always shows left axis deviation with superior orientation and counterclockwise inscription of the frontal QRS vector. Biventricular hypertrophy and prolongation of the P–R interval are usually present.

D. Cardiac Catheterization and Cineangiocardiography: Cardiac catheterization reveals arterialized blood in the right atrium. The venous catheter can be easily pushed into all cardiac chambers. Ventricular pressures are often identical; atrial pressure and pulmonary arterial pressures are elevated. Pulmonary vascular resistance is often increased. Severe increased pulmonary vascular resistance decreases the magnitude of the left-to-right shunt and may reduce arterial oxygen saturation. Cineangiocardiograms after left ventricular injection reveal a characteristic "gooseneck" deformity of the mitral valve and left ventricular outflow tract in the anteroposterior projection. Contrast material frequently regurgitates from both ventricles into both atria.

Differential Diagnosis

The ECG, vectorcardiogram, and clinical findings

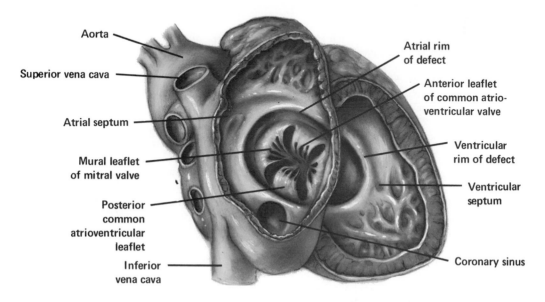

FIG 23–13. Complete persistent atrioventricular canal. The right atrium and ventricle have been cut away to illustrate the atrial defect cephalad to the atrioventricular valves and the ventricular septal defect caudad to the atrioventricular valves. The anterior and posterior atrioventricular valves are separated by a cleft. Each of the atrioventricular valves normally forms part of the mitral and tricuspid valves.

of heart failure, pansystolic murmur with loud, split S₂, and increased pulmonary arterial blood flow are sufficiently distinctive to make the diagnosis in most instances. Cardiac catheterization and cineangiocardiography confirm the diagnosis and help to define the amount of pulmonary overcirculation, the degree of pulmonary hypertension, and the severity of the anatomic lesion.

Natural History

Many infants with complete persistent atrioventricular canal die, and those that do survive have repeated episodes of heart failure and respiratory infection. Pulmonary hypertension and vascular disease generally develop during childhood in patients who survive infancy and are not treated. Patients with less severe atrioventricular canal malformations may remain well. These patients generally have diminished growth, easy fatigability, and dyspnea on exertion and frequently must take digitalis and diuretics.

Treatment

Infants with increased pulmonary arterial blood flow, pulmonary hypertension, and heart failure may benefit from pulmonary arterial banding. Patients who do not shunt blood directly from the left ventricle to the right atrium are the best candidates for banding. Patients who have direct left ventricular-right atrial shunts or severe atrioventricular valvular regurgitation are usually not helped by banding.

Infants and children who do not have pulmonary vascular disease are candidates for total correction of the anomaly using cardiopulmonary bypass with or without deep hypothermia and circulatory arrest. The repair is generally carried out through a right atriotomy. Three anatomic types of persistent atrioventricular canal defects are recognized, and the 2 most common types can be repaired using a patch (pericardium or Dacron) sutured to the cephalad margin of the ventricular septum, the atrioventricular valves, and the atrial margin of the defect. Septal portions of the mitral and tricuspid leaflets are sutured to the patch.

In the third type, some of the chordae tendineae of each atrioventricular valve arise from the opposite ventricular cavity; thus, the ventricular septal defect cannot be closed without interfering with the function of the atrioventricular valves. In many cases the mitral valve can be reconstructed, but not if the leaflet tissue is insufficient or severely malformed (poorly developed, primitive malformations that are often found in infants). Older infants and children sometimes require a mitral prosthesis. The tricuspid valve often cannot be completely repaired, but a small amount of regurgitation is generally well tolerated.

Prognosis After Operation

The mortality rate of pulmonary arterial banding during infancy for common atrioventricular canal is approximately 20%. The mortality rate for complete repair of common atrioventricular canal defects (excluding ostium primum) is 20–33%. Some patients

have residual mitral or tricuspid valvular stenosis or regurgitation, and nearly all have a residual apical systolic murmur. Complete heart block occurs in 5–10% of patients. Most surviving patients are improved, with increased exercise tolerance, reduced heart size, and reduced pulmonary vascularity. Occasional patients (5–10%) die months or years later of unexplained causes.

Hunt CE & others: Banding of the pulmonary artery: Results in 111 children. Circulation 43:395–406, 1971.

Rastelli GC & others: Surgical repair of the complete form of persistent common atrioventricular canal. J Thoracic Cardiovas Surg 55:299–308, 1968.

VENTRICULAR SEPTAL DEFECT

Essentials of Diagnosis

- Asymptomatic if defect is small.
- Heart failure with dyspnea, frequent respiratory infections, and poor growth if the defect is large.
- Grade 2–6/6 pansystolic murmur maximal at the left sternal border.
- S₂ loud with apical diastolic flow murmur and biventricular enlargement if the defect is large.

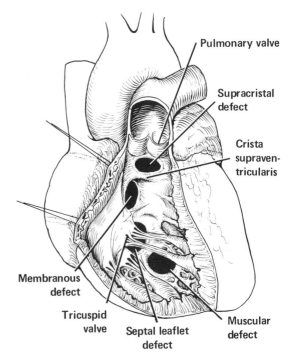

FIG 23–14. Anatomic locations of various ventricular septal defects. The wall of the right ventricle has been excised to expose the ventricular septum.

General Considerations

Approximately 85% of ventricular septal defects occur in the membranous septum, which is located just beneath portions of the right coronary and noncoronary aortic cusp adjacent to the anterior and septal leaflets of the tricuspid valve and caudad to a muscular ridge in the outflow tract of the right ventricle called the crista supraventricularis (Fig 23–14). A small number of ventricular defects occur anterior to the crista supraventricularis just beneath the pulmonary valve (supracristal defects), beneath the septal leaflet of the tricuspid valve, or in the muscular ventricular septum. Muscular septal defects (about 10% of patients) are frequently multiple and may occur in association with other types of ventricular septal defects.

Membranous or high ventricular septal defects vary in size from a few millimeters to more than 3 cm in diameter. The conduction bundle is located at the posterior and caudal margins of these defects, usually near the endocardium of the left ventricle. Occasionally, supracristal or membranous ventricular septal defects are associated with significant aortic regurgitation which is due to an abnormally formed valve or to elongation and prolapse of the right aortic cusp. Anomalies commonly associated with ventricular septal defects include patent ductus arteriosus, coarctation of the aorta, and atrial septal defect. Ventricular septal defects which are associated with pulmonary stenosis are discussed under tetralogy of Fallot. Rarely, ventricular septal defect may be associated with absence of the pulmonary valve.

Clinical Findings

A. Symptoms and Signs: The clinical features of ventricular septal defects are directly related to the size of the defect and the amount of pulmonary blood flow. The patient with a small ventricular septal defect is asymptomatic and has a normal ECG and chest film. A systolic murmur with thrill can be heard over the third and fourth left interspace, but no diastolic murmur is present at the apex. Left ventricular pressure is higher than right ventricular pressure, and pulmonary arterial blood flow is seldom more than twice systemic blood flow.

Children with moderate or large ventricular septal defects may be asymptomatic or may complain of dyspnea on exertion and easy fatigability. On physical examination, a loud pansystolic murmur with thrill is present along the lower left sternal border, and the heart is hyperactive. A soft diastolic flow murmur is present at the apex. P_2 is sometimes increased and delayed, but if pulmonary hypertension is present P_2 may be normal or decreased and the apical diastolic murmur is absent. The heart is usually enlarged; the pericardium may bulge; and growth is often slightly retarded. A few patients with associated aortic insufficiency also have a diastolic murmur in the third and fourth left sternal interspaces.

Infants with moderate or large ventricular septal defects often have severe heart failure. Failure is particularly likely if a patent ductus arteriosus is also present. Dyspnea, tachycardia, feeding problems, liver enlargement, and respiratory distress may occur 2–3 months after birth as the normally increased pulmonary vascular resistance of the newborn begins to decrease. The heart is enlarged and hyperactive and may have a gallop rhythm. A pansystolic murmur and apical diastolic murmur are present, and P_2 is loud and delayed.

B. X-Ray Findings: Chest films in patients with moderate or large ventricular septal defects show increased pulmonary vasculature with large pulmonary arteries and enlargement of both ventricles. If pulmonary vascular disease is present, the main pulmonary vessels appear very large, vessels of moderate size appear clubbed, and fine markings are reduced in peripheral lung fields. The right ventricle is greatly enlarged.

C. Electrocardiography: The ECG usually shows left ventricular hypertrophy and may show biventricular hypertrophy if pulmonary vascular resistance is moderately increased or if pulmonary blood flow is exceptionally large. If the ratio of pulmonary to systemic vascular resistance is high (> 0.75), large, notched R waves are present in the right precordial leads.

D. Cardiac Catheterization and Cineangiocardiography: The diagnosis is made or confirmed at cardiac catheterization by finding an increase in right ventricular blood oxygen saturation of more than 10%. The catheter often passes through the defect into the opposite ventricle. Ventricular pressures are equal in patients who have large ventricular septal defects and large pulmonary arterial blood flows. Right ventricular and pulmonary arterial pressures are elevated but are below systemic pressures in patients with moderate-sized ventricular septal defects. Cineangiocardiograms (particularly lateral and oblique views) demonstrate the location of ventricular septal defects and the existence of multiple or atypical defects.

Differential Diagnosis

Ventricular septal defects must be distinguished from other lesions which produce left-to-right shunts and, in infancy, from aortic or pulmonary stenosis, which produces similar murmurs. Definitive diagnosis is made by cardiac catheterization and cineangiocardiography; however, it is not always possible (nor necessary) to rule out the possibility of a small ventricular septal defect.

Natural History

Approximately 5% of infants with ventricular septal defects die in infancy from heart failure and respiratory infection. Some infants have repeated episodes of heart failure and pulmonary infections during the first year of life; however, after the first birthday, heart failure due to isolated ventricular septal defect is unusual. One of 3 developments causes the reduced incidence of heart failure after early infancy. In 25–40% of patients, the ventricular septal defect becomes smaller, and many (but not all) of these defects close spontaneously during infancy and early childhood. Few are known to close after adolescence. Patients with small ventricular septal defects and less than 1.5:1 left-to-right shunts are asymptomatic and have no risk of pulmonary vascular disease; rarely, however, they may develop bacterial endocarditis.

About 10% of infants with large ventricular septal defects develop infundibular muscular hypertrophy which reduces pulmonary blood flow.

Pulmonary vascular disease develops in 50% or more of patients with large ventricular septal defects. This dire complication may occur during the second year of life or at any time thereafter. As the arteriolar changes of pulmonary vascular disease develop, pulmonary vascular resistance increases and eventually equals or exceeds systemic resistance. In time, the flow of blood across the ventricular septal defect balances or becomes right-to-left (Eisenmenger's syndrome). These patients seldom live past age 30–40 years but may survive 15–20 years before dying of progressive hypoxia and polycythemia.

Treatment

Patients with small ventricular septal defects and pulmonary blood flow that is less than twice systemic flow have a slight risk of bacterial endocarditis but do not usually require operation.

Infants who have congestive heart failure due to ventricular septal defect and patent ductus arteriosus should have operative division of the patent ductus arteriosus. Infants who do not have patent ductus arteriosus and who have severe heart failure that cannot be controlled by medical measures should have operative closure of their ventricular septal defect. Formerly, these patients had pulmonary arterial banding.

Total correction of ventricular septal defects is most easily performed during cardiopulmonary bypass with or without deep hypothermia and circulatory arrest. High defects in the membranous septum are repaired through the right atrium and tricuspid valvular orifice. The atrial approach avoids incision and subsequent necrosis of right ventricular muscle. Over 80% of septal defects require patching with prosthetic material (Dacron or Teflon); the remainder can be closed by direct suture.

A right ventriculotomy is recommended for most other types of defects and for a technically easier repair of high septal defects. Supracristal defects can be repaired by working through a pulmonary arteriotomy and retracting the pulmonary valvular cusps. If the supracristal defect is associated with aortic regurgitation, closure of the septal defect usually improves the aortic insufficiency. Muscular septal defects are usually multiple, and these are best repaired by suturing the posterior margins of the defects to the anterior ventricular wall with mattress sutures that are tied outside the ventricle. If associated aortic insufficiency is present with a membranous septal defect, the aortic valve should be inspected and repaired through an aortotomy. A valvuloplasty, with or without plication

of one cusp, is often possible; occasionally, a deformed valve must be replaced.

All patients with ventricular septal defects must be followed closely during infancy and childhood. Although heart failure is infrequent after 1 year of age, pulmonary vascular disease may develop in any patient with a moderate or large ventricular septal defect. Change in the quality of the pulmonary second sound, increasing right ventricular hypertrophy, and changes in the chest roentgenograms suggest the onset of pulmonary vascular disease. These patients require cardiac catheterization and operation to prevent progression of pulmonary vascular disease.

Prognosis After Surgery

The mortality rate of pulmonary arterial banding for ventricular septal defects in the first year of life is 8–15%. Survivors require a second operation at which the defect is closed and the pulmonary arterial band is removed. The second operation has a mortality rate which is somewhat higher than that for uncomplicated ventricular septal defects (approximately 5%).

The mortality rate for total correction of uncomplicated ventricular septal defects in patients over 2 years of age is 1–2%. Infants who have total correction in the first months of life have a higher mortality rate, but the rate is less than the combined mortality rates of pulmonary arterial banding and subsequent closure of the ventricular septal defect. Up to 14% of patients have a residual left-to-right shunt after operation, but only a small percentage require reoperation. About 1% of patients develop permanent complete heart block, and most patients have postoperative right bundle branch block.

Nearly all patients who do not have significant pulmonary vascular disease improve postoperatively: heart size decreases and growth rate is accelerated. Successful repair of a ventricular septal defect is thought to reduce the incidence of subsequent bacterial endocarditis.

The mortality rate of total corrective operations in patients with pulmonary vascular disease is increased. The hospital mortality rate is 15–30% when the ratio of pulmonary vascular to systemic vascular resistance is greater than 0.75. Another 25% of patients die later; in 25%, pulmonary vascular disease does not change; and only 25% are improved. Pulmonary vascular resistance decreases postoperatively in 70% of patients who have a preoperative ratio of pulmonary vascular resistance to systemic vascular resistance between 0.45 and 0.75.

Barratt-Boyes BG, Simpson MM, Neutze JM: Intracardiac surgery in neonates and infants using deep hypothermia with surface cooling and limited cardiopulmonary bypass. Circulation 43 (Suppl 1):1–25, 1971.

Bloomfield DK: The natural history of ventricular septal defect in patients surviving infancy. Circulation 29:914–955, 1964.

Cartmill TB & others: Results of repair of ventricular septal defect. J Thoracic Cardiovas Surg 52:486–501, 1966.

Lillehei CW & others: Pre- and postoperative cardiac catheterization in 200 patients undergoing closure of ventricular septal defects. Surgery 63:69–76, 1968.

Mori A & others: Deep hypothermia combined with cardiopulmonary bypass for cardiac surgery in neonates and infants. J Thoracic Cardiovas Surg 64:422–429, 1972.

Stark J & others: Repair of intracardiac defects after previous constriction (banding) of the pulmonary artery. Surgery 67:536–547, 1970.

Wood P: The Eisenmenger syndrome. Brit MJ 2:701–709, 755–762, 1958.

PATENT DUCTUS ARTERIOSUS

Essentials of Diagnosis

- Patients with small or moderately large patent ducti are asymptomatic and have a continuous murmur over the pulmonary area, loud S_2, and bounding peripheral pulses.
- Poor feeding, respiratory distress, and frequent respiratory infections in infants with heart failure.
- Murmur usually systolic, sometimes continuous.
- Widened pulse pressure.

General Considerations

Normally, smooth muscle in the wall of the ductus arteriosus and increased blood oxygen tension cause the ductus arteriosus to constrict in the first days of life and to close completely with progressive fibrosis by 3 months of age. For unknown reasons, some ducti remain patent. The inside diameter of the ductus arteriosus varies from a few millimeters up to 10 mm and increases as the patient grows. With rare exceptions, the ductus arteriosus is to the left of the esophagus and trachea even when the aorta descends on the right. About 15% of patients with patent ductus arteriosus have associated anomalies, particularly ventricular septal defect or coarctation of the aorta.

Clinical Findings

A. Symptoms and Signs: Clinical findings are related to the size of the left-to-right shunt, which in turn is related to the diameter of the patent ductus arteriosus. About 15% of premature infants and a few full-term infants with large shunts develop feeding problems, heart failure, and respiratory distress in the first weeks of life, when the elevated pulmonary vascular resistance of the newborn begins to decrease. Cyanosis may occur if hyaline membrane disease, congestive atelectasis, or pneumonia occur simultaneously. A murmur may not be present initially; later (at 2–4 weeks of age), a systolic murmur may appear. The liver and heart are generally enlarged. Peripheral pulses are bounding when the left-to-right shunt is large. Some of these patients are severely ill; others develop recurrent episodes of heart failure and respiratory distress during

the first year of life. After the first year, heart failure is unusual.

Most infants and nearly all children with isolated patent ductus arteriosus are asymptomatic and have normal growth. A continuous murmur which is maximal in the second left intercostal space and widely transmitted is characteristic. An associated thrill may be present; the left ventricular impulse is increased; S_2 is loud; pulse pressure is widened; and peripheral pulses are increased.

B. X-Ray Findings: Chest films show increased pulmonary vascularity, prominent pulmonary arteries, and sometimes enlargement of the left ventricle in patients with moderate or large patent ducti. Young infants who are in heart failure may have a ground glass appearance of the peripheral lung fields, areas of atelectasis, and pulmonary infiltrates.

C. Electrocardiography: The ECG is often normal but may show left ventricular hypertrophy in older infants and children with large shunts.

D. Cardiac Catheterization and Cineangiocardiography: The catheter may pass through the ductus at catheterization. Pulmonary arterial pressures are normal or only slightly elevated in over 90% of asymptomatic patients. Pulmonary arterial pressures may approach or equal systemic pressures in symptomatic neonates. Blood oxygen saturation in the pulmonary arteries is greater than that in the right ventricle. Cineangiocardiograms demonstrate the ductus best after contrast material is injected into the aorta near the aortic isthmus.

Differential Diagnosis

In symptomatic infants, cardiac catheterization may be necessary to determine the presence of a patent ductus arteriosus and to differentiate patent ductus arteriosus from other lesions. In older patients, the classic clinical signs are sufficient to make the diagnosis.

In older infants and children, patent ductus arteriosus must be differentiated from venous hums and from the following rare lesions which produce a continuous murmur and an extracardiac left-to-right shunt: aortic-pulmonary window, ruptured sinus of Valsalva, and coronary arteriovenous fistula. Atypical location of the murmur and unusual findings on the chest film and ECG are indications for catheterization and cineangiocardiography in these patients.

Natural History

Nearly all premature infants with patent ductus arteriosus and respiratory distress die without treatment. Approximately 5% of full-term infants with untreated patent ductus arteriosus will die from heart failure and pulmonary complications in the first year of life. Another 5–10% of patients have large shunts and elevated pulmonary arterial pressures and may develop pulmonary vascular disease in late childhood or early adult life. The remainder are generally asymptomatic but have an increased incidence of subacute bacterial endocarditis at the ductus arteriosus. Adults

30–40 years of age who do not have pulmonary vascular disease often develop heart failure from the large left-to-right shunt through the ductus arteriosus.

Treatment

About two-thirds of premature infants with patent ductus arteriosus and respiratory distress can be controlled by medical means. The remaining one-third are helped by operative ligation of the patent ductus arteriosus. The mortality rate is high in both medically and surgically treated groups but is directly related to associated lesions, the severity of the pulmonary disease, and complications of therapy.

Division of the patent ductus arteriosus is recommended at any age for symptomatic infants and young children who have poorly controlled heart failure or repeated respiratory infections. The operation is contraindicated in patients with balanced or right-to-left shunts through the ductus arteriosus. Patients who have subacute bacterial endocarditis are preferably operated on after a course of antibiotics. Patients who have infected, recurrent, or aneurysmal ducti may require cardiopulmonary bypass to permit temporary occlusion of the descending thoracic aorta when the ductus is divided.

Prognosis After Surgery

In uncomplicated cases, the mortality rate from division of patent ductus arteriosus is less than 1% and approaches 0.2%. Causes of death are related to operative or postoperative hemorrhage. Operation reduces the susceptibility to subacute bacterial endocarditis.

In the first 3 months of life, division (or ligation) of a patent ductus arteriosus has a higher mortality rate. In prematures with respiratory disease, the mortality rate approaches 50%, but death is rarely due to complications of the operation. In full-term infants, the mortality rate in the first 3 months after birth is 10–15%; again, deaths are primarily due to associated pulmonary or cardiac lesions. Although approximately 10% of children or adults who have had ligation of the ductus arteriosus develop recurrence, ligation of the friable ductus in premature infants is preferable to division, and recurrence has not been observed.

Jones JC: Twenty-five years' experience with the surgery of patent ductus arteriosus. J Thoracic Cardiovas Surg 50:149–165, 1965.
Kitterman JA & others: Patent ductus arteriosus in premature infants: Incidence, relation to pulmonary disease, and management. New England J Med 287:473–477, 1972.
Rudolph AM & others: Hemodynamic basis for clinical manifestations of patent ductus arteriosus. Am Heart J 68:447–458, 1964.

AORTIC-PULMONARY WINDOW

A hole 5–30 mm in diameter between the ascending aorta and the main pulmonary artery produces a left-to-right shunt and physical findings identical with those of patent ductus arteriosus. Location of a continuous or systolic murmur in the third interspace near the left sternal border may suggest the correct diagnosis, which should be confirmed by cardiac catheterization and cineangiocardiography. Patients with large shunts have severe heart failure and are prone to develop pulmonary vascular disease at an early age. Division and closure of the aorta and main pulmonary artery during cardiopulmonary bypass produces good results in patients of all ages who do not have advanced pulmonary vascular disease.

Deverall PB & others: Aortopulmonary window. J Thoracic Cardiovas Surg 57:479–486, 1969.

RUPTURED SINUS OF VALSALVA

Rupture of the thin membranous tissue between an aortic sinus of Valsalva and an intracardiac chamber causes an immediate left-to-right shunt, a well-localized parasternal continuous murmur with associated thrill, wide pulse pressure, and increased heart size. In normal individuals, rupture is rare and generally occurs during the third or fourth decade. The cause is not known, but ruptured sinus of Valsalva occurs more frequently in patients with Marfan's syndrome or other abiotrophic diseases of connective tissue. Seventy-five percent of cases involve the right coronary sinus, which ruptures into the right ventricle (70%), right atrium (20%), or, rarely, the left ventricle or pulmonary artery. The remaining cases involve the noncoronary sinus, which ruptures into the right atrium or, less frequently, the right or left ventricle. About 20% of patients have an associated small ventricular septal defect. There are usually no symptoms, but when rupture occurs these patients suddenly develop chest pain and signs of congestive heart failure with a left-to-right shunt.

The lesion is repaired promptly by closing the fistulous opening from the right atrium, right ventricle, or aorta during temporary cardiopulmonary bypass. The operative mortality rate is less than 5%.

Paton BC & others: Ruptured sinus of Valsalva. Arch Surg 90:209–215, 1965.

LEFT VENTRICULAR-RIGHT ATRIAL SHUNT

A defect in the membranous septum near the annulus of the septal leaflet of the tricuspid valve and a perforation or cleft of the septal leaflet produces a left ventricular to right atrial shunt. The lesion is uncommon, and the size of the shunt is variable. Symptoms of heart failure may be present in infancy or may not develop until late childhood. The systolic murmur is not diagnostic. At cardiac catheterization, blood oxygen saturation is increased in the right atrium, and on cineangiocardiograms the right atrium opacifies after injection of contrast material into the left ventricle.

In symptomatic patients, the defect is closed by direct sutures from the right atrium during cardiopulmonary bypass. The operative mortality rate is less than 5%.

Barclay RS & others: Communication between the left ventricle and right atrium. Thorax 22:473–477, 1967.

CORONARY ARTERIAL FISTULA

A fistulous communication between the right (60%) or left (40%) coronary arteries and the right ventricle (90%), right atrium, or coronary sinus produces a left-to-right shunt and increased pulmonary blood flow. The involved coronary vessels are dilated, and the fistulous openings may be multiple. Many patients are asymptomatic; some develop evidence of myocardial ischemia, and others have some degree of heart failure. A continuous murmur is usually present over the heart. Angiograms are required to determine the number and location of the fistulas.

The fistulous connections are ligated at operation without interrupting the coronary artery. Cardiopulmonary bypass is sometimes required. The operative mortality rate is below 5%.

Oldham HN Jr & others: Surgical management of congenital coronary artery fistula. Ann Thoracic Surg 12:503–512, 1971.

TOTAL ANOMALOUS PULMONARY VENOUS CONNECTION

Essentials of Diagnosis

- Pulmonary congestion, tachypnea, cardiac failure, and mild cyanosis.
- Severe heart failure with mild or moderate cyanosis in infants.
- Pulmonary midsystolic murmur present with loud, fixed splitting of S_2 in some patients.
- Enlargement of right atrium and ventricle.
- Blood oxygen saturation identical in the aorta and pulmonary artery.

General Considerations

In this group of lesions, pulmonary venous blood enters the right atrium via one of several anomalous venous connections. In the right atrium, systemic venous and pulmonary blood are mixed and part of the mixed blood crosses a patent foramen ovale or atrial septal defect to reach the left heart. In approximately 25% of patients, the anomalous route of the pulmonary venous blood is not obstructed, and these patients have increased pulmonary blood flow. In the majority of patients, pulmonary venous drainage is partially obstructed; in these, pulmonary blood flow may be slightly greater—equal to or less than systemic blood flow. Since systemic and pulmonary venous blood is mixed in the right atrium, the severity of cyanosis is proportionate to the severity of the pulmonary venous hypertension and is inversely proportionate to pulmonary blood flow.

Most cases of total anomalous pulmonary venous connection can be grouped into one of 3 different types (Fig 23–15). In type I (55% of patients), the pulmonary veins enter a common vein in the transverse sinus behind the heart and drain into the right atrium by way of a persistent left vertical vein, the innominate vein, and the right superior vena cava. In type 2 (30% of patients), pulmonary venous blood enters the coronary sinus which drains into the right atrium. In type 3 (12% of patients), the common pulmonary vein behind the heart passes through the esophageal hiatus to enter the inferior vena cava, portal vein, or ductus venosus. Many mixed and complex varieties of total anomalous pulmonary venous connection have been described and carefully classified by Snellen & Bruins (see reference). Patent ductus arteriosus is the most common associated lesion.

Clinical Findings

A. Symptoms and Signs: Clinical findings vary according to the amount of pulmonary arterial blood flow and the degree of pulmonary venous hypertension. In the 25% of patients who have mild or no pulmonary venous hypertension, pulmonary arterial blood flow is greater than systemic, and symptoms and signs are similar to those found in patients with large atrial septal defects. Cyanosis is minimal.

The combination of pulmonary venous hypertension and increased pulmonary blood flow causes pulmonary congestion and severe dyspnea. These infants develop atelectasis and pneumonia and have feeding problems, but they are only mildly cyanotic. The liver often is not enlarged. The heart is usually enlarged and hyperactive, and a grade 2–4/6 systolic ejection murmur is present over the pulmonary valve. S_2 is widely split and fixed. Some patients have a tricuspid diastolic flow murmur.

Infants with severe pulmonary venous obstruction have reduced pulmonary blood flow, congestive atelectasis, severe cyanosis, and poor peripheral perfusion. The heart is usually enlarged and has a prominent right ventricular impulse. S_2 is loud and single, and the systolic pulmonary murmurs may be absent or faint.

B. X-Ray Findings: Plain chest films are diagnostic when 2 superior vena cavas cause the "snowman" or "figure-of-eight" appearance in the anteroposterior projection (type 1). In most patients, pulmonary vessels are prominent and the lungs appear congested. The heart—particularly the right atrium and ventricle—is enlarged, but in a few patients the heart may be normal in size.

C. Electrocardiography: The ECG is not diagnostic and usually indicates right atrial and right ventricular preponderance, which is normal in neonates.

D. Cardiac Catheterization and Cineangiocardiography: At cardiac catheterization, a catheter often can be passed from the right atrium into the anomalous veins and the lungs. An increase in blood oxygen saturation is found at the entrance of the pulmonary veins into the anomalous connection. Pressure differences are usually found within the anomalous veins. Both

pulmonary venous and pulmonary arterial pressures are elevated. Right atrial pressure is elevated and may exceed left atrial pressure. Right ventricular pressure is increased and in sick infants often exceeds left ventricular pressure. Blood oxygen saturation is the same in the pulmonary artery, aorta, and both ventricles and sometimes may be slightly lower in the aorta than in the pulmonary artery because of streaming from the inferior vena cava across the atrial septum. The anatomy of the anomalous veins is best determined by selective cineangiocardiography after injections of contrast material into the pulmonary veins and the common anomalous vein.

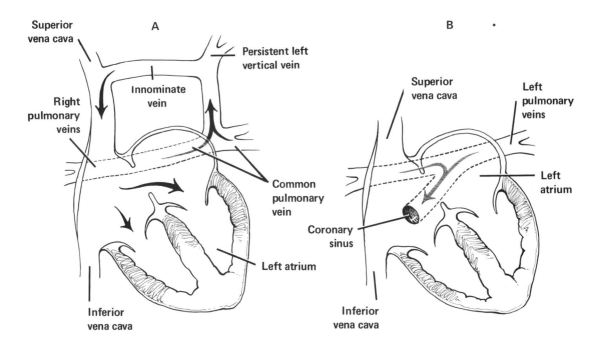

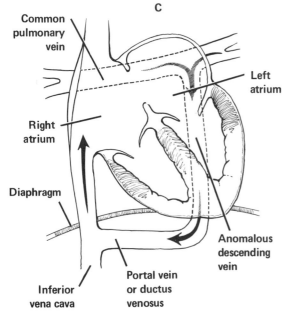

FIG 23–15. Common types of total anomalous pulmonary venous connection. *A: Type 1.* The pulmonary veins connect to a persistent left vertical vein, the innominate vein, and the right superior vena cava. *B: Type 2.* The pulmonary veins connect to the coronary sinus and the right atrium. *C: Type 3.* The pulmonary veins connect to an anomalous descending vein, a portal vein or persistent ductus venosus, and eventually the inferior vena cava.

Differential Diagnosis

Cyanotic infants with total anomalous pulmonary venous connection must be differentiated from patients with tetralogy of Fallot, transposition of the great vessels, and ventricular septal defect with associated respiratory disease. Patients with minimal cyanosis have findings which are similar to those in patients with large atrial septal defects. The anatomy and type of anomalous venous drainage must be determined by cardiac catheterization and cineangiocardiography.

Natural History

Without operation, all infants with type 3 and mixed types of total anomalous pulmonary venous connection die within a few weeks after birth. Seriously ill infants with types 1 and 2 die in infancy; fewer than 50% survive their first year. Older children and adolescents eventually develop right heart failure and pulmonary vascular disease.

Treatment

Seriously ill infants with all types of total anomalous pulmonary venous connection and pulmonary venous hypertension require emergency operation with cardiopulmonary bypass and deep hypothermia. Occasional infants with insufficient atrial septal defects may benefit from balloon septostomy performed during cardiac catheterization.

In patients with type 2 lesions, the orifice of the coronary sinus is enlarged and the atrial septal defect is patched so that all of the coronary sinus blood (and pulmonary venous return) is directed into the left atrium. In patients with types 1 and 3, an anastomosis is made between the common pulmonary vein behind the heart and the left atrium. A median sternotomy is suitable for all patients, and the anastomosis is conveniently made from the right side of the heart. After the anastomosis is completed, the anomalous vertical vein is ligated.

Prognosis After Surgery

The mortality rate of corrective operations is approximately 30–50% in infants who are less than 3 months of age. The mortality rate is highest in patients with infradiaphragmatic anomalous veins (type 3) and mixed types and in those with right ventricular pressures that are greater than systemic arterial pressures. In older infants and in children, the mortality rate is about 5%. Postoperative respiratory problems are particularly troublesome in patients with venous hypertension and congestive atelectasis. A few patients develop low cardiac output after operation.

Gersony WM & others: Management of total anomalous pulmonary venous drainage in early infancy. Circulation 43 (Suppl 1):19–24, 1971.

Gomes MMR & others: Total anomalous pulmonary venous connection. J Thoracic Cardiovas Surg 60:116–122, 1970.

Snellen HA, Bruins C: Anomalies of venous return. Chap 28, pp 416–436, in: *Paediatric Cardiology*. Watson H (editor). Mosby, 1968.

TRUNCUS ARTERIOSUS

In truncus arteriosus, a single large vessel with 4–6 semilunar valves overrides the ventricular septum and distributes all of the blood which is ejected from the heart. The main pulmonary artery (Fig 23–16A), separate right and left pulmonary arteries, or multiple pulmonary arteries originate from the ascending or descending truncal aorta and provide blood flow to the lungs. Infants develop severe heart failure unless the vessels to the lungs are small or obstructed. Most patients do not survive infancy. A few infants with well-defined pulmonary arteries have been helped by banding the main pulmonary artery or both right and left pulmonary arteries separately.

Although patients with multiple small pulmonary arteries may live to adult life, these patients are not suitable for corrective operations. Patients who have normal-sized right and left pulmonary arteries and who do not have pulmonary vascular disease can have a prosthetic conduit placed between the right ventricle and the pulmonary artery (conduit operation). The prosthetic conduit contains a homograft aortic valve to prevent pulmonary regurgitation. The ventricular septal defect is closed, and the origins of the arteries from the truncal aorta are divided during the operation (Fig 23–16B). This operation has been performed successfully in infants.

McGoon DC, Wallace RB, Danielson GK: The Rastelli operation: Its indications and results. J Thoracic Cardiovas Surg 65:65–75, 1973.

Van Praagh R, Van Praagh S: The anatomy of common aortico-pulmonary trunk (truncus arteriosus communis) and its embryologic implications. Am J Cardiol 16:406–425, 1965.

SINGLE VENTRICLE

This rare anomaly may occur as an isolated congenital heart defect but usually occurs in association with a wide variety of other severe intracardiac or extracardiac anomalies. Most commonly, the single ventricle develops from the left ventricular portion of the ventricular canal and the conus arteriosus and infundibulum of the right ventricle. Over 75% of patients have typical or atypical transposition of the great vessels, and slightly less than half have situs inversus, asplenia, or malposition of the heart. The functional pathology is directly related to associated lesions. About half of patients have aortic or pulmonary stenosis or atresia. Atresia or stenosis of an atrioventricular valve or common atrioventricular valve occurs in about half of patients with single ventricle. Atrial mixing from common atrium, atrial septal defects, or anomalous pulmonary or systemic venous drainage is common. The diagnosis of single ventricle

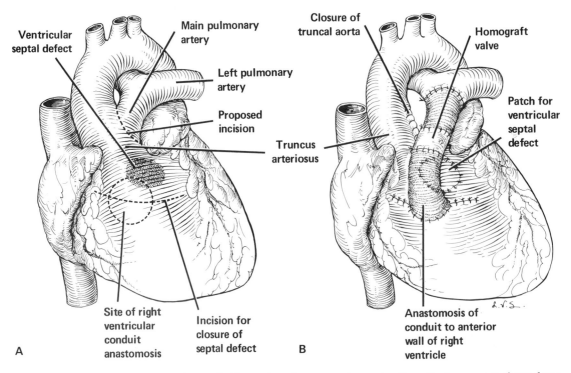

FIG 23–16. Type 1 truncus arteriosus. *A:* The main pulmonary artery arises from the truncus arteriosus downstream to the truncal semilunar valve. A ventricular septal defect is always present. *B:* The main pulmonary artery is incised from the truncus. The ventricular septal defect is closed with a patch. A conduit of Dacron which contains a homograft aortic valve is sutured to the anterior wall of the right ventricle and the distal pulmonary artery. A conduit between the right ventricle and pulmonary artery was successfully introduced by J.W. Kirklin in 1964 during correction of severe tetralogy of Fallot.

and the specific associated lesions must be made by cardiac catheterization and cineangiocardiography.

Clinical findings and prognosis are related to the relative amounts of pulmonary and systemic arterial blood flow. Surgical procedures are designed to augment (aortic-pulmonary anastomosis) or reduce (pulmonary arterial banding) pulmonary arterial blood flow. A few patients have survived into their second decade. Attempts to partition the single ventricle usually are not successful.

Lev M & others: Single (primitive) ventricle. Circulation 39:577–591, 1969.

III. CONGENITAL HEART LESIONS WHICH DECREASE PULMONARY ARTERIAL BLOOD FLOW

The combination of an obstructive lesion of the right heart and a septal defect reduces pulmonary arterial blood flow and causes some systemic venous blood to enter the systemic arterial circulation directly (right-to-left shunt). The degree of cyanosis is directly proportionate to the amount of the right-to-left shunt and inversely proportionate to the amount of pulmonary arterial blood flow. Tetralogy of Fallot is the most common lesion in this group, which also includes pulmonary atresia, tricuspid atresia, Ebstein's anomaly, and certain complex malformations with reduced pulmonary arterial blood flow. Eisenmenger's syndrome is an acquired condition in which obstruction of the pulmonary vasculature reduces pulmonary blood flow and causes blood to shunt from right to left.

Severe cyanosis stimulates red cell production, which increases blood hematocrit and hemoglobin concentration. This improves oxygen transport because blood which reaches the lungs will bind more oxygen per 100 ml. The elevated hematocrit, which may reach 80% or more, increases the viscosity of blood and may reduce certain clotting factors, particularly platelets and fibrinogen. Dehydration in patients with a very high hematocrit may cause systemic and pulmonary venous thrombosis in spite of the reduced concentration of clotting factors.

Changes in the degree of cyanosis, hypoxic spells, squatting, and clubbing are frequently associated with lesions that reduce pulmonary blood flow. Several factors may alter the degree of cyanosis by altering the ratio of pulmonary and systemic resistances. Exercise decreases systemic vascular resistance, increases systemic blood flow, and, in tetralogy of Fallot, decreases pulmonary blood flow and arterial oxygen saturation. Increased catecholamines or acidosis can also reduce pulmonary blood flow in patients with tetralogy of Fallot.

Hypoxic spells indicate severe cerebral hypoxia and are due to acute reduction of pulmonary blood flow. Spasm of the infundibular muscle is the most likely cause of hypoxic spells, which can occur without warning. Infants and young children become unconscious for varying periods of time and occasionally die. The most effective treatment is to administer oxygen and small doses of morphine, place the patient in the knee-chest position with his head down, and correct the associated metabolic acidosis.

Children who have reduced pulmonary arterial blood flow and cyanotic heart disease squat frequently. In the squatting position (sitting on the heels), systemic vascular resistance increases. The increased systemic vascular resistance decreases right-to-left shunting and temporarily increases pulmonary arterial blood flow.

Clubbing of fingers and toes develops in late infancy and early childhood and is due to proliferation of capillaries and small arteriovenous fistulas in the distal phalanges. The mechanism and teleologic advantage (if any) of clubbing are not known.

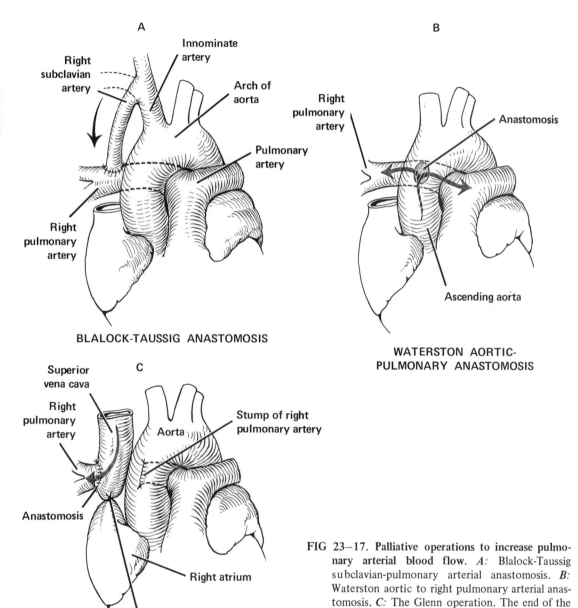

FIG 23–17. Palliative operations to increase pulmonary arterial blood flow. *A:* Blalock-Taussig subclavian-pulmonary arterial anastomosis. *B:* Waterston aortic to right pulmonary arterial anastomosis. *C:* The Glenn operation. The end of the right pulmonary artery is connected to the side of the superior vena cava, which is ligated caudad to the anastomosis.

Reduced pulmonary arterial blood flow stimulates enlargement of the bronchial and mediastinal arteries. These vessels connect with pulmonary arteries and, in some children, may provide most of the pulmonary blood flow. At birth, the ductus arteriosus is patent and provides substantial blood flow to the pulmonary arteries of patients with obstructive lesions of the right heart. Unfortunately, this useful vessel nearly always closes during the first few hours and days after birth.

Several palliative operations that shunt blood from the systemic to the pulmonary arterial circulation have been devised for infants and young children who have insufficient pulmonary arterial blood flow. The Blalock-Taussig operation connects the subclavian artery to the ipsilateral pulmonary artery with an end-to-side anastomosis (Fig 23–17A). The Waterston aortic to right pulmonary arterial anastomosis connects the posterior portion of the ascending aorta to the anterior wall of the right pulmonary artery (Fig 23–17B). The Potts operation joins the left pulmonary artery and the descending thoracic aorta by a side-to-side anastomosis. Because of the pressure difference between the systemic arterial and pulmonary circulations, these shunts increase pulmonary blood flow. The Glenn operation (Fig 23–17C) connects the superior vena cava to the right pulmonary artery in such a way that superior vena caval blood must enter the right pulmonary artery without passing through the heart.

TETRALOGY OF FALLOT

Essentials of Diagnosis

- History of hypoxic spells and squatting.
- Cyanosis and clubbing.
- Prominent right ventricular impulse, single S_2.
- Grade $1–3/6$ ejection murmur in third left intercostal space.

General Considerations

Tetralogy of Fallot is a cardiac malformation with 4 anatomic abnormalities (Fig 23–18). The lesion is due to underdevelopment of the right ventricular infundibulum (that portion of the right ventricle that is just upstream to the pulmonary valve). Parietal and septal muscular bands that attach to the crista supraventricularis (a muscular ridge between the infundibulum and the body of the right ventricle) obstruct the underdeveloped infundibulum. The ventricular septal defect is large (equal pressures in both ventricles) and is located upstream to the crista supraventricularis in the membraneous septum just caudad to the aortic valve. The aorta arises partially from the right ventricle, but the absence of muscular tissue between the aortic and mitral valves distinguishes tetralogy of Fallot from double outlet right ventricle. Right ventricular hypertrophy is the fourth anomaly of the tetrad and is a secondary development.

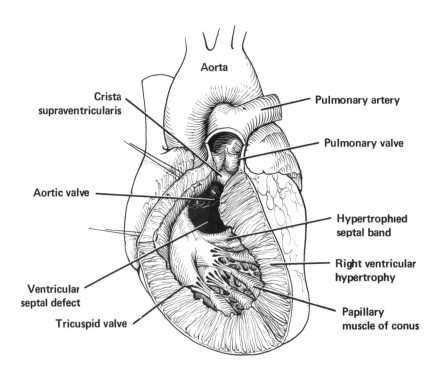

FIG 23–18. Tetralogy of Fallot. The aorta overrides the ventricular septum. A large ventricular septal defect is present, and the hypoplastic infundibulum with hypertrophied parietal and septal muscle bands obstruct blood flow to the pulmonary arteries.

The infundibular stenosis is located upstream to the pulmonary valve and downstream to the ventricular septal defect. An infundibular "chamber" may be present between the hypertrophied muscle tissue and the pulmonary valve. In approximately two-thirds of patients, the pulmonary valve is also stenotic and rarely is atretic. Occasionally, the pulmonary valvular annulus and the main pulmonary artery are hypoplastic. Occasional patients have stenotic lesions within the pulmonary arteries, usually at the junction of the right and left main pulmonary vessels. Rarely, the left pulmonary artery is absent or the pulmonary valvular cusps are rudimentary or absent.

Atrial septal defect and right aortic arch occur frequently with tetralogy of Fallot. In patients with severe obstruction, the bronchial arteries enlarge and dilate in response to the diminished pulmonary arterial blood flow. Occasionally, the anterior descending coronary artery originates from the right coronary artery and crosses the right ventricular outflow tract.

Although the functional pathology and operative treatment of ventricular septal defect with acquired infundibular obstruction are similar to those of tetralogy of Fallot, the 2 lesions differ in developmental and pathologic anatomy.

Clinical Findings

A. Symptoms and Signs: Clinical findings are directly related to the severity of the right ventricular obstructive lesion and the amount of pulmonary blood flow. Severe right ventricular obstruction or pulmonary atresia causes cyanosis in early infancy. A large patent ductus arteriosus may mask the lesion for the first few days after birth, but as the ductus constricts cyanosis increases. Infants feed poorly, tire easily, hyperventilate, and have episodic hypoxic spells. During a hypoxic spell, the infant becomes deeply cyanotic, tachypneic, and lethargic or unconscious. The heart is usually not enlarged in infants with severe tetralogy of Fallot, and murmurs often are not diagnostic. A systolic murmur may be present along the left sternal border, and in a few patients a continuous murmur of large bronchial arteries or patent ductus arteriosus may be present. The liver is not enlarged, and heart failure is absent.

Less severe right ventricular outflow obstruction and greater pulmonary arterial blood flow produce different clinical findings. Newborns do not become hypoxic and acidotic, and cyanosis may not be striking. These infants generally feed and grow well and do not have heart failure, but they do develop increasing cyanosis. Some babies develop hypoxic spells at 3—4 months of age; others do not have such spells until later, and some never have hypoxic spells. During the first year, clubbing and polycythemia develop. Later, exercise tolerance is reduced, growth rate is below normal, and squatting may occur. A systolic murmur and thrill are usually present along the left sternal border, and the pulmonary second sound is generally decreased. A continuous murmur in late infancy or childhood suggests greatly increased bronchial arterial flow

or associated patent ductus arteriosus.

B. X-Ray Findings: Chest films show reduced pulmonary vascularity, hypertrophy of the right ventricle, and little or no cardiac enlargement. Right ventricular hypertrophy elevates the apex of the heart. Central pulmonary vessels may be normal or small. In approximately 20% of patients, the aortic arch is on the right side.

C. Electrocardiography: The ECG shows right ventricular hypertrophy, which is normal in newborns. In older infants, the ECG shows moderate to severe right ventricular hypertrophy.

D. Cardiac Catheterization and Cineangiocardiography: In tetralogy of Fallot, ventricular pressures are equal and the major shunt is from right to left at the ventricular level. Occasionally, a small left-to-right ventricular shunt may also be present, and a right-to-left shunt may be present in the atria. Pressure differences are present between the body of the right ventricle and the infundibulum and may be present across the pulmonary valve and, occasionally, across a segment of the pulmonary arteries. The percentage of oxyhemoglobin in left ventricular and aortic blood is directly related to the ratio of pulmonary to systemic blood flow. Cineangiocardiograms after right ventricular injection of contrast material demonstrate the size of the right ventricle, the severity and location of the infundibular and pulmonary valvular stenoses, the size of the pulmonary valvular annulus and main pulmonary artery, and the presence of peripheral pulmonary stenosis.

Differential Diagnosis

In early infancy, severe forms of tetralogy of Fallot may be difficult to distinguish from other complex cyanotic malformations such as transposition of the great vessels with pulmonary stenosis and ventricular septal defect, severe pulmonary stenosis with patent foramen ovale, double outlet right ventricle, and tricuspid atresia. The ECG is helpful in identifying tricuspid atresia, and the absence of heart failure suggests tetralogy of Fallot or pulmonary atresia with ventricular septal defect. Cardiac catheterization and cineangiocardiography are required for accurate diagnosis. The diagnosis of tetralogy of Fallot is more easily made in older infants and children on the basis of clinical findings; however, cardiac catheterization and cineangiocardiography provide important anatomic and physiologic information which relates to the management of the patient.

Natural History

A few patients who have relatively large pulmonary arterial blood flows during childhood reach age 30—40 before increasing cyanosis, polycythemia, and clinical signs of heart failure develop. Most patients with tetralogy of Fallot do not survive past age 20; the average age at death is 12 years in patients who survive infancy. Infants with severe right ventricular outflow obstruction or pulmonary atresia usually succumb in the first few months of life during a hypoxic spell.

Progressive hypertrophy of infundibular muscle and thrombosis of pulmonary vessels during infancy and childhood increases the severity of cyanosis and polycythemia and the likelihood of a fatal hypoxic spell. Hypoxia is the cause of death in most patients who die of tetralogy of Fallot.

Infection is the second most common cause of death. Rare causes include cerebrovenous thrombosis secondary to polycythemia, cerebral abscess resulting from bacteria in venous blood passing through the shunt directly into the arterial circulation, and subacute bacterial endocarditis.

Treatment

The selection of operation for infants and children with symptomatic tetralogy of Fallot varies with the age of the patient and with the severity of the anatomic malformation. At present, palliative operations that create an anastomosis between the systemic and pulmonary arterial circulations are recommended for symptomatic infants less than 3 months of age and for older patients who have severe malformations and hypoplastic pulmonary arteries. These anatomic features increase the risk of the corrective operation, particularly in small infants.

A few infants with severe infundibular and valvular stenosis or pulmonary atresia become deeply cyanotic and acidotic shortly after birth, when the ductus arteriosus begins to close. These newborns require a shunt between the systemic and pulmonary circulation for survival. The Waterston or Blalock-Taussig anastomosis between the systemic and pulmonary circulations (Fig 23–17A and B) are recommended for these newborns.

As the infant grows, progressive muscular hypertrophy and fibrosis of the infundibulum may further restrict pulmonary arterial blood flow and threaten life. These older infants and young children who develop severe cyanosis, marked polycythemia, and hypoxic spells require operation, but the best procedure to recommend is an unsettled question. The choice is between a palliative shunt procedure or total correction of the tetralogy in infants between 3 months and 2 years of age. Increasingly, total correction is preferred if the anatomic features of the malformation are favorable for the operation.

Total correction of Fallot's tetralogy is performed during cardiopulmonary bypass. In infants, deep hypothermia and circulatory arrest are helpful. A patent ductus arteriosus or a previously constructed systemic artery to pulmonary artery shunt is closed before cardiopulmonary bypass begins. The right ventricle is opened through a transverse incision, which avoids coronary vessels. The fibrous and muscular obstruction of the outflow tract is excised widely to create an unobstructed channel to the pulmonary valve. The pulmonary valve is inspected, and incised if stenotic. Approximately 5% of patients require an outflow patch of prosthetic material to enlarge a severely hypoplastic pulmonary annulus. A homograft aortic leaflet is sometimes used during reconstruction of the pulmo-

nary annulus, but in most cases the pulmonary valve is left grossly incompetent. The infundibular resection and pulmonary annuloplasty must be sufficient to reduce the ratio between right and left ventricular systolic pressures to 0.9 or less. The ventricular septal defect is closed with a prosthetic patch. Associated atrial septal defects are also closed during the operation.

Three palliative shunt operations are used in selected patients with tetralogy of Fallot. The Waterston anastomosis between the posterior ascending aorta and right pulmonary artery can be performed at any age, but the amount of flow through the anastomosis is difficult to control. The Blalock-Taussig subclavian-pulmonary arterial anastomosis (Fig 23–17A) generally provides adequate pulmonary blood flow, but it is more difficult to perform in young infants. The Potts anastomosis (descending aorta to left pulmonary artery) is little used because it is more difficult to close at a subsequent corrective operation.

Prognosis After Surgery

A few severely cyanotic, acidotic newborns have been successfully palliated by Waterston operations in the first few hours and days of life. Postoperative complications—particularly respiratory problems—are common. Heart failure may occur postoperatively as pulmonary vascular resistance falls during the first few weeks after birth. Although some newborns are well palliated and become candidates for total correction, others develop pulmonary vascular disease or chronic heart failure if the size of the shunt increases more rapidly than somatic growth.

In older infants and young children, Blalock-Taussig or Waterston shunts have a mortality rate of about 5%. Mortality and morbidity rates are greater in infants less than 1 year of age. A successful shunt causes a continuous murmur, increases heart size, improves pulmonary vascularity, and reduces both cyanosis and the hematocrit. Over a period of 10 years, nearly a third of patients with Blalock-Taussig anastomoses will undergo stenosis or occlusion of the shunt. Arm complications and uncontrolled heart failure after Blalock-Taussig anastomoses are extremely rare; early occlusion requiring reoperation occurs in about 5% of patients.

The overall mortality rate for elective correction of tetralogy of Fallot in children is now about 5%. The mortality rate in infants less than 1 year of age is not known but is probably lower than the cumulative mortality and morbidity rates of a palliative procedure followed by a corrective operation at a later date. Right ventricular failure, heart block, arrhythmias, and infection are the most common causes of death. A previous Potts anastomosis or massive bronchial blood flow increases the operative mortality rate 2- to 3-fold.

Approximately 35% of surviving patients have no exercise limitations; 55% have no limitation of ordinary activity; and only 10% have residual disability. Many patients have some degree of pulmonary valvular regurgitation and paradoxic movement of the right ventricular outflow tract. Patients with residual disability often are found to have residual ventricular septal shunts or elevated right ventricular pressures; some of these patients have had a successful second operation.

Ceballos R, Kirklin JW: Long term anatomical results of intra-cardiac repair of tetralogy of Fallot. Ann Thoracic Surg 15:371–377, 1973.

Kirklin JW, Karp RB: *The Tetralogy of Fallot From a Surgical Viewpoint.* Saunders, 1970.

Puga FJ, DuShane JW, McGoon DC: Treatment of tetralogy of Fallot in children less than 4 years of age. J Thoracic Cardiovas Surg 64:247–253, 1972.

Starr A, Bonchek LI, Sunderland CO: Total correction of tetralogy of Fallot in infancy. J Thoracic Cardiovas Surg 65:45–57, 1973.

Taussig HB & others: Ten to thirteen year follow-up on patients after a Blalock-Taussig operation. Circulation 25:630–634, 1962.

PULMONARY ATRESIA WITH INTACT VENTRICULAR SEPTUM

Atresia or hypoplasia of the pulmonary artery associated with ventricular septal defect represents a severe malformation of tetralogy of Fallot. This lesion (also called pseudotruncus) has been discussed with tetralogy of Fallot.

Pulmonary atresia with an intact ventricular septum is usually associated with a hypoplastic or rudimentary right ventricle (type 1), but it may occur with a normal or dilated right ventricle in association with an incompetent and sometimes malformed tricuspid valve (type 2). The pulmonary valve is small and imperforate; distal pulmonary arteries are patent, and blood is shunted from right to left across the inter-atrial septum. A patent ductus is mandatory for survival, but the ductus is often small and constricts during the first few days or weeks after birth. The degree of cyanosis is inversely proportionate to the amount of pulmonary blood flow through the ductus arteriosus.

Cyanosis may be present at birth or may appear within a few days along with heart failure, hypoxic spells, and acidosis. The ECG generally shows left ventricular dominance in patients with a hypoplastic (type 1) right ventricle. Serial x-rays usually indicate a progressive increase in heart size and diminished pulmonary vasculature. The condition must be differentiated from tricuspid atresia, severe tetralogy of Fallot, severe pulmonary stenosis, and transposition of the great arteries with associated pulmonary stenosis. Cineangiocardiograms show a blind right ventricle with contrast material escaping through dilated myocardial sinusoids or through the tricuspid valve.

If the right ventricle is grossly underdeveloped, a Waterston or Blalock-Taussig anastomosis (Fig 23–17A and B) is required. If the right ventricle is small or normal in size, an attempt is made to establish a channel between the right ventricle and main pulmonary

artery by blind valvulotomy or incision of the atretic valve through the pulmonary artery. In some patients, a successful channel enhances growth of the right ventricle. Although the late mortality rate from pulmonary infection, arrhythmia, or heart failure is high, some patients have survived for many years.

Without treatment, nearly all infants die within their first year.

Dhanavaravibul S, Nora JJ, McNamara DG: Pulmonary valvular atresia with intact ventricular septum: Problems in diagnosis and results of treatment. J Pediat 77:1010–1016, 1970.

Edmunds LH Jr & others: Anastomoses between aorta and right pulmonary artery (Waterston) in neonates. New England J Med 284:464–471, 1971.

TRICUSPID ATRESIA

The tricuspid valve is completely absent in 1–2% of newborns with congenital heart disease. In the majority of patients, the great vessels are not transposed, the right ventricle is hypoplastic, a small muscular ventricular septal defect is present, and the pulmonary valve is stenotic or hypoplastic. Blood passes across the foramen ovale (or atrial septal defect if it is present), is mixed with pulmonary venous blood in the left atrium, and is pumped by the left ventricle into the great vessels. Occasionally, the ventricular septum is intact, but a large ventricular septal defect without associated pulmonary valvular obstruction is sometimes present. About 25% of patients have transposition of the great arteries.

Infants with tricuspid atresia and reduced pulmonary blood flow (80% of the total) develop cyanosis within the first week after birth. Tachypnea, dyspnea, hypoxic spells, acidosis, and feeding difficulties are additional findings. Most patients have a systolic precordial murmur. Polycythemia and clubbing develop later; liver enlargement and systemic venous hypertension may develop in older infants and children who have partial obstruction to flow at the atrial septum.

Heart size is sometimes normal, but the left heart border has a box-like contour due to left atrial enlargement on chest x-rays taken during infancy. Pulmonary vascular markings are decreased. The ECG and vectorcardiogram show left ventricular hypertrophy and left axis deviation. This finding, which is present from birth in virtually all patients with tricuspid atresia and diminished pulmonary blood flow, strongly suggests the diagnosis in cyanotic infants. At cardiac catheterization, right atrial pressure usually exceeds left atrial pressure, and blood oxygen saturation increases in the left atrium. After injection into the right atrium or systemic vein, contrast material opacifies the left atrium and ventricle and both great arteries in sequence. The right ventricle may appear only as a filling defect between the right atrium and the left ventricle. Tricuspid atresia is differentiated from tetralogy of Fallot by the ECG. Other lesions which must be included in the differential diagnosis are hypoplastic right heart, pulmonary atresia, and a variety of lesions (single ventricle, persistent atrioventricular canal, transposition of the great arteries) associated with pulmonary stenosis.

Most patients with tricuspid atresia and reduced pulmonary arterial blood flow die during a hypoxic spell within 3 months after birth as the ductus arteriosus constricts or closes. In rare types in which pulmonary arterial blood flow is adequate or increased, the prognosis is better.

Infants who have reduced pulmonary blood flow may benefit from a systemic to pulmonary arterial anastomosis. In newborns, a Waterston operation is recommended; in older infants, either a Waterston or Blalock-Taussig anastomosis is satisfactory. A balloon atrial septostomy or operative excision of the atrial septum may be required in occasional patients who have partial obstruction at the atrial septum.

Infants over 6 months of age and children are candidates for the Glenn superior vena cava to right pulmonary artery anastomosis (Fig 23–17C). This operation reduces the amount of blood which must be ejected by the left ventricle and increases pulmonary blood flow. The operative mortality is about 15% in patients over 6 months of age. Most patients are clinically improved.

A new operation recently developed by Fontan totally "corrects" tricuspid atresia. After homograft semilunar valves are placed at the ostia of both cavas in the right atrium, the right atrial appendage, with a third homograft valve, is connected to the pulmonary artery.

Deverall PB & others: Surgical management of tricuspid atresia. Thorax 24:239–245, 1969.

Edwards WS, Bargeron LM Jr: The superiority of the Glenn operation for tricuspid atresia in infancy and childhood. J Thoracic Cardiovas Surg 55:60–66, 1968.

Fontan F, Baudet E: Surgical repair of tricuspid atresia. Thorax 26:240–248, 1971.

EBSTEIN'S ANOMALY

In this malformation, the septal and posterior leaflets of the tricuspid valve are small and deformed and arise from the wall of the right ventricle below the normal tricuspid annulus. The anterior leaflet is often large and is attached to the tricuspid annulus. The malformation causes the upper portion of the right ventricle to be a part of the right atrium. This portion of the right ventricle is generally thin and contracts poorly. The downstream portion of the right ventricle is usually small, and the tricuspid valve is usually incompetent. Most patients have an associated atrial septal defect (50%) or patent foramen ovale. A minority of patients have associated pulmonary stenosis, ventric-

ular septal defect, tetralogy of Fallot, or transposition of the great arteries.

About half of patients develop right heart failure, systemic venous hypertension, hepatomegaly, arrhythmias, and cyanosis in infancy. A systolic murmur associated with a poor right ventricular impulse is often present. Associated lesions reduce life expectancy, and few of these patients survive infancy. Other patients are asymptomatic or have mild symptoms during infancy and childhood but develop progressive cardiomegaly, arrhythmias, cyanosis, and severe right heart failure in the third and fourth decades of life. Massive enlargement of the entire heart—but particularly the right atrium—may develop. The ECG characteristically shows large P waves, prolonged P–R conduction, and low voltage in the right ventricular leads. Right atrial pressure is usually increased during cardiac catheterization, and the atrial v wave is large. Most patients have a right-to-left shunt between the atria. The abnormal position of the tricuspid valve is best demonstrated by a right ventricular angiogram.

A superior vena cava to right pulmonary arterial anastomosis (Glenn operation) has provided effective palliation for some patients, but this operation is not often successful in infants. In older patients, the atrial septal defect or patent foramen ovale is closed, and an annuloplasty is performed if the anatomy of the tricuspid valve is favorable. In other patients, the tricuspid valve is not disturbed. Rarely, the tricuspid valve is replaced. Occasional patients are strikingly improved, but the overall results are generally unsatisfactory because of the inherent inability of the diseased right ventricle to contract effectively.

Kumar AE & others: Ebstein's anomaly: Clinical profile and natural history. Am J Cardiol 28:84–95, 1971.

HYPOPLASTIC RIGHT VENTRICLE

Underdevelopment of the right ventricle commonly occurs with pulmonary and tricuspid atresia and may occur with valvular pulmonary stenosis. Rarely, hypoplasia of the right ventricle may occur as an isolated lesion. The right ventricle may have a small cavity, hypertrophied ventricular walls, and a patent, deformed tricuspid valve—or may have a large cavity, thin, fibrotic ventricular walls, and an incompetent tricuspid valve. The pulmonary artery and valve are small but well formed. These lesions are part of a spectrum of right ventricular and pulmonary arterial malformations which range from tricuspid atresia and Ebstein's anomaly to pulmonary stenosis, tetralogy of Fallot, and pulmonary atresia. Older patients with thin, dilated right ventricles may benefit from superior vena cava to right pulmonary arterial (Glenn) anastomosis. An aortic to pulmonary arterial anastomosis (Waterston) is recommended for infants.

Hollman A: Underdevelopment of the right ventricle. Chap 32, pp 501–509, in: *Paediatric Cardiology*. Watson H (editor). Mosby, 1968.

IV. COMPLEX CONGENITAL HEART MALFORMATIONS

This imprecise term denotes a group of lesions which have complicated anatomic features that involve abnormal relationships between different parts of the heart and great vessels. The abnormal relationships of different subunits to each other distinguish the complex lesions from more localized defects in septation or development of specific structures. Pulmonary blood flow may be increased or decreased in complex lesions, and obstructive lesions may be present.

Most patients with complex congenital heart lesions die in infancy or early childhood, but a few live to adult life.

The principal structures of the heart and great vessels are formed and aligned between the third and seventh weeks of gestation. Normally, the straight cardiac tube develops 5 segments which are labeled (from caudad to cephalad) sinus venosus, atrial canal, ventricular canal, bulbus cordis, and truncus arteriosus. Toward the end of the third week, the segmented cardiac tube normally loops to the right (*d*-loop) and folds on itself to begin the process of septation. By the fifth week, the apex of the heart swings leftward to bring the right ventricle to an anterior position. The sinus venosus becomes part of the right atrium, and the atrial canal forms the right and left atria. At the other end, truncal ridges spirally divide the truncus arteriosus into the aorta and main pulmonary artery.

Endocardial cushions—which form the atrioventricular valves—and conal ridges of the bulbus cordis participate in the development of the ventricular septum and division of the primitive ventricular canal. In addition, the bulbus cordis forms the semilunar valves and parts of the inflow and outflow portions of the right ventricle. A part of the bulbus cordis called the conus arteriosus normally forms the parietal band and part of the free wall of the right ventricular infundibulum (outflow portion of the right ventricle immediately upstream to the pulmonary valve). After birth, the structures formed by the conus arteriosus appear to be integral parts of the right ventricle and ventricular septum, but in early fetal life the conus arteriosus may develop or fail to develop independently of other portions of the bulbus cordis. When a conus is present, it forms an integral unit with the adjacent aortic or pulmonary valve; changes in the relationship between the conus and adjacent semilunar valve do not occur. Abnormalities in the independent development of the conus arteriosus and in the looping of the cardiac tube explain the development of many complex congenital heart lesions.

Certain normal relationships deserve emphasis before individual complex lesions are considered. Normally, *d*-looping causes the aortic valve to be located to the right of the pulmonary valve. *D*-looping and subsequent shift of the apex of the heart cause the right ventricle to be located anterior to and to the right of the left ventricle. Development of the conus arteriosus beneath the pulmonary valve causes the pulmonary valve to be more cephalad in relation to the aortic valve. Normally, muscular conal tissue separates the annuli of the pulmonary and tricuspid valves. Involution of the conus arteriosus beneath the aortic valve causes the aortic annulus adjacent to the noncoronary cusp of the aortic valve to be contiguous with the annulus of the anterior leaflet of the mitral valve.

Certain rules have proved useful in the diagnostic analysis of patients with complex congenital heart lesions. With 2 rare exceptions (asplenia and polysplenia), the position of the viscera determines the location of the atria. When the stomach bubble is left and the liver is right (situs solitus), the right atrium and inferior vena cava are right-sided. In situs inversus totalis, the positions of both the viscera and the atria are reversed. The right atrium is defined as the structure receiving systemic venous blood; the left atrium is the chamber receiving pulmonary venous blood. The ventricles are designated by their structure; thus, angiocardiograms are necessary to locate the anatomic ventricles and to determine their relationship to the atria. The right ventricle is coarsely trabeculated and usually has a rounded, globular shape, whereas the left ventricle has few trabeculae and has a more conical shape, particularly in systole. The atrioventricular valves are parts of the morphologic ventricles rather than the atria.

The atria and ventricles develop independently. When the right atrium connects with the right ventricle and the left atrium connects with the morphologic left ventricle, the atria and ventricles have a *concordant* relationship. A *discordant* atrioventricular relationship exists when the right atrium connects with the left ventricle.

The direction of looping of the cardiac tube determines the location of the ventricles and nearly always the location of the aortic valve (in relation to the pulmonary valve). Thus, if the aortic valve is to the right of the pulmonary valve, a *d*-loop nearly always is present and the right ventricle is anterior to and to the right of the left ventricle. Angiocardiograms are necessary to determine conal development beneath the semilunar valves and the presence or absence of continuity between semilunar and atrioventricular valves.

The classification and terminology of complex lesions remain unsettled because many variations can exist in the positional relationships of the atria, ventricles, great arteries, cardiac axes, and heart positions. For the sake of simplicity, complex lesions can be divided into 2 large groups: malposition of the great arteries and cardiac malposition.

Malposition of the great arteries is an imprecise term that indicates an abnormal positional relationship between the 2 great arteries (aorta and main pulmonary artery). This broad definition encompasses transposition of the great arteries, double outlet ventricles, and a potpourri of rare lesions that are also designated malposition of the great arteries. Transposition of the great arteries ("typical transposition") is defined rather strictly and requires the presence of an interventricular septum, the origin of the aorta from the morphologic right ventricle, and the origin of the pulmonary artery from the left ventricle. The plane of the ventricular septum is used to determine the ventricular origin of each great artery.

Because the atria and ventricles may be concordant or discordant since the primitive cardiac tube may loop to the right or to the left, and because the conus arteriosus may be well developed or not developed beneath the aorta or pulmonary artery, a wide variety of anatomic lesions with abnormal relationships between the great arteries may exist. Many of these lesions—classified by some experts as "atypical transpositions"—do not meet the strict criteria of transposition as defined above because one great artery or ventricle is atretic, both great arteries originate from one ventricle, or the ventricular septum is absent. For this reason, typical transposition, corrected transposition, malposition of the great arteries, double outlet right ventricle, and double outlet left ventricle will be presented here under the general heading of malposition of the great arteries.

TYPICAL TRANSPOSITION OF THE GREAT ARTERIES
(*D*-Transposition)

Essentials of Diagnosis

- Situs solitus, levocardia.
- Cyanosis from birth; hypoxic spells sometimes present.
- Heart failure often present.
- Murmurs variable and not diagnostic.
- Cardiac enlargement and diminished pulmonary artery segment on x-ray.

General Considerations

Approximately 60% of all patients with transposition or malposition of the great arteries have typical transposition with situs solitus and levocardia. The lesion is more common in males. During development of the heart, the segmented cardiac tube loops to the right (*d*-loop), but the conus arteriosus beneath the pulmonary valve disappears and the conal tissue beneath the aortic valve usually (but not always) develops well. The *d*-loop and development of the subaortic conus arteriosus causes the aortic valve to be anterior to and slightly to the right of the pulmonary valve. The aorta arises from the normally placed anterior morphologic right ventricle (Fig 23–19). Involution of the subpulmonary conus arteriosus places the annuli of the

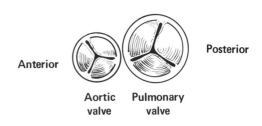

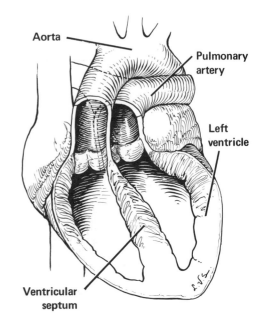

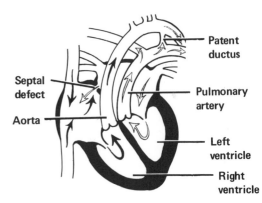

FIG 23–19. Typical transposition of the great arteries. The aorta arises from the morphologic right ventricle and is anterior to and slightly to the right of the pulmonary artery, which originates from the morphologic left ventricle. Inset at bottom illustrates the independent systemic and pulmonary circulations, which may be connected by a patent ductus arteriosus or atrial septal defect. Inset at top illustrates a common relationship of the 2 great arteries in typical transposition.

pulmonary and mitral valves in continuity. The pulmonary artery arises from the posterior left ventricle. The atria and ventricles are concordant: the right atrium empties into the right ventricle and the left atrium into the left ventricle. The coronary arteries arise from the aorta, but usually the right coronary orifice is anterior and slightly to the left.

Transposition of the great arteries causes the systemic and pulmonary circulations to be independent. Anatomic communication (ventricular septal defect, patent ductus arteriosus, atrial septal defect) between the separate circulations is required to mix oxygenated and unoxygenated blood. The degree of cyanosis is proportionate to the relative amount of oxygenated pulmonary venous blood that reaches the right ventricle and aorta. Nearly half of patients with typical transposition have an associated ventricular septal defect. The ductus arteriosus, which may mix pulmonary and systemic blood at birth, closes during early infancy in most patients. Atrial septal defects provide the third common anatomic communication between the independent circulations, but relatively few babies have large atrial septal defects. Approximately 30% of infants with transposition and ventricular septal defects also have subpulmonary stenosis within the left ventricle. About 5% of patients have subpulmonary stenosis with an intact ventricular septum. Single ventricle, persistent atrioventricular canal, total anomalous pulmonary venous connection, tricuspid atresia, and coarctation are less common anomalies associated with typical transposition of the great arteries.

Clinical Findings

A. Symptoms and Signs: Clinical findings in infancy are related to the presence or absence of a ventricular septal defect and subpulmonary stenosis. Infants with transposition and an intact ventricular septum are cyanotic at birth and develop severe cyanosis (arterial PO_2 15–30 mm Hg), acidosis, and hypoxic spells when the ductus arteriosus begins to close. Signs of heart failure—tachypnea, hepatomegaly, and cardiomegaly—are also present. Cardiac murmurs are usually not heard and, if present, are generally soft and nondiagnostic.

When a ventricular septal defect is present, cyanosis is less severe and hypoxic spells are generally absent. Heart failure may be severe, with hyperactive ventricles and severe respiratory distress. A faint systolic murmur or no murmur may be present. When transposition of the great arteries is combined with ventricular septal defect and subpulmonary stenosis, the heart is usually quiet and small and cyanosis is present without signs of heart failure. A faint or harsh systolic murmur is sometimes present over the precordium.

Older infants and children develop polycythemia and clubbing and grow slowly. The heart and liver are usually enlarged. The full clinical picture varies with specific associated lesions and previous palliative operations.

B. X-Ray Findings: In newborns, the heart may not appear enlarged and the thymic shadow may obscure the narrow mediastinal vascular pedicle. The aorta arises on the patient's right, and the pulmonary arterial segment is absent or diminished in the posteroanterior projection. After 1 or 2 weeks, cardiomegaly develops, and if pulmonary arterial blood flow is increased the lungs appear congested.

C. Electrocardiography: The ECG findings vary with the patient's age and associated lesions. In newborns, the ECG may be normal; older infants usually have some abnormal right ventricular hypertrophy. If subpulmonary stenosis is present, left ventricular hypertrophy may also be present.

D. Cardiac Catheterization and Cineangiocardiography: These studies are required to define the pathologic anatomy and physiology in patients with transposition of the great arteries. Systemic pressures are found in the right ventricle, and the catheter passes directly into the aorta. The pulmonary artery cannot be entered easily except when a large ventricular septal defect is present or when a special balloon catheter is used. In the absence of lung disease, arterial oxygen saturation in the pulmonary veins is normal. Pulmonary venous and left atrial pressures are usually elevated when pulmonary arterial blood flow exceeds systemic blood flow. Oxygen saturation of blood in the left ventricle is higher than that found in the aorta and right ventricle. Ventricular pressures are identical when a large ventricular septal defect is present. The route of the catheter and changes in blood oxygen saturation define the sites of mixing of the 2 circulations. Since the pulmonary and systemic circulations are independent, reliable calculations of shunt flows are not possible.

Cineangiocardiograms show that the aorta is located anterior to and slightly to the right of the pulmonary artery and that it fills from the right ventricle. The aortic valve is more superior than normal and is near the level of the fourth or fifth thoracic vertebra. The trabeculated, globular right ventricle is anterior to and to the right of the posterior left ventricle. Selective injections of contrast material and lateral and oblique views are necessary to demonstrate the conal anatomy and the presence of atrial and ventricular septal defects, pulmonary stenosis, patent ductus arteriosus, and other more complex cardiac anomalies.

Differential Diagnosis

In newborns, cyanosis may be caused by respiratory disease, tetralogy of Fallot, pulmonary or tricuspid atresia, total anomalous pulmonary venous connection with pulmonary venous obstruction, truncus arteriosus, Ebstein's anomaly, and atresia of the left heart. Newborns with tetralogy of Fallot usually do not develop heart failure early, and the aortic arch may be on the right. The combination of definite cyanosis and heart failure in a newborn suggests transposition of the great arteries and is sufficient indication for cardiac catheterization and cineangiocardiography.

Natural History

Without treatment, 50% of newborns with transposition of the great arteries die by 1 month of age and 90% die within 1 year after birth. Patients with intact ventricular septa have the worst prognosis, and survival beyond 1 year occurs only if a large atrial septal defect is also present. Patients with large ventricular septal defects and excessive pulmonary blood flow usually succumb during their first year from severe heart failure. Patients who have ventricular septal defect and mild or moderate subpulmonary stenosis have the best prognosis. The prognosis is particularly poor when more severe associated lesions are also present.

The combination of heart failure and severe hypoxia is the most common cause of death in infancy. Respiratory infections, systemic emboli, systemic infection, progressive pulmonary vascular disease, cerebral abscess, and occasionally cerebral venous thrombosis may cause death at any time in older infants and young children.

Patients who survive palliative procedures or operations may close their ventricular septal defects or may develop subpulmonary stenosis or pulmonary vascular disease. Approximately 15–20% of patients will close their ventricular septal defect or develop subpulmonary stenosis within the first 2 years after birth. Patients with transposition of the great arteries and increased pulmonary arterial blood flow develop pulmonary vascular disease more quickly than other patients who have increased pulmonary arterial blood flow from less complicated defects. Irreversible pulmonary vascular disease may develop within the first year after birth.

Treatment

Infants who are deeply cyanotic ($Pa_{O_2} < 35$ mm Hg) or who develop heart failure should be given oxygen and digoxin and should have cardiac catheterization. Enlargement or creation of an atrial septal defect by balloon catheter (Rashkind procedure) is recommended for virtually every patient who has transposition and who requires catheterization. The atrial septum is torn by rapidly pulling an inflated balloon from the left atrium into the right atrium. A large atrial septal defect improves blood mixing and obliterates the pressure difference between the left and right atria. A balloon septostomy is difficult to perform after 2 or 3 months of age because of increased thickness and strength of the atrial septum. These patients require either corrective or palliative operation.

Palliative operations for transposition of the great arteries include atrial septostomy (during inflow occlusion or by the Blalock-Hanlon technic), a systemic to pulmonary arterial anastomosis, or pulmonary arterial banding. Waterston or Blalock-Taussig systemic to pulmonary arterial anastomoses are performed for patients who have diminished pulmonary blood flow due to subpulmonary stenosis or a severe associated lesion (eg, pulmonary atresia). Pulmonary arterial banding may be recommended for patients who have increased pulmonary blood flows from a large ventricu-

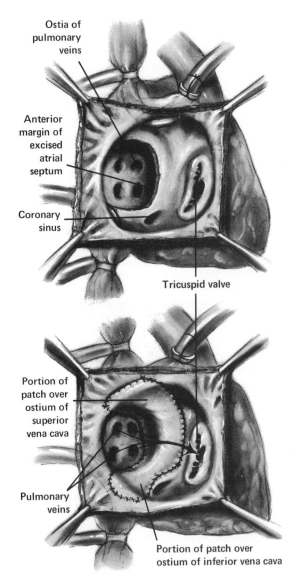

FIG 23–20. The Mustard operation. *A:* The atrial septum has been excised except for the anterior portion that contains the anterior intra-atrial conduction pathway. Pulmonary venous openings are visible at the posterior left atrial wall. *B:* A partition of pericardium or Dacron cloth is sutured around the left and right pulmonary venous openings, around the openings of the superior and inferior vena cavas, and to the anterior margin of the interatrial septum. Systemic venous blood then passes posterior to the partition toward the mitral valve. Pulmonary venous blood and blood from the coronary sinus pass anterior to the partition toward the tricuspid valve. A patch of Dacron or pericardium is often used to enlarge the right (now functional left) atrium when the atriotomy (not shown) is closed.

lar septal defect or single ventricle. Occasional patients require both atrial septostomy and either pulmonary arterial banding or a systemic to pulmonary arterial shunt. The Baffes operation, which connects the inferior vena cava to the stump of the right pulmonary vein and the distal right pulmonary veins to the right atrium, is no longer used.

Systemic venous blood can be redirected through the mitral valve, left ventricle, and pulmonary artery by insertion of a pericardial or Dacron partition in the atrium (Mustard operation; Fig 23–20). This baffle, which is sewn in place after the atrial septum is excised, redirects pulmonary venous blood into the right ventricle and aorta. This "corrective" operation converts the independent pulmonary and systemic circulations into a single circulatory system in series, but the morphologic right ventricle must support systemic blood pressure. Associated ventricular septal defects are usually closed via the atrium and tricuspid valve. Subpulmonary obstructive lesions often involve part of the mitral valve and are more difficult to relieve.

In selected patients with transposition of the great arteries, ventricular septal defect, and subpulmonary stenosis, blood flow from the left ventricle is redirected through the ventricular septal defect into the aorta by insertion of a patch within the right ventricle. A Dacron tube (conduit) that contains a homograft aortic valve is used to connect the right ventricle to the main pulmonary artery downstream to the obstruction and pulmonary valve (conduit operation; Fig 23–16B). The proximal pulmonary artery is closed. This procedure has the advantage that the morphologic left ventricle supports the systemic blood pressure and obviates the often impossible task of relieving the subpulmonary stenosis.

Prognosis After Surgery

After balloon atrial septostomy (Rashkind procedure), arterial oxygen saturation generally increases from about 40% to approximately 65%. Operative fatalities are rare, and over 80% of patients survive the initial hospitalization. The mortality rate from operative atrial septostomy is approximately 10%; the mortality rate after pulmonary arterial banding or a systemic to pulmonary arterial anastomosis is 15–20%. After palliative procedures, only 50% of patients reach 30 months of age.

The operative mortality rate of the Mustard atrial baffle operation is 5–10% in patients who do not have ventricular septal defects, subpulmonary stenosis, or severe associated anomalies. Although the mortality rate is slightly higher in infants less than 6 months of age, results are better than can be achieved with alternative procedures. The presence of an associated ventricular septal defect increases the operative mortality rate to approximately 30%. When subpulmonary stenosis is also present, the operative mortality rate for the atrial baffle procedure is about 50%. Postoperative complications include arrhythmias, partial obstruction of the superior vena cava, and pulmonary venous hypertension. Stenosis of the ostia of the pulmonary

veins and contraction of the baffle is a serious late complication that requires reoperation.

Breckenridge IM & others: Mustard's operation for transposition of the great arteries. Lancet 1:1140–1142, 1972.

Cornell WP & others: Results of the Blalock-Hanlon operation in 90 patients with transposition of the great vessels. J Thoracic Cardiovas Surg 52:525–532, 1966.

Mustard WT & others: The surgical management of transposition of the great vessels. J Thoracic Cardiovas Surg 48:953–958, 1964.

Noonan JA & others: Transposition of the great arteries: A correlation of clinical, physiologic and autopsy data. New England J Med 263:592–596, 637–642, 684–692, 1960.

Paul MH, Van Praagh S, Van Praagh R: Transposition of the great vessels. Chap 40, pp 576–610, in: *Paediatric Cardiology.* Watson H (editor). Mosby, 1968.

Rashkind WJ, Miller WW: Transposition of the great arteries: Results of palliation by balloon atrioseptostomy in 31 infants. Circulation 38:453–462, 1968.

CORRECTED TRANSPOSITION OF THE GREAT ARTERIES

Corrected transposition is a physiologic term which denotes one of 2 specific anatomic lesions. In patients with situs solitus and levocardia, this rare anomaly develops from *l*-looping of the cardiac tube and overdevelopment of the subaortic conus arteriosus. The aorta is anterior to and to the left of the posterior pulmonary artery (*l*-transposition). *L*-looping causes the morphologic left ventricle to be located anterior to and to the right of the posterior morphologic right ventricle. The lesion also occurs in patients with situs inversus and *d*-looping, with or without dextrocardia. Involution of the subpulmonary conus and development of the subaortic conus causes fibrous continuity of the pulmonary and anatomic mitral valve (functional right atrioventricular valve). The coronary arteries are inverted with the ventricles, so that the left coronary artery is anterior. When no associated lesions are present, systemic venous blood passes through the right atrium, mitral valve, and left ventricle and into the pulmonary artery. Pulmonary venous blood passes through the left atrium, tricuspid valve, and right ventricle and into the left-sided aorta. Thus, the atria and ventricles are discordant, and the ventricles and great arteries are also discordant. The normal physiologic circulation gives the lesion its name ("corrected transposition"). Unfortunately, malformations of the morphologic tricuspid valve (functional left atrioventricular valve), ventricular septal defect, arrhythmias, or subpulmonary or pulmonary valvular stenosis occur in over 90% of patients.

The clinical manifestations of corrected transpositions vary in relation to the associated lesions. Asymptomatic patients have small hearts, atrioventricular conduction delays, and occasionally mild incompetence of the anatomic tricuspid valve and very rarely may live a long life. Patients with large ventricular septal defects or tricuspid valvular incompetence (or both) develop severe heart failure and massive cardiomegaly in infancy and early childhood. Pulmonary stenosis with ventricular septal defect causes cyanosis with or without associated heart failure. Partial or complete atrioventricular heart block occurs in a high percentage of patients. More than half of patients with complicated lesions die in early childhood of heart failure or heart block.

In symptomatic patients, the posteroanterior chest film may suggest the diagnosis. The aortic knob is absent from the right mediastinal border, and the ascending aorta is displaced to the patient's left where it forms a straight left superior mediastinal border that tapers to a narrow waist. The heart may be massively enlarged, and pulmonary venous congestion may be increased. The ECG frequently shows atrioventricular conduction block. Inversion of the ventricles causes the normal q waves in the left ECG leads to be absent.

Cardiac catheterization and cineangiocardiography establish the diagnosis and the presence of associated lesions. Atrioventricular conduction disturbances occur frequently during catheterization. The passage of the catheter or angiocardiograms show the aorta anterior to and to the left of the pulmonary artery. Subaortic conal tissue pushes the aortic valve superiorly and separates the aorta and morphologic tricuspid annuli. The inverted positions of the ventricle can be determined from their anatomic characteristics. The lesion must be distinguished from typical *d*-transposition, tetralogy of Fallot, congenital mitral incompetence, and congenital heart block.

Operative management of symptomatic patients with corrected transposition is directed toward the associated lesions, but in general the results have not been satisfactory. Complete heart block with a slow ventricular rate and uncontrolled heart failure requires an implanted pacemaker with (preferably) epicardial leads. Ventricular septal defects can be closed, but technical difficulties due to the position of the coronary arteries, large size of the defects, and unknown course of the conduction bundle greatly increase the operative risk. Severe tricuspid (functional left atrioventricular valve) insufficiency requires prosthetic valve replacement. Subpulmonary stenosis is usually complicated, and a palliative systemic to pulmonary arterial anastomosis is recommended in preference to excision of the stenotic lesion.

Friedberg DZ, Nadas AS: Clinical profile of patients with congenital corrected transposition of the great arteries. New England J Med 282:1053–1059, 1970.

MALPOSITION OF THE GREAT ARTERIES

Malposition of the great arteries (excluding typical transposition, corrected transposition, and double outlet ventricles) occurs most frequently with situs inversus, dextrocardia, pulmonary atresia, single ventricle, and other severe cardiac lesions. Because of variations in the degree of conal development, direction of cardiac looping, and associated lesions, the pathologic anatomy of these lesions varies greatly. If a bilateral conus arteriosus is present, the fibrous skeletons of the semilunar valves are not in continuity with those of the atrioventricular valves. The degree of conal development beneath the 2 semilunar valves may vary; greater conal development pushes the adjacent semilunar valve cephalad and anterior. Conal development does not determine the relationship of the semilunar valves to each other; rather, this relationship is determined by the direction of cardiac looping (*d*-loop or *l*-loop).

Most patients with malposition of the great arteries do not survive infancy; however, a few patients reach childhood. The great variation in pathologic anatomy causes similar variation in circulatory dysfunction; thus, each individual must be carefully studied. The anatomic relationships of the cardiac subunits must be defined according to the diagnostic "rules" described previously. Although many lesions are inoperable, some carefully selected patients can be helped by operation.

DOUBLE OUTLET RIGHT VENTRICLE

In double outlet right ventricle, the aorta arises from the posterior wall of the right ventricle cephalad to the tricuspid valve and to the right of and posterior to the pulmonary artery (normal relationship of the great arteries). Rarely, the aorta may be directly anterior to or to the left of the pulmonary artery. As a rule, both coni arteriosi are well developed, and the semilunar valves are at the same level on the cephalad-caudad axis. A ventricular septal defect is invariably present, although in rare instances it may be small. Two variants of double outlet right ventricle are recognized depending upon the location of the ventricular septal defect beneath the aortic valve or directly beneath the pulmonary valve.

More commonly, the ventricular septal defect is located beneath the aortic valve. If associated lesions are not present, blood from the left ventricle streams through the ventricular septal defect into the aorta. These patients are acyanotic, often develop severe heart failure in infancy, and have equal pressures in the left and right ventricles. A systolic murmur is present along the left sternal border. The ECG shows right ventricular hypertrophy. Chest x-rays are not diagnostic, and the diagnosis must be made by cineangiocardiography. Cineangiocardiograms show that the aorta is displaced anteriorly and that the aortic and pulmonary valves are at the same level. Clinically, the lesion is similar to a large ventricular septal defect. If pulmonary stenosis is also present or if pulmonary vascular disease develops, the lesion must be differentiated from tetralogy of Fallot and typical transposition of the great arteries. In the absence of pulmonary vascular disease, the lesion can be corrected by placing a prosthetic tunnel between the ventricular septal defect and the aortic annulus so that the left ventricular blood passes directly into the aorta.

Occasionally, the ventricular septal defect is beneath the pulmonary valve and anterior (and cephalad) to the crista supraventricularis. Taussig-Bing malformation designates one variety of double outlet right ventricle with subpulmonary ventricular septal defect. (The aorta and pulmonary artery are positioned side by side, and a conus is present beneath each vessel.) Patients with double outlet right ventricle and subpulmonary ventricular septal defect are cyanotic from birth and often develop severe heart failure if pulmonary stenosis is not present. Left ventricular blood streams preferentially into the pulmonary artery. A loud pansystolic murmur is present along the left sternal border. Coarctation of the aorta is frequently present. Coarctation and pulmonary stenosis are the most common associated lesions with both types of double outlet right ventricle. Pulmonary vascular disease develops more rapidly in patients with subpulmonary ventricular septal defect and no pulmonary stenosis. The diagnosis is made in life on the basis of angiograms.

Pulmonary arterial banding is recommended for infants. The few patients that survive infancy without developing pulmonary vascular disease are candidates for a corrective operation. An intracardiac prosthetic tunnel is placed between the ventricular septal defect and the pulmonary annulus, and an atrial partition (Mustard operation) is inserted to direct systemic venous blood into the left atrium and ventricle.

Hightower BM & others: Double-outlet right ventricle with transposed great arteries and subpulmonary ventricular septal defect: The Taussig-Bing malformation. Circulation 39 (Suppl 1):207–213, 1968.

Kirklin JW, Harp RA, McGoon DC: Surgical treatment of origin of both vessels from right ventricle, including cases of pulmonary stenosis. J Thoracic Cardiovas Surg 48:1026–1036, 1964.

DOUBLE OUTLET LEFT VENTRICLE

Origin of both great arteries from a morphologic left ventricle is a rare anomaly. Like double outlet right ventricle, double outlet left ventricle may exist with the aorta to the right, anterior to, or to the left of the pulmonary artery, with or without a muscular conus beneath either or both great arteries. A ventricular septal defect must be present for survival. Pulmonary stenosis is usually present. Total correction by closing the ventricular septal defect and pulmonary valve and constructing a valved conduit from the right ventricle to the pulmonary artery has been performed in children. Occasionally, an intraventricular repair can

be performed by closing the ventricular septal defect so that the pulmonary artery is connected to the right ventricle.

Pacifico AD & others: Surgical treatment of double outlet left ventricle. Circulation 47 (Suppl 1), 1973.

CARDIAC MALPOSITION

Situs inversus totalis is a rare anomaly in which the stomach and other abdominal organs occupy positions which are the mirror images of normal (situs solitus). Except in asplenia and polysplenia (see below), the position of the viscera determines the location of the atrium; thus, in situs inversus, the atria are reversed and the heart is right-sided (dextrocardia). The morphologic left atrium is on the right. When the ventricles and atria are concordant, the right atrium (on the patient's left) empties into the anatomic right ventricle. If transposition is not present, the circulation is normal and the cardiac chambers and vessels are the mirror image of normal structures. If transposition is present, the aorta is anterior to the pulmonary artery in the right-sided heart.

Rather severe associated anomalies usually occur with situs inversus, dextrocardia, and malposition of the great arteries. If the atria and ventricles are discordant, transposition or malposition of the great arteries is always present and the lesion may be physiologically "corrected." In most cases, the aorta arises to the left of the pulmonary artery and severe associated anomalies are present.

Isolated levocardia is the remaining condition that occurs with situs inversus totalis. The heart is located in the left chest, and most patients have severe associated cardiac anomalies and agenesis of the left lung.

Isolated dextrocardia is the term used to designate mirror image position of the heart when the viscera are in normal position (situs solitus). Agenesis of the right lung is present in many of these patients.

Cardiac catheterization and cineangiocardiography are essential to understand the pathologic anatomy and physiology of these lesions. The diagnostic rules for locating the visceral situs, morphologic ventricles, and positions of the great vessels must be used to label each structure and chamber opacified by the contrast material.

Life expectancy is dependent upon the severity of the circulatory handicap. Some patients live to advanced age, and others can be helped by specific palliative operations to improve circulatory function. A few patients are candidates for totally corrective operations of less severe associated lesions.

Kirklin JW: Surgery for transposition, corrected transposition, and related complex anomalies. Pages 26–31 in: *Lecture Outlines, Postgraduate Course on Cardiovascular Surgery.* American College of Surgeons, 1970.

ASPLENIA & POLYSPLENIA

Absence of the spleen, midline position of the stomach and liver (indeterminate situs), distinct middle lobes of both right and left lungs, and Howell-Jolly bodies within red cells are associated with severe cardiac anomalies. About a third of such patients have dextrocardia. Single atrium, single ventricle, atrioventricular canal, transposition, pulmonary atresia, and anomalies of systemic and pulmonary venous return may occur. These patients are abnormally susceptible to bacterial infections, particularly pneumococcal infections.

Many small spleens, interruption of the hepatic portion of the inferior vena cava, absence of middle pulmonary lobes in both lungs, and absence of the gallbladder are associated with the same severe cardiac anomalies listed above with the exception of transposition.

Moller JH & others: Congenital cardiac disease associated with polysplenia. Circulation 36:789–799, 1967.

V. MISCELLANEOUS CONGENITAL HEART LESIONS

CONGENITAL HEART BLOCK

Complete atrioventricular dissociation occurs as an isolated lesion or in association with other congenital cardiac anomalies, particularly corrected transposition of the great vessels, atrial septal defect, and endocardial fibroelastosis. The cardiac rate is generally higher (40–80 beats per minute) than that which occurs in adults or in children who have complete heart block as a result of intracardiac surgery. The diagnosis is made by ECG. A few patients will develop Adams-Stokes syncopal attacks; others—particularly those with associated lesions—develop heart failure. Sudden death may occur in patients who have Adams-Stokes attacks. Digoxin is not recommended in these patients, but diuretics may help to control heart failure. Medical therapy also includes sublingual isoproterenol, but symptomatic patients are best treated with an implanted electrical pacemaker with epicardial electrodes.

CONGENITAL MITRAL INSUFFICIENCY

In children, mitral insufficiency is usually due to rheumatic valvulitis; in rare cases, however, congenital abnormalities of the mitral valve or chordae tendineae may cause mitral incompetence. Congenital mitral insufficiency usually occurs in association with other lesions such as persistent atrioventricular canal, coarctation of the aorta, anomalous left coronary artery, or corrected transposition of the great arteries. Rarely, isolated mitral insufficiency which results from deformed mitral leaflets, short, thick chordae tendineae, dilatation of the mitral annulus, or cleft leaflets may occur.

The severity of the insufficiency is variable. In severe cases, left heart failure with pulmonary venous congestion causes fatigue, poor weight gain, dyspnea, and palpitations. A pansystolic murmur is maximal at the apex and is transmitted to the left axilla. The ECG shows left ventricular hypertrophy, and chest films show cardiomegaly with left atrial enlargement and pulmonary venous congestion. The diagnosis and severity of the mitral incompetence can be assessed at cardiac catheterization; however, cineangiocardiograms do not provide sufficient detail to indicate whether or not mitral valvuloplasty is possible.

Children with poorly controlled heart failure require operation. Operation is not recommended for those with mild or moderate symptoms. Valvuloplasty and annuloplasty are preferable to valve replacement. Unfortunately, almost half of patients require valve replacement.

ANOMALOUS LEFT CORONARY ARTERY

Origin of the left coronary artery from the pulmonary artery causes myocardial ischemia and heart failure in infancy. The right coronary artery is normal and supplies blood to the entire myocardium via intracoronary collaterals. Blood flow in the anomalous left coronary artery is usually retrograde into the pulmonary artery; however, the amount of left-to-right shunting is small. The left ventricle is dilated and fibrotic, has paradoxic motion, and contracts poorly. During feeding or other activity, infants develop episodic pain, pallor, sweating, and tachypnea which suggests angina pectoris. The heart progressively enlarges, and an apical systolic murmur of mitral insufficiency occasionally develops if the papillary muscle is infarcted. The ECG often shows evidence of myocardial infarction in the left limb and precordial leads. Chest films confirm the gross cardiomegaly and pulmonary venous congestion. The diagnosis is made by cineangiocardiography. Contrast material opacifies only the right coronary artery after injection into the aortic root. The left coronary artery can often be faintly seen in late frames. An increase in oxygen saturation in the main pulmonary artery is not always found and is seldom diagnostic.

A few infants with mild symptoms can be managed medically until the aorta and left coronary artery can be connected by a saphenous vein graft (usually age 4–5 years). Most infants have severe heart failure and arrhythmias which do not respond to medical management. Recently, a subclavian-coronary anastomosis successfully established antegrade flow in the anomalous left coronary of an infant. Previously, ligation of the anomalous left coronary artery at its origin was recommended to improve myocardial blood flow from the right coronary artery. Although some infants do well after ligation of the anomalous coronary artery, both early and late mortality is high because of persistent left ventricular failure.

PULMONARY ARTERIOVENOUS FISTULA

In 50% of patients, this rare vascular anomaly is associated with multiple telangiectases (Rendu-Osler-Weber syndrome). One or more large arteriovenous fistulas that do not communicate with alveolar capillaries may occur anywhere in the lungs but are most commonly present in the lower lobes. Pulmonary arterial blood shunts through the fistula into the pulmonary veins to cause mild to moderate cyanosis. Pulmonary arterial and venous pressures are low. Occasional infants develop dyspnea, cyanosis, and right heart failure. Cyanosis, clubbing, and polycythemia are usually most pronounced in late childhood. A soft systolic or continuous murmur is occasionally present over the fistula. Chest x-rays show irregular opacified lesions in the peripheral lung fields at the site of the fistulas. The lesion is confirmed by cineangiocardiography after right ventricular or pulmonary arterial injection. Excision of the fistula is indicated in symptomatic patients and in patients with solitary lesions but is not generally recommended for patients with multiple lesions. Localized resections or lobectomy are most commonly performed.

PULMONARY ARTERIAL STENOSIS

Single or multiple stenoses of the pulmonary arteries occur commonly at the bifurcation of the main pulmonary artery but may occur anywhere between the pulmonary valve and the tertiary pulmonary arteries. About two-thirds of patients have pulmonary valvular stenosis, tetralogy of Fallot, ventricular septal defects, or patent ductus arteriosus. The stenotic lesions produce harsh systolic murmurs which are not well localized. The location of the stenotic areas is determined by observation of a pressure difference during catheterization of the main pulmonary arteries and by cineangiocardiograms after injection of contrast material into the right ventricle.

Patients without associated congenital heart lesions usually do not require operation. Supravalvular stenosis or hypoplasia of the main pulmonary artery or proximal portions of the right or left pulmonary arteries is usually treated by enlargement with pericardial or Dacron patches during correction of associated intracardiac lesions.

PERSISTENT LEFT SUPERIOR VENA CAVA

Persistence of a left superior vena cava which connects the left jugular and subclavian veins to the coronary sinus causes no symptoms but is not uncommon. The anomaly is important to the surgeon since a separate catheter must be inserted through the coronary sinus into the left superior vena cava to collect systemic venous blood during cardiopulmonary bypass. Rarely, the right superior vena cava is absent; in most cases, an innominate vein and both left and right cavas are present and each cava is adequate to carry all of the systemic venous return from the upper body.

ENDOCARDIAL FIBROELASTOSIS

This lesion is not operable, but it may occur in association with operable lesions such as coarctation of the aorta, aortic stenosis, anomalous left coronary artery, and mitral valvular disease. Hyperplasia of subendocardial elastic and collagenous tissue and proliferation of capillaries causes marked thickening of the ventricular wall and a smooth, glistening lining of the left ventricle. Trabeculae are obliterated, and papillary muscles and chordae tendineae are contracted. The disease affects principally the left ventricle and left atrium; involvement of the right heart chambers is rare.

Fibroelastosis affects 1–2% of patients with congenital heart disease and may occur primarily without other cardiac lesions. Nearly all infants die of left heart failure within the first year. No specific therapy is available.

• • •

General References

Nadas AS, Fyler DC: *Pediatric Cardiology.* Saunders, 1972.

Watson H (editor): *Paediatric Cardiology.* Mosby, 1968.

24 . . .

The Esophagus & Diaphragm

Orville F. Grimes, MD

I. THE ESOPHAGUS

Surgery of the esophagus has made significant progress in the past 25 years as improvements in anesthesia and other refinements have allowed esophageal operations to be performed with acceptable morbidity and mortality rates. Before the early 1930s, surgical procedures involving the esophagus were limited largely to the cervical and intra-abdominal segments.

ANATOMY
(See Fig 24—1.)

The esophagus is a muscular tube which serves as a conduit for the passage of food from the pharynx to the stomach. It originates at the level of the sixth cervical vertebra posterior to the cricoid cartilage. In the thorax, the esophagus passes behind the aortic arch and the left main stem bronchus, enters the abdomen through the esophageal hiatus of the diaphragm, and terminates in the fundus of the stomach. Its muscle fibers originate from the cricoid cartilage and pharynx above and interdigitate with those of the stomach below. About 2—4 cm of esophagus normally lie below the diaphragm. The junction between the esophagus and stomach is maintained in its normal intra-abdominal position by reflections of the peritoneum onto the stomach and the phrenoesophageal ligament onto the esophagus. The latter is a fibroelastic membrane which lies beneath the peritoneum, on the inferior surface of the diaphragm. When it reaches the esophageal hiatus, the ligament is reflected orad onto the lower esophagus, where it inserts into the circular muscle layer above the gastroesophageal sphincter, 2—4 cm above the diaphragm.

Three anatomic areas of narrowing occur in the esophagus: (1) at the level of the cricoid cartilage (pharyngoesophageal sphincter); (2) in the midthorax, from compression by the aortic arch and the left main stem bronchus; and (3) as it passes through the esophageal hiatus of the diaphragm (gastroesophageal sphincter).

In the adult, the length of the esophagus as measured from the upper incisor teeth to the cricopharyngeus muscle is 15—20 cm; to the aortic arch, 20—25 cm; to the inferior pulmonary vein, 30—35 cm; and to the cardioesophageal junction, approximately 40—45 cm.

The musculature of the pharynx and upper third of the esophagus is skeletal in type; the remainder is smooth muscle. Physiologically, the entire organ behaves as a single functioning unit so that no distinction can be made between the upper and lower esophagus from the standpoint of propulsive activity. As in the intestinal tract, the muscle fibers are arranged into inner circular and outer longitudinal layers.

The arterial supply to the esophagus is quite consistent. The upper end is supplied by branches from the inferior thyroid arteries. The thoracic portion receives elements from the bronchial arteries and from esophageal branches originating directly from the aorta. The intercostal arteries may also contribute. The diaphragmatic and abdominal segments are nourished by the left inferior phrenic artery and by the esophageal branches of the left gastric artery.

The venous drainage is more complex and variable. The most important veins are those that drain the lower esophagus. Blood from this region passes into the esophageal branches of the coronary vein, a tributary of the portal vein. This connection constitutes a direct communication between the portal circulation and the venous drainage of the lower esophagus and upper stomach. When the portal system is obstructed, as in cirrhosis of the liver, blood is shunted upward through the coronary vein and the esophageal venous plexus, to eventually pass by way of the azygos vein into the superior vena cava. As they become distended from the increased blood flow and pressure, the esophageal veins may eventually form varices.

The mucosal lining of the esophagus consists of stratified squamous epithelium which contains scattered mucous glands throughout. The esophagus has no serosal layer, and for this reason does not heal as readily after injury or surgical anastomosis as other portions of the gastrointestinal tract.

PHYSIOLOGY

Advances have been made in recent years in understanding the physiology and pathophysiology of the esophagus using cineradiography and measurements of intraluminal pressures. Manometric technics

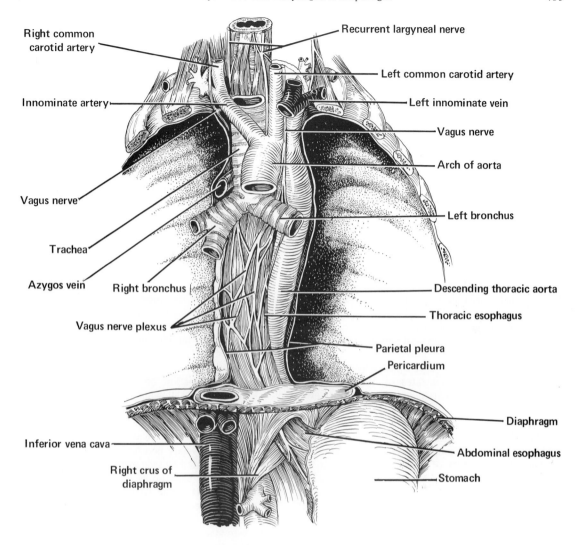

Right common carotid artery

Recurrent largyneal nerve

Innominate artery

Left common carotid artery

Left innominate vein

Vagus nerve

Arch of aorta

Vagus nerve

Left bronchus

Trachea

Azygos vein

Right bronchus

Descending thoracic aorta

Thoracic esophagus

Vagus nerve plexus

Parietal pleura

Pericardium

Diaphragm

Inferior vena cava

Abdominal esophagus

Right crus of diaphragm

Stomach

FIG 24–1. Anatomy of the esophagus.

have found valuable application in the study of a variety of diseases of the esophagus, and facilities for esophageal manometry are now available in many hospitals. The examination consists of passing into the esophagus a bundle of 2 or 3 fine polyethylene catheters each of which contains a small distal opening. Continuous perfusion of these tubes with small volumes of saline solution ensures patency of their orifices and offers a slight resistance to squeeze. The openings are situated 5 cm apart so that simultaneous recording of pressure can be made at intervals over a segment of known length. Pressures are measured in the resting state by slowly withdrawing the catheters from the stomach toward the pharynx. Pressures are recorded within the stomach, the gastroesophageal sphincter, the body of the esophagus, and the pharyngoesophageal sphincter. Additional data are obtained

during swallowing and other movements which may shed light on the suspected disorder.

Correlation of the findings of esophageal motility studies and cineradiology provides a great deal of data on which to base opinions about the causes of dysphagia and odynophagia. Measurement of intraesophageal pH and electrical potential differences may be of clinical value in some instances, but the extent of their usefulness remains to be determined.

The function of the esophagus is to transport food and fluids from the mouth to the stomach and occasionally in the reverse direction. The esophagus contains a sphincter at the junction of the pharynx and esophagus (pharyngoesophageal sphincter) and another between the esophagus and stomach (gastroesophageal sphincter). Pressures in the resting state as measured by manometry are higher in the region of these sphincters than on either side. Pressures in the mouth and pharynx are atmospheric; those within the body of the resting esophagus are slightly subatmospheric, a reflection of normal intrathoracic pressure. Pressure within the stomach is slightly greater than atmospheric.

The structures at the gastroesophageal junction normally function efficiently to prevent reflux of gastric acid and food from the stomach into the esophagus. The mechanism of gastroesophageal competence is complex and, despite intensive study, is incompletely understood at present.

The gastroesophageal sphincter comprises the lower 4 cm of esophagus, where resting pressure within the lumen normally exceeds intragastric pressure by 15−25 cm water due to tonic contraction of the esophageal musculature. The failure of excision of periesophageal structures to change the pressure indicates that it originates from the sphincter itself rather than the diaphragmatic crura or phrenoesophageal ligament. Careful dissection of the terminal esophagus has not demonstrated a separate anatomic counterpart of the special function of this area, and it is often referred to as a physiologic sphincter. However, if disease or surgical trauma injures the esophageal muscle at this point, gastroesophageal reflux may result.

The strength of the tonic squeeze by the gastroesophageal sphincter is regulated by the gastrointestinal hormones gastrin (strengthens) and secretin (weakens), but whether these are physiologic actions of these hormones is debated.

Many types of normal daily activity result in increases in intra-abdominal pressure. It was thought for years that the lack of reflux of gastric contents under these circumstances was normally due to the presence of an intra-abdominal segment of esophagus which transmitted the pressure increment to the sphincter, thus counterbalancing rises within the stomach. Later studies have now shown that pressure in the sphincter increases in response to induced rises in gastric pressure regardless of the position of the gastroesophageal junction relative to the diaphragm. For example, asymptomatic subjects with large hiatal hernias have an elevation of sphincteric pressure following abdominal compression which is quantitatively identical with that in patients whose sphincter resides below the diaphragm. The mechanism of this response has not yet been elucidated, but its rapid onset suggests a neural reflex.

When swallowing is begun, the tongue propels the bolus of food into the pharynx. Coordinated voluntary movement of the pharyngeal structures results in closure of the glottis and the nasopharynx. The glottis and pharynx rise during this maneuver, and the normal resting high-pressure zone at the pharyngoesophageal sphincter decreases, permitting entry of the food into the upper esophagus. After the food has traversed the pharynx and the pharyngoesophageal sphincter, the pharyngeal musculature relaxes and the high pressure zone returns at the pharyngoesophageal sphincter. As the bolus of food enters the esophagus, a peristaltic wave begins which travels toward the stomach at a

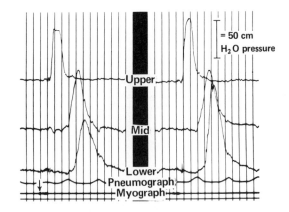

FIG 24−2. **Deglutition.** Esophageal peristaltic pressure sequence during consecutive swallows in health. The vertical lines are 1 inch apart.

speed of 4−6 cm/sec, propelling the food before it. The act of swallowing is a reflex response integrated in the medulla oblongata. When the subject is in the upright position, liquids and semisolid foods usually fall to the distal esophagus by gravity ahead of the slower peristaltic wave. The gastroesophageal sphincter relaxes in anticipation of the advancing food and peristalsis, thereby allowing the bolus to be transported into the stomach. After the food passes through, the sphincter regains its tone until another peristaltic wave arrives from above.

The term primary peristalsis denotes the wave of contraction initiated by swallowing which begins in the upper esophagus and travels the entire length of the organ (Fig 24−2). Local stimulation by distention at any point in the body of the esophagus will elicit a peristaltic wave from the point of the stimulus. This is called secondary peristalsis and aids esophageal emptying when the primary wave has failed to clear the lumen of ingested food or when gastric contents reflux from the stomach. Tertiary waves are stationary nonpropulsive contractions that may occur in any portion of the esophagus. Tertiary waves are considered abnormal, but they are frequently present in elderly subjects who have no symptoms of esophageal disease.

Incompetence of the gastroesophageal sphincter takes place normally during vomiting. During this event, the gastroesophageal junction rises above the level of the diaphragmatic hiatus. Ascent is probably the result of contraction of the longitudinal musculature of the esophagus; an additional result is effacement of the mucosal rosette. Expulsion of gastric contents by the violent contractions of the gastric antrum and abdominal wall then becomes possible. After vomiting has subsided, the structures resume their ordinary relationships with the gastroesophageal junction below the level of the diaphragm.

The buccopharyngeal and esophageal structures engaged in swallowing and transmission of food to the stomach are innervated by motor fibers from the fifth, seventh, ninth, tenth, 11th, and 12th cranial nerves.

Afferent sensory impulses are important in maintaining coordination of the motor activity.

Castell DO, Harris LD: Hormonal control of gastroesophageal-sphincter strength. New England J Med 282:886–889, 1970.

Cohen S, Harris LD: Lower esophageal sphincter pressure as an index of lower esophageal sphincter strength. Gastroenterology 58:157–162, 1970.

Cohen S, Harris LD: Does hiatal hernia affect competence of the gastroesophageal sphincter? New England J Med 284:1053–1056, 1971.

Cohen S, Lipshutz W: Hormonal regulation of human lower esophageal sphincter competence: Interaction of gastrin and secretin. J Clin Invest 50:449–454, 1971.

Davenport HW: Chewing and swallowing. Chap 1, pp 13–27, in: *Physiology of the Digestive Tract.* Year Book, 1971.

Edwards DAW: The esophagus. Gut 12:948–956, 1971.

Kaye MD, Showalter JP: Normal deglutitive responses of the human lower esophageal sphincter. Gut 13:352–360, 1972.

Lind JF & others: Responses of the gastroesophageal junctional zone to increases in abdominal pressure. Canad J Surg 9:32–38, 1966.

Lipshutz W, Cohen S: Physiological determinants of lower esophageal sphincter function. Gastroenterology 61:16–24, 1971.

Lipshutz W & others: The genesis of lower esophageal sphincter pressure: Its identification through the use of gastrin antiserum. J Clin Invest 51:522–529, 1972.

Lund WS: A study of the cricopharyngeal sphincter in man and in the dog. Ann Roy Coll Surg England 37:225–246, 1965.

Rosenow EC III: Esophageal motility. M Clin North America 54:863–873, 1970.

ESOPHAGEAL MOTILITY DISORDERS

Disturbances of the neuromuscular elements of the esophagus can result either in hypermotility or hypomotility disorders.

DIFFUSE ESOPHAGEAL SPASM

Essentials of Diagnosis

- Dysphagia, substernal pain.
- Nervous temperament, intermittency of symptoms.
- Fluoroscopic, cineradiographic, and manometric evidence of hyperperistalsis.

General Considerations

Diffuse spasm of the esophagus is accompanied by irregular uncoordinated peristaltic movements and intermittent spasm of the cardioesophageal junction. Hypermotility is probably caused by an abnormal interplay of the sympathetic and parasympathetic nerve impulses to the esophagus, although the exact cause remains obscure. It has no known relationship to the development of esophageal cancer.

Clinical Findings

A. Symptoms and Signs: Weight loss is uncommon despite the presence of dysphagia. Intermittency of symptoms is characteristic. Substernal distress varying from slight discomfort to severe, colicky pain occurs frequently. The pain often simulates that of coronary artery disease and may result in a highly nervous temperament, so that a diagnosis of psychoneurosis often is made.

B. X-Ray Findings: The esophagogram is abnormal in 60% of these patients. Fluoroscopic studies show segmental spasms, areas of narrowing, and irregular uncoordinated peristalsis. A small hiatal hernia is frequently demonstrated; less commonly, an epiphrenic diverticulum is present.

C. Manometry: Manometric studies show wide variations in pressure measurements with abolition of normal peristaltic waves. Occasionally, the lower esophagus alone may have irregular, uncoordinated muscular contractions while the proximal portions show normal peristaltic waves. More often, however, the entire esophagus is involved. Many of the patients with symptomatic diffuse spasm have a demonstrable hypersensitivity to methacholine.

Differential Diagnosis

The symptoms produced by diffuse spasm must be distinguished from those produced by heart disease, mediastinal tumors, benign and malignant esophageal tumors, and scleroderma. Although radiologic and pressure studies are diagnostically accurate, esophagoscopy should be performed to confirm the absence of intraluminal lesions such as esophagitis which often produce esophageal spasm.

Complications

Sliding hiatal hernia and epiphrenic diverticula may be secondary complications of the uncoordinated and severe contractions of the esophagus. Regurgitation and aspiration may occur, possibly leading to repeated pneumonic infections. In general, however, the condition is usually mild and does not lead to serious complications. The syndrome of gastroesophageal hypercontracting sphincter is not a separate entity from diffuse spasm, although in the latter the sphincter is usually normal.

Treatment

Antispasmodic medications are of little benefit. A soft diet taken in 5–6 small feedings daily may be required, especially when dysphagia is the most prominent symptom. Recently, a lengthy extramucous cardiomyotomy extending along the entire body of the esophagus has been used, with benefit to 50–60% of patients. The esophageal musculature is divided in a linear fashion to the level of the submucosa throughout the thoracic esophagus to include the cardioesophageal sphincter. In this way, the abnormal muscular motility affects only a portion of the circumference of the esophagus, thereby diminishing the severity of the muscular spasm of the esophagus.

Bennett JR, Hendrix TR: Diffuse esophageal spasm: A disorder with more than one cause. Gastroenterology 59:273–279, 1970.

Ellis FH Jr & others: Surgical treatment of esophageal hypermotility disturbances. JAMA 188:862–866, 1964.

Fleshler B: Diffuse esophageal spasm. Gastroenterology 52:559–564, 1967.

Garrett JM, Godwin DH: Gastroesophageal hypercontracting sphincter. JAMA 208:992–998, 1969.

Gillies M & others: Clinical, manometric, and pathological studies in diffuse oesophageal spasm. Brit MJ 2:527–530, 1967.

Kramer P & others: Oesophageal sensitivity to Mecholyl in symptomatic diffuse spasm. Gut 8:120–127, 1967.

Stiennon OA: On the cause of tertiary contractions and related disturbances of the esophagus. Am J Roentgenol 104:617–624, 1968.

Zboralski FF, Dodds WJ: Roentgenographic diagnosis of primary disorders of esophageal motility. Radiol Clin North America 7:147–162, 1969.

HYPOMOTILITY

Achalasia of the esophagus is the most common condition among the hypomotile states. Occasionally an esophagus almost totally devoid of peristalsis is encountered without true achalasia. Dysphagia results from the lack of propulsive muscular action, so that food cannot be effectively propelled downward. Perhaps because the cardioesophageal sphincter region is moderately spastic, these patients may gain some relief from esophageal bougienage.

ACHALASIA OF THE ESOPHAGUS

Essentials of Diagnosis

- Dysphagia.
- Retention of ingested food in the esophagus.
- Radiologic evidence of absent primary peristalsis, a dilated proximal esophagus, and a conically narrow cardioesophageal junction.
- Weak, uncoordinated, or absent peristalsis by manometry and cineradiography.

General Considerations

Achalasia of the esophagus is a neuromuscular disorder in which esophageal dilatation and hypertrophy occur without organic stenosis. Peristalsis is greatly diminished or absent. The musculature at the cardioesophageal junction fails to relax in response to the stimulus of food reaching this level. The circular muscle layer hypertrophies, while the longitudinal coat retains its normal thickness. Although the cause is not clearly understood, it is now generally accepted that achalasia develops on a neurogenic basis. The absence, atrophy, or disintegration of the ganglion cells of Auerbach's myenteric plexuses in many patients with achalasia lends support to this concept. The causes of the changes in the ganglia are obscure. Selective destruction of the dorsal motor nuclei of the vagus nerves in the medulla in experimental animals has produced similar changes. Achalasia affects males more often than females and may develop at any age. The peak years are 30–60. Carcinoma in association with achalasia is uncommon but occurs with greater frequency than in the general population.

Clinical Findings

A. Symptoms and Signs: Dysphagia is the dominant symptom, but weight loss is not usually marked despite the functional obstruction. The dilated esophagus is able to contain large quantities of food which only gradually pass into the stomach, largely by gravity. Pain is infrequent even though shallow ulcerations may be produced in the mucosa by the retention and disintegration of ingested food. Regurgitation is common, especially during the night while the patient sleeps in a recumbent position. Aspiration may lead to repeated bouts of pneumonia.

B. X-Ray Findings: Radiologic studies demonstrate the classic features even in early achalasia. The narrowing at the cardia has a characteristic contour. The dilated body of the esophagus blends into a smooth cone-shaped area of narrowing 3–6 cm long. On fluoroscopy the peristaltic waves are weak, simultaneous, irregular, uncoordinated, or absent. As the disease progresses, the esophagus dilates further, becomes tortuous, and, in far-advanced cases, sigmoid in shape. The lowermost segment retains the classical long linear narrowing even in the late stages of the disease. The column of barium is held up at the narrowed area because the sphincteric mechanism fails to relax normally.

C. Manometry: Manometric studies are of value in confirming the diagnosis and are more sensitive than cineradiography, although in practice both are often obtained. A motility pattern characteristic of the condition can be recognized. The cricopharyngeus pinchcock has a normal action; the body of the esophagus is devoid of primary peristaltic waves, but simultaneous disorganized muscular activity may be present. Occasionally, no peristalsis of any sort can be observed. The pressure in the gastroesophageal sphincter is greater than normal, and relaxation after swallowing is incomplete. The subcutaneous administration of methacholine, 5–10 mg, results in a forceful sustained contraction of the lower two-thirds of the esophagus which is often briefly painful. This response is a manifestation of autonomic denervation of the organ and does not occur in normal subjects. A positive response is not entirely specific for achalasia but is also noted in symptomatic diffuse spasm and suggests that the 2 conditions share some pathophysiologic characteristics. In fact, progression of typical diffuse spasm to typical achalasia has been documented, although it must be fairly uncommon.

Differential Diagnosis

Clinically and radiographically, scleroderma is the esophageal lesion which most closely mimics achalasia. In both instances, dilatation and lack of peristalsis are noted. However, in early scleroderma the long, conical, smoothly tapered region in the lower esophagus is not seen. Furthermore, the cardioesophageal sphincter in scleroderma is widely patent instead of narrowed, so that free reflux of gastric contents can frequently be observed fluoroscopically in scleroderma but is almost totally absent in achalasia. The incompetent sphincter in scleroderma results in peptic esophagitis, which often leads to distal narrowing by stricture. When this stage is reached, the radiologic appearances of achalasia and scleroderma may be identical, consisting of a widely dilated body and a narrow distal segment. Cine-radiography, manometry, and esophagoscopy may be required to differentiate the two. In scleroderma, peristalsis is usually preserved in the skeletal muscle portion of the esophagus, whereas the entire organ is affected in achalasia. The esophagus in scleroderma does not exhibit a response to methacholine.

Benign strictures of the lower esophagus and carcinoma at or near the cardioesophageal junction are important conditions to be distinguished from achalasia. In both, however, the huge dilatation of the proximal esophagus seen frequently in both achalasia and in scleroderma does not occur. Motility studies are helpful since in organic stenosis vigorous peristalsis occurs in response to the obstruction. Esophagoscopy should always be performed to aid in establishing the diagnosis and also to rule out other intraluminal esophageal conditions. Although a positive methacholine test (see above) is confirmatory when added to the classic radiographic findings, it is not exclusively diagnostic of achalasia since positive responses can be obtained in diffuse esophageal spasm and in cases of carcinoma of the upper stomach in which submucosal spread upward into the esophagus has occurred.

Complications

Small mucosal ulcerations may develop from the irritation caused by retained food, but true peptic ulceration or massive hemorrhage is rare in achalasia. Aspiration of regurgitated esophageal contents may lead to repeated episodes of pneumonitis, tracheobronchitis, and, rarely, asphyxiation. Malnutrition is rarely severe in spite of the functional obstruction at the cardia. Although carcinoma may occasionally be seen in association with achalasia, it is not yet known if earlier treatment of the esophageal stasis would prevent malignant degeneration.

Treatment

Antispasmodic drugs exert no appreciable benefit. The aim of therapy is to relieve the functional obstruction at the cardia. This can be accomplished either by forceful dilatation of the lower esophagus or by a direct surgical approach.

In order for bougienage to be successful, the dilating devices must expand the narrowed cardia in a forceful manner so that the esophageal musculature is briskly stretched and perhaps some fibers are actually divided. Although a pneumatic dilator is used most often, a hydrostatic dilator is preferred by some endoscopists. Occasionally in elderly or poor-risk patients, the cardia can be kept reasonably patent with the use of mercury-weighted (Hurst) dilators which the patient may swallow himself as necessary. The column of mercury inside the smooth-tipped rubber dilator slowly allows the instrument to pass safely through into the stomach by gravity.

Most patients are treated initially by forceful bougienage. However, the patient who has far-advanced achalasia in which the esophagus has become hugely dilated and tortuous is best treated surgically. Forceful dilatation as the first therapeutic maneuver is successful in approximately 50% of patients. An additional 35% achieve an adequate swallowing mechanism by a second forceful bougienage.

Approximately 15% of patients with achalasia will require an operative procedure either because of failure of forceful dilatation or because the esophagus is so deformed and distorted that bougienage would be extremely hazardous. Forceful dilatation is not without danger since esophageal perforation occurs in 3–5% of cases.

The extramucous cardiomyotomy of Heller provides good overall results and is now the surgical procedure used almost exclusively throughout the world. The longitudinal myotomy extends from the level of the inferior pulmonary ligament downward onto the upper stomach. The incision is about 10–12 cm long and extends no more than 1 cm in its gastric portion. Care is taken to divide all of the muscular fibers since, if a few tiny circular fibers remain undivided, dysphagia may continue. Reflux is uncommon following cardiomyotomy, and results are good to excellent in 90% of patients. In the remaining few patients, some degree of swallowing difficulty may remain—due either to an inadequate myotomy or to the extensive paralysis of the body of the esophagus.

Prognosis

Relief of obstructive symptoms can be obtained by forceful dilatation or by surgery in at least 85% of patients. A properly performed modified Heller procedure overcomes the functional obstruction and only rarely leads to esophageal reflux. The addition of vagotomy and gastric drainage operations to the myotomy procedure is unnecessary.

Cohen S, Lipshutz W: Lower esophageal sphincter dysfunction in achalasia. Gastroenterology 61:814–820, 1971.

Cohen S & others: Role of gastrin supersensitivity in the pathogenesis of lower esophageal sphincter hypertension in achalasia. J Clin Invest 50:1241–1247, 1971.

Ellis FG: The natural history of achalasia. Proc Roy Soc Med 53:663–666, 1960.

Ellis FH Jr, Olsen AM: *Achalasia of the Esophagus.* Saunders, 1969.

Grimes OF, Stephens HB, Margulis AR: Achalasia of the esophagus. Am J Surg 120:198–202, 1970.

Just-Viera JO, Haight C: Achalasia and carcinoma of the esophagus. Surg Gynec Obst 128:1081–1095, 1969.

Kramer P & others: Transition from symptomatic diffuse spasm to cardiospasm. Gut 8:115–119, 1967.

Patrick DL & others: Reoperation for achalasia of the esophagus. Arch Surg 103:122–128, 1971.

Sanderson DR & others: Syndrome of vigorous achalasia: Clinical and physiologic observations. Dis Chest 52:508–517, 1967.

Smith B: The neurological lesion in achalasia of the cardia. Gut 11:388–391, 1970.

Vantrappen G & others: Treatment of achalasia with pneumatic dilatations. Gut 12:268–275, 1971.

SCLERODERMA & RELATED PROBLEMS IN ESOPHAGEAL MOTILITY

Scleroderma and several other systemic diseases occasionally involve the esophagus. When the esophageal symptoms overshadow other manifestations of the disease, the diagnosis may sometimes be difficult.

Esophageal dysfunction occurs commonly in patients with scleroderma. The initial symptoms are usually those of reflux: regurgitation, heartburn, and, occasionally, bleeding. Dysphagia is a less common complaint until esophagitis progresses to stricture formation. The esophageal symptoms usually appear in patients with the characteristic skin changes and Raynaud's syndrome. However, a number of cases have been reported where the motility defects were noted long before other findings of the disease.

The principal abnormality is atrophy and fibrosis of the esophageal smooth muscle, resulting in progressively weakening function. The changes affect the smooth muscle portion of the esophagus and are most marked at the gastroesophageal sphincter. The motility disorder can be recognized by manometry and cineradiography as relatively specific for this disease. The most noticeable abnormality is a patulous gastroesophageal sphincter which permits free reflux of gastric contents. Primary peristaltic waves become progressively weaker as they approach the sphincter. As time passes, peristalsis becomes more and more feeble and the severe esophagitis may produce a stricture. Esophageal shortening may draw the sphincter above the diaphragmatic hiatus, producing a hiatal hernia.

Antacids and elevation of the head of the patient's bed are useful in preventing reflux esophagitis. Nothing has been found which will delay the deterioration of esophageal function. Strictures may usually be effectively treated with repeated dilatations; only rarely does resection of the strictured area become necessary.

Dysphagia commonly occurs in patients with dermatomyositis; an incidence of 60% is recognized. Motility studies show a generalized muscular defect in which weakness of the cricopharyngeus sphincteric mechanism predominates. Although the dysfunction in the body of the esophagus resembles that of scleroderma, the cardioesophageal sphincter in dermatomyositis is usually unaffected. Corticosteroids may be beneficial in controlling symptoms.

Atkinson M, Summerling MD: Oesophageal changes in systemic sclerosis. Gut 7:402–408, 1966.

Donoghue FE, Winkleman RK, Moersch HJ: Esophageal defects in dermatomyositis. Ann Otol Rhin Laryng 69:1139–1148, 1960.

McLaughlin JS & others: Surgical treatment of strictures of the esophagus in patients with scleroderma. J Thoracic Cardiovas Surg 61:641–645, 1971.

Payne WS: Surgical treatment of reflux esophagitis and stricture associated with permanent incompetence of the cardia. Mayo Clin Proc 45:553–562, 1970.

Rodman GP, Fennell RH Jr: Progressive systemic sclerosis *sine* scleroderma. JAMA 180:665–670, 1962.

Saladin TA & others: Esophageal motor abnormalities in scleroderma and related diseases. Am J Digest Dis 11:522–535, 1966.

Treacy WL & others: Scleroderma of the esophagus: A correlation of histologic and physiologic findings. Ann Int Med 59:351–363, 1963.

NEUROMUSCULAR DISTURBANCES

Disturbances in the swallowing mechanism may occur in patients with neuromuscular disorders, especially those of the myotonic type. In myasthenia gravis, the peristaltic waves have a decrease in amplitude, and, on repetitive swallowing, peristalsis disappears in the lower esophagus. In myotonia dystrophica, in which both smooth and striated muscles are involved, motor failure of the esophagus is common.

Nonspecific abnormalities in peristalsis of the esophageal musculature may occur in many central or peripheral neurologic disorders. Simultaneous waves, spasms, and weak contractions can be observed in patients with such conditions as parkinsonism, hemiplegic states, multiple sclerosis, and amyotrophic lateral sclerosis.

Fisher RA & others: Esophageal motility in neuromuscular disorders. Ann Int Med 63:229–236, 1965.

Kelley ML: Dysphagia and motor failure of the esophagus in myotonia dystrophica. Neurology 14:955–962, 1964.

PHARYNGOESOPHAGEAL DIVERTICULUM
(Zenker's Diverticulum)

Essentials of Diagnosis

- Dysphagia, pressure symptoms, and gurgling sounds in the neck.
- Regurgitation of undigested food, halitosis.
- Manual emptying of the diverticulum by the patient.

General Considerations

Pharyngoesophageal diverticulum is the most common of the esophageal diverticula, and is 3 times more frequent in men than in women. It is an acquired abnormality that arises posteriorly in the midline of the neck—above the cricopharyngeus muscle and below the inferior constrictor of the pharynx. Between these 2 muscle groups is a weakened area through which the mucosa and submucosa gradually evaginate as a result of the high pressures generated during swallowing. Zenker's diverticulum is rarely seen in patients below the age of 30, and most patients are over 60. Although the mouth of the sac is in the midline, the sac projects laterally, usually into the left paravertebral region. The body of the esophagus often shows abnormal motility patterns in patients with Zenker's diverticulum.

Clinical Findings

A. Symptoms and Signs: Dysphagia is the most common symptom and is related to the size of the diverticulum. Undigested food is regurgitated into the mouth, especially in the recumbent position, and the patient may manually massage the neck after eating to empty the sac. Swelling of the neck, gurgling noises after eating, halitosis, and a sour metallic taste in the mouth may be noted.

B. X-Ray Findings: Fluoroscopic examination demonstrates a smoothly rounded outpouching arising posteriorly in the midline of the neck.

Differential Diagnosis

The dysphagia produced by pharyngoesophageal diverticula must be distinguished from that produced by malignant lesions, although carcinoma at this level is uncommon. Achalasia of the cricopharyngeus muscle may produce symptoms similar to those of Zenker's diverticulum. Cervical esophageal webs must also be considered. However, the radiologic discovery of a smoothly rounded blind pouch is diagnostic and is rarely confused with other lesions at this level. Esophagoscopy is usually unnecessary and may be hazardous because the instrument may enter the ostium of the diverticulum instead of the true esophageal lumen. Since the diverticulum is composed only of mucosa and submucosa, it is easily perforated.

Regurgitation and aspiration may produce tracheobronchial irritation and pneumonitis. This usually occurs while in the recumbent position, as during sleep. Food may become trapped in the diverticulum and rarely may lead to perforation, mediastinitis, or a periesophageal abscess. Retained food may ulcerate the mucosa and cause bleeding. Rarely, a fistula may form between the diverticulum and the trachea as a result of infection. Pulmonary infection is the most frequent serious common complication, and many patients are first seen after experiencing repeated episodes of pneumonitis.

Treatment

Surgical removal of the diverticulum is curative. A one-stage procedure is employed. It has recently been suggested that, in addition to the diverticulectomy, the cricopharyngeus muscle should be transected; the rationale of this procedure is that spasticity of the musculature may contribute to the continuation of symptoms after excision of the diverticulum.

Prognosis

A temporary transient fistula occasionally develops postoperatively, but this will usually heal spontaneously. The mortality after surgical excision is low, and the results are good.

See references below.

EPIPHRENIC DIVERTICULUM

Essentials of Diagnosis

- Dysphagia and a sensation of pressure in the lower esophagus after eating.
- Intermittent vomiting, substernal pain.
- Typical radiologic contour.
- Disturbed motility of the lower esophagus.
- Associated hiatal hernia on occasion.

General Considerations

Epiphrenic pulsion diverticula are usually located just above the diaphragm but may occur as high as the midthorax. They are usually associated with motility disturbances, most notably achalasia and diffuse spasm, and are frequently larger than diverticula which arise elsewhere in the esophagus. Esophagitis may develop at the ostium. Peridiverticular localized mediastinitis may be seen, especially if ulceration of the mucosa of the sac occurs.

Differential Diagnosis

The appearance on x-ray films and on fluoroscopy is so distinctive that a definitive diagnosis can usually be made. Associated conditions such as benign or malignant stenoses, webs, hiatal hernia, achalasia, and other motility disorders must be ruled out. The most common condition associated with epiphrenic diverticula is achalasia or esophageal spasm below the diverticulum, and symptoms are more apt to be due to the abnormal motility than to the diverticulum itself.

Complications

Esophagitis, periesophagitis, and occasional bleeding from ulceration are the most frequent complications. Tracheobronchial aspiration of regurgitated esophageal contents is uncommon. Perforation occurs rarely.

Treatment

Most patients have minor symptoms that do not require surgery. Surgery is indicated when symptoms become progressively more severe. The operation consists of a thoracotomy, excision of the diverticulum, and correction of underlying abnormalities. A linear division of the esophageal musculature below the diverticulum should be performed in most cases because of the frequent association of epiphrenic diverticulum with diffuse spasm and achalasia. If a hiatal hernia is present, it should be repaired.

Prognosis

Surgery is successful in 80—90% of cases.

See references below.

TRACTION DIVERTICULA

Essentials of Diagnosis

- Usually an incidental radiologic finding.
- Dysphagia.
- Episodes of coughing due to fixation to the trachea or bronchus or peribronchial lymph nodes.
- Typical x-ray.

General Considerations

Traction diverticula occur in the midthoracic esophagus. Inflamed lymph nodes near the tracheal bifurcation become adherent to the esophagus, and, as fibrosis and contraction occur with healing, the esophageal wall is pulled anteriorly to form a sac. The diverticulum is at first cone-shaped, with its apex fixed to the fibrotic lymph node; later, a pulsion effect from the intraluminal pressure may be added, so that the contour becomes rounded.

Traction diverticula are usually discovered after age 40 and occur with equal frequency in both sexes. They are rarely multiple, frequently asymptomatic, and are often found during a routine gastrointestinal x-ray study.

Clinical Findings

Most diverticula of this type are asymptomatic, but occasionally the diverticulum may become inflamed and may then produce dysphagia and a sense of pulling on the tracheobronchial tree during swallowing.

Differential Diagnosis

The radiologic discovery (usually during an upper gastrointestinal fluoroscopic study) of an outpouching in the midthoracic esophagus is not likely to be misinterpreted. If associated inflammation causes narrowing of the esophageal lumen, carcinoma or benign stricture must be ruled out by esophagoscopy.

Complications

In rare instances the diverticulum may perforate into neighboring structures, causing fistula or·abscess formation. Bleeding is uncommon.

Treatment

Since most traction diverticula are asymptomatic, no specific treatment is necessary. An occasional patient may develop symptoms, in which case surgical excision is warranted.

Allen TH, Clagett OT: Changing concepts in the surgical treatment of pulsion diverticula of the lower esophagus. J Thoracic Cardiovas Surg 50:455—462, 1965.

Belsey RJ: Functional diseases of the esophagus. J Thoracic Cardiovas Surg 52:164—188, 1966.

Boyd DP, Adams HD: Esophageal diverticulum. New England J Med 264:641—645, 1961.

Ellis FH Jr & others: Cricopharyngeal myotomy for pharyngoesophageal diverticulum. Ann Surg 170:340—349, 1969.

Grimes OF, Binkley FM: Pharyngo-esophageal diverticula: Surgical treatment. California Med 87:368, 1957.

Joseph WL & others: The diagnosis and treatment of esophageal diverticula. Ann Thoracic Surg 3:375—386, 1967.

Perrott JW: Anatomical aspects of hypopharyngeal diverticula. Australian New Zealand J Surg 31:307—317, 1962.

INSTRUMENTAL PERFORATION OF THE ESOPHAGUS

Essentials of Diagnosis

- History of recent instrumentation, sudden elevation of temperature, and pain in the neck or chest.
- Leukocytosis, change of voice into bass-like tone.
- Crepitus in the neck due to extravasation of air.
- Subcutaneous emphysema (mainly in the cervical region).
- Localization of injury by fluoroscopic studies with water-soluble opaque media.
- Pneumothorax if perforation involves the thoracic esophagus.

General Considerations

Instrumental perforation during diagnostic esophagoscopy accounts for most esophageal injuries. Similar injuries may occur during gastroscopy, gastroesophageal balloon tamponade, and esophageal dilatation with various instruments. Even simple intubation of the esophagus for diagnostic or therapeutic purposes may result in perforation. Perforations are most likely to occur in the cervical esophagus. The esophagoscope may press the posterior wall of the esophagus against osteoarthritic spurs of the cervical vertebrae, causing contusion or laceration. The cricopharyngeal area is the most common point of perforation. The resistance of the muscular sphincter must be overcome in order to insert the esophagoscope into the esophageal lumen. The pressure necessary to obliterate the sphincteric tone may result in a rapid descent of the instrument to produce a tear of the esophagus.

Perforations of the intrathoracic esophagus may occur at any level but are most common at the natural sites of narrowing, ie, at the level of the left main stem bronchus and at the diaphragmatic hiatus.

Clinical Findings

A. Symptoms and Signs: Pain, fever, dysphagia, and hypotension bordering on shock are the most common early findings after perforation of the esophagus has occurred. The severity of each of these manifestations is dependent largely on the site and extent of the perforation and the rapidity of the inflammatory reaction that develops. Hyperpnea is almost always noted, but dyspnea most often indicates that the perforation has occurred in the thoracic esophagus, with laceration of the pleura to produce pneumothorax, chest pain, and a rapidly developing pleural effusion.

Cervical tenderness is a common early sign, and pain upon attempted swallowing may be severe. Crepitation in the soft tissues of the neck can almost always be demonstrated, although it may be minimal. If the thoracic esophagus is perforated, the symptoms and signs are usually limited to the chest; occasionally, crepitus is palpable in the neck but tenderness in the cervical region is not often present. Because of the escape of air into the mediastinum, a "mediastinal crunch" may be heard as the heart beats against the air-filled tissues (Hamman's sign). Shock develops earlier in thoracic perforations than in injuries to the cervical esophagus because of the rapid flooding of the mediastinum and pleural space with highly infective salivary secretions.

B. X-Ray Findings: X-ray studies are important in not only demonstrating that perforation has occurred but also in locating the exact site of the injury. In perforations of the cervical esophagus, x-ray films show air in the soft tissues, especially along the cervical spine. The trachea may be displaced anteriorly by air and fluid in the space behind the esophagus (retrovisceral space). Later, widening of the superior mediastinum may be seen. Mediastinal widening and emphysema and pleural effusion with or without pneumothorax are often present in perforations of the body of the esophagus in the thorax. Fluoroscopic examination using water-soluble opaque media should always be obtained to localize the site of the injury and to determine if associated abnormalities are present. Esophagoscopy is unnecessary except when the perforation has been caused by the ingestion of a foreign body.

Complications

Wounds of the esophagus may be fatal because regional tissues quickly become contaminated with highly virulent oropharyngeal bacteria. Fulminant mediastinitis, bronchopneumonia, pericarditis, and septicemia may occur in rapid succession. Abscess is uncommon in intrathoracic perforations because the mediastinal pleura is almost always lacerated so that the esophageal contents drain directly into the pleural space. Empyema, mediastinitis, and severe sepsis may develop if an intrathoracic perforation is not recognized and treated immediately. Since the prevertebral fascia and spaces of the neck are continuous into the mediastinum, mediastinitis may occur as a result of perforations in the cervical esophagus.

Differential Diagnosis

Wounds resulting from instrumentation are unlikely to be misinterpreted since the typical symptoms and signs occur so rapidly. When mediastinal or cervical abscesses develop slowly as a result of small tears or perforations, they must be differentiated from other masses or growths largely by fluoroscopic studies using water-soluble contrast media.

Prevention

Even in skilled hands, instrumental perforation is a recognized risk. Careful, gentle technic and the use of a lumen finder are mandatory. General anesthesia to provide complete relaxation is preferred, although the procedure can be accomplished under topical anesthesia. Many endoscopists prefer the fiberoptic instrument. Food or fluids by mouth should not be allowed for 12–24 hours or until it can be determined with absolute certainty that no injury has occurred.

Treatment

Immediate operation is advisable. Closure of the perforation and external drainage should be accomplished. Occasionally, in perforations of the cervical esophagus, simple drainage may suffice since the tears are often small and difficult to identify in the presence of inflammatory edema. Although antibiotics alone have occasionally been successful, this method of treatment is more risky than direct surgical repair and should be employed only in patients in whom a general anesthetic is strongly contraindicated.

Nonoperative management of intrathoracic perforations is extremely hazardous and rarely tried. If the perforation is contained entirely within the mediastinum and toxicity is minimal—indicating that a minor laceration has been produced—conservative therapy with nasogastric decompression and massive doses of antibiotics may be permissible.

Prognosis

With prompt operative repair, external drainage, and adjuvant antibiotics, most patients who sustain instrumental perforations of the esophagus will recover. Although intrathoracic perforations have a less favorable outlook because of the rapid development of mediastinitis and empyema, immediate operation to repair the injury is usually lifesaving.

Berry BE, Ochsner JL: Perforation of the esophagus: A 30 year review. J Thoracic Cardiovas Surg 65:1–7, 1973.

Boyd DP, Wittman CJ Jr: Some principles in treating perforation of esophagus. S Clin North America 51:567–574, 1971.

Nealon TF & others: Instrumental perforation of the esophagus. J Thoracic Cardiovas Surg 41:75, 1961.

Wychulus AR, Fontana RS, Payne WS: Instrumental perforations of the esophagus. Dis Chest 55:184, 1969.

SPONTANEOUS (POSTEMETIC) PERFORATION OF THE ESOPHAGUS
(Boerhaave's Syndrome)

Essentials of Diagnosis

- Usually in males.
- History of alcoholic debauch, excessive food intake, or both.
- Violent vomiting or retching followed by agonizing pain in the epigastrium and lower anterior thorax.
- Rigid abdomen.
- Pneumothorax, mediastinal widening, and emphysema.
- Crepitus in the neck.
- Radiographic evidence of mediastinal, pleural, or intra-abdominal air.
- Demonstration of rupture of the lower esophagus by esophagogram.

General Considerations

Spontaneous perforations often occur in patients who have had no previous esophageal disease. The rupture involves all layers of the esophageal wall and most frequently occurs in the left posterolateral aspect of the lower esophagus. The second most common site is in the midthoracic esophagus on the right side at the level of the azygos vein. The tear results from excessive pressure exerted directly upon the esophagus by violent retching and vomiting.

Clinical Findings

A. Symptoms and Signs: Shock develops rapidly. The diagnosis is suggested by a history of bouts of vomiting or retching, especially in an alcoholic male of middle age or older, followed by sudden and severe abdominal and lower chest pain. Hematemesis may occur (see Mallory-Weiss syndrome, p 457).

B. X-Ray Findings: Pneumothorax, usually on the left side, can be demonstrated on plain chest films. The rent can be localized by x-rays taken during a swallow of water-soluble contrast medium.

Differential Diagnosis

Especially if an accurate history cannot be obtained, the shock which almost always develops must be distinguished from shock due to other causes such as myocardial infarction, pulmonary embolus, ruptured intra-abdominal viscus, and sepsis. When an immediate diagnosis is not forthcoming, the patient may be thought to have either a perforated peptic ulcer or acute pancreatitis.

Treatment

Antibiotic therapy should always be employed. Immediate thoracotomy to repair the rupture is mandatory if the patient's condition permits. Ordinarily, however, primary repair is not feasible if 12 hours or more have elapsed. In these instances, drainage of the pleural space is accomplished by multiple thoracostomy tubes. In addition, bypassing of the perforated area by cervical esophagostomy and gastrostomy or jejunostomy may be lifesaving. Definitive repair can be accomplished at a later time. The ruptured area can also be sutured around a T-tube whose long arm is brought out through the lower thorax. An esophagocutaneous fistula results whose repair can be undertaken at a time of election.

Prognosis

If an early diagnosis can be made, the outlook is excellent since repair of the perforation can be accomplished with minimal contamination. However, one series showed that in only 2 of 34 patients who had spontaneous perforations was a premortem diagnosis made. In most of these, the patients were admitted in shock or severe sepsis and their problem was thought to be due to other catastrophies such as myocardial infarction, severe pancreatitis, pneumonia, or peritonitis due to a ruptured viscus.

Abbott AA & others: Atraumatic so-called "spontaneous" rupture of the esophagus. J Thoracic Cardiovas Surg 59: 67–83, 1970.

Editorial: The Boerhaave syndrome. JAMA 187:54, 1964.

Hamilton SGI: Spontaneous rupture of the esophagus. Brit J Surg 54:304, 1967.

Thompson NW & others: The spectrum of emetogenic injury to the esophagus and stomach. Am J Surg 113:13–26, 1967.

FOREIGN BODIES OF THE ESOPHAGUS

Essentials of Diagnosis

- History of recent ingestion of food or foreign material.
- Vague discomfort in the midline of the chest or neck, progressing to pain if infection develops.
- Dysphagia.
- Occasionally, respiratory distress.
- Radiographic discovery of foreign matter or of esophageal obstruction.

General Considerations

Most cases occur in children. Mentally disturbed patients often ingest foreign bodies. The esophagus may become obstructed by impactions of meat, especially in the edentulous patient. Many objects become engaged in the esophagus as it enters the superior thoracic strait. Others arrest at the level of the aortic arch, at the left main stem bronchus, or just above the cardioesophageal junction—ie, at the natural anatomic areas of narrowing.

Clinical Findings

A. Symptoms and Signs: Pain in the midline of the thorax or neck is prominent when large objects are ingested, especially when infection surrounds the foreign body. Dysphagia, varying from mild distress to complete obstruction, may occur. Pressure on the tracheobronchial tree often produces respiratory distress. In most cases, the diagnosis can be made on the basis of the history.

B. X-Ray Findings: Roentgenography, either by plain films or by the use of opaque substances, provides specific information regarding the type of foreign body and its location. Esophagoscopy is not only diagnostic but also therapeutic since the direct observation of the foreign body allows its safe removal.

Differential Diagnosis

Obstructive foreign bodies in the esophagus that cannot be identified must be differentiated from other causes of obstruction such as stenosis, caustic strictures, and tumors.

Complications

Esophageal inflammation and infection often occur around the foreign object. Perforation into the surrounding mediastinal structures may occur, leading to mediastinitis, hemorrhage from adjacent major blood vessels, or abscess formation. Neglected foreign bodies may erode through the esophageal wall to form a tracheoesophageal fistula. Late strictures may develop from the contraction of fibrous tissue incident to the inflammatory process.

Treatment

Many foreign objects will dislodge themselves and will pass through the intestinal tract without difficulty. This is especially true in children, who often ingest smooth objects such as coins and marbles. Most foreign bodies in the esophagus, however, should be removed by endoscopy following proper roentgenographic studies. Esophagotomy to remove an impacted foreign body is rarely necessary.

The use of proteolytic enzymes to dissolve a bolus of impacted meat is occasionally successful, but its dangers are significant since the esophageal wall may be injured and esophageal perforation has been reported.

Spitz L: Management of ingested foreign bodies in childhood. Brit MJ 4:469–472, 1971.

CORROSIVE ESOPHAGITIS

Essentials of Diagnosis

- History of ingestion of caustic liquids or solids.
- Burns of the lips, mouth, and tongue.
- Pain and dysphagia.

General Considerations

Ingestion of strong solutions of acid or alkali or of solid substances of similar nature produces extensive chemical burns, often leading to corrosive esophagitis. Depending upon the concentration and the length of time the irritant remains in contact with the mucosa, various pathologic changes occur. Sloughing of the mucous membrane, edema and inflammation of the submucosa, thrombosis of esophageal vessels, infection, perforation, and mediastinitis may develop if the injury is severe.

Clinical Findings

Systemic symptoms roughly parallel the severity of the caustic burns. If the damage is severe, the patient appears toxic, with high fever, prostration, and shock. Inflammatory edema of the lips, mouth, tongue, and oropharynx may cause respiratory distress. Pain on attempted swallowing may be intense. Tracheobronchitis accompanied by coughing and increased bronchial secretions is frequently noted. Complete esophageal obstruction (due to edema), inflammation, and mucosal sloughing may develop within the first few days.

The corrosive injury may be so severe that large areas of mucosa are destroyed, including that of the stomach. The burns are most often linear, but they may be patchy and irregular in outline. Many are circular and involve considerable lengths of the esophagus. Circular burns are prone to lead to early stricture. Caustic injuries tend to be more severe at the areas of anatomic narrowing of the esophagus.

Complications

Complications include perforation, bleeding, mediastinitis, tracheoesophageal fistulas, and stricture formation.

Treatment

A. Emergency Treatment: Emergency treatment consists of washing the esophagus with large volumes of water. Dilute acid or alkaline solutions may be used to neutralize the ingested liquid.

B. Medical Treatment: Broad-spectrum antibiotics are given immediately to prevent bacterial invasion of the esophageal wall. Corticosteroids are used in the acute phase to reduce fibrous tissue proliferation and thereby to decrease the possibility of stricture formation.

C. Esophagoscopy and Dilatation: Early esophagoscopy is recommended to determine the initial extent of the injury and may be repeated as necessary to assess the progress of healing. Although the procedures must be performed with extreme caution, dilatation by esophagoscopy or bougienage should be performed in patients in whom esophageal narrowing or actual stenosis appears to be developing.

D. Surgical Treatment: In spite of the prompt and efficient use of corticosteroids, antibiotics, and dilatations, the process may progress to stricture formation—especially when extensive destruction and fibrosis of the esophagus has occurred. In these instances, the esophagus must be replaced by segments of stomach, jejunum, or colon.

Prognosis

Early and proper management of caustic burns provides satisfactory results in most cases. The ingestion of strong acid or alkaline solutions with extensive immediate destruction of the mucosa produces such profound pathologic changes that the development of fibrous strictures is almost inevitable.

Cardona JC, Daly JF: Current management of corrosive esophagitis. Ann Otol Rhin Laryng 80:522–527, 1971.

Feldman M, Iben AB, Hurley EJ: Corrosive injury to oropharynx and esophagus: Eighty-five consecutive cases. California Med 118:6–9, Jan 1973.

Haller JA & others: Pathophysiology and management of acute corrosive burns of the esophagus. J Pediat Surg 6:578–584, 1971.

BENIGN TUMORS OF THE ESOPHAGUS

Essentials of Diagnosis

- Dysphagia often present but frequently mild.
- Sense of pressure in thorax or neck.
- Radiographic demonstration of intra- or extraluminal mass, smooth in outline.

General Considerations

Benign growths may arise in any layer of the esophagus. Inflammatory polyps or granulomas are occasionally associated with esophagitis and may be mistakenly interpreted as neoplastic lesions. Papillomas arising from the mucosa are either sessile or pedunculated; although they are usually small lesions, occasionally they become large enough to produce obstruction. They may slough off spontaneously into the esophageal lumen.

Leiomyoma is the most frequent benign lesion of the esophagus. Leiomyomas are intramural lesions which narrow the esophageal lumen extrinsically. The mucosa overlying the tumor is generally intact, but occasionally it may become ulcerated as a result of pressure by an enlarging lesion. Other tumors such as fibromas, lipomas, fibromyomas, and myxomas are rare.

Congenital cysts or reduplications of the esophagus (the second most common benign lesion after leiomyomas) may occur at any level, although they are most commonly in the lower esophageal segment.

Clinical Findings

Many benign lesions are asymptomatic and are discovered incidentally during upper gastrointestinal fluoroscopic examinations. Cysts and leiomyomas may be of sufficient size to appear as a density, usually round or ovoid, in the mediastinum on routine chest x-rays. Benign tumors or cysts grow slowly and become symptomatic only after sufficient encroachment into the esophageal lumen has occurred. Radiographic study of the intramural leiomyoma shows a smoothly rounded, often spherical mass which causes extrinsic narrowing of the esophageal lumen. The overlying mucosa is almost always intact. Peristalsis is not affected by leiomyomas but is often abnormal in the presence of cysts or reduplications. Spasm of the musculature adjacent to the cyst or duplication is the most common abnormality of peristalsis. Dilatation of the esophagus proximal to any of the benign lesions is rarely seen. Intraluminal growths can be recognized at esophagoscopy, and a specific tissue diagnosis should always be obtained. Attempts to biopsy intramural lesions through an intact overlying mucous membrane are hazardous because of the possibility of inducing hemorrhage into the lesion with resulting increase of its size; pressure upon the adjacent mediastinal structures may produce cardiorespiratory embarrassment.

Differential Diagnosis

Leiomyomas, cysts, and reduplications can be distinguished from cancerous growths by their classic radiographic appearance. Intraluminal papillomas, polyps, or granulomas may be indistinguishable radiographically from early carcinoma, and their exact nature must be confirmed histologically.

Complications

Cysts and duplications derive their arterial supply directly from the aorta. Hemorrhage into these lesions may occur, especially following infection, although this complication is uncommon. Adhesions which form between the cystic lesions and the adjacent esophagus often produce progressive dysphagia. Pedunculated intraluminal tumors may cause sudden obstruction by torsion of their pedicles, which is followed by edema, infection, and bleeding. In the upper esophagus, pedunculated polypoid growths may be regurgitated upward into the hypopharynx and occasionally may fall into the glottic chink and produce laryngeal obstruction.

Bleeding may occur from ulcerations of the mucosa overlying a leiomyoma. Symptoms related to benign lesions of the esophagus are usually due to the presence of the lesion itself; the severity of the dysphagia is accentuated by the development of swelling, infection, hemorrhage, or obstruction.

Treatment

Small polypoid intraluminal lesions may be

removed completely with biopsy forceps during esophagoscopy. The intramural lesions, reduplications, and cysts should be excised either by thoracotomy or through a cervical approach when located in the neck.

Deverall PB: Smooth-muscle tumours of the esophagus. Brit J Surg 55:457–461, 1968.

Schmidt HW, Clagett OT, Harrison EG Jr: Benign tumors and cysts of the esophagus. J Thoracic Cardiovas Surg 41:717–732, 1961.

Schmidt A, Lockwood K: Benign neoplasms of the esophagus. Acta chir scandinav 133:640–644, 1967.

MALIGNANT TUMORS OF THE ESOPHAGUS

Essentials of Diagnosis

- Progressive dysphagia, initially during ingestion of solid foods and later from liquids.
- Progressive weight loss and inanition.
- Classic radiographic outlines: irregular mucosal pattern with narrowing, with shelf-like upper border or concentrically narrowed esophageal lumen.
- Definitive diagnosis established by biopsy or cytology.

General Considerations

Most malignant tumors of the esophagus are carcinomas; sarcomas and carcinosarcomas are rare. Esophageal carcinoma occurs more frequently in males. The peak incidence is between 50–60 years. Malignant tumors located at the esophagogastric junction are usually adenocarcinomas. Those arising proximal to the cardia are either squamous cell carcinomas or undifferentiated lesions.

Carcinoma of the esophagus constitutes about 4% of all malignant lesions arising along the gastrointestinal tract. Twenty percent occur in the upper third, approximately 35% in the middle third, and 45% in the lower esophagus, including those developing at the cardia.

The carcinoma usually appears as a fungating growth extending irregularly into the esophageal lumen. Ulceration of its central portion is common. Annular lesions with extensive infiltration of the esophageal wall produce obstruction earlier than those which involve only a portion of the circumference of the esophagus. Regardless of their cell type, malignancies disseminate by direct invasion into surrounding mediastinal structures, through the blood stream by local vascular involvement, and by lymphatic dissemination. Lymph nodes at some distance from the primary lesion often contain metastatic deposits, and intramural extension, both upward and downward, frequently involves considerable lengths of the esophagus. Lower esophageal lesions metastasize primarily to the celiac and suprapancreatic lymph nodes. Lung, bone, liver, and brain are frequent sites of metastases.

Clinical Findings

A. Symptoms and Signs: Dysphagia is the most prominent symptom, and as a result the loss of weight is often striking. Solid foods initially cause difficulty; later, even liquids may be difficult to swallow. Weight loss, weakness, anemia, and inanition are almost always present. Pain is not common unless invasion of somatic structures occurs.

B. X-Ray Findings: Fluoroscopic studies provide a high degree of diagnostic accuracy. The malignancy appears as an irregular mass of variable size and length whose upper border is roughly horizontal and resembles a "shelf." Annular lesions appear as constricting bands with a narrowed lumen which contains an irregular mucosal outline. Dilatation of the esophagus may occur proximal to the growth, although it is not as great as that which occurs in chronic benign obstructive disease.

C. Esophagoscopy: Esophagoscopy with biopsy provides an accurate tissue diagnosis in most cases. However, the mucosa immediately proximal to the lesion may be so redundant, edematous, and inflamed that the tumor may not be directly visualized at esophagoscopy. In this case, esophageal washings to obtain cellular material are rewarding. Lesions as far distally as the midthoracic esophagus may involve the tracheobronchial tree by direct invasion. For this reason, bronchoscopy in addition to esophagoscopy is always indicated in the assessment of growths at these levels.

Differential Diagnosis

The fungating type of esophageal cancer presents a typical radiographic picture consisting of an irregular mucosal contour and the uppermost "shelf." Annular carcinomas may be mistaken for benign strictures, especially if most of the growth is largely intramural. Benign papillomas, polyps, or granulomatous masses can be distinguished from early carcinomas only on histologic examination.

Complications

Cancer of the esophagus rarely bleeds massively, although occult anemia is frequently observed. The most common complications result from invasion of important mediastinal structures such as the superior vena cava, aorta, trachea, major bronchi, and pericardium. Fatal hemorrhage, tracheal obstruction, and cardiac arrhythmias may result. A fistula may develop between the esophagus and the tracheobronchial tree and lead to aspiration pneumonitis, purulent bronchitis, and pulmonary abscesses.

Prevention

The cause of esophageal cancer is not known. Agents that have been suggested are hot liquids, alcohol, spicy foods, and tobacco. Available data do not support a cause and effect relationship with either cigarettes or pipe smoking. The incidence of esophageal cancer varies considerably throughout the world in countries with highly variable diets and customs. No basic cause has been identified in China, Japan, Russia, and Scandinavia, where the incidence is especially high.

Treatment

Esophageal carcinoma is treated by surgery, irradiation, or both. In recent years, preoperative radiation has been utilized in an effort to sterilize the soft tissues and lymphatics around the primary growth. Radiation therapy will often permit excision of an otherwise nonresectable growth and will increase the percentage of curative resections. Malignant lesions in the middle and upper thirds of the esophagus are quite likely to be nonresectable because of their propensity to invade vital nearby structures such as the aorta, pericardium, superior vena cava, and the tracheobronchial tree. Carcinomas of the lower third of the esophagus are often resected primarily; even in this area, however, preoperative radiation therapy is being given. General opinion is that radiation therapy followed by resection has improved the outlook, although the available statistics do not constitute proof.

A complete cancericidal course of radiation (5000–6000 R) is administered to the entire mediastinum, and surgery is undertaken 6–8 weeks later. Variable amounts of viable carcinoma usually remain after irradiation. Esophagogastrostomy in one stage through a 2-cavity abdominal and right thoracic approach is the most commonly employed procedure. Through an abdominal incision, an assessment is made for metastatic deposits, which occur mainly in the celiac and suprapancreatic lymph nodes and in the liver. If no metastases are found, the entire stomach is mobilized with its blood supply maintained by the right gastric and right gastroepiploic vessels. The short gastric arteries and the left gastric arteries are ligated to further free up the stomach as a pouch to be used as a replacement for the resected esophagus. A pyloroplasty completes the abdominal portion of the procedure. After the abdominal incision is closed, the patient is turned so that a right thoracotomy can be accomplished. The right-sided approach is preferable since the arch of the aorta does not obscure the operative field and also because the better exposure facilitates safe removal of the growth from adjacent structures. The esophagus and the growth are resected high in the thorax and an anastomosis is created between the transected end of the esophagus and the fundus of the stomach. The high resection prevents esophagitis and allows for the resection of as much esophagus as possible to make certain that submucosal metastatic spread of the cancer has been removed. In addition to the stomach, colon or small bowel may be used to restore intestinal continuity.

In patients with far-advanced malignancies, distant metastases, or recurrence after radiotherapy, palliation to allow the patient to swallow can be obtained by bougienage or occasionally by intraluminal plastic tubes.

Prognosis

Esophageal cancer is a dread disease, and the operative mortality is about 20%. The 3-year survival rate is approximately 5%. Carcinoma of the lower esophagus has a somewhat better prognosis than do lesions in the middle and upper thirds. The overall resectability rate is approximately 30%.

Boyd D, Kim M: Survival in carcinoma of the esophagus. S Clin North America 47:613–620, 1967.

Guernsey JM, Knudsen DF: Abdominal exploration in the evaluation of patients with carcinoma of the thoracic esophagus. J Thoracic Cardiovas Surg 59:62–66, 1970.

Gunnlaughsson G & others: Analysis of the records of 1657 patients with carcinoma of the esophagus and cardia of the stomach. Surg Gynec Obst 130:997–1005, 1970.

Humphrey CR, Clifton E: Carcinoma of the distal part of the esophagus and cardia of the stomach. Surg Gynec Obst 127:737–743, 1968.

Lawler MR & others: Carcinoma of the esophagus. J Thoracic Cardiovas Surg 58:609–613, 1969.

Nakayama K, Orihata H, Yamaguchi K: Surgical treatment combined with preoperative concentrated irradiation for esophageal cancer. Cancer 20:778–788, 1967.

Petrovsky B, Vantsian E: Our experience in the surgical management of malignant and benign esophageal tumors. Surgery 62:833–838, 1967.

ESOPHAGEAL BANDS, WEBS, OR RINGS

Congenital bands or webs may develop at any level but are more frequent in the subcricoid region. Others form in the lower esophageal segment. These bands cause dysphagia and may be treated by endoscopic dilatation in which the thin, web-like band is usually fractured, followed by complete relief of symptoms. Resection and primary anastomosis are occasionally necessary for the more fibrous unyielding concentric bands. The latter are more likely to be in the lower esophagus.

Band-like narrowing, usually associated with hiatal hernia, was described by Schatzki. Most patients are relatively free from symptoms unless the ring is less than 12 mm in diameter. Occasionally, dysphagia is severe. Endoscopy often fails to reveal the smooth concentric narrowing since the overlying mucosa is intact. Esophagitis is often present together with hiatal hernia and the Schatzki ring. Repair of the associated hiatal hernia is insufficient to control the dysphagia; the ring must be dilated or excised.

Editorial: The Paterson-Kelly lesion. Brit MJ 2:530, 1969.

Goyal RK & others: Lower esophageal ring. New England J Med 282:1298–1304, 1355–1362, 1970.

Kelley ML Jr, Frazer JP: Symptomatic mid-esophageal webs. JAMA 197:143–146, 1966.

Lam CR & others: The nature and surgical treatment of lower esophageal ring (Schatzki's ring). J Thoracic Cardiovas Surg 63:34–40, 1972.

Postlethwait RW, Sealy WC: Experiences with the treatment of 59 patients with lower esophageal web. Ann Surg 165:786–796, 1967.

COLUMNAR-LINED ESOPHAGUS WITH OR WITHOUT HIATAL HERNIA

In 1950, Barrett of England described a pathologic condition in which the lower esophagus is lined with columnar epithelium similar to that of the cardiac portion of the stomach except that acid-producing cells are not usually present. It appears to be a form of metaplasia of the epithelium for which no normal counterpart exists. The exact cause is still controversial. Some postulate a congenital basis. Others believe that the normal squamous mucosa undergoes alterations incident to peptic regurgitation. Small ulcerations due to esophagitis may heal and re-epithelize by ingrowth of a type of mucosa resembling that of the cardia. Since most of these patients have an associated hiatal hernia with esophagitis, the mucosal overgrowth theory has substance.

Although columnar-lined esophagus occasionally occurs in children and young adults, it is more commonly encountered in older people.

The most frequent complication is stricture formation at the squamocolumnar junction. Large ulcers occasionally develop, usually at the squamocolumnar junction, causing massive bleeding. Management depends upon the pathologic changes that occur. Resection may be necessary to control bleeding or to remove large, painful, penetrating ulcers. Bougienage may suffice in the elderly patient when stricture is the main complication. Operative repair of the associated hiatal hernia often allows healing of ulcers. Further laying down of fibrous tissue can also be prevented by abolishing reflux esophagitis so that the stricture that remains can be more easily dilated.

The overall results are good regardless of the type of therapy instituted.

Barrett NR: Chronic peptic ulcer of the esophagus and "esophagitis." Brit J Surg 38:175–182, 1950.

Burgess JN & others: Barrett esophagus. Mayo Clin Proc 46:728–734, 1971.

Hill LD & others: Simplified management of reflux esophagitis with stricture. Ann Surg 172:638–651, 1970.

Trier JS: Morphology of the epithelium of the distal esophagus in patients with mid-esophageal peptic strictures. Gastroenterology 58:444–461, 1970.

II. THE DIAPHRAGM
(See Fig 24–3.)

The diaphragm is a musculotendinous dome-shaped structure attached posteriorly to the first,

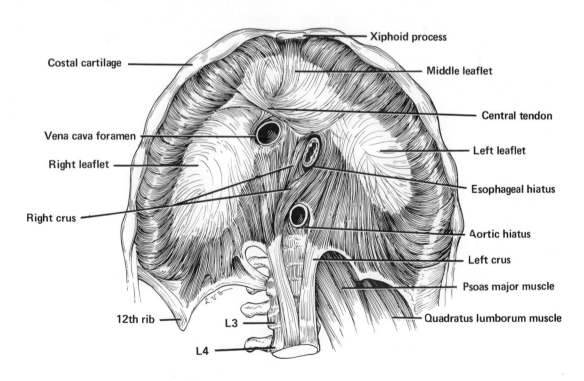

FIG 24–3. Inferior surface of diaphragm.

second, and third lumbar vertebrae, anteriorly to the lower sternum, and laterally to the costal arches. It separates the abdominal and the thoracic cavities. Through anatomic foramens, the diaphragm allows the passage of various normal structures. The aortic hiatus lies posteriorly at the level of the 12th thoracic vertebra, and through it passes the aorta, the thoracic duct, and the azygos venous system. The esophageal hiatus lies immediately anteriorly and slightly to the left at the level of the tenth thoracic vertebra and is separated from the aortic hiatus by the decussation of the right crus of the diaphragm. Through this hiatus pass the esophagus and the vagus nerves. At the level of the ninth thoracic vertebra and slightly to the right of the esophageal hiatus is the vena cava foramen, which allows passage of the inferior cava and small branches of the phrenic nerve. The phrenic arteries arising directly from the aorta supply the diaphragm along with the lower intercostal arteries and the terminal branches of the internal mammary arteries.

ESOPHAGEAL HIATAL HERNIA

Essentials of Diagnosis

- Many are asymptomatic.
- Substernal burning pain due to gastroesophageal regurgitation.
- Dysphagia due to edema and esophagitis.
- Occult bleeding is common; massive bleeding is rare.
- X-ray studies are diagnostic; esophagoscopy can show whether complications such as esophagitis, stricture, ulcers, polyps, or malignancy are present.

General Considerations

Hernias through the esophageal hiatus are the most common type, comprising at least 90% of all diaphragmatic hernias. At least two-thirds of patients are women.

There are 2 types of esophageal hiatal hernia: paraesophageal and sliding. Symptoms usually develop in adult life. Obesity, aging, and general weakening of the musculofascial structures set the stage for enlargement of the esophageal hiatus or the parahiatal defect so that herniation may eventually develop, resulting in either a paraesophageal hernia or a sliding esophageal hernia depending upon the area through which the viscera progress.

Ellis FH Jr: Esophageal hiatal hernia. New England J Med 287:646–649, 1972.

Skinner DB & others (editors): *Gastroesophageal Reflux and Hiatal Hernia.* Little, Brown, 1972.

1. PARAESOPHAGEAL HERNIA
(See Fig 24–4.)

In the paraesophageal type of diaphragmatic hernia, all or part of the stomach herniates into the thorax immediately adjacent to an undisplaced gastroesophageal junction. The intact diaphragmatic sling holds the cardioesophageal junction in its normal position, preserving the normal length of the esophagus while a pouch of stomach is transposed into the posterior mediastinum. Since the gastroesophageal sphincteric mechanism is usually normal, reflux of gastric contents does not occur. In those instances in which the paraesophageal hernia occurs in association with the sliding type, gastroesophageal reflux may occur along with other symptoms of an otherwise pure paraesophageal type The uncomplicated paraesophageal hernia accounts for less than 10% of hernias through or alongside the esophageal hiatus.

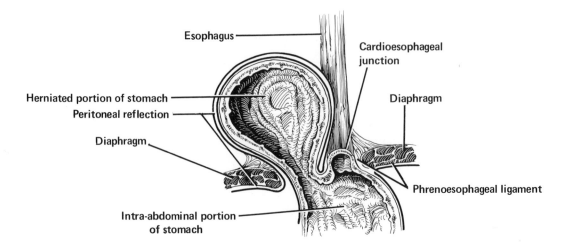

FIG 24–4. Paraesophageal hernia.

Clinical Findings

The most common symptoms of uncomplicated paraesophageal hernia usually develop in adult life and consist of gaseous eructations, a sense of pressure in the lower chest after eating, and, occasionally, palpitations due to cardiac arrhythmias. All of these are pressure phenomena caused by enlargement of the herniated gastric pouch by food displacing the fundic air bubble. As noted, heartburn due to gastroesophageal reflux is uncommon.

Complications

The most frequent complications of paraesophageal hernia are hemorrhage, incarceration, obstruction, and volvulus. The herniated portion of the stomach often becomes congested, and bleeding occurs from erosions of the mucosa. Obstruction may occur, most often at the esophagogastric junction as a result of torsion and angulation at this point—especially if a large portion (or all) of the stomach herniates into the chest. In paraesophageal hiatal hernia—in contrast to the sliding type—other viscera such as the small and large intestine and spleen may also enter the mediastinum along with the stomach.

Treatment

Since complications are frequent even in the absence of symptoms, operative repair is indicated in most cases. The usual method is to return the herniated stomach to the abdomen and fix it there by sutures to the posterior rectus sheath. The enlarged hiatus is closed snugly around the gastroesophageal junction with interrupted sutures.

Prognosis

The results of surgical management are generally good unless the diaphragmatic musculature has become weakened and tenuous.

Culver GJ & others: Mechanism of obstruction in paraesophageal diaphragmatic hernias. JAMA 181:933–938, 1962.

Hill LD, Tobias JA: Paraeosophageal hernia. Arch Surg 96:735–744, 1968.

Larson NE & others: Mechanism of obstruction and strangulation in hernias of the esophageal hiatus. Surg Gynec Obst 119:835–841, 1964.

2. SLIDING ESOPHAGEAL HERNIA
(See Fig 24–5.)

Sliding hiatal hernia comprises more than 90% of hernias in and about the esophageal hiatus. The upper stomach, along with the cardioesophageal junction, is displaced upward into the posterior mediastinum. The hernia is partially surrounded by a peritoneal sac similar to that of sliding hernia in the inguinal region. It is true that the stomach may "slide" in and out of the thorax with changes in body position, with alterations of pressure in the abdominal and thoracic cavities, and when a large meal is eaten. The term sliding refers to the anatomy of the partial peritoneal sac.

The displacement also distorts the cardioesophageal junction so that the normal competence of the gastroesophageal sphincter is compromised; reflux of gastric contents into the esophagus is a frequent phenomenon. Regurgitation is accentuated in the supine position or by any factor which increases intra-abdominal pressure such as lifting, stooping forward, straining, overeating, and the late stages of pregnancy.

Esophageal motility studies in patients with symptomatic hiatal hernia reveal abnormally low pressures in the gastroesophageal sphincter and failure of

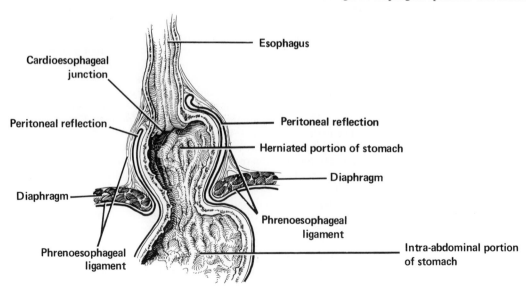

FIG 24–5. Sliding esophageal hernia.

sphincter pressure to increase sufficiently to prevent reflux following elevations in intra-abdominal pressure. It is not yet clear why a weakened sphincter develops so often in association with a hiatal hernia. Although reflux may occur in the absence of a hiatal hernia, it is common experience that a substantial majority of patients with reflux esophagitis are found to have one. Surgical procedures which correct the hernia often eliminate reflux and increase sphincteric pressure, observations which are yet to be explained by a single comprehensive theory on the origin of reflux.

Clinical Findings

A. Symptoms and Signs: In spite of the deranged anatomy in and around the cardioesophageal junction, at least 50% of these hernias are asymptomatic. Reflux of gastric contents into the esophagus accounts for most of the symptoms and complications of sliding hiatal hernia. Retrosternal and epigastric burning pain—often referred to by the patient as "heartburn"—frequently occurs after eating and while sleeping in the supine or flat lateral position. This distress is relieved partially or completely by drinking water or other clear liquids, by antacids, or, in many instances, standing up or sitting up. Patients with severe regurgitation often report that bitter or sour-tasting fluid may regurgitate as far as the throat and mouth, especially at night. They may be awakened by this phenomenon.

Dysphagia may be a prominent symptom and is due to the inflammatory edema incident to lower esophagitis. This dysphagia is never as severe as that caused by organic lesions of the lower esophagus, but its presence indicates a more advanced stage of the disease and a greater likelihood that complications will eventually develop.

In symptomatic patients, esophagoscopy should be performed to assess the severity of the esophagitis and to rule out associated conditions such as strictures, polyps, ulcers, and malignancies. Esophageal motility studies may aid in the diagnosis, and pH determinations may be necessary to determine whether or not true reflux exists.

B. X-Ray Findings: The diagnosis of sliding esophageal hiatal hernia is made by the radiographic demonstration of a portion of the stomach protruding upward through the esophageal hiatus. Repeated fluoroscopic studies may be required. The presence of hiatal hernia is often suggested on routine chest films by the discovery of a gas-filled portion of stomach above the level of the diaphragm; this is often best observed in the lateral projection, since in the anteroposterior view the cardiac shadow may obliterate the hernia outline.

Differential Diagnosis

Sliding esophageal hiatal hernia has been called "the great masquerader of the upper abdomen." Other conditions may present symptoms which mimic those of hiatal hernia, and vice versa. The symptoms caused by a variety of abdominal and intrathoracic diseases are often difficult to differentiate from each other and from those of an uncomplicated sliding hernia. Cholelithiasis, diverticulitis, peptic ulcer, achalasia, and coronary artery disease are common examples. Not infrequently, 3 conditions exist together: hiatal hernia, gallbladder disease, and sigmoid colon diverticulitis. This is sometimes called Saint's triad.

Since pain (when present) may be referred upward into the neck, shoulders, or arms, coronary artery disease—especially angina pectoris—must be considered. Bernstein's test is valuable in the differentiation. A dilute solution of hydrochloric acid is allowed to drip onto the lower esophageal mucosa to determine whether or not the substernal distress of which the patient complains can be artificially duplicated.

When anemia is present, primary blood dyscrasias must be ruled out before ascribing the anemia to the hernia.

Complications

Esophagitis is the most common complication. Derangement of the normal relationships of the cardioesophageal junction causes the sphincteric mechanism to function improperly, with the result that regurgitation of peptic juices occurs. Varying degrees of esophagitis, inflammatory edema, narrowing, and late stricture formation are common. Small, shallow ulcerations may develop as a result of the regurgitant esophagitis, and true callous ulcers may at times be observed in a long-standing neglected hiatal hernia. Carcinoma is occasionally associated with sliding hiatal hernia.

Treatment

At least 50% of sliding esophageal hiatal hernias are asymptomatic and require no treatment. An additional 30–35% of patients with these hernias can be managed by a conservative program of diet, frequent small feedings, and antacids. In addition to combating esophagitis directly, antacids raise pH in the gastric antrum and thereby increase serum gastrin levels. The gastrin may enhance gastroesophageal sphincteric squeeze, thus improving the barrier against further reflux. Anticholinergic drugs, on the other hand, weaken the sphincter and facilitate reflux; they should not be used in the treatment of this disease. About 15% will require operative repair, especially when distress is considerable or if bleeding, obstruction, or, in rare cases, strangulation occurs.

Repair can be accomplished either transthoracically or through an abdominal approach. In patients in whom intra-abdominal disease is suspected, the transabdominal approach is mandatory. In obese patients in whom healing of an abdominal wound may be poor or in patients with a shortened esophagus that requires more mobilization than can be achieved through the abdomen, a transthoracic approach is preferable. In either approach, the operative technic is similar.

Repair of sliding hernias is more complicated than

that of the paraesophageal type. The objective is to replace the cardioesophageal junction in its correct anatomic position in the abdomen and to secure it firmly in place. The enlarged hiatus is closed so that it approximates the crural columns of the diaphragm posteriorly with heavy nonabsorbable sutures. The lower esophagus is extensively mobilized so that about 5 cm of esophagus will reside in the abdomen at the conclusion of the repair. After the crura have been approximated—sometimes using the arcuate ligament in the sutures—the upper part of the lesser curvature of the stomach and the cardioesophageal junction are firmly sutured to the closed crura posteriorly.

Another effective technic—fundoplication—can be used alone or sometimes in combination with the above method. Fundoplication consists of wrapping part of the fundus around the lower 4–6 cm of esophagus and fixing it in place so that the esophagus passes through a short tunnel of stomach before it ends. Although this is a reliable technic for correcting reflux, patients may be rendered unable to belch or vomit—an uncomfortable state at times.

Pyloroplasty and vagotomy should not routinely be added to the standard hiatal hernia repair but should be reserved for patients with known peptic ulcer disease.

Prognosis

The results of operative treatment are good. The recurrence rate in sliding esophageal hernia is approximately 10%. Recurrence of symptoms is more frequent than an anatomic recurrence. The latter may be due to an inadequate technical repair initially; to excessive tension on the point of fixation of the cardioesophageal junction due to shortening of the esophagus; or to weakening of the musculofascial structures by aging, generalized muscular atrophy, or obesity.

Cohen S, Harris LD: Does hiatal hernia affect competence of the gastroesophageal sphincter? New England J Med 284:1053–1056, 1971.

Csendes A, Larrain A: Effect of posterior gastropexy on gastroesophageal sphincter pressure and symptomatic reflux in patients with hiatal hernia. Gastroenterology 63:19–24, 1972.

Dyer NH, Pridie RB: Incidence of hiatus hernia in asymptomatic subjects. Gut 9:696–699, 1968.

Garabedian M: Uses of esophageal manometry and acid perfusion in the study of gastroesophageal reflux and hiatal hernia. S Clin North America 51:589–596, 1971.

Hill LD & others: Simplified management of reflux esophagitis with stricture. Ann Surg 172:638–651, 1970.

Hill LD: Management of recurrent hiatal hernia. Arch Surg 102:296–302, 1971.

Menguy R: Acquired short esophagus with stricture. S Clin North America 50:45–55, 1970.

Polk HC Jr, Zeppa R: Hiatal hernia and esophagitis: A survey of indications for operation and technic and results of fundoplication. Ann Surg 173:775–781, 1971.

Rex JC & others: Esophageal hiatal hernia: A 10-year study of medically treated cases. JAMA 178:271–274, 1961.

Skinner DB, Booth DJ: Assessment of distal esophageal function in patients with hiatal hernia and/or gastroesophageal reflux. Ann Surg 172:627–637, 1970.

Skinner DB, Belsey RHR: Surgical management of esophageal reflux and hiatus hernia: Long-term results with 1030 patients. J Thoracic Cardiovas Surg 53:33–54, 1967.

Stilson WL & others: Hiatal hernia and gastroesophageal reflux: A clinicoradiological analysis of more than 1000 cases. Radiology 93:1323–1327, 1969.

PARASTERNAL OR RETROSTERNAL (FORAMEN OF MORGAGNI) HERNIA

Failure of fusion of the sternal and costal portions of the diaphragm anteriorly in the midline creates a defect known as the foramen of Morgagni. Normally, the diaphragm becomes fused, allowing only the internal mammary arteries and their superior epigastric branches, along with lymphatics, to pass through this area. Hernias through a persistently patent foramen are known as parasternal or retrosternal hernias or hernias through the foramen of Morgagni.

Although this condition is congenital in origin, symptoms usually do not develop until middle life or later. Most patients are women. The symptomatology is variable, but substernal fullness or pain is a major symptom. Routine chest films may show a retrosternal mass or an air-filled viscus.

Tumors of the diaphragm or in the lower anterior mediastinum may mimic a hernia through the foramen of Morgagni. Substernal pain must be differentiated from that due to coronary artery disease.

In infants, if the hernia is large and contains considerable abdominal viscera, the cardiorespiratory distress may simulate that of the more common Bochdalek's hernia and immediate repair becomes mandatory. In adults, complications are rare and many cases are asymptomatic.

Elective surgical repair is indicated in most instances to prevent complications. An emergency operation may become necessary in the newborn infant who develops progressive cardiorespiratory insufficiency. Repair of the defect by a transabdominal approach is preferable, and the results are excellent.

Thomas TV: Subcostosternal diaphragmatic hernia. J Thoracic Cardiovas Surg 63:279–283, 1972.

TRAUMATIC DIAPHRAGMATIC HERNIA

Traumatic rupture of the diaphragm may occur as a result of penetrating wounds or severe blunt external trauma. Lacerations usually occur in the tendinous portion of the diaphragm, most often on the left side. The liver provides protection to diaphragmatic injury on the right side except from penetrating wounds. Abdominal viscera may immediately herniate through the defect in the diaphragm into the pleural cavity or may gradually insinuate themselves into the thorax over a period of months or years.

Clinical Findings

The symptoms are related to the amount of viscera which herniate into the thorax. Some degree of intestinal obstruction may be present. Plain films of the chest will show either a solid mass shadow if the omentum is the primary herniated structure, or a number of fluid levels if hollow viscera herniate. Passage of a nasogastric tube into the herniated stomach above the diaphragm is diagnostic. Fluoroscopic studies often will show the stomach protruding through the diaphragmatic rent. Barium study of the colon may show irregular patches of barium in the colon above the diaphragm or a smooth colonic outline if the colon does not contain feces.

Differential Diagnosis

Traumatic rupture of the diaphragm must be differentiated from atelectasis, space-consuming tumors of the lower pleural space, pleural effusion, and intestinal obstruction due to other causes.

Complications

Hemorrhage and obstruction may occur. If herniation is massive, progressive cardiorespiratory insufficiency may threaten life. The most severe complication is strangulating obstruction or involvement of the blood vessels of the herniated viscera.

Treatment

Transthoracic repair of the ruptured diaphragm is recommended. In the asymptomatic patient in whom a definite diagnosis of a previous traumatic rupture of the diaphragm can be established—and if other conditions simulating traumatic diaphragmatic hernia can be ruled out—operative repair can be delayed until definite symptoms develop. In acute rupture of the diaphragm, associated injuries often take precedence over the diaphragmatic injury; in these instances, however, the acute traumatic tear in the diaphragm should be repaired when feasible.

Prognosis

Surgical repair of the rent in the diaphragm is curative, and the prognosis is excellent. The diaphragm supports sutures well, so that recurrence is practically unknown.

Andrus CH, Morton JH: Rupture of the diaphragm after blunt trauma. Am J Surg 119:686–693, 1970.

Childress ME, Grimes OF: Immediate and remote sequelae of traumatic diaphragmatic hernia. Surg Gynec Obst 113:573, 1961.

Ebert PA & others: Traumatic diaphragmatic hernia. Surg Gynec Obst 125:59–65, 1967.

Hood RM: Traumatic diaphragmatic hernia. Ann Thoracic Surg 12:311–324, 1971.

DUPLICATION OF THE DIAPHRAGM

Duplication—usually of the left hemidiaphragm—is rare. It is frequently associated with an anomaly of the vasculature of the lower lobe of the left lung.

TUMORS OF THE DIAPHRAGM

Primary tumors of the diaphragm are not common. The majority are benign lipomas. Pericardial cysts develop in the interval between the heart and the diaphragm and are usually unilocular and on the right side. Fibrosarcoma, the most common primary malignant diaphragmatic tumor, is extremely rare.

Benign tumors are usually asymptomatic. Since their benign nature cannot be established except by histologic study, all lesions of this type should be excised through an appropriate thoracotomy.

DIAPHRAGMATIC FLUTTER

Diaphragmatic flutter is the most common non-organic disorder of the diaphragm. The cause is not known. It is characterized by diaphragmatic contraction, either continuously or paroxysmally, at a rate of 50–300 per minute or more. Hyperventilation and respiratory alkalosis may result.

Treatment is difficult and often unsatisfactory. Injection of anesthetic solutions into the phrenic nerve may provide temporary relief. Excision of 2–4 cm of the phrenic nerve frequently is curative.

•   •   •

General References

Morson BC, Dawson IMP: *Gastrointestinal Pathology.* Blackwell, 1972.

Skinner DB & others: *Gastroesophageal Reflux and Hiatal Hernia.* Little, Brown, 1972.

Sleisenger M, Fordtran J: *Gastrointestinal Disease.* Saunders, 1973.

Smith RA, Smith RE (editors): *Surgery of the Esophagus.* Appleton-Century-Crofts, 1972.

25 ...

The Stomach & Duodenum

Lawrence W. Way, MD, & Victor Richards, MD

I. STOMACH

The stomach receives food from the esophagus and serves 4 functions: (1) It acts as a reservoir which permits eating reasonably large quantities of food at intervals of several hours. (2) Food contained in the stomach is mixed, triturated, and delivered into the duodenum in amounts regulated by its chemical nature and texture. (3) The first stages of protein and carbohydrate digestion are carried out in the stomach. (4) A few substances are absorbed across the gastric mucosa. These functions will be explained in greater detail after a description of the anatomic features of the stomach.

ANATOMY

A standard nomenclature for the parts of the stomach has not been agreed upon, and different terms are sometimes used for the same region. A descriptive terminology based upon external appearances is reflected in Fig 25–1. The **cardia**, located at the gastroesophageal junction, is so called because lesions at this site often produce symptoms suggestive of heart disease. The **fundus** is the portion of the stomach that lies cephalad to the gastroesophageal junction. The **corpus** or body of the stomach is the capacious central part; division of the corpus from the pyloric antrum is marked by the angular incisure, a crease on the lesser curvature which becomes prominent after death. The **pylorus** is the boundary between the stomach and the duodenum.

A useful system of terminology has been developed which distinguishes physiologic areas as determined by mucosal characteristics (Fig 25–1). Thus, the **cardiac gland area** is the small segment located at the gastroesophageal junction. Histologically, this mucosa contains principally mucus-secreting cells, although a few parietal cells are sometimes present. The **oxyntic gland area** is the portion covered by the mucosa containing parietal (oxyntic) cells and chief cells (Fig 25–2). Its extent in man is depicted in Fig 25–1. The boundary between this region and the adjacent pyloric gland area is reasonably sharp since the zone of transition spans a segment of

only 1–1.5 cm. The **pyloric gland area** comprises about the distal 30% of the stomach. It is important to this area contain the cells which manufacture the hormone gastrin. Mucous cells are common in the oxyntic and pyloric gland areas.

As in the rest of the gastrointestinal tract, the muscular wall of the stomach is composed of an outer longitudinal and an inner circular layer. An additional

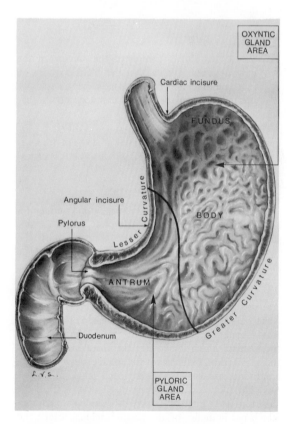

FIG 25–1. Names of the parts of the stomach. The line drawn from the lesser to the greater curvature depicts the approximate boundary between the oxyntic gland area and the pyloric gland area. No prominent landmark exists to distinguish between antrum and body (corpus). The fundus is the portion craniad to the esophagogastric junction.

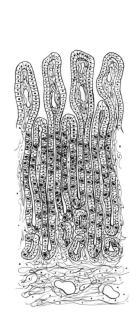

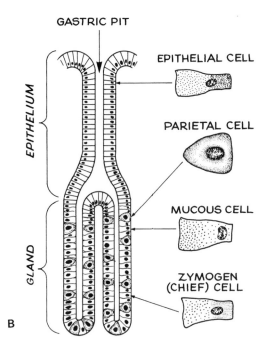

FIG 25−2. Histologic features of the mucosa in the oxyntic gland area. Each gastric pit drains 3−7 tubular gastric glands. The neck of the gland contains many mucus cells. Oxyntic (parietal) cells are most numerous in the midportion of the glands; peptic (chief) cells predominate in the basal portion. *A:* Drawing from photomicrograph of the gastric mucosa. *B:* Stylized representation of the gastric mucosa.

incomplete inner layer of obliquely situated fibers is most prominent near the lesser curvature but is of less substance than the other 2 layers.

Blood Supply

The blood supply of the stomach and duodenum is illustrated in Fig 25−3. The left gastric artery supplies the lesser curvature and connects with the right gastric artery, a branch of the hepatic artery. The greater curvature is supplied by the right gastroepiploic artery (a branch of the gastroduodenal artery) and the left gastroepiploic artery (a branch of the splenic artery). The midportion of the greater curvature corresponds to a point at which the gastric branches of this vascular arcade change direction. The fundus of the stomach along the greater curvature is supplied by the vasa brevia, branches of the splenic and left gastro-epiploic arteries.

The blood supply to the duodenum is from the superior and inferior pancreaticoduodenal arteries, which are branches of the gastroduodenal artery and the superior mesenteric artery, respectively. The stomach contains a rich submucosal vascular plexus which permits varying degrees of arteriovenous shunting. The veins from the stomach drain into the coronary veins, the gastroepiploic veins, and the splenic veins before entering the portal vein. The lymphatic drainage of the stomach partially determines the direction of spread of gastric neoplasms. Its pattern largely parallels that of the arterial supply.

Nerve Supply

The parasympathetic nerves to the stomach are shown in Fig 25−3. As a rule, 2 major vagal trunks pass through the esophageal hiatus in close approximation to the esophageal muscle. These nerves are originally located to the right and left of the esophagus and stomach during embryonic development. When the foregut rotates, the lesser curvature faces to the right and the greater curvature to the left, and corresponding shifts in location of the vagal trunks follow. Hence, the right vagus supplies the posterior gastric surface and the left the anterior surface. Approximately 90% of the fibers in the vagal trunks are sensory afferent; the remaining 10% are efferent.

In the region of the gastroesophageal junction, each trunk bifurcates. The anterior trunk sends a division to the liver which travels in the lesser omentum. The remainder of the fibers branch almost immediately on the anterior surface of the stomach. The bifurcation of the posterior trunk gives rise to fibers which enter the celiac plexus and supply the parasympathetic innervation to the remainder of the gastrointestinal tract as far as the mid transverse colon. The gastric division of the posterior trunk spreads out over the posterior gastric surface and also runs down the lesser curvature. As shown in Fig 25−3, a variable number of vagal fibers ascend with the left gastric artery after having passed through the celiac plexus. It is important to appreciate this feature when performing a selective gastric vagotomy.

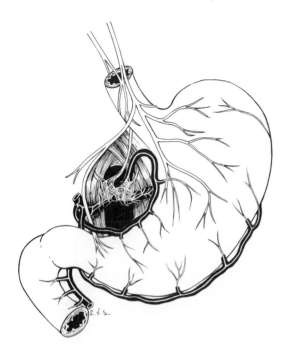

FIG 25−3. Blood supply and parasympathetic innervation of the stomach and duodenum.

The preganglionic motor fibers of the vagal trunks synapse with ganglion cells in Auerbach's plexus (plexus myentericus) between the longitudinal and circular muscle layers. Postganglionic cholinergic fibers are distributed to the cells of the smooth muscle layers and the mucosa.

The adrenergic innervation to the stomach consists of postganglionic fibers which pass along the arterial vessels from the celiac plexus.

PHYSIOLOGY

Motility

Storage, mixing, trituration, and regulated emptying are accomplished by the muscular apparatus of the stomach. Peristaltic waves originate in the fundus and pass toward the pylorus. The thickness of the smooth muscle increases in the antrum and corresponds to the stronger contractions that can be measured in the distal stomach. The pylorus behaves as a sphincter, although it normally allows a little to-and-fro movement of chyme across the junction.

An electrical pacemaker is situated in the fundal musculature near the greater curvature. Regular electrical impulses arise from this area and pass toward the pylorus in the outer longitudinal layer. The rate of discharge is about 3 per minute in man. Every impulse is not always followed by a peristaltic muscular contraction but they determine the maximal peristaltic rate. The frequency of peristalsis is governed by a variety of stimuli mentioned below. Each contraction follows sequential depolarization of the underlying circular muscle resulting from arrival of the pacesetter potential.

Peristaltic contractions are more forceful in the antrum than the body and travel faster as they progress distally. Gastric chyme is forced into the funnel-shaped antral chamber by peristalsis; the volume of contents delivered into the duodenum by each peristaltic wave depends on the strength of the advancing wave and the extent to which the pylorus closes. Most of the gastric contents which are pushed into the antral funnel are propelled backward as the pylorus closes and pressure within the antral lumen rises. Five to 15 ml enter the duodenum with each gastric peristaltic wave.

The volume of the empty gastric lumen is only 50 ml. The organ has great compliance since about 1000 ml can be ingested before intraluminal pressure begins to rise. Peristalsis is initiated by the stimulus of distention after eating. Various other factors have positive or negative influences on the rate and strength of contractions and the rate of gastric emptying. Vagal reflexes from the stomach have a facilitating influence on peristalsis. The texture of the meal participates in the regulation of emptying; small particles are emptied more rapidly than large ones which the organ attempts to reduce in size (trituration). The osmolality of gastric chyme and its chemical makeup are monitored by duodenal receptors. If osmolality is greater than 200 mOsm/liter, a long vagal reflex (the enterogastric reflex) is activated, delaying emptying. Further time within the stomach allows greater dilution by gastric juice and decreases osmolality if the gastric contents are hyperosmolar.

Humoral inhibition of gastric motility results from fat or acid in the small bowel. The former releases **enterogastrone**, an inhibitor of gastric secretion and motility. Secretin is liberated when the pH in the small bowel is below 5.0. The actions of secretin on the stomach are similar to those of enterogastrone.

Gastric Secretion

The mucosa of the stomach secretes mucus, hydrochloric acid, pepsinogen, and intrinsic factor. Secretory rates depend on the balance of stimulant and inhibitory influences. Acid and pepsin have roles in the early stages of digestion. An understanding of the mechanism of acid secretion is of particular significance to the surgeon in the rational design of operations for duodenal ulcer.

Gastric Juice

The output of gastric juice in a fasting subject varies between 500 and 1500 ml/day. After each meal, about 1000 ml are secreted by the stomach.

The components of gastric juice are as follows:

A. Mucus: Mucus is manufactured in the mucous cells of the oxyntic and the pyloric gland areas. Mucus is a heterogenous mixture of glycoproteins whose physiologic function is obscure. Mucus does not provide a barrier to the diffusion of H^+ and cannot be thought of as protective of the mucosa on that basis. It probably acts as a lubricant and may impede diffusion of pepsin.

B. Pepsinogen: Pepsinogens are synthesized in the chief cells of the oxyntic gland area (and to a lesser extent in the pyloric area) and are stored as visible granules. Cholinergic stimuli, either vagal or intramural, are the most potent pepsigogues, although gastrin and secretin are also effective. The precursor zymogen is activated when pH falls below 5.0, a process that entails severance of a polypeptide fragment from the larger molecule. Pepsin cleaves peptide bonds, especially those containing phenylalanine, tyrosine, or leucine. Its optimal pH is about 2.0. Pepsin activity is abolished at $pH > 5.0$, and the molecule is irreversibly denatured at $pH > 8.0$.

C. Intrinsic Factor: This substance is a mucoprotein which in man is secreted into the gastric lumen by the parietal cells. Intrinsic factor binds with vitamin B_{12} of dietary origin and greatly enhances absorption of the vitamin. Absorption occurs by an active process in the terminal ileum.

Intrinsic factor secretion is enhanced by stimuli that produce H^+ output from parietal cells. Pernicious anemia is characterized by atrophy of the parietal cell mucosa, deficiency in intrinsic factor, and anemia. Subclinical deficiencies in vitamin B_{12} have been described after operations that reduce gastric acid secretion, and abnormal Schilling tests in these patients can be corrected by the administration of intrinsic factor. Total gastrectomy creates a dependence on parenteral administration of vitamin B_{12}.

D. Blood Group Substances: Seventy-five percent of people secrete blood group antigens into gastric juice. The trait is genetically determined and is associated with a lower incidence of duodenal ulcer than in nonsecretors.

E. Electrolytes: The unique characteristic of gastric secretion is its high concentration of hydrochloric acid, a product of the parietal cells. As the concentration of H^+ rises during secretion, that of Na^+ drops in a reciprocal fashion. K^+ remains relatively constant at 5–10 mEq/liter. Chloride concentration remains near 150 mEq/liter and gastric juice maintains its isotonicity at varying secretory rates.

Mechanism of Gastric Acid Secretion & the Mucosal Barrier

The parietal cells secrete hydrochloric acid, which can reduce the pH within the gastric lumen to about 0.9, ie, the concentration of H^+ may reach 150 mEq/liter. This represents a concentration 10^6 times greater than is found in the blood. Despite the high concentration gradient, there is normally very little back diffusion of acid across the gastric mucosa. For this reason, one may think of the mucosa as possessing a barrier to acid diffusion, and experimental studies have outlined its properties and vulnerability to injurious agents. For example, if the mucosa is exposed to aspirin at a $pH < 3.0$, the efficiency of the barrier diminishes. Acid

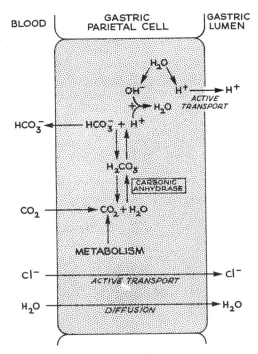

FIG 25–4. Intracellular processes in the formation of gastric hydrochloric acid.

instilled into a stomach treated in this manner escapes across the mucosa at a markedly increased rate. As it enters the submucosa, the H^+ releases tissue histamine, which dilates nearby blood vessels and increases capillary permeability. Intramural cholinergic reflexes are activated and may cause further stimulation of parietal and chief cells. Mucosal edema and bleeding may result. Counterparts of these experimental phenomena probably occur in patients and will be referred to under the discussion of stress ulcers and gastric ulcers.

Not much is known about the intracellular biochemical events that precede acid secretion. Both H^+ and Cl^- are actively transported into the gastric lumen by separate pumps which are coupled (Fig 25–4). The H^+ may be thought of as a product of the dissociation of H_2O. Carbonic acid is formed from the hydration of CO_2, a reaction which is facilitated by the large amount of carbonic anhydrase in these cells. The carbonic acid dissociates, and the resulting bicarbonate is excreted into the blood stream. Water enters the gastric lumen passively following the actively transported ions, and the secretion is isotonic or nearly so.

Gastrin

Gastrin has been extracted from the antrum, identified chemically, and synthesized. The compound originally found in antral extracts is a linear heptadecapeptide, but recent studies have shown that most of the hormone present in the circulation is about 2½ times this size. Big gastrin contains heptadecapeptide gastrin, and the 2 react identically to antigastrin antibodies. The smaller unit is probably responsible for the biologic activity of the larger one. Both types of gastrin have been identified in extracts of the antral mucosa. Gastrin is produced by specialized cells in the pyloric gland area of the stomach and in the duodenum. The jejunum contains physiologically insignificant quantities.

The C-terminal tetrapeptide of gastrin must be present for activity. In fact, this small piece can elicit the full range of actions of the entire molecule. The synthetic C-terminal pentapeptide (pentagastrin) has been used widely in Great Britain as an acid stimulant, but it is not yet available in the USA for humans.

In addition to stimulating parietal cells, gastrin has the following actions: (1) stimulation of pepsinogen secretion, (2) stimulation of pancreatic enzyme production, (3) stimulation of gastric motility, (4) enhancement of squeeze in the lower esophageal sphincter, (5) stimulation of bile flow, and (6) stimulation of protein synthesis in the gastric mucosa.

Cholecystokinin-pancreozymin (CCK) resembles gastrin by possessing the same active segment, and for this reason the 2 molecules share some physiologic actions. Their differences in biologic activity are due to the presence in CCK of a sulfated tyrosyl residue in the seventh position from the C-terminus. CCK contains 33 amino acids arranged linearly. The exact sequence has not yet been fully elucidated.

CCK stimulates pancreatic enzyme production, but gastrin has little effect on the pancreas in man. Both react with receptors on parietal cells: gastrin stimulates acid secretion; CCK is a weak stimulant when given alone, but, by competition for receptor sites, it partially blocks the action of gastrin. CCK stimulates contraction of the gallbladder, whereas gastrin has almost no effect on this organ. CCK also stimulates gastrointestinal motor activity.

Regulation of Acid Secretion

The regulation of acid secretion can be described by considering separately those factors that enhance acid production and those that depress it. The interaction of these forces results in the levels of secretion observed while fasting and after meals.

A. Stimulation of Acid Secretion: Acid production is usually presented as the result of 3 phases which are named from the locus where the stimuli impinge. The usual physiologic event that brings about increased parietal cell activity is eating a meal, and all 3 phases are excited simultaneously. Thus, the separation into phases is of value principally for descriptive purposes.

1. Cephalic phase–Stimuli which act upon the brain lead to increased vagal efferent activity and acid secretion. The sight, smell, taste, or even the thought of appetizing food may elicit this response. The effect is entirely vagally mediated and is abolished by vagotomy. The vagal stimuli have a direct effect on the parietal cells to increase acid output. Impulses via vagal fibers to the antrum release gastrin and thereby indirectly affect acid secretion. The direct parietal cell stimulation is quantitatively more important.

2. Gastric phase–The arrival of food in the stomach initiates additional processes leading to acid

secretion. Both mechanical and chemical stimuli increase gastrin release. Distention of the antrum is the major mechanical stimulus. Certain amino acids and alcohols liberate gastrin when in contact with the antral mucosa, and these stimuli comprise the chemical mechanism for gastrin release.

The presence of food in the stomach excites long vagal reflexes, impulses which pass to the CNS via vagal afferents and return to the parietal cell mucosa to evoke acid release.

A third aspect of the gastric phase involves the sensitizing effect of distention of the parietal cell area to gastrin. It is thought that distention here activates local intramucosal cholinergic reflexes which end on parietal cells.

3. Intestinal phase–The role of the intestinal phase in the stimulation of gastric secretion has been incompletely investigated. Various experiments have shown that the presence of food in the small bowel releases substances from the mucosa which evoke acid secretion from the stomach.

B. Inhibition of Acid Secretion: Without these strategically located systems which limit secretion, unchecked acid production could become a serious clinical problem. Examples can be found in the surgical literature where acid production rose after measures which eliminated these inhibitory mechanisms.

1. Antral inhibition–A reduction of pH in the antrum inhibits the release of gastrin regardless of the stimulus. When the pH reaches 1.2, it is almost completely blocked. If the normal relationship of parietal cell mucosa to antral mucosa is changed so that acid does not flow past the site of gastrin production, serum gastrin may increase to high levels with marked acid stimulation.

2. Intestinal inhibition–The intestinal mucosa produces 4 substances which inhibit acid secretion. Generically, these may be called enterogastrones because literally the word would apply to all such compounds. Two hormones, secretin and cholecystokinin (CCK), have been isolated, purified, and completely (secretin) or partially (CCK) characterized chemically. Both block the stimulating effect of gastrin on the parietal cells. Secretin, which also depresses gastrin levels, is released by the contact of acid solutions (pH < 5.0) with the intestinal mucosa. CCK is liberated by amino acids and fats.

A third substance is released by fat in the intestine. Historically, the word enterogastrone was first used to describe the inhibitory effect of fat on acid secretion, and at present its use in the narrow sense is applied to this agent. Enterogastrone has not yet been extracted in purified form.

Acid within the duodenal bulb may liberate a hormone which is confined to this small segment of the gastrointestinal tract. It has been named bulbogastrone by its discoverers and appears chemically to be a polypeptide. Bulbogastrone also blocks the action of gastrin on parietal cells.

Integration of Gastric Physiologic Function

Ingested food is mixed with salivary amylase before it reaches the stomach. The mechanisms stimulating gastric secretion are activated. Serum gastrin levels increase from a mean fasting concentration of about 75 pg/ml to 200–400 pg/ml. The peak occurs about 30 minutes after the meal. Food in the lumen of the stomach is exposed to high concentrations of acid and pepsin at the mucosal surface. Food resides in layers determined by sequence of arrival, but fat tends to float to the top. The greatest mixing occurs in the antrum. Antral contents therefore become more uniformly acidic than those in the body of the organ, where the central portion of the meal tends to remain alkaline for a considerable time, allowing continued activity of the amylase.

Peptic digestion of protein in the stomach is only about 5–10% complete. Carbohydrate digestion is more complete and may reach 30–40%. Gastric juice contains a lipolytic enzyme, but gastric digestion of triglycerides appears to be small.

The gastric contents are delivered to the duodenum at a rate that is determined by the texture of the meal, its osmolality and acidity, and its content of fat. A meal of lean meat, potatoes, and vegetables leaves the stomach within 3 hours. A meal with a very high fat content may remain in the stomach for 6–12 hours.

Berson SA, Yalow RS: Radioimmunoassay in gastroenterology. Gastroenterology 62:1061–1084, 1972.

Davenport HW: *Physiology of the Digestive Tract,* 3rd ed. Year Book, 1971.

Fisher RS, Cohen S: Physiologic characteristics of the human pyloric sphincter. Gastroenterology 64:67–75, 1973.

Grossman MI: Gastrin and its activities. Nature 228:1147–1150, 1970.

Kelley KA: Gastric motility and ulcer surgery. S Clin North America 51:927–934, 1971.

McGuigan JE, Greider MH: Correlative immunochemical and light microscopic studies of the gastrin cell of the antral mucosa. Gastroenterology 60:223–236, 1971.

Samloff IM: Pepsinogens, pepsins, and pepsin inhibitors. Gastroenterology 60:586–604, 1971.

PEPTIC ULCER

Peptic ulcers result from the corrosive action of acid gastric juice on a vulnerable epithelium. Depending on circumstances, they may occur in the esophagus, duodenum, the stomach itself, in the jejunum after surgical construction of a gastrojejunostomy, or in the ileum in relation to ectopic gastric mucosa in a Meckel diverticulum. When the term peptic ulcer was first used, it was thought that the most important factor was the peptic activity in gastric juice. Since then, evidence has accumulated which implicates the acid as the chief causative agent, and in fact it is a useful clinical axiom that if gastric juice contains no acid a (benign) peptic ulcer cannot be present. Appreciation of the central role of acid has led to the emphasis on antacid therapy as the mainstay of medical therapy of ulcers and to operations logically designed to reduce acid secretion as the major surgical approach.

It has been estimated that about 5% of the adult population in the USA suffer from active peptic ulcer disease. Males are affected 3 times as often as females. Duodenal ulcers are 10 times more common than gastric ulcers in young patients, but in the older age groups the frequency is about equal. In the USA, peptic ulcer disease annually causes about 15,000 deaths and about 15 million days lost from work. The calculated loss to the nation's economy—considering deaths, costs of hospitalization, and days of work lost—is over $1 billion a year.

In general terms, the ulcerative process can lead to 4 types of disability: (1) **Pain** is the most common of these. (2) **Bleeding** may occur due to erosion of submucosal or extraintestinal vessels as the ulcer becomes deeper. (3) Penetration of the ulcer through all layers of the affected gut results in **perforation** if other viscera do not seal the ulcer. (4) **Obstruction** may result from inflammatory swelling and scarring and is most likely to occur with ulcers located at the pylorus or gastroesophageal junction because the lumen is narrowest at those sites.

The causes, clinical features, and prognosis of duodenal ulcer and gastric ulcer are sufficiently different to suggest that they are fundamentally different diseases whose major common feature is acid-dependent ulceration.

1. DUODENAL ULCER

Essentials of Diagnosis

- Epigastric pain relieved by food or antacids.
- Epigastric tenderness.
- Normal or increased gastric acid secretion.
- Signs of ulcer disease on upper gastrointestinal x-rays.

General Considerations

Duodenal ulcers may occur in any age group but are most common in the young and middle-aged (20–45 years). They appear in men more often than women, but the incidence in men is decreasing while that in women is on the rise. Most clinicians note that fewer chronic painful duodenal ulcers are being seen but that bleeding ulcers are becoming a greater clinical problem.

About 95% of duodenal ulcers are situated within 2 cm of the pylorus, in the duodenal bulb.

Several clues are available regarding the causes of duodenal ulcer, but a satisfactory comprehensive theory remains elusive. The disease has apparently emerged as a major clinical entity in western society only since the latter part of the 19th century. An increasing incidence correlates somewhat with the increase in psychologic stresses associated with modern life. The rising prevalence in women in recent years parallels their acceptance of increased responsibilities outside the home. Duodenal ulcer is rare in most tribal African cultures, whereas in the USA the incidence in blacks equals or is greater than that in the white population.

Increased gastric acid secretion is present in many patients with duodenal ulcer. Both basal and maximal outputs are high, indicating a sustained increased drive to the parietal cells and an enlarged parietal cell mass. The latter presumably reflects a response to increased stimulation over a prolonged period. Gastrin levels in fasting patients with duodenal ulcer are slightly above those in people without ulcers. Since acid hypersecretion could normally be expected to inhibit gastrin release, the modest elevation may be significant. The traditional explanation for the hypersecretion seen in this disease is increased vagal activity, said to be a reflection of underlying psychic stresses. Empirical data to support this speculation have not been presented.

Another possible explanation for the increased acid secretion in peptic ulcer might be deficiencies in the production of enterogastrones. Several studies comparing duodenal ulcer patients with normal subjects show no differences in the response to intestinal stimulation, but this hypothesis has not yet been fully explored.

Another theoretical cause of peptic ulcer is decreased resistance of the duodenal mucosa to the action of gastric acid and pepsin. A major weakness of this theory is that it fails to account for the known acid hypersecretion. Several other clinical factors are known to be associated with enhanced susceptibility to duodenal ulcer. The disease is more common in individuals with blood group O and in those who fail to secrete blood group antigens H, A, or B in their gastric juice. An antipeptic activity of these substances may account for this relationship.

Chronic liver disease, chronic lung disease, and chronic pancreatitis have all been implicated as increasing the possibility of duodenal ulceration. Except for patients with pancreatic exocrine insufficiency who have decreased bicarbonate secretion into the duodenum, the mechanism behind the predisposition is unclear.

Fortunately, our hazy picture of the pathogenesis of duodenal ulcer has not blocked the development of effective therapies solidly based on pathophysiologic principles.

Clinical Findings

A. Symptoms and Signs: Pain is the presenting symptom in most patients with uncomplicated duodenal ulcer. It is usually located in the epigastrium and is variably described as aching, burning, or gnawing, but radiologic survey studies indicate that as many as a third of patients with active duodenal ulcer may be entirely free of gastrointestinal complaints.

The daily cycle of the pain is characteristic. The patient usually has no pain in the morning until an hour or more after breakfast. It is relieved by the noon meal, only to recur in the later afternoon. Pain may appear again in the evening, and in about half of cases it arouses the patient during the night. Food, milk, or antacid preparations temporarily relieve the discomfort.

When the ulcer **penetrates** posteriorly into the head of the pancreas, back pain is noted; concomitantly, the cyclic pattern of pain may change to a more steady discomfort, with less relief from food and antacids.

Varying degrees of nausea and vomiting accompany the pain. Vomiting may be a major feature even in the absence of obstruction. For unknown reasons, such patients are sometimes less responsive to medical or surgical therapy.

The abdominal examination may reveal localized epigastric tenderness somewhat to the right of midline. In many instances, no tenderness can be elicited.

The activity of duodenal ulcer and its accompanying symptoms typically remit and recur at intervals of several years. Relapses last for 2–4 months, but the variation is great. The natural tendency toward remission must be kept in mind when attributing improvement in symptoms to any particular therapeutic regimen.

B. Laboratory Findings:

1. Test for occult blood—Examination of the stool for occult blood should be done even in the absence of clinical or laboratory evidence of gastrointestinal bleeding.

2. Gastric analysis—The role of increased acid secretion in the production of duodenal ulcer has stimulated the development of tests for clinical assessment of gastric acid output. Although gastric analysis has been widely adopted in the investigation of patients with duodenal ulcer, the results have limited usefulness in diagnostic and therapeutic decision-making.

a. Standard gastric analysis— The standard gastric analysis consists of the following: (1) Measurement of acid production by the unstimulated stomach under basal fasting conditions; the result is expressed as H^+ secretion in mEq/hour and is termed the **basal acid output (BAO)**. (2) Measurement of acid production during stimulation by histamine, betazole (Histalog), or pentagastrin given in a dose which is maximal for this effect. The result is expressed as H^+ secretion in mEq/hour and is termed the **maximal acid output (MAO)**.

The test is performed as follows: The patient is fasted for 12 hours before the study, except that he may have water. Specifically, antacids, anticholinergic drugs, or other agents known to affect gastric secretion must be withheld. The reliability of the procedure is enhanced by having the examination performed by a specially trained technician. A nasogastric tube is passed into the stomach. Fluoroscopic verification of positioning improves results but is impractical in most

TABLE 25–1. **Mean values for acid output during gastric analysis for normals and patients with duodenal ulcer.** The upper limits of normal are: Basal (BAO), 5 mEq/hour; maximal (MAO), 30 mEq/hour.

| | Sex | Mean Acid Output (mEq/Hour) | |
		Normal	Duodenal Ulcer
Basal	Male	2.5	5.5
	Female	1.5	3.0
Maximal (betazole)	Male	30	40
	Female	20	30

instances. The stomach is emptied of its contents, which are discarded; subsequent secretions are preserved. The patient should be supine, positioned somewhat on his left side, and instructed to expectorate all saliva. Aspiration of gastric juice must be made continuously. The specimens are divided into 15-minute aliquots.

At the end of a basal hour of collection, the gastric stimulant is given by subcutaneous injection. Histamine, 0.04 mg/kg, was originally used for this purpose, but the analogue betazole hydrochloride (Histalog), 1.5 mg/kg, has largely replaced it because its side-effects are much less. Pentagastrin, the gastrin analogue, 6 μg/kg, has become the drug preferred by most British physicians, but it is not available in the USA for clinical use. Its side-effects are even less than those from betazole.

After the injection of betazole, gastric juice is collected for 1½ hours, again in 15-minute portions. Acid concentration in each 15-minute specimen is then titrated to pH 7.0. The end point may be determined with a pH meter or phenolphthalein indicator. Output (in mEq) is obtained as the product of concentration and volume of the specimen. BAO is determined as the sum of the 4 periods before betazole injection. MAO is calculated by adding the 4 highest consecutive periods after stimulation.

Interpretation of the results of gastric analysis is outlined in Table 25–1. A major limitation to the usefulness of this test derives from the observation that over half of patients with duodenal ulcer have maximal secretory values that overlap those of people without ulcers. For example, patients with acid secretory values in the normal range may have active duodenal ulcer, and the clinical course in such individuals may be indistinguishable from that of patients with hypersecretion.

The term **achlorhydria** denotes no acid (pH > 6.0) after maximal stimulation. Achlorhydria is incompatible with a diagnosis of benign peptic ulcer. In patients in whom x-ray studies have demonstrated gastric ulcer, this finding would indicate the presence of underlying gastric cancer. Malignancy in duodenal ulcers is extremely rare.

Patients with Zollinger-Ellison syndrome have elevated gastrin levels in their serum. As a result, their parietal cells are subject to maximal conditions of gastric analysis. Basal acid secretion is often greater than 15 mEq/hour, and the ratio of BAO to MAO is characteristically 0.6 or greater. Confirmation of the diagnosis requires direct measurement of elevated serum gastrin levels by immunoassay.

In the past, gastric acid output was collected during a 12-hour overnight period for clinical analysis. This method is less accurate than the basal 1-hour collection and has been abandoned. The terms "free" acid, "combined" acid, and "degrees" of acidity have been dropped from the lexicon of gastric analysis since they were confusing and without pathophysiologic significance.

b. Hollander insulin gastric analysis–This method of measuring gastric acid secretion determines the status of the vagal innervation of the stomach. The principal usefulness of the Hollander test is to detect physiologically intact vagal supply to the stomach in patients suffering from recurrent ulcer after a previous surgical vagotomy.

The patient is studied first under basal conditions as described above. Collections of gastric juice are made for 1 hour, and regular insulin, 0.2 unit/kg, is then given by rapid IV injection. A blood sample is taken for glucose determination before the insulin is given and again 30 and 60 minutes afterward. Gastric juice is aspirated for 2 hours after insulin, and each 15-minute sample is titrated to pH 7.0.

This dose of insulin should lower blood glucose below 50 mg/100 ml. The hypoglycemia activates cortical centers, resulting in increased vagal activity, and stimulates gastric secretion if gastric innervation has not been destroyed.

The interpretation of the Hollander test uses the concentrations of acid in the secreted juice rather than the quantity is milliequivalents. The standard criteria for a positive test, meaning that significant vagal innervation persists, are as follows: If the basal secretion contained no acid, a level of 10 mEq/liter after insulin is positive; if the basal secretion contained acid, an elevation of its concentration by 20 mEq/liter over basal, after insulin, is positive.

C. X-Ray Findings: Radiologic examination of the gastroduodenal region is done after the patient swallows a barium sulfate suspension. The changes induced by duodenal ulcer consist of **duodenal deformities** and an **ulcer niche**. Distortion of the normal duodenal configuration results from inflammatory swelling and scarring and leads to findings such as distortion of the duodenal bulb, eccentricity of the pyloric channel, or pseudodiverticulum formation. The ulcer itself may be seen either in profile or, more commonly, *en face*.

The reliability of x-ray diagnosis appears to be high, but accurate figures are not available to support this clinical impression. In the routine case, response to therapy should be judged mainly on symptomatic changes rather than evidence of healing demonstrated on serial x-ray examinations.

D. Special Examinations: Gastroscopy is not of

routine value in the investigation of duodenal ulcer. Its use in this disease is largely confined to patients with bleeding from the upper intestine or those who have obstruction of the gastroduodenal segment.

Differential Diagnosis

The differential diagnosis of peptic ulcer includes any other abdominal disorder that causes epigastric pain and indigestion. The most common diseases simulating peptic ulcer are (1) chronic cholecystitis, in which cholecystograms show either nonfunction of the gallbladder or stones in a functioning gallbladder; (2) pancreatitis, in which the serum amylase is elevated (not elevated in peptic ulcer disease unless the ulcer penetrates through into the pancreas); (3) functional indigestion, in which x-rays are normal; and (4) hiatal hernia, which can be seen on x-rays.

It is clear that the x-ray is the most important diagnostic adjunct in verifying the presence and character of the underlying peptic ulcer disease.

Complications

Other than the morbidity caused by pain, the common complications of duodenal ulcer are hemorrhage, perforation, and duodenal obstruction. Each of these is discussed in a separate section. Less common complications consist of pancreatitis and biliary obstruction.

Prevention

Prevention entails avoidance of ulcerogenic drugs in susceptible individuals: nicotine, alcohol, reserpine, caffeine, and other xanthines found in cola drinks. No other special dietary precautions are thought to be significant. Elimination of unusually stressful environmental factors may be helpful.

Treatment

Duodenal ulcer can be controlled by medical treatment in a substantial majority of patients. Surgical treatment is reserved for those whose ulcer disease persists in the face of an adequate medical regimen (called an **intractable** ulcer) or in whom bleeding, perforation, or obstruction develops.

A. Medical Treatment: The goals of medical treatment are to remove ulcerogenic factors and to neutralize gastroduodenal pH so that healing may occur.

1. Diet—Ulcerogenic agents must be proscribed. Nicotine, corticosteroids, reserpine, alcohol, salicylates, phenylbutazone, and caffeine and other xanthines (coffee, tea, and cola beverages) have all been shown to have theoretical or actual adverse effects in duodenal ulcer.

Food buffers gastric acid principally via the carboxyl groups in protein and the patient should be taught the importance of frequent meals of a palatable and nutritious character. A snack between each of the 3 main meals and again in the late evening is a convenient schedule during treatment of an acute ulcer.

A bland diet based on use of soft foods, including custards, creams, milk, etc, has not been shown to benefit the ulcer patient. The physician must make every attempt to enlist the patient's informed cooperation in the therapeutic program since in most instances it is the patient who makes many of the therapeutic decisions over the protracted course of the disease. In discussing dietary restrictions—which most patients assume to be the cornerstone of therapy—it is useful to point out that foods that have no injurious effects when applied to the skin of the forearm are equally well tolerated by the intestinal epithelium.

2. Antacids—Antacids are the principal drugs used in the therapy of peptic ulcer disease. The importance of therapy aimed at neutralizing gastric acid derives from the following observations: (1) in the absence of acid, benign ulcers do not appear; (2) the pH optimum for peptic activity is low, and pepsin is inactive at pH > 5.0; (3) surgical procedures that have in common the ability to lower acid secretion effectively control ulcer disease.

The criteria for adequate antacid therapy consist of selecting an effective preparation, prescribing the proper dose and dosage interval, and obtaining patient compliance with the prescribed regimen.

a. Treatment of the acute ulcer—The patient with recent onset of pain whose ulcer has been demonstrated on gastroduodenal x-rays should be treated intensively for at least 4 weeks. In addition to the dietary advice outlined above, antacids should be taken at intervals of 1 hour between meals while awake to maintain gastric pH in the range of pepsin inactivity. The hourly interval has been derived from a consideration of the rate of gastric emptying of these drugs and their neutralizing capacity. If the patient experiences pain at night, he should be instructed to take antacids one-half hour before the usual time of his discomfort. The most important time for taking antacids is the period 2–5 hours after eating. Treatment regimens that rely on self-regulated doses in response to pain and taking antacids on a 3-times-a-day schedule are irrational.

b. Chronic treatment—The patient who has once developed and healed a duodenal ulcer is prone to develop transient episodes of indigestion even in the absence of bona fide recurrent ulcers. These symptoms should be treated with antacids on a schedule sufficient to maintain comfort. Persistence of symptoms suggests recurrent ulceration, in which case hourly administration of antacids must be reinstituted after radiologic verification.

c. Choice of antacid preparation—The liquid forms of all antacids are more effective than tablets and should always be used for intensive treatment of an acute ulcer. On the other hand, for occasional dyspepsia while at work, shopping, and in other social situations, patients will find that the convenience of tablets compensates for their inferiority to liquid antacids. In such cases, the tablets should be chewed or dissolved in the mouth for maximum effect.

(1) Aluminum hydroxide gels—Some aluminum hydroxide preparations have been found to have delayed onset of activity because of their gel nature.

These drugs also adsorb antibiotics; patients with infections should never be treated simultaneously with oral antibiotics and aluminum hydroxide gel antacids. Dietary phosphorus is bound by these drugs, and they have been used therapeutically to achieve phosphorus depletion. In practice, the theoretical possibility of induced hypophosphatemia and osteomalacia is an unlikely complication of the use of aluminum gels. Most of these preparations contain enough sodium so that they would be contraindicated for patients on strict sodium restriction.

(2) **Magnesium compounds**—Magnesium oxide is probably the antacid of choice according to present knowledge. Combination with aluminum hydroxide decreases the likelihood of troublesome diarrhea resulting from therapeutically required doses. Magnesium carbonate and magnesium trisilicate are much less effective antacids and should probably be abandoned. Hypermagnesemia is a potential complication in patients with severe renal disease.

(3) **Calcium compounds**—The various forms of calcium carbonate are all effective antacids, but they possess several undesirable features. Calcium carbonate, by contrast with other antacids, increases the release of gastrin when in contact with the pyloric mucosa. This seems to account for the rebound of acid secretion which follows ingestion of calcium carbonate. However, hourly doses of the antacid keep the gastric pH in the desired range, so that these compounds can be used to good effect. Hypercalcemia can be demonstrated in about 20% of patients treated with hourly calcium carbonate. Prolonged adherence to a regimen of hourly calcium carbonate would involve a risk of renal lithiasis or milk-alkali syndrome. The constipating tendency of calcium compounds can be offset by alternating use of these drugs with magnesium oxide or magnesium hydroxide.

3. **Anticholinergic drugs**—These compounds have logical attractiveness for the treatment of peptic ulcer, but in practice they have not been shown to have therapeutic benefit. Anticholinergic drugs have theoretic value because they decrease acid secretion and delay gastric emptying. Earlier studies suggested a decreased incidence of recurrence in patients placed on anticholinergic agents after an initial remission was achieved, but attempts to repeat this observation have not been successful. They are often prescribed before bedtime to delay emptying of an evening snack.

Several anticholinergics seem to have greater gastric effect than peripheral action. Propantheline (Pro-Banthine), glycopyrrolate (Robinul), and oxyphencyclimine (Daricon) are superior to belladonna or atropine in this respect. Dosage should be sufficient to produce dryness of the mouth.

4. **Rest and sedation**—Severe anxiety calls for treatment with sedatives such as phenobarbital or diazepam, but the routine use of sedatives is not known to hasten healing of ulcers. It is occasionally necessary to recommend to the patient that he temporarily or even permanently withdraw from an anxiety-producing environment or occupation if

control of ulcer cannot be achieved otherwise.

Admission to the hospital speeds healing of gastric ulcers and may have similar value for duodenal ulcer. This action removes the patient from his environment, provides an opportunity for physical and emotional rest, and ensures greater accuracy in administration of an intensive antacid regimen. The major expense incurred by this measure demands that it be used only for those patients who do not respond to outpatient treatment or who are in imminent danger of developing complications.

5. **Gastric irradiation**—Irradiation of the parietal cell mucosa diminishes acid secretion and can be used to treat peptic ulcers in selected patients. A total dose of 1600–2000 rads is delivered to the tissues over a 10-day period. The mean secretory depression of about 50% usually appears within 3–6 weeks after completion of therapy and leads to healing of the ulcer in the majority of cases. The histologic appearance and function of the mucosa recover in a large portion of patients over several years thereafter; recurrent ulceration develops in 30% by 5 years. Hypertension due to radiation nephritis has been detected in some patients treated more than 5 years earlier by this regimen. For these reasons, this technic should be restricted to the elective treatment of elderly patients who are unacceptably poor risks for surgery.

B. Surgical Treatment: If medical management fails to control the patient's symptoms, one must first consider whether the therapeutic regimen has taken full advantage of the potential of antacids and avoidance of aggravating situations and drugs. If medical treatment has been optimal, the ulcer may be judged **intractable** and surgical treatment is indicated. There are unanswered questions regarding precise definition of the clinical state of intractability because it is difficult to conclude, for example, how many episodes of recurrence represent morbidity equivalent to that which may be expected in a large series of patients electively treated by surgery. Individual interpretation of the situation by the patient and his physician should entail a consideration of the patient's suffering, the extent to which it compromises his personal way of life, and accurate appreciation of the benefits and risks of elective surgery.

The management of hemorrhage, perforation, and obstruction due to peptic ulcer is discussed separately in later sections of this chapter. These complications frequently are manifestations of intractability in the broader sense of the word.

All of the successful surgical procedures for curing peptic ulcer are aimed at reduction of gastric acid secretion. Excision of the ulcer itself is not sufficient to relieve the problem either with duodenal or gastric ulcer; recurrence is nearly inevitable with such procedures.

The 5 fundamentally different surgical methods of treating ulcer are as follows: subtotal gastrectomy, vagotomy, antrectomy, gastrojejunostomy, and total gastrectomy. Except in special circumstances, the choice of operation today for the average patient with duodenal ulcer is between (1) vagotomy with a drainage procedure, (2) vagotomy and antrectomy, and (3) subtotal gastrectomy (Fig 25–5). However, an understanding of the physiology of gastric secretion and motility makes it possible for the surgeon to modify his technics to handle unusual findings and still control the ulcer diathesis.

1. Subtotal gastrectomy—This operation consists of resection of two-thirds to three-fourths of the distal stomach. The proximal remnant may be reanastomosed to the duodenum (**Billroth I** resection) or to the side of the proximal jejunum (**Billroth II** resection). When subtotal gastrectomy is chosen for duodenal ulcer therapy, the Billroth II is preferable because recurrent ulceration is less frequent.

When creating a Billroth II (gastrojejunostomy) reconstruction, the jejunal loop may be brought up to the gastric remnant either anterior to the transverse colon or posteriorly through a hole in the transverse mesocolon. Since either method is satisfactory, an antecolic anastomosis is elected in most cases because it is simpler. One must verify carefully that the segment of small intestine being used actually is proximal jejunum, because inadvertent gastroileal anastomosis will lead to serious malabsorption. In fact,

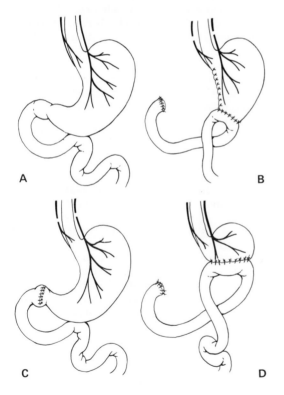

FIG 25–5. Various operations used in the treatment of peptic duodenal ulcer. *A:* Normal intact stomach. *B:* Vagotomy and antrectomy; Billroth II reconstruction. *C:* Vagotomy and (Heineke-Mikulicz) pyloroplasty. *D:* Subtotal gastrectomy; Billroth II reconstruction.

the length of the jejunal segment between the ligament of Treitz and the site of gastrojejunostomy should be as short as possible (at most, 15 cm) to avoid postoperative nutritional problems.

It appears not to matter whether the gastrojejunostomy is performed with the afferent jejunal limb at the greater curvature edge of the gastric remnant ("isoperistaltic") or at the lesser curvature ("antiperistaltic").

In most instances, the surgeon will be able to remove the ulcerated portion of duodenum in the course of the resection. However, it is not imperative that this be done, and in some cases it would be hazardous or ill-advised. The duodenal stump is closed after a Billroth II gastrectomy, and if an ulcer must be left in place it usually heals promptly.

The principal technical challenge in gastrectomy for duodenal ulcer is presented by the location of the ulcerated, inflamed duodenum at the site where the bowel must be transected. The dissection must avoid injury to the pancreas and the extrahepatic biliary ducts. After the specimen has been removed, gastroduodenal anastomosis requires a healthy cuff of duodenum about 1 cm long distal to the previous location of the ulcer. If this criterion cannot be met, a Billroth II resection provides an opportunity to reestablish gastrointestinal continuity by anastomosing healthy portions of bowel, thus avoiding the risks of anastomotic disruption. When performing the Billroth II resection, the surgeon must ensure the integrity of the duodenal closure. Occasionally, if a secure closure cannot be made with confidence, a tube should be sewn snugly into the duodenal stump and brought out through the abdominal wall as a temporary controlled decompressing fistula.

Physiologically, subtotal gastrectomy accomplishes complete removal of the major source of gastrin (the antrum) and of about half of the parietal cell area of the stomach.

The Billroth II subtotal gastrectomy has the advantages of low incidence of recurrent ulceration (about 2%) and generally good long-term outcome when all factors are taken into account. Its disadvantages are that it is a longer, more extensive surgical procedure, and it may aggravate poor nutrition in already underweight persons.

2. Vagotomy and drainage—Vagotomy has been popular for treating peptic ulcer disease for only a bit more than 2 decades, but in that period it has become the operation most often performed by the average ulcer surgeon. When vagotomy was initially done, a high incidence of symptomatic gastric stasis resulted from the loss of cholinergic innervation to the smooth muscle of the stomach. For this reason, vagotomy is now routinely accompanied by some maneuver that facilitates entry of gastric chyme into the small intestine. The drainage procedure most often selected in the USA is (Heineke-Mikulicz) **pyloroplasty**; in Great Britian, **gastrojejunostomy** is more popular. Neither gives a superior functional result, and pyloroplasty is less time-consuming. Various types of pyloroplasties are technically feasible, but their description is beyond the scope of this text.

Truncal vagotomy, the classical procedure, consists of identification of the 2 vagal trunks as they enter the abdomen on the distal esophagus and resection of a 1 or 2 cm segment of each. The cut ends are ligated with suture material, but in the past it was common to apply silver clips to the vagal stumps in the belief that this practice discouraged neural regeneration. **Selective vagotomy** has recently been introduced as a modification possessing theoretical advantages because vagal innervation of the viscera other than the stomach is preserved. The procedure entails transection of each abdominal vagus at a point just beyond its bifurcation into gastric and extragastric divisions. Thus, the hepatic branch of the anterior vagus and the celiac branch of the posterior vagus are maintained. The initial clinical trials with selective vagotomy have given promising results since positive Hollander tests and postoperative diarrhea are both somewhat less common than following truncal vagotomy. More studies are needed, however, before this technically more difficult procedure can be recommended for routine use.

In the past few years, vagal denervation limited to the oxyntic (parietal) gland area has been tested clinically under the term **superselective vagotomy**. Preservation of the vagal fibers to the antrum obviates the need for a concomitant drainage procedure, and the results in patients suggest a reduced incidence of postoperative dumping syndrome and postvagotomy diarrhea. Because sufficient experience has not been recorded to ascertain whether superselective vagotomy will be as effective in controlling peptic ulcer disease as the other methods of vagotomy, the procedure can only be recommended at this time in the context of controlled clinical trials.

Physiologically, vagotomy eliminates the direct vagal stimulant action on the parietal cells and decreases parietal cell sensitivity to gastrin. Interestingly, basal serum gastrin levels are increased because the effects of antral denervation are more than offset by the drop in gastric pH. The postprandial rise in serum gastrin is less after vagotomy. Basal and stimulated acid secretion are both reduced to about one-third of preoperative levels.

Vagotomy and a drainage procedure have the advantages of technical simplicity and preservation of the entire gastric reservoir capacity. The disadvantages are a relatively high incidence of incomplete vagotomy, and late recurrence of ulceration in about 10% of patients.

3. Antrectomy and vagotomy—This operation has been advocated as being the most physiologic approach to reduction of gastric acid secretion. Introduced on this theoretical basis, it has proved to be highly successful as predicted.

The operation entails a 50% distal gastrectomy, with the line of gastric transection carried high on the lesser curvature to conform with the boundary of the gastrin-producing mucosa. Complete removal of the antrum is important to obtain the full benefit. Vagotomy is performed as described in the preceding section. For unknown reasons, antrectomy by itself is insufficient to prevent a high recurrence rate.

After vagotomy and antrectomy, either a Billroth I or II reconstruction may be accomplished. The Billroth I type has been championed by most surgeons—in keeping with the physiologic reasoning of the early proponents of this operation.

Vagotomy and antrectomy are associated with a low incidence of marginal ulceration (2%) and a generally good overall outcome. The major disadvantage compared with vagotomy and a drainage procedure is the increased time and effort required to perform the gastric resection.

4. Gastrojejunostomy—Gastrojejunostomy was the first operation that was extensively used for the treatment of duodenal ulcer. It has been generally discarded as definitive therapy because about 20% of patients developed recurrent ulcers on the jejunal side of the stoma.

The physiologic explanation for the good results achieved with gastrojejunostomy is that it decreases the gastric phase of gastric secretion and lowers acid output.

Despite its long-term unsatisfactory results, gastrojejunostomy may still be advisable when one is forced to do as little as possible because of technical difficulties or because of the precarious condition of the patient.

5. Total gastrectomy—Complete removal of the stomach is not required to cure the usual forms of peptic ulcer disease. From the technical standpoint, the operation is of significantly greater magnitude than any form of partial gastrectomy, and short-term postoperative morbidity is greater. Nutritional difficulties are experienced by some of the patients afterward.

Total gastrectomy is the procedure of choice for patients with Zollinger-Ellison syndrome (gastrin-producing tumors). Occasionally it must be done to save a patient who is bleeding from erosive gastritis.

Complications of Surgery for Peptic Ulcer

A. Early Complications: The complications in the immediate postoperative period consist of duodenal stump leakage, gastric retention, and hemorrhage.

1. Duodenal stump leakage—Blowout of the duodenal stump is the most common cause of death after Billroth II gastrectomy. This complication can be prevented by resorting to catheter drainage of the duodenum if the degree of inflammation jeopardizes the duodenal closure. Equally important is selection of vagotomy and a drainage procedure in preference to gastric resection in any patient with a badly damaged or inflamed duodenum. Obstruction of the afferent limb of the gastrojejunostomy may contribute to this complication by increasing intraluminal pressure in the duodenum.

The clinical picture is characterized by sudden severe upper abdominal pain during the third to sixth days after surgery. The pain often radiates to the shoulder and the patient develops abdominal rigidity, high fever, and leukocytosis.

Immediate reoperation is mandatory. Drains—or, preferably, a sump suction device—should be placed in the region of the leaking duodenal closure. Attempts to resuture the duodenum at this time are unsuccessful. If the afferent loop is obstructed, this must be corrected, but not necessarily at the same time that the drains are inserted.

Large fluid and electrolyte losses through the fistula may be a clinical problem. Once drainage has been established, the patient should be managed as any case of high-output intestinal fistula. Spontaneous closure usually occurs if the patient survives the acute phase; if it does not, the fistula should be surgically closed after the condition of the patient has been stable for 4—6 weeks.

2. Gastric retention—An occasional patient is unable to tolerate oral feedings when they are started 5 or 6 days after surgery. He may become nauseated and complain of fullness and abdominal and shoulder pain, and will vomit if nasogastric suction is not reestablished. If this is due to edema of the stoma aggravated by gastric atony resulting from the vagotomy, resolution will gradually occur if the stomach is decompressed for several more days.

In some cases, organic obstruction underlies these symptoms. It may be due to a small anastomotic leak, excessive inversion of tissue at the anastomosis, perianastomotic hematoma, or anastomotic entrapment by omentum. Even in these cases, the gastric obstruction may improve with time, although as much as 3—4 weeks may be necessary.

The best rule is to handle this situation by temporization. Gastrointestinal x-ray examination following ingestion of water-soluble contrast material may suggest the functional or organic nature of the problem. If a prolonged delay is anticipated before the patient will be able to resume adequate oral nourishment, intravenous hyperalimentation is a useful adjunct. In most cases, loss of gastric tone is the principal cause. After decompression of the overdistended stomach by 48 hours of continuous aspiration, the tube should be removed and feeding begun with small amounts of palatable solid food. Intermittent aspiration at intervals of 4—8 hours is required to make certain that the stomach is not becoming overdistended. Occasionally, when no improvement has occurred after 3—4 weeks and it is clear that obstruction is present, reoperation is required.

3. Hemorrhage—Hemorrhage within 24 hours after surgery results from failure to adequately ligate the vessels in the seromuscular coats of the stomach or jejunum. Hemorrhage may also occur on the fourth to seventh postoperative days as a result of slough of tissue at the suture line and erosion into the seromuscular blood vessels. Less commonly, postoperative bleeding results from unsuspected blood dyscrasias.

Initial attempts to stop the hemorrhage consist of ice water lavage of the stomach. Blood loss should be replaced. If 1500—2000 ml of blood have been lost

and the bleeding persists, reoperation is indicated.

B. Late Complications:

1. Anastomotic ulcer (marginal ulcer, stomal ulcer, recurrent ulcer)—Recurrent ulcers form in 5—10% of duodenal ulcer patients treated by vagotomy and pyloroplasty; in 2—3% after vagotomy and antrectomy or subtotal gastrectomy; and in 15—20% after gastroenterostomy alone. Recurrence is quite unusual after gastrectomy for gastric ulcer. The ulcers nearly always develop immediately adjacent to the anastomosis on the intestinal side.

The usual complaint is upper abdominal pain, which is often aggravated by eating and improved by antacids. In some patients, the pain is felt more to the left in the epigastrium, and left axillary or shoulder pain is occasionally reported. About a third of patients with stomal ulcer will experience a major episode of gastrointestinal hemorrhage. Free perforation is much less common (5%).

a. Causes—It is often possible to explain in pathophysiologic terms why the ulcer has returned. The following causes should be considered depending on which surgical procedure was used as primary treatment.

(1) Inadequate gastric resection—The size of the gastric remnant as shown on x-rays will demonstrate with reasonable accuracy whether a full two-thirds resection has been done in the case of subtotal gastrectomy or if a complete antrectomy was done in the case of antrectomy and vagotomy.

(2) Incomplete vagotomy—When truncal vagotomy is performed for duodenal ulcer, as many as 20% of patients will have a positive Hollander test. Recurrent ulcer after vagotomy is usually found in this group.

(3) Inadequate drainage procedure—Chronic partial gastric outlet obstruction is responsible for some cases of recurrent ulcer after vagotomy and a drainage procedure. In these patients, the ulcer appears in the stomach instead of the small bowel.

(4) Retained antrum—During gastric resection, the distal line of transection should be through the duodenum so that the entire antrum is removed. If the operation has been done so that a portion of antrum remains attached to the duodenum after a Billroth II gastrectomy, the pH in the antral remnant is not affected by acid produced in the residual parietal cell mucosa. Gastrin production increases unchecked, and persistent acid stimulation leads to marginal ulceration.

(5) Loss of alkaline secretions near the anastomosis—The alkaline pancreatic and biliary secretions normally flow near the point where gastric acid enters the small bowel. If the afferent loop is especially long after a Billroth II gastrectomy, considerable absorption may occur before these juices reach the anastomosis and an ulcer may be the result. Another ulcer of similar cause follows side-to-side anastomosis of the afferent and efferent limbs of the gastrojejunostomy.

(6) Zollinger-Ellison syndrome—This condition, which is dealt with in detail in a later section, must always be considered in the differential diagnosis of stomal ulceration. Characteristic findings on gastro-intestinal x-rays or gastric analysis—or unusually severe ulcer disease—should suggest the possibility of a gastrin-producing tumor and lead to estimation of serum gastrin.

b. Diagnosis—The diagnosis is suggested initially by the patient's symptoms. Barium x-ray studies should be ordered, but the clinician must appreciate that only 50% of marginal ulcers can be demonstrated on x-rays. Thus, a negative gastrointestinal series is of little value in excluding the diagnosis. Gastroscopy should be performed if there is any question regarding interpretation of the films. In many cases, marginal ulcers can be visualized through the gastroscope that were not demonstrated by x-ray.

If the patient was treated initially by vagotomy, a Hollander gastric analysis is indicated and will usually be positive. On standard gastric analysis an elevated basal secretion of acid might suggest the Zollinger-Ellison syndrome or retained antrum. Since each of these is due to excessive gastrin, the findings on gastric analysis are similar: high basal secretion (greater than 5 mEq/hour after previous surgery) and a high ratio of basal to stimulated secretion (BAO/MAO $>$ 0.6). Gastrin immunoassay should be performed if Zollinger-Ellison syndrome or retained antrum is suspected. Retained antrum can sometimes be shown on the x-rays, but inspection of the duodenal stump during laparotomy may be necessary if the afferent loop cannot be filled with barium.

c. Treatment—Medical treatment has a low record of success for marginal ulcer. Unless some major ulcerogenic factor can be eliminated, most patients will require additional surgery.

Vagotomy alone is effective treatment for marginal ulcers which appear after subtotal gastrectomy. If the patient's original operation entailed a vagotomy, the results of the Hollander test will usually indicate incomplete vagotomy. In these cases, intact vagal fibers should be sought at laparotomy and divided. If a good-sized vagal trunk is not found, a gastric resection should be performed.

Preoperative suspicion of retained antrum should lead to examination of the duodenal stump and re-resection, depending on what is found. Retained antrum is an infrequent cause of marginal ulcer in modern practice, and elevated gastrin levels usually signify Zollinger-Ellison syndrome.

2. Gastrojejunocolic and gastrocolic fistula—A deeply eroding ulcer may occasionally produce a fistula between the stomach and colon. Most examples have resulted from recurrent peptic ulcer after an operation which included a gastrojejunal anastomosis. Rarely, spontaneous fistulas have developed between the stomach and colon from malignant gastric tumors, ulcerative colitis, or granulomatous colitis.

Severe diarrhea and weight loss are the presenting symptoms in over 90% of cases. Abdominal pain typical of recurrent peptic ulcer often precedes the onset of the diarrhea. Sometimes the pain suddenly improves at the moment the fistula is produced and

diarrhea begins. Intestinal bleeding complicates the marginal ulceration in a few patients. Bowel movements number 8–12 or more per day; they are watery and often contain particles of undigested food. The patient's breath or eructations may be unusually foul-smelling, and, although emesis is infrequent, when it does occur it may be feculent.

Malnutrition is often severe and may produce emaciation and dependent edema due to hypoproteinemia. Intestinal motility is hyperactive, and intestinal obstruction may be suggested by the combination of visible peristalsis and occasional feculent vomiting.

Laboratory studies reveal low serum proteins and manifestations of fluid and electrolyte depletion. Appropriate tests may reflect deficiencies in both water-soluble and fat-soluble vitamins.

An upper gastrointestinal series reveals the marginal ulcer in only 50% of patients who have one. In only 15% is the fistula shown on x-rays after oral ingestion of barium. The diagnosis ultimately depends on barium enema which demonstrates the fistulous tract unfailingly.

The ill effects of gastrocolic fistula are due to the enormous load of bacteria which enters the proximal intestine from the colon. Short circuit of food past the intestine via the fistula is almost never an important factor. The mechanisms by which the bacteria so severely hinder absorption include deconjugation of bile salts, production of diarrheogenic hydroxy fatty acids, mucosal damage, and undoubtedly others as yet unknown.

Initial treatment should replenish fluid and electrolyte deficits. Severely malnourished patients may benefit from a period of intravenous hyperalimentation, but surgery must be performed as soon as the patient's condition permits. Definitive surgical correction can usually be accomplished as a single procedure. In the past, procedures that diverted the fecal stream from the fistula were used to allow the patient to repair his nutritional defects before more difficult corrective operations were performed. Proximal colostomy, division of the ileum and ileosigmoidostomy, or exclusion of the fistula with colocolostomy were all effective. A single-stage correction avoids one or more additional operations and can now be accomplished safely in most cases. The involved colon and ulcerated gastrojejunal segment are excised and colonic continuity reestablished. Vagotomy, partial gastrectomy, or both are required to treat the ulcer diathesis and prevent another recurrent ulcer. Results are excellent in benign disease. The outlook for patients with malignant fistulas depends on the extent of the tumor, but in general the prognosis is poor.

3. Dumping syndrome—Symptoms of the dumping syndrome are noted to some extent by most patients who have an operation that impairs the ability of the stomach to regulate its rate of emptying, a characteristic of all procedures currently popular for treating duodenal ulcer. Within several weeks or months after surgery, dumping exists as a clinical problem in only 1 or 2% of patients. Symptoms fall into 2 categories: cardiovascular and gastrointestinal. Shortly after eating, the patient may experience palpitations, sweating, weakness, dyspnea, flushing, nausea, abdominal cramps, belching, vomiting, diarrhea, and, rarely, syncope. The degree of severity varies widely among patients, and not all symptoms are reported by all patients. In severe cases, the patient must lie down for 30–40 minutes until his discomfort passes.

The cause of dumping is not known, but a number of interesting pathophysiologic features have been described. Dumping can be elicited in normal subjects by instilling hypertonic solutions into the proximal small intestine or by mechanical distention of the jejunum. Appearance of the syndrome after gastric surgery can be explained on the basis of rapid entry of hypertonic food into the small bowel. Decreased blood volume, increased splanchnic blood flow, decreased blood pressure, and increased hematocrit can be measured by appropriate technics but are probably not directly responsible for the symptoms. The incidence of dumping correlates loosely with the amount of stomach removed, the size of the gastrointestinal anastomosis, and preoperative psychologic instability.

Diet therapy to reduce jejunal osmolality is successful in all but a few cases. The diet should be low in carbohydrates and high in fat and protein content. Sugars and carbohydrates are least well tolerated; some patients are especially sensitive to milk. Meals should be taken dry, with fluids restricted to between meals. This dietary regimen ordinarily suffices, but anticholinergic drugs may be of additional help in some patients, and others have reported improvement with serotonin antagonists.

If dumping symptoms are refractory to dietary treatment, further surgery should be considered. Good results can be achieved in about half of patients by conversion of a Billroth II to a Billroth I reconstruction. In special cases, one may elect to insert either an isoperistaltic or antiperistaltic 10 cm segment of jejunum between the gastric remnant and the duodenum. All 3 of these procedures delay gastric emptying and divert food into the less sensitive duodenum rather than the jejunum. Marginal ulcers will appear after these operations unless vagotomy is included.

Unfortunately, the term "dumping" has also been applied to an unrelated phenomenon sometimes seen in postgastrectomy patients, ie, late postprandial **reactive hypoglycemia.** This condition partially mimics early dumping syndrome, but the onset of symptoms coincides with hypoglycemia 3–4 hours after eating and the patient is relieved by eating sugar.

4. Weight loss and malabsorption—Some patients gain weight when gastrectomy relieves postprandial ulcer discomfort, but, on the average, a 5–10% loss in weight can be expected after gastric resection. Both decreased intake and decreased efficiency of digestion and absorption are responsible. Patients are usually comfortable at their lower weight and do not consider it a problem. In an occasional case, serious malnutrition complicates gastrectomy and the clinician is faced with a complicated set of variables that must be recognized and evaluated. The major factors that may contribute to malnutrition after gastrectomy are as follows:

a. Small gastric reservoir—Patients note that hunger is satisfied after smaller meals because the size of the stomach is reduced. Attempts to eat amounts equivalent to their preoperative capacity leads to uncomfortable fullness and nausea. More frequent meals may be recommended to attain increased intake.

b. Perianastomotic obstruction—Partial obstruction may occur at several points on a Billroth II anastomosis. Narrowing may follow scarring or may herald an anastomotic ulcer. Kinks and stenoses have been described at the junction of either the afferent or efferent loop with the stomach. Rarely, one of the jejunal limbs may intussuscept into the gastric remnant. The common result of these various mechanical obstructions is postprandial vomiting and pain. Patients who find that they vomit after eating voluntarily limit their intake.

The **afferent loop syndrome** in patients with a Billroth II gastrectomy consists of abdominal pain appearing 15–30 minutes after eating which is relieved suddenly by vomiting bilious fluid free of food. This is thought to be caused by partial obstruction of the afferent loop at the anastomosis and presumably is due to unimpeded passage of food from the stomach into the efferent loop, release of secretin and cholecystokinin, and stimulation of pancreatic secretion and gallbladder contraction. Bile accumulates in the afferent loop until the obstruction is suddenly overcome and the empty stomach is flooded with bile, causing vomiting. However, this classic picture is seldom present in patients who vomit after a Billroth II gastrectomy.

Standard radiologic studies with barium may be supplemented by cineradiography using a "motor meal" in attempts to delineate partial obstructions about the anastomosis.

c. Malabsorption—A decrease in the efficiency of fat absorption can be detected in most patients with a Billroth II gastrectomy. Normally, no more than 5% of ingested fat is excreted in the stool, but nearly all patients who have had a Billroth II excrete 10–15%. Steatorrhea of this degree is not usually accompanied by weight loss or diarrhea and remains subclinical in most patients after gastrectomy. Several physiologic changes created by this operation are probably additive in producing this mild steatorrhea. Decreased secretin release as a result of lowered acid production, uncoordinated arrival of food and pancreatic enzymes in the bowel, and loss of enzymes during transit along the afferent loop may all contribute to diminished lipolysis, though these defects by themselves are tolerated by most patients.

In some patients, afferent loop stasis allows excessive proliferation of bacteria and creates a variant of the **blind loop syndrome.** Most patients with symptomatic steatorrhea and malnutrition after Billroth II gastrectomy are found to have bacterial overgrowth in the afferent loop which aggravates abnormal lipolysis.

The bacteria deconjugate bile salts which then precipitate or are absorbed, making them unavailable for micellar solubilization of lipolytic products. A block in the absorption mechanism for fat is thus superimposed on the defective lipolysis. Weight loss and diarrhea may be marked and accompanied by deficiencies of fat-soluble vitamins (A, D, E, and K). Symptomatic and biochemical improvement in fat absorption often results from administration of antibiotics to lower the bacterial concentration in the afferent loop. Tetracycline and lincomycin have given the best results because they attack bacteroides, the organism that accounts for the bile salt deconjugation. Oral replacement of pancreatic enzymes may give further benefit.

Although short-term control of steatorrhea can be achieved by these means, they are too expensive and unreliable for prolonged therapy. Bacterial resistance develops to one antibiotic after another. Therefore, in the absence of major contraindications to surgery, the patient should undergo conversion of the Billroth II to a Billroth I. This procedure eliminates the afferent loop responsible for the blind loop syndrome, partially corrects the conditions which predispose to impaired lipolysis, and therefore leads to major improvement in most patients with well-documented postgastrectomy malabsorption.

5. Anemia—Iron deficiency anemia develops in about 30% of patients within 5 years after partial gastrectomy. It is caused by failure to absorb food iron bound in an organic molecule. Before this diagnosis is accepted, the patient should be checked for blood loss from the gastrointestinal tract. Slow bleeding from a marginal ulcer or an unsuspected tumor must be eliminated by appropriate endoscopic and radiologic tests. Inorganic iron—ferrous sulfate or ferrous gluconate—is indicated for treatment and is absorbed normally after gastrectomy.

Vitamin B_{12} deficiency and megaloblastic anemia appear in a few cases after gastrectomy. The usual cause is inadequate production of intrinsic factor, since addition of intrinsic factor corrects the abnormal Schilling test in most patients. In some instances, vitamin B_{12} deficiency is a manifestation of afferent loop stasis and the blind loop syndrome. In this situation, the bacteria in the intestine compete with the host for the vitamin B_{12} contained in food.

Parenteral vitamin B_{12} should be given in either case. Correction of blind loop syndrome will ordinarily be indicated because of its general adverse effects on nutrition.

6. Postvagotomy diarrhea—The daily frequency of bowel movements is increased in about two-thirds of patients who have had a vagotomy. In the great majority, this is either accepted as an improvement by the patient or is considered of no significance. About 5–10% of patients who have had a vagotomy require treatment with antidiarrheal agents at some time or another, and perhaps 1% are seriously troubled by this complication. The diarrhea may be episodic, in which case the onset is unpredictable after a symptom-free interval of weeks to months. An attack may comprise several watery movements or, in severe cases, may last for a few days. In other patients, continuous loose stools numbering 3–5 per day may be the problem.

Postvagotomy diarrhea is probably due to the effects of vagal denervation on intestinal motility, but the pathophysiology has not been fully explained. Selective gastric vagotomy has been introduced in the hope that preservation of the extragastric vagal fibers would lower the frequency of this complication. Selective vagotomy apparently does not completely prevent postoperative diarrhea, but a lower incidence has been reported in a controlled trial.

Most mild cases can be treated satisfactorily with kaolin-pectin compounds (eg, Kaopectate). Codeine or diphenoxylate with atropine (Lomotil) may be needed for severe continuous or episodic diarrhea.

Natural History, Choice of Operation, & Prognosis

Duodenal ulcer disease is characterized by exacerbations and remissions. In the average case, activity of the symptoms reaches a peak 5–10 years after the initial diagnosis and subsides slightly thereafter. Patients with severe symptoms, those who require hospitalization, and those with high acid secretion tend to do less well with medical treatment. The onset of back pain is a bad prognostic sign. Some degree of bleeding will be seen in 15%, perforation in 5%, and obstruction in less than 5%. About 20–25% of all patients who develop duodenal ulcer will eventually need surgery, and as many as 50% who have been hospitalized will come to operation.

The results of elective surgery for duodenal ulcer are satisfactory to excellent in about 90% of cases. The mortality rate following elective surgery should be less than 1% regardless of which operation the surgeon favors. For a healthy, well-nourished male undergoing elective operation, vagotomy and antrectomy combines the virtues of a low rate of recurrent ulcer with minimal early and late complications. However, if the patient's general condition is suboptimal or technical difficulties can be anticipated during gastric resection, vagotomy and pyloroplasty will minimize the immediate morbidity and mortality. This procedure offers slightly poorer long-term results than vagotomy and antrectomy or subtotal gastrectomy, principally because of the higher incidence of recurrent ulcer after vagotomy and drainage.

The most common causes of late morbidity after surgery for peptic ulcer are marginal ulcer, dumping syndrome, anemia, malnutrition, and diarrhea. Each has been discussed above.

In summary, the overall results of elective surgery for duodenal ulcer are good in 85–90% of patients. In poor-risk patients, pyloroplasty and vagotomy entail the least mortality. In good-risk patients, all 3 of the popular operations should have equally low mortality; vagotomy and antrectomy or subtotal gastrectomy might be advocated in preference to the others because their long-term results are better.

Duodenal Ulcer

Amdrup E, Jensen HE: Selective vagotomy of the parietal cell mass preserving innervation of the undrained antrum. Gastroenterology 59:522–527, 1970.

Ballinger WF II: Symposium on peptic ulceration: Pathophysiology and treatment. S Clin North America 46:233–475, 1966.

Buchman E & others: Unrestricted diet in the treatment of duodenal ulcer. Gastroenterology 56:1016–1020, 1969.

Edwards FC, Coghill NF: Clinical manifestations in patients with chronic atrophic gastritis, gastric ulcer, and duodenal ulcer. Quart J Med 37:337–360, 1968.

Fordtran JS: Acid rebound. New England J Med 279:900–905, 1968.

Fordtran JS & others: In vivo and in vitro evaluation of liquid antacids. New England J Med 288:923–928, 1973.

Fry J: Peptic ulcer: A profile. Brit MJ 2:809–812, 1964.

Hallenbeck GA: What is the best elective operation for duodenal ulcer? Canad MAJ 103:1255–1262, 1970.

Jordan PH, Condon RE: A prospective evaluation of vagotomy-pyloroplasty and vagotomy-antrectomy for treatment of duodenal ulcer. Ann Surg 172:547–563, 1970.

Jordan PH Jr: Elective operations for duodenal ulcer. New England J Med 287:1329–1337, 1972.

Kennedy T, Connell AM: Selective or truncal vagotomy? Lancet 1:899–901, 1969.

Krause U: Long-term results of medical and surgical treatment of peptic ulcer. Acta chir scandinav Suppl: 310, 1963.

McIlrath DC (editor): Symposium on acid-peptic disease. S Clin North America 51:833–1002, 1971.

Menguy R: Pathophysiology of peptic ulcer. Am J Surg 120:282–288, 1970.

Piper DW: Antacid and anticholinergic drug therapy of duodenal ulcer. Gastroenterology 52:1009–1018, 1967.

Price WE & others: Results of operation for duodenal ulcer. Surg Gynec Obst 131:233–244, 1970.

Schiff ER: Treatment of uncomplicated peptic ulcer disease. M Clin North America 55:305–315, 1971.

Wastell C (editor): *Chronic Duodenal Ulcer.* Appleton-Century-Crofts, 1972.

Marginal Ulcer

Amdrup E: Selective vagotomy of the gastric remnant for extragastric ulcer recurrence following resection. Scandinav J Gastroent 6:489–493, 1971.

Barber KW & others: Operation in one stage for gastrojejunocolic fistula. S Clin North America 42:1443–1449, 1962.

Fredens M & others: Radiography in the diagnosis of recurrent duodenal ulceration following vagotomy and pyloroplasty. Scandinav J Gastroent 6:559–561, 1971.

Stuart M, Hoerr SO: Recurrent peptic ulcer following primary operations with vagotomy for duodenal ulcer. Arch Surg 103:129–132, 1971.

van Heerden JA, Bernatz PE, Rovelstad RA: The retained gastric antrum: Clinical considerations. Mayo Clin Proc 46:25–28, 1971.

Watkin DFL, Duthie HL: Changes in the postoperative insulin test in relation to recurrent duodenal ulceration. Gut 12:303–310, 1971.

Wychulis AR, Priestely JT, Foulk WF: A study of 360 patients with gastrojejunal ulceration. Surg Gynec Obst 122:89–99, 1966.

Postgastrectomy Syndromes

Barnes AD, Williams JA: The change of bowel habits following vagotomy and pyloroplasty. Brit J Surg 54:218–220, 1967.

Buchwald H: The dumping syndrome and its treatment. Am J Surg 116:81–88, 1968.

Harvey HD: Complications in hospital following partial gastrectomy for peptic ulcer: 1936 to 1959. Surg Gynec Obst 117:211–220, 1963.

Hillman HS: Postgastrectomy malnutrition. Gut 9:576–584, 1968.

Hines JD, Hoffbrand AV, Mollin DL: The hematologic complications following partial gastrectomy. Am J Med 43:555–569, 1967.

Shultz KT & others: Mechanism of postgastrectomy hypoglycemia. Arch Int Med 128:240–246, 1971.

Wirts CW & others: The correction of postgastrectomy malabsorption following a jejunal interposition operation. Gastroenterology 49:141–149, 1965.

Woodward ER: The pathophysiology of the afferent loop syndrome. S Clin North America 46:411–423, 1966.

ZOLLINGER-ELLISON SYNDROME
(Gastrinoma)

Essentials of Diagnosis

- Severe peptic ulcer disease.
- Gastric hypersecretion.
- Elevated serum gastrin.
- Non-beta islet cell tumor of the pancreas.

General Considerations

Zollinger-Ellison syndrome consists of severe peptic ulcer disease caused by a gastrin-producing tumor (gastrinoma). More than 600 cases have been documented since the original report by Zollinger in 1955. Most have been due to non-beta islet cell adenomas or adenocarcinomas of the pancreas, but a few cases of isolated gastrinoma have been found in the submucosa of the proximal duodenum.

About a third of patients have other endocrine tumors—most commonly tumors of the parathyroid and pituitary glands. When associated with tumors in other endocrine organs, the condition is known as multiple endocrine adenomatosis (MEA) syndrome.

Clinical Findings

A. Symptoms and Signs: Abdominal pain is almost universally present as a manifestation of peptic ulceration. Diarrhea occurs in 30% of cases and is caused by hypersecretion of acid. Flooding of the duodenum with acid may destroy pancreatic lipase and produce steatorrhea, damage the small bowel mucosa, and overload the intestine with gastric and pancreatic secretions.

Hemorrhage, perforation, and obstruction are common complications. Symptoms are often refractory to large doses of antacids. The patients may drink 3 or 4 quarts of milk daily in search of relief from pain. Marginal ulcers appear after surgical procedures which would cure the ordinary ulcer diathesis.

B. Laboratory Findings: Serum gastrin levels should be obtained in any patient suspected of harboring a gastrinoma. In most laboratories, normal values by radioimmunoassay are under 200 pg/ml whereas patients with this condition have levels which usually exceed 600 pg/ml and often reach 10,000 pg/ml.

Serum calcium determinations may reveal hypercalcemia and lead to the discovery of one or more parathyroid adenomas.

Gastric analysis shows hypersecretion of > 15 mEq H^+ per hour basally in most patients who have an intact stomach. After gastrectomy, a basal collection of 9 mEq/hour would be highly suggestive. Maximal exogenous stimulation with betazole (Histalog) or pentagastrin does not increase the acid output from the already maximally secreting stomach. A ratio of basal to maximal secretion of 0.6 or more is characteristic.

C. X-Ray Findings: Upper gastrointestinal series usually shows ulceration in the duodenal bulb, although ulcers sometimes appear in the distal duodenum or proximal jejunum. The x-ray appearance is highly suggestive. The stomach contains prominent rugal folds, and secretions are present in the lumen despite the overnight fast. The duodenum may be dilated and exhibit hyperactive peristalsis. Edema may be detected in the small bowel mucosa. The barium flocculates in the intestine and transit time is accelerated.

Selective angiography can sometimes demonstrate the pancreatic tumor.

Treatment

At present, total gastrectomy with a Roux-en-Y esophagojejunostomy is the best treatment for most patients. Removal of the tumor may seem a more attractive choice at first but runs a high risk of being incomplete since 75% of patients have multiple tumor foci. (The single exception is the patient with gastrin-producing duodenal tumor; cure follows excision of these solitary lesions.) Surgical dissection frequently fails to reveal all the tumor deposits, and incomplete removal in the presence of an intact stomach has resulted in stormy exacerbations of the ulcer disease with perforation or hemorrhage in the immediate postoperative period. On the other hand, most of those who have had total gastrectomy lead a relatively normal life. Weight loss and dumping are rarely severe. Children who have had total gastrectomy for this disease have maintained normal growth curves. Lifelong parenteral vitamin B_{12} replacement is required, and supplemental oral iron should be prescribed.

Amberg JR & others: Roentgenographic observations in the Zollinger-Ellison syndrome. JAMA 190:185–187, 1964.

Ellison EH, Wilson SD: The Zollinger-Ellison syndrome updated. S Clin North America 47:1115–1123, 1967.

Sanchez RE, Longmire WP Jr, Passaro E Jr: Acid secretion and serum gastrin levels in the Zollinger-Ellison syndrome. California Med 116:1–7, June 1972.

Way LW, Goldman L, Dunphy JE: Zollinger-Ellison syndrome. Am J Surg 116:293–304, 1968.

Wilson SD, Schulte WJ, Meade RC: Longevity studies following total gastrectomy in children with the Zollinger-Ellison syndrome. Arch Surg 103:108–115, 1971.

GASTRIC ULCER

Essentials of Diagnosis

- Epigastric pain relieved by food or antacids.
- Ulcer demonstrated by x-ray.
- Acid present on gastric analysis.

General Considerations

The peak incidence of gastric ulcer is in patients age 40–60 years, or about 10 years older than the average for those with duodenal ulcer. Ninety-five percent of gastric ulcers are located on the lesser curvature, and 60% of these are within 6 cm of the pylorus. The symptoms and complications of gastric ulcer closely resemble those of duodenal ulcer.

Gastric ulcers may be separated into 2 groups with different causes and different treatments. One type occurs in patients who have had duodenal ulcer in the past and whose x-rays show duodenal deformity in addition to gastric ulcer. Acid secretion measured by gastric analysis is in the range for duodenal ulcer. The gastric ulcer is located close to the pylorus. Surgical treatment for these patients should follow the guidelines for duodenal ulcer.

Most gastric ulcers appear de novo without an earlier history of duodenal ulcer or radiologic evidence of duodenal scarring. They are usually located within 2 cm of the boundary between parietal cell and pyloric mucosa, but always in the latter. As noted above, 95% are on the lesser curvature.

Antral gastritis is universally present in gastric ulcer, being most severe near the pylorus and gradually diminishing in sections taken progressively farther from the pylorus. Regurgitation of duodenal contents into the stomach commonly occurs in patients with gastric ulcer and is associated with pyloric sphincter dysfunction characterized by failure to contract following hormonal stimulation with secretin or cholecystokinin. Experimentally, when bile and pancreatic juice in combination bathe the gastric mucosa, atrophic gastritis ensues. These findings suggest that duodenal juice weakens the mucosal resistance of the antrum and that ulceration follows the action of acid and pepsin at the site on the pyloric mucosa where they are most concentrated.

Increasingly of late, excessive ingestion of salicylates has been implicated as a cause of acute gastric bleeding and chronic gastric ulcers. Salicylates in an acid pH are known to damage the gastric mucosal barrier which normally prevents diffusion of acid out of the lumen of the stomach. The deleterious effects of salicylates have been demonstrated experimentally, and epidemiologic evidence reinforces the belief that these agents are a significant cause of gastric ulcer.

Dragstedt proposed that gastric ulcers were caused by stasis and an increased gastric phase of secretion. This arose from his observations that some patients developed gastric ulcers when vagotomy alone resulted in gastric retention. Stasis is a plausible explanation for gastric ulcers in patients with duodenal deformity and many years of duodenal ulcer disease, but seems less likely to account for those not associated with duodenal disease.

Low acid secretory levels are present with simple gastric ulcer. The low value for maximal output reflects a diminished parietal cell mass. Circulating gastrin levels are slightly higher than normal, but the difference from normal is small. The elevated gastrin seems to be a result of the higher antral pH in these hyposecretors.

A fundamental diagnostic consideration in dealing with gastric ulcer is the possibility that the niche seen on x-ray represents an ulcerated malignancy rather than a simple benign ulcer. Efforts must be expended during the *initial* stages of the work-up to establish this distinction. Despite the generally discouraging results of surgery for gastric adenocarcinoma, those whose tumors are difficult to separate from benign ulcer by x-ray have a 50–75% chance of cure after gastrectomy.

Clinical Findings

A. Symptoms and Signs: The principal symptoms are epigastric pain relieved by food or antacids, as in duodenal ulcer. Epigastric tenderness is a variable finding. Compared with duodenal ulcer, the pain in gastric ulcer tends to appear earlier after eating, often within 30 minutes. The attacks generally last longer (over 4 weeks) than those of duodenal ulcer, and the severity of symptoms is more liable to lead to loss of time from work. Vomiting, anorexia, and aggravation of pain by eating also occur with greater frequency with gastric ulcer. However, the overlap of symptoms between the 2 diseases is so great that historical information does not permit an accurate diagnosis without x-rays.

B. Laboratory Findings:

1. Gastric analysis–If gastric ulcer is accompanied by signs of active or old duodenal ulcer, the gastric analysis may show hypersecretion. If the gastric ulcer is unrelated to duodenal disease, basal and maximal acid secretion will be low or normal.

Achlorhydria is defined as absence of acid after betazole (Histalog) stimulation; pH 6.0 has been chosen as the cutoff point because this is the lowest pH found in patients with pernicious anemia who have no parietal cells. Achlorhydria is incompatible with the diagnosis of benign peptic ulcer and would imply malignancy in a gastric ulcer. About 20% of malignant

gastric ulcers will be associated with this finding.

2. Gastric cytology–Examination of cells in gastric washings should be done in all patients with gastric ulcer shortly after diagnosis. In expert hands, cytologic examination can detect 90–95% of gastric malignancies. Although the average physician may not have a laboratory available capable of quite this degree of accuracy, a positive report for malignancy is highly reliable.

C. X-Ray Findings: Upper gastrointestinal x-rays will show an ulcer usually on the lesser curvature in the pyloric area. In the absence of a tumor mass, the following suggest that the ulcer is malignant: (1) the deepest penetration of the ulcer is not beyond the expected border of the gastric wall; (2) presence of the meniscus sign, a prominent rim of radiolucency surrounding the ulcer, caused by heaped-up edges of tumor; and (3) malignancy is more common (10%) in ulcers greater than 2 cm in diameter. Coexistence of duodenal deformity or ulcer favors a diagnosis of benign ulcer in the stomach.

D. Gastroscopy: Gastroscopy should be performed as part of the initial work-up of patients with gastric ulcer to attempt to find malignant lesions. The rolled-up margins of the ulcer that produce the meniscus sign on x-ray can be distinguished from the flat edges characteristic of a benign ulcer, and a biopsy specimen may be obtained from a suspicious lesion.

Differential Diagnosis

The characteristic symptoms of gastric ulcer are often clouded by numerous nonspecific complaints. In fact, it is impossible to rely on historical information alone for diagnosis in the average patient who presents with dyspepsia as a chief complaint. Uncomplicated hiatal hernia, atrophic gastritis, chronic cholecystitis, irritable colon syndrome, and undifferentiated functional problems are distinguishable from peptic ulcer only after appropriate radiologic studies and sometimes not even then.

X-rays, gastroscopy, gastric cytology, and gastric analysis should all be performed to attempt to rule out malignant gastric ulcer. Even after the results of these tests have been considered and the ulcer is judged to be benign, about 4% will prove to be malignant.

At this point, treatment is instituted. Healing of the ulcer is desirable not only to rid the patient of his symptoms but also to demonstrate that the ulcer was in fact benign. Failure of the ulcer to heal after 6–12 weeks suggests that it may be malignant.

Complications

Bleeding, obstruction, and perforation are the principal complications of gastric ulcer. They are discussed separately under those headings elsewhere in this chapter.

Treatment

A. Medical Treatment: Medical management of gastric ulcer is the same as for duodenal ulcer. The patient should be questioned regarding the use of ulcerogenic agents, and they should be eliminated as far as possible. Detailed inquiry should be made for excessive use of salicylates. The physician may have to list each of the popular remedies which contain this compound, because patients often fail to appreciate the thrust of the questioning and deny taking aspirin when large amounts of Anacin or Alka-Seltzer are a daily habit.

The diet and antacid regimen outlined in the section on treatment of duodenal ulcer should be started if the severity of his symptoms does not require hospitalization. If symptomatic relief does not result within 1–2 weeks, hospitalization is advisable. Repeat x-rays should be obtained to document the rate of healing. After 6 weeks, healing usually has reached a plateau. At this point, treatment must be individualized according to circumstances. The medical regimen might be continued for the elderly poor-risk patient. Gastrectomy is recommended for the patient who has no contraindications to surgery. Whenever one elects to prolong medical treatment at this stage, he must understand that the failure to heal indicates a significant possibility that the ulcer is malignant. Therefore, gastroscopy and cytologic studies should be repeated.

The ulcerative process in small carcinomas may well be due to acid peptic digestion since partial healing on a regimen of antacids is common for lesions subsequently shown to be tumors. Therefore, healing should be followed to completion in all cases before the ulcer can be accepted as truly benign. Even then, a follow-up x-ray is advisable 6–12 months later as a further check on the absence of malignancy.

Carbenoxolone sodium and deglycyrrhizined licorice have both been shown by randomized clinical trials to hasten healing of gastric ulcers. These drugs are in widespread use in Europe but are not yet available in the USA.

In general, gastric ulcers are difficult to cure medically, recur frequently, and cause more severe symptoms than duodenal ulcers. In ulcers which fail to heal, malignancy cannot be excluded. For these reasons—plus the fact that gastrectomy cures gastric ulcer so efficiently—surgical treatment is advised in many of these patients.

B. Surgical Treatment: Patients with gastric ulcers located near the pylorus associated with increased acid secretion and x-ray changes similar to those of duodenal ulcer should be treated as outlined in the section on duodenal ulcer.

For patients with simple gastric ulcer not related to duodenal ulcer, a 40–50% gastrectomy and Billroth I reconstruction should be performed. The absence of duodenal disease facilitates the surgeon's task and reduces the risk of immediate postoperative complications. The recurrence rate is negligible (about 1%), and the long-term results are excellent. All late postgastrectomy problems except anemia are less common than after gastrectomy for duodenal ulcer.

Ordinarily, the ulcer is easily encompassed by the usual resection. When the ulcer is higher on the lesser curvature than the resection would otherwise extend,

it is not necessary to remove 75% or more of the stomach; in these cases, a distal gastrectomy will suffice; local excision of the ulcer allows histologic examination.

In recent years, vagotomy and pyloroplasty has been tried for gastric ulcer. The operation has led to healing, but the overall results are not as good as with gastrectomy. Unless an additional step is taken to excise the ulcer, an occasional patient will be left with a malignancy intact. Failure of the ulcer to heal or recurrent ulceration has been more frequent with vagotomy and occurs in those whose vagotomy is incomplete. Lastly, postvagotomy diarrhea complicates the course in a small percentage of cases. The place of vagotomy and pyloroplasty would seem to be in those patients who are poor risks for the additional surgical manipulation and operating time entailed in gastrectomy. Most of these are patients with acute complications from their ulcers such as hemorrhage or perforation.

Bartlett MK: The surgical treatment for gastric ulcer. S Clin North America 46:319–327, 1966.

Delaney JP & others: Gastric ulcer and regurgitation gastritis. Gut 11:715–719, 1970.

Fisher RS, Cohen S: Pyloric-sphincter dysfunction in patients with gastric ulcer. New England J Med 288:273–276, 1973.

Grossman MI: The Veterans' Administration cooperative study on gastric ulcer. Chapter 10: Resumé and comment. Gastroenterology 61:635–640, 1971.

Johnson HD: Gastric ulcer: Classification, blood group characteristics, secretion patterns, and pathogenesis. Ann Surg 162:996–1004, 1965.

Oi M & others: A possible dual control mechanism in the origin of peptic ulcer. Gastroenterology 57:280–293, 1969.

Rhodes J: Etiology of gastric ulcer. Gastroenterology 63:171–182, 1972.

Sapala JA, Ponka JL: Operative treatment of benign gastric ulcers. Am J Surg 125:19–28, 1973.

Turpie AGG, Runcie J, Thomson TJ: Clinical trial of deglycyrrhizinized liquorice in gastric ulcer. Gut 10:299–302, 1969.

Wilson WJ & others: The computer analysis and diagnosis of gastric ulcers. Radiology 85:1064–1073, 1965.

UPPER GASTROINTESTINAL HEMORRHAGE

Upper gastrointestinal hemorrhage may be mild or severe, but should always be considered an ominous manifestation that deserves thorough evaluation. Bleeding is the most common serious complication of peptic ulcer, portal hypertension, and gastritis, and these conditions taken together account for most episodes of upper gastrointestinal bleeding in the average hospital population.

The major factors that determine the diagnostic and therapeutic approach are the amount and rate of bleeding. Estimates of both should be made promptly and monitored and revised continuously until the episode has been resolved.

Hematemesis or melena is present except when the rate of blood loss is minimal. **Hematemesis** of either bright-red or dark blood indicates that the source is proximal to the ligament of Treitz. It is more common from bleeding that originates in the stomach or esophagus. In general, hematemesis denotes a more rapidly bleeding lesion, and a high percentage of patients who vomit blood require surgery. Coffee-ground vomitus is due to vomiting of blood which has been in the stomach long enough for gastric acid to convert hemoglobin to methemoglobin.

Most patients with **melena** (passage of black or tarry stools) are bleeding from the upper gastrointestinal tract, but melena can be produced by blood entering the bowel at any point from mouth to cecum. The conversion of red blood to dark depends more on the time it resides in the intestine than the site of origin. The black color of melanotic stools is probably caused by hematin, the product of oxidation of heme by intestinal and bacterial enzymes. Melena can be produced by 50–100 ml of blood in the stomach. When one liter of blood was instilled into the upper intestine of experimental subjects, melena persisted for 3–5 days, which points out that the rate of change in character of the stool is a poor guide to the time bleeding stopped after an episode of hemorrhage.

Hematochezia is defined as the passage of bright-red blood from the rectum. Bright-red rectal blood can be produced by bleeding from the colon, rectum, or anus. However, if intestinal transit is rapid during brisk bleeding in the upper intestine, bright-red blood may be passed unchanged in the stool.

Tests for Occult Blood

Normal subjects lose about 2.5 ml of blood per day in their stools, presumably from minor mechanical abrasions of the intestinal epithelium. Between 50 and 100 ml of blood per day will produce melena. Tests for occult blood in the stool should be able to detect amounts between 10 and 50 ml/day. False-positive results may be due to dietary hemoglobin, myoglobin, or peroxidases of plant origin. Iron ingestion does not give positive reactions. The various tests using guaiac, benzidine, phenolphthalein, or orthotolidine have similar specificities. The sensitivity of the guaiac test is in the desired range and is the one most commonly used at present.

Initial Management

In an apparently healthy patient, melena of a week or more suggests that the bleeding is slow. In this type of patient, admission to the hospital should be followed by a deliberate but nonemergent work-up. However, patients who present with hematemesis or sudden melena should be handled as if exsanguination were imminent until this possibility has been investigated thoroughly. The clinical approach entails a simul-taneous series of diagnostic and therapeutic steps with the following initial goals: (1) Rapidly assess the status of the circulatory system and replace blood loss as necessary. (2) Determine the amount and rate of bleeding. (3) Slow or stop the bleeding by ice water lavage. (4) Discover the lesion responsible for the episode. The last step may lead to more specific treatment appropriate to the underlying condition.

The patient should be admitted to the hospital promptly regardless of the initial apparent severity of bleeding. Historical information should be gathered about the acute problem and other major health data. Peptic ulcer, acute gastritis, esophageal varices, esophagitis, and Mallory-Weiss tear account for over 90% of cases, and questions concerning the major symptoms and predisposing factors of each may be asked in a few moments' time. The patient should be asked about salicylate intake and any history of a bleeding tendency. This information should be obtained while resuscitation is in progress if the patient requires immediate treatment.

Of the diseases commonly responsible for acute upper gastrointestinal bleeding, only portal hypertension is associated with diagnostic findings on physical examination. However, the clinician must be careful not to automatically attribute gastrointestinal bleeding in a patient with jaundice, ascites, splenomegaly, spider angiomas, or hepatomegaly to esophageal varices; over half of cirrhotic patients who present with acute hemorrhage are bleeding from gastritis or peptic ulcer. Therefore, additional diagnostic information must be obtained in these patients before specific therapy can be planned.

Blood should be drawn for cross-matching, packed cell volume, hemoglobin, creatinine, and tests of liver function. An intravenous infusion of 0.15 N NaCl solution should be started and, in the massive bleeder, a large-bore (32–36F) Ewald nasogastric tube inserted. In cases of melena, the gastric aspirate should be examined to verify the gastroduodenal source of the hemorrhage. The tube must be larger than the standard nasogastric tube (16F) so the stomach can be lavaged free of liquid blood and clots. After the gastric contents have been removed, the stomach should be irrigated with a large syringe and copious amounts of ice water or saline solution until blood no longer returns. Then the tube should be attached to continuous suction so that further blood loss can be measured. When the bleeding has stopped, the large tube may be replaced with a smaller one.

If the patient was bleeding at the time the nasogastric tube was inserted, iced saline irrigation usually stops it. If bleeding continues or if tachycardia or lowered blood pressure are present, the patient should be monitored and treated as for hemorrhagic shock. A central venous pressure line should be inserted to serve as a guide to blood replacement and an indwelling urinary catheter placed for hourly determination of urine output—an indication of tissue perfusion.

The most critical signs indicating the need for

rapid transfusion are syncope, shock, tachycardia, and hypotension. Any of these combined with a history of acute blood loss demands prompt transfusion.

In acute rapid hemorrhage, the hematocrit may be normal or only slightly lowered. A very low hematocrit without obvious signs of shock indicates more prolonged blood loss. Shock requires whole blood transfusion, but packed cells are preferable to raise a chronically low hematocrit to normal.

All of these steps can be made within 1 or 2 hours after the acutely bleeding patient has entered the hospital. In most instances, this aggressive approach will result in a patient whose bleeding is at least temporarily under control, whose blood volume has been restored to normal, and who is being adequately monitored so that recurrent bleeding can be detected immediately and its rate determined. When this stage is reached, additional diagnostic tests should be performed.

Diagnosis of Cause of Bleeding

In most cases, when the patient becomes stable enough for further evaluation, the first diagnostic measure is endoscopic examination of the upper gastrointestinal region. Extensive experience has shown that instrumental trauma to the site of bleeding is not a hazard of this procedure. Technical improvements in the available fiberoptic instruments have rendered endoscopy the most useful diagnostic test in the management of patients with bleeding from the upper digestive tract. The examination can be performed at the patient's bedside, but a more satisfactory study can usually be obtained if the patient can be moved to a special endoscopy suite. The patient should be studied as soon as practical after his condition has become stable so that the source can be identified while bleeding is still active. Thus, if it is successful, endoscopy provides a direct estimate of cause of hemorrhage rather than the indirect evidence available from barium upper gastrointestinal x-rays. Fiberoptic endoscopy has been shown to be more accurate than x-rays in demonstrating bleeding from peptic ulcers, acute gastritis, Mallory-Weiss tears, and esophagitis. The 2 methods are about equally useful in demonstrating esophageal varices, but endoscopy is more likely than x-ray to settle the question whether the varices were actually responsible for the bleeding episode.

Recently, selective angiography has been helpful in identifying the bleeding site in special cases. Insufficient experience has accumulated on which to base precise indications for the procedure. If angiography could be accomplished quickly enough so that the ongoing care of the patient was not compromised, it might perhaps be recommended routinely in cases where endoscopy failed to establish a diagnosis. Although highly skilled teams may be able to accomplish the study in less than an hour, more than this is usually required. To be of diagnostic value, angiography must be performed while the patient is still bleeding. Experimental studies show that if the rate of blood loss from a focal lesion is 0.5 ml/minute, the bleeding point can be demonstrated by selective arterial injection of the contrast material.

At present, the most clear-cut diagnostic indications for selective angiography in the work-up of a patient with gastrointestinal hemorrhage are (1) to study patients who have bled previously in whom a cause had not been determined, and (2) to demonstrate a site of bleeding beyond the ligament of Treitz. In the gastroduodenal region, this technic can demonstrate bleeding from peptic ulcers, Mallory-Weiss tears, gastritis, and tumors. Variceal hemorrhage cannot be seen, but the venous phase of the injection may show the enlarged collateral veins. In some patients, the potential value of using the angiography catheter as a route for the selective administration of vasoconstrictors may enter into the choice. However, if a standard upper gastrointestinal x-ray examination has been performed with barium sulfate, angiography is no longer possible until the barium has passed and that may take several days.

In most patients an upper gastrointestinal x-ray examination should be obtained after endoscopy has been performed. Peptic ulcers or esophageal varices may be demonstrated.

Later Management

Although a precise diagnosis of the cause of the bleeding may be valuable in later management, the patient must not be allowed to slip out of clinical control during the search for definitive diagnostic information. The indication for emergency surgery depends more on the response to immediate gastric lavage and the rate of blood loss than the specific cause of bleeding. The major exception to this rule is bleeding from esophageal varices. For varices, both nonsurgical and surgical approaches vary significantly from those pertaining to the other common causes of massive hemorrhage. Endoscopy should be performed as early as feasible in patients who seem to have varices, keeping in mind that no segment of the population is entirely free of alcoholism or other causes of portal hypertension.

The need for transfusion should be determined on a continuing basis, and blood volume must be maintained. Blood pressure, pulse, central venous pressure, hematocrit, hourly urinary volume, and amount of blood obtained from the gastric tube or from the rectum all enter into this assessment. Older notions that bleeding might subside more often if the blood volume were incompletely replenished have been rejected. However, many clinical studies have documented the tendency to underestimate blood loss and inadequately transfuse massively bleeding patients who truly need aggressive therapy. Continued bleeding at a slow rate is best followed by serial determinations of the hematocrit.

Several factors are associated with a worse prognosis with continued medical management of the bleeding episode. Most of these are not absolute indications for laparotomy, but they should alert the clinician that emergency surgery may be required.

High rates of bleeding or amounts of blood loss predict high failure rates with medical treatment. Hematemesis is usually associated with more rapid bleeding and a greater blood volume deficit than melena. The presence of hypotension on admission to the hospital or the need for more than 4 units of blood to obtain circulatory stability implies a worse prognosis; if bleeding continues and subsequent transfusion requirements exceed 1 unit every 8 hours, continued medical management is usually unwise.

Total transfusion requirements also correlate with mortality. Death is uncommon when less than 7 units of blood have been used, and the mortality rate rises progressively thereafter.

In general, bleeding from a gastric ulcer is more dangerous than bleeding from gastritis or duodenal ulcer, and patients with gastric ulcer should be always considered for early surgery. Regardless of the cause, if bleeding recurs after it had initially stopped, the chances of success without operation are low. Recurrent bleeding in the hospital is accepted by most clinicians as a clear indication for immediate laparotomy.

Lastly, patients over age 60 tolerate continued blood loss less well than younger patients and should not be permitted to bleed until secondary cardiovascular, pulmonary, or renal complications arise.

HEMORRHAGE FROM PEPTIC ULCER

Approximately 20% of patients with peptic ulcer will experience a bleeding episode, and this complication is responsible for about 40% of the deaths from peptic ulcer. Peptic ulcer is the most common cause of massive upper gastrointestinal hemorrhage, accounting for about 60% of all cases. Other causes are listed in Table 25—2. Chronic gastric and duodenal ulcers have about the same tendency to bleed, but the former produce more severe episodes. Bleeding ulcers are more common in persons with blood group O, although the reason for this association is not known.

Bleeding ulcers in the duodenum are usually located on the posterior surface of the duodenal bulb. As the ulcer penetrates, the gastroduodenal artery is exposed and may become eroded. Since no major blood vessels lie on the anterior surface of the duodenal bulb, ulcerations at this point are not as prone to bleed. Postbulbar ulcers (those in the second portion of the duodenum) bleed frequently, although ulcers in this area are much less common than those near the pylorus.

In some patients, the bleeding is sudden and massive, manifested by hematemesis and shock. In others, chronic anemia and weakness due to slow blood loss may be the only findings. The diagnosis is often suggested by a history of typical ulcer pain. In fact, the presence of a chronic ulcer has in some cases been well documented before the patient presents with acute bleeding. However, previous ulcer symptoms

TABLE 25—2. Causes of upper gastrointestinal hemorrhage.

Common Causes	Relative Incidence*	
Peptic ulcer		60%
Duodenal ulcer	40%	
Gastric ulcer	20%	
Esophageal varices		10%
Gastritis		20%
Mallory-Weiss syndrome		5%
Uncommon Causes		50%
Gastric carcinoma		
Esophagitis		
Pancreatitis		
Hemobilia		
Duodenal diverticulum		

*Considerable variation can be expected in the relative incidence between different patient populations. The incidence of gastritis as a cause of bleeding reflects the frequency of early endoscopy as a diagnostic measure.

may also be absent. Although epigastric tenderness may be present on abdominal examination, this finding is not thought to be of much diagnostic value.

In the preceding section, the management of acute upper gastrointestinal hemorrhage, the selection of diagnostic tests, and the factors suggesting the need for operation were discussed. Most patients (75%) with bleeding peptic ulcer can be successfully managed by medical means alone. Initial therapeutic efforts usually halt the bleeding. At this point, antacids should be given hourly, although some prefer to drip them continuously into the stomach through the nasogastric tube. After 12—24 hours have passed and the bleeding has clearly stopped, the patient should be fed at frequent intervals if he feels hungry. Twice daily hematocrit readings should be ordered as a check on slow continued blood loss. Anticholinergic drugs are of uncertain value and are avoided by some because their effect on the heart rate may interfere with the assessment of persistent or recurrent bleeding. Stools should be tested daily for the presence of blood, remembering that they will usually remain guaiac-positive for several days after the bleeding stops.

Since rebleeding in the hospital is attended by a mortality rate of about 25%, a policy of early surgery for those who rebleed would improve overall results. Patients who present with hematemesis and those whose hemoglobin falls below 8 g/100 ml have a higher risk of rebleeding. About 3 times as many patients with gastric ulcer (30%) rebleed compared with those with duodenal ulcer. Most instances of rebleeding occur within 2 days from the time the first episode stopped. In one study, only 3% of patients who stopped bleeding for this long bled again.

Emergency Surgery

About 25% of patients bleeding from a peptic

ulcer will require emergency surgery. Selection of those most likely to survive with surgical compared with medical treatment rests on the rate of blood loss and the other factors associated with a poor prognosis.

The patient should be brought into as good hemodynamic balance as possible. Sometimes it is not possible to entirely replace the blood deficit because bleeding is too rapid, but this is rare. Elderly patients are particularly difficult to manage because cardiac disability may make the line between too little and too much blood transfusion a fine one. Emergency treatment with digitalis may be useful at times.

The type of operation most appropriate for the emergency control of bleeding ulcer has been a subject of considerable controversy in the past 15 years. The question was whether vagotomy and pyloroplasty with suture of the bleeding site is preferable to gastrectomy. Vagotomy and pyloroplasty has the advantage of technical simplicity and therefore, perhaps, a lower operative mortality but was also thought to be less effective in preventing rebleeding. Convincing evidence has gradually accumulated to show that the overall mortality is significantly less after vagotomy and pyloroplasty and that rebleeding appears with about equal frequency after either procedure.

When laparotomy is performed, the first step should be to make a pyloroplasty incision. If a duodenal ulcer is present, the bleeding vessel should be ligated with sutures of nonabsorbable material and the duodenum and antrum inspected for additional ulcers. The pyloroplasty incision should then be closed and a truncal vagotomy performed. If the posterior wall of the duodenal bulb has been destroyed by a giant duodenal ulcer, a gastrectomy and Billroth II gastrojejunostomy would be preferable since these somewhat uncommon ulcers are especially prone to bleed again if left in continuity with the stomach. Gastric ulcers can be handled either by gastrectomy or vagotomy and pyloroplasty. A thorough search should always be made for second ulcers or other causes of bleeding.

On occasion, the bleeding point is not immediately found after the first inspection through the pyloroplasty incision. In these patients, the surgeon must consider uncommon causes of bleeding such as postbulbar ulcers, hemobilia, and bleeding esophagitis. Mallory-Weiss tears of the gastroesophageal mucosa are especially difficult to locate because they are small, unaccompanied by surrounding inflammation, and hidden within the rugae of the proximal stomach. A separate long gastrotomy and painstaking exploration are required to find these lesions.

Elective Surgery for Bleeding Ulcer

Since most patients stop bleeding under medical therapy, a plan must be made for their subsequent management. About a third of patients who bleed once do so for a second time within the next 5 years. Patients who have bled twice in the past have double the risk of rebleeding. Elective surgery can reduce the chances of additional hemorrhage to about 5–8%. The inability to achieve even better results probably re-

flects the more virulent nature of the ulcer diathesis in these patients. Early surgical treatment should generally be recommended for those who have had substantial chronic disability preceding their acute hemorrhage or for those with a giant duodenal ulcer. Young patients whose hemorrhage was the first manifestation of disease, those in whom an ulcerogenic agent is detected such as excessive salicylate ingestion, and those whose bleeding was minor might be expected to do better with good medical therapy. The large group of patients between these extremes must be individualized, since there is no proved best course. In general, they should be given vigorous medical treatment but referred for elective surgery if remissions cannot be achieved or maintained. If a second bleeding attack occurs on medical therapy, early surgery would be advisable.

Prognosis

The mortality rate for an acute massive hemorrhage is about 15% in most reported series. Careful study of the causes of death suggests that this figure could be improved by (1) more precise blood replacement—since undertransfusion can be implicated as the cause of some of the morbidity and mortality; and (2) earlier surgery in selected patients who fall into serious-risk categories—since the tendency has been to perform surgery on too few patients and to do it too late in the illness.

Allen HM & others: Gastroduodenal endoscopy: Management of acute upper gastrointestinal hemorrhage. Arch Surg 106:450–455, 1973.

Baum S, Nusbaum M: The control of gastrointestinal hemorrhage by selective superior mesenteric arterial infusion of vasopressin. Radiology 98:497–505, 1971.

Carruthers RK & others: Conservative surgery for bleeding peptic ulcer. Brit MJ 1:80–82, 1967.

Conn JH & others: Massive hemorrhage from peptic ulcer: Evaluation of methods of surgical control. Ann Surg 169:784–789, 1969.

Devitt JE, Brown FN, Beattie WG: Fatal bleeding ulcer. Ann Surg 164:840–844, 1966.

Farris JM, Smith GK: Appraisal of the long term results of vagotomy and pyloroplasty in 100 patients with bleeding duodenal ulcer. Ann Surg 166:630–639, 1967.

Foster JH, Hickok DF, Dunphy JE: Factors influencing mortality following emergency operation for massive upper gastrointestinal hemorrhage. Surg Gynec Obst 117:257–262, 1963.

Frey CF, Reuter SR, Bookstein JJ: Localization of gastrointestinal hemorrhage by selective angiography. Surgery 67:548–555, 1970.

Hallenbeck GA: Elective surgery for treatment of hemorrhage from duodenal ulcer. Gastroenterology 59:784–789, 1970.

Halmagyi AF: A critical review of 425 patients with upper gastrointestinal hemorrhage. Surg Gynec Obst 130:419–430, 1970.

Harvey RF, Langman MJS: The late results of medical and surgical treatment for bleeding duodenal ulcer. Quart J Med 39:539–547, 1970.

Malt RA: Control of massive upper gastrointestinal hemorrhage. New England J Med 286:1043–1046, 1972.

Morrissey JF: Gastrointestinal endoscopy. Gastroenterology 62:1241–1268, 1972.

Northfield TC: Factors predisposing to recurrent hemorrhage after acute gastrointestinal bleeding. Brit MJ 1:26–28, 1971.

Read RC, Huebl HC, Thal AP: Randomized study of massive bleeding from peptic ulceration. Ann Surg 162:561–577, 1965.

Schiller KFR, Truelove SC, Williams DG: Haematemesis and melaena, with special reference to factors influencing the outcome. Brit MJ 2:7–14, 1970.

Stafford ES & others: Benign gastric ulcer with life-threatening hemorrhage. Ann Surg 165:967–976, 1967.

MALLORY-WEISS SYNDROME

Mallory-Weiss syndrome is responsible for about 5% of cases of acute hemorrhage from the upper gastrointestinal region. It consists of a 1–4 cm longitudinal tear in the gastric mucosa near the esophagogastric junction which usually follows a bout of forceful retching. The disruption extends through the mucosa and submucosa but not usually into the muscularis propria. About 75% are confined to the stomach; 20% straddle the esophagogastric junction; and 5% are entirely within the distal esophagus. One-fourth of patients have a hiatal hernia.

The majority of patients are alcoholics, but the lesion may appear after severe retching for any reason. Several cases have been reported following closed chest cardiac massage.

Clinical Findings

If a good history can be obtained, it is of more diagnostic importance in this condition than in the other major causes of acute gastric bleeding. Typically, the patient first vomits food and gastric contents. This is followed by forceful retching, and then bloody vomitus. Rapid increases in gastric pressure, sometimes aggravated by hiatal hernia, undoubtedly cause the mucosal rift. Actual rupture of the distal esophagus can also be produced by vomiting (Boerhaave's syndrome; see Chapter 24), but the difference seems to depend on vomiting of food in rupture and nonproductive retching in gastric mucosal tear. During retching, the esophagogastric sphincter does not relax, and the sudden rise in pressure from abdominal and antral contraction is focused at the point where Mallory-Weiss tears appear.

The diagnosis may be strongly suspected if a typical history is obtained. Esophagogastroscopy is the most practical means of making the diagnosis before operation. Barium x-ray examination cannot demonstrate the lesion, but there have been reports on the successful use of selective angiography to show the site of bleeding.

Treatment & Prognosis

Initially the patient is handled according to the general measures prescribed for upper gastrointestinal hemorrhage. Bleeding will occasionally remain under control after cold irrigation of the stomach, but most cases will require surgical repair of the tear. The gastric balloon of the Sengstaken-Blakemore tube fails to tamponade the hemorrhage, and in several instances where it was used it was thought to further extend the tear.

If the diagnosis has been made before laparotomy, the surgeon should make a long (10–12 cm), high gastrotomy after the abdomen is opened. The tear may be difficult to adequately expose. The search must be meticulous, since in about 25% of patients there are 2 tears. A running suture of nonabsorbable material should be used to oversew the lesion. Postoperative recurrence is rare.

Atkinson M & others: Mucosal tears at the oesophagogastric junction. Gut 2:1–11, 1961.

Holmes KD: Mallory-Weiss syndrome: Review of 20 cases and literature review. Ann Surg 164:810–820, 1966.

Thompson NW, Ernst CB, Fry WJ: The spectrum of emetogenic injury to the esophagus and stomach. Am J Surg 113:13–26, 1967.

Weaver DH, Maxwell JG, Castleton KB: Mallory-Weiss syndrome. Am J Surg 118:887–892, 1969.

PYLORIC OBSTRUCTION DUE TO PEPTIC ULCER

The cycles of inflammation and repair in peptic ulcer disease may cause obstruction of the gastroduodenal junction as a result of edema, muscular spasm, and scarring. To the extent that the first 2 factors are involved, the obstruction may be reversible with medical treatment. Obstruction is usually due to duodenal ulcer and is less common than either bleeding or perforation. The few gastric ulcers that obstruct are close to the pylorus. Obstruction due to peptic ulcer must be differentiated from that caused by an antral malignancy.

Clinical Findings

A. Symptoms and Signs: The great majority of patients with obstruction have a long history of symptomatic peptic ulcer, and as many as 30% have been treated for perforation or obstruction in the past. The patient often notes gradually increasing ulcer pains over weeks or months with the eventual development of anorexia, vomiting, and failure to gain relief from antacids. The vomitus often contains food ingested several hours previously, and absence of bile staining reflects the site of blockage. Weight loss may be marked if the patient has delayed seeking medical care.

Dehydration and malnutrition may be obvious on physical examination but are not always present. A succussion splash can usually be elicited from the retained gastric contents. Peristalsis of the distended stomach may be visible on gross inspection of the

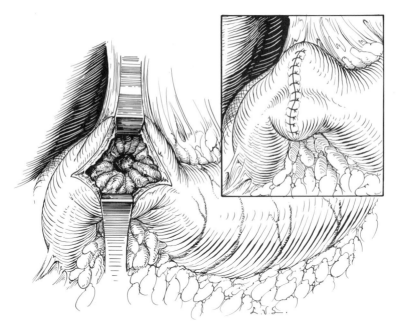

FIG 25–6. Heineke-Mikulicz pyloroplasty. A longitudinal incision has been made across the pylorus, revealing an active ulcer in the duodenal bulb. The insert shows the transverse closure of the incision which widens the gastric outlet. The accompanying vagotomy is not shown.

abdomen, but this sign is relatively rare. Most patients have upper abdominal tenderness. Tetany may appear with advanced alkalosis.

B. Laboratory Findings: A significant degree of anemia is found in about 25% of patients. Prolonged vomiting leads to a unique form of metabolic alkalosis with dehydration. Measurement of serum electrolytes shows hypochloremia, hypokalemia, hyponatremia, and increased bicarbonate. Vomiting depletes the patient of Na^+, K^+, and Cl^-; the latter is lost in excess of Na^+ and K^+ as HCl. Gastric HCl loss causes extracellular HCO_3^- to rise, and renal excretion of HCO_3^- increases in an attempt to maintain pH. Large amounts of Na^+ are excreted in the urine with the HCO_3^-. Increasing Na^+ deficit evokes aldosterone secretion, which in turn brings about renal Na^+ conservation at the expense of more renal loss of K^+ and H^+. GFR may drop and produce a prerenal azotemia. The eventual result of the process is a marked deficit of Na^+, Cl^-, K^+, and H_2O.*

C. X-Ray Findings: Plain abdominal x-rays may show a large gastric fluid level. An upper gastrointestinal series should not be performed until the stomach has been emptied because dilution of the barium in the retained secretions makes a worthwhile study impossible.

D. Special Examinations: Gastroscopy may be indicated to rule out the presence of a malignant tumor.

---

*Treatment involves replacement of water and NaCl until a satisfactory urine flow has been established. KCl replacement should then be started. Details of management are found in Chapter 12.

Treatment

A. Medical Treatment: A large (32F) Ewald tube should be passed and the stomach emptied of its contents and lavaged until clean. A large tube is necessary because particles of food cannot be withdrawn through the regular nasogastric tube. After completely decompressing the stomach, a smaller tube should be inserted and placed on suction for several days to allow pyloric edema and spasm to subside and to permit the gastric musculature to regain its tone. Anticholinergic drugs should be withheld.

The gastric aspirate should be examined for acid content and malignant cells. Absence of acid (pH > 6.0) would suggest that the block is caused by a malignancy.

After decompressing the stomach for 48–72 hours, the tube should be withdrawn and the patient given a palatable liquid diet. The tube should be passed several times at intervals of 4 hours to check the gastric residual. If less than half of the volume ingested remains, he should be continued on oral liquids. Gradual resumption of a solid diet is permitted as tolerated.

An upper gastrointestinal series should be performed at the end of the period of recovery. If a malignancy is still suspected—and especially if gastric emptying does not improve—the obstruction should be examined by gastroscopy.

B. Surgical Treatment: If 3–4 days of gastric aspiration do not result in some relief of the obstruction, the patient should be treated surgically. Persistence of nonoperative effort beyond this period in the absence of progress rarely achieves the hoped-for result and often allows the patient to deteriorate as an operative candidate.

Surgical treatment may consist either of a vagotomy and drainage procedure (Fig 25–6) or gastrectomy. Earlier fears that vagotomy in this type of patient would be complicated by delayed gastric emptying have not been realized. Either procedure is satisfactory provided gastric tonus has been restored by adequate decompression.

Prognosis

About two-thirds of patients with acute obstruction fail to improve sufficiently on medical therapy and require operation to relieve the blockage. The need for surgery in those whose acute obstruction resolves with suction may be based on the severity of persistent symptoms.

Boyle JD, Goldstein H: Management of pyloric obstruction. M Clin North America 52:1329–1337, 1968.

Howe CT, LeQuesne LP: Pyloric stenosis: The metabolic effects. Brit J Surg 51:923–932, 1964.

Kozoll DD, Meyer KA: Obstructing gastroduodenal ulcers: General factors influencing incidence and mortality. Arch Surg 88:793–799, 1964.

Kozoll DD, Meyer KA: Obstructing gastroduodenal ulcers: Symptoms and signs. Arch Surg 89:491–498, 1964.

Kozoll DD, Mittelpunkt A, Meyer KA: Obstructing gastroduodenal ulcers: Effects of treatment on morbidity and mortality. Arch Surg 91:431–442, 1965.

PERFORATED PEPTIC ULCER

Perforation complicates peptic ulcer about half as often as hemorrhage. Most perforated ulcers are located anteriorly, although occasionally gastric ulcers perforate into the lesser sac. The 15% mortality rate correlates with increased age, female sex, and gastric perforations. The diagnosis is overlooked in about 5%, most of whom do not survive.

Anterior ulcers tend to perforate instead of bleed because of the absence of protective viscera and major blood vessels on this surface. In less than 10%, acute bleeding from a posterior "kissing" ulcer complicates the anterior perforation, an association which carries a high mortality rate. Immediately after the perforation occurs, the peritoneal cavity is flooded with gastroduodenal secretions which elicit a chemical peritonitis. Early cultures show either no growth or a light growth of streptococci or enteric bacilli. Gradually, over 12 hours or more, the process evolves into a full-blown bacterial peritonitis. The morbidity and mortality are directly related to the interval between the acute event and surgical closure of the perforation.

In an unknown percentage of cases, the perforation becomes sealed by adherence to the undersurface of the liver. In such patients, the process may be self-limited, but a subphrenic abscess will develop in many.

Clinical Findings

A. Symptoms and Signs: The perforation usually elicits a sudden, severe upper abdominal pain whose onset can be recalled precisely. The patient may or may not have had preceding chronic symptoms of peptic ulcer disease. Perforation rarely is heralded by nausea or vomiting, and it typically occurs several hours after the last meal. Shoulder pain, if present, reflects diaphragmatic irritation. Back pain is uncommon.

The initial reaction consists of a chemical peritonitis caused by gastric acid or bile and pancreatic enzymes. The peritoneal reaction dilutes these irritants with a thin exudate, and as a result the patient's symptoms may temporarily improve before progressing to bacterial peritonitis. If the physician sees the patient for the first time during this symptomatic lull, he must not be misled into interpreting it as representing bona fide improvement.

The patient appears severely distressed, lying quietly with his knees drawn up and breathing shallowly to minimize abdominal motion. Fever is absent at the start. The abdominal muscles are rigid due to severe involuntary spasm. Epigastric tenderness may not be as marked as expected because the board-like rigidity protects the abdominal viscera from the palpating hand. Air escaped from the stomach may enter the space between the liver and abdominal wall, and upon percussion the normal dullness over the liver will be tympanitic. Peristaltic sounds are reduced or absent. If delay in treatment allows continued escape of air into the peritoneal cavity, this may lead to abdominal distention and diffuse tympany.

Lesser degrees of shock with minimal abdominal findings occur if the leak is small or rapidly sealed. A small duodenal perforation may leak fluid slowly which runs down the lateral peritoneal gutter, producing pain and muscular rigidity in the right lower quadrant and closely simulating appendicitis.

Perforations may be sealed by omentum or by the liver, with the later development of a subhepatic or subdiaphragmatic abscess.

B. Laboratory Findings: A mild leukocytosis in the range of 12,000/μl is common in the early stages. After 12–24 hours, this may rise to 20,000/μl or more if treatment has been inadequate. The mild rise in the serum amylase value that occurs in many patients is probably caused by absorption of the enzyme from duodenal secretions within the peritoneum. Direct measurement of fluid obtained by paracentesis may show very high levels of amylase.

C. X-Ray Findings: Plain x-rays of the abdomen reveal free air in 85% of patients. Films should be taken with the patient supine and upright. A film in the left lateral decubitus position may be a more practical way to demonstrate free air in the uncomfortable patient who cannot tolerate the upright position for long. Most patients can lie in this position for 10–15 minutes before an x-ray is taken. This allows scattered small amounts of air to accumulate between the liver and the lateral chest wall where they are more readily demonstrated. Free air in the abdomen in a patient with sudden upper abdominal pain should clinch the diagnosis.

If no free air is demonstrated and the clinical picture suggests perforated ulcer, an emergency upper gastrointestinal series should be made with a water-soluble contrast agent. If the perforation has not sealed, the diagnosis is established by noting escape of the contrast material from the lumen.

Differential Diagnosis

The differential diagnosis must include acute pancreatitis and acute cholecystitis. The former does not have as explosive an onset as perforated ulcer and is usually accompanied by a high serum amylase level. Acute cholecystitis with perforated gallbladder could mimic perforated ulcer closely but free air would not be present with ruptured gallbladder. Intestinal obstruction has a more gradual onset and is characterized by less severe pain which is crampy and accompanied by vomiting.

The simultaneous onset of pain and free air in the abdomen in the absence of trauma usually means perforated peptic ulcer. Free perforation of colonic diverticulitis or acute appendicitis are other rare causes.

Treatment

The proper diagnosis is often suspected before the patient is sent for confirmatory x-rays. Whenever a perforated ulcer is considered possible, the first step should be to pass a nasogastric tube and empty the stomach to reduce further contamination of the peritoneal cavity. Blood should be drawn for laboratory studies and an intravenous infusion of crystalloid solution started. The patient should be given high doses of antibiotics effective against a wide spectrum of enteric organisms. If the patient's overall condition is precarious due to delay in treatment, fluid resuscitation should precede diagnostic measures. X-rays should then be obtained as soon as his status will permit. The clinician must always keep in mind the penalty for delay in treating this disease.

Laparotomy and surgical closure of the perforation is the standard treatment. The suture closure should be reinforced by incorporating a healthy tab of omentum, and all fluid should be aspirated from the peritoneal cavity. Drainage is not indicated. Reperforation is rare in the immediate postoperative period.

Although the primary objective is closure of the ulcer, definitive surgery for treatment of the underlying ulcer diathesis may be done if the patient is in good condition and the perforation is early. Since more than half of patients with perforated ulcer subsequently require definitive operation, patients with a history of chronic duodenal ulcer should have a vagotomy and pyloroplasty during the initial procedure if circumstances permit.

Nonoperative treatment consists of continuous gastric suction and the administration of antibiotics in high doses. Although this has been shown to be effective therapy with a low mortality rate, it is accompanied by a high incidence of peritoneal and subphrenic abscess with substantially greater morbidity than operative closure. For this reason, it is employed only for certain selected poor-risk patients or those seen very late, with extensive peritonitis and toxemia. Even in advanced cases, operation is the best treatment if the condition of the patient permits.

Prognosis

About 15−18% of patients with perforated ulcer die, and about a third of these are undiagnosed before surgery. The mortality rate of perforated ulcer seen early is negligible. Delay in treatment, advanced age, and associated systemic diseases account for most deaths.

Burdette WJ, Rasmussen B: Perforated peptic ulcer. Surgery 63:576−585, 1968.

Cohen MM: Treatment and mortality of perforated peptic ulcer: A survey of 852 cases. Canad MAJ 105:263−269, 1971.

Felix WR Jr, Stahlgren LH: Death by undiagnosed perforated peptic ulcer: Analysis of 31 cases. Ann Surg 177:344−351, 1973.

Jordon GL, Angel RT, DeBakey ME: Acute gastroduodenal perforation. Arch Surg 92:449−455, 1966.

Nemanich GJ, Nicoloff DM: Perforated duodenal ulcer: Long term follow-up. Surgery 67:727−734, 1970.

Rees JR, Swan KG, Thorbjarnarson B: Perforated duodenal ulcer. Am J Surg 120:775−779, 1970.

Thoroughman JC & others: Free perforation of anastomotic ulcers. Ann Surg 169:790−800, 1969.

STRESS ULCER

The term stress ulcer refers to a heterogeneous group of acute gastric or duodenal ulcers which develop following trauma, sepsis, or other physiologically stressful illness. Hemorrhage is the major clinical problem, although perforation occurs in about 5%. Owing to the lack of a standard nomenclature, the literature regarding the causes and treatment of stress ulcer is difficult to interpret.

The classic problem is presented by the septic, jaundiced patient requiring ventilatory support with a respirator. Massive hemorrhage suddenly erupts from multiple shallow, linear gastric ulcers. Shock and sepsis, as in this patient, are the usual common denominators behind stress ulcers which develop in patients who entered the hospital for another illness. Despite their predilection to develop in the parietal cell mucosa, in about 30% of patients the duodenum is affected, and sometimes both stomach and duodenum are involved. At present no satisfactory theory has been proposed to explain these differences in otherwise similar patients.

Etiology

Various animal models of stress ulcer have shown

that gastric acid is a requirement and that antacids provide prophylaxis. In the human, stress ulcer is not usually associated with increased acid secretion. It is thought that damage from other sources may render the mucosa susceptible to injury by normal amounts of acid.

The concentration of acid secreted by parietal cells is 150 mEq/liter—a million times greater than the hydrogen ion concentration in blood. The ability of the stomach to secrete and hold this highly concentrated solution within its lumen depends on a physiologic barrier to back diffusion. Since this must be a feature of the mucosa itself, the efficiency of the barrier should vary in relation to mucosal health. It is not surprising, therefore, that back diffusion of acid is accelerated after various forms of mucosal injury. Disruption of the normal barrier has been shown experimentally after hemorrhage, shock, topical aspirin, alcohol, bile salts, and several other types of detergents. Aspirin and alcohol are synergistic in their damaging effects. Some of these—as well as other, as yet unknown factors—are thought to be important in the pathogenesis of some cases of gastric ulceration, both chronic and acute.

As excessive amounts of H+ enter the submucosa, they release histamine from mast cells and activate intramural cholinergic fibers (Fig 25–7). The liberated histamine leads to edema formation and probably further increases acid production. Pepsinogen is stimulated by the cholinergic activity. The result of these events is a weakened mucosa susceptible to diffuse ulceration (Figs 25–8 and 25–9).

Sepsis enhances the insult, possibly through a cholinergic mechanism or, in some cases, by causing intravascular coagulation. If a previous ulcer diathesis exists, it may also play a role. For unknown reasons, persons with blood group O are more susceptible to stress ulcers.

To what extent acute ulcers following burns (Curling's ulcer), neurosurgical problems (Cushing's ulcer), aspirin ingestion, or acute alcoholism should be lumped together with stress ulcers has been incompletely determined. Duodenal or gastric ulcers develop in 10% of burned patients, and sepsis predisposes to the complication. It seems reasonable to consider these as similar in etiology to other stress ulcers.

Cushing reported that acute gastric and duodenal ulcers developed as complications of cerebral tumors or injuries. Increased acid secretion has been detected in this type of patient, and present practice is to consider Cushing's ulcers as separate from other types of stress ulcers.

Hemorrhagic gastritis following an alcoholic binge may have common etiologic factors with stress ulcers, but the natural history is different and the response to treatment is considerably better. Most of these patients can be controlled medically. By contrast with stress ulcer, when surgery is required for alcoholic gastritis a high proportion are cured by pyloroplasty and vagotomy.

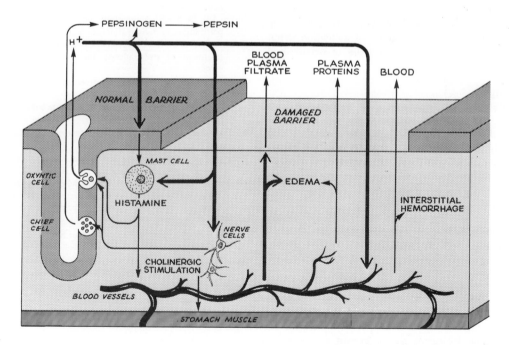

FIG 25–7. Effects of intraluminal acid on a normal or broken gastric mucosal barrier. If the barrier is intact, back diffusion of H+ is minimal and causes no harm. When the barrier is disrupted, H+ diffuses rapidly into the submucosa, histamine is released locally, and cholinergic fibers are stimulated. The consequences are increased H+ and pepsinogen secretion, stimulation of gastric motility, and production of submucosal edema and hemorrhage.

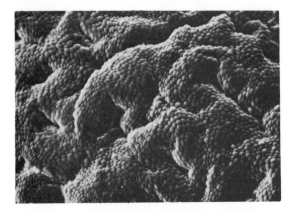

FIG 25—8. Scanning electron photomicrograph of the surface epithelium of a normal subject showing individual cells and numerous gastric pits. (Reduced from X 350.) (Courtesy of Jeanne M. Riddle.)

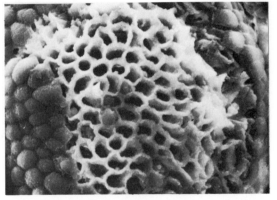

FIG 25—9. Scanning electron photomicrograph of the surface epithelium of a patient with acute gastric mucosal erosions showing a patch of cellular defoliation. Lesions such as this may account for back diffusion of H^+. (Reduced from X 1145.) (Courtesy of Jeanne M. Riddle.)

Aspirin ingestion can aggravate most types of acute and chronic ulceration. In severely ill, hospitalized patients, this drug is contraindicated because of its potentially deleterious effects on the gastric mucosal barrier and on platelet adhesiveness. However, lesions produced principally by salicylates should not be termed stress ulcers.

Clinical Findings

Hemorrhage is nearly always the first manifestation. Pain rarely occurs. Physical examination is not contributory except to reveal gross or occult fecal blood or signs of shock.

Prevention

Recent clinical experiments in high-risk patients suggest that intensive antacid therapy may prevent stress ulcers. The antacids should be given at hourly intervals or by continuous drip to maintain gastric neutrality. A milk drip will not elevate gastric pH to the desired level and should not be used as a substitute.

Treatment

Initial management should consist of gastric lavage with chilled solutions, anticholinergic drugs to block potential cholinergic links in the pathophysiology, and measures to combat sepsis if present.

Laparotomy for continued bleeding must not be delayed unless the operative risk is prohibitive. If cooling and anticholinergics fail, surgery is the only hope, since further delay is associated with a progressively increasing mortality rate.

Surgical treatment should consist of vagotomy and pyloroplasty with suture of the bleeding part or partial gastrectomy. Since most of these patients are in very poor condition, the lesser procedure is usually chosen. Partial gastrectomy that completely excises the ulcers is ideal but not commonly feasible because of

their tendency toward proximal location or diffuse distribution. Rarely, total gastrectomy has had to be used because of the extent of the ulceration and the severity of the bleeding.

Baum S, Ward S, Nusbaum M: Stress bleeding from the mid-duodenum. Radiology 95:595—602, 1970.

Davenport HW: Why the stomach does not digest itself. Sc Am 226:86—93, 1972.

Girvan DP, Passi RB: Acute stress ulceration with bleeding or perforation. Arch Surg 103:116—121, 1971.

Goodman AA & others: Symposium on the current status of the treatment of stress ulcers. Am J Surg 125:461—476, 1973.

Ivey K: Gastric mucosal barrier. Gastroenterology 61:247—257, 1971.

Ivey KJ: Acute hemorrhagic gastritis: Modern concepts based on pathogenesis. Gut 12:750—757, 1971.

Kirtley JA & others: The surgical management of stress ulcers. Ann Surg 169:801—809, 1969.

Lucas CE & others: Natural history and surgical dilemma of "stress" gastric bleeding. Arch Surg 102:266—273, 1971.

Menguy R, Gadacz T, Zajtchuk R: The surgical management of acute gastric mucosal bleeding. Arch Surg 99:198—208, 1969.

Pruitt BA, Foley FD, Moncrief JA: Curling's ulcer: A clinical-pathology study of 323 cases. Ann Surg 172:523—539, 1970.

Skillman JJ & others: Respiratory failure, hypotension, sepsis, and jaundice. Am J Surg 117:523—530, 1969.

Smith BM & others: Permeability of the human gastric mucosa. New England Med 285:716—721, 1971.

GASTRIC CARCINOMA

Carcinoma of the stomach causes 15,000 deaths in the USA annually. The incidence has dropped dramatically to one-third what it was 30 years ago. The reason for this is not known, nor is it completely understood why the incidence varies so greatly between countries. The present incidence in American males is 10 new cases per 100,000 population per year. The highest rate of 70 per 100,000 males is seen in Japan; in eastern and central European countries, it is about 40 per 100,000 per year. Carcinoma of the stomach is rare under the age of 40, from which point the risk gradually climbs. The mean age at discovery is 63.

Gastric epithelial malignancies are nearly always adenocarcinomas. Squamous cell tumors of the proximal stomach arise from the esophagus and involve the stomach secondarily. Four morphologic subdivisions are useful because they correlate loosely with the natural history and outcome:

(1) **Ulcerating carcinoma (25%).** This consists of a deep, penetrating ulcer-tumor which extends through all layers of the stomach. It may involve adjacent organs in the process. The edges are shallow by contrast with overhanging edges noted in benign ulcers.

(2) **Polypoid carcinomas (25%)** are large, bulky intraluminal growths that tend to metastasize late.

(3) **Spreading carcinoma (15%).** Superficial spreading tumor is confined to the mucosa and submucosa (carcinoma in situ). Metastases are uncommon. Linitis plastica, the other variety of spreading tumor, involves all layers with a marked desmoplastic reaction in which it may be difficult to identify the malignant cells. The stomach loses its pliability. Cure of this uncommon lesion is rare because of early spread.

(4) **Advanced carcinoma (35%).** This largest category contains the big tumors which are found partly within and partly without the stomach. They may originally have qualified for inclusion in the preceding groups but have outgrown that early stage.

Pathologists also classify gastric adenocarcinomas by the degree of differentiation of their cells. In general, rate and extent of spread correlates with lack of differentiation. Some tumors are found histologically to excite an inflammatory cell reaction at their borders, and this feature indicates a relatively good prognosis.

Extension occurs by intramural spread, direct extraluminal growth, and lymphatic metastases. Three-fourths of patients have metastases when first seen. Within the stomach, proximal spread exceeds distal. The pylorus acts as a partial barrier, but tumor is found in 25% of cases in the first few centimeters of the bulb.

Sixty percent of tumors are in the pyloric region, predominantly on the lesser curvature; 30% arise in the body, 5% at the cardia, and 5% involve the entire organ. Benign ulcers develop at the greater curvature and cardia less commonly than malignant ones. Ulcers at these points should be particularly suspect for neoplasm.

Clinical Findings

A. Symptoms and Signs: The earliest symptom is usually vague postprandial abdominal heaviness which the patient does not identify as a pain. Sometimes the discomfort is no different from other vague dyspeptic symptoms which had been intermittently present for years. However, the frequency and persistence are new.

Anorexia develops early and may be most pronounced for meat. Weight loss is the most common symptom, but when the patient is first seen by a physician it rarely amounts to more than 5–7 kg (10–15 lb). True postprandial pain suggesting a benign gastric ulcer is relatively uncommon, but one may be misled if subsequent x-rays show an ulcer. Vomiting may be present and becomes a major feature if pyloric obstruction occurs. It may be coffee-ground in appearance due to bleeding by the tumor.

An epigastric mass can be felt on examination in about one-fourth of cases. The stool will be positive for occult blood in half of these patients, and melena is seen in a few. Otherwise, abnormal physical findings are confined to signs of distant spread of the tumor. Metastases to the neck along the thoracic duct may produce a Virchow node. Rectal examination may reveal a Blumer shelf, a solid peritoneal deposit anterior to the rectum. Enlarged ovaries (Krukenberg tumors) may be caused by intraperitoneal metastases. Further dissemination may involve the liver, lungs, brain, or bone.

B. Laboratory Findings:

1. Gastric analysis—About 50% of patients with adenocarcinoma of the stomach are achlorhydric after maximal stimulation. This finding would eliminate the possibility of benign ulceration.

2. Gastric cytology—A good cytology laboratory can make the proper diagnosis in over 90% of malignant gastric tumors. False-positive reports are rare. Adenocarcinoma can be differentiated from lymphoma and squamous cell carcinoma. Only leiomyosarcomas cannot be diagnosed.

The technic involves passage of a nasogastric tube after an overnight fast. The stomach is irrigated with 100 ml of Ringer's solution, and 500 ml of acetate buffer solution (pH 5.6) containing 7 g of chymotrypsin are then instilled and allowed to remain for about 5 minutes. The fluid is withdrawn, spun down, smeared, and rapidly fixed to prevent digestion. The chymotrypsin improves collections by a mucolytic effect.

It may be difficult to obtain a satisfactory specimen from a patient with an obstructing lesion. In this case, the stomach should be lavaged and kept decompressed for 24 hours before the examination.

C. X-Ray Findings: Upper gastrointestinal series may be diagnostic for some tumors. Major diagnostic problems are posed by ulcerating tumors, a few of which may not be distinguishable radiologically from benign peptic ulcers. The differential features have been mentioned previously, but x-rays alone are insufficiently reliable to establish a diagnosis of benign ulcer. It is strongly recommended that all patients with a newly discovered gastric ulcer undergo gastroscopy, gastric analysis, and gastric cytology.

D. Gastroscopy: The quality of gastroscopic examinations has steadily improved with each new generation of fiberoptic instruments. Direct biopsy can be accomplished in many instances.

Treatment

Surgical resection is the only curative treatment. The objectives should be to remove the tumor, an adjacent uninvolved margin of stomach and duodenum, the regional lymph nodes, and, if necessary, portions of involved adjacent organs. For example, if the tumor is located in the pylorus, a curative resection would entail distal gastrectomy with en bloc removal of the omentum and, in some instances, excision of the left gastric artery and nearby lymph nodes. Reconstruction after gastrectomy may be by either a Billroth I or II procedure, but the latter is often preferable because growth of residual tumor near the pylorus would obstruct a gastroduodenal anastomosis early.

Proximal partial gastrectomy may be performed for tumors near the cardia. Total gastrectomy cannot be recommended except where the resection is curative, ie, will leave no gross tumor behind.

The propensity for proximal submucosal spread must be appreciated at surgery. It is often advisable to perform a frozen section at the proximal margin before constructing the anastomosis. If tumor is found, the gastrectomy should be extended.

Palliation is sometimes possible even though cure is not. Palliative resections may be performed for distal tumors which are obstructing or those which may soon become so. A Billroth II resection is preferable to a diverting gastrojejunostomy.

Prognosis

In the USA, the overall 5-year survival rate is about 12%. For localized tumors, the figure is 40%. In the absence of lymph node involvement, surgical cure can be predicted in two-thirds.

Death from tumor may follow dissemination to other organs or may be the result of progressive gastric obstruction and malnutrition.

Black MM & others: Prognostic significance of microscopic structure of gastric carcinomas and their regional lymph nodes. Cancer 27:703–711, 1971.

Goldsmith HS, Ghosh BC: Carcinoma of the stomach. Am J Surg 120:317–319, 1970.

Hawley PR, Westerholm P, Morson BC: Pathology and prognosis of carcinoma of the stomach. Brit J Surg 57:877–883, 1970.

Kennedy BJ: TNM classification for stomach cancer. Cancer 26:971–983, 1970.

Lilienfeld A: Epidemiology of gastric cancer. New England J Med 286:316–317, 1972.

Sakita T & others: Observations on the healing of ulceration in early gastric cancer. Gastroenterology 60:835–844, 1971.

GASTRIC POLYPS

Adenomatous polyps of the stomach are single or multiple benign tumors which occur predominantly in the elderly. Those located in the distal stomach are more apt to cause symptoms. Whenever gastric polyps are discovered, gastric malignancy must be ruled out. Many adenomatous polyps are found in stomachs which contain a separate distinct carcinoma, but it is generally agreed that benign polyps do not themselves turn malignant. Lesions with a stalk and those less than 2 cm in diameter have little risk of malignancy. The incidence of malignancy rises with increasing size.

Anemia may develop from chronic blood loss or deficient iron absorption. Over 90% of patients are achlorhydric after maximal stimulation. Deficient vitamin B_{12} absorption exists in 25%, although megaloblastic anemia is present in only a few of these. Exfoliative cytology should be performed in all patients.

Surgery is indicated for polyps greater than 2 cm in diameter or when the radiologist or cytologist suspects malignancy. Single polyps can be excised through a gastrotomy. If the polyp is found to be carcinoma at laparotomy, an appropriate type of gastrectomy is indicated. Partial gastrectomy should be performed for multiple polyps in the distal stomach. If 10–20 polyps are distributed throughout the stomach, the antrum should be removed and the fundic polyps excised. Total gastrectomy may be required for diffuse multiple polyposis, a rare condition in which the entire gastric mucosa is involved.

The patient should be followed by occasional x-rays. Recurrence is uncommon after surgery.

Marshak RH, Feldman F: Gastric polyps. Am J Digest Dis 10:909–935, 1965.

Monaco AP & others: Adenomatous polyps of the stomach. Cancer 15:456–467, 1962.

GASTRIC LYMPHOMAS

Lymphoma is the second most common primary malignancy of the stomach but comprises only 2% of the total, 95% being adenocarcinomas. Lymphomas are classified as lymphosarcomas or reticulum cell sarcomas according to cellular characteristics. Symptoms are similar to those caused by carcinoma. The tumors attain bulky proportions. X-rays demonstrate the tumor. Gastric cytology may provide the correct diagnosis. Gastric lymphomas can trap the clinician into thinking he is dealing with inoperable carcinoma, judged so because the tumor is so large. It is important to avoid this mistake since resection and postoperative radiotherapy result in 5-year survival in 50% of cases.

Loehr WJ & others: Primary lymphoma of the gastrointestinal tract. Ann Surg 170:232–238, 1969.

Naqvi MS, Burrows L, Kark AE: Lymphoma of the gastrointestinal tract. Ann Surg 170:221–231, 1969.

GASTRIC LEIOMYOMAS & LEIOMYOSARCOMAS

Leiomyomas are common submucosal growths which may cause intestinal bleeding. Leiomyosarcomas grow to a large size and often present with hematemesis. Radiologically, the tumor contains a central ulceration caused by necrosis from outgrowth of its blood supply. In most cases the tumor arises from the midportion of the stomach. It may grow into the gastric lumen, remain entirely on the serosal surface, or even become pedunculated within the abdominal cavity. Spread is by direct invasion or blood-borne metastases. Patients treated by radical resection have a 50% 5-year survival rate. The tumor is resistant to radiotherapy.

ReMine WH: Gastric sarcomas. Am J Surg 120:320–323, 1970.

GASTRITIS

Acute Gastritis

This condition has been recognized with greater frequency since the use of gastroscopy in acute upper gastrointestinal bleeding has become widespread. Ingestion of large amounts of alcohol or other injurious agents such as salicylates is an important causative factor. It is not entirely clear what important differences exist (if any) between acute hemorrhagic gastritis and acute gastric stress ulcers, although gastritis runs a milder course. The patient may experience epigastric pain, or the gastritis may be asymptomatic.

The lamina propria contains a variable number of inflammatory cells consisting principally of polymorphonuclear leukocytes. Punctate superficial mucosal ulceration may develop and occasionally leads to massive hemorrhage. When healing begins, the abnormal mucosal appearance may improve rapidly.

Diagnosis can be made by gastroscopy, sometimes supplemented by gastric mucosal biopsy.

Initial management should follow the guidelines presented for upper gastrointestinal hemorrhage. Fortunately, gastric lavage with cold solutions is usually effective in halting the blood loss. As in other conditions with acute gastric hemorrhage, the decision for operation depends on the rate of continuing hemorrhage after treatment.

Vagotomy, in addition to reducing acid secretion, has been shown to divert blood away from the gastric mucosa by opening submucosal shunts. Vagotomy with a drainage procedure would be the first effort of many surgeons. If this fails, subtotal or, in rare cases, total gastrectomy might be necessary to save the patient.

The prognosis after bleeding stops is good if intake of substances harmful to the stomach can be prevented.

Chronic Gastritis

Chronic gastritis embraces a wide variety of lesions, in some cases related only by virtue of their gastric location. Chronic atrophic gastritis of the parietal cell mucosa is found in patients with pernicious anemia who also have achlorhydria and antibodies against intrinsic factor and parietal cells. Atrophic gastritis with achlorhydria also occurs without pernicious anemia. Adenocarcinoma of the stomach is more frequent with both types compared with the normal population.

Chronic gastritis is invariably found in patients with benign gastric ulcer. It has been suggested that this is caused by regurgitation of duodenal secretions.

Croft DN: Gastritis. Brit MJ 3:164–166, 1967.

MENETRIER'S DISEASE

Menetrier's disease consists of giant hypertrophy of the gastric rugae with hypochlorhydria and excessive loss of protein. Hypoproteinemia frequently produces ascites, and chronic blood loss may be a problem. The patient complains of indigestion which responds to antacids, but treatment does not improve the gastric pathology or secondary hypoproteinemia. The hypertrophic rugae present as enormous filling defects on upper gastrointestinal series and are frequently misinterpreted as carcinoma. Partial or, sometimes, total gastrectomy is indicated for hypoproteinemia, anemia, or inability to exclude malignancy.

ACUTE GASTRIC DILATATION

Acute gastric dilatation usually follows surgery on the upper abdomen, particularly in patients who have received oxygen by nasal catheter or those who have been placed on a respirator using a face mask. Swallowed air produces gastric distention and increased intragastric pressure. As pressure exceeds that in the mucosal veins, acute bleeding may occur.

Anorexia, hiccuping, vomiting of brownish, dark-stained or bloody gastric contents, epigastric tympany, and tachycardia are important early diagnostic signs. Shock due to acute gastric dilatation can be rapidly fatal. Death may result from dehydration, bleeding, acute pulmonary edema, or aspiration of gastric contents into the tracheobronchial tree.

Treatment consists of the insertion of a nasogastric tube with decompression of the stomach and restoration of fluids and electrolytes.

PROLAPSE OF THE GASTRIC MUCOSA

This uncommon lesion occasionally accompanies small prepyloric gastric ulcers. Episodes of vomiting and abdominal pain simulate peptic ulcer disease. X-ray shows prolapse of antral folds into the duodenum. One must be alert to the presence of gastric or duodenal ulcer as the underlying cause.

Antrectomy with a Billroth I anastomosis is occasionally required for a well-authenticated case of prolapse of the gastric mucosa. Generally, conservative treatment suffices.

GASTRIC VOLVULUS

The stomach may rotate about its longitudinal axis (organo-axial volvulus) or a line drawn from the midlesser to the midgreater curvature (mesenterio-axial volvulus). The former is the most common and is often associated with a paraesophageal hiatal hernia. In other patients, eventration of the left diaphragm allows the colon to rise upward and twist the stomach by pulling on the gastrocolic ligament.

Acute gastric volvulus produces severe abdominal pain accompanied by a diagnostic triad (Brochardt's triad): (1) vomiting followed by retching and then inability to vomit, (2) epigastric distention, and (3) inability to pass a nasogastric tube. The situation calls for immediate laparotomy to prevent death from acute gastric necrosis and shock. An emergency upper gastrointestinal series will show a block at the point of the volvulus. The mortality rate is high.

Chronic volvulus is more common than acute. It may be asymptomatic or may cause crampy intermittent pain. Cases associated with paraesophageal hiatal hernia should be treated by repair of the hernia and anterior gastropexy. When due to eventration of the diaphragm, the gastrocolic ligament should be divided the entire length of the greater curvature. The colon rises to fill the space caused by the eventration, and the stomach will resume its normal position, to be fastened by a gastropexy.

Tanner NC: Chronic and recurrent volvulus of the stomach. Am J Surg 115:505–515, 1968.

Wastell C, Ellis H: Volvulus of the stomach. Brit J Surg 58:557–562, 1971.

GASTRIC DIVERTICULA

Gastric diverticula are uncommon and usually asymptomatic. Most are pulsion diverticula consisting of mucosa and submucosa only, located on the lesser curvature within a few centimeters of the esophagogas-tric junction. Those in the prepyloric region generally possess all layers and are more likely to be symptomatic. A few patients have symptoms from hemorrhage or inflammation within a gastric diverticulum, but for the most part these lesions are incidental findings on upper gastrointestinal series. Radiologically, they can be confused with a gastric ulcer.

Hughes W, Pierce WS: Surgical implications of gastric diverticula. Surg Gynec Obst 131:99–102, 1970.

BEZOAR

Bezoars are concretions formed in the stomach. Trichobezoars are composed of hair and are usually found in young girls who pick at their hair and swallow it. Phytobezoars consist of agglomerated vegetable fibers. Pressure by the mass can create a gastric ulcer which is prone to bleed or perforate.

The postgastrectomy state predisposes to bezoar formation because pepsin and acid secretion are reduced and the triturating function of the antrum is gone. Orange segments or other fruits which contain a large amount of cellulose have been implicated in most cases. Improper mastication of food is a contributing factor which can sometimes be obviated by providing the patient with well-fitting dentures. The fruit may remain in the stomach or pass into the small intestine and cause obstruction. Some surgeons routinely warn postgastrectomy patients to avoid citrus fruits.

Large semisolid bezoars of *Candida albicans* have also been found in postgastrectomy patients. It has been possible to fragment some of these with the gastroscope. The patient should also be treated with oral nystatin.

Patients with symptomatic gastric bezoars may complain of abdominal pain. Ulceration and bleeding are associated with a mortality rate of 20%.

Oral administration of papain and cellulase has been used successfully to digest the mass. This treatment must not be allowed to delay surgery and permit serious complications to develop. Symptomatic patients should be treated by operative removal of the bezoar and excision of secondary gastric ulcers.

Cain GD, Moore P Jr, Patterson M: Bezoars: A complication of the postgastrectomy state. Am J Digest Dis 13:801–809, 1968.

Jaffe BM, Sasser WF: Management of gastric persimmon bezoars. Am J Surg 114:962–965, 1967.

Pollard HB, Block GE: Rapid dissolution of phytobezoar by cellulase enzyme. Am J Surg 116:933–936, 1968.

II. DUODENUM*

DUODENAL DIVERTICULA

Diverticula of the duodenum are found in 20% of autopsies and 5–10% of upper gastrointestinal series. Symptoms are uncommon, and only 1% of those found by x-ray warrant surgery.

Duodenal pulsion diverticula are acquired outpouchings of the mucosa and submucosa, 90% of which are on the medial aspect of the duodenum. Most are solitary and within 2.5 cm of the ampulla of Vater. They are not seen in the first portion of the duodenum, where diverticular configurations are due to scarring by peptic ulceration or cholecystitis.

A few patients have chronic postprandial abdominal pain or dyspepsia caused by a duodenal diverticulum. Treatment is with antacids and anticholinergics.

Serious complications are hemorrhage or perforation from inflammation, pancreatitis, and biliary obstruction. Bile acid-bilirubinate enteroliths are occasionally formed by bile stasis in a diverticulum. Enteroliths can precipitate diverticular inflammation or biliary obstruction and rarely have caused bowel obstruction after entering the intestinal lumen.

Surgical treatment is required for complications and, rarely, for persistent symptoms. Excision and a 2-layer closure is usually possible after mobilization of the duodenum and dissection of the diverticulum from the pancreas. Removal of the diverticulum and closure of the defect is superior to simple drainage in the case of perforation. If biliary obstruction appears in a patient whose bile duct empties into a diverticulum, excision might be more hazardous than a side-to-side choledochoduodenostomy.

Luler GL & others: Perforating duodenal diverticulitis. Arch Surg 99:572–578, 1969.

McSherry CK, Glenn G: Biliary tract obstruction and duodenal diverticula. Surg Gynec Obst 130:829–836, 1970.

Neill SA, Thompson NW: The complications of duodenal diverticula and their management. Surg Gynec Obst 120: 1251–1258, 1965.

DUODENAL TUMORS

Tumors of the duodenum are rare. Carcinoma of the ampulla of Vater is discussed in Chapter 28.

Malignant Tumors

Most malignant duodenal tumors are adenocarcinomas, leiomyosarcomas, and lymphomas. They ap-

pear in the descending duodenum more often than elsewhere. Pain, obstruction, bleeding, obstructive jaundice, and an abdominal mass are the nodes of presentation.

If possible, adenocarcinomas should be resected. Pancreaticoduodenectomy is usually necessary if the tumor is localized. Biopsy and radiotherapy are recommended for lymphoma.

Surgical cure is uncommon.

Benign Tumors

These are encountered even less often than duodenal malignancies. Brunner's gland adenomas are those most likely to be symptomatic. They are small submucosal nodules which have a predilection for the posterior duodenal wall at the junction of the first and second portions. Sessile and pedunculated variants are seen. Symptoms are due to bleeding or obstruction. Leiomyomas and carcinoids may also be found in the duodenum and ordinarily are symptomatic.

Ectopic islet cell adenomas (gastrinomas) in the duodenal submucosa are responsible for a small number of cases of Zollinger-Ellison syndrome.

Bruno MS, Fein HD: Primary malignant and benign tumors of the duodenum. Arch Int Med 125:670–679, 1970.

Craig O: Duodenal carcinoma. Brit J Surg 56:39–44, 1969.

Lawrence W Jr & others: Benign duodenal tumors. Ann Surg 172:1015–1022, 1970.

ReMine WH & others: Polypoid hamartomas of Brunner's glands. Arch Surg 100:313–316, 1970.

SUPERIOR MESENTERIC ARTERY OBSTRUCTION OF THE DUODENUM

Obstruction of the third portion of the duodenum may rarely be produced by compression between the superior mesenteric vessels and the aorta. It most commonly appears after rapid weight loss following injury. Patients in body casts are particularly susceptible.

The superior mesenteric artery normally leaves the aorta at an angle of 50–60 degrees, and the distance between the 2 vessels where the duodenum passes between them is 10–20 mm. These measurements in patients with the superior mesenteric artery syndrome average 18 degrees and 2.5 mm. Acute loss of mesenteric fat is thought to permit the artery to drop posteriorly, trapping the bowel like a scissors.

Skepticism exists regarding the frequency of this condition in adults who have not experienced acute loss of weight. Most often the patient in question is a thin, nervous woman whose complaints of dyspepsia and occasional emesis are more properly explained on a functional basis. When a clear-cut example is encountered, it may actually represent a form of intestinal malrotation with duodenal bands.

*Duodenal ulcer is discussed with peptic ulcer in the preceding section.

Clinical Findings

A. Symptoms and Signs: The patient complains of epigastric bloating and crampy pain which is relieved by vomiting. The symptoms may remit in the prone position. Anorexia and postprandial pain lead to additional malnutrition and weight loss.

B. X-Ray Findings: Upper gastrointestinal x-rays demonstrate a widened duodenum proximal to a sharp obstruction at the point where the artery crosses the third portion of the duodenum. When the patient moves to the knee-chest position, the passage of barium is suddenly unimpeded. Further verification can be provided if angiography shows an angle of 25 degrees or less between the superior mesenteric artery and the aorta. However, this procedure is not recommended for routine evaluation of obvious cases.

Differential Diagnosis

Many patients whose superior mesenteric artery makes a prominent impression on the duodenum are asymptomatic, and in ambulatory patients one should hesitate to attribute vague chronic complaints to this finding.

Involvement of the duodenum by scleroderma leads to duodenal dilatation and hypomotility and an x-ray and clinical picture highly suggestive of the superior mesenteric artery syndrome. In the latter, increased duodenal peristalsis should be demonstrable proximal to the arterial blockage, whereas diminished peristalsis characterizes scleroderma. Patients with duodenal scleroderma usually have dysphagia from concomitant esophageal involvement.

Malrotation with duodenal obstruction by congenital bands can mimic this syndrome.

Treatment

Postural therapy usually suffices. The patient should be placed prone when symptomatic or in anticipation of postprandial difficulties. Ambulatory patients should be instructed to assume the knee-chest position, which allows the viscera and the artery to rotate forward off the duodenum.

Chronic obstruction may require a duodenojeju-nostomy to bypass the obstruction. Patients with various forms of malrotation may be treated by mobilizing the duodenojejunal flexure, which releases the duodenum from entrapment by congenital bands.

Louw JH: Intestinal malrotation and duodenal ileus. J Roy Coll Surg Edinb 5:101–126, 1960.

Wayne E, Miller RE, Eiseman B: Duodenal obstruction by the superior mesenteric artery in bedridden combat casualties. Ann Surg 174:339–345, 1971.

REGIONAL ENTERITIS OF THE STOMACH & DUODENUM

The proximal intestine and stomach are rarely involved in regional enteritis, although this disease has now been reported in every part of the gastrointestinal tract from the lips to the anus. Most patients with Crohn's disease in the stomach or duodenum have ileal involvement as well.

Pain can in many instances be relieved by antacids. Intermittent vomiting from duodenal stenosis or pyloric obstruction is frequent. The x-ray finding of a cobblestone mucosa or stenosis would be suggestive when associated with typical changes in the ileum. In questionable cases, verification may be obtained with the peroral suction biopsy capsule.

Medical treatment is nonspecific and consists principally of corticosteroids during exacerbations. Surgery may be indicated for disabling pain or obstruction. If localized to the stomach, a partial gastrectomy can be performed. However, when the stomach is affected, the duodenum is usually involved as well. Bypass gastrojejunostomy has provided symptomatic relief for this type of patient.

Fielding JF & others: Crohn's disease of the stomach and duodenum. Gut 11:1001–1006, 1970.

Wise L & others: Crohn's disease of the duodenum. Am J Surg 121:184–194, 1971.

●   ●   ●

General References

Davenport HW: *Physiology of the Digestive Tract,* 3rd ed. Year Book, 1971.

Harkins HN, Nyhus LM: *Surgery of the Stomach and Duodenum,* 2nd ed. Little, Brown, 1969.

Sleisenger M, Fordtran JS: *Gastrointestinal Disease.* Saunders, 1973.

26 . . .

The Liver

Lawrence W. Way, MD

Liver transplantation is still an experimental operation and is discussed in Chapter 51. The physiology of bilirubin metabolism and the diagnostic approach to the jaundiced patient are covered in Chapter 27.

SURGICAL ANATOMY

Segments

The liver develops as an embryologic outpouching from the duodenum by a process which is described in Chapter 27. The liver is one of the largest organs in the body, representing 2% of the total body weight. In classic descriptions, the liver was characterized as having 4 lobes: right, left, caudate, and quadrate. However, these traditional lobes do not describe the true segmental anatomy of the liver, which is depicted in Fig 26–1. The main lobar fissure can be thought of as represented by an oblique plane passing posteriorly from the gallbladder bed to the vena cava, dividing the anatomic right and left lobes. This primary division is to the right of the falciform ligament. The right lobe is subdivided into anterior and posterior segments by the right segmental fissure. The left lobe is subdivided into medial and lateral segments by the left segmental fissure, marked by the position of the falciform ligament.

The relationship of the liver to the other abdominal organs is shown in Fig 26–2.

Venous Blood Supply (Fig 26–3)

Both the portal and hepatic venous systems lack valves. The portal vein terminates in the porta hepatis by dividing into right and left lobar branches. The right lobar branch immediately follows the course of the segmental ducts and arteries. The left lobar branch has 2 portions: the transverse part and the umbilical part. The former is a short segment coursing through the porta hepatis. The latter descends into the umbilical fossa and supplies the medial and lateral segments of the left lobe.

The hepatic veins represent the final common pathway for the central veins of the lobules of the liver. There are 3 major hepatic veins: left, right, and middle. The middle hepatic vein lies in the major lobar fissure and drains blood from the medial segment of the left lobe and the inferior portion of the anterior

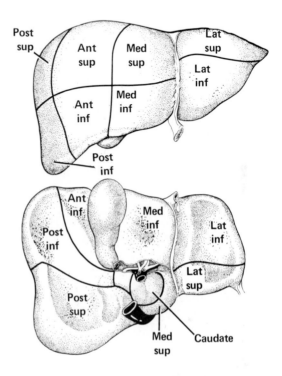

FIG 26–1. Segmental anatomy of the liver. The major lobar fissure, separating the right and left lobes, passes from the inferior vena cava through the gallbladder bed.

segment of the right lobe. The left hepatic vein drains the lateral segment of the left lobe and the right hepatic vein the posterior segment and much of the anterior segment of the right lobe. Several small accessory veins enter the inferior vena cava directly from the posterior segment of the right lobe and must be carefully ligated during a right hemihepatectomy. The middle hepatic vein usually joins the left hepatic vein before they meet the inferior vena cava.

Arterial Blood Supply

The common hepatic artery arises from the celiac axis, ascends in the hepatoduodenal ligament, and gives rise to the right gastric and gastroduodenal arteries before dividing into right and left branches in the hilum. The hepatic artery supplies approximately 25% of the 1500 ml of blood which enter the liver each

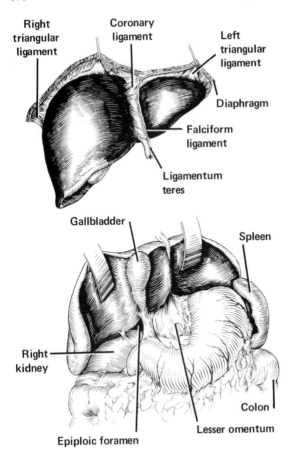

FIG 26–2. Relationships of the liver to adjacent abdominal organs.

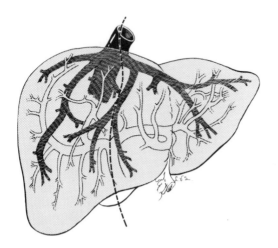

FIG 26–3. Anatomy of the veins of the liver. The major lobar fissure is represented by the dashed line. Branches of the hepatic artery and biliary ducts follow those of the portal vein. The darker vessels represent the hepatic veins and vena cava; the lighter system represents the portal vein and its branches.

minute; the remaining 75% is supplied by the portal vein. In 10% of individuals, the common hepatic artery has an anomalous origin. In the most common variants, the common hepatic or the right hepatic artery arises from the superior mesenteric artery. The left hepatic originates from the left gastric artery in 15% of subjects. The common hepatic artery divides to follow the segmental ducts. Once they enter the liver and divide, the various segmental branches are termed end arteries since they do not communicate with each other via collaterals.

Biliary Drainage

Segmental bile ducts drain each segment. The right anterior and right posterior segmental ducts unite to form the right hepatic duct, and the left lateral and left medial segmental ducts form the left hepatic duct. These lobar ducts join outside the parenchyma to form the common hepatic duct. Anatomic variations are common. In over 25% of specimens, the duct from the right posterior segment joins the left hepatic duct independently. Variations are far less common on the left side.

Lymphatics

Superficial lymphatics arise from superficial portions of the lobules and pass beneath the capsule to enter the posterior mediastinum via the diaphragm and the suspensory ligaments of the liver. Some enter the porta hepatis and others enter the coronary chain. Other lymphatics arise deep in the liver lobules and pass either with the hepatic veins along the vena cava or with the portal veins into the porta hepatis.

Elias H, Sherrick JC: *Morphology of the Liver.* Academic Press, 1969.
Goldsmith NA, Woodburne RT: The surgical anatomy pertaining to liver resection. Surg Gynec Obst 105:310–318, 1957.
Michels NA: Newer anatomy of the liver and its variant blood supply and collateral circulation. Am J Surg 112:337–347, 1966.

DIAGNOSTIC PROCEDURES

Liver Biopsy

A specimen of liver adequate for histologic diagnosis can be obtained by the percutaneous insertion of a variety of biopsy needles. The Menghini needle is preferred unless the liver substance is unusually hard, as in advanced cirrhosis or hepatic fibrosis. The Vim-Silverman needle may be needed to obtain a satisfactory specimen in these cases.

Liver biopsy is of greatest value in the diagnosis of parenchymal disease such as viral hepatitis. Tumors can often be sampled and increased accuracy can be obtained by consulting the hepatic scan before performing the biopsy. It is usually impossible to reliably differentiate among the various causes of cholestasis by histologic appearances.

The presence of a defective coagulation mechanism is a major contraindication to this procedure. It should rarely be performed if the prothrombin time is less than 50%. High-grade extrahepatic biliary obstruction may also be hazardous since bile peritonitis has followed biopsy in such instances.

The reported mortality rate is about 0.1%.

Menghini G: One-second biopsy of the liver. New England J Med 283:582–585, 1970.

Liver Scans

Scintillation scans of the liver may be performed using numerous radionuclides. At present, technetium-99m and gold-198 colloids give the best quality pictures. Lateral as well as anterior views should be routinely obtained. Space-occupying lesions in the liver such as tumors, abscesses, or cysts may be demonstrated as filling defects. Lesions with a diameter less than 2.5 cm cannot usually be detected. The accuracy of the technic is presently around 75%; 15% are false-positive and 10% false-negative. Substantial observer variation has been demonstrated in interpretation of individual scans, and they should be judged of indeterminate value unless the abnormal findings are well defined and compatible with other clinical and laboratory data.

Hepatic scans are occasionally of value to demonstrate the extent of hepatomegaly or the position of the liver in relation to a subphrenic abscess.

Castagna J & others: The reliability of liver scans and function tests in detecting metastases. Surg Gynec Obst 134: 463–466, 1972.

Ludbrook J & others: Observer error in reporting on liver scans for space-occupying lesions. Gastroenterology 62:1013–1019, 1972.

Rosenthal S, Kaufman S: Liver scan in metastatic disease. Arch Surg 105:656–659, 1973.

Arteriography

The hepatic artery may be visualized with contrast medium selectively injected through a catheter inserted percutaneously through the femoral or axillary artery. Sequential x-rays demonstrate a hepatic arterial phase, a parenchymal phase, and a portal venous phase. The procedure is useful to outline space-occupying lesions in the liver as well as abnormal vascular patterns. Since lesions smaller than the resolution of the hepatic scan can sometimes be shown, arteriography can be used as an adjunct to scanning when the results of the latter are equivocal. Advanced cirrhosis may be recognized by a characteristic corkscrew configuration of the intrahepatic vessels. Primary hepatomas and hemangiomas have distinctive vascular appearances. Metastatic tumors and adenomas vary in vascularity, but in general they have a less pronounced arterial blush than hepatomas and frequently appear as filling defects which displace the arterial vessels. Cholangiocarcinoma, cysts, and abscesses present as avascular filling defects without specific identifying

features. Angiography has been of major value in the diagnosis of hemobilia. Its use in the management of selected cases of liver trauma appears promising.

Baum S: Hepatic angiography. Chap 27, pp 444–465, in: *Progress in Liver Diseases.* Vol 3. Popper H, Schaffner F (editors). Grune & Stratton, 1970.

Pollard JJ: Abdominal angiography. New England J Med 279:1093, 1968.

HEPATIC RESECTION

Increased understanding of the anatomy and physiology of the liver has made resection of more than 50% of the organ possible with an acceptably low mortality rate. The indications for resections of major segments of the liver are relatively uncommon and include primary and secondary malignant tumors, benign tumors, traumatic rupture, cysts, and abscesses.

Removal of as much as 80–85% of the normal liver is consistent with survival. Liver function is reduced for several weeks after extensive resections, but the extraordinary regenerative capacity of the liver rapidly provides new functioning hepatocytes. Although hepatic regeneration—or, more aptly, "restorative hyperplasia"—has been the subject of intense study, the process is only vaguely understood. Normally mitoses among hepatocytes are exceedingly rare, and it has been estimated that individual cells may survive for the lifetime of the organism. However, within 24 hours after partial hepatectomy, cell replication becomes active and continues until the original weight of the organ is restored. Studies in man indicate that considerable regeneration occurs within 10 days and that the process is essentially complete by 4–5 weeks. Excised lobes are not reformed as such. Rather, the growth consists of formation of new lobules and expansion of residual lobules. The stimulus for restorative hyperplasia is known to be humoral, but it has not been further characterized.

Preoperative Evaluation

Since liver function is compromised after major hepatic resections, the decision to perform such operations must take into account the preoperative functional status. Cirrhosis with impaired function is the most commonly encountered contraindication for hepatectomy. The limited reserve of the residual cirrhotic liver after operation is usually insufficient to supply essential metabolic needs. Moreover, the cirrhotic liver possesses little capacity for regeneration. These factors prohibit resection of some primary hepatic tumors which develop in cirrhotics.

The level of serum albumin before operation should be greater than 3 g/100 ml if complications are to be avoided. If the value is lower, the patient should be prepared by parenteral albumin infusions.

Active hepatocellular disease at the time of

hepatectomy would seriously diminish the chances of postoperative recovery. Therefore, a markedly elevated SGOT (above 400 IU/liter) or demonstration of substantial necrosis or inflammation on liver biopsy would usually rule out hepatic resection until the active process subsided.

Technic of Hepatic Resections

Based upon the lobar anatomy, hepatic resections are classified as segmental or nonsegmental. Wedge resections and resectional debridement of devitalized tissue are examples of the latter. Major lobar resections must be planned in accordance with the segmental vascular anatomy (Fig 26–3). The terminology and extent of the common types of resections are depicted in Fig 26–4. The operation entails removal of a lobe or segment with its afferent and efferent vessels while avoiding injury to vessels and bile ducts supplying the residual tissue. An extended right hepatectomy–the most extensive–removes all but 15–20% of the hepatic mass.

Left lobectomy or left lateral hepatectomy can usually be performed through an abdominal incision, but procedures involving extirpation of the right lobe require a thoracoabdominal approach. The key to technical success is hemostasis. The appropriate hilar vessels are divided before beginning the dissection, and the liver tissue is then transected bluntly with the finger fracture technic or the handle of a scalpel.

The space created by removing a part of the liver must be drained with a large sump tube and numerous soft rubber drains. To be adequate, the drain must be aided by gravity by being dependent. Despite pre-

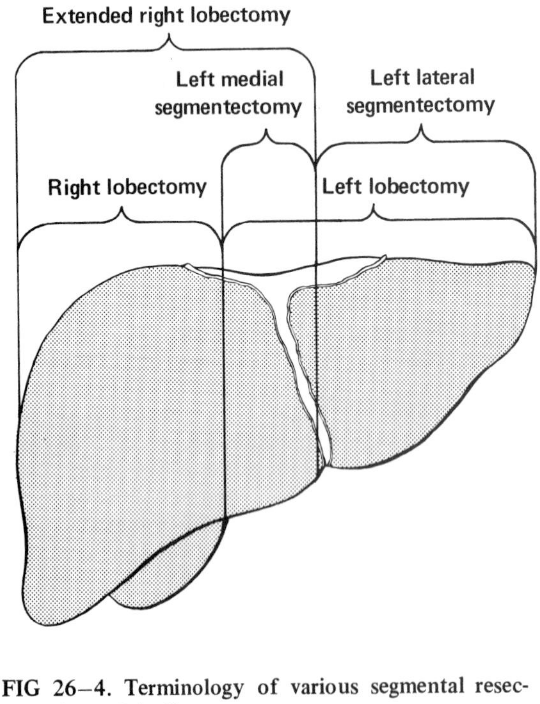

FIG 26–4. Terminology of various segmental resections of the liver.

cautions, about 20% of patients develop abscesses in or near this space and require additional operations for drainage some time in the postoperative period.

Postoperative Course

If 50% or more of the liver has been removed, the patient will require close monitoring and metabolic support for the first 1 or 2 weeks after operation.

A. Blood Glucose: The blood glucose level may fall immediately after surgery if it is not maintained by parenteral infusions. The glucose concentration should be measured twice daily for the first 2 days and 5% or 10% glucose administered intravenously in quantities sufficient to avoid hypoglycemia.

B. Plasma Protein: The serum albumin concentration drops in most patients. Hypoalbuminemia should be corrected by the intravenous route to avoid pulmonary edema or ascites. The albumin deficit presumably results from loss of functioning liver tissue plus depressed synthetic capacity of the residual liver. The usual requirement is 50–100 g of salt-poor albumin daily for about 1 week.

C. Clotting Factors: The concentrations of several clotting factors invariably drop after partial hepatectomy, but this is rarely the cause of hemorrhagic complications. The prothrombin level falls to about 50% of normal, and vitamin K must be given. Low concentrations of fibrinogen and factor IX improve spontaneously and require no treatment. Serious complications sometimes follow disseminated intravascular coagulation. This condition usually develops after severe trauma to many organs.

D. Liver Function Studies: The serum bilirubin rises to an average peak of 5–6 mg/100 ml several days after resection but usually returns to normal within 1–2 weeks. The absolute height of bilirubin is affected by the amount of blood transfused, the presence or absence of disease in the residual liver, sepsis, and trauma to other areas. The alkaline phosphatase usually remains normal after partial hepatectomy unless functioning bile ducts have been traumatized or obstructed. SGOT and serum LDH rise for several days and then return to normal levels.

Complications

Atelectasis and pneumonitis of the right lung are frequent after partial hepatectomy, especially when a thoracoabdominal approach has been used.

Fever of 39 C (102.2 F) or greater occurs in over half of patients. Fever may be due to pulmonary complications or perihepatic abscess, but in many cases no cause can be identified and convalescence in the latter patients may be otherwise unmarred. Abscess formation is a major problem in the space created by the resection and requires reexploration and drainage.

Partial hepatectomy is attended by a relatively high incidence of postoperative stress ulcers. Prophylactic antacids should be given routinely through the nasogastric tube after operation.

Liver failure may result if the residual tissue is diseased or has been compromised by prolonged ischemia during the operation. Ascites, varices, and coma are the manifestations.

Prognosis

The mortality rate is about 25% but is largely related to the underlying disease. The various prognostic factors will be discussed under the separate disease headings.

Aronsen KF & others: Metabolic changes following major hepatic resection. Ann Surg 169:102–110, 1969.

Blumgart LH & others: Observations on liver regeneration after right hepatic lobectomy. Gut 12:922–928, 1971.

Bucher NLR, Malt RA: *Regeneration of Liver and Kidney.* Little, Brown, 1971.

Foster JH & others: Recent experience with major hepatic resection. Ann Surg 167:651–668, 1968.

Mays ET: Hepatic lobectomy. Arch Surg 103:216–228, 1971.

Mercadier M, Clot JP: Experiences with anatomic hemihepatectomy and left lobectomy. Surg Gynec Obst 133: 467–471, 1971.

Pinkerton JA & others: A study of the postoperative course after hepatic lobectomy. Ann Surg 173:800–811, 1971.

Stone HH & others: Physiologic considerations in major hepatic resections. Am J Surg 117:78–84, 1969.

Tien-Yu Lin: Results in 107 hepatic lobectomies with a preliminary report on the use of a clamp to reduce blood loss. Ann Surg 177:413–421, 1973.

Tung TT, Quang ND: A new technique for operating on the liver. Lancet 1:192–193, 1963.

DISEASES & DISORDERS OF THE LIVER

HEPATIC TRAUMA

Injuries to the liver are common consequences of automobile accidents and social violence. War wounds differ in important respects from those incurred in a civilian population. Battle trauma is largely the result of penetrating high-velocity missiles. In the USA, most penetrating injuries are caused by low-velocity missiles such as handguns or knives, and the resulting hepatic damage is in most cases considerably less. By contrast, some of the most difficult to manage are wounds to pedestrians or passengers inflicted by blunt trauma in automobile accidents. In recent years, these have comprised about half of the cases of hepatic trauma seen in emergency rooms in large hospitals.

Many penetrating wounds have stopped bleeding by the time they are inspected at laparotomy. In the case of wounds caused by high-velocity missiles, devitalized liver should be debrided from along the missile tract, but this is not generally required for lacerations caused by knives or small-caliber guns.

Blunt trauma produces 2 forms of hepatic injury:

linear lacerations or stellate bursting tears. Lacerations following blunt injury usually consist of one or sometimes 2 longitudinal tears on the anterior surface oriented in a cranial-caudal direction. These are thought to be due to shearing stresses from rapid rotational deceleration. They are usually 5–15 cm long and 1 or 2 cm deep, although occasionally they may extend as deep as the large hepatic veins.

Explosive stellate injuries are most often located in the superior posterior segment of the right lobe and may be associated with one or more anterior lacerations directed inferomedially. This type of damage usually results from a direct blow over the lower right thorax and is often accompanied by rib fractures. Stellate injuries are common in pedestrians, frequently in association with head and extremity trauma. Less commonly, direct trauma may produce a contained central rupture or a subcapsular hematoma. Either of these may be responsible for delayed abdominal hemorrhage or hemobilia.

Clinical Findings

A. Symptoms and Signs: Signs of violence are usually obvious after knife or missile wounds, and diagnosis is rarely a problem (as with blunt trauma) since abdominal exploration is routine in such cases. In blunt liver injuries, the clinical presentation is often overshadowed by associated injuries to other organs. In only 10% of cases is the liver injury the only one present; head, chest, extremity, pelvic, and splenic injuries are the most common. Whenever severe blunt trauma is obvious—as manifested by extremity fractures or head injury—the physician must be on guard for ruptured abdominal organs even in the absence of abdominal signs.

The initial morbidity of liver injuries is produced by abdominal bleeding. Hypotension, shock, diminished urinary output, and abdominal distention are the usual manifestations. Many patients appear to have no important abdominal injury when first examined, and the gradual appearance of hypotension must be recognized as indicative of intra-abdominal bleeding and should never be attributed to head injury.

Abdominal examination may reveal upper abdominal muscle spasm and tenderness and occasionally hepatomegaly. Signs of fractured ribs on the right may be the initial clue to underlying hepatic damage. If positive, paracentesis would substantiate a diagnosis of intra-abdominal bleeding, but false-negatives occur and may be misleading. (See Chapter 52 for the technic of paracentesis.)

B. Laboratory Findings: The rate of blood loss is usually so rapid that anemia does not develop. Leukocytosis greater than 15,000/μl is common following rupture of the liver or spleen from blunt trauma.

C. X-Ray Findings: In most cases, x-ray evaluation is of minor importance. Hepatomegaly may be evident on plain abdominal films, or the right diaphragm may be elevated. Fractured ribs over the liver should suggest liver injury.

Hepatic scan may show filling defects in cases of

central rupture or subcapsular hematoma without active bleeding.

Angiography is not routine because it is so time-consuming. However, it may be useful to delineate the extent of central rupture and is diagnostic in hemobilia.

Treatment

If a liver injury is strongly suspected, the abdomen should be explored. The decision for laparotomy is usually automatic with penetrating injuries. After blunt abdominal trauma, signs of blood loss or a positive abdominal paracentesis are the usual indications. A conscious patient can be followed nonoperatively until definite signs develop, but patients who are unconscious following head trauma are more difficult to monitor and should be explored if there is any question of visceral injury.

The main goals of surgical therapy are to stop bleeding and excise devitalized liver tissue. Lacerations from stab wounds or blunt injury have often stopped bleeding by the time the operation is performed. Several soft rubber drains should be placed in the vicinity of the injury and brought to the exterior through a separate small incision. In the absence of active hemorrhage, these wounds should not be sutured because a closed space would be created which may be susceptible to abscess formation or hemobilia. When active bleeding is encountered, it should be controlled with catgut suture of the bleeding vessels rather than by attempting tamponade by inserting large mattress sutures to reapproximate the margins of the tear.

Devitalized liver tissue should be locally debrided until healthy bleeding parenchyma is reached. Attempts to reestablish the normal configuration of the liver by closing large defects or lacerations accomplish nothing and are apt to produce local complications.

Formal lobectomy is rarely necessary and is only used for diffuse destruction of a lobe or a major central rupture. Most cases are preferably handled by local debridement and control of bleeding with sutures.

The hilar vessels may be occluded for 10–15 minutes while bleeding points are being identified and controlled. If this fails, one should suspect either the presence of an anomalous hepatic artery which has escaped the hilar occlusion or a tear in a hepatic vein or in the suprarenal vena cava.

Bleeding from disruption of hepatic veins near their junction with the vena cava can be technically quite difficult to manage because of inadequate exposure and the fragility of the vessels.

Adequate postoperative drainage is of critical importance. If copious drainage is expected from the liver or if there is a large defect, the space should be drained with a sump tube as well as numerous soft rubber drains placed around the periphery of the hepatic wound.

Theoretically, a T-tube would prevent bile leaks by reducing biliary ductal pressure, but experience has shown a high rate of complications which, in the average case, offsets potential benefits.

A special problem is presented by massive penetrating injuries which involve the hepatic flexure of the colon as well as the liver. Resection of the colonic injury and primary anastomosis sets the stage for overwhelming subhepatic sepsis and anastomotic leakage. Therefore, this combination of injuries is preferably managed by removal of the damaged colon, construction of a temporary ileostomy and mucous fistula, and local treatment of the hepatic wound. The intestine may be reanastomosed several weeks after recovery from the initial trauma.

Postoperative Complications

With present technics, hemorrhage at laparotomy is rarely uncontrollable except with retrohepatic venous injuries. Patients who rebleed from the liver wound after initial suture ligation should be treated by reexploration and lobectomy.

Subhepatic sepsis develops in about 20% of patients and is more frequent if lobectomy has been performed. Many cases of local postoperative infection can be attributed to faulty drainage.

Hemobilia may be responsible for gastrointestinal bleeding in the postoperative period and can be diagnosed by selective angiography of the hepatic artery. Treatment consists of ligation of the artery supplying the bleeding vessel or, if that fails, segmental resection.

Bleeding from stress ulcers is a serious postoperative problem after hepatic trauma. It seems to be more common in patients who have received ancillary T-tube drainage of the common duct. All patients with liver injuries should be given antacids after operation.

Prognosis

The mortality rate of 10–15% following hepatic trauma depends largely on the type of injury and the extent of associated injury to other organs. Only 1% of penetrating civilian wounds are lethal, whereas a 30% mortality rate attends blunt trauma. The mortality rate in blunt hepatic injury is only 10% when only the liver is injured. If 3 major organs are damaged, the death rate is close to 70%.

Bismuth H: Hemobilia. New England J Med 288:617–619, 1973.

Carroll CP & others: Wounds of the liver in Vietnam. Ann Surg 177:385–392, 1973.

Fischer RP & others: The rapid right hepatectomy. J Trauma 11:742–748, 1971.

Hardy KJ: Patterns of liver injury after fatal blunt trauma. Surg Gynec Obst 134:39–43, 1972.

Lim RC Jr & others: Liver trauma. Arch Surg 104:544–550, 1972.

Longmire WP Jr, Cleveland RJ: Surgical anatomy and blunt trauma of the liver. S Clin North America 52:687–698, 1972.

Lucas CE: Prospective clinical evaluation of biliary drainage in hepatic trauma. Ann Surg 174:830–836, 1971.

Madding GF, Kennedy PA: *Trauma to the Liver,* 2nd ed. Saunders, 1971.

Mayes ET: Lobectomy, sublobar resection, and resectional debridement for severe liver injuries. J Trauma 12:309–314, 1972.

Mays ET: Hepatic trauma. New England J Med 288:402–405, 1973.

Walt AJ: The surgical management of hepatic trauma and its complications. Ann Roy Coll Surg England 45:319–339, 1969.

SPONTANEOUS HEPATIC RUPTURE

Spontaneous rupture of the liver is not common. Most cases are due to toxemia of pregnancy, but spontaneous rupture has also been reported in association with hepatic hemangioma, gallstone obstruction, primary and metastatic liver carcinoma, typhoid fever, malaria, tuberculosis, syphilis, polyarteritis nodosa, and diabetes mellitus. Rupture of the liver in the newborn is related to birth trauma in larger infants after difficult deliveries. The common course is intrahepatic hemorrhage expanding to capsular rupture.

Treatment is surgical as for traumatic rupture (see above).

PRIMARY MALIGNANT TUMORS OF THE LIVER

Primary hepatic malignancy is uncommon in the USA. However, the incidence is high in parts of the Orient and Africa, and in some regions hepatoma is the single most frequent abdominal tumor. The etiologic factors in these high-risk areas are environmental or cultural, since persons of similar racial background in the USA are at only slightly greater risk than Caucasians. About 7100 cases—distributed equally between men and women—occurred in the USA in 1972. Most arise in persons over 50 years of age, but a small number are found in children, mainly under 2 years of age.

Three cellular types are recognized: hepatocellular carcinoma (hepatoma), cholangiocellular carcinoma (cholangiocarcinoma), and a mixed form (hepatocholangioma). In children, the hepatocellular tumor is sometimes termed a hepatoblastoma because of its cellular similarity to fetal liver and the occasional presence of hematopoiesis.

Hepatomas comprise about 80% of primary hepatic malignancies. Their gross morphology allows separation into 3 classes: a **massive** form, characterized by a single predominant mass which may have small satellite nodules; a **nodular** form, composed of multiple nodules, often distributed throughout the liver; and a **diffuse** variety, characterized by infiltration of tumor throughout the remaining parenchyma.

In 70% of patients, tumor has spread outside the liver when hepatoma is first diagnosed. Metastases are almost invariably present with the nodular or diffuse forms, but 40% of the massive type are confined to the liver. The hilar and celiac lymph nodes are most commonly involved. Metastases to lung and the peritoneal surface also occur frequently. The portal or hepatic veins may be invaded by tumor, and venous occlusion may occur in either case.

Microscopically, there is little stroma between the malignant cells, and the tumor has a soft consistency. The tumor may be highly vascularized, a feature which sometimes produces massive intraperitoneal hemorrhage following spontaneous rupture. Hepatocellular function occurs in some, as indicated by the presence of bile pigment between or in the tumor cells.

Cholangiocarcinomas make up about 15% of hepatic carcinomas. They are usually well-differentiated tumors which spread invasively in the liver substance. Extrahepatic metastases are the rule by the time the tumor is detected.

The mixed tumors resemble hepatomas in their pathologic and clinical behavior.

Postnecrotic or posthepatic cirrhosis is a predisposing factor in about two-thirds of reported cases, although cirrhosis was found in only 15% in a recent large series from the USA. Most pathologists agree that hepatoma does not arise as a complication of alcoholic (nutritional) cirrhosis. Widespread infestation with liver flukes (*Clonorchis sinensis*) is at least partly responsible for the increased incidence of these tumors in the Orient, although other factors may also be important. Certain fungus products called aflatoxins have been shown to be capable of producing liver tumors experimentally. These substances have been detected in ground nuts and grain in some parts of the world where hepatomas are common. Considerable effort is being expended in an effort to clarify this relationship.

Clinical Findings

A. Symptoms and Signs: The clinical diagnosis is usually quite difficult, and until recently the majority of primary hepatic carcinomas were not diagnosed until after death. Abdominal pain and distention are the most common symptoms. The pain can be felt in the epigastrium or right upper quadrant and sometimes is associated with referred pain in the right shoulder. Weight loss is usually present, and jaundice is evident in about one-third of cases.

Hepatomegaly can be detected in 80% of cases, and a mass is palpable in most of the rest. An arterial bruit can be heard over the liver in about 25% of cases and is a useful clue to the diagnosis if acute alcoholic hepatitis can be excluded. The systolic accentuation should enable it to be easily distinguished from the venous collateral hum found in portal hypertension. In a few patients, a friction rub is present over the liver. Ascites or gastrointestinal bleeding from varices is found in about 30%. Blood in ascites is highly suggestive of hepatoma. Intermittent fever is sometimes a prominent presenting feature.

The patterns of clinical presentation are as follows: (1) rapid progression of hepatic neoplasm with pain and hepatomegaly; (2) sudden deterioration of the condition of a cirrhotic due to the appearance of hepatic failure, bleeding varices, or ascites; (3) sudden, massive intraperitoneal hemorrhage; (4) acute illness with fever and abdominal pain; (5) distant metastases; and (6) no specific clinical findings.

B. Laboratory Findings: The serum bilirubin is elevated in one-third of patients. In another 25%, serum alkaline phosphatase is increased but the serum bilirubin is normal. Since many of these patients have cirrhosis, the significance of these alterations is often difficult to assess.

C. Liver Scan: Hepatic scintiscans are abnormal in about 90% of patients.

D. Arteriography: Hepatomas are usually supplied by the hepatic artery, and in 80% of cases selective angiography demonstrates increased tumor vascularity compared with adjacent parenchyma. In about 20%, the picture is diagnostic and consists of multiple tortuous tumor vessels and an intense blush on the hepatogram phase. In some cases, the center of the tumor has become necrotic and only the peripheral areas display the dense tumor blush. Cholangiocarcinomas rarely have a substantial arterial supply and appear less vascular compared with adjacent tissue. Although 10% of metastatic adenocarcinomas show greatly increased vascularity, they do not develop the typical vessel pattern of hepatomas. Some metastatic carcinoids and hepatic hamartomas are extremely vascular, and hemangiomas display a characteristic picture of patchy vascular pooling.

Portal venograms can be obtained by observing the venous phase after splanchnic arterial injections. These may show displacement of intrahepatic portal venous branches or, in some cases, invasion or occlusion of the vein by tumor. If esophageal varices are present, they may also be seen.

E. Special Tests: Alpha-fetoprotein is an a_1 globulin normally present only in the fetal circulation. Recently, alpha-fetoprotein has been found by immunoassay in the serum of patients with primary hepatomas and a few others with testicular tumors. The antigen can be demonstrated in about 50% of Caucasian patients in the USA and in 80% of Africans or Chinese. Although at present there are numerous false-negatives, false-positive tests are rare. Thus, assay for alpha-fetoprotein has great diagnostic value if the test is positive.

F. Liver Biopsy: The diagnosis can be established by percutaneous liver biopsy in most patients if the biopsy site is selected according to the scan. Percutaneous biopsy is safe if clotting factors are normal, and early fears about implantation or dissemination of tumor during the procedure appear to have been unwarranted. The accuracy of biopsy can apparently be increased using the peritoneoscope.

Differential Diagnosis

The clinical picture is usually nonspecific.

Because of weight loss and weakness, liver cancer is most often confused with other abdominal carcinomas. Once hepatomegaly and a filling defect in the liver are found, it must be determined whether the liver harbors a primary neoplasm or metastases. Arteriography, biopsy, and serum alpha-fetoprotein determination supply data to establish the exact diagnosis in most cases. However, it may be difficult to distinguish hepatic malignancy from benign tumors or cysts or, if the patient is febrile, from liver abscess.

When complications develop suddenly in a cirrhotic patient, the possibility of hepatoma must always be considered. Numerous examples have been reported where portacaval shunts were performed for recent variceal hemorrhage in a cirrhotic patient without suspecting that a hepatoma was responsible for the portal hypertension.

In rare instances, primary hepatocellular malignancy is associated with metabolic or endocrine abnormalities such as hypoglycemic attacks, Cushing's syndrome, or virilization.

Complications

Sudden intra-abdominal hemorrhage may occur from spontaneous bleeding. Obstruction of the portal vein may produce portal hypertension, and obstruction of the hepatic veins may produce the Budd-Chiari syndrome. Liver failure is a common cause of death.

Treatment

Surgical resection is the only treatment which offers a possibility of cure. Partial hepatectomy should be considered if the tumor is localized and would be encompassed by the proposed resection. Extension of tumor into the opposite lobe or involvement of the vena cava or hepatic veins of the opposite lobe eliminates the possibility of curative resection. Cirrhosis should be considered a relative contraindication because the limited functional reserve of the diseased parenchyma greatly increases the risk of postoperative liver failure. About 75% of patients with hepatic tumors are unsuitable for resection for these reasons.

Palliation can be obtained in certain cases by selective hepatic arterial infusion of chemotherapeutic agents. Fluorouracil and methotrexate have given the best results.

Ligation of the hepatic artery has been used as treatment for hepatomas since the artery serves as the principal source of blood supply. The goal of this approach is to bring about selective ischemic necrosis of tumor. Palliation has occasionally resulted from this treatment, but residual tumor continues to multiply until the patient succumbs.

Arterial ligation and local chemotherapy have been used in combination. The hepatic artery is divided and a perfusion catheter inserted into the distal end for administration of antineoplastic drugs.

Prognosis

Despite the development in the past decade of newer technics which have permitted earlier diagnosis, there has been no appreciable improvement in survival. The average life expectancy after diagnosis is about 6 months. The patients generally die from the effects of the expanding hepatic neoplasm rather than from metastases. Fewer than 100 five-year survivors have been reported following partial hepatectomy. Several patients have survived for 2–3 years following selective perfusion of antitumor agents through the hepatic artery.

Liver transplantation could become a successful method of treatment if the problems discussed in Chapter 51 can be solved.

Alpert E & others: α-Fetoprotein in human hepatoma. Gastroenterology 61:137–143, 1971.

Curutchet HP & others: Primary liver cancer. Surgery 70:467–479, 1971.

El-Domeiri AA & others: Primary malignant tumors of the liver. Cancer 27:7–11, 1971.

Fortner JG & others: Surgery in liver tumors. Curr Probl Surg, June 1972.

Kew MC & others: Diagnosis of primary cancer of the liver. Brit MJ 4:408–411, 1971.

Lin TY: The results of hepatic lobectomy for primary carcinoma of the liver. Surg Gynec Obst 123:289–294, 1966.

Malt RA & others: Manifestations and prognosis of carcinoma of the liver. Surg Gynec Obst 135:361–364, 1972.

Rochlin DB, Smart CR: An evaluation of 51 patients with hepatic artery infusion. Surg Gynec Obst 123:535–538, 1966.

Sharpstone P & others: The diagnosis of primary malignant tumors of the liver. Quart J Med 41:99–110, 1972.

Suzuki T & others: Study of vascularity of tumors of the liver. Surg Gynec Obst 134:27–34, 1972.

METASTATIC NEOPLASMS OF THE LIVER

Metastatic malignancy is 20 times more common than primary tumors in the liver. Cancers of the breast, lung, pancreas, stomach, large intestine, kidney, ovary, and uterus account for about 75% of cases. Spread to the liver may be via the systemic circulation, portal vein, or, less often, the lymphatics. Interestingly, the cirrhotic liver, which often gives rise to primary hepatic tumors, is less susceptible than normal liver to implantation of metastases.

Over 90% of patients with hepatic metastases have tumor implants in other organs. The lung is most commonly involved and contains tumor in 30% of cases. It may be useful for the surgeon to appreciate that 10% of patients with hepatic metastases have gross tumor deposits demonstrable on hepatic section which cannot be seen or felt from the surface of the liver during laparotomy.

Weight loss, fatigue, and anorexia are the presenting general complaints. Right upper abdominal pain, ascites, and jaundice are the usual symptoms referable to the liver. The pain may radiate around the costal margin or straight through to the back. Fever without demonstrable infection is present in 15–20% of cases and bears only a loose relationship to leukocytosis.

In about two-thirds of cases, physical examination reveals hepatomegaly or a palpable metastatic tumor in the upper abdomen. Either may be tender to palpation. If portal hypertension is present, it may be manifested by abdominal venous collaterals or splenomegaly. A friction rub is sometimes heard and is always highly suggestive of hepatic tumor.

Laboratory investigation reveals a hematocrit between 30–36%. The serum bilirubin is elevated in almost half of patients, and half of these have values over 4 mg/100 ml. Sulfobromophthalein (BSP) retention is abnormal in most patients, and the alkaline phosphatase is also usually increased.

The diagnosis can be established by percutaneous liver biopsy in most cases if the hepatic scan is used to direct the site of the biopsy. Selective hepatic angiography may be diagnostic in puzzling cases. Metastatic lesions are principally supplied by the hepatic artery but on angiograms are usually shown to be less vascular than hepatomas.

Little effective treatment is available for the average patient. Partial hepatic resection may be justified for solitary metastases if there are no signs of tumor elsewhere. Partial hepatectomy is also sometimes worthwhile to extirpate a tumor invading directly from a contiguous organ.

Systemic chemotherapy does not improve survival. Recent attempts at palliation have concentrated on delivery of high levels of chemotherapeutic agents by infusion directly into the hepatic artery or portal vein. Hepatic artery ligation has also benefited some by causing necrosis of the bulk of the tumor mass.

Without treatment, the median survival time after detection of hepatic metastases is 75 days. Only 5% are alive after 2 years. Survival is slightly longer in patients with metastases from colonic cancer than in patients with metastases from pancreatic or gastric tumors.

Fenster LF, Klatskin G: Manifestations of metastatic tumors of the liver. Am J Med 31:238–248, 1961.

Foster JH: Survival after liver resection for cancer. Cancer 26:493–502, 1970.

Jaffe BM & others: Factors influencing survival in patients with untreated hepatic metastases. Surg Gynec Obst 127:1–11, 1968.

Mansfield CM & others: The influence of treatment on the survival of patients with hepatic metastases diagnosed by liver scanning. Am J Roentgenol 109:749–754, 1970.

Massey WH & others: Hepatic artery infusion for metastatic malignancy using percutaneously placed catheters. Am J Surg 121:160–164, 1971.

Murray-Lyon IM & others: Treatment of secondary hepatic tumors by ligation of hepatic artery and infusion of cytotoxic drugs. Lancet 2:172–175, 1970.

Rapoport AH, Burleson RL: Survival of patients treated with systemic fluorouracil for hepatic metastases. Surg Gynec Obst 130:773–777, 1970.

Watkins E Jr & others: Surgical basis for arterial infusion chemotherapy of disseminated carcinoma of the liver. Surg Gynec Obst 130:581–605, 1970.

BENIGN TUMORS & CYSTS OF THE LIVER*

Hemangiomas

Hemangioma is the most common of the benign hepatic tumors, and—except for the skin and mucous membranes—the liver is the most common location for hemangiomas. Females are affected more often than males in a ratio of 6:1. Histologically, hepatic hemangiomas are of the cavernous type. Most are small solitary subcapsular growths which are found incidentally during laparotomy or at autopsy. Those greater than 4 cm in diameter may cause abdominal pain or a palpable mass. Some patients have presented with hemorrhagic shock resulting from spontaneous rupture. Large congenital hemangiomas of the liver may be associated with others in the skin. Occasionally, a hemangioma may behave as an arteriovenous fistula and produce cardiac hypertrophy and congestive heart failure. Selective hepatic arteriography reveals a vascular tumor containing spaces which trap the contrast media longer than surrounding parenchyma.

Symptomatic hemangiomas should be excised. If discovered as an incidental finding during laparotomy, a hemangioma should not be biopsied or removed because difficulties with hemostasis can be extreme. Radiotherapy has been effective in limiting enlargement of unresectable tumors. Patients with congestive failure due to arteriovenous fistula have been helped by ligation of the hepatic artery.

Adenomas

Hepatic adenomas are benign tumors of well-differentiated hepatocytes contained in a circumscribed mass without lobular organization. They are found principally in women. Most are asymptomatic and are never recognized during life. Large adenomas may produce an abdominal mass and sometimes cause pain by hemorrhagic infarction. It may be difficult histologically to distinguish this tumor from a well-differentiated hepatoma.

Adenomas that produce symptoms should be resected.

Focal Nodular Hyperplasia

This lesion appears as nodules of hepatocytes surrounding an irregular accumulation of fibrous stroma and ductular endothelium. It is interrupted by fibrous septa which create a pseudolobular appearance. Whether focal nodular hyperplasia should be considered premalignant is now under debate.

Hamartomas

These are collections of hepatic cells, ductular elements, and multiple small epithelium-lined cysts. The symptomatic examples are usually discovered as abdominal masses in infancy.

*Echinococcal cysts are discussed in Chapter 10.

Cysts

Hepatic cysts are usually solitary unilocular anomalies which produce no symptoms. The occasional large cyst may present as an upper abdominal mass or discomfort. Polycystic liver disease is associated in about half of cases with polycystic renal disease. It is probably a variant of the disease called congenital hepatic fibrosis.

Large symptomatic cysts may be surgically drained. The possibility of echinococcosis (see Chapter 10) should always be ruled out by performing serologic studies before operation. Multiple cysts do not usually require treatment, but several cases have been managed by surgically creating windows between the large cysts and allowing drainage into the abdominal cavity.

Adam YG & others: Giant hemangiomas of the liver. Ann Surg 172:239–245, 1970.

Clark DD & others: Solitary hepatic cysts. Surgery 61:687–693, 1967.

Lin TY & others: Treatment of non-parasitic cystic disease of the liver: A new approach to therapy with polycystic liver. Ann Surg 168:921–927, 1968.

Longmire WP Jr: Hepatic surgery: Trauma, tumors, and cysts. Ann Surg 161:1–14, 1965.

Malt RA & others: Experience with benign tumors of the liver. Surg Gynec Obst 130:285–291, 1970.

Motsay GJ, Gamble WG: Clinical experience with hepatic adenomas. Surg Gynec Obst 134:415–418, 1972.

Park WC, Phillips R: The role of radiation therapy in the management of hemangiomas of the liver. JAMA 212:1496–1498, 1970.

Rake MO & others: Ligation of the hepatic artery in the treatment of heart failure due to hepatic haemangiomatosis. Gut 11:512–515, 1970.

Sewell JH, Weiss K: Spontaneous rupture of hemangioma of the liver. Arch Surg 83:105–109, 1961.

Shah JP & others: Hamartomas of the liver. Surgery 68:778–782, 1970.

HEPATIC ABSCESS

Hepatic abscesses may be bacterial, parasitic, or fungal in origin. In the USA, pyogenic abscesses are the most common, and amebic abscesses (see Chapter 10) are next most common. Unless otherwise specified, the following remarks refer to bacterial abscesses.

Cases are about evenly divided between those with a single abscess and those with many abscesses. Solitary abscesses affect the right lobe 5 times more commonly than the left and are particularly prone to develop in patients with diabetes mellitus. Multiple abscesses are usually distributed throughout both lobes. Therapy is usually successful for a solitary abscess which is diagnosed early and treated, whereas multiple abscesses are often incurable. Many of the latter are terminal manifestations of untreatable hepatobiliary malignancy.

In most cases, the development of a hepatic abscess follows a suppurative process elsewhere in the body. Many are due to direct spread from biliary infections such as empyema of the gallbladder or protracted cholangitis. Abdominal infections such as appendicitis or diverticulitis may spread through the portal vein to involve the liver with abscess formation. Other cases develop after generalized sepsis from bacterial endocarditis, renal infection, or pneumonitis. In 10–15% of cases, no antecedent infection can be documented ("cryptogenic" abscesses). Other rare causes include secondary bacterial infection of an amebic abscess, hydatid cyst, or congenital hepatic cyst.

In some patients, the hepatic abscess presents as an extension of an active infection; in others, months or even years may elapse between resolution of the original sepsis and the infection in the liver. Detection of the liver abscess is usually not difficult in the former, but when the primary disease and the abscess are temporally separated there is often considerable delay in diagnosis.

Clinical Findings

A. Symptoms and Signs: When liver abscess develops in the course of another intra-abdominal infection such as diverticulitis, it is accompanied by increasing toxicity, higher fever, jaundice, and a generally deteriorating clinical picture. Right upper quadrant pain may appear.

In other cases, the diagnosis is much less obvious since the illness develops insidiously in a previously healthy person. In these, the first symptoms are usually malaise and fatigue, followed after several weeks by fever. Epigastric or right upper quadrant pain is present in about half of cases. The pain may be aggravated by motion or may be referred to the right shoulder.

The course of fever is often erratic, and spikes to 40–41 C (104–105.8 F) are common. Chills are present in about 25% of cases. The liver is usually enlarged and may be tender to palpation. If tenderness is severe, the condition may be confused with cholecystitis.

Jaundice is unusual in solitary abscesses unless the patient's condition is seriously worsening. It is often present in patients with multiple abscesses and in general is a bad prognostic sign.

B. Laboratory Findings: Leukocytosis is present in most cases and is usually over 15,000/μl. A small group of patients—containing some of the most seriously ill—fail to develop leukocytosis. Anemia is present in most patients. The average hematocrit is 33%.

The serum bilirubin is usually normal except in patients with multiple abscesses or when hepatic failure has supervened. The alkaline phosphatase is often elevated even in the presence of a normal bilirubin—a pattern characteristic of segmental obstruction of the bile ducts.

C. X-Ray Findings: X-ray changes are present in the right lung in about one-third of cases and consist of basilar atelectasis or pleural effusion. The right diaphragm may be elevated and less mobile than the left.

Plain films of the abdomen are usually normal or show only hepatomegaly. In a few patients, an air-fluid level in the region of the liver reveals the presence and location of the abscess. Distortion of the contour of the stomach on upper gastrointestinal series may be seen with large abscesses involving the left lobe.

Intravenous cholangiograms and oral cholecystograms fail to outline the bile ducts and are of no diagnostic value.

Selective hepatic arteriography may add valuable supplemental information to that obtained from the scan. Abscesses smaller than the 3 cm limit of the scan may sometimes be shown. Avascularity of the defect points toward abscess rather than tumor except in the rare case where there has been extensive necrosis within the tumor.

D. Liver Scan: In the past decade, the radioactive liver scan has contributed greatly to increased diagnostic accuracy of hepatic abscesses. If several views are obtained, the site and size of a solitary abscess can be clearly established. Multiple small abscesses are usually impossible to diagnose.

Ultrasonic scans (presently under development) may simplify the differentiation of abscess from tumor.

Differential Diagnosis

In many cases, the early findings may be so vague that hepatic abscess is not even considered. The multiple other causes of malaise, weight loss, and anemia would enter into the differential diagnosis. When spiking fevers appear, the physician must consider all the causes of fever of unknown origin. Failure to entertain the possibility of hepatic abscess and to obtain the necessary hepatic scans and arteriograms leads to most errors in diagnosis. Many patients are not diagnosed until exploratory laparotomy is performed for fever and abdominal pain. Abdominal lymphoma is a common preoperative diagnosis in these cases.

After the hepatic scan has revealed an abscess, the infectious agent—amebic or bacterial—must be determined. If blood cultures are positive, a pyogenic cause can be inferred, but it is often impossible to differentiate between amebic and bacterial abscesses until after treatment has been instituted for both possibilities. Positive serologic tests would verify amebiasis, but the results may not be available for several weeks. Whenever there is doubt, the patient should receive both metronidazole for amebiasis and antibiotics for bacterial infection.

Complications

Complications result either from further dissemination of infection or from progressive impairment of liver function. Intrahepatic spread of infection may create multiple additional abscesses and is responsible for some failures after surgical treatment of an apparently solitary abscess. As the untreated abscess expands, rupture may occur into the pleural or peritoneal cavity, usually with catastrophic results. Septicemia and septic shock are common terminal complications of diffuse hepatic infection. Hepatic failure may develop in addition to uncontrolled sepsis or it may predominate over signs of infection.

Hemobilia may follow bleeding from the vascular wall into the abscess cavity. In this case, drainage of the abscess may be inadequate treatment, and lobectomy may be required to control bleeding.

Treatment

After blood cultures have been obtained, parenteral antibiotics should be administered in high doses. If the bacteria and its sensitivities have been identified, the choice of drug should be made on that basis. In the absence of such information, antibiotics should be selected according to the presumptive source of the infection. In most cases, the organism is of enteric origin. *Escherichia coli,* bacteroides, and anaerobic streptococci are most frequently recovered. Gram-positive cocci, staphylococci, or hemolytic streptococci are usually recovered if the primary infection was bacterial endocarditis or pneumonitis.

If the possibility of amebic abscess cannot be excluded, the patient should be treated with metronidazole until more definitive information becomes available. (See Chapter 10 for details of the treatment regimen for amebiasis.)

Pyogenic abscesses must be surgically drained since nonoperative management is almost uniformly fatal. Abscesses which clearly occupy the dependent posterior superior segment of the right lobe can be drained extraperitoneally through the bed of the 12th rib. In most cases, however, drainage can be more satisfactorily achieved at laparotomy. This allows inspection of the liver for possible additional undisclosed abscesses and permits preliminary exploration of other areas of the abdomen before drainage. The results of treatment in recent years suggest that it is not of major importance to establish drainage extraperitoneally as was once thought.

The contents of the abscess should be initially evacuated using a large needle or trocar attached to a suction device. Care should be taken to avoid spilling pus into the abdomen. Samples should be sent for culture and sensitivity tests and investigation for amebas. Surprisingly, some apparently pyogenic abscesses give no growth when the contents are cultured. After the cavity is emptied, an incision is made into the abscess and a large sump drain inserted which is brought out through the abdominal wall. Additional soft rubber drains should be placed in the subhepatic region. Postoperatively, the sump is left in place until the cavity begins to shrink around the tube, after which it is gradually withdrawn.

Several groups have reported that pyogenic abscesses may be definitively treated by percutaneous needle aspiration combined with specific antibiotics, but this approach has received insufficient evaluation to permit a judgment about whether it would be as successful as open drainage in the average case.

In most cases, multiple abscesses cannot be drained satisfactorily. Rarely, multiple abscesses are confined to a single lobe and can be cured by lobectomy. It has been suggested that administration of high concentrations of antibiotics through the umbilical vein may be more effective for multiple abscesses than antibiotic infusion into a peripheral vein. In any event, biliary obstruction or other causes of the sepsis must also be corrected if there is to be any hope for cure.

Prognosis

The overall mortality rate is about 40% and is related to 2 problems: delay in diagnosis of solitary abscesses and multiple abscesses for which there is no effective treatment. The appearance of jaundice and a falling serum albumin are both bad prognostic signs. Prompt diagnosis and treatment of a solitary abscess is associated with a mortality rate of about 10%.

Altemeier WA & others: Abscesses of the liver: Surgical considerations. Arch Surg 101:258–266, 1970.

Butler TJ, McCarthy CF: Pyogenic liver abscess. Gut 10:389–399, 1969.

Holt JM, Spry CJF: Solitary pyogenic liver abscess in patients with diabetes mellitus. Lancet 2:198–200, 1966.

McFadzean AJS & others: Solitary pyogenic abscess of the liver treated by closed aspiration and antibiotics. Brit J Surg 41:141–162, 1953/1954.

Pai ST, Bakk YW: Radioisotope scanning in the diagnosis of liver abscess. Am J Surg 119:330–333, 1970.

Warren KW, Hardy KJ: Pyogenic hepatic abscess. Arch Surg 97:40–45, 1968.

•   •   •

General References

Sandblom P: *Hemobilia.* Thomas, 1972.

Schiff L (editor): *Diseases of the Liver,* 3rd ed. Lippincott, 1969.

Schwartz SI: *Surgical Diseases of the Liver.* McGraw-Hill, 1964.

27 . . .

The Biliary Tract

Lawrence W. Way, MD, & J. Englebert Dunphy, MD

EMBRYOLOGY & ANATOMY

The anlage of the biliary ducts and liver consists of a diverticulum which appears on the ventral aspect of the foregut in 3 mm embryos (Fig 27–1). The cranial portion becomes the liver; a caudal bud forms the ventral pancreas; and an intermediate bud develops into the gallbladder. Originally hollow, the hepatic diverticulum becomes a solid mass of cells which later recanalizes to form the ducts. The smallest ducts—the bile canaliculi—are first seen as a basal network between the primitive hepatocytes which eventually expands throughout the liver. Numerous microvilli increase the canalicular surface area. Bile secreted here passes through the interolobular ductules (canals of Hering) and the lobar ducts and then into the hepatic duct in the hilum. In most cases, the common hepatic duct is formed by the union of a single right and left duct, but in 25% of individuals the anterior and posterior divisions of the right duct join the left duct separately. The origin of the common hepatic duct is close to the liver but always outside its substance. It runs about 4 cm before joining the cystic duct to form the common bile duct. The common duct begins in the hepatoduodenal ligament, passes behind the first portion of the duodenum, and runs in a groove on the posterior surface of the pancreas before entering the duodenum. Its terminal 1 cm is intimately adherent to the duodenal wall. The total length of the common duct is about 9 cm (3½ inches).

In 80–90% of individuals, the main pancreatic duct joins the common duct to form a common channel about 1 cm long. The intraduodenal segment of the duct is called the hepatopancreatic ampulla or ampulla of Vater—somewhat of a misnomer since the lumen is

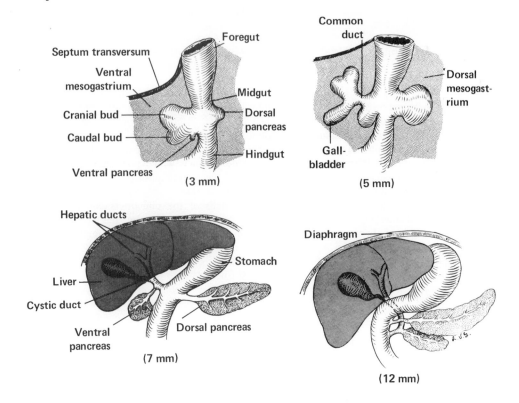

FIG 27–1. Embryonic development of the bile ducts and liver.

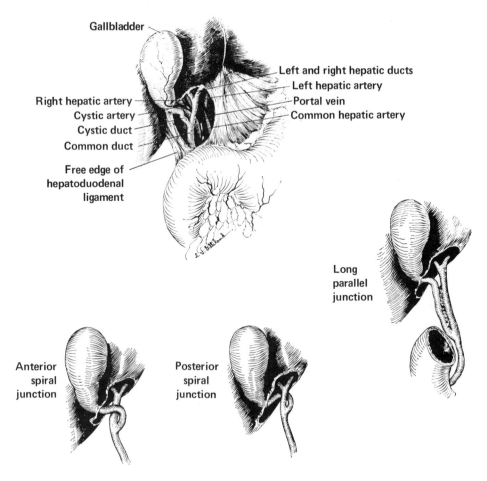

FIG 27–2. **Anatomy of gallbladder and variations in anatomy of the cystic duct.**

not wider here.

The gallbladder is a pear-shaped organ adherent to the undersurface of the liver in a groove separating the right and left lobes. The fundus projects 1–2 cm below the hepatic edge and can usually be palpated when the cystic or common duct is obstructed. It rarely has a complete peritoneal covering, but when this variation does occur it predisposes to infarction by torsion. The gallbladder holds about 50 ml of bile when fully distended. The neck of the gallbladder tapers into the narrow cystic duct which connects with the common duct. The lumen of the cystic duct contains a thin mucosal septum, the spiral valve of Heister, which offers mild resistance to bile flow. In 75% of persons, the cystic duct enters the common duct at an angle. In the remainder, it runs parallel to the hepatic duct or winds around it before joining. (Fig 27–2.)

In the hepatoduodenal ligament, the hepatic artery is to the left of the common duct and the portal vein is posterior and medial. The right hepatic artery usually passes behind the hepatic duct and then gives off the cystic artery before entering the right lobe of the liver, but variations are common.

The mucosa of the bile ducts varies from cuboidal

in the ductules to columnar in the main ducts. The gallbladder mucosa is thrown into prominent ridges when the organ is collapsed, and these flatten during distention. The tall columnar cells of the gallbladder mucosa are covered by microvilli on their luminal surface. Wide channels which play an important role in water and electrolyte absorption separate the individual cells.

The walls of the bile ducts contain only small amounts of smooth muscle, but the termination of the common duct is enveloped by a complex sphincteric muscle. The gallbladder musculature is composed of interdigitated bundles of longitudinal and spirally arranged fibers.

The biliary tree receives parasympathetic and sympathetic innervation. The former contains motor fibers to the gallbladder and secretory fibers to the ductal epithelium. The afferent fibers in the sympathetic nerves mediate the pain of biliary colic.

Kune GA: The influence of structure and function in the surgery of the biliary tract. Ann Roy Coll Surg Engl 47:78–91, 1970.

Kune GA: Surgical anatomy of the common bile duct. Arch Surg 89:995–1004, 1964.

Lindner HH, Green RB: Embryology and surgical anatomy of the extrahepatic biliary tract. S Clin North America 44:1273–1285, 1964.

PHYSIOLOGY

Bile Flow

Bile is produced at a rate of 500–1500 ml/day by secretory mechanisms in the hepatocytes and the cells of the ducts. Active secretion of bile salts into the biliary canaliculus is responsible for most of the volume of bile and its fluctuations. Na^+ and water follow passively to establish isosmolality and electrical neutrality. Lecithin and cholesterol (Fig 27–8) enter the canaliculus at rates which correlate with variations in bile salt output. It has been suggested that the coupling is due to extraction of the 2 lipids by the bile salts as they pass through the microvillous membrane. Bilirubin and a number of other organic anions—estrogens, sulfobromophthalein, etc—are actively secreted by the hepatocyte by a different transport system from that which handles bile salts.

The columnar cells of the ducts add a fluid rich in HCO_3^- to that produced in the canaliculus. This involves active secretion of Na^+ and HCO_3^- by a cellular pump which is stimulated by secretin, gastrin, and cholecystokinin. K^+ and water are distributed passively across the ducts. (Fig 27–3.)

Between meals, bile is stored in the gallbladder, where it may be concentrated at rates up to 20% per hour. Na^+ and either HCO_3^- or Cl^- are actively transported from its lumen during absorption. The changes in composition brought about by concentration are shown in Fig 27–4.

Three factors regulate bile flow: hepatic secretion, gallbladder contraction, and choledochal sphincteric resistance. When fasting, pressure in the common bile duct is 5–10 cm water and bile produced in the liver is diverted into the gallbladder. After eating, the gallbladder contracts, the sphincter relaxes, and bile is forced into the duodenum in squirts as ductal pressure intermittently exceeds sphincteric resistance. During contraction, pressure within the gallbladder reaches 25 cm water and that in the common bile duct 15–20 cm water.

Cholecystokinin-pancreozymin (CCK) is the major physiologic stimulus for gallbladder contraction and relaxation of the sphincter, but vagal impulses facilitate its action. The hormone is released into the blood stream from the mucosa of the small bowel by fat or lipolytic products in the lumen. Amino acids and small polypeptides are weaker stimuli, and carbohydrates are ineffective. Bile flow during a meal is augmented by increased turnover of bile salts in the enterohepatic circulation and stimulation of ductal secretion by secretin, gastrin, and CCK.

Bile Salts & the Enterohepatic Circulation (Fig 27–5.)

Bile salts are steroid molecules formed by hepatocytes from cholesterol. The rate of synthesis is under feedback control and can be increased a maximum of about 10-fold. Two **primary** bile salts—cholate and chenodeoxycholate—are produced by the liver cells. Before excretion into bile, they are conjugated with either glycine or taurine to enhance water solubility. Intestinal bacteria may alter these compounds to produce the **secondary** bile salts, deoxycholate and lithocholate. The former is reabsorbed and enters bile, but lithocholate is insoluble and is excreted in the stool. Bile is composed of 40% cholate, 40% chenodeoxycholate, and 20% deoxycholate, conjugated with glycine or taurine in a ratio of 3:1.

The principal function of bile salts in the intestine is to solubilize lipids and lipolytic products and facilitate their absorption. Bile salts are detergents: molecules with water-soluble and fat-soluble groups at opposite poles. In an aqueous solution they spontaneously aggregate in groups called micelles, composed of 8–10 molecules. The molecules in the micelle are arranged with the hydrophobic poles in the center and the hydrophilic groups on the surface facing the water. Micelles can solubilize lipids within their hydrophobic centers and still remain in aqueous solution.

Lecithin and cholesterol, the other major solids, are transported in bile within the micelles. Lecithin is a polar phospholipid which is incapable itself of forming micelles and is only slightly soluble in water. However, when incorporated into bile salt micelles, it expands the hydrocarbon center of the micelles and enhances their capacity to solubilize nonpolar lipids such as cholesterol.

Bile salts, lecithin, and cholesterol comprise about 90% of the solids in bile, the remainder consisting of bilirubin, fatty acids, and inorganic salts. Gallbladder bile contains about 10% solids and has a bile salt concentration between 200–300 mM/liter (Fig 27–4).

Bile salts remain in the intestinal lumen throughout the jejunum, where they participate in fat absorption. Upon reaching the distal small bowel, they are reabsorbed by an active transport system located in the terminal 200 cm of ileum. Over 95% of bile salts arriving from the jejunum are transferred by this process into portal vein blood; the remainder enter the colon, where they are converted to secondary bile salts. The entire bile salt pool of 2.5–4 g circulates twice through the enterohepatic circulation during each meal, and 6–8 cycles are made each day. The normal daily loss of bile salts in the stool amounts to 10–20% of the pool and is restored by hepatic synthesis.

Carey MC, Small DM: Micelle formation by bile salts. Arch Int Med 130:506–527, 1972.

Dowling RH: The enterohepatic circulation. Gastroenterology 62:122–140, 1972.

Hallenbeck GA: Biliary and pancreatic intraductal pressures. Chap 57, pp 1007–1025 in: *Handbook of Physiology.* Vol 2: *Secretion.* American Physiological Society, 1967.

Wheeler HO: Water and electrolytes in bile. Chap 113, pp 2409–2431 in: *Handbook of Physiology.* Vol 5: *Bile, Digestion, Ruminal Physiology.* American Physiological Society, 1968.

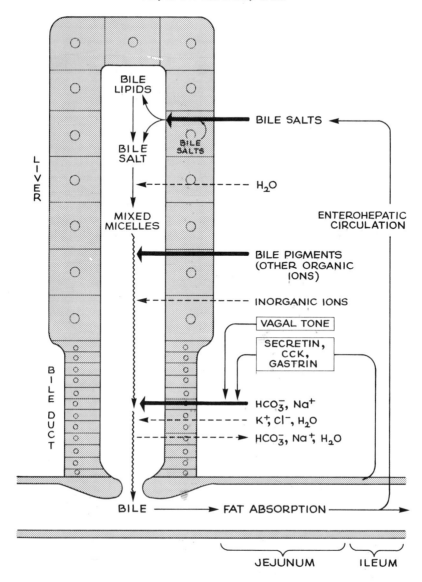

FIG 27–3. Bile formation. Solid lines into the ductular lumen indicate active transport; dotted lines represent passive diffusion.

Wheeler HO: Concentrating function of the gallbladder. Am J Med 51:588–595, 1971.

Bilirubin

About 250–300 mg of bilirubin are excreted each day in the bile, most of it from breakdown of red cells in the reticuloendothelial system. First, heme is liberated from hemoglobin, and the iron and globin are removed for reuse by the organism. Biliverdin, the first pigment formed from heme, is reduced to unconjugated bilirubin, the indirect-reacting bilirubin of the van den Bergh test. Unconjugated bilirubin is insoluble in water and is transported in plasma bound to albumin.

Bilirubin is extracted from blood by the liver cells and after entering the cytoplasm is bound to one of 2 molecules, the Y and Z proteins, for which it and several other organic anions have high affinity. Unconjugated bilirubin is then conjugated with glucuronic acid to form bilirubin diglucuronide, the water-soluble, direct bilirubin. Conjugation is catalyzed by glucuronyl transferase, an enzyme on the endoplasmic reticulum. Bilirubin diglucuronide is actively transported into the biliary canaliculus by a mechanism shared by several organic anions but separate from that responsible for excretion of bile salts.

After entering the intestine, bilirubin is reduced by intestinal bacteria to several compounds known as urobilinogens which are subsequently oxidized and converted to pigmented urobilins. The term urobilino-

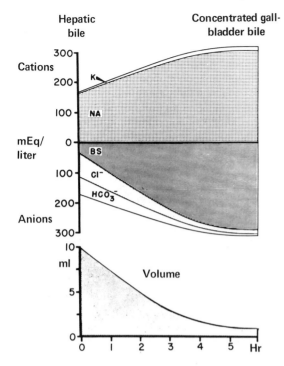

FIG 27–4. **Changes in gallbladder bile composition with time.** (Courtesy of J. Dietschy.)

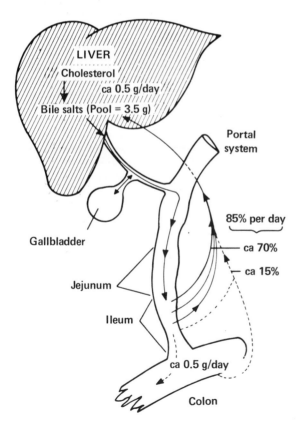

FIG 27–5. **Enterohepatic circulation of bile salts.** (Courtesy of M. Tyor.)

gen is often used to refer to both urobilins and urobilinogens.

About 300 mg of bilirubin enter the gut each day, but daily fecal urobilinogen amounts to only 200 mg. The discrepancy between bilirubin input and urobilinogen excretion has not yet been accounted for. About 1% of the intestinal pigment load is reabsorbed as urobilinogen and enters the enterohepatic circulation. The small amount of urobilinogen in the portal blood which escapes extraction and reexcretion in the bile is disposed of in the urine.

Fleischner G, Arias IM: Recent advances in bilirubin formation, transport, metabolism and excretion. Am J Med 49:576–589, 1970.
Schmid R: Bilirubin metabolism in man. New England J Med 287:703–709, 1972.

JAUNDICE

Jaundice can be categorized as prehepatic, hepatic, or posthepatic based upon the site of the underlying disease. Hemolysis is the most common form of prehepatic jaundice and is due to increased production of bilirubin. Less common prehepatic examples are Gilbert's disease and the Crigler-Najjar syndrome.

Hepatic parenchymal jaundice is subdivided into hepatocellular and cholestatic varieties. The former includes acute viral hepatitis and chronic alcoholic cirrhosis. Some cases of intrahepatic cholestasis may be indistinguishable clinically and biochemically from cholestasis due to common duct obstruction. Primary biliary cirrhosis, toxic drug jaundice, cholestatic jaundice of pregnancy, and postoperative cholestatic jaundice are the most commonly seen forms.

Extrahepatic jaundice most often results from biliary obstruction by a malignant tumor, choledocholithiasis, or biliary stricture. Pancreatic pseudocyst, sclerosing cholangitis, metastatic malignancy, and duodenal diverticulitis are less common causes.

History

The age, sex, and parity of the patient and possible deleterious habits should be noted. Most cases of infectious hepatitis occur in patients under 30 years. A history of drug addiction may suggest serum hepatitis transmitted by shared hypodermic equipment. Chronic alcoholism can usually be documented in patients with cirrhosis, and acute jaundice in alcoholics usually follows a recent binge. Obstructing gallstones or tumors are more common in older people.

Patients with jaundice due to choledocholithiasis may have associated biliary colic, fever, and chills and may report previous similar attacks. The pain in malignant obstruction is deep-seated and dull and may be affected by changes in position. Pain in the region of the liver is frequently experienced in the early stages of viral hepatitis and acute alcoholic liver injury. The patient with extrahepatic obstruction may report that his stools have become lighter in color and his urine dark.

Cholestatic diseases are often accompanied by **pruritus**—a symptom that may overshadow all others in the discomfort it causes. Pruritus may precede jaundice, but usually they appear at about the same time. The itching is most severe on the extremities and is aggravated by warm, humid weather. It is caused by an excess of bile salts in the system and correlates fairly well with amounts that can be recovered from the surface of the skin. Cholestyramine (Cuemid, Questran), an anion exchange resin, may provide dramatic symptomatic relief by binding bile salts in the intestinal lumen and preventing their reabsorption.

Physical Examination

Hepatomegaly is common in both hepatic and posthepatic jaundice. In some cases, palpation of the liver may suggest cirrhosis or metastatic malignancy, but impressions of this sort tend to be unreliable. Secondary stigmas of cirrhosis usually accompany acute alcoholic jaundice: liver palms, spider angiomas, ascites, collateral veins on the abdominal walls, and splenomegaly suggest cirrhosis. A nontender, palpable gallbladder in a jaundiced patient strongly suggests malignant obstruction of the common duct (Courvoisier's law), but absence of a palpable gallbladder is of little significance in ruling out malignancy.

Laboratory Tests

In hemolytic disease, the increased bilirubin is principally in the unconjugated indirect fraction. Since unconjugated bilirubin is insoluble in water, the jaundice in hemolysis is acholuric. The total bilirubin in hemolysis rarely exceeds 4–5 mg/100 ml because the rate of excretion increases as the total bilirubin rises and a plateau is quickly reached. Greater values suggest concomitant hepatic parenchymal disease.

Jaundice due to hepatic parenchymal disease is characterized by elevations of both conjugated and unconjugated serum bilirubin. An increase in the conjugated fraction always signifies disease within the hepatobiliary system. The direct bilirubin predominates in about half of cases of hepatic parenchymal disease.

Both intrahepatic cholestasis and extrahepatic obstruction raise the direct bilirubin, although the indirect fraction also increases somewhat. Since direct bilirubin is water-soluble, bilirubinuria develops. With complete extrahepatic obstruction, the total bilirubin rises to a plateau of 25–30 mg/100 ml, at which point loss in the urine equals the additional daily production. Higher values suggest concomitant hemolysis or decreased renal function. Obstruction of a single hepatic duct does not usually cause jaundice.

In malignant extrahepatic obstruction, the serum bilirubin is about 20 mg/100 ml, and these patients display the highest average concentrations. Obstructive

jaundice due to common duct stones often produces transient bilirubin increases in the range of 2–4 mg/100 ml, and the level rarely goes over 15 mg/100 ml. Serum bilirubin values in patients with alcoholic cirrhosis and acute viral hepatitis vary widely in relation to the severity of the parenchymal damage. Hemolysis generally increases fecal urobilinogen, and complete extrahepatic biliary obstruction reduces both fecal and urinary urobilinogen. In the presence of hepatocellular jaundice, urobilinogen reabsorbed from the intestine is poorly excreted by the diseased liver, and urinary output rises.

Fig 27–6 depicts the range of serum SGOT determinations in a variety of conditions associated with jaundice. In extrahepatic obstruction, modest rises are common, but SGOT levels as high as 1000 units have been seen (though rarely) in patients with common duct stones. In the latter patients, the high value lasted for only a few days and was associated with 10-fold increases in LDH concentrations.

Serum alkaline phosphatase comes from 3 sites: liver, bone, and intestine. In normal subjects, liver and bone contribute about equally, and the intestinal contribution is small. Hepatic alkaline phosphatase is a product of the epithelial cells of the cholangioles, and increased alkaline phosphatase associated with liver disease is the result of increased enzyme production. Alkaline phosphatase levels go up with intrahepatic cholestasis, cholangitis, or extrahepatic obstruction. Since the elevation is from overproduction, it may occur with focal hepatic lesions in the absence of jaundice. For example, a solitary hepatic metastasis or pyogenic abscess in one lobe may fail to obstruct enough to cause jaundice but usually is associated with an increased alkaline phosphatase. In cholangitis with incomplete extrahepatic obstruction, serum bilirubin may be normal or mildly elevated but serum alkaline phosphatase may be very high.

Bone disease may complicate the interpretation of abnormal alkaline phosphatase levels (Fig 27–7). If one suspects that the increased serum enzyme may be from bone, serum calcium and phosphorus and a 5'-nucleotidase or leucine aminopeptidase level should be determined. These enzymes are also produced by cholangioles and are elevated in cholestasis, but their

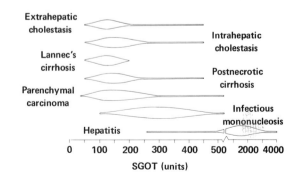

FIG 27–6. Range of SGOT values in various hepatobiliary disorders.

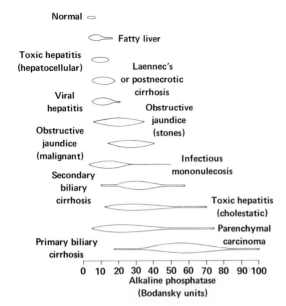

Normal ⊂

Fatty liver

Toxic hepatitis
(hepatocellular)

Laennec's
or postnecrotic
cirrhosis

Viral
hepatitis

Obstructive
jaundice
(stones)

Obstructive
jaundice
(malignant)

Infectious
mononucleosis

Secondary
biliary
cirrhosis

Toxic hepatitis
(cholestatic)

Parenchymal
carcinoma

Primary biliary
cirrhosis

0 10 20 30 40 50 60 70 80 90 100
Alkaline phosphatase
(Bodansky units)

FIG 27–7. Range of alkaline phosphatase values in various hepatobiliary disorders.

serum concentrations remain unchanged with bone disease.

Changes in serum protein levels may reflect hepatic parenchymal dysfunction. In cirrhosis, the serum albumin falls and the globulins increase. Serum globulins reach high values in some patients with primary biliary cirrhosis. Biliary obstruction generally produces no changes unless secondary biliary cirrhosis has developed. The various serum flocculation tests measure relative alterations in serum protein fractions and are markedly abnormal only in hepatocellular disease.

Javitt NB: The cholestatic syndrome–1971. Am J Med 51: 637–641, 1971.

Kaplan MM: Alkaline phosphatase. New England J Med 286: 200–202, 1972.

Lorenzo GA, Beal JM: Recent advances in obstructive jaundice. S Clin North America 51:211–221, 1971.

Popper H, Schafner F: Pathophysiology of cholestasis. Human Pathology 1:1–24, 1970.

Redman HC & others: Roentgenographic evaluation of patients with suspected obstructive jaundice. Surg Gynec Obst 131:1100–1104, 1970.

Schenker S & others: Differential diagnosis of jaundice. Am J Digest Dis 7:449–463, 1962.

Zimmerman HJ: The differential diagnosis of jaundice. M Clin North America 52:1417–1444, 1968.

GALLSTONES

Cholesterol Gallstones

It has been estimated that more than 15 million people in the USA harbor cholesterol gallstones in their gallbladders. Over 300,000 operations are per-

formed annually for this problem, and at least 6000 deaths result from the complications of gallstone disease or its treatment.

The incidence in the population increases with age. Between the ages of 50 and 65, about 20% of women and 5% of men have gallstones. The incidence in American Indian men and women is much higher than in other races, whereas blacks are less susceptible. Over 75% of American Indian women over age 40 have cholesterol stones. Until recently, cholesterol gallstones were uncommon throughout the Orient, but a higher standard of living in some areas with a change in dietary habits has been associated with a sharply increased incidence of typical cholesterol stones.

The higher incidence in females implicates hormonal factors. Before puberty, males and females are affected with equal frequency, but thereafter the incidence in females is consistently higher than in males. In general, the more times a woman has been pregnant, the greater are her chances of developing stones, and it is striking how often the first manifestations of cholelithiasis appear within a few months after delivery. The use of oral contraceptive agents may be increasing the incidence of gallstones in young women.

Cholesterol constitutes 70–95% of the solids in most gallstones except those associated with hemolysis. As noted previously, cholesterol is insoluble in water and must be transported in bile within the micelles. The ability of a mixture of bile salt and lecithin to hold cholesterol in solution can be illustrated on a triangular diagram with an ordinate for each of the 3 micellar components (Fig 27–8). Any mixture of the 3 can be represented by a single point in the triangle, and the molar percentage would always total 100%. Various mixtures of bile salt, lecithin, and cholesterol in a 10% solution (to mimic gallbladder bile) have been studied, and the region in the triangle where all the cholesterol remained in solution was plotted. Gallbladder bile from patients with cholesterol gallstones fell outside the zone of cholesterol solubility (shaded area, Fig 27–8), whereas bile from normal subjects was within the zone (clear area, Fig 27–8). Thus, stone formation occurs in bile supersaturated with cholesterol, a condition which theoretically could result from either increased cholesterol secretion or diminished cholesterol-carrying capacity. Subsequent investigations have shown that bile from patients is supersaturated as it emerges from the liver, indicating that the primary chemical abnormality exists at the site of bile secretion rather than in the gallbladder or elsewhere.

The normal bile salt pool averages 3 g, but the pool size in patients with gallstones is usually less than 2 g. The rate of bile salt secretion is reduced in patients with a shrunken pool size. The reasons for the smaller pool in patients with stones is not known; excessive external loss is not the cause. The defect appears to lie in the regulation of hepatic synthesis of bile salts.

Although the rates of hepatic excretion of bile salts, lecithin, and cholesterol are correlated, the relationship is not an exact one. In fact, with reduced

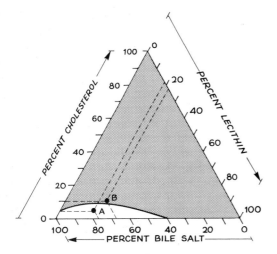

FIG 27—8. Triangular coordinates for depicting combination of bile salts, lecithin, and cholesterol. Point A represents the mean values for gallbladder bile from normal subjects: 77% bile salts, 18% lecithin, and 5% cholesterol. Point B represents the mean values for gallbladder bile from patients with cholesterol gallstones: 68% bile salts, 22% lecithin, and 10% cholesterol.

bile salt excretion, lecithin output drops more than cholesterol output does, and the final result is a change in bile composition toward cholesterol supersaturation. A diminished pool size, lower bile salt secretion, and subsequent shift in relative composition of bile are presently thought to represent important steps in the production of lithogenic bile.

Since cholesterol gallstone formation has not been successfully reproduced in vitro and since removal of the gallbladder usually cures the patient, the gallbladder must be etiologically important. It possibly supplies the nidus to crystallization, a small amount of bilirubinate or mucoprotein, contained in the center of most cholesterol stones. There is even evidence that the entire stone is laid on a complex scaffolding of mucous substances of gallbladder origin. Moreover, the gallbladder acts as an area of stasis in which precipitation of supersaturated bile would be favored, and sluggish gallbladder emptying in pregnancy may be one of the reasons that stones appear so often at this time.

Admirand WH, Small DM: The physicochemical basis of cholesterol gallstone formation in man. J Clin Invest 47:1043—1052, 1968.

Danzinger RG & others: Dissolution of cholesterol gallstones by chenodeoxycholic acid. New England J Med 286:1—8, 1972.

Heaton KW, Read AE: Gallstones in patients with disorders of the terminal ileum and disturbed bile salt metabolism. Brit MJ 3:494—496, 1969.

Maki T & others: Role of sulfated glycoprotein in gallstone formation. Surg Gynec Obst 132:846—854, 1971.

Redinger RN, Small DM: Bile composition, bile salt metabolism, and gallstones. Arch Int Med 130:618—630, 1972.

Small DM, Rapo S: Source of abnormal bile in patients with cholesterol gallstones. New England J Med 283:53—57, 1970.

Soloway RD & others: Hepatic lipid secretion and cholelithiasis. Am J Digest Dis 16:437—454, 1971.

Swell L & others: Relationship of bile acid pool size to biliary lipid excretion and the formation of lithogenic bile in man. Gastroenterology 61:716—722, 1971.

Thistle JL, Schoenfield LJ: Induced alterations in composition of bile of persons having cholelithiasis. Gastroenterology 61:488—496, 1971.

Calcium Bilirubinate Stones

Cholesterol gallstones are uncommon in Asia, where most biliary calculi are composed of calcium bilirubinate. Parasitic infestation of the biliary tree by *Ascaris lumbricoides* or *Clonorchis sinensis* is prevalent in the Orient. The disease begins when parasites create an inflammatory reaction in the ducts which becomes secondarily infected with enteric organisms. The bile of patients with calcium bilirubinate gallstones has been shown to contain high levels of the enzyme β-glucuronidase, produced by *Escherichia coli*. β-Glucuronidase deconjugates bilirubin diglucuronide to form free, insoluble bilirubin which precipitates as the calcium salt.

Maki T: Pathogenesis of calcium bilirubinate gallstone. Ann Surg 164:90—100, 1966.

RADIOLOGIC EXAMINATION OF THE BILIARY TREE

Radiography plays an important role in the evaluation of the patient with suspected disease of the biliary tree. The following types of studies are available: plain abdominal x-ray films, oral cholecystograms, intravenous cholangiograms, and percutaneous transhepatic cholangiograms.

Plain Abdominal Film

The posterior-anterior supine view of the abdomen may show gallstones in the 10 or 15% of cases where they are radiopaque. The bile itself sometimes contains sufficient calcium (milk of calcium bile) to be seen. An enlarged gallbladder can occasionally be seen as a soft tissue mass in the right upper quadrant. Indentation of an air-filled hepatic flexure may suggest gallbladder enlargement.

In several types of biliary disease, the diagnosis may be revealed by air seen in the bile ducts on a plain film. This would usually signify a fistula between the bile ducts and the intestine, whether surgically created or a spontaneous result of disease.

Oral Cholecystogram

This is the best method for obtaining radiographic

visualization of the gallbladder and its contents. Tyropanoate (Bilopaque) or iopanoic acid (Telepaque) is taken orally the night before the examination. The drug is absorbed from the intestinal tract, bound to albumin in portal blood, and extracted by the hepatocytes. It enters bile in insufficient levels to be seen radiographically until it has been concentrated within the gallbladder.

The next morning, posteroanterior and oblique supine views and an upright or a lateral decubitus film are obtained. A meal containing fat is then given, and the x-rays are repeated. The fat releases cholecystokinin, which empties the gallbladder and may outline the bile ducts.

Oral cholecystograms cannot be performed satisfactorily if the contrast agent is unabsorbed from the intestine or poorly excreted by the liver. Absorption is often impaired in acute abdominal illnesses with intestinal ileus, vomiting, or diarrhea. If the bilirubin level is over 3 mg/100 ml, hepatic excretion is not likely to be sufficient for a good study.

Intraluminal defects in the gallbladder nearly always represent gallstones. False-negative results are obtained in about 5% of tests. A normal gallbladder may not be visualized for several weeks after severe trauma or a major illness. If intestinal function is normal and hepatic excretion is unimpaired, failure to visualize the gallbladder on oral cholecystography is 95% reliable as an indication of significant gallbladder disease.

Intravenous Cholangiography

This test consists of the parenteral administration of iodipamide (Cholografin), a drug which is excreted by the hepatocyte in sufficient concentration to visualize the bile without concentration in the gallbladder. If the cystic duct is not obstructed, the gallbladder will be demonstrated as well as the bile ducts. The success of intravenous cholangiography is critically dependent on efficient hepatic excretion of the contrast agent; if the serum bilirubin concentration is greater than 4 mg/100 ml, the chances of a satisfactory examination are negligible. Between 2 and 4 mg/100 ml, the incidence of visualization is no more than 20%. In this bilirubin range, the likelihood of obtaining a useful study is greater if the bilirubin is dropping rapidly than if it is stationary or increasing.

Tomography is an essential part of the study, but even with tomography and good liver function there is a 15–20% incidence of false-negative results. Obvious strictures and stones can be missed, and a negative study does not have the same reliability as one in which a defect is demonstrated.

Intravenous cholangiography is of greatest value in (1) patients suspected of having biliary colic who have had a previous cholecystectomy, and (2) patients with acute abdominal pain in whom acute cholecystitis is suspected.

Percutaneous Transhepatic Cholangiography

Percutaneous transhepatic cholangiography may visualize the biliary tree in patients too jaundiced for satisfactory oral or intravenous studies. The examination is performed by passing a needle through the right flank into the hepatic parenchyma and a bile duct. Water-soluble contrast material is injected, and x-ray films are taken.

The technical success is related to the degree of dilatation of the intrahepatic bile ducts. Transhepatic cholangiography has been invaluable in demonstrating the obstruction in certain cases of biliary tumors, stones, and strictures. Failure to enter a duct does not prove that these conditions are absent because the ducts are not always dilated in cases where chronic cholangitis has impaired their elasticity. There is rarely any problem in obtaining a good study with malignant obstruction.

Transhepatic cholangiography should not be done in patients with active cholangitis unless the infection has been controlled with antibiotics. Septic shock has been produced by sudden inoculation of organisms from bile into the systemic circulation. Otherwise, the contraindications are the same as for percutaneous liver biopsy.

DISEASES OF THE GALLBLADDER & BILE DUCTS

CHOLELITHIASIS & CHRONIC CHOLECYSTITIS

Essentials of Diagnosis

- Episodic abdominal pain.
- Dyspepsia.
- Gallstones on cholecystography.

General Considerations

Chronic cholecystitis is the most common form of symptomatic gallbladder disease and is associated with gallstones in nearly every case. In general, the term cholecystitis is applied whenever gallstones are present regardless of the histologic appearance of the gallbladder. Repeated minor episodes of obstruction of the cystic duct cause intermittent biliary colic and contribute to inflammation and subsequent scar formation. Gallbladders from patients with gallstones who have never had an attack of acute cholecystitis are of 2 types: (1) In some the mucosa may be slightly flattened, but the wall is thin and unscarred and, except for the stones, appears normal. (2) Others exhibit obvious signs of chronic inflammation with thickening, cellular infiltration, loss of elasticity, and fibrosis. The clinical history in these 2 groups cannot always be distinguished, and inflammatory changes may also be found in patients with asymptomatic gallstones (see below).

Clinical Findings

A. Symptoms & Signs: Biliary colic, the most characteristic symptom, is caused by transient obstruction of the gallbladder by stones in the cystic duct. It usually begins abruptly and subsides gradually, lasting for a few minutes to several hours. In some patients the attacks occur postprandially, but in others there is no relationship to meals. The frequency of attacks is quite variable, ranging from nearly continuous trouble to episodes many years apart. Nausea may accompany the pain, but vomiting is not as common as in choledocholithiasis.

Biliary colic is usually felt in the right upper quadrant, but epigastric and left abdominal localization are common. In some cases pain is felt in the precordial region. The pain may radiate around the costal margin into the back or may be referred to the region of the scapula or between the scapulas. Pain on the top of the shoulder is unusual and suggests direct diaphragmatic irritation. During a severe attack, the patient usually curls up in bed, changing position frequently in search of a more comfortable position.

During an attack, the right upper quadrant may be tender. Rarely, the gallbladder is palpable.

Fatty food intolerance, dyspepsia, indigestion, heartburn, flatulence, nausea, and eructations may be associated with gallstone disease. However, they are also frequent in the general population, and their presence in any given patient may only be incidental to the gallstones. Patients with biliary colic are generally cured of the associated symptoms by cholecystectomy. However, operation for these complaints in patients without pain sometimes fails to provide relief.

B. Laboratory Findings: If a history of gallbladder colic is obtained, an oral cholecystogram will usually show stones in the gallbladder. If hepatic function and intestinal absorption are normal, failure to visualize the gallbladder after an oral cholecystogram indicates nonfunction from gallbladder disease. An intravenous cholangiogram may be ordered if malabsorption of the dye cannot be ruled out, but this is not often necessary.

Differential Diagnosis

Gallbladder colic may be strongly suggested by the history, but the clinical impression should always be verified by x-rays. Other causes of abdominal pain must be ruled out before the diagnosis is accepted. Biliary colic may simulate the pain of duodenal ulcer, hiatal hernia, pancreatitis, and myocardial infarction.

ECG and a chest x-ray should be obtained to investigate cardiopulmonary disease. It has been suggested that biliary colic may sometimes aggravate cardiac disease, but recent reviews of the relationship conclude that angina pectoris or an abnormal ECG should rarely be indications for cholecystectomy.

Right-sided radicular pain in the T6—T10 dermatomes may be confused with biliary colic. Osteoarthritic spurs, vertebral lesions, or tumors may be shown on x-rays of the spine or may be suggested by hyperesthesia of the abdominal skin.

An upper gastrointestinal series should be performed in a search for esophageal spasm, hiatal hernia, peptic ulcer, or gastric tumors. In some patients the irritable colon syndrome may be mistaken for gallbladder discomfort. Carcinoma of the cecum or ascending colon may be overlooked on the assumption that the postprandial pain of this disease is due to gallstones.

Complications

Chronic cholecystitis predisposes to acute cholecystitis, common duct stones, and adenocarcinoma of the gallbladder. The incidence of all of these complications increases the longer the stones have been present.

Treatment

A. Medical Treatment: Preliminary clinical studies have shown that oral administration of chenodeoxycholate improves the cholesterol-holding capacity of bile and over a period of 1—2 years will dissolve some gallbladder stones. Additional studies to determine the safety of this treatment are required before it can be released for general use. At present, no effective nonsurgical treatment is available for chronic cholecystitis and cholelithiasis. In some cases, symptoms follow certain foods. Avoidance of these foods may be symptomatically beneficial, but changes in diet will not reduce the risk of more serious complications.

B. Surgical Treatment: Cholecystectomy should be performed in most patients with symptoms. The procedure should be scheduled at the patient's convenience, within weeks or months after diagnosis. Active concurrent disease which increases the risk of surgery should be treated before operation. In some chronically ill patients, surgery should be deferred indefinitely.

After the abdomen is opened, the common duct is examined for the presence of stones before cholecystectomy is begun. (The indications for common duct exploration are discussed below.) An operative cholangiogram should be used as a routine check on the presence of stones in the duct.

Boquist L & others: Mortality after gallbladder surgery: A study of 3257 cholecystectomies. Surgery 71:616—624, 1972.

Edlund Y, Zettergren L: Histopathology of the gallbladder in gallstone disease related to clinical data. Acta chir scandinav 116:450—460, 1959.

French EB, Robb WAT: Biliary and renal colic. Brit MJ 3:121—135, 1963.

Gunn A, Keddie N: Some clinical observations on patients with gallstones. Lancet 2:239—241, 1972.

Haff RC & others: Biliary tract operations: A review of 1000 patients. Arch Surg 98:428—434, 1969.

Higgins JA: Nonfunctioning gallbladder. Mod Treat 5:500—504, 1968.

Price WH: Gall-bladder dyspepsia. Brit MJ 3:138—141, 1963.

Salmenkivi K: Cholesterosis of the gallbladder. Acta chir scandinav Suppl 324, 1964.

ASYMPTOMATIC GALLSTONES

Data on the prevalence of gallstones in the population of the USA indicate that only about 30% of people with cholelithiasis get to surgery. Despite several interesting studies, the natural history of asymptomatic gallstones is not completely understood. The low mortality rate from cholelithiasis suggests that the present practice of performing cholecystectomy only for those with symptoms is justified. Since there is no clear-cut evidence that unselected asymptomatic patients would benefit from cholecystectomy, it is not possible to make strong recommendations on how they should be managed. However, 3 groups are exposed to an increased risk by delay and should receive prophylactic surgery. For example, since the incidence of complications in gallstone disease increases with time, young patients with stones are more likely to develop severe manifestations if untreated. Most surgeons would recommend cholecystectomy for silent stones in people under 50–60 years of age, whereas older patients may be followed expectantly. Acute cholecystitis in patients with diabetes mellitus is accompanied by serious complications and a 10–15% mortality rate, and prophylactic cholecystectomy is strongly urged for them. Large gallstones (greater than 2 cm in diameter) are more likely to cause acute complications than small ones and should generally be removed if discovered in asymptomatic patients.

Carey JB Jr: Natural history of gallstone disease. Mod Treat 5:493–499, 1968.
Wenckert A, Robertson B: The natural course of gallstone disease: Eleven-year review of 781 nonoperated cases. Gastroenterology 50:376–381, 1966.
Wilbur RS, Bolt RJ: Incidence of gallbladder disease in "normal" men. Gastroenterology 36:251–255, 1959.

ACUTE CHOLECYSTITIS

Essentials of Diagnosis

- Acute right upper quadrant pain and tenderness.
- Mild fever and leukocytosis.
- Palpable gallbladder in one-third of cases.
- Nonvisualized gallbladder on intravenous cholangiogram.

General Considerations

In 98% of cases, acute cholecystitis results from obstruction of the cystic duct by a gallstone impacted in Hartmann's pouch. The gallbladder becomes inflamed and distended, creating abdominal pain and tenderness. The natural history of acute cholecystitis varies considerably depending on whether the obstruction becomes relieved, the extent of secondary bacterial invasion, the age of the patient, and the presence of other aggravating factors such as diabetes mellitus. Most attacks resolve spontaneously without surgery or other specific therapy, but some progress to abscess formation or free perforation with generalized peritonitis.

The pathologic changes in the gallbladder evolve in a typical pattern (Fig 27–9). Subserosal edema is the first change and is accompanied by hemorrhage and patchy necrosis of the mucosa. Polymorphonuclear leukocytes become prominent after several days have passed. Fibrosis appears near the end of the first week and is pronounced by the ninth or tenth day. Gangrene and perforation may occur as early as 3 days after onset, but most perforations occur during the second week. The edema subsides during the second week at a time when fibrosis is increasing. Lymphocytes and mononuclear cells gradually become the predominant inflammatory cells. The disappearance of the inflammatory reaction may span several months, but the acute inflammation usually resolves within 4 weeks. A moderate decrease in the fibrotic component takes place during the second to fourth month, but some scarring always remains. About 90% of gallbladders removed during an acute attack show chronic scarring, although many of these patients deny having had any previous symptoms.

The cause of acute cholecystitis is still partially conjectural. Obstruction of the cystic duct is present in most cases, but experimentally produced obstruction does not cause inflammation unless gallstones are present—nor does cholecystitis always develop after obstruction even if stones are present. Pancreatic juice, concentrated bile salts, or bacterial cultures, when injected into the gallbladders of animals with an occluded cystic duct, may produce cholecystitis. The extent to which these experiments are relevant to the pathogenesis of the disease in humans remains hazy. Bacteria can be cultured from the bile of 50% of patients with acute cholecystitis, but the frequent absence of bacteria and the lack of suppuration in

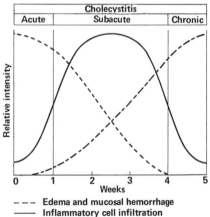

FIG 27–9. Acute cholecystitis. Changes in histopathology of the gallbladder with time.

general has led to an emphasis on nonbacterial theories of etiology.

About 2% of cases of acute cholecystitis occur in the absence of cholelithiasis. Some of these are due to cystic duct obstruction by another process such as a malignant tumor. Rarely, acute acalculous cholecystitis results from cystic artery occlusion or primary bacterial infection by *E coli,* clostridia, or occasionally *Salmonella typhosa.* Acute acalculous cholecystitis has also been reported as a complication of prolonged fasting after an unrelated operation. It has been postulated that the inflammation is caused by high concentrations of bile salts which develop in the gallbladder under these circumstances.

Clinical Findings

A. Symptoms and Signs: The first symptom is sudden abdominal pain in the right upper quadrant, sometimes associated with referred pain in the region of the right scapula. In 75% of cases, the patient will have had previous attacks of biliary colic, at first indistinguishable from the present illness. However, in acute cholecystitis the pain persists and becomes associated with abdominal tenderness. Nausea and vomiting are present in about half of patients, but the vomiting is rarely severe. Mild icterus occurs in 10%. The temperature usually ranges from 38–38.5 C (100.4–101.3 F). High fever and chills are uncommon and should suggest the possibility of complications or an incorrect diagnosis.

Right upper quadrant tenderness is present, and in about a third of patients the gallbladder is palpable in a position usually somewhat lateral to its normal one. Voluntary guarding during examination may prevent detection of an enlarged gallbladder. In others, the gallbladder is not enlarged because scarring of the wall restricts distention. If the patient is instructed to breathe deeply during palpation in the right subcostal region, he experiences accentuated tenderness and sudden inspiratory arrest (Murphy's sign).

B. Laboratory Findings: A plain x-ray of the abdomen may occasionally show an enlarged gallbladder shadow. In 15% of patients, the gallstones contain enough calcium to be seen on the plain film.

An oral cholecystogram cannot be relied on during acute cholecystitis or other acute abdominal disorders characterized by vomiting and should be postponed until 4–6 weeks after the acute attack.

Intravenous cholangiography may have diagnostic value in certain cases of acute cholecystitis. Opacification of the gallbladder excludes the diagnosis. Demonstration of contrast in the bile ducts but none in the gallbladder confirms the diagnosis of cholecystitis.

The leukocyte count is usually elevated to 12–15 thousand/μl. Normal counts are common, but if the count goes much above 15,000 one should suspect complications. A mild elevation of the serum bilirubin (in the range of 2–4 mg/100 ml) is commonly seen in acute cholecystitis. This is presumably due to secondary inflammation of the common duct by the contiguous gallbladder. Bilirubin values above this range

would most likely indicate the associated presence of common duct stones. A mild increase in alkaline phosphatase, 5'-nucleotidase, and leucine aminopeptidase may accompany the attack. Occasionally, the serum amylase concentration transiently reaches 1000 units/100 ml or more.

Differential Diagnosis

The differential diagnosis includes other common causes of acute upper abdominal pain and tenderness. An acute peptic ulcer with or without perforation might be suggested by a history of epigastric pain relieved by food or antacids. Most cases of perforated ulcer demonstrate free air under the diaphragm on x-ray. Intravenous cholangiography or emergency upper gastrointestinal series with water-soluble contrast may help in puzzling situations.

Acute pancreatitis can easily be confused with acute cholecystitis, especially if cholecystitis is accompanied by an elevated amylase. Intravenous cholangiograms would outline the gallbladder in most cases of acute pancreatitis. Sometimes the 2 diseases coexist, but pancreatitis should not be accepted as a second diagnosis without specific findings.

Acute appendicitis in patients with a high cecum may closely simulate acute cholecystitis.

Severe right upper quadrant pain with high fever and local tenderness may develop in acute gonococcal perihepatitis (Fitz-Hugh and Curtis syndrome). Clues to the proper diagnosis may be found in tenderness in the adnexa, vaginal discharge and gonococci on a gram-stained smear of the discharge, and a disparity between the patient's high fever and her general lack of toxicity.

Acute hepatitis has a more gradual onset and is accompanied by sustained elevations of SGOT and SGPT. Although the enzymes may rise in acute cholecystitis, they become normal within 24–48 hours and in all but a few cases the absolute levels do not approach those seen in hepatitis. Hepatitis is also associated with alterations in hepatic function as shown by abnormal flocculation tests.

Severe pneumonitis in the right lung or an acute myocardial infarction occasionally masquerades as an acute abdominal disorder.

Complications

The major complications of acute cholecystitis are empyema, gangrene, and perforation. Perforation may take any of 3 forms: (1) localized perforation with pericholecystic abscess; (2) free perforation with generalized peritonitis; and (3) perforation into an adjacent hollow viscus with the formation of a fistula. Although perforation may occur as early as 3 days after the onset of acute cholecystitis, most are seen in the second week. The total incidence of perforation is about 10%.

A. Localized Perforation: Pericholecystic abscess is found in most cases in which operation is delayed but the signs and symptoms do not subside. Localization is usual because the slow natural course of the disease allows time for omentum and adjacent organs to form adhesions about the inflamed gallbladder. The perforation usually appears either in the fundus or adjacent to the stone impacted in Hartmann's pouch. It often occurs on the wall of the gallbladder next to the liver, and a partly intrahepatic abscess is produced. Perforation does not usually develop unless the inflammatory process takes on a decidedly suppurative character. The patient often is more toxic than usual, with fever to 39 C (102.2 F) and a leukocyte count above 15,000/μl, but sometimes there is no correlation between the clinical signs and the development of local abscess. If the gallbladder was palpable early in the course, the mass may either become more prominent or, if the organ decompresses into the subhepatic area, may disappear. If a mass was not previously palpable, its sudden appearance may suggest an abscess.

Surgical treatment is indicated for the toxic patient as soon as he can be prepared for operation. Fluids and electrolytes and high doses of antibiotics effective against enteric organisms should be administered preoperatively.

Cholecystectomy and drainage of the contaminated subhepatic area can be performed safely in many patients. If the preoperative condition of the patient is unsatisfactory due to marked toxicity or associated disease, cholecystostomy would be preferable to cholecystectomy.

B. Free Perforation: Free perforation in acute cholecystitis develops in only 1—2% of patients. It sometimes develops early in the course of the disease because of a localized area of gangrene. It should be suspected with the advent of a sudden increase in general toxicity. Localized pain may become more diffuse and accompanied by a spread of abdominal tenderness to areas other than the right upper quadrant. Some patients report an improvement in their discomfort shortly after the rupture decompresses gallbladder tension, but it is only a brief respite.

Whenever it is suspected, free perforation must be treated by emergency laparotomy. Abdominal paracentesis may be misleading and has proved to be of little diagnostic usefulness. In general, the diagnosis is made more often than it is confirmed, but the toxic patient is usually suffering from advanced disease which is better treated by prompt surgery. Cholecystostomy should be performed and the peritoneal cavity cleansed by saline irrigation. The mortality rate depends partly on whether the cystic duct remained obstructed or the stone was dislodged after perforation. The former leads to a purulent peritonitis which is lethal in 20% of cases. In the latter, a true bile peritonitis ensues and over 50% of patients die.

C. Cholecystenteric Fistula: The acutely inflamed gallbladder may become adherent to the adjacent stomach, duodenum, or colon. If necrosis of the wall develops at the site of one of these adhesions, perforation may occur into the lumen of the adjacent viscus. This form of sudden decompression often allows the acute disease to resolve because the gallbladder is drained. If the gallbladder stones are discharged

through the fistula, they may cause mechanical obstruction of the small intestine (gallstone ileus; see below). In rare cases, patients have vomited gallstones which entered the stomach through a cholecystogastric fistula. However, in most cases the acute attack improves and the cholecystenteric fistula is clinically unsuspected.

Cholecystenteric fistulas do not usually cause symptoms unless the gallbladder is still partially obstructed by stones or scarring. Neither oral nor intravenous cholangiograms will visualize the gallbladder or the fistula, but the latter may be shown on upper gastrointestinal series, where it must be differentiated from a fistula due to perforated peptic ulcer. Malabsorption and steatorrhea have been reported in isolated cases of cholecystocolonic fistulas. Steatorrhea in this situation could be due either to absence of bile in the proximal bowel following diversion into the colon or deconjugation of bile salts in the duodenum by excess colonic bacteria.

Symptomatic cholecystenteric fistulas should be treated by cholecystectomy and closure of the fistula. The majority are discovered incidentally during cholecystectomy for symptomatic gallbladder disease.

Essenhigh DM: Perforation of the gallbladder. Brit J Surg 55:175—178, 1968.

Haff RC & others: Biliary-enteric fistulas. Surg Gynec Obst 133:84—88, 1971.

McCarthy JD, Picazo JG: Bile peritonitis. Am J Surg 116:664—668, 1968.

MacDonald JA: Perforation of the gallbladder associated with acute cholecystitis. Ann Surg 164:849—852, 1966.

Piedad OH, Wells PB: Spontaneous internal biliary fistula, obstructive and nonobstructive types. Ann Surg 175:75—80, 1972.

Rosato EF & others: Bile ascites. Surg Gynec Obst 130:494—496, 1970.

Stull JR, Thomford NR: Biliary intestinal fistula. Am J Surg 120—27—31, 1970.

Treatment

The proper treatment of acute cholecystitis is surgical once this diagnosis has been established and the condition of the patient permits operation. The patient should be admitted to the hospital and started on intravenous fluids to correct dehydration and electrolyte imbalance if present. A nasogastric tube should be inserted if the patient is nauseated or vomiting.

Analgesics should be administered for pain. Morphine and meperidine have the theoretical disadvantage of elevating biliary pressure by contracting the sphincter of Oddi. Pentazocine may be given since it does not share this action, but if relief is unsatisfactory with this drug one of the others should be prescribed.

Antibiotics are not usually required and should be reserved for patients in jeopardy of developing complications. Ampicillin, tetracycline, chloramphenicol, and cephaloridine have been recommended for the treatment of biliary infections because they are normally excreted in the bile. However, in biliary disease they are blocked from reaching the infection by this route. For the expectant treatment of acute cholecystitis of average severity, parenteral ampicillin (4 g daily) or cephaloridine (2–4 g daily) should be given. Parenteral penicillin (20 million units daily) and kanamycin (15 mg/kg daily) or penicillin and gentamicin (2–4 mg/kg daily) should be given for severe disease.

The following are the major factors that affect the timing of early surgery: (1) whether the diagnosis is established; (2) the general health of the patient as modified by coexistent disease or the present illness; and (3) signs of local complications of acute cholecystitis. The diagnosis should be clear-cut and the patient optimally prepared; if perforation is suspected, emergency surgery is indicated.

About 30% of cases satisfy the criteria for early definitive operation with little delay after admission to the hospital. An example might be a healthy young patient who is admitted within 24 hours of the onset of symptoms. If the history and physical findings are typical and if the distended, tender gallbladder is palpable, the diagnosis can be accepted. This patient might be scheduled for operation in the next open position on the surgery list. This does not mean that an emergency is present, as in the case of acute appendicitis or perforated peptic ulcer, because acute cholecystitis does not usually threaten complications within short, rigid time intervals. Left untreated, most cases would resolve without sequelae. Therefore, the operation need not be done in the middle of the night but rather under the better circumstances that prevail during the regular operating schedule with a prepared team.

In about another 30% of patients however, the correct diagnosis is not obvious. The diagnosis of acute cholecystitis based upon clinical criteria alone is in error in 5–10% of cases. In most instances these are patients whose clinical findings consist of upper abdominal pain without a palpable gallbladder. Many of the conditions listed in the section on differential diagnosis may have to be ruled out. Emergency intravenous cholangiograms can be of great value if liver function is relatively normal.

In about another 30%, the diagnosis of acute cholecystitis may be definitely established but the general condition of the patient unsatisfactory. This situation most often involves elderly patients who have been admitted to the hospital after being sick for several days. Dehydration may be severe, and the patient's cardiovascular system may be in suboptimal balance. In some cases congestive heart failure has developed, and a period of time will be required for digitalization. A wide variety of other conditions in individual patients may justify management along these lines. As a general rule, anything that may materially increase the risk of general anesthesia and laparotomy should be corrected, if possible, before cholecystectomy. Renal, pulmonary, and cardiac diseases are the most common examples.

About 10% of patients with acute cholecystitis require emergency operation. These are generally clinical situations where the disease appears to have become complicated or is about to. High fever (39 C [102.2 F]), marked leukocytosis (> 15,000/μl), or chills should alert one to the possibility that suppurative progression is occurring. The sudden appearance of generalized abdominal pain may indicate free perforation. A mass that develops in the gallbladder area where it was not felt previously may be a sign of local perforation and abscess formation. Changes of this sort are an indication for emergency laparotomy.

Since acute cholecystitis in a patient with diabetes mellitus is often a fulminating disease with a high incidence of serious complications and a mortality rate of about 15%, cholecystectomy should be considered an urgent matter in the diabetic.

Cholecystectomy is the preferable operation in acute cholecystitis and can be safely performed in the large majority of patients. Cholecystostomy is reserved for those whose general condition is precarious or when local complications are present. Nearly all patients with uncomplicated acute cholecystitis who require cholecystostomy are over 60 years of age. The decision to perform cholecystostomy should usually be made before the abdomen is opened since it depends on factors apparent during preoperative evaluation. It should rarely be the result of having initially embarked upon cholecystectomy and then attempting to get out of a difficult dissection by changing to a lesser operation; in such cases, cholecystostomy should have been the original choice.

Cholecystostomy consists of emptying the contents of the gallbladder through an incision in the fundus and then suturing a large-bore tube within the lumen for continued postoperative drainage. If possible, all gallstones should be removed, for this allows subsequent removal of the tube with a good chance that the patient will not require cholecystectomy.

After the patient has recovered, x-rays should be obtained after injecting diatrizoate (Hypaque) into the cholecystostomy tube. If the gallbladder or common duct contains stones, elective cholecystectomy should be scheduled when the patient can be optimally prepared. If the biliary tree is free of stones, the tube can be removed and the patient followed for development of new symptoms. Gallstones recur in about 50% of cases within 5 years. Many would plan routinely for cholecystectomy, but elderly patients with concomitant disease are probably managed best nonoperatively until symptoms develop. If this rule is followed, about half of such patients will need an operation.

Prognosis

The overall mortality rate of acute cholecystitis is about 5%. Nearly all of the deaths are in patients over age 60 or those with diabetes mellitus. In the older age group, secondary cardiovascular or pulmonary complications contribute substantially to mortality. Uncontrolled sepsis with peritonitis or intrahepatic abscesses are the most important local conditions responsible for deaths.

Common duct stones are present in about 15% of patients with acute cholecystitis, and some of the more seriously ill patients have simultaneous cholangitis from biliary obstruction. Acute pancreatitis may also complicate acute cholecystitis, and the combination carries a greater risk.

Patients who develop the suppurative forms of gallbladder disease such as empyema or perforation are less likely to recover. Earlier admission to the hospital and early cholecystectomy reduce the chances of these complications.

Cafferata HT & others: Acute cholecystitis in a municipal hospital. Arch Surg 98:435–441, 1969.

Crosby VG, Ziffren SE: Cholecystostomy as definitive therapy in the aged with acute cholecystitis. J Am Geriatrics Soc 13:496–500, 1965.

Dunphy JE, Ross FP: Studies in acute cholecystitis. I. Surgical management and results. Surgery 26:539–547, 1949.

Edlund Y, Olsson O: Acute cholecystitis: Its aetiology and course, with special reference to the timing of cholecystectomy. Acta chir scandinav 120:479–494, 1961.

Edlund YA & others: Bacteriological investigation of the biliary system and liver in biliary tract disease correlated to clinical data and microstructure of the gallbladder and liver. Acta chir scandinav 116:461–476, 1959.

Hoerr SO, Hazard JB: Acute cholecystitis without gallbladder stones. Am J Surg 111:47–55, 1966.

Ross FP, Dunphy JE: Studies in acute cholecystitis. II. Cholecystostomy: Indications and technique. New England J Med 242:359–364, 1970.

Scott AJ: Bacteria and disease of the biliary tract. Gut 12:487–492, 1971.

Thorpe CD: Emergency intravenous cholangiography in patients with acute abdominal pain. Am J Surg 125:46–50, 1973.

Van der Linden W, Sunzel H: Early versus delayed operation for acute cholecystitis: A controlled clinical trial. Am J Surg 120:7–13, 1970.

EMPHYSEMATOUS CHOLECYSTITIS

Emphysematous cholecystitis is a rare condition in which bubbles of gas from anaerobic infection appear in the lumen of the gallbladder, its wall, the pericholecystic space, and on occasion the bile ducts. Clostridia species are the most commonly implicated organisms, but other gas-forming anaerobes such as *E coli* or anaerobic streptococci may be found. Male patients outnumber females by 3:1, and 20% of all patients have diabetes mellitus. In contrast to the usual form of acute cholecystitis, the disease probably is a bacterial infection from the earliest moment. In many reported cases, the gallbladder contained no stones. These characteristics suggest the possibility that cystic artery occlusion and ischemia may initiate emphysematous cholecystitis.

The disease begins with sudden and rapidly progressive right upper quadrant pain. Fever and leukocytosis reach high levels quickly, and the patient is considerably more toxic than is usually the case in acute cholecystitis. On examination, a mass can usually be found in the right upper quadrant.

Plain films of the abdomen show tissue emphysema outlining the gallbladder and, in some cases, an air-fluid level in the lumen. The clinical and x-ray pictures are characteristic enough so that the diagnosis is usually obvious.

The patient should be treated with high doses of antibiotics effective against clostridia and the other species mentioned above. Emergency surgical treatment should follow the initial resuscitative measures. Cholecystectomy can be safely performed in most cases, but the most critically ill might fare better with cholecystostomy. The types of complications are the same as in other forms of acute cholecystitis, but the morbidity and mortality rates are higher.

May RE, Strong R: Acute emphysematous cholecystitis. Brit J Surg 58:453–458, 1971.

Rosoff L, Meyers H: Acute emphysematous cholecystitis. Am J Surg 111:410–423, 1966.

GALLSTONE ILEUS

Gallstone ileus is mechanical intestinal obstruction caused by a large gallstone lodged in the lumen. It is seen most often in women, and the average age is about 70 years. However, gallstone ileus may occur in any age group where cholesterol stones are found.

Clinical Findings

A. Symptoms: The patient usually presents with obvious small bowel obstruction, either partial or complete. The obstructing gallstone enters the intestine through a cholecystenteric fistula located in the duodenum, jejunum, stomach, or, rarely, the colon. Usually it is between the gallbladder and the duodenum. Oddly, a history compatible with a recent episode of acute cholecystitis can be obtained in only a third of cases. This suggests that in the others the stone may erode into the neighboring viscus by pressure necrosis rather than by producing acute cholecystitis. The gallbladder may contain one or several stones, but those that cause gallstone ileus are almost always 2.5 cm or more in diameter. The lumen in the proximal bowel will allow most of these large calculi to pass caudally until the ileum is reached. Rarely, the stone obstructs the duodenum at the site of the fistula. Obstruction of the large intestine may follow passage of a gallstone through a fistula at the hepatic flexure or may occur even after the stone has traversed the entire small bowel. Gallstone ileus of the colon is rare because the normal colonic lumen is large; most reported cases have had colonic narrowing by diverticulitis as a predisposing factor.

As the gallstone moves down the small intestine, it may temporarily block the lumen and create obstructive symptoms only to dislodge and pass farther along. This creates an intermittent or tumbling obstruction which is characteristic of gallstone ileus and is reflected clinically by intermittency of signs and symptoms. When a segment of intestine is reached where further passage is impossible, complete obstruction develops. The episodic pain and distention may last for 12–24 hours and lead the physician to optimistically predict a spontaneous resolution of the problem.

The diagnosis of gallstone ileus should always be entertained whenever small bowel obstruction is encountered in elderly patients. If the patient has never had a laparotomy that might account for adhesions and if incarceration of an external hernia can be excluded by physical examination, gallstone ileus should be high on the list. A history of recent right upper quadrant pain which preceded the bowel obstruction may provide a helpful clue, as would the tumbling type of obstruction if it can be recognized clinically.

B. Signs: In most patients the findings on physical examination are typical of distal small bowel obstruction since the stone usually becomes wedged in the ileum. Obstruction of the duodenum or jejunum may give a perplexing clinical picture because of the lack of distention. Right upper quadrant tenderness may be present in some cases, but the distended abdomen may be difficult to examine accurately. The stone can occasionally be palpated within the ileum on abdominal, pelvic, or rectal examination, but it is seldom recognized for what it is.

C. X-Ray Findings: Plain films of the abdomen may show the gallstone if it is radiopaque, and unless one is alert to the possibility of gallstone ileus the ectopic stone can be a puzzling finding. In most cases, careful examination of the film will reveal gas in the biliary tree, a manifestation of the cholecystenteric fistula. When the clinical picture is unclear, an upper gastrointestinal series may be obtained which outlines the connection between the duodenum and gallbladder. However, an upper gastrointestinal series is not recommended as a routine part of the evaluation if gallstone ileus has been diagnosed on other grounds.

Treatment

The proper treatment is emergency laparotomy and removal of the obstructing stone through a small enterotomy. The proximal intestine must be carefully inspected for the presence of a second calculus which might cause a postoperative recurrence. The gallbladder should be left undisturbed at the original operation. Although some have claimed that cholecystectomy can be performed safely at this point, it is not recommended for the following reasons: (1) the emergency operation would be converted from a simple procedure into one that may last 4–5 hours, and (2) the patient rarely obtains tangible immediate benefit from having the gallbladder out anyway. Prevention of recurrent gallstone ileus has been offered as an argument for cholecystectomy during the emergency procedure, but recurrence has been reported in

only 2% of patients, and this figure could be reduced by more careful palpation and extraction of calculi from the intestine proximal to the obstruction.

Once the patient has recovered from the operation, an elective cholecystectomy should be scheduled if the patient complains of chronic gallbladder symptoms. On this basis, cholecystectomy will be performed in about half of patients with gallstone ileus. The fistula itself is rarely the source of trouble and closes spontaneously in many patients.

Prognosis

The mortality rate of gallstone ileus remains about 15–20% largely because of the poor general condition of the elderly patients at the time of laparotomy. In many cases the patient has developed cardiac or pulmonary complications during a preoperative delay when the diagnosis was unclear. The mortality rate can be reduced by being alert for the diagnosis in appropriate circumstances because—once considered—the clinical and radiologic data can usually be pieced together.

Andersson A, Zederfeldt B: Gallstone ileus. Acta chir scandinav 135:713–717, 1969.
Raiford TS: Intestinal obstruction caused by gallstones. Am J Surg 104:383, 1962.

CHOLEDOCHOLITHIASIS

Essentials of Diagnosis

- Biliary pain.
- Jaundice
- Episodic cholangitis.
- Gallstones in gallbladder or previous cholecystectomy.

General Considerations

Gallstones may traverse the cystic duct and enter the common bile duct but are often prevented from reaching the duodenum by the narrowing in the hepatopancreatic (Vater's) ampulla. In the duct they cause symptoms by obstructing the flow of bile. Approximately 15% of patients with stones in the gallbladder are found to harbor calculi within the bile ducts. Common duct stones are usually accompanied by others in the gallbladder, but in rare cases the gallbladder is empty. The number of duct stones may vary from 1 to more than 100. Gallstones occasionally form within the ductal system de novo after prolonged ductal infection or stasis. They sometimes pass spontaneously into the duodenum. From the clinical standpoint, common duct stones should be considered potentially hazardous even when asymptomatic.

Cholangitis is a syndrome caused by bacterial infection of an obstructed biliary tree. The block to flow may be partial or, less commonly, complete. The most common predisposing causes are choledocholithiasis and biliary stricture. Involvement of the duct by neoplasm, pancreatic cysts, duodenal diverticula, or invasion by parasites is less common. The symptoms (referred to in older texts as **Charcot's triad**) are biliary colic, jaundice, and chills and fever.

Cholangitis virtually always signifies obstruction and increased biliary pressure. In the absence of obstruction, even heavy bacterial contamination of the ducts does not produce symptoms or pathologic changes. With obstruction, ductal pressure rises and bacteria proliferate and escape into the systemic circulation via the hepatic sinusoids. Experimentally, the incidence of positive blood cultures with ductal infection varies directly with the absolute height of biliary pressure—an observation that underscores the importance of decompression of the duct in the treatment of cholangitis.

The common duct may dilate to 2–3 cm proximal to an obstructing lesion, and truly huge ducts develop in patients with biliary tumors. In biliary stricture or choledocholithiasis, the inflammatory reaction restricts dilatation so that the ducts tend to be somewhat smaller. Expansion of the intrahepatic ducts also is limited by cirrhosis.

Biliary colic results from rapid rises in biliary pressure whether the block is in the common duct or neck of the gallbladder. Gradual occlusion of the duct—as in malignancy—rarely produces the same kind of pain as gallstone disease.

Clinical Findings

A. Symptoms: Choledocholithiasis may be asymptomatic or may produce sudden overwhelming toxicity with a rapid demise. The seriousness of the disease parallels the degree of obstruction, the length of time it has been present, and the extent of secondary bacterial infection.

The classic clinical manifestations are those of cholangitis: biliary colic, fever, chills, leukocytosis, and jaundice. The complete picture is not always present. Biliary colic may be the only symptom, or fever and chills may occur in the absence of pain.

Biliary colic from common duct obstruction cannot be distinguished from that caused by stones in the gallbladder. Frequent spontaneous vomiting in association with biliary colic should suggest common duct stone. The pain is felt in the right subcostal region, epigastrium, or even the substernal area. Referred pain to the tip of the right scapula or between the scapulas is common.

Choledocholithiasis should be strongly suspected if intermittent chills, fever, or jaundice accompany biliary colic. Some patients notice transient darkening of their urine during an attack even though jaundice is not evident. Light stools may also be reported during an attack.

Pruritus is usually the result of persistent longstanding obstruction. The itching is more intense in warm weather when the patient perspires and is usually worse on the extremities than on the trunk.

B. Signs: The patient may be icteric and toxic, with high fever and chills, or he may appear to be perfectly healthy. A palpable gallbladder is unusual in patients with obstructive jaundice from common duct stone because scarring of the gallbladder renders it inelastic and nondistensible. The gallbladder is palpable in rare cases of choledocholithiasis, but this usually indicates malignant obstruction. Tenderness may be present to palpation in the right upper quadrant but is not often as marked as in acute cholecystitis, perforated peptic ulcer, or acute pancreatitis. Hepatic enlargement and tenderness may occur, especially if obstruction has been present for more than several days.

C. Laboratory Findings: Leukocytosis of $15,000/\mu l$ is usually present, and values above $20,000/\mu l$ are common. A rise in serum bilirubin often appears within 24 hours of the onset of symptoms. The absolute level usually remains under 10 mg/100 ml, and most are in the range of 2–4 mg/100 ml. The direct fraction exceeds the indirect, but the latter becomes elevated in most cases. Bilirubin levels do not ordinarily reach the high values seen in malignant tumors because the obstruction is usually incomplete and transient. In fact, fluctuating jaundice is so characteristic of choledocholithiasis that it reliably differentiates between benign and malignant obstruction.

The 24-hour urinary urobilinogen will usually exceed 4 mg. Fecal urobilinogen excretion may be less than normal, but the drop is not usually great enough to be of help.

The serum alkaline phosphatase, leucine aminopeptidase, and 5'-nucleotidase levels usually rise and may be the only chemical abnormalities in patients without jaundice. When the obstruction is relieved, the alkaline phosphatase returns rapidly toward normal after brief obstruction but may remain elevated for weeks or even permanently after prolonged blockage.

Mild increases in SGOT and SGPT are often seen with extrahepatic obstruction of the ducts; rarely, SGOT levels transiently reach 1000.

D. X-Ray Findings: If the gallstones are radiopaque, they may be seen on plain films of the abdomen. Intravenous cholangiography may be successful if the patient is not jaundiced but is rarely satisfactory in the midst of an attack of cholangitis. It is better to delay the cholangiogram until the acute symptoms have subsided and the serum bilirubin has returned to normal.

Differential Diagnosis

The work-up should consider the same possibilities in differential diagnosis as for cholecystitis.

Serum amylase levels above 500 units/100 ml can be from acute pancreatitis, acute cholecystitis, or choledocholithiasis. Other manifestations of pancreatic disease should be documented before an unqualified diagnosis of pancreatitis is subscribed to.

In viral hepatitis, the SGOT and SGPT reach high levels and the indirect bilirubin fraction may predominate. A history of exposure to hepatitis and a young patient are additional clues.

Alcoholic cirrhosis or acute alcoholic hepatitis may present with jaundice, right upper quadrant tenderness, and leukocytosis. The differentiation from cholangitis may be impossible from clinical data. A history of a recent binge suggests acute liver disease. A percutaneous liver biopsy may be specific.

Intrahepatic cholestasis from drugs, pregnancy, chronic active hepatitis, or primary biliary cirrhosis may be quite difficult to distinguish from extrahepatic obstruction. Transhepatic cholangiography is required in many, but a technically unsuccessful study would leave the dilemma unresolved. If jaundice has persisted for 4–6 weeks, laparotomy and exploration of the bile duct should be performed. Most patients with intrahepatic cholestasis improve during this interval, and persistent cholestatic jaundice thus usually proves to be due to some form of extrahepatic obstruction.

Intermittent jaundice and cholangitis after cholecystectomy are compatible with biliary stricture, and the distinction may be impossible without a good cholangiogram or direct surgical exploration. The history may help, since symptoms due to stricture usually appear within several months after the cholecystectomy and cholangitis due to stones is frequently not seen for several years.

Biliary tumors usually produce jaundice without biliary colic or fever, and, once it begins, the jaundice rarely remits. The stools may be positive for occult blood when the obstruction is due to tumor.

Complications

Severe cholangitis may lead to septicemia and septic shock (see Acute Suppurative [Obstructive] Cholangitis, below). Long-standing infection can produce multiple intrahepatic abscesses. Hepatic failure or secondary biliary cirrhosis may develop in unrelieved obstruction of long duration. Since the obstruction is usually incomplete and intermittent, cirrhosis develops only after prolonged untreated disease. Acute pancreatitis is a fairly common complication of calculous biliary disease. Rarely, the stone may erode through the ampulla, resulting in gallstone ileus. Hemorrhage is also a rare complication.

Most common duct stones are discovered incidentally and treated concurrently with chronic or acute gallbladder disease. Others present as problems due to cholangitis or cholestatic jaundice.

Treatment

Patients with acute cholangitis should be treated with systemic antibiotics according to the guidelines given for acute cholecystitis (see above); this usually controls the attack within 24–48 hours. If appropriate treatment does not result in improvement after 2–4 days, surgical exploration should be seriously considered. Lack of response may indicate that suppurative cholangitis is imminent.

Once cholangitis resolves, additional attempts should be made to confirm the diagnosis. In the meantime, antibiotic treatment should be continued. An intravenous cholangiogram may reveal the cause of the

symptoms. Transhepatic cholangiography should be delayed until infection has subsided.

The patient with cholangitis and common duct stones should be scheduled for operation shortly after the attack has resolved and any other medical problems have been investigated. If the prothrombin time is abnormal, it should be corrected by parenteral vitamin K before laparotomy.

The classic indications for common duct exploration during cholecystectomy are the following: (1) preoperative jaundice, (2) demonstration of stones on intravenous or transhepatic cholangiography, (3) pancreatitis in association with the biliary disease, (4) dilated common duct ($>$ 1 cm in diameter), (5) presence of small stones in the gallbladder, (6) a palpable stone in the duct, and (7) ductal stone demonstrated by operative cholangiography. It is useful to divide these indications into absolute ones and relative ones based on their proved reliability as indications of common duct stone (Fig 27–10). Thus, the **absolute** indications are preoperative demonstration of stones by x-ray, preoperative history of cholangitis with jaundice, jaundice alone (if the bilirubin exceeds 7 mg/100 ml), palpable stone in the duct, and a positive operative cholangiogram. The **relative** indications are mild jaundice without fever and chills, small stones, and a dilated duct. The relative indications are accompanied by stones in only 20% of cases or less. When relative indications are present, the decision to explore the duct can be based upon the results of an operative cholangiogram.

After exploration of the duct is completed and all stones have been removed, a T tube is inserted. A postexploratory operative cholangiogram through the T tube should be obtained in all cases. It will often reveal overlooked stones which can be removed by reopening the duct. Cholecystectomy should be performed after the duct has been explored.

About a week after the operation, a postoperative cholangiogram should be performed through the T tube. About 3–5% of patients who have had stones removed from the duct will be found to have a residual stone on the postoperative x-ray. However, if the duct is clear, the tube should be clamped overnight to make certain that the ductal system is functional; if no symptoms appear, the tube can be pulled out the next morning.

Two methods have recently been developed for treating retained stones found on postoperative T tube cholangiograms. One technic is based on the ability of bile salt solutions to resolubilize cholesterol and is not useful for treating pigment stones. Sodium cholate solution (100 mM/liter, pH 7.5) is infused at a rate of 30 ml/hour directly into the T tube. The solution bathes the stone and passes into the duodenum. Cholestyramine resin (Cuemid, Questran), 4 g every 2 hours is given orally to bind the bile salts in the intestine and prevent diarrhea. If the retained stones are obstructing the duct, the solution can be administered into the vicinity of the stone through a small catheter passed through the lumen of the T tube and positioned under radiologic control. The cholate solution runs out

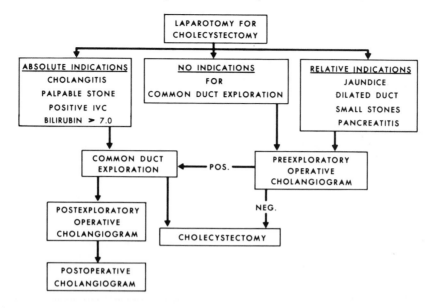

FIG 27–10. Diagnostic and therapeutic management of choledocholithiasis.

the residual lumen of the T tube. This regimen has eliminated retained stones in about two-thirds of the cases treated so far. Heparin solutions have also achieved success when used in a similar way.

If the above method fails, an attempt can be made to extract the stones with a ureteral stone basket. About 1 month should be allowed to elapse after surgery for the tract of the T tube to fully mature. The T tube is then removed in the x-ray department, and, using image intensification fluoroscopy, a ureteral stone basket is passed down the tract into the duct·and the wire cage expanded to trap the stone. The apparatus is drawn backward, and the stone will usually lodge within its grasp so that it can be extracted. Improvements in the success rate of this method can be expected with refinements in instrumentation and greater experience.

Doran FSA: The sites to which pain is referred from the common bile-duct and its implication for the theory of referred pain. Brit J Surg 54:599–606, 1967.

Way LW: Retained common duct stones. S Clin North America, Oct 1973.

Way LW & others: Management of choledocholithiasis. Ann Surg 176:347–359, 1972.

ACUTE SUPPURATIVE (OBSTRUCTIVE) CHOLANGITIS

Acute suppurative cholangitis is a severe form of biliary infection in which gross pus is present in the obstructed bile ducts. In most cases the obstruction is due to common duct stones, but examples have been reported with obstructing neoplasms, stricture, and ampullary stenosis. The evolution of suppurative cholangitis involves the same factors as the more common nonsuppurative form. The progression to pus formation and greater clinical toxicity depends on more complete biliary obstruction, more virulent organisms, lower patient resistance, or a combination of these factors.

Clinical Findings

The diagnostic pentad in suppurative cholangitis consists of abdominal pain, jaundice, fever and chills, mental confusion or lethargy, and shock. Jaundice may be mild, and the serum bilirubin is often only slightly abnormal (2–5 mg/100 ml). In some elderly patients, fever and leukocyte count may not be striking. In many instances, the significance of the mental changes goes unrecognized. For all these reasons, the diagnosis in acute suppurative cholangitis is frequently missed until it is too late to save the patient. Several studies have pointed to the positive correlation between an accurate clinical diagnosis and patient salvage.

A. Symptoms: The patients complain of severe abdominal pain, usually in the right upper quadrant but sometimes in other areas where biliary colic is referred. Fever is nearly always present and is often accompanied by chills. The temperature usually reaches levels of 39–40 C (102.2–104 F). Clinical jaundice can be detected in over half of patients.

Mental confusion, lethargy, or somnolence is a characteristic feature of suppurative cholangitis which must be appreciated as indicative of the overwhelming nature of the infection. The significance of the mental changes is often overlooked; suppurative cholangitis is not diagnosed; and insufficiently aggressive therapy leads to further deterioration in the patient's condition. Septic shock often supervenes and leads to death.

B. Signs: Physical examination of the abdomen usually reveals tenderness in the right subcostal region which may be quite marked. There may be rigidity of the abdominal wall, but this is not a frequent finding.

C. Laboratory Findings: The white blood count is usually above 15,000/μl. Serum bilirubin ranges from normal to 15 mg/100 ml. Blood cultures are nearly always positive and reveal the usual types of organisms found in biliary infections: gram-negative enteric bacilli, or, sometimes, *Staphylococcus aureus.* Thrombocytopenia develops at the height of the illness but does not contribute to complications and needs no direct therapy. Hypoglycemia appears in some patients and may be at least partly responsible for the mental changes.

Differential Diagnosis

Amebic or bacterial abscesses of the liver may cause findings similar to those of acute suppurative cholangitis. Pleural fluid above the liver in acute abscess may suggest the proper diagnosis, and hepatic scan may provide further support. In some cases, the distinction between suppurative cholangitis may be impossible without direct operative exploration.

Pylephlebitis due to sepsis remote from the liver could mimic this disorder, but pylephlebitis has become a rare condition. Knowledge of the presence of infection elsewhere in the abdomen would suggest pylephlebitis.

Treatment

The treatment of suppurative cholangitis should consist of circulatory resuscitation, preoperative preparation, and emergency laparotomy. Nonoperative treatment carries an unacceptable mortality. The most critically ill patients are those in greatest need of operation.

Initial measures are the general steps important in management of any critically ill patient with sepsis. Intravenous fluids and electrolytes should be infused. Circulatory dynamics should be monitored by a central venous pressure line and by serial determinations of blood pressure and pulse. The hourly urine output should be measured via an indwelling urinary catheter.

Parenteral antibiotics must be started as soon as possible. At present, optimal regimens for the usual causative organisms are ampicillin, 4 g IV daily, and kanamycin, 15 mg/kg IM daily, or ampicillin with gentamicin (2–4 mg/kg daily). Whole blood, albumin, plasma, and crystalloid solutions should be given to establish and maintain circulatory stability and a normal urinary flow. Digitalis or isoproterenol may be required if cardiac failure develops as it so often does in these aged patients. Some observers have suggested that intravenous administration of hypertonic glucose in amounts sufficient to correct hypoglycemia may improve the outcome.

These preoperative measures can usually be accomplished within several hours after admission to the hospital, at which point laparotomy should be performed as an emergency. The principal objective is to relieve the pressure within the common duct proximal to the obstruction. The most direct method is to perform a choledochotomy; this is more successful than attempted decompression via cholecystostomy. When the choledochotomy incision is made, pressure in the duct may cause the pus to spurt out. The duct should be irrigated with saline solution until all the pus is washed out. If the patient were moribund or rapidly deteriorating before operation, simple cleansing of the duct and insertion of a T tube would suffice. On the other hand, if the patient's condition were stable, thorough exploration and removal of the gallstones may be performed. In some patients, cholecystectomy should be done after exploration of the duct, but the life of the patient should not be jeopardized by prolonging the operation when decompression of the pus is really all that is required to treat the acute illness.

Dow RW, Lindenauer SM: Acute obstructive suppurative cholangitis. Ann Surg 169:272–276, 1969.

Hinchey EJ, Couper CE: Acute obstructive suppurative cholangitis. Am J Surg 117:62–68, 1969.

GALLSTONE PANCREATITIS

Pancreatitis is covered comprehensively in Chapter 28, but a few remarks on pancreatitis associated with biliary disease are in order here.

The diagnosis of pancreatitis may be considered with biliary disease in clinical situations where either biliary or pancreatic symptoms predominate. In the former group are patients with obvious acute cholecystitis or acute cholangitis associated with an elevated serum amylase but in whom no additional symptoms or signs point specifically to pancreatitis. The mechanism by which the amylase rises in these patients is not entirely clear because at operation the pancreas often looks normal. Intermittent obstruction of the pancreatic duct by stones in the hepatopancreatic ampulla is sometimes the cause of pancreatitis. However, when the patient presents with acute biliary disease and an increased serum amylase, common duct stones are present in less than half of cases.

On the other hand, some patients present with classic symptoms and signs of acute pancreatitis. After the acute attack subsides, gallstones can be detected in about half of these patients—either in the gallbladder alone or in the gallbladder and common duct.

Gallstones are often etiologically associated with acute pancreatitis or acute relapsing pancreatitis but rarely with chronic pancreatitis. Pancreatic calcification, steatorrhea, and chronic pain are uncommon complications of gallstone pancreatitis. Even after a number of acute attacks over many years, the pancreas usually appears normal at operation.

In acute gallstone pancreatitis, secondary complications such as hemorrhagic necrosis, pseudocyst, or abscess may ensue but are decidedly less common than after alcoholic pancreatitis. In fact, many of the most severe cases of pancreatitis are seen with alcoholism and gallstones combined as etiologic factors. This accounts for some of the variation in morbidity and mortality of gallstone pancreatitis as reported in the literature; greater morbidity is evident in series from municipal hospitals than from private hospitals.

The usual outcome of the patient with gallstone pancreatitis is complete cure if the biliary disease has been appropriately treated surgically. Cholecystectomy and common duct exploration are usually performed, although choledochotomy can sometimes be avoided if an operative cholangiogram is normal. In rare instances, pancreatitis follows fibrosis of the sphincter of Oddi. These patients have been helped by duodenotomy and sphincterotomy.

Howard JM, Ehrlich EW: Gallstone pancreatitis: A clinical entity. Surgery 51:177–184, 1962.

Searles H & others: Observations on 205 confirmed cases of acute pancreatitis, recurring pancreatitis. Gut 6:545–559, 1965.

ORIENTAL CHOLANGIOHEPATITIS

Oriental cholangiohepatitis is a type of chronic recurrent cholangitis that is prevalent in coastal areas from Japan to Southeast Asia. In Hong Kong it is the third most common indication for emergency laparotomy and the most frequent type of biliary disease. The disease is endemic in areas in Asia where parasitic infestation of the biliary tract is common. *Clonorchis sinensis* in southern regions and *Ascaris lumbricoides* to the north invade the extrahepatic bile ducts of many individuals. This apparently creates an inflammatory process that becomes secondarily infected with enteric bacilli. Calcium bilirubinate stones are formed by mechanisms described earlier in the chapter. Since malaria is prevalent in some of these areas, increased bilirubin pigment excretion may be an aggravating factor in producing stones.

Clinical Findings

The patient presents with acute abdominal pain in the right upper quadrant. Chills and high fever are usually present and jaundice develops in about half of the cases. Recurrent attacks are the rule.

On physical examination the patient may be severely toxic, but this is not invariably the case. Right upper quadrant tenderness is usually marked, and in about 80% of cases the gallbladder is palpable.

Laboratory studies show an increased bilirubin concentration and other changes typical of biliary obstruction. Leukocytosis of 15,000/μl or more is usual. Oral or intravenous biliary x-rays will not visualize during an acute attack. In Hong Kong over 90% of patients have ova for *Clonorchis sinensis* in their stool

In contrast with cholesterol cholelithiasis, which starts in the gallbladder, Oriental cholangiohepatitis is primarily a disease of the bile ducts. Only 15% of patients with Oriental cholangiohepatitis have cholecystolithiasis. The gallbladder is usually distended and palpable during an acute attack because it is not chronically scarred. It sometimes becomes secondarily infected, and gangrenous changes are found at laparotomy in about 10%. Occasionally, the distended gallbladder ruptures and leads to severe bile peritonitis.

Chronic recurrent infection often leads to biliary strictures and hepatic abscess formation. The strictures are usually located in the intrahepatic bile ducts, and for some unknown reason the left lobe of the liver is more severely involved. Intrahepatic gallstones are common, and their surgical removal may be difficult or impossible.

Treatment

Systemic antibiotics should be given for an acute attack and the patient scheduled for laparotomy. The surgical treatment consists of cholecystectomy and common duct exploration. The common bile duct may be greatly enlarged and packed with stones. Adult clonorchis worms are often found in the duct and should be removed insofar as possible. Unless side-to-side choledochoduodenostomy is performed to facilitate emptying, recurrent disease is almost inevitable. Alternatively, transduodenal sphincteroplasty has been advocated by some.

Prognosis

Although some patients can be cured, prolonged morbidity from repeated infection is common and is almost unavoidable once strictures have appeared or the intrahepatic ducts have become packed with stones.

Fung J: Liver fluke infestation and cholangio-hepatitis. Brit J Surg 48:404, 1961.

Maki T & others: A reappraisal of surgical treatment for intrahepatic gallstones. Ann Surg 175:155–165, 1972.

Ong GB: A study of recurrent pyogenic cholangitis. Arch Surg 84:63–89, 1962.

SCLEROSING CHOLANGITIS

Sclerosing cholangitis is a rare chronic disease of unknown cause which is characterized by nonbacterial inflammatory narrowing of the bile ducts.

Many of the examples of sclerosing cholangitis have been reported in patients with other chronic inflammatory diseases of postulated autoimmune origin. About 25% have had ulcerative colitis. Other less commonly associated conditions are thyroiditis, retroperitoneal fibrosis, and mediastinal fibrosis. In most cases the entire biliary tree is affected by an inflammatory process which causes irregular partial obliteration of the lumen of the ducts. The woody-hard duct walls contain increased collagen and lymphoid elements and are thickened at the expense of the lumen.

Clinical Findings

A. Symptoms and Signs: The clinical onset usually consists of the gradual appearance of mild jaundice and pruritus. There may be a vague discomfort in the right upper quadrant, but true biliary colic is uncommon.

B. Laboratory Findings: Laboratory findings are typical of cholestasis. The total serum bilirubin averages about 4 mg/100 ml and rarely exceeds 10 mg/100 ml. The serum alkaline phosphatase concentration is usually very high. SGOT and SGPT levels are normal or only slightly increased. Eosinophils are sometimes prominent histologically in biopsies of the wall of the common duct.

C. X-Ray Findings and Liver Biopsy: The diagnosis cannot be made on clinical and laboratory data alone. Oral or intravenous cholangiography will not visualize the biliary anatomy, and transhepatic cholangiograms are usually unsuccessful because the ducts are too small to be entered with the percutaneous needle. Liver biopsy may show pericholangitis and bile stasis, but the changes are nonspecific. Therefore, an exact diagnosis is usually unobtainable without surgical exploration.

Differential Diagnosis

The differential diagnosis includes other causes of chronic cholestatic jaundice without cholangitis. Primary biliary cirrhosis, toxic hepatitis, cirrhosis, chronic active hepatitis, and primary tumors of the bile ducts will all enter into consideration.

Treatment

At operation the common bile duct is found to be thick-walled and firm to hard in consistency. There may be mild inflammatory edema and enlarged lymph nodes in the hepatoduodenal ligament. The lumen is usually so small that it is difficult to locate in the center of the thickened duct. By careful dissection, a pinpoint opening can be found which contains bile. Although only a fine probe can be inserted into the lumen at first, it will usually accept gradual dilatation to a Bakes size 4–6.

After the duct is opened, an operative cholangiogram should be obtained to verify the diagnosis and to determine the extent of the disease. Narrowing exists through all or at least a large portion of the ductal system. Irregularities may be present which create an x-ray picture which has been called beading. Although most patients have generalized disease, in one-third it affects only one portion of the biliary tree and other areas appear normal. Both isolated extrahepatic or intrahepatic involvement has been described.

Sclerosing cholangitis is a diffuse process that can be closely mimicked by certain desmoplastic primary biliary malignancies. Thus, **focal** strictures of the bile duct in the absence of previous surgery will usually be discovered to be due to a malignant tumor. Malignant neoplasms sometimes cause more diffuse narrowing which may be mistaken for sclerosing cholangitis. Because of this potential diagnostic pitfall, it is always advisable to biopsy the wall of the duct whenever either of these entities is suspected.

A T tube should be placed into the common duct after the lumen has been dilated and should be left in place for an extended period after surgery (eg, 12 months). Dramatic relief of pruritus and jaundice sometimes follows this procedure, and a few patients remain free of symptoms for years.

Systemic corticosteroids have been advocated, but it is not yet certain that they have a positive effect. Nevertheless, the present practice is to begin a regimen of prednisone, 30–40 mg/day orally, shortly after laparotomy and insertion of the T tube. This dosage is maintained for several months, gradually tapered downward over a year, and the drug is then withdrawn.

Prognosis

The natural history of sclerosing cholangitis is one of chronicity and unpredictable severity. Some patients seem to obtain nearly complete remission after treatment, but this is not common. Bacterial cholangitis may develop after operation if adequate drainage has not been established. In these cases, antibiotics will be required at intervals. Most patients experience the gradual evolution of secondary biliary cirrhosis after many years of mild to moderate jaundice and pruritus. Hepatic failure, ascites, or esophageal varices are late complications and may be lethal.

Bhathal PS, Powell LW: Primary intrahepatic obliterating cholangitis: A possible variant of sclerosing cholangitis. Gut 10:886–893, 1969.

Thorpe MEC & others: Primary sclerosing cholangitis, the biliary tree, and ulcerative colitis. Gut 8:435–448, 1967.

Warren KW & others: Primary sclerosing cholangitis. Am J Surg 111:23–38, 1966.

CARCINOMA OF THE GALLBLADDER

Carcinoma of the gallbladder is an uncommon neoplasm that appears in elderly patients, 80% of whom have cholelithiasis. Cholelithiasis may be an etiologic factor, for the risk of malignant degeneration correlates with the length of time gallstones have been present. The tumor is 3 times more common in women than in men, as one would expect from the association with gallstones.

Most primary tumors of the gallbladder are adenocarcinomas which appear histologically to be scirrhous (60%), papillary (25%), or mucoid (15%). Dissemination of the tumor occurs early by direct invasion of the liver and hilar structures and by metastases to the liver and lungs. Spread is virtually certain by the time symptoms appear.

Clinical Findings

The presenting complaint is of right upper quadrant pain similar to previous episodes of biliary colic but more persistent. Obstruction of the cystic duct by tumor sometimes initiates an attack of acute cholecystitis. Other cases are first seen after obstructive jaundice has resulted from secondary involvement of the common duct, and cholangitis may be present in these.

Physical examination will usually reveal a mass in the region of the gallbladder. If the patient has acute cholecystitis, the mass may not be recognized as a neoplasm. If cholangitis is the principal symptom, a palpable gallbladder would be an unusual finding with choledocholithiasis alone and should suggest gallbladder carcinoma.

Complications

Obstruction of the common duct may produce multiple intrahepatic abscesses. Abscesses in or next to the tumor-laden gallbladder are frequent complications.

Prevention

Prevention of adenocarcinoma of the gallbladder has been offered in the past as an argument for performing cholecystectomy in patients with asymptomatic cholelithiasis. The reasoning appears to be sound if used in relation to young patients with the disease.

Treatment

Few patients are benefited by treatment. Laparotomy should be performed if the diagnosis is suspected, but spread usually rules out the possibility of a curative surgical resection. However, if conditions appear favorable, partial hepatectomy should be performed encompassing the tumor. The few reported survivors have generally had the gallbladder tumor discovered incidentally after cholecystectomy for chronic cholecystitis.

Prognosis

Radiotherapy and chemotherapy are not effective palliative agents. About 90% of patients are dead within a year after diagnosis.

Hardy MA, Volk H: Primary carcinoma of the gallbladder. Am J Surg 120:800–803, 1970.

Hart J & others: Cholelithiasis in the aetiology of gallbladder neoplasms. Lancet 1:1151–1153, 1971.

Litwin MS: Primary carcinoma of the gallbladder. Arch Surg 95:236–240, 1967.

MALIGNANT TUMORS OF THE BILE DUCT

Essentials of Diagnosis

- Cholestatic jaundice.
- Biliary colic or cholangitis (rare).
- Transhepatic cholangiogram usually diagnostic.

General Considerations

Primary malignant tumors of the bile duct are even less common than adenocarcinoma of the gallbladder. Unlike the latter, bile duct tumors are not more common in patients with cholelithiasis, and men and women are affected with equal frequency. Several hepatobiliary diseases, including malignant bile duct tumors, are found with greater frequency in ulcerative colitis, but it is not certain whether colectomy would prevent them. Chronic parasitic infestation of the bile ducts in the Orient may be responsible for the greater incidence of bile duct tumors in that area.

Most malignant biliary tumors are adenocarcinomas located in the hepatic or common bile duct. The histologic pattern varies from typical adenocarcinoma to tumors composed principally of fibrous stroma and few cells. The acellular tumors may be mistaken for benign strictures or sclerosing cholangitis if adequate biopsies are not obtained.

Clinical Findings

A. Symptoms and Signs: The illness presents with gradual onset of jaundice or pruritus. Chills, fever, and biliary colic are usually absent, and except for a deep discomfort in the right upper quadrant the patient feels well. Bilirubinuria is present from the start, and light-colored stools are usual. Anorexia and weight loss develop insidiously with time.

Icterus is the most obvious physical finding. If the tumor is confined to the common duct, the gallbladder distends and becomes palpable in the right upper quadrant. Patients with tumors of the hepatic or cystic ducts do not develop palpable gallbladders. If obstruction is unrelieved, the liver may become cirrhotic and splenomegaly, ascites, or bleeding varices become secondary manifestations.

B. Laboratory Findings: Since the duct is often completely obstructed, the serum bilirubin is usually over 15 mg/100 ml. Serum alkaline phosphatase, leucine aminopeptidase, and 6'-nucleotidase are also increased. Fever and leukocytosis are not common since the bile is sterile in most cases. Urobilinogen excretion is reduced in both urine and feces. The stool may contain occult blood, but this is more common with tumors of the pancreas or hepatopancreatic ampulla than those of the bile ducts.

C. X-Ray Findings: The upper gastrointestinal series occasionally shows impingement upon the duodenum. Oral or intravenous cholangiography is usually of no value because of the high-grade obstruction. On the other hand, transhepatic cholangiograms clearly depict the block.

Differential Diagnosis

The differential diagnosis must consider other causes of extrahepatic and intrahepatic cholestatic jaundice. Choledocholithiasis is characterized by intermittent partial obstruction and cholangitis which contrasts sharply with the unremitting but painless jaundice of malignant obstruction. Dilatation of the gallbladder characterizes tumors, whereas the gallbladder is usually too scarred to dilate with calculous obstruction.

The combination of an enlarged gallbladder with obstructive jaundice is usually recognized as due to tumor. If the gallbladder cannot be felt, primary biliary cirrhosis, drug-induced jaundice, chronic active hepatitis, metastatic hepatic malignancy, and common duct stone must be ruled out. As a general rule, whenever one is faced with cholestatic jaundice, no fever, and a normal upper gastrointestinal series, a transhepatic cholangiogram and liver biopsy should be seriously considered. If an extrahepatic tumor is present, the percutaneous cholangiogram will usually show it. If the patient is still undiagnosed after an evaluation which included an unsuccessful transhepatic cholangiogram, exploratory laparotomy is usually indicated if jaundice has been present for more than 3–4 weeks and is not improving. The chances of finding a mechanical occlusion are good.

Treatment

Jaundice appears early, but even so the tumor usually involves contiguous structures or has metastasized so that surgical cure is rarely possible. Nevertheless, laparotomy is indicated and substantial palliation may follow procedures to relieve the obstruction.

Tumors of the distal common duct should be treated by radical pancreaticoduodenectomy (Whipple procedure) if it appears that all of the tumor would be removed. Secondary involvement of the portal vein is the usual reason for unresectability for tumors in this location. If the tumor cannot be excised, bile flow should be reestablished into the intestine by means of cholecystojejunostomy, side-to-side choledochoduodenostomy, or Roux-en-Y choledochojejunostomy. The first 2 are used more often than the latter because they are technically easier.

Mid common duct or hepatic duct tumors should also be removed if possible. Otherwise, palliative procedures for unobstructing the flow of bile should be performed.

Tumors at the junction of the hepatic ducts may not be obvious to gross inspection when the abdomen is first explored. The gallbladder and common duct are normal in caliber, and the initial impression may be that the block is intrahepatic. It is important to identify these bifurcation tumors because permanent insertion of a T tube stent has resulted in survival for several years.

Prognosis

The average patient with adenocarcinoma of the bile duct may survive a year or so. Biliary cirrhosis, intrahepatic infection, and general debility with terminal pneumonitis are the usual causes of death. Palliative measures play an important role in improving the length and quality of survival even though surgical cure is rare.

Ham JM, Mackenzie DC: Primary carcinoma of the extrahepatic bile ducts. Surg Gynec Obst 118:977–983, 1964.

Klatskin G: Adenocarcinoma of the hepatic duct at its bifurcation within the porta hepatis. Am J Med 38:241–256, 1965.

Morowitz DA & others: Carcinoma of the biliary tract complicating chronic ulcerative colitis. Cancer 27:356–361, 1971.

Terblanche J & others: Prolonged palliation in carcinoma of the main hepatic duct junction. Surgery 71:720–731, 1972.

van Heerden JA & others: Carcinoma of the extrahepatic bile ducts. Am J Surg 113:49–56, 1967.

BENIGN TUMORS & PSEUDOTUMORS OF THE GALLBLADDER

Various unrelated lesions appear on the cholecystogram as projections from the gallbladder wall. The distinction from gallstones depends on whether a shift in position follows changes in posture of the patient since stones are not fixed.

Polyps

Most of these are not true neoplasms but cholesterol polyps, a local form of cholesterosis. Histologically, they consist of a cluster of lipid-filled macrophages in the submucosa. They become easily detached from the wall when the gallbladder is handled at surgery. It is not known whether cholesterol polyps are important in the genesis of gallstones. Some patients experience gallbladder pain, but whether this is related to the presence of the polyps per se or is a manifestation of functional gallbladder disease has not been established.

Inflammatory polyps have also been reported, but they are quite rare.

Adenomatous Hyperplasia

This entity presents as a slight intraluminal convexity on cholecystography which is often marked by a central umbilication. It is usually found in the fundus but may occur elsewhere. Adenomatous hyperplasia is now thought to represent a developmental abnormality and might be classified as a hamartoma rather than a neoplasm. The following synonyms for this lesion appear in the literature: adenomyomatosis, cholecystitis glandularis proliferans, and diverticulosis of the gallbladder. A number of patients with adenomatous hyperplasia have been relieved of abdominal discomfort by cholecystectomy, but the condition is probably asymptomatic in most cases.

Adenomas

These appear as pedunculated adenomatous polyps, true neoplasms which may be papillary or nonpapillary histologically. In a few cases they have been found in association with carcinoma in situ of the gallbladder.

Christensen AH, Ishak KG: Benign tumors and pseudotumors of the gallbladder. Arch Path 90:423–432, 1970.

Jutras JA, Levesque HP: Adenomyoma and adenomyomatosis of the gallbladder. Radiol Clin North America 4:483–500, 1966.

BENIGN TUMORS OF
THE BILE DUCTS

Benign papillomas and adenomas may arise from the ductal epithelium. Only 90 cases have been reported to date. The neoplastic propensity of the ductal epithelium is widespread, so the tumors are often multiple and recurrence is common after excision. The affected duct must be radically excised for permanent cure to result.

Burhans R, Myers RT: Benign neoplasms of the extrahepatic biliary ducts. Am Surgeon 37:161–166, 1971.

BILIARY STRICTURE

Essentials of Diagnosis

- Episodic cholangitis.
- Previous biliary surgery.
- Transhepatic cholangiogram often diagnostic.

General Considerations

Benign biliary strictures are caused by surgical trauma in about 95% of cases. The remainder result from external abdominal trauma or, rarely, from erosion of the duct by a gallstone. Prevention of injury to the duct depends on a combination of technical skill, experience, and a thorough knowledge of the normal anatomy and its variations in the hilum of the liver. Biliary stricture was more frequent in the past when many cholecystectomies were performed by incompletely trained surgeons.

The varieties of injury consist of transection, incision, excision of a segment, or occlusion of the duct by a ligature. The accident can sometimes be attributed to technical difficulties presented by advanced disease. The surgeon may or may not recognize immediately that he has damaged the duct. If he finds that it has been transected, an end-to-end anastomosis should be performed with insertion of a T tube through a nearby choledochotomy. However, the injury often goes unnoticed.

Clinical Findings

A. Symptoms: Manifestations of injury to the duct may or may not be evident in the postoperative period. If complete occlusion has been produced, jaundice will develop rapidly, but more often a rent has been made in the side of the duct and the earliest sign is excessive or prolonged drainage of bile from the abdominal drains.

Depending on the severity of the trauma and the amount of aggravating infection, cholangitis develops within 2 weeks or as late as a year or more after the operation. However, it is rare that more than 2 years separate the trauma and its initial symptoms.

In the typical case, the patient has episodic pain, fever, chills, and mild jaundice within a few weeks to months after cholecystectomy. Antibiotics are usually successful in controlling symptoms, but additional attacks occur at irregular intervals. The pattern of symptoms varies between patients from mild transient attacks to severe toxicity with suppurative cholangitis.

Documentation of an operative injury is sometimes available, and there may even have been previous operative procedures for stricture. When cholangitis develops in either of these types of patients, a diagnosis of recurrence of stricture is virtually certain.

B. Signs: Physical findings are not distinctive. The right upper quadrant may be tender but usually is not. Jaundice is usually present during an attack of cholangitis.

C. Laboratory Findings: The alkaline phosphatase, leucine aminopeptidase, and 5'-nucleotidase are elevated in most cases. The bilirubin fluctuates in relation to symptoms but usually remains below 10 mg/100 ml.

Blood cultures may be positive during acute cholangitis.

D. X-Ray Findings: An intravenous cholangiogram may outline the stricture if the study can be done at a time when the bilirubin is normal. In other cases, transhepatic cholangiograms have been necessary. Failure to enter the intrahepatic bile ducts when attempting a transhepatic cholangiogram would not rule out stricture as the cause of symptoms.

Differential Diagnosis

Choledocholithiasis is the condition which most often must be differentiated from biliary stricture because the clinical and laboratory findings can be identical. A history of trauma to the duct would point toward stricture as the more likely diagnosis. The final distinction must await radiologic or surgical findings in many instances. An intravenous cholangiogram or, if that fails, a transhepatic cholangiogram may answer the question. If not, laparotomy is probably indicated once episodic cholangitis has been verified.

Other causes of cholestatic jaundice may have to be ruled out in some cases.

Complications

Complications develop if the stricture is not corrected. Persistent cholangitis may progress to multiple intrahepatic abscesses and a septic death.

Other patients gradually develop portal hypertension and esophageal varices over many years. When portal hypertension has developed, operations in the hilum of the liver are bloody and technical problems are often insurmountable. A prophylactic splenorenal shunt should be performed and the stricture repair scheduled for several months later.

Treatment

Strictures of the bile duct should be surgically repaired in all but the few patients whose poor general condition dictates a nonoperative approach. Symptomatic treatment with antibiotics should be used to control acute cholangitis, but long-term antibiotic treatment is not recommended as a definitive regimen. Although the attacks may regularly respond to antibiotics, this therapy does not protect the liver from the damaging effect of the partial biliary obstruction, and, if uncorrected, secondary biliary cirrhosis or hepatic failure will gradually develop.

The surgical procedure should be selected on the basis of technical considerations presented by the individual patient. The general goals of the repair should be to reestablish biliary flow by anastomosing normal duct from the hepatic side of the stricture to either the intestine or the residual normal duct below the stricture. Excision of the strictured segment and end-to-end repair may seem the simplest solution but frequently entails more technical problems than connecting the proximal duct directly to the intestine. The duct can be reimplanted into the duodenum or a Roux-en-Y loop of jejunum. In the average case, Roux-en-Y hepaticojejunostomy is most likely to provide a suitable anastomosis without tension.

Prognosis

The death rate from biliary stricture is about 10–15%, and the morbidity is high. If the stricture is not repaired, episodic cholangitis and secondary liver disease are inevitable.

Surgical correction of the stricture is successful in about 75% of cases. Experience at centers with a special interest in this problem indicates that good results can be obtained even if several previous attempts did not relieve the obstruction. In general, therefore, if a stricture is present, the patient should be considered for correction despite a history of surgical failure.

Longmire WP Jr: Early management of injury to the extrahepatic biliary tract. JAMA 195:111–113, 1966.

Sedgwick CE & others: Management of portal hypertension secondary to bile duct strictures. Ann Surg 163:949–953, 1966.

Smith R: Strictures of the bile ducts. Progr Surg 9:147–175, 1971.

Way LW, Dunphy JE: Biliary stricture. Am J Surg 124: 287–295, 1972.

POSTCHOLECYSTECTOMY SYNDROME

This term has been used to designate the heterogeneous group of patients who continue to complain of symptoms after cholecystectomy. It is not really a syndrome and the term is confusing.

The usual reason why relief is incomplete after cholecystectomy is that the preoperative diagnosis of chronic cholecystitis was incorrect. The only symptom entirely characteristic of chronic cholecystitis is biliary colic. When a calculous gallbladder is removed in the hope that patients will gain relief from dyspepsia, fatty food intolerance, belching, etc, the operation will often leave the symptoms unchanged. The amount of scarring in the gallbladder wall correlates fairly well with the extent of symptomatic improvement after cholecystectomy; patients with vague postoperative complaints are more likely to have had a thin-walled, unscarred organ or a gallbladder without stones.

In other cases, an organic diagnosis has been overlooked during the preoperative evaluation. Pancreatitis, peptic ulcer, gastritis, or esophagitis may have actually been the origin of symptoms attributed to the gallstones. These possibilities should be reinvestigated when symptoms persist.

Choledocholithiasis or biliary stricture is sometimes responsible for abdominal pain after cholecystectomy. Liver function studies and an intravenous cholangiogram should be obtained. One normal intravenous cholangiogram does not eliminate the possibility of a common duct stone; in suspicious cases the above studies should be repeated, and in some cases a transhepatic cholangiogram is indicated.

Stenosis of the hepatobiliary ampulla, a long cystic duct remnant, and neuromas are other conditions that have been blamed for continued symptoms, but well-verified cases are uncommon.

Cattell RB & others: Stenosis of the sphincter of Oddi. New England J Med 256:429–435, 1957.

Christiansen J, Schmidt A: The postcholecystectomy syndrome. Acta chir scandinav 137:789–793, 1971.

Cole WH, Grove WJ: Persistence of symptoms following cholecystectomy with special reference to anomalies of the ampulla of Vater. Ann Surg 136:73–82, 1952.

Glenn F: Postcholecystectomy choledocholithiasis. Surg Gynec Obst 134:249–252, 1972.

● ● ●

General References

Kune GA: *Current Practice of Biliary Surgery.* Little, Brown, 1972.

Schein CJ: *Acute Cholecystitis.* Harper, 1972.

28 . . .

The Pancreas

Rayford Scott Jones, MD

EMBRYOLOGY

The pancreas first appears in embryos of 4 mm at the fourth week of gestation by the protrusion of a dorsal and a ventral pouch from the duodenal ento-derm. The dorsal pancreas grows more rapidly and by the sixth week has extended into the dorsal mesentery. The ventral pancreas grows out from the foregut along the primitive common bile duct. When the gut elon-gates and rotates, the 2 pancreatic primordia fuse; the tail, body, and part of the head of the pancreas are formed by the dorsal pancreas; the remainder of the uncinate process and head are derived from the ventral pancreas. The ductal systems of the dorsal and ventral pancreatic rudiments fuse, so that the distal dorsal duct joins the ventral duct to form the duct of Wirsung. The proximal portion of the dorsal duct becomes the accessory pancreatic duct (of Santorini) in the adult. Thus, the main pancreatic duct usually enters the duodenum with the common bile duct because of their common origin from the ventral pan-creas. The pancreatic acini develop in the third month. At about the same time, the islets of Langerhans become differentiated from the ducts of the dorsal pancreas.

GROSS ANATOMY

The pancreas is an oblong, firm, lobulated glandu-lar structure with an indistinct fibrous covering, lying obliquely across the upper abdomen retroperitoneally. It may be divided into several portions: the head, neck, body, and tail. The head of the pancreas is in contact with the left side of the duodenum and, posteriorly, the inferior vena cava, the right renal vein, and the right crus of the diaphragm. The stomach and the first part of the duodenum are anterior. The common bile duct passes in a groove in the head of the pancreas and occasionally passes through the substance of the pan-creas. Posteriorly, the neck of the pancreas lies over the superior mesenteric vein and the portal vein, while the body is in contact with the aorta; the superior mesenteric artery, the left crus of the diaphragm, the left adrenal gland, and the left kidney. The tail of the pancreas lies in the hilum of the spleen. The main pan-creatic duct (the duct of Wirsung) passes from left to right and joins the common bile duct before entering the ampulla. The accessory pancreatic duct (of San-torini) enters the duodenum approximately 2–2.5 cm proximal to the ampulla of Vater (Fig 28–1).

The blood supply of the pancreas is derived from branches of the celiac axis and the superior mesenteric artery. The superior pancreaticoduodenal artery is a branch of the gastroduodenal artery, which arises from the hepatic artery. The inferior pancreaticoduodenal artery arises from the superior mesenteric artery. The head of the pancreas is supplied by an arterial arcade formed by anastomoses between the superior and inferior pancreaticoduodenal arteries. The splenic artery supplies the body and the tail of the pancreas; the larger branches are called the dorsal pancreatic, pancreatica magna, and the caudal pancreatic arteries. The venous drainage of the pancreas parallels the arterial supply. The lymphatic drainage is into peri-pancreatic nodes which correspond in location to the direction of venous drainage (Fig 28–2).

The visceral efferent innervation of the pancreas is through the vagus and splanchnic nerves. The efferent fibers of the vagi pass to the celiac plexus through the celiac branch of the right vagus nerve to terminate in parasympathetic ganglia in the interlobu-lar septa of the gland. Postganglionic fibers then innervate the acini, islets, and ducts. The sympathetic nerves pass to the celiac plexus where they synapse with postganglionic fibers passing into the gland to innervate primarily the blood vessels. The visceral afferent fibers from the pancreas probably pass into the splanchnic nerves.

Silen W: Surgical anatomy of the pancreas. S Clin North Amer-ica 44:1253–1262, 1964.

PHYSIOLOGY

Pancreatic exocrine secretion may reach approxi-mately 1 liter per day and is a clear alkaline fluid characterized by a high inorganic electrolyte content as well as a high protein content, the protein being pre-dominantly enzymes. The flow of water and bicarbon-ate transports the pancreatic enzymes from the acini through the ducts into the duodenum. The bicarbonate

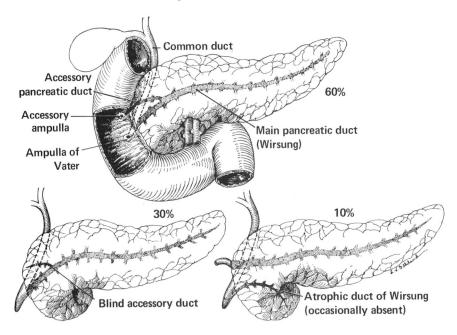

FIG 28–1. Anatomic configuration of intrapancreatic ductal system. (Reproduced, with permission, from Silen W: Surgical anatomy of the pancreas. S Clin North America 44:1253–1262, 1964.)

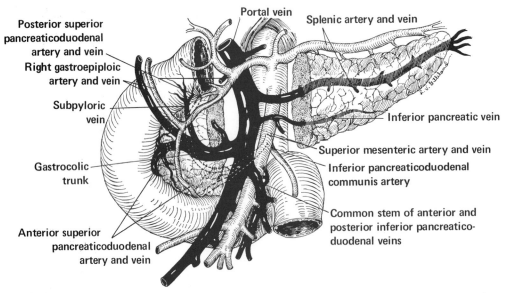

FIG 28–2. Arterial supply and venous drainage of the pancreas. (Reproduced, with permission, from Silen W: Surgical anatomy of the pancreas. S Clin North America 44:1253–1262, 1964.)

is important because most pancreatic enzymes have optimal activity at an alkaline pH.

Water & Electrolyte Secretion

The principal anion in pancreatic juice is bicarbonate. The bicarbonate concentration in pancreatic juice during secretion at low flow rates may be approximately 20 mEq/liter. As the secretory rate increases, the bicarbonate concentration of the juice increases to approximately 150 mEq/liter. As flow increases,

chloride concentration decreases, so that over a fairly wide range of flow rates there is a reciprocal relationship between chloride and bicarbonate concentrations in pancreatic juice, the sum of the concentrations of the 2 anions remaining fairly constant. Sodium and potassium concentrations in pancreatic juice are approximately the same as in plasma, while calcium concentrations vary from 0.1–5 mEq/liter.

The water, bicarbonate, and chloride of pancreatic juice are probably secreted by the centro-acinar cells. The most plausible explanation for secretion of the anions postulates that bicarbonate is secreted by the centro-acinar cells and is exchanged for chloride as the secretion passes through the ducts.

Enzyme Secretion

The protein content of pancreatic juice varies from 0.1–10% and is comprised mostly of enzymes. The proteolytic enzymes of pancreatic juice are endopeptidases or exopeptidases. The endopeptidases—trypsins, chymotrypsins, and elastases—split central peptide bonds; the exopeptidases—carboxypeptidases A and B—cleave terminal bonds of peptides or proteins. Thus, the pancreatic proteolytic enzymes act together to hydrolyze proteins to peptide fragments and then to amino acids.

The pancreatic proteolytic enzymes are secreted as inactive precursors. The intestinal mucosal enzyme enterokinase converts trypsinogen to trypsin, the active enzyme. Trypsin can activate trypsinogen and all the other proteolytic precursor enzymes. The pancreatic proteolytic enzymes are active at pH 7.5 or higher. Pancreatic juice also contains polypeptides which are trypsin inhibitors.

Pancreatic lipase is secreted in the active form and splits dietary triglycerides. Lipase activity is enhanced by Ca^{++} and bile salts.

Pancreatic amylase, also secreted in active form, hydrolyzes starch. The optimal pH for this process is about 6.9. Amylase binds Ca^{++} in large quantities, and Ca^{++} is required for amylase activity.

The synthesis of pancreatic enzymes is very rapid. Intravenously injected radioactively labeled amino acids may be found in pancreatic enzymes 1–2 minutes following injection. Such studies reveal that pancreatic enzymes may be synthesized and appear in pancreatic juice within an hour.

Control of Pancreatic Exocrine Secretion

Pancreatic exocrine secretion is stimulated by secretin, cholecystokinin, gastrin, and acetylcholine (Table 28–1). Secretin stimulates a copious secretion of water and electrolytes, principally Na^+ and HCO_3^-, from the pancreas, while cholecystokinin and acetylcholine principally stimulate pancreatic enzymes. Gas-

trin stimulates both water and enzyme output from the pancreas in dogs, but most evidence suggests it has little effect in man.

Secretin was discovered in 1902 and chemically characterized and synthesized in 1966. Secretin possesses 27 amino acid residues and has a molecular weight of 3056. The complete molecule is necessary for physiologic activity. Secretin is probably made in cells located at the base of intestinal villi.

Cholecystokinin and pancreozymin are now known to be the same 33-residue polypeptide called here cholecystokinin (CCK). The C-terminal tetrapeptide of CCK—tryptophanylmethionylaspartylphenylalanylamide—is identical to that of gastrin. Because of the similarities in structure, CCK shares many actions with gastrin but differs in potencies, having a much greater cholecystokinetic action.

Vagal stimulation causes increased pancreatic secretion by a direct cholinergic effect on the acinar cells and by releasing gastrin from the pyloric antrum. The vagi also stimulate the secretion of gastric acid, which then releases secretin from the duodenal mucosa.

The intestine regulates pancreatic secretion by releasing secretin and cholecystokinin. Secretin is released by hydrogen ions, and the amount released is dependent upon the amount of titratable acid in the lumen and the length of the intestinal segment acidified. CCK is released by fat or amino acids in the intestine. There is some evidence that the release of secretin and CCK is under cholinergic control. When CCK and secretin are administered simultaneously, potentiation of pancreatic secretion occurs.

Pancreatic Endocrine Function

The islets of Langerhans of the pancreas produce 3 hormones: insulin, glucagon, and gastrin.

A. Insulin: The first of these hormones to be observed was insulin, which is synthesized and released from the beta cells of the islets of Langerhans. Insulin is a polypeptide composed of 51 amino acid residues and is formed by an A and a B chain, linked by 2 disulfide bonds. The complete synthesis of human insulin has been accomplished and represents the first chemical synthesis of a human protein. An insulin precursor called proinsulin liberates insulin after limited treatment with trypsin. Insulin secretion occurs during hyperglycemia, protein ingestion, and intravenous administration of amino acids. Calcium is necessary for the response to hyperglycemia, although calcium does not stimulate insulin release directly. Potassium stimulates insulin secretion, but only in the presence of calcium. Sodium is necessary for insulin release in response to stimulation by glucose, leucine, tolbutamide, or glucagon. Some evidence suggests that the adenyl cyclase system may mediate insulin release. ACTH, glucagon, secretin, CCK, and gastrin also cause insulin release. CNS stimulation releases insulin and is thought to be mediated by the vagus nerve.

B. Glucagon: Glucagon is a 29 amino acid polypeptide which is secreted by the alpha cells of the islets

TABLE 28–1. Effect of primary stimulants of pancreatic secretion on flow and enzyme output.*

Stimulant	Effect on	
	Flow	Enzyme Output
Acetylcholine	+	++++
Secretin	++++	+?
Cholecystokinin	+	++++
Gastrin	+	+++

*Reproduced, with permission, from Grossman MI: Control of pancreatic secretion. In: *Symposium on the Exocrine Pancreas.* Churchill, 1971.

of Langerhans. An immunoreactive glucagon-like substance also has been identified in the gut. Glucagon is secreted in response to stimulation by pancreozymin, insulin, or amino acids. Glucagon activates hepatic phosphorylase, glycogenolysis, and gluconeogenesis. All of these actions elevate blood glucose. Glucagon also decreases hepatic glucose oxidation and incorporation into protein. Pharmacologic doses of glucagon stimulate the secretion of catecholamines from the human adrenal; this observation has prompted the use of glucagon as a provocative agent in the diagnosis of pheochromocytoma.

C. Gastrin: Recent immunofluorescent studies have detected gastrin in the islets of Langerhans. The physiologic significance of this finding is not known.

Davenport HW: *Physiology of the Digestive Tract,* 3rd ed. Yearbook, 1971.

Desnuelle P: Pancreatic lipase. Pages 2626–2636 in: *Handbook of Physiology.* Section 6, vol V. American Physiological Society, 1967.

Grossman MI: Control of pancreatic secretion. Pages 59–73 in: *Symposium on the Exocrine Pancreas.* Beck IT, Sinclair DG (editors). Churchill, 1971.

Hokin LE: Metabolic aspects and energetics of pancreatic secretion. Pages 935–953 in: *Handbook of Physiology,* Section 6, vol II. American Physiological Society, 1967.

Janowitz HD: Pancreatic secretion of fluid and electrolytes. Pages 925–933 in: *Handbook of Physiology.* Section 6, vol II. American Physiological Society, 1967.

Keller PJ: Pancreatic proteolytic enzymes. Pages 2605–2628 in: *Handbook of Physiology.* Section 6, vol V. American Physiological Society, 1967.

Mayhew DA, Wright PH, Ashmore J: Regulation of insulin secretion. Pharmacol Rev 21:183–212, 1969.

Semenza G: Pancreatic amylase. Pages 2637–2645 in: *Handbook of Physiology.* Section 6, vol V. American Physiological Society, 1967.

PANCREATITIS

The cause of pancreatitis is not known. Pancreatic ductal obstruction has been thought to be important, particularly during vigorous pancreatic stimulation. Arguments against this view are that pancreatic ductal obstruction does not exist in most patients with pancreatitis and that pancreatic ductal obstruction in man due to tumor or pancreatic ductal ligation does not usually cause pancreatitis.

Opie suggested in 1901 that the common channel formed by the union of the common bile duct and the duct of Wirsung allowed the reflux of bile into the pancreatic ductal system and initiated pancreatitis. This theory is weakened by the following: (1) Many patients with pancreatitis do not have a common channel. (2) Pressure in the pancreatic ducts is higher than in the bile ducts, making it unlikely that bile would flow into the pancreatic ducts. (3) Biliary-pancreatic reflux occurs commonly during T-tube cholangiog-

raphy without the development of pancreatitis. (4) Bile does not ordinarily activate pancreatic proteolytic enzymes.

More recent studies suggest that unconjugated bile salts may be toxic to the pancreas upon entering the pancreatic ducts. The finding of lysolecithin in the bile of patients with pancreatitis has led to the hypothesis that pancreatic phospholipase may convert biliary lecithin to lysolecithin, which may in turn damage the pancreas. Further information will be required to confirm or refute these 2 speculations.

It is generally believed that pancreatic enzymes cause the tissue destruction in pancreatitis. If so, they would require activation. A possible mechanism might be reflux of duodenal contents containing enterokinase into the pancreatic ducts during increased duodenal pressure, or the presence of a stone in the ampulla of Vater. However, most patients undergoing sphincteroplasty do not develop pancreatitis, and there is no direct evidence that duodenal juice does in fact enter the pancreatic ducts.

Bacteria are probably of minor importance in the causation of pancreatitis since acute pancreatitis can develop in germ-free animals.

Although the cause of pancreatitis is not known, there are well-defined clinical settings in which the disease occurs:

(1) Alcohol ingestion: A large proportion of patients with pancreatitis (60% in one county hospital) are alcoholics. The incidence of alcoholic pancreatitis is probably greater in larger city and county hospitals than in other institutions. Both acute and chronic pancreatitis occur in alcoholics, and most such patients will be in their 30s or 40s. Although alcohol probably stimulates pancreatic secretion, the way in which alcohol causes pancreatitis is unknown.

(2) Biliary tract disease: Cholelithiasis or choledocholithiasis are commonly associated with pancreatitis. Patients with pancreatitis due to biliary disease are generally somewhat older than those with alcoholic pancreatitis. The proportion of patients having pancreatitis associated with biliary disease varies from 30–60% depending upon the reporting institution.

(3) Hyperparathyroidism: As many as 19% of patients with primary hyperparathyroidism will develop pancreatitis. The mechanism is not understood, but it may be related to increased calcium concentration in the pancreatic juice.

(4) Familial pancreatitis: Several kindreds have been reported with pancreatitis, suggesting transmission of the disease as an autosomal dominant trait. Some of these families have also had aminoaciduria.

(5) Hyperlipidemia: Some patients with familial hyperlipidemia experience recurrent attacks of pancreatitis. The attacks in these patients are usually mild.

(6) Postoperative pancreatitis: Pancreatitis occasionally follows surgical procedures in the upper abdomen, particularly operations on the stomach or biliary system, and is fatal in about 20–40% of cases. Pancreatitis has also been reported following renal transplantation. Whether this is due to operative trauma, drugs, or other factors is not known.

(7) **Other factors:** In 10–20% of cases there is no associated predisposing condition, and these cases are called idiopathic pancreatitis. Administration of adrenal corticosteroids has been associated with pancreatitis. Pancreatitis has also complicated mumps.

1. ACUTE PANCREATITIS

Essentials of Diagnosis

- Abrupt onset of acute epigastric pain, often with back radiation.
- Nausea, vomiting, prostration, sweating.
- Abdominal tenderness and distention, fever.
- Leukocytosis, elevated serum and urinary amylase and lipase.
- History of previous episodes or alcoholic excess.
- Cholelithiasis (in many).

General Considerations

Pancreatitis is classified as acute, acute relapsing, or chronic, depending upon its natural history. Acute pancreatitis may appear as interstitial (edematous) pancreatitis or hemorrhagic pancreatitis. Acute hemorrhagic pancreatitis is the more severe form of the disease, occurs in the older age group, and is associated with an extremely high mortality rate. The pathologic features of pancreatitis are edema, the presence of inflammatory cells, hemorrhage, and necrosis. Acute pancreatitis is characterized by fat necrosis in the mesentery, omentum, and peripancreatic tissue. Fat necrosis occurs when pancreatic lipase splits fatty acids from fat which then combine with Ca^{++} to form insoluble soaps in the tissues.

Clinical Findings

A. Symptoms and Signs: The symptoms of acute pancreatitis are nausea and vomiting and severe upper abdominal pain. The onset of pain is usually rapid and it may radiate to the back. Some patients give a history suggesting biliary tract disease, and one should inquire if the patient is known to have gallstones. Many patients have a history of alcoholism and will have been on a binge before the onset of symptoms.

Physical examination usually reveals fever, tachycardia, and, in severe cases, hypotension. Patients with alcoholic pancreatitis may be inebriated and smell of alcohol. The eyes should be examined for scleral icterus. Chvostek's sign should be sought. Sometimes, there are physical findings of left pleural effusion. Inspection will reveal slight abdominal distention in most cases. One will rarely see the Grey Turner sign, a bluish discoloration in the flank, or the Cullen sign, a bluish periumbilical discoloration. These signs are associated with hemorrhagic necrosis in the abdomen or retroperitoneal area.

Palpation of the abdomen usually reveals marked epigastric tenderness. Because the pancreas is retroperitoneal in its position, abdominal rigidity is less than in a free perforation of a duodenal or gastric ulcer. Later, in severe cases, there may be marked rigidity with guarding and rebound tenderness. An upper abdominal mass is sometimes present, and the bowel sounds are usually quiet.

B. Laboratory Findings: Patients with acute pancreatitis may have an elevated hematocrit or BUN from dehydration, and leukocytosis is usually present.

An elevated serum amylase is the mainstay of the laboratory diagnosis of acute pancreatitis, and this test should be performed in all patients who present with upper abdominal pain of recent onset. The rise in serum amylase usually occurs within 24 hours of the onset of symptoms and begins to recede after several days. The test occasionally reaches high values in patients with choledocholithiasis, in which case increases in serum levels of alkaline phosphatase, leucine aminopeptidase, and bilirubin are also observed. The other conditions associated with increased serum amylase are: mumps, perforated peptic ulcer, excessive opiate administration, and strangulated intestinal obstruction.

The rate of urinary excretion of amylase also rises during acute pancreatitis. Urine should be collected over a known interval of hours and the result expressed as output per hour. This test complements measurement of serum concentrations and may be the only laboratory clue to the diagnosis. Diminished amylase excretion parallels reduction in creatinine clearance so that the status of renal function must be known when interpreting a normal urinary amylase value.

Serum lipase determination has been suggested as an alternative to amylase determination since elevations in its serum concentration are also relatively specific for pancreatitis. However, most clinical laboratories cannot perform this test within a reasonable period of time.

Mild elevations of serum bilirubin or alkaline phosphatase sometimes result from biliary obstruction by the inflammatory process in the head of the pancreas, but high levels generally indicate choledocholithiasis.

Hyperlipidemia may occur in acute pancreatitis in the absence of familial hyperlipidemia, but this phenomenon is usually transitory. Some authors believe that when hyperlipidemia occurs in alcoholic pancreatitis it may be due to fatty change in the liver.

The urine should be tested for specific gravity to aid in the assessment of dehydration.

C. X-Ray Findings: Chest x-ray may reveal left pleural effusion. Plain films of the abdomen may show signs of ileus. There is often a single dilated loop of small bowel—the so-called sentinel loop—which may suggest intestinal obstruction. There may be gas in the right and left colon with the transverse colon collapsed. If the patient has had prior attacks, pancreatic calcifications may be present. Also, one may find opaque gallstones on the plain films.

In patients with a serum bilirubin below about 3

mg/100 ml, an intravenous cholangiogram may aid in the diagnosis of biliary tract disease, particularly a common duct stone. Oral cholecystography is usually not helpful in acute pancreatitis because vomiting and ileus may prevent absorption of the contrast agent. The gallbladder may not concentrate the contrast material in acute pancreatitis. Bone lesions resembling infarcts have been reported in patients following attacks of pancreatitis.

Differential Diagnosis

Acute pancreatitis must be considered in the differential diagnosis of the acute abdomen, particularly common duct stone or perforated peptic ulcer.

Complications

Pancreatic abscess causes a rising fever, leukocytosis, and localized tenderness. Pseudocyst may develop. Diabetes mellitus is uncommon but may occur. Mild gastrointestinal bleeding may cause tests for occult blood in stool to turn positive; melena and secondary manifestations of blood loss may occur rarely.

Treatment

A. Medical Measures:

1. Fluid Replacement—One of the serious derangements occurring in patients with acute pancreatitis is fluid loss. Dehydration is caused by vomiting, loss of fluid into the bowel, retroperitoneal edema, and peritoneal as well as pleural effusion and is manifested by thirst, dry mucous membranes, poor skin turgor, and oliguria. Prerenal azotemia as well as tachycardia and hypotension may occur from the fluid deficit. Vigorous fluid replacement with saline, plasma, 5% dextrose in water, and in some instances blood, should be carried out while monitoring the central venous pressure, pulse, blood pressure, and urinary output. Serial measurements should be made of the hematocrit and serum creatinine.

2. Gastric suction—Patients with acute pancreatitis should be treated by withholding food and applying nasogastric suction. This eliminates vomiting and minimizes intestinal distention due to ileus. Nasogastric suction prevents gastric acid from entering the duodenum, although it is not known if secretin released from the duodenum aggravates acute pancreatitis.

3. Analgesics—Most patients with acute pancreatitis should receive liberal amounts of meperidine or other suitable narcotic for pain relief. In some instances, the anesthesiologist can provide pain relief by administering a celiac ganglion block or epidural anesthesia.

4. Antibiotics—The value of antibiotics in acute pancreatitis is not clearly established. Patients with coexisting cholelithiasis or choledocholithiasis may have bacterial infection and should receive antibiotics to prevent suppurative cholangitis. If the patient has a high fever and rising white blood cell counts, he should be treated with antibiotics, particularly if x-rays show a lesser sac mass.

5. Anticholinergic drugs—Anticholinergic drugs should reduce pancreatic secretion, but it is unclear whether they are of any definite therapeutic benefit. Clinical trials with the bovine trypsin inhibitor Trasylol have not revealed any significant improvement in patients receiving the drug compared with controls.

6. Calcium administration—Many patients with acute pancreatitis develop hypocalcemia, perhaps from precipitation of Ca^{++} in the abdominal fat. Alterations in the hormonal regulation of calcium may also be involved. Although it may be difficult to restore serum calcium to normal levels, the therapeutic objective should be the prevention of tetany and cardiac arrhythmias by calcium administration.

7. Observe for diabetes—Blood and urine glucose levels should be monitored, for some patients with acute pancreatitis develop diabetes.

8. Pulmonary insufficiency—Pulmonary insufficiency may occur and can be detected by monitoring of blood gas tensions.

B. Surgical Treatment: In most cases, the management of acute pancreatitis should consist of diligent supportive care as outlined above, and operation should be avoided. Surgery is indicated when the cause of the acute abdominal pain is in doubt. The clinical picture of other acute abdominal conditions may be indistinguishable from that of acute pancreatitis, and delay in abdominal exploration could be fatal.

Patients with acute pancreatitis and biliary calculi should be considered for surgical treatment, but the timing of surgery can be difficult. If the patient develops signs, symptoms, and laboratory findings of acute pancreatitis which begin to improve promptly, emergency surgery should be avoided and elective laparotomy performed when the acute episode has subsided. Other patients may develop pancreatitis which progresses with increasing jaundice and sepsis; operation is required to relieve the biliary obstruction. For additional comments on acute pancreatitis associated with cholelithiasis, see Chapter 29.

If pancreatic abscess is suspected, surgical exploration is indicated for drainage.

Prognosis

The mortality rates in acute pancreatitis vary from 8–20%. However, the mortality from acute hemorrhagic pancreatitis is approximately 80%.

See references on p 515.

CHRONIC PANCREATITIS

Essentials of Diagnosis

- Persistent or recurrent abdominal pain radiating to the back.
- Malabsorption and steatorrhea.
- Weight loss.
- Diabetes.
- Alcoholism in most.

Clinical Findings

A. Symptoms and Signs: Chronic pancreatitis is characterized by persistent or recurring abdominal pain which is usually severe, located in the epigastrium, and radiates to the back. Many patients with chronic pancreatitis develop pancreatic exocrine and endocrine insufficiency, resulting in diabetes and malabsorption, with steatorrhea.

B. Laboratory Findings:

1. Amylase—Serum and urinary amylase levels may be elevated, although repeated examinations may be necessary to demonstrate this.

2. Stool fat—Steatorrhea should be documented by measuring stool fat. If stool fat determinations are performed for 72 hours with the patient on a 100 g fat per day diet, the normal fecal fat excretion should not exceed 5 g/24 hours.

3. Secretin test—The secretin test is performed by inserting a double-lumen tube to collect the duodenal contents while aspirating gastric secretion simultaneously to prevent gastric HCl from entering the duodenum. A low rate of bicarbonate secretion in response to secretin administration is characteristic of chronic pancreatitis.

4. Serum insulin—Serum insulin measurements in patients with diabetes associated with chronic pancreatitis reveal abnormally low values that do not increase normally in response to a glucose meal or tolbutamide administration.

C. X-Ray Findings: Plain abdominal x-rays should be performed in search of pancreatic calcification. Laminagrams are helpful to clarify questionable calcifications. Pancreatic calcifications are more likely to occur in patients with alcoholic pancreatitis, pancreatitis associated with hyperparathyroidism, and familial pancreatitis than with pancreatitis associated with biliary disease. An upper gastrointestinal series may reveal deformities of the stomach and duodenum (Fig 28–3), particularly if a pseudocyst is present (Fig 28–5). Patients with chronic pancreatitis should have the biliary tract investigated by means of oral cholecystography and intravenous cholangiography. In some instances there may be partial occlusion of the common bile duct due to fibrosis of the pancreas or an inflammatory mass in the head of the pancreas.

Treatment

A. Medical Measures:

1. Alcohol—The management of chronic pancreatitis should begin with abstinence from alcohol.

2. Analgesics—The pain of pancreatitis usually requires narcotics for relief. Unfortunately, the effort to relieve pain with narcotics occasionally leads to addiction.

3. Pancreatic enzymes and diet—Patients with malabsorption should be treated by limiting fat intake and by giving supplemental pancreatic enzymes. A diet containing 40 g fat per day should be prescribed. Pancreatic enzymes should be given with meals. If clinical improvement does not occur, antacids may be helpful because lipase requires an alkaline environment for

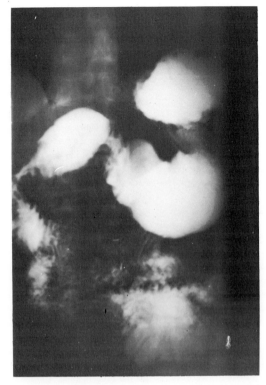

FIG 28–3. Upper gastrointestinal series illustrating persistent narrowing and stenosis of the second portion of the duodenum due to chronic pancreatitis.

optimal action and may be destroyed by gastric acid.

4. Diabetes—The diabetes associated with pancreatitis should be treated with insulin as for any other diabetic patient.

B. Surgical Measures: The variety of procedures used to treat chronic pancreatitis and its sequelae is an indication of the fact that none are curative. Since the cause is not known, it is difficult to propose curative therapy, either medical or surgical. There has been no controlled investigation of the efficacy of any surgical procedure used for the treatment of chronic pancreatitis.

1. Treatment of cholelithiasis—Acute or chronic pancreatitis requires careful diagnostic evaluation of the gallbladder and bile ducts. Patients with chronic pancreatitis should have an oral cholecystogram, an intravenous cholangiogram, or (less frequently) a percutaneous transhepatic cholangiogram. If biliary calculi are found, cholecystectomy and common duct exploration should be performed. Biliary calculi are more commonly a cause of acute or acute recurrent pancreatitis than chronic pancreatitis with calcification and steatorrhea. The elimination of cholelithiasis or choledocholithiasis prevents recurrent pancreatitis in 80–90% of patients. Unfortunately, some patients who have biliary calculi are also alcoholics, and the results of biliary surgery are less successful in these.

2. Sphincteroplasty—It has been postulated that in patients with pancreatitis the sphincter of Oddi impedes drainage of pancreatic juice into the duodenum. Although there is no convincing evidence to support this concept, division of the sphincter of Oddi has been employed to treat chronic pancreatitis. Sphincteroplasty, the most commonly used technic, is performed by incising the sphincter of Oddi for 1–2 cm up the common bile duct and suturing the duodenal mucosa to the common bile duct mucosa.

Inflammatory changes do occur in the sphincter in patients with pancreatitis; however, it is difficult to determine whether it is the cause or a result of the pancreatitis. Sphincteroplasty should not be performed for advanced pancreatitis, particularly if operative pancreatography reveals multiple strictures of the pancreatic duct. Satisfactory results are reported in about half of cases.

3. Operation to drain the pancreatic duct—Many patients with chronic pancreatitis develop dilatation of the duct of Wirsung–associated, in some instances, with multiple ductal strictures. The ductal dilatation could be due either to obstruction of the duct or to parenchymal fibrosis with contracture causing the dilatation. Some surgeons maintain that strictures of the duct of Wirsung are important in the pathogenesis of pancreatitis. This has led to the use of operations designed to decompress the pancreatic duct and facilitate drainage of pancreatic juice into the intestine. The Puestow operation is the most satisfactory one and is done by incising the pancreatic duct from the tail to the head and suturing a Roux-en-Y segment of jejunum onto the anterior surface of the gland (Fig 28–4).

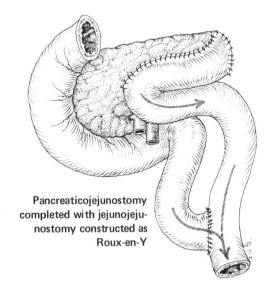

Pancreaticojejunostomy completed with jejunojejunostomy constructed as Roux-en-Y

FIG 28–4. Diagram showing pancreaticojejunostomy for the treatment of chronic pancreatitis. (Reproduced, with permission, from Silen W, Baldwin J, Goldman L: Treatment of chronic pancreatitis by longitudinal pancreaticojejunostomy. Am J Surg 106:243–258, 1963.)

4. Ablative procedures—Removal of portions of the pancreas has been employed in the treatment of a few selected patients with pancreatitis. Pancreaticoduodenectomy (the Whipple operation) has been performed, but its magnitude and significant mortality rate are especially undesirable features when treating benign disease. These objections led Child to treat chronic pancreatitis by removing the distal 95% of the pancreas, leaving a small remnant adjacent to the duodenum to avoid injury to the common bile duct and the blood supply to the duodenum. Of 32 patients operated on in this manner and followed for more than a year, 23 were well and working. There were no operative deaths. After 95% pancreatectomy, most patients will have pancreatic endocrine and exocrine insufficiency. Some patients, particularly those who continue to drink large quantities of alcohol or take narcotics, will have difficulty in managing the diabetes.

See references on p 515.

PANCREATIC PSEUDOCYSTS

Pancreatic pseudocysts are collections of fluid and sometimes bits of necrotic tissue enclosed in a fibrous capsule. The lumen usually communicates with the ductal system. Although pseudocysts arise from the pancreas and develop in the lesser peritoneal sac, they may occupy any space between the mediastinum and the pelvis. Pancreatic pseudocysts develop after episodes of pancreatitis (particularly alcoholic pancreatitis) and following pancreatic trauma.

Clinical Findings

The important clinical features of pancreatic pseudocyst are persistent abdominal pain, an abdominal mass, and elevated blood or urinary amylase levels. Upper gastrointestinal series may show anterior displacement of the stomach, widening of the duodenal loop, and duodenal deformities, perhaps with abnormalities of the duodenal mucosa (Fig 28–5). Selective arteriography is diagnostic in about 75% of cases. Pancreatic pseudocysts may at times partially obstruct the common bile duct and produce abnormalities seen on cholangiography.

Treatment & Prognosis

Pancreatic pseudocysts should be either surgically excised or drained. When drainage is employed, it is generally desirable to biopsy the pseudocyst wall to distinguish between pseudocysts and cystic neoplasms. Small pseudocysts in the tail of the pancreas may be excised safely, but opportunities for this form of therapy occur infrequently. More commonly, the appropriate treatment is drainage. If the pseudocyst is contained in a well-formed fibrous capsule and is not infected, internal drainage may be accomplished by anastomosing the cyst to the stomach, duodenum, or a

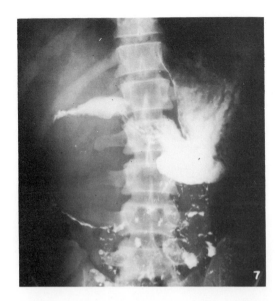

FIG 28–5. Upper gastrointestinal series illustrating widening of the duodenal loop caused by a pseudocyst in the head of the pancreas. This pseudocyst was treated by cystoduodenostomy.

Roux-en-Y loop of jejunum. It is often simple to drain pseudocysts into the stomach through the posterior gastric wall. In some instances, satisfactory drainage can be established into the duodenum. When using this technic, the surgeon must be careful to avoid injuring the common bile duct or the vessels between the head of the pancreas and the duodenum. If it is not convenient to drain the pseudocyst into the stomach or duodenum, drainage should be established into a Roux-en-Y jejunal loop. The pseudocyst must have a fibrous wall sturdy enough to hold sutures in order to accomplish internal drainage. If the wall is unsuitable for suturing, the pseudocyst should be drained externally by inserting drains, catheters, or sumps into it through the abdominal wall. External drainage of a pseudocyst may result in a pancreatic fistula, but these usually close without difficulty. Although drainage of a pancreatic pseudocyst may reduce or eliminate the mass—and in many instances relieves the pain—it does little to alter the underlying pancreatitis; if the patient continues to drink alcohol he is likely to have further attacks.

Pancreatic pseudocysts recur in 10–15% of cases. The mortality rate following drainage of pancreatic pseudocysts is approximately 10%.

Banks PA: Acute pancreatitis. Gastroenterology 61:382–397, 1971.

Brooks FP: Testing pancreatic function. New England J Med 286:300–303, 1972.

Burke EJ, Guth PH: Chronic pancreatitis. M Clin North America 54:479–492, 1970.

Creutz-feldt W, Schmidt H: Aetiology and pathogenesis of pancreatitis. Scandinav J Gastroent 5 (Suppl 6):47–62, 1970.

Dixon JA, Hillam JD: Surgical treatment of biliary tract disease associated with acute pancreatitis. Am J Surg 120: 371–375, 1970.

Glenn F, Frey C: Reevaluation of the treatment of pancreatitis associated with biliary tract disease. Ann Surg 160: 723–726, 1964.

Kalant H: Alcohol, pancreatic secretion, and pancreatitis. Gastroenterology 56:380–385, 1969.

McCutcheon AD: A fresh approach to the pathogenesis of pancreatitis. Gut 9:296–310, 1968.

Opie EL: The etiology of acute hemorrhagic pancreatitis. Bull Johns Hopkins Hosp 12:182–188, 1901.

Silen W, Baldwin J, Goldman L: Treatment of chronic pancreatitis by longitudinal pancreaticojejunostomy. Am J Surg 106:243–258, 1963.

Warren KW: Surgical management of chronic relapsing pancreatitis. Am J Surg 117:24–32, 1969.

TUMORS OF THE PANCREAS

Adenocarcinoma is the most common tumor of the pancreas and comprises about 10% of all gastrointestinal malignancies. It arises from the exocrine portion of the pancreas—usually the ductal epithelium—and occurs most commonly in the head of the organ. The incidence of these tumors rises with advancing years, and they are more common in men than in women.

Cystadenomas and cystadenocarcinomas are rare pancreatic neoplasms. Cystadenoma occurs more often in women than in men and is frequently located in the tail of the pancreas. Cystadenomas should be excised. Cystadenocarcinomas are less common than cystadenomas and also occur more often in women. They should be excised when possible.

Clinical Findings

A. Symptoms: Although there may be considerable overlap depending upon the extent of the tumor, the clinical findings vary according to its location.

1. Cancer of the head—Cancer of the head of the pancreas often presents initially with painless jaundice. Nausea, deep-seated abdominal pain, and cramping pain after eating appear later. Itching may accompany the jaundice. Nausea and anorexia are often marked, with rapid loss of weight.

2. Cancer of the body—Cancer of the body of the pancreas characteristically produces a deep-seated, poorly localized abdominal pain which is often worse at night, unrelated to meals or activity, and is easily dismissed as psychogenic in nature. Since the physical findings are often within normal limits and x-rays of the upper gastrointestinal tract show no abnormalities, additional credence may be given to psychiatric factors.

Nausea, anorexia, and severe loss of weight appear later. Jaundice is also a late sign, signifying extension to the head of the gland or liver metastasis.

3. Cancer of the tail—Cancer of the tail of the

pancreas tends to develop insidiously. Abdominal pain and loss of weight are the first symptoms. Compression of the stomach may lead to postprandial distress and vomiting. Jaundice is usually due to liver metastases.

B. Signs:

1. Jaundice and hepatomegaly—In cancer of the head of the gland, jaundice usually becomes intense. Hepatomegaly may be present in patients with long-standing obstructive jaundice. Hepatomegaly is sometimes a reflection of hepatic metastases, especially in cancers of the body or tail.

2. Epigastric mass—Examination of the abdomen may reveal a palpable mass. Patients with cancer of the body or tail of the pancreas usually have a characteristic palpable mass when first examined. Patients with carcinoma of the head often seek medical attention because of jaundice before the tumor is palpable.

3. Palpable gallbladder—When common duct obstruction has occurred, the gallbladder may be large and nontender. Such a finding in a patient with jaundice (Courvoisier's sign) suggests that the obstruction is due to a malignant tumor, and is present in over half of patients with cancer of the head of the pancreas.

4. Thrombophlebitis—Spontaneous attacks of peripheral thrombophlebitis may occur in patients with cancer of the pancreas, particularly of the body and tail.

C. Laboratory Findings: The secretin test usually reveals decreased secretion of bicarbonate in patients with carcinoma of the pancreas. This test is not sufficiently sensitive to discriminate between carcinoma and pancreatitis.

Cytologic examination of the fluid recovered from the duodenum after secretin injection frequently shows malignancy, but the diagnosis is usually apparent from other findings.

Serum amylase is not uniformly elevated. Some patients may develop diabetes. There is often an elevation of the serum alkaline phosphatase associated with biliary tract obstruction or hepatic metastasis. Some cancers of the pancreas produce alkaline phosphatase. Hematocrit and hemoglobin levels are often normal or only slightly reduced. Anemia is a late sign in cancer of the pancreas—in contrast with cancer of the ampulla of Vater.

D. X-Ray Findings: On upper gastrointestinal series, cancer of the pancreatic head may produce an enlargement of the duodenal loop, but this finding is highly variable, and it is sometimes difficult to say at what point the duodenal loop is abnormally widened. Other findings consist of alterations in the appearance of the duodenal mucosa, particularly on the medial aspect, and carcinoma of the head of the pancreas may sometimes produce effacement of the mucosa. Some tenting of the duodenum in the region of the ampulla of Vater may occur and will produce a radiographic sign called the "reverse-3" sign. Carcinomas of the pancreas may also deform the distal stomach or displace it anteriorly (Fig 28–6). Hypotonic duodenography may help to reveal abnormalities of the duodenal mucosa produced by the tumor. In some far-advanced cases,

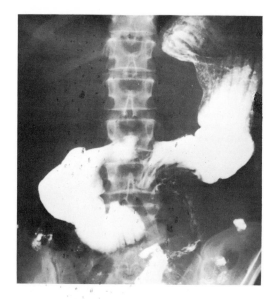

FIG 28–6. Radiograph showing invasion of the third and fourth portions of the duodenum by an adenocarcinoma of the body of the pancreas. (Courtesy of Reed Rice, Associate Professor of Radiology, Duke University Medical Center.)

there may be actual invasion of the duodenal wall by the tumor. Cancer of the tail of the pancreas may invade the kidney and renal pelvis, simulating cancer of the kidney on intravenous urograms.

Oral cholecystography or intravenous cholangiography is not ordinarily of value because the destruction of the duct will block excretion of the contrast material by the liver. Percutaneous cholangiography may circumvent this problem and reveal a tapering deformity of the distal bile duct with complete occlusion characteristic of malignant obstruction. Selective arteriography may show abnormal anatomic positions of the arteries supplying the pancreas and "cuffing" caused by compression of vessels by tumor. It is unusual for carcinoma of the exocrine pancreas to produce a tumor blush. Pancreatic scanning has been attempted with moderately successful results.

Differential Diagnosis

Cancer of the ampulla of Vater and lower end of the common bile duct (see Chapter 27) often closely simulates cancer of the pancreas. The distinguishing signs of ampullary or ductal tumor are a tendency to intermittent jaundice, anemia, and the presence of blood in the stool. Weight loss is less severe.

Treatment

Cancer of the pancreas spreads by direct extension, extension to regional lymph nodes, and by hepatic metastasis. Although the prognosis is uniformly poor since the disease has usually extended beyond the gland by the time the diagnosis is made, surgical exploration is indicated in patients with the clinical findings outlined above for 2 reasons: (1) to differentiate pancreatic adenocarcinoma from other retroperitoneal masses by direct biopsy; and (2) to palliate by relieving biliary or duodenal obstruction.

The only means available for curing pancreatic cancer is surgery and pancreaticoduodenal resection should be considered. Unfortunately, few tumors meet the criteria for curative resection, and even in these cases recurrence is common. However, in the absence of metastases or extension, palliation may be obtained by removing the tumor and relieving biliary and duodenal obstruction. Adenocarcinoma of the head of the pancreas is usually unresectable, but palliative bypass should be done for obstruction of the common bile duct or duodenum.

The most commonly employed procedure for relief of biliary obstruction in carcinoma of the pancreas is cholecystojejunostomy, but choledochojejunostomy may be necessary for patients who have had a previous cholecystectomy. The surgeon often has to decide whether to perform a gastrointestinal bypass operation when the biliary bypass is done; in general, both biliary bypass and intestinal bypass should be performed at the first operation.

Prognosis

The survival of patients treated by bypass procedures or by palliative resections for carcinoma of the head of the pancreas is usually less than 1 year.

See references on p 518.

ENDOCRINE TUMORS OF THE PANCREAS

Pancreatic endocrine tumors, although much less common than pancreatic exocrine tumors, are of interest because they produce hormones characteristic of the cell type from which the tumor originated. Four syndromes associated with functioning endocrine tumors of the pancreas have been described: hyperinsulinism, Zollinger-Ellison syndrome, hyperglycemia associated with increased serum glucagon levels, and "pancreatic cholera" (watery diarrhea, hypokalemia, and gastric hypoacidity). In the latter syndrome, a hormone responsible for the syndrome has not been identified.

Insulin-Producing Tumors (Insulinoma)

Patients with insulin-producing tumors often give a history of episodes of passing out or of "spells." Occasionally, patients with insulin-producing tumors exhibit bizarre behavior and appear to have psychiatric problems. CNS damage and even death may occur from repeated profound hypoglycemia. Patients with insulin-producing tumors often gain weight excessively because constant ingestion of food relieves the symptoms. In 1938, Whipple described 3 findings **(Whipple's triad)** which are the hallmarks of the syndrome of hyperinsulinism: (1) hypoglycemic symptoms, (2) a fasting blood glucose below 50 mg/100 ml, and (3) relief of the hypoglycemic symptoms and hypoglycemia by the administration of glucose. A fasting blood glucose below 50 mg/100 ml suggests organic hypoglycemia but does not rule out such conditions as depletion of liver glycogen or reactive hypoglycemia. An elevated fasting serum insulin level measured by immunoassay is important in the diagnosis of beta cell tumor. Tolbutamide stimulates release of insulin from the islet cells, and an augmented hypoglycemic response to the intravenous administration of tolbutamide is helpful in diagnosing hyperinsulinism, particularly when accompanied by serum insulin measurements. In some instances, selective arteriography will identify a vascular pancreatic endocrine tumor. Most patients with endocrine tumors of the pancreas fail to show a tumor blush on arteriography; nonetheless, this test should be employed, for if the tumor blush is seen it will greatly facilitate locating the tumor at surgery.

At surgery, the pancreas should be carefully palpated. If a tumor is identified, it should be excised locally and the area should be drained. Pancreatic fistula is a frequent complication of excision of pancreatic adenomas. In some instances, an adenoma may not be found on initial palpation. There is controversy about how this should be managed, but the best strategy is probably to perform a distal pancreatectomy and examine the specimen for tumor. Monitoring of blood glucose levels during operation has been used as a guide to determine whether the tumor has been removed. The technic is complicated because intravenous glucose solutions must be administered during the operation to prevent hypoglycemia. Most beta cell tumors of the pancreas are benign, but malignant tumors are occasionally encountered. Fortunately, the degree of malignancy is often very low. The main problem with these lesions is that hyperinsulinism will persist if they recur or if metastases are present. Hyperinsulinism due to recurrent or metastatic insulinomas has been treated with glucagon or diazoxide with some success. Streptozotocin, an antitumor drug toxic to the beta cells of the pancreas, has been used successfully in several cases of malignant or recurrent beta cell neoplasm. This drug must be used with care because it is also toxic to the renal tubules.

Gastrin-Producing Tumors

Zollinger-Ellison syndrome is characterized by a severe ulcer diathesis associated with marked gastric hypersecretion and a gastrin-producing islet cell tumor, usually located in the pancreas. Gastrin-producing tumors occasionally arise in the duodenum. The Zollinger-Ellison syndrome is discussed in detail in Chapter 25.

Glucagon-Producing Tumors

Rare glucagon-producing tumors have been reported, with hyperglycemia and elevated serum glucagon levels as measured by immunoassay. Following removal of the pancreatic adenoma, the hyperglycemia should subside.

Diarrheal Syndrome Associated With Nonbeta Islet Cell Tumors of the Pancreas

This syndrome is characterized by watery diarrhea, with some patients producing 8–10 liters of liquid stool a day associated with hypokalemia. Patients with this syndrome often have low gastric acid secretion and a pancreatic islet cell adenoma. The removal of the adenoma relieves the symptoms. The tumors may be benign or malignant. The mechanism of the diarrhea is unknown at the present time. The hormone secretin has been suggested to be the agent responsible for the diarrhea. Administration of a combination of glucagon and gastrin produces similar diarrhea in experimental animals. Many patients with this syndrome have parathyroid adenomas.

Following successful removal of the tumor, gastric acid levels return to normal and the diarrhea ceases.

Becker WF, Welch RA, Pratt HS: Cystadenoma and cyst-adenocarcinoma of the pancreas. Ann Surg 161:845–863, 1965.

Child CG, Frey CF, Fry WJ: A reappraisal of removal of 95% of the distal portion of the pancreas. Surg Gynec Obst 129:49–56, 1969.

Crile G: The advantages of bypass operations over radical pancreatoduodenectomy in the treatment of pancreatic carcinoma. Surg Gynec Obst 130:1049–1053, 1970.

Filipi CJ, Higgins GA: Diagnosis and management of insulinoma. Am J Surg 125:231–239, 1973.

Hartsuck JM, Brooks JR: Functioning beta islet cell tumors. Am J Surg 117:541–548, 1969.

Howard JM, Jordan GL Jr: *Surgical Diseases of the Pancreas.* Lippincott, 1960.

Jordan GL: Pancreatic fistula. Am J Surg 119:200–207, 1970.

Kraft AR, Tompkins RK, Zollinger RM: Recognition and management of the diarrheal syndrome caused by nonbeta islet cell tumors of the pancreas. Am J Surg 119:163–170, 1970.

Moldow RE, Connelly RR: Epidemiology of pancreatic cancer in Connecticut. Gastroenterology 55:677–686, 1968.

Monge JJ: Survival of patients with small carcinomas of the head of the pancreas. Ann Surg 166:908–912, 1967.

Pope NA, Fish JC: Palliative surgery for carcinoma of the pancreas. Am J Surg 121:271–272, 1971.

ReMine WH & others: Total pancreatectomy. Ann Surg 172:595–604, 1970.

• • •

General References

American Physiological Society: *Handbook of Physiology.* Section 6: Alimentary Canal. Vol 2. Waverly Press, 1967.

American Physiological Society: *Handbook of Physiology.* Section 7: Endocrinology. Vol 1. Waverly Press, 1972.

Bowers RF: Pancreatitis. Curr Probl Surg, Sept 1964.

Dixon JA, Englert E: Growing role of early surgery in chronic pancreatitis: A practical clinical approach. Gastroenterology 61:375–381, 1971.

Howat HT (editor): The exocrine pancreas. Clin Gastroenterol 1:1–256, 1972.

Margulis AR, Burhenne HJ (editors): *Alimentary Tract Roentgenology.* Part 8: The Pancreas and the Lesser Sac. Vol 2. Mosby, 1967.

Warren KW: Diagnosis and surgical treatment of carcinoma of the pancreas. Curr Probl Surg, Jan 1968.

29 . . .

The Spleen

F. William Blaisdell, MD, & Lawrence W. Way, MD

ANATOMY

The spleen is a purplish blood-filled organ lying in the left upper quadrant of the abdomen. The normal adult spleen measures 8 × 12 cm and weighs 100–150 g. It lies between the eighth to 11th ribs in the posterior axillary line. The spleen is coffee-bean- to comma-shaped and is in contact with the diaphragm posteriorly, the stomach anteromedially, the splenic flexure of the colon inferiorly, and the left kidney posteromedially (Fig 29–1). The organ develops within the primitive dorsal mesogastrium, between the stomach and the aorta. When the upper abdominal viscera rotate during fetal development, the spleen settles to the left. Except for a short segment called the phrenicosplenic ligament, the dorsal portion of its mesentery—which contains the splenic vessels—fuses with the peritoneum and the ventral portion remains as the gastrosplenic ligament. The latter contains the short gastric and left gastroepiploic vessels, which originate from the splenic artery. The presplenic fold is a thin, double peritoneal fold extending from the greater omentum to the lower splenic pole. The phrenocolic ligament is an avascular attachment which traverses the undersurface of the spleen to the diaphragm and supports the inferior pole.

Beneath the peritoneal layer, the surface of the spleen is covered by a capsule which sends finger-like projections called trabeculae into the parenchyma. In man, the capsule consists predominantly of fibroelastic tissue, although a few smooth muscle cells are present. The spleen contains 20–30 ml of red cells, or 1% of the body's total red cells. Circulation through the spleen is unimpeded; transit time averages 30 seconds and involves 50–100 ml of red cells, or 3–5% of the cardiac output.

The splenic artery, which carries blood to the spleen, promptly branches into the trabecular arteries, which enter the white pulp, or lymphatic portion of

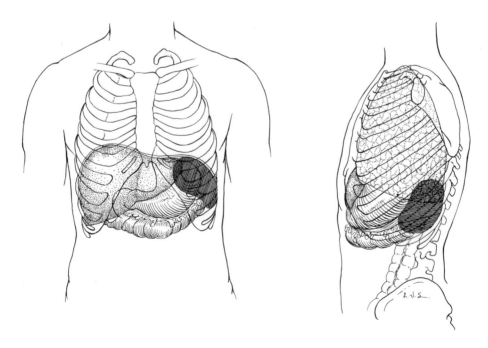

FIG 29–1. Anatomic locations of spleen.

the spleen, as central arteries. These small arteries give off (usually at right angles) short, narrow, capillary-like branches that contain mainly plasma and apparently terminate within the lymphatic sheets. This "skimming" of plasma is probably responsible for the markedly increased red cell concentration in the more distal parts of the spleen. The arteries of the white pulp eventually terminate in an open meshwork, the "marginal zone," which consists of concentric layers of flattened cells surrounding the white pulp. Abnormal cells and particulate matter are initially trapped here, but normal red cells proceed unhindered. Blood next enters the sinuses, continuous passages with a diameter of 30–40 μm, lined by potentially phagocytic reticuloendothelial cells adherent to a basement membrane. Alternating in parallel with the sinuses are partially collapsed, discontinuous passages—the so-called Billroth cords—which contain macrophages, macrocytes, and some lymphocytes. The area of sinuses and Billroth cords is called red pulp. The cords normally contain very few red cells but may become phagocytic and are capable of holding a great volume of blood. The cords communicate with the sinuses through endothelial gaps. The sinuses apparently represent a rapid flow system and the cordal pathway a slow mixing pool.

FUNCTION OF THE SPLEEN

The normal function of the spleen is indicated by its cellular composition. The predominant cells are the lymphocytes. Small lymphocytes apparently exchange with similar cells in lymphatics, lymph nodes, and marrow. The large lymphocytes contribute to antibody (immunoglobulin) formation. The reticulum cells of the spleen aid in the removal of senescent, faulty, or damaged red cells, as do reticulum cells in other parts of the body. The spleen acts as a storage site where 20–30% of the platelet pool may be sequestered during inactivity. Endogenous catecholamines may discharge platelets from this reserve into the general circulation, where they are available to initiate thrombosis. The spleen has no specialized tissue and is not essential for life.

Harker LA, Finch CA: Thrombokinetics in man. J Clin Invest 48:963–974, 1969.
Penny R & others: The splenic platelet pool. Blood 27:1–16, 1966.
Weiss L: The structure of the normal spleen. Seminars Hemat 2:205–228, 1965.
Wennberg E, Weiss L: The structure of the spleen and hemolysis. Ann Rev Med 20:29–40, 1969.

HEMATOLOGIC EFFECTS OF SPLENECTOMY

Splenectomy in a normal person is clinically of no significance. Red cell count and indices do not change. A few target cells, Howell-Jolly bodies, rare Heinz bodies, and siderocytes may appear. There may be a slight, transient leukocytosis with some eosinophilia, basophilia, and monocytosis. Platelets are usually increased—occasionally markedly so—and may stay at levels of 400–500 thousand/μl for over a year. In patients with hemolytic anemia, these abnormalities may be much more striking, and transient platelet rises to 2–3 million/μl may be seen. They are innocuous and should not be treated.

Splenectomy in very young children (under age 2) may be associated with an increased frequency of severe bacterial infections, especially pneumococcal and meningococcal. Surgery is usually deferred until the age of 4 years unless the underlying disorder (eg, hereditary spherocytosis or autoimmune hemolytic anemia) is so severe as to require transfusion or corticosteroid maintenance.

Crosby WH: Splenectomy in hematologic disorders. New England J Med 286:1252–1254, 1972.
Diamond LK: Splenectomy in childhood and the hazard of overwhelming infection. Pediatrics 43:886–889, 1969.
McBride JA & others: The effect of splenectomy on the leukocyte count. Brit J Haemat 14:225–231, 1968.
Pedersen B, Videback A: On the late effects of removal of the normal spleen. Acta chir scandinav 131:89–98, 1966.
Schwartz SI & others: Splenectomy for hematologic disorders. Curr Probl Surg, May 1971.

DISORDERS IN WHICH SPLENECTOMY IS ALWAYS INDICATED

1. INJURY TO THE SPLEEN

Essentials of Diagnosis

- History of a blow to the flank (possibly fractured rib on left side).
- Abdominal pain and tenderness.
- Pain in the left shoulder or left side of the neck.
- Tachycardia.
- Shock (late indication, or indication of major rupture).

General Considerations

Injury is the most common indication for splenectomy, and a ruptured spleen is the most common major injury after blunt abdominal trauma. In penetrating abdominal injury, surgical exploration is routine and a splenic rupture will be discovered if it has occurred.

Mortality can be attributed to delay in the diagnosis of ruptured spleen, since the diagnosis may be difficult to establish even when suspected. Associated injuries are often present which mask the signs of splenic rupture. Although abdominal pain and tenderness are usually present, the peritoneal reaction to bleeding varies greatly, and some patients will have minimal findings even when intraperitoneal bleeding is massive.

Clinical Findings

The classic findings in ruptured spleen are a history of a blow to the upper abdomen, particularly on the left side or in the left flank. It may be so slight as not to be recalled by the patient. The patient usually complains of abdominal pain which is worse in the left upper abdomen and often spreads to the left shoulder or left neck. There may be mild nausea or vomiting.

The abdominal findings are those of low-grade peritoneal irritation, ie, tenderness, mild spasm, and distention. The area of splenic dullness may be increased to percussion, or a mass may be palpable in

TABLE 29–1. Indications for splenectomy.

Splenectomy always indicated
  Splenic injury (common)
  Primary splenic tumor (rare)
  Splenic abscess (rare)
  Hereditary spherocytosis (congenital hemolytic anemia)

Splenectomy usually indicated
  Primary splenic neutropenia
  Primary splenic pancytopenia
  Chronic idiopathic thrombocytopenic purpura

Splenectomy sometimes indicated
  Autoimmune hemolytic disease
  Ovalocytosis with hemolysis
  Nonspherocytic congenital hemolytic anemias (eg, pyruvate kinase deficiency)
  Hemoglobin H disease
  Hodgkin's disease (for staging)
  Hypersplenism

Rare indications for splenectomy
  Chronic lymphatic leukemia
  Lymphosarcoma
  Hodgkin's disease
  Macroglobulinemia
  Myelofibrosis
  Thalassemia major
  Splenic artery aneurysm

Splenectomy not indicated
  Asymptomatic hypersplenism
  Splenomegaly with infection
  Splenomegaly associated with elevated IgM

the left upper quadrant. With marked bleeding, the abdomen may distend rapidly and the characteristic signs of acute blood loss, ie, tachycardia, hypotension, and shock, will appear. An important early diagnostic clue is tenderness over the ninth and tenth ribs on the left. A fractured rib in that area should arouse a strong suspicion of the possibility of a ruptured spleen.

In doubtful cases, peritoneal tap is indicated. The method and interpretation of this test are described in Chapter 52.

Plain films of the abdomen may show distortion of the gastric shadow. In doubtful cases, particularly in delayed rupture, a selective splenic arteriogram or a barium study of the stomach is indicated and may be diagnostic.

If the first clinical evidence of bleeding does not appear until more than 48 hours after injury, the rupture is termed "delayed." Roughly 5% of patients with this injury have a delay of at least this long. The longer the time between injury and the onset of bleeding, the more difficult the diagnosis.

Delayed splenic rupture is believed to evolve as follows: There is a minor rupture of the splenic pulp, but the lesion is either intraparenchymal, subcapsular, or contained within peritoneal folds. As the red cells disintegrate, the hematoma liquifies and increased osmolality of its contents attracts additional fluid. This leads to expansion of the cavity, secondary hemorrhage, and eventually rupture.

About 75% of delayed ruptures appear within 2 or 3 weeks after injury, but in rare instances months or years may pass before secondary bleeding occurs. Some patients present with anemia and a massive lesion in the left upper quadrant suggesting a retroperitoneal tumor.

The spleen may be injured during upper abdominal operations, particularly on the stomach and colon. Exposure of the esophagus for vagotomy may result in splenic injury. Traction on the gastrosplenic or splenocolic ligaments while the spleen is held in position by a retractor is one of the commonest mechanisms. Since hemostasis can rarely be obtained by suture of the injury, splenectomy is the safest policy. Careful exposure of the field with consideration to the anatomic location of the spleen will avoid these injuries.

Spontaneous rupture of the spleen may occur, particularly in association with marked splenomegaly. Delayed rupture is often the result of very minor trauma—so mild that it was not realized or was readily forgotten by the patient. In some cases, no history of trauma can be obtained.

Pregnancy predisposes to spontaneous rupture. The same is true of many diseases which cause splenomegaly, particularly malaria, lymphoma, infectious mononucleosis, and sarcoidosis. In areas where malaria is endemic, splenomegaly is common and spontaneous rupture occurs more frequently.

An abnormal development of the splenic ligaments which leaves the organ mobile instead of secured within the left upper quadrant may make it more vulnerable to rupture.

Treatment

Splenectomy is always indicated as soon as the diagnosis of splenic injury is made.

Prognosis

If the correct diagnosis is made and splenectomy is performed, the patient usually recovers without complications. Without treatment, death from hemorrhagic shock would occur in most cases.

Ballinger WF II, Erslev AJ: Splenectomy. Curr Probl Surg, Feb 1965.
Dunphy JE: Splenectomy for trauma. Am J Surg 71:450, 1946.
Lorimer WS: Occult rupture of the spleen. Arch Surg 89:434–440, 1964.
Olsen WR, Beaudoin DE: Surgical injury to the spleen. Surg Gynec Obst 131:57–62, 1970.
Shirkey AL & others: Surgical management of splenic injuries. Am J Surg 108:630–635, 1964.
Sizer JS & others: Delayed rupture of the spleen. Arch Surg 92:362–366, 1966.

2. CYSTS & TUMORS OF THE SPLEEN

Parasitic cysts of the spleen may be associated with hydatid disease (see Chapter 10). Some are asymptomatic, but usually the patient notices enlargement of the spleen. An x-ray may show calcification. Eosinophilia may be found, and serologic tests may establish the diagnosis. The treatment of choice is splenectomy.

Benign cysts of the spleen are rare. Some are believed to be congenital and others the result of infarct or delayed rupture (pseudocyst). Operative removal by splenectomy is indicated to exclude the presence of a primary tumor or other bizarre causes of splenomegaly.

Primary tumors of the spleen include lymphoma, sarcoma, and hemangiomas. These lesions are usually asymptomatic until splenomegaly becomes evident and sufficient to cause abdominal discomfort or a palpable mass. Spontaneous rupture may occur. Splenectomy is indicated if the tumor appears to be limited to that organ.

3. SPLENIC ABSCESS

Abscess of the spleen is uncommon. Unexplained sepsis and progressive enlargement of the spleen are the usual presenting manifestations. Spontaneous rupture may occur with peritonitis. Radioactive scan may help establish the diagnosis. Formerly, most abscesses of the spleen appeared during the course of malaria or typhoid fever, but bacterial abscesses originating from other types of septicemia are now more common. In 80% of cases, one or more abscesses exist in organs other than the spleen. Most cases of truly solitary splenic abscess follow trauma or invasion from an adjacent malignancy of the colon or stomach. Surgical treatment should consist either of splenectomy or drainage of the abscess depending on technical considerations.

Asbury GF: Calcified pseudocysts of the spleen. Arch Surg 76:148, 1958.
McSherry CK, Dineen P: The significance of splenic abscess. Am J Surg 103:618–623, 1962.

4. HEREDITARY SPHEROCYTOSIS

Essentials of Diagnosis

- Malaise, abdominal discomfort.
- Jaundice, anemia, splenomegaly.
- Spherocytosis, increased osmotic fragility of red cells, negative Coombs test.

General Considerations

The characteristic feature of this hemolytic disorder is the spherocyte. Under the microscope, these red cells appear smaller, thicker, more perfectly round, and more darkly red than normal cells. They are less able to mold their shape than normal cells. The red cell defect probably involves the protein structure of the membrane and leads to significant destruction only in the presence of the spleen. The spleen in a way plays a secondary role in hereditary spherocytosis. The peculiar structure of the red cells leads to their delayed passage through the meshwork of splenic cords and to further damage to their membranes. After several passages through the spleen, red cells are so severely damaged that they become nonviable and are removed permanently.

Hereditary spherocytosis is seen in all races. The incidence in Caucasians is approximately 2 per 10,000 population. It is transmitted as an autosomal dominant gene. Clinical cases are heterozygous; the homozygous form of the disease is probably not compatible with life. In about 25% of cases, no familial involvement can be demonstrated. The disorder is most commonly first recognized in children or young adults, but it may be manifest in the newborn period, when it resembles hemolytic disease of the newborn due to ABO incompatibility, or it may not be discovered until after the age of 80.

Clinical Findings

A. Symptoms and Signs: Patients may complain of easy fatigability and jaundice; the spleen is almost always enlarged and may cause left upper quadrant fullness and discomfort. Infarction may cause acute pain.

On rare occasions, an acute "aplastic" anemia develops with profound anemia and, in some cases, fever, headache, abdominal pain, and pancytopenia with hypoactive marrow. Other individuals are asymptomatic; the diagnosis is made only because the discovery of the disease in a more severely afflicted relative has led to an intensive search and laboratory testing of the blood.

B. Laboratory Findings: The red cell count is moderately decreased (3–4 million/μl). The red cells are small (MCV = 70–80 fl) and hyperchromic (MCHC = 36–40%). Spherocytes in varying numbers are seen on a Wright-stained smear. The reticulocyte count is increased.

Indirect serum bilirubin and stool urobilinogen are usually elevated; haptoglobins are often decreased or absent. The Coombs test is negative. Osmotic fragility is characteristically increased; hemolysis of 5–10% of cells may be observed at saline concentrations of 0.6% or even higher. The response may be normal in some patients, but a sample of defibrinated blood incubated at 37 C for 24 hours ("incubated fragility test") will show increased hemolysis when compared to normal blood similarly treated. Autohemolysis of defibrinated blood incubated under sterile conditions for 48 hours is usually greatly increased (10–20%, compared to a normal value of less than 5%). The addition of 10% glucose prior to incubation will decrease the abnormal osmotic fragility and autohemolysis. Red cell survival studies, using the patient's own blood labeled with ^{51}Cr, will show a greatly shortened red cell life span and sequestration in the spleen.

Differential Diagnosis

Spherocytes in large numbers occur in many patients with autoimmune hemolytic anemia. Osmotic fragility and autohemolysis are similarly increased but are less consistently improved by glucose. The positive Coombs test, negative family history, and sharply reduced survival of normal donor blood in these patients establish the diagnosis.

Complications

Gallstones composed principally of bile pigments (reflecting increased metabolism of hemoglobin) occur in up to 85% of adults and may develop even in children.

Treatment

Splenectomy is indicated in all cases of hereditary spherocytosis once the diagnosis is definitely established, even if the anemia is minimal and there is no jaundice. Preoperative transfusion is rarely necessary. When there is associated cholelithiasis, splenectomy should precede cholecystectomy unless both procedures are done at the same time. Splenectomy is usually deferred until after the first few years of life.

Prognosis

Splenectomy eliminates anemia and jaundice in over 90% of cases, but abnormal red cell morphology and abnormal osmotic fragility persist. Red cell life span is normal after splenectomy.

Jacob HS: Hereditary spherocytosis: A disease of the red cell membrane. Seminars Hemat 2:139–166, 1965.

Macpherson AIS & others: The role of the spleen in congenital spherocytosis. Am J Med 50:35–41, 1971.

DISORDERS IN WHICH SPLENECTOMY IS USUALLY INDICATED

1. PRIMARY SPLENIC NEUTROPENIA

There is considerable doubt about whether splenic neutropenia exists as a primary disease. Many cases appear to be closely related to Felty's syndrome in which the patient has severe neutropenia associated with chronic rheumatoid arthritis. If there is marked evidence of neutropenia with trapping of cells in the spleen, splenectomy usually gives good results.

2. PRIMARY SPLENIC PANCYTOPENIA

This condition is also rare, and there is some doubt about whether it exists as a separate entity. It may more appropriately be classed under the heading of hypersplenism and secondary pancytopenia. The indications for splenectomy are based on the severity of the cytopenia, recurring infections, and anemia and on evidence of destruction of cells within the spleen.

3. IDIOPATHIC (PRIMARY) THROMBOCYTOPENIC PURPURA (ITP)

Essentials of Diagnosis

- Petechiae, ecchymoses, epistaxis, easy bruising.
- No splenomegaly.
- Decreased platelet count, prolonged bleeding time, poor clot retraction, normal coagulation time.

General Considerations

ITP is a hemorrhagic disorder caused by a severe reduction in the number of circulating platelets. It often starts abruptly, involving the skin and mucous membranes with petechiae and ecchymoses. In children, it frequently follows an infection, and it usually remits spontaneously after a few weeks. It may follow the use of certain drugs, eg, diuretics or quinidine; when the drug is stopped, remission usually follows promptly in a few days. If thrombocytopenia persists for several months in the absence of any discernible cause—and if leukemia and aplastic anemia have been ruled out—some form of "autoimmunity" is probably involved and the patient becomes a candidate for surgery. Corticosteroids, while often used in the management of this disorder, do not cure it but are merely palliative.

Clinical Findings

A. Symptoms and Signs: The onset may be sudden, with petechiae, epistaxis, bleeding gums, vaginal bleeding, gastrointestinal bleeding, or hematuria. In the chronic form there may be a history of easy bruising and recurrent showers of petechiae, particularly in pressure areas. The spleen is not palpable.

B. Laboratory Findings: The platelet count is always below $100,000/\mu l$ and may be below $10,000/\mu l$. The absence of platelets on the peripheral blood smear is striking. White cells are not affected; and anemia, if present, is secondary to blood loss.

The bone marrow megakaryocytes are increased in number but not surrounded by platelets; they are abnormal, with single nuclei, scant cytoplasm, and often vacuoles. The chief value of the marrow examination is to rule out leukemia and aplastic anemia.

The bleeding time is prolonged, but coagulation time is normal. Clot retraction is poor. Prothrombin consumption is decreased in severe cases. Capillary fragility (Rumpel-Leede test) is greatly increased. An LE test and a prothrombin time should be done to look for lupus erythematosus, which may present as purpura or with bleeding due to an anticoagulant. Destruction of platelets in the spleen may be demonstrated by tagging platelets with ^{51}Cr.

Treatment

In preparation for surgery, the thrombocytopenic patient who is not purpuric needs neither corticosteroids nor transfusions, regardless of the platelet count. A patient who has constant purpura, particularly of the mucous membranes, will usually be on corticosteroids preoperatively; if not, he should receive prednisone, 40 mg daily (or equivalent), for 3 days before surgery and for about a week thereafter.

A patient who is actively bleeding may need 6 or 8 platelet packs given within 2 hours before surgery; earlier administration probably is wasted because platelet survival is only a few hours in most patients with severe thrombocytopenic purpura. Fresh blood (procured the same day) is needed at surgery if blood loss is anticipated or if the patient is anemic.

Course & Prognosis

The characteristic platelet response after splenectomy is a rise to normal levels in about 48 hours and to a peak (which may exceed 1 million/μl) usually between the sixth and tenth days. Platelet counts will level off in about 2 or 3 weeks. An initial platelet rise—even to high levels—is no guarantee that surgery has been successful. Platelet counts may fall to the preoperative level despite a good initial rise; but if the platelet count is normal 2 months after surgery it will remain normal. In some patients, platelets do not rise for about a week; then they rise gradually to acceptable levels. Others take a postoperative dip after an initial rise but return eventually to normal levels. Rises above 1 or even 2 million do not constitute a risk to the patient from thrombosis, and anticoagulants such as heparin should not be given.

Splenectomy is successful in approximately 85% of patients. In some, the remission is not complete but patients are able to get along with counts after surgery that were too low before surgery. Others can be maintained on intermittent prednisone after splenectomy when this was not possible prior to surgery. If splenectomy and corticosteroids both fail, immunosuppressive therapy may be tried.

Occasionally, it is necessary to perform splenectomy for thrombocytopenic purpura in a patient who has some other underlying disorder, eg, lupus erythematosus or another collagen disease. In such cases, the considerations for splenectomy are the same as those for patients with ITP.

Baldini M: Idiopathic thrombocytopenic purpura. New England J Med 274:1245–1251, 1301–1306, 1360–1367, 1966.

Gomes MMR & others: Indications for splenectomy in hematologic diseases. Surg Gynec Obst 129:129–139, 1969.

Karpotkin S & others: Autoimmune thrombocytopenic purpura and the compensated thrombocytolytic state. Am J Med 51:1–4, 1971.

Sandusky WR & others: Splenectomy: Indications and results in hematological disorders. Ann Surg 159:695–710, 1964.

DISORDERS IN WHICH SPLENECTOMY IS SOMETIMES INDICATED

1. AUTOIMMUNE HEMOLYTIC ANEMIA

This is an acquired form of hemolytic anemia. Patients develop antibodies to their own red cells characterized by a positive direct Coombs test. Lupus erythematosus and lymphosarcoma are sometimes underlying disorders. Occasionally a drug can be implicated as the causative agent, eg, methyldopa (Aldomet). Two-thirds of cases are of unknown origin. Bilirubin pigment gallstones are a common complication.

The onset is usually fairly acute. Patients develop symptoms of anemia, sometimes with fever and usually with jaundice. The spleen is enlarged in most patients. The diagnosis is made by demonstrating anemia, reticulocytosis, and other signs of hemolysis such as an increased indirect serum bilirubin. The direct Coombs test is positive because the patient's red cells are coated with antibody.

Splenectomy is indicated if the antibody is an IgG (warm antibody) and the disease fails to respond to corticosteroids or requires large doses for maintenance. Patients with nongamma antibody usually do not respond favorably to splenectomy. Splenectomy benefits the patient by removing a site of hemolytic antibody production as well as by removing the principal organ of red cell destruction.

Surgery achieves complete clinical remission in about 50% of cases. No special preparation is usually required; most patients will be on corticosteroids when they come to surgery, and must of course be maintained for a while on this treatment. Anemic patients can be transfused unless they also have a positive indirect Coombs test; this is because antibody excess in the serum would cause all cross-matches to be incompatible.

Gomes MMR & others: Indications for splenectomy in hematologic diseases. Surg Gynec Obst 129:129–139, 1969.

Schwartz SI & others: Splenectomy for hematologic disorders. Curr Probl Surg, May 1971.

2. HYPERSPLENISM

Essentials of Diagnosis

- Large spleen.
- Pancytopenia.
- Active marrow.

General Considerations

A great variety of hematologic disorders are associated with splenomegaly and varying degrees of cytopenia or pancytopenia. The causes are obscure, but the characteristic triad of "empty blood, full marrow, and large spleen" has caused these states to be lumped together under the unsatisfactory term hypersplenism. An exaggeration of normal splenic activity is implied. The 2 activities that may become exaggerated are sequestration and destruction of cells, especially platelets and red cells. Hypertrophy of the reticuloendothelial system, especially the Billroth cords, is a related finding.

These conditions fall under the category of diseases in which splenectomy is sometimes indicated. Determining factors in the decision to operate are the severity of the destruction of cellular elements, evidence of trapping or destruction in the spleen, and the degree of splenomegaly. In some cases, the spleen may be so massive that it incapacitates the patient, and this alone may justify its removal.

In congestive splenomegaly, stasis in the splenic vein leads to accumulation of blood in sinuses and other parts of the red pulp. Intrasplenic pressure, normally 4–16 mm Hg, doubles. The most common cause of congestive splenomegaly is cirrhosis of the liver. Thrombosis of the portal or splenic vein may be suspected if, following an abdominal injury, the spleen increases in size over a few days and is painful and tender.

Clinical Findings

A. Symptoms and Signs: Onset may be gradual and the diagnosis made on routine physical or laboratory examination. Some patients complain only of left upper quadrant discomfort or fullness; others have hematemesis. Some degree of hematemesis occurs in about half of cases.

Purpura, bruising, or diffuse mucous membrane bleeding are unusual despite low platelet counts. Severe leukopenia may be associated with recurrent infections, or with chronic leg ulcers in splenomegaly associated with rheumatoid arthritis (Felty's syndrome).

B. Laboratory Findings: The anemia is only moderate, and normocytic and normochromic. Hemoglobin values below 10 g/100 ml suggest complications: (1) iron deficiency anemia due to chronic blood loss, usually from esophageal varices secondary to portal hypertension; (2) simultaneous hemolysis in the liver; (3) "autoimmune" hemolytic anemia; or (4) relative marrow failure (as in cirrhosis). Rarely, a secondary folic acid deficiency and megaloblastic anemia may develop. Red cells in hypersplenism developing in the course of (for example) myelofibrosis or thalassemia have the characteristic morphologic abnormalities of these disorders. Despite the anemia, the body red cell mass may be normal or even increased, since the enlarged spleen pools a significant portion of the blood. Reticulocytes may be slightly elevated. The white blood count is usually 2000–4000/μl, occasionally less; the reduction involves the granulocytes, especially the polymorphonuclear cells; some "shift to the left" is common. Platelet counts are usually about 100,000/μl, occasionally as low as 50,000/μl.

Differential Diagnosis

Hypersplenism is characterized by "empty blood," "full marrow," and a large spleen.

Leukemia and lymphoma are diagnosed by marrow aspiration or lymph node biopsy and examination of the peripheral blood (white count and differential). In hereditary spherocytosis there are spherocytes, osmotic fragility is increased, and platelets and white cells are normal. The hemoglobinopathies with splenomegaly are differentiated on the basis of hemoglobin electrophoresis. Thalassemia major becomes apparent in early childhood, and the blood smear morphology is characteristic. In myelofibrosis, marrow biopsy shows proliferation of fibroblasts and replacement of normal elements. In idiopathic thrombocytopenic purpura, the spleen is normal or only slightly enlarged. In aplastic anemia, the spleen is not enlarged and the marrow is fatty.

Complications

Gastrointestinal hemorrhage due to bleeding from esophageal varices may be fatal. Granulocytopenia may cause persistent leg ulcers or overwhelming infection.

Treatment

When hematologic abnormalities are not severe or

are not associated with symptoms, no therapy is required. Splenectomy may be advisable when recurrent infections (associated with leukopenia) develop, when anemia requires repeated transfusions, or when splenic enlargement or recurrent splenic infarcts cause local discomfort.

A. Portal Hypertension: If portal-systemic shunt is indicated for patients with esophageal varices, the choice between portacaval and splenorenal shunt may be based upon considerations other than the presence or absence of hypersplenism because any procedure that lowers portal pressure tends to improve thrombocytopenia. Splenectomy alone is of lasting benefit only if the vascular obstruction is confined to the splenic vein.

B. Felty's Syndrome: This disease consists of rheumatoid arthritis, neutropenia, and splenomegaly. The reason for the neutropenia is not known, but it responds to splenectomy. Afterward, these patients are less susceptible to infection. In general, the arthritis is not affected by removal of the spleen.

C. Myelofibrosis: It was thought at one time that in myelofibrosis the spleen often performed a crucial function of extramedullary hematopoiesis and that splenectomy would lead to lethal reductions in the blood elements. Clinical trial has proved this reasoning to be false; many patients with myelofibrosis are made more comfortable by being rid of the massive spleen or by correction of anemia and thrombocytopenia. Splenectomy should be considered after treatment with drugs such as corticosteroids and busulfan has proved inadequate.

Prognosis

The prognosis is that of the underlying disorder. If there is good laboratory evidence of destruction of cellular elements in the spleen with activity of the bone marrow, the prognosis is good.

Some of the best results have followed splenectomy for Felty's syndrome, myeloid metaplasia, chronic malaria, and tuberculosis of the spleen. Less satisfactory results have been achieved by splenectomy for thalassemia major, sickle cell anemia, and the secondary hypersplenism of lymphoma and the leukemias.

The course in congestive splenomegaly due to portal hypertension depends upon the degree of venous obstruction and liver damage. Without hematemesis, the course may be relatively benign and splenectomy may not be necessary.

Amorosi EL: Hypersplenism. Seminars Hemat 2:249–285, 1965.

Gomes MMR & others: Indications for splenectomy in hematologic diseases. Surg Gynec Obst 129:129–139, 1969.

Gomes MMR & others: Splenectomy for agnogenic myeloid metaplasia. Surg Gynec Obst 125:106–108, 1967.

Holt JM, Witts LJ: Splenectomy in leukemia and the reticuloses. Quart J Med 35:369–384, 1966.

Jandl JH, Aster RH: Increased splenic pooling and the pathogenesis of hypersplenism. Am J Med Sc 253:383–397, 1967.

Sandusky WR & others: Splenectomy: Indications and results in hematological disorders. Ann Surg 159:695–710, 1964.

Sandusky WR & others: Splenectomy for control of neutropenia in Felty's syndrome. Ann Surg 167:744–751, 1968.

3. STAGING OF HODGKIN'S DISEASE

Until recently, splenectomy was performed in Hodgkin's disease principally as treatment for selected individuals with hypersplenism. In general, the results were no better than fair, because in these patients the disease was usually far-advanced.

During the past decade or so, it has been shown that many patients with Hodgkin's disease can be cured with radiotherapy. Clinical trials of a more aggressive radiotherapeutic approach have given very promising results not only when the disease is localized to the neck or mediastinum but in other cases also—eg, where abdominal and cervical involvement coexist. Spread to bone marrow and viscera other than the spleen (stage IV) indicates extension beyond the curative reach of radiation, and in these patients other treatment protocols (chemotherapy) are being tested.

With clinical evidence of disease in the upper abdomen, laparotomy and splenectomy are often helpful, particularly when the spleen is large. An enlarged spleen cannot be safely radiated because radiation exposure to the left kidney becomes technically unavoidable.

When there are no clinical signs of abdominal involvement, some groups have advocated laparotomy for accurate staging, although the value of this approach has not been firmly established. The surgical procedure in such patients should consist of splenectomy with removal of hilar lymph nodes, excisional biopsy of para-aortic lymph nodes and any others that appear abnormal, and both generous open wedge and needle biopsy of the liver.

Enright LP & others: The surgical diagnosis of abdominal Hodgkin's disease. Surg Gynec Obst 130:853–858, 1970.

Rosenberg SA, Kaplan HS: Hodgkin's disease and other malignant lymphomas. California Med 113:23–38, Oct 1970.

Trueblood HW & others: Hodgkin's disease and non-Hodgkin's lymphoma: The surgeon's role in therapy. Curr Probl Surg, Aug 1972.

4. ANEURYSM OF THE SPLENIC ARTERY

This is an uncommon problem even though this artery is the second most frequent abdominal artery to undergo aneurysmal change. It occurs twice as often in women as in men. The patients can be divided into 2 groups: (1) elderly people whose aneurysms are manifestations of atherosclerosis, and (2) young women with apparently congenital aneurysms which have a predilection for rupture during pregnancy. When a calcified atherosclerotic aneurysm is discovered in a patient over age 60, surgical excision is not indicated in the absence of symptoms or splenic enlargement. In younger patients, aneurysmectomy and splenectomy are advisable to prevent rupture. Sudden intra-abdominal hemorrhage during pregnancy suggests rupture of the splenic artery and calls for prompt laparotomy. The aneurysm is usually found within several centimeters of the hilum of the spleen.

Control of bleeding followed by excision of the aneurysm and splenectomy is the treatment of choice.

Bergner LH, Bentivegna SS: Aneurysms of the splenic artery. Ann Surg 166:767–772, 1967.

Carlisle BB, Lawler WR: Aneurysm of the splenic artery. Am J Surg 114:443–447, 1967.

5. SPLENOSIS

Splenosis is a condition in which multiple small implants of splenic tissue grow in scattered areas throughout the peritoneal surfaces. The seeding of this tissue follows dissemination after traumatic rupture of the spleen and is usually discovered much later as an incidental finding during laparotomy for unrelated causes. Histologically, the tissue can be distinguished from accessory spleens by the absence of elastic fibers or smooth muscle in the delicate capsule. Of the 70 reported cases, in only 4 patients with intestinal obstruction could the splenosis be implicated in the pathologic process. In the remainder, it apparently had no adverse effects.

Whether splenosis performs the functions of normal splenic tissue has not been settled. Aggressive attempts at surgical excision are probably not warranted.

Widmann WD, Laubscher FA: Splenosis: A disease or a beneficial condition? Arch Surg 102:152–158, 1971.

COMPLICATIONS OF SPLENECTOMY

Splenectomy is associated with few complications if the operation is competently done. If splenectomy is being carried out for conditions such as ITP, secondary bleeding may occur as a result of insufficiency of platelets. There is usually a rapid rise in platelets following splenectomy. If oozing is observed by the surgeon at operation and the platelet count fails to rise promptly after splenectomy, platelet transfusions are indicated. Major postoperative hemorrhage may be due to inadequate control of the splenic pedicle with secondary hemorrhage from the splenic artery. If the patient develops signs of intraperitoneal bleeding or unexplained hypotension postoperatively, reoperation is mandatory. In the course of mobilizing the spleen for splenectomy, the tail of the pancreas can be traumatized and pancreatitis may result. This is usually self-limited and does not require reoperation; occasionally, however, pancreatitis may be so virulent that reoperation and drainage of the left upper quadrant are indicated.

Even though the spleen has been convincingly demonstrated to be the site of hemolysis, some patients with hemolytic anemia fail to respond to splenectomy. About 25% of patients with hemolytic anemia have been shown to have accessory spleens which, if overlooked during the initial laparotomy, may undergo hypertrophy and cause clinical relapse. These accessory spleens may be anywhere in the peritoneal cavity, but most are found in the splenic hilum, in the gastrosplenic ligament, or in the omentum.

•　　•　　•

General References

Ballinger WF II, Erslev AJ: Splenectomy. Curr Probl Surg, Feb 1965.

Lennert K: *The Spleen.* Springer-Verlag, 1970.

Schwartz SI & others: Splenectomy for hematologic disorders. Curr Probl Surg, May 1971.

30 . . .

Portal Hypertension

Lawrence W. Way, MD, & F. William Blaisdell, MD

Portal hypertension is most commonly caused by cirrhosis of the liver, but various other diseases are occasionally implicated. The rise in portal pressure is usually a result of increased resistance to flow (eg, cirrhosis); rarely, massively increased portal flow is an important contributing factor. The high portal pressure stimulates expansion of rudimentary venous collaterals between the portal and systemic venous systems. The most significant is the venous plexus at the gastroesophageal junction, which drains into the azygos veins. Under the stimulus to transport greater volumes, these may develop into large fragile submucosal varices susceptible to spontaneous rupture and massive hemorrhage. This is the major complication of portal hypertension and the usual reason the surgeon becomes involved in the care of these patients. The other common clinical sequelae include ascites, hepatic encephalopathy, and secondary hypersplenism. If the surgeon can construct a large-diameter anastomosis (shunt) between the portal and systemic venous circulations, the elevated portal pressure drops and the risk of variceal hemorrhage is eliminated. However, decisions about the care of these patients are rarely simple since portacaval shunts tend to impair hepatic function and lower the threshold for encephalopathy. Potential candidates for operation must be carefully evaluated to ensure optimal surgical results.

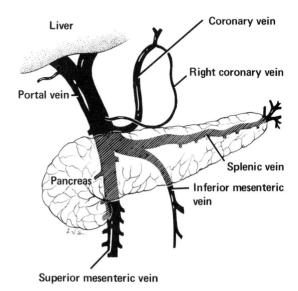

FIG 30–1. Anatomic relationships of portal vein and branches.

ANATOMY OF THE PORTAL CIRCULATION

The portal vein is formed by the confluence of the splenic and superior mesenteric veins at the level of the second lumbar vertebra behind the head of the pancreas (Fig 30–1). It runs for 8–9 cm to the hilum of the liver, where it divides into lobar branches. The coronary (left gastric) vein usually enters the portal vein on its anteromedial aspect just cranial to the margin of the pancreas in which case it usually must be ligated during the surgical construction of a portacaval shunt; in 25% of cases, the coronary vein joins the splenic vein. Other small venous tributaries from the pancreas and duodenum are less constant but must be anticipated during surgical mobilization of the portal vein.

The inferior mesenteric vein generally drains into the splenic vein several centimeters to the left of the junction with the superior mesenteric vein; not uncommonly, it empties directly into the superior mesenteric vein.

In the hepatoduodenal ligament, the portal vein lies dorsal and slightly medial to the common bile duct. A large lymph node is often encountered lateral to the vein and must be dissected off before a shunt can be performed.

PHYSIOLOGY

Total hepatic blood flow is about 1500 ml/minute and comprises 25% of the cardiac output. Two-thirds of the flow enters through the portal vein and one-third through the hepatic artery. Pressure in the portal vein is normally 10–15 cm water (7–11 mm Hg). The liver derives half of its oxygen from hepatic arterial blood and half from portal venous inflow.

Portal venous and hepatic arterial blood become pooled after entering the periphery of the hepatic sinusoid (Fig 30–2). There is evidence that sphincters

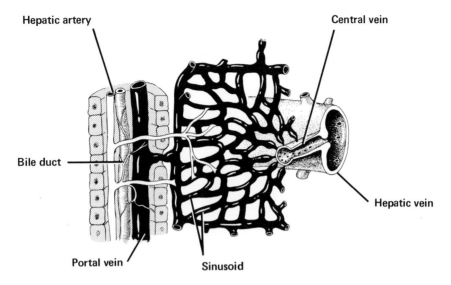

FIG 30–2. Vascular anatomy of the liver lobule.

regulate flow from the hepatic arterioles into the low-pressure sinusoids, although they have not been convincingly demonstrated by histologic technics. Flow within the sinusoids is erratic since at any given moment the blood may be stationary in as many as 40% of them. The regulatory mechanisms governing sinusoidal blood flow are not well understood, but the normal sinusoidal bed can accommodate large variations in portal flow without significant changes in portal pressure.

Sudden occlusion of the portal vein results in an immediate 60% rise in hepatic arterial flow. In a matter of weeks, total flow gradually returns toward normal. On the other hand, sudden reductions in hepatic arterial supply are not immediately met by significant increases in portal vein flow. In both normal subjects and cirrhotics, total hepatic flow and portal pressure drop following hepatic arterial occlusion. Arterial collaterals develop over the ensuing months, and arterial perfusion is ultimately restored.

Bloch EH: The termination of hepatic arterioles and the functional unit of the liver as determined by microscopy of the living organ. Ann New York Acad Sc 170:78–87, 1970.

Greenway CV, Stark RD: Hepatic vascular bed. Physiol Rev 51:23–65, 1971.

Marks C: Developmental basis of the portal venous system. Am J Surg 117:671–681, 1969.

ETIOLOGY

The causes of portal hypertension are listed in Table 30–1. In all but a few, the basic lesion is increased resistance to portal flow. Those associated with

increased resistance can be subclassified according to the site of the block as prehepatic, hepatic, and posthepatic. Cirrhosis accounts for about 85% of cases of portal hypertension in the USA, and the most common form is that due to alcoholism. Postnecrotic cirrhosis is next in frequency, followed by biliary cirrhosis. The

TABLE 30–1. Causes of portal hypertension.

I. Increased resistance to flow
  A. Prehepatic (portal vein obstruction)
    1. Congenital atresia or stenosis
    2. Thrombosis of portal vein
    3. Thrombosis of splenic vein
    4. Extrinsic compression (eg, tumors)
  B. Hepatic
    1. Cirrhosis
      a. Portal cirrhosis (nutritional, alcoholic, Laennec's)
      b. Postnecrotic cirrhosis
      c. Biliary cirrhosis
      d. Others (Wilson's disease, hemochromatosis, late schistosomiasis)
    2. Acute alcoholic liver disease
    3. Congenital hepatic fibrosis
    4. Idiopathic portal hypertension (hepatoportal sclerosis)
    5. Schistosomiasis
  C. Posthepatic
    1. Budd-Chiari syndrome
    2. Constrictive pericarditis
II. Increased portal blood flow
  A. Arterial-portal venous fistula
  B. Increased splenic flow
    1. Banti's syndrome
    2. Splenomegaly (eg, tropical splenomegaly, myeloid metaplasia)

other intrahepatic causes of portal hypertension are relatively rare in this country, although in some parts of the world hepatic schistosomiasis comprises the largest single group. Idiopathic portal hypertension appears with greater frequency in southern Asia.

Next to cirrhosis, extrahepatic portal venous occlusion is the most common cause of portal hypertension. These patients are generally younger than the cirrhotics, and many are children. Posthepatic obstruction due to Budd-Chiari syndrome or constrictive pericarditis is rare.

PATHOPHYSIOLOGY

Portal hypertension is defined as portal pressure of 20 cm water (15 mm Hg) or more.

The greater resistance to portal flow presented by the cirrhotic liver is a result of parenchymal fibrosis and changes in vascular anatomy. Portal inflow is partially obstructed by scar formation. As much as one-third of portal flow may bypass sinusoids through shunts traversing areas bridged by fibrosis between portal areas and central veins. A great deal more remains to be learned about hemodynamics through the cirrhotic liver, but it is noteworthy that the regenerative nodule is associated with a postsinusoidal* type of resistance as measured by wedged hepatic vein pressure. Regenerative nodules are supplied with blood mainly from the hepatic artery, and the escape of blood from the sinusoids of these nodules takes place through abnormal hepatic venous channels at the periphery of the nodule. An interesting phenomenon is presented by hepatic schistosomiasis which evolves through 2 pathophysiologic phases. Early in the disease, granulomas from parasitic involvement are seen in the triads, and the portal hypertension is presinusoidal. Eventually, fibrosis and regenerative nodules appear, and the block shifts to a postsinusoidal position.

Even in the absence of cirrhosis, acute alcoholism can raise portal pressure by producing centrolobular swelling and fibrosis. Sinusoidal resistance to flow is also increased by engorgement of adjacent hepatocytes with fat and resultant distortion and narrowing of the vascular pathway. Examples have been documented where the elevated portal pressure dropped with resolution of the pathologic changes.

---

*A catheter wedged in a tributary of the hepatic vein estimates the pressure in the afferent veins to the sinusoid. The gradient between the wedged pressure and that in the hepatic vein reflects resistance at any point between the wedged position and the periphery of the sinusoid. Therefore, in the absence of definite pathologic evidence for the precise location of the block, it is impossible by this technic to distinguish between a sinusoidal and postsinusoidal lesion. The literature, however, often refers with unjustified precision to cirrhosis as producing a postsinusoidal block, whereas a combination of postsinusoidal and sinusoidal resistance is actually involved.

Fluctuations in the level of portal hypertension also occur in conjunction with changes in blood volume, and patients with ascites are especially sensitive. Administration of colloid solutions to a patient with a normal or expanded blood volume could theoretically aggravate the clinical manifestations of portal hypertension.

Budd-Chiari syndrome is produced by restriction to flow through the hepatic veins or the inferior vena cava above the liver. Some cases are the result of hepatic vein thrombosis, as in polycythemia vera; tumors are occasionally implicated. In others, venous stenosis develops for unknown reasons. The posthepatic resistance in Budd-Chiari syndrome produces marked increases in sinusoidal pressure which are transmitted upstream to the portal venous blood. Sinusoidal hypertension is the factor responsible for the uniformly prominent ascites and hepatomegaly in this condition.

Total splenic blood flow is usually increased in splenomegaly regardless of the cause. Although increased portal inflow may contribute to portal hypertension in cirrhosis, it is not a decisive factor since splenectomy has no permanent effect on portal pressure. **Banti's syndrome** was originally defined as liver injury secondary to primary splenic disease, but most of the original cases actually consisted of cirrhosis as the primary disease with congestive splenomegaly. The greatly increased splenic blood flow in some cases of myeloid metaplasia and tropical splenomegaly with portal hypertension resembles the effects of an arterial-portal venous fistula, and splenectomy alone may cure the portal hypertension in some cases. Except in these terms, Banti's syndrome must be quite rare.

The average portal flow in cirrhotic patients with complications of portal hypertension is about 30% of normal, ranging from 0–700 ml/minute. On the average, hepatic arterial flow is reduced by a similar proportion. The range of portal flow rates in different patients may vary greatly; in a few, blood in the portal vein moves only sluggishly, and in rare instances the direction of flow may even be reversed so that the portal vein functions as an outflow tract from the liver. These states of low flow predispose to spontaneous thrombosis of the portal vein, an occasional complication of cirrhosis which usually renders the portal vein unsuitable for a shunt.

The obstacle to flow through the liver stimulates expansion of collateral channels between the portal and systemic venous systems. As the pathologic process develops, portal pressure increases until a level of about 40 cm water (30 mm Hg) is reached. At this point, increasing hepatic resistance, even to the point of occlusion of the portal vein, diverts a greater fraction of portal flow through the collaterals without significant increments in portal pressure.

The type of collaterals which develop depends partly on the cause of the portal hypertension. In extrahepatic portal vein thrombosis (without liver disease), collaterals (hepatopetal) in the diaphragm, in the hepatocolic and hepatogastric ligaments, etc transport blood into the liver around the occluded vein. In both cirrhosis and portal thrombosis, collaterals (hepato-fugal) appear which carry blood around the liver into the systemic circulation, and it is these that produce esophageal and gastric varices. Other common spontaneous collaterals are through a recanalized umbilical vein to the abdominal wall, from the superior hemorrhoidal vein into the middle and inferior hemorrhoidal veins, and through numerous small veins (of Retzius) connecting the retroperitoneal viscera with the posterior abdominal wall. Although spontaneous hemorrhage may occur from duodenal, cecal, or hemorrhoidal varices, only rarely does such an event present clinically as massive bleeding.

Blendis LM & others: Spleen blood flow and splanchnic haemo-dynamics in blood dyscrasia and other splenomegalies. Clin Sc 38:73–84, 1970.

Greenway CV, Stark RD: Hepatic vascular bed. Physiol Rev 51:23–65, 1971.

Moreno AH & others: Portal blood flow in cirrhosis of the liver. J Clin Invest 46:436–445, 1967.

Popper H, Hotterer F: Hepatic fibrogenesis and disturbance of the hepatic circulation. Ann New York Acad Sc 170:88–99, 1970.

Rappaport AM & others: Hepatic microcirculatory changes leading to portal hypertension. Ann New York Acad Sc 170:48–66, 1970.

CIRRHOSIS OF THE LIVER

The death rate from cirrhosis of the liver exceeds 23,000 per year in the USA. The incidence of the disease is increasing, and at present it is the third most common cause of death in men in the fifth decade of life. A variety of data indicate a causative relationship to excessive alcohol consumption, but the exact relationship remains hazy. For example, the prevalence of cirrhosis correlates with regional alcohol consumption, and the disease decreased dramatically during Prohibition. On the other hand, fewer than 10% of alcoholics develop cirrhosis, and those affected are not obviously different in other ways from those who escape the disease. Animal experiments and the effects of therapy in man indicate that protein-calorie malnutrition is an interacting factor.

Cirrhosis develops as a result of hepatocellular destruction and regeneration and scar formation. The latter may perpetuate the process by interfering with parenchymal nutrition and by contributing to portal hypertension. Hepatocellular fat deposition commonly precedes cirrhosis, but whether it is a prerequisite is not settled.

The natural history of cirrhosis is imperfectly understood because major discrepancies exist in survival statistics. Nevertheless, once the diagnosis has been established, 30% or more of patients are dead within a year. A group of cirrhotics with varices followed by the Boston Interhospital Liver Group experi-enced a 1-year mortality rate of 66%. Cirrhotics without varices may benefit substantially by returning to a nutritious diet and abstaining from alcohol. However, once bleeding has occurred, survival is only slightly improved by nonoperative therapy. Bleeding occurs in about 40% of all patients with cirrhosis, and the initial episode of variceal hemorrhage is fatal to 50–80%. At least two-thirds of those who survive their initial hemorrhage will bleed again, and the risk of dying from the second is about the same as from the first episode. It is principally for such patients that portacaval shunts are recommended.

Gabuzda FJ: Nutrition and liver disease. M Clin North America 54:1455–1472, 1970.

Garceau AJ, Chalmers TC: The natural history of cirrhosis. I. Survival with esophageal varices. New England J Med 268:469–473, 1963.

Powell WJ Jr, Klatskin G: Duration of survival in patients with Laennec's cirrhosis. Am J Med 44:406–420, 1968.

ACUTE MASSIVELY BLEEDING VARICES

About two-thirds of patients with massive bleeding from varices die as a result of the acute event. The high mortality rate reflects not only the amount and rate of hemorrhage but also the frequent presence of severely compromised liver function and other systemic disease which may or may not be related to alcoholism. Malnutrition, pulmonary aspiration and infection, and coronary artery disease are frequently coexistent factors presaging a fatal outcome. The alcoholic patient often does not cooperate during therapy, and if delirium tremens ensues even his physical control may present a major management problem.

Clinical Findings

A. Symptoms and Signs: The initial diagnostic and therapeutic management of the patient with massive gastrointestinal hemorrhage is discussed in Chapter 25. It must be emphasized that bleeding from varices cannot be accurately diagnosed on clinical grounds alone even though the history or the appearance of the patient may strongly suggest the presence of cirrhosis or portal hypertension. Most patients with bleeding varices have alcoholic cirrhosis, and the diagnosis may seem obvious in a patient with hepatomegaly, jaundice, and vascular spiders who admits to a recent alcoholic binge. Splenomegaly, the most constant physical finding, is present in 80–90% of patients with portal hypertension regardless of the cause. Ascites is frequently present. Massive ascites and hepatosplenomegaly in a nonalcoholic would suggest the rare Budd-Chiari syndrome. If cirrhosis or varices have been documented on previous examinations, hematemesis later may point toward bleeding varices.

B. Laboratory Findings: Most alcoholics with acute upper gastrointestinal bleeding have compromised liver function. The bilirubin is usually elevated; it may be normal, but BSP retention will be found if there is cirrhosis. Serum albumin is often below 3 g/100 ml. The leukocyte count may be elevated. Anemia may be a reflection of chronic alcoholic liver disease or hypersplenism as well as acute hemorrhage. The development of a hepatoma by a cirrhotic sometimes is first manifested by bleeding varices, and this possibility should be checked by testing for serum a-fetoglobulin. The prothrombin time and partial thromboplastin time may be abnormal.

C. Special Examinations:

1. Esophagogastroscopy—Emergency esophagogastroscopy is the most useful procedure for diagnosing bleeding varices and should be scheduled as soon as the patient's general condition is stabilized by blood transfusion and other supportive measures. Varices appear as 3—4 large, tortuous submucosal bluish vessels running longitudinally in the distal esophagus. The bleeding site may be visualized, but sometimes the lumen fills with blood so rapidly that the lesion is obscured. Acute hemorrhagic gastritis and Mallory-Weiss tears are 2 lesions in the differential diagnosis that can be seen on endoscopy but cannot be detected on upper gastrointestinal series.

2. Upper gastrointestinal series—A barium swallow will outline the varices in about 90% of affected patients, and if the patient's condition remains satisfactory x-rays should be performed in the acute bleeder immediately after endoscopy. If both varices and a peptic ulcer are found on x-ray, the source of the bleeding is indeterminate unless endoscopy has settled the question.

3. Measurement of portal pressure—Three methods are available for measuring portal pressure preoperatively: wedged hepatic vein pressure (WHVP), direct percutaneous splenic pulp manometry, and cannulation of the umbilical vein remnant. They all reliably reflect portal pressure with the exception that WHVP remains normal in the presence of a presinusoidal block. Since most patients have sinusoidal (or postsinusoidal) lesions and because the procedure has almost no morbidity, WHVP is usually the method of choice.

a. Wedged hepatic vein pressure (WHVP)—A catheter is passed percutaneously via the brachial or axillary vein into the vena cava and then, under fluoroscopic control, one of the hepatic veins is entered. The pressure is measured in the free hepatic vein (FHVP), and the catheter is advanced until it becomes wedged in a peripheral tributary. The reading in the wedged position measures the pressure across any resistance up to the first system of collaterals, which allows flow around the stagnated column of blood. For a catheter wedged in the hepatic vein, this point is at the periphery of the sinusoid. Subtraction of FHVP from WHVP gives the portal-hepatic pressure gradient. The normal value is about 4 cm water (3 mm Hg); a gradient above 8 cm water (6 mm Hg) is considered to represent portal hypertension; in bleeding varices, the gradient is usually greater than 20 cm water (15 mm Hg).

Although a satisfactory anatomic explanation is unavailable, it has been shown that the WHVP accurately reflects portal vein pressure (PVP) in all types of cirrhosis. If the lesion is located on the splanchnic side of the sinusoid (presinusoidal), whether it is prehepatic or intrahepatic, portal pressure is not measured by this technic. After the pressure readings are obtained, diatrizoate (Hypaque) is injected through the catheter for x-ray verification of the wedged position and to check the flow behavior of contrast refluxed into the portal vein. If portal flow is retrograde or sluggish, this suggests that portal diversion would not further impair liver function.

b. Splenic pulp manometry—Until recently, this was the best method available for determining portal pressure, but except for special cases it has largely been supplanted by hepatic vein wedged pressure. The patient should be positioned supine on an x-ray cassette changer, mildly sedated, and instructed to breathe shallowly and regularly to avoid sudden wide diaphragmatic excursions. A needle or cannula is inserted percutaneously into the estimated center of the splenic surface, which usually corresponds to a site on the skin in the eighth, ninth, or tenth intercostal space in the midaxillary line. It is best to use a plastic catheter with a metal trocar because—after insertion into the spleen—removal of the trocar allows flexibility in response to respiratory motion. Pressure readings are obtained with a water manometer using the midaxillary line as the zero reference. Fifty ml of diatrizoate are then injected over 5 seconds to visualize the portal venous system, and x-rays are taken with an automatic cassette changer every 2 seconds for 8 exposures. The quality of films is excellent, but the varices themselves are not always well opacified. This technic will usually demonstrate whether or not the portal vein is patent. When considered only from the standpoint of diagnosis, this method is less accurate than esophagoscopy or barium swallow for demonstrating varices.

Direct splenic puncture entails greater morbidity than the other methods of measuring pressure or outlining the venous anatomy. Abdominal bleeding from the splenic surface requires blood transfusion in about 5% of cases, and splenectomy is sometimes necessary. Nevertheless, this is still the best means of determining portal pressure in patients with presinusoidal block.

c. Umbilical vein cannulation—The remnant of umbilical vein passes in the falciform ligament from the umbilicus to the left branch of the portal vein. Its lumen usually remains obliterated, although in some patients spontaneous recanalization allows it to serve as a portal systemic collateral. The lumen of the obliterated vessel can be reopened with a probe and used to enter the portal circulation. This has recently been exploited as a means of measuring portal pressure and obtaining venous angiograms. The procedure can usually be done with local anesthesia and sedation. The obliterated umbilical vein is surgically located in the falciform ligament, and a dilator is forced down the lumen until the left branch of the portal vein is broken into. A catheter is inserted into the portal vein for measuring pressure and for injecting x-ray contrast medium.

Umbilical vein catheterization can be successfully performed in most patients with portal hypertension not associated with extrahepatic portal vein thrombosis. Its place in the evaluation of the average patient is not yet clear, but the procedure does provide direct access to the portal circulation and the morbidity is insignificant.

4. Selective mesenteric angiography—Selective angiography is the method most often employed preoperatively to visualize the portal vein and its tributaries. A catheter inserted percutaneously into the femoral or axillary artery is advanced into the celiac artery and, if possible, the splenic artery. Contrast medium is injected, and films are exposed during the arterial and venous phases. Complications are rare, and the quality of the x-rays is good. It is wise to routinely visualize the veins planned for use in a shunt before operation to determine their location, patency, and suitability for anastomosis.

Selective angiography does not ordinarily demonstrate active bleeding from varices. Since nearly all other causes of acute upper gastrointestinal hemorrhage can be shown by angiography, a negative examination would support the diagnosis of variceal bleeding if the patient was truly bleeding during the study.

5. Liver biopsy—In the majority of patients, the preoperative evaluation should include a percutaneous liver biopsy. It should verify the clinical diagnosis of cirrhosis but is especially important to uncover acute liver disease such as alcoholic hepatitis. Biopsy is also helpful to diagnose the less common causes of portal hypertension such as schistosomiasis, hepatic fibrosis, etc.

Treatment of Acute Bleeding

After varices have been definitely incriminated as the cause of the bleeding, specific therapy can be instituted. The therapeutic options include systemic or selective splanchnic administration of vasopressin, insertion of a Sengstaken-Blakemore tube, and emergency surgery, either variceal ligation or emergency portacaval shunt.

A. Vasopressin: Vasopressin (Pitressin) lowers mesenteric blood flow by constricting mesenteric arterioles. The action is relatively specific, since the hepatic artery is affected only slightly. In the systemic mode of treatment, 20 units of vasopressin are given intravenously over 20–30 minutes, diluted in 100–200 ml of normal saline. The reduction in flow produces a drop of 20–25% in portal venous pressure, and clinical experience suggests that this helps to stop variceal bleeding. The dose can be repeated every 3–4 hours if necessary.

More recently, vasopressin has been given directly into the superior mesenteric artery by a catheter inserted percutaneously. The drug is administered by a calibrated pump at the rate of 0.2 unit/minute in a solution containing 0.2 unit/ml. An angiogram should be obtained 15 minutes after vasopressin is begun to

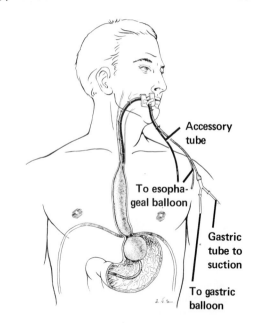

FIG 30–3. Sengstaken-Blakemore tube with both gastric and esophageal balloons inflated.

verify the interval appearance of vasospasm in the splanchnic arteries. Treatment should be continued for 48 hours after bleeding is controlled. The catheter is left in position for another 24 hours and perfused with saline. It can then be removed if there is no further bleeding. This seems to be the most promising regimen for the use of vasopressin at present. When the goal of vasopressin therapy is to slow blood loss while preparations are being made for emergency portacaval shunt, the systemic route should suffice. Vasopressin should probably not be used by either route in patients with coronary ischemia.

B. Sengstaken-Blakemore (SB) Tube: (Fig 30–3.) This tube has 2 balloons attached which can be inflated in the lumen of the gut to tamponade bleeding varices. There are 3 lumens in the tube: 2 are for filling the balloons, and the third permits aspiration of gastric contents. Since the task of placement and subsequent care is complicated and time-consuming, the SB tube should generally be used only after the diagnosis of bleeding varices has been definitely established by endoscopy. However, in some cases of massive hemorrhage, there may not be time for endoscopy and the SB tube may be used on the basis of clinical suspicion alone. However, if inflating the balloons controls the bleeding, this does not prove that it originated from varices. As a treatment device, balloon tamponade has not been regularly effective for Mallory-Weiss tears and would not be expected to affect other causes of gastroduodenal hemorrhage.

A new Davol 10F SB tube should be used, and both balloons must be checked under water for leaks. Before the tube is inserted, a standard nasogastric tube should be tied alongside with its tip located just orad to the esophageal balloon.* The patient's stomach should be emptied as completely as possible to avoid aspiration before inserting the tube. The entire assembly is then passed through the patient's mouth into his stomach. To verify that the tube has entered the stomach, inject 25–50 ml of air rapidly into the gastric balloon while listening over the epigastrium with a stethoscope. The gastric balloon is then inflated with 250–275 ml of air, and traction is applied until a snug fit is obtained between the balloon and the gastroesophageal junction. If the patient develops substernal pain while inflating the gastric balloon, stop immediately and determine that it is not in the esophagus. The position is fixed to maintain tension by taping a mouth guard to the tube (Fig 30–3). The esophageal balloon should be inflated only if bleeding continues after compression by the gastric balloon, but it will be required in most cases. The esophageal balloon should be distended with a manometer to 33–60 cm water (25–45 mm Hg), maintaining the lowest pressure that produces hemostasis.

The patient must be under continuous observation, preferably in the intensive care unit or by special nurses on the ward. A heavy pair of scissors should be kept at the bedside, and those responsible for the patient's care should be instructed to cut across the tube (which rapidly deflates the balloons) and remove it quickly if respiratory obstruction develops.

The most common serious problem is aspiration of pharyngeal secretions and pneumonitis. This has been largely obviated by tying on the additional tube which maintains the hypopharynx clear of secretions. Allowing the patient to move around in bed and to breathe comfortably also helps to preserve pulmonary function.

Another serious hazard is the occasional instance of esophageal rupture caused by inflation of the esophageal balloon. To avoid this risk, the latter should not be inflated beyond the pressures listed above. With these precautions and expert nursing care, the incidence of complications is negligible.

About 85–90% of actively bleeding patients can be controlled by the SB tube. When bleeding has been stopped, the balloons are left inflated for another 24 hours. They are then decompressed, leaving the tube in place. If bleeding does not recur in the subsequent 24 hours, the tube should be withdrawn. If an SB tube has been used but bleeding either continues or recurs with the balloons inflated, emergency surgical treatment must be considered. The return of bleeding after successful balloon tamponade should be treated by reinsertion of another tube.

Several groups which have relied heavily on the SB tube report a hospital mortality rate below 40% for acute variceal bleeding. Patients who survive may then be considered as candidates for elective portacaval shunt.

*The Edlich tube made by Davol incorporates a fourth channel for clearing the upper esophagus and will probably supplant the standard SB tube when it becomes generally available.

C. Emergency Operation: The 2 operations to control active bleeding are variceal ligation and portacaval shunt.

1. Variceal ligation—In the past this was usually performed through a left thoracotomy, but most surgeons prefer an abdominal approach because concomitant gastric varices or other causes of bleeding are easier to manage. The lumen of the lower esophagus is entered, and the varices are oversewn with a running suture of chromic catgut. When a thoracotomy is used, gastric varices can be exposed by a diaphragmatic incision and proximal gastrotomy.

Variceal ligation usually stops acute bleeding, but since it does nothing to lower portal pressure recurrent bleeding is common before the patient can be prepared for definitive portacaval shunt. For this reason, the operation is seldom used.

2. Emergency portacaval shunt—Since the bleeding is a direct consequence of elevated portal pressure, reduction of pressure by a shunt is usually successful treatment. The disadvantages of this approach are that the diagnostic work-up may have to be abbreviated in emergency circumstances; liver function is often acutely compromised; and the patient's general condition (eg, cardiac, pulmonary, and renal status) is frequently suboptimal. Despite these drawbacks, operation is sometimes necessary if bleeding continues despite tamponade or vasopressin infusion. It has been argued by some that, since the patient's overall condition so frequently deteriorates during the initial 24–48 hours of medical management, earlier surgery might be preferable for nearly all patients after initial resuscitation. This proposition needs more empirical support before being accepted.

Portacaval shunt, either end-to-side, side-to-side, or H-mesocaval, is the procedure of choice since these are easier to perform than splenorenal shunts. Angiograms are not usually available, so at laparotomy a thrombosed portal vein is occasionally discovered which is unsuitable for anastomosis. In this situation, the best operation would probably be an H-mesocaval shunt using a segment of arterial Dacron or Teflon graft.

The overall mortality for emergency shunts is about 50%. The result in the individual patient is largely determined by the quality of liver function, the extent of blood loss before and during operation, the duration of operation, and the technical result (ie, whether the shunt remains patent). In general, patients with good liver function, minimal or no encephalopathy, and mild or no ascites do well, but this describes only a minority of acute bleeders. Alcoholics seem to fare better than nonalcoholic cirrhotics since liver function in the former can be expected to improve postoperatively with restoration of good nutrition. However, patients with acute alcoholic hepatitis experience a high mortality from emergency operations and may go unrecognized preoperatively among a nonselected group of patients with bleeding varices.

There is considerable disagreement about the best way to manage the acutely bleeding patient. Each of the following 3 options has its proponents: (1) Non-operative management with vasopressin or Sengstaken-Blakemore tube for all patients initially, and emergency operation if this fails to control bleeding. (2) Emergency portacaval shunt for those who appear to be "good risks" and nonoperative management of "poor-risk" patients. (3) Emergency portacaval shunt for all patients. At present, most clinicians probably adhere to the notion that emergency surgery should be performed only after an attempt at nonoperative treatment. However, adherents to the other 2 policies report what they interpret to be improved results so that the final judgment awaits controlled clinical trials. Transesophageal ligation of varices has fallen into relative disuse because the patient is exposed to the morbidity of a major operation which often is only transiently successful in controlling the hemorrhage.

Elective Shunts

The goal of a portacaval shunt is to prevent bleeding from varices, and in these terms the operation is successful in 95% of cases. Those who rebleed usually are found to have developed thrombosis at the anastomosis. Theoretically, an elective shunt should be considered for any patient with a substantial future risk of bleeding from varices. Although about 30% of all patients with varices will bleed within 5 years, imperfect knowledge of the determining factors makes it impossible to predict the likelihood of this event in any individual patient. The principal side-effects limiting more general use of shunts are decreased liver function, increased susceptibility to encephalopathy, and an operative mortality rate of 5–10%. When making a judgment about the advisability of performing a shunt for a given patient, the physician must attempt to balance the risk of these untoward effects with that of future hemorrhage.

A. Prophylactic Shunt: Since about one-third of cirrhotics with varices who have not bled eventually die of this complication, prophylactic construction of a shunt was proposed to avoid the high mortality rate of the acute episode. Several controlled clinical trials* were performed to investigate the results of such a policy, and each showed that prophylactic portacaval shunts in unselected patients with varices did not improve longevity. The shunted group was protected from hemorrhage but experienced a completely offsetting rise in mortality from liver failure. Encephalopathy was greater among the treated group than in the controls. Unfortunately, a detailed analysis of the control groups did not turn up clues to which patients would go on to bleed without surgery. Presumably, if a high-risk group could be identified, another trial of the prophylactic shunt would be warranted.

B. Therapeutic Shunt: The results of the studies on prophylactic shunts revealed more adverse effects from the operation than had been anticipated and raised questions regarding the value of shunts in

patients who had bled previously, the so-called therapeutic shunt. Although it had long been believed that survival of these patients was prolonged by operation, controlled trials were instituted to scientifically examine the problem. The results of these studies are still incomplete, but the available data from the VA Cooperative Study, the BILG Study, and the Los Angeles-USC Study demonstrate what appears to be substantially increased longevity of those who were shunted compared with nonshunted controls. This must be considered a tentative conclusion since the data from any one of these trials have not yet achieved statistical significance. Once again, a reciprocal relationship was found between reduction of liver function following operation and the protection from bleeding. As a subgroup, those with good liver function seemed to fare even better with a shunt, but the number of patients involved was too small to allow separate statistical analysis. There was also a definite tendency in the BILG Study toward better survival with end-to-side compared with side-to-side anastomosis. Unexpectedly, the incidence of encephalopathy was about the same in the medical and surgical groups, chiefly owing to the tendency for nonshunted patients to develop this complication in conjunction with additional episodes of variceal bleeding.

These findings have added further emphasis to the need for a means of reducing portal pressure without compromising liver function. At present, the distal splenorenal (Warren) shunt is the best operative prospect. Other means being explored to improve the care of patients with varices involve development of tests which more accurately predict the hepatic effects of a shunt (eg, preoperative quantification of hepatic blood flow) and trials with operations which are technically simpler (H-mesocaval shunt).

In summary: An end-to-side shunt should generally be recommended for patients under age 60 with good liver function who have bled previously. In others, the operation may be employed, but morbidity from liver failure and encephalopathy may sometimes offset the value of a lowered portal pressure. For the latter patients, the Warren shunt may be preferable if surgery seems indicated.

Preoperative Management

After an acute hemorrhage has stopped—especially in alcoholics—the patient's condition can usually be improved by a high-calorie, high-protein diet for several weeks. If acute liver damage is present due to alcoholism, it should be allowed to subside.

Table 30–2 shows the general relationship between operative mortality and quality of liver function. The detrimental effect of a shunt on liver function is thought to be due to nutritional deprivation from loss of portal venous blood flow. Diversion of portal blood is virtually complete after portacaval shunts but is substantially less after a central splenorenal shunt or the distal splenorenal (Warren) shunt.

Tolerance of a portacaval shunt also appears related to the degree that hepatic resistance and flow

---

*VA Cooperative Study and Boston Interhospital Liver Group (BILG) Study.

TABLE 30–2. Relation of hepatic function and
nutrition to operative mortality
after portacaval shunt.

Group	A	B	C
Operative Mortality	2%	10%	50%
Serum bilirubin (mg/100 ml)	< 2.0	2.0–3.0	> 3.0
Serum albumin (gm/100 ml)	> 3.5	3.0–3.5	< 3.0
Ascites	None	Easily controlled	Poorly controlled
Encephalopathy	None	Minimal	Advanced
Nutrition	Excellent	Good	Poor

through collaterals have preoperatively reduced hepatopetal portal flow. Thus, when residual portal flow into the liver is slight, performance of a shunt would have less of an effect on hepatic nutrition and patient survival may be greater. The incidence of postoperative encephalopathy also correlates with the quantitative effect of the shunt on portal flow, and this complication is less after a central splenorenal than portacaval anastomosis. The segmental diversion of blood in the distal splenorenal shunt appears to totally avoid encephalopathy.

Unfortunately, at present the easiest shunts to perform are associated with the highest incidence of late side-effects.

Preoperative evaluation must verify the diagnosis of varices, measure portal pressure, and radiographically visualize the portal venous anatomy. Whether the blood loss in an earlier acute hemorrhage was actually from varices must be questioned since acute gastritis, peptic ulcer, and the Mallory-Weiss lesion account for more than half of the episodes of acute upper gastrointestinal bleeding in cirrhotics. Esophagoscopic visualization of bleeding varices is the most convincing evidence. If esophagoscopy and upper gastrointestinal x-rays were performed acutely and failed to reveal any abnormalities other than varices although a definitive

bleeding point was not seen, this can nevertheless be taken as fairly reliable proof. Of dubious reliability is evidence that use of an SG tube was responsible for controlling the bleeding. When nothing more is available than a history of melena or hematemesis and x-rays showing varices, other causes of the bleeding cannot be excluded with certainty. Thus, the diagnosis is often based on indirect evidence and judgment.

Measurement of portal pressure should be obtained to establish the presence and height of portal hypertension. Bleeding from varices is nearly always associated with a wedged hepatic vein-free hepatic vein pressure gradient of 15 cm water or greater. If the hepatic vein wedged pressure does not verify portal hypertension, either the diagnosis is incorrect or the block is presinusoidal. In the latter case, a direct percutaneous measurement of splenic pulp pressure should be obtained.

Selective splenic and superior mesenteric angiography is usually the best way to visualize the vascular anatomy unless a decision has already been made to measure portal pressure by splenic puncture. If the latter is necessary, a splenoportagram should be obtained simultaneously. In nearly all cases, the portal vein should be outlined angiographically before proceeding with plans for a portacaval shunt since in about 10% of cirrhotics the vein is thrombosed and cannot be used for this shunt. The behavior of contrast media in the portal vein may provide a semiquantitative impression of the rate of hepatopetal flow. The varices are often demonstrated, but angiograms are less reliable than barium swallow or esophagoscopy for the diagnosis of varices.

Optimal preoperative preparation should aim for a serum albumin above 3 g/100 ml, serum bilirubin less than 2 mg/100 ml, and a normal prothrombin time. Ascites should be absent or minimal. However, after diet therapy has been tried, nothing further is achieved by using diuretics for stable ascites. There should be no signs of encephalopathy. If these criteria cannot be met, the increased operative and late morbidity will correlate with the degree of residual hepatic dysfunction (Table 30–2).

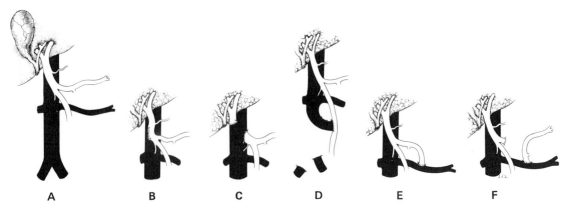

FIG 30–4. Types of portacaval anastomoses: *A:* Normal. *B:* Side-to-side. *C:* End-to-side. *D:* Mesocaval. *E:* Central splenorenal. *F:* Distal splenorenal (Warren).

Types of Shunts

Fig 30–4 depicts the various shunts in use at this time. Although they differ technically in many ways, physiologically there are only 3 different types: end-to-side, side-to-side, and distal splenorenal (Warren).

A. End-to-Side Anastomosis: The end-to-side shunt completely disconnects the liver from the portal system. The portal vein is transected near its bifurcation in the liver hilum and anastomosed to the side of the inferior vena cava. The hepatic stump of the vein is oversewn. Postoperatively, the hepatic vein wedged pressure (sinusoidal pressure) drops slightly after this procedure, reflecting the inability of the hepatic artery to fully compensate for the loss of portal inflow.

B. Side-to-Side Anastomosis: The side-to-side portacaval, mesocaval, mesorenal, and central splenorenal shunts are all physiologically similar since the shunt preserves continuity between the hepatic limb of the portal vein, the portal system, and the anastomosis. It was thought that the side-to-side portacaval shunt might permit continued hepatic perfusion with portal blood, but, in fact, flow through the hepatic limb of the standard side-to-side shunt is nearly always away from the liver and toward the anastomosis. The extent to which hepatofugal flow is produced by other types of "side-to-side" shunts listed above is not known. The physiologic consequences of this reversed flow in the average case are uncertain, but it probably accounts for the somewhat poorer results of this procedure in the BILG Study of therapeutic shunts compared with the end-to-side anastomosis.

Although ascites itself is rarely an indication for portacaval shunt, a side-to-side shunt more effectively eliminates this problem than an end-to-side shunt. The necessity for decompressing intrahepatic portal pressure makes the side-to-side shunt imperative for **Budd-Chiari syndrome.**

C. Distal Splenorenal (Warren) Shunt: The Warren shunt diverts only a section of the portal bed from the liver and preserves hepatic perfusion by blood arriving from the superior mesenteric vein. The usual method consists of transecting the mobilized splenic vein and anastomosing the splenic end to the side of the renal vein. The operation is technically difficult, and several modifications have been proposed. One involves a side-to-side anastomosis between splenic and renal veins followed by ligation of the portal (hepatic) limb of the splenic. Lastly, in some cases where mobilization of the splenic vein appeared to be hazardous, the renal vein has been transected and the end of the caval segment sutured to the side of the undisturbed splenic vein. The segment of splenic vein between the anastomosis and the portal vein is then ligated. Surprisingly, this seems to have little permanent effect on function of the kidney as long as the adrenal and other tributaries are preserved on the oversewn renal vein stump.

Choice of Shunt

In the past decade, side-to-side or end-to-side portacaval shunts have been considered the "standard" operations, the others being reserved for special appli-cation. The central splenorenal shunt was popular at one time but was eventually found to develop late thrombosis in as many as 20% of cases and was correspondingly less successful in preventing rebleeding. At present, the central splenorenal shunt is reserved by most surgeons for use when the portal vein is unavailable (eg, thrombosed).

The relatively new distal splenorenal (Warren) shunt has especially attractive physiologic advantages for patients with marginal liver function or those at special risk for developing encephalopathy. The operation is more difficult technically and cannot always be successfully accomplished. However, the Warren shunt is the procedure of choice in elderly patients who are often incapacitated by encephalopathy after the other shunts. If its early promise withstands further testing, this shunt may eventually be the one used for most patients.

The mesocaval and mesorenal shunts are useful when neither portacaval nor splenorenal anastomosis is feasible. This is most commonly seen after failure of other operations, in young children with portal vein occlusion when the splenic vein is too small, and in patients with unsuitable portal and splenic veins.

The H-mesocaval shunt has recently been advocated as worthy of more widespread trial. The operation consists of suturing a segment of prosthetic vascular graft or autogenous vein between the superior mesenteric vein and inferior vena cava, a procedure that can be accomplished quickly because the veins need little mobilization. Several reports suggest that these grafts remain patent for prolonged periods. The claim that postoperatively the patients have less encephalopathy than after end-to-side or side-to-side portacaval shunts is hard to understand and awaits substantiation. At present, the principal usefulness of this procedure is for emergency shunts where technical simplicity is especially desirable.

Complications

Encephalopathy and diminished liver function are the major complications of portacaval shunts. The incidence of peptic ulcer may be increased by the operation, but the evidence is contradictory. An increased incidence would presumably be due to the diversion of portal blood containing a gastric secretagogue of intestinal origin, normally destroyed by the liver. Hemosiderosis develops in the livers of some shunted patients over many years.

General

Boyer JL & others: Idiopathic portal hypertension. Ann Int Med 66:41–68, 1967.

Gall EA, Kierle AM: Portal systemic venous shunt: Pathological factors contributing to postoperative survival. Gastroenterology 49:656–661, 1965.

McCray RS & others: Erroneous diagnosis of hemorrhage from esophageal varices. Am J Digest Dis 14:755–760, 1969.

McDermott WV Jr: Evaluation of the hemodynamics of portal hypertension in the selection of patients for shunt surgery. Ann Surg 176:449–456, 1972.

Pitcher JL: Safety and effectiveness of the modified Sengstaken-Blakemore tube: A prospective study. Gastroenterology 61:291–298, 1971.

Reynolds TB & others: Measurement of portal pressure and its clinical application. Am J Med 49:649–657, 1970.

Takeuchi J & others: Budd-Chiari syndrome associated with obstruction of the inferior vena cava. Am J Med 51:11–20, 1971.

Warren WD & others: Preoperative assessment of portal hypertension. Ann Surg 165:999–1012, 1967.

Yale CE, Crummy AB: Splenic vein thrombosis and bleeding esophageal varices. JAMA 217:317–320, 1971.

Emergency Portacaval Shunts

Edmondson HT & others: Clinical investigation of the portacaval shunt. 4. A report of early survival from the emergency operation. Ann Surg 173:372–380, 1971.

Orloff MJ: Emergency portacaval shunt: A comparative study of shunt, varix ligation, and non-surgical treatment of bleeding esophageal varices in unselected patients with cirrhosis. Ann Surg 166:456–478, 1967.

Elective Portasystemic Shunts

Barnes BA & others: Elective portasystemic shunts: Morbidity and survival data. Ann Surg 174:76–84, 1971.

Britton RC & others: Selective portal decompression. Surgery 67:104–113, 1970.

Drapanas T: Interposition mesocaval shunt for treatment of portal hypertension. Ann Surg 176:436–448, 1972.

Jackson FC & others: A clinical investigation of the portacaval shunt. 5. Survival analysis of the therapeutic operation. Ann Surg 174:672–701, 1971.

Panke WF & others: A sixteen-year experience with end-to-side portacaval shunt for variceal hemorrhage. Ann Surg 168:957–965, 1968.

Price JB Jr & others: Operative hemodynamic studies in portal hypertension. Arch Surg 95:843–852, 1967.

Reynolds TB & others: Clinical comparison of end-to-side and side-to-side portacaval shunt. New England J Med 274:706–710, 1966.

Voorhees AB Jr & others: Portasystemic shunting procedures for portal hypertension. Am J Surg 119:501–505, 1970.

Zeppa R, Warren WD: The distal splenorenal shunt. Am J Surg 122:300–303, 1971.

EXTRAHEPATIC PORTAL VENOUS OCCLUSION

Portal vein thrombosis (in the absence of liver disease) accounts for the majority of cases of portal hypertension in childhood and for a few adults who present with an initial variceal hemorrhage. The cause is not known. Neonatal septicemia, omphalitis, umbilical vein catheterization for exchange transfusion, and dehydration have all been indicted as possible causes, but collectively they can be definitely implicated in only a minority of cases.

Most patients present for the first time with variceal hemorrhage. A few are first discovered because of splenomegaly or hypersplenism. Ascites is uncommon except transiently after bleeding and is somewhat more frequent in adults. Liver function is either normal or only slightly impaired. This protects them from encephalopathy, which in this disease is confined to the rare elderly patient.

The mortality rate for sudden massive bleeding is about 20%—much below that in other types of portal hypertension—because of the patients' good general condition and liver function.

The diagnosis can be confirmed radiologically by either splenoportography or percutaneous mesenteric angiography. The former technic allows direct measurement of portal pressure. Hepatic vein wedged pressure is normal.

Emergency treatment consists of the administration of vasopressin to reduce portal pressure and blood transfusion to restore circulating blood volume. The Sengstaken-Blakemore tube may be used in adults, but most have abandoned its use in children. If these measures fail and bleeding continues, transesophageal ligation of varices should be considered as a lifesaving measure. This will usually be successful in halting the acute episode and provide at least a month to prepare the patient for a definitive portal-systemic shunt.

In older children or adults, a central splenorenal shunt is the operation of choice. The portal vein is rarely available because of involvement by the thrombotic process. When the splenic vein is also unavailable or is too small to use, mesocaval anastomosis is the next choice. Splenectomy by itself has no long-lasting effect and has the undesirable consequence of eliminating the splenic vein from consideration for subsequent use in a shunt. Shunts in patients under 9–10 years of age have a high rate of spontaneous thrombosis, principally because of the small size of the available vessels. In this age group, it is better to attempt to pull the patient through one or more episodes of bleeding until he has grown to a more suitable size rather than to perform shunts and destroy the vessels employed. If all sites for shunts have been used and portal hypertension persists, it is sometimes necessary to perform an esophagogastrectomy to remove the source of hemorrhage. Colonic interposition is ordinarily selected to restore intestinal continuity after this operation.

Occasionally a patient is encountered who has isolated **thrombosis of the splenic vein** caused by pancreatitis or trauma. The resulting venous hypertension of the splenic veins spills over into the gastroesophageal venous plexus via the short gastric vessels; the portal and mesenteric venous pressures are normal. For these, splenectomy alone is curative.

In general, an adequate shunt is more difficult to accomplish in patients with portal vein block than in cirrhotics because of technical problems. Since they tolerate sudden blood loss much better than those with liver disease, their survival without a shunt is considerably better too.

Longstreth GS & others: Extrahepatic portal hypertension caused by chronic pancreatitis. Ann Int Med 75:903–908, 1971.

Maddrey WC & others: Extrahepatic obstruction of the portal venous system. Surg Gynec Obst 127:989–998, 1968.

Mikkelsen WP: Extrahepatic portal hypertension in children. Am J Surg 111:333–340, 1966.

Pinkerton JA & others: Portal hypertension in childhood. Ann Surg 175:870–886, 1972.

Rothwell-Jackson RL, Hunt AH: Proximal gastric resection in the treatment of bleeding gastroesophageal varices in patients with portal hypertension due to extrahepatic obstruction. Brit J Surg 57:487–494, 1970.

HEPATIC ENCEPHALOPATHY

Episodic or continuous CNS symptoms are seen in patients with chronic liver disease and are especially prone to develop after portacaval shunt. Portal-systemic encephalopathy, ammonia intoxication, hepatic coma, and meat intoxication are terms which have been used synonymously to refer to this condition.

The possible symptoms span a wide range from lethargy to coma—from minor personality changes to psychosis—from asterixis to paraplegia. A toxic action of ammonia on the CNS has been considered the most likely cause since in affected patients ammonia levels, especially in arterial blood or CSF, are elevated and experimental administration of ammonia has produced similar symptoms. Ammonia is formed in the gut— principally the colon—by the action of bacteria on urea. It is absorbed and transported in portal venous blood to the liver, where about 80% is extracted and converted to glutamine, a nontoxic storage compound. Absorbed ammonia may reach the systemic circulation in increased amounts through spontaneous portal systemic collaterals or surgically created shunts. Decreased ammonia extraction due to hepatic disease can produce the same result.

It has recently been proposed that the syndrome is actually caused by excessive exposure of the CNS to β-hydroxylated phenylethyl amines or their precursor amino acids, which displace the normal neurotransmitters norepinephrine and dopamine. These false neurotransmitters are inactive at synapses and result in CNS dysfunction. These compounds are produced in the gut by bacterial action, and thus a correlation of symptoms with ammonia levels would be expected.

Encephalopathy is a major unwanted side-effect of portacaval shunt. Since it can be socially incapacitating or even lethal, the risks in the individual patient must be carefully considered before operation. The most important factors in predicting the postoperative chance of developing this complication are the quality of liver function, the extent of reduction in hepatic parenchymal blood flow through the portal vein (ie, the extent to which the disease has already shunted portal blood), the type of liver disease, and the age of

TABLE 30–3. Factors contributing to encephalopathy.

A. Increased Systemic Ammonia Levels
1. Extent of portal-systemic venous shunt
2. Depressed liver function
3. Intestinal protein load
4. Intestinal flora
5. Azotemia
6. Constipation

B. Increased Sensitivity of CNS
1. Age of patient
2. Hypokalemia
3. Alkalosis
4. Sedatives, narcotics, tranquilizers
5. Infection
6. Hypoxia, hypoglycemia, myxedema

the patient. The contributing factors are listed in Table 30–3. Those just mentioned are patient- and disease-determined, whereas the others are at least partially under the control of the physician.

Elderly patients are considerably more susceptible—so much so that the standard shunts are rarely performed in persons over age 60. Alcoholics fare better than those with postnecrotic or cryptogenic cirrhosis, apparently due to the invariable progression of liver dysfunction in the latter.

Good liver function partially protects the patient from encephalopathy if other variables are held constant. If the liver has adapted to complete or nearly complete diversion of portal blood before operation, a surgical shunt is less apt to depress liver function further. For example, patients with thrombosis of the portal vein (complete diversion and normal liver function) do not experience encephalopathy after portal-systemic shunt.

Increased intestinal protein, whether of dietary origin or from intestinal bleeding, aggravates encephalopathy by providing more substrate for intestinal bacteria. Constipation allows greater time for bacterial action on colonic contents. Azotemia results in higher concentrations of blood urea which diffuses into the intestine, is converted to ammonia, and then reabsorbed. Hypokalemia and metabolic alkalosis aggravate encephalopathy by favoring a shift of ammonia from extracellular to intracellular sites where the toxic action occurs.

Electroencephalography is more sensitive than clinical evaluation in detecting minor degrees of involvement. The changes are nonspecific and consist of slower mean frequencies. Studies performed at different times can be compared to assess the effects of therapy.

Acute encephalopathy is often precipitated by episodes of intestinal hemorrhage. Treatment consists of removing the blood by suction and purgation, halting the bleeding if possible, and administering intestinal antibiotics (eg, neomycin). Blood volume must be maintained to avoid prerenal azotemia.

Chronic encephalopathy is treated by restricting dietary protein to 40–60 g/day, avoidance of constipation, and sometimes by continuous administration of intestinal antibiotics to reduce bacterial action. Lactalose, a disaccharide unaffected by intestinal enzymes, is sometimes useful when given orally; it lowers pH in the colonic lumen to 4.5–5.5, which favors conversion of ammonia to nonabsorbable ammonium ion and would have an analogous action on other toxic amines. If these measures are insufficient, ileostomy or colonic exclusion by ileosigmoid anastomosis is justified in carefully selected patients.

Conn HO: A rational program for the management of hepatic coma. Gastroenterology. 57:715–723, 1969.

Fischer JE, James JH: Treatment of hepatic coma and hepatorenal syndrome. Mechanism of action of L-dopa and Aramine. Am J Surg 123:222–230, 1972.

Fischer JE & others: Changes in brain amines following portal flow diversion and acute hepatic coma. Surg Forum 23:348–350, 1972.

McDermott WV Jr & others: Postshunt encephalopathy. Surg Gynec Obst 126:585–590, 1968.

Resnick RH & others: A controlled trial of colon bypass in chronic hepatic encephalopathy. Gastroenterology 54: 1057–1068, 1968.

Zieve L: Pathogenesis of hepatic coma. Arch Int Med 118:211–223, 1966.

●   ●   ●

General References

Child CG III: *The Liver in Portal Hypertension*. Saunders, 1964.

Leevy CM, Britton RC (editors): The hepatic circulation and portal hypertension. Ann New York Acad Sc 170:1–405, 1970.

Longmire WP Jr: Portal hypertension. Curr Probl Surg, July 1966.

Sedgwick CE, Poulantzas JK: *Portal Hypertension*. Little, Brown, 1967.

Warren WD, Salam AA: The treatment of esophageal varices in the patient with cirrhosis. Advances Surg 6:141–173, 1972.

31 . . .

The Acute Abdomen

J. Englebert Dunphy, MD

Acute abdominal diseases are usually manifested by pain, anorexia, nausea, vomiting, and fever. On physical examination, tenderness, muscle spasm, and changes in peristalsis are important signs. The extent to which these symptoms and findings can be correlated so as to arrive at the correct diagnosis depends upon the precision and care with which the examiner obtains the history and performs the physical examination.

HISTORY

A number of important guides to the direction in which the investigation should be pursued can be derived from the history alone provided the symptoms are carefully analyzed and evaluated. The physical examination (see next section) often supplies the critical definitive diagnostic evidence.

Mode of Onset of Abdominal Pain

If the patient is well one moment and seized with agonizing (explosive) pain the next, the most probable diagnosis is either free rupture of a hollow viscus or vascular accident. Renal and biliary colic may be very sudden in onset but are not likely to cause such severe and prostrating pain.

If the pain is rapid in onset—moderately severe at first and rapidly becoming worse—consider acute pancreatitis, mesenteric thrombosis, or strangulation of the small bowel.

Gradual onset of slowly progressive pain is characteristic of peritoneal infection or inflammation. Appendicitis and diverticulitis often start in this way.

Character of the Pain (Fig 31–1.)

It is not enough to know that the patient has abdominal pain. One must determine its exact character.

Excruciating pain not relieved by narcotics indicates a vascular lesion such as massive infarction of the intestine or rupture of an abdominal aneurysm.

Very severe pain, readily controlled by medication, is more typical of acute pancreatitis or the peritonitis associated with a ruptured viscus. Obstructive appendicitis and incarcerated small bowel without extensive infarction occasionally produce the same type of pain. The pain of biliary or renal colic is usually promptly alleviated by medication.

If the pain is **dull, vague, and poorly localized,** it is also likely to have been gradual in onset. These findings strongly suggest an inflammatory process or a low-grade infection. Appendicitis commonly presents in this fashion.

An occasional patient will say that he has no abdominal pain but only a sense of fullness, and feels that he would feel better if he could only have a bowel movement. Sometimes he has taken an enema but has had no relief despite the fact that his bowels moved. This symptom complex—the "gas stoppage sign"—is characteristic of retrocecal appendicitis. It may also be seen when the appendix is inflamed but walled off from the peritoneal cavity by omentum.

Intermittent pain with cramps and rushes is commonly seen in gastroenteritis. However, if the pain comes in regular cycles, rising in crescendo fashion and then subsiding to a pain-free interval, the most likely diagnosis is mechanical small bowel obstruction. This type of pain occurs occasionally in subacute pancreatitis. If auscultation reveals intermittent peristaltic rushes, rising in crescendo fashion and synchronous with the pain, small bowel obstruction is very likely. In the colic of gastroenteritis, on the other hand, peristaltic rushes have little or no relation to abdominal cramps.

Radiation or a shift in localization of the pain has particular significance. Pain in the shoulder follows diaphragmatic irritation due to air, peritoneal fluid, or blood. Biliary pain is often referred to the right scapula and rarely to the left epigastrium and left shoulder, simulating angina pectoris. Classically, the pain of appendicitis begins in the epigastrium and settles in the right lower quadrant. A shift or spread of abdominal pain often indicates spreading peritonitis.

Anorexia; Nausea & Vomiting

Anorexia, nausea, and vomiting are common symptoms of acute abdominal disease, and careful analysis of the character of these symptoms may be of great value in arriving at the correct diagnosis. However, there may be advanced abdominal disease without anorexia, nausea, or vomiting. If the peritoneum is well protected from infection or inflammation, as in retrocecal appendicitis or when the appendix is completely isolated by omentum, the patient may not

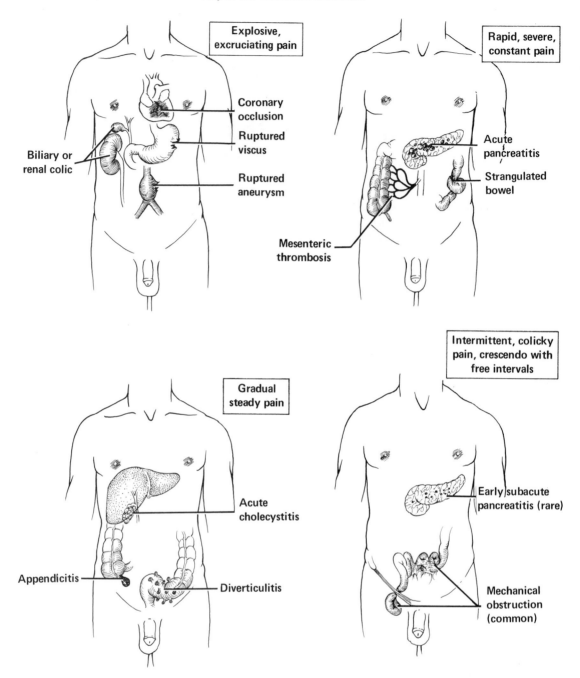

FIG 31–1. Precise identification of the nature of pain is of critical importance in differential diagnosis.

only have no anorexia but insist that he is hungry. The time of onset of these symptoms is important because, if they precede the onset of pain, gastroenteritis or some systemic illness is a much more likely diagnosis than an acute abdominal emergency requiring operation.

When nausea and vomiting are very prominent symptoms, the most likely possibilities are gastroenteritis, acute gastritis, acute pancreatitis, common duct stone, and high intestinal obstruction. In most other acute surgical emergencies, nausea and vomiting are not dominant symptoms though they may be present.

Severe vomiting with retching—particularly following a dietary indiscretion or an alcoholic bout—should immediately suggest laceration of the gastroesophageal junction (Mallory-Weiss syndrome) or an esophageal perforation (Boerhaave's syndrome; see Chapter 24). Massive hematemesis or severe pain radiating into the chest and left shoulder in association with severe vomiting and retching make these critical emergencies very likely.

Diarrhea, Constipation, & Obstipation

Some alteration of bowel function is common in most cases of acute abdominal emergencies, but the variations are extraordinary. There are several important clues. If it can be ascertained for certain that a patient has passed no gas and had no bowel movements for 24–48 hours, he has intestinal obstruction. Under these circumstances, however, there will also be either obvious distention or persistent vomiting. If the patient insists that he has not passed gas for 24–48 hours but there is no vomiting and no distention, it is likely that he has been unaware of the passage of gas. Diarrhea is the classic manifestation of gastroenteritis, but it also may be a dominant symptom of pelvic appendicitis. Bloody and repetitive diarrhea indicates ulceration of the colon. Ulcerative colitis, Crohn's disease, and bacillary and amebic dysenteries must be considered first. Although bloody diarrhea is often mentioned as a symptom of mesenteric thrombosis, it actually occurs rather rarely in this condition.

Chills & Fever

Some degree of fever is common to most acute surgical emergencies. In appendicitis, fever is not usually very high, and high fever should suggest either pylephlebitis or some other diagnosis. A very high fever with peritoneal signs in a female patient with no apparent general systemic illness is characteristic of acute pelvic inflammatory disease.

Repeated chills and fever characterize pylephlebitis and bacteremia. Their presence in suspected appendicitis strongly suggests perforation. Repeated chills and fever are most common in infections of the biliary or renal tracts. Acute cholangitis and acute pyelitis usually present with intermittent chills and fever. Chills, fever, jaundice, and hypotension indicate suppurative cholangitis—a surgical emergency.

PHYSICAL EXAMINATION

Having obtained a careful history and taken note of diagnostic possibilities along the lines suggested above, the physician proceeds to the physical examination. This must be complete, but particular emphasis is placed upon the abdominal examination. The care and the manner in which the examination is performed often establish the diagnosis. The appropriate procedural approach is outlined in Table 31–1.

Initial Abdominal Examination

The abdomen should first be inspected, looking for such striking features as the scaphoid, contracted abdomen of an early perforated viscus, the visible peristalsis of mechanical obstruction, or the soft, doughy distention of early peritonitis.

TABLE 31–1. Routine for physical examination of the acute abdomen.

(1) Inspection.	(6) Deep palpation.
(2) Cough tenderness. Examine hernial rings and male genitalia.	(7) Rebound tenderness.
(3) Feel for spasm.	(8) Auscultation.
(4) One-finger palpation.	(9) Special signs.
(5) Costovertebral tenderness.	(10) Rectal and pelvic examination.

The next step is to examine the inguinal and femoral canals in both sexes and the genitalia in the male. This must be done very gently, asking the patient to cough but causing as little discomfort as possible. In most acute inflammatory conditions, coughing will elicit pain not in the groin but in the abdomen. If the patient is then asked to point one finger to where he feels the pain, an objective localization of the lesion is obtained. With this information in hand, the examiner can proceed to examine the abdomen, deliberately avoiding the area which he now knows to be most tender.

Spasm

The next step is to establish the presence or absence of true spasm. This is done by placing the hand gently over the rectus abdominis muscle and depressing it slightly and gently, without causing pain (Fig 31–2). Properly performed, this maneuver is a comforting one to the patient. Now ask the patient to take a long breath. If the spasm is voluntary, the muscle will immediately relax underneath the gentle pressure of the palpating hand. If there is true spasm, however, the muscle will remain taut and rigid throughout the respiratory cycle. This maneuver alone is sufficient to establish the presence of peritonitis. Except for rare neurologic disorders—and, for reasons that no one understands, renal colic—only peritoneal inflammation produces abdominal muscle rigidity. In renal colic, the spasm is confined to the entire rectus muscle on one side. The distinction is important because marked rigidity of the entire length of one rectus muscle with relaxation of the opposite cannot occur in peritonitis since there is no compartmentalization of the peritoneal cavity. It is possible, however, to have segmental spasm of a rectus muscle involving only the upper or lower portion on one side, or to have segmental spasm of both rectus muscles in upper or lower abdominal peritonitis. In generalized peritonitis, both muscles are usually involved to the same degree.

Test for Abdominal Tenderness

The test for abdominal tenderness must be done with one finger and not with the entire hand (Fig 31–3). It is impossible to accurately localize peritoneal inflammation if palpation for tenderness is done with the entire hand. Careful one-finger palpation, beginning as far away as possible from the area of localized cough-elicited pain and gradually working toward it,

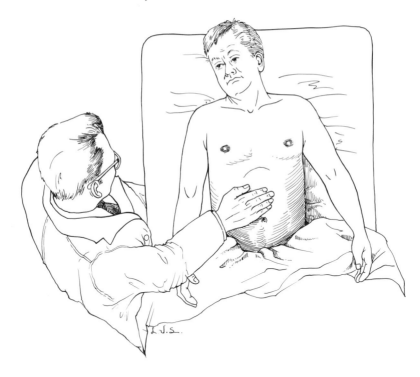

FIG 31–2. Testing for spasm.

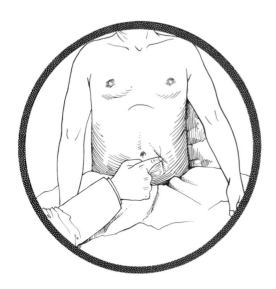

FIG 31–3. Gentle systematic palpation with one finger is the best way to localize an area of tenderness.

will usually enable the examiner to determine precisely the limitations of abdominal tenderness. In early acute appendicitis, this is often no larger than a silver dollar and sometimes smaller. Whenever there is diffuse abdominal tenderness without associated involuntary rigidity of the muscles, one should suspect gastro-

enteritis or some other inflammatory process of the intestines without peritonitis. Gastroenteritis is characteristically accompanied by diffuse abdominal tenderness with no muscular rigidity.

Percussion

In free perforation of a hollow viscus with air under the diaphragm, there may be diminished or absent liver dullness (Fig 31–4). Tympany laterally in the midaxillary line 5 cm or more above the costal margin is reliable evidence of free air. Tympany anteriorly over the liver may be due to air in distended loops of bowel.

Masses

Having established the presence or absence of muscular rigidity and localized the area of tenderness, the examiner now palpates more deeply for the presence of abdominal masses. Among the more common lesions identifiable by careful palpation in patients with acute abdominal pain are cholecystitis, appendicitis with early abscess formation, sigmoid diverticulitis, and leaking abdominal aneurysm.

Peristaltic Sounds

Auscultation is an essential part of the abdominal examination. The absence of audible peristalsis–ie, a completely silent abdomen–means diffuse peritonitis. It may be necessary to listen for as long as 2 or 3 minutes to establish the absence of peristalsis. Other manifestations of diffuse peritonitis such as rigidity

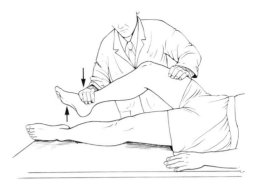

FIG 31–5. Iliopsoas sign.

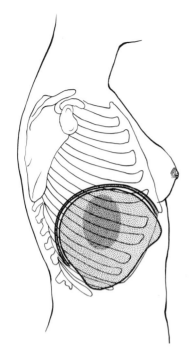

FIG 31–4. Darker shaded area shows area of de-creased liver dullness due to free air in the peri-toneal cavity.

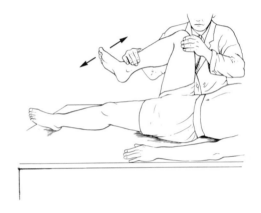

FIG 31–6. Obturator sign.

and distention are usually present also in such cases. It should be remembered that there may be persistent peristalsis in the presence of established peritonitis (see Chapter 32).

Intermittent crescendo peristaltic rushes with regular free intervals are diagnostic of acute mid small bowel obstruction. For reasons that are not entirely clear, the only other lesion that produces peristalsis of this type is early acute pancreatitis, in which the dilated sentinel loop seen on x-ray appears to undergo cyclic peristaltic contractions simulating those of acute mechanical obstruction.

In gastroenteritis, fulminating ulcerative colitis, and the dysenteries, there is abnormal high-pitched peristalsis with rushes, but these are not synchronous with the episodes of pain.

Special Signs

There are several maneuvers in physical examination which may elicit confirmatory evidence of an acute abdominal lesion:

A. Iliopsoas Sign: The patient flexes his thigh against the resistance of the examiner's hand (Fig 31–5). A painful response indicates an inflammatory process involving the psoas muscle.

B. Obturator Sign: The patient's thigh is flexed to a right angle and is gently rotated internally and externally (Fig 31–6). If pain is elicited, there is an inflammatory lesion involving the obturator internus muscle (pelvic appendicitis, diverticulitis).

C. Fist Percussion Sign: Gentle percussion with

the fist over the anterior chest wall elicits sharp pain if there is an acute inflammation involving the space between the diaphragm and liver on the right and the stomach or spleen on the left (Fig 31–7).

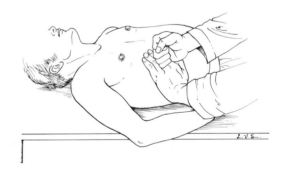

FIG 31–7. Fist percussion of lower anterior chest wall. A gentle blow will elicit pain in the presence of any inflammatory lesion involving the dia-phragm or liver on the right or the diaphragm, spleen, or stomach on the left. This sign is often positive in acute hepatitis. A negative response is rare in acute cholecystitis.

Other Examinations

The examination is completed by pelvic and rectal examination. The importance of pelvic and rectal examinations, particularly in acute pelvic appendicitis, will be discussed in Chapter 34.

LABORATORY EXAMINATION

Hematocrit, complete blood count, and urine examination should be obtained in all cases.

Blood

The hematocrit is of critical importance, reflecting in a significant way changes in plasma volume—particularly dehydration due to excessive vomiting or loss of fluids into the peritoneum or intestinal lumen. A low hematocrit may indicate preexisting anemia or bleeding.

The white blood count may be helpful if significantly elevated. However, normal or even low counts can be obtained in the presence of established peritonitis. A low blood count, particularly with lymphocytosis, may suggest viral infection or gastroenteritis. Marked leukopenia may suggest a blood dyscrasia or severe sepsis. A progressively rising white count is of considerable value and usually indicates progression of an inflammatory or septic process. A shift to the left on a blood smear may be a clue to an inflammatory reaction in the presence of a normal or only moderately elevated count.

Serum Electrolytes

Serum electrolytes are often required to document the nature and extent of fluid losses.

Serum Amylase

Serum amylase is an important test in many cases of acute abdomen. It is often an important clue to unsuspected pancreatitis. It may provide confirmatory evidence of pancreatitis. It may be moderately elevated in the presence of mesenteric thrombosis and intestinal obstruction. In some cases of perforated ulcer—particularly posterior perforations—serum amylase may be markedly elevated.

Urine

Examination of the urine is of critical importance to exclude urinary tract sepsis and diabetes. A low urine specific gravity in the presence of obvious severe vomiting may be the earliest clue to associated renal disease and require prompt evaluation of the BUN and creatinine.

Peritoneal Fluid

In obscure cases, examination of the peritoneal fluid for blood and pus may be required. This is particularly true in elderly obtunded patients in whom the physical signs are very difficult to interpret and the presence of peritonitis cannot be excluded. It may be best to tap a single quadrant of the abdomen. In other cases, particularly if intraperitoneal bleeding is suspected, insertion of a catheter is more reliable (see Chapter 52).

RADIOLOGIC EXAMINATION

Radiologic examination often provides extremely important evidence in the diagnosis of acute abdominal disease. The closest cooperation and communication between the surgeon and the radiologist is essential. Each must have maximum information available to him, and joint review of films is frequently of critical importance.

In most cases of acute abdominal disease—and in all cases in which the diagnosis is obscure—the following x-ray films should be obtained: plain films, supine and upright, of the abdomen; kidneys, ureters, and bladder (KUB); and a film of the chest. In reviewing these films, the following questions should be asked: (1) Are the outlines of the liver, spleen, kidneys, and psoas muscle clearly defined? (2) Are the peritoneal fat lines identifiable? (3) Is the gas pattern in the stomach, small bowel, and colon within normal limits? (4) Is there evidence of air outside of the bowel or beneath the diaphragm? (5) Is there air in the biliary radicals? (6) Are there abnormal opaque shadows such as gallstones, fecaliths, or calcification in lymph nodes, pancreas, aorta, or other soft tissue masses.

In addition to these studies, special contrast studies, barium swallow, judicious introduction of barium into the rectum, intravenous urograms, or intravenous cholangiograms are sometimes indicated. Rarely, a liver scan may be indicated because of suspicion of a massive fulminating hepatic abscess.

On the basis of these examinations, the following important bits of evidence may be obtained: Obliteration of the psoas shadow may indicate a retroperitoneal hematoma or an abscess (Fig 31–8). An enlarged or displaced kidney shadow may indicate a urologic lesion simulating an acute abdominal process. Enlargement of the splenic shadow with displacement of stomach or colon may suggest delayed rupture of the spleen.

Gas patterns are of particular importance. They are more readily characterized if a nasogastric tube has been passed and the stomach emptied. Residual gas and fluid within the stomach suggest pyloric obstruction. Dilated loops of small bowel with air-fluid levels and no gas in the colon are indicative of small bowel obstruction (Fig 31–9).

The position of the cecum may be a clue to appendicitis in an unusual location. Marked dilation and rotation of the cecum or sigmoid are typical of volvulus. (See Chapter 36.)

Marked dilatation of the entire colon suggests colonic obstruction. Massive dilatation of the colon in acute colitis indicates toxic megacolon.

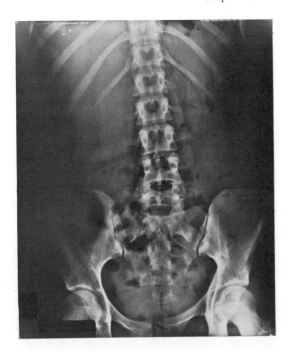

FIG 31–8. **Obliteration of the psoas shadow by a right subhepatic abscess.**

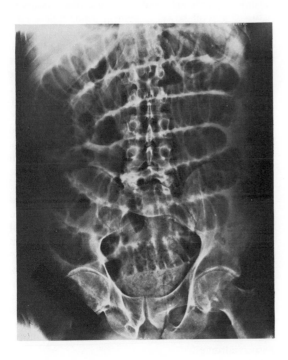

FIG 31–9. **Small bowel obstruction.** Note dilated loops of small bowel with air-fluid levels and no gas in the colon.

Distention of both small and large bowel is characteristic of ileus, peritonitis, and pseudo-obstruction of the bowel (Fig 31–10).

Free air under the diaphragm indicates a perforated viscus, most commonly seen in perforated gastric or duodenal ulcer (Fig 31–11). Massive amounts of air beneath both diaphragms suggest colonic perforation. An encapsulated air shadow outside the contours of small or large bowel may indicate localized perforation of the intestine. Air in the biliary tract is diagnostic of a free communication between some portion of the gastrointestinal tract and the biliary tree (Fig 31–12). If there is evidence of intestinal obstruction, it is characteristic of gallstone ileus.

The differentiation between distended small and large bowel may at times be difficult. In advanced cases, the clinical signs may be more reliable in the differentiation between intestinal obstruction and peritonitis.

Plain films of the abdomen may establish the diagnosis of gallstones, pancreatic calcification, retroperitoneal calcification, and vascular calcification. Such findings must be carefully correlated with the history and physical examination to establish their significance.

Rarely, a swallow of meglumine diatrizoate (Gastrografin) may be necessary to confirm or exclude a diagnosis of high intestinal obstruction or perforation of the stomach or duodenum.

Barium enema should be avoided if possible in the presence of acute abdominal disease and peritonitis. In rare cases it is required—most frequently for establishing a diagnosis of diverticulitis, sigmoid volvulus, or low partial colonic obstruction due to carcinoma.

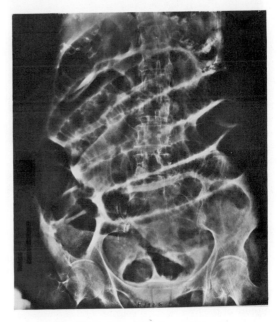

FIG 31–10. **Distention of both small and large bowel as seen in ileus and peritonitis.**

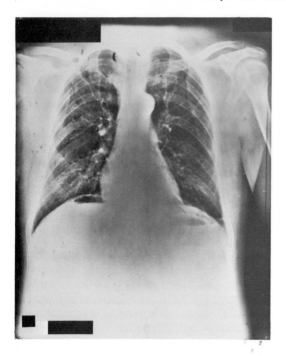

FIG 31–11. Free air under the diaphragm resulting from perforated viscus–in this case, duodenal ulcer.

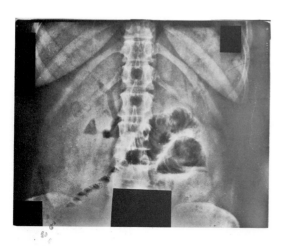

FIG 31–12. Air in the biliary tract indicating free communication between the gastrointestinal tract and the biliary tree. The common duct is well outlined.

Angiograms are being used more frequently and may be of value in obscure cases of rupture of a solid viscus such as the spleen or kidney. An angiogram may be the only way to recognize a subcapsular or central rupture of the liver.

Finally, large soft tissue masses, retroperitoneal tumors, metastatic carcinoma of the testicle, and other malignant lesions undergoing necrosis may simulate an acute abdomen. The abnormal x-ray shadows may be important in elucidating the diagnosis.

DIFFERENTIAL DIAGNOSIS OF ACUTE ABDOMEN

Although the factors in differential diagnosis of the major acute surgical conditions are discussed in relation to each particular disease elsewhere in this book, the following guides and clues should be borne in mind:

(1) Appendicitis is the commonest cause of bizarre peritoneal findings with ileus or apparent intestinal obstruction. In the presence of a suspected septic or inflammatory lesion, it should never be lower than number 2 on the list of causes.

(2) Pelvic appendicitis frequently presents with vomiting, diarrhea, and mild abdominal pain. It is easily confused with gastroenteritis. Initially, abdominal signs may be minimal and the rectal or pelvic examination may be negative. A high white count makes gastroenteritis unlikely. Repeated rectal or pelvic examinations are essential to early diagnosis.

(3) When the patient says he has no pain but only "abdominal pressure" and he is sure that passage of flatus or a good bowel movement would relieve him, remember the "gas stoppage sign" in appendicitis.

(4) Unremitting, deep-seated abdominal pain with minimal physical findings should always raise the question of a vascular lesion, particularly mesenteric vascular occlusion.

(5) Nausea, vomiting, and retching as the **dominant** symptoms suggest acute gastritis or pancreatitis.

(6) Intestinal obstruction in an old woman who has had no previous operations strongly suggests a strangulated femoral hernia. There may be no pain referred to the hernia, and the palpable sac may not be tender. Examine and reexamine the femoral rings.

(7) Upper abdominal pain (which may be so mild that the patient does not seek medical advice) followed many hours or several days later by signs of intestinal obstruction is typical of gallstone ileus. Look for an opaque gallstone and air in the biliary tract on x-ray.

(8) An acute illness characterized by jaundice, high fever with chills, and hypotension means suppurative cholangitis–a critical surgical emergency.

(9) Severe vomiting of food or gastric contents followed later by retching and hematemesis is almost diagnostic of gastroesophageal laceration (Mallory-Weiss syndrome).

Disorders which must be commonly considered in the differential diagnosis of a patient that presents with acute abdominal pain are discussed in the following paragraphs.

Myocardial Infarction

Acute myocardial infarction may simulate perforated ulcer or acute cholecystitis, particularly if the pain is epigastric. Careful examination will indicate that abdominal rigidity is absent and peristalsis is not altered. Other manifestations of coronary occlusion, including ECG changes, should promptly clarify the diagnosis.

The problem is more difficult when the patient with known coronary artery disease develops acute cholecystitis or a perforated ulcer. A palpable gallbladder is an extremely valuable finding in acute cholecystitis. In perforated ulcer, air under the diaphragm and a careful analysis of the character of the pain, together with other diagnostic criteria, usually clarify the diagnosis.

Acute Hepatitis

Acute hepatitis in its initial phases is sometimes associated with severe right upper quadrant pain and tenderness. In all instances of suspected acute cholecystitis, diffuse tenderness over the liver should immediately raise the question of acute hepatitis. Appropriate laboratory studies will make the diagnosis.

Rheumatic Fever

Rheumatic fever is not infrequently accompanied by vague, ill-defined abdominal pain simulating appendicitis. A careful history and physical examination, as described above, will indicate that no acute abdominal lesion is present.

Polyarteritis Nodosa

Many types of vasculitis may cause abdominal pain simulating acute surgical abdominal disease. At times vasculitis may involve the appendix or small bowel, so that surgery is mandatory. The diagnosis can sometimes be established by examination of the surgical specimen. In most instances, however, careful examination will indicate that there is no evidence for a progressive intraperitoneal lesion and the diagnosis can be established only by muscle or skin biopsy.

Acute Porphyria

Severe abdominal pain may accompany various forms of porphyria and porphyrinuria. A critical appraisal of the abdominal findings will usually cast doubt on the diagnosis of abdominal disease, and examination of the urine (Watson-Schwartz test) will reveal the presence of porphobilinogen.

Acute Epidemic Pleurodynia

Particularly in young people, acute epidemic pleurodynia may strongly suggest acute appendicitis. The condition appears from time to time in children's camps, and all too often the first few patients are subjected to appendectomy before the true nature of the condition is recognized. Careful examination of the abdomen is the surest way of avoiding this error. Tenderness is high and is often present over the lower thoracic wall rather than over the peritoneum.

Acute Spontaneous Pneumothorax

Acute spontaneous pneumothorax has been mistaken for acute cholecystitis. Careful physical examination again provides the answer. Chest x-ray is diagnostic.

Pneumonia, Pleurisy, & Empyema

Pneumonia, pleurisy, and empyema—or, indeed, any thoracic lesion resulting in diaphragmatic irritation—will produce right upper quadrant pain simulating an abdominal condition. Careful history and physical examination, together with appropriate x-ray studies, readily clarify the diagnosis provided the examiner bears the possibility in mind.

Lesions of the Spine

Osteoarthritis with compression of the thoracic spine and spinal nerves may produce severe, ill-defined abdominal pain simulating a variety of intraperitoneal lesions, particularly biliary colic. Some degree of involuntary rigidity of the rectus abdominis muscle may be present as an additional confusing factor. Careful analysis of the nature of the pain, its radiating character, and the presence of hyperesthesias will lead to appropriate further studies necessary to establish the diagnosis—particularly x-ray examination of the involved vertebrae.

A cord tumor may also produce radiating pain simulating biliary or renal colic.

Diseases of the Hip Joint

A variety of diseases of the hip may produce pain radiating into the right or left lower quadrant. Acute bursitis, in particular, may simulate pelvic appendicitis. Absence of true abdominal tenderness and rigidity, together with examination of the hip joint, readily clarify the diagnosis.

TREATMENT OF ACUTE ABDOMEN

When the diagnosis is in doubt and the patient is not critically ill, a conservative period of observation is in order. Analgesics for the relief of severe pain should be given without hesitation. Indeed, the evaluation of acute abdominal disease can be performed more accurately after severe pain is relieved and the cooperation of the patient obtained. What at first appeared to be very diffuse tenderness may now be better localized. Abdominal masses which could not be felt before often become obvious after moderate sedation and relief of pain.

Antibiotics should be withheld until the diagnosis is established. In obscure cases, heavy antibiotic therapy may mask progression of the disease and lead to the development of serious complications with marked morbidity.

Laboratory and physical examination should be repeated at frequent intervals.

If the diagnosis is in doubt but the patient clearly has signs of peritonitis, operation must be undertaken as soon as fluid and electrolyte imbalance has been corrected. Nasogastric suction should be initiated as soon as it is recognized that the patient has evidence of peritonitis or ileus. This is preferably done before any diagnostic measures are undertaken.

Particularly in the good-risk patient, a right or left rectus or midline incision may be preferable to a horizontal or oblique incision since the former permit more extensive exploration of the peritoneal cavity and can be adjusted more readily if the most likely diagnosis is proved to be incorrect after the peritoneal cavity is opened.

On the other hand, in the elderly, obese, poor-risk patient, it often is preferable to make a small, well-localized incision over the most likely site of the cause of the peritonitis. This can be closed and another incision made with less total risk to the patient than if a long midline or rectus incision is used. In the elderly poor-risk patient, an extensive incision is prone to infection, suppuration, and dehiscence—complications which in the elderly or poor-risk patient may prove fatal. Multiple small incisions under these circumstances are less likely to break down, and even if infection occurs dehiscence and evisceration are less likely.

•   •   •

General References

Botsford TW, Wilson RE: The acute abdomen. Vol X in: *Major Problems in Clinical Surgery*. Dunphy JE (consulting editor). Saunders, 1969.

Cope Z: *The Early Diagnosis of the Acute Abdomen,* 12th ed. Oxford Univ Press, 1963.

Hawthorne HR & others: *The Acute Abdomen and Emergent Lesions of the Gastrointestinal Tract*. Thomas, 1967.

32 . . .

The Peritoneal Cavity

J. Englebert Dunphy, MD

The abdomen is lined by a thin layer of endothelium which covers the interior of the abdominal wall (parietal peritoneum) and all of the organs within the abdominal cavity (the visceral peritoneum). As the peritoneum envelops the viscera in the course of embryologic development, numerous compartments are formed. The lesser peritoneal cavity lies behind the stomach and the lesser omentum or gastrohepatic ligament, communicating with the main peritoneal cavity through the foramen epiploicum (foramen of Winslow). (See Fig 32–1.) The endothelial surface of the peritoneum is smooth and glistening and is normally lubricated by a small amount of fluid. In its deeper layers, there is a rich network of capillaries and lymphatics.

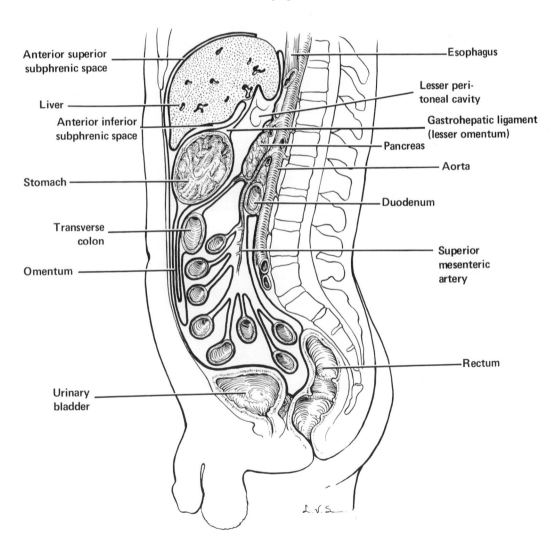

FIG 32–1. The peritoneal reflections and location of the lesser peritoneal cavity.

The peritoneum is normally quite resistant to infection. Bacteria injected into the peritoneal cavity are rapidly phagocytized and eliminated. The same quantity of bacteria injected subcutaneously or retroperitoneally would produce abscess formation or a spreading cellulitis. Bacterial peritonitis, therefore, can occur only as a result of continuous or persistent contamination or as a result of contamination with an unusually virulent bacterial strain or species. Foreign bodies also greatly reduce the resistance of the peritoneum to infection.

The omentum is a double fold of peritoneum, usually loaded with fat, which hangs from the stomach and the transverse colon as an apron over the small intestine. It is a very mobile, highly specialized tissue and plays an active role in the control of suppurative inflammation and infection within the peritoneal cavity.

ACUTE PERITONITIS

Acute peritonitis may be primary or secondary. Primary bacterial peritonitis is the result of direct hematogenous invasion of the peritoneal cavity; before the days of antibiotics, pneumococci and streptococci were not uncommonly involved in acute primary peritonitis in otherwise healthy individuals. Primary peritonitis today is most often seen in debilitated patients and is particularly common in patients with nephrosis or ascites due to any cause. The principal causes of secondary peritonitis are acute infections such as appendicitis or diverticulitis and perforations of a viscus, as in perforated duodenal or gastric ulcer or penetrating abdominal wounds.

Acute generalized peritonitis due to a ruptured viscus is characterized by severe abdominal pain, vomiting, and variable degrees of fever. Physical examination shows abdominal rigidity and absence of peristalsis. Laboratory studies show leukocytosis and hemoconcentration. Progressive abdominal distention, ileus, hypotension, and shock follow.

Peritonitis secondary to infection, as in appendicitis or diverticulitis, is more gradual in onset. Initial manifestations are those of the underlying disease, with gradual development of spreading peritonitis manifested by increasing tenderness, abdominal rigidity, and distention. In the very old and very young, peritonitis may develop insidiously, so that marked ileus and abdominal distention are present when the patient is first seen.

BACTERIAL & CHEMICAL PERITONITIS

The first result of perforation of the stomach due to peptic ulcer is chemical peritonitis, but infection soon follows. Bile, pancreatic juice, and gastric juice combined produce a severe irritation of the peritoneum, leading to profound shock which can cause death before bacterial invasion develops. The massive loss of fluid within the peritoneal cavity is comparable to that seen in an extensive burn.

Peritonitis due to bile alone has unique characteristics. If the bile is infected, as in rupture of an inflamed gallbladder, there may be profound shock and collapse. Normal, uninfected bile without pancreatic or intestinal fluid is remarkably innocuous. Bile peritonitis due to traumatic rupture of the common duct may produce a picture similar to slowly progressive ascites with very little abdominal pain.

Blood and sterile urine evoke a mild peritoneal reaction. The shock of intraperitoneal hemorrhage is due principally to loss of blood rather than peritoneal irritation. Similarly, sterile urine may produce only a mild peritoneal reaction, whereas infected urine can lead to a rapidly progressive bacterial peritonitis.

In nearly every case of peritonitis, bacterial invasion ultimately occurs. Perforation of the colon, however, produces a massive bacterial invasion of the peritoneal cavity which may lead to septicemia and overwhelming sepsis with a mixed infection, often including gas-forming organisms. Rupture of the cecum due to unrelieved large bowel obstruction, for example, produces a particularly fulminating form of peritonitis.

Depending upon the cause, peritonitis may be localized, diffuse, or generalized. Localization is dependent upon the nature of the primary lesion and the natural defenses of the host. Classically, it is seen most often in appendicitis. The omentum plays a major role in localization, but the virulence of the organisms may also determine localization or diffuse spread. The liver is an important organ in the systemic reaction to peritonitis, as bacteria picked up by the lymphatics and portal system are destroyed in the liver. In the presence of hepatic insufficiency, as in cirrhosis, this function is limited and generalized septicemia rapidly ensues. If the invading organisms are highly virulent, as is the case with clostridia, generalized septicemia may dominate the picture of peritonitis.

Clinical Findings

A. Symptoms and Signs: Regardless of the cause, abdominal pain, nausea, vomiting, and fever are present. The severity of the manifestations is directly related to the extent of the contamination. In acute generalized peritonitis, some degree of shock is always present, and shock may be profound.

There is diffuse, exquisite abdominal tenderness and board-like rigidity of the abdomen. In acute generalized peritonitis due to a ruptured viscus, the abdomen is silent from the onset. The area of liver dullness is decreased anteriorly and laterally. When peritonitis develops gradually, peristalsis may persist and be hyperactive in areas isolated from the localized area of peritoneal inflammation and infection. Without treatment, the condition rapidly progresses to marked ileus, abdominal distention, hypotension, and toxemia with ultimate respiratory, renal, and cardiac failure.

B. Laboratory Findings: There is marked leukocytosis and hemoconcentration. The serum electrolyte concentrations vary, but marked metabolic acidosis with respiratory alkalosis is a characteristic feature of bacterial or chemical peritonitis.

C. X-Ray Findings: Plain films of the abdomen show distention of both large and small bowel with fluid levels. There is a thickened appearance to loops of bowel due to the presence of fluid between loops. Air may be seen beneath the diaphragm if free perforation of a hollow viscus, as in perforated gastric or duodenal ulcer, has occurred.

D. Special Examinations: Abdominal paracentesis may be helpful in obscure cases. It is particularly valuable following nonpenetrating abdominal injury and in the aged, when symptoms and signs may be equivocal. Aspiration of the 4 quadrants of the abdomen may be carried out, but a single tap and insertion of a catheter for peritoneal lavage is more reliable, especially in cases of suspected peritonitis due to nonpenetrating trauma.

Common Surgical Causes of Peritonitis

The problem of differential diagnosis relates to the primary cause. Is it perforated ulcer? Acute pancreatitis? Mesenteric thrombosis? In more slowly progressive peritonitis, is it due to appendicitis, acute cholecystitis, or diverticulitis? The diagnosis and differential diagnosis of each of these entities are discussed in more detail elsewhere in this book.

Intestinal obstruction may produce abdominal distention and tenderness without peritonitis, but the history and physical findings usually make the diagnosis clear. The differentiation is important because, although both intestinal obstruction and peritonitis require prompt operation, a different timing and operative approach may be required.

Common Causes of Acute Peritonitis

Although each clinical entity is discussed in more detail under separate headings, a brief overview is given here. (See Fig 32–2.)

A. Acute Perforated Ulcer: Acute free perforation of the stomach or duodenum produces the classic findings of generalized peritonitis. Severe generalized abdominal pain and some degree of shock are characteristic. The abdomen is board-like, often scaphoid, and rigid throughout. Tenderness (including rectal tenderness) is diffuse. Pain often radiates to the right or left shoulder. Within a few minutes of the onset of perforation, peristalsis ceases. Air is found beneath the diaphragm in 80% of cases. In perforated duodenal ulcer, most of the air will be found on the right side. Whenever a film shows a massive amount of air on the left side of the diaphragm, a high gastric or colonic perforation should be suspected.

B. Acute Pancreatitis: Acute pancreatitis is more gradual in onset; vomiting is a more dominant feature,

and pain is progressively more severe; and hypotension and shock develop more gradually. The physical findings are also less striking in acute pancreatitis because the disease begins in a retroperitoneal organ. In the early stages, although there may be upper abdominal tenderness, spasm and rigidity are usually not present. Peritonitis due to acute pancreatitis is easily overlooked until the disease process is well established.

C. Acute Appendicitis: Acute appendicitis is the most common cause of peritonitis, but fortunately today this is usually localized rather than diffuse and generalized. Generalized peritonitis secondary to appendicitis usually develops gradually. At times, however, there is an acute exacerbation of pain, which, having arisen in the epigastrium and settled in the right lower quadrant, suddenly becomes generalized, indicating perforation. More commonly, however, when perforation occurs it is already partially walled off, and a diffusing peritonitis develops gradually over a period of hours. It is said that in no case of peritonitis should appendicitis be listed lower than second among the possible causes since it is capable—because of the varied position of the appendix—of simulating any other acute abdominal inflammatory lesion. More details are given in Chapter 34.

D. Acute Salpingitis: Acute salpingitis may produce diffuse abdominal pain and marked tenderness and spasm throughout the lower abdomen, indicative of a rapidly advancing peritoneal inflammation. The temperature is often high, but the pulse is slow and the patient exhibits a state of well-being quite out of place with the physical findings.

E. Acute Mesenteric Vascular Occlusion: Vascular lesions are characterized by severe abdominal pain with limited findings of peritonitis in the early stages. It may be exceedingly difficult to distinguish between pancreatitis and mesenteric thrombosis. Early and marked elevation of serum amylase suggests pancreatitis, but there may be an elevation of amylase in mesenteric thrombosis.

F. Acute Cholecystitis: Acute cholecystitis produces a localized peritonitis as the condition advances. In contrast to perforated ulcer and acute appendicitis, peristalsis in acute cholecystitis tends to be active and sometimes hyperactive. The finding of very active peristalsis with right upper quadrant signs is a good clue to acute cholecystitis as opposed to perforated ulcer.

G. Gallbladder Perforation: Perforation of the gallbladder may produce a diffuse, rapidly progressive form of peritonitis which simulates perforation of a duodenal or gastric ulcer. The condition is rare because gangrene of the gallbladder develops so slowly that the inflammatory process is usually walled off.

H. Trauma to Abdomen: The differential diagnosis of peritonitis is often clearly established by the history, as in penetrating or nonpenetrating abdominal wounds.

I. Acute Diverticulitis: Acute diverticulitis is a fairly common cause of peritonitis. There may be free

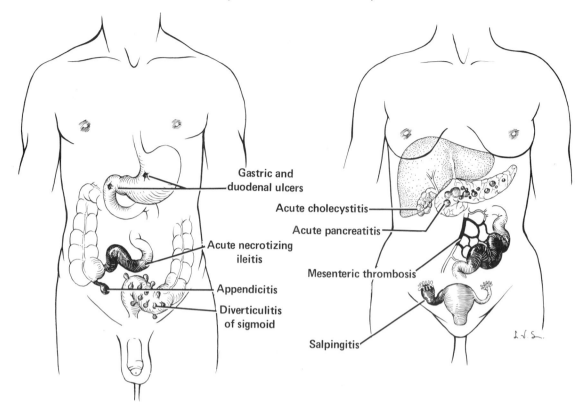

FIG 32—2. Common primary causes of peritonitis.

perforation of the diverticulum, producing a rapid diffusing peritonitis with generalized abdominal pain, tenderness, and spasm. Leakage of air from the colon may result in rapidly progressive abdominal distention with large amounts of air under the diaphragm. A massive amount of air under the left diaphragm should suggest perforated diverticulum.

More commonly, diverticulitis progresses gradually and produces signs and symptoms suggestive of left-sided appendicitis. The sigmoid loop may extend to the right side of the abdomen and closely simulate appendicitis, just as a long appendix may produce inflammatory signs on the left suggestive of diverticulitis. The details of the differential diagnosis are discussed elsewhere.

Differential Diagnosis (Nonsurgical Conditions Simulating Peritonitis)

Many systemic diseases result in marked intestinal ileus closely resembling intestinal obstruction or peritonitis. Pneumonia, particularly in the aged, is often accompanied by marked abdominal distention and ileus simulating slowly progressive peritonitis. Diaphragmatic pleurisy may also be associated with abdominal pain suggestive of acute cholecystitis or perforated ulcer.

Uremia commonly is associated with abdominal distention and ileus. Since patients with chronic renal failure may develop primary intraperitoneal diseases, such as appendicitis or perforated ulcer, the differential diagnosis may be very difficult, particularly if the history is unobtainable or unreliable. Abdominal tap may be required but is conclusive only if positive.

As discussed in the differential diagnosis of appendicitis (Chapter 34), a variety of other medical conditions may produce abdominal pain simulating early acute peritonitis.

"**Periodic peritonitis**" (**familial Mediterranean fever, familial paroxysmal polyserositis**) is a rare, obscure entity which produces all the manifestations of acute peritonitis but without any identifiable cause. The disease is characterized by recurring episodes of abdominal pain with exquisite direct and rebound tenderness. Fever (38—38.5 C [100.4—101.3 F]) and leukocytosis accompany the attack. There appears to be a familial incidence among Mediterranean populations, notably Turks, Arabs, Greeks, and Italians. Laparotomy is often performed for the first episode. At operation, the peritoneal surfaces may be inflamed and there is free fluid, but smears and cultures are negative. Although normal, the appendix should be removed to eliminate acute appendicitis in the differential diagnosis of recurrent episodes.

Complications

The principal acute complications of peritonitis

are shock, high-output respiratory failure, acute renal tubular necrosis, and hepatic failure associated with liver abscesses and pylephlebitis.

If the acute complications are prevented or corrected—and if death does not result early—the late complications are intraperitoneal abscess formation. Abscesses commonly form in the pelvis and in the subdiaphragmatic and subhepatic areas but may develop anywhere within the peritoneal cavity. The end result is intraperitoneal adhesion formation, particularly after operations for peritonitis. These adhesions are common causes of intestinal obstruction.

Abscesses and adhesions as complications of peritonitis are discussed separately below.

Prevention

Prevention depends upon early recognition and treatment. Prompt use of massive wide-spectrum antibiotic therapy also contributes to the prevention of generalized peritonitis regardless of cause.

Treatment

In early peritonitis, treatment consists of removing the cause by operation. Appendectomy, cholecystectomy, closure of perforated ulcer, and resection of gangrenous intestine are the most common surgical procedures in the control of early peritonitis. Combined with antibiotic therapy, early operation has a negligible mortality from peritonitis.

Advanced and established peritonitis also requires surgery for control in most cases. Sometimes, however, patients are seen in whom the peritonitis is localizing, and a course of cautious observation and nonsurgical treatment may be indicated.

Very rarely, especially in the aged or debilitated, the patient's condition has deteriorated to the point where anesthesia and any type of surgery would be lethal. The only hope is that antibiotics and major supportive measures will permit localization and formation of an abscess which can be drained later.

A. Preoperative Management: All patients with advanced peritonitis require a period of preoperative preparation. More complete details regarding the treatment of septic surgical shock are presented in Chapter 16. As soon as the circulation is stable and reasonable respiratory exchange has been established, operation should be performed.

1. Fluids—Correction of fluid losses and hypovolemia should be started immediately after the patient arrives in the emergency ward. Nasogastric suction should also be initiated with a moderate-sized tube.

Fluid therapy should be initiated with balanced salt solution or lactated Ringer's injection. Potassium should be restricted initially since there is likely to be poor renal function due to shock and hypovolemia.

When an adequate urinary output has been established, potassium may be given if required. Final adjustment of electrolyte administration can be made on the basis of the laboratory findings and measurement of continued fluid losses.

2. Laboratory tests—At the time fluid therapy is initiated in the emergency ward, blood should be drawn for complete blood count and serum sodium, potassium, chloride, bicarbonate, creatinine, and amylase. In critically ill patients, P_{O_2}, P_{CO_2}, and arterial pH determinations should also be obtained.

3. Urinary flow—In early or moderately advanced peritonitis, urinary catheterization should be avoided because it establishes one more portal of entry for bacteremia. In advanced peritonitis with shock and renal failure, an indwelling catheter is advisable in order to determine the hourly urinary output and to estimate fluid requirements.

4. Central venous pressure—In patients with circulatory instability, monitoring of central venous pressure may be required depending upon the severity of shock and the cardiac status of the patient. In general, central venous pressure monitoring by means of a catheter in the superior vena cava should be instituted in all critically ill patients, in moderately ill elderly patients, or in those with cardiac disease.

5. Analgesics—Narcotics and sedatives should be administered as needed to control pain. Initial sedation with morphine, 10–15 mg IM, is usually adequate, and repeated administration should be avoided in the preoperative period. If the patient is in severe pain and also in shock, morphine should be administered intravenously in small doses (1–3 mg) repeated as needed.

6. Antibiotics—Antibiotic therapy is a mainstay of treatment and should be initiated as soon as the diagnosis is made in the emergency ward. Cephalothin or ampicillin makes a useful initial form of therapy, reserving the more potent wide-spectrum antibiotics, such as kanamycin, for the postoperative period after the infectious agent has been identified and sensitivity tests obtained.

7. Oxygen—One of the most critical complications of advanced peritonitis is high-output respiratory failure. Peritonitis imposes marked increases in metabolic demands which are accompanied by proportionately increased demands for ventilation and oxygenation. Because of the marked abdominal distention, elevation of the diaphragms, and possibly associated pulmonary insufficiency from emphysema, the patient is unable to meet these expanded oxygen requirements. Oxygen therapy, assisted respiration, and, in some cases, tracheostomy may be required. Despite nasogastric suction, decompression may fail to relieve the distention sufficiently to improve the vital capacity. Consequently, operation with release of distention and decompression of the intestine may be an essential part of improving respiratory exchange. Unrecognized severe respiratory insufficiency has in the past been mistaken for the "toxemia" of peritonitis. Marked improvement of respiratory function can be expected as soon as the abdomen is opened, peritoneal fluid aspirated, and (if necessary) distended loops of bowel decompressed.

B. Operative Technic: Although the operative procedure in peritonitis is determined by the nature of the primary cause, there are several additional points in the management of generalized peritonitis which require emphasis.

1. Peritoneal toilet—At the completion of the operation, an effort should be made to remove all necrotic material and contaminated fluid from the peritoneal cavity.

2. Intestinal decompression—If there is massive intestinal distention—and particularly if the loops of small bowel contain large amounts of fluid—intestinal decompression should be employed. This may be done either by the use of a tube (the Baker tube is the most effective and can be left down postoperatively) or by aspiration of the small bowel through one or more needle points introduced through a small purse-string suture of silk, which can be tied afterward.

3. Irrigation of the peritoneal cavity—If the peritoneal cavity has been heavily contaminated with bacteria, it should be generously irrigated with balanced salt solution or lactated Ringer's solution in which kanamycin, 2–4 g/liter, has been dissolved.

4. Drainage—Drainage of the general peritoneal cavity is in most cases unnecessary, ineffective, and undesirable. Drainage should be employed only where there are localized masses of necrotic material or debris which cannot be removed, or actual abscess formation. Prophylactic drainage will not prevent the formation of intraperitoneal abscesses and may even encourage abscess formation. The principal indication for drainage is an actual or potential source of continued contamination. Wounds and inflammatory disorders of the pancreas or biliary tract are good examples. When an opening into a viscus cannot be securely closed, sump drains with continuous suction are required.

Every effort should be made to isolate the wound from the contaminated peritoneal fluid, preferably by impermeable plastic drapes. If significant contamination of the wound cannot be avoided, the skin and subcutaneous tissues should be left open. Wound closure in patients with peritonitis calls for the use of retention sutures since ileus and distention are likely complications and the risk of dehiscence is decreased.

A method of closure with retention sutures which permits the skin and subcutaneous tissues to be left open is described in Chapter 9.

5. Binders—Scultetus binders of all types should be avoided because they restrict the chest wall and compound existing respiratory insufficiency. Adhesive tapes (Fig 32–3) will provide excellent support to the wound, enable the patient to cough with less discomfort, and do not restrict the thoracic cage.

C. Postoperative Management: After operation, all of the measures instituted preoperatively should be continued. The patient should be given nothing by mouth; nasogastric suction must be continuous; and fluid and electrolyte balance must be carefully monitored. Narcotics should be used as required to control pain. An adequate dose of morphine (10–15 mg) given intramuscularly is better than repeated small doses given intravenously. Meperidine (pethidine, Demerol) is not as effective as morphine for pain.

As soon as cultures and sensitivity tests have been obtained, type-specific antibiotic therapy should be instituted.

Although the patient is usually hemoconcentrated due to fluid losses in the early phase of peritonitis, moderate degrees of anemia soon develop following correction of the hypovolemia. Transfusions of whole blood or packed red cells may have been required during the operation, and additional blood may be needed postoperatively.

Prognosis

The prognosis in all forms of peritonitis depends upon the cause. In acute peritonitis, the age of the patient and the duration of the illness before operation are critical factors. In the very young and the very old, generalized peritonitis has a grave prognosis. In early acute peritonitis, regardless of cause, the prognosis is favorable.

Prognosis is discussed in more detail under specific disease headings.

Altemeier WA & others: Intra-abdominal sepsis. Advances Surg 5:281–333, 1971.

Barabas AP: Peritonitis due to diverticular disease of the colon. Proc Roy Soc Med 64:253–254, 1971.

Clowes GHA & others: Circulating factors in the etiology of pulmonary insufficiency and right heart failure accompanying severe sepsis (peritonitis). Ann Surg 171:663–678, 1970.

Hermann G: Intraperitoneal drainage. S Clin North America 49:1279–1288, 1969.

Long WB & others: Peritonitis. J Roy Coll Surg Edinb 15:158–163, 1970.

Skillman J & others: Peritonitis and respiratory failure after abdominal operations. Ann Surg 170:122–127, 1969.

Wickstrom P & others: Intra-operative decompression of the obstructed small bowel. Surgery 73:212–219, 1973.

GONOCOCCAL PERITONITIS

Gonococcal peritonitis (discussed in greater detail in Chapter 45) has unique characteristics. It often produces severe abdominal pain, fever, and peritoneal signs without tachycardia, hypotension, or shock. Characteristically, the patient does not look ill. A unique feature is the extent of the inflammation throughout the peritoneal cavity with the formation of adhesions between the liver and diaphragm. In the early stages, acute right upper quadrant abdominal pain may occur, simulating acute cholecystitis.

TUBERCULOUS PERITONITIS

Tuberculous peritonitis is a chronic granulomatous lesion of the peritoneal cavity. It often appears as

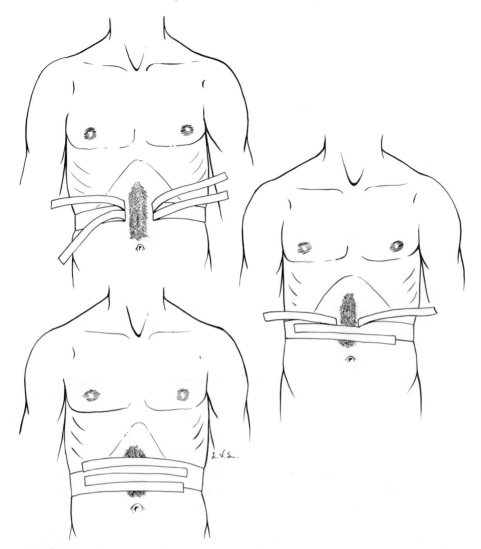

FIG 32–3. Adhesive binders after abdominal surgery, applied "Scultetus fashion" without restriction of the thoracic cage.

a primary abdominal infection without pulmonary, intestinal, or fallopian tube involvement in the early stages. The available evidence supports the concept of reactivation of a latent peritoneal focus as the most attractive explanation for most cases, although others appear as a manifestation of systemic spread of extra-abdominal infection.

The patient commonly presents with a 2- to 4-month history of weakness, night sweats, anorexia, weight loss, and abdominal distention. On physical examination, the only finding may be that of free fluid in the peritoneal cavity. At times there is a "doughy" feeling to the abdomen, and vague masses may be noted. If there are associated tuberculous lesions of the bowel, a distinct mass may be palpated, particularly in the right colon.

Paracentesis will reveal fluid which is pale or greenish-yellow. The protein content of the fluid nearly always exceeds 3 g/100 ml, and microscopy shows predominantly lymphocytes. Acid-fast bacilli are rarely identified on smear, but cultures of the ascitic fluid are positive in over 80% of cases. Percutaneous biopsy of the peritoneum is the most expeditious means of establishing the diagnosis, but diagnostic laparotomy may be necessary if that fails.

The course of the disease tends to be chronic, but the response to antituberculosis therapy is usually excellent. There is evidence that the addition of corticosteroids to the treatment regimen may lower the incidence of late intestinal obstruction from adhesive bands.

Borhanmanesh F & others: Tuberculous peritonitis. Ann Int Med 76:567–572, 1972.

Singh MM: Tuberculous peritonitis. New England J Med 281:1091–1094, 1969.

CHYLOUS PERITONITIS

Another form of chronic peritonitis is due to the presence of chyle in the peritoneal cavity. This may be of congenital origin, appearing in childhood as a chronic swelling of the abdomen.

In adults, chylous peritonitis (ascites) is usually due to obstruction of the flow of chyle by malignant tumors of the upper abdomen or thorax, although in almost half of cases no cause is uncovered. Lymphoma is a common cause, but the condition is also seen in cancer of the pancreas or stomach and in retroperitoneal sarcomas. Any abdominal neoplasm that spreads retroperitoneally may ultimately produce chylous ascites.

If chylous peritonitis is discovered at laparotomy, a retroperitoneal dissection to locate a ruptured lymph vessel is not required; the chyle leak generally seals without specific therapy.

Treatment is unsatisfactory if the primary cause is an inoperable malignant tumor. X-ray treatment, however, may result in dramatic improvement in cases of lymphoma.

Congenital chylous ascites is due to a developmental abnormality of intestinal lymphatics which may be markedly enlarged and communicate freely with the peritoneal cavity. There may be channels involving the extremities so that chyle appears in the skin ("cutaneous chylous reflux"). If ascites is minimal or absent, chylous cutaneous reflux can be corrected by an operation which divides the large incompetent lymphatic channels between the mesentery of the intestine and the lymphatics of the thigh.

Krizek TJ, Davis JH: Acute chylous peritonitis. Arch Surg 91:253–262, 1965.

GRANULOMATOUS PERITONITIS

A peculiar type of acute or chronic granulomatous peritonitis has been identified as occurring secondary to a variety of substances used in the preparation of surgical gloves. Talc produces a chronic granulomatous lesion and has not been used for some years in the preparation of surgical gloves.

More recently, substitutes for talc, particularly starch powders from corn or rice, have been used. A peculiar syndrome characterized by severe abdominal pain, fever, and marked peritoneal irritation but with a normal white blood count appears within 2–3 weeks of what has appeared to be an otherwise uncomplicated abdominal operation. The pain may be so severe and the clinical findings so disturbing that immediate laparotomy is undertaken. Experience has shown that reexploration merely aggravates the syndrome by dis-

seminating the inciting agent with reactivation of the process.

The exact cause of the reaction is not known, and it appears to be limited to a relatively small number of patients who react in a hypersensitive manner to the presence of the foreign material. Upon recognition of the syndrome, reoperation should be avoided. Good immediate results have followed corticosteroid therapy.

The condition can be prevented by carefully washing all foreign material from surgical gloves prior to operation.

Bates B: Granulomatous peritonitis secondary to corn starch. Ann Int Med 62:335, 1965.
Ignatius AJ, Hartmann H: The glove starch peritonitis syndrome. Ann Surg 175:388, 1972.
Task DA, Lasersohn JT, Hill LD: Glove starch granulomatous peritonitis. Am J Surg 120:231, 1970.

PERITONEAL ABSCESSES

Intraperitoneal abscesses are common complications of peritonitis and may also follow major abdominal operations without established peritonitis. Inadequately drained contamination, intestinal contents secondary to small leaks from anastomoses, or collections of blood and contaminated peritoneal fluid all tend to settle in dependent parts of the abdomen, and abscess formation may be a sequel. Detritus, foreign material, and necrotic tissue are more important factors in abscess formation than the mere presence of bacteria.

Common sites of abscess formation are shown in Fig 32–4. These represent dependent areas of the peritoneal cavity with the patient in the supine position. The common sites are under the diaphragm, along the undersurface of the right lobe of the liver, along the lateral gutters, and in the pelvis.

Persistent fever is the classic sign of a developing intraperitoneal abscess. As the fever following a major peritoneal insult subsides, instead of returning to normal it persists and gradually rises in a stepwise fashion. A progressively rising temperature that does not return to normal over a period of several days is typical of abscess formation. With threatened perforation or extension into adjacent structures, chills, fever, and hypotension may develop.

Midabdominal Abscesses

These abscesses may occur anywhere within the abdominal cavity from just below the transverse colon to the pelvis. The right and left gutters are the most common sites, but an abscess may form wherever a collection of foreign material or blood has occurred.

Midabdominal abscesses are particularly difficult to identify. Knowing the cause of the original peritoneal disease is of considerable help in identifying the

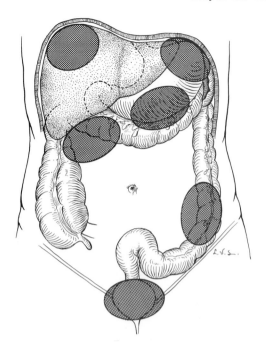

FIG 32–4. Common locations of peritoneal abscess formation.

presence of an abscess—diverticulitis being more likely to involve the left gutter and appendicitis the right gutter. Perforations from regional enteritis or ulcerative colitis may result in centrally placed abscesses.

Abscesses develop at the root of the mesentery between loops of bowel and are protected from the anterior abdominal wall by the mesentery of the small intestine.

Repeated careful and gentle examination of the abdomen, feeling for a developing mass, is the most reliable method of identifying a midabdominal abscess. Plain x-ray films of the abdomen may be helpful: A mass shadow may be identified, collections of gas or air may be seen, or persistently dilated irregular loops of bowel may indicate the presence of the abscess.

Midabdominal abscesses may subside spontaneously. Prolonged postoperative ileus is a common major complication, and continuous gastric suction, sometimes with the use of a long tube, may be required.

A progressively enlarging abdominal mass is an indication for drainage. Frequently this will be delayed for 2–3 days until the mass appears to be well localized and in close contact with the abdominal wall. On other occasions, with deep-seated midabdominal abscesses, the patient may become so ill, with high fever, chills, and hypotension, that laparotomy to find and drain the abscess becomes essential.

Open transabdominal drainage of an intraperitoneal abscess, while not ideal, can be safely done under cover of antibiotics and peritoneal irrigation. It is absolutely essential to explore the peritoneal cavity for residual abscesses if the patient is clearly deteriorating.

Huge abscesses containing more than a liter of pus may occur without significant physical findings.

Subphrenic Abscess

Subphrenic abscesses pose special problems in diagnosis and treatment. Although there is much argument about the anatomic nature of the subphrenic spaces, from a practical point of view abscesses may occur in any one of 6 areas (Fig 32–5).

On the right side (Fig 32–6), pus may be found between the liver and the diaphragm, either anteriorly (anterior superior) or posteriorly above the kidney between the liver and the diaphragm (posterior inferior) or anteriorly below the liver on the right (anterior inferior). On the left, an abscess may develop anteriorly between the left lobe of the liver, spleen, or stomach and the diaphragm (superior). Inferiorly on the left, pus may develop below the stomach anterior to the transverse colon or posteriorly in the lesser peritoneal cavity (posterior superior). The posterior space on the right is called superior by some authorities and inferior by others. The important anatomic feature is that this space is best approached through the 12th rib from behind (see below).

The recognition of subphrenic abscess and its precise localization require a combination of repeated physical and x-ray examinations. Unexplained fever after peritoneal infection of any type without evident wound infection or peritoneal abscesses should

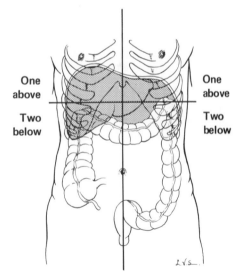

FIG 32–5. Simple scheme for remembering the subphrenic spaces. There is one space above the line on the right: the anterior superior. On the left, there is one space above the line (between the liver and the diaphragm) and 2 below: one anterior to the lesser sac and the lesser sac itself. On the right, the inferior subphrenic space extends from the bare area posteriorly to the subhepatic area anteriorly. Its posterior portion was formerly designated the posterior superior space.

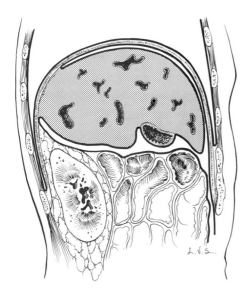

FIG 32—6. Right subphrenic spaces. The anterior superior space extends from the anterior edge of the liver to the bare area. The right inferior space extends from the bare area posteriorly to the anterior subhepatic area. Although anatomically in continuity, abscesses tend to localize either anteriorly or posteriorly.

immediately arouse suspicion of a subphrenic abscess.

The primary cause is often a clue to localization. Appendicitis commonly produces a right posterior inferior abscess. Infections of the gallbladder, stomach, and duodenum are more apt to produce anterior superior or subhepatic abscesses. Pancreatitis commonly produces a left inferior posterior abscess. Diverticulitis, particularly of the descending colon, may result in an anterior inferior abscess. Perforation of a high greater curvature ulcer and injuries or abscesses of the spleen are more apt to produce superior left-sided subphrenic abscesses lying close to the dome of the diaphragm. The old adage "Pus somewhere, pus nowhere, pus under the diaphragm" is often appropriate.

All too often, subphrenic abscesses develop insidiously, but on occasion there may be pain and tenderness anteriorly or posteriorly on the affected side. Motion of the diaphragm on the affected side is restricted, and in superior space involvement there usually is a pleural effusion. In advanced cases, there may be widening of the intercostal spaces with fullness and palpable edema.

Management with antibiotics usually suppresses the physical signs, so that a persistent spiking fever, tachycardia, and malaise are the only manifestations.

X-ray examination is of the greatest importance. Demonstration of an air-fluid level below the diaphragm with a pleural effusion above it is diagnostic. Unfortunately, this represents an advanced abscess and more commonly the only findings are fixation and elevation of the diaphragm and a pleural effusion on the involved side. Lateral films may be of great help in localizing the abscess to an anterior or posterior position.

Inferior abscesses are more difficult to recognize than superior ones and are less apt to be associated with diaphragmatic immobility and pleural effusion.

Diagnostic aspiration of suspected abscesses is very hazardous, as pus may be transferred from the abscess to the free peritoneal or pleural spaces, compounding the sepsis. If there is a large pleural effusion, it can be tapped very high, taking only a few milliliters of fluid to identify its character. In subphrenic abscess, the pleural fluid is straw-colored and sterile.

Unless recognized and treated, subphrenic abscesses may lead to septicemia and death. Rupture of the abscess into the free peritoneal or pleural cavity may occur. Direct extension into a bronchus has occurred in neglected cases.

Treatment. The treatment of subphrenic abscess is surgical. As noted earlier, however, limited infection in the subphrenic spaces with elevation and fixation of the diaphragm may resolve following antibiotic therapy.

The absolute indication for drainage is obvious progressive sepsis, often with deterioration of the general condition of the patient. Ideally, subphrenic abscesses should be identified and drained before the patient becomes gravely ill. It is often preferable to explore the subphrenic spaces surgically in order to establish the diagnosis.

The ideal treatment of subphrenic abscess is extraperitoneal and extrapleural drainage. Posterior abscesses are drained through the bed of the 12th rib on the affected side (Fig 32—7). The location of the incision is important, as it must be directly transverse and not parallel to the bed of the rib. Care must be taken to avoid entering the pleura at the inner end of the 12th rib.

Anteriorly, a subcostal incision is made and carried through the transversalis fascia. The abscess cavity is located by blunt dissection and drained without entering the peritoneal cavity (Fig 32—7).

More recently it has been shown that it is not essential to avoid a transperitoneal approach; in all cases in which the abscess cannot be identified or adequately drained by an extraperitoneal approach, transperitoneal or transpleural drainage must be employed. In transpleural drainage, it is essential that the pleura be fused or that the operation be staged. Transperitoneal operations can be performed in one stage.

The prognosis after adequate drainage of subphrenic abscesses is excellent. However, adequate drainage is often difficult to obtain, particularly in some right anterior superior and left posterior inferior abscesses. Transpleural drainage in one or 2 stages may be required in very large right superior abscesses. Repeated reoperation may be required in left posterior inferior abscess, especially when pancreatitis is the cause.

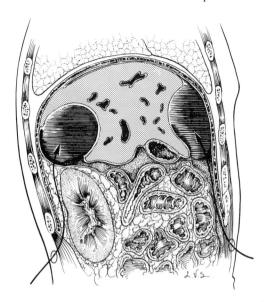

FIG 32–7. Extraperitoneal approaches to the right subphrenic spaces. An abscess in the anterior portion of the inferior space must be drained transperitoneally.

Bond DP: The subphrenic spaces and the emperor's new robes. New England J Med 275:911, 1966.

Halasz NA: Subphrenic abscesses: Myths and facts. JAMA 214:724, 1970.

Ochsner A, Groves AM: Subphrenic abscesses: An analysis of 3372 collected and personal cases. Ann Surg 98:961, 1933.

PELVIC ABSCESS

A pelvic abscess is usually readily recognized. In addition to fever, there may be lower abdominal discomfort and diarrhea. Rectal examination will disclose tenderness and a fullness in the pouch of Douglas. With a very high pelvic abscess, rectal examination may initially be negative, so that repeated daily examinations become necessary. This is essential if the patient appears seriously ill, with high fever and pulse rate.

Pelvic abscesses may subside spontaneously but most often progress to a large, tense, slightly fluctuant mass protruding into the anterior rectal wall or vagina. The onset of diarrhea is usually an indication that the abscess is mature.

Pelvic abscesses may be drained either through the rectum or vagina (Fig 32–8). Needle aspiration before introducing scissors or a clamp is a wise precaution in most cases. Drains should be left in the cavity but may be removed in several days if the clinical response is good. In general, drainage of pelvic abscess provides a very gratifying result with rapid recovery.

PERITONEAL ADHESIONS

Intraperitoneal adhesions are a late result of peritoneal trauma or peritonitis. They may occur following abdominal operations in which there was no clinical evidence of peritonitis. Adhesions may occur following peritonitis without operation–the classic example being gonococcal peritonitis (see above), which frequently results in extensive adhesions between the liver and diaphragm. Other low-grade peritoneal infections not requiring surgery (eg, tuberculosis) may produce extensive intraperitoneal adhesions.

Intraperitoneal adhesions are commonest after operations in which there is localized or generalized peritonitis. They are not the result of simple defects in peritoneal coverage. In the absence of trauma, hemorrhage, or bacterial contamination, large defects in the peritoneum heal very rapidly by metamorphosis of in situ mesodermal cells. A new peritoneal surface arises from the raw area.

The major factors contributing to intraperitoneal adhesions appear to be a combination of mechanical injury, ischemia, bacterial contamination, venous stasis, and the presence of blood. Foreign material of any kind is likely to stimulate the formation of adhesions. Talc and various starches used in the preparation of surgeons' gloves (see above) have been identified as a cause of severe postoperative peritoneal reaction with extensive adhesion formation.

Peritoneal adhesions may produce no symptoms. Very rarely, extensive adhesions may form between the abdominal wall and a loop of bowel, the stomach, or the anterior surface of the liver, producing abdominal pain. Most intraperitoneal adhesions, however, are asymptomatic until intestinal obstruction occurs.

Scrupulous surgical technic is the only way of avoiding postoperative adhesions with or without associated peritonitis. Traumatized areas of peri-

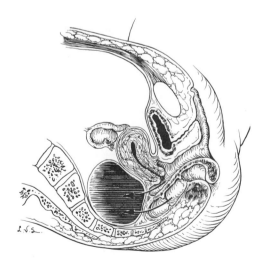

FIG 32–8. A pelvic abscess may be drained through the rectum and vagina.

toneum should be protected by interposing omentum between the area and loops of small bowel. All foreign material and blood should be carefully aspirated from the peritoneal cavity at the completion of the operation.

The management of recurrent intestinal obstruction associated with adhesions is discussed in Chapter 35.

Belzer FO: The role of venous obstruction in the formation of intra-abdominal adhesions: An experimental study. Brit J Surg 54:189, 1967.
Ellis H: The cause and prevention of postoperative intraperitoneal adhesions. Surg Gynec Obst 133:497, 1971.
Ryan JB & others: Postoperative peritoneal adhesions. Am J Path 65:117, 1971.

TUMORS OF THE PERITONEUM & RETROPERITONEUM

A variety of tumors may involve the peritoneum. In most instances, these are secondary cancerous implants from various abdominal organs—characteristically, the stomach and ovary. At times the primary lesion is small and the peritoneal seeding is disseminated widely as tiny implants. Ascites may be associated with intraperitoneal metastases, and the clinical picture may simulate chronic peritonitis due to other causes.

Diffuse abdominal carcinomatosis has a desperate prognosis except in the case of cancer of the ovary (see Chapter 45).

Pseudomyxoma Peritonei

This is a rather obscure disease which may begin by intraperitoneal dissemination of mucus and implantation of cells from a mucocele of the appendix or mucous cystadenoma of the ovary. In either case, the abdomen is filled with masses of gelatinous, partially encysted mucin. The patient may present with ascites or signs of low-grade intestinal obstruction.

At operation, huge masses of jelly-like material are easily evacuated from the abdominal cavity. The disease tends to run a chronic course, and patients are often palliated by periodic operations to remove mucin or relieve intestinal obstruction. Instillation of alkylating agents (mechlorethamine, 20 mg, or thiotepa, 60 mg) into the peritoneal cavity after removal of mucoid masses appears to have been beneficial.

With the passage of time, the disease assumes the course of a low-grade diffuse peritoneal malignancy. Distant metastases do not occur, but death ensues from malnutrition and recurrent intestinal obstruction. X-ray therapy and systemic chemotherapy have not been of benefit.

Little JM & others: Pseudomyxoma peritonei. Lancet 2:659–663, 1969.

Long RTL & others: Pseudomyxoma peritonei. Am J Surg 117:162–169, 1969.

Cysts of the Mesentery

Mesenteric cysts are rare lesions of developmental origin. They are variable in size, usually filled with straw-colored fluid, and have scant blood supply. Most mesenteric cysts are benign and can be shelled out without injury to the mesenteric blood vessels or intestine. Since the patient often presents with a fixed abdominal mass, the condition, though rare, must be carefully distinguished from retroperitoneal sarcoma. Laparotomy and excision or biopsy is essential.

Hardin W, Hardy J: Mesenteric cysts. Am J Surg 119:640, 1970.

Retroperitoneal Tumors

There are a variety of retroperitoneal tumors, usually of connective tissue origin. Fibrosarcoma, leiomyosarcoma, liposarcoma, and lymphoma may present primarily as retroperitoneal lesions. The course is usually characterized by low-grade pain or discomfort, fever, and eventually the appearance of a palpable mass on physical examination. In the early stages, x-ray studies are usually not helpful; later, as the mass enlarges, displacement of .bowel or ureters may be seen.

Rarely, the lesion proves to be benign or of such low-grade malignancy that good results follow surgical excision. In malignant lesions—except for lymphosarcoma—treatment is usually unsatisfactory. Palliation may be achieved by aggressive but incomplete removal of some liposarcomas and leiomyosarcomas. Abdominal exploration and biopsy are essential in all cases because the response to irradiation may be gratifying if a lymphoma is discovered.

Braasch JW, Mon AB: Primary retroperitoneal tumors. S Clin North America 47:663–678, 1967.
Lowman RM & others: Lumbar angiography in the diagnosis of primary retroperitoneal tumors. Surg Gynec Obst 132:597–602, 1971.
Riches E: The Gordon-Taylor tradition in the surgery of cancer with an account of paramesenteric tumors. Ann Roy Coll Surg England 42:71–91, 1968.

MESENTERIC PANNICULITIS

A bizarre form of chronic fat necrosis may involve the retroperitoneum and root of the mesentery. Histologically, the lesion is similar to that found in Weber-Christian disease and other forms of subcutaneous fat necrosis.

The course is characterized by low-grade fever, malaise, and vague recurrent abdominal pain. As in the case of other retroperitoneal tumors, x-ray studies are often negative. Sooner or later, however, an abdominal mass is palpable. Operation is usually required to establish the diagnosis, and it may be difficult to distinguish the lesion from a retroperitoneal tumor or a retroperitoneal dissection of a pancreatic pseudocyst. Biopsy will show the characteristic appearance of chronic fat necrosis.

The disease tends to be chronic and may regress spontaneously. No specific form of therapy is known.

Ogden WW & others: Mesenteric panniculitis. Ann Surg 161:864–875, 1965.

RETROPERITONEAL FIBROSIS

Retroperitoneal fibrosis usually affects the urinary tract (see Chapter 44), but on occasion it has been identified with sclerotic lesions involving the small and large bowel. It is thought to be a hypersensitivity reaction to drugs (notably methysergide) or an autoimmune process. The mesentery may be involved, and the condition may be confused with mesenteric panniculitis.

The clinical manifestations are usually those of low-grade small bowel or colonic obstruction. If retroperitoneal fibrosis is not kept in mind as a possibility, it may be mistaken for malignancy. The diagnosis can usually be established by biopsy.

Favorable results have been reported following lysis of the constricting bands and the use of corticosteroids.

Jones JH & others: Retroperitoneal fibrosis. Am J Med 48:203–208, 1970.
Mitchell RJ: Alimentary complications of non-malignant retroperitoneal fibrosis. Brit J Surg 58:254, 1971.

THE OMENTUM

The omentum may be the site of infection or tumor formations. It is also subject to torsion and frequently is involved in adhesions, producing intestinal obstruction.

Infection

The omentum is involved in all instances of peritonitis and provides an important protective mechanism against spreading peritonitis. In certain chronic diseases such as tuberculosis, the omentum may itself become infected and appear as a rolled-up tumorous mass instead of having its usual apron-like appearance.

Nonspecific inflammation of the omentum (epiploitis) may cause vague abdominal pain. At operation, the only finding is a rolled-up portion of thickened, edematous omentum. Microscopic study will show only mild inflammation. This lesion may be the result of a previous torsion.

Infarction & Torsion of the Omentum

Torsion of the omentum usually occurs when one portion of it is fixed by an adhesion or is caught in the opening of a hernia. The omentum rotates on itself, so that the blood supply becomes compressed.

Acute torsion produces severe abdominal pain, nausea, vomiting, and tenderness localized to the involved area. There may be a palpable mass. The condition is rare and is usually mistaken for some more common acute abdominal disorder such as intestinal obstruction or acute appendicitis.

At operation, the omentum will be found as a twisted mass with impaired blood supply and varying degrees of infarction. Excision is required. The prognosis is good.

Infarction of the omentum may be secondary to trauma or vascular lesions such as polyarteritis nodosa. Treatment is the same as for infarction caused by torsion.

DeLaurentis DA & others: Idiopathic segmental infarction of the greater omentum. Arch Surg 102:474–475, 1971.
Mainzer RA, Simoes A: Primary idiopathic torsion of the omentum. Arch Surg 88:974–983, 1964.

Tumors & Cysts of the Omentum

The omentum is frequently involved by secondary deposits of cancer, and at times this may appear as a primary lesion because of the small size of the original growth. More often, it is clear that the involvement is secondary to an obvious gastrointestinal carcinoma. Rarely, primary cysts or vascular anomalies of the omentum may be found incidental to operation for other disorders.

33 . . .

Hernias of the Abdominal Wall*

Harold H. Lindner, MD

A groin hernia is the protrusion of any intra-abdominal tissue or organ or combination of organs through the normally confining walls of the abdominal cavity in the region of the groin.

In 1961, Nardi noted that indirect inguinal hernia accounted for 70% of all hernias through the ventro-lateral abdominal wall; direct inguinal hernia accounted for 15% of such hernias; and femoral hernia accounted for 4%. Thus, the 3 groin hernias accounted for about 89% of all ventral abdominal wall protrusions. These figures hold not only for the USA and Great Britain but are remarkably constant in all parts of the world. Harkins has estimated that in the USA alone there are today well over a million people who have a hernia, have had a hernia repaired, or will develop a hernia at some time in the future. It thus becomes apparent that problems of the diagnosis and repair of hernia are faced very frequently by the operating surgeon and that an accurate knowledge of groin anatomy and function is essential to a good performance. Herniorrhaphy is too often considered a minor and relatively easy surgical procedure. Frequently it is performed by surgeons without adequate special training, and even in large surgical training centers it is often delegated to the junior resident without adequate senior attending control. These factors tend to cause too high a recurrence rate following hernia repair, particularly for direct hernia, recurrent hernia, and sliding hernia.

Indirect inguinal hernia is by far the most common groin hernia in infancy and childhood; direct inguinal hernia is rare in the early years of life. With increasing age, weakening of the tissues in Hesselbach's area results in a higher incidence of direct inguinal hernia, and in the age group over 55 direct inguinal hernia is the most common type of groin hernia. Moreover, the longer a patient has an indirect inguinal hernia with its resultant gradual increasing degree of stretching of tissues as it passes through the inguinal canal, the more apt he is to develop a concomitant direct inguinal hernia due to the attenuation of the transversalis fascia in Hesselbach's area.

Inguinal hernia is much more common in males than in females. Femoral hernia is more common in females than in males, but inguinal hernia is more common in females than femoral hernia.

*Additional comments on hernias in the pediatric age group are contained in Chapter 49.

ANATOMY OF GROIN HERNIA
(See Figs 33–1 to 33–4.)

The ilio-inguinal and femoral regions, commonly known as the groins, are relatively small areas of the lower ventrolateral abdominal wall and the adjacent upper mid thighs. The structures comprising these areas must be thoroughly familiar to the surgeon who wishes to understand all the varieties of inguinal and femoral hernia and the problems of their diagnosis and treatment.

Superficial Fascia (Scarpa's Fascia)

The superficial fascia of the ventrolateral abdominal wall attains its greatest thickness in the ilio-inguinal region. It fuses laterally with the external plate of the crest of the ilium and passes ventral to the inguinal ligament to fuse with the deep fascia of the upper thigh about 2.5 cm below and parallel to the inguinal ligament.

Muscles & Ligaments

The musculature of the ilio-inguinal region is composed of 3 flat, thin muscles: the external oblique, the internal oblique, and the transverse abdominal.

A. External Oblique: The external oblique is the most superficial as well as the largest and thickest of the ilio-inguinal muscles. It arises from the ventral chest wall by fleshy digitations from the lower 8 ribs; is broad, thin, and irregularly quadrilateral; and its fibers run vertically and medially from cephalad to caudad. The muscle is fleshy until it approaches a line drawn from the anterior-superior spine of the ilium to the umbilicus, at which point it forms the aponeurosis of the external oblique which covers the ilio-inguinal region deep to Scarpa's fascia. The aponeurosis is a strong, thin membranous structure whose fibers are directed inferiorly and medially.

The **subcutaneous or external inguinal ring** is a roughly triangular opening in the aponeurosis of the external oblique lying just cephalad and lateral to the pubic tubercle. The ring runs obliquely cephalad and laterally. In the male it is about 2.5 cm long from base to apex and about 1.25 cm wide. In the female it is about half this size. It is bounded inferiorly by the pubic crest and laterally and medially by its margins in the external oblique aponeurosis—called the crura of the ring. The inferior crus, or external pillar, is the

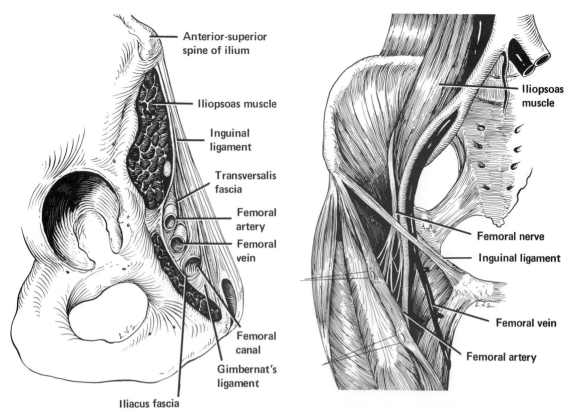

FIG 33–1. **Anatomy of the pelvis.** Internal view of structures of the subinguinal region.

FIG 33–2. Deep anatomy of the inguinal region.

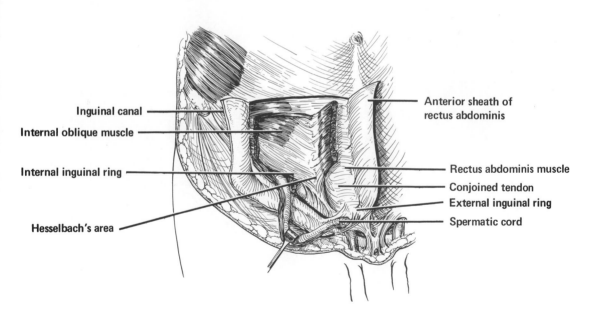

FIG 33–3. Dissection of ventrolateral abdominal wall in the ilio-inguinal region.

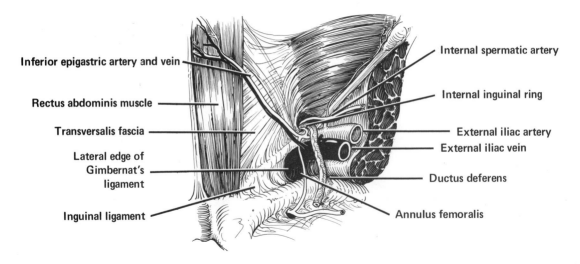

FIG 33–4. The internal inguinal ring and its relationships.

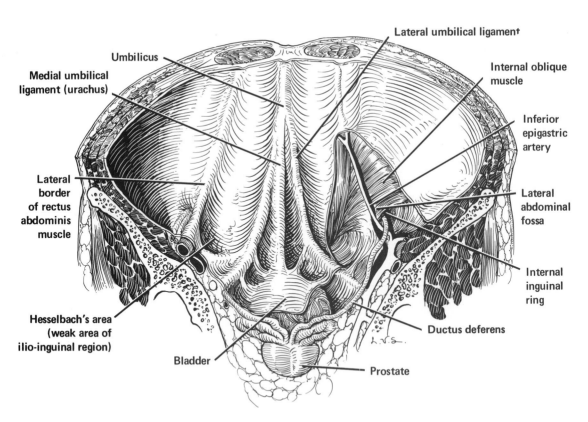

FIG 33–5. Dorsal surface of the peritoneum of the ventrolateral abdominal wall showing areas of egress of direct and indirect inguinal hernia.

stronger and more distinct of the two, being reinforced by fibers of the inguinal ligament. The ring provides egress to the spermatic cord and the ilio-inguinal nerve in the male and to the round ligament and ilio-inguinal nerve in the female. The ring is masked by a thin fascial covering—the external spermatic fascia—derived from the external oblique aponeurosis, which continues caudally along the spermatic cord or the round ligament.

The **inguinal ligament** forms the lateral inferior border of the aponeurosis of the external oblique, extending from the anterior-superior iliac spine to the pubic tubercle. It is formed as the lateral edge of the aponeurosis rolls upon itself and thickens into a cord. The ligament bows convexly downward toward the thigh. The lateral half of the ligament is thick and rounded, whereas the medial half is flattened where it is crossed by the spermatic cord. The lower end of the ligament is reflected dorsally and laterally from the pubic tubercle back along the iliopectineal line of the pubis as the **lacunar (Gimbernat's) ligament.** The lacunar ligament is about 1.25 cm long and triangular in shape, with the base directed laterally. The base is thin, concave, and sharp, and, along with the iliopubic tract of the transversalis fascia, forms the medial border of the femoral ring. The sharp, crescentic lateral border of this ligament is the unyielding noose for the strangulation of a femoral hernia.

Cooper's ligament is a strong fibrous band which extends laterally for about 2.5 cm along the iliopectineal line, starting at the lateral base of the lacunar ligament. It is used in the procedure known as Cooper's ligament repair of inguinal and femoral hernia.

B. Internal Oblique: The internal oblique muscle is thinner and smaller than the external oblique beneath which it lies. Its fibers run predominantly in a transverse direction. In the ilio-inguinal region, its fibers arise from the lateral half of the inguinal ligament, arching inferiorly and medially across the spermatic cord just below the level of the internal inguinal ring. These fibers then fuse with the lowermost arching fibers of the transverse muscle of the abdomen and insert with them into the pubic tubercle, forming the so-called conjoined tendon of the 2 muscles.

The **cremaster muscle** is a thin, attenuated muscle derived from the lowermost, superiorly arching fibers of the internal oblique, being formed by the processus vaginalis peritonei as it pushes ventrally and caudally through the internal inguinal ring. The muscle fibers with their intervening fascia become festooned along the lateral and ventral surfaces of the descending spermatic cord, forming a series of loops with their convexity facing caudally. They reach as far inferiorly as the testis and then return medially as the short arms of the loops to insert superiorly into the pubic tubercle. The cremaster muscle and fascia thus form one of the spermatic cord coverings and serve to pull the testis superiorly. This layer must be routinely identified and opened in order to properly identify an indirect inguinal hernia sac.

C. Transverse Abdominal: This muscle is the deepest and thinnest of the flat muscles of the ventrolateral abdominal wall, and, like the internal oblique, its fibers run transversely. Inferiorly, this muscle arises only from the lateral third of the inguinal ligament, well above the level of the internal inguinal ring. As a consequence, it plays little or no part in the anatomy of inguinal hernia and does not provide a covering layer to the spermatic cord. Its lowermost fibers help to form the conjoined tendon.

Transversalis Fascia

The transversalis fascia is a well-developed aponeurosis which in the ilio-inguinal region lies between the peritoneum and the deep surface of the transverse abdominal muscle superiorly, the peritoneum and the internal oblique more caudally, and, most inferiorly, the peritoneum and the aponeurosis of the external oblique. It is usually thickest and best developed over the ilio-inguinal region, and in this area has an opening in it, the **internal inguinal ring,** formed by the embryologic herniation of the processus vaginalis peritonei through the ventrolateral abdominal wall. The internal inguinal ring lies midway between the anterior-superior iliac spine and the pubic tubercle, halfway up the inguinal ligament and 1.25 cm medial to it. The ring is bounded superiorly by the arching fibers of the internal oblique muscle and below and medially by the inferior epigastric vessels. Along the medial half of the inguinal ligament the transversalis fascia passes deep to the ligament onto the medial, upper surface of the thigh. In so doing, it forms a triangular covering ventral to the femoral artery, the femoral vein, and the femoral canal. The long arm of this triangle of fascia lies laterally and is 4.5 cm long. The base of the triangle is at the inguinal ligament, while its hypotenuse runs from lateral to medial. Thus, the femoral artery is covered ventrally by the transversalis fascia for the greatest distance, whereas the femoral canal is covered for only a short distance down to the fossa ovalis. The femoral vessels, as they pass from the posterior abdomen beneath the inguinal ligament and onto the thigh along with the femoral canal, will lie on a plane deep to the transversalis fascia but superficial to the iliacus fascia. These 2 fascias fuse about the vessels forming a triangular fascial cone, the apex of which lies just deep to the fossa ovalis of the thigh.

The Peritoneum of the Ilio-inguinal Region

Over the medial third of the inguinal ligament the peritoneal envelope pulls away medially from the ligament by as much as 1.5 cm. This makes possible the use of an inguinal approach for the repair of a femoral hernia since with this approach one can draw the femoral hernia sac up from the thigh without opening the peritoneal cavity (Fig 33–5). On the deep surface of the peritoneum of the ventrolateral abdominal wall are 3 fibrous cords enfolded by peritoneum and running from the superior surface of the bladder to the umbilicus. These are of clinical interest as they serve to delineate the areas through which inguinal hernias will start their protrusion through the ventrolateral parietes. They are the medial umbilical ligament (the urachus) and the 2 lateral umbilical ligaments (the atrophied umbilical arteries). The presence of these ligaments divides the deep surface of the ventrolateral abdominal wall into 3 fossae on either side of the midline. The midline abdominal fossae lie between the medial and lateral ligaments and behind the thick rectus abdominis muscles and are of no clinical importance in inguinal or femoral hernias. The central abdominal fossae lie lateral to the lateral ligaments but medial and inferior to the inferior epigastric vessels and dorsal to Hesselbach's area. Since this is the weak area of the abdominal wall, all direct inguinal hernias leave the abdominal wall through it. The lateral abdominal fossae, lateral and superior to the inferior epigastric vessels, lie just deep to the internal inguinal ring and through them all indirect inguinal hernias will leave the abdominal cavity.

Descent of Testes (See Fig 33–6.)

During the third week of fetal life, the embryonic testis is found in the lumbar region of the posterior abdominal wall, dorsal to the posterior peritoneum and ventral to the lumbar lining fascia. Running to its superior pole are its nutrient vessels enclosed in a fold of peritoneum, the plica vascularis. During the fifth month of fetal life, the peritoneum of the ilio-inguinal region herniates out through the abdominal wall. In so doing, it forms the internal inguinal ring in the transversalis fascia, the inguinal canal, and the external inguinal ring in the external oblique aponeurosis as it passes down to the base of the scrotum. Thus, a pathway for the later descent of the testes is formed. By the sixth month of fetal life, the testes have dropped to a position approaching the preformed internal inguinal ring. Preceding the testis, attached to its lower pole, is a short cord—the gubernaculum—which persists after birth as the scrotal ligament, holding the testis loosely to the base of the scrotal sac. By the seventh fetal month, the testis has entered the internal inguinal ring; by the eighth month, it has traversed the inguinal canal and passed the external inguinal ring on its way to the scrotum. Once the testis has reached the scrotum, the ventral and dorsal walls of the processus vaginalis peritonei fuse to form the plica vaginalis. This persists distally as the tunica vaginalis testis and may persist proximally as a small peritoneal dimple just superior and deep to the internal inguinal ring. The presence of this dimple is probably responsible for the

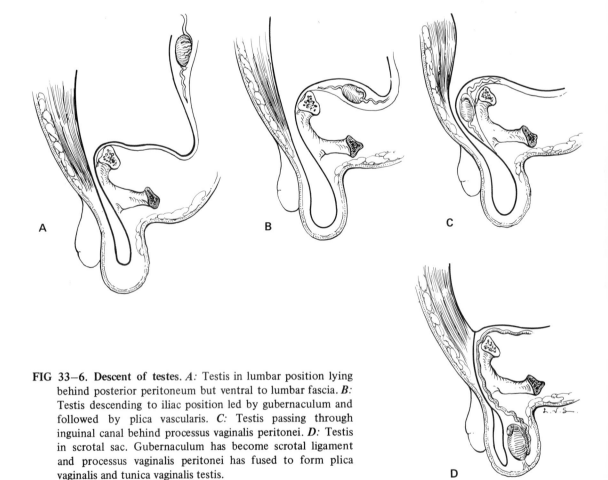

FIG 33–6. Descent of testes. *A:* Testis in lumbar position lying behind posterior peritoneum but ventral to lumbar fascia. *B:* Testis descending to iliac position led by gubernaculum and followed by plica vascularis. *C:* Testis passing through inguinal canal behind processus vaginalis peritonei. *D:* Testis in scrotal sac. Gubernaculum has become scrotal ligament and processus vaginalis peritonei has fused to form plica vaginalis and tunica vaginalis testis.

start of an acquired indirect inguinal hernia. Testicular descent and peritoneal sac fusion progress more slowly on the right side, thus accounting for the higher incidence of right-sided indirect inguinal hernias. If the distal portion of the processus vaginalis fails to fuse while the proximal portion fuses, the patient may develop hydrocele of the cord or of the testis.

The Inguinal Canal

The inguinal canal is the pathway through the ilio-inguinal area of the ventral abdominal wall formed by the passage of the processus vaginalis and the gubernaculum; the testis and spermatic cord pass through it from the abdomen to the scrotum. In both males and females, the canal also contains the ilio-inguinal nerve; in the female, it contains also the round ligament of the uterus passing to the labia majora. In running from the internal to the external inguinal ring, the canal pursues an oblique course—cephalad to caudad, lateral to medial, and dorsal to ventral. The most immediate ventral relationship of the canal is to the external oblique aponeurosis. Once this fascia is incised, the canal has been entered. Dorsally, the major relationship of the canal is to the transversalis fascia.

The Spermatic Cord (See Fig 33—7.)

The spermatic cord begins in the preperitoneal space at the level of the internal inguinal ring. This area serves as the gathering place where the structures of the cord join to pursue their course through the inguinal canal. When formed, the cord passes through the internal inguinal ring, down through the inguinal canal, out through the external inguinal ring, and down over the pubis and through the scrotal neck beyond which it is attached to the testis. The cord is composed of arteries, veins, lymphatics, nerves, fatty tissue, and the excretory duct of the testis. The coverings of the spermatic cord are as follows: (1) The internal spermatic fascia, derived from the transversalis fascia, covers the cord from the internal inguinal ring to the testis. (2) The cremasteric muscle and fascia form the middle layer of cord covering. The cremasteric muscle is derived from the lowermost arching fibers of the internal oblique muscle and is present from just beyond the internal inguinal ring to the testis. The outermost cord covering is the external spermatic fascia, derived from the external oblique aponeurosis and covering the cord only from the external inguinal ring to the testis.

ANATOMY OF THE FEMORAL TRIANGLE

Familiarity with the anatomic structures of the upper medial thigh as well as those in the ilio-inguinal region is necessary for an understanding of the diagnosis and treatment of femoral hernia. The femoral triangle is bounded superiorly by the inguinal ligament, laterally and inferiorly by the sartorius muscle, and medially by the pectineus and adductor magnus muscles. The superficial fascia of the upper thigh is continuous with Camper's fascia of the lower abdomen and consists of fatty areolar tissue. It covers the fossa ovalis, being perforated here by numerous blood and lymphatic vessels—hence the name fascia cribrosa.

Fascia Lata

Fascia lata, the lateral portion of the deep fascia of the thigh, covers the lateral and anterior two-thirds of the thigh. As this fascia swings medially in the upper thigh, it attaches superiorly to the iliac crest, to the anterior-superior iliac spine, to the entire length of the inguinal ligament, and to the body and crest of the pubis. In so doing it passes ventral to the femoral vessels and the femoral canal and lies on a more ventral plane than does the thinner fascia of the medial thigh. From the pubic tubercle, this thick fascia is reflected inferiorly and laterally as an arched margin, forming the lateral and superior borders of the fossa ovalis.

Medial Fascia

The thin medial fascia of the thigh covers the adductor group of the upper medial thigh muscles. It passes laterally, dorsal to the sheath of the femoral vessels, and forms the medial inferior border of the fossa ovalis. Since the thick lateral and superior fascia lata lies ventral to the femoral vessels and the thin medial and inferior fascia lies dorsal to them, there is an apparent aperture, the fossa ovalis, between the 2 fasciae, covered by the thin perforated fascia cribrosa. The aperture is about 2.5 cm caudal to the medial end of the inguinal ligament.

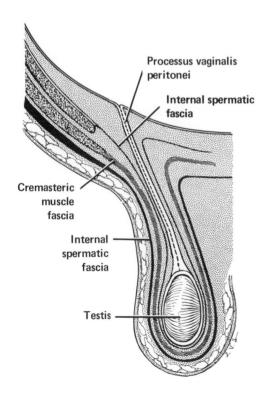

Processus vaginalis peritonei

Internal spermatic fascia

Cremasteric muscle fascia

Internal spermatic fascia

Testis

FIG 33—7. Anatomy of the scrotum and contents.

External Iliac & Femoral Arteries & Their Fascial Investments

As the external iliac artery and vein pass beneath the mid point of the inguinal ligament to become the femoral vessels, they carry with them a cone of the great lining fascia of the abdomen. This cone is formed ventrally by the transversalis fascia and dorsally by the iliacus fascia. The base of the cone lies just deep to the inguinal ligament. The fascial cone fuses with the vessel walls ventrally and dorsally, about 3 cm below the inguinal ligament and just dorsal to the superior margin of the fossa ovalis. Within this cone, 2 thin fascial septa run dorsally from the transversalis to the iliacus fascia. The lateral septum separates the femoral artery from the femoral vein; the medial one separates the femoral vein from the femoral canal. The lateral or arterial compartment is the longest; the most medial compartment, the femoral canal, lying just lateral to the lacunar ligament and the iliopubic tract of the transversalis fascia, is the shortest.

The Femoral Canal

The femoral canal lies just medial to the femoral vein on the ventral superior surface of the thigh, beginning at the level of the inguinal ligament and ending just dorsal to the superior border of the fossa ovalis. It is bounded ventrally by the transversalis fascia and dorsally by the iliacus fascia and terminates as a result of the fusion of these fasciae. It contains adipose tissue, lymphatics, and small nerves. The anulus femoralis, or the femoral ring, is the widest portion of the canal, lying just deep to the inguinal ligament. The canal faces superiorly and medially onto the abdominal cavity and laterally and inferiorly into the thigh. It is bounded ventrally by the inguinal ligament and the transversalis fascia, dorsally by the pectineus muscle and the iliacus fascia, laterally by the femoral vein, and medially by the free border of the lacunar ligament and by the iliopubic tract of the transversalis fascia.

Anson BJ, McVay CB: *Surgical Anatomy.* Saunders, 1971.

Condon RE: The anatomy of the inguinal region and its relationship to groin hernias. In: *Hernia.* Nyhus LM, Harkins H. Lippincott, 1964.

Lindner HH: *Outline of Surgical Anatomy.* Univ of California Press, 1966.

Lyttle WJ: The deep inguinal ring: Development, function and repair. Brit J Surg 57:531–536, 1970.

McVay CB: Inguinal and femoral hernioplasty. Surgery 57:615, 1965.

McVay CB: Inguinal hernioplasty: Common mistakes and pitfalls. S Clin North America 46:1089–1100, 1966.

McVay CB: The normal and pathologic anatomy of the transversus abdominis muscle in inguinal and femoral hernia. S Clin North America 51:1251–1261, 1971.

Shrock P: The processus vaginalis and gubernaculum: Their raison d'etre redefined. S Clin North America 51:1263–1268, 1971.

ETIOLOGY OF HERNIA

Indirect inguinal hernias occur in a congenitally present preformed sac, the processus vaginalis peritonei. The sac may exist simply as a small peritoneal dimple just proximal to the internal ring, or it may extend as a complete saccular structure to the base of the scrotum. Direct inguinal hernias are the result of a developed weakness of the transversalis fascia in Hesselbach's area. Femoral hernias arise due to extrusion of the adjacent peritoneal sac through the annulus femoralis, which frequently is abnormally dilated.

Factors which cause enlargement and subsequent advancement of a hernia sac are those which cause an increase in intra-abdominal pressure. Acute and chronic abdominal strain, as might be encountered in heavy exercise or lifting, is an important factor. A chronic cough or an acute coughing spell, chronic constipation with straining at stool, and prostatism with straining on micturition are important etiologic factors. Cirrhosis with an enlarged liver and ascites, pregnancy, and chronically enlarged pelvic organs may also cause hernia. Loss of tissue turgor in Hesselbach's area, associated with a weakening of the transversalis fascia, occurs with advancing age and in chronic debilitating disease. Marked obesity is another causative factor in the development of hernia.

FACTORS IN RECURRENCE AFTER OPERATIVE REPAIR

The following conditions predispose to recurrence in any hernia repair, but most particularly in repairs of the plastic type:

(1) Chronic cough which is aggravated by the surgical procedure. This may be due to prolonged recumbency, with pulmonary secretion pooling, or to the direct irritant effect of the anesthetic upon the air passages.

(2) Prostatism with straining on urination following surgery.

(3) Poor tissue turgor—in particular, poor transversalis fascia.

(4) Straining at stool in chronic constipation or with chronic painful hemorrhoids.

(5) Errors in operative technic: (a) Internal ring insufficiently tightened or cord insufficiently skeletonized. (b) Failure to appreciate sliding hernia. (c) Cooper's ligament or other plastic repair without benefit of a relaxing incision. (d) Failure to demonstrate presence of a second hernia. (e) Incomplete sac closure. (f) Dissolution of absorbable suture material.

(6) Postoperative wound infection with or without wound dehiscence.

The recurrence rate in hernioplasty can be diminished by meticulous attention to the prevention of and care and treatment of the conditions mentioned above. The operative treatment of recurrent inguinal hernia is always more difficult technically than the initial repair of a hernia and carries with it a higher percentage of recurrence (10–20%). The patient whose indirect inguinal hernia is properly repaired can, under ideal conditions, expect a cure in 95% of cases.

Marsden AJ: The results of inguinal hernia repairs: A problem of assessment. Lancet 1:461–462, 1959.

Myers RN, Shearborn EW: The problem of the recurrent inguinal hernia. S Clin North America 53:555–558, 1973.

Shuttleworth KE, Davies WH: Treatment of inguinal hernia. Lancet 1:126–127, 1960.

Zimmerman LM: Recurrent inguinal hernia. S Clin North America 51:1317–1324, 1971.

ANATOMIC MAKEUP OF HERNIA

A hernia usually consists of a sac, contents within the sac, and the sac coverings. The sac is a diverticulum of peritoneum of variable size which may or may not be occupied. The sac contents are most commonly omentum, small or large intestine (appendix), bladder, and ovary and tube. The hernia coverings will consist of those layers of the abdominal wall through which the hernia has passed.

Classification of Groin Hernia

A. Reducible: A hernia which reduces when the patient is recumbent or which can be manually returned to the abdomen by either the patient or the attending physician.

B. Irreducible or Incarcerated: A hernia which cannot be returned to the abdomen. It usually cannot be reduced either because there are adhesions between the sac and its contents or because the sac is tightly crowded with contents.

C. Obstructed: An irreducible or incarcerated hernia which contains bowel whose lumen is obstructed either by feces from within or pressure from without the sac walls. There is no interference with blood supply to the bowel at first, but this usually occurs if the incarceration persists.

D. Strangulated: Strangulation takes place in a hernia when the blood supply to the contents of the sac is compromised. Gangrene of the sac contents then occurs. This is a much more common happening in femoral than in inguinal hernia.

E. Richter's Hernia: Richter's hernia is present when only a segment of the circumference of the bowel wall becomes obstructed somewhere along the course of the hernia. It is a fairly common occurrence in both inguinal and femoral hernias but more common in femoral hernia. It can have serious implications in a hernia that is self-reducing following a Richter type of strangulation. Unless suspected, it may be overlooked at surgery and the compromised portion of

bowel may become gangrenous, rupture, and lead to peritonitis. The history of colicky abdominal pain and nausea or vomiting associated with the self-reducing hernia plus the presence of bloody fluid in the hernia sac should always call for complete abdominal exploration. Richter's hernias are reported to comprise about 0.65% of all groin hernias, about 0.7% of all femoral hernias, and about 14% of all strangulated femoral hernias.

Suture Material

Nonabsorbable material gives a definitely lower percentage of hernia recurrence when used routinely. Silk, cotton, stainless steel wire, and proline (synthetic) are the most commonly used nonabsorbable suture materials.

Bilateral Repair

In adults, bilateral hernia repair should not be performed as one procedure since it has been shown that the recurrence rate and the surgical morbidity are definitely raised if the bilateral procedure is carried out.

In children, bilateral hernia repair is the procedure of choice. Here the 2 procedures can be done under the one anesthesia, as the operating time for the simple high ligation of the hernial sac is short and the infant is spared a second anesthetic and the possibility of strangulation of the hernia on the unoperated side before it can be surgically repaired.

1. INDIRECT INGUINAL HERNIA
(See Fig 33–8.)

An indirect inguinal hernia is one which leaves the abdominal cavity via the lateral peritoneal fossa. It occurs as a consequence of the failure of proper fusion of the processus vaginalis peritonei. It enters the abdominal wall through the internal inguinal ring in the transversalis fascia and descends inferiorly, ventrally, and medially along the course of the inguinal canal in the direction of the external inguinal ring and the scrotal sac. Thus, an indirect inguinal hernia is a hernia into the spermatic cord. Its degree of completeness depends upon its distal extension relative to the position of the external inguinal ring. If it presents above the level of the ring, it is incomplete; but once it reaches or passes this ring, it becomes a complete hernia. If it reaches the scrotal sac, it is called a scrotal hernia.

Clinical Findings

A. Symptoms: If the hernia is small, there may be no symptoms. The patient will occasionally complain of a heavy dragging sensation in the groin with pain that will radiate to the ipsilateral testicle, usually in association with heavy exercise, straining, or coughing

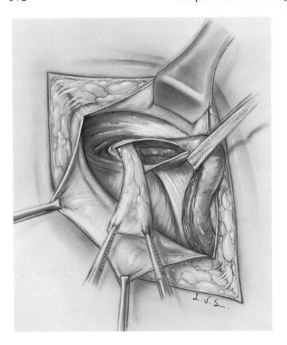

FIG 33–8. Indirect inguinal hernia. Inguinal canal opened showing spermatic cord retracted medially and indirect hernia peritoneal sac dissected free to above the level of the internal inguinal ring.

The patient may relate the first appearance of the hernial bulge to a sharp pain in the groin, or the onset of local tenderness associated with a sudden straining movement. Large indirect hernias are usually asymptomatic except for a feeling of groin or scrotal heaviness.

B. Signs: The clinical diagnosis of indirect inguinal hernia is usually not difficult. It depends upon determining whether or not a peritoneal sac exists along the course of the spermatic cord. The peritoneal sac and its contents may be visible and palpable as a protrusion in the groin, either within the inguinal canal, at the external inguinal ring, over the pubis, or within the scrotal sac. The diagnosis is particularly easy if the mass has progressed beyond the external inguinal ring to lie over the pubis or in the scrotum. A direct inguinal hernia seldom passes the level of the external inguinal ring. If the hernial bulge is not present but an indirect hernia is suspected, the patient should be examined in the standing position. The uninvolved side should be examined first so that the examiner may put the patient at ease and also observe the normal structures. The examining finger should then be inserted into the scrotal sac below its junction with the abdominal wall and carried superiorly over the pubis up to the external inguinal ring (Fig 33–9). The ring should be checked for size and the presence of abnormal tenderness. The finger is then inserted into the ring and gently up the inguinal canal and the patient is instructed to cough or strain. An impulse against the finger, traveling in the direction of the course of the canal, strongly suggests indirect inguinal hernia. An

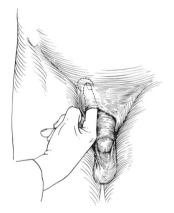

FIG 33–9. Insertion of finger through upper scrotum into external inguinal ring.

impulse which strikes the finger from a dorsal direction, accompanied by palpation of a depression in the dorsal wall of the canal, suggests the presence of a weak transversalis fascia and a direct inguinal hernia. It should be noted that a large external ring may be present without the presence of an indirect inguinal hernia. Indirect and direct inguinal hernias frequently coexist, and the examiner will on such occasions find a mass coming down the inguinal canal plus one that bulges forward into the inguinal canal. When these 2 masses coexist they are difficult to distinguish, and the proper diagnosis is usually made at surgery.

The **thumb test,** in which the thumb covers the internal inguinal ring when the patient strains, will help to differentiate between indirect and direct hernia. The direct hernia bulges forward in Hesselbach's area while the thumb is covering the exit of the indirect hernia from the abdominal wall. The hernial bulge in children and in patients who have worn trusses for a long time may be difficult to elucidate and evaluate and may require repeated examinations so that the proper diagnosis may be made. The so-called silk purse sign— increased thickness of the inguinal ligament giving a sensation like silk sliding beneath the examining finger —may help in the examination of infants and children who do not have a groin bulge.

Differential Diagnosis

It may be extremely difficult to distinguish indirect inguinal hernia from direct inguinal hernia, particularly when a direct hernia changes direction and slides down dorsal to the posterior wall of the inguinal canal (transversalis fascia). A direct inguinal hernia seldom passes the level of the external ring; thus, it is almost never a scrotal hernia.

Lipoma of the spermatic cord frequently simulates an indirect hernial sac and at times can only be differentiated at inguinal exploration.

An indirect inguinal hernia protruding at the level of the external ring may be confused with a femoral hernia. Femoral hernia usually protrudes at a point caudal to the line of the inguinal ligament. On occasion, however, after a femoral hernia has protruded through the transversalis fascia at the level of the fossa ovalis in the thigh, it may come to lie superior to the inguinal ligament.

Indirect inguinal hernia must also be differentiated from hematomas in the inguinal region, varices of the lower abdominal or upper thigh veins, abscesses in the groin secondary to breakdown of groin lymph nodes, tuberculous abscesses secondary to tuberculosis of the thoracolumbar spine which transverse down the course of the psoas major muscle, and from hydrocele of the spermatic cord. Undescended testis in the inguinal canal must also be considered.

Complications

The 2 most common complications of indirect inguinal hernia are incarceration and strangulation. When an inguinal hernia becomes incarcerated and painful, emergency surgery is usually indicated. However, in selected patients of any age who are considered especially poor operative risks for emergency surgery because of serious concomitant disease—manual reduction of the incarceration by the physician improves survival. The repair is then done electively after the patient has been properly prepared. In most cases, one can differentiate between incarceration with viable bowel and strangulation with gangrenous bowel. Treatment consists of a combination of rest, moist heat, opiates, and, sometimes, anesthesia to induce reduction. However, the risks of reducing gangrenous tissue into the abdomen by manual or self-reduction of a Richter's hernia make early exploration of the incarcerated hernia mandatory in the majority of patients.

A strangulated hernia is an incarcerated hernia in which the blood supply to the sac contents has been compromised. The clinical manifestations are localized tenderness, erythema of the overlying skin, and increase in the size of the hernia. If bowel is in the hernial sac, the symptoms of intestinal obstruction are usually present, ie, vomiting, colicky pain, and abdominal distention. An anteroposterior x-ray of the abdomen may show evidence of bowel distention with the typical stepladder pattern of the small bowel.

When the diagnosis of strangulation is made or strongly suspected, immediate surgery is called for. Patients with incarceration should be watched carefully for signs of strangulation, and the decision to operate or not must lean strongly in the direction of surgery if there is any suspicion of strangulation.

At surgery it may be found that an incarcerated hernia has reduced spontaneously, particularly under the influence of a combination of rest, moist heat, opiates, and anesthesia. The surgeon must then decide whether or not to explore the abdomen for a compromised area of bowel. The presence of bloody fluid in the hernial sac is an absolute indication for abdominal exploration. The clinical diagnosis of strangulation is based on judgment guided by the general condition of the patient, abdominal signs of peritonitis, and the elevated white blood count. Except in the preperitoneal

repair of inguinal hernia, where a fairly good abdominal exploration may be carried out via the operative approach, it is better to explore the abdomen for compromised bowel through a separate midline or rectus incision so that the abdominal contents can be properly examined and evaluated.

Treatment

All indirect inguinal hernias should be repaired as soon as feasible since a hernia always increases in extent. In addition, repair of a hernia prevents the complications of incarceration, obstruction, and strangulation, relieves groin pain and discomfort, and corrects such concomitant symptoms as constipation.

A. Major Principles of Treatment: The major principles in the repair of indirect inguinal hernia are as follows:

1. Location of the indirect hernial sac.

2. Immaculate dissection of the sac to above the level of the internal inguinal ring, with freeing of the many adjacent structures which may have become attached to the sac of the hernia.

3. Traction upon the peritoneal sac so that it may be ligated or transfixed well above the level of the internal inguinal ring.

4. Tightening of the internal ring by the use of sutures in the adjacent transversalis fascia so that the ring will not be left enlarged and predisposed to a secondary descent of an indirect hernia or the emergence of a direct hernia.

B. Types of Operation: See Surgical Repair of Inguinal Hernia, below.

C. Nonsurgical Management (Trussing): The use of a truss is recommended only when there is an extreme contraindication to operative repair. A truss holds a small inguinal hernia fairly well if the hernia is reducible. It should be affixed in the morning, before the patient arises, while the hernia is reduced. If a truss is not applied properly, it can increase the risk of strangulation. In addition, pressure of the truss upon the anatomic structures in the ilio-inguinal region tends to obliterate their identity, making later repair more difficult. Therefore, every means possible should be taken to prepare the patient for surgery so that the use of a truss will not be necessary.

Prognosis

See p 575.

Brandon WJ: Inguinal hernia: The sling operation. Brit J Surg 56:408–413, 1969.

Condon RE, Nyhus LM: Complications of groin hernia and of hernial repair. S Clin North America 51:1325–1336, 1971.

Griffith CA: The Marcy repair of indirect inguinal hernia. S Clin North America 51:1309–1316, 1971.

Kauffman HM Jr, O'Brien DP: Selective reduction of incarcerated inguinal hernia. Am J Surg 119:660–673, 1970.

Madden JL, Hakim S, Agorogiannis AB: The anatomy and repair of inguinal hernias. S Clin North America 51:1269–1292, 1971.

McVay CB: The anatomy of the relaxing incision in inguinal hernioplasty. Quart Bull Northwestern Univ M School 36:245, 1962.

McVay CB: Inguinal hernioplasty: Common mistakes and pitfalls. S Clin North America 46:1089–1100, 1966.

Palumbo LT, Sharpe WS: Primary inguinal hernioplasty in the adult. S Clin North America 51:1293–1308, 1971.

Smith RS: The use of prosthetic materials in the repair of hernias. S Clin North America 51:1387–1399, 1971.

2. DIRECT INGUINAL HERNIA
(See Fig 33–10.)

Direct inguinal hernia pushes out ventrally through Hesselbach's area, generally protruding more ventrally than inferiorly. It leaves the abdomen through the central abdominal fossa lateral to the lateral border of the rectus muscle and inferior and medial to the inferior epigastric vessels. Direct hernia is nearly always acquired, since congenital defects of the tissue of Hesselbach's area are rare. Direct inguinal hernia is due to a developed weakness in the fascia of the floor of the inguinal canal (transversalis fascia). It becomes more common with advancing age and is very infrequent in women, children, and young adults. It may follow repair of an indirect inguinal hernia or an appendectomy in which a McBurney type of incision has injured the ilio-inguinal nerve. It frequently occurs in people who have chronic long-standing wasting diseases. Predisposing factors include chronic cough, straining at stool, or heavy manual labor. It rarely is a sliding type of hernia. The bladder is an occasional occupant of its sac, particularly in men with benign prostatic hypertrophy. Direct hernia strangulates much less frequently than indirect inguinal hernia.

Clinical Findings

A. Symptoms: Most direct inguinal hernias are relatively symptomless. There may be a feeling of heaviness in the groin and a tendency toward constipation. Pain is usually present only if the hernia strangulates.

B. Signs: Direct hernia presents as a bulge in the ilio-inguinal region. It usually does not descend into the scrotum and is rarely as large as the larger of the indirect inguinal hernias. It is often difficult to distinguish clinically from an indirect hernia. The same items in differential diagnosis must be considered as for an indirect hernia. Direct hernia lies dorsal to the spermatic cord. A finger introduced into the external inguinal ring can usually be pushed dorsally toward the abdominal cavity through the weakened transversalis fascia.

Differential Diagnosis

See discussion in preceding section.

Complications

Direct inguinal hernia does not strangulate or incarcerate as often as does an indirect hernia. Occasionally, however, a direct hernia will break through the thinned-out transversalis fascia forming the floor of the inguinal canal and will be strangulated when the encircling fibers of this fascia surround its neck. A direct hernia which initially protrudes ventrally may change direction and slide caudally dorsal to the inguinal canal and the transversalis fascia. This type of hernia may strangulate dorsal to the external inguinal ring.

Treatment

Small asymptomatic direct inguinal hernias are often best left alone. Pain or progressive enlargement is an indication for operation.

Direct inguinal hernia repair presents a more complicated problem of surgical repair than indirect inguinal hernia. In direct inguinal hernia, dissection and obliteration of the sac are of less importance than the strengthening of the weakened transversalis fascia. The sac is most often not opened but is usually depressed dorsally to a position deep to the transversalis fascial repair.

In general, the major tissue used in repair of direct inguinal hernia is transversalis fascia, which can usually be found in plentiful supply deep to the rectus abdominis muscle. The anterior sheath of the rectus abdominis should be made the site of a relaxing incision to allow this transversalis fascia to be drawn laterally without undue tension.

The relaxing incision is of great value in mobilizing the inferior and lateral margins of the rectus sheath together with the accompanying fused portions of the internal oblique and transversalis abdominis muscles or their medial fascial sheaths. The incision in the rectus sheath is made in a vertical direction as close as possible to the reflexion of the aponeurosis of the external oblique and extends upward from the pubic crest for about 6–7 cm. The firm, fibrous lateral edge of the rectus muscle and sheath, along with the underlying transversalis fascia, can then be easily approximated to Poupart's or Cooper's ligament without tension.

Direct hernia is frequently accompanied by a small, asymptomatic indirect hernia. The spermatic cord must be carefully searched for this finding to prevent the development of an indirect hernia recurrence following direct hernia repair.

Surgical Repair of Inguinal Hernia

There are 4 major categories of direct hernia repair:

A. Bassini Repair: Via the usual inguinal approach, the inguinal canal is opened and a search for an indirect hernia is carried out with opening of the layers of the spermatic cord. If found, the indirect hernia is dealt with by immaculate dissection of the peritoneal sac and its high transfixion. The cord coverings are then closed and good transversalis fascia is sought beneath the lateral borders of the rectus

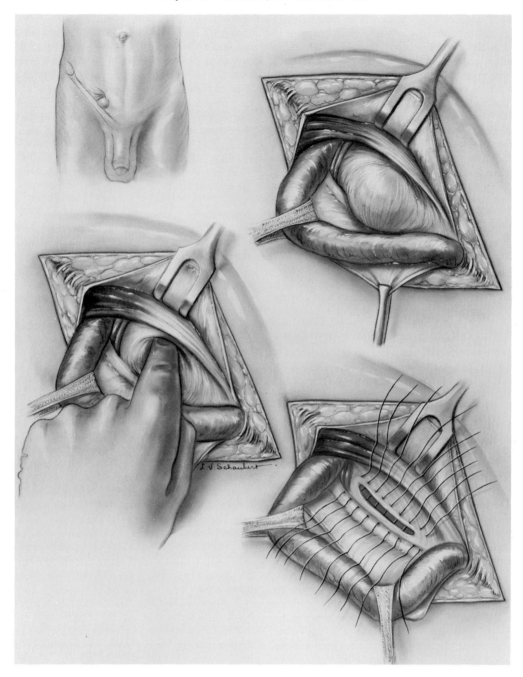

FIG 33–10. Direct inguinal hernia. *Upper left:* Location of hernia above inguinal ligament. *Upper right:* Bulging direct hernia covered with transversalis fascia and just below external oblique aponeurosis. *Lower left:* Direct hernia depressed. *Lower right:* Closure in direct hernia repair, suturing sound transversalis fascia medially to iliopubic band and to shelving edge of inguinal ligament laterally.

abdominis and conjoined tendon. Good transversalis fascia having been found, a relieving incision is made in the rectus abdominis fascia and the transversalis fascia is then sutured to the iliopubic tract of transversalis fascia and to the shelving edge of the inguinal ligament. No weakness should be allowed in this area so that direct hernia will not recur. In addition, care must be taken to place the highest sutures in such a way as to tighten the internal inguinal ring. The plastic closure is deep to the spermatic cord. The external oblique aponeurosis is then closed ventral to the spermatic cord. Care must also be taken not to superimpose the new external inguinal ring directly ventral to the tightened internal ring.

B. Classic Halsted Repair: The Halsted repair differs from the Bassini repair only in that the external oblique aponeurosis is sutured together deep to the spermatic cord, thus perhaps increasing the strength of the transversalis plastic closure and at the same time serving to place the spermatic cord in a subcutaneous position. In a patient with only a thin layer of adipose tissue, this tends to make the spermatic cord more vulnerable to external trauma.

C. Cooper's Ligament (McVay) Repair: In this procedure, good medial transversalis fascia is sutured to Cooper's ligament on the iliopectineal line of the pubis. The suturing begins just lateral to the medial inferior edge of the lacunar ligament and extends laterally to the medial border of the femoral vein. This portion of the procedure effectively repairs the lower portion of Hesselbach's area and at the same time closes the femoral ring. At the medial border of the femoral vein, a transition suture is then carried out, the transversalis fascia being sutured to the iliopubic band of transversalis fascia and to the inguinal ligament ventral to the femoral vein and artery; this suture is then continued laterally to the inferior margin of the internal inguinal ring, thus strengthening the lateral portion of Hesselbach's area. Many surgeons feel that this is the best means of strengthening the weak area of the ventrolateral abdominal wall.

D. Preperitoneal Repair: (Also called properitoneal repair, extraperitoneal repair, and posterior approach repair.) The anatomic structure known as the iliopubic transversalis fascial tract is a strong fascial band which begins laterally along the iliac crest and the anterior-superior iliac spine. It arches over the psoas muscle and the femoral vessels, where it forms a portion of the anterior femoral sheath. In its midportion it lies directly beneath the inguinal ligament but is completely separate from it. More medially, it inserts fanwise into the superior pubic ramus and into Cooper's ligament. In so doing, these fibers form the medial border of the femoral canal. Direct and indirect hernia defects are limited on their dorsal aspects by the fibers of the iliopubic tract. In both direct inguinal and recurrent direct inguinal hernia, the preperitoneal approach uses the usually untouched iliopubic tract for its repair. In addition, with this approach, sliding hernias are easily recognized and the restraining band of strangulated and incarcerated hernias can be cut easily

under direct vision. The preperitoneal space is opened through a transverse lower abdominal incision about 4 cm above the inguinal ligament. The rectus sheath is incised at its lateral border and the muscle is retracted medially so that the preperitoneal space is visualized. The transversalis fascia is incised transversely, taking care to stay out of the peritoneal cavity. This exposes the posterior wall of the inguinal canal and the area of herniation. Direct, indirect, and femoral hernia sacs can be easily visualized and reduced by traction via this exposure. Hernial defects may be closed by suture of good medial transversalis fascia to the iliopubic tract of the transversalis fascia.

Postoperative Course Following Hernia Repair

The usual hospital stay ranges from 3–7 days, and the patient who is a healthy adult is usually off work for 4–6 weeks following surgery. During the first 2 postsurgical weeks, the patient must refrain from exercise, keep his bowels open, and generally refrain from increasing his intra-abdominal pressure by coughing or straining. For the following 4 weeks, the patient gradually increases the degree of exercise, and by the sixth to eighth week should be able to perform any physical task appropriate for his age and premorbid capacity. At the end of 2 months, the ilio-inguinal region should be as strong as it will ever be.

Prognosis

A. Indirect Inguinal Hernia: The recurrence rate in adults following surgical repair of indirect inguinal hernia should be less than 2% in the hands of experienced surgeons, although some reports unfortunately describe rates as high as 10–15%. In infants and children, there should be almost no recurrences if the operation is performed properly.

The major reasons for recurrence as an indirect inguinal hernia are (1) faulty dissection of the hernial sac, (2) failure of high ligation of the hernial sac, (3) failure to tighten the internal inguinal ring about the issuing spermatic cord, and (4) failure to find the indirect sac.

If an indirect inguinal hernia recurs as a direct hernia or a femoral hernia, the recurrence is probably due to failure to recognize either of these concomitant diagnoses at the time of repair of the indirect inguinal hernia repair.

B. Direct Inguinal Hernia: There is an unusually high percentage of hernia recurrence with preperitoneal repair—in some centers, as high as 30%. This would seem to indicate the superiority of the time-tested Bassini and McVay types of repair for the treatment of direct inguinal hernia.

Repair of direct inguinal hernia carries a higher recurrence rate than does repair for indirect inguinal hernia. The rate runs from 7–10% and rates as high as 15–20% have been reported. Those factors noted above as predisposing causes of recurrence are of even more importance in direct inguinal hernia than in indirect inguinal hernia, and negligence in attention to them tends to increase the recurrence rate.

A

B

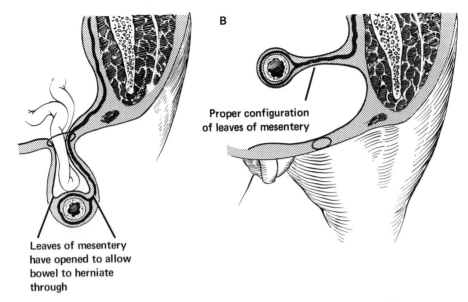

Proper configuration
of leaves of mesentery

Leaves of mesentery
have opened to allow
bowel to herniate
through

FIG 33–11. **Left-sided sliding hernia.** (After Lindner in Thorek.)

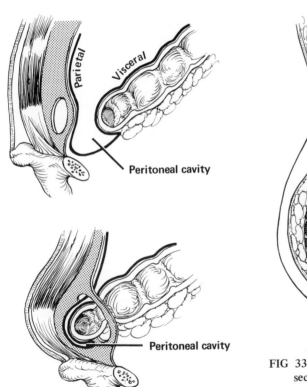

FIG 33–12. **Right-sided sliding hernia.** *Top:* Note cecum and ascending colon sliding on fascia of posterior abdominal wall. *Bottom:* Hernia has entered internal inguinal ring. Note that one-fourth of the hernia is not related to the peritoneal sac.

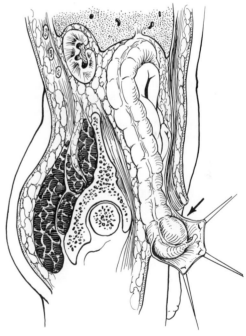

FIG 33–13. **Right-sided sliding hernia seen in sagittal section.** (After Lindner in Thorek.) At arrow, the wall of the cecum forms a portion of the hernia sac.

Not only does direct inguinal hernia have a higher recurrence rate than indirect hernia, but the recurrence rate rises with each successive attempt at repair. In second operations for direct inguinal hernia, the recurrence rate is 20—25%. Occasionally, when direct hernia recurs more than once, it becomes apparent that the transversalis fascia and the iliopubic fascial tract are of poor quality. Then and only then, one may use a foreign material to close the weakness in Hesselbach's area. Many materials may be used, either from the patient's own body (fascia lata) or of synthetic origin. Flaps from the anterior rectus sheath or from the adjacent fascia lata of the thigh brought up under the inguinal ligament have been used. More recently, relatively inert foreign material such as stainless steel, Tantalum mesh gauze, Vinyon mesh, or Marlex mesh have been used. Reported experience would indicate that Marlex mesh is the best of these materials. Prosthetic devices are contraindicated in inguinal hernia repair except when the transversalis fascia is of such poor quality or has been so attenuated by repeated inguinal surgery that it can no longer be used profitably. Foreign body reinforcement should seldom, if ever, be used in the first attempt at direct hernia repair. In cases where direct hernias have recurred one or more times and the patient is in the older age group (70 years and above), the spermatic cord may be resected in order to more effectively close Hesselbach's area.

Nyhus LM, Condon RE, Harkins HN: Clinical experiences with preperitoneal hernial repair for all types of hernia, with particular reference to the importance of transversalis fascia. Analogues. Am J Surg 100:239, 1960.
See also references under Direct Inguinal Hernia, above.

SLIDING INGUINAL HERNIA
(See Figs 33—11 to 33—13.)

This interesting and diagnostically difficult hernia comprises about 2% of all inguinal hernias. The great majority are indirect, although an occasional direct sliding hernia, with bladder as the sliding component, is encountered. A sliding hernia is one in which the wall of a viscus forms a portion of the wall of the hernia sac. The portion of the sac wall formed by the viscus may vary from as little as 2% up to 60%. On the right side, cecum or cecum and lower ascending colon form a portion of the sac wall; on the left side, sigmoid colon may form a portion of the sac wall.

Sliding hernia is much more common in males than in females and more frequent on the left side than on the right.

The development of such a hernia is intimately related to the degree of posterior fixation of the large bowel or other sliding component and its proximity to the internal inguinal ring. Thus, a partially fixed cecum which has descended too low during the third stage of gut rotation can enter the internal inguinal ring to become a sliding hernia. A nonfixed cecum in low pelvic position may enter the internal inguinal ring but would not become a sliding hernia as a portion of its wall does not form a part of the hernia sac. In addition, as a result of physiologic aging or long-standing chronic debilitating disease, the cecum and ascending colon, if partially fixed posteriorly, may slide on the tissues of the posterior abdominal wall down to the level of the internal inguinal ring and enter as a sliding hernia. On the left side of the abdomen, low position and inadequate fixation of the lower descending colon and the proximal sigmoid permit these colonic segments to slide down to and into the left internal inguinal ring, forming a sliding hernia. The ovaries and a portion of the fallopian tube can be present in sliding hernias in females. The appendix is frequently present in the right-sided sliding hernia since the cecum is its major component.

Strangulation and obstruction are no more common with sliding hernias than with other large inguinal hernias. There are no special objective signs that will distinguish sliding hernia from other inguinal hernias.

The sliding hernia may be more often only partially reducible than the usual indirect inguinal hernia.

There are no symptoms which will tend to distinguish sliding hernia from other large indirect inguinal hernias. Groin fullness, chronic constipation, and a dull groin ache may all be present in sliding hernia.

The diagnosis of sliding hernia is almost always made at surgery. The possibility should always be considered in large hernias which have suddenly appeared in the scrotal sac of an elderly man. Barium enema may be of some help in differential diagnosis. The presence of an appreciably large segment of colon in a scrotal sac is very suggestive of sliding hernia, and one must strongly suspect the diagnosis when operating on such a case. Difficulty in freeing up a large indirect hernia sac should always alert the surgeon to the possibility of a sliding hernia.

Treatment
Treatment of sliding inguinal hernia varies depending upon whether it occurs on the left or right side. The most important factor in treatment is recognition of the entity as one proceeds into the inguinal canal and opens the cremasteric fascia over the spermatic cord. As is true of all inguinal hernias, the sac will lie anteriorly, but the posterior wall of the sac will be formed to a greater or lesser degree by colon. Recognition of this is of great importance so that the surgeon will not inadvertently open the bowel when dealing with the hernia sac.

A. Small Right-Sided Sliding Hernias: The small sliding hernia is approached through the usual oblique inguinal approach. The inguinal canal is opened longitudinally and the cord coverings are dissected free from the hernia sac. The Bevan technic, which calls for a peritoneal incision on either side of the mesenteric attachment to the bowel, is then carried out. There is then a longitudinal suturing of the fusiform defect left by the peritoneal incisions. This preserves the blood supply to the bowel and allows for creation of a new mesentery, which then allows for high sac ligation. This also prevents en bloc reduction of the sliding hernia, which always predisposes to recurrence.

B. Larger Right-Sided Sliding Hernias: In large right-sided sliding hernias, the problem is to ligate the sac without bowel strangulation and with preservation of the blood supply to the bowel in order to prevent bowel necrosis. A combined abdominal-inguinal approach of the LaRoque type is carried out. In this procedure, when a large sliding hernia is discovered through the inguinal incision, a transverse muscle-splitting incision about 5 cm above the inguinal incision is made. The peritoneal cavity is entered through the transverse incision, and the sliding bowel is gently pulled back up into the abdomen to be fixed there to the posterior abdominal wall. The inguinal hernia sac is then closed at a high level and a Bassini or McVay type of hernia repair is performed, care being taken to markedly decrease the size of the internal inguinal ring to prevent the possibility of recurrence.

C. Left-Sided Sigmoid or Descending Colon Sliding Hernia: The posterior parietal peritoneum, lateral to the sigmoid wall, passes through the internal inguinal ring, resulting in an unfolding of the leaves of the mesosigmoid. If the peritoneal sac is opened anteriorly, the sigmoid is found to occupy the apex of the sac. The sigmoid should be drawn back into the peritoneal cavity through a transverse entering incision of the LaRoque type, and the leaves of the opened mesentery are then reapproximated. The sac should then be dissected high and free and transfixed. The internal ring is then tightened and Hesselbach's area strengthened with a transversalis fascia repair of the Bassini or Cooper's ligament type.

Prognosis

Sliding hernias have a high recurrence rate (15–20%). The rate appears to be higher (17–25%) when the inguinal repair route alone is used for the larger sliding hernias. With the combined abdominoinguinal route, the recurrence rate is 5–7% lower and there is a lower surgical morbidity rate.

The surgical complications most often encountered following sliding hernia repair are reflex acute dilatation of the stomach, small bowel paresis, encroachment on the circulation to the large bowel with bowel necrosis, and actual strangulation of a portion of the large bowel when attempting a high ligation of the hernia sac.

Maingot R: Operations for sliding herniae and for large incisional herniae. Brit J Clin Pract 15:993, 1961.

Ryan EA: An analysis of 313 consecutive cases of indirect sliding inguinal hernias. Surg Gynec Obst 102:45, 1956.

Williams C: Repair of sliding inguinal hernia through the abdominal (LaRoque) approach. Ann Surg 126:612, 1947.

FEMORAL HERNIA
(See Fig 33–14.)

Femoral hernia comprises about 4–6% of all groin hernias. It is an acquired hernia which is more common in women than in men. However, inguinal hernia is more common in women than femoral hernia. Women are probably more prone to develop femoral hernia because of (1) the usually wider flare of their iliac crests, resulting in a longer inguinal ligament and a wider femoral ring; (2) the increased intra-abdominal pressures which accompany pregnancy and pelvic tumors; and (3) the softening of the inguinal and pubic ligaments which occurs just prior to parturition.

Any elevation of the intra-abdominal pressure is transmitted to the femoral ring; if it is susceptible, dilatation may result from an advancing wedge of preperitoneal fat.

A femoral hernia descends inferiorly and slightly laterally through the femoral canal, to a point just deep to the superior border of the fossa ovalis, where the transversalis fascia blends with the iliacus fascia to close the femoral canal (Fig 33–14). The hernia is nearly always preceded by a greater or lesser amount of preperitoneal fat. This fat often makes a femoral hernia seem to have a larger sac and contents than it actually possesses. After the femoral hernia reaches the end of the femoral canal, it may progress to break through the transversalis fascia ventrally and pass into and through the fossa ovalis to lie in a subcutaneous position just below the medial portion of the inguinal ligament. Further movement of the hernia is usually influenced by the overhang of the sharp crescentic superior border of the fossa ovalis, which forces the hernia superiorly and laterally so that it may end up ventral to or just superior to the inguinal ligament. Thus the hernia in its full descent describes a J course. Hence, reduction by taxis is a complicated, difficult, and seldom used method of treatment.

The most common occupant of the femoral hernia sac is omentum, which is frequently incarcerated within the sac. Loops of small bowel or a portion of the urinary bladder are the next most common occupants of a femoral hernia sac.

Clinical Findings

A femoral hernia may present in a variety of ways. If it is small and uncomplicated, it usually appears as a transient, easily reducible, small bulge in the upper medial thigh just below the level of the inguinal ligament. As the hernia progresses, it enlarges and descends. In obese patients, the fat pad preceding it often becomes painful as a result of chronic irritation. If a femoral hernia incarcerates or strangulates, it is always swollen and irreducible. When femoral hernia or its preceding preperitoneal fat has completed its J course, the terminal end of the hernia will often be found lying on the abdomen just above the middle third of the inguinal ligament. When the herniated small bowel passes through a small femoral ring or through a tight hole in the transversalis fascia, it frequently strangulates in Richter fashion.

Differential Diagnosis

Femoral hernia must be distinguished from the same entities as inguinal hernia—particularly those that occur in the upper mid thigh such as a saphenous varix and femoral lymphadenopathy. Not infrequently, the diagnosis of femoral hernia will be made after an exploration for inguinal hernia. To make a certain diagnosis of femoral hernia, the transversalis fascia must be opened and the femoral ring explored. A femoral hernia that appears after an inguinal hernia repair is nearly always one that was missed at the time of the inguinal hernia procedure. The surgeon's finger placed through the internal inguinal ring via an opened indirect hernia sac will often be able to palpate the advancing femoral hernia.

Complications

The most common complications of femoral hernia are incarceration and strangulation. Fixation of either the femoral hernia sac or its preceding preperitoneal fat (or both) to the tissues of the upper thigh or lower abdomen tends to prevent reduction.

Femoral hernia is extremely prone to strangulate for the following reasons: (1) the structures forming the anulus femoralis are unyielding; (2) the transversalis fascia often forms a tight neck about the hernia as it pushes ventrally through this fascia into the fossa ovalis; (3) the upper border of the fossa ovalis is sharp

and crescentic; and (4) the hernia changes direction many times during its course.

Treatment

A. Principles: The criteria for proper femoral hernia repair are as follows (Munro):

1. Complete excision of the hernia sac.

2. Exclusion of the preperitoneal fat from the hernia repair.

3. The use of nonabsorbable sutures in the repair.

4. The repair should be immediately adjacent to the peritoneum, closing the entrance to the femoral canal.

5. The weak transversalis fascia should be repaired since it is responsible for the hernia.

6. Since Cooper's ligament gives a firm support for sutures and since it is at the proper level for repair, forming the natural line for the attachment of the transversalis fascia, it should be used in the closure (Fig 33–15).

B. Simple Repair: An oblique inguinal incision as for inguinal hernia is most often used. The inguinal canal is opened and the spermatic cord or the round ligament is isolated and retracted. The transversalis fascia is identified and opened. The hernial sac is identified and teased back through the femoral ring and then dissected free, taking care not to injure the bladder. The excess sac is cut away and the neck of the sac is transfixed at the peritoneal level. A McVay type of plastic hernia repair is then carried out, the transversalis fascia being sutured to Cooper's ligament to

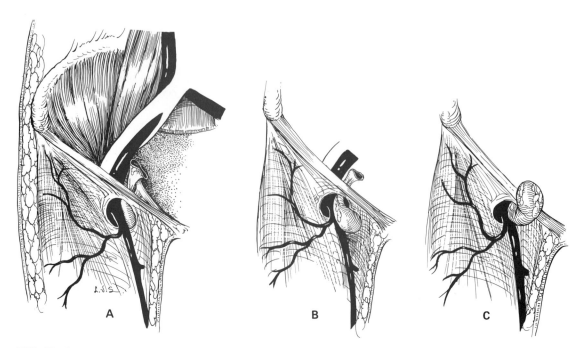

FIG 33–14. Migration of femoral hernia. *A:* Femoral hernia has passed the femoral ring and lies deep to the fossa ovalis beneath the transversalis fascia. *B:* Femoral hernia has broken through the transversalis fascia and the fossa ovalis. *C:* The sharp superior edge of the fossa ovalis has turned the hernia sac superiorly to lie ventral to the inguinal ligament and the lower abdominal wall.

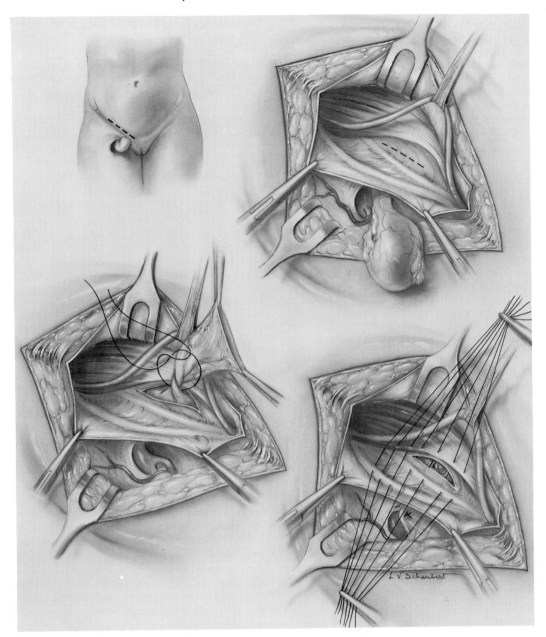

FIG 33–15. Repair of femoral hernia by McVay (Cooper's ligament) method. Note that medial sutures hook transversalis fascia to Cooper's ligament; lateral sutures hook inguinal ligament. This repair is also used for direct inguinal hernia.

reinforce the inferior portion of the floor of the inguinal canal and effectively close the femoral ring.

C. Complicated Repair: When the hernia is complicated by obstruction at the femoral ring and cannot be reduced back into the abdomen, the iliopubic tract and the lateral edge of Gimbernat's ligament must be incised cautiously to free up and reduce the hernia. If this is not enough to enlarge the neck of the femoral ring, the inguinal ligament may be divided over the neck of the sac. This is then usually sufficient to allow reduction of the hernia mass back into the abdomen. Constricting rings at the level of the breakthrough of the transversalis fascia deep to the fossa ovalis and at the level of the upper rim of the fossa ovalis can usually be cut quite easily under direct vision. It is seldom necessary to make an incision in the thigh in addition to the inguinal incision. Instead, the lower flap of the inguinal wound may be elevated and retracted in the direction of the thigh and adequate thigh exposure gained in this manner.

If the hernia sac and mass reduce under opiates or anesthesia and if bloody fluid appears in the hernia sac when it is exposed and opened, one must strongly suspect the possibility of nonviable bowel in the peritoneal cavity, possibly of the Richter hernia variety. In such cases it is mandatory to open and explore the abdomen, usually through a vertical rectus incision.

A few surgeons still prefer to repair and release femoral hernias through a thigh incision. The preperitoneal approach to femoral hernia allows good access to the femoral ring and in experienced hands is a good procedure. In addition, this exposure allows for a satisfactory exploration of the lower peritoneal cavity by simply opening the peritoneum. The possibility of the presence of an aberrant obturator artery (a branch of the external iliac rather than the internal iliac artery) running on the abdominal surface of Gimbernat's ligament near its sharp lateral edge is one of the reasons why great care must be exercised in cutting this ligament in order to release a femoral hernia strangulated at this level.

Prognosis

Before the Cooper's ligament repair was adopted, the recurrence rate in femoral hernia was 15–20%. A better understanding of the anatomy of the groin—and particularly of the importance of the transversalis fascia and its iliopubic tract—has improved the results. Recurrence rates now are about the same as for direct inguinal hernia, ie, about 7–12%. The closing of the femoral ring by suture of the transversalis fascia to Cooper's ligament is the main factor in diminishing the number of recurrences.

Lyall D, Doumanen R: Richter's hernia. Am J Surg 75:828, 1948.

Lytle WJ: Femoral hernia. Ann Roy Coll Surg Engl 21:244–262, 1957.

Lytle WJ: Femoral hernia. Brit J Hosp Med for July 1970 (pp 17–22).

McVay CB, Savage LE: Etiology of femoral hernia. Ann Surg 154:25, 1961.

McVay CB: Inguinal and femoral hernioplasty. Surgery 57:615, 1965.

REPAIR OF INGUINAL & FEMORAL HERNIAS IN THE AGED

A few special comments are in order regarding inguinal and femoral hernia in the aged.

Particularly in old men, groin hernias are one of the most frequently encountered diagnoses because of loss of muscle tone in the aged and the presence of conditions causing increased intra-abdominal pressure such as chronic bronchitis, prostatism, and chronic constipation. Hernias in aged individuals should be repaired whenever the patient's condition permits (1) to relieve discomfort and (2) to avoid the necessity for emergency hernioplasty on the elderly patient in the event of incarceration and obstruction—ie, to make the procedure an elective one, with adequate time for thorough physical evaluation, for correction of superimposed disorders (particularly benign prostate hypertrophy and chronic pulmonary disease), and for adequate preoperative build-up and maintenance. If hernias in the elderly become complicated by incarceration or strangulation, the mortality and morbidity rates are extremely high.

Elderly people withstand elective operative procedures quite well. Local anesthesia is recommended, occasionally supplemented with intravenous fentanyl-droperidol (Innovar). However, many surgeons employ general anesthesia with good results. Williams and Hale report as follows: "In comparing complications with the type of anesthesia administered, general anesthesia was associated with the highest respiratory complication rate. Spinal anesthesia was followed by the highest incidence of genitourinary complications. Local anesthesia was associated with the lowest number of complications, despite the fact that it was the procedure of choice in most of the poor risk patients."[*]

It should be remembered that removal of the spermatic cord and testicle is of distinct advantage in the closure of large or recurrent hernial defects in the aged. In older men, when there is a complete scrotal hernia with an indirect sac that is tightly fixed to cord and scrotal tissues by multiple vascular adhesions, it is better to leave the distal sac in situ. The indirect sac may be transected high in the inguinal canal and the distal sac left untouched. There is some slight danger of hydrocele occurring in these cases, but the incidence and associated disability are negligible. This procedure saves time and prevents the development of scrotal hematoma.

*Williams JS, Hale HW: The advisability of inguinal herniorrhaphy in the elderly. Surg Gynec Obst 12:100–104, 1966.

Baker JW: Abdominal wound closure in the substandard patient. Masonic Clinic Bull 1:145, 1947.

Herron PW, Jessep JE, Harkins HN: Analysis of 600 major operations in patients over 70 years of age. Ann Surg 152:686, 1960.

OTHER TYPES OF HERNIAS

UMBILICAL HERNIAS IN ADULTS
(See Fig 33–16.)

Embryology & Surgical Anatomy of the Umbilical Region

The umbilical region occupies the most central area of the anterolateral abdominal wall. The area is of great interest because of the occurrence not only of umbilical hernias of various types but also of omphalocele and gastroschisis. In addition, a number of congenital anomalies related to fetal circulation, the fetal vitello-intestinal duct, and the urachus make their presence known in this area.

Early in embryonic development, the antimesenteric border of the apex of the herniated midgut loop communicates with the yolk sac via the vitello-intestinal duct. Accompanying the duct are the vitello-intestinal vessels branching off from the termination of the superior mesenteric artery at the mesenteric border of the apex of the midgut loop. These vessels then cross the midgut apex to reach and supply the vitello-intestinal duct.

The allantois, formed as a result of an outpouching from the alimentary tube caudal to the vitello-intestinal duct, lies in the umbilicus and communicates via the urachus with the superior surface of the primitive urinary bladder.

The major blood vessels connecting the fetal to the maternal circulation run through the umbilical orifice into the umbilical stalk. These are the paired umbilical arteries and the single umbilical vein.

By the beginning of the fourth month of fetal life, the ventrolateral abdominal wall has closed in on the umbilicus. At this time, under normal circumstances, the vitello-intestinal duct has atrophied, as have also the omphalomesenteric vessels supplying the duct tract. The urachus has atrophied into a fibrous cord, and the herniated midgut loop has returned to the celomic cavity. As a consequence, the umbilical ring, which earlier was traversed by these structures, has contracted to a small orifice through which pass only the paired umbilical arteries and the umbilical vein. Following birth, blood no longer circulates in the vessels of the cord and they become fibrous. A small crust remains where the cord has been ligated and cut. This heals and epithelizes rapidly. Scarring occurs, and the urachus and the umbilical vessels draw the epithelized area against the circumference of the umbilical

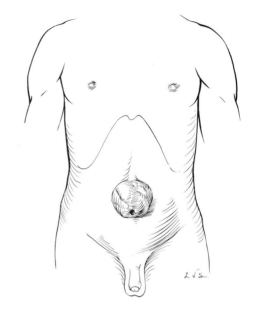

FIG 33–16. Umbilical hernia.

ring. The traction of the umbilical vein draws the scar against the superior circumference of the ring. The scar formed at the superior margin of the umbilical ring is less dense than that formed at the inferior margin where the paired umbilical arteries and the urachus exert traction on the umbilical scar. Consequently, since the superior arc of the umbilical ring is fused less tightly, it becomes the site of development of most umbilical hernias.

Etiology & Predisposing Factors

Umbilical hernia in adults occurs long after closure of the umbilical ring and is due to a gradual yielding of the cicatricial tissue closing the ring. The hernia usually presents at the superior arc of the ring, its weakest area. It occurs in females about 10 times as often as in males.

Predisposing factors include (1) multiple pregnancies with prolonged labor, (2) the ascites of liver cirrhosis, (3) obesity, and (4) the presence, over a long period, of large intra-abdominal tumor masses.

Clinical Findings

In adults, umbilical hernia does not tend toward spontaneous reduction but usually increases steadily in size. The hernia may be covered with a very thin peritoneal sac, but in long-standing hernias the sac may thicken considerably. Its outer coverings are usually so stretched as to make the hernia appear to lie in a subcutaneous position. The hernia is often lobulated in appearance. The hernia sac frequently has multiple loculations. The chief content of umbilical hernias is usually an omental mass, but small and large bowel may be present. This hernia frequently becomes strangulated, and emergency operative procedures on it are common. The necks of umbilical hernias are usually quite narrow when compared to the size of the herniated mass.

Umbilical hernias with tight rings and much herniated bowel often lead to chronic constipation and the recurrent cramping and nausea of subacute, incomplete bowel obstruction. Incarceration and strangulation are common. Very large umbilical hernias give a marked feeling of abdominal heaviness and frequently lead to backache.

Treatment

Umbilical hernia in an adult should be repaired as soon as possible after the diagnosis is made in order to avoid the necessity for emergency procedures for strangulation and incarceration. Surgical repair calls for preservation of the umbilical dimple (if possible) and a simple through-and-through fascial and peritoneal one-layer approximation. In an elderly patient with strangulation of a large umbilical hernia mass and a relatively small umbilical ring, a staged procedure may be carried out. At the first operation—because of the patient's poor condition—the constricting fascial ring is merely incised; definitive repair can then be done later.

Actually, the umbilical defect seldom involves the compartments of the rectus sheath but is a herniation through the attenuated linea alba. The best results in closure of the aponeurotic defect seem to follow suture in a transverse direction. Since the fibers of the sheaths of the 3 flat muscles of the abdominal wall run in a transverse direction as they make up the rectus sheath, transverse closure places sutures at right angles to the direction of the sheath fibers, which then are under less tension during increases in intra-abdominal pressure with respiration, defecation, etc.

Large umbilical hernia defects which cannot be closed without undue tension may be closed with an inlay of Marlex mesh.

Prognosis

Large size of the hernia, old age, debility of the patient, and the presence of any related intra-abdominal pathology are factors which may forecast a high mortality and morbidity after surgical repair. In healthy individuals, surgical repair of the umbilical defects gives good results with a low rate of recurrence.

INTERPARIETAL HERNIA

Interparietal hernias are usually of an indirect inguinal type. Rarely, however, direct or ventral hernias occasionally may be interparietal. There are 3 anatomic groups, depending upon the location of the sac, in the abdominal wall: (1) Preperitoneal: The sac lies between the peritoneum and the transversalis fascia. (Incidence 20%.) (2) Inguinal-interstitial: The sac passes through the internal ring but dissects between any of the muscle layers of the abdominal wall. (Incidence 20%.) (3) Inguinal-superficial: The sac

passes through the external ring but dissects subcutaneously. (Incidence 20%.)

Although most interparietal hernias are of one indirect inguinal type, very rarely a direct hernia or a ventral hernia may present in the same fashion.

Although the condition is rare, it is essential to recognize it because strangulation is common and the mass is easily mistaken for a tumor or abscess.

The lesion usually can be recognized on physical examination provided it is kept in mind. In most reported cases, extensive studies for intra-abdominal tumors have preceded recognition and operation. A lateral film of the abdomen will usually show bowel within the layers of the abdominal wall in cases of intestinal incarceration or strangulation.

Sometimes there are 2 sacs which are hourglass in shape. One occupies the usual position of an indirect hernia in the inguinal canal; the other component extends laterally between the layers of the abdominal wall. There is always a common opening at the internal ring.

As soon as the diagnosis is established, operation should be performed, usually through the standard inguinal approach.

Altman B: Interparietal hernia. In: *Hernia.* Nyhus LM, Harkins HN (editors). Lippincott, 1964.

Dunphy JE: Strangulated hernia. New England J Med 220:819–820, 1939.

EPIGASTRIC HERNIA
(See Fig 33–17.)

An epigastric hernia is one which protrudes through the linea alba (the midline of the anterior abdominal wall) above the level of the umbilicus. The linea alba is formed by the midline interlacing of the anterior and posterior sheaths of the rectus abdominis

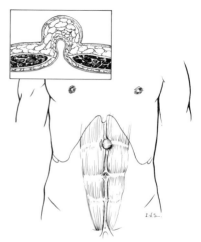

FIG 33–17. Epigastric hernia. Note closeness to midline and presence in upper abdomen. The herniation is through the linea alba.

muscles. It runs from the xiphoid process of the sternum to the symphysis pubis. In the upper third of the abdomen it is 1.25–3 cm wide and is fibrous, but as it approaches the umbilicus it narrows. Below the level of the umbilicus, it persists simply as a narrow fibrous cord. Deep to the linea alba are the transversalis fascia, a quantity of preperitoneal fat, and the peritoneum. Paired small blood vessels and nerves pierce the linea alba on either side of the midline.

There are 2 theories regarding the etiology of epigastric hernia: (1) that the hernia develops through one of the foramens of egress of the small paramidline nerves and vessels, and (2) that it develops through an area of congenital weakness in the linea alba. The latter view is supported by the observation that epigastric hernia occurs also in infants.

About 3–5% of the population have epigastric hernias. It is 3 times more common in men than in women, and most common between the ages of 20–50. About 20% of epigastric hernias are multiple, and about 80% occur just to the left of the midline.

Clinical Findings

The most common finding is a subcutaneous mass in the midline above the level of the umbilicus. Most such masses are painless and unsuspected by the patient and are frequently found on routine abdominal examination. The smaller masses most frequently contain preperitoneal fat only and are very prone to incarcerate and strangulate. These smaller hernias are therefore often tender. Larger hernias seldom strangulate and may contain, in addition to preperitoneal fat, a portion of the nearby omentum and occasionally a loop of small or large bowel.

Symptoms of epigastric hernia are many and varied and present difficult problems in diagnosis. They may range from mild epigastric pain and tenderness to deep burning epigastric pain with radiation to the back or the lower abdominal quadrants. The pain may be accompanied by abdominal bloating, nausea, or vomiting. The symptoms are usually apt to occur after a large meal and on occasion may be relieved by reclining, probably because the supine position causes the herniated mass to drop away from the anterior abdominal wall.

The diagnosis is difficult to make in the presence of an obese abdomen, since in such circumstances the presenting epigastric mass is hard to palpate. If the mass is palpable, diagnosis can often be confirmed by any maneuver that will increase intra-abdominal pressure, thus causing the mass to bulge anteriorly. Lower esophageal and upper gastrointestinal x-rays as well as cholecystography may be needed to rule out disease in these organs.

If the upper abdominal diagnostic work-up is negative but the patient has persistent pain of the sort encountered with epigastric hernia, surgical exploration of the linea alba for a possible epigastric hernia may be warranted.

Differential Diagnosis

In differential diagnosis, one must consider peptic ulcer with possible penetration or perforation, gallbladder disease, hiatal hernia, pancreatitis, and upper small bowel obstruction. On occasion it may be difficult to distinguish the hernial mass from a subcutaneous lipoma, fibroma, or neurofibroma.

Treatment

If the epigastric hernia is symptomatic or if it is larger than 0.5 cm in diameter, surgical treatment is indicated. Repair may be done through a transverse incision with direct fascial closure to eliminate the defect. Herniated fat contents are usually dissected free and removed. Intraperitoneal herniating structures are reduced, but no attempt is made to close the peritoneal sac.

Many authors feel that a liberal vertical incision is preferable since it allows the surgeon to search for multiple epigastric hernias, which are occasionally present. The fascia is then closed in a vertical fascia-to-fascia manner. The vertical incision also allows for easy intra-abdominal exploration if indicated.

The operation is best performed under general anesthesia, and postoperative nasogastric suction is usually employed as paralytic ileus is a frequent postoperative complication and may lead to a breakdown of the fascial repair as a result of pressure of the distended abdomen against the closure.

Prognosis

The recurrence rate is 15–20%. This is a higher incidence than with the routine inguinal or femoral hernia repair.

INCISIONAL HERNIA
(Ventral Hernia)

About 10% of all hernioplasties performed in large general hospitals are for repair of incisional hernias. Despite significant advances in operative technic, improved suture materials, better pre- and postoperative care, the use of reinforcing and "bridging" materials, antibiotics, etc, this iatrogenic type of hernia does not seem to be significantly decreasing in frequency. This may be partly because people are living longer so that geriatric surgery, with its high incidence of postoperative complications of all sorts, has become more frequent.

Causes & Prevention

A. Causes: Many factors contribute to the development of an incisional hernia. Any one may be the only factor responsible for the herniation, but when these causative factors are combined, the likelihood of postoperative wound weakness is greatly increased. The factors most often responsible for incisional hernia are as follows:

1. Age of the patient. Wound healing is usually slower and less solid in geriatric patients.

2. General debility of the patient. Cirrhosis, carcinoma, and chronic wasting diseases are major adverse factors.

3. Obesity. Fat patients frequently have increased intra-abdominal pressure. The presence of fat in the abdominal wound masks tissue layers and makes for a high incidence of seromas and hematomas in wounds.

4. Postoperative wound infection.

5. Type of incision used. There is much argument concerning the placement of and the direction of incisional wounds. Many surgeons feel that transverse and oblique wounds are more apt to heal well than vertical ones.

6. Postoperative pulmonary complications. These may be secondary to chronic pulmonary disease or anesthesia, or may occur as a result of lying on the operating table or on the postoperative bed for long periods.

7. Placement of drains or colostomy or ileostomy openings in the primary operative wound.

8. Failure to use nonabsorbable suture material whenever possible and suitable.

9. Failure to observe the principles of proper preoperative and postoperative nutrition. Proper attention to protein nutrition and vitamin C is of particular importance.

10. General sepsis of the patient tends to slow down wound healing.

B. Prevention: The major factors in prevention of incisional hernia are as follows:

1. Use transverse or oblique incisions when feasible.

2. Use nonabsorbable suture material in all clean wounds and in a large number of infected wounds as well.

3. Avoid undue tissue tension in wound closure.

4. Avoid dead space in wounds.

5. Ensure meticulous hemostasis.

6. Encourage weight reduction, if possible, before surgery.

7. Treat pulmonary disease before surgery and use positive pressure breathing apparatus after surgery.

8. Maintain fluid, electrolyte, and blood balance before surgery and during the postoperative period.

9. Place wound drains and colostomies and ileostomies away from the main incision whenever possible.

10. Protect wound edges, prepare the skin properly, and use prophylactic antibiotics judiciously if indicated (particularly in bowel surgery) to avoid wound infection.

11. Give cleansing enemas before surgery and initiate nasogastric intestinal suction postoperatively when indicated.

12. Use catheter drainage of bladder when indicated.

13. Use wire, heavy silk, or Dermalon retention sutures when indicated (elderly or debilitated patients, those with carcinoma, those with poor fascial and peritoneal tissues). These retention sutures should be placed 2–3 cm apart and should be tied loosely over bolsters.

14. Insist on early graded ambulation.

Early Dehiscence

Nearly all wound dehiscence is preceded by a period of serosanguineous wound drainage. This may vary in duration from a few hours to several days, but its presence is nearly always a sign of impending dehiscence and should immediately alert the operating surgeon to that possibility. The ultimate in wound weakness is complete or partial dehiscence, a breakdown of all layers of the closure except the skin, so that the intra-abdominal contents emerge into a subcutaneous position. Final breakthrough of the skin leads to evisceration. Prompt operation is mandatory in either case, with resuture of the wound, either in layers or with through-and-through retention sutures, or with a combination of both.

In contrast to the above, a surgical wound may show no postoperative indications of discomfort or drainage but (suddenly or gradually) weakens either along its entire length or in a specific area. This is due to complete or partial failure of peritoneal or fascial closure. Clinically, this wound will bulge outward with or without pain during intervals of increased intra-abdominal pressure. This hernia nearly always gradually increases in size and may become painful or show signs of partial bowel obstruction. The incidence of incarceration and strangulation of intraperitoneal contents in the wound is relatively high. These wounds often have one or 2 lengths of bowel or an area of omentum stuck to the peritoneal edge of the weakened area or areas.

Treatment

Incisional hernia should be treated by early repair. In addition to its unsightliness and the pain it causes, it is frequently the cause of bowel obstruction and is sometimes associated with chronic constipation. If the patient is unwilling to undergo surgery or is a poor surgical risk, the hernia should be supported by an elastic abdominal corset.

A. Small Hernias: Small incisional hernias usually present no difficulty in surgical repair. Many surgeons consider a direct fascia-to-fascia repair as sufficient for a satisfactory closure; others insist upon a separate peritoneal layer closure as an integral step in the repair.

B. Large Hernias:

1. **Preparation before repair**—The closure of a large incisional hernia defect is difficult and painstaking. Many large ventral hernias cannot be returned to the abdominal cavity because the intraperitoneal space has decreased in size. The repair may be preceded by a series of injections of air into the peritoneal cavity (pneumoperitoneum) to elevate the diaphragm and generally increase the intraperitoneal space. This may also be accomplished by a left-sided phrenic crush. A nasogastric tube placed prior to surgery is of assistance in closure.

2. Repair technic—Spinal anesthesia, because of its relaxant properties, is frequently used, although general anesthesia with the addition of muscle relaxants also gives excellent results. Excess and scarred skin and subcutaneous tissues over the hernia are removed. The hernia sac is then carefully dissected free from the underlying muscles and fascial tissues. The sac may be opened, particularly if there is incarceration or adhesion of intraperitoneal contents, in which case the abdominal contents are dissected free from the sac and dropped back into the abdomen. The excess sac is trimmed or, if there are no adherent intraperitoneal structures, it may be inverted (as in direct inguinal hernia) and the repair done over the inverted sac. As is true also of adult umbilical hernias of long standing, chronic ventral hernia tends to become loculated. It is essential to thoroughly clean and visualize the fascial layers about the defect to be repaired so that the closure will be a direct fascia-to-fascia repair.

Repair may be accomplished either by overlapping the fascia in a transverse manner or by lateral overlapping. Some surgeons prefer a layered closure with or without through-and-through retention sutures; others perform a through-and-through closure in one layer—similar to the closing of an evisceration.

Nonabsorbable suture material (silk, cotton, or wire) should be used in all closures, and meticulous care should be given to hemostasis and the obliteration of dead space. Where a large dead space persists, a Hemovac type of drain should be employed. The patient's own tissue should always be used if the wound can be closed without tension. If the patient's own fascial tissues are not thick and strong enough to guarantee a good closure—or if they may only be closed under tension—the use of Marlex mesh may be of help. This material may be placed directly over the peritoneal layer in a closure and serves as a bridge between good fascia on either side of the closure. The use of fascial relaxing incisions on either side of the main defect is occasionally of assistance in closure.

Defects too large to close easily are often better left without surgical repair if they are asymptomatic. The use of an abdominal support for 3—6 months after surgery may reduce the recurrence rate in ventral hernia repair.

Prognosis

The recurrence rate for incisional hernia repairs varies directly with the size of the defect to be closed. Small hernias have a recurrence rate of 2—5%; medium-sized hernias recur in 5—15% of cases; and large hernias, too often closed under tension, have a recurrence rate as high as 15—20%.

Ravitch MM: Ventral hernia. S Clin North America 51:1341—1345, 1971.

VARIOUS RARE HERNIATIONS THROUGH THE ABDOMINAL WALLS

Littré's Hernia

This consists of a herniation through one of the weak areas of the anterior abdominal wall with a Meckel's diverticulum as the sole occupant of the hernial sac. It occurs more often on the right side, more often in femoral hernia, and more often in adult males.

Treatment consists of repair of the hernia (inguinal or femoral) plus, if possible, excision of the diverticulum. If acute Meckel's diverticulitis is present, the acute inflammatory mass may have to be treated through a separate abdominal incision.

Spigelian Hernia

This is a spontaneously occurring lateral ventral hernia through the tissues of the linea semilunaris, the area where the sheaths of the lateral abdominal flat muscles join to form the rectus abdominis sheath. The crossing of the transverse fold of Douglas (linea semicircularis) by the linea semilunaris creates a weak point in the ventrolateral abdominal wall which may be further weakened by the medial turning at this point of the ascending inferior epigastric vessels. Here the vessels run dorsal to the rectus abdominis but ventral to the fold of Douglas. Thus, the crossing of these 2 lines plus the course of the inferior epigastric vessels results in Spigelian hernias at this point. These hernias always start medial to the fleshy portion of the transversus abdominis, lateral to the rectus abdominis, and caudal to the fold of Douglas. They are nearly always found above the level of the inferior epigastric vessels. Diagnosis is often difficult since the symptoms simulate those of lower quadrant abdominal disease and the hernia tends to migrate laterally between deep tissue layers. The cutaneous presentation of the mass may be quite distant from the linea semilunaris. Strangulation is frequent.

Symptoms of Spigelian hernia are difficult to elicit. There is usually discomfort at the area of hernia protrusion. The pain is usually aggravated by exertion or by elevations of intra-abdominal pressure. Recumbency will often alleviate the pain. Nausea and vomiting are occasionally associated with the pain, and the overall picture may mimic lower gastrointestinal disease, gallbladder disease, ureteral disease, or disease of the pelvic organs. The diagnosis is most easily made with the patient standing and straining; a bulge then presents in the lower abdominal area which disappears on pressure with a gurgling sound. Following reduction of the mass, the hernial orifice can usually be palpated.

These hernias are quite easily cured by adequate aponeurotic repair. The inferior epigastric vessels may be ligated without adverse effects if they interfere with the closure.

Lumbar or Dorsal Hernia (See Fig 33—18.)

These are hernias through the posterior abdomi-

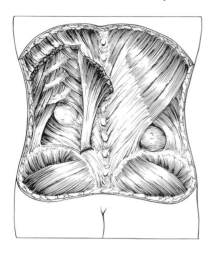

FIG 33–18. Anatomic relationships of lumbar or dorsal hernia. (Adapted from Netter.) On the left, lumbar or dorsal hernia into space of Grynfeltt. On the right, hernia into Petit's triangle (inferior lumbar space).

nal wall at some level in the lumbar region. They may occur spontaneously or following trauma or a local inflammatory process. The most common sites (95%) are the superior and inferior (Petit's) lumbar triangles. The superior triangle of Grynfeltt-Lesshaft is larger and more often involved. A "lump in the flank" is the common complaint, associated with a dull, heavy, pulling feeling. With the patient erect, the presence of a reducible, often tympanitic mass in the flank usually makes the diagnosis. Incarceration and strangulation occur in about 10% of cases. They must be differentiated from abscesses, hematomas, soft tissue tumors, renal tumors, and muscle strain.

Acquired hernias may be traumatic or nontraumatic. Severe direct trauma, penetrating wounds, abscesses, and poor healing of flank incisions are the usual causes. Congenital hernias (rare) occur in infants and are not often associated with other congenital defects. They are due to a defect that weakens the dorsolateral abdominal walls, and are usually unilateral.

Lumbar hernias increase in size and should be repaired when found. Repair is by mobilization of the nearby fascia and obliteration of the hernia defect by precise fascia-to-fascia closure.

Obturator Hernia

Herniation through the obturator canal at the upper border of the obturator membrane is more frequent in women and debilitated persons and is difficult to diagnose preoperatively. These hernias present as small bowel obstruction with cramping abdominal pain followed by nausea and vomiting. Pain or paresthesias caused by pressure on the obturator nerve may radiate to the anteromedial surface of the thigh.

The abdominal approach gives the best exposure, and these hernias should not be repaired from the thigh approach. The Cheatle-Henry approach (retropubic) gives excellent exposure. After a transverse suprapubic incision, the sheaths of the recti are split transversely, exposing the rectus abdominis and the pyramidalis muscles. The recti are separated and retracted laterally. The peritoneum is stripped off the ventrolateral abdominal wall, and the bladder is retracted dorsally to give direct visualization of the obturator foramen.

Perineal Hernia

Perineal hernia protrudes through the muscles and fascia of the perineal floor. It may be primary or acquired following perineal prostatectomy, abdominoperineal resection of the rectum, or pelvic exenteration.

These hernias are anterior or posterior to the transverse perineal muscle. They present as easily reducible perineal bulges and cause few symptoms. The anterior ones may cause dysuria; the posterior ones may cause difficulty in sitting. The perineal skin over the hernia may ulcerate.

Repair is usually done by a combined abdominal and perineal approach, with an adequate fascial and muscular perineal repair.

Sciatic Hernia

This rarest of abdominal hernias consists of an outpouching of intra-abdominal contents through the greater sciatic foramen. The diagnosis is made after incarceration or strangulation of the bowel occurs. The repair is usually made through the abdominal approach. The hernial sac and contents are reduced, and the weak area is closed by making a fascial flap of the piriformis muscle.

INTERNAL HERNIAS

Internal hernias occur into a large fossa, fovea, or foramen. The 4 major internal hernias, all extremely rare, are: (1) paraduodenal hernias, (2) hernias into the foramen of Winslow, (3) mesenteric hernias, and (4) omental hernias.

These hernias may cause chronic digestive complaints and acute or chronic intestinal obstruction.

Treatment is as follows: Attempt to reduce the hernia without opening the hernia sac, or open the anterior wall of the sac and divide any adhesions present. Perform needle decompression of dilated bowel if necessary. Reduce herniated bowel by pressure from within and traction from without. Close the hernial defect or resect the wall of the hernia area.

Great care should be taken not to injure major arteries or veins.

34 . . .

The Appendix

J. Englebert Dunphy, MD

ANATOMY & PHYSIOLOGY

In infants, the appendix is a conical diverticulum at the apex of the cecum, but with differential growth and distention of the cecum the appendix ultimately arises on the left and dorsally approximately 2.5 cm (1 inch) below the ileocecal valve. The teniae of the colon converge at the base of the appendix, an arrangement which helps to locate this structure at operation.

The position of the appendix has important clinical implications (Fig 34–1). The appendix is fixed retrocecally in 16% of adults and is freely mobile in the remainder, so that precise location varies with distention and emptying of the cecum.

Agenesis of the appendix is rare and is sometimes associated with cecal hypoplasia. True double appendix and congenital diverticula are curiosities.

The appendix is lined by columnar epithelium of the colonic type. Circular and longitudinal muscle layers are often deficient in some areas, allowing contiguity of submucosa and serosa—a fact of importance in appendiceal disease.

The appendix in youth is characterized by a large concentration of lymphoid follicles which appear 2 weeks after birth and number about 200 or more at age 15 years. Thereafter, there is progressive atrophy of lymphoid tissue, concomitant with fibrosis of the wall and partial or total obliteration of the lumen.

The function of the appendix is not known, but there is no justification for the notion that the human appendix is vestigial. Most of the lymphoid follicles of the large intestine are aggregated in the cecum in warm-blooded animals, and in a few vertebrates (including anthropoid apes and man) the lymphoid content of the colon is concentrated in the true cecal apex, the vermiform appendix.

If the appendix has a physiologic function, it is

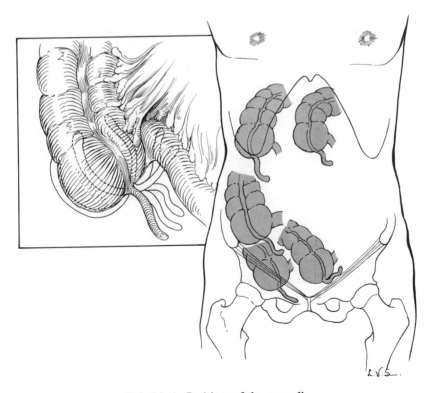

FIG 34–1. Positions of the appendix.

589

probably related to the presence of lymphoid follicles. The avian bursa of Fabricius controls the development of peripheral lymphoid tissues such as spleen and lymph nodes, and defective immunoglobulin production results from destruction of the bursa of Fabricius in young fowl. The rabbit appendix histologically resembles the avian bursa, and neonatal appendectomy in rabbits impairs their later capacity to produce antibody to various antigens. However, reports of a statistical relationship between appendectomy and subsequent carcinoma of the colon and other neoplasms in man are not supported by controlled studies and deserve little credence at this time.

Berry JA: The true caecal apex, or the vermiform appendix: Its minute and comparative anatomy. J Anat Physiol 35:83–100, 1900.

Cooper MD & others: A mammalian equivalent of the avian bursa of Fabricius. Lancet 1:1388–1391, 1966.

DeGaris CF: Topography and development of the cecum-appendix. Ann Surg 113:540–548, 1941.

Hyams L, Wynder EL: Appendectomy and cancer risk: An epidemiological evaluation. J Chronic Dis 21:391–415, 1968.

ACUTE APPENDICITIS

Essentials of Diagnosis

- Abdominal pain.
- Anorexia, nausea and vomiting.
- Localized abdominal tenderness.
- Low-grade fever.
- Leukocytosis.

General Considerations

Approximately 7% of individuals in western countries develop appendicitis at some time during their lives, and about 200,000 appendectomies for acute appendicitis are performed annually in the USA. Acute appendicitis is uncommon in parts of Africa and Asia, perhaps because of the high-residue diet ingested by inhabitants of some less well developed countries. The ingestion of cellulose-depleted foods in affluent nations alters bacterial flora, slows fecal transit, and results in smaller, firmer, and more tenacious stools which require higher intraluminal pressures. These consequences of highly refined diets may contribute to the development of various colonic diseases, including appendicitis.

The word appendicitis was introduced by Reginald Fitz in 1886; previously, the cecum was thought to be the offending part, and the disorder was called typhlitis or perityphlitis.

According to the classic concept, the pathogenesis of acute appendicitis involves bacterial infection distal to obstruction of the lumen. In approximately 70% of acutely inflamed appendices, obstruction of the proximal lumen by fibrous bands, fecaliths, tumors, para-

sites, or foreign bodies can be demonstrated; in others, lymphoid hyperplasia in response to viral disease (eg, measles) may be the cause of obstruction. Intraluminal obstruction is not found in one-third of specimens, however, and external compression by bands or kinks has been postulated to explain these cases. Another possibility is that high intraluminal pressure in the cecum—again related to the low-residue diet of western man—might functionally obstruct the appendix and allow bacterial infection to develop. It has also been suggested that acute appendicitis may begin with mucosal ulceration, perhaps viral, followed by secondary bacterial invasion. According to this hypothesis, obstruction is not fundamental to the pathogenesis of appendicitis.

As appendicitis progresses, the blood supply is impaired by bacterial infection in the wall and distention of the lumen by pus; gangrene and perforation occur at about 24 hours, although the timing is highly variable. According to some authors, gangrene implies microscopic perforation in every case.

Clinical Findings

Acute appendicitis has protean manifestations. It may simulate almost any other acute abdominal illness, and in turn may be mimicked by a variety of conditions. The surest route to accurate diagnosis is a careful history and a thorough, systematic physical examination as described in Chapter 31. Positive findings may be absent or minimal in the early stages, particularly in retrocecal, pelvic, and bizarre forms of appendicitis, and repeated physical examinations must be performed. Progression of symptoms and signs is the rule—in contrast to the fluctuating course of some other diseases in the differential diagnosis. *Localized tenderness* is the one essential physical finding that must be sought by precise one-finger palpation. Even in the very young and the elderly, sharply localized tenderness is the single most valuable finding.

A. Symptoms and Signs:

1. Classic appendicitis—Typically, the patient is awakened in the early morning by vague abdominal discomfort followed by slight nausea. He is apt to think he has eaten something the night before which has disagreed with him. The pain is persistent and continuous, but not severe, with occasional mild epigastric cramps. There may be an episode of vomiting, and within several hours the pain shifts to the right lower quadrant, becoming rather sharply localized and causing discomfort on moving, walking, or coughing. The patient has a sense of being constipated and may feel that he should take a cathartic or an enema, but if he does he experiences no relief ("gas stoppage sign").

Examination at this point will show cough tenderness, sharply localized to the right lower quadrant. There will be well-localized tenderness to one-finger palpation and possibly very slight muscular rigidity. Rebound tenderness is classically referred to the same area. Peristalsis is normal or slightly reduced. Rectal and pelvic examinations are likely to be negative.

2. Retrocecal appendicitis—Poorly localized epigastric pain heralds the onset of this form of appendicitis also. The patient is convinced he has eaten something that has disagreed with him and is apt to take a cathartic. Nausea and vomiting are mild. Because the retrocecal appendix is protected from the anterior abdominal wall, the pain remains poorly localized and the shift to the right lower quadrant may not occur. For similar reasons, the patient does not experience discomfort on walking or coughing. There may be mild diarrhea, and a retrocecal appendix lying adjacent to the ureter may cause urinary frequency or even hematuria.

Examination is deceptively unimpressive unless one-finger palpation is carried carefully into the flank, where tenderness is detected.

3. Pelvic appendicitis—Pelvic appendicitis is one of the most misleading forms of the disease. It closely simulates acute gastroenteritis and is associated with essentially no abnormal abdominal signs on physical examination until late in its course. Characteristically, the patient feels vaguely ill, with poorly localized abdominal discomfort. Nausea, vomiting, and diarrhea tend to be more prominent than in other forms of appendicitis. When the disease occurs during an epidemic of gastroenteritis, both the family and the physician are apt to assume that this is the diagnosis. Diarrhea is apt to continue because the inflamed appendix may lie against the pelvic colon.

Abdominal examination is essentially negative, and in the early phases of pelvic appendicitis both rectal and pelvic examinations may be negative. Fever is apt to be higher in pelvic appendicitis—another misleading feature of this form of the disease. The key to diagnosis is a repeat examination of the rectum and pelvis. When the examination is done within 7–8 hours of onset, there will be obvious acute tenderness; later, there may be a suggestion of fullness on palpation.

If the diagnosis is not established early, signs of peritonitis ultimately supervene, with lower abdominal rigidity, distention, and diminished to absent peristalsis.

4. Retroileal appendicitis—If the appendix lies behind the ileum, symptoms and signs are similar to those of retrocecal appendicitis. Because of difficulty in making the diagnosis, retroileal appendicitis frequently proceeds to perforation and abscess formation with appearance of a mass before the nature of the illness is appreciated.

5. Obstructive appendicitis—Obstructive appendicitis is a clinical entity characterized by severe colicky pain. Complete obstruction and invasive infection lead to vascular occlusion. Gangrene develops rapidly, and perforation occurs early in the course of the disease. The pain may be so severe that mesenteric vascular occlusion or small bowel obstruction is suspected.

6. Bizarre forms of appendicitis—The cecum may lie on the left side of the abdomen due to malrotation of the colon, and appendicitis may be mistaken for sigmoid diverticulitis. Inflamed appendices positioned in the right upper quadrant mimic acute cholecystitis or perforated ulcer. Even when the cecum is normally

situated, a long appendix may reach to other parts of the abdomen, and acute appendicitis in these circumstances may be very confusing indeed.

7. Chronic appendicitis—Chronic recurrent abdominal pain is a significant clinical problem, and when the complaints are confined to the right lower quadrant the question of chronic appendicitis is usually raised. Occasionally it is clear that the patient has recurrent acute appendicitis. Barium x-rays are not helpful, and no objective evidence establishes or refutes the diagnosis. In many patients the diagnosis is not obvious. Appendectomy in these circumstances relieves symptoms occasionally, but in general laparatomy for chronic abdominal pain is unproductive in the absence of at least one objective finding (eg, fever, mass, jaundice).

B. Laboratory Findings: Moderate leukocytosis is characteristic of appendicitis. The leukocyte count is $14,000/\mu l$ on the average and is greater than $10,000/\mu l$ in 90% of patients. In three-fourths of patients, more than 75% neutrophils are found on differential white counts. It must be emphasized, however, that one patient in 10 with acute appendicitis has a leukocyte count indistinguishable from normal, and many have a normal differential cell count.

The urine is usually normal, but a few leukocytes and erythrocytes and occasionally even gross hematuria may be noted, particularly in retrocecal or pelvic appendicitis.

C. X-Ray Findings: Although acute appendicitis may be diagnosed without radiographic studies in most young patients, plain films of the abdomen may be of value in atypical cases or in very young or very old patients.

Localized air-fluid levels, localized ileus, or increased soft tissue density in the right lower quadrant are present in 50% of patients with early acute appendicitis. Positive radiologic signs become more frequent as appendicitis progresses. Fecaliths, an altered right psoas shadow, or an abnormal right flank stripe are less common findings.

Radiologic examination may be helpful in obscure cases by disclosing evidence of other diseases which may be mistaken for appendicitis, eg, perforated peptic ulcer. Abnormal position of the cecum is an important clue which is detected in abdominal films.

Differential Diagnosis

The diagnosis of acute appendicitis is particularly difficult in the very young and in the elderly. Infants manifest only lethargy, irritability, and anorexia in the early stages, but vomiting, fever, and pain are apparent as the disease progresses. Classic symptoms are seldom elicited in aged patients, and the diagnosis is often not considered by the examining physician. The course of appendicitis is more virulent in the elderly, and perforation occurs at an earlier stage. Other types of individuals presenting diagnostic problems include muscular males (in whom the only symptom may be the "gas stoppage sensation"), pregnant women, and patients recovering from recent abdominal operations. For these reasons, appendicitis should never be lower than No. 2 on the list in the differential diagnosis of any acute abdominal condition.

The condition that is perhaps most commonly confused with appendicitis is vague gastrointestinal upset; in many cases, a specific diagnosis is never established.

A. Gastroenteritis: Gastroenteritis often simulates acute appendicitis. The differential diagnosis is especially challenging if gastroenteritis initiates inflammatory changes in appendiceal lymphoid follicles and evolves into true acute appendicitis. It is common to see a few cases of acute appendicitis in a college population in the midst of an epidemic of gastroenteritis. The history is important in differentiating these 2 conditions: vomiting occurs before the onset of pain in gastroenteritis, whereas pain is virtually always the initial symptom in acute appendicitis. Diffuse myalgias, photophobia, headache, etc may suggest a viral illness. On physical examination, tenderness is less sharply localized than in acute appendicitis.

Mesenteric lymphadenitis in children and young adults is often a diagnostic problem. This entity is discussed elsewhere in this book.

B. Female Pelvic Disorders:

1. A ruptured ovarian follicle in a young woman (mittelschmerz) may mimic acute appendicitis. A careful history usually indicates sudden onset of pain in the middle of the menstrual cycle. The pain is most severe initially and gradually subsides thereafter—a sequence not likely to occur in appendicitis. Gastrointestinal symptoms are less prominent than in appendicitis, but sharply localized right lower quadrant tenderness may be quite misleading. These patients seldom appear ill but at times a differential diagnosis is impossible and operation becomes safer than risking delay.

2. Pelvic inflammatory disease (specifically, acute salpingitis) often masquerades as appendicitis. Fever tends to be higher in salpingitis and abdominal tenderness is more diffuse, but the patient does not appear as ill. A flushed, bright-eyed, febrile female with lipstick carefully applied and lying with her hands behind her head is unlikely to have acute appendicitis even though diffuse abdominal tenderness is evident. By the time high fever and diffuse tenderness complicate appendicitis, the disease is far advanced and the patient is in desperate straits. Pelvic examination reveals a tender cervix, and demonstration of intracellular gram-negative diplococci in cervical smears clinches the diagnosis of salpingitis.

3. Twisted ovarian cyst is difficult to distinguish from acute pelvic appendicitis. Pain is severe, abdominal findings may be typical of appendicitis, and the ovarian mass may not be felt on pelvic examination because tenderness is exquisite. The cyst may be palpated by repeating the pelvic examination under anesthesia, and the appropriate incision can then be made for its removal.

4. Ectopic pregnancy may be distinguished from appendicitis by the history of menstrual irregularity, sudden onset of pain, and diffuse pelvic tenderness. Pain may be referred to the shoulder because of free blood in the peritoneal cavity, and on occasion there are signs of hypovolemic shock. Bloody fluid is usually obtained by culdocentesis.

C. Genitourinary Diseases:

1. Ureteral or renal calculi can produce right lower quadrant pain, nausea, and vomiting suggestive of retrocecal or pelvic appendicitis. A history of colicky pain radiating into the groin, findings on urinalysis, and a plain film of the abdomen often clarify the diagnosis, but an intravenous urogram is frequently required.

2. Pyelonephritis, with or without renal calculi, is also confused with appendicitis. High fever and chills are common with renal infection but infrequent in acute appendicitis. Costovertebral angle tenderness and pyuria establish the diagnosis.

D. Other Acute Surgical Emergencies: A variety of acute surgical emergencies such as perforated ulcer, acute cholecystitis, pancreatitis, diverticulitis, intestinal obstruction, Meckel's diverticulitis, and perforated carcinoma of the colon may simulate appendicitis. Differential diagnosis is discussed separately under each of these conditions. Acute regional enteritis, a nonsurgical condition, may be difficult to distinguish from appendicitis (see Chapter 35).

An additional word about Meckel's diverticulitis is appropriate at this point. Whenever right lower quadrant pain simulating appendicitis is associated with signs of mechanical small bowel obstruction, the possibility of Meckel's diverticulitis should be entertained. The point of maximal tenderness is more medial than in classic appendicitis, but the differential diagnosis may be impossible. If the appendix is found to be normal during an operation for appendicitis, the surgeon must search for Meckel's diverticulum.

E. Systemic Diseases: Any condition producing diaphragmatic irritation (eg, pneumonia) may cause right-sided abdominal pain. Connective tissue diseases which have vasculitis as a prominent feature may present with abdominal pain, and some of these patients require abdominal operation. Nonsurgical disorders associated with abdominal pain and peritoneal signs are discussed in the section on peritonitis (Chapter 32).

Complications

The complications of acute appendicitis include perforation, peritonitis, abscess, and pylephlebitis.

A. Perforation: It is unusual for the acutely inflamed appendix to perforate within the first 12 hours, although cathartics or enemas administered to children by parents may cause perforation at an early stage. Perforation may relieve pain temporarily, but the signs of advancing illness are soon apparent.

The consequences of perforation vary from generalized peritonitis to formation of a tiny abscess which may not appreciably alter the symptoms and signs of appendicitis.

B. Peritonitis: Localized peritonitis results from

microscopic perforation of a gangrenous appendix, while spreading or generalized peritonitis usually implies gross perforation into the free peritoneal cavity. Increasing tenderness and rigidity, abdominal distention, and adynamic ileus are obvious in patients with peritonitis. High fever and severe toxicity mark progression of this catastrophic illness in untreated patients. The management of peritonitis is discussed in Chapter 32.

C. Abscess: Localized perforation of the appendix leads to formation of an appendiceal abscess which is protected from the free peritoneal cavity by omentum or loops of small bowel. In retrocecal or retroileal appendicitis, an abscess is walled off by adjacent structures. If perforation is not contained, abscesses may form in any part of the peritoneal cavity.

Fever, pain, ileus, and sometimes a palpable mass are manifestations of an intraperitoneal abscess. When pus collects in the pelvis, diarrhea is a common symptom, and rectal examination discloses tenderness and fullness in the pouch of Douglas. A pelvic abscess may resorb spontaneously, may perforate into the rectum or other neighboring viscus, or may enlarge and require surgical drainage per rectum or vagina.

Subphrenic abscess is most often seen following generalized peritonitis, but retrocecal appendicitis in particular can cause subphrenic abscess in the absence of generalized peritoneal contamination. The management of subphrenic abscess is discussed in Chapter 32.

Postoperative abscesses are a significant problem. Intraperitoneal abscesses may occur anywhere but most commonly are near the surgical incision. Wound abscesses develop in 5% of primarily closed incisions after removal of an acutely inflamed appendix. If the appendix has perforated, the incidence of wound infection is greater than 30%. When skin and subcutaneous tissues are left open and delayed primary closure is accomplished several days later, the rate of wound infection is reduced to 5%. This subject is discussed further in Chapter 9.

D. Pylephlebitis: Pylephlebitis is suppurative thrombophlebitis of the portal venous system. Chills, high fever, low-grade jaundice, and, later, hepatic abscesses are the hallmarks of this grave condition, which fortunately is rare today. The appearance of shaking chills in a patient with acute appendicitis indicates bacteremia and demands vigorous antibiotic therapy to prevent the development of pylephlebitis.

Treatment

With few exceptions, the treatment of appendicitis is surgical. Early cases of acute appendicitis occasionally subside spontaneously or with the aid of antibiotics, but nonoperative treatment of acute appendicitis should be reserved for rare instances when adequate anesthesia or a competent surgeon is not available.

Some patients presenting late in the course of appendicitis with a palpable right lower quadrant mass and no signs of spreading peritonitis may be managed expectantly. If the mass is a phlegmon, it may resolve on antibiotic therapy; more often, a clearly defined abscess is ready to be drained after a few days. In some patients with appendiceal abscess, appendectomy is deferred for several weeks after the abscess is drained (interval appendectomy).

A. Preoperative Management: Antibiotics should not be administered while observing a patient with abdominal pain of uncertain cause, since antibiotics may suppress clinical signs and make the diagnosis even more difficult. Furthermore, antibiotic therapy can mask developing complications of appendicitis until the situation becomes critical. Intravenous antibiotics are indicated in patients with known perforation, abscess, or peritonitis.

Analgesics may blunt the physical findings but seldom obscure entirely the signs of progressive peritoneal irritation. When pain is severe and the diagnosis is uncertain, analgesics or sedatives may actually assist in clarifying the issue. This is particularly true when the differential diagnosis lies between appendicitis and renal colic.

Preoperative fluid therapy usually is not required in adults with early acute appendicitis, although infants must be given special attention in this regard. In advanced appendicitis with peritonitis, however, resuscitation of the patient before operation is absolutely mandatory. No matter how skillfully performed, appendectomy in a hypovolemic and hyperpyrexic patient may be fatal. Several hours are needed to replenish a severely dehydrated patient with intravenous crystalloid or colloid solutions; the volumes administered should be titrated to the patient's requirements rather than administered according to some arbitrary formula. Skin turgor, perfusion of peripheral tissues, cardiovascular signs, and urinary output are guides to adequate resuscitation. Hyperpyrexia, particularly in children, must be treated before induction of anesthesia; this is best accomplished by external cooling with alcohol sponges, ice packs, or a hypothermic blanket.

A nasogastric tube should be inserted upon admission to the emergency ward and before initiation of diagnostic studies if there is any question of peritonitis, ileus, or obstruction. Nasogastric suction decompresses the stomach and prevents further distention.

B. Anesthesia: Spinal anesthesia may be used, but most surgeons prefer general anesthesia. Care must be taken to prevent aspiration of vomitus if general anesthesia is chosen.

C. Examination Under Anesthesia: After induction of anesthesia, the surgeon should carefully repeat the abdominal, pelvic, and rectal examinations, particularly if there is the slightest doubt about the diagnosis. An ovarian cyst may be palpated in the female, or a mass indicative of carcinoma of the colon may be delineated. Such findings alter placement of the incision.

D. Operation:

1. Incision—In most cases of appendicitis, an oblique muscle-splitting incision of the type shown in Fig 34–2A should be employed. An oblique incision enables the surgeon to deal with lesions in the pelvis,

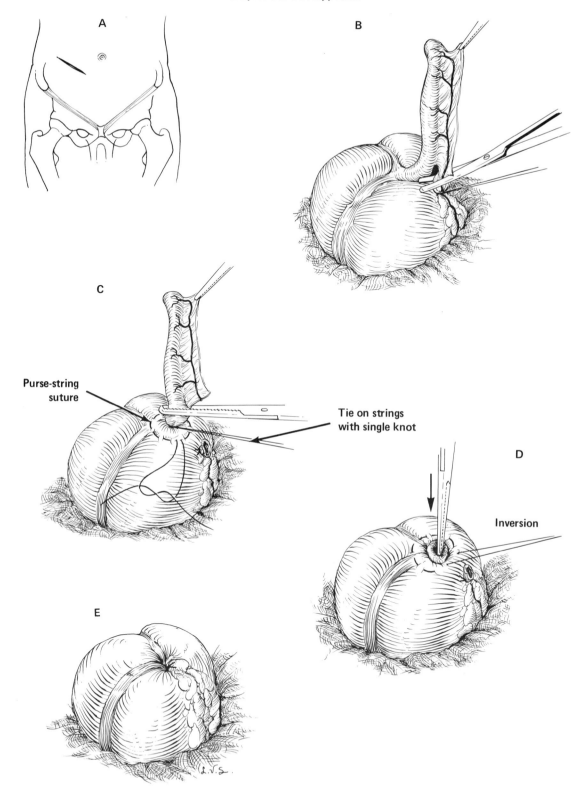

FIG 34–2. Technic of appendectomy. *A:* Incision. *B:* After delivery of the tip of the cecum, the mesoappendix is divided. *C:* The base is clamped and ligated with a simple throw of the knot. *D:* A clamp is placed to hold the knot during inversion with a purse-string suture of fine silk. *E:* The loosely tied inner knot on the stump assures that there is no closed space for the development of a stump abscess.

and it can be carried into the flank or across the rectus muscle to permit a more extensive procedure, such as resection of the right colon. A right rectus incision enters the free peritoneal cavity, and the surgeon must work from there into an area of sepsis, resulting in greater wound morbidity than with the oblique incision.

When the appendix is normal and the acute disease process is located in the upper abdomen, the appendectomy incision should be closed and a separate incision made as indicated in Fig 34–3. Whether the appendix should be removed or not depends upon the circumstances. In the presence of established peritonitis due to some other cause, appendectomy should not be done.

2. Operative approach—The technical approach to the appendix is illustrated in Fig 34–2. The appendix usually can be delivered into the incision. The mesentery is divided between clamps, and the base of the appendix is crushed with a clamp, ligated, and inverted into the cecum. The ligature at the base of the appendix should be of catgut and should be tied (as shown) with only one throw on the knot before inversion. With this technic, an abscess of the appendiceal stump cannot occur because the loose closure will open and be in free communication with the cecal lumen. The ligated base is then inverted into the cecum with a purse-string suture of fine silk or other nonabsorbable suture.

If the appendix is retrocecal or retroileal, it might not deliver easily. It is often preferable to divide the appendix, invert the stump, and remove the appendix in a retrograde fashion. Alternatively, the cecum may be mobilized prior to excision of the appendix. Although the initial incision may be kept quite small in favorable cases, the surgeon should never hesitate to enlarge the incision in either direction to provide better exposure.

If the appendix is acutely inflamed and there is local infection of the peritoneal cavity, no attempt is made to explore the rest of the abdomen. If the appendix is normal or the diagnosis is uncertain, the pelvic viscera and the distal small bowel should be inspected.

After removal of the appendix and inversion of the stump, any fluid should be aspirated from the operative field. Extensive contamination warrants the use of peritoneal irrigation with antibiotics such as kanamycin. Before closure, patency of the ileocecal valve should be ascertained, and the mesoappendix should be checked for secure hemostasis.

The peritoneal cavity should be drained if a well-defined abscess is encountered or if there is so much local necrotic material that an abscess seems likely to form. Drainage of the retroperitoneum is advisable in cases of retrocecal appendicitis with gangrene or perforation because the retroperitoneum is more vulnerable to progressive infection than is the peritoneal cavity. Generalized peritonitis or free fluid resembling pus is not an indication for peritoneal drainage.

Closure of the incision should be accomplished in layers. Whenever there is gross contamination—or if the appendix is gangrenous or perforated—the subcutaneous tissue and skin should be left open. Delayed primary closure can be carried out later by applying paper tapes or by secondary suture. Closure of skin with paper tapes instead of sutures has been shown to cause fewer wound infections in patients with early appendicitis.

E. Postoperative Management: Minimal care is required following appendectomy for simple acute appendicitis. Excessive intravenous fluid administration should be avoided during the first few hours, since bladder distention and catheterization may culminate in chronic urinary tract infection. Bowel function resumes rapidly. Skin sutures are removed on the fourth day and replaced by paper tapes. Most patients are ready for discharge on the fourth or fifth day.

The postoperative care of patients with advanced appendicitis involves intensive management of peritonitis and ileus. Nasogastric suction, antibiotics, and careful fluid and electrolyte replacement are essential. Any patient with peritonitis may develop intraperitoneal abscesses, and a search for localized collections must be made daily. The details of management and indications for drainage of abscesses are discussed as complications of peritonitis in Chapter 32.

Prognosis

Although a mortality rate of zero is theoretically attainable in acute appendicitis, 40 children per year died of appendicitis in England during the period 1963–1967, and a similar incidence of tragic outcomes is reported in the USA. The mortality rate in simple

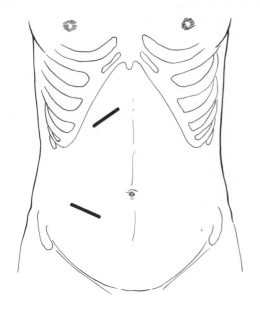

FIG 34–3. When the appendix is found to be normal, the oblique right lower quadrant incision may be closed and a similar small muscle-splitting incision made over the area of suspected disease—in this case, a lesion in the upper abdomen.

acute appendicitis is approximately 0.1% and has not changed significantly since 1930. Progress in pre- and postoperative care—particularly the emphasis on fluid resuscitation before operation, has reduced the mortality rate from perforation to about 5%. Despite declining mortality rates, postoperative infections still occur in 30–50% of patients with gangrenous or perforated appendices. Although most of these patients survive, there are many near fatalities which require lengthy hospitalization and exact an enormous toll from the patient and his family.

Further reduction of morbidity and mortality rates from appendicitis clearly rests with prevention of perforation. The greatest need for improvement lies in the diagnosis of appendicitis in young children and the elderly; in both of these groups, the incidence of perforation reaches 75% or higher. Delay by patient or parent may be unavoidable, but failure on the part of physicians to recognize the disease is disturbing. In one series of children with perforated appendices, 40% had been seen by a physician who failed to appreciate the nature of the process before perforation.

In order to minimize the incidence of perforation, it is necessary to remove a certain number of normal appendices in patients with acute illnesses suggesting appendicitis. This is not to condone careless diagnosis or ill-considered operation, but it is obviously far better to err by performing unnecessary appendectomies than to overlook the acutely inflamed appendix. It is not unreasonable to find normal appendices in 15–20% of patients operated upon with a preoperative diagnosis of acute appendicitis.

Bartlett RH & others: Appendicitis in infancy. Surg Gynec Obst 130:99–104, 1970.

Brooks DW, Killen DA: Roentgenographic findings in acute appendicitis. Surgery 57:377–384, 1965.

Burkitt DP: The aetiology of appendicitis. Brit J Surg 58:695–699, 1971.

Cantrell JR, Stafford ES: The diminishing mortality from appendicitis. Ann Surg 141:749–758, 1955.

Fock G & others: Appendiceal peritonitis in children. Acta chir scandinav 135:534–538, 1969.

Gästrin U, Josephson S: Appendiceal abscess: Acute appendectomy or conservative treatment. Acta chir scandinav 135:539–542, 1969.

Howie JGR: The place of appendicectomy in the treatment of young adult patients with possible appendicitis. Lancet 1:1365–1367, 1968.

Ingram PW, Evans G: Right iliac fossa pain in young women. Brit J 2:149–151, 1965.

Jones FC, Martin JD Jr: Present problems of acute appendicitis. Am Surgeon 38:247–250, 1972.

Magarey CJ & others: Peritoneal drainage and systemic antibiotics after appendicectomy: A prospective trial. Lancet 2:179–182, 1971.

Peltokallio P, Jauhiainen K: Acute appendicitis in the aged patient: Study of 300 cases after the age of 60. Arch Surg 100:140–143, 1970.

Pledger HG, Buchan R: Deaths in children with acute appendicitis. Brit MJ 4:466–470, 1969.

Rang EH & others: An enquiry into the incidence and prognosis of undiagnosed abdominal pain treated in hospital. Brit J Prev Soc Med 24:47–51, 1970.

Sasso RD & others: Leukocytic and neutrophilic counts in acute appendicitis. Am J Surg 120:563–566, 1970.

Sisson RG & others: Superficial mucosal ulceration and the pathogenesis of acute appendicitis. Am J Surg 122:378–380, 1971.

Stone HH & others: Perforated appendicitis in children. Surgery 69:673–679, 1971.

Thomford NR & others: Appendectomy during pregnancy. Surg Gynec Obst 129:489–492, 1969.

TUMORS OF THE APPENDIX

Benign tumors, including carcinoids, were found in 4.6% of 71,000 human appendix specimens examined microscopically. Benign neoplasms may arise from any cellular element and are usually incidental findings. Occasionally, a neoplasm obstructs the appendiceal lumen and produces acute appendicitis. No treatment other than appendectomy is indicated.

Malignant Tumors

Primary malignant tumors were found in 1.4% of appendices in the same large series. Carcinoid and argentaffin tumors comprise the majority of appendiceal malignancies, and the appendix is the commonest location of carcinoid tumors of the gastrointestinal tract. The biologic behavior of carcinoids arising in the appendix is usually benign; tumors greater than 2 cm in diameter are rare, and although local invasion of the appendiceal wall is observed in 25% of cases, only 3% metastasize to lymph nodes and only isolated reports of hepatic metastases and the carcinoid syndrome have appeared. Appendectomy is adequate therapy unless the lymph nodes are obviously involved, the tumor is greater than 2 cm in diameter, or the base of the cecum is invaded. Right hemicolectomy is the treatment of choice for these more advanced lesions.

Adenocarcinoma of the colonic type can arise in the appendix and spread rapidly to regional lymph nodes or implant on ovaries or other peritoneal surfaces. Ten percent of patients have widespread metastases when first seen. Adenocarcinoma is virtually never diagnosed preoperatively; about half present as acute appendicitis, and 15% have formed appendiceal abscesses. Right hemicolectomy should be performed if disease is localized to the appendix and regional lymph nodes. The 5-year survival rate is 63% after right hemicolectomy and only 20% after appendectomy alone, but the latter group includes patients with distant metastases at the time of diagnosis.

Mucocele

Mucocele of the appendix is a cystic, dilated appendix filled with mucin. Simple mucocele is not a neoplasm and results from chronic obstruction of the proximal lumen, usually by fibrous tissue. If the appendiceal contents distally are sterile, mucous cells continue to secrete until distention of the lumen thins the wall and interferes with nutrition of the lining cells; histologically, simple mucocele is lined by flattened, cuboidal epithelium or no epithelium at all. Simple mucocele is cured by appendectomy.

Less commonly, mucocele is caused by a neoplasm—cystadenoma, or adenocarcinoma grade 1 in the older terminology. This lesion may arise de novo or (perhaps) in a preceding simple mucocele. In cystadenoma, the lumen is filled with mucin but the wall is lined by columnar epithelium with papillary projections. Tumor does not infiltrate the appendiceal wall and does not metastasize, although it may recur locally after appendectomy. Cystadenoma is believed to undergo malignant change in some instances. Appendectomy is adequate treatment.

Pseudomyxoma Peritonei

Pseudomyxoma peritonei is a rare disorder characterized by the presence of mucinous material and epithelial cells within the free peritoneal cavity. This lesion usually arises from an ovarian neoplasm, but in some females (and in most men) it originates in the appendix. Whether simple mucocele of the appendix ever produces pseudomyxoma peritonei is unclear; more likely, only cystadenomas are responsible by seeding of cells through the intact cyst wall or by rupture.

Pseudomyxoma peritonei causes difficulty because epithelial cells implanted on peritoneal surfaces may grow autonomously in the manner of a low-grade malignancy even though the histologic appearance is benign. Invasion of abdominal viscera is rare and distant metastases are a curiosity, but pseudomyxoma peritonei has a high propensity to recur locally. Loops of small bowel become entrapped in voluminous quantities of mucin, causing recurrent bouts of intestinal obstruction. Long-term survival and even cure may be achieved by an aggressive surgical approach. All accessible pseudomyxomatous material is removed, and alkylating agents are instilled intraperitoneally. Repeated laparotomies may be necessary. External radiation therapy is of no value in this disorder. In many cases, frank carcinoma eventually develops.

Aho AJ & others: Carcinoid tumors of the appendix: Clinicopathologic and prognostic study of thirty cases. Acta chir scandinav 137:801–806, 1971.

Bernhardt H, Young JM: Mucocele and pseudomyxoma peritonei of appendiceal origin: Clinicopathologic aspects. Am J Surg 109:235–241, 1965.

Collins DC: 71,000 human appendix specimens: A final report, summarizing forty years' study. Am J Proct 14:365–381, 1963.

Flint FB & others: Adenocarcinoma of the appendix. Am J Surg 120:707–709, 1970.

Hesketh KT: The management of primary adenocarcinoma of the vermiform appendix. Gut 4:158–168, 1963.

Long RTL & others: Pseudomyxoma peritonei: New concepts in management with a report of seventeen patients. Am J Surg 117:162–169, 1969.

Melcher DH, Rayan AS: Columnar-cell (non-carcinoid) tumors of the appendix. Brit J Surg 55:693–696, 1968.

Parsons J & others: Pseudomyxoma peritonei. Arch Surg 101:545–549, 1970.

Woodruff R, McDonald JR: Benign and malignant cystic tumors of the appendix. Surg Gynec Obst 71:750–755, 1940.

• • •

General References

Brunn H: Acute pelvic appendicitis. Surg Gynec Obst 63:583–592, 1936.

Fitz PH: Perforating inflammation of the vermiform appendix, with special reference to its early diagnosis and treatment. Am J Med Sci 92:321, 1866.

Hawk JC Jr, Becker WF, Lehman EP: Acute appendicitis. III. An analysis of 1003 cases. Ann Surg 132:729, 1950.

Hoen SO: Factors in the reduction of mortality in acute appendicitis. Surgery 22:402–407, 1947.

Kazarian K, Roeder WJ, Mersheimer WL: Decreasing mortality and increasing morbidity from acute appendicitis. Am J Surg 119:681–685, 1970.

Shepherd JA: Acute appendicitis: A historical survey. Lancet 2:299–302, 1954.

Thomas DR: Conservative management of the appendix mass. Surgery 73:677–680, 1970.

35 . . .

The Small Intestine

Theodore R. Schrock, MD

The small intestine is the portion of the alimentary tract extending from the pylorus to the cecum. The structure, function, and diseases of the duodenum are discussed in Chapter 25; the jejunum and ileum are described in the present chapter.

ANATOMY

Macroscopic Anatomy

The length of the small intestine from the ligament of Treitz to the ileocecal valve depends upon the method of measurement. Autopsy specimens with the mesentery removed average 660 cm (22 feet) in length; the small bowel in life is only about 240 cm (8 feet) long, however, because the tissues are elastic and the mesenteric attachments throw the intestine into convolutions.

The upper two-fifths of the small intestine distal to the **duodenum** are termed the jejunum and the lower three-fifths the **ileum.** There is no sharp demarcation between the **jejunum** and the ileum; however, as the intestine proceeds distally, the lumen narrows, the mesenteric vascular arcades become more complex, and the circular mucosal folds become shorter and fewer in number (Fig 35—1). In general, the jejunum resides in the left side of the peritoneal cavity and the ileum occupies the pelvis and right lower quadrant.

The small bowel is attached to the posterior abdominal wall by the mesentery, a reflection from the posterior parietal peritoneum. This peritoneal fold arises along a line originating just to the left of the midline and passing obliquely to the right lower quadrant. Although the mesentery joins the intestine along one side, the peritoneal layer of the mesentery envelops the bowel and is called the visceral peritoneum or serosa.

The mesentery contains, in addition to fat, several important structures: blood vessels, lymphatics, lymph nodes, and nerves. The arterial blood supply to the jejunum and ileum derives from the superior mesenteric artery. Branches within the mesentery anastomose to form arcades (Fig 35—1), and small straight arteries travel from these arcades to enter the mesenteric border of the gut. It is important to note that the antimesenteric border of the intestinal wall is less richly supplied with arterial blood than the mesenteric side. When blood flow is impaired, the antimesenteric border becomes ischemic first. Venous blood from the small intestine drains into the superior mesenteric vein and then enters the liver through the portal vein.

Submucosal lymphoid aggregates (Peyer's patches) are much more numerous in the ileum than in

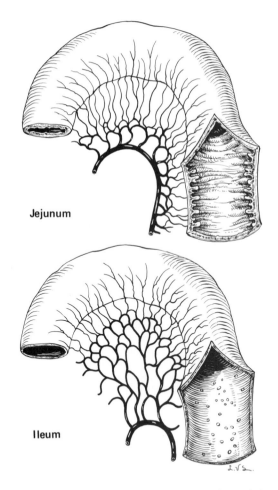

Jejunum

Ileum

FIG 35—1. Blood supply and luminal surface of the small bowel. The arterial arcades of the small intestine increase from 1—2 in the proximal jejunum to 4—5 in the distal ileum, a finding which helps to distinguish proximal from distal bowel at operation. Plicae circulares are more prominent in the jejunum.

the jejunum. Lymphatic channels within the mesentery drain through regional lymph nodes at several levels and terminate in the cisterna chyli.

Parasympathetic nerves from the right vagus and sympathetic fibers from the greater and lesser splanchnic nerves reach the small intestine through the mesentery. Both types of autonomic nerves contain efferent and afferent fibers, but intestinal pain appears to be mediated by the sympathetic afferents only.

Microscopic Anatomy

The wall of the small intestine consists of 4 layers: mucosa, submucosa, muscularis, and serosa.

A. Mucosa: The absorptive surface of the mucosa is multiplied by convolutions and projections at macroscopic, microscopic, and ultrastructural levels. Visible to the naked eye are circular mucosal folds termed plicae circulares (valvulae conniventes), which project into the lumen; they are taller and more numerous in the proximal jejunum than in the distal ileum (Fig 35–1). On the surface of the plicae circulares are delicate villi less than 1 mm in height, each containing a central lacteal, a small artery and vein, and fibers from the muscularis mucosae which lend contractility to the villus. Villi are in turn covered by columnar epithelial

cells which have a brush border consisting of microvilli 1 μm in height (Fig 35–2). The presence of villi multiplies the absorptive surface about 8 times, and microvilli increase it another 14–24 times; the total absorptive area of the small intestine is estimated at 200–500 sq m.

The columnar epithelial cells are responsible for absorption; they probably play an important role in digestion as well, since digestive enzymes are present in high concentrations in the brush border. Mucus-secreting goblet cells are also found in villi.

The crypts of Lieberkühn are situated between villi (Fig 35–3). Undifferentiated cells in the crypts are continually proliferating; some of the cells produced remain undifferentiated, but others become columnar cells and migrate to the tips of villi over a 3- to 7-day period, and still others differentiate to form new goblet cells. Paneth granular cells and argentaffin (enterochromaffin) cells are present in crypts; their functions are not known.

B. Other Layers: The submucosa is a fibroelastic layer containing blood vessels and nerves. Submucosa is the strongest component of bowel wall and must be included in intestinal sutures. The muscularis consists of an inner circular layer and an outer longitudinal

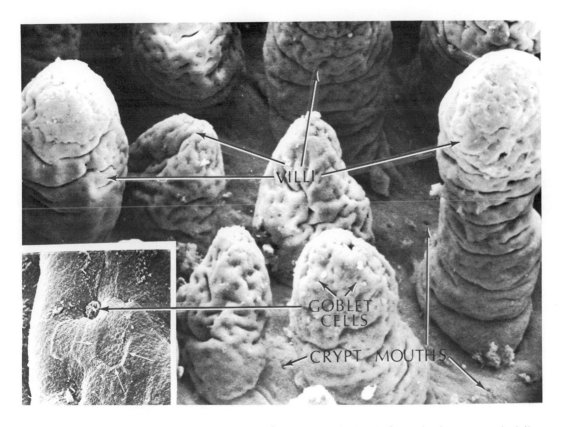

FIG 35–2. Scanning electron microscopic photo of small intestinal villi from the human terminal ileum. (Reduced from × 320.) *Inset:* Detail of a villous surface showing a mucus-filled goblet cell surrounded by polygonal absorptive epithelial cells. (Reduced from × 2100.) Epithelial cell borders are visible (white arrows). The pebbled epithelial cell surface represents closely packed microvilli seen end-on. (Courtesy of Robert L. Owen, MD, and Albert L. Jones, MD.)

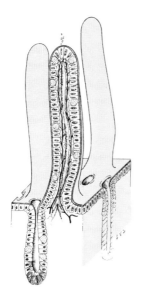

FIG 35–3. Schematic representation of villi and crypts of Lieberkühn. Villus is covered with columnar and goblet cells, and desquamating epithelial cells are seen at the tip. Lamina propria of villus contains an arteriole, a venule, and a central lacteal. The crypt contains Paneth cells and argentaffin cells at its base and mitotic cells which are responsible for epithelial renewal.

coat of smooth muscle. The serosa is the outermost covering of the intestine.

Hirsch J & others: Measurement of the human intestinal length in vivo and some causes of variation. Gastroenterology 31:274–284, 1956.

Marsh MN, Swift JA: A study of the small intestinal mucosa using the scanning electron microscope. Gut 10:940–949, 1969.

PHYSIOLOGY

The principal function of the small intestine is absorption, and a great many physiologic and biochemical mechanisms are integrated to meet this objective. The endocrine function of the small intestine is discussed in Chapters 25 and 28.

Motility

Motility of the small intestine provides for thorough mixing and slow progress of chyme through the alimentary tract. The most important type of muscular activity is the segmental contraction, which mixes chyme with digestive juices and repeatedly exposes the mixture to the absorptive surface. Eccentric contractions are confined to a segment shorter than 2 cm and do not empty the segment completely. Concentric

segmental contractions empty portions of intestine longer than 2 cm. Segmental contractions span only a few centimeters and move chyme slowly in an aboral direction.

Segmental contractions are controlled by a basic electrical rhythm (BER) arising in cells of the longitudinal muscle layer. Each segment of small intestine has a characteristic BER which is independent of nervous influences. The frequency of the BER decreases progressively from duodenum to ileum, but in intact intestine an orally located segment with a higher frequency is partially able to drive an aborally situated neighbor which has a lower frequency. Thus, in man it appears that the controlling BER is located in the duodenum near the ampulla of Vater; segmental contractions occur intermittently, in phase with the BER, at intervals which are some multiple of 3.4 seconds.

Peristalsis in the human small intestine is a short, weak, propulsive movement which travels at about 1 cm/sec for a distance of 10–15 cm before dying out. Peristaltic rushes are powerful waves of contraction which rapidly traverse the entire length of small bowel and are not normally present in man.

Extrinsic innervation modifies (but does not initiate) motility of the small intestine. Gastrointestinal hormones (especially cholecystokinin and secretin), pharmacologic agents, and pathologic states also influence motility.

Digestion & Absorption

With a few exceptions (eg, iron, calcium), the normal small intestine absorbs indiscriminately without regard to body composition. For example, absorption of fat, carbohydrate, and protein is just as complete in the obese patient as in the slender individual. Body composition is regulated through metabolic processes which dispose of substances after they have been absorbed.

A. Water and Electrolytes: Ingested fluid and salivary, gastric, biliary, pancreatic, and intestinal secretions present a total of 5–10 liters of water to the absorptive surface of the small intestine each day, and only 1–1.5 liters are discharged from the ileum into the colon. Water is absorbed throughout the intestine, but the major site of absorption after a meal is in the upper tract.

The net flow of water across the intestinal mucosa is equal to the difference between 2 opposite unidirectional fluxes: from intestinal lumen to interstitial fluid, and from interstitial fluid to intestinal lumen. Net flow of water across the mucosa follows osmotic gradients, and hypertonic solutions in the duodenum and upper jejunum are rapidly brought into ismotic equilibrium with the blood. As large complex molecules are broken down into many smaller ones, the osmotic pressure of the luminal contents increases, and isotonicity is achieved by flux of still more fluid from interstitium to lumen. Net absorption of water by simple diffusion accompanies active transport of ions and small molecules such as glucose and amino acids. If the lumen contains nonabsorbable solute, water is retained to maintain isotonicity. This is the mechanism of action of cathartics such as magnesium citrate and magnesium sulfate.

Net absorption of sodium is also determined by the difference between 2 oppositely directed fluxes. In the jejunum, a large share of net absorption accompanies active transport of hexoses; the bulk flow of water from lumen to blood associated with glucose or galactose absorption carries sodium with it—a phenomenon known as "solvent drag." Active absorption of sodium ion against a small electrochemical gradient occurs in jejunum provided that bicarbonate is present—as it usually is in the normal situation. An efficient transport mechanism for sodium is found in the ileum, where sodium is actively absorbed against steep concentration and electrochemical gradients.

The major share of chloride absorption passively follows electrical gradients from active sodium absorption, but human intestine is able to absorb chloride against an electrochemical gradient as well. Bicarbonate is absorbed by secretion of hydrogen ions into the lumen in exchange for sodium ions; one bicarbonate ion is released into the interstitial fluid for every hydrogen ion secreted, and CO_2 is generated in the lumen. This mechanism is similar to that for acidification of urine in the kidney.

Potassium diffuses passively along electrochemical gradients. Calcium is actively transported against electrochemical gradients, and most is absorbed in the duodenum. Magnesium and phosphate are absorbed by all segments of the intestine; iron is absorbed in duodenum and jejunum, primarily as the ferrous ion.

B. Carbohydrate: As much as 50% of dietary starch is digested by salivary amylase in the stomach, and the remainder is rapidly hydrolyzed by pancreatic amylase in the duodenum. The products of hydrolysis (maltose, maltotriose, and a mixture of dextrins) as well as ingested oligosaccharides are further hydrolyzed by contact with enzymes contained in the brush border of intestinal epithelial cells. The monosaccharides glucose and galactose are actively transported against a concentration gradient by a carrier-mediated mechanism. Fructose is absorbed by diffusion at a rate proportionate to its concentration within the lumen. Monosaccharides are delivered directly into portal blood from the intestinal mucosa.

Although the entire small intestine has the capacity for carbohydrate digestion and absorption, the process is so efficient that under normal circumstances complete absorption of monosaccharides occurs in the duodenum and proximal jejunum.

C. Protein: Protein entering the stomach is denatured by acid and partially digested by pepsin. This mechanism is not essential for protein digestion, and hydrolysis to polypeptides is principally by pancreatic enzymes, chiefly trypsin and chymotrypsin. Polypeptides are attacked by carboxypeptidases and aminopeptidases in or near the brush border, liberating amino acids which are absorbed by means of an active, carrier-mediated transport mechanism. More than 80% of amino acid absorption occurs in the proximal 100

cm of jejunum. Absorption of ingested protein is virtually complete, and the protein excreted in feces is derived from bacteria, desquamated cells, and mucoproteins.

D. Fat: Dietary fat is largely in the form of triglycerides, water-insoluble molecules which must be emulsified in the duodenum in preparation for attack by pancreatic lipase. Fatty acids, monoglycerides, cholesterol, lecithin, lysolecithin, protein, and bile salts are emulsifiers with varying powers. Bile salts by themselves are poor emulsifiers, but when the concentration of bile salts exceeds a certain level (the critical micellar concentration) they spontaneously aggregate with monoglycerides to form micelles. Bile salts in micelles are arranged with the fat-soluble portion of the molecule toward the center of the aggregate and the water-soluble portion at the periphery; this arrangement allows hydrophobic molecules such as free fatty acids, cholesterol, and fat-soluble vitamins to enter the micelles and thus be solubilized in an aqueous environment. Conjugated bile salts have a much lower critical micellar concentration than the unconjugated forms; when bile salts are deconjugated in the intestine (eg, by bacteria, as in blind loop syndrome), monoglycerides and free fatty acids produced by lipolysis precipitate and the efficiency of fat absorption is reduced. Pancreatic lipase is optimally active at the alkaline pH provided by bicarbonate.

Micelles in contact with the microvilli separate into their components, and monoglycerides and fatty acids diffuse through the lipoprotein plasma membrane. Absorption of these substances is completed in the jejunum. Within the endoplasmic reticulum of the mucosal cells, triglycerides and phospholipids are resynthesized and delivered to the lymph as aggregates called chylomicrons. Short- and medium-chain fatty acids are absorbed without passing through a micellar phase, and within the epithelial cells triglycerides are hydrolyzed to constituent glycerol and fatty acids which pass directly into portal blood.

Conjugated bile salts are actively absorbed in the distal ileum and return via portal blood to the liver, where they are again secreted into the bile. Disease or resection of the terminal ileum may compromise fat absorption by allowing the bile salt pool to shrink. Failure of bile salt absorption results in passage of increased amounts of these molecules into the colon, where they impair sodium and water absorption and may cause diarrhea.

E. Vitamins: Vitamin B_{12} (cyanocobalamin) is a water-soluble, high-molecular-weight cobalt compound which is absorbed intact. Other water-soluble vitamins are small enough to be absorbed by passive diffusion, but vitamin B_{12} requires a special mechanism. Dietary vitamin B_{12} complexes with intrinsic factor, a mucoprotein secreted by the gastric parietal cells. The complex is absorbed, probably by pinocytosis, in the distal ileum.

Fat-soluble vitamins—notably vitamins A, D, and K—are dissolved in mixed micelles and absorbed as other lipids are. Since they are totally nonpolar lipids, the absence of bile seriously impairs absorption of these substances.

Code CF (editor): *The Handbook of Physiology.* Section 6: *Alimentary Canal.* Waverly Press, 1967—1968.

Davenport HW: *Physiology of the Digestive Tract,* 3rd ed. Year Book, 1971.

Gray G: Carbohydrate digestion and absorption. Gastroenterology 58:96—107, 1970.

Gray G, Cooper HL: Protein digestion and absorption. Gastroenterology 61:535—544, 1971.

Schultz SG, Friezzell RA: An overview of intestinal absorptive and secretory processes. Gastroenterology 63:161—170, 1972.

SHORT BOWEL SYNDROME

Essentials of Diagnosis

- Massive small bowel resection.
- Diarrhea.
- Steatorrhea.
- Malnutrition.

General Considerations

The absorptive capacity of the small intestine is normally far in excess of need. However, when massive resection of the small intestine is performed for mesenteric vascular occlusion, midgut volvulus, strangulated internal hernia, diffuse inflammatory disease, or congenital atresias, a complex of deficiencies known as the "short bowel" or "short gut" syndrome may develop.

The clinical course following extensive resection depends on the length of bowel resected, the site of resection, and the nature of the underlying disease process. Survival of patients with only a few inches of proximal or distal small intestine has been reported, but in general the nutritional consequences of resecting more than 80% of the gut are profound. Intractable steatorrhea is likely to follow loss of 50—60% of small intestine if the terminal ileum and ileocecal valve are removed, but even a 70% resection may be well tolerated if these structures are preserved. Fistulas, abscesses, and residual intrinsic bowel disease modify the clinical course significantly, and bacterial overgrowth causing deconjugation of bile salts may aggravate fat malabsorption.

Normally, most of the dietary fat, carbohydrate, and protein are absorbed in the jejunum, yet removal of the jejunum is better tolerated than resection of an equivalent length of distal ileum. If jejunum is resected, the ileum may absorb the products of digestion. Removal of distal ileum is poorly tolerated, however, because active transport of bile salts, vitamin B_{12}, and cholesterol is localized to this region (Fig 35—4). If bile salts are not absorbed, absorption of fat is impaired even though the normal site of fat absorption in the jejunum is undisturbed. Defective absorption of calcium and fat-soluble vitamins accom-

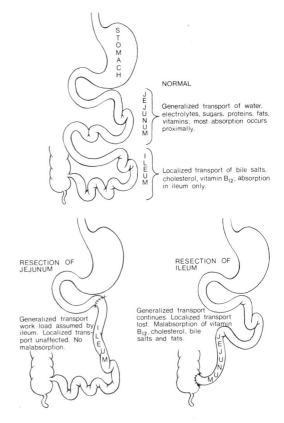

FIG 35—4. The consequences of complete resection of jejunum or ileum are predictable in part from the loss of regionally localized transport processes.

panies steatorrhea. Diarrhea is a direct consequence of distal ileal resection because unabsorbed bile salts and fatty acids enter the colon where they interfere with active transport of sodium and water. The effect of fatty acids on colonic mucosa is similar to the action of castor oil.

Major resection of the midgut may leave insufficient transport capacity to respond to the normal episodic pattern of eating. If the capacity for salt absorption is exceeded, a solute-type diarrhea results. Substances absorbed by passive diffusion, however, are absorbed in proportion to the load. This fact is taken advantage of in dietary manipulations of patients with short bowel syndrome.

Rapid transit through the short gut is partly due to the shorter distance chyme must travel, but changes in motility also contribute. Distal resections have more effect on motility than proximal ones. The mechanisms responsible for this phenomenon are unclear.

Clinical Course

A. Stages: The clinical course following massive resection of small intestine may be divided into 3 stages:

1. Stage 1—During the immediate postoperative

period, massive fluid and electrolyte losses from diarrhea are characteristic. Careful fluid and electrolyte management enables most patients to survive, and the diarrhea lessens in severity after 1–3 months.

2. Stage 2–Requirements for maintenance of nutrition take first priority after diarrhea subsides and oral feedings are begun. Steatorrhea, vitamin deficiencies, hypoproteinemia, and hypocalcemia may occur during this period.

3. Stage 3–If the therapeutic efforts in stage 2 are successful, the patient enters a final period in which a reasonably normal existence is possible with few dietary restrictions. Up to 2 years may be required in order to reach this objective.

B. Adaptation: A major feature of the progress of a patient from stage 1 to stage 3 is the phenomenon of adaptation. By mechanisms which are not understood, the intestine increases its absorptive capacity. Nutritional support during the recovery period facilitates adaptation. At least 4 components of adaptation may be listed.:

1. Villus hypertrophy occurs diffusely throughout the remaining small intestine. Doubling the length of a villus increases its absorptive area by 4-fold.

2. Hyperplasia of epithelial cells–Hyperplasia increases the numbers of epithelial cells of normal size that line the hypertrophied villi. One explanation for this process is that a greater percentage of undifferentiated cells in the crypts differentiate into absorptive cells and migrate to the tips of villi.

3. Increased work load by individual cells is probable although not all investigators agree that this phenomenon occurs.

4. New transport capacity not present in the normal state develops to some extent in gut remnants. It is unlikely, however, that this form of adaptation is adequate to compensate for loss of localized transport mechanisms such as the one for bile salts in the ileum.

C. Gastric Hypersecretion: Some patients develop gastric hypersecretion after massive small bowel resection; it is more marked after proximal resections. The outpouring of gastric juice may damage the mucosa of the proximal intestine, inactivate lipase and trypsin by lowering intraluminal pH, and present a solute load to the intestine in excess of the transport capacity of the remnant. The most attractive explanation for the increased acid production is loss of enterogastrones normally secreted by small intestine.

Treatment

A. General Measures: During the first stage, careful intravenous fluid and electrolyte therapy is essential. Patients should receive nothing by mouth until diarrhea subsides to less than 2.5 liters per day. Intravenous hyperalimentation should be used to supply nutritional needs during this period. Other important measures include control of diarrhea with codeine and maintenance of dry perianal skin to avoid anal irritation.

Initial oral feedings of isotonic fluid should be instituted while intravenous hyperalimentation is still being given. Diet is slowly advanced, and by trial and error a suitable diet for the individual patient is determined. Palatable, isotonic, calorically rich diets are not available at present, and a compromise of one of these desirable characteristics is necessary no matter what is fed. Elemental or "space diets" are far from a panacea; the earliest versions are hypertonic, the constituents require active transport mechanisms, and if the absorptive surface is inadequate they may aggravate diarrhea. Newer isotonic elemental diets are theoretically better, but patient acceptance is still a problem. Fat is added to the diet gradually and is usually maintained at less than 40 g/day. Medium-chain triglycerides may be useful because they are absorbed by passive diffusion and do not require micelle formation, although they may receive limited patient acceptance. Oral glucose reduces intestinal fluid losses in patients with cholera by potentiating active transport of sodium and water and has been successful in patients with jejunostomy; it may prove useful in other forms of short bowel syndrome.

After about 6 months, complete dependence on oral intake may be expected in patients with resection of 80% of the small bowel. Maintenance of body weight at levels 20% below normal or better, bowel habits acceptable to patients, and return to productive life are reasonable expectations.

B. Adjunctive Surgical Procedures: Many types of operations, including reversed segments and recirculating loops, have been tried in the hope of slowing transit and improving absorption. Either may produce a blind loop syndrome due to stasis. Reversed intestinal segments obstruct the bowel if too long or fail to slow transit if too short. At present, neither of these technics has a clearly established role, and, by damaging additional bowel or enhancing bacterial growth, they are likely to potentiate the malabsorption.

A small percentage of patients, usually those with peptic ulcer disease before the enterectomy, eventually require operation for gastric hypersecretion. However, vagotomy or gastrectomy could have undesirable effects, and these procedures should only be done after acid hypersecretion has been definitely implicated as a significant problem (ie, not prophylactically).

Burrington JD: Surgery after massive small bowel resection. Am J Surg 121:213–214, 1971.

Bury KD: Carbohydrate digestion and absorption after massive resection of the small intestine. Surg Gynec Obst 135:177–187, 1972.

Hardison WGM, Rosenberg IH: Bile-salt deficiency in the steatorrhea following resection of the ileum and proximal colon. New England J Med 277:337–342, 1967.

Sedgwick CE, Goodman AA: Short bowel syndrome. S Clin North America 51:675–680, 1971.

Wilmore DW & others: The role of nutrition in the adaptation of the small intestine after massive resection. Surg Gynec Obst 132:673–680, 1971.

Winawer SJ & others: Successful management of massive small-bowel resection based on assessment of absorption defects and nutritional needs. New England J Med 274:72–78, 1966.

Wright HK, Tilson MD: The short gut syndrome: Pathophysiology and treatment. Curr Probl Surg, June, 1971.

INTESTINAL BYPASS FOR OBESITY OR HYPERLIPIDEMIA

A short bowel syndrome may be created deliberately for the treatment of massive obesity, and bypass of the distal ileum has been performed experimentally in some patients with hyperlipidemia.

Intestinal Bypass for Obesity

Massively obese patients—those who weigh 2–3 times the calculated ideal—are handicapped physically, emotionally, socially, and economically. This degree of excessive weight has been termed "morbid obesity" to emphasize the life-threatening seriousness of the condition, and complications such as hypertension, diabetes, hyperlipidemia, menstrual irregularities, and Pickwickian syndrome are often encountered. The cause of morbid obesity is obscure; nonsurgical treatment is aimed at reducing caloric intake and increasing caloric expenditure. Dietary measures, exercise programs, and individual or group psychotherapy are successful in reducing body weight in some patients, but the frequent return to massive obesity once restrictions are relaxed often frustrates patients and physicians and serves in some as justification for surgical creation of malabsorption.

Intestinal bypass for refractory obesity aims to dispose of excess adipose tissue but maintain essential nutrition. The original plan was to restore intestinal continuity after ideal weight was achieved. However, because weight gain promptly returned, most surgeons now intend the procedure to be permanent although potentially reversible.

The first procedure tried was a jejunocolic shunt in which the jejunum was divided close to the ligament of Treitz and the proximal end anastomosed end-to-side to the transverse colon. Serious diarrhea and nutritional depletion led to replacement of this procedure by operations which preserve the ileocecal valve in continuity. It has not yet been settled which is the optimal technic. In the "14 and 4" operation, the jejunum is divided 14 inches (35 cm) from the ligament of Treitz, the distal stump is oversewn, and the proximal end is anastomosed end-to-side to the ileum 4 inches (10 cm) from the ileocecal valve. Insufficient weight loss in some patients has apparently been due to reflux of ileal contents into the defunctionalized segment and has prompted some surgeons to turn to an end-to-end jejunoileostomy in which the bypassed gut is joined separately to the colon and is unavailable to intestinal chyme. The overall operative mortality is 3–5% after these procedures—surprisingly low considering the magnitude of obesity and its secondary effects on cardiorespiratory function.

Without exception, these patients lose weight postoperatively. After an abrupt drop from the catabolic demands of operation, weight declines at a rate of about 4.5 kg (10 lb) a month for 6 months and less rapidly thereafter. In some cases, the weight stabilizes after a year, whereas others continue to lose for several years. Weight reduction below the calculated ideal apparently does not occur; in fact, it may plateau considerably in excess of ideal because of absorptive adaptation of the residual small intestine as in other forms of short bowel syndrome.

Diarrhea is often a problem in the early postoperative period, but in time most patients stabilize at 5 or fewer semiformed stools per day. Current operative procedures allow absorption of at least some of the bile salts by the terminal ileum, and maintenance of the ascending colon in continuity aids in absorption of water and electrolytes. Some patients complain of abdominal flatulence and borborygmus, and dietary regulation may be required to reduce the severity of these symptoms.

The transit time from stomach to cecum for a barium meal has been measured at 5–30 minutes after intestinal bypass. Metabolic studies indicate that these operations cause malabsorption of fat, cholesterol, and vitamins A, D, and K. Abnormal absorption of carbohydrate and protein varies from one series to another, and calcium, magnesium, and potassium absorption depends on the type of surgical procedure performed. Vitamin B_{12} is absorbed if some ileum is retained. The data suggest that patients tend to lose more fat than lean tissue, although atrophy of lean body mass has been observed as well.

Successful rehabilitation of some previously incapacitated patients has fostered optimism regarding these procedures by a number of surgeons. Reservations by skeptics are based on the unknown long-term effects of the drastic alterations of physiology, and it is feared that the entire spectrum of complications is yet to be observed. Of foremost concern is the sequence of fatty infiltration, cirrhosis, liver failure, and death that has been reported in a few cases following intestinal bypass. However, hepatic steatosis is almost universal in massively obese patients before treatment, and the data available at present are insufficient to allow interpretation of the effects of dietary or surgical therapy. Controlled studies are needed to answer these and related questions. Other metabolic complications which have been seen after intestinal bypass include hypocalcemia, renal calculi, and polyarthritis.

At this point, it is advisable to limit the use of intestinal bypass to a few investigative centers where patient selection and the postoperative metabolic changes can be carefully scrutinized. As yet, the optimal surgical procedure remains to be defined, and the long-term metabolic consequences must be determined before these operations can be widely applied.

Intestinal Bypass for Hyperlipidemia

Although the cause of atherosclerosis is not known, progression of the disease is stimulated by hyperlipidemia. Diet, exercise, and hypolipidemic drugs are sometimes effective, but, if serum lipid levels are not reduced by these measures, intestinal bypass may be considered to reduce the risk of atherosclerotic complications.

Bypass of the distal one-third to one-fourth of ileum lowers the cholesterol pool by 2 mechanisms: reduced absorption of cholesterol by the gut, and increased hepatic synthesis of bile salts from cholesterol to compensate for fecal loss. Oral cholestyramine (Cuemid) therapy also lowers blood cholesterol by increasing bile salt turnover and may be tried before considering ileal bypass.

Ileal bypass reduces serum lipid levels in experimental animals on atherogenic diets and also protects against the development of atherosclerotic lesions in these animals. In selected hyperlipidemic patients, it reduces serum lipid levels below the values obtained by dietary measures alone. The total body pool of cholesterol is reduced by about one-third in hyperlipidemic patients, and exchangeable cholesterol in tissues other than blood is also lowered. Physiologic improvement has been reported: symptoms of vascular insufficiency improve, work tolerance increases, xanthomas regress, and progression of coronary artery atherosclerosis appears to halt. The follow-up is too short to state with certainty that prolongation of life will also result.

A few centers are performing ileal bypass for hyperlipidemia under rigidly controlled circumstances. Until the long-term effects are known, the procedure should be considered experimental.

Braasch JW: The surgical treatment of obesity: A study in applied physiology. S Clin North America 51:667–672, 1971.

Buchwald H, Varco RL: Partial ileal bypass for hypercholesterolemia and atherosclerosis. Surg Gynec Obst 124:1231–1238, 1967.

Grundy SM, Ahrens EH Jr, Salen G: Interruption of enterohepatic circulation of bile acids in man: Comparative effects of cholestyramine and ileal exclusion on cholesterol metabolism. J Lab Clin Med 78:94–121, 1971.

Juhl E & others: Liver morphology and biochemistry in eight obese patients treated with jejunoileal anastomosis. New England J Med 285:543–547, 1971.

Morgan AP, Moore FD: Jejunoileostomy for extreme obesity: Rationale, metabolic observations, and results in a single case. Ann Surg 166:75–82, 1967.

Payne JH, DeWind LT: Surgical treatment of obesity. Am J Surg 118:141–147, 1969.

Salmon PA: The results of small intestine bypass operations for the treatment of obesity. Surg Gynec Obst 132:965–979, 1971.

Scott HW Jr & others: Experience with a new technic of intestinal bypass in the treatment of morbid obesity. Ann Surg 174:560–572, 1971.

Scott HW: Metabolic surgery for hyperlipidemia and atherosclerosis. Am J Surg 123:3–12, 1972.

Shibata HR, MacKenzie JR, Huang S: Morphologic changes of the liver following small intestinal bypass for obesity. Arch Surg 103:229–237, 1971.

Weismann RE: Surgical palliation of massive obesity. Am J Surg 125:437–446, 1973.

OBSTRUCTION OF THE SMALL INTESTINE

Essentials of Diagnosis

- Colicky abdominal pain.
- Anorexia; nausea and vomiting.
- Obstipation.
- Abdominal distention.
- Peristaltic rushes.
- Dilated small bowel on x-ray.

General Considerations

Obstruction is the most common surgical disorder of the small intestine, and a variety of lesions intrinsic or extrinsic to the intestine may obstruct the lumen.

A. Etiology:

1. Adhesions–Adhesions are the most common cause of mechanical small bowel obstruction. Congenital bands are seen in children, but adhesions acquired from abdominal operations or inflammation are much more frequent in adults.

2. Hernia–Incarceration of an external hernia is the second most common cause of intestinal obstruction. Inguinal or femoral hernias may have been present for years, or the patient may be unaware of the defect before the onset of obstructive symptoms. An incarcerated hernia may be overlooked by the examining surgeon, particularly if the patient is obese or if the hernia is the femoral type, and a careful search of the groins must be made during evaluation of every patient with acute abdominal illness. Internal hernias into the obturator foramen or foramen epiploicum (Winslow) are rare, but internal herniation is one of several mechanisms by which adhesions produce obstruction. Surgical defects–lateral to an ileostomy, for example–also provide sites for herniation of small bowel loops.

3. Intussusception–Invagination of one loop of intestine into another is rarely encountered in adults and is usually caused by a polyp or other intraluminal lesion. Intussusception is more often seen in children; an organic lesion is not required, and the syndrome of colicky pain, passage of blood per rectum, and a palpable mass (the intussuscepted segment) is characteristic.

4. Volvulus–Volvulus results from rotation of bowel loops about a fixed point, often the consequence of congenital or acquired adhesions. Onset of obstruction is abrupt, and strangulation develops rapidly. Malrotation of the intestine is a cause of volvulus in infants.

5. Foreign bodies–Foreign bodies ingested by children or emotionally disturbed adults or bezoars which form in the stomach after gastrectomy may pass into the intestine and impact the lumen.

6. Neoplasms–Intrinsic small bowel neoplasms can progressively occlude the lumen or serve as a leading point in intussusception. Symptoms may be intermittent, onset of obstruction is slow, and signs of chronic anemia are present. Neoplasms extrinsic to small bowel may entrap loops, and strategically situated lesions of the colon–particularly those near the ileocecal valve—may present as small bowel obstruction.

7. Gallstone ileus—Passage of a large gallstone into the intestine, usually through a cholecystoenteric fistula, may produce obstruction of the small bowel. Gallstone ileus is considered in detail in Chapter 27.

B. Pathophysiology: The small bowel proximal to a point of obstruction distends with gas and fluid. Swallowed air is the major source of gaseous distention because its principal component, nitrogen, is not absorbed by intestinal mucosa. Huge quantities of fluid, most of which originates in the distended segment, fill the proximal bowel. The bidirectional flux of salt and water in distended bowel is disrupted: the flow of water and solute from lumen to blood is normal, at least in the early stages, but the flux from blood to lumen is increased. Fluid and solute are therefore lost from the plasma and interstitial spaces, leading to profound hypovolemia if untreated. Reflexly induced vomiting accentuates the loss of fluid and electrolytes.

Hyperactive peristalsis and audible peristaltic rushes are manifestations of attempts by the small bowel to propel its contents past the obstruction. Bacteria proliferate in the static luminal contents, which become feculent.

Strangulation, or necrosis of the intestinal wall, develops when the mechanism of obstruction obliterates the blood supply to the involved gut. For example, in volvulus the blood vessels are occluded by the obstructing twist. If the blood supply is unobstructed initially, progressive distention can reduce blood flow through the dilated bowel and produce strangulation later. Hemorrhage into the lumen from the gangrenous mucosa exacerbates hypovolemia, and the strangulated intestine may eventually perforate.

Closed-loop obstruction, in which the lumen is occluded at 2 points, is particularly dangerous because distention with fluid is rapid and strangulation is an early threat.

The luminal contents of strangulated intestine are a toxic mixture of bacteria, bacterial products, and necrotic tissue. Some of this material is able to pass through the wall of strangulated bowel into the peritoneal cavity and is absorbed into the circulation. The importance of bacteria in strangulation is demonstrated by the marked reduction in toxicity seen in strangulation obstruction produced experimentally in germ-free animals or animals treated with antibiotics.

Clinical Findings

A. Simple Mechanical Obstruction: If blood supply to the bowel is unimpaired, the obstruction is termed "simple."

1. Symptoms and Signs—The first symptom of obstruction is cramping periumbilical abdominal pain with a crescendo-decrescendo pattern which recurs every few minutes. Anorexia and nausea and vomiting follow after an interval which varies with the level of obstruction. Gastric contents and bile are vomited initially; later, in distal obstructions, the vomitus may become feculent. Obstipation indicates that obstruction of the lumen is complete, but gas and feces present in the colon before the onset may be expelled even in complete small bowel obstruction.

Physical findings are determined by the duration and level of obstruction. Vital signs may be normal in the early stages, but with continued loss of fluid and electrolytes tachycardia, dehydration, and even hypotension are noted. The temperature is normal or mildly elevated with simple obstruction.

The abdomen is distended and mildly tender, and in thin patients peristalsis in dilated loops of small bowel may be visible beneath the abdominal wall. The magnitude of the distention depends partly on the level of obstruction. Distention may be absent in duodenal or proximal jejunal obstruction, and the cause of the vomiting and pain in this situation may go unrecognized for a while. An incarcerated groin hernia is often (but not necessarily) tender. Cramping abdominal pain is coordinated with peristaltic rushes and the high-pitched "tinkles" from churning of gas and fluid. Rectal examination is usually normal.

2. Laboratory findings—In the early stages, laboratory findings may be normal; with progression of disease, there is hemoconcentration, slight leukocytosis, and electrolyte abnormalities which depend on the level of obstruction and the severity of dehydration.

3. X-ray findings—Supine and upright plain abdominal films reveal a ladder-like pattern of dilated small bowel loops with air-fluid levels. These features may be minimal or absent in early obstruction, closed-loop obstruction, or in some cases when fluid-filled loops contain little air. The colon is often devoid of gas unless the patient has been given an enema or has undergone sigmoidoscopy. Opaque gallstones and air in the biliary tree should be looked for routinely.

B. Strangulation Obstruction: Although certain clinical features should make the surgeon suspicious of strangulation, there are no historical, physical, or laboratory findings which exclude the possibility of strangulation in complete small bowel obstruction. At least one-third of strangulating obstructions are thought to be simple before operation, a fact which underscores the unreliability of clinical assessment and the need for early operations when obstruction is complete.

1. Symptoms and signs—Shock in early obstruction is very suggestive of strangulation. When strangulation supervenes in simple obstruction, high fever may develop, previously cramping abdominal pain may become a severe continuous ache, vomitus may contain gross or occult blood, and abdominal tenderness and rigidity may appear.

2. Laboratory findings—Marked leukocytosis not accounted for by hemoconcentration alone should suggest strangulation.

3. X-ray findings—Radiographic findings are similar to those of simple obstruction. Intraperitoneal fluid is seen as a widened space between adjacent loops of dilated bowel and is often found in simple obstruction as well as in strangulation. Air-fluid levels outside the bowel indicate perforation.

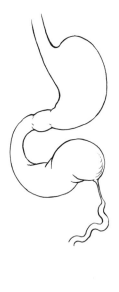 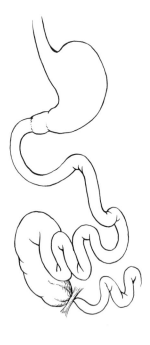 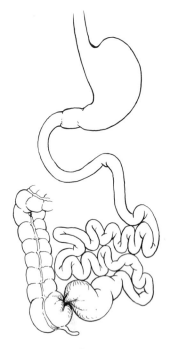

High	**Middle**	**Low**
Frequent vomiting. No distention. Intermittent pain but not classic crescendo type.	Moderate vomiting. Moderate distention. Intermittent pain (crescendo, colicky) with free intervals.	Vomiting late, feculent. Marked distention. Variable pain; may not be classic crescendo type.

FIG 35–5. Small bowel obstruction. Variable manifestations of obstruction depending upon the level of blockage of the small bowel.

C. Variations in the Clinical Findings: (Fig 35–5.) The classic picture of obstruction may be altered in high or low small bowel obstruction.

1. High obstruction—The pain is variable and often described as upper abdominal discomfort rather than cramping periumbilical pain. Profuse vomiting keeps the obstructed segment decompressed so that distention is absent, and the typical radiographic findings are not evident. The vomitus rarely develops a fecal character. Tenderness is generally minimal even with strangulation. Contrast studies may be needed to establish the diagnosis.

2. Low obstruction—Slow onset of vague abdominal discomfort, poorly localized colicky pain, and abdominal distention are typical. Vomiting may occur only hours after onset of the pain and is more often feculent. Contrast media administered orally or through a long intestinal tube may be needed to establish the diagnosis and the level of obstruction.

Differential Diagnosis

Adynamic (paralytic) ileus accompanying various inflammatory conditions in the abdomen may be difficult to differentiate from mechanical small bowel obstruction. This problem is particularly vexing in the postoperative period. Localized abdominal tenderness (eg, in the right lower quadrant with appendiceal abscess) and plain films showing uniform distribution of gas throughout the stomach, small bowel, and colon are helpful clues. Contrast studies may be required to distinguish ileus from obstruction in some patients.

Acute gastroenteritis, acute appendicitis, and acute pancreatitis can mimic simple intestinal obstruction. Serum amylase levels are generally higher in acute pancreatitis than in obstruction, but modest elevations are seen in the latter condition. Strangulation obstruction may be confused with acute hemorrhagic pancreatitis or mesenteric vascular occlusion.

Pseudo-obstruction occurs in 2 forms: (1) distention of the colon in elderly patients or those with systemic diseases, often related to fecal impaction in the left colon or rectum; and (2) chronic abdominal pain and small bowel dilatation due to abnormal motility. Pseudo-obstruction of the small intestine has been seen in mesenteric disease with disruption of extrinsic nerve supply to the gut, with collagen diseases, with diabetes mellitus, etc. In the colon it has been associated with myxedema, hypokalemia, the use of ganglionic blocking agents, etc, but most cases have no definitely established cause.

Colonic pseudo-obstruction may require decompression of the cecum to avoid perforation. The small bowel variety is best left unoperated, although radical resection has been reported with improvement of the pain and steatorrhea which often accompanies the disorder.

Treatment

Complete obstruction of the small intestine is treated by operation after a period of careful preparation. The compelling reason for operation is that strangulation cannot be excluded with certainty as long as obstruction persists, and strangulation is associated with high morbidity and mortality. The surgeon must avoid being lulled into a false sense of security by the nearly universal improvement in symptoms and signs after preparative measures are instituted. There are exceptions to the general rule that operation be performed promptly; postoperative obstruction, a history of numerous previous operations for obstruction, and abdominal carcinomatosis are situations demanding mature judgment, and judicious nonoperative management may occasionally be in the patient's best interests.

A. Preparation: In general, the longer the duration of obstruction, the longer the period of preparation required. The risk of strangulation must be weighed against the severity of fluid and electrolyte abnormalities and the need for evaluation and treatment of associated systemic diseases. Proper timing of the operation, therefore, is determined by the needs of individual patients.

1. Nasogastric suction—A nasogastric tube should be inserted immediately upon admission to the emergency ward in order to relieve vomiting, avoid aspiration, and reduce the contribution of further swallowed air to the abdominal distention. Some surgeons routinely attempt to pass a long intestinal tube to decompress the bowel below the stomach, but selective use of long tubes for those in whom operation should be delayed or avoided is probably the best policy.

2. Fluid and electrolyte resuscitation—Depending upon the level and duration of obstruction, fluid and electrolyte deficits are mild to very severe, and the period of resuscitation varies accordingly. In simple obstruction, fluid and electrolyte depletion is the principal physiologic problem directly related to the disease. A serious error is to assume that hemoconcentration induced by long-standing obstruction can be corrected by dextrose solutions alone. Fluid lost into the lumen of obstructed bowel or emptied from the stomach by vomiting and nasogastric suction is isotonic, and resuscitation should begin with infusion of isotonic saline solution. Losses of gastrointestinal fluid also entail acid-base deficits, and, since there is no neuroendocrine mechanism for correcting these deficits, the surgeon must do so. Serum electrolyte concentrations and arterial blood gas determinations are guides to electrolyte therapy; potassium is best withheld until urine output is satisfactory. The volume of fluid required and its exact electrolyte compensation must be calculated for each patient, and careful monitoring of clinical signs and attention to associated systemic diseases are imperative. Some patients—notably those with strangulation obstruction—require plasma or blood. Antibiotics should be given if strangulation is even remotely suspected.

B. Operation: Operation may commence when the patient has been rehydrated and vital organs are functioning satisfactorily. Occasionally the toxic effects of strangulation may force operation at an earlier time.

A standard groin incision is used for patients with incarcerated inguinal or femoral hernias, but other types of obstruction require an abdominal incision. Wide exposure is essential, and the position of the incision is partly dictated by the location of scars from previous operations.

Details of the operative procedure vary according to the cause of obstruction. Adhesive bands causing obstruction should be lysed; an obstructing tumor should be resected; and an obstructing foreign body should be removed through an enterotomy. Gangrenous intestine must be resected, but it is often difficult to determine whether obstructed bowel is viable or not. The loop should be wrapped in a warm saline-soaked pack and inspected for color, mesenteric pulsation, and peristalsis several minutes later. If the loop appears nonviable after 15—20 minutes, resection with end-to-end anastomosis is the safest course.

Extirpation of the obstructing lesion is not possible in some patients with carcinoma or radiation fibrosis in the pelvis. Proximal diversion by anastomosing small bowel to colon may be the best procedure in these patients.

Decompression of massively dilated small bowel loops before closure of the abdomen shortens the time for recovery of bowel function postoperatively. Decompression is accomplished by threading a long tube down from above or by needle aspiration through the bowel wall. The needle should be introduced with care to avoid contamination of the peritoneal cavity by bacteria-laden material, and the hole in the intestinal wall should be closed with a suture.

Areas of serosa which have been denuded should be repaired with fine silk sutures or reinforced by suturing an adjacent loop over the denuded portion as a serosal patch. The small bowel should be arranged in regular patterns in the hope that new adhesions will fix the bowel or mesentery to prevent recurrence. Attempts to prevent uncontrolled adhesion formation by surgically fixing the loops of bowel in a suitable relation to one another (Nobel plication procedure) have met with limited success.

Prognosis

The morbidity and mortality rates in small bowel obstruction are related to the presence or absence of strangulation more than to any other single factor. Simple obstruction has a mortality rate of 5—10%, whereas strangulation obstruction has a mortality rate of approximately 25%. When strangulation is complicated by perforation and generalized peritonitis, the outlook is even more grim. Early diagnosis and surgical correction of obstruction are essential to avoid these excessive mortality rates.

Billig DM, Jordan PH Jr: Hemodynamic abnormalities secondary to extracellular fluid depletion in intestinal obstruction. Surg Gynec Obst 128:1274–1282, 1969.

Davenport HW: *Physiology of the Digestive Tract,* 3rd ed. Year Book, 1971.

Maldenado JE & others: Chronic idiopathic intestinal pseudo-obstruction. Am J Med 49:203–212, 1970.

Miller LD, Mackie JA, Rhoads JE: The pathophysiology and management of intestinal obstruction. S Clin North America 42:1285–1309, 1962.

Silen W, Hein MF, Goldman L: Strangulation obstruction of the small intestine. Arch Surg 85:121–129, 1962.

Thomas MA & others: Strangulation obstruction in germ free dogs. Surgery 58:37–46, 1965.

Waldron GW, Hampton JM: Intestinal obstruction: A half century comparative analysis. Ann Surg 153:839–850, 1961.

Wangensteen OH: Historical aspects of the management of acute intestinal obstruction. Surgery 65:363–383, 1969.

Wright HK, O'Brien JJ, Tilson MD: Water absorption in experimental closed segment obstruction of the ileum in man. Am J Surg 121:96–98, 1971.

DIVERTICULAR DISEASE OF THE SMALL INTESTINE

1. MECKEL'S DIVERTICULUM

Meckel's diverticulum occurs in approximately 2% of infants and is the most common congenital anomaly of the gastrointestinal tract. It is due to total or partial persistence of the omphalomesenteric duct.

Meckel's diverticulum is a pouch 1–12 cm long arising on the antimesenteric border of the ileum; 90% are within 100 cm of the ileocecal valve. A fibrous vitello-umbilical cord anchors the tip of the diverticulum to the undersurface of the umbilicus in 10% of cases, and in the remainder the apex is freely mobile.

Meckel's diverticulum is a true diverticulum made up of all layers of intestinal wall. Heterotopic tissue is found in approximately 50% of all Meckel's diverticula and in 85% of symptomatic diverticula. Gastric mucosa with parietal cells is the most common heterotopic tissue and comprises 80% of cases; pancreas and mucosa of the colonic, duodenal, or jejunal type are encountered with lesser frequency.

Clinical Findings

Meckel's diverticula become symptomatic in 15–50% of cases. At least 50% of patients are under 10 years old when symptoms develop, and 80% are under age 30. Secretory activity of heterotopic gastric mucosa and obstruction by various mechanisms are the causes of symptoms in 85% of cases.

A. Symptoms and Signs:

1. Bleeding—Up to 50% of patients with symptomatic Meckel's diverticula present with painless lower gastrointestinal hemorrhage from ulceration. This is the most common cause of severe intestinal bleeding in childhood and usually is seen before age 10.

2. Intestinal obstruction—Approximately 30% of cases of symptomatic Meckel's diverticula present as small bowel obstruction, and 50% have progressed to strangulation by the time operation is performed. Several mechanisms are responsible for obstruction: volvulus around a persistent vitello-umbilical cord, intussusception of the diverticulum, entrapment of a loop of bowel beneath a mesodiverticular band, etc.

3. Acute diverticulitis—Most Meckel's diverticula are broad-based but a narrow neck can be obstructed by healing peptic ulcers, external bands, torsion, diverticuloliths, food particles, or tumors. The resulting abdominal pain, anorexia, nausea and vomiting, abdominal tenderness, fever, and leukocytosis mimic acute appendicitis. Perforation is common in acute diverticulitis.

4. Chronic abdominal pain—A few cases of chronic abdominal pain due to peptic ulceration of Meckel's diverticula have been reported.

B. Laboratory Findings: Laboratory studies reflect the mode of clinical presentation. Radiographic demonstration of Meckel's diverticulum is sometimes successful but should not be attempted in the acutely ill patient.

Treatment

Symptomatic Meckel's diverticula should be removed. Tangential excision and suture closure of the defect is usually satisfactory, but segmental resection of ileum is required for diverticula with wide bases or acute inflammation of adjacent ileum. Diverticula discovered incidentally during laparotomy for unrelated disease should be excised in children or young adults.

Prognosis

Up to 15% of patients with symptomatic Meckel's diverticula die of their disease. This high mortality rate is related to erroneous diagnosis and delayed operation leading to perforation or strangulation.

Aubrey DA: Meckel's diverticulum: A review of sixty-six emergency Meckel's diverticulectomies. Arch Surg 100:144–146, 1970.

Rutherford RB, Akers DR: Meckel's diverticulum: A review of 148 patients, with special reference to the pattern of bleeding and to mesodiverticular vascular bands. Surgery 59:618–626, 1966.

Taneja OP, Taneja S: Diseases of Meckel's diverticulum. Arch Surg 90:349–357, 1965.

2. ACQUIRED DIVERTICULA

Congenital true diverticula of jejunum and ileum (excluding Meckel's) are rare, but false diverticula are found in 1.3% of radiographic studies or autopsy series when specifically sought. These lesions are wide-mouthed sacs measuring 1–25 cm in diameter, consisting of mucosa and submucosa herniated between the mesenteric leaves at sites of vascular penetration through the wall. False diverticula are often multiple; they diminish in frequency from the ligament of Treitz to the ileocecal valve, and are associated with diverticulosis of the duodenum or colon in 30% of cases. The majority of symptomatic patients are over age 60.

Acute intestinal bleeding and diverticulitis susceptible to perforation are the chief modes of presentation. A few patients with multiple diverticula have developed malabsorption from the blind loop syndrome. Barium x-rays may outline the diverticula.

Treatment is the same as for Meckel's diverticulum except that extensively involved portions of intestine may require resection.

Altemeier WA & others: The surgical significance of jejunal diverticulosis. Arch Surg 86:732–745, 1963.

Cooke WT & others: The clinical and metabolic significance of jejunal diverticula. Gut 4:115–131, 1963.

Goldstein F & others: Diverticulosis of the small intestine: Clinical, bacteriologic, and metabolic observations in a group of seven patients. Am J Digest Dis 14:170–181, 1969.

Localio SA, Stahl WM: Diverticular disease of the alimentary tract. Part 2. The esophagus, stomach, duodenum and small intestine. Curr Probl Surg, January, 1968.

Nobles ER: Jejunal diverticula. Arch Surg 102:172–174, 1971.

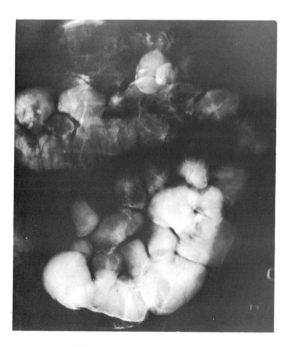

FIG 35–6. Jejunal diverticula.

CROHN'S DISEASE*
(Regional Enteritis)

Essentials of Diagnosis

- Diarrhea.
- Abdominal pain and palpable mass.
- Low-grade fever, lassitude, weight loss.
- Anemia.
- Radiographic findings of thickened, stenotic bowel with ulceration and internal fistulas.

General Considerations

Crohn's disease is a chronic inflammatory disorder affecting the gastrointestinal tract. Three to 5 new cases per 100,000 population are detected annually in Europe and the USA, and the incidence is apparently rising. Males are affected slightly more often than females. Only 25% of patients first manifest the disease after the age of 50; the peak incidence occurs between ages 20–30.

A. Etiology: The cause and pathogenesis of Crohn's disease continue to elude investigators. Some families are predisposed to the disease, suggesting a polygenic genetic influence, but the bulk of evidence favors some other mechanism than inheritance in most cases. Etiologic theories may be grouped under 4 headings:

1. Infectious—There is no direct proof that an infectious organism causes Crohn's disease, but the suspicion persists that some type of transmissible agent is responsible. If so, this organism is probably fastidious, oxygen-sensitive, and certainly difficult to culture.

2. Immunologic—The possibility that Crohn's disease results from an abnormal immunologic response to food products, ingested chemicals, or bacterial protein is under intensive study in many laboratories. The consumer in America is exposed to more than 10,000 well-defined synthetic chemicals and innumerable natural constituents of foodstuffs, and any one of these might be the elusive antigen. There is little positive evidence of a link between these materials and Crohn's disease in man, but in experimental animals it has been shown that various substances are harmful to the intestine in relatively small amounts. Crohn's disease is not caused by bovine milk or milk products, although many patients with Crohn's disease are improved symptomatically by elimination of cow's milk from the diet. Antibodies to dietary protein are found in normal people as well as in patients with disease.

Some patients with Crohn's disease have circulating antibodies to intestinal epithelium, but because these antibodies are not cytotoxic it is probable that they result from tissue damage rather than cause it. Furthermore, Crohn's disease is seen in patients with agammaglobulinemia, in whom circulating antibodies usually do not form. It is possible that cell-mediated hypersensitivity rather than circulating antibodies is an etiologic factor.

*Crohn's disease of the colon is discussed in Chapter 36.

3. **Persorption**—Various types of particulate matter—eg, starch and metallic iron—may be persorbed through intestinal epithelium and travel to other parts of the body in lymphatics and blood. A possible etiologic relationship between this phenomenon and Crohn's disease is under study, but no decisive link has been established.

4. **Psychosomatic**—Few clinicians give much credence to the theory that psychologic factors are important in the etiology of Crohn's disease, although—as might be expected in any· unpredictable chronic disease—some patients do manifest psychologic symptoms once the illness develops.

B. Pathology: Crohn's disease may affect any part of the gastrointestinal tract from the lips to the anus. The terminal ileum is the most common site, eventually becoming diseased in 80% of patients. The distribution of Crohn's disease between small bowel and colon varies from one series to another; average figures indicate that small bowel alone is involved in 50%, both small intestine and colon in 40%, and large bowel alone in 10%. Discontinuous areas of disease with patches of normal bowel between ("skip lesions") are characteristic and occur in 15—25% of patients with disease confined to the small intestine.

There are no specific microscopic features of Crohn's disease. Granulomas are seen in the bowel wall in 50—70% and in mesenteric lymph nodes in 25% of patients. The earliest lesion is thought to be hyperplasia of lymphoid follicles and Peyer's patches with later ulceration of overlying mucosa. These lesions appear grossly as tiny (pinpoint) hemorrhagic spots or clearly delimited shallow ulcers with white bases. The next stage is development of fissures, knife-like clefts beginning in mucosa over lymphoid aggregates and extending deeply into the wall. These fissures and the serpiginous linear ulcers surrounding islands of intact mucosa overlying edematous submucosa give a cobblestone appearance to the luminal surface. Crohn's disease ultimately becomes a transmural inflammatory process with thickening of the bowel wall, and it often progresses to stricture formation. The bowel and its mesentery are foreshortened in advanced cases, and on gross inspection mesenteric fat seems to have advanced on the surface of the bowel toward the antimesenteric border (Fig 35—7).

Clinical Findings

A. Symptoms and Signs: Crohn's disease has protean modes of presentation:

1. **Diarrhea**—Continuous or episodic diarrhea is the cardinal clinical feature of Crohn's disease and is noted in about 90% of patients. Stools are liquid or semisolid and characteristically contain no blood if small bowel alone is diseased. One-third of patients with colonic involvement pass blood, however, and a few individuals present with bloody diarrhea resembling that seen in ulcerative colitis.

2. **Recurrent abdominal pain**—Mild colicky pain initiated by meals, centered in the lower abdomen, and relieved by defecation is common. In patients with

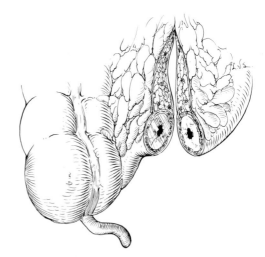

FIG 35—7. Gross appearance of Crohn's disease of the terminal ileum. Note thickened mesentery, thickened intestinal wall, and encroachment of fat over the serosal surface of the ileum. In this patient, the cecum is normal.

more advanced obstruction, pain is severe and often is associated with vomiting.

3. **Abdominal symptoms and constitutional effects**—Episodic attacks of abdominal pain and diarrhea accompanied by lassitude, malaise, weight loss, fever, or anemia is a common symptom complex. A mass is often palpable in the right lower quadrant in these patients. Occasionally, fever of unknown origin is the only clinical finding.

4. **Anorectal lesions**—Chronic anal fissures, large ulcers, complex fistulas-in-ano, or pararectal abscesses are seen in 25% of patients with Crohn's disease confined to small bowel and in 75% of those with colonic involvement. These problems may appear many years before the intestinal disease. Histologic features of Crohn's disease, including granulomas, are often found in biopsies of anorectal lesions even when the only other identifiable disease is located much higher in the gastrointestinal tract.

5. **Anemia**—Iron deficiency anemia or macrocytic anemia due to vitamin B_{12} or folate deficiency may occur in the absence of abdominal symptoms.

6. **Malnutrition**—Protein-losing enteropathy, steatorrhea, and diminished dietary intake from chronic illness contribute to malnutrition and weight loss. Children afflicted with extensive Crohn's disease fail to grow and may have severely retarded sexual maturation.

7. **Acute onset**—Acute abdominal pain and right lower quadrant tenderness mimicking acute appendicitis may be found at operation to be due to acute inflammation of the terminal ileum. In at least two-thirds of such cases, the inflammatory lesion heals spontaneously and chronic Crohn's disease never develops. This condition is discussed further in the section on mesenteric lymphadenitis.

8. Systemic complications—Any of the systemic complications described below may prompt the patient to seek medical advice.

9. Psychologic disturbances—When abdominal manifestations are absent or slight and the emotional effects are pronounced, patients may be erroneously diagnosed as suffering only from psychoneurosis.

B. Laboratory Findings: The results of laboratory tests are nonspecific and vary greatly according to the mode of presentation. Anemia and hypoalbuminemia are common. Stool often contains occult blood, and steatorrhea is quantitated by measurement of fecal fat content. Abnormal D-xylose absorption suggests extensive disease or fistula formation, since carbohydrate is normally absorbed in the upper jejunum. Numerous special studies may be obtained, including cultures of upper intestinal fluid for bacteria and determinations of intestinal enzyme levels.

C. X-Ray Findings: Radiographic studies contribute substantially to the diagnosis of Crohn's disease, although occasionally a patient with Crohn's disease may have normal bowel radiographically. The appearance of small bowel during a barium study is a composite of proliferative and destructive changes. The principal findings include thickened bowel wall with stricture ("hose-pipe"), longitudinal ulceration which is shallow at first but becomes deep and undermining, deep transverse fissures which look like spicules, and cobblestone formation (Fig 35—8). Deformity of the cecum, fistulas, abscesses, and skip lesions are additional findings of importance.

Differential Diagnosis

A. Ulcerative Colitis: Crohn's disease of the colon may be difficult to distinguish from ulcerative colitis, and approximately 5% of colons resected for inflammatory disease remain unclassified after all the evidence has been collected. This topic is covered in detail in Chapter 36.

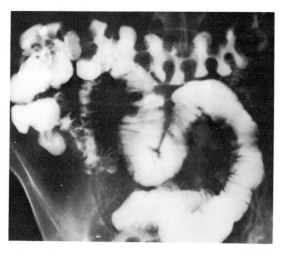

FIG 35—8. Barium x-ray showing spicules, edema, and ulcers in Crohn's disease.

B. Appendicitis: Acute ileitis may be the presenting manifestation, and differentiation from appendicitis may be impossible.

C. Tuberculosis: Tuberculosis may affect any part of the gastrointestinal tract but is uncommon beyond the cecum. Small bowel tuberculosis is discussed elsewhere in this chapter.

D. Ischemic Colitis: Differentiation may be possible by x-ray, but some cases cannot be distinguished until histologic examination of the specimen.

E. Sigmoid Diverticulitis: Some older patients may pose this diagnostic dilemma. If the sigmoid colon is involved with Crohn's disease, proctoscopic examination usually reveals abnormal rectal mucosa as well.

F. Lymphoma: Radiographic findings help differentiate lymphoma from Crohn's disease, but histologic examination of the tissue is occasionally required before the diagnosis is certain.

G. Other Diseases: Carcinoma, amebiasis, and various inflammatory conditions simulate Crohn's disease at times.

Complications

A. Intestinal: Some intestinal complications, such as obstruction, abscess, fistula, and anorectal lesions, are so common that they are regarded as part of the characteristic clinical picture. Free perforation with peritonitis, massive hemorrhage, toxic megacolon, and colonic carcinoma occur but are rare in this disease.

B. Systemic: Systemic complications are similar in Crohn's disease and ulcerative colitis. They consist of liver disease (pericholangitis), uveitis, arthritis, ankylosing spondylitis, aphthous ulcers, and skin manifestations (eg, erythema nodosum).

Treatment

Although the majority of patients with Crohn's disease come to operation eventually, initial therapy is nonoperative and surgery is reserved for the treatment of complications.

Physical rest, relief of stress, and a confiding patient-doctor relationship have favorable effects. Dietary measures such as elimination of bovine milk, low-fat diet, or a high-protein, high-calorie diet may be indicated. Temporary elimination of oral intake and intravenous hyperalimentation improve the nutritional status of severely depleted patients and may even allow healing of fistulas. Sulfonamide drugs or broad-spectrum antibiotics often improve symptoms, especially if bacterial overgrowth is prominent in diseased intestine. Adrenal corticosteroids appear to have an immediate benefit in terms of appetite, fever, and bowel symptoms in more than two-thirds of patients, but it is doubtful that corticosteroids ever bring about healing of the bowel lesion, and long-term administration of high doses has deleterious effects on the patient. Immunosuppressive therapy with azathioprine is still experimental, and apparently conflicting results have emerged from the available studies. The possibility of doing harm with this drug militates against its use except as part of a controlled trial.

In acute ileitis simulating appendicitis, appendectomy may be performed if the appendix and cecum are not involved. This eliminates the concern about appendicitis in future attacks. The involved segment or segments of small bowel should not be resected in this early uncomplicated stage.

Operation is more difficult in the presence of an acute inflammatory process, and these patients more commonly respond to corticosteroids. Chronic partial obstruction is the most common indication for operation and is a manifestation rarely affected by corticosteroids. Conservative resection of diseased small bowel with end-to-end anastomosis is the preferred surgical procedure. If an inflammatory mass adheres to vital structures, however, it may be necessary to bypass rather than resect the involved segment. In these cases, the fecal stream should be diverted completely. Extensive involvement of small bowel, either diffusely or by skip lesions, is unfavorable for curative resection. Resection is usually limited to the area responsible for the complications which prompted operation, and in occasional cases no resection at all is advisable.

Prognosis

Crohn's disease is a chronic, progressive condition. Although in the absence of surgery it usually remains confined to one segment of bowel, extension to other areas often occurs preoperatively. Disease limited to the colon may extend to the small bowel, and Crohn's disease of the small intestine may later involve the colon. The outlook is particularly discouraging for young patients and those with small bowel involvement. Remissions do occur, and in some fortunate individuals the disease seems to burn itself out spontaneously. Whether medical therapy has any long-term benefit on the course of Crohn's disease is debated.

The results of surgical treatment are partly unsatisfactory. Approximately 50% of all patients have no clinical recurrence of disease after primary resection, but the recurrence rate is high in selected groups of patients, and subclinical recurrence may be even more frequent than presently appreciated. Repeated resections have the same risk of recurrence, so that additional patients enter the "free of disease" category after each succeeding operation.

Crohn's disease does shorten life expectancy. In one study, the number of deaths—corrected for age, sex, and length of observation—was twice as large in patients with Crohn's disease as in the general population.

Banks BM & others: Morbidity and mortality in regional enteritis. Am J Digest Dis 14:369–379, 1969.

Cooke WT, Fielding JF: Corticosteroid or corticotrophin therapy in Crohn's disease (regional enteritis). Gut 11:921–927, 1970.

Dyer NH & others: The incidence and reliability of individual radiographic signs in the small intestine in Crohn's disease. Brit J Radiol 43:401–408, 1970.

Dyer NH & others: Diagnosis of Crohn's disease: A continuing source of error. Brit MJ 1:735–737, 1970.

Engel A, Larsson T (editors): *Regional Enteritis (Crohn's Disease).* Nordiska Bokhandelns Forlag (Stockholm), 1971.

Goligher JC & others: Crohn's disease, with special reference to surgical management. Progr Surg 10:1–23, 1972.

Gump FE, Lepore M, Barker HG: A revised concept of acute regional enteritis. Ann Surg 166:942–946, 1967.

Krause U & others: Crohn's disease: A clinical study based on 186 patients. Scandinav J Gastroent 6:97–108, 1971.

Kyle J: *Crohn's Disease.* Appleton-Century-Crofts, 1972.

Law DH: Regional enteritis. Gastroenterology 56:1086–1110, 1969.

Perrett AD & others: The liver in Crohn's disease. Quart J Med 40:187–209, 1971.

Sjöström B: Acute terminal ileitis and its relation to Crohn's disease. Pages 73–76 in: *Regional Enteritis (Crohn's Disease).* Engel A, Larsson T (editors). Nordiska Bokhandelns Forlag (Stockholm), 1971.

Sparberg M, Kirsner JB: Long-term corticosteroid therapy for regional enteritis: An analysis of 58 courses in 54 patients. Am J Digest Dis 11:865–880, 1966.

OTHER INFLAMMATORY & ULCERATIVE DISEASES OF THE SMALL INTESTINE

Acute Mesenteric Lymphadenitis

The cause of acute mesenteric lymphadenitis has long been regarded as infectious, but only recently has an organism been identified. Recent research also suggests the possibility that acute mesenteric lymphadenitis and acute regional enteritis may be etiologically related. Obscure, nonhemolytic coccobacilli, *Yersinia pseudotuberculosis* and *Y enterocolitica,* have been cultured from appendiceal contents, lymph nodes, and bowel wall in both children and adults with mesenteric lymphadenitis or acute regional enteritis. Yersiniae are rarely found except in these conditions, and serologic tests suggest that the bacteria have caused infection.

Acute mesenteric lymphadenitis usually occurs in children with abdominal pain, variable gastrointestinal symptoms, fever, and abdominal tenderness simulating acute appendicitis. The differential diagnosis is often difficult, although the fever is higher and the abdominal tenderness is more diffuse than in appendicitis.

If operation is performed, large, inflamed lymph nodes are encountered in the mesentery of terminal ileum. The appendix is removed, and its contents may be cultured for Yersinia organisms. Although fatal septicemia has been reported in a few cases, yersinia infections are usually self-limited. The organisms are sensitive to penicillin, tetracyclines, and other antibiotics, but treatment is not required unless the patient is severely ill.

Hubbert WT & others: *Yersinia pseudotuberculosis* infection in the United states: Septicemia, appendicitis, and mesenteric lymphadenitis. Am J Trop Med 20:679–684, 1971.

Weber J, Finlayson NB, Mark JBD: Mesenteric lymphadenitis and terminal ileitis due to *Yersinia pseudotuberculosis.* New England J Med 283:172–174, 1970.

Pseudomembranous Enterocolitis

Pseudomembranous enterocolitis is an inflammatory disease of the small bowel or colon (or both) and has even been found in the stomach. The pathologic findings include focal areas of mucosal necrosis which coalesce and deepen with formation of a characteristic pseudomembrane consisting of necrotic mucosa, cellular debris, and bacteria.

Some cases of pseudomembranous enterocolitis are caused by overgrowth of *Staphylococcus aureus* following prolonged antibiotic therapy. Oral administration of antibiotics in large doses for several days in order to prepare the colon for surgery is notorious in this regard. Other patients, however, have received no antibiotics, and indeed the disease was known before the antibiotic era; the cause in these cases is obscure.

Lethargy, weakness, fever, nausea and vomiting, diarrhea, abdominal pain and distention, and systemic toxicity are the hallmarks of the fully developed syndrome, but sudden circulatory collapse due to abrupt loss of gastrointestinal fluids may be the first manifestation.

Treatment must be instituted promptly. Massive fluid and electrolyte resuscitation, nasogastric decompression, and specific antibiotic therapy for the predominant organism in the stool are imperative. Fecal enemas to supply gram-negative bacteria have been tried in some cases of staphylococcal overgrowth. The mortality rate is nearly 100% in some series, and many deaths occur within a few hours after the first appearance of clinical signs. Adherence to strictly rational indications for the ordering of broad-spectrum antibiotics may be the best means of prevention.

Azar H, Drapanas T: Relationship of antibiotics to wound infection and enterocolitis in colon surgery. Am J Surg 115:209–217, 1968.

Birnbaum D, Laufer A, Freund M: Pseudomembranous enterocolitis: A clinicopathologic study. Gastroenterology 41:345–352, 1961.

Tuberculosis

Primary tuberculous infection of the intestine, caused by ingestion of the bovine strain of *Mycobacterium tuberculosis,* is rare in the USA. Secondary infection, due to swallowing the human tubercle bacillus, is much less common now than formerly, affecting less than 1% of patients with pulmonary tuberculosis.

The distal ileum is the most common site of involvement. The bacillus localizes in the mucosal glands and spreads to Peyer's patches, where inflammation, sloughing of tissue, and local attempts at walling off give rise to symptoms. The pathologic reaction is either hypertrophic or, more commonly, ulcerative. Hypertrophic tuberculous enteritis results in stenosis, and the symptoms and signs are those of obstruction. The ulcerative form causes alternating constipation, diarrhea, and occasionally progressive inanition. Free perforation, fistula formation, or hemorrhage may be seen in severe untreated cases.

Antituberculous chemotherapy is the mainstay of management if the diagnosis is certain, but carcinoma and regional enteritis may be difficult to exclude. surgery is required for disease resistant to chemotherapy or if complications develop. Resection is the preferred surgical procedure, and bypass is done only if abscesses or fistulas are present. The prognosis is good if the patient is operated on in the early stages of the illness.

Bentley G, Webster JHN: Gastrointestinal tuberculosis: A 10-year review. Brit J Surg 54:90, 1967.

Bacillary Dysenteries

Infection of the small bowel with *Salmonella typhosa* produces an acute illness with fever, maculopapular rash, abdominal pain, and diarrhea in the fully developed case, although symptoms are minimal in some patients. Peyer's patches become hypertrophied and the overlying mucosa may ulcerate, leading to perforation or hemorrhage. Free perforation requires operation. Hemorrhage occurs in about 15% of patients, but laparotomy is seldom necessary. The inflamed, friable bowel is treacherous to handle, and every effort should be made to avoid operation. Chloramphenicol, nasogastric suction, and intensive fluid and electrolyte management are usually successful.

Shigellosis in the adult may be confused with other diseases. Dysentery, fever, and abdominal pain are typical, and bloody diarrhea is seen in half of patients. Shigellosis is treated with antibiotics. The diagnosis is established by stool cultures and smears.

Barrett-Connor E: Shigellosis in the adult. JAMA 198:717–720, 1966.

Huckstep RL: Recent advances in the surgery of typhoid fever. Ann Roy Coll Surg England 26:207–230, 1960.

Amebiasis

Amebic ulceration of the small bowel is much less common than colonic involvement. Amebiasis is discussed in Chapter 10.

Nonspecific Ulceration

Isolated, discrete, single or multiple ulcerations of undetermined cause may occur in the small bowel. They are often on the antimesenteric border and less commonly are circumferential. The ileum is involved twice as frequently as the jejunum. Abdominal pain, perforation, hemorrhage, or obstruction may bring the condition to medical attention. Treatment is generally by surgical resection.

Alexander HC, Schwartz GF: Nonspecific jejunal ulceration in search of an etiology. Gastroenterology 50:224–230, 1966.

Guest JL: Nonspecific ulceration of the intestine. Internat Abstr Surg 117:409–416, 1963.

Shands WC, Gatting RR: Circumferential small bowel ulcers: A report of nine cases. Ann Surg 165:894–899, 1967.

Ulceration Due to Enteric-Coated Potassium

Circumferential mucosal ulcerations overlying a zone of cicatricial narrowing have been seen in patients taking enteric-coated potassium chloride. Experimental studies show that this preparation may cause venous spasm, submucosal edema, mucosal ulceration, and stenosis of the bowel. Obstruction, perforation, or hemorrhage may result. This disease has become uncommon since the cause was recognized and the use of enteric-coated potassium chloride was virtually abandoned. Resection is the treatment of choice; the results are excellent unless perforation has occurred.

Boley SJ & others: Experimental evaluation of thiazides and potassium as a cause of small-bowel ulcer. JAMA 192:763–768, 1965.

Shands WC, Gatting RR: Circumferential small bowel ulcers: A report of nine cases. Ann Surg 165:894–899, 1967.

Radiation Enteropathy

Aggressive radiotherapeutic attempts to treat abdominal or pelvic malignancy are associated with some gastrointestinal injury in nearly every case because proliferating intestinal epithelial cells are extremely radiosensitive. Degeneration of cells and edema of bowel wall may produce abdominal pain, nausea and vomiting, and sometimes bloody diarrhea during therapy or a few months later. Symptoms are minor and transient for most patients receiving radiation therapy with modern technics.

Injury to blood vessels in the bowel wall is far more serious than the early mucosal lesion. Endothelial proliferation and endarteritis gradually obliterate the vessel lumen over months or years, producing chronic intestinal ischemia. Hemorrhage, perforation, or stenosis may develop from the vascular lesion.

The incidence of significant bowel injury is dose-related and varies from 5% after 4500 rads to 30% after 6000 rads. Fixation of small bowel loops in the radiation field by adhesions from previous operations greatly increases the risk of intestinal complications.

Surgery may be required for obstruction, hemorrhage, perforation, abscess, or fistula formation. Obstructed patients often relate a long history of abdominal complaints, and obstruction is sometimes mistakenly attributed to residual or recurrent malignancy. If resection of the involved segment is not possible, bypass should be performed. It is imperative that normal bowel be used for anastomoses, because disruption of suture lines in diseased intestine is predictable and catastrophic. Irradiated bowel is friable despite its thickened appearance, and care must be taken in freeing adhesions.

The operative mortality is about 10–15%, and the prognosis thereafter depends on the extent of involvement and the presence of tumor. In one series, only 33% of 100 patients with significant gastrointestinal complications of radiation therapy were alive after 5 years. Patients with localized disease amenable to resection do very well, whereas results are discouraging with patients who have surgically untreatable fistulas or short bowel syndrome.

DeCosse JJ & others: The natural history and management of radiation induced injury of the gastrointestinal tract. Ann Surg 170:369–384, 1969.

Roswit B, Malsky SJ, Reid CB: Severe radiation injuries of the stomach, small intestine, colon and rectum. Am J Roentgenol 114:460–481, 1972.

SMALL BOWEL FISTULAS

Essentials of Diagnosis

- Fever and sepsis.
- Abdominal pain.
- Localized abdominal tenderness.
- External drainage of small bowel contents.
- Dehydration and malnutrition.

General Considerations

External fistulas of the small bowel may form spontaneously as a result of disease, but the vast majority are complications of surgical procedures with anastomotic dehiscence or injury to bowel during dissection. Fistulas are particularly prone to develop when the surgeon encounters extensive adhesions or inflamed intestine.

Clinical Findings

A. Symptoms and Signs: Postoperative fistula formation is heralded by fever and abdominal pain until bowel contents discharge through the abdominal incision. Spontaneous fistulas from neoplasms or inflammatory disease usually develop in a more indolent manner. Most fistulas are associated with one or more abscesses, which often drain incompletely with fistulization so that persistent sepsis is a common feature. Intestinal fluid escaping through the fistula may severely excoriate the skin of the abdominal wall. Fluid and electrolyte losses may be severe, especially if the fistula is large, if it is located in the upper tract, or if there is partial or complete intestinal obstruction distal to the fistula. Persistent sepsis and difficulty in nourishing the patient contribute to rapid weight loss.

B. Laboratory Findings: Routine laboratory tests reflect the severity of deficits in red cell mass, plasma volume, and electrolytes. Leukocytosis due to sepsis and hemoconcentration is common. Disease of other organs such as liver and kidneys may be detected.

C. X-Ray Findings: Abscesses and intestinal obstruction may be evident on plain abdominal films. Contrast medium administered orally, per rectum, or through the fistula (fistulogram) delineates the abnormal anatomy, including intrinsic bowel disease, and demonstrates the location and number of fistulas, the length and course of fistula tracts, associated abscess cavities, and the presence of distal obstruction. Chest films, excretory urograms, and other special studies may be indicated in certain individuals.

Complications

Fluid and electrolyte losses, malnutrition, and sepsis contribute to multiple organ failure and death unless effective therapy is instituted promptly.

Treatment

A systematic approach combining diagnostic, supportive, and operative procedures is essential in the management of patients with fistulas (Table 35–1). In few other conditions is the proper timing of operative intervention more critical.

A. Fluid and Electrolyte Resuscitation: Many fistula patients are profoundly depleted of intravascular and interstitial volume, and replacement of this fluid with isotonic saline solution takes first priority. Central venous pressure, urine output, and skin turgor are guides to the progress of volume resuscitation. Blood is sent to the laboratory for measurement of serum electrolyte concentrations, and in critical situations arterial blood pH and P_{CO_2} should be determined. Results of these studies assist in correcting electrolyte deficits and deranged acid-base balance. Fluid should be collected from fistula output, nasogastric suction, and urine for measurement of volume and electrolyte composition. Body weight is recorded daily. Fluid and electrolyte resuscitation can usually be accomplished within the first few days. Subsequent maintenance of homeostasis depends on accurately measuring fluid and electrolyte losses and replacing them.

B. Control of Fistula: Fistula drainage fluid must be collected to avoid excoriation of skin and abdominal wall tissues and to record volume losses. Temporary ostomy appliances, catheters, Karaya gum rings, and at times prone positioning on a Stryker frame have

all been used. Ingenuity and improvisation must be relied on in devising the best technic for the individual patient.

C. Control of Sepsis: Obvious and easily accessible abscesses should be drained surgically as soon as they are diagnosed. The source of sepsis is often obscure, and a continuous diligent search for the abscess or abscesses must be made by repeated physical examinations and radiologic studies until the infection is located and treated. Blind therapy with broad-spectrum antibiotics is not a substitute for surgical drainage of abscesses.

D. Delineation of Fistula: Radiographic contrast studies (see above) should be obtained as soon as practicable.

E. Nutrition: Adequate nutrition and control of sepsis make the difference between survival and demise of these patients. A useful general rule is to avoid all oral intake at the outset. Nasogastric suction may be necessary temporarily. As soon as intravascular fluid and electrolytes are restored, intravenous hyperalimentation should be instituted through a centrally positioned catheter. Occasionally, an arteriovenous fistula is constructed in an extremity in order to maintain a patient on hyperalimentation for prolonged periods. The details of hyperalimentation are described in Chapter 13.

In the long run, nutrition through the alimentary tract is preferable to parenteral technics, and feeding into the gut should begin as soon as possible. The method depends on the location of the fistula and the associated anatomy. With high fistulas, fluid may be collected proximally through one catheter and instilled distally through another. In others, a small, soft catheter attached to a tiny mercury-weighted balloon may be passed orally and threaded past the fistula. A Baron pump continuously instills blended food through the tube and provides adequate calories. Distal fistulas may not require such measures, and regular diets or special low-residue artificial diets may be given by mouth.

The greatest difficulty is presented by mid small bowel fistulas. These patients cannot be fed by any method other than intravenously.

The average patient receives treatment by both routes, with the objective being an intake (ie, a net positive balance) of 3000 Cal or more per day.

F. Operation: Although some fistulas close spontaneously, others persist despite drainage of abscesses and provision of adequate nutrition. Failure of a fistula to resolve may be caused by distal obstruction, neoplasm or foreign body at the fistula site, and extensive disruption of bowel continuity. If fistula output does not diminish on optimal treatment, operation should be undertaken. The fistulous segment should be resected, associated obstruction relieved, and continuity reestablished by end-to-end anastomosis. Bypass without resection may be indicated in some patients. The various surgical procedures are illustrated in Fig 35–9.

TABLE 35–1. Treatment of fistulas.

First:
Restore blood volume and begin correction of fluid and electrolyte imbalance.
Drain accessible abscesses.
Control fistula and measure losses.

Second:
Provide intravenous hyperalimentation.

Third:
Delineate anatomy of fistulas by radiographic studies.
Begin alimentary feedings if possible.

Fourth:
Maintain caloric intake of 3000 Calories or more per day.
Drain abscesses as they appear.
Operate if fistula fails to close.

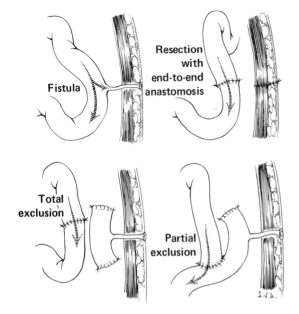

Fistula

Resection with end-to-end anastomosis

Total exclusion

Partial exclusion

FIG 35—9. Surgical procedures which may be used to remove or defunctionalize small bowel fistulas.

Prognosis

The plan of management outlined above has resulted in 90% survival of patients with external fistulas. Uncontrolled sepsis is the most important cause of death.

Chapman R, Foran R, Dunphy JE: Management of gastrointestinal fistulas. Am J Surg 108:157—164, 1964.

Halverson RC, Hogle HH, Richards RC: Gastric and small bowel fistulas. Am J Surg 118:968—972, 1969.

Nassos TP, Braasch JW: External small bowel fistulas. S Clin North America 51:687—692, 1971.

Sheldon GF & others: Management of gastrointestinal fistulas. Surg Gynec Obst 133:385—389, 1971.

ACUTE VASCULAR LESIONS OF THE SMALL BOWEL & MESENTERY

The blood supply to the gastrointestinal tract derives from the celiac, superior mesenteric, and inferior mesenteric arteries, with collateral connections to other arterial systems at either end. Venous blood from small bowel drains into the portal vein. Lesions producing acute or chronic ischemia or hemorrhage may result from intrinsic vascular disease, systemic illness, pharmacologic agents, and surgical procedures. Chronic occlusion may be amenable to vascular reconstruction and is discussed in Chapter 39.

1. ACUTE MESENTERIC VASCULAR OCCLUSION

Essentials of Diagnosis

- Severe, diffuse abdominal pain.
- Nausea and vomiting.
- Constipation or diarrhea.
- Minimal physical findings.

General Considerations

Sudden occlusion of major small bowel arteries or veins is catastrophic. It is predominately a disease of the elderly and is highly lethal. Mesenteric arterial **emboli** are most commonly from mural thrombus in an infarcted left ventricle or clot in a fibrillating left atrium in patients with mitral stenosis. **Thrombosis** of a mesenteric artery is the end result of atherosclerotic stenosis, and these patients often relate a history of intestinal angina before the acute thrombosis occurs. Other causes of acute arterial occlusion such as dissecting aortic aneurysm or fusiform aortic aneurysm are rare. Thrombosis of major mesenteric veins is associated with liver cirrhosis, abdominal sepsis, or no apparent underlying disease. In recent years, mesenteric venous thrombosis has appeared in women taking oral contraceptives.

The consequences of major vascular occlusion depend on the vessel involved, the level of occlusion, the status of other visceral vessels, the development of collaterals, and other factors. The first effect is intestinal spasm followed shortly by hemorrhagic necrosis of the mucosa, the layer most sensitive to ischemia. The mucosa ulcerates, sloughs, and bleeds. Bacteria proliferate in the ischemic segment, and infection contributes further to thrombosis of small vessels. Bacterial growth is not essential for a fatal outcome, but absorption of toxic products through the peritoneal surface is an important factor hastening the demise of untreated patients.

Ischemia progresses to full-thickness infarction of bowel wall as early as 6 hours or as long as several days after arterial occlusion. Hemorrhage into the lumen, accumulation of bloody abdominal fluid, diffuse peritonitis, and cardiovascular collapse ensue even in the absence of gross perforation.

Venous occlusions typically develop peripherally and progress insidiously, causing segmental infarction which resembles strangulation obstruction.

Clinical Findings

A. Symptoms and Signs: The most constant symptom is severe, poorly localized abdominal pain which is often unresponsive to narcotics. Nausea and vomiting and diarrhea or constipation are variable.

In the early stages there is a striking paucity of abdominal findings; in fact, pain out of proportion to the objective findings is a hallmark of mesenteric vascular occlusion. Even so, mesenteric infarction also occurs with much less severe pain, and serious illness may be recognized only later, when secondary toxicity develops. Later in the course, abdominal distention and tenderness occur. Shock and generalized peritonitis eventually develop, but by that time the opportunity for salvage has been lost. In some instances—particularly with a high venous occlusion—shock is an early finding. Stool and gastric contents may contain blood. Paracentesis does not help establish the diagnosis in the reversible stages, but later it is positive.

B. Laboratory Findings: Striking leukocytosis and some elevation of serum amylase are present. Hemoconcentration and the effects of hemorrhage into the lumen or mesentery are reflected in laboratory tests in the late stages.

C. X-Ray Findings: Plain abdominal films may be normal in the early stages of this disease. Absence of the normal amount of gas in the small intestine due to spasm of the bowel wall has been noted. Blunting of plicae, thickening of bowel wall, and rigid narrowing of the lumen with hairpin turns are all changes which may be seen on plain films and collectively are relatively specific. Later, small and large bowel may be dilated to the midtransverse colon, but this sign seldom aids in establishing the diagnosis with certainty. The appearance of gas in the portal venous system is a late sign. Selective angiography is diagnostic and should be used if the diagnosis is uncertain and the delay is justified.

Differential Diagnosis

Acute pancreatitis and strangulation obstruction of the intestine may be difficult to distinguish from mesenteric vascular occlusion. A very high serum amylase early in the disease suggests pancreatitis. Differentiation from strangulation obstruction is less important since both conditions require operation. Angiography may be definitive. Unfortunately, even surgeons with a special interest in this condition are unable to make an early diagnosis in more than half of cases; the clinical picture in these is simply nonspecific.

Treatment

Mesenteric vascular occlusion is treated surgically. Operation reveals segmental or diffuse ischemia or infarction of small bowel and colon in the distribution of the occluded vessel. If reversible ischemia is due to occlusion of the superior mesenteric artery, vascular reconstruction should be attempted. The best results are achieved in the embolic group because the embolus often lodges at the level of the middle colic artery and is accessible for removal. Thrombotic lesions of superior mesenteric artery origin require thromboendarterectomy, and patency rates are poor.

Segmental infarctions should be resected. Extensive irreversible infarction of the entire small bowel and right colon is a hopeless situation. Diffuse ischemia of bowel without frank infarction may be treated with heparin and antibiotics rather than extensive resection. In most cases, a "second look" operation should be performed 12–24 hours later to ascertain the viability of remaining bowel and to construct an anastomosis if this was not done at the first operation. Infarctions related to venous occlusion must be resected.

Prognosis

Acute mesenteric vascular occlusion is a lethal lesion if infarction is extensive; delay in performing operation and the technical difficulties of reconstructing occluded mesenteric vessels are important reasons for the grim prognosis. The mortality rate exceeds 70%, with the best results in patients with embolic occlusion or infarction localized to short segments.

Boley SJ: *Vascular Disorders of the Intestine.* Appleton-Century-Crofts, 1971.

Corter D, Einhaber A: Intestinal ischemic shock in germ-free animals. Surg Gynec Obst 122:66–76, 1966.

Friedman G, Sloan WC: Ischemic enteropathy. S Clin North America 52:1001–1012, 1972.

Marston A: Diagnosis and management of intestinal ischaemia. Ann Roy Col Surg Eng 50:29–44, 1970.

Matthews JE, White RR: Primary mesenteric venous occlusive disease. Am J Surg 122:579–583, 1971.

Ottinger LW, Austen WG: A study of 136 patients with mesenteric infarction. Surg Gynec Obst 124:251–261, 1967.

Pierce GE, Brockenbrough EC: The spectrum of mesenteric infarction. Am J Surg 119:233–239, 1970.

Scott JR & others: Acute mesenteric infarction. Am J Roentgenol 113:269–279, 1971.

Tomchik FS & others: The roentgenographic spectrum of bowel infarction. Radiology 96:249–260, 1970.

Ulano HB & others: Selective dilatation of the constricted superior mesenteric artery. Gastroenterology 62:39–47, 1972.

2. NONOCCLUSIVE INTESTINAL INFARCTION

One-half of all patients with intestinal infarction have no thrombosis of major arteries and veins. Many of these patients are hypotensive from cardiac disease or septicemia, and intestinal ischemia is caused by "low flow" through the splanchnic circulation. In a few patients, there is no systemic disease and infarction seems to be a primary phenomenon.

The clinical picture is similar to that of occlusive disease, but the onset is less often dramatic. Patchy or diffuse ischemia or infarction of bowel is variable in extent and severity. Ischemia is most pronounced on the antimesenteric border, and the mucosa is extensively involved before abnormalities are visible on the serosal surface. The major vessels are patent, but small arteries and veins may be thrombosed as the result of prolonged low flow. There are often ischemic areas in other organs such as liver and spleen.

There is no evidence that vascular reconstruction contributes to survival, and surgical procedures are limited to resection of infarcted bowel. Extensive involvement is almost uniformly fatal; efforts should be directed toward reversal of the low-flow state before frank infarction develops so that operation may be avoided. Treatment of the underlying disease is of primary importance. Infusion of glucagon or isoproterenol into the superior mesenteric artery is worth trying in these critically ill patients.

Britt LG, Cheek RC: Nonocclusive mesenteric vascular disease: Clinical and experimental observations. Ann Surg 169:704–711, 1969.

Fogarty TJ, Fletcher WS: Genesis of nonocclusive mesenteric ischemia. Am J Surg 111:130–137, 1966.

Williams LF & others: Nonocclusive mesenteric infarction. Am J Surg 114:376–381, 1967.

3. OTHER VASCULAR LESIONS

Vasculitis

Vascular lesions associated with systemic disorders such as polyarteritis nodosa or scleroderma may cause patchy infarction of the small intestine. Similar lesions have been seen recently in patients with a history of amphetamine abuse. The presenting manifestation is usually perforation with peritonitis or intraluminal bleeding. The prognosis depends on the underlying pathologic process and the severity of peritoneal contamination. These patients are often on corticosteroid therapy and do not tolerate infection well. Survivors are uncommon.

Mesenteric Apoplexy

Mesenteric apoplexy is an uncommon disorder caused by spontaneous rupture of mesenteric arteries. The more general category of **abdominal apoplexy** includes spontaneous hemorrhage into the peritoneal cavity from tumors (particularly hepatomas), the spleen, or other organs. Arteriosclerotic lesions are the cause of arterial rupture in older individuals; the superior mesenteric, right colic, and branches of the celiac artery are the usual sites. Sudden hemorrhage from congenital aneurysms occurs in younger patients; the splenic artery is most commonly involved and is particularly prone to rupture during pregnancy (see also Chapter 29).

The typical picture is sudden onset of diffuse abdominal pain followed by hypotension. A "double rupture" of splenic artery aneurysms is seen in about half of cases; bleeding initially is confined to the lesser sac, and 1–2 days later this collection breaks into the greater sac with exsanguinating blood loss. These symptoms may be confused with mesenteric vascular occlusion, rupture of an abdominal aortic aneurysm, or perforated viscus. There is diffuse abdominal tenderness and distention due to free blood in the peritoneal cavity. The diagnosis is usually clear from signs of internal blood loss and peritoneal irritation, but paracentesis is sometimes helpful.

Operation is imperative. The site of bleeding is located, and the involved vessel is ligated. Rarely, the bleeding artery can be reconstructed with autogenous or prosthetic material. If blood supply to portions of the intestinal tract is impaired, segments of bowel may have to be resected. Splenectomy with ligation of the splenic artery is preferred for patients with a ruptured splenic artery aneurysm.

Vascular Tumors & Malformations

These lesions are discussed below in the section on tumors.

GAS CYSTS
(Pneumatosis Cystoides Intestinalis)

Pneumatosis cystoides intestinalis is a rare condition characterized by the presence of gas-filled cysts in the wall and mesentery of the gastrointestinal tract. It may occur at any time of life but is most common in middle age. Most of these cysts are subserosal, but a few are submucosal; the areas of bowel most often involved (in descending order of frequency) are the proximal jejunum, the ileocecal region, and the colon. Cysts vary in size from microscopic to several centimeters in diameter.

Associated diseases of the gastrointestinal tract such as pyloric stenosis due to peptic ulcer, inflammatory bowel lesions, diverticulitis, or scleroderma are present in 85% of cases. The origin of the gas is not known but is presumed to be the intestinal lumen. Intestinal obstructive lesions producing high intraluminal pressure may be responsible in some cases.

Rarely, infection with gas-forming bacteria can produce a similar picture on x-ray. These latter patients are usually toxic and may have impaired immunologic defenses predisposing to the unusual invasion.

Symptoms are usually those of the underlying disease, and the cysts are detected incidentally on plain films of the abdomen. Rarely, perforation of a cyst, hemorrhage, obstruction, or malabsorption may bring the condition to attention.

Treatment is directed to the underlying disease. Pneumatosis itself is benign except in those infrequent cases when complications require operation. The cysts often resolve spontaneously and disappear.

Hughes DTD & others: Pneumatosis cystoides intestinalis. Gut 7:553–557, 1966.

Sawyer RB & others: Infectious emphysema of the gastrointestinal tract in the adult. Am J Surg 120:579–583, 1970.

TUMORS OF THE SMALL INTESTINE

Neoplasms of the jejunum and ileum are found in less than 1% of autopsy cases and comprise 1–5% of all tumors of the gastrointestinal tract. The terminal ileum is the favored site, followed by proximal jejunum. Approximately 85% of patients are over age 40. There is a high correlation of small bowel tumors with primary neoplasms elsewhere.

Only 10% of small bowel tumors are symptomatic. Benign lesions are 10 times as common as malignant ones, but at least 75% of symptomatic neoplasms are malignant. Obstruction and bleeding (acute or chronic) are the most frequent symptoms, and malignant tumors occasionally perforate.

1. BENIGN TUMORS

Polyps

Many varieties of intestinal tumor assume a polypoid configuration. Adenomatous or villous polyps of the type seen in the colon rarely occur in the small bowel; they are usually solitary, and cause symptoms by intussusception or bleeding.

Many "adenomas" are actually hamartomas when closely examined. These lesions are believed to be developmental abnormalities rather than neoplasms and therefore have no malignant potential. Patients with solitary lesions are free of associated anomalies. Hamartomas are multiple in 50% of cases, and 10% of these have a familial disorder characterized by diffuse gastrointestinal polyposis and mucocutaneous pigmentation (**Peutz-Jeghers syndrome**). The implications of Peutz-Jeghers syndrome are controversial. Patients may succumb to obstruction or hemorrhage from polyps, but most authors doubt that the polyps ever become malignant. Resection should be reserved for complications. Operation for bleeding is difficult because of diffuse involvement of the entire small bowel. Extensive resection is not warranted in this condition.

Gardner's syndrome is another familial disease characterized by multiple intestinal and colonic polyps, osteomas, and subcutaneous cysts or fibromas. The polyps in Gardner's syndrome are true neoplasms, and malignant degeneration is common: 8 of 13 deceased family members in Gardner's original kindred died of carcinoma of the colon.

Juvenile (retention, inflammatory) polyps are nonneoplastic accumulations of granulation tissue in small bowel or colon. Bleeding or obstruction is seen occasionally. Juvenile polyps usually autoamputate as the child approaches adolescence.

Gannon PG & others: Polypoid glandular tumors of the small intestine. Surg Gynec Obst 114:666–672, 1962.
Spiro RK: False cancer of the intestine: The inflammatory polyp. Am J Gastroenterol 52:364–369, 1969.

Vascular Tumors

Vascular tumors are multicentric in the small bowel in 55% of cases and may involve the intestine diffusely. Hemangiomas may bleed or intussuscept in children and young adults. **Hereditary hemorrhagic telangiectasia** (Rendu-Osler-Weber syndrome) is an inborn progressive tendency toward formation of dilated endothelial spaces in small bowel and other sites. Vascular malformations are not neoplasms, but they present the same diagnostic and therapeutic problems as vascular tumors.

It may be difficult to locate the bleeding point in these patients. Arteriography may help if performed during active hemorrhage, and calcified lesions may be evident on plain films. If a patient is known to have diffuse vascular lesions and the bleeding site is unknown, it is best to avoid operation if at all possible. The surgeon who is forced to operate for persistent hemorrhage and has no clues to the site of bleeding may need to use various maneuvers, including transillumination or compression of bowel between 2 glass slides. Blind resection is often followed by recurrent episodes of hemorrhage.

Monroe LS, Spencer FM: The clinical significance of hereditary hemorrhagic telangiectasia. Gastroenterology 38:906–911, 1960.

Other Tumors

Leiomyomas, lipomas, neurofibromas, fibromas, and a variety of other tumors are usually asymptomatic.

2. MALIGNANT TUMORS

Primary

Adenocarcinoma of small bowel usually arises in proximal jejunum and causes symptoms for prolonged periods before a diagnosis is made. Metastases are present in 80% at the time of operation. Segmental resection of bowel and adjacent mesentery is done when possible, but metastases deposited near the superior mesenteric artery make this a more difficult procedure than colonic resection for cancer. Five-year survival is only 25% in patients undergoing intestinal resection.

Primary lymphosarcoma or **reticulum cell sarcoma** arising in the terminal ileum may diffusely infiltrate the submucosa, producing a long rigid segment. Some patients present with fever of unknown origin, and up to one-third present with malabsorption syndrome. Sprue-like villous atrophy is often associated with lymphoma, but it is not clear whether this is cause, effect, or coincidence. Wide segmental resection, followed by radiation therapy if nodes are involved, is the treatment of choice.

Leiomyosarcoma in small bowel tends to ulcerate centrally and bleed.

Other types of primary malignant neoplasm are extremely rare.

Metastatic

Small bowel metastases are found in 50% of patients dying of malignant melanoma. Carcinomas of the cervix, kidney, breast, etc may also spread to bowel. Obstruction or hemorrhage may require operation if the patient's life expectancy is otherwise reasonably good. Significant palliation may be achieved, particularly in patients with solitary metastatic lesions.

Brookes VS & others: Malignant lesions of the small intestine. Brit J Surg 55:405–410, 1968.

Cohen A & others: Neoplasms of the small intestine. Am J Digest Dis 16:815–824, 1971.

Ebert PA, Zuidema GD: Primary tumors of the small intestine. Arch Surg 91:452–455, 1965.

Kahn LB & others: Primary gastrointestinal lymphoma: A clinicopathologic study of fifty-seven cases. Am J Digest Dis 17:219–232, 1972.

McPeak CJ: Malignant tumors of the small intestine. Am J Surg 114:402–411, 1967.

Ostermiller W & others: A clinical review of tumors of the small bowel. Am J Surg 111:403–409, 1966.

3. CARCINOID TUMORS & CARCINOID SYNDROME

The small bowel is the second most common site (after the appendix) of carcinoid tumors. About 10 times as many originate in the ileum as in the jejunum. Carcinoids occur in patients 25–45 years of age and are often associated with other primary neoplasms.

Carcinoid tumors arise from argentaffin (Kulchitsky) cells in the crypts of Lieberkühn and form yellowish, firm nodules in the submucosa; special stains may demonstrate argentaffin granules. Multiple tumors are present in 50% of cases.

Carcinoid of the small bowel should be regarded as "a malignant neoplasm in slow motion." At the time of surgical diagnosis, 40% of tumors have invaded the muscularis and 33% have metastasized to lymph nodes or liver. Fewer than 2% of primary tumors less than 1 cm in diameter metastasize, but 80% of those larger than 2 cm have spread at the time of operation. Huge metastatic deposits emanating from a minute primary are sometimes encountered.

Clinical Findings

A. Symptoms and Signs: Small tumors are usually asymptomatic. Overall, 30% of small bowel carcinoids cause symptoms of obstruction, pain, bleeding, or the carcinoid syndrome. Obstruction due to sclerosis and kinking of the bowel may be related to elaboration of vasoactive materials by metastases in the mesentery.

About 10% of patients with small bowel carcinoids present with **carcinoid syndrome**, and others develop it later. The syndrome consists of cutaneous flushing, diarrhea, bronchoconstriction, skin rash, and right-sided cardiac valvular disease due to collagen deposition. Biologically active substances secreted by carcinoids are usually inactivated in the liver, but hepatic metastases or primary ovarian or bronchial carcinoids release these compounds directly into the systemic circulation where they produce the complex of symptoms. No single substance is believed to be responsible for the entire spectrum of symptoms and a host of active materials have been implicated, including serotonin, catecholamines, histamine, 5-hydroxytryptophan, bradykinin, prostaglandins, and ACTH.

B. Laboratory Findings: Some carcinoid tumors are detected by radiographic methods. Urinary levels of 5-hydroxyindoleacetic acid (5-HIAA) can be measured in clinical laboratories, but a negative qualitative or low quantitative test does not rule out carcinoid syndrome because 5-HIAA is a metabolite of serotonin, which is only one of many mediators of the syndrome. Provocative tests of various types can be used in some patients, but full laboratory investigation of these patients is a research effort.

Treatment

All surgically accessible carcinoid tumor in small bowel mesentery and the peritoneal cavity should be removed, and repeated operations may be required. Whether this policy should be extended to include palliative resection of liver metastases is highly debatable. The tumor responds poorly to fluorouracil and other cytotoxic drugs.

Carcinoid syndrome can be treated by various pharmacologic agents designed to block the effects of active substances; this form of therapy requires definition of the responsible mediator(s) in individual patients. Among the agents sometimes used are phenothiazines, methysergide, methyldopa, corticosteroids, and adrenergic blocking drugs.

Prognosis

Carcinoid tumors grow slowly over months and years. The overall 5-year survival after resection of small bowel carcinoid is 70%; 40% of patients with inoperable metastases and 20% of those with hepatic metastases survive 5 years or longer.

A complication of advanced carcinoid that has received attention recently is intestinal infarction due to occlusion of the superior mesenteric artery by sclerosis surrounding metastatic deposits in the mesentery.

Anthony PP: Gangrene of the small intestine: A complication of argentaffin carcinoma. Brit J Surg 57:118–122, 1970.

Moertel CG & others: Life history of the carcinoid tumor of the small intestine. Cancer 14:901–912, 1961.

Sanders RJ, Axtell HK: Carcinoids of the gastrointestinal tract. Surg Gynec Obst 119:369–380, 1964.

Teitelbaum SL: The carcinoid: A collective review. Am J Surg 123:564–572, 1972.

• • •

General References

Sleisenger M, Fordtran J: *Gastrointestinal Disease.* Saunders, 1973.

Veidenheimer MC (editor): Symposium on gastrointestinal surgery. S Clin North America 51:535–828, 1971.

36...

The Large Intestine

Walter Birnbaum, MD

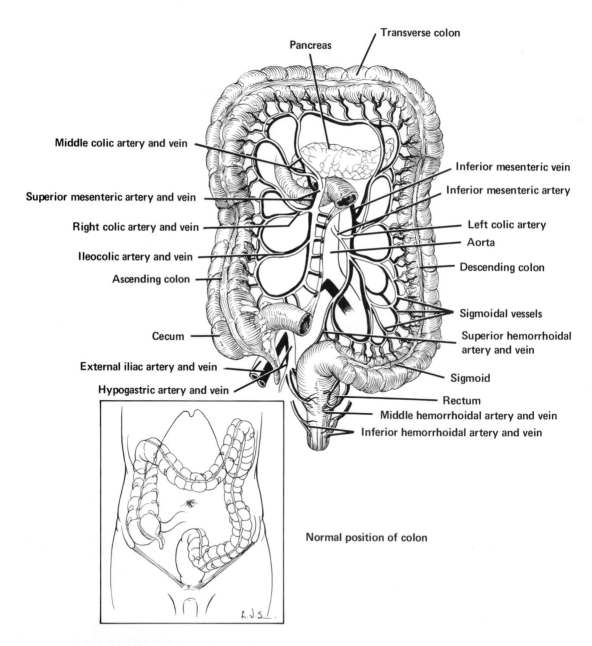

FIG 36–1. The large intestine: anatomic divisions and blood supply. The veins are shown in black. The insert shows the usual configuration of the colon.

ANATOMY

The colon extends from the end of the ileum to the rectum. Its principal anatomic divisions are the cecum, appendix, ascending colon, hepatic flexure, transverse colon, splenic flexure, descending colon, sigmoid colon, and rectosigmoid colon (Fig 36—1). Its caliber is greatest at the cecum and diminishes distally. It is sacculated, has fatty appendages (the appendices epiploicae), and is fixed in its ascending and descending portions. It has 2 muscular layers: an outer longitudinal layer and an inner circular layer. The outer longitudinal muscle coat is concentrated into 3 bands called teniae between which the longitudinal layer is imperceptibly thin. Contractions of the circular muscle occur at intervals, producing sacculations called haustra. These contractions have been observed to move longitudinally and therefore are not fixed anatomic structures. The wall is so thin that the colon distends markedly when it becomes obstructed.

The rectum is 12—15 cm in length. The longitudinal muscle, which is concentrated into the 3 teniae throughout the colon, spreads at the rectosigmoid junction and completely encircles the rectum. The lowermost portion of the rectal mucosa is required for recognition of the urge to defecate. Sacrifice of this portion of the rectum, as in some operations for malignancy, results in incontinence even though the sphincteric ring is intact.

The rectum is normally capacious and distensible. When its distensibility is lost because of surgery or disease, normal bowel habits are interfered with. Habitual use of laxatives, especially mineral oil, causes constant filling of the ampulla with a resulting vicious cycle of constipation and catharsis. The upper rectum is invested by peritoneum anteriorly and laterally, but posteriorly it is retroperitoneal up to the termination of the sigmoid colon. In females, the pelvic peritoneum—the rectouterine pouch (of Douglas)—is anterior to the rectum. Tumor masses or abscesses in this location are readily palpated on digital rectal examination.

Perforation of the rectum into the peritoneal cavity may occur at a much lower level anteriorly than posteriorly, a fact to be noted when lesions are biopsied or fulgurated or after direct trauma through the rectum. During sigmoidoscopic examination, the most difficult level to bypass with the instrument is where the intra- and extraperitoneal portions of the bowel meet. A local muscular contraction occurs here although no true sphincter has been demonstrated. The rectal valves of Houston are 3 prominent mucosal folds within the rectum, arranged spirally, 2 on the left and one on the right. Normally the valves appear thin, with sharp edges. They become thickened and blunted with inflammation. A rectal valve may hide a small lesion from endoscopic view and during sigmoidoscopy must be "ironed out" so that its superior surface can be examined.

In males, the prostate gland, the seminal vesicles, and the seminal ducts lie anterior to the rectum. The

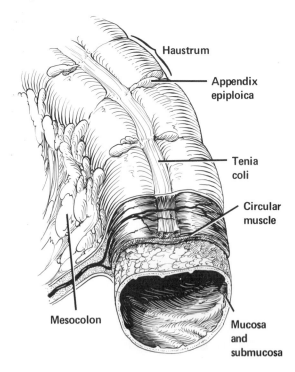

FIG 36—2. Cross-section of colon.

prostate usually is easily felt, but the seminal vesicles are not palpable unless distended because the firm, unyielding rectovesical fascia of Denonvilliers intervenes. In the female, the rectovaginal septum and uterus lie anterior and the uterine adnexa anterolateral to the rectum. The structures are easily palpated with one finger in the vagina and one in the rectum.

Blood Supply & Lymphatic Drainage

The arterial supply of the right colon, from the ileocecal juncture to approximately the mid transverse colon, is from the superior mesenteric artery through its ileocolic, right colic, and middle colic branches.

The **inferior mesenteric artery** arises from the abdominal aorta about 3.8 cm (1½ inches) above the level of the aortic bifurcation and may be covered by the lower border of the third part of the duodenum. The artery gives off the left colic and sigmoid branches and then becomes the superior hemorrhoidal artery. It passes close to the left ureter and left spermatic vessels, which are in danger during ligation of the inferior mesenteric artery. The **vasa recti** are the terminal arterial branches to the colon and run directly to the mesenteric wall or through the bowel wall to the antimesocolic border.

The colic arteries bifurcate and form arcades about 2.5 cm (1 inch) from the mesenteric border of the bowel, forming a pathway of communicating vessels called the **marginal artery of Drummond**. The marginal artery thus forms an anastomosis between the superior mesenteric and inferior mesenteric arteries. The configuration of the blood supply, however, varies greatly; the "typical" pattern is present in only 15% of individuals.

The middle hemorrhoidal artery arises on each side from the anterior division of the internal iliac artery or from the internal pudendal artery and runs inward in the lateral ligaments of the rectum. The inferior hemorrhoidal arteries are branches of the internal pudendal arteries and pass through Alcock's canal. The anastomoses between the superior hemorrhoidal vessels and those from the internal iliac arteries provide collateral circulation which is important after surgical interruption or atherosclerotic occlusion of the vascular supply of the left colon.

Veins & Lymphatics

The **veins** accompany the corresponding arteries and drain into the liver through the portal vein. There are continuous **lymphatic plexuses** in the submucous and subserous layers of the bowel wall which drain into the lymphatic channels and lymph glands that accompany the blood vessels.

Nerve Supply

The **sympathetic nerves** originate in T7–12, travel in the thoracic splanchnic nerves to the celiac plexus and then to the preaortic and superior mesenteric plexuses, from which postganglionic fibers are distributed along the superior mesenteric artery and its branches to the colon. The **parasympathetic nerves** to the right colon come from the right vagus to the celiac plexus, pass to the preaortic and superior mesenteric plexuses, and thence accompany the branches of the superior mesenteric artery to the right colon. The parasympathetic nerve supply of the left colon originates in L1–3, joins the lumbar ganglionated sympathetic chains, and leaves as the lumbar splanchnic nerves which join the preaortic plexus. The sympathetic supply is inhibitory to the bowel wall, whereas the parasympathetics contract it.

Bacon HE, Recio PM: *Surgical Anatomy of the Colon, Rectum and Anal Canal.* Lippincott, 1962.

Michels MA & others: Routes of collateral circulation of the gastro-intestinal tract as ascertained in a dissection of 500 bodies. Internat Surg 49:8–28, 1968.

Pace JL: Anatomy of the haustra of the human colon. Proc Roy Soc Med 51:934–935, 1968.

Torsoli A, Ramorino ML, Crucioli V: The relationship between anatomy and motor activity of the colon. Am J Digest Dis 13:462–467, 1968.

PHYSIOLOGY

The small bowel efficiently digests and absorbs nutrients from ingested foods and passes the residue along to the colon for further processing. The solids in the ileal effluent are largely undigested plant materials such as cellulose. The colon extracts electrolytes and water from the ileal fluid, converting it into semisolid feces which are stored until defecation is convenient. Loss of colonic function through disease or surgery results in a continuous rather than an intermittent, controlled discharge of food wastes and increases daily intestinal losses of water and electrolytes, chiefly sodium chloride. Absorption of glucose, amino acids, lipolytic products, or vitamins is not significant in the large intestine.

Flatus consists of about 70% nitrogen (N_2) and 30% a mixture of hydrogen (H_2) and carbon dioxide (CO_2). Methane (CH_4) is produced by about one-third of the adult population. The majority of flatus originates from swallowed air, the only available source for the N_2. The entire pool of intraluminal intestinal gas has been estimated to average about 100 ml in normal subjects. Much of the H_2, CH_4, and CO_2 produced in the gut is probably absorbed through the mucosa and excreted by the lungs. Increased gas production follows the ingestion of nonabsorbable carbohydrates which undergo fermentation in the presence of colonic bacteria. Such carbohydrates are found in certain fruits and vegetables, notably among the legumes. Colonic gas is potentially explosive if the lumen is opened with the electrocautery unit.

Motility

The ileocecal valve separates the ileum from the cecum. It partially regulates passage of ileal contents into the colon and serves as a barrier between them which limits colonization of the small bowel by fecal flora. Eating a meal reflexly stimulates emptying of ileal contents into the cecum.

Motor activity of the colon is classified as non-propulsive or propulsive. The former (the most frequent type) results in mixing of colonic contents, which aids in absorption of electrolytes and water. Contraction of a single haustrum, expelling its contents in either direction, is most common. The contraction may persist for a few minutes to an hour or more. When a contraction relaxes, it is often followed by another in an adjacent haustrum. This pattern, called haustral shuttling, is reduced after eating a meal, at which time it is supplanted by propulsive activity.

Propulsive movements increase postprandially and consist of 3 varieties of activity: haustral propulsion, mass propulsion, and peristalsis. Haustral propulsion results from sequential contraction at a rate of 2–3 cm/minute of adjacent haustral segments. Haustral retropulsion also occurs but is less frequent than orthograde movement. Multihaustral propulsion, or mass movement, follows systolic contraction of a segment spanning several haustra and is preceded by relaxation of the interhaustral contractions in the section of colon into which the feces are being propelled. Mass movements progress at an average rate of 5 cm/minute. Peristalsis, the least commonly observed activity, is produced by a slowly advancing contractile ring which forces the luminal contents before it. Receptive relaxation sometimes precedes the peristaltic wave.

The fecal stream itself does not move along in anything resembling orderly laminar flow. Some of the material entering the cecum flows past feces remaining from earlier periods. Portions of the stream enter the periphery of haustra, where they may fail to progress for 24 hours or more. Mixing of residue from one meal occurs with that from the past several days. In most persons with normal bowel function, residue from a meal reaches the cecum after 4 hours and the rectosigmoid by 24 hours. Mixing in the colon results in passage of residue from a single meal in movements for 3–4 days afterwards.

The urge to defecate is perceived when small amounts of feces enter the rectum and stimulate stretch receptors in the rectal wall. The sensation may be temporarily suppressed by voluntarily contracting the sphincter and pelvic diaphragm. Eventually, increased rectal filling may make the urge to defecate impossible to deny. When defecation is performed, it is aided by assuming a position with the thighs flexed so that intra-abdominal pressure can be easily increased by abdominal wall contraction. The internal and external anal sphincters relax, and the rectal or rectosigmoid contents are extruded by contraction of the colon and by increasing abdominal pressure via a Valsalva maneuver. The pelvic floor relaxes and the rectum loses its curves as the feces are discharged from the anus. Afterward, the sphincters resume their tone and the rectum remains empty until shortly before the next movement, when arrival of more feces from the sigmoid evokes the urge to defecate once again. The average interval between bowel movements in normal subjects is a little over 24 hours (but see below).

The effects on colonic motor activity of eating a meal are increased entry of ileal contents into the cecum, a shift from segmenting to propulsive motility, and a stimulus to defecate. Collectively, they comprise the "gastrocolic reflex." These effects result from the entry of food into the upper small intestine and are probably mediated by the hormone cholecystokinin.

Absorption

More than 1000 ml of ileal effluent enter the cecum each day, 90% of which is water. Colonic absorption desiccates this material, so that less than 100 ml of water is excreted in the feces each day. Table 36–1 gives average values for the electrolyte and water content of ileal effluent and feces; the difference represents normal colonic absorption. Figures are also given for the estimated maximal absorptive capacity of the colon. The capacity for absorption is several times greater in the right half than in the left half of the colon.

Absorption of sodium is accomplished by an active transport mechanism. Chloride and water absorption is passive along electrical and osmotic gradients established by the sodium pump. Colonic absorption of sodium and chloride removes 95% of that presented by the ileum. Mineralocorticoids increase absorption of sodium by the colon. Normally, sodium absorption is so efficient that a person can stay in balance on as little as 5 mEq in the daily diet. Colectomy imposes an obligatory minimal daily intake of 80–100 mEq of sodium to offset losses from the ileostomy.

A small amount of bicarbonate is secreted into the colonic lumen in exchange for chloride. Potassium enters feces chiefly by passive diffusion but also via secretion in mucus. Excessive mucus production in some forms of diarrhea or by certain tumors such as villous adenomas may lead to substantial potassium losses in the stool.

Normal formed feces are composed of 70% water and 30% solids; almost half of the fecal solids are bacteria; the remainder is food waste and desquamated colonic epithelium.

If the diet contains a large amount of cellulose or other residue, food passes through the intestinal tract more rapidly. The average interval between bowel movements is a little over 24 hours but may vary in normal subjects from 2 or 3 days to 8–12 hours. There is much undue apprehension concerning "constipation" in bowel-conscious western civilization. The symptoms of constipation are due mostly to anxiety and not to the discredited concept of absorption of "toxic substances." A change in bowel habits, however, demands investigation to rule out organic disease. Diarrhea may be debilitating and can be fatal, as in cholera. Infants tolerate diarrhea poorly. Large amounts of potassium, sodium, and water may be lost, resulting in dehydration, hypovolemia, and shock. Parasympathetic stimulation evokes mucinous secretion which varies greatly during emotional tension and may produce myxorrhea. Excessive secretion of mucus may deplete protein and electrolytes, eg, in ulcerative colitis and villous tumors.

TABLE 36–1. Mean values for electrolyte and water balance in the normal colon. A plus (+) sign indicates absorption from the colonic lumen; a minus (−) sign indicates secretion into the lumen.

	Ileal Effluent		Fecal Fluid		Colonic Absorption (per 24 hours)	
	Concentration (mEq/liter)	Quantity (per 24 hours)	Concentration (mEq/liter)	Quantity (per 24 hours)	Normal	Maximal Capacity
Na^+	120	180 mEq	30	6 mEq	+178 mEq	+400
K^+	6	10 mEq	67	5 mEq	+5 mEq	−30
Cl^-	67	100 mEq	20	1.5 mEq	+98 mEq	
HCO_3^-	60	90 mEq	80	6 mEq	+84 mEq	
H_2O		1500 ml		75 ml	+1425 ml	+3000

The cells of the mucosa of the colon normally proliferate rapidly and are completely replaced every 3 or 4 days. Cellular kinetics are markedly altered by a variety of abnormal conditions.

Connell AM: The movements of the alimentary tract. Practitioner 203:571–575, 1969.

Hagihara PF, Griffen WO Jr: Physiology of the colon and rectum. S Clin North America 52:797–805, 1972.

Holdstock DJ, Misiewicz JJ: Factors controlling colonic motility. Gut 11:100–110, 1970.

Phillips SF: Absorption and secretion by the colon. Gastroenterology 56:966–971, 1969.

Ritchie JA: Colonic motor activity and bowel function. Gut 9:442–456, 502–511, 1968.

Ritchie JA: Movement of segmental constrictions in the human colon. Gut 12:350–355, 1971.

Ritchie JA & others: Propulsion and retropulsion of normal colonic contents. Am J Digest Dis 16:697–704, 1971.

MICROBIOLOGY

Over 99% of the normal fecal flora is anaerobic. The most prevalent anaerobe is *Bacteroides fragilis;* the second most prevalent is *Lactobacillus bifidus.* Other anaerobes include clostridia and anaerobic cocci of various types. The major aerobic fecal flora are coliforms and enterococci. Of these *Escherichia coli* is predominant, with a count of 10^7 per gram of wet feces. The colon is sterile at birth, but the bacterial flora is established soon afterward.

The brown color of stool is due to bile pigments which are acted upon by bacteria. The amines indole and skatole are responsible for the characteristic fecal odor.

Conversion of bilirubin to urobilinogen takes place in the intestine through the activity of the intestinal flora. Conjugated bile acids are deconjugated by the large bowel flora, and only free bile acids are found in the feces. The steroid nucleus is also changed by colonic bacteria so that cholic acid is converted to deoxycholic and chenodeoxycholic acid to lithocholic. Deoxycholic acid is absorbed from the colon for reexcretion in bile, but the insoluble lithocholic acid is excreted in feces. It has been suggested that a carcinogen responsible for cancer of the colon may be produced by the action of bacteria on bile acids.

Daikos G, Kontomichalou P, Bilalis D: Faecal flora changes after oral antibiotics. Proc Roy Soc Med 62:260, 1969.

Dubos RJ, Savage DC, Schaedler RW: The indigenous flora of the gastrointestinal tract. Dis Colon Rectum 10:23, 1967.

Finegold SM: Intestinal bacteria. California Med 110:455, 1969.

Fink S, Mais RF: Cell-mediated immune reaction to colon altered by bacteria. Gut 9:629–632, 1968.

Nichols RL, Gorbach SI, Condon RE: Alteration of intestinal microflora following preoperative mechanical preparation of the colon. Dis Colon Rectum 14:128–133, 1971.

ROENTGENOLOGIC EXAMINATION

Plain films of the abdomen depict the distribution of gas in the intestines, calcifications, tumor masses, and the size and position of the liver, spleen, and kidneys. In the presence of acute intra-abdominal disease, additional erect, lateral, and oblique projections and lateral decubitus views are helpful.

The lumen of the colon can be visualized radiographically by instilling a suspension of barium sulfate through the anus (barium enema) (Fig 36–3). Adequate preparation of the bowel is imperative before barium enema examination so that the colon will be as free as possible of fecal material and gas. Although many rectal lesions can be visualized by barium enema, x-rays are not as accurate here as with lesions above the rectosigmoid. Proctosigmoidoscopy is the best method for inspecting the rectum. Postevacuation films reveal the mucosal pattern and small lesions. Double contrast (pneumocolon, air contrast) studies are useful to demonstrate small intraluminal lesions such as polyps. This is accomplished by allowing a coat of radiopaque barium to remain on the mucosa and filling the lumen with radiolucent air. The peroral double contrast enema, in which barium is given by mouth and air injected through the anus, is of value to identify abnormalities of the cecum and ascending colon.

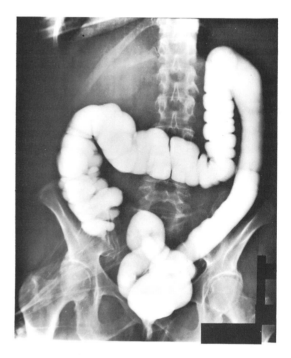

FIG 36–3. Roentgenogram of normal colon. The colon has been rendered radiopaque by a barium enema.

Fainsinger MH: The avoidance of complications in barium-enema studies. Dis Colon Rectum 13:31–33, 1970.

Margulis AR, Goldberg HI: The current status of radiologic technique in the examination of the colon: A survey. Radiol Clin North America 7:27–42, 1969.

FIBEROPTIC COLONOSCOPY

With the development of fiberoptic colonoscopes, endoscopic examination of the colon beyond the range of the proctosigmoidoscope has become a reality. The 105 cm colonoscope can reach the transverse colon; the 186.5 cm instrument can reach the ascending colon and the ileocecal valve. The instrument is flexible, and its tip may be advanced in any direction by guiding it with controls on the handle.

The procedure may be decisive in establishing a correct diagnosis in patients in whom barium x-ray studies are inconclusive. Endoscopic excision of polyps beyond the reach of the rigid proctosigmoidoscope can be accomplished with the snare-cautery unit and laparotomy avoided. Biopsy and cytologic study are possible under direct vision.

Considerable training, experience, and skill are required before colon fiberoscopy can be used effectively and safely. It is not now a procedure for general use, as is the proctosigmoidoscope.

Overholt BF: Flexible fiber optic sigmoidoscopy. Cancer 28:123–126, 1971.

Sugarbaker PH, Vineyard GC: Fiberoptic colonoscopy: A new look at old problems. Am J Surg 125:429–431, 1973.

DISEASES OF THE COLON & RECTUM

COLONIC OBSTRUCTION

Essentials of Diagnosis
- Abdominal pain.
- Constipation or obstipation.
- Nausea and vomiting (late).
- Abdominal distention and sometimes tenderness.
- Characteristic x-ray findings.

General Considerations
Twenty-five percent of intestinal obstructions in adults occur in the large bowel. Obstruction may be of 4 types: simple, strangulating, paralytic, and closed loop. Mechanical obstructions occur predominantly in the distal portion of the colon. However, early disten-tion may be most marked in the cecum and the ascending colon because they have thinner walls and a larger luminal caliber than the descending and sigmoid segments (Laplace's law). If the cecum, as measured on x-ray, reaches a diameter greater than 10 cm (4 inches), perforation may be imminent. This usually occurs in the area of lowest blood supply on the anterior surface.

The treatment plan must recognize that most of the gas in the distended colon is derived from swallowed air. Large amounts of fluid accumulate from

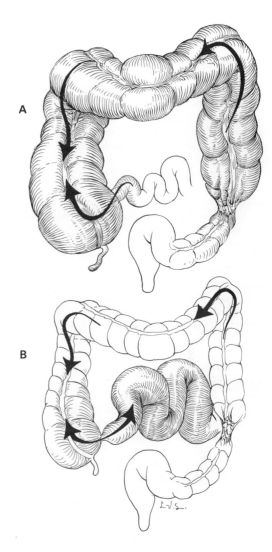

FIG 36–4. **The role of the ileocecal valve in obstruction of the colon.** The obstruction is in the upper sigmoid. *A:* The ileocecal valve is competent and has been closed by back pressure. Reflux from the colon into the ileum is prevented. A "closed loop" between the obstruction and the valve has resulted. *B:* The ileocecal valve is incompetent. Reflux into the ileum is permitted. The colon is relieved of some of its distention and the small bowel has become distended.

hypersecretion by the distended bowel and from ileal effluent, but electrolyte abnormalities from large bowel obstruction are usually less severe than those in small bowel obstruction.

Clinical Findings

A. Symptoms and Signs: Simple mechanical obstruction of the colon may develop insidiously. Deep, visceral, crampy pain from obstruction of the colon is usually referred to the hypogastrium. Lesions of the fixed portions of the colon (cecum, hepatic flexure, splenic flexure) may cause pain which is felt immediately anteriorly. Pain originating from the sigmoid is often located to the left in the lower abdomen. Severe, continuous abdominal pain suggests strangulation or peritonitis. Borborygmus may be loud and coincident with cramps. Constipation or obstipation is a universal feature of complete obstruction. The colon distal to the obstruction may empty after the initial symptoms, but no flatus or stool is passed thereafter. Vomiting is a late finding and may not occur at all if the ileocecal valve prevents reflux. If reflux decompresses the cecal contents into the small intestine, the symptoms of small bowel as well as large bowel obstruction appear. Feculent vomiting is a late manifestation.

Physical examination discloses abdominal distention and tympany. Peristaltic waves may be seen if the abdominal wall is thin. High-pitched, metallic tinkles, which may be associated with rushes and gurgles, may be heard on auscultation. Localized tenderness or a tender, palpable mass may indicate a strangulated closed loop. Signs of localized or generalized peritonitis suggest gangrene or rupture of the bowel wall. Fresh blood may be found in the rectum in intussusception and in carcinoma of the rectum or colon. Sigmoidoscopy may disclose a neoplasm.

B. X-Ray Findings: The distended colon frequently creates a "picture frame" outline of the abdominal cavity. The colon can be distinguished from the small intestine by its haustral markings, which do not cross the entire lumen of the distended colon. Barium enema will confirm the diagnosis of colonic obstruction and identify its exact location. However, barium enema may be dangerous if the vascular supply is compromised, and the increased risk associated with perforation of the colon by the barium is such that the procedure should be omitted under these circumstances. Barium must not be given orally in the presence of suspected colonic obstruction.

Differential Diagnosis

A. Small Versus Large Bowel Obstruction: X-ray may be required to make the differential diagnosis. Large bowel obstruction is frequently slow in onset, causes less pain, and does not cause vomiting in spite of considerable distention. Elderly patients with no history of abdominal surgery or prior attacks of obstruction will most frequently have carcinoma of the large bowel.

B. Paralytic Ileus: The distinguishing features of

paralytic ileus are signs of peritonitis or a history of trauma to the back or pelvis. The abdomen is silent and without cramps. There may be tenderness. Plain films show dilated bowel (see Chapter 31).

Complications

Delay in treatment may lead to progressive impairment of the blood supply of the bowel wall with frank ischemic necrosis, perforation, and peritonitis. Although rupture of the cecum is not a common complication of closed loop obstruction of the left colon, when it does occur the mortality rate is high.

Treatment

If strangulation is suspected, emergency operation is required.

Obstructing lesions of the cecum produce a clinical picture of small bowel obstruction. With adequate preoperative decompression of the small bowel, a one-stage resection of the right colon with ileotransverse colostomy is possible. If the patient's condition is not satisfactory, a bypassing end-to-side ileotransverse colostomy with exteriorization of the distal segment of ileum can be done, to be followed by subsequent resection of the right colon. If the lesion is nonresectable, a side-to-side ileotransverse colostomy may be performed. Loop ileostomy should be avoided if possible.

Obstructions of the ascending colon, the hepatic flexure, and the right half of the transverse colon are best decompressed by cecostomy (Fig 36–5). When the ileocecal valve is competent and neither the terminal ileum proximal to the obstruction nor the transverse colon distal to the obstruction are dilated or edematous, an emergency right hemicolectomy and anastomosis of the ileum to the transverse colon may be performed.

In the case of **obstructing lesions distal to the splenic flexure** either cecostomy or transverse colostomy will provide decompressive treatment.

Cecostomy is a simple operation which can be done under local anesthesia and is the operation of choice in aged, poor-risk patients with marked distention. It provides adequate decompression if the distal colon is not packed with feces, and complete diversion of the fecal stream is not necessary. Cecostomy has the advantage that it does not interfere with subsequent extensive resection of the left colon. **Transverse colostomy**, on the other hand, completely diverts the fecal stream and produces more adequate decompression. Transverse colostomy is preferable to cecostomy (1) in obstruction due to diverticulitis, (2) for removal of impacted barium or feces proximal to the obstruction, and (3) in case of failure of a cecostomy to provide decompression.

Prognosis

The prognosis depends upon the age and general condition of the patient, the extent of vascular impairment of the bowel, the presence or absence of perforation, and the promptness of surgical management.

A

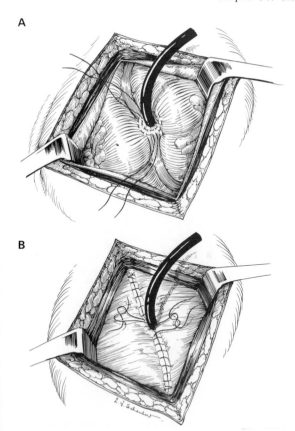

B

FIG 36–5. Cecostomy. *A:* A tube has been inserted through the wall of the cecum into its lumen and secured with a purse-string suture. *B:* Peritoneal closure. The cecum is fixed to the peritoneum.

Balslev I, Jensen H-E, Nielsen J: The place of cecostomy in relief of obstructive carcinoma of the colon. Dis Colon Rectum 13:207–210, 1970.

Schulman NH, Prithan HG, Polin SG: Decompression of the colon with complete diversion of the fecal stream by an in situ colonic catheter. Surgery 67:918, 1970.

CANCER OF THE COLON & RECTUM

Essentials of Diagnosis

Right Colon

- Persistent right abdominal discomfort.
- Dyspeptic symptoms.
- Unexplained anemia.
- Palpable abdominal mass.
- Occult blood in feces.
- Characteristic x-ray findings.

Left Colon

- Change in bowel habits.
- Gross blood in stool.
- Obstructive symptoms.

- Characteristic sigmoidoscopic findings.
- Characteristic x-ray findings.

Rectum

- Rectal bleeding.
- Alteration in bowel habits.
- Sensation of incomplete evacuation.
- Intrarectal palpable tumor.
- Sigmoidoscopic findings.

General Considerations

Cancer of the colon and rectum accounts for more cases of cancer in the total population than any other site except the skin. In men, the incidence is exceeded only by lung and skin cancer, and in women only by breast, uterus, and skin cancer. Colon cancer is more frequent than rectal cancer in both sexes. Women have more cancer of the colon than males, and men slightly more cancer of the rectum. In 1971 there were 75,000 new cases of cancer of the colon and rectum in the USA. The incidence increases with age; it begins to rise at age 40 and reaches a peak at 60–75 years. In 1971 there were about 46,000 deaths from cancer of the colon and rectum of which 35,700 were due to cancer of the colon. The death rate from colonic cancer is highest in the developed countries and lowest in the underdeveloped countries. Predisposing factors are familial polyposis, ulcerative colitis, villous adenomas, and possibly adenomatous polyps.

The distribution of cancers of the colon and rectum is shown in Fig 36–6.

Ninety-five percent of malignant tumors of the colon and rectum are adenocarcinomas: medullary, scirrhous, papillary, villous, or mucoid. The remainder are carcinoids (argentaffinoma), sarcomas of various types, malignant lymphomas, malignant melanoma, and adenoacanthoma. Adenomas frequently are found in a colon that also harbors a carcinoma.

Multiple synchronous cancers of the colon and rectum—ie, 2 or more carcinomas which occur simul-

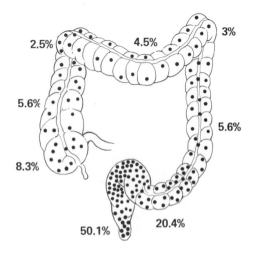

FIG 36–6. Distribution of cancer of the colon and rectum.

taneously—are found in 5% of patients. Metachronous cancer, which is a new primary independent lesion in a patient who has had a previous resection for cancer, has a similar incidence.

Cancer of the colon and rectum spreads in the following ways:

A. Colon:

1. Direct extension—Extension by contiguity occurs as the lesion penetrates the outer layers of the bowel. Direct submucosal extension along the bowel wall with invasion of the intramural lymphatic network rarely exceeds 5 cm from the tumor edge. Depending upon the site of the lesion in the bowel, neighboring structures may be involved directly: the liver, the greater curvature of the stomach, the small bowel, the bladder, the vagina, the kidneys and ureters, the tail of the pancreas, and the spleen. Subacute perforation with inflammatory attachment of the bowel to an adjacent viscus may be indistinguishable from direct invasion on gross examination. By direct extension, the growth may encircle the bowel, usually in the left colon. It takes about 1 year for a tumor to encircle three-fourths of the circumference of the bowel.

2. Hematogenous metastasis—The tumor may invade colonic veins and be carried via portal venous blood to the liver to establish hepatic metastases. Tumor embolization also occurs through lumbar and vertebral veins to the lungs and elsewhere. Venous invasion occurs in 15–35% of cases even though it does not always cause distant metastases. An attempt is made to avoid producing hematogenous metastases during operation by ligating the major veins before manipulating the tumor.

3. Regional lymph node metastasis—This is the most common form of tumor spread (Fig 36–7). The nodes adjacent to the tumor must be removed in curative operations. Fifty to 60 lymph nodes can usually be identified in the average specimen and some nodal involvement will be found in over half of the specimens. Regional nodes are not necessarily involved in a progressive or orderly fashion: positive nodes may be found at some distance from the primary site with normal nodes intervening. The size of the lesion bears no relationship to the degree of nodal involvement. The more anaplastic the lesion, the more likely that lymph node metastasis will occur.

4. Gravitational metastasis—"Seeding" may occur when the tumor has extended through the serosa and tumor cells are carried to distant points of the peritoneal cavity, eventually producing general abdominal carcinomatosis. The rectovesical or rectouterine pouches are usually involved, and on digital rectal examination can be felt as a hard shelf ("Blumer's shelf") and, later, as a "frozen pelvis." Because metastasis to the ovaries occurs in 3–4% of cases, bilateral oophorectomy should be performed when the bowel is resected in postmenopausal patients.

B. Rectum:

1. Direct extension—Longitudinal extension usually does not exceed 6 cm. Lateral extension into the contiguous viscera occurs when the growth has ex-

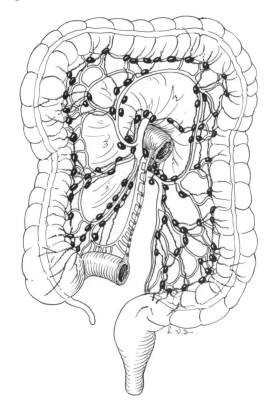

FIG 36–7. Lymphatic drainage of the colon. The lymph nodes (black) are distributed along the blood vessels to the bowel. Metastasis of cancer of the colon to these regional lymph nodes is the most common form of spread of this malignant tumor.

tended through the bowel wall. Cancer of the rectum may invade the vaginal wall, along the levators, the prostate, or to the sacrum.

2. Lymphatic spread—Cancer first involves the lymph nodes adjacent to the tumor and then spreads successively to the more proximal lymph nodes; occasionally it spreads to nodes outside the normal continuity. Retrograde lymphatic spread occurs in 5% of cases, and then only when the cancer is far advanced. The lymphatic chain from the rectum is along the superior hemorrhoidal, iliac, and inferior mesenteric arteries and the aorta.

3. Hematogenous metastases—In 15% of cases, it will have spread through the portal veins to the liver when first diagnosed. Metastasis to the lungs occurs less frequently. The brain and spine may also be involved.

4. Perineural spread—Cancer may spread by perineural invasion. When it does so, the rate of local recurrence is high.

Clinical Findings

A. Symptoms and Signs: The symptoms of carcinoma of the colon depend upon the anatomic location of the lesion, its type and extent, and upon complications such as perforation, obstruction, or hemorrhage. Early carcinoma is asymptomatic, and diagnosis depends upon routine examination.

The symptom complex of cancer of the **right colon** is different from that of the left. On the right, the caliber of the bowel is 2½ times that of the left, the content is fluid, carcinoma tends to be large and fungating, and the bowel wall is thinner and more distensible. There may be persistent right abdominal pain or discomfort. The pain may be postprandial and mistakenly interpreted as being due to gallbladder disease. Patients often present with pallor, fatigability, weakness, dizziness, dyspnea, and cardiac palpitations due to severe anemia. Unexplained microcytic hypochromic anemia should always raise a question of cecal carcinoma. Blood may not be visible in the stool but may be detected by tests for occult blood. In about 10% of cases, the first sign of the disease is discovery by the patient or physician of a mass in the right abdomen. A change in bowel habits is less marked than when the left colon is involved. Obstruction is uncommon but may occur, especially with lesions of the ileocecal junction or hepatic flexure.

The **left colon** has a smaller lumen than the right and the feces are solid here. Tumors of the left colon are usually scirrhous and tend to encircle the bowel and create obstruction. There may be changes in bowel habits with alternating constipation and increased frequency of defecation (not true watery diarrhea). The stool may be streaked or mixed with blood, which may either be bright red or dark. Mucus is often passed mixed with blood or blood clots. Symptoms of partial obstruction with colicky abdominal pain or complete obstruction may be the presenting picture.

Complete obstruction may occur without previous symptoms, or there may be an antecedent history of increasing constipation, diminution in stool caliber, and increasing abdominal distention with pain or discomfort. Nausea and vomiting are usually absent if the ileocecal valve is competent and prevents reflux into the ileum. When the valve is competent, a closed loop is created, and distention of the right colon may even produce cecal perforation. If the ileocecal valve is incompetent, nausea and vomiting may occur with distention of the small bowel.

In **cancer of the rectum,** the most common presenting symptom is the passage of blood with bowel movement. Whenever rectal bleeding occurs, even in the presence of an obviously benign lesion such as hemorrhoids, coexisting cancer must be ruled out. Bleeding is usually persistent; it may be slight or (rarely) copious. Blood may or may not be mixed with stool or with mucus. There may be tenesmus without diarrhea, and the patient may have a feeling of incomplete defecation. Pain is noticeably absent except in advanced stages of the disease or when the carcinoma involves the anal canal. Cancer of the rectosigmoid may produce obstruction, but cancer of the rectum rarely does.

Marked weight loss, cachexia, jaundice, and enlargement of the liver are indications of metastatic cancer. Perforation causes localized or generalized peritonitis. General physical examination is important to determine the extent of the local disease and to reveal distant metastases. The groin and supraclavicular areas should be carefully palpated for metastatic nodules. Enlarged, firm nodes should be biopsied. Examination of the abdomen may disclose a palpable mass, enlargement of the liver, ascites, or enlargement of the abdominal wall veins if there is portal obstruction. Anemia may be obvious. Jaundice indicates hepatic metastases.

Seventy-five percent of cancers of the colon and rectum are within reach of the examining finger or the sigmoidoscope. Most rectal cancers can be felt digitally as a flat, hard, oval or encircling tumor, which may be nodular on the surface. Its extent, the size of the lumen at the site of the tumor, and the degree of fixation should be noted. Blood may be found on the examining finger. Vaginal and rectovaginal examination will yield additional information on the extent of the tumor. The size of the prostate gland should be noted.

B. Laboratory Findings: Urinalysis, red and white blood counts, and hemoglobin determination must be done. Serum proteins, calcium, bilirubin, serum alkaline phosphatase, serum glutamic oxaloacetic transaminase (SGOT), and serum lactic dehydrogenase (LDH), and prothrombin time should be determined. Chest films and ECG should be taken routinely.

Abnormal amounts of **carcinoembryonic antigen (CEA)** can be found by radioimmunoassay of the sera of patients with cancer of the colon and in fetal colonic tissue. At first believed to be specific for cancer of entodermal origin, CEA has been detected in the sera of patients with several other nonentodermal malignancies and in some with ulcerative colitis who have no neoplasm. In localized cancer of the colon, the test for CEA is positive in only one-fifth of cases. Reversal from a positive to a negative CEA test following resection of the growth does not exclude residual tumor. The test is strongly positive in all instances of metastatic cancer of the colon. It is expensive and as yet has no role in patient management.

In carcinoma of the lower sigmoid and rectum excretory urography is necessary to determine whether obstruction of the ureters has occurred. If a history of decreased size or force of the urinary stream, nocturia, or urinary incontinence is obtained or if obstruction or displacement of the ureters or bladder is found by x-ray, further urologic evaluation should include urethral calibration, cystoscopy, or cystometry depending on the specific findings.

C. Special Examinations:

1. **Proctosigmoidoscopy**—The typical rectal cancer is raised, red, bleeding slightly, and ulcerated. The size of the rectal lumen should be noted. If possible, the sigmoidoscope should be passed through the lumen at the site of the lesion for higher inspection. Associated polyps may be seen. Mobility of the lesion can be determined by manipulation with the instrument.

When the lesion is above the reach of the procto-sigmoidoscope, a bloody discharge may be seen coming from above; streaks of blood may be seen in the stool; or the test for occult blood may be positive. A biopsy of the lesion should be taken through the instrument.

2. Colonoscopy—With the fiberoptic instrument, lesions can be inspected at any level in the colon, but this examination need only be performed when the x-ray diagnosis is inconclusive.

3. Cytology—Experimental studies suggest that cytologic examination of colonic washings may help in distinguishing between benign and malignant lesions, but a practical clinical method for performing cytology has not been devised.

D. X-Ray Findings: Barium enema x-ray examination is the most important means of diagnosing cancer of the colon. The length of involvement is usually 2–5 cm, and the bowel wall is stiffened at the site of the lesion. A fixed filling defect is present, and the mucosal pattern is destroyed. An annular carcinoma produces a "napkin ring" or "apple core" defect (Fig 36–8).

Localized spasm of the bowel may mimic carcinoma on x-rays. If the barium enema examination

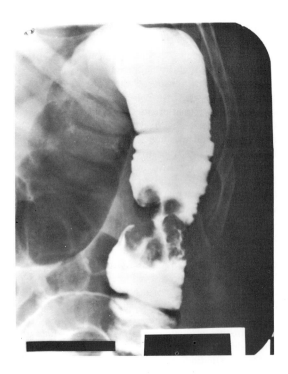

FIG 36–8. Barium enema roentgenogram of an encircling carcinoma of the descending colon presenting an "apple core" appearance. Note the loss of mucosal pattern, the "hooks" at the margins of the lesion due to undermining by the growth, the relatively short (6 cm) length of the lesion and its abrupt ends.

shows nothing abnormal but symptoms are suggestive, the examination should be repeated once or twice. If there is evidence of carcinoma of the colon, particularly on the left, barium should not be administered by mouth since it may precipitate acute intestinal obstruction.

X-ray diagnosis should not be relied upon to detect cancer of the rectum. Such growths are preferably diagnosed by palpation and endoscopy.

The value of radioactive scans of the liver in the diagnosis of hepatic metastases is discussed in Chapters 8 and 26.

Differential Diagnosis

Pain in the right side of the abdomen due to carcinoma may simulate appendicitis. When the cancer obstructs the colon, even though the obstruction is on the left, the pain may be most acute over the distended cecum.

Differentiation from diverticulitis may be difficult clinically and even at operation. Lesions in the ascending colon or hepatic flexure may cause mild obstruction resulting in postprandial pain in the right upper quadrant which can be confused with biliary colic.

Unexplained microcytic hypochromic anemia may be due to cancer of the right colon; unless repeated barium enemas are done, valuable time may be lost in ineffectual medical treatment. Colonoscopy may disclose small lesions not seen on x-ray examination.

Cancer of the colon and rectum should head the list of differential diagnoses when rectal bleeding of any type occurs. Even in the presence of large bleeding hemorrhoids, concomitant cancer must be ruled out. Differentiation from ulcerative colitis is made on the basis of sigmoidoscopic and x-ray examinations.

Prevention

Both physician and patient may be responsible for delay in diagnosis. Many patients complaining of rectal bleeding, severe constipation, or abdominal crampy pain have been treated symptomatically or even operated upon for benign rectal conditions.

Chronic ulcerative colitis has malignant potentiality. Malignancy almost always develops in untreated familial polyposis. If it is found in an individual, all other members of the family must be examined. There is often a family history of cancer of the colon and rectum, and this fact should bear weight in the clinical evaluation.

Treatment

The accepted treatment of cancer of the large bowel is wide surgical resection of the lesion and its regional lymphatics after adequate preparation of the bowel. The choice of operation is determined by the site of the tumor, its local spread, and regional lymph node drainage. During operation, care must be taken not to contribute to spread of the tumor. Unnecessary palpation of the tumor should be avoided so that tumor cells will not be released into the portal circulation. The blood vessels that supply the involved segment of the colon must be divided and ligated early in the operation. The cancer may exfoliate tumor cells which may be seeded on the peritoneum or into the lumen of the colon.

Recurrence of colon cancer at the suture line is due to shedding of cells into the lumen of the bowel and their implantation. To avoid it, the bowel should be tied tightly with an encircling tape on each side of the lesion and the 2 ends of the bowel irrigated before anastomosis. The irrigating fluid commonly employed is distilled water, although some prefer half-strength Dakin's solution (0.25% sodium hypochlorite) or 1:500 bichloride of mercury.

At the time of operation, the abdomen should be explored to determine the presence or absence of multiple primary carcinomas of the colon, distant metastases, resectability of the tumor, and associated abdominal disease.

The extent of resection of the colon, blood vessels, and lymph nodes for cancers in various locations and the methods of restoration of continuity are shown in Fig 36–9.

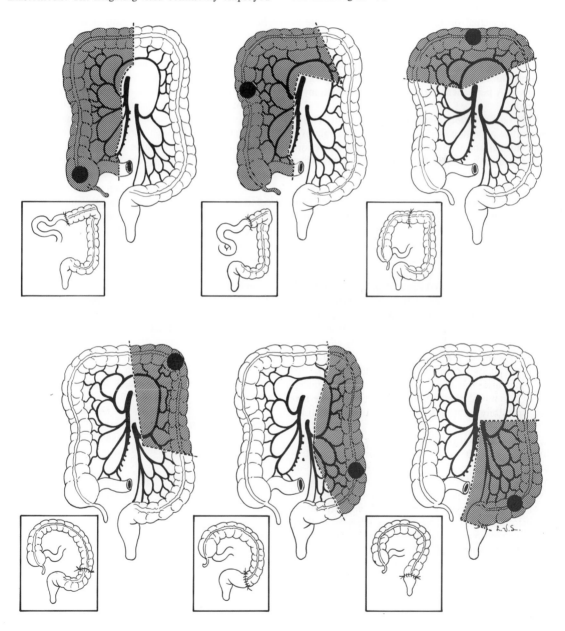

FIG 36–9. Extent of surgical resection for cancer of the colon at various sites. The cancer is represented by a black disk. Anastomosis of the bowel remaining after resection is shown in the small insets. The extent of resection is determined by the distribution of the regional lymph nodes along the blood supply. The lymph nodes may contain metastatic cancer.

For cancer of the rectum, the choice of operation depends on the height of the lesion, the gross extent of the tumor, and its degree of cellular differentiation. An adequate excision requires at least a 5 cm segment of rectum below the growth or sometimes complete excision of the rectum; removal of as much of the rectal tissue as is anatomically feasible at the level of the growth; and removal of at least 10 cm of normal bowel proximal to the growth along with the lymph node-bearing tissue. Although preservation of the anal sphincter is highly desirable, the primary goal of the operation is ablation of the malignancy. Avoidance of a colostomy is of secondary importance.

The principal operations for rectal tumors are as follows:

(1) Abdominoperineal resection of the rectum: The distal sigmoid, rectosigmoid, and rectum are removed through a combined abdominal and perineal approach. A permanent terminal sigmoid colostomy is required.

(2) Low anterior resection of the rectum: This is the curative operation of choice provided a margin of 5 cm of normal bowel can be resected below the lesion, or as a palliative operation to avoid colostomy when there are demonstrable metastases in the liver. The lesion and adjacent bowel are removed through an abdominal incision. The descending colon is anastomosed to the distal rectum, thus avoiding a colostomy.

This type of resection is contraindicated for primary operable cancer in the distal rectum or for extensive carcinoma with local spread.

(3) "Pull-through" operations: The rectum is removed and the proximal sigmoid pulled through the anal canal and anastomosed to a few centimeters of preserved rectal mucosa. However, because of technical difficulties, complications, and variable degrees of continence, these procedures are not widely employed.

(4) Palliative procedures: Other, more limited operations or palliation such as the Hartmann procedure, in which the bowel with its contained malignancy is removed through the abdomen with permanent colostomy but without removal of the distal rectum, are at times indicated.

(5) Local treatment of some cancers of the rectum by radon seed implantation and electrocoagulation has a place in a small proportion of patients who are marginal operative risks because of advanced age, serious associated disease, or blindness; those who are inmates of institutions and dependent on custodial care; or those who are adamant in their refusal of colostomy. The place of such limited procedures in the control of carcinoma of the rectum is under study. At present, total surgical excision is regarded as the procedure of choice in good-risk patients.

Treatment of Complications

A. Obstruction: In cases of acute obstruction due to carcinoma, surgical decompression is required in addition to other preparatory measures before definitive operation can be safely undertaken. Acute large bowel obstruction requires immediate surgical decompression because of the danger of perforation, especially of the cecum. Upper intestinal intubation is only an adjunct and will not suffice by itself. Cecostomy will relieve the obstruction unless there is a large amount of fecal material distal to the cecum. In this case, transverse colostomy is better and, with obstructive cancer of the left colon, will allow resection of the tumor in defunctionalized bowel (Fig 36–10). Transverse colostomy, however, requires a formal closure with resection of the exteriorized bowel and end-to-end anastomosis of the remaining transverse colon.

B. Perforation: Perforation of cancer of the colon should be dealt with by resection of the involved segment, exteriorization of the transected proximal end of the bowel, and exteriorization or closure of the distal end. Secondary anastomosis may be possible after an interval of 3 months. If a localized abscess has formed due to perforation, it must be drained and a proximal, diverting colostomy established, with the intent of subsequent resection of the segment in which the tumor lies. Although perforation of a carcinoma is attended by a considerable early mortality and an unfavorable long-term prognosis, in some instances resection may result in cure.

C. Direct Extension: When carcinoma of the colon has spread by contiguity to adjacent viscera such as the uterus, small intestine, spleen, urinary bladder or other viscera, resection of the involved viscus along with the resected portion of the colon should be done en bloc.

Prognosis

Cancer of the colon and rectum has the highest survival following surgical resection of any cancer of the gastrointestinal tract. One of the best methods of determining prognosis is the use of the Duke classification (Fig 36–11 and Table 36–2), which depends on the degree of direct extension through the bowel wall and the presence or absence of lymph node involvement.

Ten to 15% of lesions are not resectable at the time of operation. Twenty-five percent of patients may have resectable lesions but have liver metastases or

TABLE 36–2. Duke's classification of cancer of the colon.

Type	Extent	5-Year Survival (%)
A	Limited to mucosa	100
B1	Into muscularis mucosae with negative nodes	66
B2	Through entire wall with negative nodes	54
C1	Limited to wall with positive nodes	43
C2	Through all layers with positive nodes	22
D	Distant metastases	0

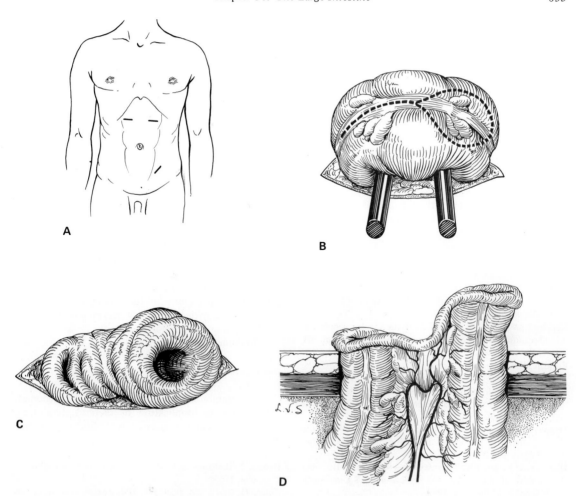

FIG 36-10. Diverting loop colostomy. *A:* Common incisions for loop colostomy. *B:* The loop has been exteriorized over short rods which prevent retraction. The dotted line depicts the incision used to open the bowel. *C:* Double-barreled appearance after the incision has been made. *D:* Cross-sectional view of the colostomy in relation to the abdominal wall.

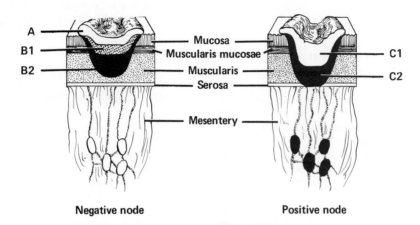

FIG 36-11. Modified Duke's classification of cancer of the rectum. In type A, the lesion is confined to the mucosa. In type B, the lesion extends through the muscularis mucosae without involving lymph nodes. In type C1, the lesion is limited to the wall with positive nodes. In type C2, the lesion extends through all wall layers with positive nodes.

peritoneal carcinomatosis. Hence, operation for cure can be performed on only about 60% of those who come to surgery. There has been little improvement in this figure over the past 20 years despite intensive efforts to educate the public about the early symptoms of this disease. The average delay between onset of symptoms and definitive therapy is about 10 months. The degree of differentiation of the tumor and the finding of intravascular tumor cells histologically also have a bearing on the prognosis.

In cancer of the rectum, the prognosis correlates with the degree of penetration of the bowel wall, the extent of regional lymph node involvement, and the degree of differentiation of the tumor cells.

If the patient is free of disease at 5 years, he is unlikely to develop a recurrence.

The operative mortality rate is 1–4%.

Calabrese CT, Adam YG, Volk H: Geriatric colon cancer. Am J Surg 125:181–184, 1973.

Cole WH: Cancer of the colon and rectum. S Clin North America 52:871–882, 1972.

Copeland AM, Jones RS, Miller LD: Multiple colon neoplasms: Prognostic and therapeutic implications. Arch Surg 98: 143–148, 1969.

Corman ML & others: Colorectal carcinoma at the Lahey Clinic, 1962 to 1966. Am J Surg 125:424–428, 1973.

Crile G Jr, Turnbull RB Jr: The role of electrocoagulation in the treatment of carcinoma of the rectum. Surg Gynec Obst 135:391–396, 1972.

Dunphy JE, Broderick E: A critique of anterior resection in the treatment of cancer of the rectum and pelvic colon. Surgery 30:106, 1951.

Higgins GA, Dwight RW: The role of preoperative irradiation in cancer of the rectum and rectosigmoid. S Clin North America 52:847–858, 1972.

Hight D, Kjartannsson S, Barillas AE: Importance of early diagnosis in the treatment of carcinoma of the colon and rectum. Am J Surg 125:304–307, 1973.

Turnbull RB Jr: Cancer of the colon: The five- and ten-year survival rates following resection utilizing the isolation technique. Ann Roy Coll Surg Engl 46:243, 1970.

OTHER TUMORS OF THE COLON & RECTUM

Carcinoids may occur in any part of the gastrointestinal tract but are most common in the appendix and small bowel. Carcinoids of the cecum and colon are uncommon, but compared with carcinoids elsewhere in the gut they have the highest incidence of metastases. Rectal carcinoids are usually asymptomatic. Lesions less than 2 cm in diameter behave as if they were benign, whereas larger ones are usually accompanied by metastases. Small rectal carcinoids should be excised locally, but large ones require wide excision.

Lipomas are among the most frequent of the benign nonepithelial tumors and are usually asympto-

matic but may cause intussusception or obstruction if they occur at the ileocecal valve.

Leiomyomas are much less common in the colon than in the stomach and small intestine. In the colon they are less apt to cause exsanguinating hemorrhage such as occurs in the upper gastrointestinal tract. It is not possible to predict with certainty whether a benign leiomyoma will or will not become a leiomyosarcoma.

Hemangiomas are rare in the colon. They are usually multiple and may cause bleeding which is difficult to diagnose. Selective mesenteric arteriography may reveal the lesion.

Lymphosarcomas are the most common of the noncarcinomatous malignant tumors of the large bowel and are usually of the reticulum cell type.

Benign lymphomas, while uncommon are the most frequent nonepithelial benign tumors of the rectum. They form sessile and sometimes pedunculated polyps. They are usually solitary but may be multiple. Diffuse lymphoid hyperplasia which produces a cobblestone appearance of the rectum is occasionally seen in young patients. Lymphomas may be associated with lymphoid tumors elsewhere in the body.

Endometriomas sometimes involve the subserosal, muscular, and submucous tissues of the rectosigmoid and rectum. They are associated with endometriosis of the ovary.

Uncommon benign tumors include hemangiomas, enterocystomas (duplication of rectum), teratomas, and neurofibromas associated with Recklinghausen's disease.

Dawson I: Hamartomas in the alimentary tract. Gut 10:691–694, 1969.

Kuiper H, Gracie WA Jr, Pollard HM: Twenty years of gastrointestinal carcinoids. Cancer 25:1424, 1970.

Naqvi MS, Burrows L, Kark AE: Lymphoma of the gastrointestinal tract: Prognostic guides based on 162 cases. Ann Surg 170:221–231, 1969.

Rosato FE, Anderson JR, Andrus P: Carcinoids of the large intestine. Dis Colon Rectum 13:211–214, 1970.

Wychulis AR, Beahrs OH, Woolner LB: Malignant lymphoma of the colon: A study of 69 cases. Arch Surg 93:215–225, 1966.

POLYPS OF THE COLON & RECTUM

Essentials of Diagnosis

- Usually asymptomatic.
- Passage of blood per rectum.
- Possible family history.
- Sigmoidoscopic, colonoscopic, or radiologic discovery of polyps.

General Considerations

By definition, polyps are "pedunculated growths arising from a mucous surface." The term is sometimes used incorrectly as synonymous with adenomatous

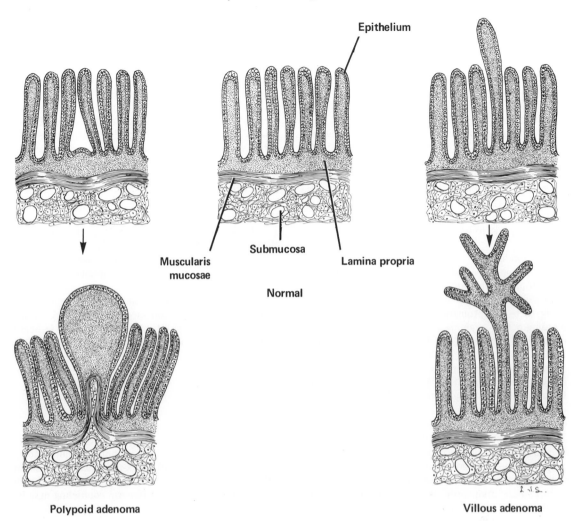

FIG 36–12. Origin of benign, lobulated, polypoid adenoma (left) and papillary (villous) adenoma (right).

polyps. However, on microscopic examination, polypoid lesions may prove to be (1) benign sessile or pedunculated adenomas; (2) papillary (villous) adenomas characterized on histologic examination by fronds of papillary tissue (Fig 36–12); (3) colonic polyps showing only hypertrophy of normal colonic mucosa; (4) adenomas with histologic changes marking the transition to polypoid carcinoma or focal carcinoma; (5) polypoid carcinomas that grossly resemble adenomatous polyps except that they tend to be more firm, with a more irregular surface, and microscopically are cancer; (6) inflammatory polyps (or pseudopolyps), usually associated with ulcerative colitis; (7) juvenile polyps—stroma-filled hamartomas with cyst-like glands in the center, often infiltrated by eosinophils—usually seen in children; and (8) other less common lesions such as pedunculated lipomas, myomas, and fibromas.

Estimates of incidence range from 7–50%, the higher figure including small polyps found at autopsy. The incidence of polyps detected on routine barium enema ranges from 1–10%. Polyps are frequently multiple. After the age of 20, the incidence of adenomatous polyps increases with each decade. The average age of patients with benign polyps is about 10 years less than that of cancer patients. The most common sites of polyps are the rectum and sigmoid colon, with the descending colon, splenic flexure, transverse colon, hepatic flexure, and ascending colon following in order of decreasing frequency.

About 25% of papillary (villous) adenomas are known to evolve into cancer, but there is controversy about whether or not adenomatous polyps are precancerous lesions. The arguments supporting the view that simple adenomas become cancer may be summarized as follows: (1) One-fourth of patients with cancer of the colon also have polyps. (2) The distribution in the colon and rectum of polyps and cancer is similar. (3) Patients with familial polyposis die of cancer before age 40 unless the colon is removed surgically. (4) Benign polyps seen through the sigmoidoscope have, at a later date, become typical carcinomas.

(5) Inclusion bodies in the cytoplasm of polyps and cancer are identical. (6) Cancers smaller than 1.5 cm in diameter are rarely discovered, whereas small polyps are frequent, suggesting that the smaller polyps ultimately grow into larger cancers.

The contrary arguments are as follows: (1) Long-term follow-up studies have shown that most adenomatous polyps do not become malignant. (2) If all adenomatous polyps became malignant, the incidence of cancer of the colon would be much higher. (3) Histologic study of cancers arising in polyps rarely show benign adenoma and cancer together. (4) Polyps are more evenly distributed throughout the colon than are cancers. (5) The sex incidence is not the same for adenomas as for cancer. (6) Lesions less than 1.5 cm in size rarely prove to be cancer.

Clinical Findings

A. Symptoms and Signs: Many adenomas are asymptomatic. The larger the polyp, the more likely it is to cause symptoms. Polypoid carcinomas are more likely to be symptomatic than benign polyps. Rectal bleeding occurs in about 40% of cases. In general, the more distal the lesion, the brighter red the blood. It may be on the surface of the stool or mixed with the feces, and may appear intermittently or occur with every bowel movement but is rarely profuse. At times it may be detected only by testing for occult blood.

Larger benign tumors may produce tenesmus, constipation, or increased frequency of bowel movement, although alterations in bowel habits are more common in the presence of frank carcinoma. Large polypoid tumors may induce peristaltic cramps or varying degrees of intussusception. Intussusception occurs more frequently with benign or low-grade malignant lesions because infiltrating carcinomas are more likely to fix the bowel and mesentery and prevent intussusception. Occasionally, a polyp on a very long pedicle will prolapse through the anus. This is particularly true of juvenile polyps in children. Adenomas should be thought of as a source of unexplained blood loss.

Juvenile polyps are more likely to be symptomatic, causing rectal bleeding, prolapse of the tumor, or abdominal cramps and pain. They may autoamputate by torsion of the pedicle and be passed in the stool.

General physical examination must be done but will yield little information except in Peutz-Jeghers and Gardner's syndromes. On rectal examination, a polyp may be felt. Sigmoidoscopic examination may disclose polyps of the rectum, a polyp prolapsing from above, or evidence of bleeding beyond the reach of the instrument. Since polyps are often multiple and often occur synchronously with cancer, further investigation of the colon is mandatory even if a lesion is found by sigmoidoscopy. Fiberoptic colonoscopy is proving to be one of the most reliable methods of detecting and removing colonic polyps.

B. X-Ray Findings (Barium Enema): The colon must be thoroughly cleansed before x-ray examination.

Small polyps may be obscured by a dense barium mixture. Thinner barium and high kilovoltage technics have successfully demonstrated very small polyps. A polyp causes a rounded translucent filling defect with smooth, sharply defined margins. The presence or absence of a pedicle may be determined. The post-evacuation roentgenogram is important since a thin layer of barium usually remains on the polyp. Polyps smaller than 0.5 cm in diameter usually cannot be detected on x-ray. The use of double-contrast examination is of value in that the polyp, coated by barium, forms a positive shadow as it projects into the lumen filled with radiolucent air.

Differential Diagnosis

Inflammatory polyps or pseudopolyps occur in chronic ulcerative colitis, are usually multiple, have a different x-ray appearance, and are associated with the symptoms and other findings characteristic of that disease.

Many artifacts seen on barium enema x-ray examination may be confused with polypoid filling defects. These include bits of feces, oil and air bubbles, diverticula, indenting appendices epiploicae, calcified lymph nodes, and many others. Colonoscopy is essential in doubtful situations before operation is performed.

Prevention

Since the pathogenesis of adenomatous polyps of the colon is not known, no particular preventive measure can be taken. However, annual sigmoidoscopic examination after age 40 and x-ray examination when indicated may discover early polypoid lesions which can be removed surgically. Genetic counseling may be of value in familial polyposis.

Treatment

Most pedunculated polyps of the colon can be removed through the colonoscope or sigmoidoscope using a snare and electrocautery. Sessile polyps are less amenable to this technic because of the danger of perforating the bowel. If endoscopic removal is not possible, laparotomy will be required.

One must balance the risk of operation against the possibility of a polyp's being or becoming malignant. The reasons for removal of polyps requiring laparotomy are that (1) about 20% of them are cancer rather than benign adenomas; (2) many cause symptoms ascribable to the adenoma itself; (3) about 10% of adenomas, including papillary adenomas, will develop into cancer if left alone; and (4) sessile lesions are more likely to be cancer.

The decision to operate will depend upon the size of the lesion, the presence or absence of a pedicle, the presence or absence of symptoms, and the age and physical condition of the patient. The chance of cancer increases significantly as the size of the tumor increases. The possibility of cancer in a polyp smaller than 1.5 cm in diameter is less than 2%. The overall operative mortality from removal of a colonic polypoid lesion is also about 2%. Therefore, when the operative risk exceeds risk of cancer, smaller polyps may be treated conservatively and followed by periodic x-ray examination to see if they are enlarging. If the lesion is cancer, it will steadily increase in size.

If, on palpation through the bowel wall, the lesion is felt to be sessile or hard, segmental resection should be done. If the lesion is soft, pedunculated, single, and benign on frozen section and if the "surgical margin" is adequate, simple colotomy and polypectomy will suffice. If all of these criteria are not met, segmental resection with anastomosis should be done.

When multiple polyps in different segments of the colon are found, subtotal colectomy should be done, especially in young, good-risk patients.

Prognosis

Recurrence at the site of surgical excision of adenomas is rare. Since new adenomas frequently develop with the passage of time, periodic follow-up endoscopic and radiographic examinations must be done for an indefinite period. In general, follow-up examination should be scheduled every 3 months for 1 year, twice the following year, and annually thereafter.

Familial polyposis of the colon is a rare but important disease because colonic malignancy develops between ages 20–40 in nearly all patients. The sex incidence is equal. In affected families, half the children inherit the abnormality while the remainder are normal; it is a heterozygous autosomal dominant trait. Multiple polyps carpet the colon and rectum throughout. These vary in size and configuration. Total colectomy eliminates the risk of cancer; however, after subtotal colectomy and ileorectal anastomosis, the polyps often disappear from the rectum and the patient may be followed with a substantially lower risk of developing cancer. If the polyps do not regress and biopsy shows marked cellular atypia, the distal rectum should be removed and a permanent ileostomy established. Most authorities today favor an initial trial of subtotal colectomy and low ileorectal anastomosis, especially in adolescents.

Gardner's syndrome is a rare form of familial polyposis inherited in an autosomal dominant pattern. In addition to multiple polyps of the colon, there are soft tissue masses (especially desmoid tumors) and osteomas of the skull or mandible. Treatment is the same as for familial polyposis.

Peutz-Jeghers syndrome is an uncommon, autosomal dominant, congenital disease in which multiple adenomatous polyps appear in the stomach, small bowel, and colon. Affected individuals have melanotic pigmentation of the skin and mucous membranes, especially about the lips and gums. The polyps are not precancerous and should be removed only if they cause symptoms.

Other rare syndromes have been reported in which polyps of the bowel were associated with tumors of the endocrine glands.

Bolt RJ: Sigmoidoscopy in detection and diagnosis in the asymptomatic individual. Cancer 28:121–122, 1971.

Dozois RR & others: The Peutz-Jeghers syndrome: Is there a predisposition to the development of malignancy? Arch Surg 98:509–517, 1969.

Dunphy JE, Patterson WB, Legg MA: Etiologic factors in polyposis and carcinoma of the colon. Ann Surg 150:488, 1959.

Louw JH: Polypoid lesions of the large bowel in children with particular reference to benign lymphoid polyposis. J Pediat Surg 3:195–209, 1968.

Paradny R, Kark AE: Adenomas of the colon. Am J Gastroenterol 50:186–194, 1968.

Simpkins KC, Young AC: The radiology of colonic and rectal polyps. Brit J Surg 55:731–735, 1968.

Veidenheimer MC, Connolly JM, Legg MA: Carcinoma in colonic and rectal polyps. Dis Colon Rectum 13:194–200, 1970.

Welch CE: *Polypoid Lesions of the Gastrointestinal Tract.* Saunders, 1964.

Williams JL, Wightman JAK: Familial polyposis of the colon. Brit J Surg 53:780–783, 1966.

DIVERTICULAR DISEASE OF THE COLON

Essentials of Diagnosis

- Acute abdominal pain and fever.
- Constipation or frequency of defecation.
- Dysuria.
- Left lower quadrant abdominal tenderness and mass.
- Characteristic radiologic findings.

General Considerations

Diverticula, or outpouchings, may occur along the entire gastrointestinal tract. They are most common in the colon, where there may be only a few though in most cases many are present. When uninflamed, the condition is known as diverticulosis; when inflammation occurs, it is called diverticulitis. Since it is often difficult to differentiate diverticulosis from diverticulitis clinically, the general term diverticular disease is preferred.

Diverticular disease becomes more frequent with advancing age. The incidence below age 35 is low. In the USA, as shown by routine barium enema x-ray examinations, the incidence is about 10% at age 40 and about 65% by age 85.

Diverticular disease is somewhat more common in women than in men. The incidence is considerably higher in North America and Europe than in the Orient and Africa. When it does occur in Orientals, it is more common on the right side of the colon. An unusually high incidence of the disease occurs in some families.

The pathogenesis is not completely understood. Experimentally in rats, lifetime low-residue diets result in colonic diverticula whereas normal high-bulk diets prevent their development. It has been suggested that the relatively low-residue diet consumed by those living in Europe and North America may be responsible for the higher incidence there in contrast to other parts of the world where higher-bulk diets are consumed.

It was once believed that obesity, endomorphic diathesis, and weakening of the bowel wall with advanced age were etiologic factors, but these hypotheses have not proved tenable. Functional disturbances of neural and muscular elements of the colon appear to play an important part in the pathogenesis. The distal colon and sigmoid are the most frequent location of diverticula even when more proximal segments are also involved. The descending, transverse, and ascending colon and the cecum are involved in decreasing order of frequency. At times the entire colon is extensively involved. Irritability of the sigmoid promotes muscular spasm, muscle thickening, increased intraluminal pressure, and the development of diverticula. Muscular thickening and shortening in both muscle layers occurs early and consistently. There is a relative increase in the number of ganglionic cells. It is possible that segmental contraction of interhaustral rings forms compartments in which intraluminal pressure may become very high. Segmental areas of high pressure may be responsible for diverticula formation.

Colonic diverticula consist of herniations of the mucosa and submucosa through the muscular layer, which is markedly attenuated or absent in the wall of the diverticulum (Fig 36–13). They often develop at the point where blood vessels pass through the bowel wall. They may have a narrow neck and may vary from a few millimeters to several centimeters in diameter. Fecal matter becomes inspissated in the diverticulum and cannot be emptied because of the narrow opening and lack of musculature. On examination of a segment of colon removed surgically for "diverticulitis," the principal finding is usually muscle hypertrophy with induration and some congestion in the pericolic fatty tissue without microscopic evidence of inflammation.

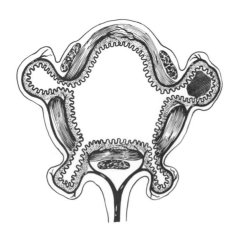

FIG 36–13. Cross-section of the colon depicting the sites where diverticula form. Note that the antimesenteric portion is spared.

Inflammation results from rupture of a diverticulum with peridiverticulitis, manifested by intramural or extramural abscesses, edema, and inflammation of the adjacent peritoneum, small intestine, bladder, and other surrounding structures. Fistulas into adjacent structures may occur.

A. Symptoms and Signs:

1. Diverticulosis—Uncomplicated diverticulosis may be asymptomatic or may present with the symptoms of "irritable colon," ie, frequent, small, hard bowel movements with crampy abdominal pain. The patient may suffer mildly in this fashion for years without developing complications. Often, however, diverticulosis is found on barium x-ray studies for a suspected polyp or carcinoma, with no history of abnormal colonic function except bleeding.

In approximately 80% of all cases of massive lower gastrointestinal hemorrhage, diverticulosis is the only abnormality found on barium enema. In a high proportion of such cases, bleeding is coming from a small artery in the wall of a diverticulum.

2. Diverticulitis—Although, as previously noted, mildly symptomatic diverticulosis and diverticulitis are difficult to distinguish, once an infectious complication develops the disease becomes chronic with episodes of exacerbation and remission. Diverticulitis may simulate appendicitis, salpingitis, endometriosis, ovarium tumors, infarction of an epiploic appendage, ulcerative colitis, cystitis, and retroperitoneal tumors.

In most cases, the disease presents somewhat like acute appendicitis but on the left side of the abdomen. In the acute attack, there is tenderness and often a palpable mass in the left lower quadrant. In contrast to appendicitis, the tenderness is likely to be more diffuse, but without signs of rapidly progressive peritonitis. A mass is often palpable early in an attack.

Constant mild to severe left lower quadrant abdominal or suprapubic pain is present and may be associated with cramps. Defecation or the passage of flatus may bring mild relief. Either constipation or increased frequency of defecation rather than actual diarrhea occurs. Partial obstruction with abdominal distention gradually ensues. There may be progressive enlargement of a mass in the left lower quadrant.

In some cases, the inflammatory signs are not marked but a palpable mass with tenderness and signs of large bowel obstruction are present, so that carcinoma of the left colon seems the more likely diagnosis.

Since the sigmoid colon often lies close to the bladder, the adjacent inflammation may produce dysuria and frequency of urination. These may progress to the development of a colovesical fistula with severe cystitis, pneumaturia, and fecaluria. If perforation occurs into the vagina, the resulting colovaginal fistula will be manifested by feculent vaginal drainage.

In all cases of diverticulitis, occult blood may be found in the stool if searched for carefully. Occasionally, gross bleeding makes the differential diagnosis between carcinoma and diverticulitis difficult. Massive hemorrhage. however, is more likely to occur in diverticulosis without inflammation or infection.

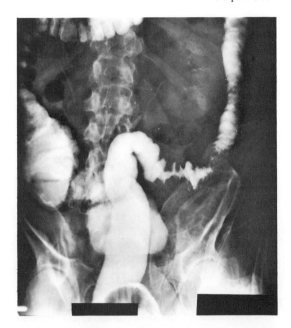

FIG 36–14. Barium enema roentgenogram showing upper sigmoid colon involved by diverticulitis. Note the long segment of narrowing, the spasm, and the deformity.

At times the progress of diverticulitis is so insidious that vague abdominal pains associated with an abscess in the groin or pneumaturia is the initial presentation. The mildness of the left lower quadrant pain in association with a large fixed mass may suggest lymphoma or retroperitoneal tumor.

B. X-Ray Findings: While barium enema is most useful in the detection of diverticular disease, it is not accurate in determining whether or not inflammation is present. Barium enema should not be done early in acute diverticulitis or if there are marked peritoneal signs and suspected perforation.

In the incipient stage of diverticular disease, x-ray may show only segmental spasm and muscle thickening. Later, diverticula appear either in a localized segment of the sigmoid or scattered diffusely throughout the colon (Fig 36–14). As spasm and muscular thickening become advanced, one sees multiple diverticula with a deformed haustral pattern, sharp serrations along the outline of the bowel ("saw-tooth appearance"), and narrowing of the lumen. These signs are not the result of inflammation, and may persist after an acute attack has subsided. Reliable features of active inflammation are (1) an abscess cavity or sinus tract outside the colonic wall communicating with the lumen; (2) intramural sinuses; (3) extramural abscesses which do not fill with barium but which cause eccentric impressions on the bowel wall; (4) flattening of the colonic mucosa from pressure by an extracolonic mass; (5) fistulas into the bladder or vagina; (6) fixation of the bowel; (7) restricted distensibility or "stiffening"

of the bowel; and (8) edema of the mucosa or of the wall of adjacent small bowel.

Intravenous urography may reveal distortion or partial obstruction to the ureter or compression of the bladder by the inflammatory mass.

C. Special Examinations: Sigmoidoscopy is sometimes helpful. The instrument usually cannot be passed beyond the rectosigmoid because of acute angulation and fixation at that level with a decrease in size of the lumen. Erythema and edema as well as spasm may be noted. A purulent discharge can sometimes be seen coming down from above. Rarely, the mouth of the diverticulum with a fecalith in it may be seen.

Differential Diagnosis

As noted earlier, diverticulitis may be protean in its manifestations. It may simulate any of the inflammatory lesions of the lower abdomen, particularly appendicitis and pelvic inflammatory disease. In many instances, a history of previous bowel symptoms provides a clue to diverticulitis rather than appendicitis or salpingitis. In the more silent forms of diverticulitis with a mass which compresses the bowel or bladder on x-ray, the final diagnosis may not be resolved until laparotomy.

With mild diverticulitis associated with bleeding, the differentiation from bleeding colonic polyps may be difficult.

The most difficult differential diagnosis is between carcinoma and diverticulitis. The differentiation is sometimes impossible until the bowel has been removed and examined by the pathologist.

Complications

In uncomplicated diverticulosis, massive hemorrhage may be severe; it is usually self-limited but may be exsanguinating.

Diverticulitis. Acute perforation through the overlying peritoneum results in localized or generalized peritonitis. The differentiation from other forms of visceral perforation may be extremely difficult. The presence of a very large amount of free air associated with acute peritonitis should suggest the possibility of a perforated diverticulum.

Slower perforation results in localized abscesses contained by adjacent omentum, bowel, or the leaves of the mesentery. Obstruction is usually slow and incomplete. Acute small bowel obstruction may result from the attachment of a loop of ileum to an inflamed sigmoid.

Fistula, especially in males, usually involves the bladder. Urinary frequency, dysuria, fecaluria, and pneumaturia are symptoms of vesicocolic fistula. Fistulas may also occur to the ureter, urethra, abdominal wall, vagina, uterus, perineum, cecum, and small bowel. A retroperitoneal perforation may dissect along the psoas muscle and present in the thigh.

Treatment

A. Medical Treatment: Uncomplicated diverticular disease should be managed medically. Diet should contain the normal amount of bulk except during an acute attack, when it should be restricted to liquids or parenteral feeding.

Parenteral antibiotics such as penicillin and streptomycin in combination, chloramphenicol, tetracyclines, kanamycin, and ampicillin are indicated during acute attacks for short periods only. Morphine should be avoided since it increases spasm; meperidine or pentazocine should be used for relief of pain if narcotics are required. After acute manifestations have subsided, additional bulk-forming hemicellulose (1 rounded teaspoonful in a full glass of cold water twice a day) is given. Antispasmodics may be helpful. Dioctyl sodium sulfosuccinate (Colace, etc) is helpful in keeping the stool soft. Hot abdominal packs may be utilized.

B. Surgical Treatment: Ideally, recurrent symptomatic diverticulitis should be treated surgically before the development of the major complications—abscess, free perforation, fistula, or obstruction. Unfortunately, the disease often progresses so insidiously that a major complication is the first sign of the disease requiring hospitalization.

1. Massive hemorrhage—See below.

2. Abscess—Localized abscess is the most common presenting form of diverticulitis. It may vary in extent from a simple limited intramural dissection with localized inflammation to the development of a massive abscess filling the pelvis and exerting pressure on the rectum and bladder. Rarely, when completely localized to the colonic wall, acute diverticulitis may be treated by a single stage resection and anastomosis.

Large abscesses usually require drainage and simultaneous diversion of the fecal stream by colostomy. A direct attack upon the involved bowel is often possible. If extensive abscess formation is found, the lesion can be resected, the distal segment closed, and a proximal colostomy performed (Hartmann procedure).

3. Obstruction—Significant degrees of colonic obstruction associated with abscess formation are best treated by proximal colostomy. If there is any question of perforation of the bowel, the colostomy should be performed in the descending rather than the transverse colon; otherwise, copious amounts of feces between the transverse colostomy and the site of the perforation will enter the peritoneal cavity. In this situation also, a Hartmann type of procedure may occasionally be preferable. In poor-risk patients, a staged procedure is clearly best.

4. Perforation—Free perforation with generalized peritonitis is rare. It requires emergency operation with mobilization and exteriorization of the perforated segment. If this is not possible, a Hartmann procedure should be performed (Fig 36–15). In either case, excision or exteriorization of the site of a free perforation has given better results than suture-closure of the perforation and proximal colostomy.

5. Fistula—Fistula into the bladder or vagina, when associated with abscess formation, is best treated by staged operations. Transverse colostomy followed later by resection and anastomosis and then by sub-

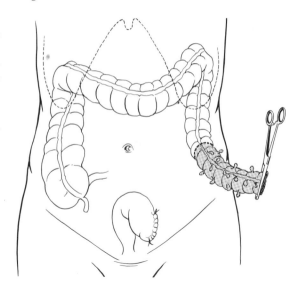

FIG 36–15. Two-stage (Hartmann) resection for diverticulitis of the colon. *Stage I:* The affected segment (shaded) has been divided at its distal end and brought out through the abdominal wall. It will then be removed by transection at its proximal margin (dotted line), leaving a healthy colostomy stoma of the surface of the abdomen. The upper end of the rectosigmoid stump has been sutured closed. Alternatively, it could have been exteriorized without closing it. *Stage II:* The divided ends of the bowel will be mobilized and anastomosed.

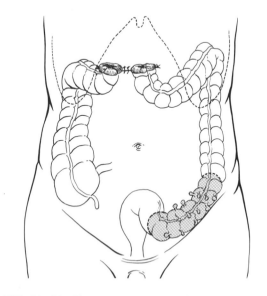

FIG 36–16. Three-stage procedure for resection of a segment of the colon involved by diverticulitis. *Stage I:* Transverse colostomy. *Stage II:* Resection of the involved segment (shaded) (lines of resection indicated by dotted lines) and anastomosis of healthy ends. *Stage III:* Closure of transverse colostomy.

sequent closure of the colostomy is the procedure of choice (Fig 36–16).

At times, fistulas are sharply localized and not associated with extensive inflammation or abscess formation. Under these circumstances, a one-stage resection may be undertaken.

6. Diverticula involving the right colon—About 1% of surgically treated diverticula occur in the cecum. Because of the similarity in the symptoms and signs, the most common preoperative diagnosis is appendicitis. In cecal diverticulitis, nausea and vomiting may not occur, diarrhea is more common than constipation, and melena occurs occasionally. At operation, the lesion is often thought to be malignant. Upon surgical exploration, if an easily recognizable inflamed diverticulum (often containing a fecalith) is found, simple excision of the diverticulum and closure should be done. If a more extensive indurated mass which cannot be differentiated from carcinoma is discovered, right colectomy is the procedure of choice.

Prognosis

About 15% of all patients with diverticular disease will develop diverticulitis, and about 25% of these will require surgical treatment. The prognosis in diverticulitis is related to age, the severity of the disease, and the occurrence of complications. The operative mortality rate is 3–5%. In properly selected cases, the outlook following operation is good.

Bahabozorgui S, DeMuth WE Jr, Blakemore WS: Diverticulitis of the ascending colon. Am J Surg 115:295–300, 1968.

Behringer GE, Albright NL: Diverticular disease of the colon: A frequent cause of massive rectal bleeding. Am J Surg 125:419–423, 1973.

Eusebio EB, Eisenberg MM: Natural history of diverticular disease of the colon in young patients. Am J Surg 125:308–311, 1973.

Parks TG: Rectal and colonic studies after resection of the sigmoid for diverticular disease. Gut 11:121, 1970.

Parks TG, Connell AM: Motility studies in diverticular disease of the colon. Gut 10:534–542, 1969.

Parks TG & others: Limitations of radiology in the differentiation of diverticulitis and diverticulosis of the colon. Brit MJ 2:136, 1970.

Sawyer KC, Sawyer RB, Waggener HU: The pathogenesis of diverticulosis coli. Dis Colon Rectum 12:49–57, 1969.

MASSIVE LOWER GASTROINTESTINAL HEMORRHAGE

Massive lower gastrointestinal hemorrhage should be suspected whenever copious amounts of bright-red blood are passed by rectum without signs of hypotension or shock. Although bright-red blood may be passed by rectum in large amounts from upper gastrointestinal bleeding, the bleeding in such cases is usually so copious that shock is present. The most common causes of massive lower gastrointestinal hemorrhage—in addition to diverticulosis—are ulcerative colitis, superficial ulcers, and vascular anomalies of the distal small bowel and right colon, polyps of the colon, benign ulcers of the cecum, and ulcerative ectopic gastric mucosa in a Meckel's diverticulum. A variety of bizarre intestinal hemangiomas are being identified by means of angiography. Massive hemorrhage is rare in carcinoma.

Evaluation of massive rectal hemorrhage should include aspiration of the stomach to rule out upper gastrointestinal bleeding, sigmoidoscopic examination to exclude extensive local inflammatory lesions or neoplasms, and emergency x-ray studies. When the clinical diagnosis of massive lower gastrointestinal hemorrhage seems well established, selective angiography appears to be the most reliable means of identifying the site of the bleeding. Barium enema may be required, particularly where there is a suggestion of carcinoma. The differentiation from massive upper gastrointestinal hemorrhage may be so difficult that gastroscopy, duodenoscopy, and an upper gastrointestinal series may be required.

In most cases, massive lower colonic hemorrhage ceases spontaneously and permits interim evaluation. At times, however, as in upper gastrointestinal bleeding, the hemorrhage is exsanguinating, and the same criteria for emergency operation should be employed as in upper gastrointestinal bleeding. Preoperative angiography should be done whenever possible, since otherwise it may be extremely difficult to localize the site of bleeding.

Recently, continuous infusion of vasopressin into the artery supplying the bleeding point has shown great therapeutic promise. The vasoconstrictor is administered through a catheter passed percutaneously and positioned selectively in the orifice of the appropriate vessel.

At operation, the colon is found to be massively distended with blood and localization of the bleeding point by operative colonoscopy and isolation of loops of bowel between clamps is hazardous and often unrevealing.

If the site of the bleeding has not been identified by angiography, subtotal colectomy with ileorectal anastomosis is the procedure of choice. If there is extensive diverticulosis, the resection should be started on the left side of the colon and, in poor-risk patients, may be terminated if the bleeding site is found. If no diverticula are present, the likelihood of mucosal erosions, benign ulcers, or hemangiomas is great and—since these lesions are more common on the right side—the resection should be started by removing the right colon. Again, if the bleeding point is not identified, subtotal colectomy is the operation of choice.

In patients in whom the hemorrhage stops spontaneously and no cause can be found, operation should not be done. Twenty-five to 50% of these patients may return with recurrent bleeding. Prompt angiographic study should be undertaken in hopes of identifying the bleeding point.

Albo RJ & others: Management of massive lower gastrointestinal hemorrhage. Am J Surg 112:264–272, 1966.

Judd ES: Massive bleeding of colonic origin. S Clin North America 49:977–989, 1969.

VOLVULUS

Essentials of Diagnosis

- Colicky abdominal pain, usually with persistence of pain between spasms.
- Vomiting.
- Abdominal distention.
- Cecal volvulus may simulate low small bowel obstruction.
- Usually older age groups.
- Characteristic x-ray findings.

General Considerations

Rotation of a segment of the intestine on an axis formed by its mesentery may result in partial or complete obstruction to the lumen and may be followed by varying degrees of circulatory impairment of the bowel (Fig 36–17). In the colon, volvulus usually occurs in the sigmoid or, less frequently, in the cecum.

Sigmoid volvulus is twice as common in males as it is in females, whereas in cecal volvulus the reverse is true. Predisposing factors in cecal volvulus include a hypermobile cecum due to incomplete embryologic fixation of the ascending colon and (often) distention due to partial obstruction of the left colon. In sigmoid volvulus, elongation of the sigmoid and a high-residue vegetable diet may be implicated. Mentally ill, elderly, or bedridden patients have a propensity to develop volvulus. As the bowel twists about the mesentery, it forms a closed loop obstruction as the entry and exit points of the twist engage. Gaseous distention occurs within the loop. The veins may become obstructed, and the impaired circulation may cause rupture. The mortality rate is great if the process is allowed to reach the stage of gangrene and peritonitis.

Clinical Findings

A. Cecal Volvulus:

1. Symptoms and signs—The symptoms of cecal volvulus begin abruptly, with severe, intermittent colicky pains in the right abdomen which eventually become continuous. Nausea, vomiting, and dehydration follow. Passage of gas and feces per rectum decreases to the point of obstipation. There is often a history of milder but similar attacks.

2. X-ray findings—The diagnosis is seldom made without x-ray examination. X-rays show a dilated cecum which may be anywhere in the abdomen but often is located in the epigastrium. A single fluid level is present which may resemble gastric dilatation. However, large amounts of gas or fluid cannot be aspirated from the stomach, and the x-ray picture is not changed by this maneuver. The dilated segment may appear ovoid and may change position on repeated x-rays. After a short time, the findings of small bowel obstruction appear because the volvulus obstructs the ileocecal valve.

B. Sigmoid Volvulus:

1. Symptoms and signs—In volvulus of the sigmoid there are intermittent cramp-like pains, increasing in severity as obstipation becomes complete. Abdominal distention may be marked. There may be a

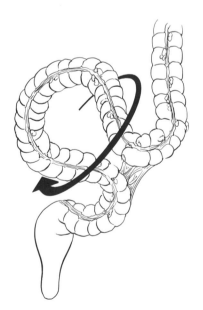 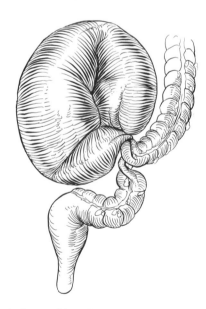

FIG 36–17. Volvulus of the sigmoid colon. A clockwise twist is shown although the twist is counterclockwise in most cases of sigmoid volvulus.

history of transient attacks in which spontaneous reduction of the volvulus has occurred.

2. X-ray findings—On a plain film of the abdomen a single greatly distended loop of bowel which has lost its haustral markings is usually seen rising up out of the pelvis, frequently as high as the diaphragm. The distended loop may assume a "coffee bean" shape. In cecal volvulus, the concavity of the "coffee bean" points toward the right lower abdominal quadrant and in sigmoid volvulus it points toward the left lower quadrant. On barium enema a "bird's beak" or "ace of spades" deformity with spiral narrowing of the upper end of the lower segment is pathognomonic (Fig 36–18). Between attacks, barium enema may reveal localized sigmoid megacolon.

Differential Diagnosis

The causes of obstruction of the colon include carcinoma, fecal impaction, diverticulitis, incarcerated hernia, intussusception, and adhesions. The obstruction caused by diverticulitis is usually incomplete. In the USA, sigmoid volvulus is the second most common cause (following adenocarcinoma) of complete obstruction of the colon.

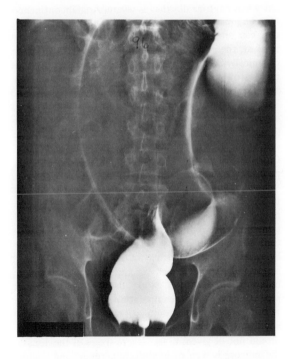

FIG 36–18. Volvulus of the sigmoid colon. Roentgenogram with barium enema taken with the patient in the supine position. Note the massively dilated sigmoid colon. The distinct vertical crease, which represents juxtaposition of adjacent walls of the dilated loop, points toward the site of torsion. The barium column resembles a bird's beak or ace of spades because of the way in which the lumen tapers toward the volvulus.

Complications

Early diagnosis and treatment are imperative because of the danger of closed loop obstruction and the high incidence of circulatory damage to the bowel wall. In cases of colonic volvulus with perforation, a mortality rate of about 50% can be expected. Delay may be due to incorrect diagnosis or to attempts at proximal decompression by gastric intubation or cecostomy, neither of which would relieve the closed loop obstruction.

Treatment

In **cecal volvulus**, early operation is the treatment of choice. Untwisting the loop with fixation or plication procedures has often been followed by recurrence of the volvulus. If the patient's clinical condition permits, right hemicolectomy with ileotransverse colon anastomosis is desirable. If the bowel is gangrenous or the patient's condition is poor, exteriorization of the involved segment and obstructive resection may be preferable. Reduction of the volvulus and fixation by cecostomy may be lifesaving in aged, poor-risk patients, but volvulus may recur.

In **sigmoid volvulus**, the distended sigmoid may be deflated by passing a soft rectal tube through a sigmoidoscope into the twisted loop. This maneuver is contraindicated if there are signs of strangulation or perforation. The tube should be inserted while the patient is in the knee-chest position. Occasionally, when the knee-chest position is assumed, detorsion of the loop occurs spontaneously. The tube should be left in the sigmoid and secured by tape or sutures to the perianal skin. If the tube must be forced to enter the obstructed loop, the bowel may be perforated. After the bowel is decompressed with the tube, surgical resection of the sigmoid should be scheduled as soon as the patient's condition permits and the intestine can be thoroughly cleansed (usually in 4–6 days). Discharge from the hospital before the sigmoid is removed imposes a high risk of recurrent volvulus, but elderly patients may be treated expectantly after initial decompression and sigmoidectomy performed only if recurrence appears. Exteriorization or obstructive resection of the involved loop is the procedure of choice if emergency laparotomy is indicated for strangulation. If the distal segment of the involved bowel is too short to be brought out onto the abdomen, it may be transected and closed and the upper segment alone brought out as a single-barreled colostomy. Primary resection is rarely justified during emergency operations.

Prognosis

The prognosis depends on the amount of circulatory impairment of the involved loop and the general condition of the patient. Strangulation can be avoided by rapid diagnosis and treatment. Under the most favorable circumstances and with the employment of proper surgical measures, recurrence is almost nil and operative mortality is low. With delay in diagnosis and ill-conceived operation, recurrences are common and the mortality rate high.

Hines JR, Geurkink RE, Bass RT: Recurrence and mortality rates in sigmoid volvulus. Surg Gynec Obst 124:567, 1967.

Kerry RL, Ransom HK: Volvulus of the colon: Etiology, diagnosis, and treatment. Arch Surg 99:215–222, 1969.

Krippaehne WW, Vetto RM, Jenkins CC: Volvulus of the ascending colon. Am J Surg 114:323–332, 1967.

Prather JR, Bowers RF: Volvulus of the sigmoid: Surgical indications. Resident Physician 14:39–48, 1968.

NONSPECIFIC COLITIS

In recent years, nonspecific colitis has been divided into 2 types on the basis of pathologic and clinical manifestations: (1) idiopathic mucosal colitis (ulcerative colitis) and (2) granulomatous colitis (Crohn's disease). There are, however, morphologic features and characteristics of clinical behavior which are common to both, and, since the cause is not known in either case, a sharp distinction between the 2 cannot always be made.

1. IDIOPATHIC MUCOSAL ULCERATIVE COLITIS*

Essentials of Diagnosis

- Bloody diarrhea.
- Lower abdominal cramps.
- Fever, weight loss, anemia.
- No stool pathogens.
- Specific findings on sigmoidoscopy and roentgenography.

General Considerations

Ulcerative colitis is an inflammatory disease of the colon characterized by bloody diarrhea and a tendency to remissions and exacerbations. It usually begins between 20 and 30 years of age, but may have its onset in any age group. Its incidence is about equal in both sexes. In at least 2% of cases there is a family history of the disease. Ulcerative colitis is more frequent in Jews. It is infrequent in persons with Rh-negative blood. The cause is not known, though infections and immunologic, nutritional, and psychologic factors have all been postulated. Chronic ulcerative colitis may follow an attack of acute infective enterocolitis in a previously healthy person. There is some evidence that autoimmune reactions occur in ulcerative colitis, possibly related to a lipopolysaccharide colonic antigen. The theory that the disease is a primary psychologic disturbance is not generally accepted; however, stressful episodes may precede relapses or aggravate the diarrhea.

*See also Granulomatous Colitis, p 650.

The disease initially involves the mucosa, with inflammatory changes in the crypts of Lieberkühn and the formation of crypt abscesses. In the early stages, hyperemia and mucosal granularity occur; as the disease progresses (at an extremely variable rate), multiple, ragged ulcerations occur. The mucosa may be denuded, sometimes leaving islands of residual epithelium hanging as "pseudopolyps." It usually starts in the rectum and sigmoid colon and may spread to involve the entire colon rapidly or over the course of years. It characteristically stops short at the ileocecal valve but may involve the terminal ileum. In these cases it is not known whether the disease is primary in the ileum or whether ileal involvement is due to reflux from the colon to cause a "backwash ileitis." If the inflammation is severe, it may penetrate through the muscularis mucosae to the deeper layers of the bowel.

Clinical Findings

A. Symptoms and Signs: The onset is often insidious, with recollection of loose or frequent stools only after accentuation of symptoms. Infrequently, the patient presents for the first time during a fulminating attack. A relapse commonly occurs following a prolonged remission or superimposed on low-grade continuous symptoms. Nocturnal diarrhea is usually present when daytime diarrhea is severe. Anal incontinence may be present. A history of intolerance to dairy products can often be obtained. When symptoms are most marked, the picture is that of a febrile, pale, acutely or chronically ill patient who is passing frequent discharges of watery stool, mucus, blood, and pus with abdominal cramps, rectal urgency, and tenesmus. There are varying degrees of weight loss and protein, water, electrolyte, and vitamin depletion. If the symptoms are mild, the clinical picture varies from one of malnutrition to that of almost complete normality. Constipation, possibly due to spasm, is sometimes the presenting symptom.

On physical examination, the abdomen may be tender, especially in the left lower quadrant. The colon may be palpable or distended. There may be rebound tenderness; this sign does not always represent perforation. The anus is often secondarily inflamed and may be fissured, tender, and spastic. The rectal mucosa may feel normal or gritty. The examining gloved finger may be covered with mucus, blood, or pus. If the disease is mild, general physical examination may be normal.

Sigmoidoscopic examination is essential and usually establishes the diagnosis. A preexamination enema should not be given. In less severe stages of the disease, the mucosa is seen to be dull, hyperemic, and friable, so that the touch of a cotton swab results in oozing of blood. Patches of mucus may be adherent to the mucosa. In a more advanced stage, the friability of the mucosa is marked and there are petechial hemorrhages with mucus, pus, and fibrin presenting a yellow or greenish color adherent to the mucosa. Superficial ulcers are seen. In severe stages, the mucosa is edematous and oozes freely and blood is mixed with the mucus and pus.

The apparent severity of what is seen with the sigmoidoscope does not necessarily parallel the radiographic findings nor the symptoms. With healing, the mucosa appears granular, edema subsides, and inflammatory polyps of various sizes may be seen. There may be stricture formation. Rectal biopsy of the mucosa is helpful in confirming the diagnosis and establishing the severity of the disease.

B. Laboratory Findings: Hypochromic, microcytic anemia is usually present. In acute disease, polymorphonuclear leukocytosis may be present. The sedimentation rate is elevated. There may be hypoproteinemia and electrolyte disturbances.

C. X-Ray Findings: In acutely symptomatic patients, a plain film of the abdomen must be taken to detect dilatation of the colon. Barium enema examination will reveal the extent of colonic involvement but should not be performed early in an acute attack. It must be done carefully—often without preliminary catharsis. In acute cases, the involved area shows mucosal irregularity which varies from fine serrations to a rough, ragged appearance due to deep undermined ulcers. As the disease progresses, secondary thickening and rigidity of the muscle cause narrowing and shortening of the involved portion. Normal haustrations are gradually effaced (Fig 36–19). Pseudopolyposis may be seen and signifies severe ulceration. Periproctitis is

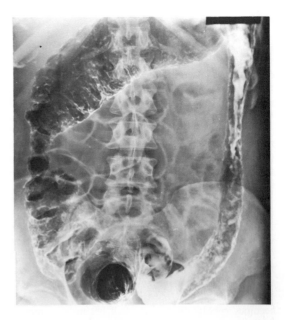

FIG 36–20. Roentgenogram of ulcerative colitis. Note dilatation of the transverse colon, the multiple irregular densities in the lumen which represent pseudopolyps, the thickening of the wall of the descending colon and the loss of haustral markings.

indicated by a widening of the space between the sacrum and rectum.

Toxic dilatation in acute attacks tends to occur in the transverse colon. The bowel wall is thickened, and air within the dilated segment may outline irregular nodular pseudopolyps which project into the lumen (Fig 36–20). Barium enema examination is especially hazardous and contraindicated with toxic dilatation and may precipitate this complication if performed in severely ill patients with acute colitis.

Strictures, which are not typical of the inflammatory process, should be presumed to be neoplastic in patients with chronic ulcerative colitis of long duration.

Differential Diagnosis

Differentiation from bacillary dysentery and amebic dysentery cannot be made on clinical grounds alone, and cultures must be taken for specific stool pathogens. Rectal strictures must be differentiated from lymphogranuloma venereum by history and the Frei or complement fixation test. Functional diarrhea, intestinal neoplasms and diverticulitis must be differentiated on the basis of the history and the sigmoidoscopic and x-ray findings.

The differentiating features of mucosal idiopathic ulcerative colitis and granulomatous transmural colitis are listed in Table 36–3.

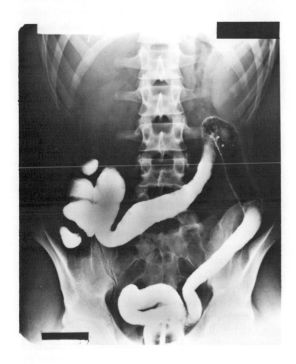

FIG 36–19. Nonspecific ulcerative colitis. Barium enema roentgenogram of colon. Note shortening of colon, loss of haustral markings ("lead pipe" appearance) and fine serrations at the edges of the bowel wall which represent multiple, small ulcers.

Complications

Systemic complications consist of (1) skin lesions such as erythema nodosum, erythema multiforme, or pyoderma gangrenosum; (2) pustular dermatitis; (3) aphthous ulcers of the mouth; (4) uveitis; (5) arthralgias, especially of the hips, knees, and ankles; (6) pericholangitis and cholestasis; and (7) cirrhosis of the liver.

Anorectal complications consist of (1) ischiorectal abscess; (2) fistula in ano and rectovaginal fistula (although these occur less frequently than in granulomatous colitis); and (3) incontinence following destruction of the sphincteric mechanism.

Perforation of the colon in acute cases may result in diffuse peritonitis or localized pericolic abscesses.

A serious complication is the marked dilatation which occurs during a severe attack. In **toxic dilatation** ("toxic megacolon"), the patient is very ill, with high fever, leukocytosis, dehydration, hypoproteinemia, and a hugely distended abdomen. A segment of the colon (usually the transverse) or the entire colon becomes greatly dilated; its wall becomes extremely thin and fragile; and the inflammation extends from the mucosa through the bowel wall to the serosa. Hypokalemia, opiates, anticholinergic drugs, barium enema, and corticosteroids have been implicated as inciting factors.

Massive hemorrhage is uncommon but is a life-threatening complication when it does occur.

Cancer of the colon develops in 10–30% of cases of over 10 years' duration. It may occur at any site in the rectum and colon, and may be multicentric and aggressively malignant.

Treatment

A. Conservative Measures: Bed rest is necessary during the acute phase and may substantially reduce intestinal cramping and diarrhea. The diet should be bland. During the acute phase, elimination of milk, milk products, and wheat may reduce the diarrhea; these foods may be added to the diet when the disease process has improved. Understanding and reassurance of the patient is necessary. Mild sedation is often necessary for nervousness.

Care should be taken in the administration of antiperistaltic agents (anticholinergics, opiates) because they may produce dilatation of the colon during an acute severe attack. Narcotics should be avoided except for severe diarrhea. Corticotropin, adrenocorticosteroids, and the sulfonamides are the best drugs for control of the disease. The hospitalized patient may be given corticotropin (ACTH) as an intravenous drip (20–40 units over a period of 8 hours), or 80–100 units of corticotropin gel subcut. Alternatively, hydrocortisone (100–300 mg/day), prednisone or prednisolone (20–80 mg/day), or equivalent may be given. If response to corticotropin is satisfactory, the dosage may be reduced to oral therapy with prednisone (20–40 mg/day) and gradually reduced at weekly intervals over a period of 1–3 months. Long-term suppression of ulcerative colitis with these agents

leads to hyperadrenocorticism, osteoporosis, toxic psychosis, peptic ulcer, hypokalemia, and hyperglycemia.

Topical therapy with hydrocortisone enemas allows long-term treatment with corticosteroids with minimal side-effects and is the best treatment once the attack has been brought under control. Give hydrocortisone hemisuccinate (100 mg) or prednisolone-21-phosphate (20 mg) in 100 ml of saline once or twice daily by slow rectal drip or retention enema; or hydrocortisone in oil (100 mg/60 ml) every night as a retention enema. The patient should preferably lie on his left side with the buttocks elevated. Hydrocortisone is the least expensive and can be prepared for home use by mixing 1.6 g of hydrocortisone powder in one quart of vegetable oil. Sixty ml of the well-shaken mixture is instilled in the rectum with a 60 ml bulb syringe.

Sulfonamides are not curative, but chronic administration may reduce the incidence of recurrence and severity of individual attacks. Give either (1) salicylazosulfapyridine (Azulfidine), 2–8 g/day orally, or (2) sulfisoxazole (Gantrisin), 2 g/day orally.

B. Surgical Treatment:

1. Indications—

a. Emergency—Emergency operation is indicated in the following circumstances: (1) development of abdominal physical signs suggesting perforation of the bowel; (2) sudden deterioration in the general condition of the patient; (3) persistent massive hemorrhage from the bowel which does not subside with bed rest and transfusions; (4) acute toxic dilatation of the colon unresponsive to 48–72 hours of treatment.

Surgery should be scheduled for any adult suffering from a severe attack who fails to respond to intensive conservative treatment within 2–3 days, or for younger patients who fail to respond in 4–5 days. A severe attack may be defined as one in which there is diarrhea of 6 or more bowel movements a day, gross blood in the stool, fever, tachycardia, leukocytosis, and anemia. The necessity for operation, however, cannot be arbitrary; each case must be evaluated individually.

b. Chronic debilitating ulcerative colitis—When patients become "bowel cripples," unable to maintain nutrition, and suffer economic loss and are confined to bed for long periods, colectomy results in dramatic improvement.

c. Perianal and perirectal infections may be crippling, and local surgical methods result in worsening of the local process more often than not. Removal of the colon may be necessary for rehabilitation.

d. Carcinoma of the colon or rectum—Carcinoma complicating ulcerative colitis often defies early diagnosis since the symptoms are similar. The infected, scarred bowel interferes with the interpretation of the barium enema, and cancer often infiltrates along the bowel wall rather than growing into the lumen.

e. Obstruction is a rare complication and occurs more frequently in granulomatous colitis.

f. Severity of the distant complications such as arthritis, uveitis, and skin manifestations may serve as an indication for surgery.

g. Impaired growth and development in children.

2. Surgical procedures–Total proctocolectomy with permanent ileostomy, usually performed in one stage, is the operation of choice in the great majority of cases. If the condition of the patient does not permit resection of the most distal segment, abdominoperineal resection of the rectum may be performed later. Impotence in men may result from the abdominoperineal resection but is not likely if the dissection is kept close to the bowel.

Subtotal colectomy with ileorectal anastomosis may be considered if there is relative sparing of the rectum by the disease. Earlier reports of good results with this operation probably included many cases of granulomatous colitis, and it is applicable at most to 10–15% of patients.

Prognosis

The course is characterized by remissions and exacerbations over a period of many years. With conservative treatment of "high-risk" groups, ie, those who have repeated severe attacks, those with total involvement of the colon, children, and those over 60 years of age, early mortality is 10–40% and the cumulative expected mortality over 20 years is nearly 60%. Death is due to the complications of acute attacks, cancer, and liver failure. Most patients do not fall into these high-risk groups and respond well to modern methods of conservative management, although permanent and complete cure on medical therapy is unusual.

The operative mortality is under 5% for elective surgery and under 25% in acute cases. Over 90% of surviving patients report good health following operation.

Anton HC: Radiological signs of ulcerative colitis. Gut 10:74, 1969.

Bargen JA, Aylett SO: Treatment of ulcerative colitis. Postgrad Med 45:176–180, 1969.

Edwards FC, Truelove SC: The course and prognosis of ulcerative colitis. I. Short-term prognosis. II. Long-term prognosis. III. Complications. IV. Carcinoma of the colon. Gut 4:299–315, 1963; 5:1–22, 1964.

TABLE 36–3. Comparison of various features of ulcerative colitis with those of granulomatous colitis.

	Ulcerative (Mucosal) Colitis	Granulomatous (Transmural) Colitis
Signs and symptoms		
Diarrhea	Marked.	Present; not severe.
Gross bleeding	Characteristic.	Infrequent.
Perianal lesions	Infrequent.	Frequent; may precede diagnosis of intestinal disease.
Toxic dilatation	Yes.	Rare.
Carcinoma	Frequent.	Rare.
Systemic manifestations (arthritis, uveitis, pyoderma, hepatitis)	Common.	Infrequent.
X-ray studies	Confluent, diffuse.	Skip areas.
	Tiny serrations (crypt abscess), coarse mucosa, mucosal tags.	Longitudinal ulcers, transverse ridges, "cobblestone" appearance.
	Concentric involvement.	Eccentric involvement ("fingerprinting").
	Rare internal fistulas.	Internal fistulas and sinus tracts (occasionally).
	Colon only involved; usually worse on left.	Any portion of intestinal tract may be involved.
Morphology		
Gross	Confluent involvement.	Segmental involvement with or without skip areas.
	Rectum usually involved.	Rectum often not involved.
	Mesentery not involved; nodes enlarged.	Thickened mesentery; pronounced lymph node enlargement.
	Widespread ragged superficial ulceration.	Large longitudinal ulcers; lateral fissures.
	Inflammatory polyps (pseudopolyps) common.	Inflammatory polyps not prominent.
	No thickening of bowel wall.	Thickened bowel wall.
Microscopic	Inflammatory reaction usually limited to mucosa and submucosa; only in severe disease are muscle coats involved.	Chronic inflammation of all layers of bowel wall; damage to muscle layers usual.
	No sarcoid reaction.	Foreign body giant cells and tubercle formation (sarcoid reaction).
Natural history	Exacerbations, remissions; may be explosive, lethal.	Indolent, unrelenting, crippling; seldom lethal.
Treatment		
Response to medical treatment	Good response in 80% of cases.	Difficult to evaluate; seldom controlled.
Type of surgical treatment and response	Coloproctectomy with ileostomy; rectum can rarely be preserved.	Partial or complete colectomy with or without ileorectal anastomosis; rectum can often be preserved.

Goligher JC: The surgical treatment of ulcerative colitis. Postgrad MJ 44:708–719, 1968.

Goligher JC, Hoffman DC, deDombal FT: Surgical treatment of severe attacks of ulcerative colitis, with special reference to the advantages of early operation. Brit MJ 5:703–706, 1970.

Tompkins RK & others: Reappraisal of rectum-retaining operations for ulcerative and granulomatous colitis. Am J Surg 125:165–175, 1973.

Watson DW: The problem of chronic inflammatory bowel disease. California Med 117:25–41, July 1972.

Wright R: Ulcerative colitis. Gastroenterology 58:875–897, 1970.

2. GRANULOMATOUS COLITIS

Granulomatous colitis (Crohn's disease, regional colitis, transmural colitis) is now believed to be a separate entity from idiopathic mucosal ulcerative colitis. It is segmental. Noncaseating granulomas are found microscopically, and the inflammatory process is usually most evident in the proximal ascending colon and rectosigmoid colon.

The consistent distinguishing feature between ulcerative colitis and Crohn's disease is the mucosal location of the inflammatory process in the former and the transmural involvement in the latter. Serositis, occurrence of inflammatory masses, and the tendency to fistulization (Table 36–3) are other points of difference.

The most common presenting symptoms are diarrhea, crampy abdominal pain, and weight loss. Anal fistula or perianal abscess may antedate intestinal symptoms by years. The disease commonly occurs in younger people but may develop even after age 50. Stool examination is mandatory to exclude amebic and bacterial infections. Sigmoidoscopic examination may disclose characteristic granulomatous changes. Biopsy of the mucosa and submucosa may be diagnostic. The radiographic features include sparing of the rectum, involvement of the ileum, "skip areas" in the ileum or colon (or both), internal fistula, eccentric mucosal involvement, transverse fissures, and longitudinal ulcerations.

Medical management is the same as for ulcerative colitis. Sulfonamides and corticosteroids are not as effective in patients with granulomatous disease of the bowel as in those with ulcerative colitis, but these drugs appear to be of sufficient value to warrant their use in the initial medical management.

The effectiveness of medical versus surgical treatment of granulomatous colitis cannot yet be assessed. Since many of the available data on granulomatous colitis are based on highly selected groups of surgical cases, with pathologic specimens as the main source of the diagnosis, it has not yet been possible to accumulate sufficient data on the natural course of the disease and its prognosis.

Complications such as fistula, abscess, and stricture with obstruction necessitate surgery more frequently than in ulcerative colitis. Furthermore, surgery is more readily considered in granulomatous colitis because the distal colon is less often involved and it is possible to excise the diseased portion and perform an anastomosis, thereby restoring intestinal continuity.

Bypass operations (side-to-side anastomosis) and exclusion operations have not proved useful. Surgical treatment is now aimed at total excision of the involved segment of the bowel; the length of bowel to be removed depends upon the extent of the disease. Thus, ileectomy and right hemicolectomy with ileocolic anastomosis, or subtotal colectomy with ileorectal anastomosis, or total colectomy with ileostomy may be required.

Removal of the rectum may cause impotence in men unless the dissection is carried out close to the bowel. Fistulas and local inflammation and edema may make this difficult in Crohn's disease.

Carcinoma is rare in transmural colitis.

Recurrence following surgery is common if a segmental resection and anastomosis has been performed. Recurrence is rare in the ileum after total colectomy and ileostomy. If the ileum is involved at the time surgery is performed, the chance of recurrence elsewhere in the small bowel or colon or at the anastomosis is considerably higher than if the disease is confined to the colon.

Edwards H: Crohn's disease: An inquiry into its nature and consequences. Ann Roy Coll Surg Engl 44:121–139, 1969.

Glotzer DJ & others: Comparative features and course of ulcerative and granulomatous colitis. New England J Med 282:582–587, 1970.

Jones JH: Colonic cancer and Crohn's disease. Gut 10:651–654, 1969.

Lennard-Jones JE: Crohn's disease. Natural history and treatment. Postgrad MJ 44:674–679, 1968.

Schaupp WC, Gallagher DM, Scarborough RA: Regional colitis in lesions of the colon and rectum. Dis Colon Rectum 10:6, 1967.

Zetzel L: Granulomatous (ileo)colitis. New England J Med 282:600–605, 1970.

PNEUMATOSIS COLI

Pneumatosis coli is characterized by multiple cystic collections of gas in the wall of the bowel. It has a characteristic x-ray appearance. On endoscopic examination, superficial bleb-like cysts resembling adenomas are seen.

The cause is not known, and in most instances spontaneous resolution occurs. Rarely, this disorder has been associated with necrotizing ulcers of the bowel wall leading to perforation and peritonitis.

Unless signs of peritoneal irritation develop, operation is not indicated.

RADIATION (FACTITIAL) PROCTITIS

Exposure to radium, ^{60}Co, and x-ray employed in the treatment of malignant lesions of the pelvis, especially cancer of the cervix, uterus, bladder, and prostate, often causes reaction to the adjacent bowel. With the advent of high-voltage x-ray and ^{60}Co irradiation, skin effects are minimal and no longer limit the depth dose as was the case with 200–400 kv x-ray therapy.

The rectal mucosa is much more sensitive to irradiation than normal vaginal mucosa.

There may be no demonstrable external abnormalities or areas of skin change at the site of the x-ray exposure. On digital rectal examination, the anal canal may be tender and spastic. Induration of the rectal mucosa may be palpable, and the crater of an ulcer may be felt.

Proctosigmoidoscopy in the first few weeks after exposure shows the mucosa to be red and edematous and to bleed easily with slight trauma. It later becomes indurated and then flat, pale, and atrophic, and develops persistent telangiectasis. When ulcers occur, they are grayish, well defined, and oval or circular. Barium enema x-ray examination is helpful in the study of mucosal abnormalities and possible fistulas. It may reveal an annular filling defect due to stricture.

The rectosigmoid may be involved, resulting in a stenosing ulcerative lesion closely resembling cancer. Stenosis may not develop for months or years after treatment.

Small increments of radiation therapy to multiple fields, megavoltage doses, and cobalt therapy reduce the incidence of injury to the rectum and sigmoid colon when irradiation treatment is required. Direct exposure of bladder, bowel, and ureters must be avoided where possible. Special shield applicators for radium insertion and positioning of the patient should be used.

A low-residue diet, rectal instillations of warm oil, antispasmodics, and sedatives are indicated, as well as bed rest if necessary. Rectal instillation of hydrocortisone as in the treatment of ulcerative colitis may be helpful. Hydrocortisone (alcohol), 1.6 g in 1 liter of sesame oil, is shaken well and 60 ml of the mixture are injected into the rectum at bedtime with a rubber syringe. Bleeding often demands iron therapy or blood replacement. Colostomy may be indicated for patients with severe hemorrhage, intractable pain, or fistulas. Resection of the affected portion of the intraperitoneal bowel may be performed when the lesion is very localized and there is obstruction. Healing of irradiated tissue, including bowel, is notoriously poor. Rectal strictures should not be dilated since they often retrogress spontaneously.

It may take 1–2 years for the reaction in the bowel to reach a plateau, during which time bleeding continues. A stricture with partial obstruction may occur during healing. If the neoplastic disease has been eradicated, most patients will recover in time.

Nance FC, Persson AV, Piker JF: Radiation injuries to the lower gastrointestinal tract. Am Surg 34:21–25, 1968.

Quan SHQ: Factitial proctitis due to irradiation for cancer of the cervix uteri. Surg Gynec Obst 126:70–74, 1968.

COLONIC ENDOMETRIOSIS

Endometriosis undoubtedly affects the intestines far more than is reported, but it often does not cause sufficient symptoms to come to the physician's attention. Ectopic endometrium most commonly occurs in the ovaries, the posterior cul-de-sac, the pelvic peritoneum, the sacro-uterine ligaments, and on the peritoneal surface of the rectum and rectosigmoid. It may become locally invasive. In the colon, invasive endometrial tissue proceeds to the muscularis and submucosa and then spreads in a layer in all directions. Severe rectosigmoid obstruction is rare. The gross appearance may resemble carcinoma. A localized endometrioma may form.

Endometriosis of the colon or rectum should be suspected if there are irregularities of bowel function or rectal bleeding at the time of the menstrual period or if the patient has metrorrhagia, menorrhagia, dysmenorrhea, or deep dyspareunia. Pelvic examination may elicit severe tenderness and some degree of fixation of the pelvic organs and retroversion of the uterus, or there may be firm, tender nodules and enlarged ovaries. Sigmoidoscopy may be difficult if there is a tender mass causing fixation of the rectum or pelvic colon. Implants may be present on just the serosal surface of the upper portion of the rectum or lower colon, or may involve the entire wall of the intestine. If the mucosa is involved, ulceration and bleeding may occur. Stricture of varying degrees may be observed by endoscopy.

It is unusual to make a diagnosis by biopsy. X-ray examination is helpful but not always diagnostic.

The most common lesion confused with endometriosis of the rectum or colon is carcinoma. In endometriosis, barium enema shows a long filling defect with tapered irregular borders; the mucosa is intact; the filling defect is inconstant; and there is fixation of the bowel, which is tender on palpation. In carcinoma, the filling defect is short and has sharp irregular margins; the mucosa is ragged and "moth-eaten"; the filling defect is constant; and fixation and tenderness are often not present.

The history is very important. Cyclic colonic bleeding or obstruction in premenopausal women should be regarded as endometriosis until proved otherwise. Failure to appreciate this may result in an unnecessary resection of the rectum (see Chapter 45).

Treatment varies depending upon the severity of the symptoms and the degree of involvement. Removal of the ovaries usually causes regression of established lesions. In women up to age 40, the ovaries should be preserved. Progesterone-type hormones can reduce the size of lesions and hold them in check, but endometriosis recurs when they are withdrawn. Androgens may exert a similar but lasting influence. Localized endometriosis of the anterior rectosigmoid may be easily excised. Local resection may be indicated if obstruction has occurred.

The outcome has been satisfactory in those instances in which resection of the colon was necessary.

Lewis MI, Rio F: Colonic endometriosis. Dis Colon Rectum 12:137–141, 1969.

DISEASES OF THE APPENDICES EPIPLOICAE

The appendices epiploicae are tabs of fat attached to the teniae and are most numerous in the cecum and the transverse and sigmoid colon. Each contains an artery which loops through the appendage and continues into the antimesenteric border of the bowel. They may contain diverticula.

The most common pathologic process encountered is infarction, and abdominal pain, localized to the involved area, is the chief symptom. The onset is usually sudden, but chronic and recurrent cases are reported also. There may be moderate fever and leukocytosis. The condition may simulate appendicitis. Physical examination reveals evidence of localized peritonitis. A mass may be palpable. X-ray examination is nonspecific. Treatment is invariably surgical because of the uncertainty of preoperative diagnosis. The offending epiploica is amputated.

Infarction and separation of epiploicae account for some of the free fibrous or calcified intraperitoneal bodies which may be diagnosed by x-ray as calculi.

Indentation of the wall of the bowel by an appendix epiploica may simulate a sessile polypoid tumor.

If it is necessary to remove redundant fatty appendices epiploicae in preparing the ends of resected bowel for anastomosis, care must be taken not to ligate the structure too close to the bowel and occlude its nutrient artery since local bowel necrosis will result.

Ghosh S, Bilton JL: Torsion and infarction of the appendices epiploicae. Dis Colon Rectum 11:457, 1968.
Swain VA, Young WF, Pringle EM: Hypertrophy of the appendices epiploicae and lipomatous polyposis of the colon. Gut 10:587–589, 1969.

*   *   *

INTESTINAL STOMAS
(Colostomy & Ileostomy)

Colostomy

A colostomy is an opening of the large bowel onto the surface of the abdomen. Colostomies may be double-barreled, in which both ends of the bowel are exteriorized; or single-barreled, in which one end of the bowel is brought out. The colostomy may be temporary, in which event it is subsequently closed; or it may be permanent. Colostomies are made for the following purposes: (1) for decompression of an obstructed, distended colon; (2) to protect a distal anastomosis following segmental resection; (3) to divert the fecal current in preparation for resection of an inflammatory or obstructive lesion or following traumatic injury; (4) to serve as an artificial anus when the distal segment of the colon or rectum is removed; or (5) for obstructive resection in which the diseased portion of the bowel is exteriorized and amputated.

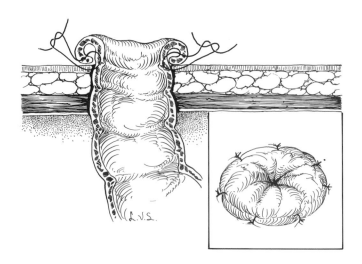

FIG 36–21. Terminal single-barreled colostomy. The margins of the stoma are everted and fixed to the skin with sutures.

The indications for cecostomy versus transverse colostomy have been discussed earlier in this chapter.

The most common permanent colostomy is sigmoid colostomy made at the time of combined abdominoperineal resection for cancer of the rectum (Fig 36–21). Such a colostomy is quite compatible with a normal life. The surgeon must instruct the patient carefully in the postoperative period concerning the care of the colostomy and diet. A low-residue diet is prescribed at first and gradually liberalized over a period of a few weeks until eventually the only restrictions are for foods which cause diarrhea.

The colostomy should be managed by irrigation daily or every other day, although some individuals have regular bowel movements without irrigation. It is important that the colostomy be routinely emptied at a regular time and that loose stools be avoided. Irrigation is performed by inserting a catheter into the stoma and instilling 1500 ml of water, 500 ml at a time, from a bag held at shoulder height. Many commercial colostomy kits make care simple and convenient. A small disposable tissue pad worn over the colostomy—held in place by an elastic belt or ordinary girdle or underpants—is usually all the protection required during the day. Excellent pamphlets describing colostomy care are available for the patient's use. Transverse colostomy, because of the more liquid feces, can sometimes be cared for in this fashion, but in most cases the patient must wear a pouch over the stoma.

The overall complication rate of colostomies is 20%, but most of these are minor; 15% of the complications require operative correction. Complications occur much more frequently in children than in adults. Serious complications, which can usually be avoided by attention to technical details, include prolapse, necrosis, retraction, paracolostomy hernia, and stenosis. Description of the technical pitfalls in colostomy construction is beyond the scope of this text.

Perforation of the colostomy may occur during irrigation or barium enema x-ray examination, especially if there is a paracolostomy hernia or diverticulosis. It may result from inserting the irrigating tube too far, from having the irrigating water pressure too high, or from overdistention of the balloon at the end of the catheter while administering a barium suspension. The irrigating tube need be inserted in the stoma for only 2.5 cm or less. A plastic olive-shaped (Laird) tip may be attached to the end of the irrigating tube. This tip fits snugly in the stoma and allows irrigation without penetrating the lumen. The container holding the irrigating water should be no higher than the patient's shoulders. Perforation above the peritoneum is treated expectantly. An infection of the abdominal wall may occur. Signs and symptoms of peritonitis indicate that intraperitoneal perforation has occurred and emergency exteriorization of the perforated portion of the colostomy with revision is required.

Less serious complications include diarrhea, skin irritation, and fecal impaction. Diarrhea is treated by excluding specific causative foods. If that fails, a low-residue diet, pectin-kaolin mixtures (15–30 ml after each diarrheic stool), or diphenoxylate with atropine (Lomotil), 2.5 mg 3–4 times a day as needed, may be tried.

Ileostomy

Permanent ileostomy is performed most commonly after total colectomy for ulcerative colitis. As much normal ileum must be preserved as possible, so that absorption of water, electrolytes, and nutrients is maximal. The optimal position of the stoma is the right lower abdominal quadrant (Fig 36–22).

The stoma protruding 4 cm above the surface of the skin is everted upon itself and the cut edge is sutured to the skin for healing of mucosa to skin; in this way the ileostomy is surgically "matured." Before the development of this simple step, it was necessary to wait for the stoma to "mature" spontaneously; during the process, severe adynamic ileus sometimes occurred.

A properly fitted ileostomy appliance is cemented to the skin over the stoma immediately after operation so that irritation of the skin by the ileal effluent will not occur. Many commercial appliances are available. The ileostomy appliance has an opening at the bottom so that it can be drained without removing it.

The typical ileostomate can usually enjoy a normal diet, avoiding only foods that cause diarrhea or excessive odor or gas, and can lead an active social, occupational, and sexual life. Pregnancy need not be avoided in women with ileostomies. Specially trained enterostomal therapists can offer valuable initial training and advice. "Ostomy Clubs" are active in many localities.

Immediately after its construction, the ileostomy usually puts out 1–2 liters per day, but this drops off to an average of 500 ml/day after a month or two (Table 36–1). This fluid and electrolyte output continues even during fasting and must be replaced. Thus, the ileostomy patient loses 60–100 mEq of NaCl and 500–700 ml of water per day via the stoma. The patient should be counseled to salt his food liberally, but supplemental salt tablets are necessary only if losses suddenly increase. Urinary output should be at least 1000 ml/day, and unless the patient deliberately consumes extra water the amount taken to satisfy thirst is usually somewhat below the optimal level—a situation which probably accounts for the increased incidence of renal stones in these patients. When the ileostomy output has reached a stable level several months after its construction and the patient has been rehabilitated in his normal environment, it is advisable to measure urinary output for several days and adjust water intake upward if necessary to achieve an output of 1 liter of urine daily.

Any situation that endangers fluid and electrolyte balance is hazardous to the ileostomy patient. Exercise is permissible, but heavy work under a hot sun could be risky if the increased salt and water needs are not anticipated. Diarrhea poses a similar problem. Diuretics must also be prescribed with caution.

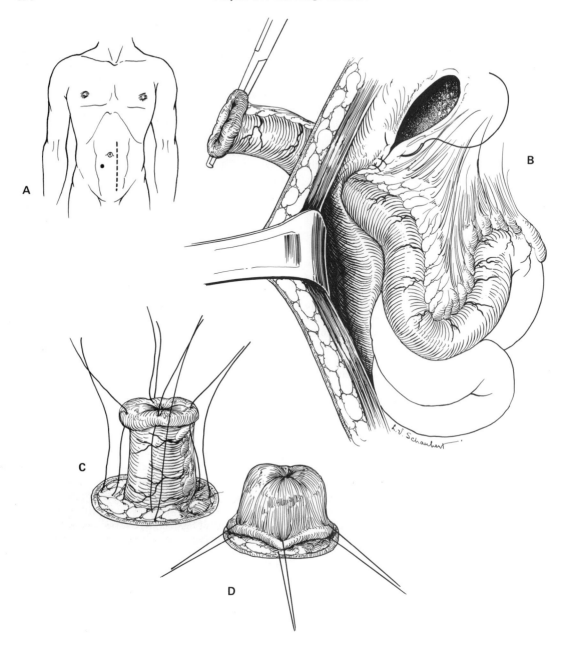

FIG 36−22. Ileostomy after colectomy. *A:* Abdominal incision for colectomy indicated by the dotted line and the site of the ileostomy by the black dot. *B:* The ileum has been brought through the abdominal wall. *C and D:* The ileostomy stoma has been everted and its margins sutured to the edges of the wound.

Complications are reported in 30−75% of ileostomies; 25% require operative correction. The complications include the following:

(1) Intestinal obstruction: Obstruction may be due to adhesive bands, volvulus, or paraileostomy herniation of bowel.

(2) Retraction or stenosis: This rarely occurs now when the ileostomy is everted at the time of its construction.

(3) Stomal narrowing: This is often amenable to correction by a minor local plastic operation.

(4) Ileostomy dysfunction: This consists of profuse output of a watery, foul-smelling discharge from the ileostomy associated with loss of appetite, cramping abdominal pain, and visible peristalsis. It is due to partial obstruction of the ileum, although the mechanical derangement may not be obvious. Treatment should consist of intravenous fluid and electrolytes and gentle insertion of a catheter into the ileostomy to improve egress of the luminal contents. If the condition persists, the ileostomy may require revision. In some cases, inflammation confined to the ileum adjacent to the stoma has been considered a primary process, but this must be rare.

(5) Prolapse: This is uncommon if the mesentery has been sutured to the parietal peritoneum and the stoma everted. It may require operative revision of the ileostomy.

(6) Periileostomy abscess and fistula: These may follow either mucosal perforation by sutures or pressure necrosis from the ileostomy apparatus.

(7) Urinary calculi: Uric acid stones are increased after ileostomy and are probably the result of chronic dehydration due to inadequate fluid intake. Even healthy patients with ileostomies who have no history of urolithiasis have a more acid urine and a higher concentration of uric acid in the urine than do normal persons who do not have ileostomies.

(8) Peristomal skin irritation: This complication may be minimized by applying a properly fitting ileostomy apparatus immediately postoperatively and by protecting the skin with karaya powder and karaya rings.

(9) Offensive odors: Odors can be avoided by good appliance hygiene, commercial odor preventives, and, in some individuals, by avoiding certain foods such as onions, fish, eggs, and coffee.

(10) Diarrhea: If excessive, this may result in hypokalemia, dehydration, and cardiac arrhythmia and lethargy.

American Cancer Society, 219 E. 42nd Street, New York, N.Y. 10017. Care of your colostomy. 1967.

Biermann HJ, Tocker AM, Tocker LR: Statistical survey of problems in patients with colostomy or ileostomy. Am J Surg 112:647, 1966.

Harrower HW: Management of colostomy, ileostomy, and ileal conduit. S Clin North America 48:941–943, 1968.

Hertz RE, Spiro H: Colostomy perforation. Surgery 60:590, 1966.

Hollister Company, Inc, 211 East Chicago Avenue, Chicago, Illinois 60611. Managing your ileostomy. 1971.

Lane DG: Ileitis following ileostomy. Dis Colon Rectum 13:143–146, 1970.

Rowbotham JL: The stoma rehabilitation clinic. Dis Colon Rectum 13:59–61, 1970.

Roy PH & others: Experience with ileostomies. Am J Surg 119:77, 1970.

PREOPERATIVE PREPARATION OF THE COLON

Since the colonic lumen must be opened during many operations, efforts must be made to prevent infection by emptying the bowel preoperatively and reducing the number of infective organisms. Mechanical cleansing by means of purgation and enemas is effective for this purpose. A controversy exists concerning whether antibiotics should be given preoperatively in addition to mechanical preparation.

In situations where operation is urgent, rapid preparation of the bowel can be obtained by mechanical cleansing combined with neomycin, 1 g orally for 2–4 days, or kanamycin (see Chapter 10).

Tumor implantation at the line of anastomosis may be increased by the use of intestinal antibiotics, but the practical significance of this experimental observation has not been established.

If contamination of the wound and peritoneal cavity is anticipated—as in acute diverticulitis or toxic megacolon—broad-spectrum antibiotics should be administered parenterally before operation.

Nichols RL, Condon RE: Antibiotic preparation of the colon: Failure of commonly used regimens. S Clin North America 51:223–232, 1971.

Nichols RL, Condon RE: Preoperative preparation of the colon: Collective review. Surg Gynec Obst 132:323–337, 1971.

Sellwood RA, Burn JL, Waterworth PM: A second clinical trial to compare two methods for preoperative preparation of the large bowel. Brit J Surg 56:610–612, 1969.

Swinton NW & others: Symposium: Preoperative evaluation of the surgical patient. Dis Colon Rectum 13:175–194, 1970.

• • •

General References

Bacon HE, Recio PM: *Surgical Anatomy of the Colon, Rectum, and Anal Canal.* Lippincott, 1962.

Chadwick VS & others: Mechanism for hyperoxaluria in patients with ileal dysfunction. New England J Med 289:172–176, 1973.

Goligher JC & others: *Surgery of the Anus, Rectum and Colon,* 2nd ed. Thomas, 1967.

Morson BC, Dawson IMP: *Gastrointestinal Pathology.* Blackwell, 1972.

Morson BC (editor): *Diseases of the Colon, Rectum and Anus.* Appleton-Century-Crofts, 1969.

Sletsenger M, Fordtran J: *Gastrointestinal Disease.* Saunders, 1973.

Truelove SC, Reynell PC: *Diseases of the Digestive System,* 2nd ed. Davis, 1970.

Turell R (editor): Symposium on diseases of the colon and anorectum. S Clin North America 52:795–1091, 1972.

37 . . .

The Anorectum

Walter Birnbaum, MD

SURGICAL ANATOMY & PHYSIOLOGY

The anal canal is derived from the proctodeum, an invagination of the ectoderm. The rectum is of entodermal origin. Because of the difference in their origins, the arterial and nerve supply and the venous and lymphatic drainage differ in the 2 structures, as do their linings also. Thus, the rectum is lined with glandular mucosa and the anal canal with anoderm, a continuation of the external stratified epithelium. It is incorrect to speak of anal "mucosa." The marginal zone between the rectum and the anal canal contains transitional cells. The anal canal and adjacent external skin are generously supplied with somatic sensory nerves and are highly susceptible to painful stimuli; the rectal mucosa has an autonomic nerve supply and is relatively insensitive to pain. Pain is not an early symptom in patients with rectal neoplasm.

Venous drainage above the anorectal juncture is through the portal system; drainage of the anal canal is through the caval system. This distribution is important in understanding the modes of spread of malignant disease and infection and the formation of hemorrhoids. The lymphatic return from the rectum is along the superior hemorrhoidal vascular pedicle to the inferior mesenteric and aortic nodes, but the lymphatics from the anal canal pass ventrally to the inguinal nodes.

The **anal canal** is about 3 cm long and points toward the umbilicus (Fig 37–1). It forms a distinct angle with the rectum in its resting state. During defecation, the angle straightens out. At the superior boundary of the anal canal is the **anorectal juncture** (pectinate line, mucocutaneous juncture or dentate line). Here there are 8–12 **anal crypts** whose openings face cephalad. From each of the crypts a tubular duct extends distally; at the distal end of the duct is a small glandular structure. Anorectal fistulas originate in the crypts. Adjacent to the crypts are 5–8 tiny anal papillae. They become enlarged in inflammatory conditions. The rectal mucosa is red and glistening. The modified skin of the anal canal closely resembles the external skin but is thinner and contains no hair follicles. The white line of Hilton runs around the circumference of the anal canal and represents the intersphincteric line. It is easily palpable.

The **anorectal sphincteric ring** encircles the anal canal. Posteriorly and laterally it is composed of the fusion of the internal sphincter, longitudinal muscle, the central portion of the levators (puborectalis), and components of the external sphincter. Anteriorly it is weaker because the puborectalis muscle passes directly ventrally and takes no part in the formation of the ring there. Thus, the anorectal ring is more distinctly palpated with the examining finger posteriorly. Knowledge of the detailed anatomy of these structures is important in treating rectal abscesses and fistulas since complete surgical division may result in incontinence. The subcutaneous portion of the external sphincter acts as a corrugator of the perianal skin. The internal sphincter is composed of smooth involuntary muscles; the remaining muscles are striated voluntary ones.

Supporting Structures

The **puborectalis** forms a muscular sling around the rectum to give it support and to act synergistically

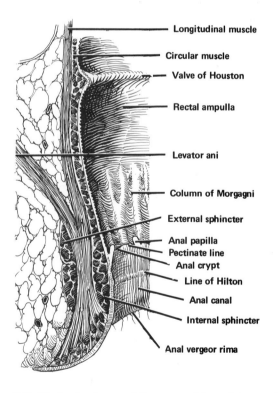

FIG 37–1. Anatomy of the anorectal canal (coronal section). (Semidiagrammatic.)

- Longitudinal muscle
- Circular muscle
- Valve of Houston
- Rectal ampulla
- Levator ani
- Column of Morgagni
- External sphincter
- Anal papilla
- Pectinate line
- Anal crypt
- Line of Hilton
- Anal canal
- Internal sphincter
- Anal vergeor rima

in defecation. The rectum is supported by the **fascia of Waldeyer**, a heavy, avascular layer of the parietal pelvic fascia, the **lateral ligaments** through which pass the middle hemorrhoidal vessels, and the posterior **mesorectum**, which assists in fixing the rectum to the anterior surface of the sacrum (see Rectal Prolapse).

Arteries

The **superior hemorrhoidal artery** is a direct continuation of the inferior mesenteric artery. It divides into 2 main branches, left and right. The right branch again bifurcates. These 3 terminal divisions probably account for the characteristic location of internal hemorrhoids, ie, 2 in each of the right quadrants and one in the left lateral quadrant.

The **middle hemorrhoidal artery** arises on each side from the anterior division of the internal iliac artery or from the internal pudic artery and runs inward in the lateral ligaments of the rectum. The **inferior hemorrhoidal arteries** are branches of the internal pudic arteries and pass through Alcock's canal. The anastomoses between the superior and inferior vascular arcades provide collateral circulation which is of importance after surgical interruption or atherosclerotic occlusion of the vascular supply of the left colon.

Veins

The **superior hemorrhoidal veins** originate in the internal hemorrhoidal venous plexus and pass cephalad to the inferior mesenteric veins and thence to the portal venous system. They have no valves. Rectal cancer may be disseminated by venous embolism to the liver, and septic emboli may cause pylephlebitis. The inferior hemorrhoidal veins drain into the internal pudic veins and so to the internal iliac and caval system. Varices of the hemorrhoidal veins produce hemorrhoids.

Lymphatics

The **lymphatics** of the anal canal form a fine plexus draining into larger collecting vessels leading to the inguinal lymph nodes, whose efferents lead to the external iliac or common iliac lymph nodes. The lymphatics of the rectum above the level of the anorectal line accompany the veins to the superior hemorrhoidal vascular pedicle and thence to the inferior mesenteric and aortic lymph nodes. Posterior to the rectum lie the nodes of Gerota. The radical operations for eradication of cancer of the rectum and anus are based upon the lymphatic anatomy. Infections about the anus may result in inguinal lymphadenopathy.

Nerves

The **nerve supply** of the rectum is derived from the sympathetic and parasympathetic systems. The sympathetic fibers are derived from the inferior mesenteric plexus and the hypogastric (presacral) nerve, which arises by 3 roots from the second, third, and fourth lumbar sympathetic ganglia. The parasympathetic supply (nervi erigentes) is derived from the second, third, and fourth sacral nerves. Injury to these nerves during operation may cause bladder dysfunction and sexual impotence.

Becerra & others: Electromyography in ano-rectal diseases. Dis Colon Rectum 10:282–287, 1967.

Long CL, Gyiger JW, Kinney JM: Absorption of glucose from the colon and rectum. Metabolism 16:413–418, 1967.

McColl I: The comparative anatomy and pathology of the anal glands. Ann Roy Coll Surg Eng 40:36–67, 1967.

Shepherd JJ, Wright PG: The response of the internal anal sphincter in man to stimulation of the presacral nerve. Am J Digest Dis 13:421–427, 1968.

Torsoli A, Ramorino ML, Crucioli V: The relationship between anatomy and motor activity of the colon. Am J Digest Dis 13:462–467, 1968.

Wilson PM: Anchoring mechanisms of the anorectal region. South African MJ 41:1127–1132, 1138–1143, 1967.

DISEASES OF THE RECTUM & ANUS

PRURITUS ANI

The perianal skin has a "maximum readiness to itch." Pruritus ani is due to a wide variety of causes and is not in itself a clinical entity.

Etiology

Note: Contrary to popular belief, hemorrhoids are not a cause of pruritus ani.

A. Dermatologic: Psoriasis, seborrheic dermatitis, atopic eczema, lichen planus, etc.

B. Contact Dermatitis: Due to the use of local anesthetics (all "-caine" preparations must be suspected), topical antihistamines, various ointments, suppositories, douches, aromatic and other chemical substances used in soap.

C. Fungal: Dermatophytosis, candidiasis, etc.

D. Bacterial: Secondary infection due to scratching.

E. Parasitic: Pinworms (*Enterobius vermicularis*) and, less commonly, scabies or pediculosis.

F. After Oral Antibiotic Therapy: Especially tetracyclines.

G. Systemic Diseases: Diabetes (usually candidiasis), liver disease, etc.

H. Proctologic Disorders: Skin tags, cryptitis, draining fistulas or sinuses, etc.

I. Neoplasms: Intradermal carcinoma (Bowen's disease), extramammary Paget's disease, etc.

J. Hygiene: Poor hygiene with residual irritating feces or overmeticulous hygiene with excessive use of soap and rubbing.

K. Warmth and Hyperhidrosis: Due to a tight girdle, jockey shorts, warm bedclothing, obesity, climate.

L. Occupational: Exposure to constant high temperatures.

M. Allergy: Although pruritus may occur following the ingestion of certain foods, it is doubtful that a true allergy is a causative agent.

N. Psychogenic: The importance of the anxiety-itch-anxiety cycle varies from trivial to overwhelming. The significance of this area as an erotic zone in its relation to pruritus ani is not firmly established.

O. Idiopathic.

Clinical Findings

A. Symptoms and Signs: Itching of the anogenital area may be related to sleeping, defecation, warmth, activity, ingestion of certain foods, or activity. It may vary from intermittent and mild to constant and severe. The clinical manifestations are consistent with the underlying cause. Skin changes may be minimal. Characteristic changes may be masked by excoriation caused by scratching and secondary infection. There may be erythema, fissuring, maceration, lichenification, thickening and fibrosis of the skin, changes suggestive of fungal infection, the presence of pinworms (seen with the endoscope), and lesions elsewhere on the body.

The etiologic diagnosis is based upon a careful history and physical examination and appropriate laboratory tests. Characteristic lesions must be searched for elsewhere on the body. The use of oral or topical medication and the patient's hygienic habits should be determined.

B. Laboratory Findings: Urinalysis may reveal diabetes mellitus. Direct microscopic examination or culture of tissue scrapings may reveal yeasts, other fungi, or parasites. The "Scotch Tape" test may be used to disclose pinworm ova. In the case of persistent pruritus which does not respond to treatment, a biopsy must be taken to detect unusual but important malignant or premalignant lesions.

Complications

Complications include local secondary infection, dermatitis medicamentosa, and those associated with loss of sleep and persistent severe discomfort.

Prevention

The use of any kind of soap directly applied to the perianal area during bath or shower is interdicted. Self-medication with anesthetic or antihistamine ointments must be avoided. Scratching leads to secondary infection and should be inhibited, as should vigorous rubbing with harsh toilet tissue. Clothing should be loose. For men, the "boxer" type of underpants is preferred. Women should avoid elastic girdles or body stockings which press the buttocks together. Bedclothing should be light. Systemic causes should be treated. Spices (especially peppers) and citrus fruits (especially grapefruit) should be avoided.

Treatment

Soft, moistened paper tissue or cotton or soft cloth impregnated with glycerin and witch hazel, should be used to clean thoroughly after bowel movements. Instruct the patient regarding the harmful effects of scratching, rubbing, and the use of soap. Hydrocortisone acetate, 1% in Emulsion Base applied sparingly 4 times daily, is usually most effective. Iodochlorhydroxyquin (Vioform), 3%, may be added as a fungicide. Moisture may be combated by liberal and frequent dusting with nonmedicated talcum powder. Acute inflammation may be alleviated by the use of 1:20 aluminum acetate solution. A protective ointment of aluminum hydroxide (Protegel) as a protective coating is helpful when there is anal seepage. Surgical correction of anal infection should be performed only when indicated. Specific dermatologic conditions are often best managed by dermatologists. Parasitic infestations must be treated specifically.

X-ray treatment and surgical operations or injections designed to create permanent local anesthesia are rarely if ever indicated.

Prognosis

The prognosis depends upon the underlying cause. In most cases dramatic relief can be achieved, but some cases are persistent and recurrent.

Anogenital itching. Med Lett Drugs Ther 8:30–31, 1966.

Davis C: Pruritus ani. MJ Australia 1:600–601, 1969.

Granet E: Pruritus ani. GP 36:89–93, 1967.

Lochridge E Jr: Pruritus ani-perianal psoriasis. South MJ 62:450–452, 1969.

Marks MM: The influence of the intestinal pH on anal pruritus. South MJ 61:1005–1006, 1968.

FECAL IMPACTION

Hardened or putty-like stool in the rectum or colon becomes progressively more dehydrated as·it fails to pass. If not removed, it can cause partial or complete intestinal obstruction. It may result from painful anorectal disease, the abuse of bulk laxatives, residual barium from x-ray study, low-residue diet, starvation, drug-induced stasis (especially codeine and anticholinergic drugs), prolonged bed rest, and muscular hypotonicity (especially in senility), and may occur postoperatively in patients in whom the colon and rectum were not evacuated before operation.

Clinical Findings

The manifestations of fecal impaction consist of a history of small or absent bowel movements for several days, constant bearing down sensations, bowel urgency, and lower abdominal cramps. There may be signs of bowel obstruction. The impacted feces can be digitally palpated.

"Paradoxic diarrhea" consists of the passage of small amounts of watery stool forced around the impaction by spasm.

Differential Diagnosis

Unless the molded mass is identified by the examining finger, a misdiagnosis of rectal abscess or tumor may be made. After the impaction has been relieved, endoscopic examination of the rectum should always be made to ensure that an inflammatory or neoplastic process has not been missed.

Complications

Neglected impaction may rarely result in complete bowel obstruction, erosion of the impaction through the bowel wall, peritonitis, ulceration, and even death.

Prevention

In patients in whom an impaction is likely to occur, careful attention should be given to the regularity of their bowel habits. Mild laxatives or enemas are ordered when indicated. This is particularly true in postobstetric, postoperative, and cardiac patients; patients confined to bed for long periods; and elderly and mental patients.

Treatment

The impaction must be broken up as thoroughly as possible by placing the finger in the rectum anteriorly and breaking up the mass by pressing it against the sacrum. This is followed by an oil retention enema or by 5 ml of 1% dioctyl sodium sulfosuccinate (Doxinate) in 30 ml of mineral oil. The oil should be allowed to remain in the rectum for 8 hours, preferably overnight. The next morning this should be followed by a sodium phosphate or plain water enema, repeated if necessary. (Hydrogen peroxide enemas should never be used.) At the same time, a magnesium or sodium phosphate cathartic should be given by mouth.

If these methods fail, the impaction should be removed under anesthesia in the hospital.

Abella ME, Fernandez AT: Large fecalomas. Dis Colon Rectum 10:401–404, 1967.

Braasch JW: Fecal impaction of the colon. Lahey Clin Found Bull 13:60–63, 1963.

Lal S: Some unusual complications of fecal impaction. Am J Proct 18:226–231, 1967.

COCCYGODYNIA

Fracture or deformity of the coccyx is caused by falling to a sitting position or by striking the coccyx against a hard object. This may result in persistent pain and tenderness. However, pain referred to the "tailbone" or coccygeal area is most frequently related to chronic anal infection, parturition, poor sitting posture, or osteoarthritis. The discomfort is greatest after sitting for long periods on a soft seat such as after a long automobile ride or watching television. "Proctalgia fugax" consists of a sudden severe lancinating or cramp-like pain of brief duration in the rectal or coccygeal region. It may occur at any time and often awakens the patient at night. Examination discloses tenderness and spasm of the coccygeus and levator muscles.

Persistent coccygodynia is often the basis of workmen's compensation or personal injury legal claims.

Clinical Findings

When actual fracture or displacement of the coccyx has occurred, the coccyx will be tender when it is palpated externally. With the examining index finger in the rectum and the coccyx grasped between it and the external thumb, displacement, deformity and pain on motion (particularly acute anterior angulation) can be demonstrated. Radiographic studies should also be diagnostic.

In cases not due to trauma, there is no localized tenderness of the coccyx and movement of it is not painful. However, as the intrarectal examining finger is swept laterally from the coccyx and lower sacrum, the coccygeus, levator, and piriformis muscles can be felt to be spastic and tender, usually more so on the left than on the right. Intrarectal digital pressure upon the involved muscle will reproduce the symptoms.

Differential Diagnosis

Anal fissure causes pain during bowel movement, but coccygodynia is not related to defecation. With fissure, tenderness and spasm on examination are localized to the anal canal rather than to the retrorectal musculature. Rectal abscess is identified by the signs of an inflammatory mass and more acute symptoms.

Treatment

When there is no demonstrable bony injury, the sitting posture should be corrected so that the patient sits erect and on a hard, flat surface. A hard seat should be used when driving an automobile. Soft cushions should be avoided.

Intrarectal digital stretching or massage of the involved muscles is often dramatically helpful. When there has been actual injury to the coccyx, warm baths, diathermy, sedation, local anesthetic injections, and special cut-out seat pads may be helpful.

Coccygectomy for intra-articular fracture or deformity is only rarely indicated and may be followed by persistence of symptoms due to chronic spasm of the involved muscles.

Prognosis

Coccygodynia is characteristically a condition of long standing and may persist for periods up to many months, or, rarely, years when appropriate therapy is not undertaken.

Paradis H, Marganoff H: Rectal pain of extrarectal origin. Dis Colon Rectum 12:306–312, 1969.

Peilling LF, Swenson WM, Hill JR: The psychologic aspects of proctalgia fugax. Dis Colon Rectum 8:372–376, 1965.

Stern SF: Coccygodynia among the geriatric population. J Am Geriatrics Soc 15:100–102, 1967.

Thiele GH: Coccygodynia: Cause and treatment. Dis Colon Rectum 6:422–435, 1963.

ANAL FISSURE
(FISSURE-IN-ANO, ANAL ULCER)

Essentials of Diagnosis

- Rectal pain related to defecation.
- Bleeding.
- Constipation.
- Sentinel pile.
- Spasm of sphincters.
- Anal tenderness.
- Ulceration of anal canal.
- Stenosis.
- Hypertrophic anal papilla.

General Considerations

Acute fissures of the anal canal are longitudinal tears. Most lesions called anal fissures are actually chronic elliptic or round ulcers which, when examined upon partial eversion of the anus, appear to be longitudinal cracks. They may be extremely painful.

Anal ulcers are usually single and occur in the posterior midline or, less commonly, in the anterior midline. They may occur first in the lower portion of the anal canal or may involve its entire length. Ulcers tend to occur in the posterior midline position because of the acute angulation between the anal canal and the rectum and the lack of support of the subcutaneous portion of the external sphincter.

The superficial bundle of the external sphincter arises from the coccyx and bifurcates as it comes forward to surround the anus. The subcutaneous bundle completely surrounds the canal so that it forms an unsupported bar overlying the Y formed by the bifurcation of the superficial bundle (Fig 37–2). When this bar loses its elasticity or is unduly stretched, the overlying anoderm is disrupted.

Infection of the adjacent crypt results in chronic inflammation and then fibrosis of these structures. Edema of the anal papilla adjacent to the crypt occurs with enlargement and fibrosis of the papilla so that it becomes a firm, whitish, finger-like or rounded, polypoid, smooth structure. It is then called a "hypertrophic papilla." Hypertrophic papillae are not neoplastic but are often confused with adenomatous polyps. External to the anal ulcer, the adjacent skin likewise is involved in chronic inflammatory changes and interference with its lymphatic drainage. A fibrotic nubbin of skin forms at the anal verge. This is termed a "sentinel pile" because it stands as a "sentinel" just below the ulcer. Thus, the "fissure triad" has been formed: (1) the ulcer itself, (2) the hypertrophic papilla, and (3) the sentinel pile (Fig 37–3). Although infants normally may pass stools of suprisingly large caliber without pain, they may develop acute linear fissures with diarrhea or as a result of passing hard feces. Fissures may occur as a result of excessive straining at stool, habitual use of cathartics (especially mineral oil), chronic diarrhea, avulsion of an anal valve, childbirth trauma, laceration by a sharp foreign body, or iatrogenic trauma such as the passage of a large speculum or by prostatic massage. Usually no cause can be definitely identified.

Fissures of the perianal skin may be associated with pruritus ani and are the result of chronic dermatitis.

Clinical Findings

A. Symptoms and Signs: Pain may be severe and is described as tearing, burning, or cutting. It occurs during passage of stool, then usually subsides somewhat and becomes more severe when secondary sphincteric spasm occurs. Fissures are characterized by their chronicity, with periods of exacerbation and remission over a number of years. Bleeding is bright red, not mixed with the stool, usually noted on the toilet tissue, and small in amount. Constipation

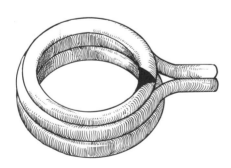

FIG 37–2. Model of external sphincter ani showing its 3 components. The usual site of a posterior anal fissure is indicated.

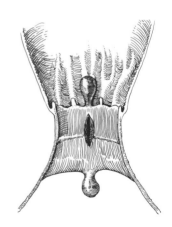

FIG 37–3. Diagram of the anorectum showing the fissure or ulcer triad.

develops as a result of fear of defecation, which is so frequently postponed that regular bowel habits become disrupted. During periods of healing, pruritus may occur.

The sentinel pile can be observed externally. Gentle eversion of the anus may reveal the inferior portion of the ulcer. Application of a topical anesthetic should precede a very gentle digital examination to ascertain the site of the ulcer, the degree of induration and stenosis, etc. There is often marked spasm of the sphincters.

B. Special Examinations: A small caliber anoscope can be introduced with pressure on the side of the anal canal opposite the lesion. The hypertrophic papilla, ulcer, and associated lesions can then be seen. Sigmoidoscopic examination should be deferred (but not omitted) until it can be done painlessly.

Differential Diagnosis

Other anal ulcerations which must be differentiated from fissure include the primary lesion of syphilis, malignant epithelioma, tuberculous ulceration, and ulceration associated with blood dyscrasias and granulomatous enteritis higher in the intestinal tract. Each of these lesions has its own characteristics, but any lesion not in the midline nor displaying the typical findings outlined above should be investigated by means of further diagnostic tests. Anal fissure often occurs concomitantly with internal hemorrhoids and may be overlooked. Internal hemorrhoids are not painful; when pain occurs, fissure must be suspected. The persistence of pain following hemorrhoidectomy is frequently due to a missed fissure.

Treatment

A. Medical Treatment: Warm sitz baths for 10 or 15 minutes after each bowel movement or as often as necessary for discomfort will give temporary relief. The water should be comfortably warm, not hot, and just deep enough to sit in. Deep, hot, frequent sitz baths may be enervating. Topical application of anesthetic ointments injected sparingly with a "pile pipe" on the end of an ointment tube is helpful. Suppositories are of no value unless they are inserted into the anal canal and held by the fingers until they have melted. Otherwise, the suppository slips into the rectal ampulla or higher and is ineffective in coating the ulcer in the anal canal.

Divulsion of the canal under local or general anesthesia so as to disrupt the sphincteric fibers has its advocates; it does give temporary relief but is generally regarded as poor surgical practice.

Topical application of 50% phenol in oil is anesthetic, produces a coating of protein coagulum, and may interrupt the pain-spasm-pain cycle until healing occurs. Mild silver nitrate solution is also used.

Diarrhea or constipation must be corrected. Mineral oil is to be avoided. Stool softeners are of value only when the feces are desiccated and hard. Proper diet and regular bowel habits usually suffice to correct constipation.

B. Surgical Treatment: When conservative measures fail, surgical correction is in order. Operation consists of (1) block excision of the crypt, the hypertrophic papilla, the ulcer and its margins, the sentinel pile, and an adjacent segment of skin for "drainage," (2) superficial division of the underlying · fibrotic sphincter; and (3) covering the orad portion of the wound with normal mucosa. Postoperatively, the surgical wound must be followed closely to ensure healing "from within outward."

Prognosis

Anal ulcers tend to become chronic with alternate periods of healing and exacerbation. They do not become malignant. Surgical treatment is highly successful.

Georgoulis B: Pain caused by anal fissure. Proc Roy Soc Med 62:260, 1969.

Goligher JC: An evaluation of internal sphincterotomy and simple sphincter-stretching in the treatment of fissure-in-ano. S Clin North America 45:1299–1304, 1965.

Mazuji MK, McGivney JQ: Etiology of anterior anal ulcer in the female. Virginia M Month 95:523–524, 1968.

Notaras MJ: Lateral subcutaneous sphincterotomy for anal fissure: A new technique. Proc Roy Soc Med 62:713, 1969.

Sanan DP, Singh A: Results of sphincter dilatation under local anesthesia in anal fissure: Report of 100 cases. Dis Colon Rectum 11:470–472, 1968.

Vantrappen G, Goethals C, Hendrickx H: Treatment of complicated anal fissures by sclerosing injections and fissurectomy. Dis Colon Rectum 10:365–368, 1967.

ANORECTAL ABSCESS

Essentials of Diagnosis

- Persistent throbbing rectal pain.
- External evidence of abscess such as palpable induration and tenderness may or may not be present.
- Systemic evidence of infection.

General Considerations

Anorectal abscess results from the invasion of the pararectal spaces by pathogenic microorganisms. A mixed infection usually occurs, with *Escherichia coli, Proteus vulgaris,* streptococci, and staphylococci predominating. Anaerobes are often present.

The incidence is much higher in men. The most common cause is infection extending from an anal crypt into one of the pararectal spaces. Less commonly, abscesses superficial to the corrugator muscle may result from infection of hair follicles, sebaceous and sweat glands of the skin, abrasions due to scratching, infection of a perianal hematoma, as a complication of deep anal fissure, infection of a prolapsed internal hemorrhoid, or following sclerosing injection of hemorrhoids. Deeper abscesses usually

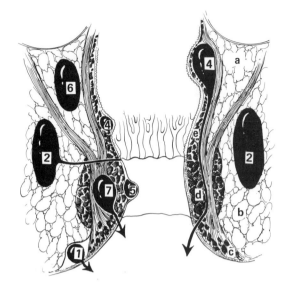

FIG 37—4. Composite diagram of acute anorectal abscesses with arrows indicating the chronic fistulous stage. (a) Pelvirectal or supralevator space. (b) Ischiorectal space. (c) Perianal or subcutaneous space. (d) Marginal or mucocutaneous space. (e) Submucous space. Numbers designate abscesses as enumerated in text below. (Retrorectal abscess is not shown.) Arrows indicate fistulous tracts.

arise in the crypts but may also result from trauma, foreign bodies, etc. (See Anorectal Fistulas, below.)

Abscesses are classified according to the anatomic spaces they occupy (Fig 37—4): (1) Perianal abscess lies immediately beneath the skin of the anus and the lowermost part of the anal canal. (2) Ischiorectal abscess occupies the ischiorectal fossa and is actually uncommon, although the term is often improperly used to describe most anorectal abscesses. (3) Retrorectal (deep postanal) abscess is situated in the retrorectal space. (4) Submucous abscess is situated in the submucosa immediately above the anal canal. (5) Marginal abscess is situated in the anal canal beneath the anoderm. (6) Pelvirectal (supralevator) abscess lies above the levator ani muscle and below the peritoneum. (7) Intermuscular abscess lies between the layers of the sphincter muscles. A lateral abscess may extend through the triangle just posterior to the anal canal and pass around to the opposite side to form a horseshoe abscess. Abscesses may extend from the supralevator space down through the levator into the ischiorectal fossa to form an "hourglass" abscess.

Rectal abscesses frequently contain a large quantity of foul-smelling pus.

Abscesses are the precursors of anorectal fistulas.

Clinical Findings

Superficial abscesses are the most painful, with pain related to sitting and walking but not necessarily to bowel movement. Inspection discloses the characteristic evidence of external swelling with redness, induration, and tenderness. Deeper abscesses will cause toxic symptoms, but localized pain may not be severe. External inspection shows no swelling. Digital rectal examination reveals the tender swelling and, on bidigital examination with the index finger in the rectum and the thumb external, the abscess may be readily felt. High pelvirectal abscesses may cause minimal or no rectal symptoms, may be associated with lower abdominal pain, and may be the source of fever of undetermined origin.

Complications

Unless the abscess is evacuated promptly by surgery or ruptures spontaneously, it will extend into other adjacent anatomic spaces. Rarely, an anaerobic infection will spread extensively without respect for anatomic planes of cleavage.

Treatment

The treatment of pararectal abscesses is prompt incision and adequate drainage. Suppuration will almost always have occurred when the diagnosis is first made. One should not await "pointing" of the abscess externally. Antibiotics are of limited value, may only serve to mask the infection temporarily, and may result in the outgrowth of resistant organisms. Warm sitz baths and analgesics are palliative.

Prior to operation, the patient should be advised that after the abscess is drained he may have a persistent fistula. The operation for drainage may be a one-stage or 2-stage procedure. If, under anesthesia, the primary origin of the abscess can be found and if the tract connecting it to the abscess can be incised without division of a significant portion of the sphincteric ring, the abscess can be adequately drained externally and fistulotomy performed at the same time. A second operation for fistula will then be avoided. If the fistulous tract is deep, only the abscess should be drained and fistulectomy performed after the cavity completely heals and support is provided for the sphincteric ring. The wound should not be packed since this may result in a broad scar which may interfere with sphincteric closure of the anal canal, resulting in leakage or partial incontinence.

The wound should be inspected at frequent intervals to make certain that it heals from the "bottom up" and bridging of the wound is discouraged.

Prognosis

Abscesses that rupture spontaneously or are drained surgically without removal of the offending fistulous connection will frequently recur until the underlying cause is removed.

Goligher JC, Ellis M, Pissidis AG: A critique of anal glandular infection in the etiology and treatment of idiopathic anorectal abscesses and fistulas. Brit J Surg 54:977—983, 1967.

Hill JR: Fistulas and fistulous abscesses in the anorectal region; personal experience in management. Dis Colon Rectum 10:421–434, 1967.

Lindell TD, Fletcher WS, Krippaehne WW: Anorectal suppurative disease: A retrospective review. Am J Surg 125:189–194, 1973.

Kott I, Urca I: Perianal abscess as a presenting sign of leukemia. Dis Colon Rectum 12:338–339, 1969.

Smith ND: Perirectal abscesses and fistulas. J-Lancet 84:145–148, 1964.

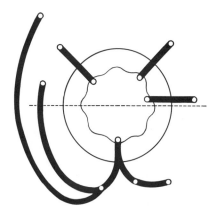

FIG 37–5. Salmon-Goodsall rule.

ANORECTAL FISTULAS

Essentials of Diagnosis

- Chronic purulent discharge from a para-anal opening.
- Tract which may be palpated or probed leading to rectum.

General Considerations

By definition, a fistula must have at least 2 openings connected by a hollow tract—as opposed to a sinus, which is a tract with but one opening. Most anorectal fistulas originate in the anal crypts at the anorectal juncture. The crypt becomes injured or infected (cryptitis), the infection extends along one of several well-defined planes, and an abscess occurs. When the abscess is opened or ruptures, a fistula is formed. The fistula may be subcutaneous, submucosal, intramuscular, or submuscular. It may be anterior or posterior, single, complex, or horseshoe.

Fistulas are usually due to pyogenic infection or, less commonly, due to granulomatous disease of the intestine or tuberculosis. Those that do not originate in the crypts may result from diverticulitis, neoplasm, or trauma. Cryptogenic fistulas which have their secondary (external) opening posterior to an imaginary line passing transversely through the center of the anal orifice usually have their primary (internal) opening in a crypt in the posterior midline. When the secondary (external) opening is anterior to the transverse line, the primary (internal) opening is usually in a crypt immediately opposite the secondary opening (Salmon-Goodsall rule; Fig 37–5).

Clinical Findings

A. Symptoms and Signs: The chief complaint is intermittent or constant drainage or discharge. There is usually a history of a recurrent abscess which ruptured spontaneously or was incised surgically. On inspection, one or more secondary openings can be seen. There may be a pink or red elevation exuding purulent material, or it may have healed over. In granulomatous disease or tuberculosis, the margins may be violaceous and the discharge watery. On palpation, the cord-like tract can be felt and its course, both in relation to the sphincters and to its primary orifice, can often be determined. A probe can be inserted into the tract to determine its depth and direction. However, this maneuver should be terminated if it is painful; under these circumstances it is best completed under anesthesia at the time of operation. Bidigital examination is helpful.

Anorectal fistulas in infants are congenital, may cause abscesses, are more common in boys, and are anterior, straight, and superficial. The treatment is the same as in adult fistulas. Rectovaginal fistulas may be congenital, may follow radiotherapy, pelvic surgery or vaginal repair, obstetric delivery, or may occur in association with malignancy. The most common complaint is the passage of flatus or feces per vagina. The lesion can usually be seen by vaginal inspection, but the aperture may be so small or so well concealed in folds of mucosa that it is not easily discovered. In these instances, a vaginal pack saturated with methylene blue solution may allow the dye to be detected in the rectum.

B. Special Examinations: Anoscopic inspection of the crypts may reveal the primary opening, which at times will discharge pus. Gentle probing of the primary opening with a short crypt hook may be confirmatory. Associated lesions must also be noted. Sigmoidoscopic examination must be done. Roentgen fistulography in fistulas which are suspected of being noncryptogenic or extensive is a valuable diagnostic adjunct. A thin, radiopaque liquid such as diatrizoate (Hypaque) is injected through the external opening, and stereoscopic or multiplane x-ray films are taken. A radiopaque marker may be inserted into the anal canal to localize the inner limit of the sphincters and the position of the anal orifice. A barium enema x-ray study is indicated if the fistula is thought to arise in the sigmoid colon, and an upper gastrointestinal study is done if regional enteritis is suspected.

Differential Diagnosis

Hidradenitis suppurativa is a disease of the apocrine sweat glands characterized by the formation of multiple, deep perianal sinuses. Other sites of predilection are the axillas and the inguinal and pubic areas. There may be scrotal or labial involvement.

Pilonidal sinus with a tract leading into the perianal area may resemble a fistula. The direction of the tract on palpation or probing, the presence of another opening in the sacrococcygeal area, and the possible presence of tufts of hair may establish the diagnosis, although the differentiation may be difficult.

Granulomatous disease (regional enteritis) of the small or large bowel is associated with anorectal fistulas in a high percentage of cases. The fistula is often the first manifestation of proximal disease and may precede it by months or even years. Such fistulas are indolent in appearance and have pale granulations and characteristic microscopic findings.

Tuberculous fistulas are now uncommon. They too have an indolent appearance and are usually associated with pulmonary, glandular, or osseous tuberculosis elsewhere in the body.

Infected comedones, infected sebaceous cysts, chronic folliculitis, and **bartholinitis** are other dermal sources of draining sinuses. The history, the location of the sinus in relation to the anus or vulva, and the absence of an anorectal source are helpful in the diagnosis. Examination under anesthesia may be necessary.

Rectorectal dermoid cysts, more common in females, form chronic perianal sinuses.

Coloperineal fistulas may occur in diverticulitis of the sigmoid colon. Whenever a probe can be passed deeply into a perianal fistula and sigmoidal diverticular disease coexists, the intracolonic origin of the fistula should be suspected and can be proved by fistulography.

Sinuses from trauma and foreign bodies are not uncommon. The foreign body may gain entrance from the outside by penetration or from within the canal from the ingestion of a sharp piece of bone, etc. A nonabsorbable suture remaining from perineorrhaphy or episiotomy or a piece of drainage tubing may act as a foreign body.

Urethroperineal fistulas are often traumatic in origin, resulting from urethral instrumentation or direct external trauma. Rectourethral fistulas may be congenital or may follow urethral instrumentation or prostatectomy. The chief complaint is pneumaturia or fecaluria. Small, recent fistulas may close spontaneously, or urinary diversion by cystostomy and repair may be required.

Less common causes of perianal sinuses and fistulas are **tubo-ovarian abscess, actinomycosis, osteomyelitis,** and **carcinoma.** In these instances the history, physical findings, x-ray examination, and laboratory studies will provide the differential diagnosis.

Complications

Without treatment, chronically infected fistulas may be the source of systemic infection. Although carcinoma develops rarely in a chronic, untreated anorectal fistula, many such cases have been reported and effective removal of the fistula is a prophylactic measure against such an eventuality.

Treatment

Small acute fistulas may heal spontaneously, but in most cases the only effective treatment is by fistulotomy (commonly termed fistulectomy). The following principles must be observed: (1) The primary opening must be found. (2) The fistulous tract or tracts must be identified completely. (3) The tract must be unroofed throughout its entire length so that the fistulous "tunnel" is converted into an open "ditch" throughout its entire course. (4) The wound must be constructed so as to make certain that the cavity will heal from within outward. Fistulotomy should never be performed in the presence of chronic diarrhea, active ulcerative colitis, or active granulomatous enterocolitis since delayed wound healing may present a severe problem. When the clinical manifestations of the enteric disease appear to be under control, operation may be performed although prolonged wound healing is to be expected.

A 2-stage operation is indicated only when the fistula passes deep to the entire anorectal ring so that all the muscles must be divided in order to extirpate the tract. This need rarely be done. If the deeper portions of the sphincteric ring and the levator ani muscles are left intact and there is an adequate nerve supply, incontinence will not occur.

Frequent follow-up examination of the wound following fistulotomy is of great importance to make certain that bridging and re-formation of the fistula does not occur.

Prognosis

The recurrence rate following fistulotomy is high for the following reasons: (1) the primary opening of the fistula is not removed; (2) collateral tracts are missed; (3) the operation is inadequate for fear of creating incontinence; (4) there is a mistaken diagnosis; and (5) postoperative care is inadequate.

Dunphy JE, Pikula J: Fact and fancy about fistula-in-ano. S Clin North America 35:1469, 1954.

Heaton JR, Cohen RS: Complicated para-anal fistulas of obscure origin. Dis Colon Rectum 8:437–440, 1965.

Heidenreich A & others: Cancer in anal fistulas: Report of two cases. Dis Colon Rectum 9:371–376, 1966.

Jackman RJ: Anorectal fistulas: Current concepts. Dis Colon Rectum 11:247–255, 1968.

Manganaro JA, Fields M: Intestinal tuberculosis with fistula in ano. Internat Surg 46:578–581, 1966.

Mazier WP: The treatment and care of anal fistulas: A study of 1000 patients. Dis Colon Rectum 14:134–144, 1971.

Wilson E: Skin grafts in surgery for anal fistula. Dis Colon Rectum 12:327–331, 1969.

HEMORRHOIDS*

Essentials of Diagnosis

- Rectal bleeding, protrusion, and vague discomfort.

*See also Thrombosed External Hemorrhoid (next section).

- Mucoid discharge from rectum.
- Possible secondary anemia.
- Characteristic findings on external anal inspection or anoscopic examination.

General Considerations

A hemorrhoid is a varicose dilatation of the veins of the superior or inferior hemorrhoidal venous plexuses, or both. Dilated, chronically infected veins of the superior hemorrhoidal plexus are called internal hemorrhoids and originate above the level of the anorectal juncture immediately above the anal canal. They are covered by redundant mucous membrane and lie in a bed of loose areolar tissue. Those of the inferior hemorrhoidal plexus are termed external hemorrhoids, are situated below the anorectal juncture, and are covered by anal epithelium or external skin. The 2 plexuses anastomose freely, forming internal and external hemorrhoids in continuity known as interno-external hemorrhoids or mixed hemorrhoids. They contain the terminations of the superior hemorrhoidal arteries. They occur in 3 primary or "cardinal" positions—right anterior, right posterior, and left lateral posterior—depending upon how the artery divides and terminates. Smaller, secondary "satellite" hemorrhoids may develop between the primary hemorrhoids (Fig 37–6).

Since the superior hemorrhoidal venous plexus drains into the portal venous system, which contains no valves, the erect position of man greatly increases the pressure within the hemorrhoidal veins and thus predisposes to hemorrhoidal disease. Hemodynamic studies, clinical features, and the rarity of the disease in quadrupeds support this hypothesis. The importance of heredity as a predisposing cause of hemorrhoids is difficult to evaluate accurately because of the high incidence of the disease. However, when severe hemorrhoidal disease is found in young patients, there is frequently a strong family history, suggesting a hereditary background.

There is good evidence that the principal cause of hemorrhoids is chronic anal infection since chronic periphlebitis and an inflammatory reaction commensurate with the severity of the disease are usually found. Abnormalities of the microcirculation with demonstrable arteriovenous communication have also

been implicated as causes of hemorrhoids.

Pregnancy is by far the most common cause of hemorrhoids in young women. The increased incidence of hemorrhoids during pregnancy is thought to be due to the steadily increasing pressure exerted on the iliac veins by the enlarged, gravid uterus, causing increased venous pressure within the middle and inferior hemorrhoidal veins, which are tributaries of the internal iliac (hypogastric) veins. These hemorrhoids are not to be confused with the thrombosed external hemorrhoids (see below) occurring in pregnancy. After pregnancy, the hemorrhoids tend to subside, although they may become progressively worse with subsequent pregnancies or with advancing age.

Although the hemorrhoidal vessels do constitute one of the avenues of collateral circulation from the portal venous system, true hemorrhoids rarely if ever are a result of portal hypertension or obstruction due to hepatic cirrhosis. Large, bleeding rectal varices do occur in hepatic cirrhosis, but these are not hemorrhoids.

The question of the pathogenesis of hemorrhoidal disease often arises in medicolegal, health insurance, workmen's compensation, and military matters. Hemorrhoidal disease which is already present may be responsible for constipation or, indeed, may reflexly alter bowel habits, but hemorrhoids are not produced by constipation. Sedentary occupations, sitting on hard cold surfaces, straining at work or play, prolonged standing, catharsis, diarrhea, and climate or psychic factors are no longer believed to cause hemorrhoids. Such factors may, indeed, produce thrombosed external hemorrhoids.

Clinical Findings

A. Symptoms and Signs: Patients will frequently complain of "hemorrhoids" regardless of what their rectal symptoms may be.

Bleeding is usually the first symptom. It is bright red, unmixed with the stool, and may vary in quantity from streaks on the toilet tissue to amounts sufficient to be noticed in the bowl water. It may actually spurt or, when prolapse occurs, stain the underclothing. Protracted hemorrhoidal bleeding may result in marked secondary anemia. Prolapse occurs at first only with defecation and spontaneously reduces itself. At a later stage, the hemorrhoids must be reduced manually by the patient after defecation. Still later, they protrude with walking, prolonged standing, or other exertion, and, finally become permanently prolapsed. Mucoid discharge is most marked when the piles are permanently prolapsed and soiling of the clothing is noted. Irritation of the perianal skin may occur as a result of the constant leakage of mucus. However, persistent pruritus ani is not a symptom of hemorrhoidal disease. Pain occurs only when there is an acute attack of prolapse with inflammation, congestion, and edema or when there is a coexisting painful lesion.

On external inspection the subcutaneous external varices may be seen in their characteristic distribution. If the internal hemorrhoids are prolapsed, the

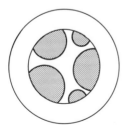

FIG 37–6. The usual arrangement of primary and secondary internal hemorrhoids. The anal canal as seen with the patient in the lithotomy position.

redundant covering of red, moist mucosa will be observed. The 3 major masses with sulci in between can be noted. Whitish epithelium often extends up onto the mucosa of the internal hemorrhoid in an irregular fashion ("creeping epithelium") due to chronic trauma of the mucosa.

Internal hemorrhoids are not palpable unless they are inflamed or thrombosed. However, digital examination must be done to detect tenderness or spasm from a concomitant painful lesion and to rule out the presence of a palpable tumor.

B. Special Examinations: Internal hemorrhoids, unless prolapsed, can be seen only with the anoscope. The anoscope is introduced for its full length, and the hemorrhoids will bulge into its lumen as it is slowly withdrawn. If the patient is then instructed to bear down, the hemorrhoids will follow the instrument to the outside if they are prolapsible. Other abnormalities at this level should likewise be noted. It is imperative that proctosigmoidoscopic examination also be carried out to detect the presence of inflammatory or malignant disease at a higher level which may have been responsible for symptoms attributed to the hemorrhoids.

Differential Diagnosis

Rectal bleeding, the most common symptom of internal hemorrhoids, also occurs with carcinoma of the colon and rectum, diverticular disease, adenomatous polyps, ulcerative colitis, and other less common diseases of the colon and rectum. Sigmoidoscopic examination must therefore constitute a part of the routine examination for hemorrhoids. Barium enema x-ray studies must be done in all patients over 40 years of age with rectal bleeding even when the source of the hemorrhage appears to be obviously of hemorrhoidal origin.

Mucosal rectal prolapse (common in children) presents as a circle of mucosa around the entire circumference marked by radial furrows and without varices.

In its later stages, procidentia of the rectum also forms a circle of protruding bowel, greater anteriorly, with the lumen pointing posteriorly, with concentric mucosal folds and without the characteristic "cardinal" positions of hemorrhoids with intervening sulci. The double, full thickness of the protruding wall can be felt upon bidigital palpation. When the procidentia is reduced, it can usually be prevented from redescending with straining by light pressure of the examining finger on the anterior wall of the rectum. Hemorrhoids and procidentia may coexist.

Perianal and intra-anal condylomas and anorectal tumors are so characteristic in their appearance that differentiation should not be difficult. Thrombosed external hemorrhoid (perianal hematoma) is described below. External skin "tabs" or "tags" which are the result of previous marginal thromboses, pregnancy, rectal surgery, or perianal dermatitis are not true hemorrhoids. The "sentinel pile" usually seen in the midline signifies an adjacent fissure (see above).

Complications

The hemorrhoids may become prolapsed and irreducible (incarcerated) as a result of inflammation, intravascular thrombosis, congestion, and edema. This condition is sometimes erroneously termed "strangulation" on the assumption that the irreducibility is due to the constriction of the hemorrhoids by the sphincteric ring. However, digital examination will show that there is actually some relaxation of the anal canal in this condition. Although the hemorrhoids may appear dark because of the underlying thrombosis, the mucosa is still viable. Ulceration and secondary infection may supervene.

Gangrene occurs following occlusion of the terminal nutrient artery supplying the hemorrhoid. The mucosa becomes black, finely wrinkled, loses its sheen, and appears dead. Sloughing occurs following hemorrhoidal ischemia.

Septic embolism via the portal system to form liver abscess has occurred but is rare. Severe secondary anemia may occur due to intermittent large hemorrhages or the persistent loss of small amounts of blood.

Treatment

Asymptomatic hemorrhoids require no treatment. Pruritus and pain are not symptoms of uncomplicated hemorrhoids. Straining at stool or diarrhea should be avoided to minimize bleeding and prolapse.

Prolapsed, irreducible, thrombosed, inflamed, or gangrenous hemorrhoids may be treated either conservatively or by immediate operation. Surgery offers the most rapid relief of symptoms and the shortest convalescence. Internal hemorrhoids requiring operative removal during pregnancy should be removed during the second trimester. Hemorrhoids appearing at delivery or immediately postpartum should not be treated surgically until sufficient time has elapsed to determine whether they will persist.

A. Medical Treatment: Suppositories and rectal ointment are of limited value in the treatment of uncomplicated internal hemorrhoids except for their transient anesthetic and astringent effects. If prolapsed hemorrhoids are reducible, they should be replaced within the rectum by gentle pressure. The patient is then instructed to lie down and reduce the protrusion whenever necessary. Following reduction, the associated external edema will soon subside. When the piles have been replaced, they may be kept in position by firm compresses and the patient should be confined to bed for a few days. In the acute stage, the patient should be put to bed and cold compresses of either water or witch hazel are applied. After the acute reaction has subsided, warm compresses or warm (not hot) sitz baths are in order. Sedation should be given as required.

In some instances, a spontaneous "cure" will be caused by fibrosis.

B. Injection Treatment: Injection treatment is a form of sclerotherapy in which an irritating chemical solution is injected submucosally into the areolar tissue surrounding the internal hemorrhoidal varices. The scarring which results from the inflammatory reaction effects, in varying degrees, obliteration of the hemorrhoidal varices. Recurrences are reported in about 50% of cases of early hemorrhoids and with increasing frequency in the more advanced stages of hemorrhoidal disease.

The advantages of the injection method are that it will control bleeding due to minor internal hemorrhoids which are not severe enough to require operation; it may be used as a "therapeutic test" to rule out another, higher source of bleeding in the presence of hemorrhoids; it is useful in the palliative treatment of hemorrhoids in persons who refuse surgery or are poor surgical risks; and it avoids surgery in patients who are cured by this means.

To be suitable for sclerotherapy, hemorrhoids must be early, uncomplicated, and internal.

Several types of sclerosing agents are used; 5% phenol in sesame oil is a satisfactory choice. Quinine urea hydrochloride, 5% aqueous solution, is also an effective agent. The injection is made with a 10 ml Luer-Lok syringe to which is attached a special long angulated hemorrhoidal needle. Through the anoscope, the needle is inserted into the upper pole of the hemorrhoid into the submucosal space. Aspiration is attempted to ensure that the needle is not within the lumen of a vessel. Enough of the solution (usually 1–5 ml) is then injected so that the hemorrhoid is distended but not blanched. One hemorrhoid at a time is usually injected, with subsequent injections of other hemorrhoids at intervals of 3 or 4 days.

Complications of injection treatment include sloughing, infection, acute prostatitis, and sensitivity to the injected material. If the procedure is properly done, however, such complications are rare.

C. Rubber Band Method: Using a special "gun," a rubber band may be placed so as to encircle the base of the hemorrhoid and strangulate it. This method has limited popularity.

D. Surgical Treatment: Surgical excision of all redundant mucosa and hemorrhoidal tissue produces an excellent long-term result. There are several methods of accomplishing this objective. For technical details, the reader should consult texts on operative technic.

Prognosis

Recurrence is extremely rare after a properly executed hemorrhoidectomy.

Clark CG, Giles GR, Goligher JC: Results of conservative management of internal hemorrhoids. Brit MJ 2:12–13, 1967.

Eisenhammer S: Proper principles and practices in the surgical management of hemorrhoids. Dis Colon Rectum 12:288–305, 1969.

Ganchrow MI & others: Hemorrhoidectomy revisited: A computer analysis of 2,038 cases. Dis Colon Rectum 14:128–133, 1971.

Granet E: Hemorrhoidectomy failures: Causes, prevention and management. Dis Colon Rectum 11:45–48, 1968.

Rowe RJ: Symposium: Management of hemorrhoidal disease. Dis Colon Rectum 11:127–136, 1968.

THROMBOSED EXTERNAL HEMORRHOID
(Perianal Hematoma)

This common lesion is not a true hemorrhoid but rather a subcutaneous hematoma or small venous aneurysm. It is caused by the rupture of one of the subcutaneous external hemorrhoidal veins close to the anal verge—usually external to it or in the anal canal. It is characterized by a painful, tense, smooth, bluish, sessile elevation beneath the skin. Varying in size from a few millimeters to several centimeters in diameter, it may be multilobular, and there may be several such lesions. The rupture through the vein wall is usually not complete, so that a thin layer of adventitia covers the clot. Recurrence is frequent. The hematoma follows a sudden increase in the intravenous pressure and usually occurs after episodes of heavy lifting, coughing, sneezing, athletics, straining at stool, or parturition. The disorder occurs most frequently in otherwise healthy young persons and is not related to hemorrhoidal disease.

Pain is greatest at the onset and gradually subsides in 2–3 days as the acute edema subsides. Spontaneous rupture frequently occurs, with disgorgement of the thrombus and considerable bleeding. Spontaneous resolution will occur without treatment.

Symptoms may be alleviated by warm sitz baths, applications of petrolatum to minimize friction on walking, and mild sedation. If examined within the first 48 hours, the course may be shortened and immediate relief obtained by either evacuation of the thrombus or by complete excision ("external hemorrhoidectomy") under local anesthesia. When evacuating the thrombus, an ellipse of skin should be removed to prevent agglutination of the skin edges and re-formation of an underlying clot. After the clot has begun to organize it cannot be evacuated, so that it is best, when the lesion is first seen 48 hours or more after onset, to employ conservative measures. No attempt should be made to "reduce" the thrombosed external hemorrhoid since it belongs in an external position.

It is important to differentiate this lesion from a prolapsed internal hemorrhoid. The pathology and methods of treatment are entirely different in the 2 conditions.

ANAL STENOSIS

Stenosis or narrowing of the anal canal may be a postoperative event (particularly following hemorrhoidectomy), a congenital variation, a senile change, or due to the habitual use of laxatives (particularly mineral oil). It may also result from chronic inflammatory disease such as fissure-in-ano or extensive electrocoagulation in the anal canal. It is characteristically caused by an annular subepithelial fibrosis. The most common symptom is increased straining at defecation associated with a small caliber stool and a sense of incomplete evacuation. There may be pain and bleeding due to simple fissuring. Examination reveals an unyielding narrowing of the anal canal.

Anal stenosis must be differentiated from strictures of the rectum due to lymphogranuloma venereum, malignancy, ulcerative colitis, and congenital stricture.

Definitive treatment is invariably surgical; digital or instrumental dilatations are of no avail and may even worsen the condition because of trauma. The operation consists of division of the stenotic bundle followed by mobilization, advancement, interposition, and transverse suture of the proximal rectal mucosa. The results are good.

Laird DR & others: Anoplasty—what, when, how, why: Symposium. Dis Colon Rectum 12:179—189, 1969.
Turell R: Postoperative anal stenosis. Surg Gynec Obst 90:231, 1950.

PILONIDAL DISEASE

Essentials of Diagnosis

- Acute abscess or chronic draining sinuses in the sacrococcygeal area.
- Pain, tenderness, induration.

General Considerations

Pilonidal disease is characterized by a pit or sinus of variable depth lined by epithelium or granulation tissue which may lead to a cavity, often containing hair, which is liable to form abscesses and secondary sinuses. It is usually caused by trauma and the penetration of hair into the subcutaneous tissues. The hair acts as a foreign body and nidus for the development of infection.

In about 10% of cases, pilonidal disease is of congenital origin. It also occurs in the finger webs of barbers as a result of implanted hair and in the umbilical region as result of improper hygiene. The male/female sex incidence is 3:1, usually in hirsute white individuals of dark complexion. In hirsute young men with pilonidal disease the hair of the eyebrows frequently meets above the bridge of the nose.

Pilonidal disease is rare in blacks and is unknown among Orientals and American Indians. It becomes clinically manifest coincident with the increase of hair growth and activity of the sebaceous glands at puberty. In most cases symptoms are first noticed at age 20—25. It is commonly seen in military personnel and has been called "jeep disease" because of its frequent relationship to riding in mechanized vehicles.

Clinical Findings

The lesion is usually asymptomatic until it becomes acutely infected. The symptoms and findings of acute suppuration are similar to those of acute abscesses in other locations. The inflammatory process may spontaneously subside or progress until relief is obtained by spontaneous rupture or surgical drainage. After drainage has occurred, the purulent discharge may cease completely or, more commonly, may recur intermittently with drainage from one or many sinus openings, each communicating with the parent sinus or cyst. On examination, one or several midline or excentric cutaneous openings in the skin of the sacral region are found. One or several hairs can often be seen projecting from the openings. A probe may be passed into the sinuses for distances of several millimeters to many centimeters.

Pilonidal disease rarely may extend anterior to the coccyx or sacrum.

Differential Diagnosis

The midline postanal dimple commonly noted in infants is rarely the precursor of pilonidal disease. The external openings of anal fistulas are usually closer to the anus, not necessarily in the midline, have a palpable tract extending toward the rectum, and may have a demonstrable internal opening at the anorectal juncture and a history of rectal abscess. Passage of a probe in the tract may indicate its course. Occasionally, however, the differentiation may be difficult.

Osteomyelitis can be demonstrated by x-ray study.

Furuncle or carbuncle may be associated with similar lesions elsewhere on the skin and present a rounded, mound-like appearance surrounded by a whitish-yellow "head" whereas the infected pilonidal cyst is more flattened and blends into the surrounding tissues. X-ray fistulograms made by injecting a radiopaque substance in the external opening may be helpful in delineating the extent of the pathology.

Complications

Untreated pilonidal infection may result in the formation of multiple, sometimes long, draining sinuses. Rarely, malignant degeneration has occurred.

Treatment

Treatment of the acute abscess is by incision and drainage. This may often be accomplished under local anesthesia. If the abscess cavity is small and superficial, unroofing and packing it open may result in complete healing. As a rule, however, a chronic draining sinus persists which must be surgically extirpated by excision and primary closure or, preferably, by an "open" technic and marsupialization. The variety of closed methods which have been described testifies to their unacceptable recurrence rate and to superiority of the open technic. Two open methods may be described briefly as follows:

(1) The sinuses and all of their ramifications are opened over a grooved director. The sinus tracts are then completely exteriorized by circumcising the overhanging skin edges. Finally, the intact skin edge is sutured to the edge of the sinus tract and a pressure

dressing is applied until the following day.

(2) The area involved by the disease is excised with an elliptical skin incision carried down through the subcutaneous tissue to the posterior sacrococcygeal fascia and the block of tissue is dissected from the fascia. The edges of the wound are then sutured to the fascia and a pressure dressing is applied.

The pressure dressing may be removed on the second postoperative day and the sutures in a week. Daily warm sitz baths are then begun. The wound is inspected every 5–7 days so that bridging-over may be prevented.

Healing time depends upon the size of the defect, but is usually 3–6 weeks. The patient is entirely ambulatory throughout the treatment.

Prognosis

The recurrence rate following surgical correction varies with the method and after-care. With the open method, the recurrence rate is 5–10%.

Flannery BP, Kidd HA: A review of pilonidal sinus lesions and a method of treatment. Postgrad MJ 43:353–358, 1967.

Miller RJ: Pilonidal disease: A logical approach. Postgrad Med 41:382–385, 1967.

O'Neal RM, Grabb WC: Pilonidal disease. Univ Michigan Med Cent J 32:270–273, 1967.

Sherry JK: Primary closure of pilonidal sinus. Surg Gynec Obst 126:986–994, 1968.

Swinton NW, Samaan ST: Pilonidal sinus disease. Hosp Med 4:12–19, 1968.

Zimmerman K: Pilonidal disease. Dis Colon Rectum 13:330–332, 1970.

FOREIGN BODIES IN THE RECTUM

Swallowed foreign bodies such as chicken or fish bones, toothpicks, false teeth, pins, etc may become lodged at the anorectal juncture. Psychotic persons may swallow all manner of objects. Foreign bodies are swallowed sometimes for the purpose of concealment. Foreign bodies such as gallstones, fecaliths, urinary calculi, vaginal pessaries, orthopedic appliances, or surgical sponges or instruments may erode into the rectum. Foreign bodies may be introduced intentionally into the rectum for purposes of concealment, sexual stimulation, as a prank, for self-therapy, or from impalement. Enema tips and thermometers, broken or intact, are among the most common. The list of foreign bodies so introduced is long and often bizarre.

Clinical manifestations will depend upon the size and shape of the foreign body, its duration in situ, and the presence of infection or perforation. The occurrence of sudden excruciating pain during defecation should arouse suspicion of a perforating foreign body. Constant pain and tenesmus are almost invariably present. Bleeding will occur if there is concomitant trauma. There may be severe sphincteric spasm and tenderness.

Digital rectal and proctoscopic examinations are usually diagnostic, although very small foreign bodies may be difficult to palpate. X-ray examination is helpful only when the foreign body is radiopaque.

The diagnosis may be missed if, as is often the case, the patient does not admit to insertion of the foreign body. Sharp small foreign bodies which lodge in or tear the anal crypts and cause marked pain and spasm may be missed, leading to an erroneous diagnosis of fissure, cryptitis, or proctitis. Fecal impaction must be differentiated.

Complications include pararectal infection, intra- or extraperitoneal rupture of the bowel, injury to the sphincters, and fistulization to adjacent viscera.

Removal of foreign bodies in the rectum is often difficult because they tend to slip through the tight sphincteric ring into the commodious ampulla and are then difficult to grasp and to extract. Special procedures include the use of gauze coverage, rubber tubing, a corkscrew for soft objects, a tonsil-type snare, etc. The ingenuity and skill of the operator are often taxed. A hole may be bored through the foreign body in order to overcome the suction which opposes withdrawal. Such procedures are best done under the complete relaxation of spinal anesthesia. Sphincterotomy may be necessary. Simultaneous external pressure upon the abdomen is sometimes helpful.

Small foreign bodies may be extracted with a speculum under regional anesthetic. Foreign bodies eroding into the rectum from the uterus, vagina, bladder, prostate, or bowel are best removed and subsequent treatment of the residual fistula delayed until after the acute inflammatory reaction has subsided. If perforation of the bowel has occurred, closure and complementary colostomy must be done. Foreign bodies may be passed spontaneously in the purulent material of a pararectal abscess. Enemas should not be used with the hope of "flushing out" the object.

In neglected cases, extensive necrosis and gangrene of the buttocks and perirectal tissues may develop. Radical debridement then becomes a life-saving procedure.

Jansen AAJ: Foreign body in the rectum. New Zealand MJ 70:174–175, 1969.

Lowicki EN: Accidental introduction of giant foreign body into the rectum: case report. Ann Surg 163:395–398, 1966.

Sachdev YV: An unusual foreign body in the rectum. Dis Colon Rectum 10:220–221, 1967.

Stone HH, Martin JDJ: Synergistic necrotizing cellulitis. Ann Surg 175:702, 1972.

RECTAL PROLAPSE

Essentials of Diagnosis

- Protrusion of the rectum through the anus.
- Partial or complete fecal incontinence.
- Bleeding and discharge.

General Considerations

The causes of rectal prolapse are often obscure. It is far more common in women than in men, and is common in mentally ill patients—perhaps as a result of their tendency to strain excessively at stool. Extensive injury to or weakening of the puborectalis sling due to surgery, trauma, neurologic defects, senility, large rectal or sigmoidal polyps, wasting diseases, or nutritional deficiency may be responsible. Secondary muscular weakness is produced by the prolapse itself.

Errors in diagnosis and treatment are partially due to failure to differentiate the 4 types:

(1) **Mucosal prolapse:** Transient, minor prolapse of just the rectal mucosa frequently occurs in otherwise normal infants and may be alarming to the parents. In adults, however, mucosal prolapse is persistent and may grow progressively worse.

(2) **Procidentia:** This consists of complete prolapse of the entire thickness of the rectum along with the peritoneum as a sliding hernia. In children, it is thought to be due to the flatness of the sacrum (so that the rectum forms a vertical straight tube), the reduction of the supporting fat of the ischiorectal fossa, and weakness of the supporting ligaments of the rectum. It may be associated with other congenital anomalies such as exstrophy of the bladder. In adults, procidentia associated with a deep cul-de-sac represents a sliding hernia in which the anterior rectal wall and the peritoneal sac attached to it first protrude externally. As the muscular supports become weaker, there is complete procidentia of the entire circumference. The lateral suspensory ligaments of the rectum are attenuated or absent. The levators ani are separated, and the rectovaginal septum is shortened or absent. Prolapse of the uterus with cystocele may be present. The anterior hernial sac may contain omentum or small bowel. Abnormal anterior displacement of the rectum due to elongation of the mesorectum is probably the primary causative factor.

(3) **Eversion of the rectal and anal wall:** This is due to deficiency of the pelvic musculature. It contains no peritoneal pouch and is a complete circumferential protrusion of the full thickness of the lower anorectum.

(4) **Prolapse of a colonic intussusception:** This rare type consists of a protrusion of the intraabdominal colon through the anus while the rectum remains in its normal position.

Clinical Findings

A. Symptoms and Signs: A mass protrudes from the rectum during defecation or even during walking. At first the mass reduces spontaneously, but with time it becomes more difficult to reduce. Soiling of the clothing occurs from discharge, bleeding, and fecal incontinence. The musculature becomes progressively weaker until it is completely atonic and complete fecal incontinence results. In mucosal prolapse, the protrusion is relatively small, is symmetrical about the circumference, the mucosal folds are arranged in a radial fashion and, by palpating the thickness of the protrusion between the thumb and index finger, the 2 apposed thicknesses of mucosa can be recognized. With procidentia of the sliding hernia type, the protrusion may reach a considerable length. The anterior wall will be larger than the rest of the circumference because of its contained hernial sac; the lumen will be directed posteriorly and will be off center; the mucosal folds will be arranged in a circular fashion; and palpation of the thickness of the protrusion anteriorly will disclose the double·full thickness of the bowel wall and its hernial sac. Intussusception is recognized by the deep sulcus between the intussusceptum and the rectal wall.

It is essential that the prolapse be demonstrated. Examination in either a standing or squatting position with the patient straining is required if the full extent of the prolapse is to be demonstrated. The extent of weakness of the pelvic musculature and sphincteric ring should be evaluated by observing their tonus, their ability to contract voluntarily, and by palpation.

B. Special Examinations: Sigmoidoscopy and barium enema x-ray examination of the colon must be done to search for intrinsic disease. A lateral x-ray or cineradiography may disclose the anterior displacement of the rectum away from the sacrum.

Neurologic examination is necessary to rule out primary neurologic disorders.

Differential Diagnosis

Prolapsing internal hemorrhoids are recognizable by their varicose appearance and separation into discrete masses. They may be associated with some degree of mucosal prolapse as well. Large hypertrophic anal papillae, fibromas, and rectal polyps are solitary, circumscribed, and of firmer consistency.

Complications

The prolapsing mucosa frequently shows signs of superficial infection, ulceration, and edema. Irreducibility is uncommon. Gangrene or rupture of the anterior wall of the rectum with extrusion of the small bowel is rare and now occurs only in places remote from medical aid.

Treatment

A. Medical Treatment: In children, conservative treatment is most satisfactory; recurrences in adult life occur only rarely. When there is underlying mental deficiency, neurologic disorder, or incurable chronic disease, surgical correction may be required. Underlying nutritional or febrile disorders should be corrected and the causes of straining eliminated. Defecation in a recumbent position is recommended, and the buttocks should be strapped firmly together between bowel movements. Stool softeners and enemas may be necessary.

B. Surgical Treatment: In adults, conservative measures are rarely sufficient, and operative treatment is nearly always required. At least 50 procedures have been described, which testifies to the imperfection of all of them.

The operation must be properly chosen for the

particular type of prolapse present.

The most effective operations in current use are as follows:(1) For simple mucosal prolapse, operation consists of excision of diamond-shaped segments of mucosa in each of 4 quadrants with apposition by suture of the apices of the diamonds so as to foreshorten the protruding mucosa. (2) For complete procidentia, perineal operations or proctosigmoidectomy are recommended in which the outer layer of the intussusception is circumcised and the intussuscipiens, including the intraperitoneal sigmoid colon, is drawn externally until it is taut up to its point of fixation at its juncture with the descending colon. The anterior hernial sac is then sutured closed in a high position. The diastasis of the puborectalis is repaired. The redundant bowel is amputated, and an anastomosis is made between the inner and outer walls of the bowel. (3) Abdominal operation consists of mobilization and elevation of the rectum below the peritoneum, excision of the redundant peritoneum from the pouch of Douglas, repair of the levator muscles, reconstruction of the pelvic floor at a high level, and resection of the redundant pelvic colon when indicated. (4) Elevation and posterior fixation of the rectum to the sacrum to correct its anterior displacement, either by direct suture or by the use of a Teflon mesh sling. (5) A combination of both the perineal and abdominal operations. (6) In eversion of the rectum due to pelvic floor weakness, a Teflon or fascial sling encircling the lower portion of the rectum posteriorly and attached anteriorly to the pubic bone provides an effective means of support. (7) In patients who are very old or in poor general condition, a Thiersch-Jackman wire may be used. This consists of a stainless steel braided wire which encircles the sphincteric ring.

In all types, the muscles supporting the rectum can be strengthened to some degree by exercising the sphincteric mechanism.

Prognosis

Success rates are highest when the operation has been properly chosen for the particular type of prolapse. In general, the recurrence rate is high, although individual surgeons who have properly performed an appropriate operation have reported from 75—100% successes. When muscle deficiency is great, improvement following postoperative exercising of the sphincters is insignificant. There are conflicting reports concerning the effectiveness of electric stimulation.

Bordén B, Snellman B: Procidentia of the rectum studied with cineradiography. Dis Colon Rectum 11:333—347, 1968.

Dunphy JE, Pikula JV: Rectal prolapse. In: *Diseases of the Colon and Anorectum.* Turell R (editor). Saunders, 1969.

Khubchandani IT, Bacon HD: Complete prolapse of the rectum and its treatment. Arch Surg 90:337, 1965.

Moore HD: Complete prolapse of the rectum in the adult. Ann Surg 169:368—375, 1969.

Nigro ND: An evaluation of the cause and mechanism of complete rectal prolapse. Dis Colon Rectum 9:391—398, 1966.

Ripstein CB, Lanter B: Etiology and surgical therapy of massive prolapse of the rectum. Ann Surg 157:259, 1963.

Ripstein CB: A simple effective operation for rectal prolapse. Postgrad Med 45:201—204, 1969.

Wilson E: Thiersch's operation. Australian New Zealand J Surg 38:239—243, 1969.

FECAL INCONTINENCE

Essentials of Diagnosis

- Loss of voluntary control of passage of feces through anus.
- Fecal soiling of clothing.

General Considerations

Anal incontinence may result from injuries or diseases of the spinal cord, congenital abnormalities, accidental injuries to the rectum and anus, procidentia, senility, fecal impaction, extensive inflammatory processes, lymphogranuloma venereum, malignant tumors, stricture, and deformities following obstetric, dilational, and operative procedures. The extent to which gas, liquid feces, or semisolid feces can be controlled may be used as a measure of the severity of the lesion. Postobstetric or postoperative incontinence may not become manifest until many years after the causative incident, when senile hypotonicity of the pelvic musculature occurs.

An understanding of the detailed anatomy and physiology of the anorectum is essential for a proper approach to the prevention and repair of anal incontinence. Rectal incontinence is more than "a simple affair of a purse-string pulled by the cerebral cortex." The rectum is a capacious, distensible organ which forms a (usually empty) reservoir. The "anal ring" is a composite muscle consisting of the various bundles of the external sphincter, the internal sphincter, the prolongation of the longitudinal layer of the rectum, and the puborectalis portion of the levator ani muscles. The levators support the anal canal only posteriorly and laterally, leaving an area of comparative weakness anteriorly, where it is more vulnerable to injury. The central portion of the levator acts as a sphincter. Maintenance of the acute angulation of the anorectal juncture is also important in effecting normal evacuation.

There is a cerebral inhibitory control over the spinal cord reflex for both defecation and micturition. Destruction of the second, third, and fourth sacral segments or cauda equina results in loss of reflex evacuation. Sensory incontinence may result after removal of the lowermost portion of the rectum, as in some types of operations for cancer.

Clinical Findings

In neurogenic incontinence there is atony of the pelvic musculature with laxity of the anal canal, insensibility to tactile stimulation, inability to contract the anorectal musculature voluntarily, and absence of the anal reflexes. In traumatic or postoperative incontinence, the actual defect in the circumference of the anorectal ring with scarring can be seen and palpated. A clue to the site of the defect is the loss of corrugation or wrinkling of the perianal skin due to the defect in the underlying subcutaneous corrugator ani muscle. With extensive inflammatory or malignant disease, rigidity of the rectal outlet is readily identifiable. There may be some degree of rectal prolapse.

Prevention

At the time of surgical operation on the anorectum, forceful dilatation and inadvertent division of the sphincters must be avoided. In operations for fistula, a sufficient portion of the anorectal ring must remain to allow control. Postoperative packing must be avoided. Obstetric injuries to the sphincters must be immediately recognized and promptly repaired.

Treatment

A. Medical Measures: For mild degrees of incontinence, nonsurgical measures may suffice. These include a low-residue, bland diet and anticholinergic drugs to reduce intestinal motility; daily enemas with a device to allow for retention of the irrigating fluid; and daily exercises of sphincteric contraction. Patients with neurogenic incontinence may be trained to initiate defecation by digital stimulation of the anal canal. If not immediately corrected, repair of obstetric tears should be delayed for 6 months or more after parturition.

Methods of continuous electrical stimulation of the sphincters by an implanted electronic device are in the process of development.

B. Surgical Treatment: When anal incontinence is associated with rectocele and cystocele, colpoperineoplasty is essential. Methods of surgical repair of defects in the sphincteric ring include "reefing" operations; fascial slings using fascia lata or transplantation of the gracilis muscle from the medial side of the thigh; "pullout wire" reapposition, encircling the anus with a silver or stainless steel wire; and the "classical" method in which the divided ends of the muscles are reapposed.

Prognosis

Conservative measures as outlined above are frequently all that is required. Operative results are good if surgery is performed before atony of the muscle occurs. Concomitant irritability of the bowel, neurogenic, inflammatory, or neoplastic disease, or other anatomic defects make for a poor prognosis.

Birnbaum WD: Fecal incontinence. In: *Diseases of the Colon and Anorectum.* Turell R (editor). Saunders, 1969.

Birnbaum WD, Sproul G: The treatment of fecal incontinence. S Clin North America 35:1487–1496, 1955.

Fecal incontinence. Brit MJ 3:72, 1969.

Gaston EA: Recent advances in the study and restoration of fecal incontinence. Dis Colon Rectum 10:213–219, 1967.

Jackman RJ: Fecal incontinence: Nonsurgical treatment. JAMA 166:1281–1285, 1958.

Scharli AF, Kiesewetter WB: Defecation and continence: Some new concepts. Dis Colon Rectum 13:81–107, 1970.

MALIGNANT TUMORS OF THE ANAL CANAL & PERINEUM

Basal cell epithelioma is uncommon, usually arises at the anal verge, occurs 3 times as frequently in males as in females, and is similar to the more frequent "rodent ulcer" seen on exposed skin surfaces. All chronic, indurated growths at the anal margin should be suspect. A wide excisional biopsy of the suspicious area should be done which will not only allow a diagnosis but will effect a cure if adequate normal tissue margins are obtained. Local excision is the treatment of choice for anal basal cell epithelioma because of its nonmetastasizing nature. Irradiation therapy can also be used as the primary treatment, but surgical excision is preferable because of the undesirable side-effects of radiation in the anal region.

Perianal Bowen's disease (intraepidermal carcinoma, carcinoma in situ) is a rare, chronic, slowly maturing tumor. Two or 3% of the growths will become infiltrative and metastasize. Other malignant tumors are often present elsewhere in the body. The disease is manifested as a dull red, spreading, irregular, plaque-like, eczematoid, weeping lesion of the skin which is usually pruritic. It must be considered in the differential diagnosis of pruritus ani. The diagnosis is made by biopsy, and the distinguishing histopathologic feature is the presence of intraepidermal, haloed, multinucleated "giant" Bowen cells. Treatment is by local excision with adequate margins of normal skin.

Extramammary Paget's disease of the anus (epidermotrophic carcinoma) is a rare mucinous carcinoma involving the external anogenital area that occurs most commonly in women over age 50. It probably arises in the apocrine glands with secondary intradermal metastases. It is a malignant, extremely slowly growing tumor that may metastasize late. It must be differentiated from neurodermatitis, psoriasis, Bowen's disease, basal cell cancer, squamous cell cancer, and unpigmented melanoma. Treatment consists of wide excision with microscopic control since the margins of excision may appear to be grossly normal.

Cloacogenic cancer of the anorectal junction (transitional cell, basaloid, basosquamous carcinoma) arises from embryologic remnants that have persisted in the cloacogenic zone just above the dentate line where the glandular mucosa of the rectum meets the stratified epithelium of the anal canal. It occurs twice as frequently in females as in males. The history of discomfort and possibly of bleeding is often a short one. The growth is usually of an "iceberg" type, with the bulk of the tumor in the deeper tissues and only the surface presenting in the anal canal. Early, rapid metastatic spread is common. Microscopically, the appearance is strikingly similar to that of papillary transitional cell tumors seen at the vesical neck and posterior urethra. Treatment consists of early, radical abdominoperineal resection of the rectum.

Anorectal malignant melanoma is rare. Growth is dynamic, with a tendency for early spread, rapid metastasis, and a very high rate of recurrence even after radical surgery. This is the most lethal of the tumors occurring at the anorectal juncture. Most are pigmented, but about a third are amelanotic. When pigmented, the lesion can simulate a thrombosed or strangulated hemorrhoid; when amelanotic, it can resemble a mucosal rectal polyp or internal hemorrhoid. The current treatment of choice is radical abdominoperineal resection of the rectum. Additional dissection of aorto-ileopelvic and bilateral inguinal lymph nodes has not materially improved the survival rate. Primary irradiation has proved ineffective. Perfusion chemotherapy may possibly improve the survival rate.

Epidermoid carcinoma of the anorectum (squamous cell carcinoma) comprises 3–5% of cancers of the rectum and anus. It occurs twice as frequently in females as in males. Leukoplakia, lymphogranuloma venereum, chronic fistulas, and irradiated anal skin are potential predisposing causes. Most of these tumors are histologically moderately well differentiated, but occasional ones are poorly differentiated. The degree of differentiation is inversely proportionate to the rate of growth, infiltration, and metastasis. Direct extension into the perianal tissues and sphincter muscles is frequent. Epidermoid carcinomas arising in the anal canal metastasize along the lymphatics of the rectum to the perirectal and mesenteric lymph nodes as well as to the inguinal lymph nodes. Hepatic metastases via the portal venous system occur in about 10% of cases. Carcinomas arising external to the anus metastasize to the inguinal lymph nodes either across the perineum to the superficial inguinal lymph nodes or along the middle hemorrhoidal lymphatics to the hypogastric and obturator lymph nodes and from there to the external

iliac and inguinal lymph nodes. Unsuspected epidermoid carcinoma is occasionally discovered in the specimens from hemorrhoidectomy. When hemorrhoids are removed surgically, they should be marked to show their position in the circumference of the rectum and must always be examined microscopically.

Rectal bleeding is the most common' presenting symptom. Local pain, change of bowel habits, sensation of a lump, tenesmus, soilage, perianal itching, or a feeling of moisture also may occur.

Surgery is the treatment of choice. The type of operation indicated is dependent upon evaluation of the clinical features of the tumor. Wide local excision may be done for small superficial lesions which are located at or below the mucocutaneous juncture. Large tumors which penetrate the anal sphincters or which originate above the mucocutaneous line and involve the rectum should have a combined abdominoperineal resection of the rectum with a wide perineal phase of excision to include the levator muscles as well as the contents of the ischiorectal fossae. In the female patient, posterior vaginectomy may also be indicated. Extramesenteric pelvic lymph node dissection is indicated whenever it can be done with little difficulty in good-risk patients as part of combined abdominoperineal resection.

The simultaneous appearance of an inguinal metastasis in a patient whose primary tumor is as yet untreated is an ominous sign. Subsequent appearance of an inguinal metastasis portends a somewhat better outlook. When inguinal lymph nodes are not clinically involved on initial examination, bilateral radical groin dissection should not be done as a prophylactic measure. The poor salvage rate of this procedure must be weighed against the significant morbidity usually attended with bilateral radical groin dissection. Frequent, careful follow-up examination of the inguinal lymph nodes with prompt therapeutic groin dissection when indicated is preferable.

The prognosis of squamous cell carcinoma of the anorectum has improved markedly in recent years. An overall 5-year nonrecurrence rate of greater than 50% can now be anticipated.

• • •

General References

Morson BC: Rectal biopsy in inflammatory bowel disease. New England J Med 287:1337–1339, 1972.

Ross ST (editor): Symposium on anorectal diseases. Mod Treat 8:861–979, 1971.

Turell R (editor): Symposium on diseases of the colon and anorectum. S Clin North America 52:795–1091, 1972.

Waite VC & others: Symposium: Complications of colonic and rectal surgery. Dis Colon Rectum 16:1–28, 1973.

38...

The Adrenals

Thomas K. Hunt, MD

Operations on the adrenal glands are performed for hyperadrenocorticism (Cushing's disease or Cushing's syndrome), ectopic ACTH-producing tumors, primary hyperaldosteronism, pheochromocytoma, and, less commonly, other adrenocortical tumors.

These conditions are usually characterized by hypersecretion of one or more of the adrenal hormones.

Adrenalectomy is also useful in the management of metastatic breast and prostatic carcinoma.

The biochemical pathways of adrenal secretions are described in many sources.

Anatomy & Surgical Principles

The anatomy of the adrenals (Fig 38–1) is quite constant. The right gland lies posterior and lateral to the vena cava and superior to the kidney. The left gland lies medial to the superior pole of the kidney, just lateral to the aorta, and immediately posterior to the superior border of the pancreas. An important surgical feature is the remarkable constancy of the adrenal veins. The right adrenal vein is usually 2–5 mm long and several millimeters wide and joins the anterior face

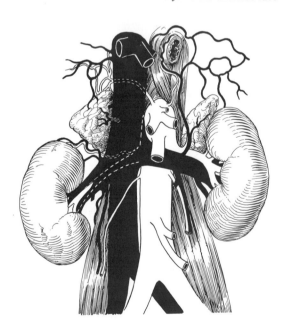

FIG 38–1. Anatomy of the adrenals showing venous return.

of the adrenal gland to the posterolateral aspect of the vena cava. The left adrenal vein is usually several centimeters long and travels almost straightly inferiorly, joining the lower pole of the gland to the left renal vein after receiving the inferior phrenic vein. The adrenal arteries are small, multiple, and inconstant.

The normal combined weight of the adrenal glands is 7–12 g.

The major principles of adrenal surgery are as follows:

(1) The diagnosis must be absolutely firm before operation is undertaken. The surgeon must be free to conduct an exhaustive search if the expected pathology is not found in the adrenal area and must be prepared to take definitive action even if the lesion is not grossly apparent. For example, he must be so confident of the preoperative diagnosis of hyperaldosteronism that even when the adrenals appear normal he can perform a total or subtotal adrenalectomy knowing that he will cure the patient.

(2) Since the gross pathology is often subtle, the surgeon must work with complete hemostasis and must be familiar with adrenal pathology in its most subtle forms.

(3) The patient must be carefully prepared so that he will be able to withstand the metabolic problems caused by his disease and his operation. Preparation of the patient is explained in the body of the chapter.

(4) The surgeon and his consultants must be ready to detect and treat any metabolic crisis occurring during operation or afterward.

Adrenal operations are done from various surgical approaches. The anterior or transperitoneal approach through a long vertical midline incision or a bilateral subcostal incision is used for pheochromocytoma and is the approach of choice for other potentially bilateral diseases of the adrenals. This approach permits adequate exposure of most of the retroperitoneum. Unfortunately, the postoperative period is painful and the patient has ileus and is exposed to the risk of poor healing such as evisceration. Poor wound healing is fairly common in patients with Cushing's syndrome (Table 38–1).

The posterior approach, performed through incisions on each side of the spine with the patient lying prone, is somewhat better tolerated postoperatively but gives only limited exposure. In this retroperitoneal operation, poor healing does not have the potential of evisceration. The posterior approach can be made through many incisions with approaches varying from transpleural to those through the bed of the 11th or 12th rib with the patient in a lateral or semilateral position. The latter are also retroperitoneal and well tolerated and give excellent exposure. A lateral approach through the bed of the 12th rib, exposing the adrenals retroperitoneally, is useful for known unilateral conditions or for bilateral conditions in obese patients.

DISEASES OF THE ADRENALS

PRIMARY HYPERALDOSTERONISM

Essentials of Diagnosis

- Hypertension, polyuria, polydipsia, muscular weakness, tetany.
- Hypokalemia, alkalosis, renal damage.
- Elevated, autonomous urinary aldosterone level and low plasma renin level under carefully controlled conditions.
- Tumors usually too small to be visualized by x-ray.

General Considerations

Primary hyperaldosteronism is renin-independent aldosterone hypersecretion in hypertensive, nonedematous patients. The syndrome was first recognized in the early 1950s by Conn, who found that it was usually caused by an adrenal tumor and could be cured simply by excision of the tumor.

Adrenal adenoma is the cause of primary hyperaldosteronism in about 85% of cases. About 90% of adenomas are unilateral, and most of these are 1–2 cm in diameter. The adenoma has a characteristic chromate-yellow color on section.

On examination by light microscopy, most tumors appear to be adenomas of the zona fasciculata, although the electron microscopic characteristics more closely resemble the zona glomerulosa. About 5% of adenomas are multiple, occurring in the same gland or in both glands. About 15% of patients—particularly those with atypical clinical syndromes—have bilateral adrenal hyperplasia.

Aldosterone is the most potent mineralocorticoid hormone secreted by the adrenal cortex. Its major functions are to regulate the electrolyte composition of the body, fluid volume, and blood pressure. In contrast to other adrenal steroids, its major control is by the renin-angiotensin system.

In clinical disorders of aldosterone secretion, the major problem is overproduction. These disorders can be classified as (1) primary hyperaldosteronism due to adrenal disease, usually tumor; (2) secondary hyperaldosteronism, usually in the hypertensive nonedematous patient; and (3) hyperaldosteronism in the edematous patient. Only primary hyperaldosteronism will be discussed here.

Clinical Findings

Hypertension and hypokalemia are the findings which most often lead to investigation of hyperaldosteronism.

A. Symptoms and Signs: The usual clinical symptoms are muscle weakness, polydipsia, nocturia, and headache. Carpopedal spasm and paresthesias sometimes occur from metabolic hypokalemic alkalosis. Hypertension is usually moderate and rarely malignant. The patient may have signs of advanced hypertension but rarely has severe retinopathy. Although extracellular fluid volume is usually higher than normal, edema is almost never seen until severe renal failure occurs. There are no other characteristic physical findings.

B. Laboratory Findings: One of the major sites of aldosterone action is in the distal nephron, where it facilitates the exchange of sodium for potassium and hydrogen ions whereby sodium is retained and potassium is lost. Therefore, when aldosterone secretion is chronically elevated, body potassium and hydrogen fall (alkalosis), total body sodium rises, and hypertension eventually results. Thus, the most expedient way to identify patients with primary hyperaldosteronism is to demonstrate hypokalemia. This can be accomplished by giving patients who are not taking diuretics or potassium 2 g of sodium chloride during each meal for 4 days. If hypokalemia is provoked by this salt-loading procedure or if spontaneous hypokalemia occurs, measurement of urinary aldosterone is then indicated.

In primary hyperaldosteronism, the plasma renin level is low. The diagnostic value of this finding, taken by itself, is somewhat limited because of the high incidence (25%) of reduced plasma renin activity in patients with essential hypertension. However, a **high** renin measurement is of great value in eliminating the possibility of primary aldosteronism. In aldosteronism due to hyperplasia, renin values often are in an intermediate range.

Aldosterone secretion rates are high and autonomous, ie, they are not suppressed by fludrocortisone, desoxycorticosterone acetate (DOCA), or plasma volume expansion. Administration of DOCA, 10 mg IM every 12 hours for 3 days, is useful in distinguishing primary from secondary hyperaldosteronism. When urine aldosterone excretion is not reduced into the normal range by this test (or by fludrocortisone), the hypersecretion is probably caused by an aldosterone-producing adenoma.

Differential Diagnosis

Secondary hyperaldosteronism in hypertensive patients can be caused by a number of disorders, particularly malignant hypertension, renovascular hypertension, and the recent use of diuretics or birth control pills. Consequently, patients who are taking estrogens (particularly birth control pills) must cease taking the medication for at least 2 months before valid measurements of renin or aldosterone can be made. Increased plasma renin activity is characteristic of all such cases, and the administration of DOCA can distinguish the hyperreninemia and hyperaldosteronism induced by these secondary factors since aldosterone levels will fall into the normal range when DOCA is given.

Complications

Progressive cardiorenal failure secondary to hypertension is the most common complication. In rare cases, almost complete muscular paralysis occurs when serum potassium becomes very low. Patients with heart disease may have arrhythmias because of low serum potassium, especially if they are taking digitalis. Stroke is a common and serious complication.

Treatment

A. Medical Treatment: The only cure for this disease is excision of hyperfunctioning adrenal tissue. Even so, unless hypokalemia or hypertension is unusually severe, there is little urgency about operation. Patients with mild disease can be managed with spironolactone and methyldopa, but the side-effects, particularly impotence and postural hypotension, are relatively severe. Escape from treatment is common.

B. Preoperative Care: Preoperative preparation is important since hypokalemic, alkalotic patients tend to develop serious cardiac arrhythmia under anesthesia. The optimal preparation includes withdrawal of antihypertensive medication for about 7 days unless hypertension is severe. Sodium is restricted, and potassium chloride (up to 120 mEq/liter/day in addition to regular diet) is administered in the immediate preoperative period until serum potassium is normal. If hypertension is severe, spironolactone can be safely given up to a few days before surgery.

C. Surgical Treatment: The usual operation is bilateral adrenal exploration and removal of the adenomatous adrenal gland. This operation can be done through an anterior transabdominal approach or through a posterior retroperitoneal approach, using separate incisions to expose each adrenal. The anterior approach is usually made through a bilateral subcostal incision. Most adenomas are found on the left side.

Localization of adenomas can often be accomplished by determining the plasma aldosterone levels in the right and left adrenal vein. A clear difference between the 2 sides is of great value, but a negative study does not necessarily rule out unilateral adenoma. Adrenal venography can be helpful but is difficult and relatively hazardous. [131]I-19 iodocholesterol scans can localize large adenomas. The small but appreciable incidence of multiple adenomas and the 10–20% incidence of hyperplasia make bilateral adrenal exploration mandatory if localization is not absolutely sure.

Only 2 cases of aldosterone-producing heterotopic adrenocortical adenoma have been described; one was in the kidney and the other in the ovary.

When hyperplasia is the cause, bilateral total or subtotal adrenalectomy is done, leaving only a small remnant of the left gland. The right gland usually is totally removed; reoperations on the right adrenal gland are particularly hazardous because the gland adheres to the vena cava. The left gland can be subtotally (approximately 70%) removed. In a few patients, the glands will appear grossly normal on close inspection. Signs of hyperplasia are subtle and consist of a "mealy appearance" of the cortex. The experienced surgeon can usually recognize hyperplasia. The surgeon must then remove the right gland and closely examine it for tiny adenomas or signs of hyperplasia. If none exist, the major portion of the left gland is also removed. Obviously, the surgeon must be absolutely confident of the diagnosis before undertaking this operation.

For adrenocortical steroid maintenance therapy after total adrenalectomy, see Hyperadrenocorticism.

D. Postoperative Care: Unilateral adrenalectomy can be accomplished without administration of corticosteroids pre- or postoperatively. The patient tends to carry forward his preoperative increased total body salt and hypervolemia. Blood losses are small; therefore, no more than normal water needs must be met in the postoperative period, and saline is not given unless there is some specific reason for giving it. Potassium is rarely given postoperatively. If large amounts of saline are given after operation, bladder decompensation and atelectasis are likely to occur.

Rare cases have been described in which glucocorticoid deficiency has followed unilateral adrenalectomy. A few patients have temporary aldosterone deficiency postoperatively because the normal adrenal gland has been suppressed by the hyperfunctioning adenoma. The signs of hypoaldosteronism are continuing weight loss, undue fall in blood pressure, and hyperkalemia. In these cases it is usually necessary to give fludrocortisone, 0.1 mg/day orally, until the other adrenal gland has regained its ability to secrete aldosterone. The patient can usually be weaned from this drug within a month after operation.

Blood pressure does not always fall immediately after resection of an adenoma; this may occur slowly over a period of 1–6 months after operation. When an obvious adenoma is removed, the postoperative blood pressure response is usually excellent. When hyperplasia is the cause—as it often is in young men with atypical syndromes—blood pressure response occurs but the patient usually retains some hypertension and may need medical treatment.

The patient usually notes an increase in strength and stamina after a successful operation. The response to operation usually parallels the preoperative pressor response to spironolactone.

Prognosis

Hyperaldosteronism usually follows a prolonged and subtly changing course. In untreated cases, death often results from stroke and cardiac and renal failure. The weakness is sometimes so severe and the hypokalemia so difficult to treat that operation becomes particularly desirable for relief of symptoms.

If operation is successful, the patient's condition usually returns to normal. Progressive hypertension due to hyperaldosteronism is halted when the hyperaldosteronism is cured. Unfortunately, if renal impairment has occurred, it is not reversed by operation.

Silen WS & others: Management of primary aldosteronism. Ann Surg 164:600–610, 1966.

Slaton PE, Schambelan M, Biglieri EG: Stimulation and suppression of aldosterone secretion in patients with an aldosterone-producing adenoma. J Clin Endocrinol 29: 239–250, 1969.

PHEOCHROMOCYTOMA

Essentials of Diagnosis

- "Spells" or "attacks" of headache, visual blurring, severe sweats, vasomotor changes in a young adult, weight loss.
- Hypertension, often paroxysmal ("spells") but frequently sustained.
- Postural tachycardia and hypotension; cardiac enlargement.
- Elevated urinary catecholamines or their metabolites.

General Considerations

Pheochromocytomas are tumors of the adrenal medulla and related chromaffin tissues elsewhere in the body which release epinephrine or norepinephrine (or both), resulting in sustained or episodic hypertension and other symptoms of excessive catecholamine secretion.

Clinical Findings

A. Symptoms and Signs: The clinical findings of pheochromocytoma are so variable that some investigators recommend investigation for pheochromocytoma in all patients with newly discovered hypertension regardless of symptoms. Nevertheless, pheochromocytoma is a rare disease. The "classical" patient with pheochromocytoma has episodic hypertension associated with pallor and subsequent flushing, palpitations, headache, excessive perspiration, nervousness, and anxiety. An important feature is the triad of palpitations, headache, and sweating occurring simultaneously. The symptoms are what one would expect from an injection of epinephrine.

The physical examination is usually unremarkable unless the patient is observed during an attack. Pheochromocytomas can cause sustained hypertension with or without obvious symptoms of excessive catecholamine secretion. In this case, the usual signs are tachycardia, retinopathy, signs of hypermetabolism, emotional lability, and weight loss. Clinical findings may mimic hyperthyroidism even to the point of exophthalmos. Excess secretion of epinephrine raises blood glucose and therefore may mimic diabetes. Patients with pheochromocytoma are usually thin.

Pheochromocytomas in adults are usually benign. Multiple tumors are present in about 10% of cases. Only a rare patient will never be hypertensive. In children, hypertension is less prominent, and many children (reported to be as many as 50%) will have multiple or extra-adrenal tumors. Malignancy is also more common in children.

Pheochromocytomas often occur in patients with neurofibromatosis. The condition may be familial and is also associated with medullary cancer of the thyroid. Pheochromocytoma can also be a part of the polyendocrine adenoma syndrome.

On pathologic examination, these tumors are quite uniform. They are reddish-brown and vascular. They feel firm but may be multicystic. Cells in any single tumor vary in size and shape. The cytoplasm is finely granular. Nuclei are round or oval, with prominent nucleoli. Mitoses are frequent, and necrotic areas are common. Ganglion-like cells are often seen. Veins and capsules may be invaded, even in clinically benign tumors. Size varies widely from a few grams to a reported high of 3600 g, more than twice the size of the normal adult liver. The average is about 100 g. The only reliable signs of malignancy are the presence of metastases or infiltrative invasion of surrounding tissues.

B. Laboratory Findings: The laboratory plays a very important part in the diagnosis. Several tests, including urinary 3-methoxy-4-hydroxymandelic acid ("VMA") determination, are available for screening. If these are positive, urinary assay for the individual catecholamines, epinephrine and norepinephrine, is indicated. Serum catecholamine determination can be of particular value. Direct measurement of epinephrine and norepinephrine in the urine or blood is the single most important laboratory test.

"Normal" values for catecholamines are difficult to define. Minor degrees of stress will cause considerable elevation of catecholamines even in a normal patient. There is considerable overlap between the values in some patients with intermittently secreting tumors and normal patients under stress.

Suppression or excitation tests are rarely necessary. If they must be done because of equivocal laboratory findings, the glucagon test is the safest method of stimulation and phentolamine (Regitine) the safest and most definitive method of suppression. *All excitation or suppression tests are hazardous and should be used only if essential for diagnosis.* In a sustained hypertensive crisis, cautiously used phentolamine can be both diagnostic and therapeutic.

Note: When the biochemical diagnosis is made, medical treatment should be started before further diagnostic measurements are taken (see Treatment, below). Preoperative localization of the tumors then becomes part of the sequence of treatment.

C. X-Ray Findings: X-ray findings include a solid tumor or displacement of a kidney shadow, both of which are often detectable on plain films of the abdomen. Nephrotomograms obtained during an intravenous urogram may show displacement of a kidney and an adrenal mass, and arteriograms show prominent feeding vessels and tumor blush. Arteriography is particularly helpful.

Differential Diagnosis

The differential diagnosis includes all causes of hypertension, with essential hypertension, renal hypertension, hyperaldosteronism, Cushing's syndrome, and hyperthyroidism leading the list. Hyperthyroidism and pheochromocytoma have many features in common. The differential diagnosis is easier if episodic hypertension is present.

Acute anxiety attacks mimic the symptoms, but anxiety rarely produces severe hypertension.

Labile essential hypertension is ruled out when clearly elevated catecholamine levels are detected.

Carcinoid syndrome may be mistaken for pheochromocytoma. In taking the history and making the differential diagnosis, the physician should remember that the pheochromocytoma attack mimics the symptoms of an injection of epinephrine.

Mild cases may be very difficult to diagnose. In labile hypertension, blood or urinary catecholamine levels should be checked several times during episodes of hypertension before the possibility of pheochromocytoma is discarded.

Hypertension in pregnancy is usually ascribed to toxemia. Unfortunately, a number of cases of pheochromocytoma, some of them fatal, have occurred in pregnant women.

Complications

Complications of this disease are usually the sequelae of hypertension, ie, stroke, renal failure, myocardial infarction, and cardiac decompensation. Sudden ventricular arrhythmia from release of catecholamines is probably responsible for many deaths. In patients not treated preoperatively with alpha-adrenergic blocking agents, postoperative hypotension is common, requiring catecholamine infusion and blood volume expansion to maintain tissue perfusion. This rarely occurs in properly managed patients.

Treatment

A. Medical Treatment: *Note:* Treatment with adrenergic blocking agents should be started as soon as the biochemical diagnosis is established. The purpose is to prevent the paroxysms of hypertension and also to correct the characteristic blood volume deficiency which is due to prolonged vasoconstriction. All of the alpha-adrenergic blocking agents have been used to treat this syndrome. Phentolamine (Regitine) and phenoxybenzamine (Dibenzyline) are the most frequently used drugs. Phentolamine has been effective in doses up to 600 mg/day orally. Because of its longer action, phenoxybenzamine in doses of about 10–30 mg orally is now preferred by most authorities. These drugs have complex actions and are potentially dangerous. References in the reading list should be consulted for the details of their use.

Propranolol (Inderal), a beta-adrenergic blocking agent, is often useful when cardiac arrhythmias and severe tachycardia are prominent features of the disease. Sedatives and tranquilizers are also useful in treating the very real anxiety that often accompanies pheochromocytoma.

The aims of preoperative therapy are (1) to restore the blood volume, which has been depleted by excessive release of catecholamines, and (2) to relieve the patient of the danger of a severe attack with all its potential complications. Blood volume is characteristically decreased about 15% in pheochromocytoma. Close control of symptoms is necessary in order to keep blood volume normal. Even 15 minutes of hypertension due to release of catecholamines can significantly reduce blood volume.

Once treatment is well established, localization of the tumor by angiography is safe and extremely useful. The tumor or tumors are located by the characteristic enlargement of feeding vessels and tumor blush. Another good method for localization is tomography in conjunction with intravenous urography. A third method is by measuring epinephrine and norepinephrine levels at various levels along the vena cava. If the secretion is predominantly norepinephrine, with normal or decreased epinephrine levels, extra-adrenal tumor becomes a possibility. Extra-adrenal tumors lack the methylating enzyme needed to convert norepinephrine to epinephrine (Fig 38–2). When epinephrine levels are elevated, the tumor is almost always in or

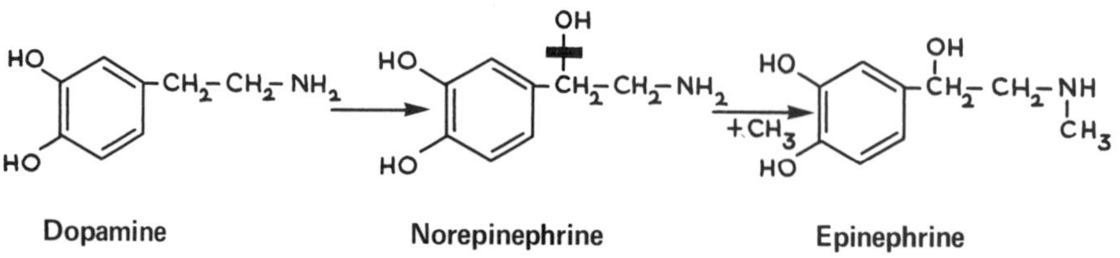

FIG 38–2. Sequence of catecholamine synthesis from dopamine. The more primitive extra-adrenal pheochromocytomas lack the methylating enzyme necessary to convert norepinephrine to epinephrine. Thus, when norepinephrine levels are high and epinephrine levels are normal or low, extra-adrenal tumor becomes a good possibility.

near the adrenal area. In any case, 90% of pheochromocytomas in adults are in the adrenal areas. Thus, if the tumor secretes epinephrine, aggressive attempts to localize it preoperatively are not called for since the likelihood is great that it will be in the adrenal area.

B. Surgical Treatment: The definitive treatment of pheochromocytoma is by surgical excision. In most cases, the tumor is relatively small and is confined to the adrenal area. The transabdominal approach is almost always used unless the tumor has been localized elsewhere. Multiple tumors are more likely to be found by the transabdominal approach.

The anesthesiologist should rely on an arterial catheter and ECG for constant monitoring of arterial pressure and heart action. Phentolamine and propranolol should be immediately available to treat the excessive hypertension and cardiac arrhythmias which often occur when the tumor is manipulated. The surgeon usually tries early in the procedure to divide the major venous tributaries draining the tumor to avoid unnecessary metabolic crises. Most anesthesiologists use nitrous oxide and muscle relaxants for anesthesia, although many other agents have been recommended.

The major surgical problems arise in excising large malignant tumors and in detecting multiple and ectopic tumors. Both adrenals should be explored thoroughly before the operation is concluded. About 10% of tumors will be multiple or bilateral (a larger percentage in children). About 7% will be malignant. Extra-adrenal pheochrome tumors are usually found along the abdominal aorta and in the organ of Zuckerkandl. However, tumors have been reported in widely scattered sites such as the genital organs, the mediastinum, the neck, and even the skull.

The well-prepared patient seldom needs treatment with drugs during surgery, and the well-prepared surgeon seldom fails to find all the functioning tumor. It is best to pretreat the patient in such a way that he still develops a pressor reaction to manipulation of the tumor at surgery since this allows detection of ectopic and multiple tumors. Blood pressure will almost always fall when all functioning tissue has been removed. If the patient has been properly prepared with alpha-blockers, the pressure fall will not be a problem. If the patient has not been properly prepared, ie, if blood volume is not increased preoperatively by blocking agents, postoperative hypotension will be a severe problem.

Prognosis

The outlook for patients with untreated pheochromocytoma is grim. The operative mortality rate has dropped to less than 5% since the introduction of drug therapy, but it is higher for malignant tumors. Second tumors in the remaining adrenal have been reported to occur years after excision of the primary pheochromocytoma. The results of surgery for benign disease are most gratifying.

The outlook for patients with malignant tumors (about 7%) is highly variable. Some patients have had long symptom-free intervals after excision of malignant tumors. X-ray therapy will sometimes control symptoms caused by metastases. The various blocking agents can also be used in palliative therapy with good results. However, death usually occurs a short time after the appearance of metastases.

Ross EJ & others: Preoperative and operative management of patients with pheochromocytoma. Brit MJ 1:191–198, 1967.

Sheps SG, Maher FT: Histamine and glucagon tests in diagnosis of pheochromocytoma. JAMA 205:79, 1968.

Sjoerdsma A & others: Pheochromocytoma: Current concepts of diagnosis and treatment. Ann Int Med 65:1302–1326, 1966.

HYPERADRENOCORTICISM
(Cushing's Disease & Cushing's Syndrome)

Essentials of Diagnosis

- Buffalo obesity, easy bruisability, psychosis, hirsutism, purple striae, acne, impotence or amenorrhea, and moon facies.
- Osteoporosis, hypertension, glycosuria.
- Elevated, autonomous 17-hydroxycorticosteroids, low serum potassium and chloride, low total eosinophils, and lymphopenia.
- Special x-ray studies may reveal a tumor or hyperplasia of the adrenals.

General Considerations

Cortisol and corticosterone are the most abundant glucocorticoids in man. Cushing's syndrome is due to hypersecretion of these hormones. It may be due to bilateral adrenal hyperplasia from increased stimulation by ACTH (corticotropin) or ACTH-independent adrenocortical tumors. Excess ACTH may be produced by pituitary overactivity, pituitary tumors (described by Harvey Cushing), or extrapituitary ACTH-producing tumors in the lung, pancreas, or ovary. Cushing's syndrome not dependent on ACTH may be caused by an autonomous adrenocortical benign adenoma or malignant carcinoma.

The sex incidence of Cushing's syndrome is 10 females to one male. The peak incidence is in the third and fourth decades, although the span ranges from infancy to the eighth decade. The natural history of the disease varies widely from mild stationary patterns to rapid progression and death. Complications are severe and often fatal. The diagnosis is complex, and the choice of treatment often depends on a precise clinical and biochemical appraisal.

Clinical Findings

A. Symptoms and Signs: (Table 38–1 and Fig 38–3.) The classic description of Cushing's syndrome includes truncal obesity, hirsutism, moon facies, acne, buffalo hump, purple striae, hypertension, and diabetes. However, other signs and symptoms are com-

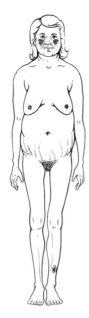

FIG 38–3. Major clinical features of Cushing's syndrome.

monly seen, and the most striking single feature is
weakness. The constellation of weakness and other
features is also seen after prolonged and excessive
administration of adrenocortical steroids or ACTH.

As in other diseases of the adrenals, the syndrome
is somewhat different in children, the most consistent
finding being cessation of growth. The most common
cause in children is malignant adrenal tumor, but
benign tumors and bilateral hyperplasia have been
described.

TABLE 38–1. Estimated frequency of
manifestations of Cushing's syndrome.

	Percentage
Obesity	90
Hypertension	80
Evidence of diabetes with normal fasting blood glucose	80
Centripetal distribution of fat	80
Weakness	80
Muscle atrophy in upper and lower extremities	70
Hirsutism	70
Menstrual disturbance or impotence	70
Purple striae	70
Plethoric facies	60
Osteoporosis	50
Easy bruisability	50
Acne or skin pigmentation	50
Mental changes	50
Edema	50
Headache	40
Poor wound healing	40
Leukocytosis with lymphopenia	Frequent

For the surgeon, some of the important findings
are obesity (which only rarely surpasses 90 kg [200
lb]) and muscular weakness, both of which have predictive value in relation to the likelihood of postoperative pulmonary difficulties. Other important features
are acne and diabetes, which indicate susceptibility to
infection; and atrophic skin and easy bruisability,
which forecast a difficult operation and poor wound
healing.

Pituitary tumors and tumors producing ectopic
ACTH usually secrete melanotropins (MSH) as well as
ACTH. Therefore, increased skin pigmentation is an
important feature of Cushing's syndrome due to excess
ACTH.

B. Pathologic Examination: The pathologic features of the gland itself also vary widely. The gross
changes in adrenal hyperplasia may be subtle and often
are called micronodular. Adrenal weights vary from
normal (7–12 g combined weight) to as much as 70 g
for both glands, combined; the usual combined adrenal
weight in hyperadrenocorticism is below 25 g.

In a few patients, pituitary tumors are the cause
of adrenal hyperplasia. These tumors are usually
benign and may be basophilic, acidophilic, or chromo-
phobic.

Adrenal adenomas in Cushing's syndrome range in
weight from a few grams to over 100 g, are usually
larger than aldosterone-producing adenomas, and are
very rare in males. The typical cells usually resemble
those of the zona fasciculata. Variable degrees of
anaplasia are seen, and differentiation of benign from
malignant tumors is often difficult.

Adrenal malignancies are frequently highly undifferentiated and spread by direct invasion or via the
blood stream. Since they tend to invade surrounding
structures, they are technically difficult to remove.

In a few cases, ectopic adrenal tissue has been the
source of excessive cortisol secretion. This tissue has
been found in a wide variety of locations, but most
commonly is near the abdominal aorta.

Occasionally, the important pathologic finding is
a nonendocrine, ACTH-secreting neoplasm. By far the
most common example is cancer of the lung. This
ectopic ACTH syndrome has also been associated with
tumors of the pancreas, thymus, prostate, esophagus,
colon, and other organs. Even an appendiceal carcinoma has been identified as ACTH-producing. Most
such tumors have in common their derivation from
embryonic entoderm and, in particular, their origin
from tissues derived from branchial clefts.

Cushing's syndrome sometimes results from ovarian tumors. These are usually malignant and are associated with adrenal hyperplasia and consequently represent a form of ectopic ACTH syndrome.

C. Laboratory Findings: Normally there is a daily
rhythmic variation of plasma ACTH elevation followed
by cortisol secretion. Levels are highest early in the
morning, decline gradually during the day, and are
lowest in late evening. Cortisol also regulates the rate
of pituitary ACTH secretion through the servomecha-
nism whereby an elevation of the cortisol level turns

off the ACTH that was responsible for the rise. In Cushing's syndrome, circadian rhythm is abolished and total secretion of cortisol is increased. The excess circulating cortisol leads to elevated plasma and urinary 17-hydroxycorticosteroids and 17-ketogenic steroids.

When Cushing's syndrome is suspected, a dual approach to diagnosis is taken. The diagnosis is established first, and the cause is then determined.

1. Overnight dexamethasone suppression test— Dexamethasone suppression is the first test in screening the patient suspected of having Cushing's syndrome. Normal subjects produce up to 30 mg of cortisol a day. Dexamethasone, 1 mg orally (equivalent to about 30 mg of cortisol), will suppress ACTH secretion in normal subjects and cortisol production will stop. In Cushing's syndrome, regardless of the cause, this amount of dexamethasone will not suppress increased ACTH secretion or excessive autonomous production of cortisol by an adrenocortical tumor. At exactly 11:00 pm, the patient is given 1 mg of dexamethasone and 100 mg of pentobarbital by mouth. The latter is added to ensure a good night's rest. A fasting plasma sample for cortisol determination is drawn the following morning. A basal plasma sample is required for evaluating the suppression if the patient is receiving estrogen therapy. Normal women receiving estrogens (eg, birth control pills) will have increased cortisol-binding globulin and thus will show high basal values of plasma cortisol. In normal and obese subjects, the morning plasma cortisol level will be suppressed to less than 5 $\mu g/100$ ml. Patients who are taking estrogens will have a greater than 50% suppression of baseline. Patients with Cushing's syndrome will not suppress below 12 $\mu g/100$ ml. Since 1 mg of dexamethasone contributes almost nothing to the cortisol in plasma, suppression of endogenous circulating cortisol is easily demonstrated. Its absence indicates fixation of pituitary ACTH production or cortisol overproduction by the adrenals (Cushing's disease). Partial suppression may occur in patients with acromegaly or thyrotoxicosis, chemically depressed patients, and those who are chronically ill or under chronic physical stress. Ordinarily, these conditions are clinically evident.

2. Twenty-four hour dexamethasone suppression test— If, in patients who are noncushingoid in appearance but are suspected of having Cushing's disease, complete cortisol suppression does not occur, the more cumbersome small-dose test of Liddle is required. A 24-hour urine collection for baseline urinary 17-hydroxycorticosteroid determination is taken on the first day. Starting on the second day, the patient takes 0.5 mg of dexamethasone orally every 6 hours for a total of 8 doses (through the third day). On the third day, a second 24-hour urinary 17-hydroxycorticosteroid determination is made. In normal patients, the 17-hydroxycorticosteroid level will be suppressed to below 4 mg in 24 hours. In patients with Cushing's disease, the 17-hydroxycorticosteroid level will not be suppressed.

3. Free urinary cortisol test— If, after the above

procedures, a firm diagnosis of hyperadrenocorticism still cannot be established or ruled out, the free urinary cortisol test is indicated. This test directly measures the physiologically active form of circulating cortisol and is the most sensitive and reliable means of diagnosing Cushing's syndrome. Free urinary cortisol will exceed 120 $\mu g/24$ hours only in hyperadrenocorticism.

4. Urinary 17-hydroxycorticosteroid excretion test— Because the free urinary cortisol test is not yet generally available, the physician may have to resort to a more readily available test which indirectly measures cortisol secretion. The urinary 17-hydroxycorticosteroid excretion follows the diurnal variation of plasma 17-hydroxycorticosteroid. Normal daily secretion (in milligrams) can be estimated by dividing body weight in kilograms by 7.5. For example, a subject weighing 90 kg (200 lb) should excrete about 12 ± 2 mg in 24 hours, which is the upper limit of normal in most laboratories. However, elevation may occur in association with obesity, thyrotoxicosis, acromegaly, emotional disturbances, and surgical stress, and the tests described above are necessary to rule out true hyperadrenocorticism.

Etiologic Diagnosis

Once the diagnosis of hyperadrenocorticism has been established, it becomes necessary to differentiate between ACTH-dependent adrenal hyperplasia and ACTH-independent adrenocortical tumor. Measurement of plasma ACTH levels is the most direct means of determining whether hyperadrenocorticism is ACTH-dependent. This most direct method is now becoming more widely available.

The **metyrapone test** is generally available and determines whether the pituitary is secreting ACTH (as in most cases of hyperplasia) or whether it has been suppressed (as in tumor). Metyrapone (Metopirone) blocks the conversion of the inactive precursor, deoxycortisol, to cortisol. If pituitary ACTH secretion is preserved, as in hyperplasia, it will respond to falling levels of cortisol with increased output and a secondary increase in urinary 17-hydroxycorticosteroid. If pituitary ACTH is suppressed, as in autonomous adrenocortical tumor, there will be no increase in 17-hydroxycorticosteroid in response to metyrapone. A 24-hour urine collection for basal 17-hydroxycorticosteroid is made on the day before the test. Beginning at 7:00 am on the day of the test, another 24-hour urine collection is started and 750 mg of metyrapone are given by mouth starting at 7:00 am and every 4 hours thereafter for a total of 6 doses. In bilateral hyperplasia due to overproduction of pituitary ACTH, there will be at least a doubling of urinary 17-hydroxycorticosteroid in response to the metyrapone test. An extrapituitary ACTH-producing tumor can give a positive response to metyrapone at times. This condition may be distinguished from a pituitary tumor by x-ray findings and clinical characteristics—eg, hypokalemic alkalosis with very high corticosteroid production and clinical characteristics of Cushing's syndrome typifies the ectopic ACTH syndrome. An enlarged pituitary fossa will be found in Cushing's disease due to pituitary tumor.

Patients with autonomous adrenocortical tumors do not respond to the administration of metyrapone; instead, the level of urinary 17-hydroxycorticosteroid on the day of the test remains unchanged or is lower than basal levels.

The exogenous corticotropin stimulation test is not a discriminating test. In bilateral hyperplasia as well as in some benign adrenocortical tumors, marked elevations of urinary 17-hydroxycorticosteroid occur after corticotropin is given intramuscularly or intravenously. Conversely, no response usually occurs in patients with adrenocortical carcinoma.

If, after this, a chemical diagnosis of adrenal tumor is made, x-ray examination is valuable. A simple tomogram of the suprarenal area often shows a unilateral adrenocortical tumor with typical contralateral adrenal atrophy. ^{131}I-19 iodocholesterol scanning is proving very useful in localizing adenoma and demonstrating greatly enlarged glands.

When the laboratory investigation is well planned, the problems of differential diagnosis are minimized. Before surgery is undertaken, there should be no doubt of the diagnosis.

Complications

The severe or terminal complications are most often those of hypertension (renal failure, strokes, etc), diabetes (hyperglycemia, insulin reactions, infections), or severe, debilitating muscular wasting and weakness. Cancer of the adrenals and uncontrolled tumors of the pituitary gland also have their characteristic complications.

Treatment of Cushing's syndrome also leads to numerous complications. **Nelson's syndrome** is due to pituitary oversecretion after adrenalectomy for bilateral hyperplasia of hypothalamic or pituitary origin. This includes hyperpigmentation, headaches, exophthalmos, and heightened sex hormone effects. Findings of pituitary enlargement are usually present, and blindness may result.

Treatment

Cushing's syndrome can be treated in several ways, including surgical or irradiation attack upon the pituitary, adrenals, or both; or by attempts to modify the synthesis of adrenal hormones.

A. Medical Treatment: Mitotane (o,p'DDD, Lysodren) is a DDT derivative which is toxic to the adrenal cortex. It has been used with modest success in treatment of adrenal hypersecretory states, especially adrenal cancer. Unfortunately, serious side-effects are common at effective doses.

Temporary control of Cushing's disease is possible with metyrapone (see above) and aminoglutethimide, both of which inhibit steps in steroid biosynthesis. Eventual escape from control is the rule in ACTH-dependent Cushing's syndrome, but temporary control (usually for months) may be advantageous in preoperative preparation. Complete medical adrenalectomy in

benign adrenocortical tumors is often possible when immediate surgery is contraindicated—eg, in patients with myocardial infarction.

B. Surgical Treatment: Even though operation is the treatment of choice, patients with severe Cushing's syndrome are poor risks for surgery. Complications are common, with wound infection, hemorrhage, peptic ulceration, and pulmonary problems heading the list.

1. Pituitary ablation—The pituitary can be excised (rarely done for Cushing's syndrome) or irradiated. Irradiation is effective for pituitary ablation and is applicable in 20–65% of patients (depending on the series reported) in whom pituitary dysfunction is the cause of the syndrome. However, it takes 8–18 months or even longer before significant effects are achieved—too long for patients with rapidly progressive disease. Enlarging pituitary tumors are usually best removed by surgical excision. Recurrences after radiotherapy are common.

Cryohypophysectomy has been tried with limited success. Implantation of ^{90}Y seeds is currently under evaluation.

2. Adrenalectomy—The safest and surest treatment of Cushing's syndrome due to bilateral hyperplasia is bilateral total adrenalectomy. Various surgical approaches can be used: transabdominal, bilateral flank, or transpleural. The manifestations of excessive cortisol secretion subside rapidly after surgery. Total extirpation necessitates total adrenal replacement therapy, but if patients are chosen properly this is a small price to pay for relief of Cushing's syndrome.

Subtotal resection is still preferred by a few surgeons, but the results are difficult to predict. We do not recommend it because it leaves inadequate adrenocortical reserve, often with a fixed high output of cortisol secretion. Furthermore, Cushing's disease recurs in about 40% of patients after partial resections.

In rare cases, for very poor risk patients, the surgeon may elect to do adrenalectomy in 2 stages through flank incisions.

For malignant tumors resection is the treatment of choice. Unilateral adrenalectomy is preferred 'for benign adenomas, which are rarely bilateral.

C. Postoperative Maintenance Therapy: After total adrenalectomy, lifelong corticosteroid maintenance therapy becomes necessary. The following schedule is commonly used: No cortisol is given until the adrenals are removed during surgery. On the first day, give 100 mg IM of cortisol phosphate or hemisuccinate every 8 hours. (If the patient is not doing well and is in shock, give intravenously.) In the next 24 hours after surgery, give 50 mg IM every 8 hours. Thereafter, the dose should be tapered downward as tolerated.

The higher doses are sometimes maintained if the patient has had severely elevated levels preoperatively.

As the hydrocortisone dose falls below 50 mg/day, it is wise to add fludrocortisone, 0.1 mg daily orally to avoid excessive electrolyte losses. The usual maintenance doses are about 20–30 mg of hydrocortisone and 0.1 mg of fludrocortisone daily. (More than half the dose is given in the morning.)

Prognosis

The prognosis for patients with benign Cushing's syndrome is quite good after adrenalectomy. The clinical manifestations begin to subside in several weeks, and complete cure is the rule. The major long-term problems are recurrence due to retained adrenal tissue (about 10%) and Nelson's syndrome, which occurs in about 15% of patients with hyperplasia of the pituitary associated with an ACTH-producing pituitary tumor.

When the syndrome is due to malignant disease, the prognosis is as grave as that of the tumor causing it. Unfortunately, by the time Cushing's syndrome occurs secondary to ectopic ACTH-producing cancers, the tumor is almost always beyond surgical curability. Palliation can occasionally be achieved by adrenalectomy when Cushing's syndrome is the principal clinical problem.

Lieberman LM & others: Diagnosis of adrenal disease by visualization of human adrenal glands with [131]I-19 iodocholesterol. New England J Med 285:1387–1392, 1971.

Orth DN, Liddle GW: Results of treating Cushing's syndrome. New England J Med 285:243–247, 1971.

Pavlatos FC, Smilo RP, Forsham PH: A rapid screening test for Cushing's syndrome. JAMA 193:720–723, 1965.

Smilo RP, Forsham PH: Diagnostic approach to hypofunction and hyperfunction of the adrenal cortex. Postgrad Med 46:146–152, 1969.

Sparks LL & others: Experience with a rapid oral metyrapone test and the plasma ACTH content in determining the cause of Cushing's syndrome. Metabolism 18:175–192, 1969.

Welbourn RB, Montgomery DAD, Kennedy TL: The natural history of treated Cushing's syndrome. Brit J Surg 58:1–16, 1971.

VIRILIZING & FEMINIZING TUMORS OF THE ADRENAL GLANDS

Virilizing adrenal tumors are rare. Congenital adrenal hyperplasia is the most common cause of virilization. Ovarian tumors, testicular tumors, and adrenal carcinoma must be distinguished from this group.

Under the influence of pituitary ACTH, the adrenal cortex secretes a number of weakly androgenic hormones. They contribute several milligrams to the total 24-hour urinary output of 17-ketosteroids. Virilization of adrenal origin is caused by overproduction of these androgens and their subsequent partial conversion to testosterone. The excessive levels of adrenal androgens are reflected in marked increases in urinary excretion of 17-ketosteroids. Testosterone, the most potent androgen, is not a 17-ketosteroid. Thus, marked virilization with normal or only slightly elevated urinary 17-ketosteroid excretion suggests that the excess testosterone originates in the ovary. Virilization may also be caused by specific deficiency of one or more of the enzymes necessary for normal formation of cortisol and mineralocorticoids. It may be associated with

Cushing's syndrome, as in adrenocortical carcinoma, or may be due to androgenic hyperactivity associated with excess testosterone production—a condition occurring only in females.

The 3 major patterns of congenital virilizing adrenal hyperplasia are simple virilism, virilism with hypertension, and virilism with renal sodium loss. Simple virilism is caused by a partial defect in synthesis of 21-hydroxycorticosteroids. As a result, a precursor of cortisol, 17-hydroxyprogesterone, accumulates and its metabolites pregnanetriol and 11-ketopregnanetriol appear in large amounts in the urine. When the defect in 21-hydroxylation becomes more severe, synthesis of aldosterone is impaired and renal sodium loss occurs. In the third type, 11-hydroxylation is incomplete, DOC concentration increases, and renal sodium conservation and hypertension occur.

Virilization by the adrenal occurs because of oversecretion of androgens—principally testosterone—which is due to excessive ACTH secretion in response to the block in hydrocortisone synthesis. Amelioration is easily achieved by administration of small quantities of hydrocortisone.

Virilization caused by tumor is distinguished by the following: (1) it does not occur early in life, (2) there is no increase of pregnanetriol or of DOC in the urine and no salt wasting, and (3) treatment with hydrocortisone or ACTH has no effect on androgen excretion or secretion. Therefore, excision is necessary.

Feminization as a result of adrenal disease is almost always due to adrenal tumors, most of which are malignant. The only known treatment is excision.

Clinical Findings

A. Symptoms and Signs: (Fig 38–4.) The clinical findings are the usual ones of virilization: sexual pre-

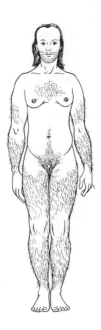

FIG 38–4. Woman with adrenogenital syndrome.

cocity, acne, increased hirsutism, male physique, male hair pattern and baldness, and, in males, increased libido. In females, the principal manifestations are atrophy of secondary sex characteristics, decreased libido, hirsutism, and acne. Rapid growth may occur in prepubertal females. Hypertension may accompany tumor-induced virilization.

These tumors are frequently large and are often palpable.

Feminization due to estrogen-secreting tumors also follows standard patterns as outlined above.

B. Laboratory Findings:

1. ACTH stimulation test—17-Ketosteroid, pregnanetriol (or 17-KGS), and 17-hydroxycorticosteroids are estimated in 24-hour urine samples collected in the basal state and after stimulation with ACTH given intravenously for 8 hours. With inhibition of normal cortisol and mineralocorticoid formation by an enzymatic block in the adrenal cortex, there is a resulting lack of restraint of production of ACTH by the pituitary. This leads to secondary increase in various cortisol and aldosterone precursors of different androgenic potency which is reflected in elevated urinary 17-ketosteroid and pregnanetriol (or 17-KGS) levels. In an adult with adrenogenital syndrome due to 21-hydroxylase deficiency, the urinary 17-hydroxycorticosteroid level is low or normal, 17-ketosteroids are moderately elevated, and the pregnanetriol characteristically exceeds the upper normal limit of 2 mg/day. ACTH stimulation markedly accentuates this difference: pregnanetriol levels increase several times, 17-ketosteroid levels usually more than double, and the 17-hydroxycorticosteroid remains the same or increases minimally.

2. Dexamethasone suppression test—Dexamethasone suppression differentiates androgenic adrenal hyperplasia from adrenocortical carcinoma (characterized by very high levels of 17-ketosteroids and pregnanetriol in the basal state). 17-Ketosteroids, pregnanetriol, and 17-hydroxycorticosteroids are estimated in 24-hour urine samples collected in the basal state and after suppression with dexamethasone, 2 mg orally every 6 hours for 8 doses (2 days). In the absence of carcinoma, excretion will be suppressed to very low levels on the second day of suppression.

In cases of marked androgenicity with normal or only slightly elevated urinary 17-ketosteroids, a search must be made for the site of production of excess plasma testosterone. In normal females, plasma testosterone should not exceed 0.06 μg/100 ml. If the basal level is higher than this, the suppression by dexamethasone should reduce it by more than 50% unless one is dealing with testosterone excess derived from the ovary or an independent tumor of the adrenal cortex.

Differentiation of adrenal tumors from those that arise in the ovary or testis is based on physical examination and culdoscopy or may require laparotomy. The adrenal tumor can also often be localized by nephrotomography or arteriography since it is usually large.

The diagnosis of feminizing tumors of the adrenal depends on recognition of the syndrome, identification of increased urinary or plasma estrogens, and exclusion of ovarian or testicular feminizing neoplasms.

Differential Diagnosis

The differential diagnosis includes testicular and ovarian tumors and other causes of ovarian dysfunction such as Stein-Leventhal syndrome, Cushing's syndrome, adrenal hyperplasia with virilization, and exogenous sex steroid administration.

Treatment

Treatment consists of excision of the tumor. Complications of the operation are relatively uncommon. Tumors are rarely bilateral or ectopic.

Prognosis

The prognosis is generally good after operation for virilizing tumors. Feminizing tumors are usually large and malignant; therefore, the prognosis is guarded.

Glenn F, Peterson RE, Mannix H Jr: *Surgery of the Adrenal Gland.* Macmillan, 1968.

Solomon SS & others: Feminizing adrenocortical carcinoma with hypertension. J Clin Endocrinol 28:608–612, 1968.

NONENDOCRINE TUMORS OF THE ADRENAL GLANDS

The most common nonendocrine adrenal tumor is neuroblastoma. It occurs only in children and is discussed in Chapter 49.

Nonfunctioning cancers of the adrenal cortex in the adult present as malignant masses. Fewer than 100 have been reported.

About 200 adrenal cysts have been reported. They may become quite large but are rarely malignant. They can usually be decompressed and removed by the abdominal route.

PALLIATIVE ADRENALECTOMY

Bilateral adrenalectomy is a widely recognized (though infrequently applicable) palliative treatment for metastatic breast carcinoma in both sexes. It is also effective in some patients with metastatic cancer of the prostate gland.

All patients with metastatic cancer of the breast or prostate are potential candidates for bilateral adrenalectomy. However, the criteria for selection of patients are somewhat uncertain and the subject of considerable controversy at present. In general, the best candidates for bilateral adrenalectomy are patients who have responded to previous endocrine manipulation, usually oophorectomy. Patients who respond to adrenalectomy usually have had at least a 2-year tumor-free interval after the original mastectomy, and the first recurrence is in the area of the mastectomy or in bone.

About 30% of all premenopausal patients with breast cancer will have an objective remission following oophorectomy. About half of this group will have an objective remission after adrenalectomy. Only about 20% of patients who have not responded to oophorectomy will respond to adrenalectomy. Attempts to base the selection of patients for adrenalectomy on measurements of endocrine function have not yet proved successful enough for widespread use.

In terms of tumor response, adrenalectomy and hypophysectomy are about equally effective, but the side-effects of bilateral adrenalectomy are usually more tolerable.

The rationale of endocrine ablation is to decrease circulating estrogen levels. Oophorectomy in premenopausal women or in women no more than 1 year past the menopause usually reduces estrogen levels by about 50%. The remaining estrogen is produced by the adrenals, and the adrenal component sometimes increases in the postmenopausal period. Therefore, adrenalectomy can be expected to reduce circulating estrogen levels to zero if total oophorectomy has already been done. If estrogen excretion tests are available, it is wise to measure urinary estrogens before adrenalectomy to determine (1) whether total oophorectomy has in fact been done, and (2) that estrogen levels are high enough so that regression of the tumor can be expected if they are reduced to zero.

High doses of cortisone will also lower estrogen levels. However, they also produce Cushing's syndrome and cause many complications, including peptic ulcer, bleeding diatheses, and osteoporosis. Bilateral adrenalectomy remains the procedure of choice when further endocrine ablation procedures can be expected to produce remission of disease.

The posterior surgical approach is generally considered preferable. Tumor implants in the abdomen can make the anterior approach very difficult, and the posterior approach is somewhat better tolerated by these usually debilitated patients.

Postoperative complications are usually the result of metastatic breast cancer. Pathologic fractures may occur during manipulation under anesthesia, and pleural effusion secondary to tumor implants is common.

If patients are selected properly, about half can be expected to respond with objective remission that lasts several months or more. Replacement therapy is both easy and safe in these patients. The patient with surgically induced addisonism who takes maintenance corticosteroids is no more difficult to manage than the diabetic who takes insulin.

Prognosis is also a function of the preoperative state of the patient. Adrenalectomy done in desperation for a patient with terminal disease is frequently fatal. Patients with pleural effusion, restricted pulmonary function, and extensive soft tissue metastases are poor operative risks.

●　　●　　●

General References

Egdahl RH: Surgery of the adrenal gland. New England J Med 278:939–949, 1968.

Egdahl RH: Some recent advances in endocrine surgery. Am J Surg 118:363–367, 1969.

Glenn F, Peterson RE, Mannix H Jr: *Surgery of the Adrenal Gland*. Macmillan, 1968.

39 . . .

The Arteries

Edwin J. Wylie, MD, & William K. Ehrenfeld, MD

ATHEROSCLEROSIS

The degenerative processes that characterize atherosclerosis appear in 2 forms. One consists of diffuse destruction and weakening of the arterial media, which may cause dilatation and elongation of any of the major arteries of the body. The process may be exaggerated in places, with the production of focal aneurysms. The other degenerative process principally involves the intima without weakening the media. The degeneration is diffuse but in some areas may be apparent only on microscopic examination, and grossly visible disease may be localized to short segments. Intimal atheromas produce focal arterial narrowing which may progress to total occlusion of the lumen. The obstructive lesions have a predilection for the arterial wall adjacent to arterial bifurcations. In extremities there is often symmetry in the distribution of lesions between the 2 sides.

Progressive narrowing of the arterial lumen at any given site stimulates the development of collateral circulation about the obstructed segment. Stenosis of more than 50% of the lumen reduces arterial pressure beyond the stenotic zone. This creates a pressure gradient compared with the proximal branches and causes blood in nearby branches to return to the parent artery beyond the stenotic zone. With time, the sizes of the collateral vessels expand to accommodate greater flow.

When the stenosis approaches total occlusion, the sharply reduced blood flow eventually leads to thrombosis. The clot propagates in the stagnant column of blood both proximally and distally to the first major tributary. Persistent flow at these sites halts the propagation of clot. The end result is a totally occluded segment bypassed by a collateral system (Fig 39–1). Since resistance to flow in the collaterals is greater than that in the normal primary system, total collateral flow may be less than normal and unresponsive to increased distal demand. Clinical ischemia is related to the overall effectiveness of the collateral system. The development of additional occlusions further reduces blood flow. Severe chronic ischemia is nearly always accompanied by multiple sites of occlusion of the major vessels proximal to the affected tissues.

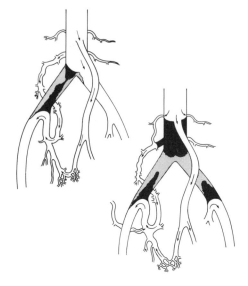

FIG 39–1. Development of collateral channels in response to occlusion of the right common iliac artery and the terminal aortic bifurcation.

PERIPHERAL ATHEROSCLEROTIC OCCLUSIVE DISEASE

Essentials of Diagnosis
- Intermittent claudication; rest pain.
- Impotence.
- Bruit over constriction.
- Decreased pulsation, thickening of arteries.
- Pallor, cyanosis, and coldness.
- Necrosis and atrophy.

General Considerations
Peripheral occlusive atherosclerosis is predominantly a disease of the lower extremities. In the arms, arterial lesions are largely confined to the subclavian and axillary arteries, and symptoms, if present at all, are limited to fatigue of the forearms with extremes of exertion. In the lower extremities, obstructive lesions are usually confined to segments of the arterial system from the infrarenal aorta to a few centimeters beyond the origins of the terminal branches of the popliteal artery (Fig 39–2). The symptoms are related to the location and number of obstructed arterial segments.

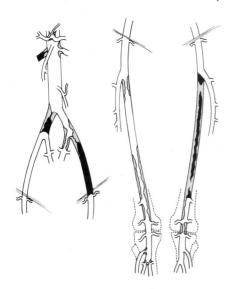

FIG 39—2. Common sites of stenosis and occlusion of the visceral and peripheral arterial systems.

Clinical Findings

A. Symptoms:

1. Intermittent claudication—Intermittent claudication is muscular pain or fatigue in muscles of the lower extremity caused by exertion (eg, walking) and relieved by rest. The pain is a deep-seated ache which gradually progresses to a degree that halts further exertion. It is completely relieved after 2—5 minutes of inactivity. It is distinguished from other pains in the extremities in that some exertion is always required before it appears, it does not occur at rest, and it is relieved in the standing position. The pain appears first in the dominant muscle group in the ischemic zone but may spread to other muscle groups in the same zone. The distance a patient can walk varies with the rate of walking, the level of incline, and the degree of arterial obstruction. The average patient with obstruction in a single arterial segment can walk 90—180 meters (100—200 yards) on a level terrain at an average pace before pain appears. The presence of additional lesions may reduce his walking tolerance to less than 18 meters (20 yards).

Claudication produced by obstruction in the superficial femoral-popliteal arterial segment is localized to the calf muscles. Occlusions proximal to the origin of the profunda femoris extend the pain to involve the thigh. Gluteal pain is added by lesions in or proximal to the hypogastric arteries. When obstruction occurs in this more proximal level, claudication is often described as extreme fatigability of the entire lower extremity. Similar symptoms, but involving both lower extremities, may be caused by occlusion of the distal aorta. An occasional patient may describe transient numbness of the extremity accompanying the pain and fatigue of claudication.

Muscular fatigue or pain may also occur from arterial lesions in the arms, but the disability is minor except in persons whose occupations require prolonged muscular activity of the arms, ie, carpenters. The term claudication is not strictly appropriate since this word derives from Latin *claudicare,* meaning to limp.

2. Impotence—Inability to attain or maintain a penile erection is produced by lesions which obstruct blood flow through both hypogastric arteries and is most commonly found in association with obstruction of the terminal aorta.

3. Rest pain—Ischemic rest pain is a continuous burning pain usually confined to the forefoot. In accord with the gravitational influence on blood flow, it is aggravated by elevation of the extremity or even by bringing the leg to the horizontal position. Thus it appears at bed rest and if severe may prevent sleep. The patient obtains relief by returning the foot to the dependent position. It occasionally may extend to involve the entire foot but never to a level proximal to the ankle. In its extreme form, narcotics may be required for relief. Rest pain indicates an advanced stage of ischemia.

4. Sensation—Although the patient may experience subjective numbness in the extremity, except when actual tissue necrosis has developed, sensory abnormalities are generally not present on examination. If decreased sensation is found in the foot, one should suspect a peripheral neuropathy, often of diabetic origin.

B. Signs:

The physical findings of peripheral atherosclerosis are related to changes in the peripheral arteries and to tissue ischemia.

1. Bruits—A bruit is the sound produced by the turbulence of blood flowing through an irregular arterial lumen usually due to stenosis. It is heard only during systole and is transmitted distally along the course of the artery. Thus, when a bruit is heard through a stethoscope placed over a peripheral artery, stenosis is present at or proximal to that level. The pitch of the bruit rises as the stenosis becomes more marked.

2. Arterial palpation—Thickening and rubbery firmness of the arterial wall is easily palpable in vessels near the surface of the extremity, ie, the brachial, common femoral, and superficial femoral arteries. Decreased amplitude of the pulse denotes proximal stenosis. Occasionally, collateral flow is sufficient to produce a pulse distally even when an artery is completely occluded. The differentiation between stenosis and occlusion, in this circumstance, is made by the presence of a bruit in the former.

3. Pallor—Pallor of the foot (or of the hand in cases of upper extremity disease) on elevation of the extremity uniformly accompanies clinically significant arterial obstruction. Lesser degrees of elevation are necessary to produce pallor in patients with advanced lesions. The rate of return of color when the extremity is returned to a dependent position is proportionate to the efficiency of the collateral circulation.

Exercise in a normal individual increases the pulse rate or amplitude without producing arterial bruits or peripheral color change. Exercise will sometimes produce peripheral pallor, an audible bruit, and decrease in pulse strength in an individual who complains of claudication but has no abnormal findings at rest. The findings indicate an otherwise inapparent stenosis. A typical example is seen in the patient with mild claudication of the entire lower extremity from minimal iliac stenosis who has normal peripheral pulses without bruits while at rest. If the patient is made to walk briskly and is reexamined after claudication appears, a bruit will be heard over the femoral triangle and the foot will be pale, with decreased or absent pulses.

4. Cyanosis—In advanced stages of atherosclerotic occlusion, the skin of the foot displays a peculiar ruborous cyanosis on dependency. During the delay while blood reaches the foot, hemoglobin is deoxygenated and the color of the blood when it reaches the capillary circulation is similar to that usually found in the venous side of the circuit. The concurrent vasodilatation due to ischemia causes blood to suffuse the cutaneous plexus, imparting a particularly livid appearance to the skin.

5. Temperature—With chronic ischemia, the temperature of the skin of the foot approaches that of its surroundings. The examiner can best detect a fall in skin temperature by palpating with the back of his hand against the sole of the foot.

6. Necrosis—Tissue necrosis first becomes apparent in the most distal portions of the extremity, often at a site where pressure from a shoe or position in bed causes additional ischemia. Necrosis often is the sequel to mechanical trauma or local infection which increases the local metabolic needs of tissues. Necrosis halts proximally at a line where the blood supply is adequate to maintain viability.

7. Atrophy—Moderate to severe degrees of chronic ischemia produce gradual muscle atrophy and loss of strength in the ischemic zone. A frequently associated complaint is reduction of joint mobility in the forefeet.

C. X-Ray Findings: Calcification in the walls of atherosclerotic arteries is often visible by standard x-ray technics. Calcification in the arterial wall may occur, however, without narrowing of the arterial lumen; for this reason, it is not an index of the functional status of the artery.

Arteriography supplements the physical findings by defining precisely the degree and site of arterial occlusion and the status of the arteries in the collateral circulation and of the primary arterial tree both proximal and distal to the diseased segment. The safest and most thorough technic for investigation of occlusive disease in the lower extremities is injection of contrast media into the abdominal aorta by the translumbar route followed by exposure of successive films to visualize the arteries of the abdomen and lower extremities.

Treatment & Prognosis

A. Upper Extremities: Symptoms are rarely severe enough to require operations on the arteries for vascular insufficiency in the upper extremities. Cervi-

cothoracic sympathectomy usually relieves fatigability or coldness, and the viability of fingers or hands is rarely in question.

B. Lower Extremities: The objectives of management of atherosclerotic occlusive disease in the lower extremities are the relief of disability and the prevention of leg loss. Vasodilating or anticoagulant drugs are generally of no value. When disability is minimal (claudication well tolerated) and arteriography demonstrates one or more isolated lesions with unimpaired, well-functioning collateral channels, expectant treatment is all that is required. Under these circumstances, the patient is counseled on foot care and the need for avoiding infection or mechanical and thermal trauma.

Severe disability or impending gangrene requires surgical revascularization if anatomically feasible. The method selected depends upon the location and distribution of arterial lesions and is influenced by associated pulmonary or cardiothoracic disease.

1. Arterial reconstruction—Direct revascularization operations are applicable for patients with obstructive lesions located anywhere from the abdominal aorta to the terminal branches of the popliteal artery providing there is demonstrable patency of the arteries immediately distal to the segment to be revascularized. The favored operations for occlusion in the aortoiliac-common femoral segments are (1) endarterectomy or (2) arterial bypass grafts of knitted Dacron (Fig 39–3). Long-term success can be expected provided the patient is left with a widely patent arterial tree to and including the profunda femoris artery. In most clinical situations, revascularization to the common femoral artery is generally adequate even when additional occlusive lesions are present in the femoropopliteal segment.

The most successful operation for occlusive disease in the femoropopliteal segment is bypass grafting using a reversed segment of the saphenous vein. If a saphenous vein of adequate size (diameter exceeding 3–4 mm) is not available, the cephalic vein from the arm may be used. The immediate results with endarterectomy are nearly comparable, but the frequency of late occlusion is higher (Fig 39–4). The frequency of late closure with synthetic grafts is even higher. In general, the durability of reconstructive operations in the femoral and popliteal segments is considerably less than for similar operations in the aortoiliac segment. The reasons are the lesser volume of blood flow through the femoral artery, the smaller caliber of the arteries at this level, and the higher incidence of advanced atherosclerosis in the outflow arteries. For these reasons, many surgeons limit direct operation at this level to situations where leg salvage is the principal objective.

Bypass operations, in which grafts are brought to arteries beyond the popliteal artery, are occasionally successful. Information on the long-term patency of these grafts is not yet available.

2. Lumbar sympathectomy—Lumbar sympathectomy is seldom indicated as the only method of treatment for patients with occlusion of major arteries in

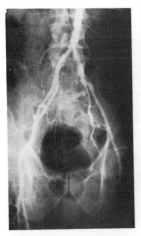
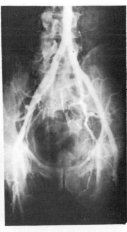

FIG 39–3. *Left:* Aortogram showing atherosclerotic occlusive disease of the infrarenal aorta and iliac arteries. *Right:* Postoperative aortogram showing wide patency after aortoiliac endarterectomy.

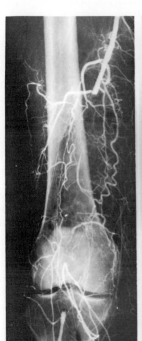
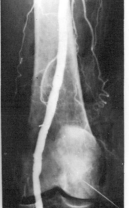
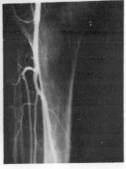

FIG 39–4. *Left:* Femoral arteriogram showing occlusion of the superficial femoral and proximal popliteal arteries. *Right:* Femoral arteriogram showing patency of the femoral and popliteal arteries after endarterectomy. (Reproduced, with permission, from Morton DL, Ehrenfeld WK, Wylie EJ: Significance of outflow obstruction after femoropopliteal endarterectomy. Arch Surg 94:592, 1967.)

the lower extremities. This approach is reserved for circumstances in which revascularization operations are not technically applicable and where experience indicates that it would benefit the patient. Sympathectomy is of greatest value (1) for patients in the early stage of advanced ischemia whose primary complaint is mild nocturnal rest pain and (2) for the treatment of chronic ulceration of the leg due to arterial insufficiency. Sympathectomy is ineffective in the management of gangrene of the toes or foot and does not lower the required level for amputation.

Many surgeons routinely combine lumbar sympathectomy with arterial reconstructive operations which entail a laparotomy. Sympathectomy causes dilatation of the peripheral arteries, decreasing peripheral resistance. This increases flow through the reconstructed segment and perhaps decreases postoperative thrombosis.

3. Amputation–Amputation is required for the management of peripheral gangrene and intractable rest pain whenever arterial reconstruction cannot be successfully performed. Amputation of the toes or the forefoot at the transmetatarsal level is successful in the rare circumstance of distal gangrene where there is adequate blood supply in the remainder of the foot.

Dale WA (editor): *Management of Arterial Occlusive Disease.* Year Book, 1971.

Edwards EA: Acute peripheral arterial occlusion. JAMA 223:909–912, 1973.

Humphries AW, Young JR, McCormack LJ: Experiences with aortoiliac and femoropopliteal endarterectomy. Surgery 65:48–58, 1969.

Linton RR, Wilde WL: Modifications in the technique for femoropopliteal saphenous vein bypass autografts. Surgery 67:234–248, 1970.

Morton DL, Ehrenfeld WK, Wylie EJ: The significance of outflow obstruction after femoropopliteal endarterectomy. Arch Surg 94:592–599, 1967.

Mundth ED & others: Quantitative correlation of distal arterial outflow and patency of femoropopliteal reversed saphenous vein grafts with intraoperative flow and pressure measurements. Surgery 65:197–206, 1969.

Najafi H & others: Aortoiliac reconstruction in patients 32 to 45 years of age. Arch Surg 101:780–784, 1970.

Noon GP & others: Distal tibial arterial bypass. Arch Surg 99:770–775, 1969.

Skinner JS, Strandness DE Jr: Exercise and intermittent claudication. Circulation 36:15–22, 1967.

Wylie EJ: Thromboendarterectomy for arteriosclerotic thrombosis of major arteries. Surgery 32:275–282, 1952.

ATHEROSCLEROTIC ANEURYSM

An atherosclerotic aneurysm is a true aneurysm appearing as a focal fusiform arterial dilatation. It is found, in descending order of frequency, in the distal abdominal aorta, the popliteal artery (Fig 39–5), the common femoral artery, the arch and descending por-

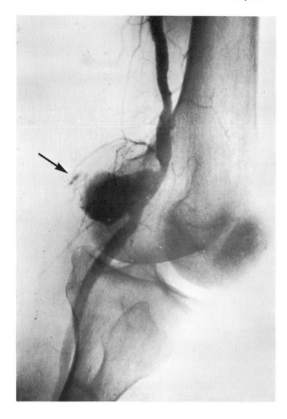

FIG 39–5. Arteriogram showing aneurysm of the popliteal artery (arrow).

tions of the thoracic aorta, the carotid arteries, and other peripheral arteries. As the aneurysm enlarges, mural thrombus is deposited on its interior surface owing to eddy currents and stagnant flow. The functional lumen of the artery may remain unchanged and may appear relatively normal on arteriograms—a factor which limits their usefulness in diagnosis.

1. INFRARENAL ABDOMINAL ANEURYSM

Over 99% of aneurysms of the abdominal aorta are caused by atherosclerosis. Most of these involve the segment of the aorta between the takeoff of the renal arteries and the aortic bifurcation but may include variable portions of the common iliac arteries. Rupture and exsanguination is the major complication.

Clinical Findings

A. Symptoms and Signs: An intact abdominal aneurysm rarely produces more than minimal symptoms. The patient is usually aware of little more than a

painless, throbbing mass. Severe pain in the absence of rupture characterizes the rare inflammatory aneurysm which is surrounded by 2–4 cm of perianeurysmal inflammatory reaction.

The sole physical finding is usually a palpable fusiform or globular pulsatile abdominal mass. With smaller aneurysms, this mass is centered in the upper abdomen just above the umbilicus, the normal location of the infrarenal portion of the abdominal aorta. Larger aneurysms bulge distally into the abdomen below the umbilicus and proximally into the space behind the rib cage. The aneurysm may be slightly tender to palpation. Severe tenderness is found only in inflammatory aneurysms or after rupture has occurred.

C. X-Ray Findings: Plain films of the abdomen in anteroposterior, lateral, and oblique projections reveal calcification in the outer layers of over 90% of atherosclerotic abdominal aneurysms. This allows assessment of its size and proximal extent. Aortography is indicated whenever suprarenal involvement of the aorta or associated visceral artery occlusion is suspected. Suprarenal aneurysms are usually associated with dilatation of the descending thoracic aorta, detectable on posteroanterior and right posterior oblique chest x-rays.

Treatment

Since most uncomplicated abdominal aneurysms are asymptomatic, the principal indication for elective operation is to prevent rupture. Rupture rarely occurs until the diameter of the aneurysm exceeds 6 cm; operation for aneurysms smaller than 6 cm is advised only in young patients with a long life expectancy.

Operation consists of replacing the aneurysmal segment with a synthetic fabric graft. Tubular or bifurcation grafts of knitted Dacron are preferred. The proximal anastomosis is usually made to the transected aorta proximal to the aneurysm, 3–6 cm distal to the origin of the renal arteries. The site of the distal anastomosis is determined by the extent of aneurysmal involvement of the iliac arteries. In most circumstances, the iliac arms of a bifurcated graft are anastomosed to the distal ends of the transected common iliac arteries. The graft is generally placed in the lumen of the incised and isolated aneurysm, the outer layers of which are sutured around the graft after the anastomoses are completed (Figs 39–6 and 39–7).

2. SUPRARENAL AORTIC ANEURYSMS

Aneurysms of the segment of aorta between the diaphragm and the renal arteries are rare and are usually associated with similar changes in the thoracic and infrarenal aorta. When they do occur, the 3–6 cm segment at the level of the renal arteries is frequently less dilated, and a dumbbell-shaped aneurysm results. The risk of rupture of the suprarenal segment is not appreciable until its diameter exceeds 7–9 cm. Symptoms are rare unless rupture occurs.

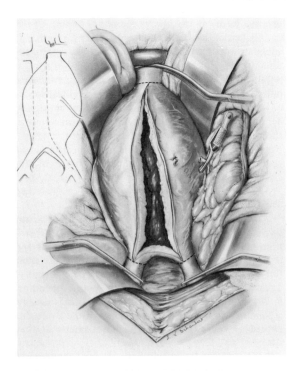

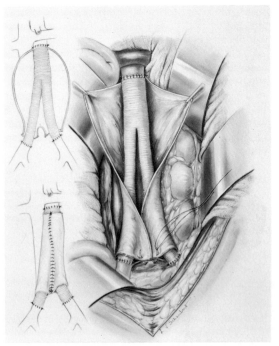

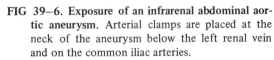

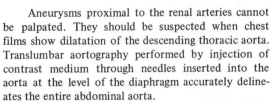

FIG 39–6. **Exposure of an infrarenal abdominal aortic aneurysm.** Arterial clamps are placed at the neck of the aneurysm below the left renal vein and on the common iliac arteries.

FIG 39–7. **Replacement of an aortic aneurysm with a synthetic bifurcation graft.** The laminated clot within the aneurysm has been removed and the outer wall is closed over the graft.

Aneurysms proximal to the renal arteries cannot be palpated. They should be suspected when chest films show dilatation of the descending thoracic aorta. Translumbar aortography performed by injection of contrast medium through needles inserted into the aorta at the level of the diaphragm accurately delineates the entire abdominal aorta.

Resection and graft replacement of the upper abdominal aorta is an operation of far greater magnitude and risk than operations on the infrarenal aorta. A thoracoabdominal approach is necessary, and provision must be made for reimplantation of the celiac axis and the superior mesenteric and renal arteries. At this time, the risks of operation for asymptomatic aneurysms at this level less than 7–9 cm in diameter are probably greater than the risk of rupture.

3. RUPTURED AORTIC ANEURYSM

With increasing size, lateral pressure within the aneurysm may eventually lead to spontaneous rupture of the aneurysmal wall. Although immediate exsanguination may ensue, there is usually an interval of several hours between the first episode of bleeding, consisting of a self-limited extravasation into the subadventitia or periaortic tissue, and later retroperitoneal rupture.

Clinical Findings

A. Symptoms and Signs: Most aortic aneurysms are asymptomatic until rupture begins with sudden severe abdominal pain which occasionally radiates into the back. Faintness or syncope results from blood loss. Pain may lessen or faintness may disappear after the first hemorrhage, only to reappear and progress to shock if bleeding continues.

When bleeding remains contained in the periaortic tissue, a discrete, pulsatile abdominal mass can be felt. In contrast with an intact aneurysm, the ruptured aneurysm at this stage is exquisitely tender. As bleeding continues—usually into the retroperitoneum—the discrete mass is replaced by a poorly defined mid-abdominal fullness, often extending toward the left flank. Shock becomes profound, manifested by peripheral vasoconstriction, hypotension, and anuria.

B. X-Ray Findings: Immediate operation should be performed without pausing to obtain x-rays.

Treatment & Prognosis

Immediate laparotomy is mandatory whenever aortic rupture is suspected. If operation can be performed during the first phase, the mortality rate is only slightly greater than for elective aneurysmectomy. When massive bleeding has produced shock, the operative mortality exceeds 50%. Without operation, however, the outcome is uniformly fatal.

The operation is identical to that for unruptured

aneurysms except for the necessity of gaining immediate control of the aorta proximal to the aneurysm to halt bleeding.

The early local complications of abdominal aortic aneurysmectomy are those of any arterial reconstructive operation, ie, arterial thrombosis and hemorrhage. In experienced hands, these are negligible. Disruption of arterial suture lines with false aneurysm formation is a rare late complication. The use of synthetic suture material instead of silk has resulted in a sharp decrease in the incidence of false aneurysms.

DeBakey & others: Aneurysm of abdominal aorta: Analysis of results of graft replacement therapy one to eleven years after operation. Ann Surg 160:622–639, 1964.

Foster JH & others: Comparative study of elective resection and expectant treatment of abdominal aortic aneurysm. Surg Gynec Obst 129:1–9, 1969.

Klippel AP, Butcher HR: The unoperated abdominal aortic aneurysm. Am J Surg 111:629–631, 1966.

Stoney RJ, Wylie EJ: Surgical treatment of ruptured abdominal aneurysms: Factors influencing outcome. California Med 111:1–4, 1969.

Szilagyi DE & others: Contribution of abdominal aortic aneurysmectomy to prolongation of life: Twelve-year review of 480 cases. Ann Surg 164:678–699, 1966.

Szilagyi DE, Elliott JP, Smith RF: Clinical fate of the patient with asymptomatic abdominal aortic aneurysm and unfit for surgical treatment. Arch Surg 104:600–606, 1972.

4. FEMORAL & POPLITEAL ANEURYSMS

Atherosclerotic aneurysms of the common femoral and popliteal arteries tend to thrombose and produce distal ischemia. Unlike aortic aneurysms, rupture is rare. Occlusion results from fragmentation of the mural thrombus lining the aneurysmal sac, an event which may partly be due to the mobility of the adjacent hip or knee. Thrombus may occlude the lumen at the aneurysm or embolize downstream into smaller arteries in the leg or foot.

Clinical Findings

A. Symptoms and Signs: Until thrombosis occurs, symptoms are usually minimal or absent. The patient is aware of a throbbing mass when the aneurysm is in the groin, but popliteal aneurysms are usually undetected by the patient. Rarely, popliteal aneurysms will produce symptoms by compressing the popliteal vein or tibial nerve. In most patients, the first symptom is produced by the ischemia of acute arterial occlusion. The pathologic findings range from rapidly developing gangrene to only moderate ischemia which slowly lessens as collateral circulation develops. Symptoms from recurrent embolization to the leg are often transient; sudden ischemia may appear in a toe or part of the foot, followed by slow resolution, and the true diagnosis may be elusive. Recurrent ischemic episodes due to occlusion of small arteries in the leg in patients over age 50 are almost always embolic in origin.

Palpation of local arterial enlargement is generally adequate for diagnosis. Since popliteal aneurysms are usually bilateral, the diagnosis of thrombosis of a popliteal aneurysm is often aided by the palpation of a pulsatile aneurysm in the contralateral popliteal space.

B. X-Ray Findings: Arteriography may not demonstrate the aneurysm accurately because mural thrombus reduces the apparent diameter of the lumen. Nevertheless, arteriography is advised—especially when operation is considered—to define the status of the arteries distal to the aneurysm.

Treatment

Immediate operation is indicated when acute thrombosis has caused pregangrenous ischemia. Operation may not be necessary if ischemic changes are reversible and lessening. Early operation is indicated for recurrent peripheral embolization. The evidence is unclear regarding the advisability of routine operation in the absence of symptoms, but operation is usually recommended if the external diameter of the aneurysm exceeds 3 times the normal arterial diameter at that site.

The standard surgical treatment for both femoral and popliteal aneurysms has been resection with graft replacement. Recently, however, popliteal aneurysms have been more satisfactorily managed by exclusion and bypass graft. In this procedure, the popliteal artery distal to the aneurysm is transected and the proximal end oversewn. A graft is then interposed from the side of the distal superficial femoral artery to the transected distal end of the popliteal artery. The undissected aneurysm is left in place. As with other arterial grafting operations in the extremities, the saphenous vein or an autologous artery is preferred for the graft to one of synthetic material.

Prognosis

The long-term patency of bypass grafts for femoral and popliteal aneurysms depends on the adequacy of the outflow tract. Late graft occlusion is less common than in similar operations for occlusive disease.

Edmunds LH Jr, Darling RC, Linton RR: Surgical management of popliteal aneurysms. Circulation 32:517–523, 1965.

Edwards WS: Exclusion and saphenous vein bypass of popliteal aneurysms. Surg Gynec Obst 128:829–830, 1969.

Inahara T: Aneurysms of the common femoral artery: Reconstruction with the mobilized external iliac artery. Am J Surg 111:759–763, 1966.

Wychulis AR, Spittell JA Jr, Wallace RB: Popliteal aneurysms. Surgery 68:942–952, 1970.

LARGE ARTERY OCCLUSIVE DISEASE

ACUTE PERIPHERAL ARTERIAL OCCLUSION

Essentials of Diagnosis

- Abrupt onset of ischemia with coldness, numbness, and occasionally pain.
- Late pain (12–18 hours later).

General Considerations

Sudden total occlusion of a previously patent artery supplying an extremity is usually a dramatic event characterized by abrupt and severe distal ischemia. Tissue viability depends on the extent to which flow is maintained by collateral circuits or surgical intervention. The clinical manifestations are those of ischemia of nerves, muscle, and skin. When ischemia persists, motor and sensory paralysis, muscle infarction, and cutaneous gangrene become irreversible in a matter of hours. A line of demarcation develops between viable and nonviable tissue. Flow in the distal arteries is reduced progressively by propagating intraluminal thrombus, and surgical restoration of blood flow to the ischemic portion of the extremity eventually becomes impossible.

Ischemia after occlusion of the superficial femoral or brachial arteries beyond their respective profunda branches is often followed by progressive recovery. Recovery after brachial occlusion reaches its maximum within 2–4 days; from femoral occlusion, within 2–4 months. The terminal aorta and common femoral artery are 2 sites where collaterals are inadequate to supply distal needs. Sudden occlusion of these arteries is generally followed by severe, progressive ischemia culminating in gangrene.

Acute arterial occlusion may be caused by an embolus, thrombosis, or trauma. Embolic occlusion results from dislodgement of a blood clot or a tumor fragment into the blood stream. The former usually originate from the left atrium in patients with atrial fibrillation or from an intraventricular mural thrombus in patients with recent myocardial infarction. Tumor emboli are rare, the most common being fragments of a cardiac myxoma.

Sudden thrombosis of an atherosclerotic peripheral artery may be difficult to differentiate clinically from embolic occlusion. The usual mechanism is hemorrhagic dissection beneath an atherosclerotic plaque.

Traumatic occlusion may be due to numerous causes, eg, contusion or laceration by a bone after a fracture or dislocation, penetrating injuries, and—commonly in recent years—as a complication of arterial catheterization.

Clinical Findings

Coldness, numbness, and occasionally pain in the ischemic zone are the first complaints and are followed by loss of motor function. Late pain, appearing after 12–18 hours, is the result of swelling of infarcted muscle confined in fascial compartments.

Pallor appears first but is replaced by mottled cyanosis after a few hours as deoxygenated blood gradually suffuses the extremity. Cutaneous hypesthesia slowly progresses to anesthesia, and function is lost in muscles supplied by the ischemic nerves. When these changes persist beyond 12 hours, gangrene is inevitable. If collateral flow increases, it becomes evident by return of warmth and pinkness of the skin and a lessening of the sensory deficit. When collateral flow has reached its maximum, the signs and symptoms are those of chronic occlusion of the involved artery. When reversible ischemia has been severe and protracted at the onset, normal sensory function may not return for 6 months.

Tense swelling and acute tenderness of a muscle belly—a common occurrence in the gastrocnemius following superficial femoral artery occlusion—generally denotes irreversible muscle infarction.

The level of demarcation of ischemic changes suggests the site of arterial occlusion. Since collaterals always supply the tissues just beyond the occlusion, the demarcation is as follows:

Site of Occlusion	Line of Demarcation
Infrarenal aorta	Mid abdomen
Aortic bifurcation and common iliac arteries	Groin
External iliacs	Proximal thigh
Common femoral	Lower third of thigh
Superficial femoral	Upper third of calf
Popliteal	Lower third of calf

Treatment & Prognosis

Immediate anticoagulation by intravenous heparin slows the development of distal thrombosis and allows time for assessment of adequacy of collateral flow and preparation for operation if indicated. Nonoperative management is best for many emboli to major arteries in the upper extremities and for some in the lower extremities but only when skin color improves or neural function returns within 3 hours after occlusion. If the initial ischemia recedes, the decision for removal of the embolus is based upon an estimate of the disability that will be produced by chronic occlusion of the involved artery. Chronic occlusion of the axillary or brachial arteries is usually well tolerated, whereas chronic occlusion of lower extremity vessels causes claudication at best.

If advanced ischemia persists, the embolus must be removed within 8–12 hours after the occlusion. Successful embolectomy requires removal of the embolus and the "tail" of thrombus which extends distally or proximally from it. If operation is not performed within the first 8–12 hours, the ramifications of this thrombus into arterial branches usually cannot be extracted and revascularization is impossible. Late thrombectomy (after 18 hours) is successful only when propagation of thrombus has been arrested by collateral blood flow reentering the vessel distal to the embolus.

Embolectomy may be performed through an arteriotomy at the site of the embolus or, most commonly, by extraction with a balloon (Fogarty) catheter inserted through a proximal arteriotomy.

Traumatic arterial occlusion (see also Chapter 17) must also be corrected within a few hours to avoid gangrene. Management of the arterial injury is often only one part of an operation which includes repair of other traumatized structures. The general principles in treatment of the arterial injury are as follows:

(1) Restore patency of the distal arterial tree (remove distal thrombus by retrograde "milking" of the extremity or passage of a balloon catheter).

(2) Suture simple arterial lacerations or anastomose cleanly transected arteries.

(3) Replace extensively damaged arterial segments by grafting: Use synthetic fabric for replacing large vessels in uncontaminated wounds; use autologous tissue (vein or artery) to replace small vessels or if the wound is contaminated.

Fogarty TJ, Cranley JJ: Catheter technic for arterial embolectomy. Ann Surg 161:325–330, 1965.

Fogarty TJ & others: A method for extraction of arterial emboli and thrombi. Surg Gynec Obst 116:241–244, 1963.

Thompson JE & others: Arterial embolectomy: A 20-year experience with 163 cases. Surgery 67:212–220, 1970.

SMALL ARTERY OCCLUSIVE DISEASE

This section deals with occlusive diseases involving the small (< 3 mm diameter) arteries in the extremities. As a group, their clinical manifestations are similar, but they can usually be distinguished without difficulty from conditions involving larger arteries.

Collateral flow around small vessels is functionally superior to that following more proximal occlusions. For example, gradual occlusion of a digital artery may be asymptomatic, and even the findings after acute thrombosis may resolve in a matter of hours or days. It follows, therefore, that chronic ischemia is almost always the result of occlusion of multiple small arteries.

PERIPHERAL EMBOLI

Recurrent multiple emboli to small arteries can arise from atrial fibrillation, prosthetic cardiac valves, proximal arterial aneurysms, or arterial mural thrombus from atherosclerosis or compression by a cervical rib.

The patient experiences sudden pain, cyanosis, or coldness in the affected digits which improves over several days only to reappear, perhaps in a different hand or foot. With each succeeding episode, recovery is slower and less complete.

Physical examination reveals focal ischemia of one or more digits. The **Allen test** demonstrates the ischemic zone clearly. This is performed by having the patient rapidly open and close his fist with the arm elevated while the examiner compresses the brachial artery at the elbow. The arm is then lowered and the brachial compression released. The normal color response is a sudden suffusion of the hand and fingers with bright-red blood. When vasoconstriction is present, color return is slow and progresses through the forearm to the fingers. If digital arterial occlusion is present, the skin normally supplied by the occluded artery remains pale for several seconds after color has returned to the rest of the hand and fingers. A proximal source for the emboli should be sought. Angiography will visualize causative lesions in major arteries.

Once discovered, the source of the emboli should be surgically corrected if possible. Sympathectomy is usually performed. Chronic anticoagulation may be necessary if more definitive surgical treatment is not possible.

Crane C: Atheromatous embolism to lower extremities in arteriosclerosis. Arch Surg 94:96–101, 1967.

Hoye SJ & others: Atheromatous embolization: A factor in peripheral gangrene. New England J Med 261:128–130, 1959.

Perdue GD Jr, Smith RB: Atheromatous microemboli. Ann Surg 169:954–959, 1969.

THROMBOANGIITIS OBLITERANS

Thromboangiitis obliterans (Buerger's disease) is characterized by multiple segmental occlusions of small arteries in the extremities distal to the brachial and popliteal arteries. Migratory phlebitis is frequently present. The disease occurs almost exclusively in young adult cigarette-smoking males and is believed to represent an allergic response to nicotine. Contrary to former belief, it is not confined to Jews.

Symptoms consist of slowly developing digital pain, cyanosis, and coldness, progressing eventually to necrosis and gangrene. Claudication in the muscles of the foot may be the first symptom.

Examination shows an irregular pattern of digital ischemia. The Allen maneuver (see above) demonstrates delayed filling of affected digital arteries and rapid filling in adjacent vessels.

Arteriography, although rarely necessary to confirm the diagnosis, shows discrete zones of total arterial occlusion in one or more arteries combined with apparently uninvolved arterial segments.

It is essential that the patient stop smoking to avoid progression of the disease. Sympathectomy dramatically improves collateral blood flow and is advisable in all but the least symptomatic patients. Consideration of amputation should be postponed until the effect of sympathectomy has been observed since advanced lesions often heal completely. Amputation is indicated for persisting pain or gangrene and can be performed adjacent to the line of demarcation with satisfactory primary healing.

The disease may become dormant if the patient can stop smoking, but this is unfortunately difficult to achieve in many who ultimately develop gangrene of additional digits.

Brown H & others: Thromboangiitis obliterans. Brit J Surg 56:59–63, 1969.

McKusick VA & others: Buerger's disease: A distinct clinical and pathologic entity. JAMA 181:5–10, 1962.

Szilagyi DE, DeRusso FJ, Elliott JP: Thromboangiitis obliterans: Clinico-angiographic correlations. Arch Surg 88:824–835, 1964.

Wessler S & others: A critical evaluation of thromboangiitis obliterans: The case against Buerger's disease. New England J Med 262:1149–1159, 1960.

ERGOTISM

Ergotism was once common due to ingestion of rye containing the fungus ergot. At present the condition appears only rarely as an idiosyncratic reaction to ergotamine. Segmental occlusion of small arteries produces a clinical picture similar to that of thromboangiitis obliterans. Improvement may occur if the drug is withdrawn early in the disease. The lower extremities are usually the first involved. The femoral pulses are normal, but more distal pulses are absent. Gangrene develops first in the toes. Lumbar sympathectomy is the only treatment other than ergot withdrawal.

SCLERODERMA

In scleroderma, digital ischemia due to perivascular fibrosis and intimal thickening produces slowly progressive coldness, numbness, and pain which affects the fingers symmetrically. It can be distinguished from thromboangiitis obliterans by its symmetry, slow progression, and associated fingertip atrophy. The characteristic skin changes are evident on physical examination in addition to signs of ischemia. The Allen test shows poor filling throughout the hand and fingers. Sympathectomy and amputation are the only available surgical treatments. Temporary healing of ischemic skin changes and subjective relief of discomfort are frequent after sympathectomy.

Norton WL, Nardo JM: Vascular disease in progressive systemic sclerosis (scleroderma). Ann Int Med 73:317–324, 1970.

VASOCONSTRICTIVE DISORDERS

Vasoconstrictive disorders are characterized by abnormal lability of the sympathetic nervous system which affects the arterial and venous side of the capillary bed to reduce cutaneous blood flow. Sluggish flow of deoxygenated blood causes cutaneous cyanosis, coldness, numbness, and pain.

Raynaud's phenomenon can be precipitated by exposure to cold. It consists of sequential pallor, cyanosis, and rubor after a cold stimulus and is the visible manifestation of vasoconstriction, sluggish flow, and reflex vasodilatation. The term **Raynaud's disease** has been applied to disorders associated with the above findings but in whom no specific cause, such as scleroderma, is discovered. Digital gangrene may appear as small vessel occlusion is added to the vasoconstrictive process.

ACROCYANOSIS

Acrocyanosis is a common chronic, benign vasoconstrictive disorder which is largely restricted to young females. It is characterized by persistent cyanosis of the hands and feet. Numbness and pain accompany its more severe form. The changes disappear with exposure to a warm environment. Examination in a cool room shows diffuse symmetric cyanosis, coldness, and occasionally hyperhidrosis of hands and feet. Cyanosis of the skin of the calf, thigh, or forearm usually displays a reticulated pattern and has been called **livedo reticularis** and **cutis marmorata**. The peripheral pulses may diminish in the cold but return to normal with rewarming. Demonstration of the absence of arterial occlusion by the Allen test confirms the diagnosis of a purely vasoconstrictive disorder.

The patient usually benefits by wearing warm gloves or socks when exposed to extremes of cold. When genuine disability from chronic pain or coldness results, sympathectomy gives dramatic relief. Vasodilating drugs are of little benefit.

POSTPOLIOMYELITIS VASOCONSTRICTION

Chronic vasoconstriction confined to an extremity affected by poliomyelitis may develop many years later. Pain and coldness are often severe, and cutaneous ulcers may develop, particularly in the skin of the lower legs. Sympathectomy for the more severe forms gives excellent symptomatic relief and causes rapid healing of cutaneous ulceration.

Holmes TW Jr, Gilfillan RS, Cuthbertson EM: Sympathectomy in the release of vasoconstriction: Similarities of response in cerebral palsy and poliomyelitis. Surgery 61:129–136, 1967.

POSTTRAUMATIC VASOMOTOR DYSTROPHY

Contusing injuries to the distal arms or legs—often complicated by bony fracture—are occasionally the precipitating incident to a prolonged and often intractable pain syndrome. When accompanied by chronic cyanosis or coldness due to vasoconstriction, the term **posttraumatic vasomotor dystrophy** is applied. The syndrome is more common in the lower extremities and frequently follows ankle fractures. Diffuse pain and tenderness through the foot and ankle develop out of proportion to the degree of injury. Mild edema is common. The patient's resistance to weight-bearing or movement of the foot and ankle leads to bony atrophy and joint fixation. When x-ray shows additional punched-out areas of bony rarefaction, the term **Sudeck's atrophy** is applied.

Management requires vigorous physical therapy. Sympathectomy is occasionally useful in overcoming the vasomotor symptoms.

CAUSALGIA

Causalgia is a unique pain syndrome largely confined to the upper extremities and was originally thought to result from injury to a major peripheral nerve, usually the median nerve. However, it has been observed following penetrating or contusing injuries to the hand or arm without demonstrable nerve injury. The pain usually begins days or weeks after the original injury. Severe increases in the pain may be provoked by lightly touching the extremity, vibrating the bed, or even extraneous noises. Examination reveals cyanosis, coldness, and glossiness of the skin.

Sympathectomy sometimes relieves the pain.

Baker AG, Wineganer FG: Causalgia. Am J Surg 117:690–694, 1969.

Mayfield FH: *Causalgia.* Thomas, 1951.

Mitchell SW, Morehouse GR, Keen WW: *Gunshot Wounds and Other Injuries of Nerves.* Lippincott, 1964.

. . .

SYMPATHECTOMY

The sympathetic nervous system consists of 2 ganglionated chains of neurons coursing longitudinally along each side of the spinal column. Fibers are sent to the prevertebral ganglia and the mixed plexuses. The ganglia are divided into cervical, thoracic, lumbar, and sacral paravertebral components. The first 3 or 4 ganglia comprise the superior cervical ganglion; the fifth and sixth represent the middle cervical ganglion; and the seventh and eighth combine into the first thoracic to form the "stellate ganglion."

The thoracic is the most regular component with regard to representation by separate segments. There are 12 separate ganglia. In the lumbar segment, 3–5 ganglia may be present. The sacral-paravertebral portion is a continuation of the lumbar segment into the pelvis. The splanchnic nerves are derived from the thoracic sympathetic trunk.

The postganglionic fibers in the extremities supply smooth muscle of small vessel walls, sweat glands, and piloerector muscles. The sympathetic innervation is vasoconstrictor. Its functions include the regulation of the economy of body heat. Sympathetic denervation is then confirmed if increased warmth and redness, dryness of skin, and inability to have "gooseflesh" occur.

Indications for Sympathectomy

A. Nonarterial Disease: Sympathectomy may be of benefit in numerous nonarterial disease states, eg, hyperhidrosis, acrocyanosis, posttraumatic dystrophy, and some cases of frostbite and causalgia.

B. Arterial Disease: Sympathectomy is of benefit in Raynaud's disease, Buerger's disease, and connective tissue diseases that cause Raynaud's phenomenon. It has fallen into disrepute for the therapy of hypertension. Sympathectomy is occasionally helpful in occlusive disease due to atherosclerosis. Many surgeons perform lumbar sympathectomy as an adjunct to aortoiliac and femoral and popliteal artery reconstructive operations.

The operation removes vasoconstrictor tone and increases skin blood flow. Higher flow rates are thought to increase the chances of arterial patency and help sustain a collateral circulation. In addition, drying of the skin diminishes the chance for infection.

Types of Sympathectomy

A. Cervical Sympathectomy: Denervation of the upper extremity is achieved by division and resection of the cervicothoracic ganglia and trunks. If resection does not include the inferior cervical ganglion, sympathetic innervation to the eye is preserved.

B. Lumbar Sympathectomy: Denervation of the lower extremity is achieved by division and resection of the lumbar ganglia and trunks. Resection of the L4 ganglion alone is usually adequate, and extensive sympathetic resection is rarely worthwhile.

Results of Sympathectomy

Sympathectomy lowers peripheral resistance by reducing tone in the arterioles, venules, and capillaries to the skin and subcutaneous tissues. Whether sympathectomy increases blood flow to muscle is disputed. Unilateral cervicothoracic or lumbar sympathectomy in a normal resting subject increases blood flow to the extremity by 400%, and even greater increases occur when excessive vasomotor tone was present preoperatively. Smaller responses may occur (1) if the peripheral vessels are incapable of vasodilatation (scleroderma), (2) if an "auto-sympathectomy" already exists as a result of profound chronic ischemia, or (3) if arterial occlusion prevents greater flow. Lumbar sympathectomy only affects the vessels distal to the knee.

Claudication caused by obstructive arterial lesions in the aorto-popliteal segments responds variably to sympathectomy. Walking tolerances may be slightly increased, and pain usually subsides more rapidly after cessation of walking. The relatively slight effect of sympathectomy on claudication is explained by the theory that muscular ischemia during exercise produces maximal vasodilatation in the muscular arterial branches and that sympathectomy does not increase it further.

Sympathectomy is rarely effective for severe chronic rest pain or for toe or forefoot gangrene due to extensive proximal arterial disease. In both situations, sympathectomy cannot increase blood supply sufficiently to relieve pain or to promote healing of gangrene. Gangrenous ulcers proximal to the ankle generally respond favorably.

When digital gangrene is the result of segmental small artery occlusion (as with peripheral emboli or Buerger's disease), sympathectomy often provides dramatic relief. As might be expected, syndromes associated with profound cutaneous vasoconstriction without occlusion are often markedly improved by sympathectomy.

Palumbo LT, Lulu DJ: Anterior transthoracic upper dorsal sympathectomy. Arch Surg 92:247–257, 1966.

Ruberti U, Edwards EA, Ottinger L: Changes in the peripheral pulses after sympathectomy for arteriosclerosis. Surgery 47:105–114, 1960.

Shackelford RT: Henry's anterior, transthoracic extrapleural upper dorsal sympathectomy. Am Surgeon 32:853–856, 1966.

Szilagyi DE & others: Lumbar sympathectomy: Current role in the treatment of arteriosclerotic occlusive disease. Arch Surg 95:753–761, 1967.

OCCLUSIVE CEREBROVASCULAR DISEASE

Essentials of Diagnosis

- Episodic ataxia, diplopia, blurring of vision.
- Stroke.
- Bruits over common carotids or subclavians.

General Considerations

The origin of symptoms in about 80% of patients with occlusive cerebrovascular disease is an atherosclerotic lesion in a surgically accessible artery in the neck or mediastinum (Figs 39–8 and 39–9). Less common causes are arterial emboli, fibromuscular dysplasia, dissecting aneurysm, and Takayasu's arteritis. The syndromes are sometimes associated with cerebral infarction through either of 2 mechanisms.

Cerebral infarction can be produced by a sudden decrease in blood supply which, if it drops below a critical level, causes cellular death within minutes. This event is manifested by a fixed or advancing neurologic deficit. It can result from local arterial thrombosis, cerebral embolization, or sudden decrease in cardiac output, all of which are complications of stenosis of the internal carotid artery.

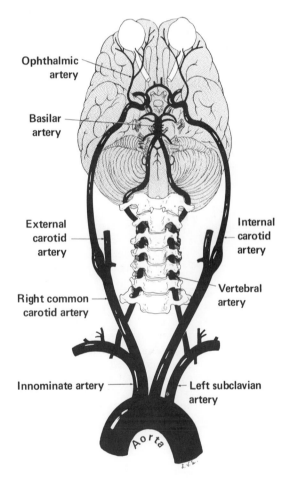

FIG 39–8. Diagram of arterial blood supply to the eyes and brain. (Reproduced, with permission, from Wylie EJ, Ehrenfeld WK: *Extracranial Occlusive Cerebrovascular Disease: Diagnosis and Management.* Saunders, 1970.)

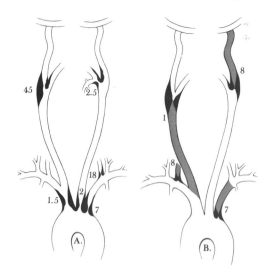

FIG 39–9. Diagram showing common sites of stenosis and occlusion of the extracranial cerebral vasculature. (Reproduced, with permission, from Wylie EJ, Ehrenfeld WK: *Extracranial Occlusive Cerebrovascular Disease: Diagnosis and Management.* Saunders, 1970.)

Except for the internal carotid, isolated occlusion of an extracranial artery does not produce infarction or a neurologic deficit since collateral flow is usually adequate. When occlusion occurs in the internal carotid, the usual cause is an atherosclerotic lesion just distal to the common carotid bifurcation. Contralateral hemiplegia often results.

Embolization is the second mechanism of cerebral infarction from carotid lesions. The atherosclerotic plaque ulcerates, and atheromatous debris and blood clot accumulates on its surface and may dislodge to produce cerebral infarction when they reach the brain. Most lesions of this sort occur at the origin of the internal carotid, but the innominate artery and ascending aorta are sometimes implicated.

Neurologic dysfunction without infarction may be produced in 2 ways: (1) Cerebral embolization by small (microembolic) fragments which only temporarily impede arterial flow; and (2) transient reduction in cerebral perfusion short of that required to give irreversible ischemia.

Since most microemboli originate from an ulcerative lesion in the internal carotid artery, neurologic dysfunction is confined to the carotid territory and appears as momentary paresis or numbness of the contralateral arm or leg. This is called a **transient ischemic attack (TIA).** A TIA from microembolization to the retinal artery may consist of temporary loss of vision (amaurosis fugax) in all or part of the visual field in the ipsilateral eye. Emboli may be visible in the retinas of some patients as small bright flecks of cholesterol. The diagnosis of TIA rests on the transient dysfunction and is supported by finding a bruit at the bifurcation of the common carotid artery on the appropriate side. In the absence of surgical treatment, many patients with TIAs will eventually develop permanent neurologic or visual impairment either from dislodgement of a macroembolus or thrombotic occlusion of the internal carotid artery.

Cerebral ischemia sufficient to produce neurologic dysfunction is usually caused by lesions in the extracranial arteries which are amenable to surgery

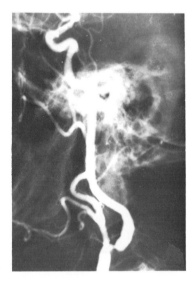
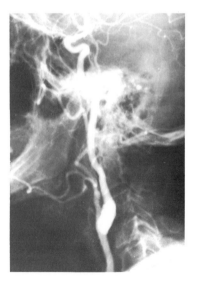

FIG 39–10. *Left:* Preoperative carotid arteriogram showing stenosis of the proximal internal carotid artery. *Right:* Postoperative carotid arteriogram showing restoration of normal luminal size following endarterectomy. (Reproduced, with permission, from Wylie EJ, Ehrenfeld WK: *Extracranial Occlusive Cerebrovascular Disease: Diagnosis and Management.* Saunders, 1970.)

(Fig 39–10), but episodic symptoms may sometimes be precipitated by maneuvers which impair blood flow in otherwise unobstructed collateral arteries—eg, rising from a supine to an upright position (producing momentary postural hypotension) or hyperextension or rotation of the neck.

Clinical Findings

A. Symptoms: Obstruction of the proximal subclavian or vertebral artery may produce episodic ataxia, diplopia, bilateral blurring of vision, and drop attacks, symptoms caused by reduction of blood flow in the basilar artery. Internal carotid stenosis may cause only recurrent faintness or "lightheadedness" without motor or sensory changes unless hypotension is unusually severe. Innominate artery obstruction may cause symptoms in either the vertebrobasilar or carotid territories or both.

Persistent (but reversible) symptoms may occur with any of the lesions just described. Notable are subtle mentation or memory deficits and chronic decrease of vision. The former are frequently seen in patients with bilateral internal carotid lesions—the latter as a unilateral complaint in patients with common carotid occlusion.

Since many hemodynamic symptoms are mild and infrequent, the decision to surgically relieve arterial obstruction often depends upon the surgeon's assessment of the natural history of the specific lesion. In this regard, occlusion or stenosis of the innominate,

subclavian, or vertebral arteries can be considered benign, whereas occlusion of the common or internal carotid artery poses a much greater threat.

B. Signs: Reduced pulses, audible bruits, and asymmetry of pressure in the brachial arteries reveal the presence of most clinically important lesions in the extracranial arteries. The following may exist without clinical signs: occlusion of the internal carotid artery, occlusion and (frequently) stenosis of the vertebral arteries, and ulceration without stenosis in any artery.

1. Palpation—Of the cerebral vessels, only the pulse of the common carotid artery can be felt with certainty. The internal carotid artery is not palpable, either externally or from within the oropharynx. Although the subclavian pulse cannot be reliably evaluated, a weakened axillary pulse usually indicates a subclavian artery lesion.

2. Bruits—Bruits over both subclavian and common carotid arteries generally denote stenosis of the aortic valve. A bruit localized to one artery indicates a stenosis at or proximal to the point where it can be heard. A bruit with maximal intensity high in the neck indicates stenosis at the common carotid bifurcation. Bruits caused by stenosis at the origin of the vertebral artery, if heard at all, are most prominent over the lower portion of the trapezius muscle at the back of the neck. Bruits due to proximal subclavian stenosis are most audible above the midpoint of the clavicle and are transmitted into the axilla. Innominate artery stenosis produces a bruit heard along the full length of

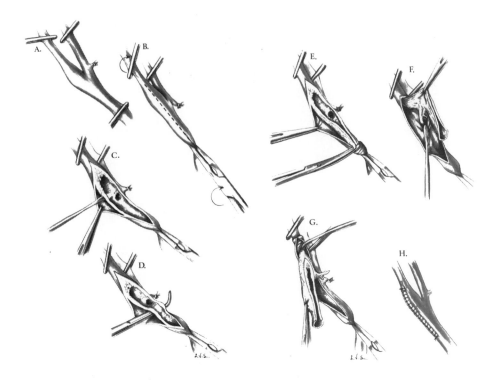

FIG 39–11. Technic of carotid endarterectomy. (Reproduced, with permission, from Wylie EJ, Ehrenfeld WK: *Extracranial Occlusive Cerebrovascular Disease: Diagnosis and Management.* Saunders, 1970.)

the right common carotid and right subclavian arteries.

3. Brachial blood pressures—A discrepancy between the blood pressures in the 2 arms indicates arterial stenosis or occlusion proximal to the brachial artery on the side of reduced pressure.

C. X-Ray Findings: Cerebral arteriography is indicated whenever a lesion is suspected which might require operation. The procedure provides valuable ancillary information about collateral blood supply, other unsuspected stenoses, and occasionally a CNS lesion. The ideal study visualizes both the vertebral-basilar and carotid systems and their intracranial branches.

Treatment

The objectives of operative treatment are to prevent stroke or relieve an existing disability, and these may be accomplished by improving blood flow or removing a source of microemboli. There is no effective medical treatment in most cases.

Surgery is only performed for syndromes not involving cerebral infarction because restoration of normal blood flow and arterial pressures to an infarcted area often causes hemorrhage into the infarct. Most surgical candidates have an accessible lesion in the neck or mediastinum, either causing transient cerebral ischemia or threatening to cause a stroke. Carotid lesions found in patients who have had a previous stroke should be considered for correction. Asymptomatic healthy patients are candidates for surgery when severe stenosis is present and life expectancy is long.

Endarterectomy is the preferred technic for the removal of atherosclerotic lesions at the common carotid bifurcation, in the orifices of the right vertebral and subclavian arteries, and in the innominate artery (sternum splitting approach) (Fig 39–11). The left vertebral artery is difficult to approach through the neck, and obstruction at its orifice is more easily managed by transplanting the vertebral artery to the side of the adjacent left common carotid artery. Obstruction at the origins of the left common carotid artery and left subclavian artery would require an open thoracotomy for endarterectomy. However, thoracotomy and its risks can be avoided by dividing the common carotid low in the neck and transplanting it to the distal cervical portion of the left subclavian artery. Lesions in the proximal subclavian artery causing the "subclavian steal" syndrome can be managed by inserting a bypass graft from the left common carotid to the subclavian artery distal to the lesion (Fig 39–12).

Variations of Occlusive Cerebrovascular Disease

Primary disease in the extracranial arteries other than atherosclerosis is rare. **Takayasu's arteritis** is an obliterative arteriopathy principally involving the aortic arch vessels which often affects young females. Surgery may be necessary to alleviate symptoms due to low cerebral perfusion. Bypass grafts may occasionally be adaptable to overcome the obstructive process.

Dissecting aneurysms of the aorta may extend into the arch branches, producing obstruction and cerebral symptoms. These are discussed in Chapter 23. Rarely, localized dissection can occur in the internal carotid artery with subsequent narrowing or obliteration.

Fibromuscular dysplasia, a disease of young adult

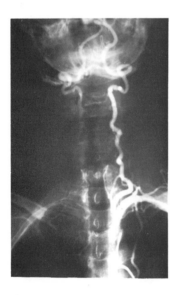 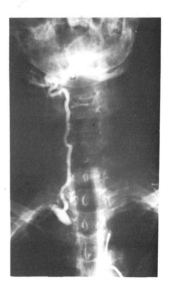

FIG 39–12. *Left:* Arteriogram showing selective injection of the left subclavian artery. There is antegrade flow in the ipsilateral vertebral artery and retrograde flow in the contralateral vertebral artery. *Right:* A later film in this sequence shows filling of the right subclavian artery by retrograde flow in the right vertebral artery. There is proximal occlusion of the right subclavian artery causing the "subclavian steal" syndrome. (Reproduced, with permission, from Wylie EJ, Ehrenfeld WK: *Extracranial Occlusive Cerebrovascular Disease: Diagnosis and Management.* Saunders, 1970.)

females, occasionally involves one or both internal carotid arteries. When symptomatic, these lesions can be managed either by internal dilatation or resection and graft replacement.

Acute embolic obstruction of the extracranial arteries usually involves the carotid bifurcation and produces hemiplegia due to cerebral infarction. As with other conditions causing cerebral infarction, surgical removal of the obstructing lesion is contraindicated.

Prognosis

Postoperatively, late restenosis or occlusion is rare. The morbidity from operation consists mainly of neurologic deficits and occurs in less than 2%. The operative mortality for all extracranial cerebrovascular operations in our personal experience is less than 1%.

DeBakey ME & others: Cerebral arterial insufficiency: One- to eleven-year results following arterial reconstructive operation. Ann Surg 161:921–945, 1965.

Ehrenfeld WK, Hoyt WF, Wylie EJ: Embolization and transient blindness from carotid atheroma. Arch Surg 93:787–794, 1966.

Fisher M: Transient blindness associated with hemiplegia. Arch Ophth 47:167–203, 1952.

Julian OC & others: Ulcerative lesions of the carotid artery bifurcation. Arch Surg 86:803–809, 1963.

Reivich M & others: Reversal of blood flow through the vertebral artery and its effect on cerebral circulation. New England J Med 265:878–885, 1961.

Wylie EJ, Ehrenfeld WK: *Extracranial Occlusive Cerebrovascular Disease: Diagnosis and Management.* Saunders, 1970.

RENOVASCULAR HYPERTENSION

Essentials of Diagnosis

- Hypertension.
- Suspicion of renal artery involvement.

General Considerations

Hypertension may result from any process which causes prolonged ischemia of one or both kidneys. Ischemia presumably causes an increase in numbers and activity of juxtaglomerular cells which leads to increased renin production. Assay of renal vein plasma for renin is used in the selection of patients for operation since a large difference in plasma renin levels between one or both kidneys and the vena caval plasma supports a renal cause for the hypertension.

The most common causes of renovascular hypertension are stenosis or occlusion of the renal arteries by atherosclerosis or fibromuscular dysplasia. Less common causes are emboli, dissecting aneurysm, hypoplasia of the renal arteries, and stenosis of the suprarenal artery. Atherosclerosis characteristically produces stenosis at the orifice of a main renal artery and is more prominent in males over age 45. The process is bilateral in over 35% of cases.

Fibromuscular dysplasia usually involves the middle and distal thirds of the main renal artery (Fig 39–13). It often extends into the renal artery branches and involves both renal arteries in 50% of cases. Arterial stenosis is caused by one or more concentric rings of medial hyperplasia which project into the arterial lumen as a perforated diaphragm. The arteriographic deformity often resembles a chain of beads. The disease is largely confined to women, and the onset of hypertension is usually before age 45.

Clinical Findings

A. Symptoms and Signs: Most patients are asymptomatic, but irritability, headache, and emotional depression are seen in a few. Persistent elevation of the diastolic pressure is usually the only abnormal physical finding. A bruit is frequently audible to one or both sides of the midline in the upper abdomen. Other signs of atherosclerosis may be present when this is the cause of the renal artery disease.

B. Diagnostic Studies: When the process is unilateral, divided urinary excretion studies show decreased volume from the involved kidney, reduction in sodium concentration, and increase in concentration of substances not subject to tubular reabsorption, eg, creatinine, para-aminohippurate, and inulin. Renin in renal vein plasma is higher from the affected kidney. These studies depend upon comparison of the functions of the 2 kidneys and are less useful when both kidneys are involved or when the patient has only one kidney.

Comparative measurements of renal blood flow are considered by some to be a more specific test for renovascular hypertension than measurements of urinary excretion. The most commonly used methods employ radioactive iodohippurate sodium or technetium 99m pertechnetate and are described in Chapter 8.

C. X-Ray Findings: Intravenous urography with rapid injection and rapid sequence exposure is a common screening test which also depends upon comparison of the 2 kidneys. The ischemic kidney has delayed

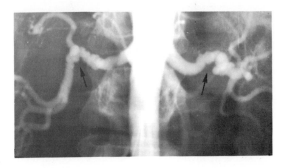

FIG 39–13. Renal arteriogram showing bilateral fibromuscular hyperplasia of the renal arteries (arrows).

appearance of dye in the calyces and hyperconcentration in the later films as water is extracted by the tubules. The nephrogram phase may show a small kidney on the affected side.

Renal arteriography is the only method that delineates the occlusive lesion. The Seldinger technic, with retrograde passage of a catheter from the femoral arteries, is preferred. Renal arteriography should be performed if the diastolic blood pressure exceeds 110 mm Hg, other clinical criteria are consistent with renovascular hypertension, and long life is otherwise expected.

Treatment

Surgical treatment consists of nephrectomy or revascularization of the renal artery. The indications for arterial reconstruction are influenced by the extent of disease in the renal arteries, the degree of associated arterial disease, the response to medical control of hypertension, the patient's life expectancy, and the anticipated morbidity of the operation. Nephrectomy should be considered when arterial repair is impossible or especially hazardous and the disease is unilateral.

Endarterectomy is effective in the management of atherosclerotic lesions and is most easily accomplished by a transaortic approach. When there is extensive intimal degeneration in the aorta (eg, associated aneurysmal disease in the aorta), a fabric bypass graft may be used as a sidearm from the aortic prosthesis.

Bypass grafting is the preferred method in patients with fibromuscular dysplasia of the renal artery. Autologous grafts using a segment of saphenous vein or hypogastric artery are advised (Fig 39–14).

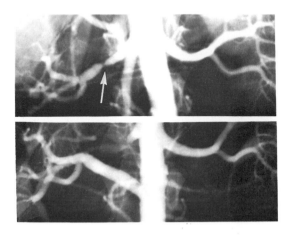

FIG 39–14. *Top:* Preoperative renal arteriogram of a patient with stenosis of the midportion of the right renal artery (arrow). *Bottom:* Postoperative renal arteriogram after renal artery bypass with an autograft of the hypogastric artery. (Reproduced, with permission, from Wylie EJ, Perloff DL, Stoney RJ: Autogenous tissue revascularization technics in surgery for renovascular hypertension. Ann Surg 170:416, 1969.)

Instrumental dilatation of the diseased renal artery may be effective in relieving stenosis in selected patients.

Prognosis

Operations for revascularization of the renal artery are successful in lowering blood pressure in over 90% of patients with fibromuscular hyperplasia. Operation for atherosclerotic stenosis results in improvement or cure in about 60%.

Dustan HP & others: An evaluation of treatment of hypertension associated with occlusive renal arterial disease. Circulation 27:1018–1027, 1963.

Foster JH & others: Hypertension and fibromuscular dysplasia of the renal arteries. Surgery 65:157–165, 1969.

Morris GC Jr & others: Late results of surgical treatment for renovascular hypertension. Surg Gynec Obst 122:1255–1261, 1966.

Thomas CS Jr, Brockman SK, Foster JH: Variability of the pressure gradient in renal artery stenosis. Surg Gynec Obst 126:339–346, 1968.

Wylie EJ, Perloff DL, Stoney RJ: Autogenous tissue revascularization techniques in surgery for renovascular hypertension. Ann Surg 170:416–428, 1969.

Wylie EJ, Perloff D, Wellington JS: Fibromuscular hyperplasia of the renal arteries. Ann Surg 156:592–609, 1962.

GASTROINTESTINAL ISCHEMIA SYNDROMES

The celiac axis, the superior and inferior mesenteric arteries, and the 2 internal iliac arteries are the principal sources of blood supply to the stomach and intestines. The anatomic collateral interconnections between these arteries are numerous and may become quite large. Single or even multiple occlusions are generally well tolerated because collateral flow is readily available (Fig 39–15). With the exception of the superior mesenteric artery, even acute occlusion of any one of them rarely causes significant visceral ischemia. This section deals with the diagnosis and management of the syndromes that are produced by acute or chronic obstruction of these visceral arteries. The related syndrome of bowel ischemia that may result from an acute systemic hypotensive episode is described in another section. (See also Chapter 35.)

ACUTE OCCLUSION

The most common causes of acute occlusion of the visceral arteries are embolism (usually of cardiac origin), thrombosis of an atheromatous artery, and acute aortic dissection. Symptoms of vascular insuffi-

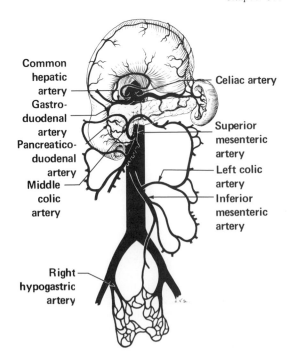

Common
hepatic
artery
Gastro-
duodenal
artery
Pancreatico-
duodenal
artery
Middle
colic
artery

Celiac artery

Superior
mesenteric
artery

Left colic
artery

Inferior
mesenteric
artery

Right
hypogastric
artery

FIG 39—15. Visceral arterial circulation and interconnections.

ciency are those of intestinal infarction, usually in the distribution of the superior mesenteric artery. When infarction results from arterial thrombosis, there is often a preceding history of intermittent postprandial abdominal pain (intestinal angina). The rapid appearance of diffuse, continuous, severe abdominal pain is a uniform complaint. This is usually followed by vomiting and diarrhea. The early findings are diffuse abdominal tenderness, muscle guarding without board-like rigidity, and absence of peristalsis. Abdominal distention occurs late. Shock, when present, signifies widespread and advanced necrosis of bowel. Leukocytosis appears within 2—5 hours of the onset of pain and signifies advancing hemorrhagic infarction.

Immediate laparotomy is indicated if there is a reasonable suspicion of the diagnosis since a revascularization procedure is feasible only early, before bowel ischemia becomes irreversible. An embolus usually lodges at the first major arterial bifurcation and may be removed. Retrograde "milking" of the mesenteric vessels may be required to remove distal propagating thrombus. Occlusion by thrombosis of the superior mesenteric artery is usually superimposed upon a chronic atherosclerotic lesion at the orifice of the artery. Thromboendarterectomy of the occluded segment or a bypass graft may restore arterial flow. If prolonged ischemia has resulted in irreversible necrosis of the intestine, resection of the infarcted intestinal segment is indicated.

Successful revascularization of acute occlusions of visceral arteries is rare, and intestinal resection of infarcted bowel is usually indicated. When viability of

remaining bowel is in doubt, a "second look" operation hours later may be necessary to more accurately delineate the extent of further resection.

CHRONIC OCCLUSION

Chronic occlusion of either the celiac or superior mesenteric arteries is caused by atherosclerosis or external compression by ligamentous or neural bands. When atherosclerosis is the cause, the usual lesion is a collar of thickened intima in the orifice of the visceral artery. Associated atherosclerosis in the aorta and its other branches is frequent.

Visceral ischemia due to external compression of visceral arteries is a syndrome that has only recently been described. The celiac artery is customarily involved where compression is by the median arcuate ligament of the diaphragm. Women 25—50 years of age are most commonly affected.

Clinical Findings

The principal complaint is postprandial abdominal pain, which has been labeled abdominal or visceral angina. Pain characteristically appears 15—30 minutes after the beginning of a meal and lasts for an hour or longer. It occasionally is so severe and prolonged that opiates are required for relief. It is a deep-seated steady ache in the epigastrium, occasionally radiating to the right or left upper quadrant. Weight loss results from reluctance to eat. Diarrhea and vomiting have been described but in our experience are rare. An upper abdominal bruit may be heard in over 80% of patients.

Arteriography (by retrograde catheter injection whenever possible) in the anteroposterior and lateral projections demonstrates both the arterial lesion and the patterns of collateral blood flow (Fig 39—16).

Treatment

When the obstruction is atherosclerotic, surgical revascularization of the superior mesenteric or the celiac axis (or both) may be performed either by endarterectomy or graft replacement (Fig 39—16). External compression of the celiac artery by the median arcuate ligament may be relieved by simple division of the ligament in 50% of cases. In the remainder, residual stenosis may persist and must be relieved by instrumental arterial dilatation or by resection of the stenotic segment and graft replacement.

Prognosis

Surgery for atherosclerotic visceral artery insufficiency almost always results in relief of symptoms if a technically adequate operation is accomplished. If operation in these patients is not performed, death will often occur from inanition or massive bowel infarction.

Patients with median arcuate ligament compression respond favorably to operation in the majority of

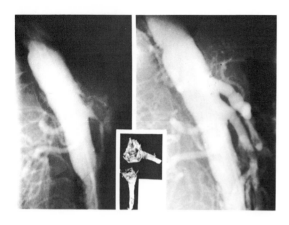

FIG 39–16. *Left:* Preoperative visceral arteriogram showing severe stenosis of the celiac and superior mesenteric arteries. *Right:* The postoperative visceral arteriogram shows wide patency of the celiac and superior mesenteric arteries after transaortic endarterectomy. The inset shows the atherosclerotic stenotic lesions removed by endarterectomy.

instances. Because of the greater difficulty of clinical diagnosis, some of these patients may not improve even though a technically adequate operation is accomplished.

Marable SA & others: Celiac compression syndrome. Am J Surg 115:97–102, 1968.
Rob D: Surgical diseases of the celiac and mesenteric arteries. Arch Surg 93:21–32, 1966.
Stoney RJ, Wylie EJ: Recognition and surgical treatment of visceral ischemic syndromes. Ann Surg 164:714–722, 1966.

THORACIC OUTLET SYNDROME

The term thoracic outlet syndrome refers to the variety of disorders caused by abnormal compression of arterial, venous, or neural structures in the base of the neck. Numerous mechanisms for compression have been described, including cervical rib, anomalous ligaments, hypertrophy of the scalenus anticus muscle, and positional changes which alter the normal relation of the first rib to the structures that pass over it. This has prompted the confusing assortment of names related to the assumed mechanism, ie, **cervical rib, scalenus anticus, costoclavicular,** and **hyperabduction syndromes.** The term **shoulder-hand syndrome** developed from the observation that the hand and forearm are the usual site of symptoms from compression at the base of the neck and shoulder.

Symptoms rarely develop until adulthood. For this reason, it has been assumed that an alteration of normal structural relationships which occurs with advancing years is the primary factor. Even anomalous cervical ribs seem well tolerated during childhood and adolescence.

Inclusion of these syndromes in discussions of vascular disease originates from a former view that many of the symptoms were the result of intermittent compression of the subclavian or axillary arteries. This assumption was reinforced by the frequent finding that certain postural manipulations could produce depression of the radial pulse. The present view holds that whereas transient circulatory changes may indeed occur, the primary cause of symptoms in most patients is intermittent compression of one or more trunks of the brachial plexus. Thus, neurologic symptoms predominate over those of ischemia or venous compression.

Most patients associate their symptoms with certain positions of the shoulder girdle. These may occur from prolonged hyperabduction, as in house painters, hairdressers, and truck drivers. Others may relate their symptoms to the downward traction of the shoulder girdle produced by carrying heavy objects. Numbness of the hands often wakes the patient from sleep.

Clinical Findings

A. Symptoms and Signs: Symptoms consist of pain, paresthesias, or numbness in the distribution of one or more trunks of the brachial plexus (usually in the ulnar distribution). These symptoms can be elicited by specific positions of the arm. Peripheral sensory or motor deficits are rare and usually indicate severe compression of long duration. Muscular atrophy may be present in the hand. The radial pulse can be weakened by abduction of the arm with the head rotated to the opposite side (**Adson's test**), though pulse reduction by this maneuver often occurs in completely asymptomatic persons. Dilatation of the superficial veins of the arm usually indicates axillary vein thrombosis, a complication of chronic venous compression. Peripheral cyanosis and coldness from vasoconstriction occur rarely.

B. X-Ray Findings: X-rays of the neck are of value only in the diagnosis of cervical rib or an elongated transverse process at C5 or C6. The demonstration of subclavian or axillary artery stenosis by arteriograms with the arm in abduction has minimal usefulness since similar changes may be produced in asymptomatic patients.

Treatment

Most patients benefit from postural correction and a physical therapy program directed toward restoring the normal relation and strengthening the structures in the shoulder girdle. Surgical technics for decompression of the thoracic outlet are reserved for patients who have not responded after 3–6 months of conservative treatment. Resection of an anomalous cervical rib may give dramatic relief. Resection of the first rib is the best method for decompressing the space at the thoracic outlet. The transaxillary approach is preferred.

Prognosis

When the correct diagnosis is made, resection of the first rib gives dramatic relief of symptoms.

Roos DB: Transaxillary approach for first rib resection to relieve thoracic outlet syndrome. Ann Surg 163:354–358, 1966.

Sanders RJ, Monsour JW, Baer SB: Transaxillary first rib resection for the thoracic outlet syndrome. Arch Surg 97:1014–1023, 1968.

Urschel HC Jr, Razzuk MA: Management of the thoracic-outlet syndrome. New England J Med 286:1140–1143, 1972.

ARTERIOVENOUS FISTULAS

Arteriovenous fistulas may be congenital or acquired. Abnormal communications between arteries and veins occur in many diseases and may affect vessels of all sizes. Their effects depend upon the degree of communication present. In congenital fistulas, the systemic effect is often not great because the degree of communication, though diffuse, is small. Larger acquired fistulas enlarge rapidly and may ultimately produce cardiac failure. Cardiac dilatation and heart failure may result when shunting is excessive, prolonged, or untreated. Overloading of the venous side of the circulation may ultimately cause venous insufficiency.

Congenital fistulas are often noted in infancy or childhood. When a limb is involved, muscle mass or bone length may be increased. Arteriovenous malformations frequently involve the brain, visceral organs, or lungs. Gastrointestinal hemorrhage may occur. Pulmonary lesions cause polycythemia, clubbing, and cyanosis.

Acquired fistulas result from injuries that produce artificial connections between adjacent arteries and veins and may be the result of trauma or disease. Penetrating injuries are the most common cause, but fistulas are sometimes seen after blunt trauma. Connective tissue disorders (eg, Ehlers-Danlos syndrome), erosion of an atherosclerotic or mycotic arterial aneurysm into adjacent veins, communication with an arterial prosthetic graft, and neoplastic invasion are other causes.

Clinical Findings

A. Symptoms and Signs: The time of onset and the presence or absence of associated disease should be determined. A typical continuous machinery murmur can be heard over most fistulas and is often associated with a palpable thrill and locally increased skin temperature. Proximally, the arteries and veins dilate and the pulse distal to the lesion diminishes. There may be signs of venous insufficiency and coolness distal to the communication on the involved extremity.

B. X-Ray Findings: Precise delineation of arteriovenous fistulas can only be done with appropriate arteriograms. The use of selective catheter injection technics has permitted accurate radiologic diagnosis.

Treatment

Not all arteriovenous connections require operation. Small peripheral fistulas may be observed and frequently will never cause difficulties. Some fistulas close spontaneously, often as a result of venous thrombosis. Some are surgically inaccessible.

The indications for surgery include hemorrhage, expanding false aneurysm, severe venous or arterial insufficiency, cosmetic deformity, and heart failure.

Numerous technics are available. These include the classic quadruple ligation, amputation, en bloc excision, and repair of the fistula with reconstruction of the involved arteries and veins. Iatrogenic embolization with beads or muscle has recently been recommended for inaccessible or inoperable fistulas. Quadruple ligation of both proximal and distal artery and vein ensures obliteration of the fistula. This technic depends upon collateral blood flow to compensate for the arterial ligation and preserve tissue viability.

Since the introduction of refined vascular surgical technics in recent years, primary repair is being attempted more often. The arterial repair is most important since venous ligation can usually be done with impunity.

En bloc resection is reserved for diffuse arteriovenous malformations, though hemostasis may be difficult. Congenital arteriovenous fistulas are amenable to surgical management only when en bloc resection of all tissue involved in the fistula can be accomplished. When the fistulous connections involve substantial portions of an extremity, local arterial ligation is invariably followed by recurrence, and only temporary palliation can be expected. Amputation may be a last resort to control unmanageable peripheral fistulas.

Prognosis

The results of surgery vary according to the extent, location, and type of fistula. In general, traumatic fistulas have the most favorable prognosis. Congenital fistulas are more difficult to eradicate because of the numerous arteriovenous connections usually present. These fistulas have a high propensity for recurrence, and most surgeons are reluctant to operate unless the surgical indications are urgent.

Cross FS & others: Congenital arteriovenous aneurysms. Ann Surg 148:649–665, 1958.

DeBakey ME & others: Arteriovenous fistula involving the abdominal aorta: Report of four cases with successful repair. Ann Surg 147:646–658, 1958.

Holman E: *Arteriovenous Aneurysm*. Macmillan, 1937.

Szilagyi DE & others: Peripheral congenital arteriovenous fistulas. Surgery 57:61–81, 1965.

AMPUTATION OF THE LOWER EXTREMITY IN ARTERIAL OCCLUSIVE DISEASE
Wesley S. Moore, MD

Arterial reconstruction is the preferred treatment for reversible ischemic lesions of the lower extremity. However, when the arterial disease is not amenable to reconstruction—or when the ischemic changes are irreversible—amputation of the lower extremity must be done. The indications for amputation are gangrene, uncontrolled infection, or rest pain.

General Principles

(1) The goal of amputation is to treat the lower extremity ischemia and to rehabilitate the patient to his preischemic ambulatory status.

(2) The amputation should be designed to remove the least amount of viable tissue but should be done at a level which has a blood supply sufficient to ensure a reasonable chance of primary healing.

Preoperative Preparation

A. Control of Infection: When a patient has wet gangrene or acute bacterial infection of the foot, infection should be treated before elective amputation. Culture and sensitivity data should be obtained and the patient started on appropriate antibiotic therapy. If cellulitis and lymphangitis are treated successfully, elective amputation with primary closure can be safely performed. If infection cannot be controlled by local measures and antibiotics, major debridement of the infected tissue may be necessary. Effective debridement may require supramalleolar open guillotine amputation of the foot. This is an effective method of preparing for below-the-knee amputation. Guillotine debridement above the level of lymphangitis is not necessary because open supramalleolar amputation removes the source of infection and provides drainage through the open end of the stump. This form of radical debridement, combined with antibiotic therapy, will effectively prepare the patient for below-the-knee amputation within 2 or 3 days.

B. Vascular Supply: One method of making certain that amputation can be successfully carried out at the most distal level possible is to establish good inflow to the profunda femoris artery. Diminution of the femoral pulse on the affected side is evidence of reduced profunda femoris blood flow. However, a good pulse does not in itself guarantee adequate inflow to the profunda femoris since a high-grade obstruction of the iliac system in conjunction with a tandem stenotic lesion of the orifice of the profunda femoris artery can produce a femoral pulse of normal quality. Therefore, when time permits, angiography should be performed before amputation to determine the adequacy of arterial inflow to the profunda femoris artery. If inflow disease of the vessel is found and corrected, the amputation may be successfully performed at a more distal level.

C. Sympathectomy: It has been suggested that lumbar sympathectomy will improve blood supply to the skin of the lower extremity and facilitate primary healing at a distal amputation level. This contention has not been proved and at the present time cannot be recommended.

Determination of Amputation Level

The amputation level depends upon the extent of tissue necrosis and the quality of the blood supply immediately proximal to the infected or gangrenous part. The circulatory status at the level of proposed amputation can also be evaluated by determining the presence and quality of peripheral pulses, the level to which dependent rubor reaches, and the capillary refill time. The condition of the skin and skin appendages should be examined for distribution of hair, ischemic nail changes, thickness of skin, and amount of subcutaneous tissue at the level of proposed amputation. Angiography of the distal aorta and its branches down to and including the tibial vessels is helpful in establishing the location of major arterial occlusions and the patterns of collateral circulation. The temperature of the skin at the level of proposed amputation can be used to evaluate circulation. Quantitation of capillary circulation by isotope clearance at the proposed site of amputation is currently undergoing investigation. However, the information obtained is still inexact, and the site of amputation is often based upon the experience of the surgeon.

Amputation for Acute Arterial Occlusion

Amputation of the acutely ischemic limb deserves special attention. The timing of amputation will be determined partly by the success or failure of arterial reconstruction. Also influencing this decision will be the duration of arterial occlusion before reconstruction and evidence of massive limb swelling after reestablishment of arterial blood flow. In general, if only a slight amount of ischemic or necrotic tissue results from acute arterial occlusion, amputation should be deferred until there is a clear demarcation between viable and nonviable skin. This also permits the development of collateral blood supply to viable tissue. However, if extensive tissue is involved, delayed amputation runs the risk of systemic toxicity from ischemic by-products in marginally vascularized tissue. The anticipation of systemic toxicity—or its actual manifestations as evidenced by deterioration of vital signs, confused mentation, hemoglobinuria, or failing renal function—is an indication for emergency amputation. Emergency amputation after acute arterial occlusion must be carried out at a higher level than if collateral circulation and demarcation were allowed to develop. However, the disadvantage of amputation at a higher level must be balanced against the life-threatening danger of delayed amputation if a large amount of ischemic tissue is present.

TOE AMPUTATION

Indications

Toe amputation is indicated for infection or gangrene limited to the distal or middle phalanx of one or more toes, associated with sharp demarcation and good circulation in the proximal skin.

Contraindications

(1) Gangrene or infection extending toward the metatarsal crease with an indistinct line of demarcation.

(2) Extensive ischemic disease of the foot involving the tissue through which the incision for toe amputation would be made. This includes rest pain, atrophy of the skin and subcutaneous tissue, or dependent rubor.

Procedure

Toe amputation can be accomplished by surgical excision or autoamputation. If there is dry gangrene with distinct demarcation and no evidence of infection, the safest method is to allow autoamputation of the gangrenous toe (or toes) to take place. The patient must be instructed regarding care of the ischemic foot, eg, separation of the toes, hygiene, avoidance of hot water, and meticulous drying between the toes following washing. With time, epithelization will take place under the ischemic eschar. When epithelization is complete, the gangrenous phalanx will autoamputate, leaving a well-healed epithelized stump. This process usually takes several months.

In toe amputation, a circular incision is made proximal to the line of demarcation, down to bone. The bone is divided and rongeured back far enough to permit transverse closure of the skin with careful coaptation of the skin edges.

Advantages Over Amputation at a Higher Level

The operative procedure is simple and produces no major deformity or interference with the patient's gait.

Disadvantages

Failure to heal may produce a spreading space infection which may require amputation at a considerably higher level.

Results & Postoperative Considerations

The functional result is excellent. No prosthesis, specific gait training, or rehabilitation is required.

TRANSMETATARSAL AMPUTATION
(See Fig 39–17.)

Indications

(1) Gangrenous changes in 3 or more toes.

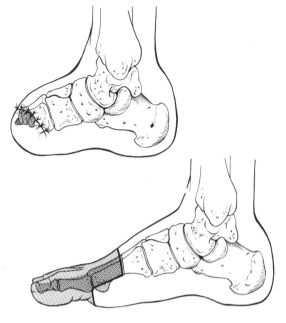

FIG 39–17. Transmetatarsal amputation.

(2) Gangrene extending past the metatarsal crease on the anterior aspect of the foot but sparing plantar skin.

(3) Contiguous osteomyelitis of the metatarsal head with good plantar skin and good circulation.

This amputation is most successfully applied to diabetic patients with gangrene due to necrotizing infection but with good peripheral circulation confirmed by the presence of pedal pulses.

Contraindications

(1) Neuropathy of plantar skin, resulting in anesthesia.

(2) Dependent rubor of the forefoot involving the area of proposed skin incision.

(3) Rest pain of the forefoot, suggesting more extensive ischemia.

(4) Infection extending into the metatarsal spaces.

(5) The absence of pedal pulses is a relative contraindication for amputation, but this contraindication can be negated by evidence of good collateral circulation as manifested by absence of skin atrophy, the presence of hair, and a normal amount of subcutaneous tissue.

Procedure

The forefoot is amputated at the midmetatarsal level. A long, full thickness, posterior skin flap is brought up over the divided surface of the metatarsals and sutured to the anterior skin. The anterior skin is incised at the same level as metatarsal bone division. The plantar skin flap can be thinned by excision of tendon and fascial structures, but the plantar muscles and subcutaneous tissues are left intact so that blood supply to the skin flap is undisturbed. Edge-to-edge coaptation is obtained between posterior skin and anterior skin using interrupted vertical mattress sutures. Particular care is taken to avoid trauma to the skin edges. Handling of skin edges with forceps is not permitted.

Advantages Over Amputation at a Higher Level

Amputation at this level does not require a prosthesis. The gait will be reasonably normal, and walking will not require unusual (or additional) effort.

Disadvantages

Amputation at this level often fails in the absence of pedal pulses.

Results & Postoperative Considerations

The functional result is excellent. The only prosthetic requirement is a shoe insert consisting of a spring steel plantar shank with an attached piece of wood or plastic simulating the forefoot, which will fill out the tip of the shoe. Minimal gait training is required.

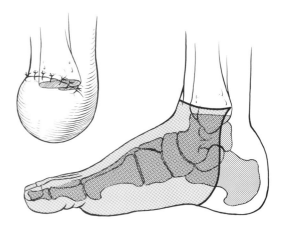

FIG 39—18. Syme's amputation.

by a carefully applied plaster cast to achieve immobilization.

Advantages Over Amputation at a Higher Level

(1) A Syme amputation produces an end weight-bearing stump, giving greater stability during ambulation.

(2) The patient can use a simple cup slipper as a prosthesis to wear around the house. This is easily and quickly applied, and a definitive prosthesis is not needed except for cosmetic effect.

Disadvantages

(1) The cosmetic prosthesis is more difficult to fit than a below-the-knee prosthesis. The Syme prosthesis is less cosmetic in appearance than the below-the-knee prosthesis because of increased width of the ankle required to accommodate the amputation stump.

(2) Amputation at this level often fails to heal in the absence of pedal pulses.

SYME'S AMPUTATION
(See Fig 39—18.)

Indications

The indications for the Syme amputation are gangrene or infection (or both) that involves the forefoot but spares the heel. This amputation is most successfully used in patients with diabetes mellitus and gangrene caused by necrotizing infection but who have a good peripheral blood supply as manifested by the presence of one or both pedal pulses.

Contraindications

(1) Neuropathy of the skin of the heel, manifested by anesthesia.

(2) Evidence of inadequate blood supply, demonstrated by rubor of the entire foot, ulceration about the ankle or heel, or atrophic skin changes extending to the area of proposed incision.

Procedure

The foot is disarticulated at the ankle mortise by dividing the collateral ligaments and carefully filleting the calcaneus from the heel pad to avoid damage to the blood supply from the posterior tibial artery. The weight-bearing surface is prepared by cutting off the tips of both malleoli so that the distal portion of the tibia and fibula become a continuously flat surface in the same plane as the articular surface of the tibiofibular synostosis. The heel pad is brought up and sutured to the anterior skin by a single-layer closure with vertical mattress sutures to obtain perfect edge-to-edge skin closure. The heel pad must be stabilized to prevent medial or lateral dislocation. This is best accomplished

Results of Postoperative Considerations

The functional result is excellent. A cup slipper is used for wear around the house. The formal prosthesis consists of a foot attached to a laminated plastic shell that fits around the calf and stump. Minimal gait training is required.

BELOW-THE-KNEE AMPUTATION
(See Fig 39—19.)

Indications

Amputation below the knee is the method most frequently used for ischemic disease in major amputation centers. Gangrene or infection of the foot in conjunction with a good blood inflow to the profunda femoris artery will result in a high rate of primary healing. A popliteal pulse is desirable (but not necessary) for satisfactory healing.

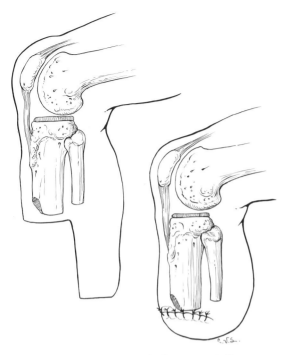

FIG 39—19. Below-the-knee amputation.

Contraindications

(1) Gangrene or ulceration at the level of proposed skin incision.

(2) Hemiparesis on the side of the amputation. Below-the-knee amputation on the side of a hemiparesis causes spastic flexion contracture of the stump, preventing satisfactory prosthetic rehabilitation.

(3) A knee flexion contracture greater than 20 degrees that cannot be improved by physical therapy.

Procedure

Below-the-knee amputation is best performed by using a long posterior skin flap. The posterior skin is thicker and has a better blood supply than the corresponding anterior skin at the calf level. The optimum length of the tibia is 10 cm measured from the tibial tuberosity. The fibula is divided 6 mm shorter than the tibia. The fascia is closed with interrupted absorbable sutures, and the skin is meticulously approximated with vertical mattress sutures to obtain exact edge-to-edge coaptation.

In patients with a satisfactory blood supply (evidenced by bleeding at operation), there may be an advantage to stabilizing the anterior and posterior muscle groups. This is accomplished by suturing the anterior tibial and gastrocnemius-soleus muscles to bone through holes drilled in the anterolateral and posterior aspects of the tibia. The sutured muscles are then amputated flush with the end of the bone. A tourniquet should never be used in amputations for ischemic disease.

Advantages Over Amputation at a Higher Level

(1) Below-the-knee amputation will result in a higher rate of prosthetic rehabilitation, and less energy is required to walk than with an above-the-knee amputation. This is of particular importance to elderly patients. The presence of a knee joint will assure prosthetic rehabilitation if the patient was ambulatory before amputation. This includes patients who may ultimately require bilateral below-the-knee amputation.

(2) The mortality rate for below-the-knee amputation is considerably less than that for above-the-knee amputation in geriatric patients.

Results & Postoperative Considerations

The functional result is excellent. Ambulation and prosthetic rehabilitation have been made possible by advances in prosthetic technology. Some younger patients can even engage in sports with a below-the-knee prosthesis. Elderly patients confined to bed who are not suitable candidates for ambulation find that the presence of a knee joint helps them to turn and to transfer their weight.

The artificial leg for the below-the-knee amputee is a patellar tendon weight-bearing prosthesis. This has an excellent design and mechanical capability. The prosthesis is lightweight and is easily managed by the elderly patient with limited strength.

Prosthetic rehabilitation with below-the-knee amputation is quite successful. Patients easily achieve a good gait pattern after proper training.

KNEE DISARTICULATION
(See Fig 39—20.)

Indications

Knee disarticulation is indicated for ulceration, infection, or gangrene at a level that precludes a high below-the-knee amputation in patients with good arterial inflow to the profunda femoris artery and adequate viable skin to cross over the disarticulated femur.

Contraindications

Ulceration of anterior skin over the tibial tuberosity.

Procedure

A knee disarticulation operation is most easily performed with the patient prone and the knee flexed. A long, total anterior flap is used because of the better quality of the prepatellar skin in this area. The patella is not excised but is pulled into an articulated position of flexion over the femoral condyles and fixed in that position by suturing the patellar tendon to the posterior capsule of the knee joint. Disarticulation is accomplished by division of the collateral ligaments and joint capsule after separation of the attachment of the patellar tendon to the tibial tuberosity. The anterior

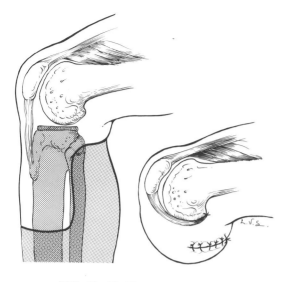

FIG 39—20. Knee disarticulation.

skin flap is brought over the end of the stump and sutured to the posterior skin with interrupted vertical mattress sutures.

Advantages Over Amputation at a Higher Level

(1) The knee disarticulation amputation produces an end weight-bearing stump which provides greater stability during ambulation.

(2) The knee disarticulation prosthesis is lighter and easier to handle than the prosthesis used for above-the-knee amputation. Gait training—particularly for the geriatric amputee—is considerably easier than gait training with above-the-knee amputation.

(3) More patients will obtain prosthetic ambulatory rehabilitation on a knee disarticulation prosthesis than with an above-the-knee prosthesis.

Results & Postoperative Considerations

The ambulatory result of the knee disarticulation is almost as good as that of the below-the-knee amputation. The knee disarticulation prosthesis consists of an artificial distal leg and foot combined with a leather thigh lacer that is articulated with the use of external hinges to simulate knee joint motion.

Rehabilitation is excellent. The training period for ambulation and the gait obtained with a knee disarticulation are almost comparable to those of the below-the-knee amputation.

ABOVE-THE-KNEE AMPUTATION

Until recently, lower extremity amputation for ischemia was usually performed above the knee; below-the-knee amputation was rare. This practice was reversed when it was recognized that most patients with vascular disease can heal at the below-the-knee level and benefit from a superior functional result and lower immediate morbidity and mortality.

Indications

The indications for above-the-knee amputation include healing failure of below-the-knee or disarticulation amputation and extensive ischemic damage from an acute embolus or thrombus, resulting in destruction of tissue distal to the knee joint.

Contraindications

The principal contraindication to above-the-knee amputation is the possibility of obtaining a better functional result with a more distal amputation.

Procedure

The site of amputation is usually in the mid or distal thigh. Either a circular skin incision or equal anterior or posterior flaps are developed. Bone division is performed at a level proximal enough to permit a transverse fascial and skin closure.

Advantages Over Amputation at a Higher Level

(1) The operation is easy to perform.

(2) Primary healing is the rule.

(3) Hip disarticulation is rarely required for ischemic disease.

Disadvantages

(1) Above-the-knee amputation has a higher mortality rate than amputation at the lower level.

(2) The energy required for ambulation on an above-the-knee prosthesis is considerably greater than with amputation at the lower level.

(3) The ability to achieve prosthetic rehabilitation in the elderly debilitated patient is less likely with an above-the-knee amputation than with an amputation at the lower level.

Results & Postoperative Considerations

The functional result is fair. Ambulation on a prosthesis is possible after extended training provided the patient is in reasonably good health and has adequate strength. If prosthetic rehabilitation is not possible, crutches or a wheelchair must be used.

The artificial limb used for the above-the-knee amputee is an ischial weight-bearing prosthesis with a mechanical knee joint.

Rehabilitation after above-the-knee amputation is much less satisfactory than is the case with amputation at a lower level, particularly in geriatric patients. In relatively healthy patients, after a period of extensive physical therapy and gait training, a suitable gait—often supplemented with a cane or a crutch—can be achieved.

•   •   •

COMPLICATIONS OF AMPUTATION

The early complications of amputation are necrosis of the stump, infection, and hematoma formation. Later complications include flexion contracture of the next proximal joint, edema of the stump, or the development of a painful neuroma due to improper handling of the nerve or nerves at the time of amputation. Morbidity and mortality after amputation are often due to pulmonary complications such as pneumonia and pulmonary embolization due to venous thromboembolic disease. Myocardial infarction is also a major cause of morbidity and mortality. These complications are seen more frequently after amputations above the knee than after amputations at a more distal level.

IMMEDIATE POSTOPERATIVE PROSTHESIS

This relatively new technic has been used as an adjunct to amputation in an attempt to facilitate early ambulation, improve healing, decrease the morbidity and mortality, and shorten the period of prosthetic rehabilitation. Immediate application of a prosthesis can be achieved at any amputation level but has been most frequently used in below-the-knee amputation.

A plaster of Paris cast is applied to the stump in the operating room after the amputation is completed. A pylon device and prosthetic foot are incorporated into the cast, which enables the patient to ambulate. Prosthetic gait training begins on the first or second postoperative day and continues during the healing phase of amputation.

Advocates of this technic claim that it has several advantages over conventional amputation with a soft dressing:

(1) Prevention of edema. With the stump in a rigid dressing, the external support prevents edema, thus promoting healing in marginally vascularized tissue. Prevention of edema also accelerates rehabilitation by eliminating the need to wait for stump maturation and shrinkage before fitting a permanent prosthesis.

(2) Reduction of postoperative pain by wound immobilization.

(3) Prevention of knee flexion deformity by knee immobilization.

(4) Protection of the wound from external trauma.

The method also leads to earlier ambulation, with the following advantages:

(1) Fewer pulmonary complications. Pulmonary embolism and pneumonia—major causes of morbidity and mortality following amputation—are the result of prolonged immobilization. Immediate ambulation apparently reduces the incidence of these complications.

(2) Weight-bearing with limited stump compression contributes to control of edema.

(3) Rehabilitation is accelerated by gait training in the early postoperative period. Since there is no prolonged period of bed rest, the patient does not forget how to walk. He is able to maintain strength and muscle tone by continuing to be ambulatory immediately after operation.

(4) Immediate ambulation provides psychologic benefits to the patient adjusting to amputation. When the amputee realizes that he is able to walk on the day following operation, his attitude toward amputation changes. He begins to think positively and starts to work toward rehabilitation on an artificial limb.

The immediate postoperative prosthesis appears to have several advantages in the management of patients following amputation. However, because a prosthetist trained in immediate fitting technics is necessary, this procedure may have to be reserved for centers that perform a large number of amputations.

●　　●　　●

General References

Burgess EM, Romano RL: The management of lower extremity amputees using immediate postsurgical prostheses. Clin Orthop 57:137, 1968.

Committee on Prosthetic-Orthotic Education: *The Geriatric Amputee: Principles of Management.* National Academy of Sciences, 1971.

Cranley JJ: *Vascular Surgery.* Vol 1. *Peripheral Arterial Diseases.* Harper & Row, 1972.

DeBakey M (editor): Symposium on vascular surgery. S Clin North America 46:823–1071, 1966.

Fairbairn JF II, Juergens JL, Spitell JA (editors): *Allen-Barber-Hines Peripheral Vascular Diseases,* 4th ed. Saunders, 1972.

Holling HE (editor): *Peripheral Vascular Diseases.* Lippincott, 1972.

Kappert A, Winsor T: *Diagnosis of Peripheral Vascular Disease.* Davis, 1972.

Lim RC Jr & others: Below-knee amputation for ischemic gangrene. Surg Gynec Obst 125:493–501, 1967.

Moore WS, Hall AD, Wylie EJ: Below knee amputation for vascular insufficiency. Arch Surg 97:886–893, 1968.

Prosthetic and Sensory Aids Service: *The Management of Lower-Extremity Amputations.* Publication No. TR 10–6. Veterans Administration, Aug 1969.

Sarmiento A, Warren WD: A re-evaluation of lower extremity amputations. Surg Gynec Obst 129:799, 1969.

Thompson RC, Del Blanco TL, McAllister FF: Complications following lower extremity amputation. Surg Gynec Obst 120:301–304, 1965.

Warren R, Kihn RB: A survey of lower extremity amputations for ischemia. Surgery 63:107–120, 1968.

Wheelock FC: Transmetatarsal amputations and arterial surgery in diabetic patients. New England J Med 264:316–320, 1961.

40 . . .

The Veins & Lymphatics

John M. Erskine, MD

VARICOSE VEINS

Essentials of Diagnosis

- Dilated, tortuous superficial veins in the lower extremities.
- May be asymptomatic or may be associated with fatigue, aching discomfort, or pain.
- Edema, pigmentation, and ulceration of the skin of the distal leg may occur.

General Considerations

The major factor predisposing to the development of varicose veins is an inherent abnormality of valvular competence which ultimately leads to distention, dilatation, and greater valvular incompetence. Pigmentation and thinning of the skin and chronic edema with fibrosis of the subcutaneous tissues ultimately ensue—especially of the lower leg just above the medial malleolus. Chronic or recurring dermatitis or ulcerations in these areas may result.

Pregnancy, prolonged standing, and perhaps obesity and aging aggravate the pathophysiologic process.

Secondary varicosities can develop as a result of damage or obstruction to the deep venous system following thrombophlebitis. Obstruction of the iliac veins or vena cava (surgical ligation, tumor, fibrosis) can result in varicosities in the extremity. Arteriovenous fistulas (congenital or acquired) may also lead to regional varicosities. Congenital venous malformations in the extremity may have the appearance of varicose veins without the usual anatomic distribution.

The long saphenous vein and its tributaries are most commonly involved, but dilatation of the short saphenous vein is also common. In women, the varicose saphenous system may connect with the vulval venous plexus. There are often incompetent perforating veins between the deep and superficial veins in the thigh and lower leg. (Fig 40–1A–D.)

Clinical Findings

A. Symptoms: The severity of the symptoms caused by varicose veins is not necessarily correlated with the number or size of the varicosities; occasional patients with minimal varicosities complain of many symptoms, and patients with extensive involvement often have few complaints. Aching or burning discomfort, fatigue, or pain in the leg brought on by standing is the most common complaint. These symptoms gradually subside when the legs are elevated, and the individual is generally more comfortable in the morning than later in the day. Aching pain or cramps in the calf which appear during walking and subside during rest are caused by arterial insufficiency and should not be ascribed to varicosities; vein surgery is generally contraindicated if significant arterial insufficiency is also present. Itching may occur if an associated eczematoid dermatitis is present.

B. Signs: Dilated, tortuous, elongated veins beneath the skin in the thigh and leg are usually visible when the patient is standing; in very obese patients, inspection may fail to disclose the presence and extent of varicose veins, and palpation and percussion over the vein to elicit a fluid wave along the course of the vein proximal and distal to the point of percussion may be of more value. If the varicosities are of long duration, brownish pigmentation, thinning of the skin, and even a weeping dermatitis may be present above the ankles, particularly on the medial aspect. Swelling may occur, but signs of severe chronic venous stasis such as extensive swelling, fibrosis, pigmentation, and ulceration of the lower leg usually denote the postphlebitic state.

C. Special Examinations:

1. The Brodie-Trendelenburg test–(Fig 40–2.) The affected leg is elevated and the veins emptied by gravity. A tourniquet is then applied around the upper thigh sufficiently tight to constrict the saphenous vein but not the femoral artery or vein. The patient then stands upright, and the degree of filling of the saphenous varicosities is noted with the tourniquet in place and again when it is removed. The results and their interpretations are as follows:

a. With the tourniquet in place, the varicosities remain collapsed throughout a 30-second period; upon release of the tourniquet, the long saphenous vein and the varicosities rapidly fill with blood from above. *Interpretation:* These findings suggest that the valves in the saphenous vein at the saphenofemoral junction are incompetent but the valves of the communicating veins are intact and functioning. (Fig 40–1C.)

b. The varicosities fill within 30 seconds with the tourniquet in place. Upon release of the tourniquet, no increased filling of the veins is observed. *Interpretation:* The filling is due to incompetence of the communicating veins and no retrograde flow has taken place through the saphenofemoral junction. (Fig 40–1D.)

c. The varicosities fill rapidly with the tourniquet

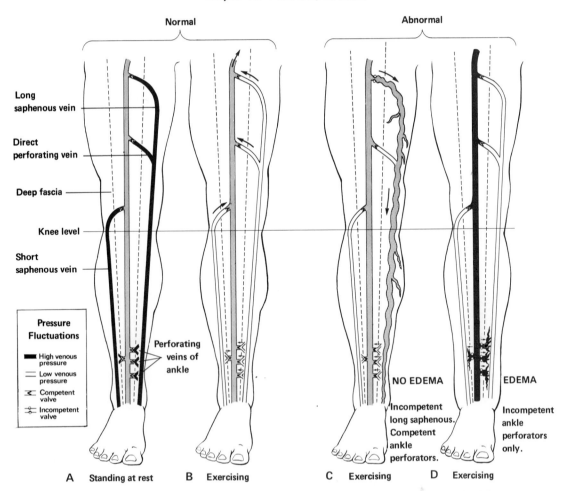

FIG 40–1. Normal venous physiology during standing (A) and walking (B), and abnormalities during exercise (C, D). Pressure in the superficial veins is diminished (if the valves are competent) by the pumping action of the muscles, which facilitates venous return to the heart (B). When the proximal valves are incompetent, the superficial veins become varicose, but competence of the valves in the distal communicators maintains the integrity of the muscle pump, and pressure remains high in the superficial veins even during exercise (C). If the valves of the leg communicators are incompetent, the muscle pump is ineffective even when the valves in the thigh are competent, and the venous pressure at the ankle remains high even during exercise (D). This produces edema, diapedesis of red cells, poor tissue nutrition, and, ultimately, ulceration (postphlebitic syndrome).

in place but become even further distended when the tourniquet is released. *Interpretation:* The valves at the saphenofemoral junction as well as the valves of one or more communicating veins are incompetent. (Fig 40–1C and D.)

d. If varices in the leg fill within less than 30 seconds with the tourniquet at the mid-thigh level but remain relatively empty with the tourniquet at the level of the knee, an incompetent short saphenous vein should be suspected.

e. With the tourniquet in place, and again with it removed, there is only slow filling of the veins from below. *Interpretation:* The valves of both the saphenous and communicating system of veins are competent and varicose veins are not present. (Fig 40–1A.)

Differential Diagnosis

Primary varicosities should be differentiated from those secondary to the following: (1) Chronic venous insufficiency of the deep system of veins (see below). (2) Extrinsic or occlusive retroperitoneal venous obstruction. (3) Arteriovenous fistulas (congenital or acquired). A bruit is present and a thrill is often palpable. (4) Congenital venous malformations. These are noted at birth or soon after. Phlebography is often of value in defining the extent of the malformation.

Complications

If thin, atrophic, pigmented skin has developed at the ankle, secondary ulcerations may occur—often as a result of little or no trauma. An ulcer will occasionally extend into the varix and the resulting fistula will

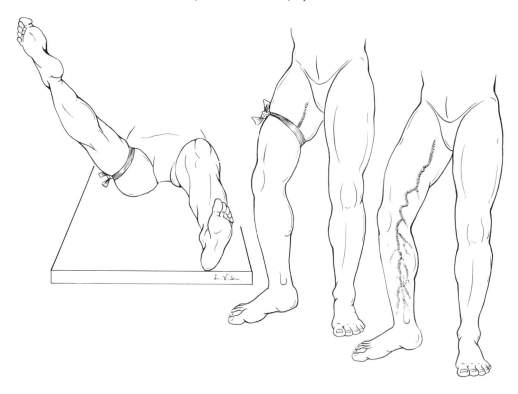

FIG 40–2. Positive Brodie-Trendelenburg test. Blood refluxes into the varicosities through incompetent valves at the saphenofemoral junction when the tourniquet is released. Absence of distal filling while the tourniquet is in place for 30 seconds indicates that the valves of the communicating veins between the superficial and the deep systems are competent. (Fig 40–1C.)

result in profuse hemorrhage. This should be controlled by elevation of the leg and local pressure on the bleeding point.

Thrombophlebitis may develop in the varicosities, particularly in pregnant or postpartum women or those taking oral contraceptives. Local trauma or prolonged periods of sitting may also lead to superficial venous thrombosis. Extension into the deep venous system by way of the perforating veins or through the saphenofemoral junction may occur. (See Thrombophlebitis, Superficial and Deep, below.) Stasis dermatitis. may also be a problem. (See Chronic Venous Insufficiency.)

Prevention

Individuals with a strong family history of varicose veins, particularly if their work involves a great deal of standing or if they become pregnant, should use elastic stockings to protect their veins from overdistention during long periods of sitting or standing.

Treatment

A. Nonsurgical Treatment: Elastic stockings (medium or heavy weight) supporting the proximal foot and the leg to just below the knee and intermittent elevation of the legs constitute the therapeutic approach in most elderly patients, in those that refuse or wish to defer surgery, and sometimes in women with mild or moderate varicosities who are going to have more children. Individuals with very early varicosities—particularly those with a strong family history of varicosities—may also benefit from the use of elastic stockings.

B. Surgical Treatment: The surgical treatment of varicose veins entails the interruption or removal of the varicosities and the incompetent perforating veins. Accurate delineation and division of the latter is required to prevent recurrence. The initial procedure is transection and ligation of the long saphenous vein at its junction with the femoral vein combined with ligation of the 5 or 6 tributaries joining the terminal 1–10 cm of this vein. Ligation of the saphenous vein at its junction with the femoral vein is important for the following reasons: (1) to eliminate a cul-de-sac which might act as the source of a propagating thrombus into the common femoral vein; and (2) to make certain that all the tributaries that could act as the origin of recurrent varicosities are ligated. These tributaries, which vary greatly in their anatomic pattern, are the superficial circumflex iliac, epigastric, and external pudendal veins, the deep external pudic vein, and, a few centimeters distally, the lateral and medial superficial femoral cutaneous tributaries.

Additional surgical procedures employed after the high ligation depend on the following: (1) The distribution of the varicosities and of the incompetent perforating veins (if present). (2) The possible involvement of the short saphenous vein with varicosities. (3) The age and general condition of the patient. (4) The basic condition of the deep venous system (see Chronic Venous Insufficiency, below). (5) The presence of significant arterial occlusive disease in the leg.

Preoperatively, the course of the varicosities and the location of incompetent perforators must be carefully marked with an indelible solution which will last through a thorough surgical skin preparation.

Ulcerations and stasis dermatitis should be treated and allowed to heal before vein surgery, particularly if stripping procedures are to be used. Skin grafting of the ulcer or the wound created by excision of the ulcer is occasionally necessary.

The surgical procedures available are as follows.

1. **Stripping**–The long saphenous veins are usually removed, although in the poor-risk or elderly patient ligation of the long saphenous at the saphenofemoral junction without stripping is an acceptable compromise. The veins are removed from the ankle to the proximal end, generally with an internal stripper. A general anesthetic is required, at least for the stripping phase of the procedure. Bleeding from the tributaries after stripping is controlled by pressure. Ligation of secondary varicosities associated with incompetent perforations or significant collateral veins should be included with the stripping procedure.

2. **Ligation**–

a. Multiple distal ligations of the tributaries of the saphenous vein and the incompetent perforators may be employed in older patients, in those with minimal varicosities, or in those undergoing treatment for recurrence following a previous stripping procedure. The entire procedure can be done under local anesthesia and is associated with less morbidity than the stripping procedures; however, there is a higher incidence of recurrent varicosities.

b. Multiple incompetent perforators can sometimes be exposed and ligated deep to the deep fascia through a long longitudinal incision in the leg.

C. **Sclerotherapy:** Sclerotherapy of residual small varicosities following definitive varicose vein surgery is occasionally necessary. This method of treatment is ancillary to surgical eradication and is of use in varices remaining after surgery, small recurrent varices, and in varicosities of very superficial, thin-walled veins. It should not be employed as the primary treatment of well-established varicose veins; in the presence of infection, arteriosclerosis, or thrombophlebitis; or in allergic or pregnant individuals.

The chemically caused thrombus must be small in order to encourage adhesions of opposing traumatized vein intima and thus obliteration of the venous channel. Sodium tetradecyl sulfate (Sotradecol), 3%, is currently favored and is more effective when used as a foam as follows: (1) 0.5 ml of the solution and 0.5 ml of air are aspirated into a small syringe and a foam is formed by shaking the mixture. (2) With the leg dependent and after aspirating 0.25 ml more air into the

syringe, the 25 gauge needle is inserted into the vein. (This can be verified by observing blood flow into the syringe and the injection of the small amount of air in the syringe to be sure there is no paravenous emphysema.) With the needle thus definitely in the vein, the foam and solution are injected and the needle is removed. (3) After injection, the leg is placed in a horizontal position, a gauze pad is placed over the vein, and a blood pressure cuff is inflated for 5 minutes to 10 mm Hg above the patient's diastolic pressure. (4) An elastic bandage is then applied from the foot to the knee with a thin foam rubber pad to occlude the vein which has been injected.

Prognosis

Varicose vein surgery is major surgery which should be done only by surgeons who have a thorough knowledge of the anatomy of the region and the principles involved. The most common causes of recurrent varicosities are failure to detect and ligate all perforating veins, failure to remove a varicose short saphenous system, inadequate dissection and ligation of the tributaries of the great saphenous vein at its junction with the common femoral vein, and failure to recognize and ligate (when possible) communicating veins between the pelvic venous plexus and the medial and posterior thigh veins. Wound infections and deep thrombophlebitis can complicate the surgery, and arterial injuries have resulted in loss of limb.

Recurrent varicosities do occur in spite of surgery which is properly performed in approximately 10% of patients. The venous pathogenetic defect may allow varicosities to develop in the remaining superficial veins, and additional surgery may be necessary–though usually not until years have passed.

Carter BN II, Johns TNP: Recurrent varicose veins: Anatomical and physiological observations. Ann Surg 159:1017–1023, 1964.

Dodd H, Cockett FB: *The Pathology of the Veins of the Lower Limb.* Livingstone, 1956.

Hershey FB, Calman CH: Pp 247–268 in: *Atlas of Vascular Surgery,* 2nd ed. Mosby, 1967.

Massell TB, Raphael HA: Causes and prevention of failure in varicose vein operations. California Med 118:1–5, May 1973.

Sherman RS: Varicose veins. S Clin North America 44:1369–1381, 1964.

THROMBOPHLEBITIS

Venous thrombosis may arise as a complication of many different clinical conditions, and it can also develop in individuals who have been active and in good health. The thrombotic process, once established, is generally quite similar, though the initiating causes may be quite variable–eg, exposure of subendothelial tissue by local trauma to the endothelium of the vein, a variety of intravascular stimuli affecting the blood (antigen-antibody complexes, viruses, bacteria, and endotoxins).

Within a few days, the thrombus becomes adherent to the vein wall and secondary inflammation develops. There is less danger of an embolus at this stage, though there may still be a free-floating tail in a more proximal vein. Ultimately, the thrombus is invaded by fibroblasts, resulting in scarring of the wall of the vein and destruction of its valves. Central recanalization may occur with restoration of blood flow, although directional control is permanently lost because valves do not regain competency. The resulting venous stasis and altered hemodynamic forces cause dependent edema and ultimately the other distressing sequelae of the postphlebitic leg (see below).

1. THROMBOPHLEBITIS OF THE DEEP VEINS
(See Fig 40–3.)

Essentials of Diagnosis
- There may be no clinical manifestations.
- Pain or discomfort may be present in the involved extremity.
- Swelling of the calf or the entire lower extremity may be present.
- Calf tenderness and a positive Homans sign may be elicited.
- Tachycardia, fever, and anxiety may be present.

General Considerations

Thrombophlebitis of the deep veins of the lower extremity develops most commonly in individuals who have sustained severe trauma, those that have undergone major surgery or are in the early postpartum period, and those that are suffering from acute or chronic cardiac disease or strokes. The thrombosis apparently develops during the major surgical procedure or in the first 24 hours following operation (or trauma), and thrombosis, which can be minimal and limited to the deep calf veins, occurs in 30–50% of these patients. Other conditions that predispose to this complication are age, malignancy, prolonged immobilization, prior episodes of thrombophlebitis, obesity, prolonged periods of sitting (such as long airplane or automobile trips), and birth control pills. Fractures of the long bones of the lower extremity commonly lead

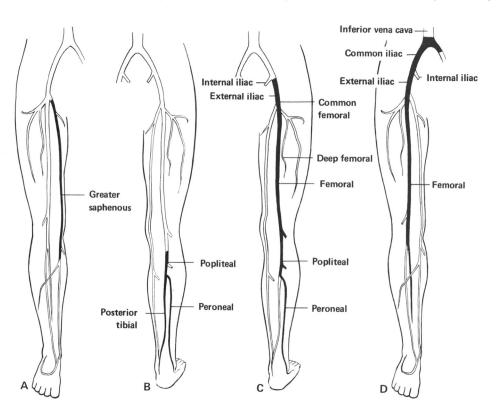

FIG 40–3. Common patterns of venous thrombosis. *A:* Superficial thrombophlebitis. *B:* The most common form of deep thrombophlebitis. *C and D:* Deep thrombophlebitis from the calf to the iliac veins. These patterns produce phlegmasia alba dolens or, if more complete, phlegmasia cerulea dolens. The usual locations of thrombosis in milk leg are shown in C. (Reproduced, with permission, from Haller JA Jr: *Deep Thrombophlebitis: Pathophysiology and Treatment.* Vol 6 in: *Major Problems in Surgery.* Dunphy JE [consulting editor]. Saunders, 1967.)

to venous thrombosis, and the uninjured leg is involved almost as frequently as the injured one (though swelling is more frequent in the injured leg).

The local manifestations are related to the venous stasis or obstruction which results from the presence of the thrombus (swelling, fullness of the superficial veins) and the inflammatory reaction in the vein wall and the perivenous tissue to the thrombus (pain and local tenderness). The thrombosis is asymptomatic in about 50% of cases and may occur in more than one vein in the same extremity. Even when the thrombotic process is very extensive, there may be no local clinical manifestations, and emboli may go to the lung from a leg which is clinically normal and without any manifestations of thrombophlebitis.

Clinical Findings

There may be no symptoms or signs in the extremity, particularly in the early stages.

A. Symptoms: An aching discomfort, a "tight" feeling, or a definite pain may be noted in the calf or the thigh or the entire extremity. This may be noted only when walking or when contracting the calf muscles. A feeling of anxiety is not uncommon.

B. Signs: Typical findings, though quite variable, are as follows: Tenderness and induration or spasm in the calf muscles, slight swelling of the ankle and calf (as noted by careful measurements of the circumference of both legs at the same levels), pain in the calf resulting from forceful dorsiflexion of the foot by the examiner (Homans' sign), slight fullness of the superficial veins, warmth of the affected leg when both legs are exposed to room temperature for a few minutes, slight fever, and tachycardia. When the femoral and iliac veins are involved there may be tenderness over these veins and when a significant obstruction has developed, swelling in the entire extremity may be marked (phlegmasia alba dolens). This extremity may become pale and cool, with diminished pulsations, if reflex arterial spasm is superimposed. If major venous obstruction develops, it may become slightly or markedly cyanotic (phlegmasia cerulea dolens). Venous collaterals may appear over the trunk. Very significant fluid loss into such an extremity may occur; gangrene may even develop.

C. Laboratory Findings: Phlebography of the deep venous channels in the lower extremity may reveal thrombi in one or more of the major venous channels, but some major veins that may contain thrombi such as the profunda femoris and the internal iliac will not be defined. Because the clinical diagnosis of thrombophlebitis is difficult and sometimes inaccurate—and because the treatment is both prolonged and relatively expensive—it may be advisable in cases where the diagnosis is uncertain to confirm the diagnosis by phlebography before starting treatment. Ultrasound may be used to detect deep venous occlusion and may prove to be a safe, simple, and rapid screening procedure to detect thrombosis in the larger veins in high-risk patients. Thrombosis in the small calf veins may not be detected by either of these procedures. The skin

temperature may be slightly higher in the involved extremity. Isotope scanning technics using radioactive iodine-labeled fibrinogen have been used and are accurate in the early detection of a developing thrombosis, and there may be more general use of the test in the future.

Differential Diagnosis

Calf muscle strain or contusion may be difficult to differentiate from thrombophlebitis; phlebography may be required to determine the true diagnosis.

Cellulitis may be confused with thrombophlebitis, but there is usually an associated wound, and inflammation of the skin is more marked with infection.

Obstruction of the lymphatics or the iliac vein in the retroperitoneal area from tumor or irradiation may lead to unilateral swelling, but it is usually more chronic and painless. Bilateral leg edema is more apt to be due to heart or renal disease. An acute arterial occlusion is more painful, the distal pulses are absent, there is usually no swelling, and the superficial veins fill slowly when emptied.

Complications

A. Postphlebitic Venous Incompetence: (See Chronic Venous Insufficiency, below.) This complication occurs commonly as a consequence of destruction of the venous valves. The saphenous as well as the deep veins may be involved.

B. Gangrene: Necrosis of skin and even the deeper tissues may develop on rare occasions, particularly in individuals with associated arterial occlusive disease and in those in whom extensive thrombosis has almost completely occluded the veins in the extremity.

C. Pulmonary Embolism: Fragmentation of the thrombus in the leg or pelvic veins with embolization to the lungs is a common and dangerous complication of venous thrombosis. This is discussed in Chapter 22.

Prevention

Preventive measures during major surgical procedures are undoubtedly of great importance and should include elevation of the patient's legs by 15 degrees during the operation. Simple measures that involve inconvenience but no risk to the patients should be used whenever possible. They include the following:

A. Postoperative Care: Leg exercises (active or passive) should be carried out at frequent intervals, particularly in patients confined to bed (stroke and cardiac patients), immediately after a long surgical procedure (when the patient is in the recovery room), and throughout the postoperative, posttrauma, or postpartum period. Early ambulation should be ordered whenever possible. The foot of the bed should be elevated to 15–20 degrees to encourage venous drainage from the legs, and elevation of the head of the bed and the segment of the bed beneath the knees should be minimized. Elastic stockings or bandages on the lower legs (particularly in patients with a history of thrombophlebitis or in those with varicose veins) may help prevent venous stasis.

TABLE 40–1. Prothrombin depressants. Oral dosages (as single doses) and duration of effect.

	1st Day	2nd Day	Usual Daily Maintenance and Range	Approximate Time to Peak Effect (Days)	Approximate Duration of Effect (Days)
Dicumarol	200–400 mg	100–200 mg	100 mg (25–150)	2–3	4
Warfarin (Coumadin, Panwarfin, Athrombin-K)	30–50 mg	10–15 mg	7.5 mg (5–15)	1–2	2–3

Brief but regular periods of walking during long airplane and automobile trips should be encouraged. Venous thrombosis and pulmonary embolism do occur during such times even in active, healthy adults.

B. Treatment of Predisposing Conditions: Hypovolemic shock, dehydration, anemia, infections, and congestive heart failure should be recognized and treated promptly and aggressively, particularly in older patients and those with cancer. Birth control pills should be discontinued for at least several weeks prior to elective surgery.

C. Anticoagulants: Prophylactic anticoagulant agents may be employed in the categories of patients most likely to develop thromboembolic complications, and there is growing evidence that the incidence can be significantly reduced by drugs.

1. Prothrombin depressants–(Table 40–1.) If started soon after severe injury and hospital admission and maintained through the period of immobilization, these agents can lower the incidence of thromboembolic problems in high-risk patients. Few bleeding complications occur when the drugs are used carefully. A therapeutic effect is generally not achieved until the third day. Venous thrombosis and embolism can occur in spite of such measures.

2. Dextran 40–Dextran affects platelet adhesiveness and imparts a coating of similar electrical charge on the erythrocytes, platelets, and endothelial cells lining the vessels, causing them to repel each other. It also dilutes the clotting factors and improves blood flow. It produces no bleeding tendency if limited to 15 ml/kg/24 hours, and the usual dose is 7–10 ml/kg/24 hours. The incidence of thrombophlebitis may be reduced if 500 ml of 6% solution are given each day over a period of 6–8 hours, starting before surgery in high-risk patients and continuing on a daily basis for 3 days and then every other day until the convalescent period is finished. Dextran may be safer than warfarin or heparin in the early postoperative or posttrauma period, when bleeding complications can occur. Only in excessive amounts will it interfere with normal clotting mechanisms, and yet it may reduce the postoperative and posttrauma hypercoagulability. It should not be used in patients with cardiac or renal failure or in those with known preexisting coagulopathy or hypersensitivity to the drug. It potentiates the effect of heparin and the antiprothrombin drugs and should thus be used with these drugs with great caution and with reduced dosage of the drugs. It should not be

used after massive transfusions.

3. Heparin–Heparin in low doses (5000 units subcut every 8–12 hours) has been demonstrated by radioactive isotope scanning technics to have significant prophylactic efficiency in high-risk surgical and medical patients. Even when started preoperatively and continued for 7–9 days following surgery, the incidence of serious hemorrhagic complications does not appear to be increased.

Treatment

A. Local Measures: Place the patient at bed rest with the foot of the bed elevated 15–20 degrees and the head of the bed in the horizontal position to encourage venous return (with pillows as desired under head and shoulders). After 5–10 days, when the local inflammation has resulted in a more adherent thrombus–and provided the swelling and local symptoms have largely subsided–walking but not standing or sitting is permitted.

Elastic bandages or stockings are used on the foot and leg both during the initial treatment and in the subsequent months (until all tendency toward swelling of the leg has permanently disappeared).

B. Anticoagulants: Anticoagulants should be started immediately in most patients with deep thrombophlebitis with or without pulmonary embolism. The incidence of pulmonary embolism complicating thrombophlebitis is significantly reduced by adequate anticoagulant therapy. Progression of the local thrombosis is halted, and the local symptoms subside as the acute inflammatory reaction in the vein wall subsides.

Contraindications to the use of anticoagulants are active ulcerative diseases of the gastrointestinal tract, blood dyscrasias, severe liver or kidney disease, subacute bacterial endocarditis, severe hypertension, open ulcerative wounds, and very recent surgery (particularly on the CNS or eye). The oral agents are contraindicated during pregnancy and lactation.

Heparin is the drug of choice, at least during the initial phase of treatment, and anticoagulation should be continued for at least 10 days for venous thrombosis and 21 days if pulmonary embolism has occurred. Treatment should be continued for at least 3 days after all local pain and tenderness in the extremity have subsided, most or all of the swelling has disappeared, and ambulation has been fully established. The rate of subsidence of symptoms is variable, and occasional cases are quite refractory to therapy, so that treatment lasting many weeks or months may be necessary. This is particularly true in individuals who develop the thrombosis without any antecedent injury or operation, in those with a history of prior episodes of thrombophlebitis, and in those who have had one or more emboli. A prothrombin depressant drug is generally used for such long-term management, and the heparin is discontinued when the prothrombin time has been prolonged to the therapeutic range.

Though dextran 40 has been used as the primary drug in patients with acute thrombosis, it probably should be reserved for prophylactic rather than therapeutic uses (see above). It may be more specifically indicated as the therapeutic agent in the very recent postoperative patient who would probably hemorrhage if given heparin.

1. Heparin—Heparin, which inactivates thrombin before the thrombin can act on fibrinogen, is generally used during the first phase of anticoagulant therapy because of its rapid action and relative efficiency, and many prefer to use heparin throughout the course of therapy. Others use heparin until the symptoms and signs of thrombophlebitis have largely or completely subsided (for the first 7—14 days) and then shift to the prothrombin depressant drugs for the final phase (stopping heparin when the prothrombin time has been depressed to the therapeutic range, generally a matter of 3 or 4 days).

The whole blood partial thromboplastin time (WBPTT), the activated clotting time (ACT), or the Lee-White clotting time (LWCT) and the prothrombin time should be determined before initiating heparin therapy. The normal pretreatment range for the WBPTT test is 55—75 seconds; for the ACT, 80—130 seconds (at 37 C); and for the LWCT, 6—15 minutes (mean, 10 minutes).

The dose required to establish a therapeutic range may vary considerably with individuals or even with the same patient at different stages of therapy. (Smaller doses are often sufficient later in the period of treatment.) The therapeutic dose must be determined by laboratory determinations, and several measurements may be necessary before the proper dose is ascertained. One test each day, with the blood sample drawn 30—60 minutes before the next anticipated heparin dose, is usually all that is necessary once the general dose range for an individual has been determined. The therapeutic range as determined by the WBPTT or the ACT test is 1½—2 times the baseline pretreatment value; if the LWCT is the test used, the therapeutic range is 2—4 times the baseline pretreatment value. A test near the lower limits of the therapeutic range immediately prior to the next scheduled heparin dose is desired; if it is close to the upper limit of the range or above, further heparin should be delayed until the effect of the previous dose has diminished. The dosage regulation must be done with great care in patients who have had recent surgery or injuries; aspirin ingestion in the week prior to treatment may also add to the risk of hemorrhagic complications because of the effect on platelet function.

Several methods of administration are available:

a. Deep subcutaneous—For the adult of average size, sodium heparin, 6000—8000 units every 6 hours, is a convenient starting dose. After several days of therapy, the required dose usually drops to a range of 4000—6000 units. Some prefer an 8-hour schedule with somewhat larger doses (10,000—12,000 units), and some use still a larger dose (14,000—20,000 units) on a 12-hour schedule. Hematomas at the injection site can be expected.

b. Intravenous—Intermittent intravenous injections of sodium heparin may be used. The usual initial dose is 5000 units followed by an individualized dose of 5000—8000 units every 4 hours. Occasionally, a continuous intravenous infusion may be used, beginning with 10,000 units in 1 liter of 5% glucose at 15—25 drops/minute and altering the rate of flow depending on frequent laboratory determinations (approximately every 4 hours). Control is more difficult by this route, but its use is sometimes worthwhile in a patient manifesting extreme thrombotic tendencies and in those that must be anticoagulated very rapidly with a large dose—eg, the patient who has just had a massive pulmonary embolism. The postembolic reflex bronchial constriction appears to be blocked by large doses of heparin in the range of 15,000 units initially and 80—100 thousand units in the first 24 hours. There is clinical evidence that some patients that would otherwise die in the first few hours after a massive pulmonary embolism will survive if vigorously treated with these very large doses of heparin in the first 24—48 hours.

2. Prothrombin depressants—(Table 40—1.) The prothrombin depressants differ from each other in rapidity of onset and duration of effect. Although the actual rates are dependent upon dose, approximate values for comparison are given in Table 40—1. Dicumarol and warfarin are the most widely used drugs in this group.

A good therapeutic effect has been achieved when prothrombin activity has fallen to at least 25%, preferably between 10 and 20%, or when the prothrombin time is 2—2½ times the control. At the beginning of treatment, daily prothrombin activities should be determined and the subsequent dose withheld until the report is received. In well-stabilized patients, weekly or even monthly determinations may be adequate.

The usual starting doses and maintenance doses of the common antiprothrombin drugs are shown in Table 40—1. Patients with initial activities below 80—100% should receive smaller doses.

Interaction of these drugs with other drugs does occur, and careful clinical and laboratory supervision of patients on oral anticoagulants is mandatory when other medications are being given.

3. Treatment of bleeding and overdosage—The principal danger of anticoagulant therapy is abnormal bleeding. In bleeding due to heparin excess, the coagulation time can be rapidly returned to normal by administering 1% protamine sulfate in physiologic saline intravenously to neutralize the heparin. Give a dose in mg equal to 0.01 of the number of units of heparin administered. If there is active hemorrhage, fresh blood may also be used.

Bleeding due to excess prothrombin depressants is more difficult to control, for the prothrombin activity rises slowly after therapy is discontinued.

Phytonadione (Mephyton and Aqua-Mephyton) is indicated in patients receiving the prothrombin depressant drugs who must have the prothrombin activity returned to normal—either because they are bleeding (spontaneously or from trauma) or because emergency surgery is necessary. To correct excessive hypoprothrombinemia, with or without a minor hemorrhage and when continued anticoagulant therapy is anticipated, 5–10 mg orally may be enough. Severe hemorrhage should be treated by the slow, intravenous administration of the drug in a dose of 10–40 mg; if the liver is normal, a safe range may be achieved in 4–24 hours. (Repeated injections may be required over 2–3 days.) Fresh blood transfusion may also be indicated if active hemorrhage is present to restore blood volume and replace clotting factors during the latent period of phytonadione's action.

C. Surgical Measures:

1. **Venous ligation or plication procedures**—When the risk of pulmonary embolism is great in an individual with known or suspected thrombophlebitis and when anticoagulants are contraindicated or are thought to be inadequate, venous ligation or plication may be indicated in the following circumstances: (1) When there is a significant danger of hemorrhage from a large, fresh wound, an active peptic ulcer, or ulcerative colitis. (2) When a very large pulmonary embolus has already occurred, and it is thought an additional embolus (even a small one) will be fatal. (3) When there have been multiple small emboli over a period of time, and pulmonary insufficiency is developing. (4) When there is septic pelvic phlebitis. (5) When pulmonary embolism has occurred while the patient has been well anticoagulated. (6) Occasionally, in conjunction with a distal thrombectomy or a pulmonary embolectomy.

Venous interruption may be performed at the level of the inferior vena cava or the femoral vein.

a. **Inferior vena cava**—This is the procedure of choice in most cases when ligation is indicated and the preferred level is just below the renal veins because at this point there is less chance of thrombosis above the point of ligation. Some prefer total interruption of the vena cava with ligature; others advocate partial interruption (plication) by means of a plastic clip which reduces the channel to a number of separate 2–3 mm channels, thus allowing continued flow through the cava but trapping any large embolus. (Such an embolus will result in total caval occlusion, and propagation of thrombus through the small channels with subsequent emboli from above the clip may occur in about 15% of cases.) Postoperative emboli occur in 4–15% even in patients whose cavas have been ligated (from above the ligature or through the ovarian or testicular vein); for this reason, the ovarian veins should be ligated at the time of caval interruption in women. The operative

mortality is high (10–15%). Additional postoperative thrombosis in the leg veins may be a major acute or long-term problem; dextran in the early postoperative period (shifting later to heparin) together with elevation of the legs may reduce this problem.

b. **Femoral vein**—Femoral vein ligation is occasionally indicated and may be adequate if there is clinical and x-ray evidence that the thrombosis is in the calf and lower thigh. Suture plication of the common femoral vein, reducing the channel into 3 smaller lumens, is now being advocated as a means of filtering out possible emboli without producing the extensive thrombosis of the veins in the lower extremity distal to the point of ligation which has occasionally resulted in a very significant accentuation of the acute thrombotic process in the extremity. Because of the high incidence of bilateral thrombophlebitis, even when there is no clinical evidence of involvement of both legs, the procedure should usually be carried out on both legs, and, because the deep femoral vein may be the source of the emboli, the common rather than the superficial femoral is generally ligated. This can be carried out under local anesthesia. Anticoagulant therapy should be continued in the postoperative period.

Phlegmasia alba and cerulea dolens. Acute iliofemoral thrombophlebitis characteristically produces an extensive painful swelling of the limb with pallor and varying degrees of mottling. The term phlegmasia alba dolens applies to the more common white, painful swelling. In extreme cases, there may be extensive cyanosis progressing to gangrene (phlegmasia cerulea dolens).

Treatment may involve the following: (1) Immediate intravenous heparin anticoagulant therapy using liberal doses of the drug. (2) The marked edema should be combated by elevating the legs to 45 degrees. (3) Associated arterial insufficiency may force a modification of this approach, and a translumbar sympathetic block (before the heparin is started) may be of value. (4) Active fluid replacement is often necessary to correct for the fluid, plasma protein, and electrolyte loss into the extremity and to treat the shock that may exist. (5) Diuretics and digitalis are indicated in cardiac patients. (6) Antibiotics are indicated in the cyanotic form because of the danger of infection in the cutaneous bullae or gangrene that may develop.

These measures will generally result in a gradual reversal of the process, although the edema may subside very slowly and a relatively prolonged hospital stay may be required.

Thrombectomy, a procedure which is still under clinical investigation, is advocated as a means of prompt decompression of obstructed iliac and femoral veins and of establishing flow through them. Half the patients with phlegmasia cerulea dolens develop superimposed gangrene and almost a third die; in this condition, the procedure may not only save the limb but also the life of the patient.

If extensive ileofemoral thrombosis has been present for less than 48 hours, the thrombus can usually be removed through a common femoral venotomy under local anesthesia with the patient heparinized. The proximal thrombus may be forced out when the patient performs the Valsalva maneuver. Fogarty venous (balloon-tipped) catheters may aid in clearing out the proximal thrombus, or catheter suction using a large syringe may be of value. The distal thrombus will generally be extruded if forceful manual compression of the calf and thigh is carried out or if a heavy rubber compression bandage is applied. Elevation of the leg (wrapped with elastic bandages) and continued heparin therapy to prevent rethrombosis and possible embolus are most important.

Postoperative embolus, though possible, is not frequent, and the extreme swelling and discomfort in the extremity generally subside rapidly. Liberal blood replacement is necessary, and wound hematomas and secondary infection are a hazard. Rethrombosis, though often not associated with the major swelling that initially developed, leads to poor results in at least one-third of cases.

Prognosis

With adequate treatment, the patient usually recovers from the acute thrombophlebitis within 2–4 weeks. The prognosis is good once the danger of pulmonary embolism has passed, but massive pulmonary embolus during the first 2–3 weeks may occur. Recurrent episodes of phlebitis may occasionally occur in spite of good local and anticoagulant management, and there may be associated emboli. Chronic venous insufficiency often occurs within 5–10 years.

Atik M & others: Pulmonary embolism: A preventable complication. Am Surgeon 34:888–894, 1968.

Bertelsen S & others: Phlegmasia coerulea dolens. Acta chir scandinav 134:107–114, 1968.

Freeark RJ & others: Post-traumatic venous thrombosis. Arch Surg 95:567–575, 1967.

Gallus AS & others: Small subcutaneous doses of heparin in prevention of venous thrombosis. New England J Med 288:545–551, 1973.

Haller JA Jr: *Deep Thrombophlebitis: Pathophysiology and Treatment.* Saunders, 1967.

Hershey FB & others: Phlebography in diagnosis and management of venous disease of the legs. M Clin North America 51:161–174, 1967.

Hume M, Sevitt S, Thomas DP: *Venous Thrombosis and Pulmonary Embolism.* Harvard Univ Press, 1970.

Martard JF & others: Thromboembolism: A manifestation of the response of blood to injury. Circulation 42:1–21, 1970.

Mosher KM: *Pulmonary Thromboembolism.* Year Book, 1973.

Negous D & others: [121]I-labeled fibrinogen in the diagnosis of deep-vein thrombosis and its correlation with phlebography. Brit J Surg 55:835–839, 1968.

Sevitt S & others: Venous thrombosis and pulmonary embolism: Clinicopathological study in injured and burned patients. Brit J Surg 48:475–489, 1961.

Skinner DB & others: Anticoagulant prophylaxis in surgical patients. Surg Gynec Obst 125:741–746, 1967.

THROMBOPHLEBITIS OF SUPERFICIAL VEINS

Thrombophlebitis in the superficial veins may occur spontaneously, as in pregnant or postpartum women or in individuals with varicose veins or thromboangiitis obliterans; or it may follow trauma, as after a blow to the leg. It is sometimes the result of venous infusion of irritating solutions. In the migratory or recurrent form, thromboangiitis should be suspected. It may also be a manifestation of abdominal malignancy such as carcinoma of the pancreas and may be the earliest sign. Superficial thrombophlebitis is usually not associated with thrombosis in the deep leg veins.

The long saphenous vein is most often involved. Pulmonary emboli are infrequent but do occur.

Clinical Findings

The patient usually experiences a dull pain in the region of the involved vein. Local findings consist of raised, indurated, firm, red, and tender inflammation over a superficial vein and involving adjacent subcutaneous tissue and skin. The process may be localized, or it may involve most of the long saphenous vein and its tributaries (Fig 40–3). The inflammatory reaction generally subsides in 1–2 weeks; a firm cord may remain for a much longer period. Edema of the extremity is absent.

Differential Diagnosis

The linear rather than circular nature of the lesion and its distribution along the course of a superficial vein serve to differentiate superficial phlebitis from erythema nodosum, erythema induratum, panniculitis, and fibromyositis.

Treatment

If the process is well localized and not near the saphenofemoral junction, local heat and bed rest with the leg elevated are usually satisfactory. Phenylbutazone (Butazolidin), 100 mg 3 times daily for 5 days, will sometimes aid in the resolution of the inflammatory process.

If the process is very extensive or shows a tendency to proceed upward toward the saphenofemoral junction—or if it is near the saphenofemoral junction initially—ligation and division of the saphenous vein at the saphenofemoral junction is indicated. The inflammatory process usually regresses following this procedure, though removal of the involved segment of vein (stripping) may result in a more rapid recovery.

Anticoagulant therapy is seldom indicated but may be used when the disease is progressing rapidly or when involvement of the deep system seems imminent.

Prognosis

The course is generally benign and brief, and the prognosis depends on the underlying disease. When phlebitis of a saphenous vein extends to the deep veins, pulmonary embolism may occur.

CHRONIC VENOUS INSUFFICIENCY

Essentials of Diagnosis

- A history is often obtained of phlebitis, a leg injury, or an illness requiring a prolonged period in bed.
- Chronic ankle edema is the earliest sign.
- Subcutaneous fibrosis, stasis pigmentation or dermatitis, and often varicosities develop later.
- Ulceration at or above the ankle (stasis ulcer) is a common late complication.

General Considerations

Chronic venous insufficiency generally results from changes secondary to deep thrombophlebitis, although a definite history of phlebitis is often not obtainable. It can also occasionally occur as a result of neoplastic obstruction of the pelvic veins or congenital or acquired arteriovenous fistula.

When insufficiency is secondary to deep thrombophlebitis (postphlebitic syndrome, the valves in the deep venous channels and sometimes in the perforating veins have been damaged or destroyed. These recanalized, valveless, irregular veins are functionally inadequate, and the venous blood is not effectively pumped out of the legs as it is in an individual with normal veins by the contracting calf muscles when the patient walks. Thus, unlike the normal situation in which the venous pressure falls when the leg muscles are contracting, the venous pressure in the postphlebitic lower extremity remains high at all times, ie, when the individual is walking as well as when he is sitting or standing. The tissues normally tolerate very well the intermittent rises of venous pressure that occur on standing or sitting provided there are also periods when the pressure is reduced by the muscular activity of walking or by elevation of the extremity. The subcutaneous tissues and skin of the leg and ankle do not tolerate the continuous and prolonged elevation of venous pressure that occurs as a result of impairment of the venous pumping mechanism in the postphlebitic lower extremity. In addition, veins that have not recanalized and have remained occluded add to the chronic high venous pressure, and those that are open but have been damaged are inelastic and act as a passive conduit. Ultimately, secondary changes occur: (1) Incompetence of the valves in the communicating channels between the deep and the superficial veins may develop. The continuously high venous pressure in the deep system is then transmitted to the superficial veins, frequently resulting in secondary varicosities (Fig 40–1D). Venous blood in the deep system may be forcefully extruded into the superficial veins during calf muscle contraction, accentuating the effects of the persistently high venous pressures on the superficial veins and the surrounding subcutaneous tissue and overlying skin. (2) The normal resorption of extracellular fluid into the venous end of the capillaries does not take place. The loss of normal capillary fluid exchange ultimately results in chronic edema in the lower leg and foot; protein is deposited in the extracellular space; and fibrosis and loss of elasticity of the skin and subcutaneous tissue develops. The skin ceases to function as an adequate protective barrier, and chronic dermatitis or ulcerations occur in the leg and ankle area.

Clinical Findings

Chronic venous insufficiency is characterized by progressive edema of the leg and secondary changes in the skin and subcutaneous tissues. The edema diminishes at night. The usual symptoms are itching, a dull discomfort made worse by periods of standing, and pain if an ulceration is present. The skin is usually thin, shiny, atrophic, and cyanotic and often brownish pigmentation develops. Eczema is frequently present, and there may be large areas of superficial weeping dermatitis. The subcutaneous tissues are thick and fibrous. Recurrent ulcerations are common, usually just above the ankle, on the medial or anterior aspect of the leg; healing results in a thin scar on a fibrotic base which breaks down with minor trauma. Varicosities are often present and are usually associated with incompetent perforating veins which are often close to or just proximal to the ulceration. (See Fig 40–1D.)

Differential Diagnosis

The leg edema present in chronic heart, kidney, or liver failure is usually bilateral and is generally associated with clinical or laboratory evidence of the basic disease.

Lymphedema is generally brawny and does not diminish promptly with elevation of the legs. A low-grade cellulitis may be present, and varicosities, pigmentation, and ulcerations are absent.

Patients with primary varicose veins may develop lower leg changes very similar to those of chronic venous insufficiency; venography may occasionally be necessary to differentiate the 2 disorders if the diagnosis cannot be made on the basis of the history and local findings.

Extensive ulcerations of the leg (particularly the lower third and ankle area) are most often venous in origin, but other causes include arterial inadequacy, bacterial and mycotic infections, tumors, blood diseases, and trauma. Ulcerations secondary to arterial insufficiency are generally more painful then those of venous origin (particularly when the leg is elevated); chronic swelling is usually not present; and the pedal pulses are absent.

Complications

Renewed episodes of acute thrombophlebitis may occur in individuals with chronic venous insufficiency, particularly after operations. Extra precautions should be taken during the postoperative period to prevent such reoccurrences.

Prevention

Prevention of deep thrombophlebitis is basic in

the prevention of chronic venous insufficiency. The adequate care of acute thrombophlebitis may minimize damage to the valves and thereby avoid the postphlebitic syndrome in later years. The individual who has recovered from acute thrombophlebitis should be advised that symptoms of venous insufficiency may appear after several years. The dangers of chronic leg edema should be emphasized, and the patient should be given detailed instructions about how to counteract its development by using elastic stockings, by intermittent periods of elevation of the legs, and by elevating the foot of the bed with blocks or elevating the lower portion of the mattress with pillows underneath the mattress. Long periods of sitting or standing should be avoided. If there is a tendency to develop edema, well-fitting heavy duty elastic stockings which extend from the mid foot to just below the knee should be used permanently during the day and evening.

Treatment

If adequate preventive measures have not been initiated or followed and stasis ulceration has developed, more active and aggressive treatment is necessary. Control of the persistent high venous pressures and the secondary edema is the basic goal. Initially, this can be achieved by bed rest with the legs elevated 12–18 inches above the level of the heart to facilitate return of venous blood and edema. Later, a well-fitted, semirigid boot-like support on the foot and leg (Gelcast, Gauztex, Viscopaste) may allow the individual to work while dermatitis or ulcerations heal. These boots must be changed every 1–2 weeks, and care must be taken to pad the bony prominences and the ulcer. After healing has occurred, the more convenient heavy duty lower leg elastic stocking usually will prevent a recurrence of ulcers if the patient is diligent in his self-care.

A. Stasis Dermatitis: Eczematous eruptions may be acute or chronic, and the local treatment varies accordingly.

1. Acute weeping dermatitis—Wet compresses of boric acid solution (1 tbsp/liter of water), potassium permanganate solution (100 mg/liter of water), or aluminum acetate buffered solution (Burow's solution) (2 tablets per liter of water) should be applied for 1 hour 4 times daily. Compresses are followed with 0.5% hydrocortisone cream in a water-soluble base (neomycin may be incorporated into this cream). Systemic antibiotics are indicated if active infection is present.

2. Subsiding or chronic dermatitis—Continue the hydrocortisone cream for 1–2 weeks or until no further improvement is noted. Cordran Tape, a plastic, corticosteroid-impregnated tape, is a convenient way to apply both medication and dressing.

Apply zinc oxide ointment with ichthammol (Ichthyol), 3%, 1–2 times a day, cleaned off as desired with mineral oil. Application of carbolfuchsin (Castellani's) paint to the toes and nails 1–2 times a week may help control dermatophytosis and onychomycosis. Undecylenic acid and zinc undecylenate (Desenex) powder, ointment, or aerosol may also be used.

B. Ulceration: Stasis ulcers will heal in the ambulatory patient through the use of the semirigid boot which must be changed every 10–14 days, and this approach is often satisfactory or may be necessary in the individual who cannot stop work. More rapid healing can usually be achieved—especially if the ulcer is large and associated with sloughing tissue, crusts, and chronic infection (usually multiple strains of bacteria of low virulence, particularly staphylococci and pseudomonas)—if the ulcer is treated with compresses of isotonic saline solution or buffered aluminum acetate solution. Frequent changes will clean the ulcer bed, encourage free drainage, and eliminate the need for surgical debridement. Bacteriologic studies are generally of no value, and antibiotics are seldom indicated. Bed rest with the leg elevated is an important part of this treatment. The ulcer will become shallower as edema fluid is removed from the leg; the edges will become clean; and healthy granulation tissue will appear in the base after a few days. An ulcer thus prepared (if less than 2–3 cm in diameter) will generally heal in a couple of weeks without grafting. Larger ulcers can be covered with split thickness skin grafts to shorten the overall healing time. Recurrent ulcerations are common unless varicosities and incompetent perforating veins neighboring the ulcer are eliminated and elastic stockings or bandages are used permanently on the leg. Occasionally, the ulcer is so large, scarred, and avascular that it is better to totally excise the ulcer and skin-graft the surgical wound.

C. Secondary Varicosities: Efficient and long-term external pressure over secondary varicosities of the leg will reduce the high pressure in these veins and force the blood to flow through the deep system of veins. External elastic support is necessary anyway to counteract the tendency toward edema formation.

Surgical ligation and division of the incompetent perforator veins in the leg and their associated varicose veins in the area of maximum tissue damage or ulceration is a more efficient way to eliminate the persistent high venous pressure. If the valves in the proximal end of the long saphenous vein are also incompetent (as determined by the Brodie-Trendelenburg test; see discussion in the section on varicose veins and Fig 40–2), a high saphenous ligation and stripping may also be necessary to diminish the persistent venous hypertension. The decision must be individualized depending on the local findings. Patency of the deep venous channels must be present if all or part of the main superficial veins are ligated or removed. Inadequate capacity of the deep system may be suggested by marked varicosities of the superficial veins, in which case phlebography should be performed and obstruction of most or all of the deep veins may be demonstrated. If there is any question of the capacity of the deep system, venography should be performed. If significant obstruction exists, superficial vein surgery should not be done.

Some surgeons prefer to ligate the incompetent communicating veins at the level of the deep fascia. Others use a subfascial approach to locate and divide these veins—a particularly effective approach if they are numerous (Linton procedure). A long longitudinal incision in the posterior aspect of the lower leg is usually necessary.

No surgical procedure will eliminate the need for external elastic support throughout life for all patients with symptomatic chronic venous insufficiency, though the amount of support required to prevent edema will vary.

Prognosis

Individuals with chronic venous insufficiency often have recurrent problems, particularly if measures to counteract persistent venous hypertension, edema, and secondary tissue changes are not conscientiously adhered to throughout life.

Field P, Van Boxel P: The role of the Linton flap procedure in the management of stasis dermatitis and ulceration in the lower limb. Surgery 70:920–926, 1971.

Haeger K: The treatment of the severe post-thrombotic state. A comparison of some surgical and conservative methods. Angiology 19:439–449, 1968.

Linton RR: Modern concepts in the treatment of the post-phlebitic syndrome with ulcerations of the lower extremity. Angiology 3:431–439, 1952.

Lofgren KA, Lofgren EP: Extensive ulcerations in the postphlebitic leg. S Clin North America 49:1033–1043, 1969.

Sarjeant TR: Surgical anatomy in the treatment of venous stasis. S Clin North America 44:1383–1402, 1964.

LYMPHEDEMA

Primary lymphedema is due to congenital developmental abnormalities of the lymphatics. Secondary lymphedema results from obstruction of the proximal lymphatics by trauma, regional lymph node resection or irradiation, or extensive involvement of regional nodes by malignant disease or filariasis.

The secondary dilatation of the lymphatics that occurs in both forms leads to incompetence of the valves in the lymphatics with progressive stasis of protein-rich fluid in the interstitial spaces. Recurrent attacks of lymphangitis and cellulitis, common in all forms and almost always the result rather than the cause of the edema, may add to the lymphatic obstruction and incompetence and in turn to the accumulation of edema fluid. This fluid stimulates fibroblastic proliferation, and a brawny, relatively nonpitting edema with thickened skin and subcutaneous tissue ultimately results. Stasis pigmentation, ulcerations, and varicosities do not occur.

Lymphangiography and radioactive isotope studies on the rate of uptake of subcutaneously injected material are sometimes useful in defining the specific lymphatic defect.

Primary lymphedema appears in childhood or early adult life in 80% of cases, usually in females. The earlier it develops, the greater the lymphatic defect and the worse the prognosis. In some cases, other congenital malformations may be present or there may be a familial incidence. The lymphatic channel may be absent (aplasia), small (hypoplasia), or varicose (hyperplasia). Soft pitting edema of the foot and ankle is usually the first manifestation. Later, the entire leg and often the opposite leg also may become involved. The arms are very rarely affected. Minor injury or infection may initiate swelling in a limb with marginal lymphatic reserve. Increased weight and fatigue in the limb is the usual complaint. Pain is rarely present.

Secondary lymphedema. In the leg, secondary lymphedema is most common after radical groin dissections, particularly if the external iliac nodes as well as those in the femoral triangle have been removed. It may occur after extensive irradiation of lymph nodes involved with malignant disease in the femoral, iliac, or aortic areas. The usual dependent position of the leg accentuates the drainage defect, resulting in progression of the edema and secondary changes.

In the arm, secondary lymphedema is generally the result of radical mastectomy for carcinoma of the breast. Significant swelling develops in at least 12% of patients. Although the extent of the axillary dissection, particularly along the vein, is closely related to this complication, there seems to be some variation in the ability of an individual to regenerate lymphatics and establish collateral pathways. Postoperative infection, fibrosis, and radiotherapy may impair regeneration of lymphatics.

Treatment

A. Conservative Measures: There is no very satisfactory treatment for lymphedema, but the following measures should be instituted: (1) Flow of lymph out of the extremity, with a decreased stasis, can be enhanced by intermittent elevation of the extremity. If the lower extremities are involved, the foot of the bed can be elevated on 8–12 inch blocks, or pillows may be placed beneath the mattress at the foot of the bed. Elastic bandages or carefully fitted heavy duty elastic stockings should be employed, and massage toward the trunk, either by hand or by means of pneumatic pressure devices, may be helpful. (2) Cellulitis can be a serious problem and very difficult to control. Stringent measures should be adopted to prevent infection of minor wounds or trichophytosis of the toes. Once infection starts, it should be treated by strict bed rest with elevation as well as with antibiotics. Intermittent prophylactic antibiotics may be indicated in patients with recurrent attacks of cellulitis. (3) Intermittent courses of diuretic therapy, especially in those with premenstrual or seasonal exacerbations of symptoms, may be useful.

B. Surgical Treatment: Surgery is indicated in severe cases when conservative management fails to control the size of the limb or when recurrent attacks of infection cannot be prevented by other measures. It is not indicated for cosmetic reasons since postoperative improvement in appearance is minor. Surgical treatment is often attended by a significant postoperative morbidity rate.

Many operative approaches have been tried, either to bridge the lymphatic obstruction with lymphatic-bearing tissue transferred from elsewhere or excision of the edematous skin and subcutaneous tissue with skin grafts applied to the deep fascia. The results have generally been very disappointing, particularly in patients with primary hypoplasia of the lymphatics. The most promising procedure thus far devised involves the establishment of direct anastomotic connections between the superficial obstructed lymphatics and the subfascial uninvolved lymphatics for the whole length of the limb. This can be achieved by removing a strip of epidermis for the length of the involved extremity and then constructing a longitudinal flap of the underlying dermis and subcutaneous tissue which is folded inward deep to the fascia and close to the lymphatics that accompany the major vessels of the extremity. In addition to the lymphatic communications that develop, lymphaticovenous communications may also form to add to the drainage of the congested superficial lymphatics. This operation appears to offer a reasonable solution to a notoriously difficult problem, and satisfactory or good functional results are achieved in 75% to 90% of properly selected patients.

In patients with primary hyperplasia or ectasia of the lymphatics and in those with abnormal communications between the mesenteric lymphatics and those in the pelvis and extremity (resulting in chylous cutaneous reflux), ligation of the incompetent lymphatics in the femoral or iliac area may be successful.

Amputation of a markedly involved extremity may occasionally be the best solution and is mandatory if secondary lymphangiosarcoma develops.

Prognosis

Prolonged nonoperative management of chronic lymphedema will, in most cases, prevent progressive involvement and disability but will seldom completely cure the problem except in cases with minimal involvement. New surgical methods, when used in patients with marked involvement and limitation of function or who have had repeated attacks of cellulitis, will yield satisfactory functional but not cosmetic results in most cases. Ligation of incompetent channels provides the best results, but cases in which this can be done are rare. Lymphangiosarcoma, a highly malignant tumor, may occasionally develop in an extremity with long-standing lymphedema.

Battezzati M, Donini I, Marsili E: The morphologic and physiologic basis for a new classification of lymphoedema. J Cardiovas Surg 8:52–61, 1967.

DeRoo T: The value of lymphography in lymphedema. Surg Gynec Obst 124:755–765, 1967.

Gough MH: Primary lymphoedema: Clinical and lymphangiographic studies. Brit J Surg 53:917–925, 1966.

Kinmonth JB & others: Primary lymphoedema: Clinical and lymphangiographic studies of a series of 107 patients in which the lower limbs were affected. Brit J Surg 45:1–10, 1958.

Love L, Kim SE: Clinical aspects of lymphangiography. M Clin North America 51:227–248, 1967.

Smith RD, Spitell JA Jr, Schirger A: Secondary lymphedema of the leg: Its characteristics and diagnostic implications. JAMA 185:80–82, 1963.

Taylor GW: The surgical management of primary lymphoedema. Proc Roy Soc Med 58:1024, 1965.

Thompson N: The surgical treatment of chronic lymphoedema of the extremity. S Clin North America 47:445–503, 1967.

Tough JS: Advances in plastic surgery. Practitioner 197:536, 1966.

● ● ●

General References

Fairbairn JF II & others: *Peripheral Vascular Disease,* 4th ed. Saunders, 1972.

Haeger K: *Venous and Lymphatic Disorders of the Leg.* Lippincott, 1966.

Haller JA Jr: *Deep Thrombophlebitis: Pathophysiology and Treatment.* Saunders, 1967.

Hershey FB, Calman CH: Chap 15, pp 247–279 in: *Atlas of Vascular Surgery,* 2nd ed. Mosby, 1967.

41 . . .

Neurosurgery & Surgery of the Pituitary

Charles B. Wilson, MD*

DIAGNOSIS & MANAGEMENT OF DEPRESSED STATES OF CONSCIOUSNESS

Many neurosurgical disorders—eg, trauma, brain tumor, ruptured intracranial aneurysm—produce alterations in consciousness. In approaching the unconscious patient, the priorities are emergency care, etiologic diagnosis, and definitive treatment.

Deterioration of consciousness may be instantaneous (as in cerebral concussion) but more often occurs in an orderly sequence from lethargy (sleepy, indifferent) to obtundation (dull and inactive—examiner must speak loudly to gain attention) to semicoma or stupor (no response to voice but reacts to painful stimuli) to coma (unresponsive to any external stimulus). As a rule, decerebrate rigidity of recent onset is accompanied by stupor. Crude responsiveness is retained in akinetic mutism.

Differential Diagnosis

Initially, the examiner may be able to fit a suspected pathologic process into one of the following categories: trauma, increased intracranial pressure, cerebrovascular accident, cerebral hypoxia, poisoning, metabolic disorder, or infection. The history is often sufficient to establish the diagnosis. However, the epileptic or the alcoholic may have a subdural hematoma; the diabetic may have meningitis; and the hypertensive patient may have struck his head when felled by a cerebrovascular accident.

In the absence of historical and physical clues, the following diagnostic studies must be done: complete blood count and the differential white count, urinalysis, blood chemistries (glucose, BUN, sodium, chloride, CO_2), x-rays of the skull and chest, ECG, and, if physical or x-ray signs of increased intracranial pressure are absent, lumbar puncture. if the opening pressure is not > 300 mm water, fluid should be removed for cell count, glucose, and protein. Bloody CSF should be centrifuged to determine the character of the supernatant; CSF containing many white cells should be cultured for bacteria and fungi. In the presence of elevated CSF pressure, fluid should be removed slowly and in the smallest volume needed for diagnosis. (*Note:* Headache and nuchal rigidity may be due to posterior fossa tumor rather than meningitis.)

*Individual sections contributed by others as noted in the text.

Complications

Immediate threats are airway obstruction, aspiration of vomitus, atelectasis, and pneumonia.

Management

Maintain an unobstructed airway by whatever measures are required: positioning of the head and jaw, endotracheal intubation, or tracheostomy. Prevent aspiration of vomitus by emptying the stomach, nasogastric suction, and placing the patient in a lateral or semiprone position. Prevent atelectasis by hourly changes in position, humidification of inspired air, and intermittent positive pressure breathing.

Specific treatment is discussed under appropriate headings elsewhere in this chapter.

Plum F, Posner JB: *The Diagnosis of Stupor and Coma.* Davis, 1966.

PHYSIOLOGY & MANAGEMENT OF INCREASED INTRACRANIAL PRESSURE

The skull contains brain, CSF, and blood vessels (Fig 41–1). At normal intracranial pressure (120–180 mm water), these 3 components maintain volumetric equilibrium. Increased volume of one component will elevate the intracranial pressure unless the volume of the other 2 components decrease proportionately (Monroe–Kellie doctrine). Because compensatory volumetric changes have physical and physiologic limits, the ability of the skull's contents to resist a rise in intracranial pressure can be exceeded by a change in volume that is either too sudden or too large. Common examples of a significant volumetric change in one or more of the 3 normal intracranial components are cerebral edema (brain), hydrocephalus (CSF), and venous obstruction (blood vessels).

An intracranial mass (eg, tumor or hematoma) represents a fourth component, and its introduction initiates compensatory adjustments: (1) intracranial veins are compressed; (2) CSF volume is reduced by an increased rate of absorption (and, at elevated pressures, by a reduced rate of production); and (3) the brain adjusts by a poorly understood reduction of intra- and extracellular volume. Infants and small children have an additional compensatory mechanism—an expand-

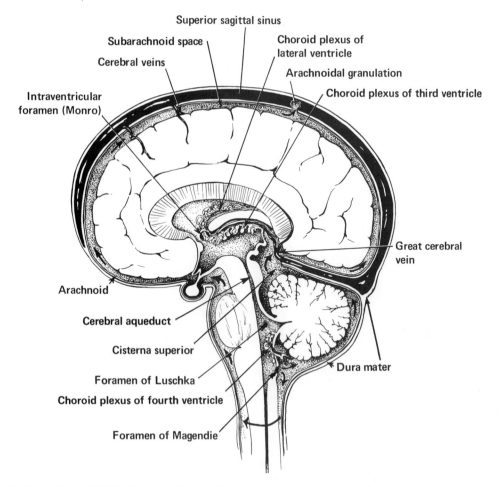

Superior sagittal sinus

Subarachnoid space

Cerebral veins

Choroid plexus of lateral ventricle

Arachnoidal granulation

Choroid plexus of third ventricle

Intraventricular foramen (Monro)

Great cerebral vein

Arachnoid

Cerebral aqueduct

Cisterna superior

Foramen of Luschka

Choroid plexus of fourth ventricle

Foramen of Magendie

Dura mater

FIG 41–1. Circulation of CSF. (Redrawn from original drawings by Frank H. Netter, MD, which first appeared in Ciba Clinical Symposia, © 1950. Reproduced with permission.)

able skull. The younger the child, the greater the capacity of the skull to enlarge as shown by the massive craniomegaly of infantile hydrocephalus.

Increased intracranial pressure indicates failure or exhaustion of these compensatory mechanisms. When the rise in pressure occurs slowly, the intracranial contents can accommodate large volumetric shifts with only slight elevation of pressure. Compensatory adjustments are less effective when the rise occurs rapidly.

In response to unevenly distributed forces within the skull, semisolid brain tissue can be deformed and displaced as a hernia. The openings through or across which it may herniate are the incisure of the tentorium cerebelli; the foramen magnum; and beneath the less restrictive midline partition, the falx cerebri, which partly bisects the supratentorial cavity. Herniation may lead to compression of specific structures some of which, such as the brain stem, are essential to life.

Clinical Findings

A. Acutely Elevated Intracranial Pressure: The pathophysiologic consequences of acutely elevated intracranial pressure are a rise in systolic blood pres-

sure, bradycardia, and a fall in respiratory rate. This triad usually signifies hematomas of arterial origin, eg, epidural hematoma and ruptured aneurysm.

B. Chronically Elevated Intracranial Pressure: Chronically elevated intracranial pressure, such as that due to hydrocephalus or benign brain tumor, is far more common than acute elevations and causes little change in vital signs except as a terminal event. Common manifestations are headache, papilledema, diplopia, and dulling of intellect. The headache is usually present on awakening and relieved by vomiting. Papilledema causes blurred vision. The diplopia (due to sixth nerve palsy) is the most common false localizing sign and is probably attributable to the nerve's long course and the sharp angle at which it penetrates the dura to enter the cavernous sinus. These nonspecific clinical manifestations provide no indication of the cause of the increased intracranial pressure.

1. Tentorial herniation—The tentorium forms a rigid partition between the cerebral hemispheres (supratentorial compartment) and the cerebellum and brain stem (infratentorial compartment, posterior fossa). The tentorial opening (incisura tentorii) lies in a

TABLE 41–1. Clinical manifestations of tentorial herniation.

Compressed Structure	Clinical Manifestation
Cranial nerve III	Ipsilateral mydriasis
Midbrain: physiologic (functional) transection	Decerebrate rigidity
Reticular formation	Coma
Ipsilateral cerebral peduncle	Contralateral hemiparesis
Contralateral cerebral peduncle	Ipsilateral hemiparesis (false localizing sign)*
Cerebral aqueduct (of Sylvius)	Headache and vomiting due to acute hydrocephalus
Posterior cerebral artery	Contralateral hemianopsia (false localizing sign)*

*This sign is the consequence of herniation and does not indicate the localization of the primary process; in this sense, the sign falsely localizes the primary lesion.

plane at a right angle to the upper end of the clivus. The incisure contains the following structures: (1) centrally, the midbrain; (2) anteriorly, the bifurcation of the basilar artery; (3) laterally, the posterior cerebral arteries; (4) anterolaterally, the third nerves in their course from the interpeduncular fossa to the cavernous sinus; and (5) immediately lateral to the third nerves, the medial 2–4 mm of the temporal lobes (uncus). A unilateral supratentorial mass displaces the brain medially beneath the falx cerebri (see below) and downward through the tentorial incisure. The medial aspect of the temporal lobe is displaced into the incisure, deforming and compressing its contents.

Death follows descending impairment of brain stem function. The process becomes irreversible when hemorrhage occurs into the midbrain and pontine tegmentum.

2. Foraminal (cerebellar) herniation—The cerebellar tonsils lie dorsolateral to the medulla just above the foramen magnum. A mass in the posterior fossa displaces the cerebellar vermis upward into the incisure and—of greater clinical significance—forces the cerebellar tonsils downward into the foramen magnum. Acting as a wedge, the tonsils may compress the medulla. The hallmark of medullary compression is respiratory failure: slow and irregular breathing followed by respiratory arrest. Earlier impaction of the foramen magnum by the cerebellar tonsils causes nuchal rigidity. Posterior fossa masses obstruct the flow of CSF and cause hydrocephalus. Attacks of decerebrate rigidity ("cerebellar fits") reflect increased supratentorial pressure secondary to hydrocephalus. Consciousness is often retained until respirations fail.

Subfalcial herniation (displacement of the cingulate gyrus beneath the free edge of the rigid falx cerebri) has no obvious clinical correlate but assumes great importance in the radiologic localization of supratentorial masses.

Differential Diagnosis

The diagnosis of increased intracranial pressure as such is relatively easy. The etiologic diagnosis, however, must be based on the history, physical and neurologic examination, radiologic studies—including skull x-rays, angiography, brain scan, pneumoencephalography, and ventriculography—EEG, and echoencephalography. *Caution:* Lumbar puncture rarely provides essential information when increased intracranial pressure is known or suspected to be present and, by lowering intraspinal pressure, may precipitate fatal foraminal or tentorial herniation. In the presence of known or suspected intracranial hypertension, lumbar puncture is justifiable only when examination of the fluid (as opposed to measurement of the CSF pressure) is necessary in order to decide on therapy—eg, in meningitis or subarachnoid hemorrhage. When the provisional diagnosis is brain tumor, lumbar puncture is often deferred.

Treatment

Ideally, increased intracranial pressure should be corrected by specific measures directed at the cause. When this is not possible, intracranial pressure can be reduced by several means.

Emergency measures include intravenous hyperosmotic solutions of urea and mannitol and corticosteroids to reduce cerebral edema; hyperventilation; and drainage of hydrocephalic ventricles.

Definitive measures include establishing a CSF shunt; bony decompression, usually by removal of bone lying underneath the temporalis muscle (subtemporal decompression); and, if possible, removal of the mass.

Prognosis

Two factors determine the outcome: the degree and duration of increased intracranial pressure and the underlying cause. The first factor is modified by the presence or absence of a mass (eg, hematoma, tumor) with its attendant shift of intracranial structures. Increased intracranial pressure without a mass (eg, diffuse cerebral edema, hydrocephalus) is better tolerated than equivalent pressure elevation accompanied by a mass.

The long-term prognosis depends upon the nature of the surgical lesion (eg, evacuated hematoma versus incompletely removed tumor).

Cushing H: Some experimental and clinical observations concerning states of increased intracranial tension. Am J Med Sc 124:375, 1902.

Howell DA: Upper brain-stem compression and foraminal impaction with intracranial space-occupying lesions and brain swelling. Brain 82:525, 1959.

Jennett WB, Stern WE: Tentorial herniation, the midbrain and the pupil: Experimental studies in brain compression. J Neurosurg 17:598, 1960.

Weintraub CM: Bruising of the third cranial nerve and the pathogenesis of midbrain hemorrhage. Brit J Surg 48:62, 1960.

Youmans JR, Neely WA: Sequelae of acute increase in intracranial pressure. J Trauma 3:386, 1963.

NEUROSURGICAL DIAGNOSTIC PROCEDURES

CONTRAST STUDIES

Although plain x-rays of the skull and spine are valuable, they often do not provide the information needed. The examiner should then consider using one or more contrast studies.

Myelography

Myelography is useful principally in the study of the spinal canal, although injection of a contrast medium such as iophendylate (Pantopaque) into the subarachnoid space has recently been used to delineate the cerebellopontine angle and the internal auditory meatus in the posterior fossa. By this technic, contrast medium is introduced into the lumbar subarachnoid space via lumbar puncture. The patient is tilted at various angles, the contrast medium (heavier than CSF) flows by gravity, and x-rays are obtained in desired projections at the appropriate level. The defects produced in the dye column by the various pathologic entities can be characterized, in general, as extradural, intradural-intramedullary, or intradural-extramedullary. Unless a complete block is present, the contrast medium should be removed (if feasible) at the completion of the study. Air may be used instead of contrast medium but is generally helpful only when hydromyelia is suspected. Contrast medium myelography should not be done in the presence of a bloody spinal tap because of the reported increased risk of aseptic arachnoiditis.

Diskography

This technic has been used to study intervertebral disk disease. It consists of introducing contrast material—usually sodium diatrizoate (Hypaque)—into the disk space via a spinal needle and taking x-rays to see if extravasation occurs outside the space. In the author's opinion, this is not a reliable means of determining disk abnormality.

Angiography

The arterial and venous systems of the brain and spinal cord can be visualized by the intra-arterial injection of a water-soluble iodinated contrast medium. Angiography, if done, is generally performed before other contrast studies. The contrast material may be injected via a femoral catheter introduced by the Seldinger technic. All the cranial vessels may be studied separately, including the external and internal carotid arteries. Such a study may demonstrate displacement of vessels, pathologic vessels, occlusion of vessels, abnormality of the vessel wall, or avascular areas. The risk of neurologic sequelae following angiography has been reduced by the newer contrast media and technics but has not been eliminated, particularly in patients with cerebrovascular disease.

Pneumoencephalography (Fig 41–2 a and b.)

In performing pneumoencephalography, the basal cisterns and ventricular system of the brain are gradually filled with increments of air introduced via a lumbar puncture needle. The study is hazardous in the patient with increased intracranial pressure and may precipitate respiratory arrest. Such an occurrence is rare if, after the initial injection of a small volume of air, tomograms are taken to demonstrate the position

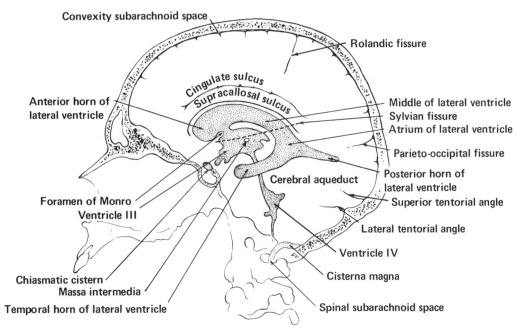

FIG 41–2a. Lateral encephalogram. (Reproduced, with permission, from Chusid JG: *Correlative Neuroanatomy & Functional Neurology,* 15th ed. Lange, 1973.)

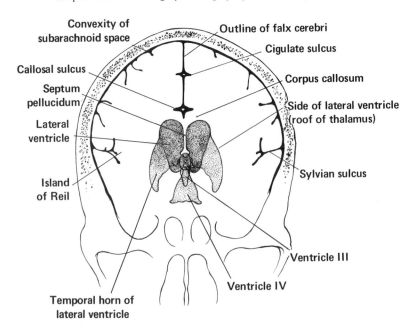

FIG 41–2b. Anteroposterior encephalogram. (Reproduced, with permission, from Chusid JG: *Correlative Neuroanatomy & Functional Neurology*, 15th ed. Lange, 1973.)

of the cerebellar tonsils. If the tonsils are herniated, the procedure should be terminated.

Pneumoencephalograms are particularly helpful in the study of posterior fossa lesions, sellar and suprasellar lesions, and atrophic processes. When tomography is done during this study, the value of the study is greatly enhanced. Pneumoencephalography may produce transient headache, nausea, vomiting, and vertigo.

Ventriculography

In the presence of increased intracranial pressure, cerebellar tonsillar herniation, or both, contrast study of the ventricular system may be necessary in place of pneumoencephalography. Such a study is carried out via a bur hole made off the midline at the coronal or lamboidal suture. Air may then be introduced by ventricular puncture in exchange for CSF. The lateral ventricles and the third ventricle can usually be filled quite satisfactorily by this technic, but visualization of the cerebral aqueduct and the fourth ventricle is often inadequate unless a positive contrast agent is used instead of air. As a rule, the basal cisterns and the subarachnoid space over the hemispheres are not satisfactorily visualized. Definitive surgical treatment nearly always follows ventriculography, since a patient with a demonstrable lesion deteriorates rapidly from the effects of injected air on the dynamics of the intracranial fluid. Ventricular taps can produce cerebral hemorrhage, porencephalic cysts, seizures, or infection, and should be done only when clearly necessary. Occasionally, such taps are done for decompression, for obtaining ventricular fluid for analysis, or to introduce a therapeutic agent.

ELECTRICAL STUDIES

Electromyography (EMG)

EMG is helpful in the diagnosis of neuromuscular disorders, particularly in determining the anatomic site of a lesion on an individual peripheral nerve or in separating a diffuse peripheral neuropathy from a single root or nerve lesion. It is sometimes useful in identifying the specific root involved. In conjunction with muscle biopsy, it is frequently helpful in the diagnosis of muscle diseases.

Electroencephalography (EEG)

EEG records the electrical activity of the brain. It is perhaps most useful in identifying and localizing seizure disorders, but abnormal or localizing signs may also be seen in brain abscess, subdural hematomas, brain tumors, metabolic disorders, and degenerative diseases of the CNS. Although it is a diagnostic procedure without risk, its usefulness to the neurosurgeon is limited.

ISOTOPE STUDIES

Isotopes of arsenic, copper, mercury, and other elements have been used for brain scanning, but technetium 99m pertechnetate has the most desirable characteristics. The intravenously injected isotope is preferentially taken up in the brain where the blood-brain barrier has been disturbed, and this area of isotope concentration shows up as a "hot spot" on the scan readout. With high-speed repetitive scanning, it is also possible to determine intracranial vascular flow patterns.

The flow characteristics of CSF can be studied by isotope cisternography, which involves the lumbar injection of radioiodinated serum albumin (RISA) and scanning during its course through the subarachnoid space. Such a study provides useful information in certain cases of hydrocephalus.

ECHOENCEPHALOGRAPHY

By passing an electrical current through a crystal, a beam of ultrasound can be produced which is then directed from one side of the skull to the other. Some of the sound waves are deflected by the midline structures in the area of the third ventricle, and a characteristic deflection is produced on the recording apparatus. This is a rapid, safe, and easy method of detecting a shift of midline structures—information that is particularly helpful in acute head injuries or other conditions causing a shift of the midline such as brain tumor, cerebral infarct, cerebral hemorrhage, subdural collections, and brain abscesses.

Alexander E: Lumbar puncture. JAMA 201:316–317, 1967.

Brinker RA, King DL, Taveras JM: Echoencephalography. Am J Roentgenol 93:781–790, 1965.

Holt EP: Fallacy of cervical discography: Report of 50 cases in normal subjects. JAMA 188:799–801, 1964.

Howard FM Jr: The electromyogram and conduction velocity studies in peripheral nerve trauma. Clin Neurosurg 17:63–76, 1969.

McAfee JG & others: Tc-99m pertechnetate for brain scanning. J Nuclear Med 5:811–827, 1964.

Taveras JM, Wood EH: *Diagnostic Neuroradiology.* Williams & Wilkins, 1964.

CRANIOCEREBRAL TRAUMA
Roland K. Perkins, MD

Most head injuries seen in the emergency room are closed injuries, ie, the brain and its coverings have not been penetrated and there is no evidence of compound skull fracture. The major diagnostic difficulty, then, is recognition of, localization of, and determination of the extent of intracranial damage.

Head injuries may be induced by many forces, the most common being low-velocity impacts (such as those received in a car accident), direct blows from a solid object, and high-velocity wounds from missiles. In civilian practice, low-velocity impacts are most frequent. About 60% of all injuries due to traffic acci-

dents involve the head, and in fatal accidents the percentage rises to 70%. In two-thirds of these fatal cases, the injuries to the head are the cause of death. At autopsy following head injury, about 35–50% of patients have intracranial hemorrhage. If an individual is comatose after an accident, there is an estimated 50% chance of intracranial hemorrhage with or without brain damage.

Sudden acceleration or deceleration of the intracranial mass may cause injuries due to compression (pushing material together), tension (tearing material apart), or shearing (sliding portions of material over other portions). These may occur singly or in any combination.

With a localized head injury, the forces spent upon local areas of the skull and its underlying brain may give rise to complications, including those of hemorrhage and infection, but the mortality rate is low. With generalized head injuries, the force, if severe, will move or deform the entire skull, accelerate or squeeze the entire brain, and transmit this distortion to the vital central core and brain stem.

Pathology

Injuries may be limited to the scalp, the skull, or the brain; they may involve only 2 of these or all 3.

A. Scalp: The scalp consists of 5 layers: epidermis, dermis, fat, galea, and the subareolar area. From a practical standpoint, it consists of the epidermis and galea. The rigidity of these 2 layers holds open the many blood vessels in the fatty layer between them. Because it is unyielding, blunt injuries tend to burst rather than squash the scalp.

B. Skull: Skull fractures can be classified as simple (linear and depressed) or compound. A skull fracture does not necessarily provide an index to the severity of head injuries, since fatal damage to the brain may follow a closed head injury without evidence of fracture. A skull fracture does, however, indicate that a severe blow to the head has been sustained.

1. Simple skull fractures—If the fracture overlies the groove of the middle meningeal artery or one of the dural venous sinuses, extradural or subdural hemorrhage must be suspected and the patient must be evaluated immediately for signs that may suggest the need for operative intervention.

2. Basilar skull fractures—These are often not seen on x-rays. A linear fracture that extends into an accessory nasal sinus or into mastoid air cells is really a compound fracture since it is in communication with the external surfaces of the body.

3. Depressed skull fractures and compound skull fractures—These are often obvious clinically, but x-ray confirmation is essential. Palpation of the intact scalp is often misleading because of subgaleal edema and hematoma.

C. Brain: Direct brain injury may cause concussion, contusion, or laceration. These may occur singly but are more commonly seen in various combinations. With contusion and laceration or subsequent pressure from a hematoma, the brain often becomes edematous. Although the mechanism of brain swelling is not clearly understood, it is related to increased vascular permeability; in severe head injuries at least, superimposed hypoxia plays a role.

1. **Concussion**—Concussion is a clinical syndrome characterized by immediate and transient impairment of neural function due to mechanical forces applied to the head. The term was formerly restricted to an injury resulting in loss of consciousness. At present, an injury which has caused no loss of consciousness but only a brief period of mental confusion is referred to as a mild concussion. The terms moderate and severe concussion imply a longer period of unconsciousness. Amnesia for the events preceding the injury is termed retrograde amnesia. In cerebral concussion, there is little or no demonstrable permanent pathologic change in the brain.

2. **Cerebral contusion (bruise)**—This term implies a structural alteration of the brain. A localized external or cortical blow usually produces slight direct cortical injury. Contusions frequently occur along the base of the posterior frontal lobes and at the tips of adjacent temporal lobes. Trauma to the underlying neuroglia may produce local edema. Injuries to surface vessels usually produce only local hematoma, although there may be some ischemia. Subcortical and deep injuries are more devastating and involve larger structural masses.

3. **Brain laceration**—Laceration of the brain usually occurs at the point of application of substantial force to the head or directly opposite that point ("contrecoup").

Clinical Findings

The state of consciousness is by far the most important measure of the patient's condition, and the importance of frequent checks on the state of consciousness cannot be overemphasized. If the patient does not respond to a command, his responses should be tested with painful stimuli such as pinprick of the extremities.

An adequate airway should first be guaranteed; if an aid to breathing is needed, an endotracheal tube is preferred. The vital signs are recorded. The ears, nose, and mouth should be examined for spinal fluid and blood. Although occasionally very large scalp lacerations can bleed copiously enough to produce shock, shock does not usually occur with an uncomplicated head injury. Thus, if shock is present and cannot be attributed to hemorrhage from a scalp laceration, its cause must be sought promptly. Temporary control of scalp bleeding can be accomplished with a pressure dressing.

It should be kept in mind that even with external signs of trauma there may be underlying pathologic entities as well, such as drunkenness, epilepsy, insulin shock, and secondary cardiac problems. Determination of the degree to which one of these entities and the head trauma contribute to the patient's condition is imperative.

Any medication recently given the patient should be noted. The use of narcotics, particularly morphine, should be avoided in head injuries because such patients are highly susceptible and because the drug may mask changes in the state of consciousness and in the neurologic signs, particularly the pupils. Narcotics also tend to depress respiration.

A. Symptoms and Signs:

1. **Neck signs**—Contusions overlying the carotid vessels in the neck and the pulsations of these vessels should be noted.

2. **Headache**—Severe unilateral headache may be a sign of an expanding intracranial lesion.

3. **Retrograde amnesia**—A significant period of retrograde amnesia indicates a definite cerebral injury. The longer the period of amnesia, the more severe the injury is likely to be. If there is no retrograde amnesia, the degree of cerebral injury is likely to be slight even though there is major skull damage. However, absence of retrograde amnesia does not mean that extradural or subdural hematoma will not develop.

4. **Eye signs**—The size and responsiveness of the pupils should be noted and the fundi examined. In most head injuries with increased intracranial pressure, papilledema does not develop in less than 12–18 hours. However, early ophthalmoscopic examination establishes a baseline and may reveal retinal hemorrhages.

Third nerve paresis can result from immediate injury to the nerve or an abrupt increase in intracranial pressure. However, if the pupils are the same size just after the injury and subsequently start to dilate, a progressive lesion is present which requires immediate diagnosis and treatment. Third nerve involvement in a fully awake and oriented patient generally means direct damage to the nerve in the orbit, in the superior orbital fissure, or in the cavernous sinus. A tiny, nonreactive pupil in a comatose or semicomatose patient suggests primary involvement of the brain stem.

Conjugate deviation of both eyes usually indicates a lesion of the opposite frontal lobe (adversive fields). Spontaneous nystagmus indicates damage to the cerebellum or vestibular connections. Skew deviation of the eyes occurs in injuries to the brain stem; local damage to the orbit or to the ocular muscles can also produce deviation of the eyes.

5. **Muscle examination**—Facial weakness may be evaluated by exerting pressure over the supraorbital ridge. In alert patients it is possible to estimate the strength of muscles in the extremities; in drowsy or semicomatose patients this is often possible only by administering painful stimuli. The most common motor sign of craniocerebral trauma is hemiparesis or hemiplegia. Abnormal posturing also occurs—most frequently decerebrate rigidity (extreme rigidity of all 4 extremities, with adduction and rotation of the upper extremities on painful stimulation). Decerebrate rigidity immediately after injury generally indicates direct injury to the brain stem, although occasionally a rapidly developing intracranial hematoma can cause identical postural changes secondary to compression of the brain stem by a herniated temporal lobe.

B. Lumbar Puncture: Lumbar puncture has no role in the diagnosis of head injuries. Even at a later stage, lumbar puncture **should never be done** where there is suspicion of increased intracranial pressure or of brain shift, such as transtentorial herniation or herniation at the foramen magnum.

Some degree of subarachnoid bleeding is common in head injury. The spinal fluid pressure may also rise with an expanding intracranial hematoma or with brain swelling. However, since a large subdural hematoma may exist without increasing spinal fluid pressure, a finding of normal spinal fluid pressure does not rule out the possibility of an expanding intracranial hematoma.

C. Special Diagnostic Studies: Various special diagnostic studies are of value in assessing the type and site of acute head injury and its intracranial complications. However, it is important to keep in mind that the patient's clinical state determines what diagnostic studies can and should be performed. For example, with a rapidly expanding hematoma, the sequence of events may be too rapid to permit angiography. Bur holes, on the other hand, can be made quickly and allow exploration of the epidural and subdural spaces as well as evacuation of a hematoma if found. Bur holes are placed bilaterally in the frontal, temporal, and parietal regions.

1. Skull x-rays—X-rays should be obtained as soon as the patient's general condition permits. They may show a linear or depressed fracture or a fracture line crossing one of the major vascular structures, which will suggest the possibility of an expanding intracranial hematoma. A fracture extending into a sinus warns of the danger of ascending intracranial infection. A shift of the pineal gland (which is calcified and radiopaque in 70% of persons after age 20) 3 mm or more to either side of the midline suggests an expanding intracranial lesion. Skull x-rays may show a preexisting intracranial abnormality.

2. Echoencephalography—The echoencephalogram may demonstrate midline shifts, indicating the presence of an extracerebral or an intracerebral mass. Bilateral lesions do exist, however, and, unless markedly asymmetric, will not shift midline structures.

3. Brain scan—Radioactive brain scan is becoming increasingly useful in the diagnosis of intracranial injuries such as cerebral contusion and extra- or intracerebral hematoma.

4. Cerebral angiography—Angiography has the distinct value of accurately localizing intra- and extracerebral hematomas. The venous phase of the angiogram may show obstruction of the venous sinuses by fracture fragments, and the arterial phase may reveal partial or complete occlusion of the carotid artery or one of its branches.

5. Air contrast studies—These are not often used in evaluating acute head injuries since angiography is more accurate and safer in the presence of an expanding lesion. There are times, however, when tapping the ventricle and evaluating ventricular size and position may be of value.

Differential Diagnosis

The history of a blow to the head usually makes the cause of the unconsciousness evident, although a concomitant pathologic state may exist. Without a history of head trauma, other causes of the unconscious state must be kept in mind, including cardiac conditions, cerebrovascular accidents, and diabetic, hepatic, alcoholic, or drug-induced coma. An expanding intracranial tumor may have been responsible for a seizure with subsequent fall and head injury.

Cerebral fat embolism, which may follow fracture of a long bone, may mimic extradural hemorrhage, subdural hematoma, or midbrain injury. With cerebral fat embolism, fat globules usually appear in the urine 2–6 days after the fracture. The optic fundi should be examined for emboli, small hemorrhages, white exudates, and edema. Petechiae should be sought in the conjunctivas and on the skin of the chest and arms. A sudden rise in temperature without evidence of pneumonia suggests the possibility of cerebral fat embolism.

The progression of clinical signs of traumatic internal carotid artery thrombosis following a blow to the neck may suggest an expanding intracranial lesion. The diagnosis is made by angiography; palpation of the vessels of the neck is of little aid.

Complications

The complications of trauma to the head include vascular lesions (hemorrhage, thrombosis, fistula formation), infections (meningitis, abscess, osteomyelitis), rhinorrhea, otorrhea, pneumatocele, leptomeningeal cysts, cranial nerve injuries, and focal brain lesions.

A. Hemorrhage: Intracranial hemorrhage may occur within the extradural, subdural, or subarachnoid spaces, or within the brain. Extradural and subdural hemorrhage are discussed below as separate entities.

1. Subarachnoid hemorrhage—Blood in the spinal fluid is a common finding with head injuries. The bleeding usually arises from the superficial cortical vessels, particularly the communicating veins that drain into the sinus. Large amounts of blood within the subarachnoid space may be tolerated well and require no specific treatment. Initially, the patient may have severe headache, restlessness, nuchal rigidity, fever, and a positive Kernig sign.

Acute subarachnoid hemorrhage is not a surgical lesion, and spinal fluid drainage is rarely of benefit. Subsequently, if the hemorrhage has been massive, arachnoiditis may interfere with absorption of CSF, and this may require shunting of the fluid to another site where it can be reabsorbed.

2. Subdural hygroma—Subdural hygroma is an accumulation of spinal fluid in the subdural space, usually through a fine tear in the arachnoid created by a craniocerebral injury. The spinal fluid is trapped in the subdural space and cannot be absorbed. Patients with subdural hygromas are usually suspected of having subdural hematomas, and the fluid is identified and removed by surgical exploration.

3. Intracerebral hemorrhage—Intracerebral hematomas may result from injury to a cerebral vessel with major hemorrhage or from a coalescence of smaller subcortical hemorrhages. These hematomas produce no clear-cut clinical picture but may present as an expanding intracranial lesion. They are often associated with cortical lacerations and contusion, and the patient's condition either becomes stable after a few days or deteriorates. The most common sites are in the anterior temporal lobe and the frontal lobe. Angiography establishes the diagnosis.

Hematomas large enough to cause symptoms and signs should be evacuated.

B. Carotid Cavernous Fistula: A carotid cavernous fistula is a channel which shunts blood from the internal carotid artery into the cavernous sinus. The traumatic carotid cavernous fistula results from a tear in one of the small intracavernous carotid branches. The symptoms usually arise within the first month and include headache, retro-orbital pain, blurred vision, diplopia, and often a bruit. The eye becomes proptotic, and the conjunctivas and eye muscles are extremely edematous. The eye is often immobile. Papilledema and engorgement of the retinal veins are usually present.

The fistula is demonstrated by cerebral angiography. Digital pressure upon the carotid artery in the neck often abolishes or diminishes the bruit. Treatment is directed toward reducing the arterial supply to the fistula; it often involves a combination of cervical and intracranial carotid ligations. More recently, technics to create thrombosis within the cavernous sinus have also been used.

C. CSF Leak: CSF rhinorrhea and otorrhea indicate a fistulous communication between the subarachnoid space (or ventricular system) and the nose or ear, respectively. This fistulous connection can serve as a path for spreading infection; the longer the leak persists, the greater the risk of infection. This can lead to meningitis, brain abscess, or both.

The fluid is characterized by the presence of glucose, which is not present in mucous secretions, and this helps to establish the diagnosis.

CSF rhinorrhea can result from a fracture which communicates with any of the paranasal sinuses. The most common site is a fracture through the cribriform plate extending into an ethmoid sinus. If the leak persists beyond 2 weeks, intracranial repair is indicated. Occasionally, early infection is encountered, and antibiotic therapy may cure both the infection and the leak. However, months later, the patient may abruptly develop meningitis, usually pneumococcal. Surgical repair should be done after antibiotic treatment.

CSF otorrhea or otorrhagia occurs most frequently in association with fractures through the petrous portion of the temporal bone with a dural tear in the middle or posterior fossa. In most cases, the leak seals off spontaneously; if it does not, surgical repair is necessary.

D. Cranial Nerve Palsies: The olfactory nerves are often torn at the cribriform plate, and traumatic olfactory palsies seldom recover. The prognosis is generally poor in an optic nerve lesion where there has been immediate complete blindness. Partial lesions may be followed by recovery of visual function as edema subsides. Palsies of the third, fourth, and sixth cranial nerves usually improve following trauma, although they may remain complete. Recovery, if it occurs, may take 6–9 months. Facial palsies may occur immediately or several days after trauma. Recovery of a delayed facial palsy is generally the rule; the prognosis is not as good if the palsy occurs at the moment of injury. If there has been no return of function within 6–8 weeks, intratemporal decompression of the facial nerve should be considered. If the nerve has been irreversibly damaged, a facial nerve anastomosis can be done, utilizing either the hypoglossal or the spinal accessory nerve. If deafness occurs following auditory nerve damage, improvement is usually slight.

E. Posttraumatic Cerebral Syndrome: The posttraumatic cerebral syndrome is more common after serious head injuries but may be produced by relatively mild ones. The patient complains of headache, difficulty in concentration, dizziness, memory defects, giddiness, and fatigability. Personality changes are common. The symptoms are more pronounced and prolonged in patients with a preexisting or underlying emotional problem. In almost all instances, these symptoms clear within a few months and rarely last more than a year.

F. Posttraumatic Epilepsy: Patients may develop seizures during the initial phase of a head injury. This may be due to an expanding intracranial hematoma as well as to brain swelling. These seizures do not mean, however, that the patient will develop posttraumatic epilepsy. The incidence of seizures following closed head injuries is reported to be 3–6%. The incidence following penetrating injuries is much higher (20–50%). In most cases, the epileptic seizures begin within 2 years after injury, and most of these patients are still subject to seizures after 5 years.

Treatment

A. Emergency Measures: The first requirement is to ensure an adequate airway, with tracheal intubation and respiratory assistance if necessary. Hypoxia is decidedly detrimental to the patient with head injury.

Any external hemorrhage should be controlled, and shock must be treated. Intravenous fluids and blood should be given as required.

The patient's clinical situation should be assessed —particularly his state of consciousness. The type and severity of the nervous system injury should be determined as accurately as possible. In addition, a general examination should be done to ascertain the type and degree of associated injuries.

B. General Measures: If the patient's condition is rapidly deteriorating and there is a possibility that an expanding intracranial hematoma is present, bur hole exploration should be done without delay.

A prominent factor in most severe head injuries is cerebral swelling or edema, occurring as a consequence of increased vascular permeability. Hypoxia due to decreased respiratory exchange also contributes to cerebral swelling. In general, this should be treated by intravenous urea or mannitol, and corticosteroid injections; the value of intravenous injections of hypertonic agents is limited and temporary. *Caution:* The use of any of these agents before a definitive diagnosis has been established could allow further expansion of an intracranial hematoma.

Antibiotic treatment should be instituted in contaminated compound wounds and in basal skull fractures.

Anticonvulsant medication is given if seizures occur. However, it must be remembered that seizures may be the sign of a rapidly expanding intracranial lesion that requires immediate treatment by operation.

Progressive deterioration of the patient's condition is an indication for exploratory bur holes or for angiography, depending upon the rate of progression and the patient's overall condition. This deterioration may be manifested by progressive impairment of the state of consciousness, progression of neurologic signs, or evidence of increased intracranial pressure. Compound fractures of the skull and penetrating wounds of the brain are clear-cut indications for operation.

C. Specific Measures:

1. Scalp wounds—Bleeding can usually be controlled with a simple pressure dressing or, in the case of arterial bleeding, by means of firm finger pressure along the edges of the wound or by a hemostat attached to the galea. The hemostat is allowed to hang down over the skin to hold the galea firmly against the skin and compress the bleeding vessels. With simple wounds, debridement and control of hemorrhage are the important considerations. These wounds should be closed as soon as possible unless they overlie a depressed fracture or a wound that penetrates the skull.

Scalp hair must be shaved over a generous margin about the wound. The wound should be thoroughly cleansed and the edges approximated either with buried galeal sutures and removable superficial sutures or with a vertical mattress suture utilizing stainless steel wire. Buried sutures should not be used for infected wounds.

2. Depressed skull fractures—Depressed bone fragments beneath intact scalp usually require elevation, depending upon the anatomic area and the degree of depression. As a general rule, depressions of 0.4 cm or more over the motor and speech areas should be elevated. Unless there are untoward neurologic signs, however, elevation can be delayed until optimal surgical facilities are available.

3. Compound skull fractures—To prevent infection, debridement and repair should be undertaken as soon as possible after injury. The patient with a depressed compound skull fracture should be taken to a hospital with complete neurosurgical facilities and treated by a surgeon with adequate neurosurgical training.

Emergency treatment consists of applying a sterile compression dressing. The wound should not be closed, and no attempt should be made to remove any foreign body protruding from the wound until the patient is in the operating room and all preparations have been made for craniotomy. If the fragments are depressed into the transverse or sagittal sinus, their removal may cause alarming hemorrhage at the edge of the bone opening. Thus, adequate access to control the sinus distally and proximally must be made before such a depressed fragment is elevated. Mature judgment is required in deciding whether bone fragments should be removed or realigned.

If the dura is torn, the opening is enlarged to allow inspection and debridement of the brain. The brain substance may contain foreign bodies such as bone, hair, and microorganisms.

4. Linear or stellate undepressed fractures—These can be treated by simple closure of the skin wound after a thorough cleansing. If there is suspicion of a coexistent intracranial hemorrhage, the epidural and subdural spaces may need to be explored concurrently.

Prognosis

The prognosis and course are related to the severity and site of cranial injury. The longer the period of unconsciousness, the poorer the prognosis—although in children recovery from a severe injury may be quite gratifying. The early development of a decerebrate state implies a poor prognosis. The prognosis is exceedingly poor in an adult who presents in coma with dilated fixed pupils and signs of brain stem injury.

The full extent of clinical recovery cannot usually be ascertained for 6–12 months. Postconcussion symptoms may persist for a long period.

See references on p 737.

EXTRADURAL HEMORRHAGE

The most common cause of extradural hematoma is fracture-induced laceration of a branch of the middle meningeal artery. This artery is liable to injury where it lies within a groove in the inner table of the temporal bone. Extradural bleeding may also result from laceration of the dural sinuses; fractures that cross the superior sagittal sinus or the transverse sinus are particularly liable to cause extradural bleeding.

Extradural hemorrhage may be produced by a minor blow to the head, and there may have been no period of unconsciousness. An initially unconscious patient may have a "lucid interval"—ie, he may become more alert and then progressively less so—but this classic sign is not invariably present. The hematoma rapidly increases in size and compresses the cerebral cortex, producing contralateral hemiparesis or hemiplegia. As the hemisphere is further compressed, the medial portion of the temporal lobe is forced through the tentorial incisure (compressing the third cranial nerve and producing dilatation of the pupil on the same side) and the brain stem is shifted to the opposite side of the tentorial notch. If compression of the brain stem becomes severe enough, venous hemorrhages into the stem will lead to irreversible neurologic deficit or death. (Fig 41–3.)

Extradural hematoma carries a mortality of approximately 50%, principally because it often is not recognized until irreversible changes have occurred within the brain. Thus, it is important to realize that a serious hemorrhage may develop even though the blow to the head was minor. The patient with a history of blow to the head leading to unconsciousness for even a brief interval should have a thorough neurologic examination and skull x-rays. If the x-rays show a fracture, careful monitoring of the conscious level and the vital signs is indicated. If the patient is admitted in deep coma with findings—dilated pupils, decerebrate rigidity, hemiplegia—indicating the possibility of an extradural clot, immediate placement of bur holes is justified. Since the majority of extradural clots occur in the temporal area, this should be the site of initial exploration.

Extradural hematomas may also be seen in the posterior fossa. Trephination over the posterior fossa is justified in a patient with an occipital contusion or laceration plus a fracture traversing the transverse sinus or entering the foramen magnum with further impairment of consciousness and no signs of a supratentorial lesion that would account for the symptoms.

SUBDURAL HEMATOMA

The symptoms that develop from subdural bleeding depend in large measure on the speed and the

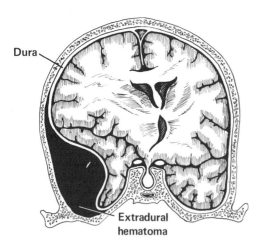

FIG 41–3. Extradural hemorrhage. (Reprinted from *Hosp Med* 1:9, October, 1965, by permission of the authors and Wallace Laboratories.)

magnitude of the initial hemorrhage. A subdural hematoma may be acute, subacute, or chronic depending on the type and size of the blood vessel torn. The latter factors determine the rapidity of the bleeding.

Acute Subdural Hematoma

In general, the symptoms and signs of acute subdural hematoma may be those of rapid and massive compression of the brain. The term acute is usually reserved for a hematoma that develops within 24 hours, although some authors have suggested that a lesion developing within a 3-day period after injury should also be designated as acute. The hemorrhage can result from lacerations of the pia with arterial bleeding as well as from laceration of the veins that bridge from the cortex to the sagittal sinus. Acute subdural hematoma is accompanied by diffuse cerebral swelling, which further increases intracranial pressure.

The mortality rate in patients with acute subdural hematoma is approximately 80–90%. Treatment consists of removal of the hematoma. Unfortunately, this often does not produce significant clinical change because the major neurologic deficit is produced by extensive cerebral contusion, laceration, or both.

Subacute Subdural Hematoma

Subdural hematomas that are detected within 1–10 days after injury are termed subacute. They may be associated with contusion and laceration of the brain. The majority of these hematomas result from laceration of veins that traverse the subdural space. Their neurologic signs develop more gradually than those of acute subdural hematomas, and in many cases are masked by the signs of contusion and laceration of the brain.

Evacuation of the clot may improve the patient's condition, but the degree of ultimate recovery depends upon the extent of underlying brain damage.

Chronic Subdural Hematoma

Chronic subdural hematomas become symptomatic from 10 days to 3 months after injury—an interval of 6 weeks is common. The symptomatology may be very insidious and may occur after a seemingly minor traumatic incident has been forgotten. The history is usually one of progressive mental or personality changes with or without focal signs and symptoms.

The hemorrhage usually results from trauma to the veins that bridge from the cortex to the sagittal sinus. Since venous bleeding is under low pressure, it arrests spontaneously before becoming large enough to compress the brain. A membrane forms around the clot, and, as the protein molecules disintegrate, osmotic pressure increases so that blood serum or CSF is drawn through the semipermeable membranes, causing further expansion of the encapsulated hematoma. (Fig 41–4.)

Chronic subdural hematomas are most common in infants and in adults past middle age. Because of the slow and insidious development of symptoms, the

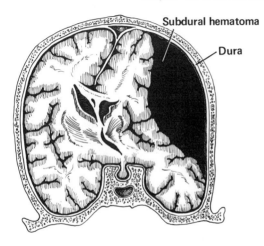

FIG 41—4. Subdural hemorrhage. (Reprinted from Hosp Med 1:9, October, 1965, by permission of the authors and Wallace Laboratories.)

patient's behavior is all too often explained on a psychiatric rather than a physical basis. Skull x-rays often show a shift of the pineal gland, although 20% of hematomas are bilateral and may be unassociated with a shift in midline structures. The spinal fluid pressure may or may not be elevated. EEG may show slowing on the side of the hematoma and depressed voltage. An echoencephalogram will often disclose a shift of midline structures. A definitive diagnosis is made by angiography. The brain scan of a subdural hematoma is usually diagnostic.

Chronic subdural hematoma is usually found in the frontoparietal region. This lesion must be strongly suspected in the middle-aged person with a history of head injury who has shown a progressive personality change, headache, and mental dulling. Treatment consists of evacuation of the hematoma via bur holes.

Brock S: *Injuries of the Brain and Spinal Cord and Their Coverings,* 4th ed. Springer, 1960.

Clare FB, Bell HS: Extradural hematomas. JAMA 177:887–891, 1961.

Craigmile TK: Operative treatment of acute craniocerebral injuries. S Clin North America 49:1425–1434, 1969.

Evans JP: *Acute Head Injury,* 2nd ed. Thomas, 1963.

Evans JP & others: A summary of current concepts of the dynamics of head injury. Tr Am Neurol A 94:256–258, 1969.

Finney LA, Walker AE: *Transtentorial Herniation.* Thomas, 1962.

Gurdjian ES, Webster JE: *Head Injuries.* Little, Brown, 1958.

McKissock W, Richardson A, Bloom WH: Subdural haematoma: A review of 389 cases. Lancet 1:1365–1369, 1960.

Morley TP, Hetherington RF: Traumatic cerebrospinal fluid rhinorrhea and otorrhea, pneumocephalus, and meningitis. Surg Gynec Obst 104:88–98, 1957.

Rowbotham GF: *Acute Injuries of the Head,* 4th ed. Williams & Wilkins, 1964.

Schneider RC: Craniocerebral trauma. In: *Correlative Neurosurgery,* 2nd ed. Kahn EA & others. Thomas, 1969.

Shulman K, Ransohoff J: Subdural hematoma in children. J Neurosurg 18:175–181, 1961.

Zülch KJ: Neuropathology of intracranial hemorrhage. Progr Brain Res 30:151–165, 1968.

• • •

SPINAL TRAUMA
Charles B. Wilson, MD

The spine supports the head and trunk, allows a wide range of mobility, and protects neural structures contained within it. Impairment of spinal stability and mobility is an orthopedic problem and is discussed in Chapter 46; this section is concerned only with the neurologic aspects of spinal injuries. All spinal injuries, however, should be managed by the neurosurgeon and the orthopedist in collaboration.

Spinal injuries damage neural structures by encroaching upon the spinal canal and intervertebral foramens. The injuries to be considered here are fractures of the vertebral body and neural arch; dislocations, partial or complete, unilateral or bilateral, with or without x-ray fracture; and lateral or posterior herniation of intervertebral disk fragments. Neurologic involvement ranges from mild and transient to severe and permanent. Injuries of the cervical and thoracic spine may involve spinal cord and local nerve roots; injuries from T11 through L1 involves the conus, local nerve roots, and nerve roots of the cauda equina; and injuries below L1 involve nerve roots only (Fig 41—5).

Clinical Findings

Spinal injury may be unsuspected, particularly in the patient sustaining other more obvious injuries—eg, cerebral concussion, blunt abdominal trauma, facial fractures. Spinal injury should be considered in the presence of the following findings: (1) all acute injuries to the head and jaw; (2) pain in occiput, spine, or limbs; (3) weakness of one or more limbs; (4) spinal deformity; (5) paralysis of accessory muscles of respiration, with diaphragmatic breathing; and (6) manifestations of "spinal shock" such as ileus, priapism, hyper- or hypothermia, and low blood pressure.

Caution: Extreme care must be exercised in transporting or examining a patient with a suspected spine injury.

A. Symptoms and Signs: Isolated injury of the spinal nerve roots causes motor and sensory loss in corresponding myotomes and dermatomes. The characteristic pain of nerve root injuries may be intensified by the slightest movement.

1. Total loss of spinal cord function—There are 3 types of manifestations: (1) **motor** (immediate areflexia and flaccid paralysis; in time, reflexes return and spasticity replaces flaccidity); (2) **sensory** (absence of sensation below the injured segment; sacral sensation must be examined because, in otherwise complete transection, it may be spared); and (3) **autonomic** (urinary retention due to detrusor paralysis, paralytic

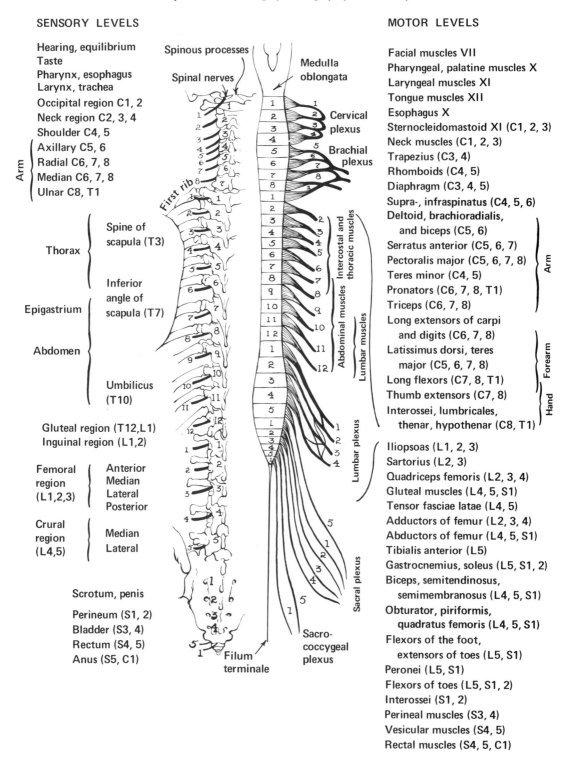

FIG 41–5. Motor and sensory levels of the spinal cord. (Reproduced, with permission, from Chusid JG: *Correlative Neuroanatomy & Functional Neurology*, 15th ed. Lange, 1973.)

ileus, anhidrosis below the injury, mild hypotension secondary to vasomotor paralysis, and, with high injuries, fever caused by failure to dissipate body heat). The early depression of motor and autonomic function goes by the unfortunate term "spinal shock."

2. Regional injury—

a. Cervical—

(1) C1—2—Because spinal cord injury at this level causes fatal respiratory paralysis, patients reaching a hospital alive have either no or minimal neurologic damage. Dislocation at C1—2 (almost always associated with odontoid fracture) causes pain in the neck and occiput, rigidity or rotation of the neck, and abnormal prominence of the C2 spine. The signs and symptoms of "hangman's fracture," a bilateral pedicle fracture of C2 with C2—3 dislocation, are similar.

(2) C4—T1—Quadriparesis or quadriplegia occurs in varying degrees, the extent being determined by the severity of injury and the level involved. Lesions at C4 involve the entire upper limb; lower injuries spare the proximal muscles.

(3) Hyperextension—Extreme hyperextension of the neck narrows the anteroposterior diameter of the spinal canal and, if intraspinal osteophytic spurs (spondylosis) are present, the cord may be injured. Because the greatest damage occurs centrally within the cord, sparing of the posterior columns and disproportionate involvement of the hands are characteristic.

b. Thoracolumbar—Except for simple compression fractures of the vertebral body without neurologic impairment, high and mid thoracic injuries are uncommon. In the less common but more serious thoracolumbar injuries, paralysis due to lesions of lower motor neurons is immediately and permanently flaccid. The extent of lower limb involvement is determined by the level of injury, but all thoracolumbar injuries cause paralysis of bowel and bladder.

B. X-Ray Examination: Although invaluable in diagnosis, x-ray examination of a spinal injury may cause further damage (perhaps fatal) if care is not taken. Any patient with a suspected or known spinal injury should be moved onto the x-ray table by 2 or more persons standing *on one side,* their arms beneath his body. Moving in unison, they should lift him onto the table while 2 more persons (one at his head and one at his feet) exert gentle traction to maintain alignment. The patient should not be turned to a lateral position; lateral views are taken across the x-ray table. When injury to the cervical spine is suspected, the head and neck should be immobilized in the neutral position before x-rays are taken. This can be done by placing sandbags alongside the head, strapping the head to a spine board with a forehead strap, applying an adjustable cervical collar, or by cervical halter traction. The C7—T1 junction must be visualized, which may require pulling the supine patient's arms directly downward or taking a "swimmer's view" exposure. The patient with a thoracolumbar injury is easily immobilized on a board.

Myelography may be indicated when neurologic

changes are present but the spine films are normal. Acute rupture of an intervertebral disk may injure the spinal cord, nerve roots, or both, without fracture or dislocation of the spine. Acute disk rupture is suspected when plain spine x-rays do not explain observed neurologic deficits, and in this circumstance myelographic verification of a ruptured disk precedes its surgical removal.

Complications

Quadriplegic patients have an ineffective cough and reduced tidal volume secondary to paralysis of accessory muscles of respiration, so that tracheostomy is indicated in selected cases. Frequent but less threatening early complications involve the skin (pressure sores), bladder (urinary tract infection), and paralyzed muscles (contractures and deformity).

Prevention

Inexpert handling at the scene of the accident and during transportation to the emergency department may cause or aggravate neurologic damage, and movement of the victim with known or suspected spinal injury should await arrival of trained personnel. Prevention of further injury during x-ray examination is discussed above.

Training leading to certification of ambulance personnel and standardization of ambulance vehicles and equipment would prevent many serious and permanent sequelae of spine injuries.

Treatment

The objectives of treatment are to protect undamaged neural structures, to restore function to reversibly damaged structures, to correct spinal alignment, and to achieve permanent spinal stability. Early supportive care is of great importance. This includes attention to the skin, bladder, paralyzed and paretic muscles, and nutrition. The quality of early care determines the speed with which active rehabilitative measures can be started.

A. Immediate Care: An adequate airway must be established and maintained. The injured spinal segment must be immobilized while a search for associated injuries—particularly injuries involving anesthetic areas —is carried out.

1. Care of the skin—Pressure sores (decubitus ulcers) may develop with astonishing rapidity. As soon as a diagnosis of cord transection is made, it is essential to change the position of paralyzed parts at least every 2 hours. Stabilization of cervical spine injury by traction is a critical component of early change in position (see Chapter 9).

2. Vesical paralysis and ileus—These require insertion of a urethral catheter and a nasogastric tube.

3. Cervical—All cervical injuries with fracture or dislocation of vertebrae are managed by skeletal traction, usually by means of Crutchfield tongs placed in line with the mastoid tips. Dislocations are reduced gradually with up to 16 kg (35 lb) of traction. Nonoperative management requires 6 weeks of continuous traction followed by 12 weeks of external support (by brace or plaster cast); fractures of C1 and C2 require traction for twice as long.

Three surgical procedures have been applied to cervical fractures: (1) Laminectomy for decompression of the spinal cord and nerve roots, the accepted indication being progression of neurologic deficit. (2) Posterior fusion, either at the time of laminectomy or later, because of spinal instability. All odontoid fractures may be treated by early fusion of C1—3. (3) Anterior removal of intervertebral disk and involved bone, exploration of the spinal canal, and interbody fusion. This should be considered for cervical injuries below C2 with or without neurologic deficit. It permits early activity, allows removal of intraspinal disk and bone fragments, and assures a stable undeformed spine. Hyperextension injuries without fracture require neither traction nor operation.

4. **Thoracolumbar**—All thoracolumbar and lumbar fractures with neurologic deficit should be treated by decompression and exploratory laminectomy. Internal fixation with or without fusion is often done by the orthopedist at the same time. Conus injuries seldom improve following decompression, but the cauda equina roots may regain function.

3. **Disk rupture**—Operative removal of a ruptured disc at any level should follow localization of the lesion by myelography.

B. **Special Care of Missile Injuries:** High-velocity missiles can damage the spinal cord without entering the spinal canal. Missiles that enter or traverse the spinal canal produce open wounds of the spinal cord and cauda equina that must, in every instance, be debrided. Laminectomy with exploration of the damaged structures has 2 objectives: to prevent infection and to ensure optimal conditions for recovery. Unlike other traumatic forces, missile injuries do not produce spinal instability.

C. **Long-Term Care (Rehabilitation):** Unfortunately, facilities for the care of paraplegic and quadriplegic civilians are at present sadly inadequate. A critical part of rehabilitation is bladder training, the goal being a catheter-free patient with sterile urine. Repeated bouts of pyelonephritis and dilatation of the collecting system are indications for urinary diversion.

Prognosis

Although physiologic transection of the cord (total paralysis and anesthesia below the site of damage) is indistinguishable from anatomic transection immediately after injury, a thorough neurologic examination 24 hours after injury permits an accurate prognosis. There is early return of some function following concussion of the cord. If total interruption of cord function is documented 24 hours after injury, the spinal cord has been irreversibly damaged and any slight recovery will be functionally insignificant. Any evidence of voluntary motor or sensory function below the level of injury indicates an incomplete injury with the potential for incomplete to near-complete recovery. Testing of sacral sensation is particularly

important because of the prognostic implications of sacral sparing as an indication of incomplete transection.

The long-term prognosis in severe spinal injury is intimately related to renal function because uremia is the major cause of death.

Alexander E Jr, Davis CH Jr, Forsyth HF: Reduction and fusion of fracture dislocation of the cervical spine. J Neurosurg 27:588, 1967.

Aufranc OE, Jones WN, Harris WH: Thoracic spine fracture with paralysis. JAMA 189:1018, 1964.

Bailey RW: Fractures and dislocations of the cervical spine: Orthopedic and neurosurgical aspects. Postgrad Med 35:588, 1964.

Bertrand G: Management of spinal injuries with associated cord damage. Postgrad Med 37:249, 1965.

Bray EA, Miller JA, Bouzard WC: Traumatic dislocation of the cervical spine. J Trauma 3:569, 1963.

Jane JA, Evans JP, Fisher LE: An investigation concerning the restitution of motor function following injury to the spinal cord. J Neurosurg 21:167, 1964.

Kaufer H, Hayes JT: Lumbar fracture-dislocation. J Bone Joint Surg 48A:712, 1966.

Norrell H, Wilson CB: Early anterior cervical fusion for injuries of the cervical spine. JAMA 214:525—530, 1970.

Nyquist RH, Bors E: Mortality and survival in traumatic myelopathy during nineteen years, from 1946 to 1965. Paraplegia 5:22, 1967.

TRAUMATIC PERIPHERAL NERVE LESIONS
Barton A. Brown, MD

Regardless of cause, peripheral nerve injuries fall into 3 categories: neurotmesis, in which both the axons and the investing sheaths are disrupted; axonotmesis, in which the axons are interrupted but the sheath remains intact; and axonapraxia, in which both axons and nerve sheaths are intact but there is a failure of conduction. The types of injuries may be compression (from casts, tourniquets, bandages, entrapment), lacerations (by sharp objects, missiles, fractures), contusions (by blunt trauma, either chronic or acute), stretch, ischemia, and injection.

The peripheral nerves contain sensory and motor fibers, most of which are myelinated. Each axon is surrounded by an endoneurial connective tissue tube; groups of axons are bound together by perineurium; and the resultant fascicles are enmeshed in the epineurium, which is bounded by the external nerve sheath.

Depending upon its severity, trauma may produce edema, swelling, and variable disruption of the axonal and connective tissue elements, and distal wallerian degeneration. Resolution of the acute process results in scar formation within the nerve and for variable distances above and below the site of injury. If the nerve has been completely divided, no immediate prediction can be made of the extent of scarring.

In a divided nerve, the proximal end will develop a neuroma composed of connective tissue and tangled axons. The distal free end will have an end bulb of connective tissue. If the injured nerve retains its continuity, scar tissue may develop within the nerve and cause constriction of the axons with resultant dysfunction.

Clinical Findings

Sensory, motor, and reflex changes will depend upon the peripheral nerve involved and the level of involvement. A standard neuroanatomy textbook should be available for review of specific motor and sensory innervation and possible anatomic variations.

A history of remote as well as recent trauma should be elicited. In neurologic diagnosis, the history suggests the type of pathology while the neurologic examination localizes the lesion. A complete neurologic examination must be done, with emphasis on the nerves involved. Motor, sensory, and reflex deficits must be correlated to determine severity and distribution of involvement. Electromyography and nerve conduction studies establish a baseline for monitoring subsequent recovery.

Differential Diagnosis

An accurate history and a meticulous examination are the key elements. The history will help differentiate traumatic neuropathies from those of infectious origin (diphtheria, mumps, influenza, pneumonia, meningitis, malaria, syphilis, typhoid, typhus, dysentery, tuberculosis, gonorrhea) or toxic or metabolic origin (diabetes, rheumatic fever, gout, leukemia, vitamin deficiency, polyarteritis nodosa, drug reaction, heavy metals, carbon monoxide).

Complications

Causalgia is a dysesthetic, severe burning pain in the distribution of a nerve with a partial lesion. Hyperpathia, trophic changes, and vasomotor hyperactivity are characteristic. (Minor stimuli may produce severe exacerbations of the pain.) Although spontaneous remissions may occur, sympathetic blocks and sympathectomy are specific diagnostic and therapeutic procedures.

"Reflex sympathetic dystrophy" or "minor causalgia" sometimes occurs, usually in relation to painful osteoporosis or Sudeck's atrophy. The major complaint is hyperesthesia. Treatment consists of sympathetic blocks and active physical therapy.

Treatment

When a peripheral nerve has been severed, reanastomosis by suture is the appropriate treatment. Primary suture should be attempted only in wounds that are clean, seen immediately, caused by knife or razor, and devoid of adjacent tissue damage. In the remainder of cases, the nerve ends should be tagged and secondary suture undertaken when the wound has completely healed, adjacent tissue reaction has subsided, and infection has cleared. After a delay of 3 weeks or more, the extent of intraneural scarring can be determined at the time of secondary suture, and the nerve ends should be resected until normal tissue is reached. Delayed repair greatly enhances the chances for functional recovery. If removal of scarred ends leaves a gap that is too large to be bridged, the limb can be flexed until the gap is closed. After healing, the sutured nerve can be stretched over a period of months by placing the limb in a series of gradually straightened casts. Frozen irradiated homografts offer a means of bridging extensive nerve defects, but all the problems of rejection have not yet been solved and chance of success is limited.

Nerve injuries in continuity—whether loss of function is complete or incomplete—should be explored if they do not improve within 6 weeks after injury. Intra- and extraneural scar tissue at the site of the lesion often causes axonopraxia or prevents axonal regrowth by virtue of its constricting effects. External and internal neurolyses via microsurgical technics are indicated. Some of these lesions would improve spontaneously if left alone for more than 6 weeks, but the disadvantage of continued denervation outweighs the risk of surgical exploration.

Some lesions resulting from contusion or compression are improved by neurolysis. The same is true of some injection neuropathies (depending upon the substance injected).

Prompt institution of physical therapy for improvement of muscle function and maintenance of joint range of motion is indicated. The denervated portion of the limb is subject to muscle atrophy and fibrosis, joint stiffness, motor end plate atrophy, and trophic skin changes. The longer the denervation persists, the less likely it is that a good functional result will be achieved. Physical therapy is the best means of minimizing the complications of denervation.

Prognosis

Grading of sensorimotor function from 0–5 is helpful in documenting progress. Most improvement occurs during the first year, but the maximum may not be reached for 3–4 years. The younger the patient, the better the prognosis; injuries with minimal adjacent tissue damage have a better prognosis than those with widespread tissue damage such as war wounds. Proximal lesions recover less well than distal ones. Intraoperative factors such as axial orientation of the nerve, proper coaptation, suture material, hemostasis, and suture line tension are important determinants of the end result. Electromyography and nerve conduction studies are helpful guides during the recovery period. Healing in a damaged peripheral nerve is slow (approximately 1 mm/day), and the patient must be prepared for this. He must understand that his role in treatment is an active one, and his motivation must be maintained.

Brown BA: Internal neurolysis in treatment of traumatic peripheral nerve lesions. California Med 110:460–462, 1969.

Brown HA, Brown BA: Treatment of peripheral nerve injuries. Rev Surg 24:1–8, 1967.

Campbell JB: Peripheral nerve repair. Clin Neurosurg 17:77–98, 1969.

Chusid JG: *Correlative Neuroanatomy & Functional Neurology,* 15th ed. Lange, 1973.

Sunderland S: *Nerves and Nerve Injuries.* Williams & Wilkins, 1968.

BRAIN TUMORS

Essentials of Diagnosis

- Headache.
- Progressive neurologic deficit.
- Convulsions, focal or generalized.
- Increased intracranial pressure.
- Organic mental changes.

General Considerations

Although by custom tumors are considered either benign or malignant, *all* brain tumors are malignant in the sense that they may lead to death if not treated. By compression or invasion of neighboring structures, brain tumors cause specific signs of localizing value. Most brain tumors, either by virtue of their bulk or by obstructing the flow of CSF, eventually produce increased intracranial pressure which may have no localizing value.

Among adults, 70% of brain tumors originate above the tentorium cerebelli; the remainder occupy the infratentorial compartment (posterior fossa). In children, the majority of tumors are infratentorial. Age and site are correlated with tumor type in Table 41–2. The frequency of major tumor types is indicated in Table 41–3.

Meningiomas and nerve sheath tumors are more common in females than in males; most glial tumors—particularly medulloblastomas—have a predi-

TABLE 41–2. Frequency of brain tumor types according to age and site.

Age	Cerebral Hemisphere	Intrasellar and Parasellar	Posterior Fossa
Childhood and adolescence	Ependymomas; less commonly, astrocytomas.	Astrocytomas, craniopharyngiomas.	Astrocytomas, medulloblastomas, ependymomas.
Age 20–40	Meningiomas, astrocytomas; less commonly, metastatic tumors.	Pituitary adenomas; less commonly, meningiomas.	Acoustic neuromas, meningiomas, hemangioblastomas; less commonly, metastatic tumors.
Over age 40	Glioblastoma multiforme, meningiomas, metastatic tumors.	Pituitary adenomas; less commonly, meningiomas.	Metastatic tumors, acoustic neuromas, meningiomas.

TABLE 41–3. Frequency of major types of brain tumors.

Intracranial Tumors*		Frequency of Occurrence
Gliomas		50%
Glioblastoma multiforme	50%	
Astrocytoma	20%	
Ependymoma	10%	
Medulloblastoma	10%	
Oligodendroglioma	5%	
Mixed	5%	
Meningiomas		20%
Nerve sheath tumors		10%
Metastatic tumors		10%
Congenital tumors		5%
Miscellaneous tumors		5%

*Exclusive of pituitary tumors.

lection for males, and pineal tumors occur almost exclusively in young males. Other primary tumors attack the sexes equally.

Classification

A. Gliomas: Tumors composed of glial cells constitute 50% of intracranial neoplasms. The neuroglia, once thought to serve only as a supporting structure, contains complex cellular elements involved with important functions such as the blood-brain barrier, myelin metabolism, and neuronal metabolism. Astrocytes and oligodendroglia are present throughout the CNS, whereas ependymal cells are confined to the ventricular cavities and the central canal. Medulloblastomas are included among gliomas, although a medulloblast is a theoretically bipotential cell (neuroglial and neuronal).

1. Astrocytomas—These slowly invasive tumors are widely distributed throughout the brain at all ages. Among younger patients, they involve predominantly 3 sites—optic nerves and hypothalamus, brain stem, and cerebellar hemispheres—typically as a cyst containing a relatively small neoplastic nural nodule.

2. Oligodendrogliomas—These slowly growing tumors rarely arise outside the cerebral hemispheres. They are tumors of adult life and calcification within the tumor is often seen on x-ray.

3. Ependymomas—Ependymomas are uncommon in adults. In the cerebral hemispheres, they may extend intracerebrally, whereas in the fourth ventricle they show less tendency to invade deeply into adjacent neural tissue. Papillomas of the choroid plexus may be considered to be a special type of ependymoma; their ability to "overproduce" CSF is doubtful.

4. Glioblastoma multiforme—Biologically and histologically, these are malignant astrocytomas (and are sometimes classified as astrocytoma grade III–IV). Mean survival from the date of diagnosis is slightly over 6 months—in contrast to 2–5 years for the tumors described above. Most occupy the cerebral hemisphere in adults, and the remainder occur in the brain stems of children. Characteristic features include tumor tissue with necrosis, new vessel formation, spontaneous hemorrhage, and associated cerebral edema.

5. Medulloblastomas–Predominantly tumors of infancy and childhood, medulloblastomas are highly malignant tumors arising in the cerebellar vermis. Distinctive features are their extreme radiosensitivity and their tendency to seed down the spine in the CSF.

B. Nonglial Tumors: These tumors arise from various tissues. They are biologically benign and compress rather than invade adjacent brain.

1. Meningiomas–These are firm, generally globular tumors readily separable from compressed neural tissues. Because of their slow rate of growth, meningiomas often attain massive proportions. Believed to originate from arachnoid granulations, they have a broad base along the dura (including the dural partitions, the falx cerebri, and the tentorium cerebelli), often extend into bone, and derive a portion of their blood supply from extracerebral arteries, eg, the external carotid branches. Preferred sites are along the length of the superior sagittal sinus (parasagittal; Fig 41–6), over the cerebral convexities, beneath the frontal lobe (olfactory groove and tuberculum sellae; Fig 41–7), along the sphenoid wing, and within the posterior fossa (cerebellopontine angle and clivus). The tendency of meningiomas to involve the orbit explains the frequent occurrence of exophthalmos (sphenoid wing; Fig 41–8).

Figures 41–6 to 41–12 are reproduced, with permission, from Scarff: *Classic Syndromes of Brain Tumor.* Annual Clinical Conference of the Chicago Medical Society, 1953.

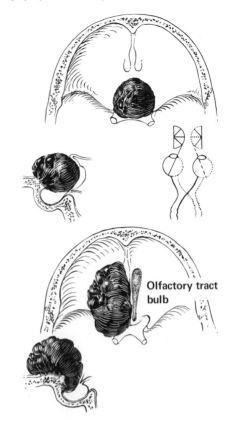

FIG 41–7. *Top:* Meningioma of tuberculum sellae. Failing vision, primary optic atrophy bitemporal hemianopsia, but no endocrine disturbance and no enlargement of the sella turcica in middle-aged persons. ***Bottom:*** Olfactory groove meningioma. Ipsilateral anosmia and primary optic atrophy; contralateral papilledema.

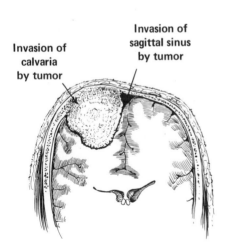

FIG 41–6. Parasagittal meningioma. Disturbances of cerebral function, depending on localization. Focal hyperplasia and hypervascularization of the overlying bones.

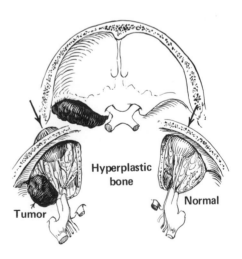

FIG 41–8. Retro-orbital meningioma. *Early stage:* Unilateral exophthalmos, slowly progressing (months to years). Increased density (in x-rays): retro-orbital plate, ipsilateral side.

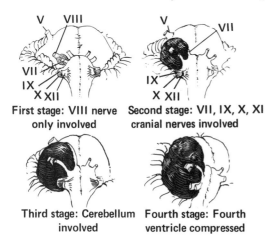

First stage: VIII nerve only involved

Second stage: VII, IX, X, XI cranial nerves involved

Third stage: Cerebellum involved

Fourth stage: Fourth ventricle compressed

FIG 41–9. Acoustic neurinoma. *First stage:* Tinnitus; later, deafness and disturbances of equilibrium. *Second stage:* Weakness of facial muscles, pain in face, dysphasia and dysarthria. *Third stage:* Ataxia and incoordination. *Fourth stage:* Evidence of increased intracranial pressure.

2. Nerve sheath tumors (Fig 41–9)—These tumors are termed acoustic neurinomas because they originate almost exclusively in the eighth cranial nerve. From its point of origin within the internal auditory canal, this slowly growing tumor expands the auditory meatus as it extends into the angle formed by the cerebellum and pons. At the time of diagnosis it typically compresses the fifth cranial nerve, the pons, the cerebellum, and the fourth ventricle. The seventh cranial nerve is stretched remarkably, but its function is usually little affected. Patients with multiple neurofibromatosis are liable to develop sheath tumors of the eighth nerve, but the vast majority of patients harboring acoustic tumors have no stigmas of this disease.

3. Craniopharyngiomas (Fig 41–10)—Arising from remnants of Rathke's pouch, this typically cystic tumor extends from the sella turcica to involve the optic nerves, the hypothalamus, and the third ventricle. Fluid within this tumor resembles motor oil in appearance. Most craniopharyngiomas contain calcified areas which can be seen on x-ray and become symptomatic in childhood. Some, however, first appear in mid and late adult life.

4. Congenital tumors—

a. Epidermoid tumors—These consist of a mass of desquamated epithelium produced by a simple epithelium-lined cyst. Intracranially, they occur most frequently in the parasellar region and at the cerebellopontine angle.

b. Intracranial dermoids—These tumors are rare. Most occupy the posterior fossa.

c. Teratomas—These tumors (also rare) arise most commonly in the pineal gland.

d. Chordomas—These tumors originate from notochordal remnants along the clivus. Like the more common sacrococcygeal chordomas, they grow slowly.

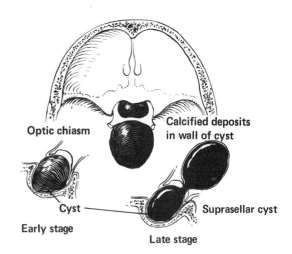

Optic chiasm

Calcified deposits in wall of cyst

Cyst

Early stage

Suprasellar cyst

Late stage

FIG 41–10. Craniopharyngioma. *Early stage:* Failing vision, primary optic atrophy, bitemporal field defects, endocrine disturbances (hypopituitarism), suprasellar calcification (80%) in children and adolescents. *Late stage:* Headache, nausea, and vomiting.

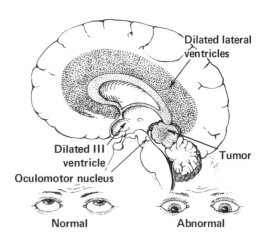

Dilated lateral ventricles

Dilated III ventricle

Oculomotor nucleus

Tumor

Normal

Abnormal

FIG 41–11. Pinealoma. Symptoms and signs of increased intracranial pressure, without lateralizing signs. Limitation of upward gaze. Abnormal pupillary reactions.

e. Pineal tumors (Fig 41–11)—Almost all pineal tumors are either true teratomas or atypical teratomas. The latter are germinomas identical with testicular seminomas and ovarian dysgerminomas. Germinomas may originate in the hypothalamus, where they have been termed (incorrectly) "ectopic pinealomas."

5. Metastatic tumors—Carcinoma of the lung in males and carcinoma of the breast in females account for almost 70% of all metastases within the skull; other primary tumors are other supradiaphragmatic tumors (eg, thyroid), renal carcinoma, and malignant melanoma. The distribution of metastatic tumors is determined by blood flow in different areas, and the frequency in a particular site is roughly proportionate to its mass. One-third of brain metastases are solitary. Metastatic tumors provoke varying degrees of surrounding brain edema.

Clinical Findings

Brain tumors may produce general and focal signs either singly or together. General signs relate to increased intracranial pressure. Local signs may be irritative (convulsive) or destructive (paralytic). The temporal evolution (rate of progression) of neurologic signs correlates with each tumor's rate of growth.

The manifestations of intrinsic supratentorial tumors are related to the site involved. Frontal tumors may cause personality changes, with loss of interest, facetiousness, and moral laxity. Tumors involving the posterior frontal region may produce contralateral mono- or hemiparesis. Temporal lobe tumors may cause behavior disorders, often accompanied by superior quadrantanopsia or uncinate seizures. Parietal lobe tumors may cause contralateral hemisensory disturbances and homonymous hemianopsia. Occipital tumors may produce homonymous visual field defects characteristically consisting of unformed visual hallucinations. Tumors in the dominant hemisphere may cause disorders of communication (asphasia); nondominant cerebral hemispheric lesions may cause apraxia. Extrinsic supratentorial tumors cause similar disturbances appropriate to their location. Frontal meningiomas unsuspected during life may be discovered on postmortem examination of inmates of state mental institutions. Subfrontal meningiomas should be suspected in the presence of mental deterioration accompanied by anosmia and optic atrophy. Tumors in the region of the sella turcica may involve the optic chiasm (visual loss), hypothalamus (endocrine abnormalities), or foramen interventriculare (hydrocephalus). Intraventricular tumors usually present with signs of intracranial hypertension.

Posterior fossa tumors have characteristic patterns. Brain stem tumors cause multiple cranial nerve palsies (usually fifth through seventh) and later involve motor and sensory long tracts. Tumors in the cerebellar vermis produce truncal ataxia and those in the cerebellar hemisphere an ipsilateral limb ataxia and hypotonia. Tumors originating within the fourth ventricle often produce hydrocephalus without clinical involvement of neighboring structures; and extrinsic tumors occupying the cerebellopontine angle may involve the fifth, seventh, and eighth cranial nerves in association with cerebellar deficits and, in later stages, hydrocephalus through deformity of the fourth ventricle.

Differential Diagnosis

Because brain tumors can cause focal neurologic signs and increased intracranial pressure, many conditions may be simulated by a brain tumor.

During infancy and childhood, an unexplained convulsion usually indicates the onset of idiopathic epilepsy, whereas in later life a convulsion is often the initial manifestation of a brain tumor. Neurologic examination, skull x-rays, EEG, and radioisotopic brain scan will serve to select patients for more definitive radiologic procedures such as angiography and pneumography.

Brain tumors may mimic cerebrovascular disease, and glioblastomas and metastatic tumors in particular cause confusion in this regard. A careful inquiry into antecedent symptoms may disclose evidence suggestive of tumor, but the diagnosis is often not suspected until the patient's course indicates deterioration rather than improvement.

Chronic subdural hematomas and brain abscesses may pursue a course similar to that of a tumor. Without a history of head injury or a source of infection, the diagnosis may be unsuspected until disclosed by angiography or operation.

Increased intracranial pressure has many causes. In the pediatric age group, the list includes lead encephalopathy, acute glomerulonephritis, administration of antibiotics to infants predisposed to increased intracranial pressure, and downward adjustment of dosage in patients being given long-term corticosteroid therapy. The history usually makes the diagnosis.

Pseudotumor cerebri (idiopathic brain swelling, benign intracranial hypertension) typically affects adolescent and young adult females, and the cause is probably an endocrine imbalance. A similar "benign brain edema" occurs in women receiving oral contraceptives and in certain patients with Addison's disease and hyperparathyroidism. Again, the history, neurologic examination, and special neuroradiologic tests such as angiography should distinguish these patients from those with increased intracranial pressure caused by brain tumor.

Complications

Missed or late diagnosis may lead to irreversible brain damage, which is all the more tragic in the case of a favorably situated benign tumor. Injudicious lumbar puncture may precipitate fatal temporal lobe or tonsillar herniation.

Treatment

Total removal is the surgeon's goal in the treatment of most extrinsic tumors (meningiomas, nerve sheath tumors, craniopharyngiomas, colloid cysts, and epidermoids) and cerebellar hemangioblastomas. If the location, size, and vascularity of the tumor precludes safe extirpation, subtotal removal may be all that can be done. With the exception of cystic cerebellar astrocytomas containing a mural tumor nodule, glial tumors in the cerebral hemispheres and cerebellum are rarely curable by operation alone, and the surgeon's objective becomes radical subtotal removal within the limits determined by the tumor's location—eg, dominant hemisphere, motor area. Postoperative radiation therapy in the range of 5000 rads over the course of 5–6 weeks is then delivered to the residual tumor. In patients with medulloblastoma, the spinal axis is also irradiated because this tumor frequently seeds throughout the CSF.

Tumors of the brain stem and pineal regions are usually treated by irradiation alone on the basis of clinical and x-ray diagnosis. Although pineal tumors can be removed, their marked radiosensitivity and the high risk of operation argue for radiotherapy, usually preceded by placement of a CSF shunt for hydrocephalus.

Under certain circumstances, solitary metastatic tumors are suitable for surgical extirpation. Their radiosensitivity varies.

Chemotherapy has been used with variable and modest success for recurrent glioblastomas and medulloblastomas.

Prognosis

Surgically removable tumors can be cured, and this group includes the majority of meningiomas and nerve sheath tumors, epidermoids, colloid cysts, small craniopharyngiomas, and many cerebellar astrocytomas and hemangioblastomas. Although low-grade gliomas are not highly radiosensitive, long survival is possible when operation and irradiation are combined. Some glioblastomas appear to be radiosensitive, but survival beyond 18 months is uncommon. For medulloblastomas treated by operation and irradiation, the 5-year survival rate is 40%.

Bickerstaff ER, Howell JS: The neurological importance of tumours of the glomus jugulare. Brain 76:576–593, 1953.

Cushing H, Eisenhardt L: *Meningiomas: Their Classification, Regional Behaviour, Life History, and Surgical End Results.* Thomas, 1938.

Kernohan JW, Sayre GP: Tumors of the central nervous system. Fascicle 35 in: *Atlas of Tumor Pathology.* Armed Forces Institute of Pathology, 1952.

Pulec JL: A system of management of acoustic neuroma based on 364 cases. Tr Am Acad Ophth 75:48–55, 1971.

Revilla AG: Differential diagnosis of tumors at the cerebellopontile recess. Bull Johns Hopkins Hosp 83:187–212, 1948.

Wilson DH, Gardner J, McCormack LJ: Life history and treatment of meningiomas within the lateral ventricles. Surg Gynec Obst 112:299–304, 1961.

Zülch KJ: Pp 187–199, 204–206 in: *Brain Tumors: Their Biology and Pathology.* Springer, 1957.

TUMORS OF THE SPINAL CANAL

Essentials of Diagnosis

- Symptoms and signs consistent with a single lesion.
- Progressive involvement.
- Manifestations of pressure on the cord, intraspinal roots, or surrounding tissues, including the vertebral column.

General Considerations

Neoplasms of the spinal canal may be intrinsic within the spinal cord; may originate from spinal roots within the spinal subarachnoid space or from the meninges pressing upon the roots, the cord, or both; or may originate outside the dura, pressing there upon the extradural root structure and transdurally upon the contents of the spinal theca. The last are almost always metastatic tumors.

In general, primary intramedullary tumors are not as likely to be painful as intrathecal extramedullary growths, which may shift with position to painfully displace the roots, or as the extradural tumors, which may involve the roots outside the dural canal. However, any neoplasm within the vertebral column and any neoplasm involving the spinal canal may cause pain.

Clinical Findings

A. Symptoms and Signs: Intramedullary lesions may interrupt the fiber pathways that cross the midline as well as axial pathways to produce bilateral sensory disturbances that are confined to a few segments. More extensive intramedullary lesions may cause more extended sensory disturbances but with sacral sparing—this related to the disposition of the axial pathways in the cord.

Neoplasms involving the roots are likely to be painful and usually produce signs of actual root dysfunction in the appropriate distribution of the nerve root. As a tumor enlarges, there may be dysfunction of the long tracts due to direct pressure as well as to involvement of the vascular supply to the cord, the latter especially at certain unpredictable root levels. Long tract dysfunction and local pain are common with extradural lesions secondary to neoplastic disease of the vertebral column.

A thorough and meticulous clinical neurologic examination is imperative. Both the intramedullary and extramedullary growths may manifest their level by involving either bilateral or unilateral motor and sensory pathways. Demonstration of both a motor and a sensory level strongly supports the presumptive diagnosis and is a basis for advising contrast x-ray investigation.

B. Laboratory and Special Examinations: Lumbar puncture should be planned under circumstances that permit introduction of positive contrast material (usually iophendylate [Pantopaque]) during the same procedure. Neither of these studies should be done unless arrangements have been made to proceed with surgery if the signs and symptoms increase rapidly during or immediately following the studies.

With the patient in the lateral position and the vertebral column horizontal, an 18–20 gauge needle is inserted into the lumbar sac, usually at L4 or L5. The needle should not be smaller than 20 gauge if manometric studies are to be done.

When an intraspinal space-occupying lesion is suspected, the Queckenstedt test (jugular compression) is mandatory. At the time of the puncture, an assistant can manually compress the veins of the neck or (Cone-Grant technic) wrap a child's sphygmomanometer cuff around the neck and increase the pressure to 10, 20, 30, and 40 mm Hg for 10 seconds, abruptly interrupting cuff pressure at the end of each 10-second interval and noting the rise of spinal fluid pressure and the rate of fall to the original level.

C. X-Ray Findings: When an intraspinal growth is suspected, x-rays of the vertebral column in the appropriate region are obtained; these should include films of the foramens as well as anteroposterior and lateral views. Stereoscopic views of the vertebral column, especially in the anteroposterior direction, may be of value.

If the Queckenstedt test indicates or the clinical course suggests a major block, only a small amount of contrast material should be injected initially. The radiologist can then determine the degree to which the spinal subarachnoid space is obstructed. If the block seems to be complete or almost complete, the contrast material should be left in place since withdrawal may precipitate rapid advance of symptoms even to complete permanent transverse myelopathy.

If there is no significant spinal subarachnoid block, contrast material should be injected to show the dorsal surface of the canal in the thoracic region as well as the ventral surface of the canal generally. This is especially true when a vascular lesion is suspected, since many of the vascular masses lie on the dorsal surface of the thoracic cord.

Differential Diagnosis

The differential diagnosis may include inflammatory transverse myelopathy, acute degenerative disease of the cord, peripheral neuropathy, radiculomyelopathies, and hemorrhagic or occlusive vascular lesions of the cord.

Complications

Spinal tumors may result in permanent motor and sensory paralyses. Ascending urinary tract infection is the most common secondary complication, ultimately resulting in nephritis and uremia. Another major complication is trophic dysfunction in the lower portion of the trunk and in the legs (pressure sores and the like) with its associated morbidity.

Treatment

Treatment of spinal canal neoplasia is surgical. It is imperative that the cause be identified as soon as there is evidence of spinal cord or spinal root dysfunction. Surgical decompression must be done as soon as possible, since recovery of function after the cord is compressed is sharply limited, particularly when compression is acute. This is especially true when compression is secondary to metastatic disease. Care of the patient with metastatic disease can be severely compromised if the evidence of metastasis to the spinal canal is ignored during the early phase. The patient who is able to control his lower extremities and his bowel and bladder sphincters will have less pain and will generally be an easier patient to care for than one who has lost these functions. This is true even when

death is expected within a few months.

The affected area is approached by laminectomy. Extramedullary tumors should be removed completely if possible—tumors of the meninges and of the roots are usually, though not always, completely resectable. Some intramedullary tumors can be resected; those that are cystic often may be drained. Cysts of the cord, such as hydromyelia, behave as tumors and frequently can be drained. Metastatic and the rare intrinsic extradural tumors, after having been decompressed, should be treated by the method appropriate to the nature of the neoplasm—radiation, chemotherapy, or hormonal therapy.

If complete transverse myelopathy has occurred, appropriate supportive care to the tissues below the level of involvement is imperative. An effort should be made to minimize the development of ascending urinary tract infection.

Prognosis

If clinically evident neurologic destruction progresses slowly, the prospects for improvement are generally better than when it progresses rapidly since the cord adjusts to slowly developing lesions much more satisfactorily than to those that progress with great speed. Under any circumstance, the earlier the diagnosis can be made and the earlier definitive therapy can be done, the better the outlook for improvement or at least for a stabilization of loss of function.

Bailey IC: Dermoid tumors of the spinal cord. J Neurosurg 33:676–681, 1970.

Pool JL: The surgery of spinal cord tumors. Clin Neurosurg 17:310–330, 1969.

TUMORS OF PERIPHERAL NERVES
Edwin B. Boldrey, MD

Essentials of Diagnosis

- A mass along the course of a peripheral nerve.
- Evidence of motor or sensory dysfunction confined to a single peripheral nerve.
- Pain in the distribution of a single peripheral nerve.

General Considerations

Peripheral nerve tumors may be benign or malignant. The most common benign tumor is the nerve sheath tumor, variously called perineurial fibroblastoma, neurilemmoma, schwannoma, or neurofibroma. These tumors displace the major portion of the nerve to one side and can often be totally or almost totally excised. Nerve sheath tumors are more common in patients with Recklinghausen's disease than in the general population. With chronic trauma—particularly in patients with Recklinghausen's disease at puberty—these tumors may become malignant, metastasizing to other portions of the body and invading surrounding tissues.

The true schwannoma—a tumor of verifiable Schwann cells (fortunately rare)—has a high potential for malignancy, particularly in patients with Recklinghausen's disease.

When a neurofibroma is present, the neoplastic activity in the sheath is generalized; in any histologic preparation, a wide spectrum of connective tissue, endoneurial cells, and axonal fibers will be seen. These are diffuse growths and usually cannot be excised; they may spread along all branches of any particular nerve in a plexiform fashion. Neurofibromas are almost invariably a part of the Recklinghausen disease complex.

Nerve sheath tumors may be less than 1 mm in diameter, and these usually occur on the smaller nerves. They may be quite painful. In deeper structures, nerve sheath tumors may grow to substantial size—eg, as extensive as the entire sciatic nerve in the thigh, extending from the ischium to the popliteal space.

Clinical Findings

The symptoms and signs are those of peripheral nerve dysfunction, either irritative or paralytic. The nature and distribution of this dysfunction show that it is related to a specific nerve rather than to a root, tracts in the cord, or cerebral disease. The diagnostic problem is determining the final common pathway.

Differential Diagnosis

Peripheral neuropathies may mimic peripheral nerve tumors, but a tumor that produces symptoms ordinarily is large enough to be palpated. Generalized sensitivity along the nerve pathway is more common in neuritis than in dysfunction secondary to tumor mass.

Treatment

If possible, sheath tumors should be removed. Some response to radiation therapy has been reported for certain types of nonremovable sheath tumors, but on the whole they must be regarded as resistant to irradiation and other forms of nonsurgical therapy. When an invasive malignant sheath tumor exists in an extremity, amputation of the extremity may be advisable unless the malignancy is so advanced that the likelihood of long-term survival is slight under any circumstances.

In Recklinghausen's disease, removal of peripheral nerve tumors is confined to those that cause clinical signs and symptoms such as pain or sensorimotor loss. Tumors that do not cause apparent clinical dysfunction should usually be left alone unless they cause exceptional cosmetic deformity or lie beneath pressure points, eg, at the beltline.

Prognosis

The prognosis for life is good with most peripheral tumors. Multiplicity and recurrence plus a tendency to produce motor or sensory deficits usually result in moderate morbidity.

PITUITARY TUMORS
Robert J. Seymour, MD

Essentials of Diagnosis

- Signs and symptoms referable to abnormal endocrine function and compression of the optic chiasm.
- Headache, easy fatigability, and diminished libido; sweating and paresthesias in acromegalic patients.
- Visual field changes are usual with chromophobe adenomas; acral and facial changes are usual with acidophilic tumors.
- Hypopituitarism is usual with chromophobe adenomas; elevated serum growth hormone and abnormal glucose tolerance test in acromegalic patients; Cushing's syndrome may be seen with ACTH-secreting tumors.
- Sella turcica enlarged on skull x-rays.

General Considerations

Classically, the cells in the adenohypophysis are divided into (1) granular chromophils, which are either acidophilic (35%) or basophilic (15%); and (2) agranular chromophobes (50%). Recent studies indicate a more diverse cell population, and a specific cell type for each hormone can be designated on the basis of granule size and special histochemical reactions. Nevertheless, pituitary tumors are still classified as chromophobe, acidophilic, and basophilic adenomas. Together, they account for 10–15% of all intracranial tumors. About 80% are chromophobes, and most of the remainder are acidophils. Basophilic adenomas are rare.

Clinical Findings

Chromophobe tumors of the pituitary cause symptoms by compressing adjacent structures, by altering pituitary function, or by doing both (Fig 41–12). Suprasellar extension causes visual field changes, first in the upper temporal quadrants and progressing to bitemporal hemianopsia. As the tumor grows, visual acuity diminishes and optic disk pallor develops. Occasionally, the tumor grows laterally to produce a cavernous sinus syndrome with facial numbness and extraocular muscle palsies. Rarely, the tumor may extend into the temporal lobe or hypothalamus.

Cushing's syndrome is occasionally the initial sign of an ACTH-secreting chromophobe adenoma. Following adrenalectomy, the sella enlarges and skin pigmentation is striking (Nelson's syndrome). Less commonly, Nelson's syndrome is associated with a basophilic adenoma.

Pituitary tumors commonly produce hypopituitarism, manifested by amenorrhea, sterility, loss of libido, easy fatigability, loss of body hair, and fine-

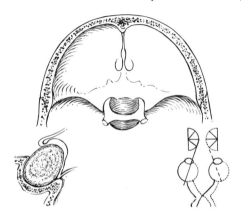

FIG 41–12. Pituitary adenoma (chromophobe type). Failing vision, primary optic atrophy, bitemporal hemianopsia, endocrine disturbances, and enlargement of sella turcica.

ness of the skin. On rare occasions, sudden bleeding occurs in a pituitary tumor, producing "pituitary apoplexy" and precipitous rather than slowly evolving clinical signs. The patient suddenly becomes blind and hypotensive and develops acute fluid and electrolyte imbalances.

The clinical manifestations of eosinophilic adenomas result from the systemic effects of elevated serum growth hormone. Headache, typical facial and acral changes, easy fatigability, paresthesias of the extremities, increased sweating, and decreased sexual function occur in acromegaly. Gigantism is added when the tumor occurs before epiphyseal closure. Occasionally there are ophthalmologic findings, signs of hypopituitarism, or both. As with all pituitary tumors, the sella is often enlarged.

Pituitary, adrenal, thyroid, and gonadal function are depressed in patients with chromophobe adenomas. In acromegaly, serum growth hormone is elevated and cannot be suppressed by glucose.

Differential Diagnosis

The characteristic appearance of the acromegalic patient makes the diagnosis a simple one. It is confirmed by assaying the serum growth hormone. Although patients with chromophobe adenomas usually present a fairly characteristic clinical picture, the following pathologic entities can simulate chromophobe tumors: craniopharyngioma, aneurysms of the internal carotid artery, suprasellar meningiomas, optic chiasm gliomas, dilatation of the third ventricle in hydrocephalus, mucoceles of the sphenoid sinus, and encephaloceles.

Without histologic verification, a tentative diagnosis can be established by tomograms of the sella, angiography, and pneumoencephalography with tomography. All patients suspected of harboring a pituitary tumor should be investigated by means of contrast studies and evaluations of endocrine function.

Treatment

Chromophobe adenomas must be treated, because their pressure on contiguous structures is progressive. Treatment often requires craniotomy to decompress the optic nerves and chiasm. Postoperative irradiation is indicated since tumor removal is seldom complete. Irradiation alone is not adequate because a significant number of pituitary tumors are cystic, and even after extensive study the responsible lesion may prove to be something other than a tumor. Furthermore, the effects of radiation are delayed and cannot produce the prompt decompression that is necessary if vision is to be preserved. In at least two-thirds of patients, vision will be improved by decompression alone; in about one-third, it will be unchanged. A recurrence rate of 5–15% is reported.

Acromegaly should always be treated because the cardiovascular effects of excess growth hormone shorten the life span. Transsphenoidal cryohypophysectomy is probably the most satisfactory method of treatment. Conventional and supervoltage irradiation are not applicable. Heavy particle irradiation offers an alternative to the surgical procedure but is not widely available. By the transsphenoidal approach, pituitary and adrenal function are usually preserved. Nelson's syndrome may also be treated satisfactorily by this technic.

Adams JE & others: Transsphenoidal cryohypophysectomy in acromegaly: Clinical and endocrinological evaluation. J Neurosurg 28:100–104, 1968.

Chamlin M, Davidoff LM: Ophthalmologic criteria in diagnosis and management of pituitary tumors. J Neurosurg 19:9–18, 1962.

Correa JN, Lampe I: The radiation treatment of pituitary adenomas. J Neurosurg 19:626–631, 1962.

Rovit RL, Berry R: Cushing's syndrome and the hypophysis. J Neurosurg 23:270–295, 1965.

Russell DS, Rubinstein LJ: *Pathology of Tumours of the Nervous System.* Williams & Wilkins, 1963.

Svien HJ, Colby M: *Treatment for Chromophobe Adenoma.* Thomas, 1967.

CERVICAL DISK DISEASE
Edward S. Connolly, MD

Essentials of Diagnosis

Subjective

- Pain in the suboccipital, cervical, interscapular, thoracic, and shoulder areas and in the upper extremities.
- Discomfort aggravated by neck movements and Valsalva's maneuver.
- Paresthesias and dysesthesias in the cervical dermatomes.

Objective

- Lower motor neuron signs in the upper extremities manifested by weakness, fasciculations, depression of deep tendon reflexes, and dermatome sensory changes.

- Upper motor neuron signs in the lower extremities manifested by spasticity, weakness, and a positive plantar extensor sign.
- Spastic neurogenic bladder.
- Straightening of cervical curve, limitation of cervical movements, and paraspinous muscle spasm.
- Radiologic evidence of collapsed disk spaces and formation of osteophytes.
- Myelographic evidence of extradural cervical mass.

General Considerations

Cervical intervertebral disk disease is a general term used to describe degeneration of the cervical intervertebral disk that may develop into 3 separate clinical and pathologic entities. Perhaps the most common is the "hard disk," in which osteophytes arising from the anterior margin of the intervertebral foramen narrow the foramen and compress a cervical nerve root. The second most common is the "soft disk," in which herniation of the nucleus pulposus through a rupture in the posterior or posterolateral aspect of the annulus fibrosus compresses the spinal cord, the nerve root, or both. The third type is cervical spondylosis, characterized by bony spurs that form on the superior and inferior aspects of the posterior surface of the vertebral bodies to produce a washboard effect or so-called bar disk. These compress the spinal cord, causing spasticity in the lower segments but frequently without pain or discomfort in the neck.

Clinical Findings

A. Symptoms and Signs: The onset of symptoms and signs of "soft disk" may be acute or insidious. Acute symptoms may follow trauma or may be unrelated to trauma. Neck and radicular discomfort occur simultaneously; spinal cord symptoms are rare. There is usually limitation of neck motion with tenderness over the brachial plexus and straightening of the normal cervical lordosis. Decrease in a deep tendon reflex is common with or without weakness in the muscles supplied by the compressed root. There is also hypesthesia or hyperesthesia in the dermatome pattern of the affected root. With "hard disks," episodes of cervical discomfort recur over many months or years before radicular symptoms occur. Interscapular aching and suboccipital headaches are common complaints. Following the onset of radicular symptoms, the signs of a "hard disk" are indistinguishable from those of a "soft disk." The signs and symptoms of cervical spondylosis are those of progressive spastic paraparesis with some limitation of neck motion, mild to moderate sensory changes in the lower extremities, and a cervical dermatome pattern.

B. X-Ray Findings: Plain x-rays of "soft disks" may be within normal limits (except for straightening of the cervical lordosis) or may demonstrate narrowing of a disk space. X-rays of "hard disks" show osteophytic formation at the appropriate neural foramen with disk narrowing. This is usually best seen on oblique views. In cervical spondylosis there is usually x-ray evidence of osteophytes and disk narrowing at multiple levels, and in most cases the sagittal diameter of the cervical spinal canal is congenitally narrow.

Myelography in "soft disks" may show no abnormality, but more commonly, there is a small ventral extradural defect obliterating a nerve root cuff. In "hard disks" the myelogram usually demonstrates a root cuff defect. In cervical spondylosis, the myelogram shows bar-like ventral defects at the disk space, usually occurring at multiple levels and sometimes associated with apparent widening of the cord shadow on the anteroposterior projection.

Differential Diagnosis

Cervical disk disease must be differentiated from inflammatory diseases affecting the soft tissues and joints of the pectoral girdle, such as subdeltoid and subacromial bursitis, Tietze's syndrome, and cervical sprains; cervical rib and scalenus anticus syndrome, nerve entrapment syndromes in the upper extremities such as carpal tunnel syndrome and tardy ulnar palsy; coronary insufficiency and angina pectoris; neoplasms of the pulmonary apex, eg, Pancoast tumors; neoplasms of the brachial plexus; neoplasms of the cervical cord and medullocervical junction; fractures, dislocations, or subluxations of the cervical spine; and inflammatory disease of the cervical theca such as arachnoiditis, sarcoidosis, and Pott's disease.

Complications

Permanent damage to the nerve roots and spinal cord may occur, with loss of motor and sensory function. This is particularly true in cervical spondylosis, in which both direct pressure on the spinal cord and compression of its vascular supply may produce a severe irreversible myelopathy with spastic paraplegia or quadriplegia and loss of sphincteric control.

Treatment

A. Conservative Measures: Initially, cervical disk disease should be treated conservatively unless there is evidence of spinal cord compression or severe motor loss in an extremity secondary to root compression. In these situations, prompt surgical decompression is indicated.

Adequate conservative therapy for patients suffering from radiculitis involves immobilization of the neck with mild traction exerted on the neck in a neutral position. This is usually best achieved with continuous or interrupted (2 hours in and 1 hour out) halter cervical traction. Salicylates, other analgesics, tranquilizers with muscle-relaxing properties, and local heat are frequently used in combination with traction. *Caution:* Since improper traction may produce increased discomfort and additional muscle spasm, cervical traction must be applied correctly and be checked repeatedly by the physician with daily counseling of the patient about the importance of proper alignment of the traction to provide a neutral pull. Cervical traction may be applied so that the neck is held neutral in both the sitting and supine positions. The weight used generally ranges from 2–5 kg (5–10 lb) depending on the size of the patient.

B. Surgical Treatment: There are 2 methods of treating cervical disk disease surgically: (1) posterior decompression of the nerve roots, spinal cord, or both; and (2) anterior decompression of nerve roots, spinal cord (or both) with or without fusion. Neither can be designated as **the** correct procedure. The choice is based on consideration of a particular patient's anatomic lesions. It may occasionally be necessary to use both an anterior and a posterior approach.

Prognosis

Seventy-five percent of patients will recover following an adequate trial (10–14 days) of conservative therapy even though some will continue to have cervical or interscapular discomfort or mild paresthesias and some will have recurrence of their radicular symptoms on return to full activity status. In some cases, these patients can be managed for years with intervals of cervical traction and a cervical collar, but many will require surgical therapy. For the 25% who do not respond to conservative therapy, operation is required.

Improvement follows operative treatment of hard and soft cervical disks in approximately 80% of patients. Surgical treatment of cervical spondylosis with myelopathy results in improvement in 65% of cases and arrest of progression in most of the remainder.

Cloward RD: New method of diagnosis and treatment of cervical disc disease. Clin Neurosurg 8:93–132, 1962.

Connolly ES, Seymour RJ, Adams JE: Clinical evaluation of anterior cervical fusion for degenerative cervical disc disease. J Neurosurg 23:431–437, 1965.

Guidetti B, Fortuna A: Long-term results of surgical treatment of myelopathy due to cervical spondylosis. J Neurosurg 30:714–721, 1969.

Haft A, Shenkin HA: Surgical end results of cervical ridge and disk problems. JAMA 186:312–315, 1963.

Odom GL, Finney W, Woodhall B: Cervical disk lesions. JAMA 166:23–28, 1958.

Roaf JE: Surgical treatment of patients with cervical disk lesions. J Trauma 9:327–338, 1969.

Robinson RA: The results of anterior interbody fusion of the cervical spine. J Bone Joint Surg 44A:1569–1587, 1962.

Spurling RG: *Lesions of the Cervical Intervertebral Disc.* American Lecture Series. Thomas, 1956.

LUMBAR DISK DISEASE
Norman L. Chater, MD

Essentials of Diagnosis

- History of back injury (common).
- Low back pain (usual).
- Signs of root compression, eg, sciatica.
- Pain aggravated by activity and relieved by bed rest.
- Abnormal straight leg raising test.
- Neurologic findings are variable and usually mild.

General Considerations

Intervertebral disk disease takes 3 forms: (1) degeneration of the nucleus pulposus without demonstrable protrusion; (2) degeneration and protrusion or bulging behind a weakened annulus fibrosus which, if posterior or posterolateral, may cause pressure on adjacent nerve roots; or (3) extrusion or herniation of the nucleus pulposus through a rent in the annulus, again commonly associated with nerve root compression. The predominant precipitating factor in all is acute or repeated trauma.

Clinical Findings

Over 90% of problems arise from the L4–5 and L5–S1 intervertebral areas and most of the remainder at L3–4. Lumbar disk disease rarely involves higher levels.

A. Symptoms and Signs: Pain is usually chronic and of long standing, but the onset may be acute when associated with frank herniation. There may be back pain, leg pain, or both. The radiation of low back pain into the buttock, posterior thigh, and calf is usually the same with disease at the L4–5 or L5–S1 interspaces. This radiating pain may be aggravated by coughing, sneezing, or the Valsalva maneuver. Bending or sitting accentuates the discomfort, whereas lying down characteristically relieves it. Most commonly, the pain is described as aching, but it frequently has a sharp or shooting element.

Numbness of the legs is present in fewer than one-third of patients. Rarely, bowel and bladder sphincteric disturbances are noted.

Palpation over the buttock (less frequently, over the vertebral spines) usually reveals tenderness over the sciatic notch or nerve. The paravertebral musculature may be in spasm. Straight leg raising produces back or leg pain that may be accentuated by further stretching of the sciatic nerve (by foot dorsiflexion or palpation in the popliteal fossa). Pain produced when the leg opposite the affected side is raised is highly suggestive of disk herniation.

Weakness of the anterior leg (with the extensor hallucis longus being the first affected) is a common finding, especially with L4–5 disease. Weakness of the gastrocnemius when testing strength in the standing position is difficult to evaluate because of pain. Weakness of the quadriceps may occur with L3–4 herniation. Atrophy may be present in long-standing cases.

Sensory patterns are extremely variable. Hypesthesia on the dorsum of the foot is common; sensory deficit on the outside of the foot is more frequent with L5–S1 disease, and deficit on the medial aspect of the foot is more frequent with L4–5 disease.

Comparison of knee and ankle reflexes is important. Depression of the ankle jerk is common with L5–S1 disease but is also present in a significant number of cases of L4–5 disease. The knee jerk may be depressed in L3–4 disease.

B. X-Ray Findings: Plain films of the lumbosacral spine should be taken to identify congenital or acquired bony changes. The common narrowing of the disk spaces occurs in asymptomatic patients with the same frequency as in symptomatic patients and therefore has no diagnostic value.

Myelography is diagnostic in 70–80% of cases and is important in localizing the disease and ruling out intraspinal tumors. Sufficient iodized oil to cover the lower disk spaces in the semi-upright position is injected into the subarachnoid space, and posteroanterior, lateral, and oblique pictures are then taken. It must be remembered that both false-positive and false-negative findings occur.

Contrast material may be injected directly into the disk space with the diffusion monitored radiographically (discography). A normal disk will usually accept less than 0.5 ml, whereas a degenerated disk will accept 2–3 ml. Diskography is used infrequently because the finding of disk degeneration has no consistent relationship to symptoms.

C. Special Examinations: Electromyography may demonstrate denervation of the muscles in the appropriate nerve root distribution and can be used as an adjunct to difficult diagnosis. Electromyography alone is not diagnostic.

Some physicians use segmental epidural block with local anesthetics as an aid in identifying single or multiple root irritations and in distinguishing between a peripheral or a central source of pain.

Differential Diagnosis

Back pain with radiation to the leg has many causes: (1) bony abnormalities such as spondylolisthesis, spondylosis, or the "narrowed" lumbar canal; (2) primary and metastatic tumors of the cauda equina or the intrapelvic region; (3) inflammatory disorders, including abscess, arachnoiditis, and rheumatoid spondylitis; (4) degenerative lesions of the spinal cord and peripheral neuropathies; and (5) peripheral vascular occlusive disease.

Treatment

A. Conservative Measures: A trial of conservative treatment is indicated in all patients who do not demonstrate progressive weakness or sphincteric disturbance. This consists of bed rest with local heat; analgesics and skeletal muscle relaxants; pelvic traction, partially immobilizing the patient, which helps relieve muscle spasm; physical therapy and graded exercise in chronic cases or after an acute episode subsides; corset or back brace to act as an immobilizer and to allow patients with a musculoskeletal component to return earlier to activity, or a body cast or plastic jacket in cases where chronic pain is relieved by immobilization.

B. Surgical Treatment: Surgical treatment is indicated in patients with progressive neurologic deficits and chronic disabling pain. Acute onset of symptoms associated with weakness or sphincteric disturbance must be treated with all expediency to curtail or reverse permanent deficit.

A simple laminotomy is made at the appropriate interspace, with care being taken to protect the nerve root and dura. If actual herniation has occurred, the surgeon should attempt to remove this in one piece and should diligently search for other extruded portions. In the absence of herniation, the surgeon makes a window in the ligamentous annulus and removes all degenerated material from the interspace. Some surgeons recommend that a fusion be done primarily or as a secondary procedure in chronic cases where immobilization has relieved symptoms.

Prognosis

Surgical results vary greatly. The best results are obtained in the patient with true extrusion of disk material where compensation for injury is not a factor. Emotional factors play a great part in the results and must be carefully evaluated before operation is undertaken.

Brown HA, Pont MD: Disease of lumbar discs: Ten years of surgical treatment. J Neurosurg 20:410–417, 1963.

Gurdjian ES & others: Herniated lumbar intervertebral discs: An analysis of 1776 operated cases. J Trauma 1:158–176, 1961.

Mixter WJ, Barr JS: Rupture of the intervertebral disc with involvement of the spinal canal. New England J Med 211:210–215, 1934.

Raaf J: Some observations regarding 905 patients operated upon for protruded lumbar intervertebral disc. Am J Surg 97:388–399, 1959.

Raaf J: Removal of protruded lumbar intervertebral discs. J Neurosurg 32:604–611, 1970.

Spurling RG: *Lesions of the Lumbar Intervertebral Disc With Special Reference to Rupture of the Annulus Fibrosus With Herniation of the Nucleus Pulposus.* Thomas, 1953.

PEDIATRIC NEUROSURGICAL PROBLEMS
Byron C. Pevehouse, MD

Most neurosurgical problems in infancy and childhood are due to 4 causes: congenital malformation, neoplasm, infection, and trauma. Infection and trauma are adequately discussed in other sections of this chapter and will not be considered in this section.

Congenital malformations occur in the nervous system more frequently than in any other organ system and are exceeded only by prematurity as a cause of death in infants. In most cases, no specific cause can be demonstrated, although a number of teratogenic factors have been recognized:

(1) Maternal infections such as rubella, toxoplasmosis, cytomegalic inclusion disease, and syphilis.

(2) Drugs ingested by the mother during a critical period of gestation, eg, thalidomide, LSD, methotrexate.

(3) Ionizing radiation (x-rays, radioisotopes) to the mother.

(4) Maternal anesthesia.

(5) Systemic disease, electrolyte imbalance, and dietary deficiencies.

Even the "genetic" anomalies such as spina bifida, anencephaly, and Down's syndrome probably result from a complicated interplay of genetic predisposition and various intrauterine factors.

The gross structural neonatal abnormalities that can be repaired surgically include the following: (1) malformations of the skull or spine, (2) incomplete formation of the neural tube, (3) disturbances of CSF circulation and absorption, and (4) vascular malformations.

1. MALFORMATIONS OF THE SKULL OR SPINE

Craniosynostosis is defined as premature closure of one or more cranial sutures, producing deformity of the skull. Primary craniosynostosis, which is always present at birth, must be differentiated from the secondary approximation and fusion of sutures in microcephaly and that which sometimes follows operative procedures on the skull or treatment to reduce increased intracranial pressure.

Compensatory growth of the craniosynostotic skull occurs parallel to the plane of the fused suture. When the process involves 2 or more sutures, growth and development of the brain are affected, particularly during the first year of life when the brain ordinarily triples its weight.

In order of diminishing incidence, the following malformations occur: fusion of the sagittal suture results in a long, narrow head (scaphocephaly); of a coronal suture, a broad, shortened head with flattened forehead (brachycephaly); of both sagittal and coronal sutures, a high, pointed head (oxycephaly); and of the metopic suture, a vertical midline prominence of the forehead (trigonocephaly).

Treatment consists of excision of the fused suture and insertion of a polyethylene film barrier to prevent rapid reclosure. This should be done as early as possible (before significant cranial deformity is present) and is probably ineffective after the patient is 2 years old.

Numerous other skeletal anomalies involve the base of the skull and cervical spine with various signs related to compression of the cerebellum, medulla, spinal cord, or adjacent nerves:

Basilar impression—upward displacement of the cervical spine into the base of the skull—results in reduced capacity of the posterior fossa and stenosis of the foramen magnum.

Arnold-Chiari malformation—caudal displacement of the cerebellum and medulla through the foramen magnum into the cervical canal—is often associated with hydrocephalus or myelomeningocele.

Klippel-Feil deformity—improper segmentation and fusion of elements of the cervical spine—is associated with abnormalities of the spinal cord.

Atlanto-occipital fusion—fusion of the atlas to the foramen magnum.

Diastematomyelia—bony spicule projecting through the middle of the spinal canal to divide the meninges and spinal cord into 2 compartments; other skeletal anomalies are usually present.

2. INCOMPLETE FORMATION OF THE NEURAL TUBE

Such defects originate during the third and fourth week of fetal life; they may be small and concealed or may be exposed and involve large areas of spinal cord, meninges, spine, overlying muscles, and skin. The most frequently involved anatomic level is the lumbosacral area; the least frequently involved is the thoracic area.

Spinal bifida occulta is a defect in fusion of the spinous processes and laminas which is present in about 25% of all children. It usually has no clinical significance.

Meningocele consists of herniation of meninges through a spina bifida without abnormality of the spinal cord or nerve roots.

Myelomeningocele is protrusion of nerve roots or cord elements along with the meninges. It occurs about 7 times more often than simple meningocele and always causes some degree of neurologic deficit. Findings range from mild weakness and slight sphincteric disturbance to complete sensory and motor paralysis below the lesion and no control of bowel or bladder function. Hydrocephalus is associated with at least 80% of lumbosacral myelomeningoceles; Arnold-Chiari malformation is typically present.

Encephalocele with cranium bifidum is a much less common midline protrusion of meninges through the skull. It is usually occipital or at the base of the nose.

Treatment of all such defects includes early repair of the meningeal lesion to prevent meningitis, to preserve maximal neurologic function, and to facilitate nursing care. Supportive appliances should be provided if paralysis is present. Early recognition and control of hydrocephalus is essential.

Improved means of treating such problems have increased the number of children who survive and have greatly improved their condition. Musculoskeletal abnormalities require close attention to prevent contractures, joint dislocation, and deformities and to provide as much physical independence as the neurologic deficit and intelligence permit. Urologic problems, also either congenital or paralytic, represent the greatest threat to life after the second year of age, usually from chronic pyelonephritis.

3. DISTURBANCES OF CSF CIRCULATION & ABSORPTION

A considerable portion of CSF originates in the choroid plexus of the lateral and fourth ventricles, passes through the internal channels, and out the foramens of the fourth ventricle into the subarachnoid spaces and thence over the cerebral hemispheres to be absorbed through the arachnoidal villi into the venous circulation. Hydrocephalus, the "backing up" of flow and dilatation of the ventricles, can result from any of the 3 following disturbances in this normal pattern of flow: (1) excess production of CSF, as by a papilloma of the choroid plexus; (2) obstruction of pathways of flow, either internal or external to the brain; and (3) inadequate absorption of CSF through the arachnoidal villi.

Obstruction of the internal channels—ie, the foramen interventriculare, the third ventricle, the cerebral aqueduct, the fourth ventricle, or the outlet foramens —produces a noncommunicating hydrocephalus, so-named because dye injected into the lateral ventricle cannot be recovered 20 minutes later by lumbar subarachnoid puncture. Internal or noncommunicating hydrocephalus is commonly congenital, with atresia or "forking" of the aqueduct or inadequate opening of the fourth ventricle foramens with massive enlargement of the fourth ventricle (Dandy-Walker syndrome). Other causes include neoplasms that obstruct the channels at any level and ependymal reaction subsequent to ventricular hemorrhage or infection.

Obstruction of the external pathways or diminished absorption of CSF will produce a communicating hydrocephalus, in which dye can be recovered from the lumbar caudal sac after ventricular injection but CSF flow into the venous circulation is retarded, resulting in an excess volume of CSF within the skull. External or communicating hydrocephalus usually results from arachnoiditis involving the basal cisterns and subarachnoid spaces over the cerebrum, subsequent to meningitis, hemorrhage, or occasionally a tumor at the tentorium.

Hydrocephalus is treated by removal of the obstruction or opening of the channel for normal flow, excision of a choroid plexus papilloma, or bypass of CSF around the obstruction via a shunt of silicone rubber tubing. A lumbar subarachnoid-peritoneal shunt is usually effective in communicating hydrocephalus; in noncommunicating hydrocephalus, ventriculoatrial or ventriculoperitoneal shunt is necessary, usually with a valve mechanism to control the rate of CSF flow. Complications are frequent, including obstruction of the tubing, displacement by growth, intravenous or cardiac thrombus, acute or chronic septicemia, and pulmonary hypertension.

4. VASCULAR MALFORMATIONS

Collections of abnormal blood vessels, ranging in size from a large mass to a microscopic crypt, usually provide a direct arteriovenous shunt. The involved vessels have thin walls with defective muscular and elastic layers and thus frequently bleed. The hemorrhage may be minimal or massive. It is usually not fatal in children, but is often repeated during later life. Other symptoms include epileptic seizures and intellectual deterioration due to ischemia of the cortex. A loud bruit can be heard over the cranium in many cases. The diagnosis is suggested by the history and confirmed by bloody spinal fluid, skull x-rays, and cerebral angiography. Treatment depends on the patient's symptoms, his age and condition, and the size and location of the malformation. If feasible, total excision is preferred, but not if it would produce a severe neurologic deficit.

A saccular aneurysm at the bifurcation of the arteries that form the circle of Willis is a frequent cause of subarachnoid hemorrhage in the young adult but is rarely symptomatic in childhood or infancy. Aneurysm of the great cerebral vein (of Galen) is more common in the pediatric patient, with obstruction of the aqueduct causing hydrocephalus, a loud cranial bruit, and signs of high-output cardiac failure.

•   •   •

NEOPLASMS

Neoplasms of the CNS are the most common solid tumors of childhood, exceeded only by neoplastic disease of the hematopoietic system. Twenty percent of pediatric neural tumors are located in the spinal cord and 80% in the brain. Of the latter, 60% are in the posterior fossa and 40% in the supratentorial area (Table 41–4).

Brain Tumors

Brain tumors produce symptoms (1) by occupying space, obstructing spinal fluid pathways, or both,

TABLE 41–4. Types of CNS tumors in children.

Cell Type	Incidence	Supratentorial	Posterior Fossa
Medulloblastoma	30%	. . .	Midline cerebellum
Astrocytoma	30%	Occasional	Cerebellar hemisphere
Ependymoma	10%	Rare	Fourth ventricle
Pontine glioma	10%	. . .	Pons
Craniopharyngioma	4%	Suprasellar	. . .
Dermoid tumors and teratoma	3%	Rare	Rare
Other gliomas	8%	Uncommon	Uncommon

thereby increasing intracranial pressure; and (2) by direct invasion or compression of neural tissues.

In infants and children, the symptoms and signs of increased intracranial pressure are vomiting, headache, papilledema, mental dysfunction, personality changes, and abducens nerve palsy. Symptoms and signs of direct brain involvement are ataxia, incoordination, nystagmus, weakness of extremities, seizures, and head tilt to the side of the lesion (cerebellar). (See section on brain tumors for further details.)

The object of treatment is always total removal of the neoplasm, but in childhood this is possible in only a few types (cerebellar astrocytoma, hemangioblastoma, dermoid cyst, craniopharyngioma, unilateral optic nerve glioma). The remaining types are partially resected, CSF pathways are reopened or bypassed, and radiation therapy or chemotherapy is given postoperatively.

Spinal Cord Tumors

Spinal cord tumors are uncommon, and early diagnosis is most important. Spinal tumors comprise congenital tumors such as dermoids, lipomas, teratomas, and neurofibromas; gliomas such as astrocytomas and ependymomas; medulloblastomas which seed from primary brain tumors; and extradural metastatic tumors such as neuroblastomas and lymphosarcomas.

The manifestations of spinal cord tumors usually include pain in the spine, weakness of the legs or disturbances of gait, torticollis or scoliosis, impairment of bowel or bladder function, numbness of one or more limbs, local tenderness, and paravertebral muscle spasm.

Plain films of the spine are abnormal in 65% of children with spinal cord tumor. Electromyography will differentiate diffuse peripheral nerve and muscle disorders. Contrast myelography is the definitive test to confirm and localize an intraspinal mass lesion.

Treatment begins with operative biopsy followed by removal if possible. For those tumors that are radiosensitive and clearly cannot be excised—or those that are obviously metastatic—radiation therapy is the treatment of choice.

Foltz EL, Shurtleff DB: Five-year comparative study of hydrocephalus in children with and without operation. J Neurosurg 20:1064, 1963.

Gardner JW: Myelocele: Rupture of the neural tube. Clin Neurosurg 15:57–79, 1967.

Matson DD, Ingraham FD: *Neurosurgery of Infancy and Childhood,* 2nd ed. Thomas, 1969.

Matson DD: Surgery of posterior fossa tumors in childhood. Clin Neurosurg 15:247–264, 1967.

Shillito J Jr, Matson DD: Craniosynostosis: A review of 519 surgical patients. Pediatrics 41:829–853, 1968.

INTRACRANIAL ANEURYSMS
Edwin B. Boldrey, MD

Essentials of Diagnosis

- Evidence of intracranial hemorrhage (headache, stiff neck, etc).
- Evidence of progressive involvement of cranial nerves, or of fiber pathways or major ganglionic centers of the cerebrum, cerebellum, or brain stem.
- Angiographic demonstration of aneurysmal sac.

General Considerations

There are 5 types of intracranial aneurysm: congenital, most commonly involving the vessels of the circle of Willis (Fig 41–13); arteriosclerotic, mycotic, traumatic, and dissecting. Congenital aneurysms vary in size from a few millimeters to 4–5 cm in diameter, and they are smoothly or irregularly globoid. The others are markedly variable in size and configuration; fortunately, they are less common.

Above the age of 40 years, the incidence of intracranial aneurysm is greater in females by a ratio of 3:2; below the age of 40, the incidence is greater in males.

The location of congenital aneurysm leading to intracranial hemorrhage is, in order of frequency (Fig 41–14): (1) anterior cerebral-communicating arteries, (2) internal carotid-posterior communicating arteries, (3) middle cerebral artery, (4) terminal bifurcation of internal carotid artery, (5) vertebral-basilar system, and (6) distal anterior cerebral artery. Multiple aneurysms occur in 14–20% of patients and may be scattered widely or clustered.

Ruptured intracranial aneurysm is the most common single cause of subarachnoid intracranial hemorrhage after the third decade of life (51%). One-third of hemorrhages from aneurysm occur during periods of rest, and another third during general activity. A variety of acutely stressful activities, such as lifting, bending, straining at stool, etc account for the remainder.

When an intracranial aneurysm of any type ruptures, the severity of clinical symptoms will usually be directly related to the amount of bleeding. Major hemorrhage may be followed by impairment of consciousness, coma, respiratory paralysis, and death. Minimal bleeding may produce only a sudden, severe headache, often with neck stiffness and usually with nausea and vomiting.

Clinical Findings

A. Symptoms and Signs: The classic history is that of sudden, severe headache with nausea, vomiting, and often prostration. The process may advance to coma, respiratory paralysis, and death within minutes or within the first few days. With less serious bleeding, there is stiffness of the neck, pain in the back, and photophobia.

Hemorrhage from the internal carotid artery may

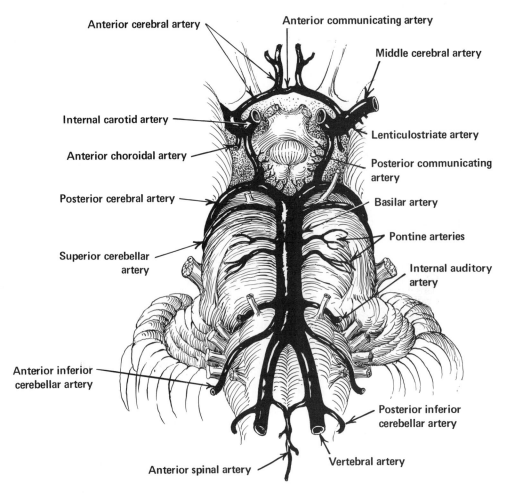

FIG 41–13. Circle of Willis and principal arteries of the brain. (Reproduced, with permission, from Chusid JG: *Correlative Neuroanatomy & Functional Neurology,* 15th ed. Lange, 1973.)

cause paralysis of function of the second through sixth cranial nerves. Ruptured aneurysm from the middle cerebral artery may be followed by contralateral hemiparesis. Ruptured aneurysms of the posterior circulation may produce brain stem as well as cerebellar signs and paralysis of the cranial nerves below the trigeminal nerve. Aneurysms of the anterior communicating arteries frequently bleed into the cerebral tissue and the ventricles, the latter usually being fatal. Middle cerebral aneurysms frequently bleed into the temporal and frontal lobes.

In approximately 10% of ruptured intracranial aneurysms, blood in a significant amount does not reach the subarachnoid space. Subhyaloid ocular hemorrhages may be found in association with intracranial hemorrhage.

Intracranial aneurysms can manifest themselves by virtue of their size. Enlargement of an aneurysm without hemorrhage may produce only cranial nerve palsies, or intrinsic nuclear or fiber tract dysfunction. The problem of identification is that of any intracranial space-occupying mass.

B. Lumbar Puncture: Proof of subarachnoid intracranial hemorrhage is the demonstration of blood in the CSF by lumbar puncture. The spinal fluid is uniformly bloody, and, within hours, the supernatant will be xanthochromic. With the passage of time, white blood cells increase in the fluid—a sign of meningeal irritation. *Caution:* Withdrawal of spinal fluid in the presence of spontaneous subarachnoid hemorrhage should be done with great care since the abrupt removal of large amounts may precipitate secondary hemorrhage. On the other hand, repeated lumbar puncture may help to identify or confirm suspected secondary bleeding.

C. Cerebral Angiography: Cerebral angiography is a most important diagnostic procedure and must be done in all cases of spontaneous subarachnoid hemorrhage unless there is an obvious compelling contraindication. It should be done as soon as the patient's condition permits and the necessary equipment and personnel are available. Ideally, the angiogram should show both carotid arteries and the vertebral-basilar system. At times, the intracranial portion of both

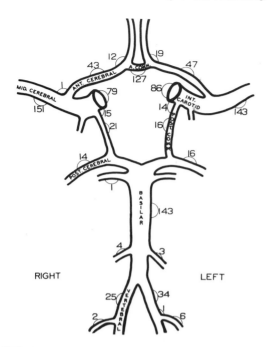

FIG 41–14. Location of intracranial aneurysms in 1023 cases. (Reproduced, with permission, from McDonald & Korb: Arch Neurol Psychiat 42:298, 1939.)

vertebral arteries can be demonstrated following injection of one vertebral artery in which case direct injection of the second artery may not be necessary. If the initial angiogram is within normal limits, it may be repeated in 4–6 weeks; about one-fifth of these second arteriograms will demonstrate an aneurysm.

Differential Diagnosis

Although there is seldom serious question about the diagnosis when the clinical symptoms and signs are as described above, intracranial neoplasms will occasionally bleed into the subarachnoid space. There are also other vascular sources of hemorrhage such as vascular hypertension, intracranial arteriovenous malformations, and inflammatory intracranial vascular disease. Occasionally, acute meningitis will mimic the clinical signs of spontaneous subarachnoid hemorrhage, but examination of the spinal fluid will clarify the issue.

Treatment

A. Medical Treatment: Nonoperative treatment consists of absolute bed rest with or without the use of hypotensive agents. This is usually continued for 4–6 weeks, with subsequent gradual resumption of activity over a similar period of time.

B. Surgical Treatment: Surgical treatment consists of a direct attack upon the aneurysm by clipping the base, wrapping the aneurysm with foreign materials to reinforce the wall, isolating the aneurysm by proximal and distal clipping of the parent vessel, or, for certain

carotid aneurysms, by ligating the cervical carotid artery. The location and size of the aneurysm, the condition of the patient, and the preference of the surgeon will determine which procedure is used.

In general, most neurosurgeons advocate a direct intracranial approach to ruptured aneurysms. Other factors being equal (eg, location of aneurysm), the results depend upon the patient's condition at the time of operation. Except for the removal of intracerebral and subdural hematomas, aneurysm surgery is preventive, ie, aimed at the prevention of further bleeding.

Prognosis

Irreversible damage occurring at the time of initial rupture will remain as a fixed deficit. If the aneurysm is successfully treated, the patient's long-term outlook depends upon the damage caused by initial and subsequent hemorrhage and on whether complications of surgical treatment develop.

The accumulated mortality from ruptured intracranial aneurysm is reported to be approximately 10% during the first 24 hours, 20% within the first 5 days, 30% within the first 9 days, 40% within the first 16 days, and 50% within 29 days. Secondary subarachnoid hemorrhage occurs most frequently between days 3–11, with a peak on the seventh day. The mortality rate during second episodes of subarachnoid hemorrhage is approximately 42%. With ruptured aneurysms of the posterior (ie, vertebral-basilar) circulation, secondary bleeding is less frequent during the first 2 weeks after initial hemorrhage.

Forbus WD: On origin of miliary aneurysms of superficial cerebral arteries. Bull Johns Hopkins Hosp 47:239–284, 1930.
Sahs AL: *Intracranial Aneurysms and Subarachnoid Hemorrhage: A Cooperative Study.* Lippincott, 1969.

CONGENITAL ARTERIOVENOUS MALFORMATIONS OF THE BRAIN

Essentials of Diagnosis

- Spontaneous subarachnoid or intracerebral hemorrhages.
- Convulsive seizures.
- Progressive signs of cerebral, cerebellar, or brain stem dysfunction.
- Subjective or objective bruits.

General Considerations

Arteriovenous malformations vary greatly in size. They may be smaller than 1 cm in diameter or may involve an entire cerebral hemisphere. They may be supplied by a single small artery or by all vessels entering the cranium.

Arteriovenous malformations and congenital aneurysms may occur in the same patient. Bilateral malformations are not rare—particularly in the deeper structures of the brain, including the basal ganglia.

The intracranial hemorrhage secondary to arteriovenous malformation usually occurs during the first 3 decades of life and is seldom encountered after the fourth decade. Mortality from the first intracranial hemorrhage is about 10%, which is less than that from intracranial aneurysm. Second episodes occur in approximately 23% of patients, and the mortality rate in this group is about 12%. The time between the first and second hemorrhages may be days or years; in the latter case, convulsive seizures commonly intervene.

Arteriovenous malformations may enlarge by dilatation of connecting vessels, producing the signs and symptoms of an intracranial space-occupying mass.

Clinical Findings

The clinical findings of intracranial hemorrhage due to arteriovenous malformations are the same as those of subarachnoid or intracerebral hemorrhage due to other causes.

A bruit over the cranium strongly suggests an angioma but is not pathognomonic of angioma. Occasionally, brain scans may be helpful in identifying large arteriovenous angiomas. EEG may show focal changes in the affected cerebral hemisphere.

Differential Diagnosis

See section on Intracranial Aneurysms.

Treatment

When possible, arteriovenous angiomas are excised; ligation of extracranial vessels has proved to have very limited value. In some instances, however (eg, interhemispheric angiomas), the likelihood of secondary hemorrhage may be reduced if the main feeding vessel is clipped even though the lesion cannot be extirpated. This should be done as close to the lesion as possible.

No matter what is or is not done, the possibility always exists that a convulsive state will develop.

If surgery is indicated, the timing depends upon the condition and the desires of the patient, the location of the lesion, and the size of the malformation.

Prognosis

When the lesion is surgically extirpated, the prognosis for life is good but the morbidity rate (especially the development of seizures) is significant. The operative mortality rate is directly related to the size and location of the malformation.

INFECTIOUS DISEASES OF THE CNS*
Edward S. Connolly, MD

PYOGENIC MENINGITIS

Essentials of Diagnosis

- Fever, headache, mental confusion, nausea and vomiting, and diplopia.
- In infants: fever and failure to thrive.
- Nuchal rigidity, a positive Kernig or Brudzinski sign, and petechial rash.
- Elevated white blood count with shift to the left, elevated sedimentation rate, elevated CSF pressure and protein, decreased CSF glucose, CSF leukocytosis.
- Organisms on CSF culture or smear.

General Considerations

Approximately 70% of cases of bacterial meningitis are caused by 3 organisms: *Neisseria meningitidis, Diplococcus pneumoniae,* and *Haemophilus influenzae. H influenzae* is the commonest cause in children. Less frequent causative organisms are coliforms (except in infants), staphylococci, streptococci, pseudomonas, and proteus. These organisms usually invade the CNS via the blood from a systemic infection, although they may produce meningitis by direct invasion via CSF leaks and fistulas, by direct extension from overlying osteomyelitis, and from foreign bodies and at time of operation.

Clinical Findings

A. Symptoms and Signs: The cardinal signs of meningitis are fever, headache, mental confusion, and nuchal rigidity. Very young, elderly, or debilitated patients may have a low-grade fever and anorexia, and may be irritable. An extremely fulminating course may begin with acute onset of fever and headaches and progress to unconsciousness, seizures, and death within 24 hours. There is usually a history of an upper respiratory tract infection followed by malaise, headache progressing to mental confusion, nausea and vomiting, and a stiff neck. A petechial rash (if present) is usually an indication of meningococcal infection. Fever usually varies from 38–40 C (100.4–104 F).

B. Laboratory Findings: The white count is elevated above 10,000/μl and the differential count shows a preponderance of immature polymorphonuclear cells.

C. Lumbar Puncture: The CSF is usually cloudy and under increased pressure; it usually contains many polymorphonuclear leukocytes, an elevated protein content, a low glucose content, and organisms visible on a gram-stained smear. CSF culture is usually positive if the patient has not been receiving antibiotics.

*Rabies is discussed in Chapter 10.

Differential Diagnosis

Pyogenic meningitis must be differentiated from subarachnoid hemorrhage, "aseptic meningitis" secondary to echovirus or chemical hypersensitivity, granulomatous or yeast meningitis, Behçet's syndrome (recurrent oral and genital lesions with recurrent ocular lesions), and neoplastic meningeal involvement.

Complications

The major complications of pyogenic meningitis are seizures, cranial nerve palsies, hemiparesis, infantile subdural effusion (particularly from *H influenzae*), mental retardation, hydrocephalus, coma, adrenal crisis, etc. These complications usually affect infants and children, whereas adults are usually left with few or no residual deficits.

Treatment

Type-specific antibiotic therapy is the treatment of choice. Intravenous ampicillin, 300 mg/kg/day, is effective against *D pneumoniae, H influenzae,* and *N meningitidis* and may be given while CSF culture and sensitivity tests are being performed. Intravenous hydration and correction of electrolyte imbalances, anticonvulsants, salicylates and hypothermia if necessary to control fever, and correction of corticosteroid deficiency are all part of treatment. Antibiotic therapy should be continued until the patient is afebrile and free of meningeal signs and his CSF has returned to normal. He should be observed in the hospital for 48–72 hours after the completion of antibiotic therapy.

Subdural effusions and hydrocephalus may require drainage and shunting procedures.

Prognosis

The mortality of pyogenic meningitis remains in the range of 30%, with the majority of fatalities occurring in infants and in elderly or debilitated patients. *D pneumoniae* is the most lethal of the 3 major causative organisms.

Meningitis recurs most frequently if CSF leakage is present or if treatment has been inadequate.

BRAIN ABSCESS

Essentials of Diagnosis

- History of sinusitis, otitis, systemic pulmonary infection, or congenital heart defect.
- Headache, localized neurologic signs.
- High-voltage, slow-wave focus on EEG.
- Angiographic evidence of a mass lesion creating a vascular halo.
- Positive brain scan.

General Considerations

Brain abscesses usually occur secondary to some focus of infection outside the CNS—chronic middle ear infection with mastoiditis being the most common source. Infections of the nasal cavity and its accessory sinuses, chronic suppurative diseases of the lungs and pleura, congenital heart disease, acquired valvular heart disease, and retained foreign objects from trauma are other sources. The organisms most commonly responsible are staphylococci, streptococci, and pneumococci, although abscesses have been reported as a result of infection with almost every known bacterium.

Abscesses arising from sinusitis usually occur in the frontal lobes, whereas those arising from middle ear disease occur in the posterior temporal lobe or cerebellum. Hematogenous abscesses are usually found in the distribution of the middle cerebral arteries.

Clinical Findings

A. Symptoms and Signs: The usual presenting symptom is headache followed (in order of frequency) by decrease in sensorium, drowsiness, confusion and stupor, generalized or focal seizures, nausea and vomiting, and focal motor, sensory, or speech disorders. There is usually a low-grade fever (38–39 C [100.4–102.2 F]).

B. Laboratory Findings: Blood and CSF studies may be within normal limits, but more commonly there is a mild polymorphonuclear leukocytosis, mildly increased CSF pressure with an occasional neutrophil, and mildly elevated CSF protein.

C. X-Ray Findings: Skull films may show evidence of mastoiditis, sinusitis, or a pineal shift.

D. Special Examinations: EEG may show a high-voltage, slow-wave focus. Brain scans are usually positive. Angiography demonstrates a mass lesion with a circular halo blush.

Differential Diagnosis

Brain abscess must be differentiated from brain tumor, cerebral infarction, intracranial thrombophlebitis, subdural empyema, extradural abscess, and encephalitis.

Complications

The major complication of brain abscess is rupture, usually into the ventricles, leading to acute ventriculitis and meningitis. Other complications may include obstruction of CSF pathways, transtentorial herniation, seizures, hemiparesis, and mental deficiency.

Prevention

Correct management of otitis media, mastoiditis, sinusitis, and other systemic infections usually prevents brain abscesses.

Treatment

The most desirable method of treatment of brain abscess is systemic administration of type-specific antibiotics and total surgical extirpation if the abscess is in an accessible location. Drainage and secondary excision or marsupialization are sometimes necessary. While sensitivity tests on the organisms of the abscess are being completed, the patient should be treated with an antibiotic that is effective against the suspected causative organism—eg, the ear flora if the patient has mastoiditis. Anticonvulsants should be used as a supportive measure, and eradication of the primary source of infection is essential. If the abscess is tapped, type-specific antibiotics and a radiopaque substance are instilled, the latter allowing visualization of the contraction and migration of the abscess.

Prognosis

Mortality due to brain abscess remains between 25–50% despite antibiotic therapy.

LESS COMMON PYOGENIC INFECTIONS

Epidural Abscess

Epidural abscess in the cranial or spinal epidural space produces focal neurologic deficit by pressure on the underlying neural tissues. In the cranium, it is usually secondary to adjacent osteomyelitis; in the spine, it is usually metastatic from a remote infection in the pelvis or lower extremities.

Treatment consists of immediate drainage of the pus followed by appropriate treatment of the primary infection with antibiotics and operation.

Subdural Abscess

Subdural abscess or empyema, a serious complication of (usually) frontal sinusitis, progresses rapidly and has a high mortality rate. Immediate surgical drainage and antibiotic therapy are indicated. There is a significant incidence of hydrocephalus among survivors, necessitating a shunt procedure following eradication of the infection.

Cerebral Thrombophlebitis

Cerebral thrombophlebitis is a complication of meningitis, epidural and subdural abscesses, and thrombophlebitis of facial veins. The lateral, cavernous and superior sagittal sinuses are most commonly involved, producing neurologic deficit by venous infarction. If marked cerebral edema is associated, then treatment with glucocorticoids and diuretics as well as operative decompression should be considered.

CLOSED DISK SPACE INFECTIONS FOLLOWING REMOVAL OF LUMBAR INTERVERTEBRAL DISK

Closed disk space infection is seen in approximately 1–3% of patients following lumbar laminectomy with diskectomy, and is thought to be due to pyogenic infection confined to the disk space. Symptoms usually occur 1–2 weeks or longer after opera-

tion. Preoperative sciatica has usually resolved when the patient complains of severe pain localized in the back and thighs, aggravated by any motion. The patient may run a low-grade fever or be afebrile; the white count may be normal or slightly elevated. The erythrocyte sedimentation rate is usually over 50 mm. Radiographic signs usually appear in 4 weeks and consist of destruction of the vertebral end plates and narrowing and eventual bony fusion of the disk space.

Treatment consists of immobilization and analgesics. Antibiotics do not enhance therapy.

TUBERCULOUS MENINGITIS

Tuberculous meningitis is a more insidious disease than the common pyogenic meningitides. It is most common in children and debilitated patients and in patients with active pulmonary tuberculosis.

Clinical Findings

A. Symptoms and Signs: Tuberculous meningitis is characterized by gradual onset of headache, easy fatigability, anorexia, irritability, and low-grade fever. Few if any signs of neurologic or meningeal involvement are seen early; later, all of the signs characteristic of clinical meningitis may become evident, followed by coma and death.

B. Laboratory Findings: The tuberculin skin test is usually positive but may be negative in an overwhelming infection just prior to death. The spinal fluid pressure is usually normal or only slightly elevated. The CSF shows mild lymphocytosis, mildly elevated protein, and low glucose. Cultures sometimes require incubation for weeks before the bacteriologic diagnosis can be confirmed.

Treatment

Triple therapy with streptomycin, isoniazid, and aminosalicylic acid—along with proper hydration and nutrition—are the cardinal principles of treatment. If associated with a tuberculoma or hydrocephalus secondary to arachnoidal adhesions, surgical removal of the mass lesion and shunting of the hydrocephalus are indicated.

Prognosis

If the diagnosis is made early in the disease—prior to the appearance of major neurologic symptoms—the prognosis is excellent; if made late, the prognosis for full recovery is poor. Because of the insidious nature of the disease, diagnosis is frequently delayed, and most series show a mortality rate of approximately 50%.

TUBERCULOSIS OF THE SPINE
(Pott's Disease)

The spinal cord dysfunction usually seen with far-advanced vertebral tuberculous lesions progresses rapidly to paraplegia or quadriplegia within a few weeks. The thoracic cord is most commonly involved, followed by the cervical cord and the lumbar cord segments. Radiographically, there is usually destruction of one or more intervertebral disks, apposition of the adjacent vertebral bodies, and destruction of one or more vertebral bodies. Soft tissue swelling is usually evident around the affected area, and a soft tissue mass of varying size is commonly present. A total extradural type block may be seen myelographically 1–2 levels below the obvious bony changes.

Treatment consists of (1) streptomycin, 1 g IM 4 times a day; aminosalicylic acid, 3 g orally 4 times a day; and isoniazid, 100 mg orally 3 times a day; (2) surgical drainage of the abscess via an anterior or lateral approach; and (3) immobilization of the affected area, eg, with skeletal tongs if in the cervical area, with a circulo-electric bed or Stryker frame if in the thoracic or lumbar area. Posterior laminectomy has no place in the treatment of Pott's disease.

COCCIDIOIDOMYCOSIS MENINGITIS

Meningeal infection with *Coccidioides immitis* occurs in the course of a disseminated infection. The neurologic manifestations usually follow an antecedent respiratory infection and may be either acute or chronic. Headache, fever, meningeal signs, and transient focal neurologic deficits are characteristic. A severe adhesive arachnoiditis may occur, producing hydrocephalus. Examination of CSF usually demonstrates increased pressure and protein, mildly decreased glucose, and leukocytosis. Organisms may be cultured from the fluid, but the coccidioidal complement fixation test is the most consistent pathognomonic test.

Treatment is with systemic, intraventricular, and intrathecal amphotericin B (Fungizone). Amphotericin B is given intravenously in 5% glucose in distilled water (not saline), beginning with 0.55 mg/kg/day and increasing by increments of 0.1 mg/kg to 1.5 mg/kg/day. Intraventricular instillation is best done through an Ommaya reservoir; the drug is mixed in equal parts with 5% distilled water and started at a dose of 0.2 mg/kg and increased by 0.1 mg increments per treatment to 1 mg 3 times a week. A similar dosage and schedule is used for intrathecal injection.

NEUROSYPHILIS

Treponema pallidum affects the CNS in essentially 4 clinicopathologic entities: acute syphilitic meningitis, meningovascular syphilis, general paresis, and tabes dorsalis. The diagnosis depends upon a positive reagin test for syphilis in the CSF. False-positive findings in the CSF are extremely rare as compared to those in serum.

Treatment is with benzathine penicillin G, 9 million units IM, given as 3 million units at 7-day intervals; or with PAM (procaine penicillin G with 2% aluminum monostearate), 9.6 million units IM given as 1.2 million units at 3-day intervals.

POLIOMYELITIS

Poliomyelitis affects the motor neurons of the anterior horns, primarily those in the spinal cord but also those in the brain stem and cortex.

Treatment is mainly supportive, aimed at preventing complications. As in most viral diseases, prevention by vaccination is the best treatment.

HERPES ZOSTER (SHINGLES)
AND HERPES SIMPLEX INFECTION

Herpes zoster is caused by a virus that has a predilection for the posterior root ganglia, posterior roots, and posterior gray horns of the spinal cord. The ganglion most often involved is the fifth thoracic ganglion; of the cranial nerves, the gasserian and geniculate ganglia are most commonly affected. The most significant complications are postherpetic pain, corneal ulceration and scarring, and persistent facial palsy.

Surgical treatment of postherpetic pain has included undercutting of the affected cutaneous distribution, posterior rhizotomy, cordotomy, medullary tractotomy, thalamotomy, and leukotomy. None of these procedures are particularly effective.

Herpes simplex encephalitis produces an acute necrotizing hemorrhagic leukoencephalitis. It has an abrupt onset characterized by fever, headache, drowsiness, and convulsions. Temporal lobe signs such as dysphasia, olfactory hallucinations, and psychomotor activity are common. X-ray contrast studies, brain scans, and EEG may demonstrate a mass in one temporal lobe. CSF studies usually show increased pressure and pleocytosis; routine cultures of CSF are negative. When a temporal lobe mass is present, surgical exploration of the lobe is indicated with brain biopsy and external decompression. A portion of brain tissue should be cultured. The characteristic Cowdry type A intranuclear inclusion bodies may be seen histologically, and the herpes simplex virus may be isolated in the culture.

Carpenter RR, Petersdorf RG: The clinical spectrum of bacterial meningitis. Am J Med 33:262–275, 1962.

Fetter BF, Klintworth GK, Hendry WS: Pp 74–88 in: *Mycoses of the Central Nervous System.* Williams & Wilkins, 1967.

Garfield J: Management of supratentorial intracranial abscesses: A review of 200 cases. Brit MJ 2:7–11, 1969.

Hoffman HJ, Hendrick EB, Hiscox JL: Cerebral abscesses in early infancy. J Neurosurg 33:172–177, 1970.

Kiser JL, Kendig JH: Intracranial suppuration: A review of 139 consecutive cases with electronmicroscopic observations on three. J Neurosurg 20:494–511, 1963.

Krayenbühl HA: Abscess of the brain. Clin Neurosurg 14:25–44, 1966.

MacGee EE, Cauthen JC, Brackett CE: Meningitis following acute traumatic cerebrospinal fluid fistula. J Neurosurg 33:312–316, 1970.

Page LK, Tyler HR, Shillito J: Neurosurgical experiences with herpes simplex encephalitis. J Neurosurg 27:346–352, 1967.

Pilgaard S: Discitis (closed space infection) following removal of lumbar intervertebral disk. J Bone Joint Surg 51A: 713–716, 1969.

Sullivan CR: Diagnosis and treatment of pyogenic infection of the intervertebral disk. S Clin North America 41:1077–1086, 1961.

Swartz MN, Dodge PR: Bacterial meningitis: A review of select aspects. New England J Med 272:725–730, 779–787, 842–848, 898–902, 954–962, 1003–1010, 1965.

Tuli SM: Treatment of neurological complications in tuberculosis of the spine. J Bone Joint Surg 51A:680–692, 1969.

Victor M, Banker BQ: Brain abscess. M Clin North America 47:1355–1370, 1963.

Wilkinson HA & others: Central nervous system tuberculosis: A persistent disease. J Neurosurg 34:15–22, 1971.

Witorsch P & others: Intraventricular administration of amphotericin B. JAMA 194:699–702, 1965.

MOVEMENT & PSYCHOPATHOLOGIC DISORDERS RESPONSIVE TO SURGERY
John E. Adams, MD

PARKINSON'S DISEASE

Parkinson's disease is the most common of the various disorders of movement and posture. However, such disorders are not clear-cut entities but constitute a spectrum of abnormal postures, states of muscle tone, and movements varying from hypotonic flaccidity to extreme muscular contraction and from akinesia (inability to initiate movement) to relentless violent movements capable of producing exhaustion and death. The extremes of such a spectrum would be from the severe akinesia of advanced Parkinson's disease—rendering the patient incapable of voluntary movement and thereby preventing any degree of self-care—to the wild, uncontrollable movements of Huntington's chorea.

Clinical Findings

Parkinson's disease is characterized by 3 main disturbances in movement and posture: tremor, rigidity, and bradykinesia or akinesia. The tremor is characteristically of the pill-rolling type that begins in the distal upper extremities and progresses proximally as time passes. It is usually abolished by voluntary movement. Rigidity involves both the agonist and antagonist muscles of the extremity and, when severe, literally immobilizes the arm or leg. The bradykinesia or akinesia is represented by a gradually worsening stooped posture, shuffling gait, festination, or a tendency to fall forward; poverty of speech to the point where the voice becomes only a whisper; difficulty in swallowing, etc.

Treatment

In its early stages, parkinsonism is treated medically and is primarily the concern of the internist or neurologist. The treatment of tremor in medically unresponsive patients is surgical and the operation should be done relatively early before the tremor becomes incapacitating.

Stereotaxic surgery is a technic for reaching subcortical or deeper intracerebral structures via electrodes or probes that are guided to the site by a 3-dimensional coordinate system attached to the skull. This technic allows creation of subcortical lesions with minimal trauma to overlying cortex. In patients with Parkinson's disease, the lesion formerly was placed in the medial portion of the globus pallidus and improvement occurred in about 50% of cases. At present, most surgeons make a small lesion (5 mm in diameter) in the ventrolateral nucleus just posterior to the posterior ventrolateral nucleus of the thalamus. If correctly placed, this lesion will effectively stop a tremor in the contralateral hand and arm in well over 80% of cases. Rigidity is likewise improved. The disabling hypokinetic symptoms of parkinsonism are not benefited by such a thalamotomy, and at times may even be made worse.

Levodopa (Larodopa, Dopar) is very effective in the treatment of the akinetic aspects of the disease, although it may have little effect on tremor. A combination of surgical thalamotomy and levodopa would seem to provide the most effective approach to therapy at the present time.

Other movement disorders that will respond to a lesion in the same thalamic area are dystonia musculorum deformans, essential cerebellar tremors, hemiballismus, chorea, etc. Stereotaxic destruction of the dentate nucleus has recently been used effectively in the treatment of such disabling conditions as choreoathetosis.

EPILEPSY

Epilepsy may be defined as an uncontrolled paroxysmal discharge of an aggregate of neurons within the brain. These neurons are most frequently within the cerebral cortex but may be subcortical. The unrestrained discharge may remain focal, or it may spread to adjacent areas of cortex and may ultimately involve both hemispheres as well as diencephalic and brain stem structures. The clinical characteristics of the seizure are related to the site of origin of the discharge: a diencephalic origin is manifested by unconsciousness as the initial event in a seizure, and a discharging focus in the motor area will produce a seizure initiated by clonic contractions of the appropriate portion of the body (face, hand, arm, etc). It is obvious, therefore, that the clinical manifestations of seizure discharges are greatly variable and may involve essentially all bodily systems. For practical purposes, however, all epilepsy may be considered focal in origin, and this constitutes the basis for the surgical treatment of the disease.

Only intractable cases are treated surgically. About 15–20% of all epileptic patients cannot be controlled by medical therapy and are candidates for surgical excision of the epileptogenic focus if it can be localized and is accessible. Stereotaxic placement of depth electrodes is a new technic for recording from and possibly locating subcortical epileptogenic foci.

PSYCHIATRIC DISORDERS

Small, carefully placed stereotaxic lesions have replaced the much more disabling and destructive frontal lobotomy in the treatment of certain psychiatric disturbances. Patients with obsessive compulsive behavior can be dramatically improved by small lesions in the cingulum. In rare instances, a severe anxiety neurosis that cannot be managed by more conservative methods will be improved by small lesions placed in the white matter just anterior to the dorsal medial thalamic nucleus.

Cooper IS: *Involuntary Movement Disorders.* Harper, 1969.

Spiegel EA, Wycis HT (editors): *Advances in Stereo-encephalotomy.* Part I: *Methodology and Extrapyramidal Systems.* Part II: *Pain, Convulsive Disorders, Behavioral and Other Effects of Stereoencephalotomy.* Karger (New York), 1965, 1966.

Van Manew J: *Stereotatic Methods and their Applications in Disorders of the Motor System.* Thomas, 1967.

PAIN
Yoshio Hosobuchi, MD

Pain is a symptom resulting from the stimulation of specialized nerve endings. The psychologic effect of pain varies according to individual factors and the patient's cultural and ethnic background.

Pain may serve as a warning of some disease or abnormal condition in the body, eg, ureteral colic or angina pectoris, or it may be a pathologic derangement of the pain conduction system itself, eg, thalamic pain following a vascular accident in that area.

Pain is the major cause of suffering in the terminal stage of malignancy. Terminal cancer pain usually originates from malignant invasion of the intercostal nerves, brachial and lumbosacral plexuses, or osseous structures. Pain may be particularly severe if the malignancy is situated at the orifices of the body, where it is increased by ingestion or excretion.

Useful pain warns of abnormal body function and aids in diagnosis of that dysfunction. Useless pain is triggered by diseases, mostly neoplastic or degenerative, about which little can be done. Many neurosurgical procedures are available to alleviate severe forms of useless pain by interruption of pain conduction pathways.

In the not too distant future, surgical procedures for relief of pain will be relegated to the annals of medical history. However, until this urgently desired goal is achieved, the neurosurgeon must assume responsibility for relief of pain in many patients. The extent to which our operative technics (eg, stereotactic surgery) should be used for the treatment of pain is no longer limited by technical factors as much as by our incomplete understanding of the mechanisms and central representations of pain.

Surgery is indicated in the management of pain when the cause defies more direct treatment and when the severity of the pain justifies a major operative procedure. Experience has shown that operation should be considered when a patient requires more than codeine by mouth (or its equivalent) for relief of chronic pain. Patients with a life expectancy shorter than 2 months should rarely be subjected to a neurosurgical pain-relieving operation. While not an absolute contraindication to operation, established narcotic addiction complicates surgical management and reduces the chances of obtaining a satisfactory result. Emotional instability—more often a lifelong pattern than the response to illness—constitutes a relative contraindication to operation on pain pathways.

SURGICAL ANATOMY

Because the peripheral nerves usually have mixed components, distal division of a peripheral nerve for control of pain is a poor procedure unless the nerve is purely sensory. At the level of the spinal roots, however, the peripheral nerves are clearly divided into motor and sensory components, and the posterior (sensory) root can be sectioned without loss of motor strength. Because of sensory overlap, several adjacent posterior roots must be divided to control a small area of pain. Posterior rhizotomy must be done carefully at the cervical and lumbar levels to preserve proprioceptive fibers; a limb without proprioception is quite useless despite its intact muscle strength.

Within the spinal cord, pain and proprioceptive fibers diverge, the proprioceptive fibers ascending the posterior column. The pain fibers synapse in the posterior horn of the cord and then decussate to the opposite anterolateral region to form the lateral spinothalamic tract. Since the motor fibers traverse the corticospinal tracts, it is possible to divide the lateral spinothalamic tract without losing motor or proprioceptive function. Such a division in the upper thoracic (T2–3) or upper cervical (C2–3) areas is known as cordotomy. Previously a procedure requiring laminectomy, it is now easily performed, especially in the cervical area, by a simple percutaneous stereotaxic approach with local anesthesia. Percutaneous cervical cordotomy is of particular value in providing pain relief to severely ill patients who are not good candidates for open surgical cordotomy. If the pain is located bilaterally or in the midline, as is often the case with neoplasm of the rectum, bladder, and uterus, bilateral cordotomy may be required.

In the medulla, the descending sensory tract of the trigeminal nerve and the spinothalamic tract are located superficially and are accessible for surgical ablation. Because of their proximity to each other, it is difficult to make a lesion in one tract without affecting the other. In addition, if the restiform body is damaged during the procedure, ipsilateral ataxia will result.

Enthusiasm for mesencephalic tractotomy has increased with the recent advances in stereotactic procedures. With this technic, extremely discrete lesions can be made in the still superficially located spinothalamic tract, in the quintothalamic tract, or in both, after stimulation studies via chronically implanted electrodes have determined the appropriate area. This procedure is quite effective for the control of pain involving the face or upper half of the body, although it is often followed by transient abnormal oculomotor activity. Another approach to pain in this area of the head—eg, pain from carcinoma of the mouth, pharynx, and larynx—involves denervation of pertinent cranial nerves. Complete denervation of the fifth nerve, the nervus intermedius of the seventh nerve, the ninth nerve, and the upper part of the tenth nerve is often required to assure good results.

Chronic intractable pain or pain originating from a thalamic disorder can be treated stereotactically. Lesions placed in the main sensory thalamic nuclei, although producing complete analgesia and anesthesia of the contralateral half of the body, do not always relieve pain. Carefully placed lesions in the nucleus centrum medianum and the parafascicularis of the thalamus (the nonspecific midline projection nuclei) usually do relieve pain although they fail to produce any sensory disturbance. Lesions placed in the posteromedian portion of the thalamus encompassing the probable terminations of the multisynaptic spino-

thalamic pain pathways are effective in relieving pain, as are similar lesions placed in the tegmentum of the mesencephalon. In general, however, these operations are best reserved for patients with a short life expectancy since the pain pattern frequently recurs after a few months or a few years.

Psychosurgery (eg, frontal lobectomy or leukotomy, cingulotomy) has been used in relief of intractable pain, although the results are unpredictable. Frontal lobectomy especially is losing support among neurosurgeons.

CEPHALIC NEURALGIA

Trigeminal Neuralgia

Trigeminal neuralgia is characterized by paroxysmal attacks of severe stabbing pain in the distribution of one or more branches of the trigeminal nerve. The maxillary and mandibular divisions are most often affected. The pain lasts for only a few seconds and may be triggered by talking, eating, or merely touching the affected area of the face. It is usually unilateral and occurs in the middle-aged and especially the elderly patient. Trigeminal neuralgia in patients under age 30 is quite unusual. Most patients respond well to medical management by carbamazepine (Tegretol). For those who cannot tolerate the medication or who do not respond to it, surgery is the ultimate method of treatment. Peripheral nerve block can be accomplished with alcohol or other substances injected at the foramen ovale or in the pterygopalatine fossa; the immediate effect of alcohol block is good, but it is usually only temporary. The overall results of supraorbital or infraorbital nerve avulsion are unsatisfactory. Probably the most satisfactory neurosurgical treatments of trigeminal neuralgia are intracranial decompression or massage of the trigeminal ganglion or trigeminal rhizotomy in either the middle or posterior fossa.

Glossopharyngeal Neuralgia

Sharp stabbing pain similar to that of trigeminal neuralgia may occur at the root of the tongue, radiating down the throat and to the ear. The pain can be triggered by swallowing or by touching the pharynx. Cocainization of the area temporarily blocks the pain and serves as a diagnostic test. Section of the glossopharyngeal nerve and the upper vagal fibers in the posterior fossa will alleviate the pain.

Nervus Intermedius Neuralgia

The postero-inferior margin of the external auditory meatus is thought to be innervated by the nervus intermedius of the facial nerve. Characteristic paroxysmal pain occurring in this area can be relieved by section of the nerve at the cerebellopontine angle.

POSTINFECTION PAIN

Postherpetic Neuralgia

Vesicular eruption of herpes zoster infection along the distribution of the cutaneous nerves is often followed by a continuous, intense burning pain in the area that is also hyperesthetic to touch. Undercutting of the involved skin or posterior rhizotomy is practically always unsatisfactory. Anterolateral cordotomy or quintothalamic medullary tractotomy for facial postherpetic neuralgia is successful in less than 70% of cases. The failure of these procedures is thought to be due to the involvement of secondary and tertiary sensory neurons by herpesvirus.

Pain of Tabes Dorsalis

The lancinating pain of tabes dorsalis frequently seen in the lower extremities responds well to carbamazepine (Tegretol). If the patient cannot tolerate the medication, anterolateral cordotomy is the procedure of choice.

PAIN FOLLOWING INJURIES TO PERIPHERAL NERVES

Long-standing severe pain after laceration or contusion of the peripheral nerves is associated with the formation of perineuronal or intraneuronal scarring. Simple excision of neuromas in areas of traumatic or postoperative fibrosis has consistently failed to abolish such pain. Neurolysis rarely helps except in cases of compression of the median nerve by the carpal ligament, but in these cases the results are excellent.

Proximal neurotomy is likely to be rewarding when the nerve can be divided high enough to include all the branches that enter the scar below. Posterior rhizotomy is often successful provided a sufficient number of roots can be sacrificed to prevent sensory overlap. For pain in the extremities, this operation has been limited to the roots of the ulnar, lateral femoral, cutaneous, and either the fifth lumbar or first sacral nerves, in order to retain proprioception.

Anterolateral cordotomy has been followed by early success in nearly all cases, but more than a third of cases have failed to maintain permanent analgesia.

PAIN FOLLOWING AMPUTATION

At the time of amputation, chemical injection of the severed nerve ends has proved useless in preventing postamputation pain. Most general surgeons and orthopedists agree that the best routine procedure is to cut the nerve trunks high and let their ends retract into a deep bed of healthy muscle. In the case of painful bulbs, a single resection is recommended. If the more simple procedures fail to produce relief, anterolateral cordotomy is the only alternative.

In the more difficult problem of phantom limbs, effective analgesia by cordotomy has seldom eliminated awareness of the ghost extremity, and pain often recurs when the effect of cordotomy wears off. Postcentral resection of the sensory cortex has usually failed, but extensive undercutting of the parietal lobe is worthy of trial if it can be done in the nondominant hemisphere. Frontal lobotomy has also been ineffectual unless carried out to the extent that it produces psychologic deterioration. The value of thalamotomy is too premature to be assessed, but this may well prove to be the procedure of choice.

White JC, Sweet WH: *Pain and the Neurosurgeon.* Thomas, 1969.

● ● ●

General References

Jennett WB: *An Introduction to Neurosurgery.* Mosby, 1970.
Kahn EA & others: *Correlative Neurosurgery,* 2nd ed. Thomas, 1969.

Mullan S: *Essentials of Neurosurgery for Students and Practitioners.* Springer-Verlag, 1961.

42...

Otolaryngology

Herbert H. Dedo, MD, & Francis A. Sooy, MD

I. THE EAR

EAR INFECTIONS

1. PERICHONDRITIS & CHONDRITIS OF THE PINNA

Perichondritis or chondritis of the pinna may occur spontaneously or following trauma, ear surgery, or frostbite. It is manifested by swelling, pain, tenderness, and discoloration (redness) of the pinna.

Treatment consists of systemic antibiotics, incision and drainage to release any blood or pus, and insertion of cotton packing in the crevices of the pinna to suppress fluid collection in the subcutaneous space. The antibiotics most often used are penicillin. A mastoid dressing is then applied so as to exert moderate pressure on the cotton. If blood or pus is allowed to collect adjacent to the cartilage and is not removed, infection can destroy the cartilage, produce fibrosis, and leave a severely deformed "cauliflower" ear.

2. EXTERNAL OTITIS

External otitis—superficial infection of the skin of the ear canal—causes itching or pain and is usually due to local trauma from water, cotton swabs, or other foreign bodies. Hearing is not impaired unless the ear canal has swelled shut. There may be minimal discharge.

Treatment consists of cleaning the ear canal with suction and administering antibiotic-corticosteroid ear drops for 5–7 days. If the skin of the ear canal is severely swollen, a cotton wick saturated with antibiotic-corticosteroid ointment should be placed in the ear canal for 48 hours to squeeze out the edema before the ear drops are administered.

Systemic antibiotics and analgesics may be necessary.

3. ACUTE SUPPURATIVE OTITIS MEDIA

The presenting complaint is usually pain—except in infants, in whom the first symptom may be fever. This disease is more common in children than adults and is usually caused by obstruction of the eustachian tube by an upper respiratory infection, which causes the adenoid to enlarge. Allergy is occasionally a causative factor. Conductive hearing loss is usually present because pus has collected behind the eardrum. Examination of the ear shows a reddened and, in the later stages, bulging tympanic membrane. If the tympanic membrane has ruptured (Fig 42–1), thick, purulent discharge will be found in the external ear canal.

Treatment is with oral penicillin G, erythromycin, or tetracycline. Oral decongestants should be given to shrink the nasal and eustachian tube membranes.

If there is significant pain from the bulging eardrum, myringotomy should be done (Fig 42–2), both for immediate pain relief and to release the pus before it erodes a hole in the eardrum that is too large to heal. The incision should be made in the posterior-inferior quadrant of the drum, midway between the umbo and

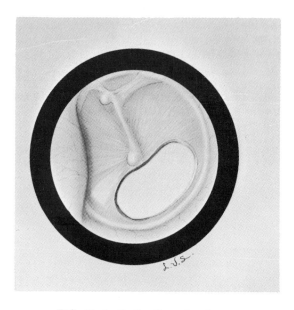

FIG 42–1. Perforation of eardrum.

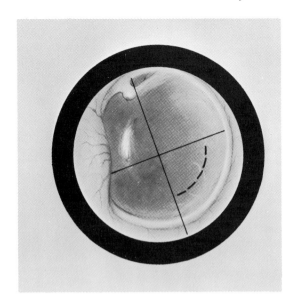

FIG 42–2. Site of myringotomy.

the rim, to avoid injury to the incus and stapes, which are in the posterior-superior quadrant.

In children, if acute otitis media recurs 2 or 3 times a year, tonsillectomy and adenoidectomy should be done to improve the function of the eustachian tube and thus decrease or prevent future ear infections.

4. SEROUS OTITIS MEDIA

Serous otitis media is characterized by sterile serous fluid in the middle ear. The patient is aware of a stuffy feeling in his ear, occasionally accompanied by gurgling when he moves his head, and has a conductive hearing loss. Pneumatic otoscopy demonstrates either that the middle ear is completely filled with fluid (manifested by a dull and immobile tympanic membrane) or that there is some fluid behind the tympanic membrane. In adults with unilateral serous otitis media—especially if they are Chinese—cancer of the nasopharynx must be ruled out by nasopharyngeal examination.

Serous otitis media is treated with antibiotics and decongestants. If the fluid persists for more than 4 weeks in a patient between the ages of 18 months and puberty, tonsillectomy, adenoidectomy, and myringotomy (Fig 42–2) with suction removal of the middle ear fluid should be done. In infants and adults, myringotomy, suction removal, and placement of Teflon collar button tubes should be done under general anesthesia. Nasal allergy and sinusitis should be treated if present. If the fluid recurs after tonsillectomy and adenoidectomy, myringotomy should be done and the collar button tubes placed. The tubes are ordinarily extruded by the body after several months,

but if the serous otitis media persists they may be replaced—except in infants in whom tonsillectomy and adenoidectomy become feasible because they are over 1 year of age.

5. CHRONIC OTITIS MEDIA

The presenting symptoms of chronic otitis media are chronic or recurrent ear discharge and pain. Examination shows a perforation in the eardrum with thick yellow or white discharge in the external canal. Chronic infection of the middle ear is usually the result of chronic mastoid infection or abnormal function of the eustachian tube. The latter cause can be eliminated in some children by tonsillectomy and adenoidectomy and by control of sinus infection, if present, with antibiotics and decongestants. Allergy of the respiratory system should be treated if present.

Local treatment of chronic otitis media includes administration of ear drops (1% boric acid in 80% ethyl alcohol), or antibiotic solutions such as Cortisporin Otic or powders and frequent suction cleansing of the ear canal and middle ear.

If the infection cannot be controlled or if complications such as meningitis, brain abscess, lateral sinus thrombosis, seventh nerve paralysis, or labyrinthitis develop, modified radical or radical mastoidectomy is required. Once the infection is controlled and the ear remains clean and dry for 3–6 months, myringoplasty may be done to close the perforation in the eardrum. Successful closure is possible in 70% of patients, and reconstruction technics now available for the ear drum and ossicular chain improve hearing in 50% of patients—ie, each patient has a 70% chance of closure and a 50% chance of hearing again.

6. MASTOIDITIS

The presenting complaints are ordinarily pain and tenderness behind the ear, occasionally a swelling on the mastoid, discharge from the middle ear, sagging of the posterior-superior ear canal, fever, or any of the complications of chronic otitis media mentioned previously. Ear examination shows mastoid tenderness, ear discharge, a protuberant pinna, or mastoid swelling (from a subperiosteal abscess). Roentgenograms of the mastoid show breakdown of the septa (from the osteomyelitis) and cloudiness (from the pus).

Acute mastoiditis is a complication of infection of the middle ear since the mucous membrane of the mastoid is always infected when the middle ear is infected. If untreated, osteomyelitis may result. Antibiotics are effective, and emergency mastoidectomy is only occasionally necessary to remove the pus and infected bone.

Chronic mastoiditis may follow acute mastoiditis and otitis media. The chronic drainage of pus from the ear can often be controlled by mastoidectomy to remove the diseased bone. If a cholesteatoma (a squamous epithelial sac that has grown inward from the skin of the ear canal or drum) develops, it will gradually erode the bone surrounding the antrum. Cholesteatomas can drain pus for years as they gradually enlarge until a complication such as meningitis, brain abscess, seventh nerve paralysis, labyrinthitis, or lateral sinus thrombosis occurs. Mastoidectomy should be done under the following circumstances and the cholesteatoma removed or the sac opened to the surface: whenever a cholesteatoma has been demonstrated (by keratin debris in the attic or middle ear space or by bony erosion on roentgenograms); whenever one of the above complications of chronic ear discharge appears; or whenever a fistula test is positive.

EIGHTH NERVE DISORDERS

1. HEARING LOSS

Differentiation between conductive hearing loss and sensorineural hearing loss is essential because each is treated differently. The patient with a significant conductive hearing loss will hear the 512 Hz tuning fork more clearly when it is vibrating on his mastoid bone than when it is moved 5 cm (2 inches) in front of the ear on the same side (**Rinne's test**). When it is placed on his forehead immediately above his nose or on his upper incisors (**Weber's test**), he will hear it best in the ear with the greater conductive hearing loss. Conversely, the patient with a sensorineural hearing loss will hear the tuning fork better during the Rinne test when it is vibrating in front of his ear and will hear the tuning fork better in the Weber test with his better ear. For any patient with a clinically significant hearing loss, an audiogram, including tests for pure tone and speech, should be obtained (1) to confirm the diagnosis, (2) to measure the amount of hearing loss in decibels at the different frequencies, and (3) to determine the amount of distortion (loss of discrimination or understanding of words). A normal audiogram is shown in Fig 42–3.

CONDUCTIVE HEARING LOSS

Perforation of the Eardrum

Diagnosis is made by examination with an ear speculum and a pneumatic otoscope. If discharge is present, it must be controlled (see Chronic Otitis

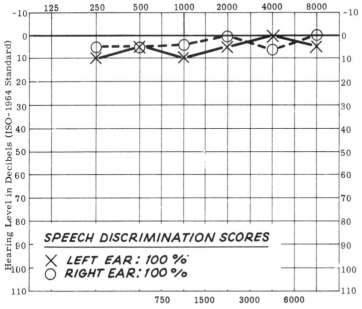

Air Conduction
 O Right ear (red)
 X Left ear (blue)
 △ Right ear with_____db
    masking in left
 □ Left ear with_____db
    masking in right
Bone Conduction
 > Right ear (red)
 < Left ear (blue)
 ▶ Right ear with_____db
    masking in left
 ◀ Left ear with_____db
    masking in right
    No response at maximum
 ↓ limits of audiometer

SPEECH DISCRIMINATION SCORES

X LEFT EAR : 100 %
O RIGHT EAR: 100 %

To convert the above readings based on the 1964 ISO reference thresholds to readings based on the 1951 ASA reference thresholds, subtract the following (rounded) difference in dB:

125	250	500	1000	2000	4000	8000
10	15	15	10	10	5	10

FIG 42–3. Normal hearing.

Media) for 3 months with suction, cleaning, and ear drops (or, if necessary, with mastoidectomy) before the hole in the eardrum is closed by myringoplasty. Several materials have been used successfully in closing tympanic perforations; a favored one at present is a pedicle graft of canal wall skin, usually supplemented by a temporalis fascia graft for large or anterior perforations. Initial reports of results from homograft eardrum and ossicle transplants have been encouraging.

Otosclerosis

Otosclerosis is manifested by a progressive conductive hearing loss that begins at or after puberty without evidence of eardrum or middle ear disease (Fig 42—4). The eardrum is intact and mobile when tested with pneumatic otoscopy, and there is no evidence of previous infection that might have resulted in necrosis of the ossicular chain.

Treatment is by stapedectomy. After a flap of posterior canal wall skin is elevated in continuity with the posterior-superior eardrum, the stapes can be seen fixed in the oval window by formation of otosclerotic bone around the edges of the footplate. This bony mass is removed in fragments and the ossicular chain is reconstituted—eg, by placing a piece of vein from the patient's hand over the oval window as a diaphragm and then placing a stainless steel wire prosthesis, approximately 4.5—5 mm long, crimped around the long process of the incus and reaching down to the surface of the vein. This procedure can dramatically reduce or eliminate the conductive hearing loss in properly selected patients.

Ossicular Chain Disruption

A diagnosis of ossicular chain disruption is made when a patient has a conductive hearing loss and a history of significant chronic infection, head trauma, or ear trauma. The most common disruptions are necrosis of the long process of the incus and absent stapes crura. The hearing loss is usually in the range of 45—55 db unless a partial reconstitution with fibrous tissue or a cholesteatoma has occurred.

Treatment consists of reconstruction of the ossicular mechanism with one of a variety of natural and artificial prostheses through an exploratory tympanotomy approach to the middle ear.

Adhesions in the Middle Ear

Middle ear adhesions are the probable diagnosis in a patient with conductive hearing loss and a retracted and immobile tympanic membrane as demonstrated by pneumatic otoscopy. The diagnosis can be confirmed by exploratory tympanotomy, using the stapedectomy approach described above. If any air space exists in the anterior-superiod middle ear, a layer of Silastic sheeting can be placed between the drum and the promontory in an attempt to reestablish the middle ear space. The results are variable.

SENSORINEURAL HEARING LOSS

The most common causes of significant sensorineural hearing loss are advancing age, trauma from prolonged exposure to sound above 90 db, viral or bacterial infections, **Ménière's syndrome** (sensorineural hearing loss, tinnitus, and vertigo), vascular obstruction, diabetes, or prediabetes. Typical audiograms are shown in Figs 42—5 and 42—6.

The only treatment is preventive since, with the exception of those accompanying Ménière's syndrome, these hearing losses are irreversible and some tend to be progressive. Rehabilitation can be achieved with a hearing aid if necessary. The ear should be examined to rule out correctable diseases such as chronic infection and otosclerosis.

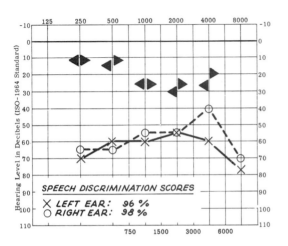

FIG 42—4. Bilateral severe conductive hearing loss due to otosclerosis.

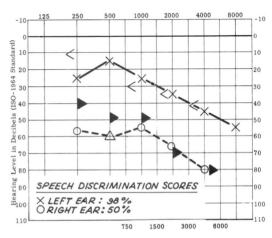

FIG 42—5. Mild left high-frequency and severe right sensorineural hearing loss (latter due to internal auditory meatus tumor).

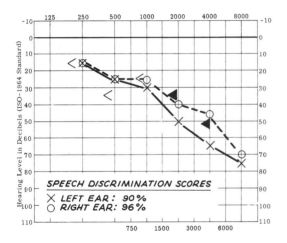

FIG 42−6. Bilateral high-frequency sensorineural hearing loss.

2. VERTIGO

Because the patient with vertigo ordinarily complains of "dizziness," the physician must be careful to distinguish between true vertigo, faintness (which is more apt to signify orthostatic hypotension), and a floating sensation (more apt to signify hyperventilation syndrome). True vertigo (a sensation of rolling or spinning in relationship to the environment) is evaluated on the basis of (1) the history, (2) audiograms—including special audiologic studies (Békésy and SISI [small increment sensitivity index] tests) to ascertain whether the lesion is cochlear or retrochlear, (3) tests of vestibular function (caloric or electronystagmographic), and (4) roentgenograms of the internal auditory meatus to detect any erosion by an eighth nerve tumor. If a defect of the labyrinthine system is diagnosed, it is treated medically (low-salt diet; no caffeine, tobacco, or alcohol; and chlorpheniramine maleate). The patient with acute vertigo (as well as the patient with severe sudden unilateral sensorineural hearing loss) should be hospitalized and given an intravenous histamine drip twice daily for 5 days. (This consists of giving histamine phosphate, 2.75 mg in 250 ml of 5% dextrose in water. Administer twice daily at a rate that achieves flushing.) If the patient is still incapacitated by the vertigo after 3 months, surgical decompression or section of the vestibular nerve (if useful hearing persists) or destruction of the labyrinth is done.

3. TINNITUS

The patient with tinnitus hears a constant or intermittent ringing, humming, or buzzing sound not caused by a source external to the ear. The cause is not known. When it accompanies otosclerosis, it disappears in 80% of patients after stapedectomy. In other patients, the tinnitus may disappear with the treatment regimen outlined above for vertigo. If tinnitus persists for more than 6 months in spite of treatment, the patient must learn to live with it. He can minimize it at bedtime by placing a noisy clock or radio near his bed.

BENIGN TUMORS & FOREIGN BODIES OF THE EAR

Osteomas

Osteomas are rounded, bony-hard protuberances that develop under the skin of the ear canal adjacent to the drum. They are usually asymptomatic and are detected during routine ear examination. They should be removed if they obstruct 75−90% of the ear canal since further growth will cause hearing loss and infection from obstruction.

Granulomas & Polyps of the Ear Canal

These growths, ordinarily the result of chronic otitis media, are soft, pink, friable masses usually projecting through a perforation in the eardrum. They require surgical removal via a tympanotomy or mastoidectomy incision.

Internal Auditory Meatus Tumor (Schwannoma)

This is a benign tumor of the sheath of the eighth nerve which tends to erode bone and may eventually create enough pressure on the seventh and eighth nerves to cause complete loss of function. It can enlarge until it compresses the fifth, sixth, and ninth nerves and the brain stem, causing death. Early diagnosis and surgical removal may avoid these complications.

Foreign Bodies in the Ear Canal

Most foreign bodies in the ear canal can be removed with a ring curet, a 90 degree angle hook, or an alligator forceps. If the object is firmly fixed, it should be removed under local or general anesthesia since the patient's movements in response to pain can result in injury to the eardrum and the ossicular chain.

MALIGNANT TUMORS OF THE EXTERNAL EAR

Basal cell carcinoma, squamous cell carcinoma, and occasionally melanoma can occur in the pinna, external ear canal, or middle ear. They should be suspected in the presence of a lesion that persists for over 2 weeks. They should be removed surgically if that can be done. If the eardrum or the mastoid has been invaded, mastoidectomy or total resection of the temporal bone may be necessary. If the tumor cannot be removed completely, radiation therapy is required.

MALIGNANT TUMORS OF THE MIDDLE EAR

Squamous Cell Carcinoma

Squamous cell carcinoma, although rare, should be suspected in any patient with unexplained ear pain or ear pain more severe than the physical findings would seem to justify. It may appear as a mass in the ear canal or middle ear. Roentgenograms may show erosion. The diagnosis is made by tympanotomy and biopsy. Treatment consists of temporal bone resection if feasible; otherwise, radiation therapy is required. The 5-year cure rate is very low.

GLOMUS JUGULARE TUMOR

Glomus jugulare is a tumor that usually arises from the jugular bulb and spreads upward into the middle ear space and posteriorly into the mastoid bone. If it is not controlled, it will progressively paralyze the nerves of the jugular foramen (cranial nerves IX, X, and XI) and then nerves VII, VIII, and XII. The diagnosis is based on the appearance of a pink mass behind the eardrum which compresses with pneumatic otoscopy and then pulsates back to full size when the air pressure is released. In some cases, the diagnosis is based on the concurrence of tinnitus or signs of cranial nerve defects with roentgenographic enlargement of the jugular foramen and, in more advanced cases, erosion of the temporal bone. Carotid arteriography and retrograde jugular venography are used to outline the extent of the tumor and to evaluate the patency of the contralateral sigmoid sinus. The tumor somewhat resembles an inflammatory polyp, and, because it will bleed profusely if cut, no "ear polyp" should be biopsied or removed in the physician's office.

Surgical removal of glomus jugulare may be feasible, but the procedure is quite difficult. Occasionally, some degree of palliation is achieved by radiation therapy in inoperable cases.

CONGENITAL DEFECTS OF THE EAR

Atresia of the External Ear & Ear Canal

This disfiguring congenital defect is uncommon. Since the results of surgical correction to improve hearing are modest, unilateral defects should not be so treated. The external ear can be reconstructed with plastic surgery or with a prosthesis if the patient desires. If the defect is bilateral, if roentgenograms of the mastoid show an air-filled middle ear space and some pneumatization of the mastoid, and if some development of the external ear exists, surgical reconstruction of the ear canal can be achieved by mastoid-

ectomy and skin graft. If hearing is thus improved and the ear can be kept dry, a hearing aid can be placed in the reconstructed ear canal. If this is not feasible, a bone conduction hearing aid can be placed on the mastoid bone behind the ear. Normal hearing will not be achieved, but significant improvement often results. A hearing aid is more a hindrance than a help if the hearing is normal in the other ear.

Preauricular Sinus or Cyst

The sinus (measuring 1 mm in diameter and 5–10 mm or more in depth) or cyst is located just anterior to the upper helix. Excision is indicated to stop discharge.

SEVENTH NERVE PALSY

Paralysis of the facial (seventh) nerve immobilizes the muscles of expression on that side of the face. There is loss of both voluntary and involuntary contraction; the eye fails to close; the forehead cannot be wrinkled; and that side of the mouth droops. Paralysis can result from trauma that injures or fractures the base of the skull or from surgical procedures on the parotid gland, the middle ear, the mastoid, or in the area of the brain stem in the posterior fossa. It can also be caused by viral infections (Ramsay Hunt syndrome with herpes zoster or other neurotropic viral infections), pressure on the seventh nerve in the posterior fossa by tumors of the cerebellopontine angle or internal auditory meatus, or diabetes or prediabetes. When the cause is not known, it is called **Bell's palsy**. Some cases of Bell's palsy may be the result of vascular spasm causing nerve edema, most often in the vertical portion near the stylomastoid foramen.

The diagnostic work-up must include a careful history; ear, nose, and throat examination; pure tone, speech, and special audiograms; roentgenograms of the mastoid to detect any erosion of the internal auditory meatus or in the area of the antrum or attic; a 5-hour glucose tolerance test to exclude diabetes and prediabetes; and a caloric test. Electromyographic or nerve conduction studies (or both) may be done but are of limited value in predicting the outcome of facial nerve paralysis. Loss of voluntary muscle potentials immediately and response to external electrical stimulation 3–7 days later occur after both anatomic (surgical or traumatic) or physiologic interruption of the nerve. This does not mean that facial nerve function will not return spontaneously in 1–16 weeks; spontaneous recovery occurs in approximately 80% of cases of Bell's palsy.

Treatment consists of removing identifiable causes such as cholesteatoma or tumors of the internal auditory meatus, or of treating the infection or diabetes. The treatment of Bell's palsy is still controversial; statistical data support the effectiveness of early treatment with corticosteroids to reduce edema in the nerve—eg, dexamethasone. Surgical decompression (through the mastoid) should be done (1) if function has not returned within 3 months after the onset of Bell's palsy; (2) if the nerve is paralyzed after head trauma with roentgenographic evidence of a fracture in the area of the nerve; or (3) if the nerve is damaged during a mastoid or middle ear operation. If a damaged segment of the nerve cannot be decompressed, a section of the great auricular nerve may be grafted in its place. If function has not returned by 9 months after decompression or grafting, anastomosis of the facial nerve to the hypoglossal nerve may be done. This latter procedure will not result in return of involuntary function, but the patient will have better tone in the facial muscles at rest and, with practice, will be able to move his face. He does this by pressing his tongue against his teeth to send impulses along the 12th nerve into the face through the anastomosis and the seventh nerve.

CEREBROSPINAL FLUID OTORRHEA & ENDAURAL ENCEPHALOCELE

CSF leakage or brain herniation into the temporal bone occurs most commonly after mastoidectomy. It is usually manifested by clear watery discharge from the ear; a polyp or a pink, pulsating, enlarging mass in a mastoid bowl; or meningitis. The diagnosis is confirmed by analysis of the fluid for protein and sugar and by dye tests (indigo carmine or 5% fluorescein injected via lumbar puncture to see if it appears in the discharge). If it does not close spontaneously within 2 weeks of onset, the dural defect needs to be closed surgically from below via the mastoid with a muscle graft or via craniotomy with fascia.

Dedo HH, Sooy FA: Endaural brain hernia (encephalocele): Diagnosis and treatment. Laryngoscope 80:1090–1099, 1970.

Saunders WH, Paparella MM: *Atlas of Ear Surgery.* Mosby, 1968.

II. NOSE, PARANASAL SINUSES, & FACE

INFECTIONS OF THE NOSE, PARANASAL SINUSES, & FACE

1. SINUSITIS

Sinusitis is usually preceded by nasal allergy or by a bacterial or viral upper respiratory infection. In the acute stage, there is severe pain in the maxilla or forehead. The diagnosis is based on an aching facial pain associated with or preceded by purulent nasal drainage or upper respiratory tract infection and the appearance of mucopus in the nose. If paranasal sinus x-rays show fluid partially or completely filling one or more of the sinuses (Fig 42–7), it is probably pus and should be treated with antibiotics and a decongestant.

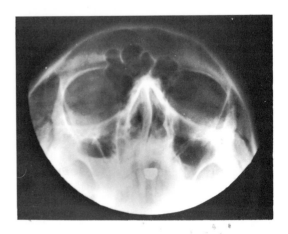

FIG 42–7. Sinus x-ray showing air-fluid (pus) level in maxillary sinuses (20% on left; 50% on right).

Maxillary Sinusitis

When pus is demonstrated in the maxillary sinus, it should be washed out by antral irrigation—passing a trocar through the lateral wall of the inferior nasal meatus into the maxillary sinus and running water through the needle, into the sinus, and out the ostium. This should be done only after the patient has taken antibiotics for 48–72 hours to minimize the incidence of osteomyelitis in the maxilla. Care must be taken to avoid passing the trocar into the orbit. If nasal polyps are present, they should be removed when the acute (pain) phase has passed (see below). If 3 or 4 antral irrigations 4–7 days apart do not control the infection, a Caldwell-Luc operation (Fig 42–10) should be done to remove the diseased membrane from the sinus and to create a permanent opening for drainage from the antrum into the nose.

Acute or Chronic Ethmoidal, Sphenoidal, or Frontal Sinusitis

This infection is suggested by pain and tenderness between and above the eyes. It is diagnosed by x-ray and can often be cured by controlling any concurrent maxillary sinusitis with antibiotics, decongestants, and Proetz displacements (displacement of air in the sinus with a topical vasoconstrictor). If these fail and no maxillary sinusitis exists, treatment is by exenteration of the ethmoid or sphenoid sinuses (or both), either via the antrum (Caldwell-Luc operation; Fig 42–10) or via an external Lynch incision between the medial canthus of the eye and the bridge of the nose. Any object obstructing the drainage of the frontal sinus duct should be created with a flap of mucosa from the nasal septum to prevent future accumulations of pus in the frontal sinus (Sewell operation). If drainage of the frontal sinus cannot be established, all mucous membrane must be removed from the frontal sinus and the space obliterated either with fat or by removing its anterior wall.

Montgomery WW: Surgery of the frontal sinuses. Otol Clin North America 4:97–126, 1971.
Ogura JH, Watson RK, Jurema AA: Frontal sinus surgery: The use of mucoperiosteal flap for reconstruction of a nasofrontal duct. Laryngoscope 70:1229–1243, 1960.

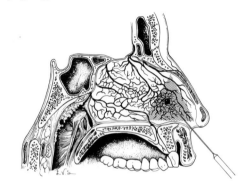

FIG 42–8. Cauterization to control bleeding in Kiesselbach's area.

2. FOLLICULITIS

Folliculitis, an infection of a hair follicle at the anterior nasal choana, is characterized by pain, swelling, redness, and tenderness of the anterior nose. Treatment is with local warm compresses and local applications of antibiotic and corticosteroid ointment. Systemic antibiotics are given for significant swelling or spreading cellulitis. Incision and drainage are done if an abscess appears. Folliculitis should be treated vigorously as soon as it is detected because cavernous sinus thrombosis has been known to result from infection in the face between the mouth and the eyes.

EPISTAXIS

Spontaneous nosebleed most commonly occurs from Kiesselbach's triangle on the septum just inside the anterior nares. The patient himself can usually control a minor nosebleed by pinching his nostrils together or by placing a cotton plug in the bleeding nostril. If this is not successful, apply a cotton pressure pack soaked with a local vasoconstrictor such as epinephrine, 1:1000, or phenylephrine, 0.25%, to the bleeding area for 5 minutes and then cauterize the bleeding vessel with silver nitrate or a chromic acid bead (Fig 42–8). Cautery should not be used in patients taking anticoagulants or in patients with leukemia, thrombocytopenic purpura, or other bleeding problems. The best treatment in patients with bleeding problems is insertion of a wedge of salt pork in the nostril for 4 or 5 days. (Start with a piece 2 × 2 × 4 cm and carve off just enough so it can be inserted.) When the pork is removed, it does not stick to the nasal membrane, thereby breaking loose the newly formed clot.

Bleeding from the middle portion of the nose that cannot be controlled by cautery requires treatment with an anterior nasal pack left in place for 6–9 days.

Bleeding from the posterior part of the nose usually requires both a posterior and an anterior pack, placed after local anesthesia and shrinkage of the nasal

membranes with tetracaine, 2%, and epinephrine, 1:1000, applied with cotton swabs. The posterior pack is installed by passing a catheter posteriorly along the floor of the nose and out the posterior choana into the pharynx where it can be grasped through the mouth with a hemostat (Fig 42–9). Two of the 3 strings on the posterior pack are tied to the pharyngeal end of the catheter, and both are brought back out through one anterior naris and tied over a bolster. The anterior nose is then packed with half-inch gauze.

Note: A posterior pack must always have a third string attached to it extending downward along the posterior pharyngeal wall. When the pack is removed (after 4–7 days), the third string should be grasped with a locked hemostat to prevent the pack from falling into the larynx and asphyxiating the patient when the 2 anterior strings have been cut.

If anterior and posterior packing still fails to arrest bleeding in the posterior or superior part of the nose, ligation of the anterior ethmoid, internal maxillary, or external carotid arteries—singly or in any combination—is required.

DEVIATED SEPTUM

Deviated nasal septum can result from trauma during birth or later or from progressive, differential growth of the septum and the rest of the nose. It is corrected by straightening the deformed portions and removing the permanently deformed cartilage and bone of the septum through an incision in the anterior septal mucosa (nasal septoplasty).

BENIGN TUMORS & FOREIGN BODIES OF THE NOSE, PARANASAL SINUSES, & FACE

Rhinophyma

Rhinophyma is a swelling of the tip of the nose caused by proliferation of the connective tissue and

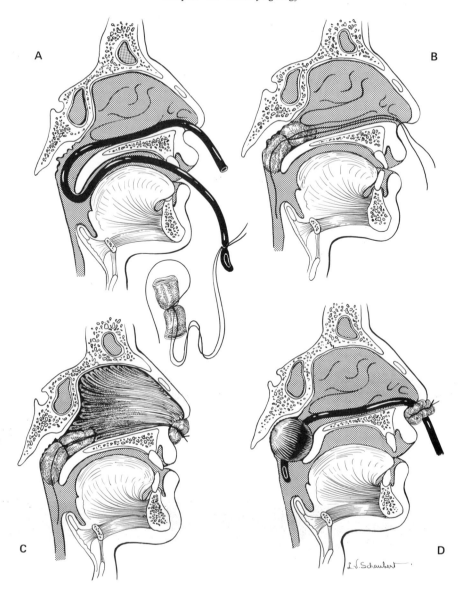

FIG 42–9. Packing to control bleeding from the posterior nose. *A:* Catheter inserted and pack attached. *B:* Pack drawn into position as catheter is removed. *C:* Strip tied over a bolster to hold pack in place. *D:* Alternative method using balloon catheter instead of gauze pack.

glands in the skin. Treatment is by excision of the affected skin down to the basal layer.

Nasal Polyps

Nasal polyps can cause nasal and sinus obstruction. They are usually associated with allergy, although intensive therapy for nasal allergy, including the use of corticosteroids, does not abolish them and rarely prevents their recurrence. Nasal polyps should be removed surgically. If infection has resulted from their obstruction of sinuses, drainage procedures such as a Caldwell-Luc operation (Fig 42–10) or a fronto-ethmoidectomy are required.

Mucocele of the Sinus

Mucocele is usually manifested by pain or swelling over a paranasal sinus. If a paranasal sinus is chronically and totally obstructed, mucous secretion gradually accumulates under sufficient pressure to erode the surrounding bone. In the frontal sinus, such erosion can expose the dura and lead to meningitis and brain abscess, especially if the mucocele becomes infected (mucopyocele). The pain results from progressive pressure and irritation of surrounding structures.

Treatment consists of surgical removal of the mucocele and reestablishment of drainage from the involved sinuses as described above for acute sinusitis.

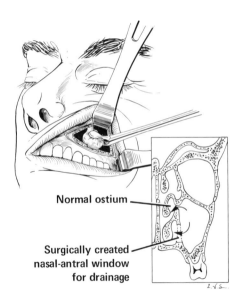

Normal ostium

Surgically created
nasal-antral window
for drainage

FIG 42–10. Caldwell-Luc nasal polypectomy.

Juvenile Angiofibroma of the Nasopharynx

Recurrent nasal bleeding or chronic nasal obstruction is the usual sign of this locally invasive but usually nonmetastasizing tumor, which occurs most frequently in teen-age boys. It arises from the periosteal layer of the basilar process of the occipital bone (the posterior superior nasopharynx) and progressively erodes into the sphenoid sinus, the posterior nose, the pterygomaxillary fossa, the maxillary sinus, and rarely, into the brain.

Radiation therapy has not been effective. The tumor should be removed via a transpalatal route.

Nasal Foreign Bodies

A foreign body must be suspected in any patient with unilateral nasal secretion or unilateral reduction in the nasal airway. The object should be removed with appropriate forceps or hooks. Vegetable material such as a bean should be removed as rapidly as possible because it swells.

CHRONIC NASAL CONGESTION & DISCHARGE

Vasomotor Rhinitis

This diagnosis is made in a patient with no evidence of infection who has recurrent episodes of copious, thin nasal drainage precipitated by cold air or by eating hot or cold foods and whose sinus roentgenograms show no significant abnormalities. Decongestants and reassurance are used for treatment but are not entirely satisfactory.

Cerebrospinal Fluid Rhinorrhea

Unilateral, clear, watery nasal discharge which increases during the Valsalva maneuver must be regarded as CSF until proved otherwise. The most common cause of CSF leakage is head trauma. Chemical tests for glucose and protein (to identify the fluid) and dye studies (to indicate the site of a bony and dural defect) may be useful. The defect must be closed surgically if it does not close spontaneously within 2 weeks after onset. Frontal and sphenoid leaks are best approached from below by the otolaryngologist. Ethmoid defects are best closed via craniotomy by the neurosurgeon.

McCoy G: Cerebrospinal rhinorrhea: A comprehensive review. Laryngoscope 73:1125, 1963.

Chemical Rhinitis

The chronic use of nasal drops or sprays causes the nasal membranes to swell severely and drain continuously. Treatment consists of stopping the local nasal medication and administering oral decongestants for 2–3 weeks to allow the membranes to return to normal.

CONGENITAL ABNORMALITIES OF THE NOSE

Anterior choanal atresia is rare but is obvious when it occurs. Posterior choanal atresia should be suspected in any newborn who has difficulty breathing. The diagnosis is made by holding the baby's mouth closed and seeing if a piece of cotton held in front of each nostril moves. If there is still doubt, the inability to pass a catheter through each nostril into the pharynx will substantiate the diagnosis. If both posterior nares appear to be closed, the baby's respiration should be assured by holding his mouth open with an oral airway or, if necessary, by inserting an endotracheal tube. Definitive diagnosis is made by placing a few drops of radiopaque material in each anterior naris while the baby is supine and taking a lateral roentgenogram of the skull to see if the material has entered the nasopharynx.

To establish an immediate airway, a temporary opening is made with a mastoid curet through the mucosal—often bony—membrane that extends from the posterior end of the hard palate to the sphenoid basiocciput. This opening is kept patent by placing a segment of No. 16 or No. 18F Portex endotracheal tube through it. When the baby's general condition permits, transnasal resection of the obstruction and resection of the posterior end of the nasal septum should be done under general anesthesia using the operating microscope. If this fails—and in older children or in adults with unilateral posterior choanal atreaia—surgical repair is best done via the transpalatal route. This route permits the surgeon to use the nasal septal mucosa on the uninvolved side to epithelize part of the raw portion left after removal of the unilateral posterior choanal atresia, thereby minimizing the chances of stenosis.

III. MOUTH, PHARYNX, & SALIVARY GLANDS

INFECTIONS OF THE MOUTH, PHARYNX, & SALIVARY GLANDS

Glossitis & Pharyngitis

The presenting symptom is mouth or throat pain. The membranes of the mouth or pharynx are injected and may have a white coating. Bacterial glossitis or pharyngitis is treated with systemic antibiotics; candida infections (thrush) are treated with topical nystatin (1%).

Tonsillitis

Acute tonsillitis is diagnosed on the basis of sore throat and fever in a patient with injected, enlarged tonsils—often with an exudate or white crypts on their surfaces. Tonsillitis is differentiated from diphtheria by the absence (in tonsillitis) of extension of this surface coating onto the soft palate and anterior pillars and by culture of a throat smear. Treatment is with antibiotics and, if necessary, analgesics. The tonsils should be removed if tonsillitis recurs more than 3 or 4 times a year in a child or more than once or twice a year in an adult. In children, the adenoids should also be removed at this time since they become infected whenever the tonsils do.

Other indications for tonsillectomy and adenoidectomy in children include recurrent otitis media, chronic otitis media, obstruction of the nasopharynx by enlarged adenoids, and subacute bacterial endocarditis or chronic glomerulonephritis resulting from recurrent or chronic streptococcal infections of the pharynx or tonsils.

Sialitis (Infection of the Salivary Glands)

The swelling and pain of acute infection of the parotid or submandibular (submaxillary) glands usually respond rapidly to treatment with antibiotics and warm compresses. Culture of Stensen's duct secretion should be done. Staphylococci are often the cause of parotid gland infection, especially in elderly or severely debilitated people. If a gram-stained smear or culture shows coagulase-positive *Staphylococcus aureus,* methicillin should be given. If the infection does not respond to antibiotic therapy, incision and drainage should be carried out. Multiple incisions made parallel to the course of the facial nerve and its branches may be required.

Infection can often be prevented by the maintenance of good hydration, so that there is an adequate salivary flow to prevent retrograde infection via Stensen's duct. When the parotid gland must be removed—as in cases of chronic recurrent infection, often associated with calculi—care must be taken to preserve the facial nerve.

Abscesses

Abscesses of the floor of the mouth or of the peritonsillar, pharyngeal, or parapharyngeal spaces are usually the result of tooth or tonsillar infection and are manifested by swelling and pain. While still in the cellulitis stage, they may be controlled by antibiotics and warm compresses. If rapid resolution does not occur, incision and drainage should be done.

BENIGN TUMORS OF THE MOUTH & PHARYNX

Papilloma

Small papillomas resembling warts can occur anywhere in the mucosa of the pharynx but are most common on the soft palate. They do not ordinarily become malignant.

Alveolar Ridge Tumors

These tumors (embryonic rests of teeth) appear as mandibular or maxillary lumps and are diagnosed by biopsy. Treatment is usually by surgical excision after the extent of the tumor has been delineated radiographically and after biopsy has proved it not to be a carcinoma.

Leukoplakia

Localized "white spots" less than 5–10 mm in diameter which persist longer than 2 weeks should be biopsied. Extensive oral leukoplakias should be observed and, if ulcers or piled up areas develop, these should be biopsied.

Hemangioma & Lymphangioma

Hemangiomas and lymphangiomas can occur anywhere in the buccal or pharyngeal mucosa. In the tongue, they can be so large at birth that they interfere with breathing and swallowing. Hemangiomas are purplish; lymphangiomas tend to be the color of the overlying mucous membrane. Diagnosis should be by biopsy since a sarcoma or lymphoma may resemble these tumors. Surgical treatment is by excision if feasible, although extensive hemangiomas and lymphangiomas often cannot be removed completely since they do not remain encapsulated.

Palatal Exostosis (Torus Palatinus)

Palatal exostosis is a malformation composed of knobby, bony, submucosal nodules projecting downward from the midline of the hard palate. It results from the overriding of the 2 palatal bones when they come together in the midline in the embryo. It does not become malignant and need not be removed unless it interferes with the fitting of an upper dental plate.

TRAUMA TO THE MOUTH, PHARYNX, & SALIVARY GLANDS

Perforation of the soft palate often occurs when a child falls on an object, such as a pencil, that he is carrying in his mouth. It should not be sutured. If cellulitis develops, it should be treated with antibiotics. A small laceration of the tongue should not be closed with sutures, but more extensive lacerations should be closed with interrupted 3–0 chromic gut sutures to minimize scarring.

Perforations of the hard palate or around the eyes may be intracranial as well. The penetrating object should not be removed until the depth of penetration has been ascertained—with roentgenograms if possible—and until neurosurgical assistance is available.

The location, number, and extent of mandibular fractures should be determined by x-ray. Any teeth in the fracture line should be removed to help prevent infection. After the fracture has been reduced, fixation can be achieved by intraoral wiring, an external prosthesis, or wiring at the side of the fracture through an external incision.

IV. LARYNX, HYPOPHARYNX, & TRACHEA

INFECTION

Infection of the epiglottis, larynx, or trachea (acute epiglottitis or laryngotracheobronchitis, ie, "croup") causes airway obstruction in children but only hoarseness in adults because the adult airway at the glottic level is so much larger than the minimum space required for breathing. Cultures have usually shown gram-positive organisms or *Haemophilus influenzae*. Treatment is with ampicillin, corticosteroids, and cold mist. In children, close observation in the hospital for 72 hours is necessary so that endotracheal intubation and tracheotomy (Fig 42–13) can be done immediately if the airway obstruction becomes too severe or if the effort of breathing tires the child too much.

AIRWAY OBSTRUCTION (TRACHEOTOMY)

In addition to the infections discussed above, airway obstruction can occur as a result of trauma to or congenital deformities of the nose or larynx, tumors, or paralysis of one or both vocal cords at birth. The most rapid way to establish an airway when the obstruction lies above the midpoint of the trachea is to install an endotracheal tube via the mouth or nose. A laryngoscope is used to visualize the vocal cords and the endotracheal tube is then passed into the upper trachea. The patient should then be taken immediately to the operating room where a tracheotomy can be done under local or general anesthesia while the patient is oxygenated through the endotracheal tube. Sometimes it is necessary to perform a bedside tracheotomy, but when possible it is better to move the patient to the operating room.

The indications for tracheotomy include airway obstruction above the mid trachea or the need for prolonged assisted ventilation. Whenever there is infection in the larynx, an endotracheal tube should not be used any longer than necessary to do a tracheotomy because of the high incidence of mucosal injury and stenosis that results.

To establish a tracheotomy (Fig 42–11), a 5 cm collar incision is made 5–10 mm below the inferior edge of the cricoid cartilage. Dissection is carried down to the surface of the strap muscles, and vertical dissection is then carried between the strap muscles the anterior surface of the cricoid, the thyroid isthmus, and the trachea. The isthmus of the thyroid is mobilized by blunt dissection and pushed cranially to expose the upper tracheal cartilages. A square (2 × 2 or 3 × 3 mm) segment of the third or fourth tracheal ring is excised, and the opening is enlarged by incising the membrane for 2–3 mm above and below the ring from which the segment was removed. Hemostasis is achieved with clamps and gut ligatures. The smallest tracheotomy tube that will permit adequate ventilation of the patient (rather than the largest one that can be forced into the trachea) is then installed. The largest tube that should be used in an adult male is a No. 6; in an adult female, No. 5. Children 6–10 years old usually do well with No. 3 tracheotomy tubes; and younger children and infants require a No. 1–2. A low-pressure balloon-cuffed tube may be used if assisted ventilation or prevention of aspiration is necessary. The incision is closed with one or 2 sutures at each end, care being taken not to close the incision under the face plate of the tracheotomy tube since this can result in subcutaneous emphysema, pneumomediastinum, and pneumothorax. A 10 × 10 cm (4 × 4 inch) sponge is cut two-thirds of the way up the center and placed under the face plate; the cloth tapes attached to the face plate are then tied tightly enough to prevent the tube from coming out of the trachea without being so tight that they occlude the external jugular vein. If a low-pressure balloon-cuffed tube is

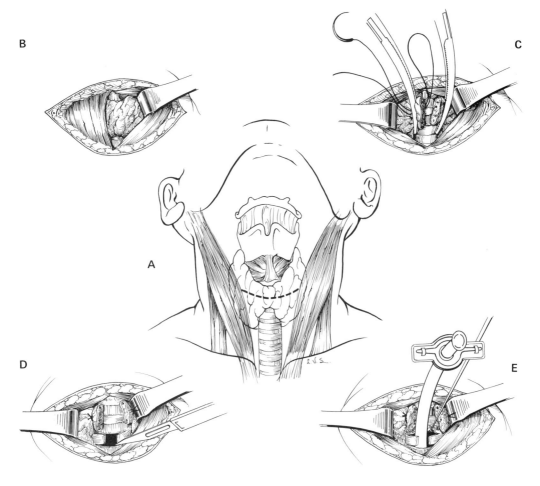

FIG 42—11. Technic of tracheotomy. *A:* Collar incision one fingerbreadth below cricoid from sternocleidomastoid to sternocleidomastoid. *B:* Vertical line of dissection down to thyroid isthmus, cricoid, and anterior trachea. *C:* If the thyroid isthmus cannot be mobilized to expose the third or fourth ring, it should be divided as shown. *D:* Square segment removed from third or fourth tracheal ring with horizontal extension incision in membrane above and below this ring. *E:* Smallest possible (not largest possible) tracheotomy tube is installed (adult male, No. 6; adult female, No. 5; 10-year-old, No. 3; infant, No. 1 or No. 0).

used, the balloon should be inflated only until the airway becomes airtight when the tracheotomy tube is temporarily occluded. It should be completely deflated 4 times per day and reinflated only until the airway again becomes airtight when the tube is occluded. Overinflation of a balloon cuff causes tracheal necrosis and stenosis.

Postoperative roentgenograms of the chest (posteroanterior and lateral views) should be taken to show whether the tube fits the trachea properly and to rule out pneumothorax. The tracheotomy tube should not be removed until it can be plugged continuously for 48 hours without impairing respiratory function.

BENIGN TUMORS & FOREIGN BODIES OF THE LARYNX, HYPOPHARYNX, & TRACHEA

All tumors and foreign bodies of these structures cause hoarseness and occasionally airway obstruction.

Singer's Nodules

Singer's nodules are small projections from the free edge of the cord, each resembling a grain of sand. They usually occur at the junction of the anterior and middle thirds of the true vocal cords and are caused by singing or shouting, especially during an episode of laryngitis. The patient should avoid shouting, singing, smoking, and drinking alcohol. Removal of the nodule, if required, is by direct laryngoscopy with the newer types of large-opening fiberoptic laryngoscopes such as the Jako-Dedo, which utilize the operating microscope to improve visualization and facilitate precise removal.

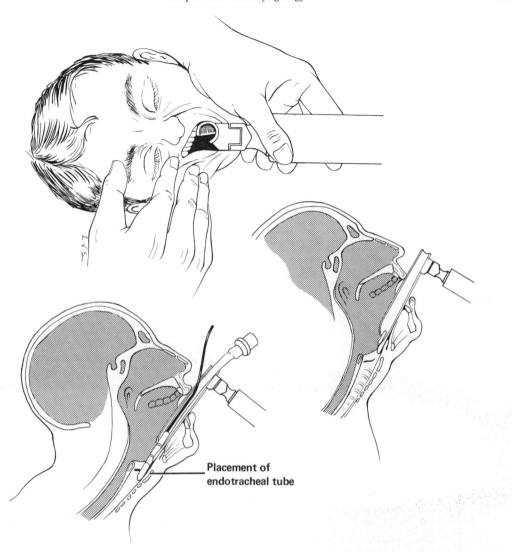

FIG 42–12. Technic of laryngoscopy.

Placement of
endotracheal tube

Granulomas

Granulomas appear on the posterior third of the vocal cord, usually as a result of injury to the mucosa over the arytenoid cartilage. The most common causes of injury are endotracheal intubation and excessive shouting, singing, or throat clearing. Granulomas appear as pink or purple (and later white) rough masses. Early, when they are sessile, they should not be removed because they will return and grow larger than before. Treatment is by avoidance of further vocal trauma and removal of the tumor when its base has become pinched into a narrow stalk.

Polyps of the Vocal Cord

Polyps usually occur as a late stage in granuloma of the arytenoid portion of the cord. Like granulomas, they should be removed only when they have a narrow stalk. The term "polypoid cords" refers to cords that are thickened in the membranous portion and, in

extreme cases, resemble floppy elephant ears. Some polyps may be due to vocal abuse, excessive use of tobacco or alcohol, diabetes, or hypothyroidism.

Treatment consists of resting the voice and eliminating the underlying problem. If the polypoid cord persists, the mucous membrane should be stripped from the vocal cord, care being taken not to remove tissue deeper than Rinke's space to avoid injuring the thyroarytenoid muscle fibers themselves.

Papilloma of the Larynx

Laryngeal papilloma occurs more commonly in children than in adults. Treatment is by surgical removal after placement of a low-pressure balloon-cuffed tracheotomy tube to protect the airway, simplify anesthesia, and prevent blood from reaching the lower trachea during the operation. Because they keep returning, removal should be repeated at 6-week intervals. Removal should be thorough each time but not so deep that the underlying normal tissue is injured. The surgical instruments should not be passed into the lower trachea or bronchi below the point where the airway can be protected by a tracheotomy tube.

Laryngeal Web

This thin membrane, usually formed between the true cords, can occur as a congenital deformity or after laryngeal trauma. It is diagnosed by inspection via direct laryngoscopy. It is treated by division and placement of a tantalum keel by the laryngofissure (McNaught) or endolaryngeal (Haslinger) technic.

Hemangioma

Subglottic hemangioma is a pink or purple mass which usually occurs in infants and causes airway obstruction which increases dramatically during crying (because the Valsalva effect causes venous obstruction and distention). Diagnosis is made by direct laryngoscopy under general anesthesia, using inspection and palpation but not biopsy. Tracheotomy may be necessary to maintain the airway until spontaneous regression occurs, usually about age 6–12 months. Radiation therapy is not given because of the high incidence of subsequent thyroid carcinoma.

Chondroma

These hard, white, submucosal, subglottic masses cause airway obstruction in infants which, like other fixed obstructions, increases with crying. The diagnosis is based on inspection via direct laryngoscopy under general anesthesia. Tracheotomy may be necessary to maintain an adequate airway until differential growth or surgical resection via laryngofissure provides an adequate laryngeal breathing space.

Foreign Bodies

Foreign bodies of the hypopharynx or trachea usually require removal with a bronchoscope and special instruments under general anesthesia. When the foreign body is in the upper trachea, the bronchoscope should be introduced quickly through the larynx and used to push the foreign body into the right main stem bronchus to reestablish the airway. The best treatment is prevention, and this is best done in children by keeping them away from tiny toys or toys that can be separated into tiny parts and by not letting them eat nuts or hard candies until their molar teeth have appeared.

MALIGNANT TUMORS OF THE LARYNX, HYPOPHARYNX, & TRACHEA

Malignant tumors of the throat structures are manifested by hoarseness, pain, and, in later stages, obstruction of the airway. Ninety-five percent of carcinomas of the larynx are squamous cell. The diagnosis is made by means of indirect laryngoscopy, direct laryngoscopy, and palpation of the neck to determine the extent of the lesion, plus biopsy of the lesion via direct laryngoscopy for microscopic diagnosis. *Note:* Squamous cell carcinoma should be suspected in any patient with hoarseness that lasts for over 2 weeks. Evaluation of these patients includes general physical examination, routine laboratory studies of blood and urine, ECG, and evaluation of other major systems. A chest x-ray is necessary to rule out metastasis to the lung. Early diagnosis permits conservation of the voice with removal of the tumor by partial laryngectomy.

Radiation treatment with 4500 rads over a 5-week period and supraglottic laryngectomy 3–4 weeks later (sparing the vocal cords and hence the voice) is feasible for tumors in the upper larynx and hypopharynx (1) if they are in the vallecula, epiglottis, false cord, or piriform sinus; (2) if they do not reach more than 5 mm above the vallecula, do not involve the true cord, and do not extend within 1 cm of the apex of the piriform sinus and 1 cm of the apex of the inter-arytenoid notch; and (3) if they stop 5 mm above the anterior commissure. If they extend lower than this, treatment is with full-course radiation therapy (6500 rads over 6–7 weeks).

If a tumor persists or recurs and the patient's general condition permits, treatment is by total laryngectomy and radical neck dissection under the following circumstances: (1) if the tumor does not extend more than 5 mm up the base of the tongue, into the posterior pharyngeal wall, or below the upper edge of the cricopharyngeus muscle; and (2) if there is no evidence of distant metastases.

Carcinoma limited to the true vocal cord is treated by full-course radiation therapy (6000–6500 rads over 6–7 weeks), with vertical hemilaryngectomy or laryngectomy and radical neck dissection being reserved for persistence or recurrence.

Radiation therapy plus surgery is indicated for the following: (1) fixation of a vocal cord by tumor; (2) transglottic (false and true cord) lesions; (3) subglottic lesions (ie, those that extend more than 1 cm below the free edge of the cord); and (4) large lesions involving the piriform sinus. The dosage is 5500 rads in 6 weeks. Laryngectomy and radical neck dissection are done 4–6 weeks later.

Dedo HH: Supraglottic laryngectomy indications and techniques. Laryngoscope 78:1183, 1968.

LARYNGEAL PARALYSIS

Vocal cord paralysis can occur as a result of surgical or external trauma; malignancy in the base of the skull, neck, or chest; or infection. In 30% of cases, the cause is not known. Work-up should include esophagography and roentgenograms of the chest and the base of the skull to check for malignancy if the cause is uncertain.

If the vocal cord is paralyzed as a result of malignancy or operation, immediate Teflon injection may be performed under topical anesthesia to move the paralyzed cord to the midline. This will improve the voice and minimize or stop aspiration during swallowing. If the cause is not clear, Teflon injection to improve the voice or swallowing should be deferred for 6 months because function may return spontaneously.

STENOSIS OF THE LARYNX & TRACHEA

Stenosis of the larynx and trachea is usually due to infection, external trauma such as a blow to the neck, or internal trauma from balloon cuffs of the tracheostomy tubes. If there has been severe trauma to the neck, the possibility that the larynx has been fractured or that the trachea has been transected should be considered even though the skin remains intact. The airway obstruction from such an injury may not become apparent until 3–4 days after the trauma. Suspicion that such a severe injury has occurred is heightened if there is hoarseness, hemoptysis, significant soreness in the anterior neck, or any suggestion of airway obstruction. When airway obstruction is abrupt and severe, an endotracheal tube should be placed and the trachea and larynx explored through an anterior neck incision. If the trachea has been transected, it should be anastomosed with interrupted 3–0 Tefdek sutures. Fracture of the thyroid cartilage should be reduced and the segments fixed with 2–0 chromic gut sutures. If the mucosa of the interior of the larynx has been lacerated, a laryngofissure should be done and the

lacerations closed with interrupted 4–0 plain gut sutures. If the airway is not so severely occluded that it requires a tracheostomy, laryngeal edema and infection should be treated with systemic corticosteroids and antibiotics. Follow-up examination by indirect laryngoscopy after 24–72 hours should then permit more precise evaluation of the extent of the injuries in the larynx.

Laryngeal Stenosis

Stenosis of the larynx requires repair via a laryngofissure using tantalum keel or skin graft and stent or mucosal advancement flaps.

Dedo HH, Sooy FA: Surgical repair of late glottic stenosis. Ann Otol Rhin Laryng 77:435, 1968.

Tracheal Stenosis

Internal trauma to the trachea can occur from endotracheal tubes; removal of large windows to insert tracheostomy tubes; and overinflation of balloon cuffs on endotracheal and tracheostomy tubes. Treatment is by dilatation for up to 6 dilatations. Stenoses such as those caused by balloon cuffs can occasionally be successfully treated with prolonged stenting or a skin graft plus stenting, but often require segmental resection of the trachea with (1) release of the superior attachments of the larynx to permit it to drop downward and (2) upward mobilization of the mediastinal trachea to permit primary anastomosis of the tracheal stumps.

Dedo HH, Fishman NH: Laryngeal release and sleeve resection for tracheal stenosis. Ann Otol Rhin Laryng 78:285, 1969.

• • •

General References

Ballenger JJ (editor): *Diseases of the Nose, Throat and Ear,* 11th ed. Lea & Febiger, 1969.

Block GE (editor): Symposium on head and neck surgery. S Clin North America 53:1–276, 1973.

DeWeese DD, Saunders WH: *Textbook of Otolaryngology,* 3rd ed. Mosby, 1968.

Gaisford JC: Reconstruction of head and neck deformities. S Clin North America 47:295–322, 1967.

Lore JM Jr: *An Atlas of Head and Neck Surgery.* Saunders, 1962.

Maccomb WS, Fletcher GH: *Cancer of the Head and Neck.* Williams & Wilkins, 1967.

Ryan RE & others: *Synopsis of Ear, Nose and Throat Diseases,* 3rd ed. Mosby, 1970.

Shambaugh GE Jr: *Surgery of the Ear,* 2nd ed. Saunders, 1967.

43...

Ophthalmology

Daniel G. Vaughan, MD

OCULAR EMERGENCIES

It is not necessary to refer every patient with an eye disease to an ophthalmologist for treatment. In general, sties, bacterial conjunctivitis, superficial trauma to the lids, corneas, and conjunctivas, and superficial corneal foreign bodies can be treated just as effectively by the surgeon or family physician as by the ophthalmologist. More serious eye disease such as the following should be referred as soon as possible for specialized care: iritis, acute glaucoma, retinal detachment, strabismus, contusion of the globe, and severe corneal trauma or infection.

In the management of acute ocular disorders it is most important to establish a definitive diagnosis before prescribing treatment. The maxim, "All red eyes are not pink-eye," is a useful one; and the physician must be alert for the more serious iritis, keratitis, or glaucoma (Table 43–1). The common practice of prescribing "shotgun" topical antibiotic combinations containing corticosteroids is to be discouraged, prin-cipally because of the inherent danger of indiscreet steroid treatment.

This chapter is an attempt to summarize the basic principles and technics of diagnosis and management of common ocular problems, with special emphasis on ocular emergencies, particularly those caused by trauma.

Ocular emergencies may be classified as true emergencies and urgent cases. A true emergency is defined as one in which a few hours' delay in treatment can lead to permanent ocular damage or extreme discomfort to the patient. An urgent case is one in which treatment should be started as soon as possible but in which a delay of a few days can be tolerated.

FOREIGN BODIES

If a patient complains of "something in my eye" and gives a consistent history, he usually has a foreign body even though it may not be readily visible. Almost

TABLE 43–1. Differential diagnosis of common causes of inflamed eye.

	Acute Conjunctivitis	Acute Iritis*	Acute Glaucoma†	Corneal Trauma or Infection
Incidence	Extremely common	Common	Uncommon	Common
Discharge	Moderate to copious	None	None	Watery or purulent
Vision	No effect on vision	Slightly blurred	Markedly blurred	Usually blurred
Pain	None	Moderate	Severe	Moderate to severe
Conjunctival injection	Diffuse; more toward fornices	Mainly circum-corneal	Diffuse	Diffuse
Cornea	Clear	Usually clear	Steamy	Change in clarity related to cause
Pupil size	Normal	Small	Moderately di-lated and fixed	Normal
Pupillary light response	Normal	Poor	None	Normal
Intraocular pressure	Normal	Normal	Elevated	Normal
Smear	Causative organisms	No organisms	No organisms	Organisms found only in corneal ulcers due to in-fection

*Acute anterior uveitis.
†Angle-closure glaucoma.

all foreign bodies, however, can be seen under oblique illumination with the aid of a hand flashlight and loupe.

Note the time, place, and other circumstances of the accident. Test visual acuity before treatment is instituted as a basis for comparison in the event of complications.

Conjunctival Foreign Body

A foreign body of the upper tarsal conjunctiva is suggested by pain and blepharospasm of sudden onset in the presence of a clear cornea. After instilling a local anesthetic, evert the lid by grasping the lashes gently and exerting pressure on the midportion of the outer surface of the upper lid with an applicator. If a foreign body is present, it can be easily removed by passing a sterile wet cotton applicator across the conjunctival surface.

Corneal Foreign Body

When a corneal foreign body is suspected but is not apparent on simple inspection, instill *sterile* sodium fluorescein into the conjunctival sac and examine the cornea with the aid of a magnifying device and strong illumination. The foreign body may then be removed with a sterile wet cotton applicator. An antibiotic should be instilled, eg, polymyxin B-bacitracin (Polysporin) ointment. It is not necessary to patch the eye, but the patient must be examined in 24 hours for secondary infection of the crater. If the nonspecialist cannot remove the corneal foreign body in this manner, it should be removed by an ophthalmologist. If there is no infection, a layer of corneal epithelial cells will line the crater within 24 hours. It should be emphasized that the intact corneal epithelium forms an effective barrier to infection. Once the corneal epithelium is disturbed, the cornea becomes extremely susceptible to infection.

Early infection is manifested by a white necrotic area around the crater and a small amount of gray exudate. These patients should be referred immediately to an ophthalmologist.

Untreated corneal infection may lead to severe corneal ulceration, panophthalmitis, and loss of the eye.

Intraocular Foreign Bodies

Foreign bodies which have become lodged within the eye should be identified and localized as soon as possible. They usually cause extensive damage to the eye upon entry, and the degree of ocular injury is increased by leaving the foreign body in place.

In unusual cases, a metallic foreign body can enter the eye, cause minimal initial damage, and be overlooked by the physician. A patient using a hammer and chisel may be struck by a small particle of either instrument which enters his eye at high speed and with minimal symptoms. Complications arising weeks to years later may lead to loss of the eye. The important diagnostic points are to obtain a history of pounding "steel on steel" and to order an x-ray. The anterior

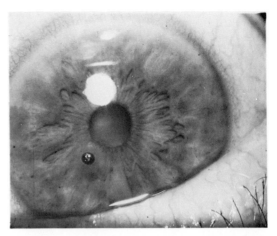

FIG 43–1. Metallic corneal foreign body. (Courtesy of A. Rosenberg.)

portion of the eye, including the cornea, iris, lens, and sclera, should be inspected with a loupe or slit lamp in an attempt to localize the entry wound. Direct ophthalmoscopic visualization of an intraocular foreign body may be possible. An orbital x-ray must be taken to verify the presence of a radiopaque foreign body.

An intraocular foreign body should be removed as soon as possible, preferably through the wound of entry. In the case of a foreign body with magnetic properties, the sterilized tip of a magnet held in the wound of entry can result in a quick and dramatic removal of the foreign body.

TRAUMATIC CATARACT

Traumatic cataract (Fig 43–2) is most commonly due to a metallic intraocular foreign body striking the lens. BB shot is a frequent cause; less frequent causes include arrows, rocks, overexposure to heat ("glass-blower's cataract"), x-rays, and radioactive materials. Most traumatic cataracts are preventable. In industry, the best safety measure is a good pair of safety goggles.

The lens becomes white soon after the entry of the foreign body since the interruption of the lens capsule allows aqueous and sometimes vitreous to penetrate into the lens structure. The patient is often an industrial worker who gives a history of striking steel upon steel. A minute fragment of a steel hammer, for example, may pass through the cornea and lens at high speed and lodge in the vitreous, where it can usually be seen with the ophthalmoscope (Fig 43–3).

The patient complains immediately of blurred vision. The eye becomes red, the lens opaque, and there may be intraocular hemorrhage. If aqueous or vitreous escapes from the eye, the eye becomes extremely soft. Complications include infection, uveitis, retinal detachment, and glaucoma.

The cataractous lens should be removed after the inflammation subsides and it is certain that no further absorption of lens material is taking place. In people

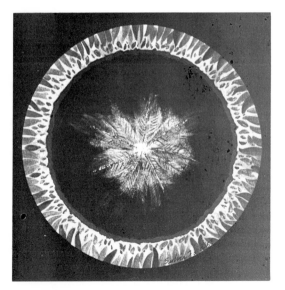

FIG 43–2. Traumatic "star-shaped" cataract in the posterior lens. This is usually due to ocular contusion and is only detectable through a well-dilated pupil. (From Cordes F: *Cataract Types,* 3rd ed. American Academy of Ophthalmology and Otolaryngology, 1954.)

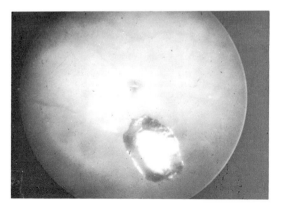

FIG 43–3. Ophthalmoscopic view of intraocular metallic (iron) foreign body in vitreous.

under the age of 25 or 30, the lens material in a traumatic cataract will often absorb almost completely over a period of months without surgery. A thin membrane may remain, in which case discission (needling) may be necessary to improve vision.

The lens material may clog the anterior chamber angle, interfering with aqueous outflow and causing glaucoma. If glaucoma occurs and cannot be controlled medically, the lens must be removed without delay. Most eye surgeons are now using a combination of irrigation and aspiration for traumatic cataract in younger people.

LACERATIONS

Note: Tetanus prophylaxis is indicated whenever penetrating eye or lid injury occurs.

Lacerations are usually caused by sharp objects (knives, scissors, a projecting portion of the dashboard of an automobile, etc). Such injuries are treated in different ways depending upon whether there is prolapse of tissue.

Lacerations Without Prolapse of Tissue

If the eyeball has been penetrated anteriorly without gross evidence of prolapse of intraocular contents, and if the wound is clean and grossly free from contamination, it can usually be repaired by direct interrupted sutures of fine silk or catgut.

Lacerations With Prolapse

If only a small portion of the iris prolapses through the wound, it should be grasped with a forceps and excised at the level of the wound lip. If uveal tissue has otherwise been injured, the possibility of sympathetic ophthalmia must be kept in mind during the period of recovery.

If the wound has been extensive and loss of contents has been great enough that the prognosis for useful function is hopeless, evisceration or enucleation is indicated as the primary surgical procedure.

Lacerations of the Lids

Many lacerations of the lids do not involve the margins and may be sutured in the same way as other lacerations of the skin (Fig 43–4). If the margin of the eyelid is involved, special technics are required to prevent notching of the lid margin.

Rarely, extreme edema of the tissues prevents apposition of the wound for primary closure and the repair must be delayed (secondary repair) until the edema has subsided. Local debridement and irrigation, with use of antibiotics, should be carried out until it is possible to approximate the edges of the wound.

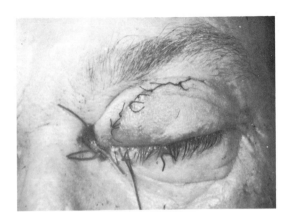

FIG 43–4. Complete laceration of upper lid and upper and lower canaliculi. Large sutures used in repair of severed canaliculi and medial canthal tendon.

Lacerations of the lids near the inner canthus frequently involve the canaliculi. If these are not repaired, permanent strictures with epiphora will result. Small polyethylene tubes are usually placed in the canaliculi at the time of repair and left in place until healing occurs.

Canaliculus repair should be performed immediately since later repair is much more difficult.

NONPENETRATING INJURIES OF THE EYEBALL

Corneal Abrasions

Abrasions of the cornea do not require surgical treatment. The wound should be cleansed of imbedded foreign material. In order to facilitate the examination, the pain associated with abrasions of the cornea can be relieved by instillation of a local anesthetic such as 0.5% tetracaine (Pontocaine) solution, but routine instillation of a local anesthetic by the patient must not be permitted since it may delay the diagnosis of complications and is conducive to further injury. Antibiotic ointment, eg, polymyxin B-bacitracin (Polysporin), helps prevent bacterial infection. An eye bandage applied with firm pressure lessens discomfort and promotes healing by preventing movement of the lids over the involved area. The dressing should be changed daily and the wound inspected for evidence of infection or ulcer formation.

Corneal abrasions cause severe pain, and if not treated properly they may lead to recurrent corneal erosion. They rarely become infected.

Contusions

Contusions of the eyeball and its surrounding tissues are commonly produced by traumatic contact with a blunt object. The results of such injury are variable and are often not obvious upon superficial examination. Careful study and adequate follow-up are indicated. The possible results of contusion injury are hemorrhage and swelling of the eyelids (ecchymosis, "black eye"), subconjunctival hemorrhages, edema or rupture of the cornea, hemorrhage into the anterior chamber (hyphema), rupture of the root of the iris (iridodialysis), traumatic paralysis of the pupil (mydriasis), paralysis or spasm of the muscles of accommodation, traumatic cataract, dislocation of the lens (subluxation and luxation), vitreous hemorrhage, retinal hemorrhage and retinal edema (most common in the macular area, called commotio retinae, or Berlin's traumatic edema), detachment of the retina, rupture of the choroid posteriorly, and optic nerve injury.

Many of these injuries cannot be seen on casual external observation. Some, such as cataract, may not develop for many days or weeks following the injury.

Except for those involving rupture of the eyeball itself (see below), most of the immediate effects of contusion of the eye do not require immediate definitive treatment. However, any injury severe enough to cause intraocular hemorrhage involves the danger of secondary hemorrhage from the broken vessel, which may cause intractable glaucoma and loss of the eye.

Rupture of the Eyeball

Rupture of the eyeball may be direct, at the site of injury, or may occur indirectly as a result of sudden increase in intraocular pressure, causing the wall of the eyeball to tear at one of the weaker points. Common sites of rupture are the limbus and the area around the optic nerve. Anterior ruptures can be repaired surgically by interrupted sutures of fine silk if the intraocular contents have not become deranged in a manner that will prohibit useful function of the eye. If this is the case, evisceration or enucleation is indicated. If either of these procedures is required, implantation of a plastic sphere is useful as a space-filler and to aid in movement of an artificial eye.

CHEMICAL CONJUNCTIVITIS & KERATITIS

Chemical burns are best treated by thorough irrigation of the eyes with saline solution or water immediately after exposure. It is wise not to try to neutralize an acid or alkali by using its chemical counterpart, as the heat generated by the reaction may cause further damage. If the chemical irritant is an alkali, the irrigation should be continued longer since alkalies are not precipitated by the proteins of the eye, as acids are, but tend to linger in the tissues, producing further damage long after exposure. A local anesthetic solution is instilled before the irrigation in order to relieve pain. The pupil should be dilated with sterile 5% homatropine or 0.2% scopolamine solution to prevent synechia formation.

Corticosteroid ointment is placed in the affected eye often enough to relieve pain and irritation. The frequency of instillation depends upon the severity of the burn. The patient must be watched carefully for such complications as symblepharon, corneal scarring, closure of the puncta, and secondary infection.

ULTRAVIOLET KERATITIS
(Actinic Keratitis)

Ultraviolet burns of the cornea are usually caused by exposure to a welding arc or to the sun when skiing ("snow blindness"). There are no immediate symptoms, but about 12 hours later the patient complains of agonizing pain and severe photophobia. Slit lamp examination after instillation of sterile fluorescein shows diffuse punctate staining of both corneas in the exposed areas.

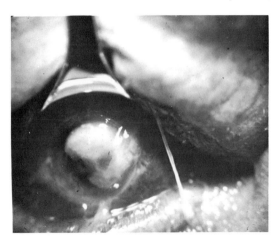

FIG 43–5. Pseudomonas corneal ulcer of right eye. Evisceration was done.

Treatment consists of local corticosteroid therapy, systemic analgesics, and sedatives as indicated. All patients recover within 24–48 hours without complications.

ORBITAL INJURY

There are many types of injury to the bony orbit. Only blowout fracture will be considered here.

Blowout Fracture
Isolated orbital floor or "blowout" fracture, without concurrent orbital rim fracture, usually follows blunt injury to the eye. Orbital contents herniate into the maxillary sinus, and the inferior rectus or inferior oblique muscle may become incarcerated at the fracture site.

Signs and symptoms are pain and nausea at the time of injury and diplopia on looking up or down. Diplopia may occur immediately or within a few days. Enophthalmos may not be present until the orbital reaction clears. The fracture site is best demonstrated by antral roof deformation on Waters' view x-rays or laminograms. There is limited movement of the eye even with forced ductions.

If the fracture is large or the muscle imbalance is great, prompt surgical reduction is imperative. If the vertical imbalance is small, surgery can be delayed a few days or weeks as long as steady improvement is noted. The orbital floor fracture is most commonly repaired using the Caldwell-Luc approach.

INFECTIONS OF THE EYE

1. BACTERIAL CORNEAL ULCER

Corneal ulcers constitute a medical emergency. The typical gray, necrotic corneal ulcer is preceded by trauma, usually a corneal foreign body. The eye is red with lacrimation and conjunctival discharge, and the patient complains of blurred vision, pain, and photophobia.

Prompt treatment is essential to prevent complications. Otherwise, visual impairment may occur as a result of corneal scarring or intraocular infection.

Corneal ulcers may result from many causes including bacterial, viral, fungal, and allergic. Only the most serious types will be discussed here.

Pneumococcal ("Acute Serpiginous") Ulcer
Diplococcus pneumoniae is the commonest bacterial cause of corneal ulcer. The early ulcer is gray and fairly well circumscribed.

Since the pneumococcus is sensitive to both sulfonamides and antibiotics, local therapy is usually effective. If untreated, the cornea may become perforated. Concurrent dacryocystitis, if present, should also be treated.

Pseudomonas Ulcer
A less common but much more virulent cause of corneal ulcer is *Pseudomonas aeruginosa* (Fig 43–5). The ulceration characteristically starts in a traumatized area and spreads rapidly, frequently causing perforation of the cornea and loss of the eye within 48 hours. *Ps aeruginosa* usually produces a pathognomonic bluish-green pigment.

Early diagnosis and vigorous treatment with polymyxin and gentamicin locally are essential if the eye is to be saved.

2. HERPES SIMPLEX KERATITIS

Corneal ulceration caused by herpes simplex virus is more common than any type of bacterial corneal ulcer. It is almost always unilateral, and may affect any age group of either sex. It is often preceded by trauma, upper respiratory tract infection with fever, and facial "cold sores."

The commonest finding is of one or more dendritic ulcers (superficial branching gray areas) on the corneal surface (Fig 21–6). These are composed of clear vesicles in the corneal epithelium; when the vesicles rupture, the area stains green with fluorescein. Although the dendritic figure is its most characteristic

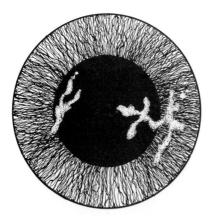

FIG 43—6. Herpes simplex keratitis with dendritic figures.

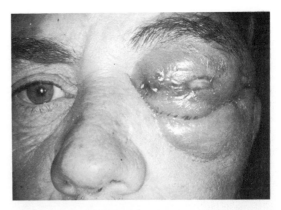

FIG 43—7. Orbital cellulitis. Abscess draining through upper eyelid.

manifestation, herpes simplex keratitis may appear in a number of other configurations.

Treatment consists of mechanical removal of the virus-containing corneal epithelium without disturbing Bowman's membrane or the corneal stroma. This is best done by an ophthalmologist.

Frequent instillation of idoxuridine drops is used by many ophthalmologists in preference to removing the corneal epithelium.

3. ACUTE IRITIS
(Nongranulomatous Uveitis, Endogenous)

Most cases of nongranulomatous uveitis are apparently of spontaneous onset, but there is a fairly close correlation with rheumatoid spondylitis. The iris and ciliary body are primarily affected, but occasional foci are found in the choroid. Exacerbations parallel the rheumatic process.

The onset is acute, with marked pain, redness, photophobia, and blurred vision. A circumcorneal flush, caused by dilated limbal blood vessels, is present. Fine white keratic precipitates (KPs) on the posterior surface of the cornea can be seen with the slit lamp or with a loupe. The pupil is small, and there may be a collection of fibrin with cells in the anterior chamber. If posterior synechias are present, the pupil will be irregular and the light reflex will be absent.

Local corticosteroid therapy tends to shorten the course. Warm compresses will decrease pain. Atropine, 2%, 2 drops in the affected eye, will prevent posterior synechia formation and alleviate photophobia. The frequency of instillation will depend upon the severity of the symptoms and may vary from once a day to several times a day. Recurrences are common, but the prognosis is good.

4. ORBITAL CELLULITIS

Orbital cellulitis is manifested by an abrupt onset of swelling and redness of the lids, often accompanied by proptosis (Fig 43—7). Fever is common. It is usually caused by a pyogenic organism. Immediate treatment with systemic antibiotics is indicated to prevent brain abscess or rapid increase in the orbital pressure causing subsequent embarrassment of the blood supply to the eye. The response to antibiotics is usually excellent.

DIPLOPIA

Double vision is due to muscle imbalance or to paralysis of an extraocular muscle as a result of inflammation, hemorrhage, trauma, tumefaction, or infection of the third, fourth, or sixth nerves. The sixth nerve is most commonly affected.

ANGLE-CLOSURE (ACUTE) GLAUCOMA

Acute glaucoma can occur only with the closure of a preexisting narrow anterior chamber angle. If the pupil dilates spontaneously or is dilated with a mydriatic or cycloplegic, the angle will close and an attack of acute glaucoma is precipitated; for this reason, it is a wise precaution to examine the anterior chamber angle before instilling these drugs (Fig 43—8). About 1% of people over age 35 have narrow anterior chamber angles, but many of these never develop acute glaucoma.

A quiet eye with a narrow anterior chamber angle may convert spontaneously to angle-closure glaucoma. The process can be precipitated by anything that will

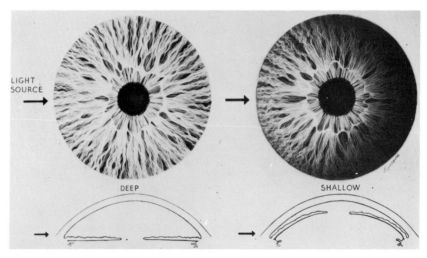

FIG 43–8. Estimation of depth of the anterior chamber by oblique illumination (diagram). (Courtesy of R. Shaffer.)

dilate the pupil, eg, indiscriminate use of mydriatics or cycloplegics by the patient or the physician. The cycloplegic can be administered in the form of eyedrops or systemically, eg, by the anesthetist ordering scopolamine or atropine prior to a general surgical procedure. Increased circulating epinephrine in times of stress can also dilate the pupil and cause acute glaucoma. Sitting in a darkened movie theater can have the same effect.

It should be emphasized that about 95% of patients with glaucoma have the open angle (chronic) type and are in no danger of converting to angle-closure glaucoma. This is particularly important to understand when doing a general surgical procedure on a patient with open angle glaucoma. It is quite safe to give them scopolamine, atropine, or other anticholinergic drugs as a part of their premedication. Acute glaucoma is usually precipitated by these drugs in patients with narrow anterior chamber angles without previous glaucoma history.

Patients with acute glaucoma seek treatment immediately because of extreme pain and blurring of vision. The eye is red, the cornea is steamy, and the pupil is moderately dilated and does not react to light. Intraocular pressure is elevated.

Acute glaucoma must be differentiated from conjunctivitis and acute iritis.

Peripheral iridectomy within 12–48 hours after onset of symptoms will usually result in a permanent cure. Untreated acute glaucoma results in complete and permanent blindness within 2–5 days after onset of symptoms. Before surgery, the intraocular pressure must be lowered by means of miotics instilled locally and osmotic agents and carbonic anhydrase inhibitors administered systemically.

OCCLUSION OF THE CENTRAL RETINAL ARTERY

This uncommon unilateral disorder (the ocular equivalent of coronary thrombosis) occurs only in older people. Occlusion may be the result of thrombin formation on a preexisting plaque or may be due to subintimal hemorrhage with resultant displacement of the plaque. Spasm of the artery is often a complicating factor. Emboli may occur. There is a sudden, painless, complete loss of vision in the affected eye. Ophthalmoscopic examination soon after onset reveals segmentation of the blood in the veins and arterioles as a

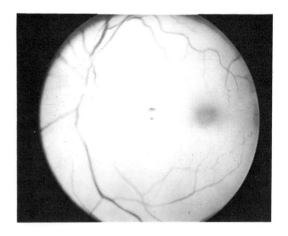

FIG 43–9. Twenty-four hours after closure of the central retinal artery, left eye. The disk is pale; the macula is edematous and ischemic. The fovea appears as a cherry-red spot because of its choroidal blood supply showing through.

result of the absence of retinal blood flow. The disk is pale, and there is marked retinal edema in the posterior pole associated with a cherry-red spot in the macula (Fig 43–9). If the occlusion is complete, total light perception is permanently lost and the pupil will not react directly to light (although the consensual pupillary light reflex is normal).

If the patient is seen within 30–60 minutes after onset, an effort should be made to restore blood flow through the obstructed artery by vigorous massage of the eyeball or paracentesis of the anterior chamber followed by systemic administration of a rapid-acting vasodilator, eg, tolazoline (Priscoline), 75 mg IV.

Because the retina can survive hypoxia longer than brain tissue, the prognosis is not hopeless if treatment is instituted promptly. If treatment is delayed for over 30–60 minutes, the visual prognosis is all but hopeless and the value of any type of treatment is questionable.

RETINAL DETACHMENT

Essentials of Diagnosis

- Blurred vision in one eye becoming progressively worse. ("A curtain came down over my eye.")
- No pain or redness.
- Visible detachment ophthalmoscopically.

General Considerations

Detachment of the retina is usually spontaneous but may be secondary to trauma. Spontaneous detachment occurs most frequently in persons over 50 years old. Predisposing causes such as aphakia and myopia are commonly present.

Clinical Findings

As soon as the retina is torn, a transudate from the choroidal vessels, mixed with vitreous, combines with abnormal vitreous traction on the retina and the force of gravity to strip the retina from the choroid. The superior temporal area is the most common site of detachment. The area of detachment rapidly increases, causing corresponding progressive visual loss (Fig 43–10). Central vision remains intact until the macula becomes detached.

On ophthalmoscopic examination, the retina is seen hanging in the vitreous like a gray cloud. One or more retinal tears, usually crescent-shaped and red or orange, are always present and can be seen by an experienced examiner.

Differential Diagnosis

Sudden partial loss of vision in one eye may also be due to vitreous hemorrhage or thrombosis of the central retinal vein or one of its branches.

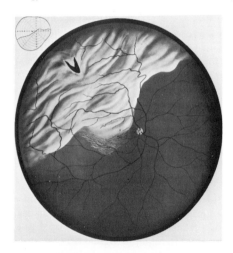

FIG 43–10. Retinal detachment and retinal tear 6 days after onset. (From Arruga: *Detachment of the Retina.* Salvat, 1936.)

Treatment

All cases of retinal detachment should be referred immediately to an ophthalmologist. If the patient must be transported a long distance, his head should be positioned so that the detached portion of the retina will recede with the aid of gravity. For example, a patient with a superior temporal retinal detachment in the right eye should lie on his back with his head turned to the right. Position is less important for a short trip.

Retinal detachment is a true emergency if the macula is threatened. If the macula is detached, permanent loss of central vision usually occurs even though the retina is eventually successfully reattached by surgery.

Treatment consists of drainage of the subretinal fluid and closure of the retinal tears by diathermy or scleral buckling (or both). This produces an inflammatory reaction which causes the retina to adhere to the choroid. Photocoagulation is of value in a limited number of cases of minimal detachment. It consists of focusing a strong light from various sources through the pupil to create an artificial inflammation between the choroid and the retina.

The main use of the photocoagulator and laser is in the prevention of detachment by sealing small retinal tears before detachment occurs.

Cryosurgery is also being used effectively in the treatment of retinal detachment. A supercooled probe is applied to the sclera to cause a chorioretinal scar with minimal scleral damage. This decreased scleral damage (as compared with diathermy) makes the operation less hazardous and, because scar formation is minimal, greatly facilitates reoperation. Cryosurgery may eventually replace diathermy completely.

Prognosis

About 85% of uncomplicated cases can be cured with one operation; an additional 10% will need repeated operations; the remainder never reattach. The prognosis is worse if the macula is detached, if there are many vitreous strands, or if the detachment is of long duration. Without treatment, retinal detachment almost always becomes total in 1–6 months. Spontaneous detachments are ultimately bilateral in 20–25% of cases.

VITREOUS HEMORRHAGE

Hemorrhage into the vitreous is an uncommon but serious disorder. It is usually due to traumatic rupture of a retinal vessel but may be related to diabetes mellitus, hypertension, perivasculitis, or retinal detachment. One or both eyes may be affected, depending upon the cause.

There is a sudden and complete loss of vision in the affected eye. The fundus reflection is absent, but the anterior chamber, cornea, and lens are clear.

The visual prognosis is guarded no matter what the cause, since the blood often remains in the vitreous for months. If the vitreous clears after a long period, the retina will usually have been damaged by prolonged intimate contact with blood elements. *Note:* These patients should be observed periodically, as the hemorrhage occasionally clears dramatically in a few days or weeks to reveal a retinal detachment. If this happens, vision may be restored by surgical reattachment of the retina.

HORDEOLUM

Hordeolum is a common staphylococcal abscess which is characterized by a localized red, swollen, acutely tender area on the upper or lower lid. Internal hordeolum is a meibomian gland abscess which points to the skin or to the conjunctival side of the lid; external hordeolum or sty (infection of the glands of Moll or Zeis) is smaller and on the margin.

The primary symptom is pain. The severity of the pain is directly related to the amount of swelling.

Warm compresses are helpful. Incision is indicated if resolution does not begin within 48 hours. An antibiotic or sulfonamide instilled into the conjunctival sac every 3 hours is beneficial during the acute stage. Without treatment, internal hordeolum may lead to generalized cellulitis of the lid.

CHALAZION

Chalazion is a common granulomatous inflammation of a meibomian gland characterized by a hard,

nontender swelling on the upper or lower lid. It may be preceded by a sty. The majority point toward the conjunctival side.

If the chalazion is large enough to impress the cornea, vision will be distorted. The conjunctiva in the region of the chalazion is red and elevated.

Treatment consists of excision by an ophthalmologist.

DACRYOCYSTITIS

Dacryocystitis is a common infection of the lacrimal sac. It may be acute or chronic and occurs most often in infants and in persons over 40. It is usually unilateral and is always secondary to obstruction of the nasolacrimal duct.

Adult Dacryocystitis
The cause of obstruction is usually unknown, but a history of trauma to the nose may be obtained. In acute dacryocystitis the usual infectious agent is one of the staphylococci; in the chronic form, *Diplococcus pneumoniae* or, occasionally, *Haemophilus influenzae* is found. Mixed infections do not occur.

Acute dacryocystitis is characterized by pain, swelling, tenderness, and redness in the tear sac area; purulent material may be expressed. In chronic dacryocystitis, tearing and discharge are the principal signs. Mucus or pus may be expressed from the tear sac.

Acute dacryocystitis responds well to antibiotic therapy, but recurrences are common if the obstruction is not surgically removed. The chronic form may be kept latent by using antibiotic eye drops, but relief of the obstruction is the only cure.

Infantile Dacryocystitis
Normally the nasolacrimal ducts open spontaneously during the first month of life. Occasionally, one of the ducts fails to canalize and a secondary pneumococcal dacryocystitis develops. When this happens, forceful massage of the tear sac is indicated, and antibiotic or sulfonamide drops should be instilled in the conjunctival sac 4–5 times daily. If this is not successful after a few weeks, probing of the nasolacrimal duct is indicated regardless of the infant's age.

STRABISMUS

Any child under age 7 with strabismus should be seen without delay to prevent the occurrence of or to treat the beginning of amblyopia. In adults the sudden onset of strabismus usually follows head trauma, intracranial hemorrhage, or brain tumor.

About 5% of children are born with or develop a malfunction of binocular coordination known as strabismus. In descending order of frequency, the eyes may deviate inward (esotropia), outward (exotropia), upward (hypertropia), or downward (hypotropia). The cause is not known, but fusion is lacking in almost all cases. If a child is born with straight eyes but has inherited "weak fusion," he may develop strabismus.

Clinical Findings

Children with frank strabismus first develop diplopia. They soon learn to suppress the image from the deviating eye and the vision in that eye therefore fails to develop. This is the first stage of amblyopia ex anopsia.

Most cases of strabismus are obvious, but if the angle of deviation is small or if the strabismus is intermittent, the diagnosis may be obscure. The best method for detecting strabismus is to direct a light toward each pupil from a distance of 1–2 feet. If the corneal reflection is seen in the center of each pupil, the eyes can be presumed to be straight at that moment.

As a further diagnostic test ("cover test"), cover the right eye with an opaque object ("cover") and instruct the patient to fix his gaze on the examining light with the left eye. If fusion is weak, covering the right eye will disturb the fusion process sufficiently to allow the right eye to deviate, and this can be observed behind the cover. The right eye may swing back into alignment when the cover is removed (phoria). In obvious strabismus, the covered eye will maintain the deviated position after the cover is removed (tropia). Ask the patient to follow the examining light with both eyes to the right, left, up, and down to rule out extraocular muscle paralysis. If there is a history of deviation but it cannot be demonstrated, the patient should be reexamined in 6 months.

Prevention

Amblyopia due to strabismus can be detected by routine visual acuity examination of all preschool children. Visual acuity testing is best done with an illiterate E card close to the fourth birthday by the child's mother, but is often performed in the physician's office as a routine procedure. Treatment by occlusion of the good eye is simple and effective.

The prevention of blindness by these simple diagnostic and treatment procedures is one of the most rewarding experiences in medical practice.

Treatment

The objectives in the treatment of strabismus are (1) good visual acuity in each eye; (2) straight eyes, for cosmetic purposes; and (3) coordinate function of both eyes.

The best time to initiate treatment is around the age of 6 months. If treatment is delayed beyond this time, the child will favor the straight eye and suppress the image in the other eye; this results in failure of visual development (amblyopia ex anopsia) in the deviating eye.

If the child is under 7 years of age and has an amblyopic eye, the amblyopia can be cured by occluding the good eye. At 1 year of age, patching may be successful within 1 week; at 6 years it may take a year to achieve the same result, ie, to equalize the visual acuity in both eyes. Prolonged patching seldom impairs vision in the good eye. Surgery is usually performed after the visual acuity has been equalized.

Prognosis

The prognosis is more favorable for strabismus which has its onset at age 1–4 than for strabismus which is present at birth; better for divergent (outward deviation) than for convergent strabismus; and better for intermittent than for constant strabismus.

OTHER DISEASES OF THE EYE

OCULAR TUMORS

Many tumors of the ocular adnexa can be completely excised if they are diagnosed in an early stage. Malignant intraocular tumors (except of the iris) nearly always require enucleation.

OPTIC NERVE PATHOLOGY

Optic nerve disorders such as optic neuritis, optic atrophy, and papilledema are very serious and may indicate accompanying intracranial or systemic disease. The patient should be examined from a neurologic as well as an ophthalmologic standpoint.

SYMPATHETIC OPHTHALMIA
(Sympathetic Uveitis)

Sympathetic ophthalmia is a rare, severe bilateral granulomatous uveitis. The cause is not known, but the disease may occur at any time from 1 week to many years after a penetrating injury near the ciliary body. The injured (exciting) eye becomes inflamed first and the fellow (sympathizing) eye second. Symptoms and signs include blurred vision with light sensitivity and redness.

The best treatment of sympathetic ophthalmia is prevention by removing the damaged eye. Any severely injured eye (eg, one with perforation of the sclera and ciliary body, with loss of vitreous and retinal damage) should be enucleated within 1 week after the injury.

Every effort should be made to secure the patient's reasoned consent to the operation. In established cases of sympathetic ophthalmia, systemic corticosteroid therapy may be helpful. Without treatment, the disease progresses gradually to bilateral blindness.

CHRONIC GLAUCOMA

Antiglaucoma therapy should be instituted without delay in order to decrease the intraocular pressure and preserve the remaining visual field.

UNILATERAL EXOPHTHALMOS OF RECENT ORIGIN

The most common cause of bilateral exophthalmos is hyperthyroidism, although it may also appear after thyroidectomy. Unilateral exophthalmos may be due to an orbital tumor, cavernous sinus thrombosis, or atrioventricular shunt from the internal carotid artery to the cavernous sinus. These disorders are treatable.

.   .   .

TECHNICS USED IN THE TREATMENT OF OCULAR DISORDERS

Instilling Medications

Place the patient in a chair with his head tilted back, both eyes open, and looking up. Retract the lower lid slightly and instill 2 drops of liquid into the lower cul-de-sac. Have the patient look down while finger contact on the lower lid is maintained for a few seconds. Do not let him squeeze his eye shut.

Ointments are instilled in the same general manner.

Self-Medication

The same technics are used as described above, except that drops should usually be instilled with the patient lying down.

Eye Bandage

Most eye bandages should be applied firmly enough to hold the lid securely against the cornea. An ordinary patch consisting of gauze-covered cotton is usually sufficient. Tape is applied from the cheek to the forehead. If more pressure is desired, use 2 or 3 bandages. The black eye patch is difficult to sterilize and therefore is seldom used in modern medical practice.

Water Compresses

A clean towel or washcloth soaked in warm tap water is applied to the affected eye 2–4 times a day for 10–15 minutes.

Removal of a Superficial Corneal Foreign Body

Record the patient's visual acuity, if possible, and instill sterile local anesthetic drops. With the patient sitting or lying down, an assistant should direct a strong light into the eye so that the rays strike the cornea obliquely. Using either a loupe or a slit lamp, the physician locates the foreign body on the corneal surface. He may remove it with a sterile wet cotton applicator or, if this fails, with a spud, holding the lids apart with the other hand to prevent blinking. An antibacterial ointment (eg, Polysporin) is instilled after the foreign body has been removed. It is preferable not to patch the eye, but the patient must be seen on the following day to make certain healing is under way.

PRECAUTIONS IN THE MANAGEMENT OF OCULAR DISORDERS

Use of Local Anesthetics

Unsupervised self-administration of local anesthetics is dangerous because the patient may further injure an anesthetized eye without knowing it.

Pupillary Dilation

Cycloplegics and mydriatics should be used with caution. Dilating the pupil can precipitate an attack of acute glaucoma if the patient has a narrow anterior chamber angle.

Local Corticosteroid Therapy

Repeated use of local corticosteroids presents several serious hazards: herpes simplex (dendritic) keratitis, fungal overgrowth, open angle glaucoma, and cataract. Furthermore, perforation of the cornea may occur when the corticosteroids are used for herpes simplex keratitis.

Contaminated Eye Medications

Ophthalmic solutions must be prepared with the same degree of care as fluids intended for intravenous administration.

Tetracaine (Pontocaine), proparacaine (Ophthaine, Ophthetic), physostigmine, and fluorescein are most likely to become contaminated. The most dangerous is fluorescein, as this solution is frequently contaminated with *Pseudomonas aeruginosa,* an organism which can rapidly destroy the eye. Sterile fluorescein filter paper strips are now available and are recommended in place of fluorescein solutions.

Plastic dropper bottles are becoming more popular each year. Solutions from these bottles are safe to use in uninjured eyes. Whether in plastic or glass containers, eye solutions should not be used for long periods of time after the bottle is first opened. Two weeks is a reasonable time to use a solution before discarding.

If the eye has been injured accidentally or by surgical trauma, it is of the greatest importance to use sterile medications supplied in sterile, disposable, single use eye-dropper units.

Fungal Overgrowth

Since antibiotics, like corticosteroids, when used over a prolonged period of time in bacterial corneal ulcers, favor the development of secondary fungal corneal infection, the sulfonamides should be used whenever they are adequate for the purpose.

Sensitization

A significant portion of a soluble substance instilled in the eye may pass into the blood stream. This suggests that an antibiotic instilled into the eye can sensitize the patient to that drug and cause a hypersensitivity reaction upon subsequent systemic administration.

•   •   •

General References

Allen JH: *May's Manual of Diseases of the Eye,* 24th ed. Williams & Wilkins, 1968.

Arruga HM: *Ocular Surgery,* 3rd ed. Blakiston-McGraw, 1962. [Translated from the Spanish by Hogan and Chapparo.]

Beard C, Quickert MH: *Anatomy of the Orbit: A Dissection Manual.* Aesculapius, 1969.

Becker B: *Current Concepts in Ophthalmology.* Vol. 3. Mosby, 1972.

Duke-Elder WS: *Diseases of the Eye,* 15th ed. Williams & Wilkins, 1970.

Ellis PP, Smith DL: *Handbook of Ocular Therapeutics and Pharmacology,* 3rd ed. Mosby, 1969.

Havener WH: *Atlas of Cataract Surgery.* Mosby, 1972.

Havener WH: *Ocular Pharmacology,* 2nd ed. Mosby, 1970.

Helveston EM: *Atlas of Strabismus Surgery.* Mosby, 1972.

Hogan MJ, Zimmermann LE: *Ophthalmic Pathology: An Atlas and Textbook,* 2nd ed. Saunders, 1962.

Hughes WF: *Year Book of Ophthalmology, 1972.* Year Book, 1972.

Keeney AH: *Ocular Examination: Basis and Technique.* Mosby, 1970.

King JH, Wadsworth JAC: *An Atlas of Ophthalmic Surgery,* 2nd ed. Lippincott, 1970.

Kolker AE, Hetherington J: *Becker-Shaffer's Diagnosis and Therapy of the Glaucomas,* 3rd ed. Mosby, 1970.

Leopold IH (editor): *Symposium on Ocular Therapy.* Vol 6. Mosby, 1969.

Martin-Doyle JLC: *A Synopsis of Ophthalmology,* 4th ed. Williams & Wilkins, 1971.

May's Manual of the Diseases of the Eye, 24th ed. Williams & Wilkins, 1968.

Moses RA: *Adler's Physiology of the Eye: Clinical Application,* 5th ed. Mosby, 1970.

Newell FW: *Ophthalmology: Principles and Concepts,* 2nd ed. Mosby, 1969.

Scheie HG, Albert DM: *Adler's Textbook of Ophthalmology,* 8th ed. Saunders, 1969.

Trevor-Roper PD: *Lecture Notes on Ophthalmology,* 4th ed. Blackwell, 1971.

Vaughan D, Asbury T, Cook R: *General Ophthalmology,* 6th ed. Lange, 1971.

Walsh FB, Hoyt WF: *Clinical Neuro-ophthalmology,* 3rd ed. Williams & Wilkins, 1969.

44...

Urology

Donald R. Smith, MD, & Emil A. Tanagho, MD

DEVELOPMENT OF THE GENITOURINARY TRACT & ANOMALIES OF DEVELOPMENT

Embryologically, the genital and urinary systems are intimately related. Associated anomalies are commonly encountered.

THE KIDNEYS

The kidneys pass through 3 embryonic phases (Fig 44–1): (1) The **pronephros** is a vestigial structure that disappears completely by the fourth week except

for its primary duct. (2) The primary duct gains connection to the **mesonephros** tubules and becomes the mesonephric duct. While most of the mesonephric tubules degenerate, the mesonephric duct persists; where it bends to open into the cloaca, the ureteral bud develops, starts to grow cranially, and meets the metanephric blastema. (3) This forms the **metanephros**, which is the final phase. During cephalad migration and rotation, the metanephric tissue progressively enlarges, with rapid internal differentiation into small vesicular masses that will later differentiate into uriniferous tubules. Simultaneously, the cephalad end of the ureteral bud expands within the metanephros to form the renal pelvis. Numerous outgrowths from the renal pelvic dilatation develop, branch and rebranch, and finally connect to the differentiating metanephric

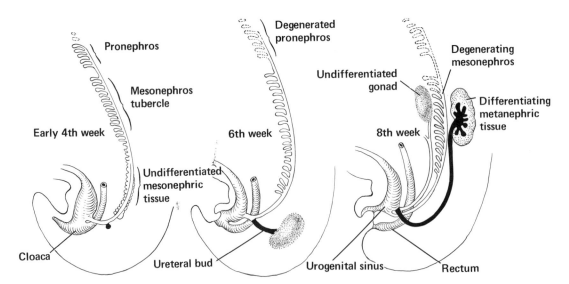

FIG 44–1. Schematic representation of the development of the nephric system. Only a few of the tubules of the pronephros are seen early in the fourth week, while the mesonephric tissue differentiates into mesonephric tubules that progressively join the mesonephric duct. The first sign of the ureteral bud from the mesonephric duct is seen. At 6 weeks, the pronephros has completely degenerated and the mesonephric tubules start to do so. The ureteral bud grows dorsocranially and has met the metanephrogenic cap. At the eighth week there is cranial migration of the differentiating metanephros. The cranial end of the ureteric bud expands and starts to show multiple successive outgrowths.

The illustrations in this chapter are from Smith DR: *General Urology,* 7th ed. Lange, 1972.

vesicular masses, establishing continuity of the secreting and collecting ducts.

Failure of the metanephros to ascend leads to ectopic kidney; failure to rotate during ascent causes a malrotated kidney. Horseshoe kidney results from fusion of the 2 metanephric masses.

Bifurcation of the ureteral bud results in a bifid ureter. Development of an accessory bud leads to a duplicated ureter, commonly meeting the same nephric mass; rarely, each bud has a separate metanephric mass, resulting in supernumerary kidneys. Failure of a ureteral bud to develop results in a solitary kidney and a hemitrigone.

BLADDER & URETHRA

Subdivision of the cloaca (the blind end of the hindgut) into a ventral (urogenital sinus) and a dorsal (rectum) segment is completed during the seventh week and initiates the early differentiation of the urinary bladder and urethra. The urogenital sinus receives the mesonephric duct and gradually absorbs its caudal end so that by the end of the seventh week the ureteral bud and mesonephric duct have independent openings. The former migrates upward and laterally. The latter moves downward and medially, and the structure in between (the trigone) is formed by the absorbed mesodermal tissue, which maintains direct continuity between the 2 tubes (Fig 44–2).

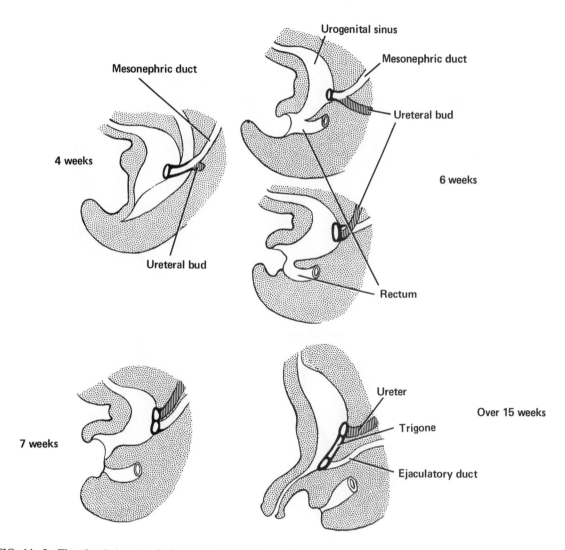

FIG 44–2. The development of the ureteral bud from the mesonephric duct and their relationship to the urogenital sinus. The ureteral bud appears at the fourth week. The mesonephric duct distal to this ureteral bud will be gradually absorbed into the urogenital sinus, resulting in separate endings for the ureter and the mesonephric duct. The mesonephric tissue that is incorporated into the urogenital sinus will expand and form the trigonal tissue.

The fused müllerian ducts also meet the urogenital sinus at Müller's tubercle. The urogenital sinus above Müller's tubercle differentiates to form the bladder and part of the urethra in the male (supramontanal part of the prostatic urethra) or the bladder and the whole urethra in the female. Below it, the urogenital sinus differentiates into the inframontanal part of the prostatic urethra and the membranous urethra in the male or the distal vagina and vaginal vestibule in the female. The rest of the male urethra is formed by fusion of the urethral folds on the ventral surface of the genital tubercle. In the female, the genital folds remain separate and form the labia minora.

Failure of cloacal division results in persistent cloaca. Incomplete division is more frequent and results in rectovesical, rectourethral, or rectovestibular fistulas (usually with imperforate anus or anal atresia). Development of genital primordia in an area more caudal than normal results in complete or incomplete epispadias. A more extensive defect results in vesical exstrophy. Failure of the urethral folds to fuse leads to various grades of hypospadias.

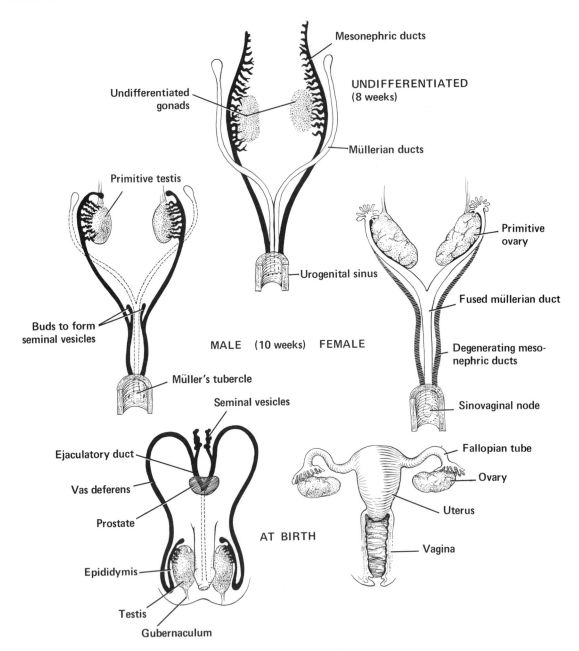

FIG 44–3. Transformation of the undifferentiated genital system into the definitive male and female systems.

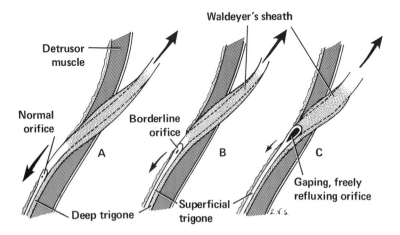

FIG 44–4. Ureterovesical reflux. The length and fixation of the intravesical ureter and the appearance of the ureteral orifice depend upon the muscular development and efficiency of the lower ureter and its trigone. The normal appearance is shown in *A*. Moderate muscular deficiency leads to the appearance shown in *B*. Marked deficiency results in a golf hole distortion of the submucosal ureter as shown in *C*.

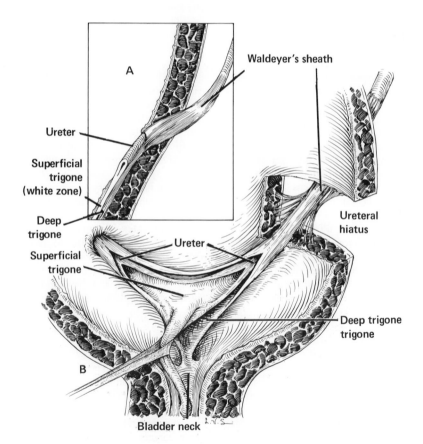

The ureteral muscle extends downward and becomes the superficial trigone.

Waldeyer's sheath extends downward and becomes the deep trigone.

FIG 44–5. Normal ureterotrigonal complex. *A:* Side view of ureterovesical junction. Waldeyer's muscular sheath invests the juxtavesical ureter and continues downward as the deep trigone, which extends to the bladder neck. The ureteral musculature becomes the superficial trigone, which extends to the verumontanum in the male and stops just short of the external meatus in the female. *B:* Waldeyer's sheath is connected by a few fibers to the detrusor muscle in the ureteral hiatus. This muscular sheath, inferior to the ureteral orifices, becomes the deep trigone. The musculature of the ureters continues downward as the superficial trigone. (Adapted from Tanagho EA, Pugh RCB: Brit J Urol 35:151–165, 1963.)

The prostate develops at the end of the 11th week as 5 groups of outgrowths of urethral epithelium both above and below the entrance of the mesonephric duct. These form the 5 lobes of the prostate. The developing glandular element incorporates within it the differentiating mesenchymal cells surrounding that segment of the urogenital sinus. These form the muscular stroma and capsule of the prostate.

THE GONADS

Each embryo is at first morphologically bisexual; the development of one set of sex primordia and the gradual involution of the other are determined by the sex type of the gonad, which starts to be differentiated during the seventh week (Fig 44–3). If the gonad develops into a testis, the germinal epithelium grows into radially arranged, cord-like masses that differentiate later into seminiferous tubules. If it develops into an ovary, it becomes differentiated into a cortex and a medulla; the cortex later differentiates into ovarian follicles containing ova.

The testis remains at the abdominal end of the inguinal canal until the seventh month. It then passes through the inguinal canal to the scrotum, guided by the primary attachment of the gubernaculum. The ovary undergoes internal descent to enter the pelvis.

Lack of complete testicular descent is known as cryptorchidism; descent to an abnormal site is known as testicular ectopia. In the male, the genital duct system develops from the wolffian duct, which differentiates into epididymis, vas deferens, seminal vesicles, and ejaculatory ducts. In the female, the genital duct system develops from the müllerian ducts, which fuse at their caudal ends and differentiate into the fallopian tubes, uterus, and most of the vagina.

The external genitalia start to differentiate by the eighth week. The genital tubercle and the genital swellings develop into the penis and scrotum in the male and the clitoris and labia majora in the female.

With the breakdown of the urogenital membrane in the seventh week, the urogenital sinus achieves a separate opening on the undersurface of the genital tubercle. The expansion of the infratubercular part of the urogenital sinus will form the vaginal vestibule and distal part of the vagina. The 2 folds on the undersurface of the genital tubercle unite in the male to form the penile urethra; in the female, they remain separate to form the labia minora. Their failure to fuse in the male leads to hypospadias, which is usually associated with incomplete formation of the prepuce with a dorsal hood and a ventral penile curvature. It is never proximal to the bulbous urethra, and continence is always preserved. Epispadias is a milder form of bladder exstrophy. Dorsal penile curvature, if extensive, can extend to the bladder neck and is frequently associated with incontinence. A rudimentary penis or a hypertrophied clitoris is seen with pseudohermaphroditism.

·   ·   ·

Allan FD: *Essentials of Human Embryology*. Oxford Univ Press, 1960.

Arey LB: *Developmental Anatomy: A Textbook and Laboratory Manual of Embryology*, 6th ed. Saunders, 1954.

Patten BM: *Human Embryology*, 2nd ed. Blakiston, 1953.

Stephens FD: *Congenital Malformations of the Rectum, Anus and Genitourinary Tracts*. Livingstone, 1963.

APPLIED ANATOMY OF THE GENITOURINARY TRACT: GROSS & MICROSCOPIC

The Kidneys

The kidneys are paired organs lying retroperitoneally in the posterior abdomen and separated from the surrounding renal fascia by perinephric fat. The renal vascular pedicle enters the renal sinus; the vein is anterior to the artery, and both are anterior to the renal pelvis. The renal artery divides in the renal sinus into anterior and posterior branches that undergo further subdivisions with variable extents of distribution. They are end arteries. The venous tributaries anastomose freely and usually drain into one renal vein. Accessory vessels are not uncommon.

The Renal Parenchyma

The renal parenchyma consists of over 1 million functioning units (nephrons) and is divided into a peripheral cortex containing secretory elements and a central medulla containing excretory elements. The nephron starts as Bowman's capsule, which surrounds the glomeruli and leads to a long tubular structure consisting of proximal and distal convoluted tubules with the loop of Henle in between; it ends in a collecting duct that opens at the tip of a papilla into a minor calyx.

The Renal Pelvis & Calyces

The renal pelvis and calyces are within the renal sinus and function as the main collecting reservoir. The pelvis, which is partly extrarenal and partly intrarenal (but could be totally extra- or intrarenal), branches into 3 major calyces that in turn branch into several minor calyces. These calyces are directly related to the renal parenchyma; they receive the tips of the medullary pyramids (the papillae) and act as a receiving cup to the collecting tubules. The pelvicalyceal system is a highly muscular structure; the musculature runs in every direction and is directly continuous between the pelvis and the various calyces, helping to synchronize their contractile activity.

The Ureter

The ureter connects the renal pelvis to the urinary bladder. It is a small, muscularized tube; its muscle fibers lie in an irregular helical arrangement and are meant primarily for peristaltic activity. Ureteral musculature is directly continuous with the renal pelvis cranially and with the vesical trigone distally.

The pelvic and ureteral blood supply is segmental, arising from the renal, spermatic or ovarian, and vesical arteries—with rich subadventitial anastomosis.

The Bladder

The bladder is primarily a reservoir with a mesh-work of muscle bundles that not only change from one plane to the other but also branch and join each other to constitute a synchronized organ. Its musculature is directly continuous with the urethral musculature, and this functions as a urethral sphincteric mechanism in spite of the lack of a true circular sphincter.

The ureters enter the bladder postero-inferiorly through the ureteral hiatus; after a short intravesical submucosal course, they lose their lumen and become continuous with the trigone, which is superimposed on the bladder base though deeply connected to it.

The Urethra

The female urethra is about 4 cm long and is muscular in its proximal four-fifths. This musculature is arranged in an inner longitudinal coat which is continuous with the inner longitudinal fibers of the bladder, and an outer circular coat which is continuous with the outer longitudinal coat of the bladder. These outer circular fibers comprise the sphincteric mechanism. The striated external sphincter surrounds the middle third of the urethra.

In the male, the prostatic urethra is heavily muscular and sphincteric. The membranous urethra is within the urogenital diaphragm and is surrounded by the striated external sphincter. The penile urethra is poorly muscularized and traverses the corpus spongiosum to open at the tip of the glans.

The Prostate

The prostate surrounds the proximal portion of the male urethra; it is a fibromuscular, glandular, cone-shaped structure about 2.5 cm long and weighing about 20 g. It is traversed from base to apex by the urethra and is pierced posterolaterally by the ejaculatory ducts that converge to open at the verumontanum on the floor of the urethra.

The prostatic glandular elements drain through about 12 paired excretory ducts that open into the floor of the urethra above the verumontanum. The prostate is surrounded by a thin capsule, derived from its stroma, which is rich in musculature, and part of the urethral musculature and the sphincteric mechanism. A rich venous plexus surrounds the prostate, especially anteriorly and laterally. Its arterial blood supply is from the inferior vesical, internal pudendal, and middle hemorrhoidal arteries. Its lymphatic drainage is into the hypogastric, sacral, vesical, and external iliac lymph nodes.

The Testis

The testis is a paired organ surrounded by the tunica albuginea and subdivided into numerous lobules by fibrous septa. The extremely convoluted seminiferous tubules gather to open into the rete testis, where they join the efferent duct to drain into the epididymis.

Arterial supply is via the internal spermatic artery; venous drainage is through the pampiniform plexus, which drains into the spermatic veins. The right joins the vena cava and the left joins the renal vein.

The lymphatics drain into the lumbar lymph nodes.

Cussen LJ: The structure of the normal human ureter in infancy and childhood. Invest Urol 5:179–194, 1967.

Hutch JA, Rambo ON Jr: A study of the anatomy of the prostate, prostatic urethra and the urinary sphincter system. J Urol 104:443–453, 1970.

Layton JM: The structure of the kidney from the gross to the molecular. J Urol 90:502–515, 1963.

Osathanondh V, Potter EL: Development of human kidney shown by microdissection. IV. Development of tubular portions of nephrons. V. Development of vascular pattern of glomerulus. Arch Path 82:391–402, 403–411, 1966.

Tanagho EA, Smith DR: The Anatomy and function of the bladder neck. Brit J Urol 28:54–71, 1966.

PHYSIOLOGY OF THE URINARY SYSTEM

The Kidneys

The kidneys maintain and regulate homeostasis of body fluids by the following mechanisms:

A. Glomerular Filtration: This is dependent on glomerular capillary arterial pressure minus plasma colloid osmotic pressure plus capsular resistance. The resultant glomerular filtration pressure (about 35 mm Hg) forces protein-free plasma through the capillary filtering surface into Bowman's capsule. Normally, about 130 ml of plasma are filtered every minute through the extremely rich renal circulation; every drop of plasma recirculates through the kidney and is subjected to the filtration process once every 27 minutes.

B. Tubular Reabsorption: About 99% of the filtered volume will be reabsorbed through the tubules together with all the valuable constituents of the filtrate (chlorides, glucose, sodium, potassium, calcium, and amino acids). Urea, uric acid, phosphates, and sulfates are also reabsorbed to varying degrees. The process of reabsorption is partly passive (by diffusion) and partly active. Reabsorption of water and electrolytes is under control of adrenal, pituitary, and parathyroid hormonal influence.

C. Tubular Secretion: This helps (1) to eliminate and thus maintain plasma levels of certain substances, or (2) to exchange valuable ions from the filtrate for less desirable ions in the plasma (eg, sodium ion from the urine for a hydrogen ion in the plasma). Failure of adequate secretory function leads to the acidosis commonly encountered in chronic renal disease.

The Uretero-pelvicalyceal System

This system is one continuous tubular structure with adequate musculature which is imperceptibly moving from one segment to the other to maintain anatomic continuity and physiologic synchrony at various levels. Waves of contraction starting from the renal pelvis or occasionally from the calyces usually proceed in antegrade (anterograde) fashion toward the urinary bladder. These peristaltic waves occur at a rate of about 5–8 per minute, involve 2–3 cm segments at a time, and usually proceed at the velocity of 3 cm/second. Frequency, amplitude, and velocity are influenced by urine output and flow rate. Ureteral filling is primarily passive; ureteral emptying is primarily active. Ureteral peristaltic activity is essential in order to transport urine across points of resistance (eg, ureterovesical junction) and to prevent retrograde flow.

The Ureterovesical Junction

The ureterovesical junction allows free flow of urine from the ureter to the bladder and at the same time prevents retrograde flow. The continuity and the specific muscular arrangement of the intravesical ureter and the trigone provide a muscularly active valvular mechanism that can efficiently adapt itself to the variable phases of bladder activity during filling and voiding.

Progressive bladder filling leads to firm occlusion of the intravesical ureter against retrograde flow and increased resistance to antegrade urine flow due to trigonal stretching. During voiding, trigonal contraction completely seals the intravesical ureter against any antegrade flow of urine and definitely against any retrograde flow.

The Urinary Bladder

The urinary bladder functions primarily as a reservoir that can accommodate variable volumes without increasing its intraluminal pressure. When the bladder reaches full capacity voluntarily, the detrusor muscle contracts uniformly and maintains its contraction until the bladder is completely empty. Funneling of the bladder outlet with progressive downward movement of the dome ensures complete emptying.

The vesical sphincteric mechanism is primarily a smooth muscle sphincter in the male prostatic urethra and in the proximal four-fifths of the female urethra. There is no purely circular sphincteric entity, but there are abundant circularly oriented muscle fibers which are directly continuous with the outer coat of the detrusor muscles. The sphincter has the same nerve supply as, and reacts simultaneously with, the detrusor. It maintains urethral closure by its passive tone, yet when it shares detrusor contraction it does not hinder voiding.

There is another voluntary striated sphincter which is part of the urogenital diaphragm and surrounds the midurethra in the female and the membranous urethra in the male. It is not essential for continence, though it adds to urethral resistance. Its pathologic irritability or spasticity can lead to obstructive manifestations.

Ganong WF: Formation and excretion of urine. Section 8, pp 506–538, in: *Review of Medical Physiology,* 5th ed. Lange, 1971.

Harper HA: *Review of Physiological Chemistry,* 13th ed. Lange, 1971.

Maxwell MH, Kleeman CR (editors): *Clinical Disorders of Fluid and Electrolyte Metabolism.* Blakiston-McGraw, 1962.

Milne MD: Diseases of the kidney and genito-urinary tract. In: *Biochemical Disorders in Human Disease,* 2nd ed. Thompson RHS, King EJ (editors). Academic Press, 1964.

Welt L: *Clinical Disorders of Hydration and Acid-Base Equilibrium,* 3rd ed. Little, Brown, 1971.

Wesson LG Jr: *Physiology of the Human Kidney.* Grune & Stratton, 1969.

Windhager EE: Kidney, water and electrolytes. Ann Rev Physiol 31:198, 1969.

VESICOURETERAL REFLUX

The main function of the ureterovesical junction is to offer free drainage from the ureter to the bladder and at the same time to prevent every drop of urine that passes through from refluxing back. Anatomically, the ureterovesical junction is well equipped for this function. Although the ureter seemingly ends at the ureteral orifice, all of its musculature actually continues uninterrupted into the base of the bladder to form the superficial trigone. The intravesical ureter is of purely longitudinal muscle fibers. The roof fibers split at the ureteral orifice and sweep on either side to meet the floor fibers and continue as one sheet, the superficial trigone. The terminal 4–5 cm of the ureter are surrounded by a musculofascial sheath (Waldeyer's sheath) which follows the ureter through the ureteral hiatus; after its fibers split on the roof of the ureter, they sweep to the sides and continue in the base of the bladder as the deep trigone (Fig 44–4).

Both the superficial and the deep trigones are superimposed on the detrusor muscle. The deep trigone, which is closely adherent to the detrusor, forms the link between the ureteral mesodermal structures and the detrusor endodermal structure through interchange of a few muscle fibers. Direct continuity between the ureter and the trigone offers an efficient, muscularly active, valvular function. Any stretch of the trigone (with bladder filling) or any trigonal contraction (with voiding) leads to firm occlusion of the intravesical ureter, thus increasing resistance to flow from above downward and perfectly sealing the intravesical ureter against any retrograde flow (Fig 44–5).

Etiology & Classification

Vesicoureteral reflux may be classified according to cause as follows:

(1) Primary reflux (developmental ureterotrigonal weakness).

(2) Reflux secondary to infravesical obstruction, neurogenic dysfunction, iatrogenic causes, and inflammation, especially specific infection (eg, tuberculosis).

(3) Reflux due to congenital ureteral anomalies—ectopic orifices, duplicated ureters, or ureterocele.

Primary reflux is by far the most common type, and is consistently associated with some degree of developmental muscular deficiency in the trigone and terminal ureter. The severity of reflux is proportionate to the degree of this muscular deficiency.

Secondary reflux and congenital types are relatively rare. In most such cases there is also an underlying muscular deficiency, especially in cases of inflammation. Aside from specific infections (tuberculosis, schistosomiasis), nonspecific infections can never lead to reflux unless there is an underlying muscular deficiency in a marginally competent valve.

Reflux is harmful to the upper urinary tract for the following reasons: (1) It leads to postvoiding residual urine that encourages infection. (2) It carries infection from the bladder to the kidney. (3) It permits the relatively high intravesical pressure to be transmitted to the renal papillae and calyceal fornices leading to interstitial extravasation of sterile or infected urine. (4) It has serious hydrodynamic effects since it increases the load of urine to be transported by the ureter and also subjects the weak pelvi-ureteral musculature to high intravesical pressures, leading to stasis, dilatation, and tortuosity. (5) It can encourage stone formation, papillary necrosis, or secondary ureteropelvic junction obstruction.

Reflux is the commonest cause of pyelonephritis and is found in about 50% of children presenting with urinary tract infection. It is present in over 75% of patients with radiologic evidence of chronic pyelonephritis. Inability to demonstrate reflux does not exclude its presence.

In primary reflux, the patient usually presents with symptoms of pyelonephritis or cystitis. Vague abdominal pain is not uncommon. Renal pain and pain with voiding are relatively rare. Pyelonephritis is not uncommonly asymptomatic and the patient may present with azotemia and advanced renal failure due to bilateral renal parenchymal damage with pyelonephritic or hydronephrotic changes. In males, who are relatively protected from infection, reflux is frequently detected late as an incidental finding with a variable degree of renal parenchymal damage.

In secondary reflux, manifestations of the primary disease (neurogenic, obstructive, etc) are usually the presenting symptoms.

Clinical Findings

A. Symptoms and Signs: With acute pyelonephritis, costovertebral angle tenderness may be present. In cases of obstruction or neurogenic deficit, palpable hydronephrotic kidney or a distended bladder may be found.

B Laboratory Findings: Urine examination usually reveals infection. PSP excretion is diminished if there is some vesical or ureteral residual urine or damaged kidneys.

C. X-Ray Findings: The intravenous urogram may be normal but usually reveals pyelonephritic changes or ureteropyelectasis. Dilatation of the lower ureters is commonly seen in mild cases.

Voiding cystourethrography gives conclusive evidence of reflux and should be done in every case of recurrent urinary tract infection. It may also reveal distal obstruction as with posterior urethral valves or spastic external sphincter syndrome in girls (commonly seen with distal urethral stenosis).

Endoscopic examination and evaluation of the trigonal development and the position and configuration of the ureteral orifice is the most helpful means not only of diagnosis but also of assessing prognosis and reversibility. Cineradiography, chromocystoscopy, lipoidal cystography, and radioisotope studies are adjunctive diagnostic measures.

Differential Diagnosis

Ureteral stasis and dilatation due to trigonal hypertrophy are seen in infravesical obstruction or neurogenic lesions.

Functional ureteral obstruction is due to abundance of circularly oriented muscle fibers. It is commonly seen in the lower end, where the muscle fibers act as a partially obstructive sphincteric segment.

Spastic striated external sphincter syndrome can also perpetuate urinary tract infection.

Treatment

In primary reflux, treatment of infection, dilatation of any distal urethral stenosis, and proper evaluation for degree of trigonal ureteral muscular deficiency and the chances of reversibility are the essential preliminary management steps. Not every refluxing orifice requires surgical repair. The improvement in voiding dynamics achieved by conservative management may be all that is needed in borderline valve incompetence. If infection is kept suppressed, reflux may never recur. One-third of cases of reflux are cured in this way. In another third of cases, advanced ureteral or pyelonephritic changes have occurred together with severe ureteral orifice deformity, indicating immediate surgical intervention.

Most of the cases in the remaining third will come to surgical repair after repeated conservative trials to control urinary tract infection and to stop progression of the renal damage have proved inadequate.

Spontaneous reversal of ureteral orifice incompetence occurs only in marginally incompetent valves due to the relief of an existing insult—commonly urinary tract infection or abnormal voiding dynamics.

In obstructive secondary reflux (eg, posterior urethral valves) release of obstruction may cure reflux. Occasionally, reimplantation is still required. In neurogenic reflux, urinary diversion usually is the wisest choice. In congenital reflux, ectopic orifices, duplication with ureterocele, and other congenital malformations, nothing short of reimplantation will cure the reflux.

The aim of surgery is to excise the muscularly weak terminal ureter, provide proper ureterotrigonal fixation, and give adequate posterior support to an intravesical ureter about 2.5 cm long. There are 3 main approaches to achieve this repair:

A. Suprahiatal Repair: (Politano-Leadbetter, Paquin.) A new ureteral hiatus is developed about 2.5 cm above the original one, and the ureter, after passing through a submucosal tunnel, is sutured to the cut edge of the trigone at the level of the original orifice.

B. Infrahiatal Repair: The original hiatus is maintained and, after discarding the weak terminal ureter, the ureter is advanced through a 2.5 cm submucosal tunnel to end closer to the internal meatus.

C. Supra-infrahiatal Repair: A combination of the above.

Prognosis

The prognosis is good both for those who are treated conservatively and for those requiring surgery. The success rate of surgical repair (no reflux, clearance of infection, and no obstruction) is about 90%.

The ultimate prognosis depends on the severity of kidney damage and the degree of ureteral decompensation and atony. In advanced cases, where neither one is reversible, the prognosis is not favorable. These cases constitute about 30% of cases now coming to kidney transplant.

Hutch JA, Amar AD: Vesicoureteral reflux. Malformations, vol 7-1 in: *Encyclopedia of Urology.* Aiken CE & others (editors). Springer-Verlag, 1968.

Leadbetter WF: Surgical management of simple reflux: Indications, objectives, techniques, follow-up and results. Pages 157–163 in: Proceedings of a workshop on ureteral reflux in children. National Academy of Sciences-National Research Council, Washington, DC, 1967.

Lyon RP, Marshall S, Tanagho EA: The ureteral orifice: Its configuration and competency. J Urol 102:504–509, 1969.

Smith DR: Vesicoureteral reflux and other abnormalities of the ureterovesical junction. Chap 10 in: *Urology,* 3rd ed. Campbell MF, Harrison JH (editors). Saunders, 1970.

Tanagho EA: Surgical revision of the incompetent ureterovesical junction: A critical analysis of techniques and requirements. Brit J Urol 42:410–424, 1970.

Tanagho EA, Guthrie TH, Lyon RP: The intravesical ureter in primary reflux. J Urol 101:824–832, 1969.

OBSTRUCTIVE UROPATHY

Obstruction is one of the most important pathologic entities affecting the urinary tract, since it eventually leads to decompensation of the muscular conduits and reservoirs, back pressure, and atrophy of renal parenchyma; it also invites infection and stone formation, which cause additional damage to the organ involved and can ultimately end in complete unilateral or bilateral destruction of the kidneys.

Both the level at which the obstruction occurs and the degree of obstruction are important to an understanding of the pathologic consequences of this group of disorders.

(1) Level of obstruction: Any obstruction at or distal to the internal meatus leads to back pressure effects on both kidneys. Obstruction at or proximal to the ureteral orifice leads to unilateral damage unless the lesion involves both ureters simultaneously.

(2) Degree of obstruction: Complete obstruction leads to rapid decompensation of the system proximal to the site of obstruction with immediate muscular failure. For example, acute retention occurs if the obstruction is distal to the bladder, and anuria occurs if obstruction involves both ureters. Partial obstruction leads to gradual progressive muscular hypertrophy followed by gradual dilatation, decompensation, and hydronephrotic changes.

Etiology

Urinary tract obstruction may be congenital or acquired.

A. Congenital:

1. Meatal stenosis, urethral strictures, posterior urethral valves; ureterovesical and ureteropelvic junction obstruction (various causes).

2. Neurologic deficits.

B. Acquired:

1. Urethral strictures, inflammatory or traumatic.

2. Bladder outlet obstruction (benign prostatic hypertrophy or cancer of the prostate).

3. Vesical tumors.

4. Neurogenic bladder.

5. Extrinsic ureteral compression (tumor, retroperitoneal fibrosis, enlarged lymph nodes).

6. Ureteral or pelvic stones.

7. Ureteral strictures.

8. Ureteral or pelvic tumors.

Pathogenesis

Regardless of its cause, acquired obstruction leads to the same changes in the various segments in the urinary tract, depending on its severity and duration. Congenital obstruction, though basically similar to the acquired type, produces its effect while the system is still in the phase of differentiation and development; its effect may go beyond simple obstruction, leading to other anomalous renal development or kidney dysplasia.

A. Urethral Changes: Proximal to the obstruction, the urethra dilates and balloons. A urethral diverticulum may develop, and dilatation and gaping of the prostatic and ejaculatory ducts may occur.

B. Vesical Changes: Early, the detrusor and trigonal thickening and hypertrophy compensate for the outlet obstruction and lead to complete bladder emptying. This change leads to progressive development of bladder trabeculation, cellules, saccules, then diverticula. Beyond a certain phase, bladder decompensation occurs and is characterized by the above changes, plus variable amounts of residual urine. Trigonal hypertrophy leads to secondary ureteral obstruction due to increased resistance to flow through the intravesical ureter. With the detrusor decompensation and residual urine accumulation, there is stretching of the hypertrophied trigone, which appreciably increases ureteral obstruction. This is the mechanism of back pressure on the kidney in the presence of vesical outlet obstruction (while the ureterovesical junction maintains its competence). Catheter drainage of the bladder relieves trigonal stretch and improves drainage from the upper tract.

A very late change with persistent obstruction (more frequently encountered with neurogenic dysfunction) is decompensation of the ureterovesical junction, leading to reflux, which aggravates the back pressure effect on the upper tract by exposing it to abnormally high intravesical pressures—in addition to favoring the onset or persistence of urinary tract infection.

C. Ureteral Changes: The first noted change is a gradually progressive increase in ureteral distention. This increases ureteral wall stretch, which in turn increases contractile power, and ureteral hyperactivity and hypertrophy develop. Because the ureteral musculature runs in an irregular helical pattern, stretching of its muscular elements leads to lengthening as well as widening. This is the start of ureteral decompensation, where tortuosity and dilatation become apparent. These changes can progress, leading to marked ureteral dilatation and lengthening, and the ureter becomes atonic with infrequent or completely absent peristalsis.

D. Pelvicalyceal Changes: The renal pelvis and calyces, being subjected to progressively increasing volumes of retained urine, progressively distend. The pelvis first shows evidence of hyperactivity and hypertrophy and then progressive dilatation and atony. The calyces show the same changes to a variable degree depending on whether the renal pelvis is intra- or extrarenal. In the latter, the calyceal dilatation may be minimal in spite of marked pelvic dilatation. In the intrarenal pelvis, calyceal dilatation and renal parenchymal damage are maximum. The successive phases seen with obstruction are rounding of the fornices, followed by flattening of the papillae and finally clubbing of the minor calyces.

E. Renal Parenchymal Changes: With progressive pelvicalyceal distention, there is parenchymal compression against the renal capsule. This, plus the more important factor of compression of the arcuate vessels as a result of the expanding distended calyces, results in a marked drop in renal blood flow. This phenomenon leads to progressive parenchymal compression and ischemic atrophy. Lateral groups of nephrons are affected more than central ones, leading to patchy atrophy with variable degree of severity. The glomeruli and proximal convoluted tubules suffer most of this

ischemia. Associated with the increased intrapelvic pressure there is progressive dilatation of the collecting and distal tubules with compression and atrophy of tubular cells.

Clinical Findings

A. Symptoms and Signs: These vary according to the site of obstruction:

1. Infravesical obstruction—Infravesical obstruction leads to difficulty in initiation of voiding, a weak stream, and a diminished flow rate with terminal dribbling. Burning and frequency are common associated symptoms. A distended or thickened bladder wall may be palpable. Urethral induration of a stricture, benign prostatic hypertrophy, or cancer of the prostate may be noted on rectal examination. Meatal stenosis and impacted urethral stones are readily diagnosed.

2. Supravesical obstruction—Renal pain or renal colic and gastrointestinal symptoms are commonly associated. Supravesical obstruction may be completely asymptomatic when it develops very gradually over a period of several weeks or months. An enlarged kidney may be palpable. Costovertebral angle tenderness may be present.

B. Laboratory Findings: Evidence of urinary infection, hematuria, or crystalluria may be seen. Impaired kidney function is noted by diminished PSP excretion and elevated BUN and serum creatinine, with the ratio well above the normal 10:1 relationship because of significant urea reabsorption.

C. X-Ray Findings: Radiologic examination is usually diagnostic in cases of stasis, tumors, and strictures. Dilatation and anatomic changes occur above the level of obstruction, whereas distal to the obstruction the configuration is usually normal. This helps in localizing the site of obstruction. Combined antegrade visualization by intravenous urograms and retrograde visualization by ureterograms or urethrograms, depending on the site of obstruction, is sometimes needed to demonstrate the extent of the obstructed segment. In supravesical obstruction, demonstration of stasis and delayed drainage is essential to establish and measure the severity of obstruction.

D. Special Examinations: Instrumental calibration of sites of obstruction is also valuable.

Complications

The most important complication of urinary tract obstruction is renal parenchymal atrophy as a result of the back pressure effect.

Urinary tract obstruction predisposes to infection and stone formation, and infection added to obstruction leads to rapid kidney destruction.

Treatment

The aim of therapy is relief of the obstruction—eg, in acute urinary retention, treatment consists of bladder drainage by a catheter. Surgery is often necessary. Simple urethral stricture may be managed conservatively by dilatation. Urethrotomy or urethroplasty may be required. Urethral valves must be ruptured. Benign prostatic hypertrophy and obstructing bladder tumors require surgical removal.

Impacted stones must be either removed or bypassed by a catheter to be surgically removed later or given a chance to pass spontaneously.

Ureteral or ureteropelvic obstruction requires surgical revision and plastic repair, either by ureterovesicoplasty, ureterolithotomy, ureteroureteral anastomosis, bladder flaps to bridge a gap in the lower ureter, transureteroureteral anastomosis, or ureteropyeloplasty.

Preliminary drainage above the obstruction is sometimes needed to improve kidney function. Occasionally, permanent drainage and diversion by cutaneous ureterostomy, ileal or colonic loop diversion, or permanent nephrostomy are required.

Prognosis

The prognosis depends on the cause, site, duration, and degree of kidney damage and renal decompensation. In general, relief of obstruction leads to improvement in kidney function except in seriously damaged kidneys, especially those destroyed by inflammatory scarring.

Barnett JS, Stephens FD: The role of the lower segmental vessels in the aetiology of hydronephrosis. Australian New Zealand J Surg 31:201–213, 1962.

Culp OS.& others: Hydronephrosis and hydroureter in infancy and childhood: A panel discussion. J Urol 88:443–450, 1962.

Earlam RJ: Recovery of renal function after prolonged ureteric obstruction. Brit J Urol 39:58–62, 1967.

Green N, Fingerhut AG, French S: Mechanism of renovascular backflow: A pathophysiologic study. Radiology 92:531–536, 1969.

Johnston JH: The pathogenesis of hydronephrosis in children. Brit J Urol 41:724–734, 1969.

Kelalis PP & others: Ureteropelvic obstruction in children: Experience with 109 cases. J Urol 106:618–622, 1971.

Krohn AG & others: Compensatory renal hypertrophy: The role of immediate vascular changes in its production. J Urol 103:790–794, 1970.

Smart WR: Chap 55 in: *Urology*, 3rd ed. Campbell MF, Harrison JH (editors). Saunders, 1970.

Tanagho EA, Meyers FH: Trigonal hypertrophy: A cause of ureteral obstruction. J Urol 93:678–683, 1965.

Tanagho EA, Smith DR, Guthrie TH: Pathophysiology of functional ureteral obstruction. J Urol 104:73–88, 1970.

Williams DI, Hulme-Moir I: Primary obstructive megaureter. Brit J Urol 42:140–149 1970.

GENITOURINARY TRACT TUBERCULOSIS

Specific infections of the urinary tract are those (tuberculosis, actinomycosis, and syphilis) that cause a specific pathologic tissue reaction and usually have a distinctive clinical course. Only tuberculosis will be discussed here.

Tuberculosis is the most important and the most commonly missed type of specific genitourinary infection. It should always be considered in any case of pyuria without bacteriuria or in any resistant urinary tract infection that does not respond to treatment.

Genitourinary tuberculosis is always secondary to pulmonary infection though in many cases the primary focus has already healed or is in a subclinical form. Infection occurs via the hematogenous route. The kidneys and (less commonly) the prostate are the principal sites of urinary tract involvement, though all other segments of the genitourinary system can be affected.

Pathology

Renal tuberculosis usually starts as a tuberculoma that gradually enlarges, then caseates, and later ulcerates and breaks through the pelvicalyceal system. Caseation and scarring are the principal pathologic features of renal tuberculosis. In the ureter, tuberculosis usually leads to stricture, periureteritis, and mural fibrosis.

In the bladder, the infection is characterized by areas of hyperemia and a coalescent group of tubercles followed by ulcerations around the involved ureteral orifice. Bladder wall fibrosis and contracted bladder are the end results.

Urethral involvement in the male (uncommon) leads to urethral stricture, usually in the bulbous portion. Periurethral abscess and fistula are common complications.

Genital tuberculosis involves the prostate, seminal vesicles, and epididymides, either separately or in association with renal involvement. Tubercle formation with later caseation and fibrosis is the basic pathologic feature, leading to enlargement, nodulation, and irregular consistency of the prostate and to fibrosis and distention of the seminal vesicles. Induration, thickening of the epididymis, and beading of the vas deferens are characteristic findings.

Clinical Findings

A. Symptoms and Signs: The patient commonly presents with lower urinary tract irritation, usually with pyuria. Less common manifestations are hematuria, renal pain, and renal colic.

B. Laboratory Findings: Sterile pyuria is the rule. The organism can be identified on an acid-fast stain of the centrifuged sediment of a 24-hour urine specimen, by culture, or by guinea pig inoculation.

C. X-Ray Findings: Radiologic findings of motheaten, caseous cavities or bizarre irregular calyces, strictures in straight, rigid, moderately dilated ureters, and a contracted bladder with vesicoureteral reflux are all suggestive evidence.

D. Special Examinations: Cystoscopy will show typical findings of tuberculous cystitis.

Treatment

A. Medical Treatment: Tuberculosis must be treated as a generalized disease. Once the diagnosis is established, medical treatment for at least 2 years is indicated whether or not surgery is required also. Whenever possible, medical treatment should be continued for at least 3 months before surgery is undertaken. In addition to general supportive measures, specific antituberculosis therapy should be given.

B. Surgical Measures: In unilateral renal lesions, nephrectomy is indicated. In bilateral disease that has seriously damaged one kidney and is in an early stage in the other, unilateral nephrectomy still should be considered; in localized polar lesions, partial nephrectomy may be done.

In epididymal involvement, epididymectomy plus contralateral vasectomy or bilateral epididymectomy should be done, depending on whether involvement is unilateral or bilateral.

Prognosis

Tuberculous involvement of other structures in the genitourinary tract must be treated medically.

Lattimer JK & others: Current treatment of renal tuberculosis. J Urol 102:206, 1969.

Mangelson HL, Saunders JC, Brosnan SA: Urogenital tuberculosis. J Urol 104:309–314, 1970.

NONSPECIFIC URINARY TRACT INFECTIONS

General Considerations

Nonspecific urinary tract infection is the second most common type of infection in humans and is encountered in about 75% of patients seen by urologists.

These infections are caused by a variety of pyogenic bacteria, and the pathologic tissue response is not specific to the offending organism. The commonest organisms are gram-negative bacteria, particularly *Escherichia coli.* Less common are *Aerobacter aerogenes, Proteus vulgaris* and *P mirabilis, Pseudomonas aeruginosa,* and *Streptococcus faecalis.*

The ascending route of infection is by far the most common. Infection by this route is a common occurrence encountered in young girls and in women during active sexual life. It is related to the short length of the female urethra and the perineal bacterial flora. In males, ascending infection is usually a consequence of urethral instrumentation. Infection may be contained in the bladder if there is a competent ureterovesical junction. Otherwise, ascending infection can reach the kidney, leading to pyelonephritis (see below).

Descending or hematogenous infection is relatively uncommon. When it occurs, it is usually in association with local urinary tract disorders—most commonly, obstruction and stasis; less commonly, trauma, foreign bodies, or tumors.

Lymphatic spread occasionally occurs from the large bowel or from the cervix and adnexa in the female through the perivesical and periureteral lymphatics.

Direct extension to the urinary bladder of nearby inflammatory processes—eg, appendiceal abscess or a pelvic abscess—may occur.

Predisposing Factors

Urinary tract infection is usually initiated or maintained because of certain predisposing factors:

A. General Systemic Factors: Examples include diabetes, debilitation, and prolonged illness. These disorders probably favor urinary tract infection by interfering with normal bladder and body defense mechanisms.

B. Local Factors: Any of the following local conditions predisposes to a urinary tract infection: obstruction, organic or functional; stasis (residual urine); vesicoureteral reflux; foreign bodies, especially catheters and stones; tumors or any necrotic tissue; and trauma, especially to the kidneys.

Classification of Nonspecific Urinary Tract Infection

A. Upper Urinary Tract Infection: Acute or chronic pyelonephritis, papillary necrosis, and renal carbuncle are the most common types.

B. Lower Urinary Tract Infection: Cystitis and urethritis, including gonorrheal urethritis.

C. Genital Infection: Prostatitis, epididymitis, seminal vesiculitis, and orchitis.

Hinman F Jr: Bacterial elimination. J Urol 99:811–825, 1968.

Hodson CJ, Wilson S: Natural history of chronic pyelonephritic scarring. Brit MJ 2:191–194, 1965.

Kunin CM: The natural history of recurrent bacteriuria in school girls. New England J Med 282:1443–1448, 1970.

Kunin CM, McCormack RC: Prevention of catheter-induced urinary tract infections by sterile closed drainage. New England J Med 274:1155–1161, 1966.

Stamey TA, Pfau A: Urinary infections: A selective review and some observations. California Med 113:16–35, Dec 1970.

Stamey TA & others: Recurrent urinary infections and nothing else. J Urol 106:441–442, 1971.

1. ACUTE & CHRONIC PYELONEPHRITIS

Except in the presence of stasis, foreign bodies, or trauma, pyelonephritis is an ascending type of infection. Pathogenic organisms usually reach the kidney from the bladder via an incompetent ureterovesical junction.

Clinical Findings

A. Symptoms and Signs: In the acute attack, pain is present in one or both loins. Young children commonly present with ill-localized abdominal pain. Irritative lower urinary tract symptoms may be associated. Chills and fever are common. In chronic pyelonephritis, dull aching pain in the loins may be present; however, there are usually no symptoms.

B. Laboratory Findings: Pyuria and bacteria on stained smear are consistent findings. In acute attacks, the sedimentation rate is elevated. Urine culture identifies the organism.

C. X-Ray Findings: In acute attacks, only minimal changes such as delayed function and poorer concentration are usually noted. In chronic cases, typical calyceal deformities with evidence of peripheral scarring can usually be seen. Evidence of stasis may be apparent. Cystography usually reveals reflux.

Complications

If the diagnosis is missed in the acute stage, the infection may become chronic. Both acute and chronic pyelonephritis lead to progressive renal scarring and destruction and may result in a small, atrophic, scarred, nonfunctioning kidney.

Treatment

Specific therapy should be given to eradicate the infecting organism after proper identification and sensitivity testing. Symptomatic treatment is indicated for pain and bladder irritability. Rest and adequate urinary output are required. Failure to simultaneously identify and treat predisposing factors is the principal cause of failure of therapy or chronicity and ultimate renal failure.

Prognosis

The prognosis is good with adequate treatment of both the infection and its predisposing cause, depending on the degree of preexisting renal parenchymal damage.

Freedman LR: Chronic pyelonephritis at autopsy. Ann Int Med 66:697–710, 1967.

Heptinstall RH: Pathology of end-stage kidney disease. Am J Med 44:656–663, 1968.

Hodson CJ: The radiology of chronic pyelonephritis. Postgrad MJ 41:477–480, 1965.

Kimmelstiel P: The nature of chronic pyelonephritis. Geriatrics 19:145–154, 1964.

Symposium on pyelonephritis. J Infect Dis 120:1–140, 1969.

Williams DI: Urinary tract infection. Brit MJ 1:1043–1046, 1965.

Zinner SH, Kass EH: Long-term (10–14 years) follow-up of bacteriuria of pregnancy. New England J Med 285:820–824, 1971.

2. PAPILLARY NECROSIS

This disorder consists of ischemic necrosis of the renal papillae or of the entire pyramid. Excessive ingestion of analgesics, sickle cell trait, diabetes, obstruction with infection, and vesicoureteral reflux with infection are common predisposing factors.

The symptoms are usually those of chronic cystitis with recurring exacerbation of pyelonephritis. Renal pain or renal colic may be present. Azotemic manifestations may be the presenting symptoms. In acute attacks, localized loin tenderness and generalized toxemia may occur. Laboratory findings consist of pyuria, occasionally glycosuria, and acidosis. Impaired kidney function is shown by diminished PSP excretion and elevated serum creatinine and BUN. X-ray usually shows impaired function and poor visualization in advanced cases; evidence of ulceration, cavitation, or linear breaks in the base of the papillae and negative shadows due to sloughed papillae may be seen. Retrograde urograms may be needed for proper visualization if kidney function is markedly impaired.

Preventive measures consist of proper management of diabetic patients with recurrent infection and avoidance of chronic use of analgesic compounds containing phenacetin and aspirin.

Intensive antibacterial therapy may be needed, yet it is commonly unsuccessful in eradicating infection. Little can be done surgically except to remove obstructing papillae and correct predisposing factors (reflux, obstruction) if identified.

In severe cases, the prognosis is poor. Kidney transplant might be considered.

Lindvall N: Renal papillary necrosis. A roentgenographic study of 155 cases. Acta radiol, Suppl 192, 1960.

Longacre AM, Popky GL: Papillary necrosis in patients with cirrhosis: A study of 102 patients. J Urol 99:391–395, 1968.

Murray RM, Lawson DH, Linton AL: Analgesic nephropathy: Clinical syndrome and prognosis. Brit MJ 1:479–482, 1971.

Nanra RS, Kincaid-Smith P: Papillary necrosis in rats caused by aspirin and aspirin-containing mixtures. Brit MJ 3:559–561, 1970.

3. RENAL CARBUNCLE

Renal carbuncle is usually due to a hemolytic staphylococcal infection which spreads to the kidney by the hematogenous route from a pyogenic skin lesion. The onset may be acute, with high fever and definite localization. In occasional cases, low-grade fever and general malaise are the presenting symptoms. Localized costovertebral angle tenderness and a palpable kidney mass may be present. The mass may be evident on intravenous urograms or renal angiograms. The urine is not infected until the abscess breaks into the pelvicalyceal system.

If organism sensitivity can be established by appropriate tests (blood and urine cultures and sensitivity tests), treat with the proper antibiotic. Local drainage or even heminephrectomy may be indicated.

Fair WR, Higgins MH: Renal abscess. J Urol 104:179–183, 1970.

Moore CA, Gangai MP: Renal cortical abscess. J Urol 89:303–306, 1967.

4. CYSTITIS

Cystitis is more common in females and is usually an ascending infection. In the male, it usually occurs in association with obstruction, prostatitis, foreign bodies, or tumors. The urinary bladder is normally capable of clearing itself of infection unless an underlying pathologic process interferes with its defensive mechanisms.

In the acute phase, the principal symptoms of cystitis are burning on urination, frequency, urgency, and hematuria; low-grade fever and suprapubic, perineal, and low back pain may be present. In chronic cystitis, irritative symptoms are usually milder.

Evidence of prostatitis, urethritis, and vaginitis may be present. Laboratory findings, in addition to hematuria, consist of bacteriuria and pyuria. Urine culture identifies the organism. Cystoscopy is not advisable in the acute phase. In chronic cystitis, evidence of mucosal irritation may be present.

In any recurrent lower urinary tract infection, a complete urologic work-up is indicated. Instrumentation is contraindicated in the acute phase but essential in chronic or recurrent cases to identify the predisposing factor.

Specific antibacterial therapy is given according to the results of sensitivity testing of recovered organisms. Sterilization of urine is preferably followed by a variable period of suppressive medication depending upon the predisposing factor or the chronicity and recurrence of the disease.

In children with cystitis due to distal urethral stenosis, dilatation is required. Prolonged suppressive medication is usually indicated in cases associated with voiding dysfunction.

In women with recurrent postcoital cystitis, prosuppressive medication (eg, sulfonamides) on the night of intercourse and the following day and immediate postcoital voiding usually help in preventing recurrences.

5. URETHRITIS

Nonspecific urethritis is not uncommon in both men and women. It usually occurs as an ascending bacterial infection in women and is associated with prostatitis in men. Viral and chemical urethritis may also be encountered.

Urethral discharge and a burning sensation with urination are commonly the presenting symptoms. The onset of symptoms is usually related to intercourse. Examination reveals meatal congestion and tenderness along the urethra. The first glass of urine usually shows urethral discharge, bacteriuria, and pyuria. The midstream urine is clean unless there is associated cystitis or prostatitis.

Treatment consists of giving specific antimicrobial therapy. The best combination is one of the tetra-cyclines and a sulfonamide.

If prostatitis is the underlying factor, prostatic massage is indicated after the acute phase has subsided. Urethral stricture should be treated. Empirical urethral dilatation may help in the female with urethritis. Infected periurethral glands may have to be properly drained or fulgurated.

Gonorrheal Urethritis

Gonorrhea is usually transmitted through sexual contact. *Neisseria gonorrhoeae* is a gram-negative organism commonly seen as intracellular diplococci. It can be identified on a stained smear of discharge or urine sediment or, if necessary, by culture.

A purulent yellow or brown urethral discharge starting 3–4 days after sexual contact is the first symptom. Burning and pain along the urethra and meatal inflammation are common. The first glass of urine is cloudy but midstream urine is clear.

Penicillin and tetracycline each cure over 90% of cases. A combination of the 2 is more effective. Simultaneous treatment of the partner is essential. Prolonged therapy is indicated in the presence of gonorrheal prostatitis, seminal vesiculitis, epididymitis, or cystitis. Inadequate treatment can lead to periurethritis, periurethral abscess, and urethral strictures.

Conger KB: Gonorrhea and nonspecific urethritis. M Clin North America 48:767–772, 1964.

Csonka GW: Non-gonorrheal urethritis. Brit J Ven Dis 41:1–8, 1965.

Shepard MC: Nongonococcal urethritis associated with human strains of "T" mycoplasmas. JAMA 211:1335–1340, 1970.

6. PROSTATITIS

Prostatitis commonly follows ascending urethral infection and inadequately treated urethritis. Occasionally it is due to hematogenous infection. It is most commonly seen in young adults but also occurs in young children and more frequently in association with benign prostatic hyperplasia.

Symptoms of acute prostatitis consist of perineal pain, urethral discharge, marked irritative urinary symptoms, and fever. The prostate is tender, enlarged, and usually firm. Fluctuation may be elicited if there is abscess formation. In chronic prostatitis, mild perineal pain, low backache, or mild irritative symptoms are common. The prostate is usually enlarged, firm, and irregular. Prostatic massage (contraindicated in the acute phase) leads to copious discharge. Laboratory findings consist of bacteria and pus in the urethral discharge, the prostatic smear, or the first glass of urine. Leukocytosis is present in the acute phase.

Specific antibacterial therapy should be given according to culture and sensitivity testing. The response is usually good in the acute phase but not so gratifying in chronic cases. Diffusion of antibiotics in prostatic acini is very poor.

Prostatic massage is helpful in chronic cases. Regular sexual intercourse is advisable.

Bourne CW, Frishetti WA: Prostatic fluid analysis and prostatitis. J Urol 97:140–144, 1967.

Morrisseau PM, Phillips CA, Leadbetter GW Jr: Viral prostatitis. J Urol 103:767–769, 1970.

Stamey TA, Meares EM Jr, Winningham DG: Chronic bacterial prostatitis and the diffusion of drugs into prostatic fluid. J Urol 103:187–194, 1970.

Trapnell J, Roberts M: Prostatic abscess. Brit J Surg 57:567–569, 1970.

7. EPIDIDYMITIS

Common causes of epididymitis include urethral instrumentation, chronic prostatitis, and reflux of sterile urine into the ejaculatory ducts. In acute cases there is usually a history of preceding instrumentation, catheterization, chronic prostatitis, or severe straining. The symptoms are sudden pain in the scrotum, rapid unilateral scrotal enlargement, and marked tenderness that extends over the spermatic cord and is relieved by lifting the testis. In the chronic phase there is usually minimal local tenderness and pain, with irregular nodular enlargement of the epididymis. Hydrocele may be associated. Laboratory findings reveal pyuria, bacteriuria, and marked leukocytosis.

Nonspecific epididymitis must be differentiated from torsion of the testis, testicular tumor, and tuberculous epididymitis.

In the acute phase, treatment consists of infiltrating the spermatic cord with 20 ml of 1% procaine hydrochloride. Pain, fever, and swelling usually subside gradually. Antibiotics (tetracycline) are helpful. Scrotal support, rest, and hot sitz baths and sedation are indicated. Chronic prostatitis should be treated if present.

Acute attacks usually resolve in 2–3 weeks with treatment; exacerbations can be controlled by treating the predisposing factor. Chronic epididymitis usually never resolves completely; it has no consequences except, occasionally, sterility in bilateral cases.

Lyon RP, Bruyn HB: Treatment of mumps epididymo-orchitis. JAMA 196:736–738, 1966.

Smith DR: Treatment of epididymitis by infiltration of the spermatic cord with procaine hydrochloride. J Urol 46:74–76, 1941.

CALCULOUS DISEASE

1. RENAL STONE

Essentials of Diagnosis

- Flank pain, hematuria, pyelonephritis, previous stone passage; high vitamin D, milk, and alkaline intake.
- Renal tenderness.
- Urinalysis shows red cells and sometimes white cells and bacteria in the urine.
- Stone visualized on urography.

General Considerations

Most stones are composed of calcium salts (oxalate, phosphate, magnesium-ammonium phosphate—the latter secondary to urea-splitting organisms). Most calcium stones are idiopathic (idiopathic hypercalciuria), and hypercalciuria encourages stone formation in hyperparathyroidism, immobilization, high calcium or vitamin D intake, and dehydration. An alkaline urine increases the insolubility of calcium.

The less common metabolic stones, cystine and uric acid, usually form secondary to hypersecretion of these substances. Uric acid stones are radiolucent. Stones that obstruct the ureteropelvic junction lead to hydronephrosis and infection.

Clinical Findings

A. Symptoms and Signs: If the stone obstructs the ureteropelvic junction or a calyx, moderate to severe renal pain will be noted, often accompanied by nausea, vomiting, and ileus. Hematuria is common. Symptoms of infection, if present, will be exacerbated. Nonobstructive calculi are usually painless. This includes staghorn calculus, which may form a cast of all calyces and the pelvis. In the symptomatic patient, there may be costovertebral angle tenderness and a quiet abdomen. Infection secondary to obstruction may lead to high fever, prostration, and abdominal muscle rigidity.

B. Laboratory Findings: With acute infection, leukocytosis is to be expected. With renal insufficiency, anemia may be noted. Urinalysis may reveal red and white blood cells and bacteria. A pH of 7.6 or higher implies the presence of urea-splitting organisms. A pH consistently below 5.5 is compatible with the formation of uric acid or cystine stones. Crystals of uric acid or cystine in the urine are suggestive. A Sulkowitch test may reveal evidence of hypercalciuria, which is observed with hyperparathyroidism, essential hypercalciuria, and disseminated osseous metastases.

Determination of serum calcium and phosphorus may afford evidence of hyperparathyroidism, in which the tubular reabsorption of phosphate is diminished. An elevated serum uric acid is compatible with uric acid lithiasis. Significant cystinuria may be found. Hyperchloremic acidosis suggests renal tubular acidosis with secondary renal calcifications. Total renal function will be impaired only if the stones are bilateral, and particularly if infection is a complication.

C. **X-Ray Findings:** About 90% of calculi are radiopaque (calcium, cystine). Excretory urography is necessary to place them in the excretory tract and also affords a measure of renal function (Fig 44–6). An acutely obstructed kidney may only show increasing density of the renal shadow without significant radiopaque material in the calyces. A nonopaque stone (uric acid) will show as a "negative" shadow since it displaces the contrast medium.

Bone disease due to metastatic carcinoma or Paget's disease may account for hypercalciuria.

D. **Stone Analysis:** If a stone has previously been passed or the present one is recovered, its chemical nature should be analyzed. Such knowledge may be significant when planning a regimen of prevention.

Differential Diagnosis

Acute pyelonephritis may start with acute renal pain, thus mimicking a renal stone. Urinalysis reveals infection, and urograms fail to reveal a calculus.

Renal tumor may bleed into its own substance, causing acute pain simulating obstructing stone. Urograms make the differentiation.

Renal tuberculosis is complicated by stone in 10% of cases. Pyuria without bacteriuria is suggestive. Urography reveals the motheaten calyces typical of tuberculosis.

Papillary necrosis may cause renal colic if a sloughed papilla obstructs the ureteropelvic junction. Excretory urography will settle the issue.

Renal infarction may cause renal pain and hematuria. Evidence of a cardiac lesion, nonfunction of the kidney on urography, and absence of evidence of calculus help in differentiation. Infarction may be established by angiography.

Complications

The presence of a stone lowers the resistance of the kidney to infection, although in many instances the infection is primary. A stone lodged in the ureteropelvic junction leads to progressive hydronephrosis. A staghorn calculus, as it grows, may destroy renal tissue by pressure, although the infection that is usually present also contributes to renal damage.

Prevention

An effective preventive regimen depends upon stone analysis and chemical studies of the serum and urine.

A. **General Measures:** Ensure a high fluid intake to keep solutes well diluted. Combat infection, relieve stasis or obstruction, and advise the patient to avoid prolonged recumbency. For calcium stone formers, stop vitamin supplements (vitamin D) and medications containing calcium salts. Eliminate alkalies from the diet (by reducing the intake of fruit and vegetables) to produce an acid urine in which calcium is most soluble.

B. **Specific Measures:**

1. **Calcium stones**—Remove parathyroid tumor, if present. Eliminate dairy products (milk, cheese) from the diet. Calcium is most soluble in acid urine (below pH 6.0). Give cranberry juice, 200 ml 4 times a day; ascorbic acid, 1 g 4 times a day; and potassium acid phosphate (see below). In renal tubular acidosis, however, give alkali to reduce urinary calcium excretion.

To convert "stone-forming" to 'non-stone-forming" urine, give 2.5 g of neutral sodium (or potassium) phosphate daily in divided doses. Potassium acid phosphate, 4–6 g/day, is also effective.

Thiazide diuretics such as hydrochlorothiazide (HydroDiuril), 50 mg twice a day, decrease the calcium content in the urine.

2. **Oxalate stones (calcium oxalate)**—Prescribe phosphate (see above) and limit calcium intake.

3. **Metabolic stones (uric acid, cystine)**—These substances are most soluble at a pH of 7.0 or higher. Give 50% citrate solution, 4–8 ml 4 times a day; check urine pH with paper indicator. For uric acid stone formers, limit purines in the diet and give allopurinol

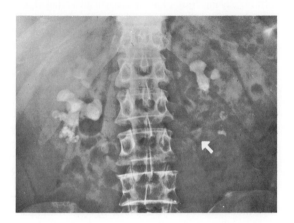 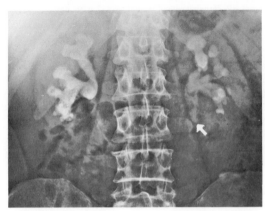

FIG 44–6. Bilateral staghorn calculi and left upper ureteral stone. *Left:* Plain film. Arrow points to ureteral stone. *Right:* Excretory urogram showing bilateral impaired function.

(Zyloprim), 300 mg every 12 hours. Patients with mild cystinuria should receive a low-methionine diet. For severe cystinurics, give penicillamine (Cuprimine), 30 mg/kg/day orally in divided doses. This regimen should reduce urinary cystine to safe levels. Penicillamine should be supplemented with pyridoxine, 50 mg/day orally.

Treatment

A. Conservative Measures: No intervention is indicated for a small, asymptomatic stone trapped in a calyx. A conservative approach should be utilized for coralliform (staghorn) stones—particularly if bilateral—in an older individual with impaired renal function since function is not apt to improve after their removal, the recurrence rate is significant, and infection is difficult to eradicate. Stones secondary to renal tubular acidosis should be treated with alkalies. Give 50% solution of sodium (or potassium) citrate, 4–8 ml 4 times a day. Secondary stones are apt to be small and may pass spontaneously.

Combat infection. Urea-splitting organisms significantly contribute to development and growth of stones (triple phosphate).

Metabolic stones may cease to grow or even dissolve on specific medication.

B. Surgical Measures: Removal of the stone is indicated for disabling pain, progressive hydronephrosis, or infection that resists chemotherapy. If the kidney is badly damaged and its mate is normal, nephrectomy may be indicated.

Prognosis

The recurrence rate of renal stone is significant unless rigorous attention is paid to prophylaxis. The danger from stone is the progressive destruction of the kidney by obstruction and infection.

Herrin JT: The child with urolithiasis: Practical considerations in diagnosis and management. Clin Pediat 10:306–308, 1971.

Symposium on urinary stone. Am J Med 45:654–783, 1968.

Yendt ER: Renal calculi. Canad MAJ 102:479–489, 1970.

2. URETERAL STONE

Essentials of Diagnosis

- Severe ureterorenal colic.
- Hematuria.
- Nausea, vomiting, and ileus.
- Stone, usually obstructive, on excretory urography.

General Considerations

Stones passing down the ureter originate in the kidney. They are ordinarily obstructive and are therefore a threat to renal function. Complicating infection may occur. Most stones entering the ureter will pass spontaneously.

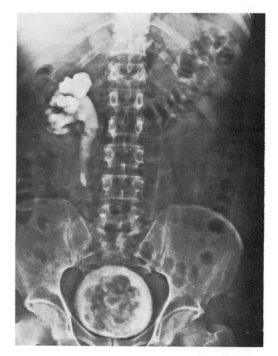

FIG 44—7. Excretory urogram showing right ureteral stone causing hydronephrosis. Large irregular filling defect from unsuspected vesical neoplasm.

Clinical Findings

A. Symptoms and Signs: The pain usually comes on abruptly and is felt in the costovertebral angle; it tends to radiate into the ipsilateral lower abdominal quadrant. Nausea, vomiting, and abdominal distention are common. Gross hematuria is usual. When the stone approaches the bladder, symptoms resembling those of cystitis are experienced. Should the kidney be infected, the resulting obstruction will lead to its exacerbation.

The patient is usually in such agony that only the intravenous injection of an opiate will give relief. There is tenderness in the costovertebral angle. Spasm of the ipsilateral abdominal muscles is present. Peristalsis is minimal; abdominal distention is usual. Fever indicates a complicating renal infection.

B. Laboratory Findings: Same as for renal stone.

C. X-Ray Findings: Excretory urograms are essential. The plain film may reveal an opacity in the region of the ureter, but proof that it is indeed a stone depends on seeing it within the ureteral lumen (Fig 44—7). This procedure depicts the degree of obstruction and the size and position of the stone, observations that permit judgment as to treatment. If the stone is nonopaque, it will show as a negative shadow in the ureter, which is dilated above it; ureteral tumor or a blood clot will give a similar finding. If the diagnosis is still in doubt, cystoscopy, ureteral catheterization, and retrograde urography may be indicated.

Differential Diagnosis

Passage of crystals down the ureter may cause colic. Urograms are usually normal. The presence of crystals in the urine may be significant.

A tumor of the kidney or renal pelvis may bleed. Passage of a blood clot will cause symptoms typical of stone. Urograms may reveal a radiolucent area in the ureter surrounded by the radiopaque urine.

Primary tumor of the ureter may become obstructive and cause pain and hematuria. The urogram will reveal the ureteral filling defect with secondary obstruction. Urinary cytology will reveal malignant transitional cells.

Acute pyelonephritis may be associated with pain as acute as that seen with stone. Pyuria and bacteriuria are found. Stone is absent on urography.

A sloughed papilla coursing down the ureter may cause colic and will afford a urogram compatible with uric acid stone. Evidence of papillary sloughs, however, will be noted.

Complications

If obstruction from the ureteral stone is prolonged, progressive renal damage may ensue. Bilateral stones may cause anuria, requiring immediate establishment of drainage with indwelling ureteral catheters or removal of the stones.

Infection may supervene, but most renal infections are iatrogenic, ie, introduced at the time of stone manipulation.

Prevention

See section on renal stone.

Treatment

A. General Measures: Most ureteral stones will pass spontaneously—particularly those 0.5 cm in diameter or less. Once the diagnosis has been established, pain should be relieved by suitable opiates given intravenously, eg, morphine, 8 mg.

B. Specific Measures: Should the stone cause intractable pain, lead to progressive hydronephrosis, or be complicated by acute infection, removal is indicated. Cystoscopic manipulation is highly successful for stones in the lower ureter. Surgical removal is at times necessary.

Prognosis

About 80% of ureteral stones pass spontaneously. Periodic plain films of the abdomen or excretory urograms will portray progress of the stone and any renal damage that might develop.

Fox M, Pyrah LN, Draper FP: Management of ureteric stone: A review of 292 cases. Brit J Urol 37:660–667, 1965.

3. VESICAL STONE

Primary vesical calculi are rare in the USA but are common in Southeast Asia. The cause is probably dietary. Secondary stones usually complicate vesical outlet obstruction with residual urine and infection; 90% of those affected are men. They are common in vesical schistosomiasis or in association with radiation cystitis. Foreign bodies in the bladder may act as nuclei for the precipitation of urinary salts. Most stones are calcific; some are composed of uric acid.

Clinical Findings

A. Symptoms and Signs: Symptoms typical of obstruction distal to the bladder are elicited. There may be sudden interruption of the stream, associated with urethral pain if a stone occludes the bladder neck during voiding. Hematuria is not uncommon. Vesical distention may be noted; evidence of urethral stricture or an enlarged prostate is usually found.

B. Laboratory Findings: Pyuria and bacteriuria are almost always present; hematuria is usual. The PSP excretion is depressed because of residual vesical urine.

C. X-Ray Findings: Vesical calculi are usually radiopaque. Excretory urograms will reveal that the stones are indeed intravesical; residual urine is usually depicted on the postvoiding film.

D. Instrumental Examination: Arrest of a sound or endoscope may lead to the diagnosis of urethral stricture. The catheter may uncover residual urine. Cystoscopy will visualize the stones and, in addition, reveal an obstructing prostate.

Differential Diagnosis

A pedunculated vesical tumor may suddenly occlude the vesical neck during voiding. Cystoscopy leads to definitive diagnosis.

Extravesical opacifications may simulate stones on a plain film. Cystoscopy will make the differentiation.

Complications

Vesical infection is worsened by the presence of a stone, which defeats attempts at sterilization of the urine. A small stone may lodge in the urethra, causing complete urinary obstruction. It must be removed.

Prevention

Prevention requires relief of the primary obstruction, removal of the stones, and sterilization of the urine.

Treatment

A. Specific Measures: Small stones can be removed or crushed transurethrally. Large stones will require suprapubic transvesical removal. The obstructive lesion must also be corrected.

Chemical dissolution is feasible, but it fails to attack the cause. Frequent instillation of hemiacidrin (Renacidin), with the catheter clamped off for 1 hour, may prove successful.

B. General Measures: Analgesics for pain and anti-microbials for control of infection can be utilized until the stones can be removed.

Prognosis

The recurrence rate of vesical stone is low if the obstruction and infection are treated.

Aurora AL, Taneja OP, Gupta DN: Bladder stone disease of childhood. I. An epidemiologic study. II. A clinico-pathologic study. Acta paediat scandinav 59:117–184, 385–398, 1970.

Gharib R: Lithiasis in the urinary tract of children. Clin Pediat 9:157–164, 1970.

Reuter HJ: Electronic lithotripsy: Transurethral treatment of bladder stones in 50 cases. J Urol 104:843–848, 1970.

4. NEPHROCALCINOSIS

Nephrocalcinosis is a precipitation of calcium in the tubules, parenchyma, and, occasionally, the glomeruli. Its presence implies some renal impairment, often severe. Stones may be found in the calyces and pelvis. The common causes are primary hyperparathyroidism, high milk-alkali ingestion, high vitamin D intake, and secondary hyperparathyroidism which develops secondary to severe renal damage associated with hyperchloremic acidosis. Calcifications may also be seen in the skin, lungs, stomach, spleen, corneas, and around the joints.

There are no specific symptoms. If the patient is a child, he may merely fail to thrive. Stones or sand may be passed. The complaints are usually those of the primary disease. Physical examination may reveal an enlarged parathyroid gland, corneal calcifications, and pseudorickets.

The urine may be infected. In renal tubular acidosis, the pH is fixed between 6.0–7.0. The Sulkowitch test is strongly positive in hyperparathyroidism, both primary and secondary. Tests of renal function are depressed; uremia is common. Hypercalcemia and hypophosphatemia are seen with primary hyperparathyroidism; secondary hyperparathyroidism may be associated with a low serum calcium and an elevated serum phosphate. Hyperchloremic acidosis and hypokalemia accompany renal tubular acidosis.

A plain x-ray will reveal punctate calcifications in the papillae of the kidneys. Calyceal or pelvic stones may also be noted. This calcification may have to be differentiated from renal tuberculosis and medullary sponge kidney.

The complications include renal damage caused by the calcifications and renal and ureteral calculi. Chronic renal infection may complicate the primary disease.

The primary cause should be treated, if possible (eg, parathyroidectomy). Discontinue vitamin D, give a low-calcium diet, and force fluids. With hyperchlore-mic acidosis, replace base to decrease hypercalciuria; give a 50% solution of potassium citrate, 4–8 ml 4 times a day, in order to alkalinize the urine.

If nephrocalcinosis is secondary to primary renal disease, the outlook is poor. If the cause is correctable and renal function is fairly good, the prognosis is more favorable.

Dretler SP & others: The physiologic approach to renal tubular acidosis. J Urol 102:665–669, 1969.

Pyrah LN, Hodgkinson A: Nephrocalcinosis. Brit J Urol 32:361–373, 1960.

TRAUMA

1. INJURIES TO THE KIDNEY

Essentials of Diagnosis

- History or evidence of trauma, usually local.
- Hematuria.
- Mass in the flank.
- Failure of visualization of kidney or urinary extravasation on excretory urography.

General Considerations

Renal injury is not common, but it is potentially serious and is often accompanied by injury to other organs or structures. The most common causes are athletics and industrial or automobile accidents. The degree of injury may range from mere bruising to complete laceration of the parenchyma or even rupture of the renal pedicle.

Clinical Findings

A. Symptoms and Signs: Gross hematuria following trauma means injury to the urinary tract. Pain and tenderness over the renal area may be significant, but they could be due to injury to osseous or muscular structures. Shock is common with multiple injuries or brisk bleeding from a lacerated kidney. It is accompanied by oliguria. Nausea, vomiting, and abdominal distention (ileus) are the rule. Bruising may be noted over the costovertebral area. A mass in the flank may represent extravasation of blood, urine, or both. This is best judged by percussion. Other injuries should be sought.

B. Laboratory Findings: Serial hematocrit determinations will give clues to persistent bleeding. Hematuria is to be expected.

C. X-Ray Findings: A plain film may reveal a large area of grayness in the region of the injured organ. Bowel gas may be displaced from that area. Evidence of fractures may be noted. Excretory urograms (high dose of radiopaque medium in the face of hypotension) may show a reasonably normal kidney if mildly contused, or extensive extravasation of the radiopaque material with laceration. Nonfunction suggests the possibility of injury to the vascular pedicle. The greatest value of excretory urograms lies in demonstrating that the contralateral kidney is normal; emergency removal of the injured kidney would then be feasible. Retrograde urograms are seldom necessary. Angiography may prove useful in selected cases.

Differential Diagnosis

Bony fractures or contusion of soft tissues in the region of the kidney may cause confusion. Hematuria might be secondary to vesical injury. The absence of a perirenal mass and normal urograms and radioisotope scans would rule out renal trauma.

Complications

A. Early: The most important complication is continuing perirenal hemorrhage, which can reach the stage of exsanguination. Serial hematocrit, blood pressure, and pulse determinations are essential. Evidence of an enlarging mass in the flank implies persistent bleeding. In the majority of cases, bleeding stops spontaneously, probably as a result of the tamponade effect of the perirenal fascia. Secondary bleeding 1 or 2 weeks later is occasionally observed. Spontaneous infection of the perirenal hematoma may occur.

B. Late: Excretory urograms should be obtained 3–6 months after surgery to observe for progressive hydronephrosis from ureteral obstruction or progressive atrophy due to vascular injury; this may cause hypertension.

Treatment

A. Emergency Measures: Treat shock and hemorrhage with blood transfusions. Bed rest is indicated until hematuria stops.

B. Surgical Measures: Most injured kidneys cease to bleed and heal without surgical intervention. Persistent bleeding requires exploration. A laceration may be sutured; nephrectomy or partial nephrectomy may be indicated.

C. Complications: Perinephric infection requires drainage. Nephrectomy or repair of secondary ureteral obstruction may be necessary.

Prognosis

Most injured kidneys heal spontaneously, although the patient must be examined at intervals for the onset of hypertension (renal ischemia) or progressive hydronephrosis due to secondary ureteral stricture.

Lang EK & others: Arteriographic assessment of injury resulting from renal trauma: An analysis of 74 patients. J Urol 106:1–8, 1971.

Morrow JW, Mendez R: Renal trauma. J Urol 104:649–653, 1970.

Morse TS & others: Kidney injuries in children. J Urol 89:539–547, 1967.

Vermillion CD, McLaughlin AP, Pfister RC: Management of blunt renal trauma. J Urol 106:478–484, 1971.

2. INJURIES TO THE URETER

Essentials of Diagnosis

- Anuria, prolonged ileus, or flank pain following pelvic operation.
- Onset of urinary drainage through wound or vagina.
- Demonstration of urinary extravasation or ureteral obstruction by urography.

General Considerations

Most ureteral injuries follow extensive operations in the pelvis, eg, gynecologic procedures. A few follow cystoscopic ureteral manipulation. One ureter may inadvertently be sutured without evident complications, although progressive hydronephrosis develops. Division of the ureter will cause urinary extravasation, which usually results in a urinary fistula.

Clinical Findings

A. Symptoms and Signs: If the accident is not recognized at surgery, the patient may complain of flank and lower abdominal pain on the injured side. Ileus may be marked. Pyelonephritis may develop. Later, urine may drain through the wound or vagina. Anuria following pelvic surgery means bilateral ureteral ligation until proved otherwise. Rebound tenderness may be found if urine leaks into the peritoneal cavity. Leakage of urine into the deep vagina may be noted.

B. Laboratory Findings: Tests of renal function will be normal unless both ureters are occluded.

C. X-Ray Findings: Excretory urograms may show evidence of ureteral occlusion. Extravasation of radiopaque fluid may be seen in the region of the ureter. Retrograde urography will depict the site and nature of the injury (Fig 44–9).

Differential Diagnosis

Peritonitis may be mimicked if urine leaks into the peritoneal cavity. Excretory urography will reveal the ureteral involvement.

Oliguria may be due to dehydration, transfusion reaction, or bilateral incomplete ureteral injury. A survey of fluid and electrolyte intake and output, including serial body weights, should prove definitive. Total anuria implies bilateral ureteral injury and indicates the need for urologic investigation.

Vesicovaginal and ureterovaginal fistulas may be confused. Methylene blue solution instilled into the bladder will stain the vaginal urine in the former. Cystoscopy will visualize the vesical defect. Retrograde urography should reveal the ureteral fistula.

Complications

These include urinary fistula, ureteral stenosis with hydronephrosis, renal infection, peritonitis, and uremia (with bilateral injury).

Prevention

In the presence of large pelvic masses wherein the

ureters may be dislocated, preoperative indwelling ureteral catheters should be placed for easy identification at surgery.

Treatment

A. Accident Recognized at Surgery:

1. Ureteral division—Repair of a ureter inadvertently cut during surgery consists of anastomosis of the ends over an indwelling T tube or 2 catheters; reimplanting the ureter into the bladder if the injury is juxtavesical; or implanting the end of the injured ureter into the side of the other ureter.

2. Ureteral ligation—Remove the suture. To prevent late necrosis, excise the injured segment and anastomose the ureteral ends over a splint.

B. Accident Discovered After Surgery: Early intervention is recommended. Depending on the findings, the following procedures may be utilized: end-to-end anastomosis, reimplantation into the bladder, transureteroureterostomy, and replacement of a long ureteral segment with an isolated ileal segment. Nephrectomy may be indicated if the contralateral kidney is normal.

Prognosis

The results are best if the injury is recognized at the time of surgery. Late repair, if severe periureteral fibrosis has developed is less likely to afford a good outcome.

Carlton CE Jr, Scott R Jr, Guthrie AG: The initial management of ureteral injuries: A report of 78 cases. J Urol 105:335–340, 1971.

Lee RA, Symmonds RE: Ureterovaginal fistula. Am J Obst Gynec 109:1032–1035, 1971.

3. INJURIES TO THE BLADDER

Essentials of Diagnosis

- History of trauma (including surgical and endoscopic).
- Fracture of the pelvis.
- Suprapubic pain and muscle rigidity.
- Hematuria.

General Considerations

The most common cause of vesical injury is external force over a full bladder. Rupture of the organ is seen in 15% of patients with pelvic fracture. The bladder may be inadvertently opened during pelvic surgery or injured by cystoscopic maneuvers, eg, transurethral resection of vesical tumor. If intraperitoneal, free extravasation of blood and urine will supervene, leading to signs of peritonitis. If extravesical, a mass will develop in the pelvis.

Clinical Findings

A. Symptoms and Signs: There is usually a history of local trauma. Hematuria is to be expected. Low abdominal pain is the rule. With severe trauma, the patient may be in shock. There is suprapubic tenderness and muscle rigidity. With intraperitoneal extra-

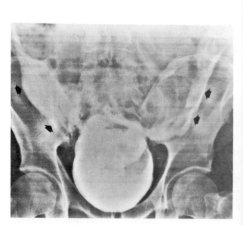
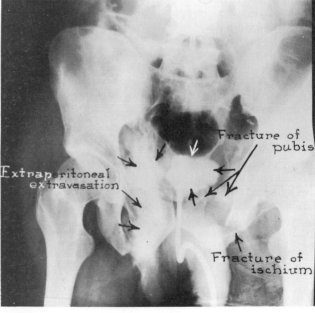

FIG 44–8. Vesical injuries. *Left:* Retrograde cystogram showing intraperitoneal extravasation. Note radiopaque material in both lumbar gutters. *Right:* Retrograde cystogram showing extraperitoneal rupture of the bladder secondary to fracture of the pelvis.

vasation, rebound tenderness may be elicited. With extraperitoneal injury, a mass may be felt or percussed in the suprapubic area.

B. Laboratory Findings: Progressive bleeding may be reflected by a falling hematocrit. Hematuria is to be expected if the patient can void at all.

C. X-Ray Findings: A plain film may reveal fracture of the pelvis. An extraperitoneal collection of blood and urine may be revealed by a large gray area in the vesical area. Excretory urograms will survey the kidneys for damage. Extravasation of radiopaque fluid may be noted in the extravesical space or peritoneal cavity. The bladder may be compressed by a surrounding mass. A cystogram will almost always reveal escape of the fluid outside the bladder (Fig 44–8).

Differential Diagnosis

Renal injury is also associated with trauma and usually presents with hematuria. Excretory urograms show changes compatible with trauma; the cystogram is negative.

Injury to the membranous urethra can mimic extraperitoneal rupture of the bladder. With avulsion of the urethra, a catheter will be arrested in its passage. A urethrogram will reveal the site of injury.

Treatment

A. Emergency Measures: Treat shock and hemorrhage.

B. Specific Measures: For extraperitoneal rupture, drain the site of injury and insert a cystostomy tube. For intraperitoneal rupture, close the rent transperitoneally and drain the bladder by cystostomy. Injury to other organs should be sought.

Prognosis

Early diagnosis and treatment lead to a low morbidity and mortality.

Cullum PA: Rupture of the male bladder and posterior urethra following external violence. Brit J Surg 54:258–265, 1967.

Flaherty JJ & others: Relationship of pelvic bone fracture patterns to injuries of urethra and bladder. J Urol 99:297–300, 1968.

4. INJURIES TO THE URETHRA

Membranous Urethra

This injury is commonly associated with pelvic fracture. Urinary extravasation and bleeding are periprostatic and perivesical. Urethral bleeding may be noted. With complete avulsion, voiding will lead to urinary extravasation. A suprapubic mass may develop. Rectal examination may reveal upward dislocation of the prostate.

The degree of bleeding may lower the hematocrit.

If the patient can void, the urine will be found to contain red cells. A plain x-ray film usually reveals a fractured pelvis. A retrograde urethrogram will show extravasation at the site of injury. If a catheter can be passed to the bladder, the injury is minor.

Differentiation from vesical injury is made by urethrography and cystography. Injury to the bulbous urethra leads to perineal extravasation; injury to the membranous portion causes extravasation above the urogenital diaphragm (Fig 44–11).

Bleeding may be severe, requiring prompt replacement. Late complications include urethral stricture at the site of healing and impotence as a result of damage to local nerves.

If a catheter passes readily to the bladder, it should be left in for 10–14 days. If the urethra is completely avulsed, the area should be exposed surgically and the ends of the urethra anastomosed over a catheter. Postoperative urethrograms should be made in search of evidence of late stricture. There is no treatment for the impotence.

The prognosis must be guarded because of the frequent occurrence of late stricture, which will require appropriate therapy.

Bulbous Urethra

Injuries to the bulbous urethra may occur as a result of instrumentation or, more commonly, falling astride an object. Urethral contusion may merely cause a perineal hematoma without injury to the urethral wall. Laceration will lead to urinary extravasation.

A history of perineal injury can usually be obtained. Local pain and some urethral bleeding are to be expected. Sudden swelling in the perineum may develop on attempt at urination. Examination reveals a perineal mass; extravasation of blood and urine involves the penis and scrotum and may spread onto the abdominal wall.

A catheter may pass to the bladder if the injury is minor but not if a severe laceration is present. The latter can be demonstrated by urethrography.

If the patient can void well and the perineal hematoma is small, no treatment is necessary. If the caliber of the urinary stream diminishes later, the urethra should be explored for stricture. If the injury is more severe and a catheter can be passed to the bladder, it should be left in for 10 days. Drainage of a large hematoma may be indicated.

If a catheter cannot be passed, surgical repair over an indwelling catheter will be necessary. If urinary extravasation is extensive, drainage will be required. If infected, appropriate antibiotics should be administered. If the patient has suffered multiple injuries and is in a state of shock, suprapubic cystostomy should be considered. Later, repair can be accomplished.

The only serious complication is stricture, which will require urethral dilatations.

Pendulous Urethra

External injury to this portion of the urethra is not common since the penis tends to "ride with the blow." The erect organ, however, is not so protected. Most trauma to this area is secondary to instrumentation. As a rule these injuries are mild, although a few may be complicated by stricture.

Some urethral bleeding and penile swelling are to be expected. The history of local injury is clear. A urethrogram may reveal the site and degree of injury.

If voiding is normal, no treatment is required. A large hematoma may be an indication for drainage. If a catheter cannot be passed, surgical repair over an indwelling catheter should be done.

Blumberg N: Anterior urethral injuries. J Urol 102:210–213, 1969.

Gibson GR: Impotence following fractured pelvis and ruptured urethra. Brit J Urol 42:86–88, 1970.

Kaiser TF, Farrow FC: Injuries of the bladder and prostatomembraneous urethra associated with fracture of the bony pelvis. Surg Gynec Obst 120:97–112, 1965.

Reid RE, Herman JR: Rupture of the bladder and urethra: Diagnosis and treatment. New York J Med 65:2685–2696, 1965.

5. INJURIES TO THE PENIS

The penis may be injured by a penetrating object or by a blow when the organ is erect. A constricting steel washer or rubber band can lead to gangrene. The skin of the penis may be avulsed if caught in machinery. The corpora cavernosa may be ruptured, leading to considerable extravasation of blood which can spread to the penis, scrotum, perineum, and abdominal wall. Occasionally, the urethra may be injured as well.

Constricting bodies must be removed. Avulsion of skin may require grafting. If a corpus cavernosum has been ruptured, suture of its tunica albuginea will be necessary.

Kendall AR, Karafin L: Repair of the denuded penis. J Urol 98:484–486, 1967.

Meares EM Jr: Traumatic rupture of the corpus cavernosum. J Urol 105:407–408, 1971.

6. INJURIES TO THE TESTIS

Because of their mobility, the testes are seldom injured. If traumatized, pain is severe and there may be nausea and vomiting. Shock may result. The organ may be merely contused, but can undergo complete rupture, in which case bleeding into the tunica vaginalis occurs, leading to marked swelling. In case of doubt, exploration should be done and lacerations closed. A few testes, seriously injured, may later undergo atrophy.

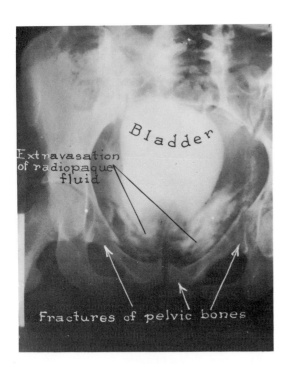 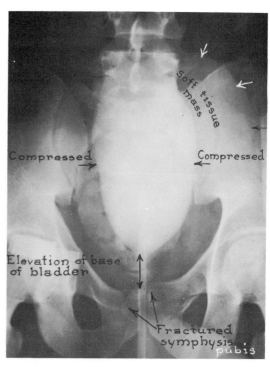

FIG 44–9. Injury to the membranous urethra. *Left:* Retrograde cystogram showing periprostatic extravasation; laceration of membranous urethra with fracture of pelvis. *Right:* Retrograde cystogram showing elevation and lateral compression of bladder due to periprostatic and perivesical extravasation of blood and urine; laceration of membranous urethra from fracture of pelvis.

Merricks JW, Papierniak FB: Traumatic rupture of the testicle. J Urol 103:77–79, 1970.

TUMORS OF THE GENITOURINARY TRACT

1. TUMORS OF THE KIDNEY*

Essentials of Diagnosis

- Painless gross hematuria.
- Enlarged, firm kidney.
- Urographic evidence of vascular renal tumor.

General Considerations

Benign renal tumors are rare. Although lymphomatous or metastatic tumors occasionally involve the kidneys, by far the most common malignant neoplasm is adenocarcinoma. Adenocarcinoma arises from renal tubular cells, and as it expands it displaces calyces, blood vessels, and the renal pelvis. It is these characteristics that lead to urographic diagnosis. Later, the renal vein and even the vena cava may be occluded by tumor cells. Intraperitoneal organs may be displaced or invaded by the tumor.

The tumor has a pseudocapsule, and its cells resemble tubular cells. This tumor most commonly metastasizes to the liver, lungs, long bones, and regional lymph nodes.

Clinical Findings

A. Symptoms and Signs: Painless gross hematuria is the most common symptom. Pain is a late manifestation and is apt to be caused by hemorrhage into the tumor. The patient may discover a flank mass. Symptoms from metastasis may be the primary complaint, eg, loss of weight, anemia, bone pain (at times with spontaneous fracture), and pulmonary difficulties.

If the tumor is large, it may be easily palpable. It is nontender, firm, and may be nodular. With local invasion, it is fixed on respiration. Swelling over a bone may represent a metastasis. The liver may be enlarged and nodular.

B. Laboratory Findings: Gross or microscopic hematuria is usual. Erythrocytosis is seen in a few patients, and anemia is usually present in advanced disease. Total renal function is usually normal. The sedimentation rate is elevated in most cases. Hypercalcemia is at times observed.

C. X-Ray Findings: A plain abdominal film may reveal an enlarged kidney or a definite bulge of one portion. Osseous metastases may be seen on a skeletal series. Excretory urograms show evidence of a space-occupying lesion typified by bending and displacement of calyces, and possibly an indentation of the renal

*Wilms's tumor is discussed in Chapter 49, Pediatric Surgery.

pelvis (Fig 44–10). Visualization may be poor if most of the kidney is involved or if the renal vein is occluded by tumor. In the latter instance, retrograde urograms may be needed to afford necessary calyceal detail.

Nephrotomography may reveal increased density of the mass because of its vascularity. A cyst, from which tumor must be differentiated, will be revealed by lack of opacification. Angiography, particularly by the selective technic, will reveal typical tumor vessels

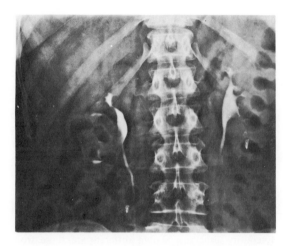

FIG 44–10. Adenocarcinoma of the kidney. Excretory urogram. Distortion of the pelvis and the middle and lower calyces of the right kidney. The left kidney is normal.

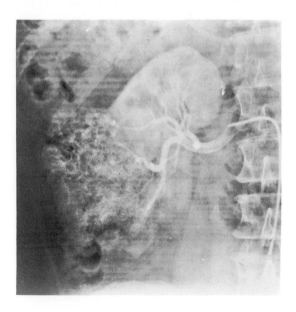

FIG 44–11. Adenocarcinoma of the kidney. Selective renal angiogram showing marked vascularity of mass in lower portion of right kidney typical of malignant tumor.

in the capillary phase and increased opacification in the venous phase (Fig 44–11). Venacavography and selective renal phlebography will portray invasion of these structures.

A chest film is essential since pulmonary metastases are common.

D. Isotope Scanning: The ^{203}Hg scan will portray a tumor as a "cold" area but does not differentiate from cyst. The gamma camera, however, will reveal the vascularity of the mass with ^{99m}Tc infusion.

E. Instrumental Examination: If the patient has gross hematuria when seen, immediate cystoscopy should be performed to identify the source of bleeding (renal or vesical).

Differential Diagnosis

Other renal lesions may present as a mass in the flank, including hydronephrosis and polycystic disease. Radiographic technics afford differentiation.

Renal cyst causes urographic changes similar to tumor, but steps taken to reveal vascularity of the mass (nephrotomography, angiography) lead to the proper diagnosis. In case of doubt, the cyst can be aspirated, then filled with radiopaque fluid. If the fluid is bloody, tumor should be expected. If clear, it should be subjected to cytologic study.

Lesions that also cause hematuria are stone; renal pelvic, ureteral, and vesical neoplasm; and tuberculosis. Excretory urograms should differentiate these from renal parenchymal tumor. In the case of vesical tumor, cystoscopy will be definitive.

Complications

These are usually related to local invasion or metastases. A few patients develop hydronephrosis from ureteral compression or hypertension from interference with renal blood supply. Occlusion of the renal vein may cause findings compatible with the nephrotic syndrome.

Treatment

A. Nephrectomy: In the absence of demonstrable metastases, radical nephrectomy is indicated.

B. X-Ray Therapy: These tumors are ordinarily radioresistant, but radiotherapy may have value in the palliative treatment of osseous metastases.

C. Chemotherapy: The administration of medroxyprogesterone (Depo-Provera), 1000 mg/week IM), may have some palliative effect, but in general chemotherapy has been disappointing.

Prognosis

About 35% of nephrectomized patients are alive at 5 years, but metastases may become evident 10–15 years later. The prognosis is poor if the renal vein is involved by tumor.

Aron BS, Gross M: Renal adenocarcinoma in infancy and childhood: Evaluation of therapy and prognosis. J Urol 102:497–503, 1969.

Cox CE & others: Renal adenocarcinoma: 28-year review, with emphasis on rationale and feasibility of preoperative radiotherapy. J Urol 104:53–61, 1970.

Folin J: Angiography in renal tumors: Its value in diagnosis and differential diagnosis as a complement to conventional methods. Acta radiol, Suppl 267, 1967.

McCoy RM, Klatte EC, Rhamy RK: Use of inferior venacavography in the evaluation of renal neoplasms. J Urol 102:556–559, 1969.

Rafla S: Renal cell carcinoma: Natural history and results of treatment. Cancer 25:26–40, 1970.

Wagh DG, Murphy GP: Hormonal therapy in advanced renal cell carcinoma. Cancer 28:318–321, 1971.

Warren MM, Kelalis PP, Utz DC: The changing concept of hypernephroma. J Urol 104:376–379, 1970.

2. TUMORS OF THE RENAL PELVIS

Histologically, these tumors are similar to those seen in the ureter and bladder. They comprise about 10% of renal neoplasms. Benign tumors are very rare. Satellite tumors may involve the ureter. The rare epidermoid carcinoma is associated with chronic infection, and often with calculi. Such tumors may obstruct the ureteropelvic junction. The more malignant types may invade the renal parenchyma. These tumors metastasize to regional lymph nodes. Almost all are transitional cell carcinomas. The metabolites of tryptophan are suspect as carcinogenic agents.

Clinical Findings

A. Symptoms and Signs: Gross painless hematuria is the usual initial symptom. There may be flank pain if the tumor is obstructive.

B. Laboratory Findings: Hematuria is to be expected. Cytologic study discloses malignant cells in the urine in a high percentage of cases.

C. X-Ray Findings: Excretory or retrograde urograms will show a space-occupying lesion in the pelvis displacing the radiopaque medium (Fig 44–12). Secondary ureteral growths may be seen.

D. Instrumental Examination: Cystoscopy must be done immediately if there is gross hematuria so that its source can be identified. Such examination may reveal satellite tumors near the ureteral orifice.

Differential Diagnosis

Adenocarcinoma of the kidney usually presents with hematuria also, but urography should show the intrarenal position of the mass.

A nonopaque renal stone (ie, uric acid) may simulate renal pelvic tumor on urograms. Cytology is negative. The differential diagnosis may be made only at the operating table.

Renal tuberculosis may show an obliterated calyx, thus simulating an invasive pelvic neoplasm. Other calyces, however, may show ulceration. Sterile pyuria and a positive urine culture for tubercle bacilli will make the differentiation.

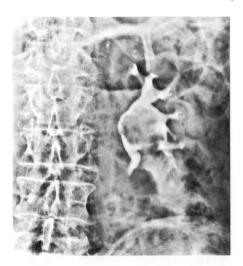

FIG 44–12. Excretory urogram showing space-occupying lesion of left renal pelvis. Transitional cell carcinoma.

Complications

Rarely, hemorrhage may be so severe as to require immediate nephrectomy. Obstruction may lead to secondary infection.

Treatment

Nephroureterectomy plus removal of a cuff of bladder around the ureteral orifice should be done, for satellite tumors in the ureter and bladder may develop later. These tumors are somewhat resistant to radiotherapy.

Prognosis

With low-grade malignancies, the cure rate is about 75%. The outlook is poor with the more anaplastic neoplasms.

Grabstald H, Whitmore WF, Melamed MR: Renal pelvic tumors. JAMA 218:845–854, 1971.

Poole-Wilson DS: Occupational tumours of the renal pelvis and ureter arising in dye-making industry. Proc Roy Soc Med 62:93–94, 1968.

Schapira HE, Mitty HA: Tumors of the renal pelvis: Clinical review with emphasis on selective angiography. J Urol 106:642–645, 1971.

3. TUMORS OF THE URETER

Tumors of the ureter are seldom benign. They may be found in association with transitional cell tumors of the renal pelvis or bladder. Carcinogens are suspect as the etiologic factor (see Tumors of the Bladder, General Considerations). Transitional cell carcinomas range from a low to a high grade of malignancy.

The latter are invasive and most commonly metastasize to regional lymph nodes, lungs, and liver.

Clinical Findings

A. Symptoms and Signs: Micro- or macrohematuria is the most common symptom. Should the tumor produce obstruction, renal pain may be noted. Local examination is usually unrewarding; a large hydronephrotic kidney might be palpable.

B. Laboratory Findings: Hematuria is usually found. Anemia may be noted if bleeding has been severe or if metastases are widespread. Tests of renal function are normal if the disease is unilateral.

C. X-Ray Findings: Excretory urograms portray a space-occupying lesion in the ureter (Fig 44–13). The ureter may be dilated proximal to that point. Evidence of tumor of the renal pelvis should also be sought. A chest film should be examined for evidence of metastasis. If the kidney is nonfunctioning, a retrograde ureterogram is essential to delineate the lesion.

D. Instrumental Examination: Any patient who presents with gross hematuria should immediately undergo cystoscopy to identify the source of bleeding. Bloody efflux from a ureteral orifice requires further study of the upper urinary tract. Occasionally, the

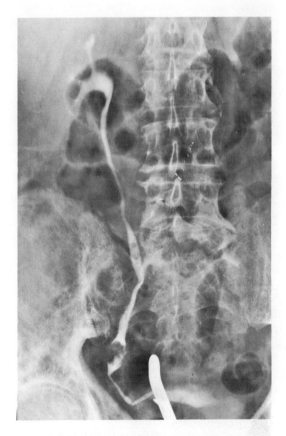

FIG 44–13. Retrograde urogram showing "negative" shadow caused by transitional cell carcinoma of the lower right ureter without evidence of obstruction.

tumor can be seen protruding from the ureteral orifice.

E. **Urinary Cytology**: Cytologic examination of urine sediment shows cancer cells in well over 90% of patients with transitional cell tumors (renal pelvis, ureter, bladder).

Differential Diagnosis

A radiolucent ureteral stone can mimic the signs and symptoms of ureteral tumor. The excretory (or retrograde) urogram will reveal a "negative" shadow in each. Cytology is negative with stone. At times, the definitive diagnosis is made at the operating table.

Ureteral stenosis—usually due to external compression by a blood vessel or lymph nodes involved by cancer—may cause similar symptoms, signs, and x-ray findings. Negative cytology and evidence of a primary site of metastases should lead to the differentiation.

Complications

Hydronephrosis may develop secondary to an obstructing tumor. The stasis that results may lead to infection.

Treatment

In the absence of metastases, complete nephroureterectomy plus removal of the periureteral vesical area is indicated in order to prevent "seeding" of the ureter below the lesion and in the bladder. Nephroureterectomy may be needed even in advanced cases if pain or severe hematuria becomes disabling.

Prognosis

The outlook for the patient with a tumor of low-grade malignancy is good. Those with highly malignant tumors seldom live 2 years after definitive surgery.

Bloom NA, Vidone RA, Lytton B: Primary carcinoma of the ureter: A report of 102 new cases. J Urol 103:590–598, 1970.

Hawtrey CE: Fifty-two cases of primary ureteral carcinoma: A clinical-pathologic study. J Urol 105:188–193, 1971.

4. TUMORS OF THE BLADDER

Essentials of Diagnosis

- Hematuria.
- Symptoms of cystitis.
- Renal pain.
- Positive urinary cytology.
- Cystoscopic visualization and positive biopsy.

General Considerations

Most vesical neoplasms are transitional cell in type. Both the prognosis and the type of treatment indicated depend upon the degree of differentiation of the cells and the depth of penetration of the tumor in the bladder. Low-grade tumors (I and II) tend to be superficial, whereas grade III and IV tumors are more invasive and are usually found in the muscle layer. The higher the grade and the more invasive, the poorer the prognosis. Low-grade superficial tumors respond well to transurethral technics; high-grade invasive tumors require radiotherapy or radical surgery or both.

Most vesical tumors develop in the posterior half of the bladder (trigonal region). Occlusion of a ureteral orifice, leading to hydronephrosis, is therefore not uncommon. An ulcerated tumor not only tends to bleed but may become secondarily infected. Even some of the low-grade tumors tend to "seed" in other parts of the bladder.

Rarer tumors include squamous cell carcinoma, adenocarcinoma (in a urachal remnant), and rhabdomyosarcoma (mostly in children).

It has long been established that prolonged exposure to certain industrial aromatic amines is associated with a high incidence of vesical neoplasia. Recent work suggests that multiple transitional cell tumors are probably caused by carcinogens, particularly tryptophan, which is changed in the urinary tract to orthophenols which have proved to be carcinogenic in dogs and mice. Smoking increases the amount of these substances in the urine. On cessation of smoking, the levels return to normal.

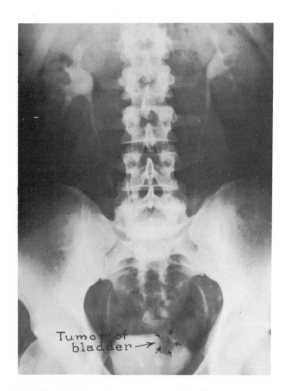

FIG 44–14. Excretory urogram showing space-occupying lesion (transitional cell carcinoma) on the left side of the bladder; the upper tracts are normal.

Clinical Findings

A. Symptoms and Signs: Gross hematuria is the most common complaint. Secondary infection leads to symptoms of cystitis. Should the tumor involve the vesical neck, symptoms of urinary obstruction may supervene. Extravesical extension may cause constant suprapubic pain. If the tumor occludes a ureteral orifice, renal pain may develop; if both are overgrown, uremia results.

In most cases, nothing abnormal is found on physical examination. An extensive tumor may be palpable suprapubically, vaginally, or rectally. Bimanual palpation (abdominovaginal or rectal) may reveal a palpable mass and evidence of fixation (invasion). This is best done under anesthesia.

B. Laboratory Findings: Anemia (secondary to uremia or hemorrhage) may be present. Red cells are usually found in the urine. Pyuria and bacteriuria are common. Renal function tests are normal unless bilateral ureteral obstruction has developed.

C. X-Ray Findings: Excretory urograms are usually normal, but the tumor may be depicted as a "negative" shadow (Fig 44–14). Ureteral occlusion will be reflected by the presence of hydroureteronephrosis. Vesical angiography may prove helpful in judging the presence of invasion of the extravesical tissues.

D. Instrumental Examination: Cystoscopy is the definitive test since the tumor is readily visualized (Fig 44–15). Biopsy is mandatory.

E. Cytology: Papanicolaou preparations are almost diagnostic.

Differential Diagnosis

Vesical neoplasm is differentiated from other causes of hematuria by cystoscopy, urography, and cytologic examination.

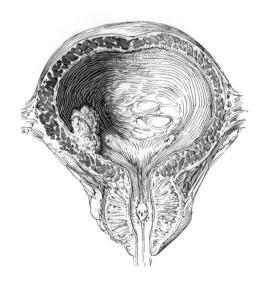

FIG 44–15. Transitional cell (papillary) carcinoma of the bladder with minimal invasion of the bladder wall.

Complications

Secondary vesical infection is common when the tumor becomes ulcerated. Hydroureteronephrosis is the product of invasion of the intravesical ureter. The degree of hemorrhage may become a problem.

Prevention

Contact with analine dyes should be limited to 3 years, during which time urinary cytologic studies and periodic cystoscopy are indicated.

Treatment

A. Surgical Measures: Most single or multiple superficial tumors can be cured by deep saucerization of the vesical wall with the resectoscope. However, this method will fail if the tumor has invaded deeply. Wide partial cystectomy may be utilized for tumors involving the dome. Total cystectomy (with removal of the prostate) may be indicated for papillomatosis and for high grade invasive tumors. Urinary diversion is then necessary, eg, uretero-ileal cutaneous conduit or ureterosigmoidostomy.

B. Radiation Therapy: The more undifferentiated the tumor, the more radiosensitive it is. Radiotherapy is particularly useful for high-grade invasive neoplasms. A dosage of 6000 rads given over a period of 6 weeks preserves vesical function. If recurrence of the tumor is discovered 3 months after therapy, total cystectomy is feasible.

C. Chemotherapy: The effects of parenterally administered chemotherapeutic agents have been disappointing. Superficial low-grade tumors may be controlled or even disappear with thiotepa instillations. Sixty mg are dissolved in 30–60 ml of normal saline. Instillations by catheter are made weekly for 4–6 weeks. Monthly treatment should then be given for 6–10 months. Before each instillation, a white cell and platelet count should be obtained. If the white count is less than $4000/\mu l$ or the platelets below $100,000/\mu l$, treatment should be deferred until the hemogram improves.

Prognosis

Superficial, well-differentiated tumors may recur or new papillomas may appear. Periodic urinary cytologic examination and cystoscopy should be done for at least 3 years. The low-grade tumors afford the best prognosis. The more undifferentiated invasive tumors are controlled by cystectomy or radiation therapy in 15–20% of cases.

Barnes RW & others: Control of bladder tumors by endoscopic surgery. J Urol 97:864–868, 1967.

Caldwell WL, Bagshaw MA, Kaplan AS: Efficacy of linear accelerator x-ray therapy in cancer of the bladder. J Urol 97:294–303, 1967.

Jarman WD, Kenealy JC: Polypoid rhabdomyosarcoma of the bladder in children. J Urol 103:227–231, 1970.

Lerman RI, Hutter RV, Whitmore WF Jr: Papilloma of the urinary bladder. Cancer 25:333–342, 1970.

Poole-Wilson DS, Barnard RJ: Total cystectomy for bladder tumours. Brit J Urol 43:16–24, 1971.

Powel-Smith CJ, Reid EC: Preoperative irradiation and radical cystectomy in carcinoma of the bladder. Cancer 25:781–786, 1970.

Rubin P & others: Cancer of the urogenital tract: Bladder cancer. JAMA 206:1761–1776, 2719–2728, 1968.

Veenema RJ & others: Thiotepa bladder instillations: Therapy and prophylaxis for superficial bladder tumors. J Urol 101:711–715, 1969.

Whitmore WF Jr & others: Preoperative irradiation with cystectomy in the management of bladder cancer. Am J Roentgenol 102:570–576, 1968.

5. BENIGN PROSTATIC HYPERPLASIA

Essentials of Diagnosis

- Prostatism: hesitancy, slow stream, terminal dribbling, frequency.
- Residual urine.
- Acute urinary retention.
- Uremia in advanced cases.

General Considerations

The cause of benign prostatic enlargement is not known, but it is probably related to estrogen-androgen imbalance. Hyperplasia of the prostatic lobes causes increased outflow resistance, largely by upsetting the mechanism for opening and funneling the vesical neck at the time of voiding. This creates a need for a higher intravesical voiding pressure to accomplish voiding, which in turn causes hypertrophy of the vesical and trigonal muscles. This may lead to the development of vesical diverticula, which represent outpocketings of vesical mucosa through the detrusor muscle bundles. Hypertrophy of the trigone causes an abnormal degree of traction upon the intravesical ureter, leading to its functional obstruction and resulting in hydroureteronephrosis. In late cases, ureterovesical reflux may develop.

Stagnation of urine leads to the complication of infection; the onset of cystitis will exacerbate the obstructive symptoms. Pyelonephritis will only occur if there is reflux of infected urine from the bladder.

The lobes that most commonly undergo enlargement are the 2 lateral lobes and the subcervical lobe.

The prostate of the young adult has an anatomic capsule like an apple peel. In the man with prostatic enlargement, there is a thick "surgical" capsule similar to an orange peel composed of peripherally compressed prostatic tissue. This permits intracapsular enucleation of the enlarged lobes (Fig 44–16).

Clinical Findings

A. Symptoms and Signs: Typically, the patient notices hesitancy and loss of force and caliber of the stream. Terminal dribbling is particularly disturbing. The complication of infection increases the degree of obstructive symptoms and is often associated with burning on urination. Acute urinary retention may supervene. This is associated with severe urgency,

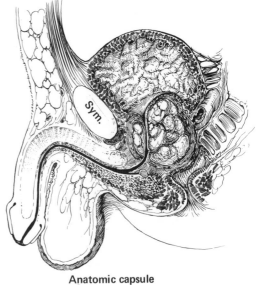

Anatomic capsule

Posterior prostatic lobe

FIG 44–16. Pathogenesis of benign prostatic hyperplasia. Enlarged prostate enclosed by relatively thick "surgical" capsule which is composed of the posterior prostatic lobe.

suprapubic pain, and a palpable bladder.

The size of the prostate is not of diagnostic importance since the correlation between the size of the gland and the degree of symptoms and amount of residual urine is poor.

B. Laboratory Findings: Urinalysis may reveal evidence of infection. The PSP test may show an excretion curve compatible with residual urine or impaired renal function. The serum creatinine may be elevated in cases with prolonged severe obstruction.

C. X-Ray Findings: Excretory urograms are usually normal but may show hydroureteronephrosis if significant obstruction is present. This is usually due to an abnormal pull on the intravesical ureters by the hypertrophied trigonal muscle; these changes usually revert to normal after prostatectomy. An indentation into the inferior surface of the bladder from the enlarged gland may be seen.

D. Instrumental Examination: The presence of residual urine may be discovered if the patient is catheterized immediately after voiding. Endoscopy will reveal secondary vesical changes (eg, trabeculation) and enlargement of prostatic lobes.

Differential Diagnosis

Neurogenic bladder may offer a similar syndrome. A history suggesting a neurogenic difficulty may be obtained. Neurologic deficit involving S2—4 is particularly significant.

Cancer of the prostate also causes symptoms of vesical neck obstruction. Such a patient may have, in addition, symptoms and signs of osseous metastases. Typically, the cancerous gland is stony hard. Serum acid phosphatase is elevated in advanced cases. Serum alkaline phosphatase is usually increased if the tumor has spread to bone.

Acute prostatitis may cause symptoms of obstruction, but the patient is septic and has infected urine. The prostate is hot and exquisitely tender.

Urethral stricture diminishes the caliber of the urinary stream. There is usually a history of complicated gonorrhea or local trauma. A retrograde urethrogram will show the stenotic area. A stricture arrests the passage of an instrument.

Complications

Obstruction and residual urine lead to vesical and prostatic infection which may be difficult to eradicate. In the few patients with vesicoureteral reflux, pyelonephritis may ensue.

The obstruction may lead to the development of vesical diverticula. Infected residual urine may contribute to the formation of calculi.

Functional obstruction of the intravesical ureter, caused by the hypertrophic trigone, may lead to hydroureteronephrosis.

Treatment

The criteria for operative intervention are impairment of or threat to renal function and symptoms disturbing enough so that the patient demands relief. Because the degree of obstruction progresses slowly if at all in most patients, conservative treatment is usually adequate.

A. Conservative Measures: Regular intercourse or masturbation is the best means of relieving prostatic congestion. If this is not feasible, periodic prostatic massage (3 or 4 times at 2-week intervals) will relieve the congestion and cause some alleviation of symptoms. Should symptoms increase, another series of massages can be given. Treatment of prostatitis may reduce prostatic edema. The resolution of a complicating cystitis will usually afford some relief. In order to protect vesical tone, the patient should be cautioned to void as soon as the urge develops. Forcing fluids over a short period of time, leading to rapid vesical filling, decreases vesical tone and is a common cause of sudden acute urinary retention.

Catheterization is mandatory for acute urinary retention. In most cases, spontaneous voiding will result. If it does not, a catheter should be left indwelling for 3 days while detrusor tone returns to maximum. If this fails, surgery is indicated. If the patient is a very poor operative risk, cryosurgery or a permanent catheter may be necessary.

B. Surgery: Four methods of prostatectomy are available to the surgeon: transurethral, retropubic, suprapubic, and perineal. The type of approach should be left to the judgment of the urologist. The mortality rate is low for all (1—4%). Sexual potency is threatened only when the perineal route is used.

Cryosurgery has its proponents in the poor-risk patient. The place for this procedure in the treatment of the obstructing prostatic hypertrophy remains to be evaluated.

Prognosis

Most patients receive considerable relief following conservative treatment. If, on follow-up, symptoms increase or renal function begins to diminish, surgery is warranted.

Blandy JP: Benign prostatic enlargement. Brit MJ 1:31—35, 1971.

Finestone AJ, Rosenthal RS: Silent prostatism. Geriatrics 26:89—92, 1971.

Gill W & others: An experience with cryoprostatectomy. Surg Gynec Obst 131:877—884, 1970.

Green NA: Cryosurgery of the prostate gland in the unfit subject. Brit J Urol 42:10—20, 1970.

6. CARCINOMA OF THE PROSTATE

Essentials of Diagnosis

- Symptoms of vesical neck obstruction.
- Stony hard prostate.
- Osteoblastic osseous metastases.
- Anemia.

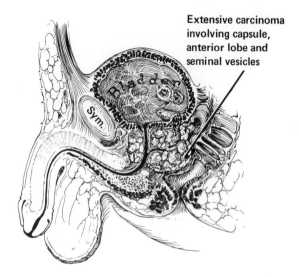

Extensive carcinoma involving capsule, anterior lobe and seminal vesicles

FIG 44—17. Advanced carcinoma of prostate; trabeculation of bladder wall.

- Elevated serum acid phosphatase in advanced cases.

General Considerations

Prostatic cancer is rare before age 60. The cause is not known. Androgens stimulate its growth; estrogens retard it. Most malignancies arise in the posterior lobe, which does not undergo benign enlargement. The early hard lesion is usually found in the lateral sulcus of one lobe. As it progresses, it involves the entire gland and the seminal vesicles (Fig 44–17). Metastasis to the pelvic lymph nodes and the bones of the pelvis is common.

Clinical Findings

A. Symptoms and Signs: The presenting symptoms in 95% of men with prostatic malignancy are due to obstruction, infection, or both. (See Benign Prostatic Hyperplasia, above.) Some patients have symptoms due to metastases also when first seen—eg, low back pain radiating down one or both legs. In a few cases, only the latter are present at onset.

Rectal examination may reveal an isolated hard nodule in the prostate, usually in one of the lateral margins. In advanced cases, the entire gland may be stony hard and fixed. The seminal vesicles may be involved. Signs of metastases include a nodular liver, pathologic fracture, and paraplegia due to sudden collapse of a vertebral body.

B. Laboratory Findings: Anemia may be found in patients whose bone marrow has been replaced by tumor or those with uremia. Urinalysis may reveal infection. In the early stages, renal function is normal, but if ureteral occlusion develops or if there is residual urine, the PSP will be depressed. Serum creatinine may be elevated. Serum acid phosphatase levels are usually increased when the tumor has extended outside its capsule. In the presence of osseous metastases, the alkaline phosphatase is elevated, reflecting osteogenic activity.

C. X-Ray Findings: A chest film may show evidence of metastases to hilar nodes, lungs or ribs. A plain film of the abdomen may reveal osseous spread. The common sites include the pelvic bones, lumbar spine, and femoral heads. Excretory urograms may show hydroureteronephrosis from vesical neck or ureteral obstruction.

D. Isotope Studies: A total body scan may show increased uptake of ^{18}F in areas of bony metastases even before the osteograms reveal such evidence.

E. Instrumental Examination: Passage of a catheter will measure the amount of residual urine. Cystoscopy will reveal the degree of prostatic encroachment and secondary vesical changes, eg, trabeculation. Invasion of the trigone is a late sign.

F. Biopsy: The diagnosis in advanced cases may be established on tissue removed by transurethral resection or needle biopsy. With small localized lesions, these methods may fail. Aspiration of marrow from the iliac crest may reveal tumor cells even though osteograms are normal.

Differential Diagnosis

Benign prostatic hyperplasia lacks the hard areas exhibited by cancer. Bone films and serum phosphatases are normal.

Hard nodules may be caused by scarring secondary to chronic infection, tuberculosis, or calculi. Evidence of tuberculosis, or stones seen in an x-ray of the prostatic area, may be of help. Biopsy should be definitive.

Complications

Significant vesical neck or ureteral obstruction may lead to uremia. Edema of a leg may develop from compression of the iliac vein by metastases to regional lymph nodes. Spontaneous fractures may occur.

Treatment

A. Curative Measures: In the patient with an isolated nodule, and in the absence of demonstrable metastases, radical prostatectomy may lead to cure.

B. Palliative Measures: Antiandrogen therapy has an excellent palliative effect on advanced prostatic cancer, but it has been suggested that estrogens are apt to increase the incidence of thromboembolic phenomena. It is probably best to reserve it for the most advanced cases, eg, urinary retention, osseous metastases. Bilateral orchiectomy (which can be combined with estrogen therapy) is an excellent palliative procedure.

In late cases, medical adrenalectomy—accomplished by the administration of corticosteroids—may afford temporary relief from the pain of metastatic bone lesions. Destruction of the pituitary by the local injection of ^{90}yttrium or by cryotherapy may afford a remission.

Transurethral prostatic resection may be necessary to relieve prostatic obstruction. Cryosurgery has its advocates. Radiation therapy to the gland is being accepted with increasing enthusiasm. The prostate is apt to shrink, thus relieving obstructive symptoms. X-ray therapy to painful osseous metastases may relieve pain.

Prognosis

Radical prostatectomy cures more than 70% of the patients suitable for this operation, but it should be limited to men with a reasonable life expectancy. After age 70, palliative therapy will afford as good a result as radical surgery. This means that only about 5% of patients with prostatic malignancy are curable. Careful rectal examination, seeking suspicious areas of induration, in all men over age 50 is mandatory if this cure rate is to be improved.

Bailar JC III, Byar DP: Estrogen treatment for cancer of the prostate: Early results with 3 doses of diethylstilbestrol and placebo. Cancer 26:257–261, 1970.

Dow JA: The technique of cryosurgery of the prostate. J Urol 105:286–290, 1971.

Corriere NJ Jr, Cornog JL, Murphy JJ: Prognosis in patients with carcinoma of the prostate. Cancer 25:911–918, 1970.

Gilbertsen VA: Cancer of the prostate gland: Results of early diagnosis and therapy undertaken for cure of the disease. JAMA 215:81–84, 1971.

Grant DC & others: Radiation therapy in the treatment of carcinoma of the prostate. J Urol 105:411–415, 1971.

Rubin P: Cancer of the urogenital tract: Prostatic cancer. JAMA 209:1695–1705, 1969.

Rubin P: Cancer of the urogenital tract: Prostatic cancer: Advanced and metastatic. JAMA 210:1072–1081, 1969.

7. SARCOMA OF THE PROSTATE

Sarcoma of the prostate is rare. Half of cases occur in boys under age 5. The tumor is highly malignant and metastasizes to the pelvic and lumbar lymph nodes, lungs, liver, and bone. Symptoms are those of obstruction to urination. The prostate is found to be enlarged. Cystography or excretory urography may show superior displacement of the bladder or encroachment of the tumor into the bladder. Endoscopy will reveal the growth and allows biopsy.

Total prostatocystectomy has cured a few cases. The neoplasm is relatively radioresistant.

Lemmon WT Jr, Holland JM, Ketcham AS: Rhabdomyosarcoma of the prostate. Surgery 59:736–744, 1966.

8. TUMORS OF THE URETHRA

Malignant tumors of the urethra are uncommon. They occur most often in women. Those arising distally are squamous epitheliomas which metastasize to the inguinal nodes. The deeper tumors are transitional cell in type and spread to the lymph nodes in the pelvis. Bleeding on urination or bloody spotting is noted. The growth may be visible at the meatus. The more proximal tumors may cause obstructive symptoms as well. The diagnosis is established by biopsy.

In the female, distal tumors will require resection. In men, penile amputation is necessary. For the most proximal neoplasms, urethrocystectomy is indicated. In general, these tumors are radioresistant.

The prognosis is fair to poor.

Guinn GA, Ayala AG: Male urethral cancer: Report of 15 cases including a primary melanoma. J Urol 103:176–179, 1970.

Zeigerman JH, Gordon SF: Cancer of the female urethra: A curable disease. Obst Gynec 36:785–789, 1970.

9. TUMORS OF THE TESTIS

Essentials of Diagnosis

- Painless, enlarged, firm testis developing between the ages of 18–35.
- Midline abdominal mass (lymph nodes).
- Gynecomastia.

General Considerations

With rare exceptions, all tumors of the testis are malignant. Most are observed between the ages of 18–35. Those containing trophoblastic cells are highly malignant and are associated with gynecomastia and increased levels of urinary chorionic gonadotropins. Most arise from germ cells; seminomas, embryonal carcinomas, and malignant teratomas are the most common. Choriocarcinoma is rare. Testicular tumors metastasize to the lumbar and mediastinal lymph nodes and lungs. Probably 30–40% of patients will have metastases when first seen.

The rarest testicular tumors are Sertoli cell and interstitial cell tumors, and most of these are benign.

Clinical Findings

A. Symptoms and Signs: These tumors usually present as a painless enlargement, although the onset may be painful if spontaneous bleeding occurs. With endocrine-functioning tumors, gynecomastia may be the initial complaint. Symptoms due to metastases include a supraclavicular or upper midline abdominal mass (lymph nodes) or loss of weight and anorexia.

Examination reveals a symmetrically enlarged, firm, nontender organ. Secondary hydrocele is noted in 10% of cases. Gynecomastia may be present. A midline abdominal mass or enlarged Virchow's nodes are evidence of metastases.

B. Laboratory Findings: Analysis of a preoperative sample of urine for chorionic gonadotropins is essential since their elevation reflects a poor prognosis (choriocarcinoma).

C. X-Ray Findings: A chest film may reveal pulmonary or hilar node metastases. Excretory urograms are indicated in all cases to note whether the upper ureter is deviated by the presence of metastases to the lumbar lymph nodes (Fig 44–18). Lymphangiography will reveal evidence of metastases to these nodes.

Differential Diagnosis

Hydrocele presents as a scrotal enlargement. The mass feels cystic and transilluminates. Some tumors, however, are associated with secondary hydrocele. This should be aspirated if the testicle cannot be properly palpated.

Spermatocele is a small cystic mass lying free above the testis. Aspiration will reveal dead sperms.

Should the tumor bleed spontaneously, it may present as a painful swelling, thus being confused with acute epididymitis. The latter usually presents with fever and pyuria. In the early stages, the enlarged, tender epididymis can be delineated from the normal testis. Confusion in this differentiation is a common cause of delayed diagnosis.

Complications

These arise from metastasis. A ureter may be occluded by lumbar nodes, leading to hydronephrosis.

Treatment

A. Surgery: If tumor cannot be ruled out, the testis should be removed. Orchiectomy is performed through an inguinal incision and the spermatic cord divided at the internal ring. The testicle is then delivered from the scrotum and removed. Radical resection of the retroperitoneal lymph nodes is indicated in all cases of embryonal carcinomas, teratocarcinomas, and, possibly, choriocarcinomas. In some, inoperability is discovered.

B. X-Ray Therapy: Radiotherapy is indicated in all cases. Seminomas are highly radiosensitive. For the other types of tumors, radiotherapy is given following lymph node resection. Some surgeons give half the radiation before node dissection and the rest after surgery. X-ray to the mediastinum and neck for prophylactic reasons is probably beneficial.

C. Chemotherapy: Antitumor chemotherapy is utilized in the palliation of metastatic cancer with demonstrable benefit. Triple drug therapy is favored. This usually consists of an alkylating agent (eg, chlorambucil), an antimetabolite (eg, methotrexate), and the antitumor antibiotic dactinomycin. (See Chapter 50.)

Prognosis

Except in the case of seminomas, which are the least malignant and the most radiosensitive testicular tumors, the presence of metastases implies a poor prognosis. In teratocarcinoma or embryonal carcinoma, the 5-year survival is 50%. With few exceptions, patients with choriocarcinoma are dead at 2 years despite intensive therapy.

Castro JR, Gonzalez M: Results in treatment of pure seminoma of the testis. Am J Roentgenol 111:355–359, 1971.

Dykhuizen RF & others: The use of cobalt 60 telecurietherapy or x-ray therapy with and without lymphadenopathy in the treatment of testis germinal tumors: A 20-year comparative study. J Urol 100:321–328, 1968.

Jacobs EM: Combination chemotherapy of metastatic testicular germinal cell tumors and soft part sarcomas. Cancer 25:324–332, 1970.

Johnson DE, Kuhn CR, Guin GA: Testicular tumors in children. J Urol 104:940–943, 1970.

McCullough DL, Carlton CE, Seybold HM: Testicular tumors in infants and children: Report of 5 cases and evaluation of different modes of therapy. J Urol 105:140–148, 1971.

Rubin P & others: Cancer of the urogenital tract: Testicular tumors. JAMA 213:89–106, 1970.

Skinner DG, Leadbetter WF: The surgical management of testis tumors. J Urol 106:84–93, 1971.

Smithers D, Wallace ENK, Wallace DM: Radiotherapy for patients with tumours of the testicle. Brit J Urol 43:83–92, 1971.

Walsh PC & others: Retroperitoneal lymphadenectomy for testicular tumors. JAMA 217:309–312, 1971.

10. TUMORS OF THE PENIS

Almost all penile tumors are malignant and usually involve the prepuce and glans. The incidence is higher in the uncircumcised. With rare exceptions, these are squamous cell epitheliomas. They metastasize to the inguinal lymph nodes; the iliac nodes may then become involved.

A nodular or warty growth is noted on the inner side of the foreskin or on the glans. Ulceration and secondary infections are common. If the foreskin cannot be retracted, a dorsal slit of the prepuce is essential for diagnosis and biopsy. Matted enlarged inguinal nodes may represent either metastasis or secondary infection from the tumor. Biopsy is necessary for the establishment of the diagnosis.

In differential diagnosis, syphilitic chancre must be considered. The demonstration of the specific organism (and biopsy) should settle the issue. Chancroid may present as an ulcerating lesion. The demonstration of *Haemophilus ducreyi* is diagnostic. Condylomata acuminata are soft warty growths of viral origin. If doubt exists, biopsy is indicated.

After establishing the diagnosis by biopsy, amputation of the penis at least 2 cm proximal to the lesion must be done, though very small tumors may be curable with radiotherapy. In the presence of inguinal

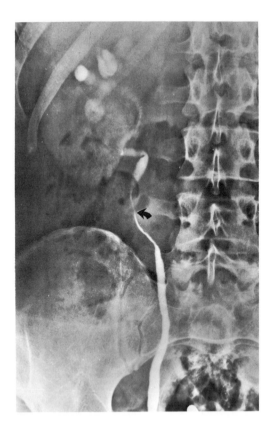

FIG 44–18. Carcinoma of the testis. Retrograde bulb ureterogram showing hydronephrosis and ureteral deviation at L4 secondary to metastases in right lumbar lymph nodes.

lymph node involvement, node dissection should be considered, for these are radioresistant.

The prognosis is fairly good in the absence of metastases.

Alexander LL & others: Radium management of tumors of the penis. New York J Med 71:1946–1950, 1971.

Das Gupta TK: Radical groin dissection. Surg Gynec Obst 129:1275–1280, 1969.

Dehner LP, Smith BH: Soft tissue tumors of the penis. Cancer 25:1431–1447, 1970.

Hanash KA & others: Carcinoma of the penis. J Urol 104:291–297, 1970.

NEUROGENIC BLADDER

Myoneural Anatomy

The urinary bladder and its involuntary sphincter develop and differentiate from the tubular urogenital sinus. The differentiation of the encasing mesenchymal cells forms the musculature of the detrusor and urethral sphincter. They are one and the same continuous structure with the same innervation.

Innervation

The innervation of the bladder and its involuntary sphincter is through the autonomic nervous system. The motor supply to the bladder and the sphincter is parasympathetic via the pelvic nerves, which arise from S2–4. These fibers carry also the stretch sensory receptors to the same spinal cord center (S2–4).

The sensory supply for pain, touch, and temperature is carried via the sympathetic fibers arising from the thoracolumbar segments (T11–L2).

Motor and sensory supply of the trigone is via the thoracolumbar sympathetic fibers.

The striated external sphincter as well as the entire urogenital diaphragm receive their motor and sensory innervation from the somatic fibers arising from S2–4 (via the pudendal nerve).

It is clear that S2–4 are the origin of the motor supply to the bladder musculature, to the involuntary sphincter, and to the striated external sphincter. The trigone is the only structure that is partly independent in its innervation. This is why segment S2–4 is called the spinal cord center for micturition. It is located at the level of the T12 and L1 vertebral bodies. There is connection between the spinal cord center and the midbrain and cerebral cortex. Through these connections, inhibition and control of the spinal cord reflexes can be maintained. Any injury above the level of the T12 vertebral body will leave the spinal cord center intact, leading to an upper motor neuron lesion; injuries at the spinal cord center or below will lead to a lower motor neuron lesion.

Myoneurophysiology

The primary functions of the urinary bladder are to act as a reservoir, maintain urinary continence, and prevent vesicoureteral reflux. Intact myoneural elements are essential for these functions. The primary reservoir function is possible through the particular detrusor muscular arrangement and because of the accommodation phenomenon. The normal bladder can accommodate variable volumes (up to 400 ml) without increasing intravesical pressure. We perceive bladder fullness through increases in intravesical pressure. Until this happens, we have no perception of the actual volume in the bladder.

Overdistention and stretch initiate detrusor activity that can be controlled and inhibited by the high cortical centers or can be allowed to progress to active detrusor contraction associated with voiding. Normally, voiding detrusor contraction is maintained until the bladder is completely empty unless voluntarily interrupted or inhibited.

Normally, before voiding starts, there is relaxation of the pelvic floor and the striated external sphincter. This leads to a drop in the bladder base, funneling of the bladder outlet, and appreciable lowering of urethral resistance. This is shortly followed by active detrusor contraction, generating a rise in intravesical pressure to about 20–40 cm water and resulting in a flow rate of about 15–25 ml/second. The detrusor contraction is maintained until the bladder is completely empty, when the pelvic floor and striated external sphincter contract, elevating the bladder base and increasing urethral closure pressure, and terminating voiding. Intact nerve pathways are essential for these synchronized activities to occur.

Cystometry

Cystometry is a simple method for testing the above functions and gives information about: residual urine, bladder capacity, the accommodation phenomenon and its extent, sensation of fullness, and effective detrusor contraction. A simple water cystometer and a normal cystometrogram are shown in Fig 44–19.

Classification & Clinical Findings

Neurogenic bladder can be divided into 2 main groups depending on the site of the lesion in relation to the spinal cord center (S2–4): upper motor neuron lesions (above the spinal cord center) and lower motor neuron lesions (at or below the spinal cord center).

A. Upper Motor Neuron Lesions (Spastic): Lesions above the voiding reflex arc are most commonly due to trauma. Although the reflex arc is intact, it has lost the inhibitory control of the higher centers. Both motor and sensory fibers are commonly involved. There is loss of accommodation and, frequently, uninhibited detrusor contraction. The bladder outlet is usually funneled. The striated external sphincter and pelvic floor are spastic. Detrusor contractions, though they can generate abnormally high intravesical pressure, are not effective in producing adequate urine flow (because of the spastic external sphincter) and are incapable of maintaining the contraction, so that there is always some residual urine. Bladder capacity is

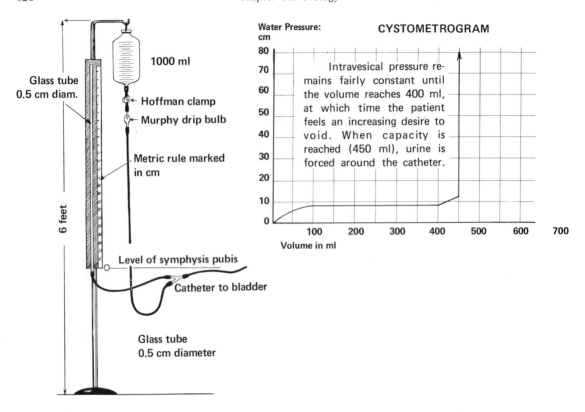

FIG 44–19. Cystometry. *Left:* A simple water manometer. *Right:* Normal cystometrogram. As fluid is slowly introduced into the bladder, the detrusor gradually relaxes to accept increasing amounts of fluid without change in intravesical pressure. At a volume of 400 ml, the patient felt an urge to avoid. Shortly thereafter, an involuntary contraction of the detrusor occurred which was reflected in a sharp increase in intravesical pressure.

reduced. Detrusor contraction and mass reflexes can be initiated from certain trigger areas.

There is marked detrusor thickening and hypertrophy, together with trigonal hypertrophy, that initially leads to functional obstruction at the ureterovesical junction. Later, decompensation of the ureterovesical valve and reflux accentuates renal back pressure and pyelonephritic damage.

Fig 44–20 is a typical cystometrogram of a spastic upper motor neuron lesion.

B. Lower Motor Neuron Lesions (Flaccid): Any lesion involving the spinal cord center (S2–4), cauda equina, sacral roots, or peripheral nerves leads to atonic or flaccid lower motor neuron involvement. Trauma is the most common cause, but tumors, ruptured intervertebral disks, and meningomyelocele may cause this type of neurogenic bladder also. Again, both motor and sensory fibers are usually affected. Damage of the stretch receptors results in loss of sense of fullness. Accordingly, bladder capacity progressively increases.

Detrusor contractions are primarily on a myogenic basis, as the bladder has lost its connection to the spinal cord center (Fig 44–21). They are usually weak and unsustained. In spite of diminished outflow resis-

tance (funneled bladder neck and flaccid external sphincter), flow rates are inadequate and bladder emptying is incomplete, resulting in relatively large amounts of residual urine. Bladder thickening and trabeculation and trigonal hypertrophy develop but are less apparent because of the overstretching. Trigonal hypertrophy, augmented by the stretch caused by the large residual, lead to functional obstruction of the ureterovesical junction. Decompensation and reflux occur relatively late in comparison to spastic upper motor neuron lesions.

Differential Diagnosis

Cystitis, interstitial cystitis, and organic obstruction are occasionally confused with neurogenic bladder, but associated neurologic lesions usually make the diagnosis of neurogenic bladder easy. However, psychosomatic disturbances such as spastic external sphincter, incomplete voiding, retention, or incontinence should always be considered.

Complications

Common complications include urinary tract infection, stone formation, and incontinence. The most serious consequences of these lesions is the

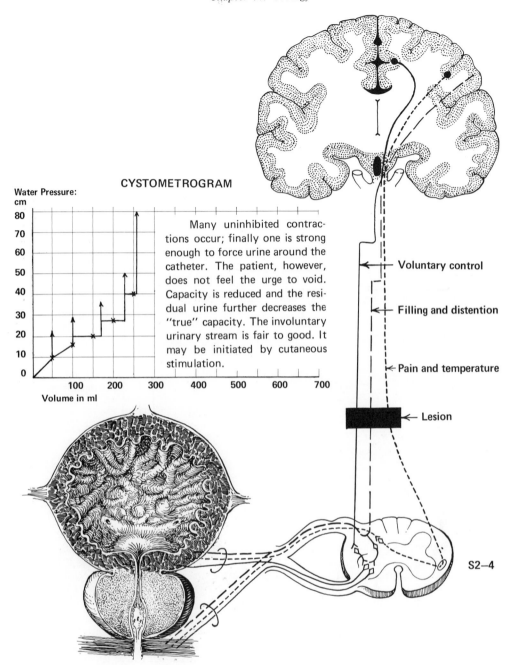

CYSTOMETROGRAM

Water Pressure: cm

Many uninhibited contractions occur; finally one is strong enough to force urine around the catheter. The patient, however, does not feel the urge to void. Capacity is reduced and the residual urine further decreases the "true" capacity. The involuntary urinary stream is fair to good. It may be initiated by cutaneous stimulation.

Volume in ml

Voluntary control

Filling and distention

Pain and temperature

Lesion

S2–4

FIG 44–20. Complete spastic neurogenic bladder. Caused by a more or less complete transection of the spinal cord above S2. Cystometric study of a typical case shows function after recovery from spinal shock. (Modified after Nesbit, Lapides, & Baum: *Fundamentals of Urology.* Edwards, 1953.)

hydrodynamic back pressure on the kidneys, causing hydronephrosis with or without infection and resulting ultimately in trigonal hypertrophy—aggravated by stretch if there is residual urine—and decompensation of the ureterovesical junctions.

Treatment

Immediately following spinal cord injury there is

a shock phase which may last a few weeks to 2–3 years. The bladder is completely dissociated from any nervous control and thus has no sensation and is completely inactive.

Treatment is aimed at avoiding the aforementioned complications in the hope of partial or complete recovery. During the shock phase, continuous closed drainage should be maintained by urethral cath-

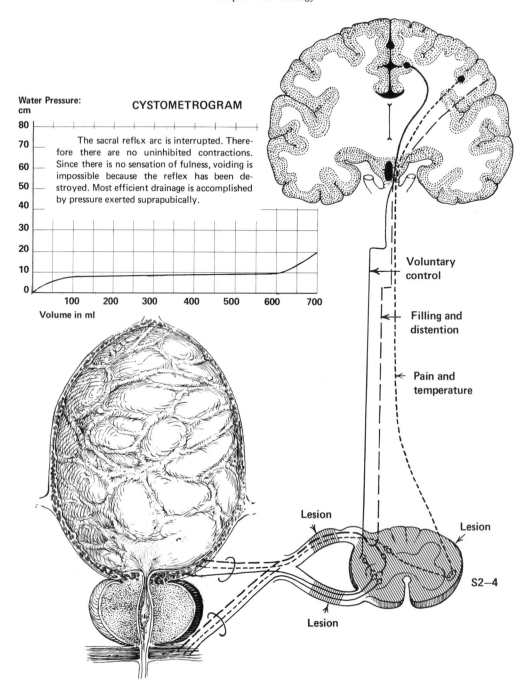

Water Pressure: cm

CYSTOMETROGRAM

The sacral reflex arc is interrupted. Therefore there are no uninhibited contractions. Since there is no sensation of fulness, voiding is impossible because the reflex has been destroyed. Most efficient drainage is accomplished by pressure exerted suprapubically.

Volume in ml

Voluntary control

Filling and distention

Pain and temperature

Lesion

Lesion

S2–4

Lesion

Lesion

FIG 44–21. Flaccid neurogenic bladder. Caused by a lesion of the sacral portion of the cord or of the cauda equina. Cystometric study of a typical case shows function after recovery from spinal shock. (Modified after Nesbit, Lapides, & Baum: *Fundamentals of Urology.* Edwards, 1953.)

eter or suprapubic cystostomy until bladder activity resumes.

Control of infection and maintenance of a high fluid intake are important. Dietary measures (low-calcium diet, increased fluid intake, etc) and early ambulation are helpful in prevention of stone formation.

Urinary incontinence alone is occasionally an indication for diversion in the female. In the male, the use of external penile collecting devices is helpful.

A. Spastic Neurogenic Bladder: In the spastic neurogenic lesions, bladder rehabilitation is the aim. Residual urine should be minimized by diminishing urethral resistance by means of transurethral resection of the prostate or incision of the spastic external sphincter, or by unilateral or bilateral blocking or excision of the pudendal nerves.

Functional capacity can be increased by eliminating infection. Anticholinergics—eg, methantheline bromide (Banthine), 50—100 mg 4 times daily, or propantheline bromide (Pro-Banthine), 15—30 mg 4 times daily—increase functional capacity. Trigger areas should be used to initiate voiding. Conversion to a flaccid lower motor neuron lesion can be achieved by subarachnoid injection of absolute alcohol or by anterior and posterior rhizotomy. If decompensation of the ureterovesical junction and deterioration of the upper urinary tract occur, urinary diversion is indicated.

B. Flaccid Neurogenic Bladder: In the flaccid neurogenic bladder, functional capacity can be improved by manual compression (Credé) and by diminishing resistance of the bladder outlet (transurethral resections of the bladder neck). The patient should be instructed to void on a time schedule to avoid wetness. Continuous drainage by a urethral catheter or a suprapubic cystostomy should be employed when necessary. Decompensation of the ureterovesical junction and deterioration of the upper urinary tract require urinary diversion.

Prognosis

Decompensation of the ureterovesical junction and persistence of infection are the most serious consequences of neurogenic bladder. Spastic neurogenic bladders deteriorate more rapidly than lower motor neuron lesions. Proper timing of surgical intervention is essential for preservation of kidney function.

Bors EH, Commar AE: *Neurological Urology: Physiology of Micturition: Its Neurological Disorders and Sequelae.* University Park Press, 1971.

Chapman WH & others: A prospective study of the urinary tract from birth in patients with meningomyelocele. J Urol 102:363—366, 1969.

Currie RJ & others: External sphincterotomy in paraplegics: Technique and results. J Urol 103:64—68, 1970.

Emmett JL, Love JG: Vesical dysfunction caused by protruded lumbar disk. J Urol 105:86—91, 1971.

Halverstadt DB: Electrical stimulation of human bladder 3 years later. J Urol 106:673—677, 1971.

Manfredi RA, Leal JF: Selective sacral rhizotomy for the spastic bladder syndrome in patients with spinal cord injuries. J Urol 100:17—20, 1968.

Marchetti LJ, Gonick P: A comparison of renal function in spinal cord injury patients with and without reflux. J Urol 104:365—367, 1970.

Morales P: Neurogenic bladder in traumatic paraplegia. New York J Med 68:2031—2037, 1967.

DISORDERS OF THE KIDNEYS

POLYCYSTIC KIDNEYS

Polycystic kidney disease is a familial disorder that involves not only the kidneys but sometimes the liver and pancreas as well. The renal cysts are thought to be due to failure of union of the collecting and convoluted tubules. As the cysts enlarge, pressure is exerted on normal tissue, leading to its gradual destruction. The diagnosis is usually made during investigation for the cause of hypertension or uremia discovered in the third or fourth decade. The sex incidence is about equal. Flank pain may be noticed if bleeding occurs into a cyst; hematuria may then occur. Examination reveals bilateral nodular enlargement of the kidneys.

The urine often shows red blood cells and evidence of infection. Serum creatinine or BUN measures the degree of renal insufficiency. Urograms reveal the enlarged kidneys, with marked bending and elongation of the calyces that are bent around large cysts (Fig 44—22).

Surgery is not warranted unless a large extrarenal cyst obstructs the upper ureter. Therapy is medical.

Bernstein J: Heritable cystic disorders of the kidney: The mythology of polycystic disease. P Clin North America 18:435—444, 1971.

Ivemark BI, Lagergren C, Lindvall N: Roentgenologic diagnosis of polycystic kidney and medullary sponge kidney. Acta radiol 10:225—235, 1970.

Lazarus JM & others: Hemodialysis and transplantation in adults with polycystic renal disease. JAMA 217:1821—1824, 1971.

Lieberman E & others: Infantile polycystic disease of the kidneys and liver. Medicine 50:277—318, 1971.

SIMPLE RENAL CYST

Simple cyst of the kidney is usually unilateral and single, but it may be multiple and bilateral. Whether this disorder is congenital or acquired is not clear. By compression, the cysts can destroy adjacent parenchyma. They contain fluid that resembles (but is not) urine. A few harbor cancer on their walls. Most cysts are diagnosed after the age of 40 years.

Flank pain may be the presenting symptom, though most renal cysts are found incidentally on urography done for other purposes. A mass may be felt in the renal area and must be differentiated from tumor. Urinalysis and tests of renal function are normal. Excretory urograms reveal a mass in the kidney that distorts adjacent calyces. Nephrotomography will show that the mass is avascular (in contradistinction to tumor). Angiography shows similar findings, including

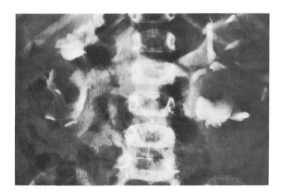

FIG 44–22. Polycystic kidneys. Excretory urogram in a child showing elongation, broadening, and bending of the calyces around cysts. Good renal function.

the absence of capillaries in the area of the mass. A technetium gamma camera scan will also demonstrate the absence of blood vessels in the cyst.

Simple cyst must be differentiated from adenocarcinoma of the kidney. Nephrotomography, angiography, and the technetium scan usually make the differentiation. If the presumptive diagnosis is cyst, a needle can be introduced into the mass. Clear fluid implies a cyst; it should be subjected to cytologic study. In polycystic disease the cysts are multiple and bilateral and renal insufficiency is to be expected.

Complications are rare, but bleeding into the cyst or infection of a cyst may occur.

Unless the patient is a poor surgical risk, cysts should be explored, for a few will be associated with cancer requiring nephrectomy. The extrarenal portion of a cyst should be resected.

Bernstein J: Heritable cystic disorders of the kidney: The mythology of polycystic disease. P Clin North America 18:435–444, 1971.

Deliveliotis A, Zorzos S, Varkarakis M: Suppuration of solitary cyst of the kidney. Brit J Urol 39:472–478, 1967.

Genert JE, Stein J, Bischoff AJ: Solitary renal cysts: Experience with 100 cases. J Urol 100:251–253, 1968.

Weitzner S: Clear cell carcinoma of the free wall of a simple renal cyst. J Urol 106:515–517, 1971.

MEDULLARY SPONGE KIDNEY

Cystic dilatation of the renal collecting tubules is occasionally seen. It represents a congenital ectasia of these tubules, which may be complicated by the development of microcalculi. The lesion is often bilateral and may involve all calyces.

There is an increased incidence of infection in such kidneys. Symptoms include those typical of pyelonephritis or stone. Hematuria is not uncommon.

Excretory urograms reveal the dilated distal tubules as a "blush."

There is no specific treatment. Infection must be combated. In the presence of calculi, a prophylactic regimen should be prescribed. (See Calculous Disease, above.)

Pyrah LN: Medullary sponge kidney. J Urol 95:274–283, 1966.

RENAL FUSION

The metanephric tissue may form one renal mass occupying one flank, or it may lie ectopically in the pelvis. The most common anomaly, however, is horseshoe kidney with the renal poles joined inferiorly. These anomalous kidneys are fed by many aberrant arteries, one of which is apt to compress the upper ureter and lead to hydronephrosis. Complicating infection is not uncommon.

There are usually no symptoms unless complications arise, in which case pain from obstruction or symptoms of infection may appear. An enlarged renal mass may be felt, and the isthmus of a horseshoe kidney may be palpable. Urography establishes the diagnosis (Fig 44–23). In the case of a "cake" kidney, both ureters will be shown to arise from their own calyceal system in the renal mass. The renal masses of a horseshoe kidney lie on the psoas muscles, and their inferior calyces point medially into the isthmus.

No treatment is necessary unless there is evidence of obstruction or infection.

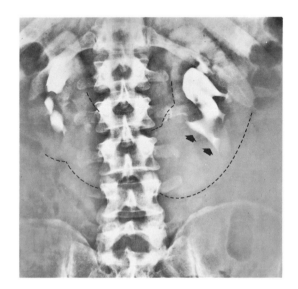

FIG 44–23. Excretory urogram showing horseshoe kidney with expansion of left side of isthmus and compression of lower left calyceal system. Surgical diagnosis: adenocarcinoma.

Gregoir W: Conservative surgery in horseshoe kidney. Urol Internat 16:129–138, 1963.

ANEURYSM OF THE RENAL ARTERY

Aneurysm of the renal artery is relatively rare. It results from weakening of its wall by arteriosclerosis, periarteritis nodosa, or trauma. Some are congenital. If the aneurysm causes stenosis of the artery, hypertension may ensue secondary to ischemia. Plain x-ray film may reveal a ring-like calcification in its wall (Fig 44–24). Angiography is diagnostic.

Because there is a significant incidence of spontaneous rupture of these lesions, their repair or removal by heminephrectomy must be considered. Nephrectomy may be necessary, particularly if emergency intervention for bleeding is necessary. A few of these patients will become normotensive after definitive surgery.

Cerny JC, Chang C-Y, Fry WJ: Renal artery aneurisms. Arch Surg 96:653–662, 1968.

Hogbin BM, Scorer CG: Spontaneous rupture of an aneurism of the renal artery with survival. Brit J Urol 41:218–221, 1969.

RENAL INFARCTION

The common causes of occlusion of the renal artery are subacute bacterial endocarditis, atrial or ventricular thrombi, arteriosclerosis, polyarteritis nodosa, and trauma. Multiple emboli are common and lead to patchy renal ischemia. Occlusion of a main renal artery will cause atrophy of a portion or all of the kidney.

The patient may suffer from flank pain, or the lesion may be silent. Hematuria is common. Excretory urograms may reveal no excretion of radiopaque material or may only opacify a portion of the kidney. With complete occlusion of the main renal artery, a ureteral catheter will drain no urine, yet the retrograde urogram will reveal normal anatomy. Renal angiography makes the diagnosis by revealing occlusion of the artery or arterioles; a renal scan will show similar findings. This disease may be mimicked by ureteral stone, but urograms and angiograms will differentiate them. Following renal infarction, hypertension may develop secondary to renal ischemia; it may later resolve spontaneously.

If the diagnosis is made promptly, endarterectomy should be considered. Otherwise, anticoagulation therapy should be instituted. If permanent hypertension develops, definitive treatment of the arterial occlusion or nephrectomy should be performed.

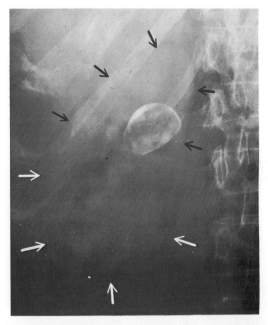

FIG 44–24. Intrarenal aneurysm of renal artery. Plain film showing calcified structure over the right renal shadow.

Fergus JN, Jones NF, Thomas ML: Kidney function after arterial embolism. Brit MJ 4:587–590, 1969.

Goldsmith E & others: Embolectomy of the renal artery. J Urol 99:366–370, 1968.

Grablowsky OM & others: Renal artery thrombosis following blunt trauma: Report of four cases. Surg 67:895–900, 1970.

Lang EK, Mertz JHO, Nourse M: Renal arteriography in the assessment of renal infarction. J Urol 99:506–512, 1968.

THROMBOSIS OF THE RENAL VEIN

Thrombosis of the renal vein affects both infants and adults. In infants, it is apt to complicate ileocolitis. In the adult, it may be secondary to renal infection or ascending thrombosis of the vena cava. There is usually flank pain and a palpable kidney. If secondary to infection, the patient is septic and urinalysis reveals pus cells and bacteria. The patient with bilateral involvement is found to have renal insufficiency. Nephrotic syndrome may develop. Excretory urograms show delayed and impaired opacification in an enlarged kidney. The calyces are elongated. Later, the kidney may become atrophic. Renal angiography reveals stretching and bowing of arterioles. Selective renal venography will demonstrate the thrombus (Fig 44–25).

If the diagnosis of unilateral infected renal vein thrombosis can be established, nephrectomy should be done. In bilateral disease, anticoagulant therapy is

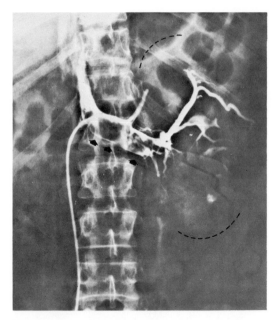

FIG 44–25. Thrombosis of renal vein. Selective left renal venogram showing almost complete occlusion of vein. Veins to lower pole failed to fill. Note large size of kidney.

required. A few cases of successful thrombectomy have been reported.

Alexander F, Campbell WAB: Congenital nephrotic syndrome and renal vein thrombosis in infancy. J Clin Path 24:27–40, 1971.

Mauer SM & others: Bilateral renal vein thrombosis in infancy: Report of a survivor following surgical intervention. J Pediat 78:509–512, 1971.

Rosenman E, Pollak VE, Pirani CL: Renal vein thrombosis in the adult: A clinical and pathologic study based on renal biopsies. Medicine 47:269–335, 1968.

Wegner GP & others: Renal vein thrombosis: A roentgenographic diagnosis. JAMA 209:1661–1667, 1969.

DISEASES OF THE RETROPERITONEUM

RETROPERITONEAL FIBROSIS

One or both ureters may be compressed by a chronic inflammatory process, usually of unknown cause, which involves the retroperitoneal tissues of the lumbosacral area. Patients treated for migraine with methysergide (Sansert) may develop this fibrosis. Sclerosing Hodgkin's disease has been found to be an occasional cause. The symptoms include renal pain, low backache, and the syndrome of uremia. Some patients present with complete anuria. Urinary infection is unusual. If both ureters are obstructed, the serum creatinine will be elevated.

Excretory urograms show hydronephrosis and a dilated ureter down to the point of obstruction. The ureters are displaced medially in the lumbar area. Retrograde ureterograms show a long segment of ureteral stenosis, although a catheter passes easily through it. If anuric, indwelling ureteral catheters should be placed as a temporary measure. Definitive treatment consists of lysis of the ureters and implantation into the peritoneal cavity. Those caused by the ingestion of methysergide may resolve on cessation of the drug. Resolution of the lesion has been reported following the administration of corticosteroids.

Bianchine JR, Friedman AP: Metabolism of methysergide and retroperitoneal fibrosis. Arch Int Med 126:252–254, 1970.

Cerny JC, Scott T: Non-idiopathic retroperitoneal fibrosis. J Urol 105:49–55, 1971.

Mitchinson MJ, Withycombe JFR, Jones RA: The response of idiopathic retroperitoneal fibrosis to corticosteroids. Brit J Urol 43:444–449, 1971.

Morandi LP, Grob PJ: Retroperitoneal fibrosis: Response to corticosteroid therapy. Arch Int Med 128:295–298, 1971.

Packham DA, Yates-Bell JG: The symptomatology and diagnosis of retroperitoneal fibrosis. Brit J Urol 40:207–222, 1968.

PERINEPHRIC ABSCESS

Perinephric abscess can arise secondary to a staphylococcal infection of the kidney, but in most cases it is a complication of advanced chronic renal infection. The abscess is enclosed within the perirenal fascia. There may be a long history of repeated attacks of urinary infection. In the rare staphylococcal type, a history of an antecedent skin infection may be elicited. Most patients with abscess are septic, but a few may present with no more than mild flank pain. Tenderness over the kidney is to be expected. A flank mass may be palpable. The diaphragm on the affected side may be elevated and fixed. Urograms show obliteration of the psoas shadow and scoliosis of the spine with its concavity on the side of the abscess. Calculous pyonephrosis may be noted. The lower pole of the kidney may be displaced laterally.

The history and physical findings may be consistent with infected hydronephrosis. Excretory urograms should make the differentiation. Considerable compression of the abscess upon the ureter may lead to hydronephrosis. Later, after definitive treatment retroperitoneal scarring may cause ureteral stenosis.

If seen early, those cases secondary to staphylococcal infection of the kidney may resolve with appropriate antimicrobial therapy. When a frank abscess is present, surgical drainage is indicated. If the kidney is badly damaged, nephrectomy should be done. If the kidney is not removed, serial urograms should be obtained in search of secondary ureteral stenosis that might require repair.

Salvatierra O Jr, Bucklew WB, Morrow JW: Perinephric abscess: A report of 71 cases. J Urol 98:296—302. 1967.

DISEASES OF THE URETERS

DUPLICATION

Complete or incomplete (Y-type) duplication of the ureters is not uncommon. It presupposes 2 renal pelves in the renal mass. Most are observed in females. The Y-type ureter seldom causes trouble. With complete duplication, the ureter from the upper renal pole opens closest to the bladder neck (Fig 44—26). The ureter to the lower pole thus has a relatively short intravesical segment and is therefore prone to reflux. Most ureteroceles in children involve the ureter from the superior pelvis, leading to hydroureteronephrosis. This ureter may open ectopically at the bladder neck or in the urethra and frequently exhibits reflux. If it opens at the vestibule, it is obstructed. Duplication is significant only if it leads to pyelonephritis or hydronephrosis, evidence of which is found on excretory urograms. Vesicoureteral reflux may require repair of the incompetent ureterovesical junction. Obstruction to the upper pole ureter often indicates the need for heminephroureterectomy.

Amar AD, Chabra K: Reflux in duplicated ureters: Treatment in children. J Pediat Surg 5:419—430, 1970.

Gross M, Chait A: Renal duplication with hydronephrotic segment. Am J Roentgenol 101:728—731, 1967.

Lundin E, Riggs W: Upper urinary tract duplication associated with ectopic ureterocele in childhood and infancy. Acta radiol 7:13—24, 1968.

URETEROCELE

A ureterocele is a ballooning of the submucosal ureter into the bladder. This cyst-like structure has a pinpoint orifice and is therefore obstructive, leading to hydronephrosis. If large enough, it may obstruct the vesical neck. It is most common in little girls, and always involves the ureter draining the upper renal pole of a duplicated system. Because of its position and size, it may cause the other ipsilateral ureterovesical junction to become incompetent (reflux).

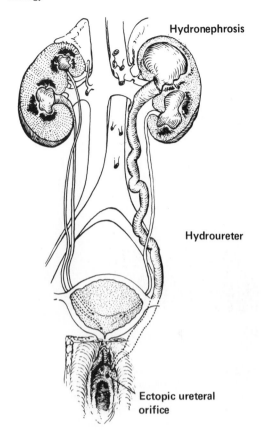

FIG 44—26. Duplication of ureters and ectopic ureteral orifice. Complete duplication with obstruction to one ureter with ectopic orifice on left. The ureter with the ectopic opening always drains the upper pole of the kidney.

Symptoms are usually those of pyelonephritis or obstruction. Excretory urograms may show a negative shadow in the bladder cast by the ureterocele (Fig 44—27). The ureter and renal pole so obstructed reveal marked dilatation. A cystogram may show reflux into the second ureter going to the lower pole of the kidney.

Small, mildly obstructive ureteroceles can be destroyed transurethrally. The large ones seen in childhood require transvesical excision and, usually, reimplantation of both ureters into the bladder to prevent reflux. If the kidney tissue obstructed by this cyst is badly damaged, nephroureterectomy (or heminephrectomy with ureteral duplication) is necessary.

Clark CW, Leadbetter GW Jr: General treatment, mistreatment and complications of ureteroceles. J Urol 106:518—520 1971.

Johnston JH, Johnson LM: Experiences with ectopic ureteroceles. Brit J Urol 41:61—70, 1969.

Stephens FD: Caecoureterocele and concepts on the embryology and aetiology of ureteroceles. Australian New Zealand J Surg 40:239—248, 1971.

Tanagho EA: Anatomy and management of ureteroceles. J Urol 107:729—736, 1972.

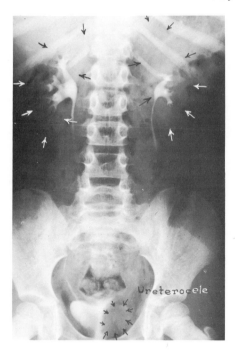

FIG 44–27. Ureterocele. Excretory urogram in a girl 8 years old, showing a space-occupying lesion on the left side of the bladder caused by ureterocele. Absence of calyceal system in the upper portion of the left kidney implies duplication of the ureters and pelves and nonfunction (advanced hydronephrosis) of the upper pole; its dilated ureter drains into the obstructing ureterocele and displaces the visualized ureter laterally just below the kidney.

ECTOPIC URETERAL ORIFICE

In rare instances, the ureter may drain into the urethra, vestibule, seminal vesicle. or vagina. If the orifice lies proximal to the external urinary sphincter, no incontinence ensues, but vesicoureteral reflux is common. Should it drain into the vagina or at the vestibule, there is continuous leakage of urine apart from voiding. Most ectopic orifices involve the ureter draining the upper pole of a duplicated system, and most are observed in the female. Hydroureteronephrosis of the involved segment is to be expected.

Symptoms are those of infection or obstruction. If the orifice is distal to the external sphincter, constant wetness is noticed. Such an orifice may be seen beside the urethral orifice or in the roof of the vagina on endoscopy. Excretory urograms will reveal hydroureteronephrosis, usually involving the upper renal segment. Cystography may show reflux into the ectopic orifice. If the hydronephrotic segment is only moderately damaged, the ureter can be divided and reim-

planted into the bladder. Usually, however, heminephroureterectomy is necessary.

Grossman H, Winchester PH, Muecke EC: Solitary ectopic ureter. Radiology 89:1069–1072, 1967.
Williams DI, Royle M: Ectopic ureter in the male child. Brit J Urol 41:421–427, 1969.

CONGENITAL STENOSIS OF THE URETER

The common sites of congenital ureteral stricture are the ureteropelvic and ureterovesical junctions. Ureteral dilatation down to the bladder level is most often caused by vesicoureteral reflux. True stenosis at this point is uncommon; when it does occur, a sphincter-like muscle bundle is found in the juxtavesical ureter. The common symptoms are renal pain from obstruction and symptoms due to pyelonephritis. Excretory urograms depict the dilatation above the ureterovesical junction. There is no reflux on cystography. Treatment consists of division of the ureter just proximal to the obstruction with reimplantation of the ureter into the bladder.

Ureteropelvic obstruction is much more common than stricture at the ureterovesical level. Urographic studies in patients with vesicoureteral reflux are apt to reveal pseudostenosis at the ureteropelvic junction. Some of these become truly obstructive. Symptoms include renal pain and those of renal infection. Excretory urograms show varying degrees of hydrocalycosis with a ureter of normal caliber below the site of obstruction. (If the ureter is dilated below the ureteropelvic junction, such changes suggest reflux as the cause.) Even on late films, much of the contrast medium is retained in the kidney. Cystography should also be done in order to rule out reflux, since repair of the ureterovesical junction usually causes the pseudostenosis to disappear.

If the kidney appears to have functional potential, surgical repair of the stenotic area should be accomplished. Nephrectomy may be indicated if damage is severe.

Allen TD: Congenital ureteral strictures. J Urol 104:196–204, 1970.
Smart WR: Surgical correction of hydronephrosis. Pages 2198–2239 in: *Urology,* 3rd ed. Campbell MT, Harrison JH (editors). Saunders, 1970.
Tanagho EA, Smith DR, Guthrie TH: Pathophysiology of functional ureteral obstruction. J Urol 104:73–88, 1970.

ACQUIRED STENOSIS OF THE URETER

Acquired ureteral stenosis is not so common as the congenital types. Causes include (1) ureteral injury (surgical, traumatic, radiation therapy), (2) compression of the ureter by lymph nodes harboring cancer, (3) prolonged pressure by an aberrant blood vessel, (4) tuberculous or bilharzial ureteritis, (5) retroperitoneal fibrosis, (6) aneurysm of the aorta or following aortofemoral bypass grafts, (7) ureteropelvic obstruction secondary to reflux, (8) occlusion of the uretero-vesical junction by infiltrating cancer of the bladder, (9) and functional obstruction of the ureterovesical junction secondary to hypertrophy of the trigone developing from obstruction distal to the bladder neck.

Symptoms are usually those of obstruction to urine flow from the kidney, though many are silent. An unsuspected lesion is often discovered on excretory urography.

Therapy consists of treatment of the cause, eg, prostatectomy or resection of the stenosed segment with end-to-end anastomosis.

Graham JB, Abad RS: Ureteral obstruction due to radiation. Am J Obst Gynec 99:409–412, 1967.

Kerr WS Jr & others: Idiopathic retroperitoneal fibrosis: Clinical experiences with 15 cases, 1957–1967. J Urol 99:575–584, 1968.

Lang EK, Nourse M: The roentgenographic diagnosis of obstructive lesions of the ureter. J Urol 101:812–820, 1969.

Tanagho, EA, Meyers FH: Trigonal hypertrophy: A cause of ureteral obstruction. J Urol 93:678–683, 1965.

DISORDERS OF
THE URINARY BLADDER*

VESICAL FISTULAS

Vesical fistulas may be congenital or acquired. Congenital fistulas usually involve the urachus. Acquired fistulas may be secondary to trauma (physical, surgical, or obstetrical), malignant tumors, or inflammatory lesions. The most common types of vesical fistulas are vesicovaginal, vesicointestinal, and vesicocutaneous. Vesicovaginal fistulas are commonly secondary to obstetrical trauma due to obstructed labor. They occur rarely as a complication of tumor infiltration from the cervix or the bladder. Vesicointestinal fistulas are commonly due to malignant lesions of the bowel or the bladder. They also occur secondary to inflammatory pelvic lesions in association with diverticulitis, pelvic abscess, or appendicular abscess. Vesicocutaneous fistulas are common after cystostomy in the presence of bladder outlet obstruction, bladder malignancy, or foreign bodies.

Vesicovaginal fistulas must be differentiated from ureterovaginal fistulas, vesicorectal fistulas from ure-

*Urinary stress incontinence in women is discussed in Chapter 45.

throrectal fistulas, and vesicocutaneous fistulas from either ureterocutaneous or urethrocutaneous fistulas.

Treatment is essentially that of the primary cause plus temporary proximal drainage and excision of the fistulous tract.

Aldrete JS, Re Mine WH: Vesicocolic fistula: A complication of colonic cancer. Arch Surg 94:627–634, 1967.

Boronow KC: Management of radiation induced vaginal fistulas. Am J Obst Gynec 110:1–71, 1971.

Hutch JA, Noll LE: Prevention of vesicovaginal fistula. Obst Gynec 35:924–927, 1970.

Moir JC: Vesicovaginal fistula: Thoughts on the treatment of 350 cases. Proc Roy Soc Med 59:1019–1022, 1966.

Pugh JI: On the pathology and behavior of acquired non-traumatic vesicointestinal fistula. Brit J Surg 51:644–657, 1964.

DISORDERS OF THE SCROTUM, TESTIS, & SPERMATIC CORD*

SCROTAL LESIONS

Congenital scrotal lesions include congenital (unilateral or bilateral) hypoplasia of the scrotum in association with cryptorchidism (see below) and bifid scrotum with extensive hypospadias. **Acquired lesions** may consist of scrotal abscess, sebaceous cysts, lymphedema (parasitic, traumatic, idiopathic), or gangrene. These are not specific for the scrotum, and each follows general rules of clinical course and management for similar disorders elsewhere.

HYDROCELE

Congenital hydrocele is due to a patent processus funicularis communicating with the peritoneal cavity. In infantile hydrocele, the processus vaginalis and funicularis are obliterated at the peritoneal cavity connection. Hydrocele of the cord is due to accumulation of fluid in the processus funicularis while it is obliterated at both the peritoneal and the testicular ends. In hydrocele of the tunica vaginalis (the commonest type), the hydrocele only surrounds the testis. Acute hydrocele results from trauma, inflammation, torsion, and sometimes neoplasm. Chronic or idiopathic hydrocele is of unknown cause.

Hydrocele is manifested by scrotal swelling, which is cystic and translucent. In the communicating types, it enlarges during the day and diminishes upon

*Cryptorchidism is discussed in Chapter 49.

lying down. It is usually painless unless secondary to trauma, torsion, infection, or tumor.

Congenital types may heal spontaneously or may require surgical repair. In secondary hydrocele, treat the primary underlying cause. Chronic idiopathic hydrocele may require surgical repair, or no treatment.

SPERMATOCELE

Spermatocele is a retention cyst of an aberrant tubule of the rete testis or head of the epididymis. The cyst is distended with a whitish milky fluid that contains sperm. Cysts are usually at the superior pole of the testis or between it and the epididymis. They are usually soft, with the feeling of not being fully distended.

No therapy is needed unless the patient is concerned, in which case aspiration or surgical excision may be done.

VARICOCELE

Varicocele is due to an impediment in the deep venous drainage of the scrotal contents, leading to dilatation, tortuosity, and distention of the pampiniform plexus. It is more common on the left side since on that side the testicular vein is more subject to venous stasis because of its right angle drainage into the renal vein, absent or incompetent valves, or compression by the pelvic colon.

Mild degrees are commonly asymptomatic, but a dragging scrotal sensation and occasionally sexual neurosis may be associated. Varicocele may lead to low fertility in some men.

Asymptomatic varicocele is best left alone unless its possible effect on fertility is a matter of concern. Symptomatic varicocele can be corrected surgically, either by ligating the external spermatic vein at the level of the internal inguinal ring or by a direct scrotal approach and isolation and ligation of individual vessels.

Clarke BG: Incidence of varicocele in normal men and among men of different age groups. JAMA 198:1121–1122, 1966.

Kiska EF, Cowart GT: Treatment of varicocele by high ligation. J Urol 83:713–715, 1960.

McGowan AJ, Howley TF: Experiences with the extrusion operation for hydrocele. J Urol 101:366–367, 1969.

TORSION OF THE SPERMATIC CORD

Torsion of the spermatic cord is most common in adolescent boys. A twist in the spermatic cord interferes with testicular blood supply. If torsion is complete, testicular gangrene may occur. The cause is unknown, but an underlying anatomic abnormality (spacious tunica vaginalis, loose epididymo-testicular connection, undescended testis) is usually present.

Clinical findings consist of lower abdominal and scrotal pain and scrotal swelling of sudden onset. There may be a history of previous attacks in young adolescents. These findings warrant a diagnosis of torsion until it can be disproved on examination. The testis is swollen, tender, and retracted. The pain is not relieved by testicular support. The cord above the swelling is normal.

Torsion must be differentiated from orchitis, epididymitis, and pain due to testicular trauma. If the diagnosis cannot be established by examination and history, exploration is required.

Torsion of the spermatic cord is a surgical emergency. Unless the testis is definitely gangrenous and there is a long history of neglected exploration, try to conserve the testis. Orchiopexy on the other side is always necessary because of the common incidence of bilateral congenital anomaly and the possibility that torsion will occur on that side at a later time.

Lyon RP: Torsion of the testicle in childhood. A painless emergency requiring contralateral orchiopexy. JAMA 178:702–705, 1961.

Parker RM, Robison JR: Anatomy and diagnosis of torsion of the testicle. J Urol 106:243–247, 1971.

Skoglund RW, McRoberts JW, Ragde H: Torsion of the spermatic cord: A review of the literature and an analysis of 70 new cases. J Urol 104:604–607, 1970.

PENILE & URETHRAL LESIONS

HYPOSPADIAS

The hypospadiac penis presents with a urethral orifice proximal to the usual site. It may be coronal, midshaft, penoscrotal, or midscrotal. In the case of the latter, the scrotum is bifid. The penis is bent ventrally distal to the ectopic meatus (Fig 44–28). In many cases, this may preclude intercourse. The midscrotal hypospadiac penis may resemble female external genitalia with an enlarged clitoris and labia. Buccal smears are indicated in this group, a few of which may be found to have a rudimentary uterus and vagina (pseudohermaphroditism). The urinary sphincters are normal. The incidence of cryptorchidism is high.

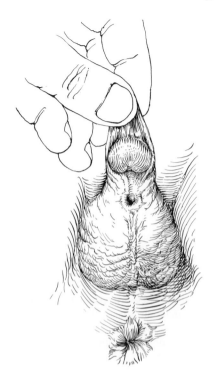

FIG 44–28. Hypospadias, penoscrotal type. Redundant dorsal foreskin which is deficient ventrally; ventral chordee.

If it is obvious that the degree of hypospadias will make intercourse difficult or impossible (due to the degree of chordee) and that the position of the urethral orifice will not allow the boy to stand to urinate or to deposit semen deep in the vagina in adulthood, surgical correction of the chordee and, later, urethroplasty is indicated. These operations are highly successful and should be completed before school age.

Culp OS: Struggles and triumphs with hypospadias and associated anomalies: Review of 400 cases. J Urol 96:339–351, 1966.
Fuqua F: Renaissance of urethroplasty: The Belt technique of hypospadias repair. J Urol 106:782–785, 1971.
Smith DR: Repair of hypospadias in the preschool child: A report of 150 cases. J Urol 97:723–730, 1967.

EPISPADIAS

Epispadias is a rare congenital anomaly which is also always present in association with bladder exstrophy; it is considered a milder degree of the latter.

The urethra opens on the dorsum of the penis with deficient corpus spongiosum and loosely attached corpora cavernosa. If the defect is extensive, it can reach up to the bladder neck and is associated with complete incontinence. The pubic bones are separated, as in exstrophy. Marked dorsiflexion of the penis is usually present.

Treatment consists of correction of penile encurvature, reconstruction of the urethra, and reconstruction of bladder neck in incontinent cases. If these measures fail, urinary diversion may be indicated.

Burkholder GV, Williams DI: Epispadias and incontinence: Surgical treatment of 27 children. J Urol 94:674–679, 1965.
Michalowski E, Modelski W: The surgical treatment of epispadias. Surg Gynec Obst 117:465–468, 1963.

URETHRAL FISTULAS

Urethral fistulas may be urethrovaginal, urethrorectal, or urethrocutaneous. The first and second types are commonly traumatic (obstetrical or surgical); rarely, congenital or due to malignant infiltration. Urethrocutaneous fistulas commonly complicate urethral trauma, stricture, periurethral abscesses, and surgery. Urethral tumor is a rare cause.

Treatment consists of correction of any underlying disease (if feasible), and excision of all fistulous tracts and proximal diversions.

Culp OS, Calhoun HW: A variety of rectourethral fistulas: Experiences with 20 cases. J Urol 91:560–571, 1964.
Gray L: Urethrovaginal fistulas. Am J Obst Gynec 101:28–35, 1965.

POSTERIOR URETHRAL VALVES

Posterior urethral valves are folds of mucosa, seen only in males, which originate at or are attached at some point to the verumontanum. The embryologic bases are indefinite. They are partially obstructive and thus lead to variable degrees of back pressure damage to the urinary bladder and upper urinary tract. Progressive renal damage may occur as a result of hypertrophy, trabeculation, diverticula formation, bilateral hydroureter, or hydronephrosis, with early obstruction at the ureterovesical junction because of trigonal hypertrophy and later development of reflux. Dilatation and obstruction of the prostatic urethra are always present.

Manifestations consist of difficult voiding a weak urinary stream, an abdominal mass that represents a distended or hypertrophied bladder, and in some cases palpable kidneys. Urinary incontinence and urinary tract infection may occur in young boys. Laboratory findings include elevated BUN and serum creatinine, diminished PSP excretion, and evidence of urinary infection. Urograms show evidence of bladder thickening and trabeculation, hydroureter, hydronephrosis, and reflux. Demonstration of urethral valves on retrograde urethrograms or, preferably, voiding cystourethrograms establishes the diagnosis. Endoscopic visualization of valves and evidence of bladder changes are also usually seen.

Posterior urethral valves must be differentiated from neurogenic dysfunction, tumors, and meatal stenosis. If meatal stenosis and phimosis are excluded, any lower urinary tract obstructive disorder in a newborn or young boy should be considered posterior urethral valves until proved otherwise.

Treatment consists of destruction of the valves by overstretching, either by means of dilators through a perineal urethrotomy or by endoscopic fulguration or resection. Supravesical drainage (bilateral nephrostomy or bilateral loop ureterostomy) may be required to improve markedly impaired kidney function. Bilateral ureterovesicoplasty may be needed for a persistently obstructed or refluxing ureterovesical junction. Permanent urinary diversion is sometimes required.

The prognosis depends upon the original degree of kidney damage and the success of efforts to prevent or treat infection. In early cases, the prognosis is quite favorable.

Hendren WH: Posterior urethral valves in boys: A broad clinical spectrum. J Urol 106:298–307, 1971.

Waldraum RS, Marshall VF: Posterior urethral valves: Evaluation and surgical management. J Urol 103:801–809, 1970.

Waterhouse K: The dilated posterior urethra. I. Male. J Urol 91:71–75, 1964.

Williams DI, Eckstein B: Obstructive valves in the posterior urethra. J Urol 93:236–246, 1965.

URETHRAL STRICTURE

Congenital urethral strictures are common at the meatus, rare in the penile urethra. Acquired strictures may be due to external trauma and rupture, or to instrumentation; may be inflammatory, due to gonorrhea (most common), tuberculous urethritis, or schistosomiasis; or, rarely, may be a complication of malignancy. The common presenting symptoms are dysuria, weak stream, bifurcation of the urinary stream, urinary retention, and urinary tract infection. Evidence of scarring due to trauma or induration and perineal fistula may be seen. Urethral calibration reveals the degree of narrowing. A retrograde urethrogram will delineate the site and degree of stricture. A voiding cystourethrogram may show its proximal extension.

Urethral stricture must be differentiated from bladder outlet obstruction due to prostatism, impacted urethral stones, urethral foreign bodies, and tumors.

Treatment consists of repeated dilatation, internal urethrotomy for limited annular strictures, and urethroplasty for extensive stricture.

Helmstein K: Internal urethrotomy: Modifications in the operative technique. Acta chir scandinav, Suppl 340, 1965.

Jessen C: Resection of urethral stricture and end-to-end anastomosis. Scandinav J Urol Nephrol 4:87–91, 1970.

Katz AS, Waterhouse K: Treatment of urethral stricture in man by internal urethrotomy: A study of 61 patients. J Urol 105:807–809, 1971.

Turner-Warwick R: The repair of urethral strictures in the region of the membranous urethra. J Urol 100:303–314, 1968.

PRIAPISM

Priapism is a rare disorder that consists of prolonged erection, usually painful, which is unassociated with sexual stimulation. The blood in the corpora cavernosa becomes sludge-like rather than clotted. About 25% of cases are associated with leukemia, metastatic carcinoma, or sickle cell anemia. In most cases the cause is unclear.

If the erection does not subside in a few hours, ice water enemas may lead to resolution. If not, evacuation of the sludged blood of the corpora with a needle and syringe, followed by lavage with an anticoagulant, or controlled hypotension and systemic anticoagulation should be tried. If these methods fail, anastomosis of the saphenous vein to the ipsilateral corpus cavernosum should be done, and the earlier the better.

Even though one of these methods relieves the erection, inability to achieve an erection thereafter is a common sequence.

Harrow BR: Simple technique for treating priapism. J Urol 101:71–73, 1969.

Howe GE & others: Priapism: A surgical emergency. J Urol 101:576–579, 1969.

Seeler RA: Priapism in children with sickle cell anemia: Successful management with liberal red cell transfusions. Clin Pediat 10:418–419, 1971.

DISORDERS OF THE FEMALE URETHRA

DISTAL URETHRAL STENOSIS

The female urethra is muscular in its entire length except for the terminal 0.5 cm, where there is a dense collagen deposition which probably acts as a point of fixation for the urethral musculature. This collagenous ring is a normal histologic finding in the female urethra. Abnormal abundance of this collagenous tissue may encroach on the urethral lumen. This tissue seems to be under the influence of female hormones and becomes quite soft at puberty. This distal urethral segment receives its sensory supply from the pudendal nerve; any irritation to this area (commonly by infection) leads to reflex spasm of the striated external sphincter, which in turn leads to variable symptoms of irritative, obstructive voiding with urethrovesical reflux, washing urethral bacteria into the bladder and thus initiating or perpetuating lower urinary tract infection.

Urethral dilatation (up to 36F), rupture of the distal urethral ring, and clearance of infection relieve the urethral spasm. Normal voiding dynamics are restored, and urinary tract infection is cleared in most of these cases.

A marginally competent ureterovesical junction might become incompetent in the face of the abnormally high voiding pressure caused by the sphincter spasm. Where the latter is relieved, reflux may spontaneously disappear.

Lyon RP, Marshall S: Urinary tract infections and difficult urination in girls: Long-term follow-up. J Urol 105:314–317, 1971.

Lyon RP, Tanagho EA: Distal urethral stenosis in little girls. J Urol 93:379–387, 1965.

Tanagho EA & others: Spastic striated external sphincter and urinary tract infection in girls. Brit J Urol 43:69–82, 1971.

URETHRITIS & PERIURETHRITIS

Urethritis in the female may be acute or chronic. Acute urethritis is commonly gonorrheal in origin. Chemical urethritis is occasionally acquired from exposure to bubble bath crystals. Chronic urethritis is a common problem in females because the female urethra is always exposed to pathogenic bacteria due to its anatomic location; the distal part of the urethra is always infected. Urethral trauma, instrumentation, and increase in the number of pathogenic organisms lead to flare-up of infection and overt, manifest urethritis. Urethritis usually precedes cystitis.

Hormonal changes associated with menopause cause vaginal and urethral mucosal changes which lead to irritative symptoms and increased susceptibility to inflammatory flare-ups. Repeated labor and coital trauma can lead to periurethral fibrosis, which again can lead to irritative lower urinary tract symptoms even in the absence of any bacterial infection.

Urethritis usually causes irritative lower urinary tract symptoms similar to those of cystitis and, occasionally, functional obstructive symptoms. Examination may reveal urethral discharge, marked tenderness, or congested everted mucosa at the external meatus. Thickening and induration along the urethra, associated vaginal mucosal changes, and evidence of cervicitis and vaginitis may be present. Endoscopic examination may reveal obstruction, congested mucous membranes, infected urethral glands with pus exuding from their ducts, or inflammatory polyps around the internal meatus. Urethral calibration rarely reveals obstruction. Resistance of the spastic external sphincter may be noted.

Treatment consists of removal of the underlying cause, if possible. Estrogen cream or diethylstilbestrol suppositories are indicated for senile urethritis. Surgical treatment consists of urethral dilatation and opening and draining of infected periurethral ducts. Correction of vaginitis, cervicitis, and cervical erosions helps in ameliorating symptoms.

Marshall S, Lyon RP, Schieble J: Nonspecific urethritis in females. California Med 112:9–10, June 1970.

Quinlivan LG: The treatment of senile vaginitis with low doses of synthetic estrogens. Am J Obst Gynec 92:172–174, 1965.

URETHRAL CARUNCLE

Urethral caruncle, commonly seen after menopause, represents granulomatous overgrowth of the posterior lip of the external meatus. It is usually painful to touch, during intercourse, and with urination. The most important consideration is to exclude malignancy.

Treatment is local excision.

Marshall FC, Uson AC, Melicow MM: Neoplasms and caruncles of the female urethra. Surg Gynec Obst 110:723–733, 1960.

URETHRAL DIVERTICULUM

Urethral diverticulum commonly presents as recurrent lower urinary tract infection. It should be suspected whenever urinary infection fails to resolve with treatment. Symptoms consist of urinary dribbling and cystic swelling in the anterior vaginal wall during voiding. If diverticulum is suspected, it can usually be seen during panendoscopy and visualized radiographically on a voiding cystourethrogram with the external meatus occluded, or by using special catheters.

Treatment consists of transvaginal surgical excision, taking care not to injure the urethral sphincter during dissection.

Hoffman MJ, Adams WE: Recognition and repair of urethral diverticula. Am J Obst Gynec 92:106–109, 1965.

Spence HM, Duckett JW Jr: Diverticulum of female urethra: Clinical aspects and presentation of a simple operative technique for cure. J Urol 104:432–437, 1970.

Widholm O, Rynänen VA: Diverticulum of the female urethra. Acta obst gynec scandinav 46:107–117, 1967.

between deficiency of maturation and obstruction of the conduction system.

Treatment

A. Hormonal Therapy: Appropriate therapy should be instituted for hypothyroidism. Hyperadrenocorticism should be suppressed with corticosteroids, which will lead to increase in the number of sperms and a higher percentage of normal forms. There is some evidence that the administration of human gonadotropins may be of value in hypopituitarism.

Small doses of androgen (eg, 5–10 mg/day) may improve motility if the sperm count is high. Androgens may also be helpful if the count is normal but the volume of ejaculate is low. If the quality of the semen is very poor, testosterone, 50 mg IM 3 times a week, should be given for 3 months; this will result in complete azoospermia. On cessation of the drug, a "rebound" phenomenon may occur.

B. General Measures: The patient should abstain from intercourse for a few days before his wife's fertile period. Obesity should be treated.

C. Surgical Measures: Vasovasostomy is indicated for men who have had previous vasoligation. Epididymovasostomy should be done for epididymal occlusion. Ligation of the spermatic vein is indicated in the presence of varicocele; fertility will be restored in half of this group.

Prognosis

The poorer the quality of the semen, the poorer the outlook. When the count is under 1 million/ml, there is little room for optimism.

MALE INFERTILITY

A couple can be judged infertile if conception does not occur after 12 months of adequate cohabitation. About 10% of marriages are barren, and spermatogenic deficiencies are responsible in at least 40% of cases. The common causes are (1) deficiencies in maturation of germ cells (the most common), (2) obstruction to the conduction system, (3) hypothyroidism, (4) hyperadrenalism, (5) the formation of sperm antibodies, and (6) varicocele.

A history of mumps, cryptorchidism, testicular trauma, varicocele, or epididymitis may prove significant. Evidence of endocrinologic abnormality should be sought. The scrotal contents should be carefully examined for testicular size and consistency, scarring of the epididymides, and the presence of intact vasa deferentia. The finding of varicocele is of the greatest importance, for its treatment offers the best hope for reversal of infertility.

Analysis of the semen is the most important laboratory test. The specimen should be obtained after at least 4 days of abstinence from intercourse. Most fertile men have at least 50 million sperms/ml, 70% of which are motile. A differential count, judging morphology, should be done; at least 70% of the sperms in most fertile men are normally formed.

A test of thyroid function and an estimate of urinary pituitary gonadotropins and 17-ketosteroids should be obtained. A buccal smear should be taken for nuclear chromatin analysis. If chromatin mass is positive, the patient has Klinefelter's syndrome. In the face of azoospermia, testicular biopsy will differentiate

Agger P: Scrotal and testicular temperature: Its relation to sperm count before and after operation for varicocele. Fertil Steril 22:268–297, 1971.

Dubin L, Amelar RD: Etiologic factors in 1294 consecutive cases of male infertility. Fertil Steril 22:469–474, 1971.

Garduno A, Mehan DJ: Testicular biopsy findings in patients with impaired fertility. J Urol 104:871–877, 1970.

Kolodny RC & others: Sperm-agglutinating antibodies and infertility. Obst Gynec 38:576–582, 1971.

•   •   •

General Bibliography

Boyarsky S (editor): *Urodynamics.* Academic Press, 1971.

Campbell MF, Harrison JH (editors): *Urology,* 3rd ed. Saunders, 1970.

Dodson AI (editor): *Urological Surgery.* Mosby, 1950.

Emmett JL (editor): *Clinical Urography: An Atlas and Textbook of Roentgenologic Diagnosis,* 3rd ed. Saunders, 1971.

Federman DD (editor): *Abnormal Sexual Development.* Saunders, 1967.

Glenn JF, Boyce WH (editors): *Urologic Surgery.* Hoeber, 1969.

Graves FT (editor): *The Arterial Anatomy of the Kidney.* Williams & Wilkins, 1971.

Hinman F Jr (editor): *Hydrodynamics of Micturition.* Thomas, 1971.

Lowsley OS, Kirwin TJ (editors): *Clinical Urology,* 3rd ed. Williams & Wilkins, 1956.

Nowinski W, Goss RJ: *Compensatory Renal Hypertrophy.* Academic Press, 1970.

Pitts RF (editor): *Physiology of the Kidney and Body Fluids.* Year Book, 1963.

Smith DR: *General Urology,* 7th ed. Lange, 1972.

Stamey TA (editor): *Renovascular Hypertension.* Williams & Wilkins, 1963.

Stephens FD (editor): *Congenital Malformations of the Rectum, Anus and Genitourinary Tracts.* Livingstone, 1963.

Youssef AF (editor): *Gynecological Urology.* Thomas, 1960.

45 . . .

Gynecology

Edward C. Hill, MD

CONGENITAL ANOMALIES OF THE FEMALE REPRODUCTIVE SYSTEM

Congenital defects of the female reproduction system arise as a result of abnormal embryologic development of the müllerian ducts and urogenital sinus. The most common defects are imperforate hymen, septate or double vagina, transverse septum of the vagina, congenital absence of the vagina, and duplication defects of the uterus.

An adequate physical examination will detect or at least arouse a suspicion of defective development. Examination under anesthesia and exploration of the uterus with a sound will often provide additional valuable information. An intravenous urogram should be done in all cases because one-third to one-half of cases are associated with anomalies of the urinary tract such as absent kidney, horseshoe kidney, and duplication of the collecting system. Injury to the urinary tract can result from failure to recognize associated urinary tract anomalies during corrective surgery.

Congenital anomalies of the genitourinary tract must be distinguished from primary amenorrhea due to endocrine disorders, leiomyomas of the uterus, and ovarian tumors. Errors in diagnosis have resulted in unnecessary surgery, particularly when a preoperative diagnosis of leiomyoma uteri is made in a case of uterus didelphys or bicornuate uterus. Laparoscopic examination may be of considerable value in an evaluation of the patient with a suspected anomaly of the genitourinary tract.

Minor anomalies of the reproductive tract require only explanation and reassurance. For example, a small vaginal septum, bicornuate uterus, or even a complete uterus didelphys usually will not interfere with coital or reproductive function and will cause no significant symptoms.

Imperforate Hymen

Imperforate hymen is often not recognized until puberty, when, despite the appearance of menstrual symptoms, bleeding fails to occur. Examination at this time will reveal a bulging, imperforate hymen. Rectal examination may demonstrate a large, cystic pelvic mass representing a distended vagina (hematocolpos) and even a cystically enlarged uterus (hematometra). Urinary obstruction has been reported due to a large hematocolpos resulting from menstruation behind an imperforate hymen.

Imperforate hymen is treated by cruciate incisions of the mucous membrane (hymenotomy), releasing the trapped menstrual discharges and correcting the hematocolpos and hematometra. Antibiotics should be given when there is a significant hematocolpos and hematometra in order to prevent secondary infection.

Duplication of the Vagina

Duplication of the vagina may occur with or without a single or a double uterus. There may be a double vagina, a double cervix, and a single uterus. The duplication may be only partial and take the form of a longitudinal septum, in which case excision may be required in the event that there is soft tissue dystocia in labor. Complete duplication of the vagina usually requires no treatment.

Occasionally, the duplication takes the form of a rudimentary vagina which fails to communicate with the second vagina or the outside. This may result in the formation of a hematocolpos at the time of menarche, with an apparent paravaginal cystic mass as a presenting sign. The finding of old blood upon incising such a tumor should lead to the correct diagnosis. A separate cervix and corpus will be found at the top of this space. Marsupialization of the rudimentary vagina with the primary vagina is the usual method of management.

Transverse Septum of the Vagina

A transverse vaginal septum usually is incomplete. If imperforate, it may be mistaken for congenital absence of the vagina.

Transverse vaginal septa are treated by excision.

Absence of the Vagina

Absence of the vagina usually is associated with absence of the uterus. Often there is a very small lower vagina, representing that portion that develops from the urogenital sinus. The condition is commonly not recognized until the physician is consulted because of primary amenorrhea in a teen-ager.

Congenital absence of the vagina is managed by construction of an artificial vagina. This should be deferred until the patient has a desire and a need for a functioning vagina. A variety of technics have been described, but those utilizing skin grafts placed in an artificially created channel between the bladder and the rectum have been the most widely used. Artificial vaginas can be constructed from the labia majora or by using isolated segments of the large intestine.

Construction of an artificial vagina will allow girls to develop satisfactory social and sexual relationships with members of the opposite sex. The psychologic benefits are as important as the physical ones.

Duplication Defects of the Uterus

Duplication defects of the uterus are most often detected in the course of investigation for habitual abortion or for repeated premature labor. They may vary from a simple midline septum in a single uterus to a complete duplication of the corpus and cervix. Uterine anomalies of this type can often be detected during the third trimester of pregnancy because of the characteristic abdominal outlines of the uterine fundus and persistent malpresentations of the fetus. Manual exploration of the uterine cavity immediately postpartum will demonstrate a uterine septum or a double horn. Hysterosalpingography is essential to an accurate diagnosis.

If there is a history of repeated fetal loss due to abortions or premature labor, the surgical correction of uterine anomalies is warranted in the hope of improving the patient's fertility. The classic operation for bicornuate uterus is that described by Strassman in which the horns are incised transversely anterior to the insertion of the fallopian tubes and then closed in a longitudinal direction. The septate uterus is corrected either by excising a midline wedge, removing the septum, or merely incising the septum and suturing the margins, thus constructing a single cavity. Subsequent pregnancies after operations for such uterine anomalies should be delivered by cesarean section in order to avoid the risk of uterine rupture in labor. This ideally is done approximately 10 days prior to the expected date of confinement as the risk of rupture increases with approaching term and with labor.

When uterine anomalies are responsible for a poor obstetric history with high fetal wastage, one can expect significant improvement following surgical correction. Fortunately, most patients with abnormalities of the uterus have no significant obstetric problems and require no therapy.

Capraro VJ & others: Improved fetal salvage after metroplasty. Obst Gynec 31:97–103, 1968.

Crosby WM, Hill EC: Embryology of the müllerian duct system: Review of present day theory. Obst Gynec 20:4, 507–515, 1962.

Semmens JP: Abdominal contour in the third trimester: An aid to diagnosis of uterine anomalies. Obst Gynec 25:779–786, 1965.

BACTERIAL INFECTIONS OF THE FEMALE REPRODUCTIVE SYSTEM

Chancroid

Chancroid is an acute ulcerative (soft chancre) lesion of the vulva with secondary involvement of the inguinal and femoral lymph nodes caused by *Haemophilus ducreyi.* It is transmitted through coitus and has an incubation period of 2–14 days. The lesion first appears as a papule which rapidly becomes a large pustule. This breaks down, ulcerates, and forms satellite lesions. The regional nodes become enlarged and painful, and chills, fever, and malaise develop. Leukocytosis is usually present. The diagnosis is confirmed by finding the organism in a smear of the exudate, although a culture may be required.

The skin test for chancroid (suspension of the organism) becomes positive within 3–5 weeks of an acute infection and remains positive for life. It is, therefore, of limited value.

The sulfonamides are the drugs of choice, eg, sulfadiazine, 1 g 4 times daily for 7 days. Streptomycin, 1–2 g daily IM for 7 days, may be used as an alternative.

Large, painful, fluctuant buboes may be aspirated, but prompt antibiotic therapy usually allows prompt regression.

Syphilis

The primary lesion of syphilis in women is often a transient, painless, small ulcer on the cervix or the labia. Because this lesion does not take the usual classic form of a chancre, it is often overlooked. The disease usually is transmitted by coitus and is due to the spirochete *Treponema pallidum,* which can be recognized in a darkfield examination of serum obtained from the lesion. Most often, however, the diagnosis is made on the basis of a positive serologic test. The *Treponema pallidum* immobilization test may be helpful in the diagnosis.

Penicillin is the antibiotic of choice. Procaine penicillin with 2% aluminum monostearate in oil (PAM), 2.4 million units IM initially and then 1.2 million units IM every other day for 4 doses, has been found to be effective.

Gonorrhea

Neisseria gonorrhoeae is transmitted by sexual intercourse. It may involve the lower genital tract as a suppurative process involving the Bartholin glands, Skene's ducts, or the cervix. Only in prepubertal girls does it involve the vaginal mucosa since cornified squamous epithelium of the adult vagina resists infection. After infection of the lower tract it may spread via the endometrial surface, following a menstrual period, to the fallopian tubes, where it produces an acute salpingitis, sometimes leading to pelvic peritonitis, tubo-ovarian abscess, chronic salpingitis, and tubal obstruction with bilateral hydrosalpinx. The incidence of subsequent sterility is very high.

If the infection involves only the lower tract, there may be no or few symptoms unless a Bartholin abscess develops, in which case there is a large, painful swelling in the posterior aspect of the labium majus. Acute gonorrheal cervicitis is seen as a mucopurulent exudate from an inflamed cervix. With tubal involvement, which is almost always bilateral, there is lower abdominal pain of a colicky nature, malaise, and fever. There may be signs of acute peritonitis with tenderness, rigidity, rebound tenderness, and ileus. The white blood cell count and the sedimentation rate are moderately elevated. Pain in the right upper quadrant of the abdomen is an unusual manifestation due to spread of infection in a cephalad direction up the right "peritoneal gutter." Violin string adhesions between the liver and parietal peritoneum may result.

Pain and tenderness may closely simulate the findings in acute cholecystitis (Fitz-Hugh and Curtis syndrome).

The diagnosis of gonorrhea is made by finding the typical gram-negative intracellular diplococci in smears or in anaerobic culture (Thayer-Martin V.C.N. media). Disease of the upper tract and the pelvic peritoneum must be distinguished from acute appendicitis, ovarian cysts, tubal pregnancy, endometriosis, diverticulitis, tuberculous salpingitis, and pedunculated leiomyomas of the uterus.

Penicillin is the antibiotic of choice. Tetracycline is used in penicillin-resistant disease.

Bartholin abscess should be incised and drained. Marsupialization or excision of Bartholin cysts may be required if the duct remains obstructed and the cyst is large or symptomatic. Tubo-ovarian abscesses require incision and drainage. This can usually be accomplished through the vagina via the cul-de-sac. Tuboplastic procedures are done for the relief of sterility in chronic tubal obstruction. Chronic salpingo-oophoritis often requires a total abdominal hysterectomy and bilateral salpingo-oophorectomy.

Reznichek RC & others: Gonorrhea today (problems of diagnosis, management, treatment). California Med 115:32–37, Aug 1971.
Waters JR, Raulston TM: Gonococcal infection in a prenatal clinic. Am J Obst Gynec 103:532–536, 1969.

Tuberculosis

Tuberculous infection of the fallopian tubes with secondary involvement of the endometrium (and, rarely, the cervix) is an uncommon disease in the USA, accounting for 5–10% of cases of salpingitis. It is usually secondary to tuberculous infections elsewhere, such as the lung or the urinary tract.

The process may be asymptomatic, with infertility the only complaint. Symptoms, when they occur, are those of low-grade fever, weight loss, fatigue, and menstrual irregularities. There may be palpable adnexal masses.

The diagnosis may be made upon finding a granulomatous lesion in the endometrium at the time of dilatation and curettage for menstrual irregularity. The acid-fast organisms are difficult to demonstrate in histologic sections, and culture or guinea pig inoculation of endometrial tissue or the menstrual discharge often is necessary. Chest x-ray, sputum studies, acid-fast smears, cultures, and guinea pig inoculation of the urine should be done as well.

Treatment of advanced genital tuberculosis consists of medical therapy with isoniazid, aminosalicylic acid (PAS), and streptomycin for at least 6 months followed by total abdominal hysterectomy and bilateral salpingo-oophorectomy. Mild cases may be treated medically in the hope of relieving infertility, but close follow-up is mandatory.

Schaefer G: Diagnosis and treatment of female genital tuberculosis. Internat Surg 48:240–258, 1967.
Sutherland AM: Treatment of genital tuberculosis in women. Geneesk gids 45:362–386, 1967.

Granuloma Inguinale

Infection with *Calymmatobacterium (Donovania) granulomatis* is seen in the USA most often in the southern states. It is transmitted through sexual intercourse and begins as a small vulval papule which then becomes a small area of beefy-red granulomatous tissue. This process spreads superficially and eventually involves the entire perineum, extending into the inguinal areas. Secondary infection is common.

The symptoms are pain, burning, itching, and discharge from the involved area. Smears or biopsies stained with Wright's stain or hematoxylin-eosin stain will show the characteristic Donovan inclusion bodies within large mononuclear cells.

Treatment is with tetracycline, 500 mg orally 4 times daily for.1 week and then 250 mg 4 times daily for an additional 2 weeks.

Lymphogranuloma (Lymphopathia) Venereum

Lymphogranuloma venereum (LGV) is caused by infection with one of the chlamydia group of gram-negative, obligately intracellular bacteria (not by a "large virus," as formerly believed). It is transmitted by coitus and is manifested initially as a small vulval vesicle which appears 1–3 weeks after exposure. This soon disappears but is followed in another 2–3 weeks by an inguinal lymphadenitis which progresses to bubo formation, ulceration, and breakdown. The perirectal lymphatics frequently are similarly involved. Healing often leads to inguinal scarring, rectal stricture, and vulval elephantiasis.

The Frei skin test has been used to confirm the diagnosis and becomes positive about 1 week after the enlargement of the inguinal lymph nodes. It is nonspecific for LGV infection and will be positive in individuals previously infected with other members of the psittacosis group. Therefore, it is diagnostic only if it is negative in the acute phase of the disease and then becomes positive. A positive complement fixation test with a rising titer is also diagnostic.

Treatment is with sulfadiazine, 1 g orally 4 times daily for 3 weeks, or tetracycline, 500 mg orally 4 times daily for 1 week followed by 250 mg 4 times daily for an additional 2 weeks.

VIRAL INFECTIONS OF THE FEMALE REPRODUCTIVE SYSTEM

Condylomata Acuminata (Venereal Warts)

These are usually multiple papules seen on the skin of the vulva and the mucous membranes of the vagina and cervix. They are of viral origin and are usually associated with a vaginal discharge and irritation.

Treatment is with podophyllin applied topically in a 25% solution of compound tincture of benzoin, or by electrocoagulation.

Graber EA & others: Simple surgical treatment for *condyloma acuminatum* of the vulva. Obst Gynec 29:247–250, 1967.

Herpes Progenitalis

Herpes progenitalis is caused by *Herpesvirus hominis* type 2 and is venereally transmitted. It is characterized by the appearance of clusters of small, painful, erythematous vesicular lesions on the vulva. Examination may also demonstrate these in the vagina and on the portio vaginalis of the cervix. The vesicles often proceed to ulceration; with coalescence, large, painful ulcers of the vulva, vagina, and cervix may develop.

The diagnosis can be made cytologically by finding characteristic "ground glass" inclusions in mono- or multinucleated giant cells from the squamous epithelium.

There appears to be a relationship between herpes progenitalis and carcinoma of the cervix, as antibodies to herpesvirus type 2 have been found significantly more often in women with cervical cancer than in matched control groups. Whether this is merely a coincidental factor transmitted sexually or an etiologic relationship has not yet been established.

There is no specific treatment. The discomfort may be relieved with moist compresses of aluminum subacetate followed by topical application of fluocinolone acetonide (Synalar) cream, 0.025%.

Because of the risk of severe systemic disease in infants delivered vaginally, a patient with an acute infection near term in pregnancy should be delivered by cesarean section.

Josey WE & others: Genital herpes simplex infection in the female. Am J Obst Gynec 96:493–501, 1966.
Naili ZM & others: Genital herpetic infection: Association with cervical dysplasia and carcinoma. Cancer 23:940–945, 1969.
Rawls WE & others: Herpesvirus type 2: Association with carcinoma of cervix. Science 161:1255–1256, 1968.
Yen SSC, Reagen JW, Rosenthal MS: Herpes simplex infection in the female genital tract. Obst Gynec 25:479–492, 1965.

TRICHOMONAS VAGINALIS VAGINITIS

Trichomonas vaginalis vaginitis is caused by a motile flagellated protozoon which produces a vaginal inflammation characterized by a profuse, thin, foamy, yellowish discharge, local burning, and itching. The diagnosis is made by finding the organism in a wet mount smear from the vagina.

Treatment with metronidazole (Flagyl), 250 mg orally 3 times daily for 10 days, is usually successful. It may be necessary to treat the patient's sexual partner concomitantly in order to prevent recurrent infections. Numerous topical agents are available for use in the vagina, and until the teratogenicity of metronidazole has been ruled out the drug should not be used in the pregnant patient.

CANDIDIASIS
(Moniliasis)

Candida albicans, a yeast organism, is the cause of candidal vaginitis, seen often in diabetics, pregnant patients, and women using oral contraceptives. Candidal infections also occur as a complication of antibiotic therapy, with suppression of the normal bacterial flora and overgrowth by yeast organisms. Candidal vaginitis and vulvitis are characterized by intense itching and inflamed skin and mucosa. Frequently there is a clinging, cheesy-white exudate, although this finding may be absent. Intense pruritus is the primary symptom. The diagnosis is made by finding spores or mycelia on a wet mount smear preparation to which a few drops of 10% potassium hydroxide are added or by culturing the organism on Nickerson's medium.

Office treatment consists of cleansing the vagina of the curd-like exudate and applying a 2% aqueous solution of gentian violet. Nystatin (Mycostatin) vaginal tablets are used by the patient each night at bedtime for 2–3 weeks. Nystatin cream is also available for use on the irritated vulval skin.

MENSTRUAL DISORDERS

AMENORRHEA

Amenorrhea may be primary (a delay of the menarche beyond age 17) or secondary (a cessation of menstrual function of several months' or years' duration occurring after the development of normal, cyclic menstruation). True primary amenorrhea may be due to an abnormality in function or disease of the ovary, pituitary, or hypothalamus. Congenital anomalies of the uterus and vagina as a cause of primary amenorrhea are discussed above.

Clinical Findings

A. Primary Amenorrhea:

1. Congenital anomalies—
2. **Ovarian agenesis and dysgenesis—**
   a. Short stature.
   b. Webbing of neck.
   c. Cubitus valgus.
   d. Infantile external genitalia.
   e. Absent sex chromatin on buccal smear.
   f. Most have a chromosomal karyotype of 45,X, but mosaic patterns (45,X/46,XX or 45,X/46,XX/47,XXX) are encountered.
3. **Hermaphroditism—**
   a. Ambiguous external genitalia with enlarged clitoris and urogenital sinus into which vagina and urethra open.
   b. Normal breast development.
   c. Menstruation may occur.
   d. Sex chromatin present in buccal smear.
   e. Chromosomal karyotype usually 46,XX.
   f. Ovarian and testicular tissue combined in a single gonad (ovotestis).
4. **Testicular feminization syndrome—**
   a. Female habitus with relatively large hands and feet.
   b. Normal breast development.
   c. Scant or absent pubic and axillary hair.
   d. Normal external genitalia.
   e. Hypoplastic vagina ending in a short, blind pouch.
   f. Absent or rudimentary uterus and tubes.
   g. Sex chromatin absent in buccal smear.
   h. Chromosomal karyotype is 46,XY.
   i. Gonads are testes which lie in abdomen, pelvis, or inguinal canal.

B. Secondary Amenorrhea:

1. **Pregnancy—**
   a. Signs and symptoms of pregnancy.
   b. Positive chorionic gonadotropin test.
2. **Menopause—**
   a. Hot flashes.
   b. Familial history of early menopause.
   c. Elevated pituitary gonadotropin.
3. **Psychogenic—**
   a. Traumatic experience or psychologic disturbance.
   b. Usually temporary (less than 6 months).
4. **Following oral contraceptives.**
5. **Stein-Leventhal syndrome—**
   a. Obesity.
   b. Hirsutism.
   c. Bilaterally enlarged ovaries.
6. **Pituitary insufficiency or failure (depressed pituitary gonadotropins)—**
   a. Following traumatic labor or delivery (Sheehan's syndrome).

   b. Pituitary tumors (headache and visual disturbances).

Treatment

A. Primary Amenorrhea:

1. Congenital anomalies—
2. Ovarian agenesis and dysgenesis—
   a. Cyclic estrogen-progestin therapy to simulate normal menstrual cycle and develop secondary sex characteristics.
   b. Plastic surgery if webbing of neck is severe.
3. **Hermaphroditism—**
   a. Surgical removal of contradictory sex organs and reconstruction of those compatible with sex in which patient has been reared.
4. **Testicular feminization syndrome—**
   a. Excision of gonads.
   b. Cyclic estrogen therapy.

B. Secondary Amenorrhea:

1. **Pregnancy—**Obstetrical care.
2. **Menopause—**Replacement estrogen therapy given cyclically to relieve menopausal symptoms.
3. **Psychogenic—**
   a. Usually self-limited.
   b. Cyclic estrogen-progestin therapy in the anxious patient.
4. **Following oral contraceptives—**Same as for psychogenic amenorrhea.
5. **Stein-Leventhal syndrome—**
   a. Clomiphene citrate (Clomid).
   b. Human gonadotropin therapy.
   c. Bilateral wedge resection of ovaries if failure to respond to above.
6. **Pituitary insufficiency or failure—**
   a. Replacement therapy (corticosteroids, thyroid, estrogens).
   b. Treatment of pituitary tumors.

ABNORMAL UTERINE BLEEDING

Abnormal uterine bleeding may occur at any age. In the newborn it is frequently related to removal of the infant at birth from the influence of maternal estrogen which has produced endometrial proliferation in the baby's uterus. During the reproductive years, it may occur as **hypermenorrhea**, excessive or prolonged bleeding at the normal time of menstruation; **polymenorrhea**, bleeding which occurs more frequently than every 3 weeks; or **intermenstrual bleeding**, which occurs during the interval between normal menstrual periods.

Hypermenorrhea may be due to such organic conditions as uterine leiomyoma, endometrial polyps, and blood dyscrasias, or it may be related to a functional disturbance such as irregular shedding of the endometrium, presumably due to faulty regression of the corpus luteum of the ovary. Polymenorrhea may be related to early ovulation with a shortened proliferative phase, which frequently is secondary to hypothyroidism. One of the most frequently encountered problems is the completely acyclic and sometimes heavy and prolonged bleeding of the anovulatory patient, leading to so-called **dysfunctional uterine bleeding**. This condition is seen most often in adolescents and in premenopausal women and is due to a failure in regular ovulatory function by the ovaries. The endometrium is proliferative in type at a time in the menstrual cycle when it would show secretory changes had ovulation occurred. In many instances there is, after a period of time, the development of endometrial hyperplasia, either of the cystic glandular or adenomatous pattern, due to the prolonged stimulus of estrogen on the endometrium without the modifying influence of progesterone. Intermenstrual bleeding may be due to the slight drop in estrogen titer associated with ovulation, in which event it occurs quite regularly at about midcycle. Other causes of intermenstrual bleeding which occurs at any time during the cycle are polyps, submucous leiomyomas, blood dyscrasias, genital tuberculosis, and cancer of the cervix, uterine corpus, or fallopian tube. Complications of pregnancy should not be overlooked as a cause of abnormal bleeding in women of the reproductive age.

Postmenopausal bleeding (vaginal bleeding which occurs a year or more following the menopause) is due to cancer in about 40% of cases. The exogenous administration of estrogenic substances, including their use in cosmetic preparations, is another important cause of this type of abnormal bleeding. Atrophic changes, polyps, trauma, blood dyscrasias, hypertensive cardiovascular disease, and estrogen-producing tumors of the ovary are less frequent causes. The bleeding may be represented by a scant brownish vaginal discharge, or it may be frank, profuse, bright-red bleeding. Because it looms so large in the etiology of postmenopausal bleeding, cancer should be considered the cause until proved otherwise.

Clinical Findings

In the assessment of any type of menstrual disorder, the following points should be considered:

(1) Careful documentation of the menstrual history and an accurate record of the temporal relationship of the abnormal bleeding to the menstrual cycle are necessary. A special menstrual calendar kept by the patient or a basal body temperature graph can be very helpful in this regard.

(2) A history of hormonal medication or cosmetics containing hormones.

(3) A general medical history and physical examination may lead to the correct diagnosis of hypothyroidism, blood dyscrasia, genital tuberculosis, etc.

(4) A carefully performed pelvic examination often will reveal vaginal, cervical, uterine, or adnexal pathology.

(5) Cytologic examination is essential in all

patients, and the specimen should be collected prior to the introduction of lubricating jelly into the vagina.

(6) A complete blood count and measurement of red cell indices will reflect the degree of iron deficiency secondary to acute or chronic blood loss. Additional blood studies may be necessary when blood dyscrasias are suspected.

(7) Thyroid function studies may be indicated.

(8) Dilatation and curettage of the uterus with biopsies of the cervix often are required to establish the cause of abnormal menstrual bleeding. This should be done at an appropriate time in the menstrual cycle—eg, after the 16th day of the cycle if anovulatory bleeding is suspected, or on the fourth or fifth day if the working diagnosis is irregular shedding of the endometrium. Curettage will reveal unsuspected endometrial polyps or submucous myomas. Fractional curettage and cervical biopsies are recommended if malignancy is suspected.

Treatment

Acute, massive blood loss should be treated by recording the central venous pressure, placing the patient in the Trendelenburg position, and replenishing the circulating blood volume with intravenous fluids and whole blood transfusions.

Dilatation and curettage is the most effective method of controlling bleeding from the endometrial cavity.

In chronic blood loss due to hypermenorrhea produced by leiomyomas, total menstrual suppression may be achieved by the continuous administration of an estrogen-progestin preparation (see section on endometriosis). The oral administration of iron may obviate blood transfusion in the preparation of the patient for a definitive surgical procedure.

After organic causes have been excluded, the dysfunctional bleeding of the teen-ager and the premenopausal woman is treated with cyclic progestin therapy (aqueous progesterone, 50 mg IM on the 25th day, or norethindrone acetate, 5 mg orally daily from the 20th to the 25th days of the cycle).

Severe, intractable bleeding of a dysfunctional nature may require hysterectomy, but this is rare.

Postmenopausal bleeding of nonneoplastic cause may require estrogen therapy if due to atrophic changes. Curettage is curative if due to endometrial hyperplasia or polyps. Endometrial carcinoma is a contraindication to estrogen therapy and is treated by total abdominal hysterectomy and bilateral salpingo-oophorectomy with or without preoperative radiation therapy (see malignant disease of the uterine corpus).

DeCosta EJ: Menstrual problems: Dysfunctional uterine bleeding. JAMA 193:950–952, 1965.

Greenblatt RB & others: Spectrum of gonadal dysgenesis: Clinical cytogenetic and pathologic study. Am J Obst Gynec 98:151–172, 1967.

Jones GS: Endocrine problems of the adolescent. Maryland MJ 16:45–48, 1967.

Lang W & others: Pediatric and adolescent gynecology. Ann New York Acad Sc 142:547—834, 1967.

Lorencz AB: Managing gynecologic problems in the adolescent. GP 36:83—89, December 1967.

* * *

CERVICITIS

Essentials of Diagnosis

- Leukorrhea.
- Intermenstrual bleeding may occur.
- Sense of pelvic heaviness and backache.
- Dyspareunia.
- Cervix may show old, healed obstetric lacerations and appear elongated and enlarged.
- Cervical eversion or ectopy is common.

General Considerations

Acute cervicitis is caused by acute gonorrheal infection or occurs in association with trichomonal or candidal vaginitis. Chronic cervicitis (very common) is usually the aftermath of pregnancy and vaginal delivery. After the trauma of cervical effacement and dilatation, the cervix often heals with islands of ectopic, mucus-secreting columnar epithelium on the portio vaginalis of the cervix. This cervical "ectopy" or "eversion" without the healed lacerations and deformities of the cervix is also common in young nulligravidas (15—20%) and is related to a dislocation of the squamocolumnar junction onto the portio vaginalis; it is often asymptomatic and is of no clinical significance except in the occasional instance of excessive mucus production.

Clinical Findings

A. Symptoms and Signs: In acute cases the cervix is acutely inflamed and there is a purulent exudate; gonorrhea should be suspected. Chronic cervicitis may be mild and asymptomatic. In symptomatic cases, a copious vaginal discharge is the most common presenting complaint. In severe, deep-seated infections, there may be a low-grade pelvic cellulitis (parametritis) with a sense of heaviness in the pelvis, low backache, and dyspareunia. Postcoital bleeding may be present. The cervix appears distorted by old, healed obstetric lacerations and is reddened, boggy, and edematous. Nabothian cysts are frequently seen and are due to obstruction of the cervical tunnels, clefts, and crypts lined by mucus-secreting columnar epithelium. Endocervical and ectocervical polyps are commonly present.

B. Laboratory Findings: Cytologic smears demonstrate numerous pus cells and may show epithelial dysplasia. Cervical biopsy shows a leukocytic infiltrate in the subepithelial stroma and often squamous metaplasia and cystic dilatation of the glandular spaces. A gram-stained smear from a patient with acute gonorrheal cervicitis will often show the typical diplococci.

Culture in an atmosphere of reduced oxygen tension may be required in chronic cases.

Differential Diagnosis

Early cervical cancer may present similar symptoms and signs and must be excluded before proceeding with treatment. A negative cytologic smear does not rule out malignant disease. Multiple, representative punch biopsies from the "transformation zone" of the cervix are required.

Complications

Infertility may result from chronic cervical inflammation, which produces an environment unfavorable to penetration of the cervical mucus by spermatozoa.

Treatment

Acute gonorrheal cervicitis is best treated with penicillin. Tetracycline or kanamycin may be used in penicillin-resistant cases or in individuals who are allergic to penicillin. Treatment of nonspecific cervicitis is indicated even in asymptomatic cases because of the possible relationship between chronic cervicitis and carcinoma of the cervix. Mild degrees of cervicitis can be treated effectively with office cauterization, either chemically, with 20% silver nitrate solution on cotton-tipped applicators, or by light radial cauterization with the nasal-tipped thermal cautery or electrocautery. For the deeply involved, deformed cervix, hospitalization is required for electroconization of the cervix under anesthesia. Trachelorrhaphy (plastic repair) of the obstetrically deformed cervix may be necessary in an occasional patient with secondary infertility due to chronic cervicitis. Cryosurgery (freezing) of chronic cervicitis has been used recently with good results.

Cervical polyps usually can be removed in the office. These should be examined by a pathologist for evidence of malignancy.

Prognosis

Cure of acute cervicitis can usually be accomplished within a few days. Chronic cervicitis usually is more resistant and may require several weeks or months of treatment.

Collins RJ & others: Cryosurgery of human uterine cervix. Obst Gynec 30:660—667, 1967.

Keys TF & others: Single-dose treatment of gonorrhea with selected antibiotic agents. JAMA 210:857—861, 1969.

Ostergard DR, Townsend DE, Herose FM: The treatment of chronic cervicitis by cryotherapy. Am J Obst Gynec 102:426—432, 1968.

Saylor LF: The physician's role in venereal disease control. California Med 114:114—116, May 1971.

ADENOMYOSIS

Essentials of Diagnosis

- Multiparous patient 35–50 years of age.
- Hypermenorrhea, polymenorrhea, or intermenstrual bleeding with dysmenorrhea or dyspareunia.
- Uterus slightly to moderately enlarged, symmetric and globular.
- May be tender to palpation, particularly in premenstrual phase of cycle.

General Considerations

Adenomyosis—formerly called "internal endometriosis"—occurs when fingers of endometrium extend into the myometrium to a depth greater than 2 low-power microscopic fields. It may be a focal or a diffuse process and not infrequently involves the entire thickness of the myometrium. The pathogenesis is not known, but the theory of direct growth of the basal layer of endometrium into the myometrium is widely accepted. Estrogen has been implicated as a stimulus to the development of adenomyosis, and the symptomatic improvement which occurs with the menopause supports this concept. The disease is seen most often in the decade which precedes the menopause.

Clinical Findings

A. Symptoms and Signs: The preoperative diagnosis of adenomyosis is very difficult, and the diagnosis is usually not made until pathologic examination of a uterus which has been removed because of hypermenorrhea, polymenorrhea, or intermenstrual bleeding occurring just prior to menses. Because it may be associated with endometriosis (see next section), there may be an acquired dysmenorrhea and dyspareunia. The condition should be suspected if one or more of these symptoms occurs in a multiparous woman age 35–50. Examination will reveal a slightly to moderately enlarged, symmetric, mobile uterus with a finely granular external surface.

B. Special Examinations: Hysterography may be helpful in confirming the clinical diagnosis.

Differential Diagnosis

Adenomyosis must be distinguished principally from leiomyomas of the uterus. Although the symptoms may be quite similar, the palpatory findings should enable the careful observer to make the correct diagnosis. Hysterography is necessary in doubtful cases.

Other disorders which may be confused with adenomyosis are chronic subinvolution of the uterus (benign, idiopathic uterine hypertrophy), endometriosis, chronic salpingitis, and cancer of the endometrium.

Treatment

Total hysterectomy with or without bilateral salpingo-oophrectomy is curative. Hormonal therapy—estrogen alone, progesterone alone, or estrogen-progesterone combinations—has not been successful and has actually caused exacerbations of symptoms. If the symptoms are not severe and more serious conditions such as endometrial carcinoma or submucous leiomyomas have been excluded, symptomatic treatment in anticipation of the menopause constitutes rational therapy.

Prognosis

Adenomyosis is a self-limited process that undergoes spontaneous regression, becoming asymptomatic after the menopause.

An analogous condition, endolymphatic stromal myosis (stromal endometriosis), although histologically benign, clinically behaves as a low-grade malignancy. In this condition, connective tissue cells resembling those of the endometrial stroma infiltrate the lymphatic and venous spaces of the myometrium. This process may extend into the vessels of the broad ligament, in which event local recurrence is possible following hysterectomy. Metastases to the ovary, peritoneal surfaces, and lung have been reported, but only rarely. This disease, usually of the postmenopausal years, is very rare and should not be confused with adenomyosis.

Mahfouz N: Adenomyosis and endometriosis. J Internat Fed Gynaec Obst 5:28–38, 1967.

ENDOMETRIOSIS

Essentials of Diagnosis

- History of progressive dysmenorrhea and dyspareunia.
- Patient (often nulligravid and infertile) 20–40 years of age.
- Symptoms of rectal or bladder pain at menses, rarely with blood in feces or urine at the time of menstruation.
- Tender, shotty nodules in cul-de-sac.
- Enlarged, adherent ovary.
- Constricting lesion of large intestine on barium enema.
- Typical findings at peritoneoscopy (laparoscopy or culdoscopy).

General Considerations

In endometriosis, functioning endometrial tissue is present in ectopic sites other than the myometrium (see Adenomyosis, above). The areas most often involved are the ovaries, the cul-de-sac peritoneum, the uterosacral ligaments and rectovaginal septum, the sigmoid colon, the pelvic peritoneum, and the small intestine (Fig 45–1). Malignancy may develop in areas of ovarian endometriosis. Ectopic endometrium has been found in the umbilicus, in abdominal scars, and (rarely) in the breasts, the extremities, the pleural

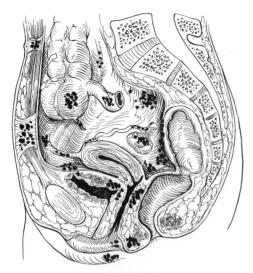

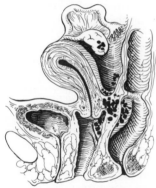

FIG 45–1. Endometriosis.

cavity, and the lungs.

The histogenesis of endometriosis involves 3 different mechanisms: (1) Sampson's theory of retrograde menstruation and implantation; (2) lymphatic and venous dissemination; and (3) müllerian metaplasia of coelomic epithelium. Most cases of endometriosis probably develop as a result of the retrograde passage of bits of menstrual endometrium through the lumens of the fallopian tubes into the peritoneal cavity. Here they implant on the surface of the ovaries and fall by gravity into the cul-de-sac (pouch of Douglas), where they implant and respond to the cyclic hormonal influences of the menstrual cycle, shedding and bleeding at the time of menstruation. Conditions which favor the passage of the menstrual discharge in this direction—eg, cervical stenosis, uterine retroflexion, and uterotubal insufflation—particularly in the menstrual or premenstrual phase of the cycle, are considered predisposing conditions.

Endometriosis is primarily a disease of women in the higher socioeconomic levels and is uncommon in black women. It occurs only after the onset of regular menstruation, but is rarely encountered in patients with anovulatory cycles.

Endometriosis is commonly associated with in-fertility, but it is not known which comes first. It becomes quiescent during pregnancy and hormonally induced pseudopregnancy. Multiparity—particularly if childbearing starts early in menstrual life—appears to protect against the development of endometriosis.

Clinical Findings

A. Symptoms and Signs: Endometriosis has protean manifestations. Some patients with extensive disease with large, bilateral ovarian endometriomas may remain essentially asymptomatic, whereas others with small peritoneal implants may be incapacitated with pain. Characteristically, the disease is first manifest as dysmenorrhea developing in the 20s or 30s. This progresses, with increasing severity, to pain which is associated not only with menstruation but also during several days preceding menses, often accompanied by dyspareunia and rectal tenesmus. There may be a continuous, vague sense of lower abdominal and pelvic discomfort throughout the menstrual cycle which is markedly exaggerated during menstruation. Some women complain of low back pain and of painful defecation associated with the menstrual period. This symptom is quite characteristic of cul-de-sac and rectovaginal septum involvement.

Menstrual aberrations are reported in fewer than 50% of patients with endometriosis, and these are probably related to associated conditions such as endometrial polyps or leiomyomas as much as to interference with ovarian function by the endometriotic process.

Bladder involvement may be signified by a suprapubic bearing-down type of pain with or without dysuria and hematuria at the time of menstruation. Involvement of the bladder mucosa is quite rare. If an endometriotic implant involves the peritoneum overlying the ureter, the resulting tissue reaction may produce hydroureter and hydronephrosis with flank and lower abdominal pain.

Implants on the sigmoid colon or rectum may produce signs of partial obstruction of the large bowel, recurring with the menstrual periods.

Occasionally, rupture of a large ovarian endometrial cyst presents symptoms of an acute abdominal emergency with all the signs and symptoms of peritonitis.

B. Pelvic Examination: Rectovaginal bimanual pelvic examination is vital to the detection of pelvic endometriosis since this is the only way the cul-de-sac, the area of the uterosacral ligaments, and the posterior wall of the uterine corpus can be adequately palpated. Moreover, the ovaries, when they are involved, frequently are prolapsed and adherent to the posterior leaf of the broad ligament lateral to the cul-de-sac and are best felt by the rectal finger. An examination performed during the days just preceding the menstrual period is most likely to provide the best opportunity for palpation of the characteristic shotty nodules in the pouch of Douglas, since this is the stage of the menstrual cycle when they are under the full stimulus of the ovarian hormones.

Bilateral, tender, fixed ovarian cystic masses 5–10 cm in diameter are significant findings.

C. Special Examination: Culdoscopic examination can be performed if the diagnosis is in doubt but should be done only if the cul-de-sac is free of obstructing masses. Otherwise, laparoscopic examination is often quite helpful in establishing a diagnosis of endometriosis in a patient in whom the symptoms are suggestive but the signs are minimal or absent. A finding of characteristic raspberry or blueberry implants or of the powder-burn marks of scarred endometriosis is most valuable. Biopsy of such lesions will establish the diagnosis. Laparotomy is occasionally necessary.

Differential Diagnosis

Endometriosis may mimic chronic salpingitis with bilateral tubo-ovarian masses, ovarian carcinoma, twisted ovarian cyst, appendicitis, ectopic pregnancy, diverticulitis, and carcinoma of the rectosigmoid colon. A detailed history, a carefully performed physical examination, and the use of diagnostic x-ray and laparoscopy or culdoscopy will be helpful in the differential diagnosis. Biopsy of suspicious lesions of the intestine prior to resection will be helpful in avoiding needless bowel resections when endometriosis simulates carcinoma of the gastrointestinal tract.

Complications

Infertility is a common problem in patients with endometriosis and occurs in about three-fourths of women with this disease.

Bowel obstruction does not develop often, but it may occur when there is intestinal involvement by endometrial implantation involving either the small or large bowel. A mechanical ileus may result from the numerous dense adhesions which form as a result of the inflammatory reaction in response to cyclical bleeding from peritoneal implants.

Rupture of a large endometrial cyst of the ovary usually produces an acute, widespread peritoneal reaction with signs and symptoms of an acute surgical emergency.

Scarring around the ureter may cause obstruction, with the development of hydroureter and hydronephrosis, and this may explain many cases of idiopathic hydronephrosis seen in women during the reproductive years.

Ovarian carcinoma has been known to develop in endometriomas and usually takes the form of adenocarcinoma resembling serous cystadenocarcinoma of the ovary. Adenoacanthomas and endometrial stromal sarcomas have been reported, but these are rare.

Prevention

Early, repeated pregnancy appears to prevent the development of endometriosis.

Assuming that retrograde passage of endometrial tissue through the fallopian tubes is the primary method of implantation, one should avoid repeated injections into the endometrial cavity such as gas insufflation for determination of tubal patency or the intro-

duction of radiopaque media for the purpose of x-ray delineation of the uterine cavity and tubal lumen (hysterosalpingography), particularly at or near the menstrual period.

Cervical stenosis should be corrected in order to allow free passage of the menstrual discharge into the vagina.

There is suggestive evidence that long-term contraceptive pill users are less likely to develop endometriosis, particularly if the pill contains a small amount of estrogen in combination with a potent progestin.

Treatment

Therapy may be medical, surgical, or a combination of both methods. Treatment should be tailored to fit the circumstances with respect to the age of the patient, her symptoms, her desire for children, and the extent of the disease. Therapy may vary, therefore, from mere observation, reassurance, and analgesia if necessary, to complete surgical removal of the uterus, tubes, and ovaries.

A conservative approach is recommended for the patient who is symptom-free or only mildly symptomatic with minimal pelvic findings such as slightly tender cul-de-sac nodules. Regular examinations should be carried out at intervals of not more than 6 months. Evidence of progression of the disease—either in the form of increasing symptomatology, infertility, or the development of pelvic masses—requires more specific treatment.

A. Hormonal Treatment: The induction of anovulation and amenorrhea has been successful in bringing about regression in a high percentage of patients with endometriosis. This may be accomplished in several ways:

1. Estrogens alone—Give diethylstilbestrol in increasing doses, beginning on the first day of the menstrual period with 1 mg/day orally and increasing every 3 days by 1 mg until 5 mg/day are being given. The patient is then instructed to take one-fourth of a 25 mg tablet, increasing this by one-fourth tablet every 3 days to 100 mg/day. This method has the side-effects of nausea early in the course of treatment, breast tenderness, and occasional breakthrough bleeding with endometrial hyperplasia.

2. Androgens alone—Methyltestosterone, 5–10 mg sublingually daily, will be effective in some patients, but side-effects such as acne, voice changes, and hirsutism in sensitive patients are drawbacks. Doses in excess of 300 mg/month are not recommended. In the therapeutic dose range, ovulation and menstruation are not inhibited by androgens; their effect is probably a direct one on the endometrial implants rather than a suppression of the anterior pituitary.

3. Progestins—Norethynodrel, norethindrone, hydroxyprogesterone caproate, and medroxyprogesterone are the agents most commonly used. They are most often used in combination with an estrogen (to prevent breakthrough bleeding). One such combination—norethynodrel, 2.5 mg, with mestranol, 0.1 mg (Enovid-E), may be given in the following schedule: 2.5 mg/day for 1 week, 5 mg/day for 1 week, and 10 mg/day for 2 weeks, increasing by 2.5 mg each time there is breakthrough bleeding. The production of a pseudopregnancy state through hormonal therapy is maintained for 6—12 months and is effective in about 80% of patients. It is useful as a preoperative adjunct for 6 weeks to soften areas of scarred endometriosis and to make the surgical procedure somewhat easier. The most frequent indication for the prolonged use of these compounds is for recurrent endometriosis following a conservative operation. Side-effects are nausea, breast tenderness, fluid retention, and breakthrough bleeding.

Hormonal therapy is not indicated in patients with unproved endometriosis or uterine leiomyomas or in individuals with a history of breast cancer, thrombophlebitis, pulmonary embolus, or liver disease.

B. Surgical Treatment: The surgical approach to endometriosis may be designed to improve fertility, to prevent further progression of the disease with preservation of the ovaries, or to cure the disease by removal of the uterus and the adnexal structures.

1. Conservative surgery—Preservation of childbearing function by removal or cauterization of implants, freeing up of tubal adhesions, presacral neurectomy for the relief of pain, and uterine suspension is indicated in the young woman who desires to have children. It is not recommended in the patient with extensive endometriosis involving the intestines.

2. Modified radical surgery—This involves the removal of the uterus, excision or fulguration of endometrial implants, and preservation of the ovaries. This approach may be considered in the younger woman who has no desire to retain her childbearing function but is not near the menopause. It carries the risk of recurrence, but without the uterus the risk is small.

3. Definitive surgery—This requires the removal not only of the uterus but of the tubes and ovaries as well. Since endometriosis is dependent upon ovarian function for its continued growth and development, total hysterectomy and bilateral salpingo-oophorectomy should be done in patients with extensive disease, particularly those with bowel involvement. It is critically important not to mistake bowel implants for cancer. Unnecessary abdominoperineal resections have been performed in young women for unrecognized endometriosis.

Oral estrogen replacement therapy in the form of diethylstilbestrol, 0.25—0.5 mg/day, ethinyl estradiol, 0.02—0.05 mg/day, or conjugated estrogens, 0.625—1.25 mg/day, interrupting the cycle for 5—7 days each month, may be given without danger of exacerbating the endometriotic process. The use of estrogen-progestin combinations is not recommended.

Gunning JE, Moyer D: Effect of medroxyprogesterone acetate on endometriosis in the human female. Fertil Steril 18:759—774, 1967.

Molitor JJ: Adenomyosis: A clinical and pathologic appraisal. Am J Obst Gynec 110:275—284, 1971.

Samuelson S, Sjövall A: Diagnostic value of laparoscopy in ovarian endometriosis. Acta obst gynec scandinav 47:350—360, 1968.

Ulfelder H: Endometriosis. Postgrad Med 40:146—152, 1966.

TUBAL PREGNANCY

Essentials of Diagnosis

- Cramping, colicky, or steady lower abdominal pain.
- Missed period or menstrual irregularity.
- Vaginal bleeding.
- Tender adnexal mass.
- Signs of intraperitoneal bleeding (culdocentesis).
- Slight uterine enlargement.

General Considerations

Ectopic pregnancy occurs once in every 150—200 pregnancies. The fallopian tube is the most frequent site of an ectopic pregnancy (95%), and the ampulla or isthmic portion of the tube is the section usually involved. Interstitial (cornual) pregnancies are infrequent but significant because profuse, exsanguinating intraperitoneal bleeding occurs at the time of rupture. Ectopic pregnancies are seen also in the peritoneal cavity (abdominal pregnancy), ovary, and cervix; because they are extremely rare, only tubal pregnancy will be discussed here.

Tubal pregnancy is the result of implantation of the fertilized ovum into the wall of the fallopian tube, an event probably related to a delay in the transfer of the egg through the tubal lumen. Preexisting disease affecting the tubes (salpingitis, appendicitis, endometriosis, and pelvic operations, particularly tuboplastic procedures) predisposes to tubal pregnancy, but tubal pregnancy is not infrequent in patients with no such history.

With implantation of the ovum, there is vascular engorgement and trophoblastic invasion with resultant weakening of the wall of the fallopian tube. Rupture of the tube frequently follows, often with massive bleeding into the peritoneal cavity. The pregnancy, on the other hand, may separate from the implantation site into the lumen of the tube and then be extruded through the fimbriated extremity into the peritoneal cavity together with a considerable amount of blood (tubal abortion). In either event there may be sufficient acute blood loss to produce the clinical picture of hypovolemic shock.

Regardless of the implantation site in the fallopian tube, uterine enlargement with decidual change in the endometrium occurs because of the influence on the uterus of pregnancy levels of estrogen and progesterone.

Clinical Findings

The symptoms and signs of tubal pregnancy are extremely variable, and this disease is not infrequently overlooked or misdiagnosed because of the atypical clinical picture.

A. "Classical" Findings: Classically, in a ruptured tubal pregnancy the history is of 1–2 missed menstrual periods with accompanying presumptive symptoms of pregnancy (tender breasts, urinary frequency, nausea). Mild to moderate vaginal bleeding then ensues, followed, after an interval of a few days, by the onset of unilateral lower abdominal pain—at first cramping or colicky and then steady, becoming generalized through the lower abdomen. Referred shoulder pain results from irritation of the diaphragm by the intraperitoneal blood. Syncope often occurs due to hypotension.

Examination reveals a pale, cold, clammy, apprehensive patient with a rapid, thready pulse and hypotension. The abdomen is tender throughout, with rigidity and rebound tenderness. These findings are often more pronounced on the affected side. Rarely there is a bluish discoloration around the umbilicus (Cullen's sign). Dark blood is often present in the vagina, issuing from the cervical canal. Marked tenderness throughout the entire abdomen can be elicited, and displacement of the cervix digitally produces considerable discomfort in the abdomen. The uterus is slightly to moderately enlarged and soft. A tender adnexal mass may be palpated, and there is often a feeling of fullness in the cul-de-sac. Culdocentesis reveals the presence of nonclotting blood in the peritoneal cavity.

Hemoglobin and hematocrit are below normal values, and a moderate leukocytosis is present. The pregnancy test may or may not be positive.

B. "Atypical" Findings: The majority of tubal pregnancies (60–85%) do not fit this typical picture and manifest themselves in more subtle ways. There may be no history of menstrual irregularity or presumptive symptoms of pregnancy. The abdominal pain may be mild and vague. Physical findings often are confusing with some pelvic tenderness but no palpable adnexal mass. The uterus may or may not be enlarged and softened. Slow hemorrhage into the peritoneal cavity may circumvent the clinical picture of surgical shock. A gradually falling hematocrit may be the only real clue to bleeding. For these reasons, tubal pregnancy often is a diagnostic enigma, and it is necessary to be alert to the possibility and to properly investigate suspected cases in order to avoid a tragic outcome.

Culdocentesis is particularly helpful in proving the presence of free blood in the peritoneal cavity, but it may be negative in an unruptured tubal pregnancy or if a blood clot obstructs the lumen of the needle.

A decidual cast from the uterus passed through the vagina or curettings which demonstrate decidua but no evidence of trophoblast on careful pathologic examination are suggestive of ectopic pregnancy. Laparoscopy may be very helpful in establishing the correct diagnosis.

Differential Diagnosis

Early intrauterine pregnancy with or without threatened abortion and pelvic inflammatory disease are the conditions most often confused with ectopic pregnancy. The cramping pain of a threatened or inevitable intrauterine abortion is usually suprapubic rather than unilateral. There is no adnexal structure suggestive of tubal pregnancy; little pain is present in the adnexal area or on cervical motion; and culdocentesis shows no blood in the peritoneal cavity. Laparoscopy reveals normal adnexal structures. Acute appendicitis may simulate a tubal pregnancy on the right side. A diagnosis of appendicitis is suggested by nausea and vomiting of acute onset, absence of a significant menstrual history or vaginal bleeding, a higher white blood count, and culdocentesis negative for blood but perhaps productive of a small amount of fluid which has a high white blood count. Acute salpingitis, particularly when the symptoms and signs are more pronounced on one side, may be confused with ectopic pregnancy. In this condition, there is usually some evidence of bilateral disease. There are no symptoms or signs of pregnancy, and culdocentesis may show inflammatory elements rather than blood in the peritoneal cavity. A corpus luteum cyst of the ovary with rupture and bleeding into the peritoneal cavity may closely simulate a ruptured tubal pregnancy and often requires laparotomy for the differential diagnosis. Laparoscopy may be diagnostic.

Complications

The complications of tubal pregnancy are those of shock due to hemorrhage, infection, and sterility.

Prevention

Prompt diagnosis and treatment of unruptured ectopic pregnancy will prevent the often massive intraperitoneal hemorrhage associated with rupture. Unruptured ectopic pregnancy must be considered whenever a patient is presumed to be pregnant and an adnexal mass is palpated which is thought to be separate from the ovary on that side. Only prompt investigation regarding the nature of the mass will circumvent the possibility of a ruptured tubal pregnancy.

Treatment

Ideally, treatment is surgical, with excision of the implant and preservation of the fallopian tube before rupture occurs.

Ruptured tubal pregnancy is a surgical emergency. Immediate transfusion and operation are imperative. The surgical procedure usually performed is unilateral salpingectomy or salpingo-oophorectomy, although it may be possible to preserve the fallopian tube in unruptured pregnancies and in cases of tubal abortion.

Prognosis

The prognosis is good if the diagnosis is made promptly and appropriate therapy given. Death may result from hemorrhage or infection in neglected cases.

Breen JL: A 21-year survey of 654 ectopic pregnancies. Am J Obst Gynec 106:1004–1019, 1970.

Cepraro UJ & others: Cul-de-sac aspiration and other diagnostic aids for ectopic pregnancy: 22-year analysis. Internat Surg 53:245–250, 1970.

Kleiner GJ, Roberts TW: Current factors in causation of tubal pregnancy. Am J Obst Gynec 99:21–28, 1967.

Webster HD & others: Ectopic pregnancy: 17 year review. Am J Obst Gynec 92:23–34, 1965.

INCOMPETENCE OF PELVIC SUPPORT
(Uterine Prolapse, Cystourethrocele, Rectocele, Enterocele, Prolapse of Vagina After Hysterectomy)

Essentials of Diagnosis

- Parous woman.
- Complaints of "bearing down" or "falling out" sensation in the pelvis, mass protruding from vaginal introitus, stress incontinence of urine, and difficulty in evacuating rectum.
- Physical findings of defective perineal body, bulge of anterior vaginal wall with loss of urethrovesical angle, bulge of posterior vaginal wall due to defect in rectovaginal septum or hernia sac between rectum and vagina (enterocele), descent of uterus in pelvis, and protrusion of vagina (following hysterectomy).

General Considerations

An understanding of pelvic floor relaxation with its sequelae of cystourethrocele, rectocele, enterocele, and uterine (or vaginal) prolapse requires a thorough knowledge of the anatomic relationships of the pelvic viscera and their supporting tissues. Almost invariably, these conditions result initially from stretching and tearing of the connective tissues of the pelvis during delivery. The supporting structures are weakened, and this is followed by the slow, insidious additional loss of strength brought about by the gravitational forces of the erect position over the years and the sudden, intermittent increases of pressure from above (intra-abdominal pressure) associated with lifting, coughing, straining, sneezing, etc. Finally comes the additional insult of loss of tone due to the hormonal withdrawal associated with the menopause.

These conditions are rarely seen in nulligravidas, in whom they are thought to be related to congenital anomalies (spina bifida occulta).

The levator ani muscle forms the basic portion of the floor of the pelvis. It is trough-shaped and perforated in its thickened, central portion (pubococcygeus) by the urethra, vagina, and rectum. The fascia covering the superior surface of this muscle is continuous with the endopelvic fascia as well as the cardinal and uterosacral ligaments supporting the uterus. The fascia covering the inferior surface of the levator ani muscle is in continuity with that of the obturator internus and the urogenital diaphragm (Fig 45–2). The urogenital

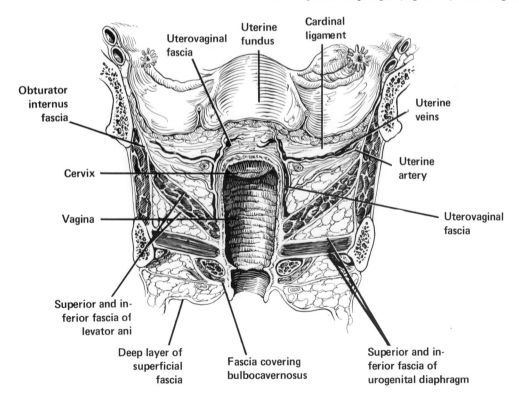

FIG 45–2. Ligamentous and fascial support of pelvic viscera.
(Redrawn after Frank Netter: Ciba Symposium.)

diaphragm (triangular ligament) bridges that portion of the perineum anterior to the ischial tuberosities, between the descending rami of the pubis. It is composed of the deep transverse perineal muscle and its investing superficial and deep fascia and is penetrated by the urethra and the vagina. It forms a secondary but less important support for these structures.

In obstetric injuries to the pelvic floor there is often damage to the investing endopelvic fascia and the supporting ligaments of the uterus as well as to the levator sling, so that combinations of anatomic defects often are encountered rather than a single one—ie, prolapse of the uterus in combination with cysto-urethrocele, rectocele, and enterocele.

Stress incontinence represents the involuntary loss of urine from the urethra with increases in intra-abdominal pressure such as that which occurs with coughing, straining, sneezing, laughing, etc. It can be demonstrated clinically during pelvic examination by asking the patient to cough. Stress incontinence should be carefully distinguished from another common type of involuntary loss of urine, ie, urgency incontinence. The latter condition usually is related to inflammatory conditions in and around the bladder trigone, producing bladder irritability, and the patient experiences the loss of urine with bladder filling and the desire to void. The 2 conditions may occur simultaneously. Surgical correction of stress incontinence may produce a temporary urgency incontinence until the postoperative inflammatory reaction subsides. Other types of urinary incontinence such as the overflow type of neurogenic bladder must also be recognized.

Anatomically, the bladder and urethra are supported by the muscles of the pelvic floor and the endopelvic fascia. The intraluminal hydrostatic pressure relationships are all-important to an understanding of the mechanism of stress incontinence and its correction. In the nulliparous woman, the proximal urethra is held high and is subjected to the same intra-abdominal pressure changes as those affecting the bladder. Thus, with coughing, straining, sneezing, etc, the greater "closure pressure" of the proximal urethra (50—135 cm water) over that of the intravesical pressure (10—60 cm water) is maintained, and the patient remains continent. In the multipara with pelvic floor relaxation, however, descent of the posterior wall of the bladder neck and urethra produces a funneling effect (loss of the posterior urethrovesical angle). The proximal urethra no longer maintains a higher closing pressure with stress, and incontinence occurs. Most operations for the correction of urinary stress incontinence are designed to reconstruct the posterior urethrovesical angle and prevent funneling of the bladder neck and proximal urethra, restoring the increased "closing pressure" of the urethra over the hydrostatic pressure within the bladder during stress.

A cystocele of significant degree may be present without stress incontinence, and the overzealous surgeon may, in correcting the cystocele, straighten out the posterior angle, produce a funneling of the bladder neck and urethra, and thus cause an iatrogenic stress incontinence.

Clinical Findings

Mild degrees of pelvic floor relaxation are found in many multiparous women without significant symptoms. Prolapse of the uterus varies in degree depending upon the level of the uterus in the pelvis. In a first degree prolapse, the cervix does not protrude through the vaginal introitus. Second degree prolapse is manifest by the presence of the cervix outside the vagina, whereas in third degree prolapse (procidentia) the entire uterus comes through the introitus covered by the everted vagina.

Descent and bulging of the anterior wall of the vagina indicates the presence of a cystocele, urethrocele, or both, whereas a similar anatomic defect in the posterior wall signifies that a rectocele or enterocele (or both) exists. All of these conditions can be demonstrated during examination with the patient in the lithotomy position by asking her to bear down or strain. However, the existence of an enterocele can best be demonstrated by performing a rectovaginal examination with the patient in the standing position. The hernia is felt between the rectal and vaginal fingers.

The symptoms of pelvic floor incompetence are those of a dragging sensation or sense of "falling out" of the pelvic organs, a mass protruding from the vagina (which may be a cystocele, rectocele, cervix, or all 3), stress incontinence, repeated urinary tract infections due to sacculation of the bladder and a high residual urine, and difficulties in defecation, occasionally requiring digital compression of the posterior vaginal wall.

Differential Diagnosis

Prolapse of the uterus must be distinguished from hypertrophy and elongation of the cervix due to chronic inflammation. Sounding of the cervical canal to the level of the internal os will accomplish this.

Urethral diverticula may simulate cystourethrocele, producing a bulge of the anterior vaginal wall. The diverticulum is usually palpable as a discrete mass, and pressure against the mass often expresses purulent material from the urethral meatus. Endoscopic and urethrocystographic examinations confirm the diagnosis.

Treatment

The asymptomatic patient requires no treatment, and it is best to defer therapy in such a patient or one with only mild symptoms until she requests correction for the relief of symptoms.

A. Nonoperative Treatment: The postmenopausal woman with mild to moderate anatomic defects may become symptom-free after the administration of estrogen—either topically, in the form of creams or suppositories, or systemically, by oral tablets or intramuscular injections of a long-acting estrogen preparation. Programmed, active exercises of the pelvic floor musculature (Kegel exercises) may prove helpful in relieving symptoms of mild degree.

Pessary support of the descending pelvic structures will provide temporary relief of symptoms and is useful in the surgical high-risk patient.

B. Surgical Treatment: The operation performed most often for the correction of pelvic floor relaxation with multiple anatomic defects is vaginal hysterectomy with anterior colporrhaphy (urethral suspension, plication of the bladder neck, and cystocele repair) and posterior colporrhaphy (rectocele [and enterocele] repair with perineoplasty).

Special operations devised for severe degrees of incompetence and for recurrent defects following surgical correction are as follows: Pereyra and Marshall-Marchetti procedures for stress incontinence; Le Fort operation or partial colpocleisis for the elderly, poor-risk patient with uterine prolapse; total colpocleisis or sacral suspension for prolapse of the vagina following total hysterectomy; Moskowitz procedure or obliteration of the cul-de-sac for enterocele.

Prognosis

The surgical correction of these conditions results in complete relief of symptoms and no recurrence of the defect in about 85% of patients. Obesity, chronic cough, and straining contribute to recurrences. Overlooking an enterocele at the time of repair is a frequent cause of failure of surgical correction.

Beck RP & others: Surgical results in the treatment of pressure equalization stress incontinence. Am J Obst Gynec 100:483–489, 1968.

Enhorning G & others: Urethral closure studied with cineroentgenography and simultaneous bladder-urethra pressure recording. Surg Gynec Obst 118:507–516, 1964.

Hodgkinson CP: Stress urinary incontinence in the female. Surg Gynec Obst 120:595–613, 1965.

Pereyra AJ, Lebherz TB: Combined urethrovesical suspension and vaginourethroplasty for correction of urinary stress incontinence. Obst Gynec 30:537–546, 1967.

Ullery JC, Villalon R: Urinary tract injuries in obstetrics and gynecology. West Virginia MJ 64:127–132, 1968.

Ward JH & others: Diagnosis and treatment of urethral diverticula in the female. Surg Gynec Obst 125:1293–1300, 1967.

URINARY TRACT FISTULAS

Urinary tract fistulas are of several varieties: vesicovaginal (most common), ureterovaginal, and urethrovaginal. They occur most often as a result of accidental injury to the urinary tract at the time of pelvic surgery or because of ischemic necrosis resulting from an impaired blood supply. The latter can occur either following radiation therapy for carcinoma of the reproductive organs (especially the cervix) or as a result of prolonged impaction of the fetal head during labor in obstetrics.

Total abdominal hysterectomy is the operation most often complicated by the development of vesicovaginal fistula, which may also occur as a result of tumor invasion of the vesicovaginal septum.

Clinical Findings

A. Symptoms and Signs: Constant urinary incontinence is the cardinal symptom. Urine can be seen usually coming through an opening in the vagina. In vesicovaginal and ureterovaginal fistulas, the vaginal ostium is at or near the vault closure, whereas the urethrovaginal fistula opens along the anterior wall of the vagina. If the urethrovaginal fistula involves the distal urethra, the patient may remain continent and lose urine into the vagina only at the time of voiding.

A communication between the urinary bladder and the vagina can be demonstrated by instilling sterile milk or a dye (methylene blue or indigo carmine) into the bladder via a catheter and watching it come through into the vagina on speculum examination. If leakage of urine into the vagina cannot be colored in this fashion, the defect probably is ureteral and can be demonstrated by giving the patient methylene blue tablets by mouth and finding a blue stain on a cotton pledget placed in the vagina.

B. Urologic Examination: Cystoscopy and x-ray studies of the urinary tract will localize the urinary tract opening of the fistulous tract. Occasionally, the fistulous tracts are branching or multiple.

Prevention

Close attention to surgical technic, recognition of urinary tract injuries, and their proper repair at the time of surgery will prevent most of the fistulas which are the result of urinary tract injury.

Treatment

Urinary tract fistulas rarely close spontaneously. They must be repaired surgically, but sufficient time should elapse (4–6 months) to allow for resolution of edema and inflammatory reaction. Otherwise, attempts at repair are doomed to failure. The use of cortisone has been recommended as an anti-inflammatory agent to shorten this waiting period. Control of the urine leakage from the vaginal vault pending surgical repair often is possible by introducing a small rubber menstrual cup (Tassette) to which is attached a catheter and a leg bag urinal (Fig 45–3). Urinary tract infections should be treated with appropriate urinary antiseptic agents before surgical correction.

Ureterovaginal fistulas are repaired by performing a uretero-ureterostomy or by implanting the severed ureter into the bladder (uretero-neocystostomy).

The abdominal (suprapubic) and vaginal approaches are used to repair vesicovaginal fistulas, and a number of technics are available (layer closure, partial colpocleisis). Regardless of the method used, the principles of repair are the same: meticulous technic, using fine suture material; approximation of broad surfaces without tension; and maintenance of bladder decompression postoperatively until healing has occurred.

Falk HC: Prevention of vesicovaginal fistula in total hysterectomy for benign disease. Obst Gynec 29:865–868, 1967.

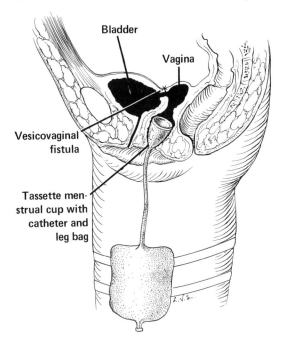

Bladder

Vagina

Vesicovaginal
fistula

Tassette men-
strual cup with
catheter and
leg bag

FIG 45–3. Vesicovaginal fistula with menstrual cup and leg bag.

Higgins CC: Ureteral injuries during surgery. JAMA 199:82–88, 1967.

Moir JC: Vesicovaginal fistula: Thoughts on the treatment of 350 cases. Proc Roy Soc Med 59:1019–1022, 1966.

RECTOVAGINAL FISTULAS

Rectovaginal fistulas are seen most often as a result of obstetric injury, surgical procedures, cervical cancer, or radiation therapy. The symptoms are those of incontinence of flatus or feces through the vagina. The vaginal ostium usually can be demonstrated by speculum examination, and a probe passed through the fistulous tract can be palpated by the rectal finger.

Low rectovaginal fistulas near the vaginal introitus should be repaired after the surrounding inflammatory reaction and edema have subsided. This may require 3–4 months. Those that are found high in the vagina—particularly fistulas resulting from radiation therapy—are often best managed with an initial diverting colostomy which is then closed 2–3 months after a successful repair.

Prior to surgical repair of a rectovaginal fistula, the bowel should be prepared with a low-residue diet, enteric antibiotics, and cleansing enemas.

Fistulas which occur as a result of malignancy are not amenable to surgical repair. A diverting colostomy may give the patient considerable comfort.

Lescher TC, Pratt JH: Vaginal repair of simple rectovaginal fistula. Surg Gynec Obst 124:1317–1321, 1967.

CORRECTION OF INFERTILITY DUE TO TUBAL ABNORMALITIES

A married couple may be considered infertile if a pregnancy does not occur after 1 year of normal coital activity without contraceptives. About 15% of marriages are infertile, and in approximately 40% of these there is a significant male factor (low sperm count, impaired motility, or anomalous forms). Chronic salpingitis is the single most common cause of sterility in women, although endometriosis and peritubal adhesions from previous appendicitis (with rupture) may be causative factors.

Clinical Findings

There may or may not be palpable adnexal pathology. Tubal insufflation with carbon dioxide (Rubin's test) demonstrates some impairment in tubal patency. If several Rubin tests done during the week following menstruation and prior to ovulation reveal nonpatency, a hysterosalpingogram should be obtained. This may reveal an obstruction at the cornu, hydrosalpinx, fimbrial occlusion, or peritubal adhesions. Peritoneoscopy (culdoscopy, laparoscopy) with the passage of a dye through a uterine cannula while the fallopian tubes are under vision is also an excellent diagnostic method.

Treatment

Tuboplasty operations are designed to reestablish tubal patency. These surgical procedures are more successful if the obstruction is localized with little damage to the fallopian tube as a whole (fimbrial adhesions, previous tubal ligation). Reestablishment and maintenance of tubal patency has been more successful with the development of inert plastic materials for splinting and protecting the tube from adhesions during the healing process. Salpingolysis, reimplantation of the tube into the uterus, end-to-end anastomosis, and fimbrial salpingostomy are the operations usually performed.

Prognosis

An overall pregnancy incidence of about 20% is reported following tuboplasty, but about one in 10 of these is a tubal pregnancy. The best results (26%) are achieved following cornual reimplantation when the remainder of the tube is anatomically and physiologically normal.

Crane M, Woodruff JD: Factors influencing the success of tuboplastic procedures. Fertil Steril 19:810–820, 1968.

Mulligan WJ: Results of salpingostomy. Internat J Fertil 11:424–430, 1966.

Rock J, Mulligan WJ, Easterday CL: Polyethylene in tuboplasty. Obst Gynec 3:21–29, 1954.

Siegler AM: Salpingoplasty: Classification and report of 115 operations. Obst Gynec 34:339–344, 1969.

TUMORS OF THE FEMALE GENITAL TRACT

CARCINOMA OF VULVA

BENIGN TUMORS OF THE VULVA & VAGINA

Hidradenoma

Hidradenomas are small, discrete, firm, mobile structures in the subcutaneous tissues of the labia or perianal region. These sweat gland tumors are benign but may be mistaken for a malignancy because of an adenomatous microscopic pattern.

Treatment consists of local excision.

Sebaceous Cysts

Sebaceous cysts are small, raised, discrete, white, cystic structures in the skin of the labia majora or minora which contain white sebaceous material. They may become infected, producing small abscesses.

Most sebaceous cysts require no therapy. If they cause discomfort, simple excision is indicated.

Bartholin Cyst

Bartholin cysts cause swelling deep in the tissues of the posterior portion of the labium majus. The cysts vary in size from 1 cm in diameter to several centimeters. The larger masses tend to bulge into the vestibule of the vulva and the lower vagina. They may be asymptomatic or may produce local pressure symptoms and dyspareunia. Secondary infection occurs frequently, producing a large, painful abscess.

Bartholin abscesses with surrounding cellulitis should be treated with antibiotic therapy followed by incision and drainage. Symptomatic cysts and low-grade abscesses should be either marsupialized (in order to retain the mucus-secreting gland) or surgically excised.

Gartner Duct Cysts

These occur as small round or fusiform cystic swellings, often bilateral, beneath the mucosa of the anterolateral wall of the vagina. They arise from remnants of the vaginal portion of the mesonephric (wolffian) duct and contain a clear serous fluid. They are usually asymptomatic and discovered in the course of a routine physical examination. Occasionally they reach 5–6 cm in size.

Small asymptomatic cysts require no therapy. Larger masses should be surgically excised.

Endometriosis

Small, bluish, cystic elevations of the vaginal mucosa representing ectopic endometrial tissue are seen most often in the posterior fornix (as an extension of cul-de-sac endometriosis) or in episiotomy scars.

Vaginal endometrial implants are treated by local excision or fulguration. (See section on pelvic endometriosis.)

Essentials of Diagnosis

- Patient in postmenopausal age group.
- Long history of vulval irritation with pruritus, local discomfort, and slightly bloody discharge.
- Early lesions may appear as chronic vulval dermatitis.
- Late lesions appear as a lump in the labium, a large cauliflower growth, or a hard ulcerative area in the vulva.
- Biopsy is necessary to make the diagnosis.

General Considerations

The vast majority (90–95%) of vulval malignancies are squamous cell carcinomas, and these tumors represent about 5% of all cancers of the female reproductive tract. Other types of vulval malignancy are Bartholin gland carcinoma (adenocarcinoma), Paget's disease of the vulva, basal cell carcinoma, malignant melanoma, and metastatic carcinoma from the cervix, endometrium, ovary, or elsewhere. Rarely, sarcomas are found arising primarily in the vulva soft tissues.

Squamous cell carcinoma is frequently associated with leukoplakia (50–70%), which, in the vulva, is considered a premalignant change only when associated with epithelial dysplasia. A history of syphilis with or without associated granuloma inguinale or lymphogranuloma venereum is a frequent finding in vulval cancer.

The area most often involved is the labium majus. The clitoris is the second most often involved.

Metastasis to the regional lymph nodes (inguinal, femoral, iliac, and obturator) occurs in about 35–60% of invasive lesions. Because of bilateral lymph drainage, the nodes on the contralateral side may be involved (Fig 45–4). There is a high incidence of second primary malignancies in these patients, particularly in the cervix, endometrium, and breast.

Clinical Findings

In situ carcinoma (Bowen's disease) of the vulva usually is found in areas of "leukoplakia." The early lesion is a small, elevated, superficial papillary or ulcerated lesion with underlying subcutaneous induration. Late cancers present either as large, fungating, infected tumors or as shallow ulcers with indurated margins. The larger the primary lesion, the greater the chance of lymph node involvement; but palpatory evidence is misleading, as regional node enlargement may be related to secondary infection in these tumors. Furthermore, metastatic disease in the lymph nodes may not be palpable. There may be submucosal spread of the tumor cephalad to involve the vagina and urethra, or there may be involvement of the posterior vulva with invasion of the anus and rectum.

Differential Diagnosis

Chronic hypertrophic and atrophic skin condi-

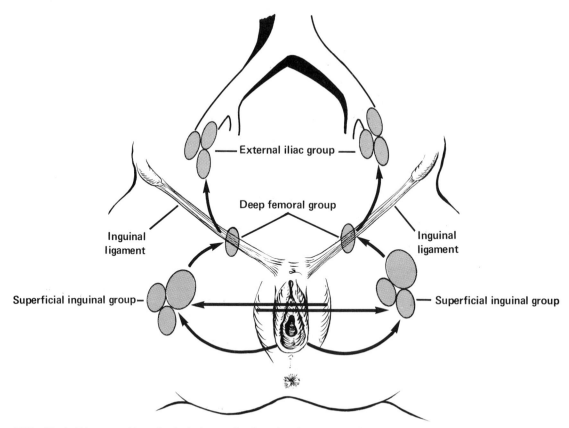

FIG 45—4. Diagram of lymphatic drainage of vulva, showing capacity for bilateral node involvement. (From Way S: Carcinoma of the vulva, in: *Progress in Gynecology.* Meigs JV, Sturgis SS [editors]. Vol 3. Grune & Stratton, 1957.)

tions may or may not be associated with vulval malignancy. Multiple biopsies are necessary to establish the correct diagnosis. Granulomatous venereal lesions of the vulva may be clinically suspicious, and biopsy of the involved area is mandatory. The Frei and complement fixation tests may be helpful, but it must be remembered that granulomatous disease and cancer of the vulva may occur simultaneously.

Prevention

Simple vulvectomy in cases of lesions which show epithelial dysplasia will prevent the subsequent development of invasive carcinoma. Likewise, the discovery and removal (by simple vulvectomy) of intraepithelial carcinoma of the vulva is effective prophylaxis for the invasive form of the disease. Toluidine blue in 1% solution applied to the vulval skin and mucosa and then decolorized with 1% acetic acid solution has been effective in determining the extent of the neoplastic epithelial change.

Treatment

Radical vulvectomy with bilateral superficial and deep groin dissection is the most widely accepted form of therapy. Radiation therapy is used in the inoperable lesions.

Prognosis

Adequate surgery is very effective in a high percentage of patients, even when there is evidence of spread to the inguinal and femoral nodes. Eighty-six percent 5-year cure rates are reported when the nodes are not involved, and a 50% salvage is possible in the presence of lymph node involvement if the surgical procedure has been adequate.

Collins CG & others: Cancer involving the vulva. Am J Obst Gynec 87:762–772, 1963.

McKelvey JL, Adcock LL: Cancer of the vulva. Obst Gynec 26:455–466, 1965.

Way S: Carcinoma of the vulva. Am J Obst Gynec 79:692–697, 1961.

CARCINOMA OF THE VAGINA

Carcinoma in situ of the vagina occurs either as a direct extension of the process from the portio vaginalis of the cervix or as a separate area in a "neoplastic field." It should be suspected whenever carcinoma in situ or invasive carcinoma of the vulva or cervix is present, and it may appear in the vagina many months or years after successful treatment of either of these 2 conditions. Carcinoma in situ of the vagina is diagnosed by biopsying Schiller-positive areas* of the vagina after finding neoplastic or dysplastic cells in the vaginal cytologic specimens.

Treatment is by local excision of involved areas when they are few and small. Extensive involvement of the vaginal mucosa may require vaginectomy with complete colpocleisis in the elderly, sexually inactive patient or with skin graft construction of an artificial vagina in the patient who wishes to retain coital function.

Invasive squamous cell carcinoma of the vagina, arising primarily from the vagina, is an unusual lesion, most cancers of the vagina being extensions from an epidermoid carcinoma of the cervix. The lesion is most often ulcerative, with a cauliflower configuration being less common. There is a firm induration surrounding the ulcerative lesion, and these are easily palpated, whereas a small, soft, papillary lesion may be missed. The upper third of the vagina is the site in about 75% of patients. In many cases the only symptom is a bloody vaginal discharge, and the diagnosis is made by biopsy.

Treatment is by radiation therapy or radical surgery. Unfortunately, these tumors grow rapidly and insidiously, and in over 50% of patients it has penetrated the vaginal wall at the time of the initial examination. Involvement of the bladder and rectum is common. As a result, the overall 5-year survival figures are in the range of 20–30%.

Recently adenocarcinoma of the vagina arising in teen-age girls has been described, apparently arising in areas of vaginal adenosis (probably müllerian duct remnants). There appears to be a relationship between the appearance of this tumor in these young patients and the administration of diethylstilbestrol to their mothers during the fetal life of the patient.

The International Classification of Carcinoma of the Vagina is as follows:

Stage	0	Carcinoma in situ.
Stage	I	Carcinoma is confined to the vaginal wall.
Stage	II	Carcinoma involves the subvaginal tissue but not the pelvic wall.
Stage	III	Carcinoma extends to the pelvic wall.
Stage	IV	Carcinoma extends beyond the true pelvis or involves the mucosa of the bladder or rectum (biopsy proof is required).

Metastatic carcinoma of the vagina is much more common than primary carcinoma, the most frequent sources being the cervix, vulva, bladder, urethra, rectum, endometrium, and ovary.

Rare primary tumors of the vagina are sarcoma

(mixed mesodermal tumors, including sarcoma botryoides of infants, fibrosarcoma, leiomyosarcoma, hemangiosarcoma), adenocarcinoma arising from mesonephric (Gartner's) duct or müllerian duct remnants, embryonal carcinoma, and malignant melanoma. Radical surgical removal offers the best hope of cure for the majority of these neoplasms.

Frick HC II, Jacox HW, Taylor HC Jr: Primary carcinoma of the vagina. Am J Obst Gynec 101:695–703, 1968.

Goperlud DR, Keettel WC: Carcinoma of the vulva. Am J Obst Gynec 100:550–553, 1968.

Herbst AL & others: Adenocarcinoma of the vagina: Association of maternal stilbestrol therapy with tumor appearance in young women. New England J Med 284:878–881, 1971.

Kottmeier HL (editor): *Annual Report on the Results of Treatment in Carcinoma of the Uterus and Vagina,* vol 14. Stockholm, 1967.

TUMORS OF THE FALLOPIAN TUBE (ADENOCARCINOMA)

Benign tumors of the fallopian tubes are very rare. Primary carcinoma of the tube is the most common malignant lesion, but it is rarely encountered, comprising less than 1% of female reproductive cancers.

Postmenopausal vaginal bleeding is the usual presenting complaint. There may be a history of intermittent, profuse, serous, yellow or bloody vaginal discharge (hydrops tubae profluens). An adnexal mass may or may not be palpable.

The diagnosis of primary carcinoma of the fallopian tube is rarely made preoperatively. Total abdominal hysterectomy and bilateral salpingo-oophorectomy is the treatment of choice in operable lesions. Tumors which are inoperable yet confined to the pelvic structures should receive radiation therapy—followed by operation if there is a favorable response as judged by increased mobility and diminution in tumor size. Radical hysterectomy and bilateral pelvic lymph node dissection have been advocated as possibly a more curative procedure than simple hysterectomy and bilateral salpingo-oophorectomy.

If the disease is confined to the tube, the prognosis is quite good. Unfortunately, most of these tumors are advanced at the time of discovery, and the overall 5-year cure rate is in the range of 10–20%.

Green TH, Scully RE: Tumors of the fallopian tube. Clin Obst Gynec 5:886–906, 1962.

Sedlis A: Primary carcinoma of the fallopian tube. Obst Gynec Surv 16:209–226, 1961.

*After application of Lugol's solution, the area of carcinoma does not take up the iodine stain.

CANCER OF THE CERVIX

Essentials of Diagnosis

- May be asymptomatic.
- Vaginal discharge.
- Intermenstrual bleeding.
- Suspicious or positive cytologic examination.
- Biopsy diagnosis is essential.

General Considerations

Carcinoma of the cervix is the most common cancer in the female reproductive tract and second only to carcinoma of the breast as the most frequent malignancy in women.

Early sexual activity, promiscuity, parity, and chronic inflammation are predisposing factors. Epithelial dysplasia of the cervical epithelium is probably a precursor.

The vast majority of cervical cancers are squamous cell (95%); the remainder consist of adenocarcinomas, mixed carcinomas (adenosquamous), and rare sarcomas (mixed mesodermal tumors, lymphosarcomas).

The earliest squamous cell carcinoma is confined to the epithelial layers (carcinoma in situ, intraepithelial carcinoma, preinvasive carcinoma), and it is thought that the disease remains confined to the mucous membrane for several years before invading the subjacent stroma. Carcinoma in situ occurs most frequently during the decade between 30 and 40 years of age, whereas invasive carcinoma is encountered most often in women between 40 and 50.

Following penetration of the basement membrane and involvement of the cervical stroma, the disease spreads by direct contiguity to the vagina and the adjacent parametrium, and via the lymphatic channels (which are abundant in this area) to the regional lymph nodes of the pelvis (iliac and obturator) and to the periaortic lymph nodes.

Estimating the extent of the malignant process is extremely important in determining the mode of therapy and in estimating the prognosis. This is judged clinically and is defined according to the Clinical Classification of the International Federation of Gynecology and Obstetrics as follows:

Stage	0	Carcinoma in situ; intraepithelial carcinoma.
Stage	I	Carcinoma strictly confined to the cervix (extension to the corpus should be disregarded).
	IA	Cases of early stromal invasion (preclinical carcinoma).
	IB	All other cases of stage I.
Stage	II	The carcinoma extends beyond the cervix but has not extended onto the pelvic wall. The carcinoma involves the vagina, but not the lower third.
	IIA	No parametrial involvement.
	IIB	Parametrial involvement.
Stage	IIIA	The tumor involves the lower third of the vagina.
	IIIB	The carcinoma has extended onto the pelvic wall. On rectal examination there is no cancer-free space between the tumor and pelvic wall.
Stage	IV	The carcinoma has extended beyond the true pelvis or has involved the mucosa of the bladder or rectum.

It is known from an examination of surgical specimens that the probability of lymph node metastasis increases according to the local extent of the disease, being approximately 15% in stage I, 30% in stage II, and 45% in stage III. About 80% of patients with stage IV cancer have lymph node involvement.

Clinical Findings

A. Carcinoma in Situ: Carcinoma in situ does not cause symptoms. However, the majority of patients with this condition have an area of redness (erythroplakia) on the portio vaginalis of the cervix which is indistinguishable from chronic cervicitis. In fact, the 2 conditions often coexist. Fifteen to 20% of patients with carcinoma in situ have no visible lesion. Cytologic examination (Papanicolaou) of a representative specimen collected from the squamocolumnar junction (transformation zone) of the cervix will demonstrate severely dysplastic or frankly malignant cells in 95% of women with this stage of disease.

The Schiller test, using Lugol's solution (see p 861, *note*), is often helpful in demonstrating areas of abnormal epithelium, even in cervixes which appear normal on gross inspection, because of the lack of glycogen in these cells and their failure to take up the stain. The test is not specific for neoplasm since areas of ectopy, cervicitis, atrophy, and dysplasia are also iodine-negative. A sharply demarcated border of nonstaining is more suggestive of epithelial neoplasia.

Colposcopic examination of the cervix has been useful in detecting areas of dysplasia and carcinoma in situ. This method is based primarily upon changes which occur in the capillary vascular pattern of the cervix associated with epithelial proliferation.

Punch biopsy is required in all cases in which there is a visible area of redness or an iodine-negative area. A knife cone biopsy and curettage of the endometrial cavity should be done in the following circumstances:

1. No visible lesion; no iodine-negative zone; cytologic examination indicates dysplasia or malignant cells.

2. Punch biopsies of a visible lesion (erythroplakia) or an iodine-negative zone demonstrate dysplasia or carcinoma in situ.

3. Punch biopsies and cytologic examination do not agree; eg, biopsy demonstrates chronic cervicitis, cytology indicates dysplasia or carcinoma.

B. Invasive Carcinoma: Invasive carcinoma of the cervix usually produces symptoms. Intermenstrual or postcoital bleeding is often the first symtom. A watery vaginal discharge, occasionally blood-streaked, may be the only symptom. Pain is a manifestation of far-advanced disease. In most patients with invasive cancer, inspection of the cervix reveals an ulcerated or papillary lesion of the cervix which bleeds on contact. The cytologic examination almost always demonstrates exfoliated malignant cells, and biopsy reveals the invasive nature of the lesion. An occasional endocervical, endophytic lesion will produce enlargement of the cervix without becoming evident on the portio vaginalis.

Differential Diagnosis

Chronic cervicitis can be distinguished from cancer of the cervix only by multiple negative cytologic and biopsy examinations. Polyps of the cervix should be examined by a pathologist to exclude malignant change. It may be very difficult to distinguish severe dysplasia of the cervical epithelium from carcinoma in situ. These now are considered different stages of the same basic process. One pathologist's dysplasia will be another's carcinoma in situ, and more rigid pathologic criteria are needed in order to differentiate the 2 conditions. Lesser degrees of dysplasia usually cause no diagnostic problem.

Complications

The complications are those due to the spread of the disease or secondary to treatment. Obstruction of the ureter, resulting in hydroureter, hydronephrosis, and uremia, occurs with advancing disease. Bilateral obstruction of the ureters leads to failure of kidney function and death.

Involvement of the iliac and obturator lymph nodes may lead to lymphatic obstruction with lymphedema of the lower extremity.

The lumbosacral plexus of nerves may become infiltrated by tumor, causing pain in the low back, hip, and leg.

Vesicovaginal and rectovaginal fistulas occur as a result of tumor involvement of these structures or as complications of radiation therapy. A cloaca may result from massive slough of necrotic tumor tissue. Widespread metastases to lung, liver, brain, and bone may occur.

Complications of radiation therapy such as cystitis, colitis, and proctitis are not uncommon but are usually only transitory problems in modern treatment centers. Castration is an unavoidable complication of radiation therapy. Severe radiation damage to the bladder and rectum may result in hemorrhage, fistulas, and strictures. Radiation necrosis of the cervix and diffuse radiation pelvic fibrosis are rare complications.

The complications of surgery are hemorrhage, infection, thromboembolism, and fistula (ureterovaginal, vesicovaginal, rectovaginal) formation.

Prevention

Invasive cancer of the cervix can be prevented by detecting and properly treating chronic cervicitis, cervical dysplasia, and carcinoma in situ of the cervix. Annual cytologic and pelvic examinations with appropriate therapy have proved to be effective in the prevention of this disease.

Treatment

The proper treatment of cervical cancer requires individualization of therapy for each patient according to the clinical circumstances.

A. Carcinoma in Situ: Carcinoma in situ is most often treated by total hysterectomy with an adequate margin of normal adjacent vaginal mucosa. When the lesion is confined to the cervix and can be removed in its entirety, conization of the cervix may be considered definitive therapy in a young woman who desires to retain her childbearing potential. Close cytologic follow-up is necessary in order to ensure that this form of therapy has, indeed, been adequate.

B. Invasive Carcinoma: In general, invasive carcinoma is best treated by irradiation under the cooperative management of a radiotherapist and a gynecologist experienced in the treatment of cancer. Both internal (radium) and external sources (x-ray, cobaltous chloride Co 60, betatron, linear accelerator) should be employed. Radical pelvic surgery (radical hysterectomy, exenteration procedures) may be indicated in certain cases of invasive carcinoma complicating pregnancy, mixed adenosquamous carcinomas, or recurrent or persistent cancer following radiation therapy.

Prognosis

The earlier the disease is treated, the better the prognosis. Carcinoma in situ is almost 100% curable. The best results in stage I cancer of the cervix approach a 90% 5-year survival rate. For stage II, the figure drops to 60%; for stage III, to 30%; and for stage IV, to less than 10%.

Brunschwig A: Surgical treatment of cancer of the cervix: Stage I and II. Am J Roentgenol 102:147–151, 1968.

Devereux WP, Edwards CL: Carcinoma in situ of the cervix: Applicability of diagnostic and treatment methods in 632 cases. Am J Obst Gynec 98:497–508, 1967.

Fox CH: Biologic behavior of dysplasia and carcinoma in situ. Am J Obst Gynec 99:960–974, 1967.

Kottmeier HL (editor): *Annual Report on the Results of Treatment in Carcinoma of the Uterus and Vagina.* Vol 14. International Federation of Obstetrics and Gynecology. Stockholm, 1967.

LEIOMYOMAS OF THE UTERUS

Essentials of Diagnosis

- Often asymptomatic.
- Palpable, irregular enlargements of the corpus uteri.

- Abnormal uterine bleeding (hypermenorrhea or intermenstrual bleeding).
- Vague pelvic discomfort or pressure on neighboring pelvic organs (urinary frequency, constipation).
- Enlargement of uterine cavity (sounding).
- X-rays may demonstrate calcifications within myomas.
- Laparoscopy (peritoneoscopy) may be useful in difficult diagnostic cases.

General Considerations

Leiomyomas of the uterus are found in approximately 20% of all white women and 50% of black women. The cause is not known. Most are asymptomatic. They probably arise from the smooth muscle of the myometrium, and they grow in response to the stimulus of estrogen as evidenced by an increased growth rate during pregnancy and a cessation of growth with the menopause. They are usually multiple and, depending upon the direction of growth, may remain within the myometrium (intramural), distend the external surface of the uterus (subserous), or come to lie beneath the endometrium (submucous). Other types of myomas are intraligamentous (between the leaves of the broad ligament), parasitic (detached from the uterus and deriving blood supply from other abdominal organs), and cervical. Myomas may vary in size from tiny "seedlings" to massive tumors filling the entire abdomen and pelvis.

On cut section, leiomyomas are well circumscribed, solid tumors with a pseudocapsule of compressed myometrium and a pearly-gray whorled appearance.

Leiomyomas are subject to various degenerative changes, probably as a result of interference with the blood supply to various segments of the tumor: hyaline and cystic degeneration, calcification, carneous degeneration (during pregnancy), and, rarely, malignant change (sarcoma).

Clinical Findings

A. Symptoms and Signs: The majority of leiomyomas produce no symptoms and are discovered in the course of a routine pelvic examination. Symptoms, when they occur, are those of an enlarging tumor, causing abdominal distention, discomfort, urinary frequency, constipation, and hypermenorrhea. Submucous myomas may cause intermenstrual bleeding, at times alarmingly profuse. They may also become pedunculated and extrude through the cervix into the vagina.

Palpation of the uterus reveals an irregularly enlarged structure which, if large enough, may be felt on abdominal examination. They are usually nontender, but they may become painful in the event of carneous degeneration or torsion of the pedicle of a pedunculated subserous myoma.

A rapidly growing myoma suggests the possibility of sarcomatous change within the tumor (leiomyosarcoma).

B. Laboratory Findings: Anemia may result from acute or chronic blood loss.

C. X-Ray Findings: X-rays may demonstrate the typical calcifications. Hysterography or exploration of the uterine cavity with a curet will define submucous tumors.

Differential Diagnosis

Enlargement of the uterus by a large, soft myoma (cystic degeneration) may mimic the pregnant uterus or vice versa. A history of amenorrhea suggests pregnancy, as does the appearance of any of the presumptive signs of pregnancy such as secondary breast changes, Montgomery follicles, and a positive Chadwick or Hegar sign. A pregnancy test should be done in all suspected cases. Pregnancy may occur in a myomatous uterus.

Solid ovarian tumors and pedunculated subserous myomas pose a problem in differential diagnosis. In ovarian neoplasm there is a distinct separation between the adnexal mass and the uterus. If examination (under anesthesia if necessary) does not provide sufficient information to allow differentiation, laparoscopy or culdoscopy may be helpful.

Complications

Hemorrhage from a submucous myoma or prolonged hypermenorrhea often results in secondary iron deficiency anemia. Rapid growth of myomas and degenerative changes may occur in women taking oral contraceptives. Torsion of the pedicle of a pedunculated subserous myoma may result in necrosis and present the picture of an acute abdominal emergency.

Infertility may be secondary to myomas. Abortion, premature labor, prolonged labor, and postpartum hemorrhage due to uterine atony are encountered in pregnancy complicated by myomas. These tumors infrequently obstruct the birth canal, producing a soft tissue dystocia.

Treatment

Small, asymptomatic myomas require no therapy. Examination every 6 months to observe the rate of growth is recommended. Myomectomy should be done in the young woman who desires preservation of childbearing function should symptoms or infertility require treatment. Hysterectomy is the treatment of choice in most patients with symptoms or in the asymptomatic woman who harbors a rapidly growing myoma. Myomectomy usually requires laparotomy and, in terms of postoperative morbidity, is a more hazardous operation than hysterectomy.

Prognosis

Myomectomy may not cure the condition, and the risk of recurrence should be accepted by the patient before proceeding with the operation. Hysterectomy is curative.

Miller NF, Ludvici PP: On the origin and development of uterine fibroids. Am J Obst Gynec 70:720–740, 1955.

Parks J, Barter RH: The myomatous uterus complicated by pregnancy. Am J Obst Gynec 63:260–271, 1952.

Wilson JR: Premenopausal pelvic neoplasms. Hosp Med 3:15–32, 1967.

ENDOMETRIAL CARCINOMA

Essentials of Diagnosis

- Postmenopausal bleeding.
- Uterus frequently not enlarged.
- Uterine enlargement and pain are signs of advanced disease.
- Vaginal cytology fails to detect a high percentage of cases.
- Endometrial biopsy or curettage is required to confirm the diagnosis.

General Considerations

Endometrial carcinoma is primarily a disease of postmenopausal women, with a peak incidence in the decade from 55–65 years of age. It also occurs in premenopausal women, particularly those with prolonged anovulation. Evidence suggests that prolonged unopposed (by progesterone) estrogen stimulation of the endometrium may be a predisposing factor in the development of endometrial carcinoma. The coincidence of obesity, hypertension, and diabetes in many patients with this disease is indicative of an underlying endocrine disorder.

Benign cystic hyperplasia progressing to adenomatous hyperplasia and then adenomatous hyperplasia with anaplasia and, finally, neoplasia has been demonstrated as a preliminary sequence in a number of patients with endometrial carcinoma.

Although cancer of the endometrium has been produced in laboratory animals through the continuous administration of estrogen, there is no conclusive evidence that estrogens cause cancer in women.

Carcinoma of the endometrium probably has an in situ (intraepithelial) first stage, followed by invasion of the surrounding endometrial stroma before it involves the underlying myometrium. Fortunately, deep myometrial penetration, extension beyond the corpus of the uterus, lymph node involvement, and distant metastases occur relatively late in the disease, so that most lesions are detected early.

The International Classification (clinical staging) of endometrial cancer is as follows:

Stage	0	Histologic findings suspicious of malignancy, but malignancy not proved.
Stage	I	The carcinoma is confined to the corpus.
Stage	II	The carcinoma has involved the corpus and cervix.
Stage	III	The carcinoma has extended outside the uterus but not outside the true pelvis.
Stage	IV	The carcinoma has extended outside the true pelvis or has obviously involved the mucosa of the bladder or rectum.

Clinical Findings

Postmenopausal bleeding is the primary symptom and should be considered to be caused by malignancy until proved otherwise. About 40% of women with vaginal bleeding following the menopause will have reproductive tract cancer, and in the vast majority of these cases the malignancy is endometrial. Cervical stenosis with pyometra or hematometra is highly suggestive of endometrial carcinoma. Pain is not a common symptom, but there may be mild uterine cramping, particularly if there is any degree of stenosis of the cervix. Vaginal cytology is positive in 40–80% of cases. Endometrial biopsy will almost always detect an endometrial carcinoma, as will cytologic sampling of the endometrial cavity also. Curettage first of the endocervix and then of the endometrial cavity, with careful examination under anesthesia is considered the most definitive method of diagnosing and clinically staging the disease. Myometrial involvement is suspected if the corpus is enlarged.

Differential Diagnosis

Other causes of postmenopausal and intermenstrual bleeding such as vaginitis, cervicitis, polyps, cervical cancer, and hormonal therapy must be considered. (See section on menstrual disorders, above.)

Complications

Endometrial carcinoma which is histologically poorly differentiated may disseminate relatively early in the course of the disease. Metastatic spread to the vagina, regional pelvic and para-aortic lymph nodes, ovaries, lungs, liver, brain, and bone may occur.

The most frequent site of recurrence following treatment for endometrial carcinoma is the vaginal vault.

Prevention

There is presumptive evidence that cyclic progesterone therapy will reduce the possibility of endometrial carcinoma in the anovulatory patient. Detection and adequate therapy of the precursors of the disease (polyps, hyperplasia, and carcinoma in situ of the endometrium) will prevent the subsequent development of endometrial carcinoma.

Treatment

Total hysterectomy and bilateral salpingo-oophorectomy is recommended in the patient with a well-differentiated tumor in a small uterus without cervical involvement.

In less well differentiated tumors or if the disease extends beyond the endometrium, preoperative irradiation therapy, either with intrauterine and intravaginal radium or by full pelvic external radiation, should be given prior to hysterectomy. Radical hysterectomy with bilateral pelvic lymph node dissection can be used in carefully selected patients who are in good general condition in stage II carcinomas.

The application of multiple small dose radium capsules (Heyman packing technic) to the endometrial cavity, supplemented by intravaginal radium and full pelvis external therapy, is the treatment of choice in patients who are considered poor surgical risks.

Disseminated endometrial carcinoma is treated with large dose progestin therapy (hydroxyprogesterone caproate or medroxyprogesterone) which produces satisfactory remission of the metastatic disease in about 35% of cases. Subjective improvement is noted in the majority of patients so treated.

Barter RH & others: Place of curettage in diagnosis of carcinoma of the endometrium. Am J Obst Gynec 100:696–702, 1968.

Copenhaver EH, Barsamian M: Management of adenocarcinoma of the endometrium. S Clin North America 47:723–735, 1967.

Kottmeier HL (editor): *Annual Report on the Results of Treatment in Carcinoma of the Uterus and Vagina.* Vol 14. International Federation of Obstetrics and Gynecology. Stockholm, 1967.

Nolan JF & others: Value of preoperative radiation therapy in stage I carcinoma of the uterine corpus. Am J Obst Gynec 98:663–674, 1967.

SARCOMAS OF THE UTERUS

Uterine sarcomas are relatively rare. They may arise in preexisting leiomyomas, from the myometrium itself, or from the endometrial stroma. Mixed tumors (carcinosarcoma, mixed mesodermal tumors) containing both epithelial and connective tissue malignant cells are also encountered.

Sarcomas of the uterus metastasize via the blood stream and lymphatics as well as spread by direct contiguity. The lungs are a frequent site of metastatic disease.

In patients in whom the tumor is confined to the pelvic organs, treatment consists of total hysterectomy and bilateral salpingo-oophorectomy.

The outlook for patients with uterine sarcoma is variable. Sarcomas arising in preexisting myomas carry a relatively good prognosis, whereas those of mixed mesodermal origin are almost invariably fatal within 2 years.

Radiation therapy and chemotherapy have not been successful in treating uterine sarcomas. Mixed mesodermal tumors with predominantly adenocarcinomatous elements may respond to palliation with large doses of progestins.

Ober WB, Tovell HMM: Mesenchymal sarcomas of the uterus. Am J Obst Gynec 77:246–268, 1959.

Stearns HC, Sneeden VD: Leiomyosarcoma of the uterus. Am J Obst Gynec 95:374–380, 1966.

Thornton WN Jr, Carter JP: Sarcoma of the uterus: A clinical study. Am J Obst Gynec 62:294–302, 1951.

Webb GA: Uterine sarcomas. Obst Gynec 6:38–50, 1955.

OVARIAN TUMORS

Essentials of Diagnosis

- Adnexal mass palpated during pelvic examination.
- Rupture of a cyst or a twisted pedicle may produce symptoms of an acute abdominal emergency.
- Abdominal distention and symptoms of pressure on surrounding organs are manifestations of a large tumor or of ascites due to peritoneal seeding.
- Plain films of the abdomen and pelvic pneumography often are helpful. Because the ovaries are a frequent metastatic site for bowel malignancy, x-ray studies of the small and large intestine are indicated when one suspects ovarian malignancy.
- Peritoneoscopy (laparoscopy or culdoscopy) is often useful.
- Paracentesis with cytologic examination of ascitic fluid.
- Chest x-ray will demonstrate pulmonary disease and pleural fluid.
- Culdocentesis with cytologic examination of a small amount of peritoneal fluid (which is present under normal circumstances) may detect very early lesions.

General Considerations

Because of their complex embryologic and histogenetic development, the ovaries are a source of a greater variety of tumors, both benign and malignant, than any other organ in the body. Ovarian tumors may be frankly benign, frankly malignant, or somewhere in between; they may be solid or cystic, or there may be mixed types; and they may be functional (producing sex steroids) or nonfunctional. Of the greatest clinical significance is the fact that, whether benign or malignant, they are often clinically silent until late in the course of their development.

Benign cysts of the ovary may be functional (follicle or corpus luteum cysts) or proliferative (dermoid, serous, and mucinous cystadenomas). The more frequent solid benign tumors are fibromathecomas, fibroadenomas, and the Brenner tumors. Endometriosis is a frequent cause of cystic enlargement of the ovary (see section on endometriosis, above).

The common malignant tumors are serous and mucinous cystadenocarcinoma, endometrioid carcinoma, and undifferentiated solid adenocarcinoma. Less common are the hormone-producing neoplasms: granulosa-theca cell tumors, arrhenoblastomas, and adrenal cell rest tumors. These have variable degrees of malignancy. Rarely encountered are tumors of germ cell origin, ranging from the dysgerminoma, the homologue of the testicular seminoma, to the highly malignant teratocarcinoma. Metastatic carcinoma from the gastrointestinal tract (Krukenberg's tumor), breast, pancreas, and kidney must always be considered whenever there is bilateral malignant disease of the ovaries.

Follicle cysts result from failure of a number of developing ovarian follicles to undergo atresia (regression) during the second half of the menstrual cycle. Usually they appear as multiple cystic structures filled with clear serous fluid, but they may be single. Rarely do they cause the ovary to become larger than 6–7 cm in diameter.

Corpus luteum cysts, likewise, do not become very large; they are single cysts, resulting from failure of the corpus luteum to regress, and they often contain an amber or brown serous fluid or they may be filled with blood.

Dermoid cysts (benign cystic teratomas) are common, comprising about 20% of all ovarian tumors in mature women. Occasionally they are bilateral (8–15%). They may vary from a few millimeters to more than 20 cm in diameter, and the external appearance is one of a smooth, glistening, thick-walled, pearly-gray cyst. When opened, they are found to contain a thick sebaceous material and hair. Occasionally, bone structures and teeth are found. In fact, almost any tissue may be found on microscopic examination. A rare but interesting type is the benign cystic teratoma composed largely of thyroid tissue (struma ovarii) which, if functional, may give rise to hyperthyroidism. Current thinking regarding the histogenesis of these tumors is that they develop from an autofertilization of haploid germ cells. Malignant change is rarely encountered in dermoid cysts.

Serous, endometrioid, and mucinous cystic tumors (cystomas, cystadenomas, cystadenocarcinomas) arise from the surface epithelium of the ovary. The serous variety is the most common (20% of benign tumors and 40% of malignant tumors). They may become very large—particularly those of the mucinous type—and may fill and distend the entire abdomen. They may be unilocular or multilocular. If they contain small papillary excrescences, the likelihood of malignancy is greater. Although mucinous tumors of a benign type are about as frequent as the serous variety, malignant mucinous tumors are less common (10% of ovarian cancers). Endometrioid carcinomas are the second most frequent variety (24% of ovarian cancers).

Granulosa-theca cell tumors and **arrhenoblastomas** arise from the ovarian stroma. They frequently retain the ability to secrete sex hormones (estrogen, androgen), producing the systemic effects associated with these steroids—feminization or masculinization, as the case may be. The granulosa-theca cell tumors are the most frequent of the hormonally active tumors, constituting about 4–6% of ovarian malignancies. About two-thirds are benign in their clinical behavior. Arrhenoblastomas are rare and usually manifest themselves first by producing defeminization (amenorrhea, atrophy of the breasts) and then masculinization (deepening of the voice, hirsutism, clitoral hypertrophy). Like granulosa-theca cell tumors, the majority are benign, the reported incidence of malignancy being about 20%.

The clinical staging of ovarian malignancy recommended by the International Federation of Gynecology and Obstetrics is as follows:

Stage	I	Growth limited to the ovaries.
	IA	One ovary, no ascites.
	IB	Both ovaries, no ascites.
	IC	One or both ovaries, with ascites.
Stage	II	Growth involving one or both ovaries with pelvic extension.
	IIA	Extension or metastasis to the uterus or tubes only but not other pelvic organs.
	IIB	Extension to other pelvic organs.
Stage	III	Growth involving one or both ovaries with abdominal spread.
Stage	IV	Growth involving one or both ovaries with distant metastases outside the peritoneal cavity.

Clinical Findings

Cystic enlargements of one or both ovaries are a frequent finding on routine pelvic examination of young women in the reproductive age group. In general, these are nonneoplastic and cause no symptoms. They rarely become larger than 8 cm in diameter and usually regress without treatment. Torsion of the pedicle with consequent strangulation may occur, producing abdominal pain of sudden onset, nausea and vomiting, a tender abdominopelvic mass, peritoneal irritation, slight fever, and moderate leukocytosis. Dermoid cysts are particularly apt to twist in this fashion. Because they are usually filled with sebaceous material and may contain tooth structures, these may be diagnosed by x-ray.

Cystic enlargements of the ovary in women of menopausal or postmenopausal age should be regarded as malignant until proved otherwise. Nodularity of an ovarian tumor (palpated on pelvic examination) is presumptive evidence of malignancy, as is associated ascites also. It is often impossible to determine the benign or malignant nature of an ovarian tumor until laparotomy. Papillarity of the external surface, adherence to surrounding structures, and peritoneal implants are signs of malignancy. Psammoma bodies seen on x-ray may arouse suspicion of a papillary process. If there is any doubt at the time of surgery, the tumor should be removed without spilling its contents into the peritoneal cavity and submitted to a pathologist in the operating room for gross examination and frozen section microscopic analysis of any suspicious areas. These cystic enlargements may represent simple cysts, serous or mucinous cystadenomas, or cystadenocarcinomas with serous, mucinous, endometrioid, or mesonephric duct epithelium.

Solid enlargements of the ovary may be benign. Fibroma-thecoma tumors of the ovary comprise about 5% of benign ovarian neoplasms. They are smooth, rounded, firm, mobile masses, usually unilateral and relatively small. An infrequent accompaniment of these solid, benign ovarian tumors is the development of ascites and hydrothorax (Meigs' syndrome). The ascites in these benign tumors is believed to be related to fluid seepage from the tumor into the peritoneal cavity with subsequent transfer to the pleural cavity via the diaphragmatic lymphatics.

Tumors with solid as well as cystic areas palpated at the time of pelvic examination are highly suspicious of malignancy, and the diagnosis is virtually certain if there are, in addition, nodulations in the cul-de-sac, an upper abdominal mass (omental cake), and ascites.

Differential Diagnosis

Ovarian enlargements must be distinguished from pedunculated uterine myomas, hydrosalpinx, tubal tuberculosis, diverticulitis, tumors of the colon, pelvic kidney, retroperitoneal tumors, and metastatic disease from distant sites. In most instances the correct diagnosis can be made if an accurate medical history is obtained, a careful physical examination performed, and judicious use is made of ancillary diagnostic procedures such as radiology, cytology, and peritoneoscopy.

Prevention

Bilateral salpingo-oophorectomy at the time of hysterectomy for benign uterine disease in women over age 40 is advocated by many to prevent the possible development of ovarian cancer. Estrogen replacement should be given to forestall menopausal symptoms, osteoporosis, and atherosclerosis. The detection and removal of potentially malignant ovarian tumors (serous cystadenoma, granulosa-theca cell tumors, dysgerminomas, arrhenoblastomas) may prevent the subsequent development of ovarian cancer, particularly if both ovaries are removed. Problems arise when one encounters such neoplasms in young women who wish to retain their childbearing potential. In such patients, a conservative approach with very careful follow-up examinations is probably best.

Treatment

Cystic enlargements of the ovary suspected to be physiologic (follicle and corpus luteum cysts) require only repeat examinations at intervals of 4–6 weeks to ascertain that they are regressing.

Many benign neoplasms can be treated by simple excision, conserving the ovary. Dermoid cysts, endometriomas, simple serous cysts, and para-ovarian cysts (broad ligament cysts arising from mesonephric duct remnants) can be managed in this fashion. The proper management of ovarian neoplasms obviously requires an intimate knowledge of the gross appearance of ovarian tumors.

Cystadenomas and solid tumors of the ovary should, in younger women, be removed by unilateral salpingo-oophorectomy. The tumor should be opened in the operating room, and frozen-section examination of any solid or papillary areas should be done before the incision is closed.

In women approaching the menopause or older, and in any patient in whom there is bilateral disease, total hysterectomy and bilateral salpingo-oophorectomy are indicated.

When the disease extends beyond the ovaries into the pelvis or abdomen, abdominal hysterectomy and bilateral salpingo-oophorectomy are done if surgically feasible. The omentum is removed if it contains metastatic deposits. Postoperative radiation therapy is then given. If surgical removal of the uterus, tubes, and ovaries is not possible, a biopsy is taken and radiation therapy is administered. It is not uncommon to find, following irradiation, that surgical removal of the internal genitalia can then be done.

Disseminated disease is best treated with chemotherapy, the polyfunctional alkylating agents—mechlorethamine (Mustargen) and its analogues, thiotepa, chlorambucil (Leukeran), and others—being the drugs of choice. These agents are toxic, and close attention—particularly to the hematopoietic function—must be maintained during treatment.

Small bowel obstruction due to tumor occasionally requires surgical treatment, but this should not be done in a patient in the terminal stage of the disease.

Prognosis

The outlook for patients with benign ovarian neoplasms is excellent. The prognosis for those with malignant disease is poor, primarily because most of them are discovered when the disease is far-advanced. The overall cure rate for ovarian cancer is no more than 30%. For stage IA disease, however, 5-year survival rates of 80–85% can be achieved.

Burns BC Jr & others: Management of ovarian carcinoma: Surgery, irradiation and chemotherapy. Am J Obst Gynec 98:374–386, 1967.

Graham JB, Graham RM: Cul-de-sac puncture in the diagnosis of early ovarian carcinoma. J Obstet Gynaec Brit Common 74:371–378, 1967.

Gray LA, Barnes ML: Endometrioid carcinoma of ovary. Obst Gynec 29:694–701, 1967.

Long RTL & others: Variations in survival among patients with carcinoma of the ovary: Analysis of 253 cases according to histologic type, anatomic stage and method of treatment. Cancer 20:1195–1202, 1967.

Munnell EW: The changing prognosis and treatment in cancer of the ovary: Report of 235 patients with primary ovarian carcinoma, 1952–1961. Am J Obst Gynec 100:790–805, 1968.

Santesson L: Suggested classification of ovarian tumors. Presented at meeting of The Cancer Committee of the International Federation of Gynecology and Obstetrics, Stockholm, August 24–26, 1961. In: Kottmeier HL: Malignant tumors in the female pelvis, in: *Cancer of the Uterus and Ovary.* MD Anderson Hospital. Year Book, 1969.

Weingold AB & others: Factors affecting the survival of patients with ovarian carcinoma. Bull New York Acad Med 43:829–842, 1967.

Wilson JR: Premenopausal pelvic neoplasms. Hosp Med 3:15–32, August 1967.

HYDATIDIFORM MOLE & CHORIOCARCINOMA

Essentials of Diagnosis

- Presumptive symptoms of pregnancy.
- Vaginal bleeding.
- Uterus disproportionately large for duration of pregnancy.
- Absence of fetus.
- Passage of grape-like vesicles.
- High serum or urine levels of chorionic gonadotropin.

General Considerations

Hydatidiform mole represents hydropic changes in the placental villi of a pregnancy which is developing in the absence of an embryo (blighted ovum). The swelling of the villi is related to the absence of a fetal circulation and is often accompanied by varying degrees of trophoblastic proliferation. There is a tendency to myometrial penetration which may progress to frank, deep invasion of the uterine wall (chorioadenoma destruens), and a small percentage (about 5%) of hydatidiform moles are followed by the highly malignant choriocarcinoma.

The frequency of hydatidiform mole is about 1:1500–2000 pregnancies in the USA and about 1:450–650 pregnancies in the Far East. Hydatidiform mole is also more common in women over 40 years of age.

Clinical Findings

The usual picture is one of a presumed threatened abortion with a missed menstrual period, nausea, breast changes, and urinary frequency followed by vaginal bleeding. This may go on for several weeks with little or no abdominal pain. Examination reveals a uterus which is disproportionately large for the duration of the pregnancy. There may be bilateral cystic enlargement of the ovaries (theca lutein cysts). Preeclamptic toxemia may develop in women with large moles, and molar pregnancy should be suspected in any patient who develops hypertension, edema, and proteinuria in the first half of pregnancy.

Serum and urinary chorionic gonadotropin levels are unusually high and persist at high levels beyond the 12th week, when in normal pregnancy there is usually a significant drop. X-ray studies are helpful, and amniography (transabdominal injection of radiopaque material) may confirm the diagnosis. Ultrasound (B-scan) has also been useful.

In many cases the diagnosis is not made until the patient spontaneously aborts the molar pregnancy.

Differential Diagnosis

Threatened abortion is the diagnosis most often entertained in the presence of a mole. Multiple pregnancy must be considered because it may produce unusually high levels of chorionic gonadotropin. If a fetal skeleton is visible on x-ray (at 16 weeks) or if a fetal heartbeat can be heard, the patient almost certainly does not have a mole.

Complications

About 15% of moles become locally invasive (chorioadenoma destruens), which carries the danger of hemorrhage due to penetration of the vascular uterine wall or pelvic infection from perforation.

About 5% of moles are followed by choriocarcinoma, a highly malignant tumor. Although this cancer may occur after normal pregnancy, abortion, or ectopic pregnancy, about half of them develop from an antecedent hydatidiform mole. Metastases are found in the lungs, liver, CNS, bone, vagina, and vulva.

Treatment

Once the diagnosis of a molar pregnancy has been established, the uterus should be emptied. This is done by dilatation and curettage if the uterus is smaller than a 12-week pregnancy. Larger moles are better evacuated by the administration of an oxytocin solution intravenously; this is then followed by careful curettage to ensure complete removal of the molar tissue. All specimens are examined pathologically for evidence of proliferative activity of the trophoblast, which serves as an index to the probability of malignant change.

The suction method of uterine evacuation has been used successfully in the removal of larger moles; however, abdominal hysterotomy is used to remove moles as large as a 5-month pregnancy, with curettage of the endometrial cavity through the hysterotomy wound. Lutein cysts of the ovaries, which occur in about a third of molar pregnancies, will regress following removal of the mole and should not be surgically excised.

All patients with hydatidiform mole should be examined frequently following evacuation of the uterus for the possible development of chorioadenoma destruens or choriocarcinoma. They should be given effective contraceptive advice and advised not to become pregnant for at least a year. Persistence of chorionic gonadotropin in the serum 4–6 weeks after a molar pregnancy is presumptive evidence of active trophoblastic tissue. Disappearance of the hormone followed by a later reappearance, particularly with rising titers, is strongly suggestive of choriocarcinoma if pregnancy can be ruled out.

The usual treatment of chorioadenoma destruens is total abdominal hysterectomy. Methotrexate, a chemotherapeutic agent which competes with folic acid in cellular metabolism, has been very effective in controlling not only invasive moles but choriocarcinoma as well. It is given in courses of 15–25 mg/day for 5 days. It is an extremely cytotoxic agent and is preferably given by someone skilled in its use (see

Chapter 50). Other effective chemotherapeutic agents useful in methotrexate-resistant tumors are dactinomycin (Cosmegen), chlorambucil (Leukeran), and vinblastine (Velban).

Prognosis

The prognosis for cure in hydatidiform mole and chorioadenoma destruens is excellent. Before the anticancer drugs became available, the outlook for choriocarcinoma was very poor. Five-year remission rates in the range of 80% or better are now being reported.

Hammond CB & others: Primary chemotherapy for non-metastatic gestational trophoblastic neoplasms. Am J Obst Gynec 98:71–78, 1967.

Llewellyn-Jones D: Management of benign trophoblastic tumors. Am J Obst Gynec 99:589–594, 1967.

Tow WSH, Cheng WC: Recent trends in treatment of choriocarcinoma. Brit MJ 1:521–523, 1967.

. . .

CELIOSCOPY IN GYNECOLOGY

The development of fiber optics has stimulated the use of 2 technics for the visualization of the internal organs of reproduction: culdoscopy and laparoscopy. The first utilizes the knee-chest position and can be performed with either local or conduction (caudal or spinal) anesthesia. Laparoscopy is usually performed with the patient in the Trendelenburg position or in the dorsal recumbent position under general anesthesia. Both depend upon the introduction of a pneumoperitoneum, atmospheric air usually being used in culdoscopy and either carbon dioxide or nitrous oxide in laparoscopy. In addition to the value of these technics diagnostically, certain operative and manipulative procedures can be carried out. Each method has its advantages and disadvantages and its proponents and opponents.

Culdoscopy can be performed under local anesthesia after preoperative sedation. Although CO_2 or N_2O pneumoperitoneum can be used, air is usually allowed to enter the peritoneal cavity through a posterior vaginal fornix/cul-de-sac puncture. Visualization is carried out transvaginally, and the view of the pelvic organs is somewhat more restricted than that seen through the laparoscope. The procedure is contraindicated whenever a lesion such as endometriosis, chronic salpingitis, or a tumor occupies the cul-de-sac. It cannot be done in the presence of vaginal atresia.

Laparoscopy has the disadvantage of requiring endotracheal anesthesia and operating room facilities. It affords a better view of the pelvic contents and allows a greater variety of manipulative and minor operative procedures than does culdoscopy. It is contraindicated in patients with cardiac or respiratory insufficiency, abdominal hernias, large abdominal tumors, or advanced pregnancy and in patients with a likelihood of disseminated abdominal malignancy. Previous abdominal surgery is not an absolute contraindication, and the procedure can be done safely in patients with abdominal surgical scars provided certain safeguards are observed in the introduction of the pneumoperitoneum and the placement of the trocar through the anterior abdominal wall.

Riva HL & others: Further experience with culdoscopy: An analysis of 2850 cases. JAMA 178:873–877, 1961.

Siegler AM: Trends in laparoscopy. Am J Obst Gynec 109:794–809, 1971.

Steptoe PC: *Laparoscopy in Gynaecology.* Livingstone, 1967.

● ● ●

General References

Anderson Hospital and Tumor Institute: *Cancer of the Uterus and Ovary.* Year Book, 1969.

Corscaden JA: *Gynecologic Cancer.* Williams & Wilkins, 1962.

Fluhmann CF: *The Cervix Uteri and Its Diseases.* Saunders, 1961.

Graham JB, Sotto LSJ, Paloucek PP: *Carcinoma of the Cervix.* Saunders, 1962.

Gray LA (editor): *Dysplasia, Carcinoma in Situ and Micro-Invasive Carcinoma of the Cervix Uteri.* Thomas, 1964.

Green TH Jr: *Gynecology: Essentials of Clinical Practice.* Little, Brown, 1965.

Kraus FT: *Gynecologic Pathology.* Mosby, 1967.

Meigs JV, Sturgis SH (editors): *Progress in Gynecology.* Vol 4. Grune & Stratton, 1963.

Pack GT, Ariel IM (editors): *Tumors of Female Genitalia.* Harper, 1962.

Rovinsky JJ (editor): *Davis' Gynecology and Obstetrics.* Harper, 1968.

Steptoe PC: *Laparoscopy in Gynaecology.* Livingstone, 1967.

Taylor ES: *Essentials of Gynecology,* 4th ed. Lea & Febiger, 1962.

46...

Orthopedics

Floyd H. Jergesen, MD

OSTEOMYELITIS

Osteomyelitis is an acute or chronic infection of bone and is classified according to origin as primary or secondary, according to microbial flora, and according to course as acute, subacute, or chronic.

Primary osteomyelitis is caused by direct implantation of microorganisms into bone and is usually localized to that site. Open (compound) fractures, penetrating wounds (especially those due to firearms), and surgical operations on bone are the most common causes. Operative treatment is usually necessary; treatment with antimicrobial drugs is adjunctive.

Secondary or **acute hematogenous osteomyelitis** is usually due to spread through the blood stream. Occasionally, secondary osteomyelitis may result from direct extension of infection in contiguous soft tissues or from septic arthritis in an adjacent joint.

1. ACUTE PYOGENIC OSTEOMYELITIS
(Secondary or Hematogenous Osteomyelitis)

Essentials of Diagnosis

- Pain, tenderness, swelling, and limitation of joint motion.
- Fever, chills, malaise, and sweating.

General Considerations

About 95% of cases of acute secondary osteomyelitis are caused by pyogenic organisms, usually a single strain. Secondary contamination during treatment may produce a mixed infection.

Acute hematogenous osteomyelitis occurs predominantly during the period of skeletal growth, with the peak incidence during childhood. About 75% of cases in children are due to staphylococci; group A streptococci are the next most common pathogen; and the remainder of cases are caused by a wide variety of organisms. Preexisting infection of another organ system is present in about half of cases. Males are affected

about 4 times as frequently as females. The tibia and femur are the most commonly involved of the long bones.

The initial lesion may become progressive or chronic, or the infection may resolve with or without treatment.

If the initial lesion is not controlled, spread of infection causes bony destruction that differs in infancy, childhood, and adulthood due to the vascular supply of bone. During infancy, terminal ramifications of the nutrient artery perforate the growth plate and end in the cartilaginous precursor of the epiphysis. This may explain both the frequency of complicating septic arthritis during infancy and subsequent disturbances of growth. There may also be rapid spread of infection throughout the entire length of the bone, but involucrum formation is not characteristic.

At about 18 months of age, the epiphyseal plate becomes a vascular barrier. The blood flow on the metaphyseal side of the growth plate reverses its direction, forming loops that empty into the large sinusoidal veins where the rate of blood flow is slower. This may explain the frequency of metaphyseal infections in the long bones during childhood. Initial localization of infection in cancellous bone is rapidly followed by edema which causes increased intraosseous pressure. Suppuration follows edema, and the escape of exudate beneath the periosteum causes elevation with disruption of vascular channels. The inflamed periosteum starts to produce a shell-like layer of new bone which can be identified by x-ray. Disturbance of blood supply to the inner surface of the cortex from thrombosed branches of nutrient vessels leads to necrosis of compact bone and sequestration. Because the epiphysis is separated from the metaphysis by the growth plate, it is protected from direct involvement.

In adulthood, metaphyseal and epiphyseal vessels communicate across the scar of the previous growth plate, and microorganisms can enter the epiphysis through the nutrient artery. This permits organisms to reach the subchondral bone of joints and precipitate a complicating septic arthritis. Since the periosteum of adults is rather fibrous and adherent, extensive subperiosteal abscess formation is not a prominent feature. However, periosteal inflammation can be identified by demineralization and absorption of the cortex. Involucrum formation and extensive cortical sequestration are not uncommon in adulthood. Involvement of the diaphysis, chronic infection of the marrow, and abscesses of the soft tissues surrounding bone are more common sequelae in adults.

Clinical Findings

A. Symptoms and Signs: In infants and children, the onset is often sudden, with marked toxicity; an insidious onset may produce more subtle symptoms. Voluntary movement of the extremity is inhibited. Tenderness followed by swelling and redness are the local manifestations.

The onset in adults is likely to be less striking than in infants and children. Generalized symptoms of bacteremia may be absent, and vague, shifting, or evanescent local pain may be the earliest manifestation. Limitation of joint motion may be marked, especially in patients with spine involvement or when lesions are near joints.

B. Laboratory Findings: Identification of the causative organism is often possible by blood culture. The ESR and white count are often elevated.

C. X-Ray Findings: (Fig 46–1.) Significant changes in bone cannot be identified by x-ray before 7–10 days after onset in infants and 2–4 weeks after onset in adults, but extraosseous soft tissue swelling adjacent to the infection may appear within 3–5 days after the onset of symptoms. Xeroradiography may demonstrate subtle changes in extracortical soft tissues that are not apparent on routine x-ray films. If antimicrobial therapy was started early, x-ray changes in bone may not appear for 3–5 weeks. Subperiosteal new bone formation is a late manifestation of healing.

D. Special Examinations: Exudates may be recovered for culture by aspiration of extraosseous tissues in areas of tenderness or directly from the involved bone. In severe infections of more than 2 days' duration, material for culture and smear is usually obtained during open surgical treatment.

Differential Diagnosis

Acute local infections of bone must be differenti-

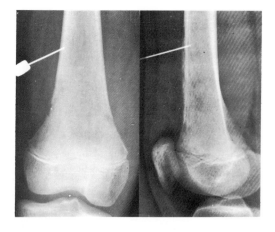

FIG 46–1. Pyogenic osteomyelitis in a 9-year-old girl 5 weeks after onset of symptoms.

ated from the prodromal stages of acute exanthems and from traumatic injuries.

Acute hematogenous osteomyelitis must be differentiated from suppurative arthritis, rheumatic fever, cellulitis, tuberculosis, mycotic infections, and Ewing's sarcoma. The pseudoparalysis associated with acute osteomyelitis in infancy may simulate poliomyelitis. When symptoms are mild, osteomyelitis may initially mimic Legg-Perthes disease.

Complications

Delayed diagnosis or inadequate early treatment can lead to chronic osteomyelitis. Other complications include soft tissue abscess formation, septic arthritis, and metastatic infections to other organs. Pathologic fracture may occur at sites of extensive bone destruction.

Treatment

A. General Measures: Toxic patients require intravenous administration of fluid and electrolytes. Accompanying anemia should often be corrected by blood transfusion. Immobilization of the affected extremity by splinting, plaster encasement, or suspension in an orthopedic apparatus is advisable for relief of pain and protection against pathologic fracture.

B. Specific Measures: Although antibiotics are of great benefit, they are not usually curative. The mainstay of therapy is surgery. Treatment must be individualized, and only broad guidelines will be given here.

1. Operative treatment—During the first 2–3 days after the onset of acute infection, open surgical treatment can be avoided in many cases, especially in infants and children. If vigorous general care and appropriate antibiotic therapy are instituted promptly, the progress of the local lesion may be controlled and spread of the infection halted before suppuration and significant tissue destruction have occurred.

If an abscess has formed beneath the periosteum or has extended into the soft tissues of infants and children, it should be drained at least once daily by aspiration. Pain and fever that persist longer than 2–3 days after initiating aspiration and antimicrobial therapy suggest spread. Surgical decompression of the medullary cavity by drilling or limited fenestration should be done promptly with the hope of minimizing progression of bone necrosis. Subsequent treatment of the local lesion may be by open or closed technics. Open treatment of the wound by packing requires multiple dressing changes, which are painful and frequently cannot be accomplished except under general anesthesia. Closed wound treatment with intermittent suction drainage provides egress of exudates and minimizes the likelihood of secondary contamination. Antibiotics can be given topically through the drainage tube in concentrations that systemically would be toxic.

Radical surgical technics such as extensive guttering and diaphysectomy should be reserved for the treatment of chronic osteomyelitis.

2. Antibiotics—(See Chapter 10.) Antibiotic therapy is aided by identification of the organism and its antibiotic sensitivities. Since acute infections in children are usually due to staphylococci or β-hemolytic streptococci, appropriate systemic antibiotics for these organisms should be administered without waiting for culture reports. Chemotherapy should be continued for about 2–3 weeks after the patient becomes afebrile or repeated wound cultures fail to show growth.

Course & Prognosis

The mortality rate in treated acute osteomyelitis is about 1%, but morbidity continues to be high. If effective treatment can be instituted within 48 hours after onset, prompt recovery can be expected in about two-thirds of cases. Chronicity and recurrence of infection are likely when treatment is delayed.

Capitanio MA, Kirkpatrick JA: Early roentgen observations in acute osteomyelitis. Am J Roentgenol 108:488–496, 1970.

Jergesen F, Jawetz E: Pyogenic infections in orthopaedic surgery. Am J Surg 106:152–163, 1963.

Martin CM & others: Initial, presumptive therapy for serious acute gram-negative rod infections: Preliminary report of a controlled clinical trial. Trans New York Acad Sc (Series II) 29:589–605, 1967.

Waldvogel F, Medoff G, Swartz MN: Osteomyelitis: A review of clinical features, therapeutic considerations and unusual aspects. New England J Med 282:198–206, 260–266, 316–322, 1970.

2. SALMONELLA OSTEOMYELITIS & ARTHRITIS

Infection of bones and joints occurs as a complication in less than 1% of cases of typhoid fever. The precise diagnosis depends upon recovery of *Salmonella typhi* from the osteoarticular focus, and treatment is essentially the same as for other salmonella infections and osteomyelitis in general.

In otherwise healthy patients, the bone lesion of salmonellosis is more likely to be solitary and may exhibit any of the protean gross pathologic manifestations of acute or chronic pyogenic osteomyelitis. In infants and children, it commonly affects the metaphysis of a major long bone, especially the lower femur, proximal humerus, or distal tibia. In the adult, in addition to the shafts of long bones, the lesion may be found in the metaphyses or epiphyses; other probable locations include the ribs and spine.

Infants and children with sickle cell disease complicated by antecedent episodes of marrow thrombosis and bone infarction can present a somewhat different picture since there is a tendency toward diaphyseal involvement, multiple foci, and a propensity toward symmetric localization.

The principles of surgical treatment are the same as for pyogenic osteomyelitis.

Constant E & others: Salmonella osteomyelitis of both hands and the hand-foot syndrome. Arch Surg 102:148–151, 1971.

Engh CA & others: Osteomyelitis in the patient with sickle-cell disease. J Bone Joint Surg 53A:1–15, 1971.

Waldvogel FA & others: Osteomyelitis: A review of clinical features, therapeutic considerations and unusual aspects. New England J Med 282:316–321, 1970.

3. BRUCELLA OSTEOMYELITIS & ARTHRITIS

Osteoarticular infection due to brucellae is not common in the USA. The manifestations include chronic osteomyelitis, pyogenic arthritis, synovitis, and bursitis. In the USA, *Brucella abortus* and *B suis* are the usual organisms, but *B melitensis*, is more common worldwide. Adult men employed in the meat processing or dairy industries and persons who ingest unpasteurized milk products are most likely to be infected.

The osteoarticular lesions appear histologically as caseating or noncaseating granulomas. The lesion caused by *B suis* is more likely to be suppurative and caseous than those caused by other species; the similarity to sarcoidosis and tuberculosis has also been emphasized.

General treatment measures are those applicable to any chronic pyogenic infection, modified when acute symptoms of septicemia are present. Tetracycline, streptomycin, or chloramphenicol is used systemically, although penetration of the bony foci is incomplete.

Kelly PJ & others: Brucellosis of the bones and joints. JAMA 174:347–353, 1960.

Serre H & others: Sacro-iliitis due to brucellosis. Sem Hôp Paris 46:3311–3317, 1970.

4. CHRONIC PYOGENIC OSTEOMYELEITIS

Essentials of Diagnosis

- Pain, tenderness, swelling, edema, and redness of overlying skin.
- Sinus tract formation.

General Considerations

Chronic pyogenic osteomyelitis may occur as a consequence of acute infection or may appear as an indolent, slowly progressive process with no striking symptoms. Recurrent infection is manifested by exacerbation of symptoms with or without drainage after a quiescent period of days, weeks, or years. Chronic osteomyelitis at the site of healed or unhealed fracture is discussed under the treatment of fractures.

Clinical Findings

A. Symptoms and Signs: Symptoms may be so mild and the onset so insidious that there is little or no disability, but recurrent fever, pain, and swelling are common. There may be a history of injury. The infection may communicate through a sinus to the skin surface with periodic or constant discharge of pus.

B. Laboratory Findings: Leukocytosis, anemia, and acceleration of the ESR are inconstant and cannot be relied upon.

C. X-Ray Findings: (Fig 46–2.) Architectural alterations of bone depend upon the stage, extent, and rate of progress of the disease. Destruction of bone may create diffuse areas of radiolucency. Bone necrosis, apparent as areas of increased density, is due in part to increased absorption of calcium from surrounding vascularized bone. Involucrum and new bone formation are healing responses which may be identified beneath the periosteum or within bone. Subperiosteal

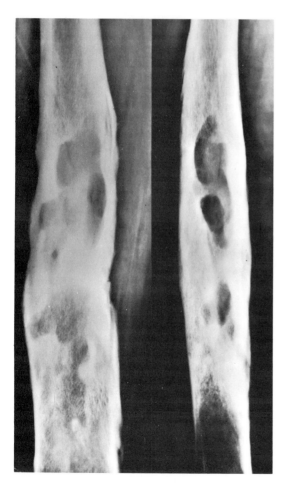

FIG 46–2. Chronic pyogenic osteomyelitis of the lower femur due to *S aureus* in a 38-year-old woman. This patient had numerous clinical exacerbations with 17 operations over a period of 35 years.

new bone may be seen as a lamellar pattern. Progressive resorption of sclerotic bone and reformation of the normal trabecular pattern also suggest healing.

Tomography may be helpful in identifying deep areas of bone destruction. Sinograms made with aqueous radiographic media may aid in localization of sequestra or points of persistent infection and will demonstrate the course of sinus tracts. Occasionally, bone scanning with radioisotopes will localize otherwise occult infection.

D. Special Examinations: The causative organisms should be cultured and drug sensitivity studies performed. Culture of exudates from sinus orifices may be misleading because skin contaminants are likely to be present. More reliable specimens can be obtained by taking samples of suspected tissue at operation or by deep aspiration at a distance from sinus tracts.

Differential Diagnosis

Chronic pyogenic osteomyelitis should be differentiated from benign and malignant tumors; from certain forms of osseous dysplasia; from fatigue fracture; and from specific infections discussed later in this section.

Complications

The most common complication is persistence of infection and acute recurrences. Persistent infection may cause anemia, weight loss, weakness, and amyloidosis. Chronic osteomyelitis may disseminate to other organs.

Acute exacerbations can be complicated by serious effusions in adjacent joints or by frank purulent arthritis.

Constant erosion and progressive destruction of bone cause structural weakening which occasionally leads to pathologic fracture.

Before epiphyseal closure, osteomyelitis can produce overgrowth of a long bone from chronic hyperemia of the growth plate. Focal destruction of an epiphyseal plate can create asymmetric growth.

Rarely, after many years of drainage, squamous cell carcinoma or a fibrosarcoma arises in persistently infected tissues.

Treatment

A. General Measures: During the quiescent phase, no treatment is necessary and the patient lives an essentially normal life. Minor exacerbations accompanied by drainage may be managed adequately with dressing changes. More acute episodes may require immobilization, bed rest, local heat, and mild analgesics.

B. Medical Measures: Occasionally, when the drug sensitivities of the causative organism are known, systemic antibiotic therapy without surgical intervention is advantageous. This is especially true during the early phase of a recurrence without external drainage or abscess formation.

Copious drainage and clinical and x-ray evidence of progressive bone destruction and sequestration require more aggressive treatment.

C. Surgical Treatment: Soft tissue abscesses without sequestration can be treated adequately by operation and open or closed drainage. Similar treatment may also suffice for **Brodie's abscess,** a rare walled-off infection of bone. Removal of a sequestrum with drainage of the abscess cavity often permits rapid healing. With the exception of the fibula, metatarsals, and possibly the metacarpals, diaphysectomy should be avoided if possible because the resected shaft will not regenerate. More extensive and long-standing infections may require more radical surgery such as diaphysectomy or amputation.

Course & Prognosis

Even after vigorous treatment, recurrence of infection is likely. This is usually due to incomplete removal of all areas of infected soft tissue scar or necrotic and unseparated bone.

Dymling JF, Wendeberg B: External counting of ^{85}Sr and ^{47}Ca in localized bone infections. Acta orthop scandinav 36:8–20, 1965.

Gordon SL & others: Recurrent osteomyelitis: Report of four cases culturing L-form variants of staphylococci. J Bone Joint Surg 53A: 1150–1156, 1971.

Jergesen F, Jawetz E: Pyogenic infections in orthopaedic surgery. Am J Surg 106:152-163, 1963.

Johnson LL Kempson RL: Epidermoid carcinoma in osteomyelitis. J Bone Joint Surg 47A:133–145, 1965.

West WF & others: Chronic osteomyelitis. I. Factors affecting the results of treatment in 186 patients. JAMA 213:1837–1842, 1970.

SPECIFIC INFECTIONS OF BONES & JOINTS

MYCOTIC INFECTIONS OF BONES & JOINTS

Fungal infections of the skeletal system are usually secondary to a primary infection in another organ system, frequently the lower pulmonary tract. Although skeletal lesions have a predilection for the cancellous extremities of long bones and the bodies of vertebrae, the predominant lesion—a granuloma with varying degrees of necrosis and abscess formation—does not produce a characteristic clinical picture.

Rhangos WC, Chick EW: Mycotic infections of bone. South MJ 57:664–674, 1964.

Schwarz J, Salfelder K: Diagnosis of surgical deep mycoses. Surg Gynec Obst 128:252–274, 1969.

SYPHILIS OF BONES & JOINTS

Syphilitic arthritis or osteitis may occur during any stage of congenital or acquired infection. Neurotrophic arthropathy (Charcot's joints) can be caused indirectly by syphilitic disease of the spinal cord.

In **infancy,** congenital syphilis typically causes epiphysitis and metaphysitis. Radiologically, a zone of sclerosis appears adjacent to the growth plate but is separated from another similar zone by one of rarefaction. Partial replacement of the rarefied bone by inflammatory tissue precedes suppuration, which may in turn allow epiphyseal displacement because of structural weakening. Focal periosteal thickening of the anterior fontanel causes Parrot's nodes.

Congenital syphilis causes periostitis and osteoperiostitis in **childhood** and **adolescence.** Bone involvement is frequently symmetric, and periosteal proliferation along the tibial crest causes the classic "saber shin." A painless bilateral effusion of the knees (Clutton's joints) is a rare manifestation.

In **adults,** gumma formation is a tertiary manifestation. This granulomatous process is characterized by localized destruction of bone accompanied by surrounding areas of sclerosis. Extensive destruction with accompanying rarefaction may cause pathologic fracture. Periostitis in the adult is likely to occur in the bones of the thorax and in the shafts of long bones. The x-ray picture of syphilitic osteitis in the adult is not diagnostic, but bone production is generally more pronounced than bone destruction.

Osteoarticular lesions due to other causes must be differentiated from syphilis. Serologic studies will usually provide confirmatory evidence. Biopsy is not necessary to establish a direct diagnosis, but it may differentiate a gumma from other lesions. A favorable response to penicillin treatment supports the diagnosis.

The only local treatment necessary is immobilization to provide comfort or protection from fracture if the bone is seriously weakened. Lesions of bones and joints respond promptly to adequate chemotherapy.

Fleming TC & others: Congenital syphilis. J Bone Joint Surg 53A:1648–1651, 1971.

Johns D: Syphilitic disorders of the spine. J Bone Joint Surg 52B:724–731, 1970.

Slapinker S, Minnaar deV: Syphilitic disease of the long bones in the Bantu. J Bone Joint Surg 33B:578–583, 1951.

TUBERCULOSIS OF BONES & JOINTS

Essentials of Diagnosis

- Pain, tenderness, swelling, limitation of joint motion.
- Known primary infection in another organ system.

General Considerations

Infection of the musculoskeletal system with

Mycobacterium tuberculosis is usually caused by hematogenous spread from the respiratory or gastrointestinal tract. Tuberculosis of the thoracic or lumbar spine may be associated with an active lesion of the genitourinary tract.

Clinical Findings

A. Symptoms and Signs: The onset of symptoms is generally insidious. Pain in an involved joint may be mild and accompanied by a sensation of stiffness. It is commonly accentuated at night. Limping and restriction of joint motion are seen. As the disease progresses, the joint becomes fixed by muscle contractures, organic destruction of the joint, and healing in soft tissues and bone.

Local findings during the early stages may be limited to tenderness, soft tissue swelling, joint effusion, and increase in skin temperature about the involved area. As the disease progresses without treatment, muscle atrophy and deformity become apparent. Abscess formation with spontaneous external drainage leads to sinus formation. Progressive destruction of bone in the spine, especially in the thoracolumbar region, may cause a gibbus.

B. Laboratory Findings: The diagnosis rests upon recovery of acid-fast bacilli from joint fluid, tissue exudates, or tissue specimens. Biopsy of the lesion or of a regional lymph node may demonstrate the characteristic histologic picture but does not differentiate tuberculosis from other nontuberculous mycobacterial lesions.

C. X-Ray Findings: (Fig 46–3.) The earliest

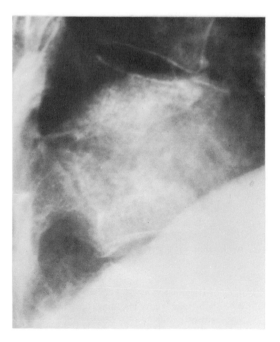

FIG 46–3. Tuberculosis of the lower thoracic spine in an 82-year-old woman. Note extensive destruction and collapse of the bodies of the vertebras adjacent to the eleventh thoracic disk.

changes of tuberculous arthritis are soft tissue swelling and distention of the capsule by effusion. Subsequently, bone atrophy causes thinning of the trabecular pattern, narrowing of the cortex, and enlargement of the medullary canal. As joint disease progresses, destruction of cartilage causes narrowing of the joint cleft and focal erosion of the articular surface, especially at the margins. Extensive destruction of joint surfaces causes deformity. As healing takes place, osteosclerosis becomes apparent around areas of necrosis and sequestration. Where the lesion is limited to bone, especially in the cancellous portion of the metaphysis, the x-ray picture may be that of single or multilocular cysts surrounded by sclerotic bone. As intra-osseous foci expand toward the limiting cortex and erode it, subperiosteal new bone formation takes place.

D. Special Examinations: Exudates for culture may be collected by aspiration, or representative tissues may be removed by either percutaneous or open biopsy.

Differential Diagnosis

Tuberculosis of the musculoskeletal system must be differentiated from other subacute and chronic infections, rheumatoid arthritis, gout, and occasionally from osseous dysplasia. Infections caused by nontuberculous mycobacteria can be differentiated only by laboratory procedures.

Complications

Destruction of bones or joints may occur in a few weeks or months if adequate treatment is not provided. Deformity due to joint destruction, abscess formation with spread into adjacent soft tissues, and sinus formation are common. Paraplegia is the most serious complication of spinal tuberculosis. As healing of severe joint lesions takes place, spontaneous fibrous or bony ankylosis follows.

Surgical Treatment

In acute infections where synovitis is the predominant feature, treatment can be conservative, at least initially; immobilization by splint or plaster, aspiration, and chemotherapy may suffice. A similar approach is used for infections of large joints of the lower extremities in children during an early stage. It may also be used in adults either as definitive treatment of mild infections or before operation. Synovectomy may be valuable for less acute hypertrophic lesions of tendon sheaths, bursas, or joints.

Various types of operative treatment are necessary for chronic or advanced tuberculosis of bones and joints. The advent of effective drug treatment has broadened the indications for synovectomy and debridement at the expense of more radical surgical procedures such as arthrodesis and amputation. Even though the infection is active and all involved tissue cannot be removed, supplementary chemotherapy may permit healing to occur. In general, arthrodesis of weight-bearing joints is preferred when function cannot be salvaged. Reconstructive arthroplasty to restore function has not proved reliable in eradicating disease and is not recommended at present.

Allen AR, Stevenson AW: A ten-year follow-up of combined drug therapy and early fusion in bone tuberculosis. J Bone Joint Surg 49A:1001–1003, 1967.

Falk A: A follow-up study of the initial group of cases of skeletal tuberculosis treated with streptomycin, 1946–1948. J Bone Joint Surg 40A:1161–1168, 1958.

Friedman B: Chemotherapy of tuberculosis of the spine. J Bone Joint Surg 48A:451–474, 1966.

Hodgson AR & others: The pathogenesis of Pott's paraplegia. J Bone Joint Surg 49A:1147–1156, 1967.

Kelly & others: Infection of synovial tissues by mycobacteria other than *Mycobacterium tuberculosis*. J Bone Joint Surg 49A:1521–1530, 1967.

Martin NS: Pott's paraplegia: A report on 120 cases. J Bone Joint Surg 53B:596–608, 1971.

Neville CH Jr & others: Is surgical fusion still desirable in spinal tuberculosis? Clin Orthop 75:179–187, 1971.

Palmer CE, Edwards LB: Identifying the tuberculous infected. JAMA 205:167–169, 1968.

Tull SM & others: Early results of treatment of spinal tuberculosis by triple drug therapy. Clin Orthop 81:56–70, 1971.

Wilkinson MC: Tuberculosis of the hip and knee treated by chemotherapy, synovectomy, and debridement. J Bone Joint Surg 51A:1343–1359, 1969.

PYOGENIC ARTHRITIS

Pyogenic arthritis (suppurative, infectious, or septic arthritis) is an acute or chronic inflammation of joints which may be caused by a variety of microorganisms, especially cocci or enteric gram-negative bacilli. Classification can be based on the mechanism of introduction of the pathogen or the microbial etiology.

Primary pyogenic arthritis can be the result of direct implantation of microorganisms into joints through penetrating wounds or can complicate open surgical procedures (eg, arthrocentesis or intra-articular drug therapy). Joint infections that follow open surgical operations are discussed under acute pyogenic arthritis.

Secondary pyogenic arthritis is generally blood-borne; it can also result from direct extension from an adjacent focus of osteomyelitis or from an extra-articular soft tissue infection.

Chronic pyogenic arthritis can be a sequel to unsuccessful treatment of an acute infection. It may also follow open operations on joints, especially those involving surgical implants. Under other circumstances, the course may be indolent, and infection may be subclinical.

1. ACUTE PYOGENIC ARTHRITIS

Essentials of Diagnosis

- Acute onset of pain.
- Restriction of joint motion.
- Local tenderness, swelling, warmth.
- Fever, chills, and malaise.
- Recovery of the pathogen from the joint cavity.

General Considerations

Pyogenic cocci—staphylococci, streptococci, pneumococci, and meningococci—are the most frequent pathogens. Gonococcal arthritis is discussed separately in the following section. Enteric gram-negative bacilli, especially *Escherichia coli*, may produce infection in adults. *Haemophilus influenzae* is a frequent pathogen in children 6 months to 2 years of age.

In acute hematogenous arthritis, the larger joints (knee, hip, elbow, shoulder, and ankle) are more commonly involved. The presence of a nearby acute or chronic infection of bone or soft tissue may secondarily involve a joint. Infections of other organ systems, eg, skin, respiratory tract, and genitourinary tract, are possible sources of blood-borne infections. Although a single joint is generally involved in adults, multiple joints may be involved by hematogenous arthritis in children. Antecedent trauma to the area may be misleading.

The initial reaction is an acute synovitis. The intra-articular fluid during this phase may show a few polymorphonuclear leukocytes. Later, the synovial fluid changes to pus and edema, and cellular infiltration occurs in the subsynovial soft tissues. Destruction of cartilage follows, especially at the point of contact of opposing joint surfaces. Continued infection may produce destruction of synovia and capsular components as well as cartilage and bone. Following successfully treated early infections, there may be no permanent sequelae, but extensive tissue destruction after severe infections can only be partially repaired and fibrous or complete bony ankylosis may result.

Clinical Findings

A. Symptoms and Signs: Systemic disease or another serious infection may distract attention from the infected joint. Migratory polyarthralgia or multiple joint symptoms may be misleading. Systemic symptoms include fever, chills, and malaise. Pain is generally progressive and is usually accentuated by active or passive joint motions. The patient tends to limit motion of the involved joint. Local tenderness and warmth are present over the joint and are often accompanied by soft tissue swelling and joint effusion.

B. Laboratory Findings: Examination of joint fluid is crucial. During the incipient stage of infection, the fluid may be grossly clear or only slightly turbid, but it tends to become purulent as the infection progresses. The white cell count is likely to be greater than 50,000/μl, with more than 90% polymorphonuclear neutrophils. The fasting blood glucose level is usually more than 50 mg/100 ml above that of the synovial fluid. The acid mucin clot tends to fragment or disintegrate. The sedimentation rate is almost invariably accelerated.

The morphologic and staining characteristics of the pathogen on Gram stain alone may suggest the appropriate antibiotic. Culture of the blood and synovial fluid establishes a definitive diagnosis and provides specific information on antibiotic sensitivities.

C. X-Ray Findings: The appearance of significant x-ray findings depends in part on the virulence of the infection. X-ray changes lag behind the clinical and pathologic process. During the first 2 weeks, the joint capsule can be seen on x-ray to be distended by effusion. As the inflammatory reaction spreads, demarcation between capsule and fat becomes obliterated. Increase in intra-articular pressure from effusion may cause widening of the joint cleft in hip infections, especially in infants, where subluxation can occur. Comparative x-rays of the opposite normal joint can aid in the identification of subtle changes. With persistent hyperemia and disuse, demineralization of subchondral bone occurs adjacent to the joint cleft and extends centrifugally. Trabecular detail is progressively lost and the compact subchondral bone appears accentuated. Destruction of cartilage is reflected by narrowing of the width of the joint cleft until subchondral bone is in apposition.

Complications

Chronic pyogenic arthritis may follow delay in diagnosis or inadequate treatment. Joint infections can disseminate to other sites either via the blood stream or directly.

Differential Diagnosis

Acute pyogenic arthritis must be differentiated from other acute arthropathies (eg, rheumatic fever, rheumatoid arthritis, gout and pseudogout, and gonococcal arthritis). Hematogenous osteomyelitis, rheumatic fever, and epiphyseal trauma may mimic acute septic arthritis in childhood.

Acute pyogenic arthritis may complicate other types of preexisting joint disease, notably rheumatoid arthritis or neurotrophic arthropathy. Concomitant or recent systemic treatment with corticosteroids may cloud the diagnosis, especially during the prodromal stage, by modification of physical signs. Polyarthralgia may occur in systemic viral infections or allergic reactions, but other features of pyogenic arthritis are lacking. Acute infections or inflammations of periarticular structures (eg, septic bursitis and tenosynovitis, osteomyelitis, cellulitis, and acute calcific tendinitis) may be difficult to differentiate. Transient synovitis of the hip in infancy and childhood may be especially difficult to distinguish from bacterial infection, and culture of aspirated joint fluid may be the only method of differentiation.

Treatment

A. General Measures: Analgesics and splinting of the involved joint in the position of maximum comfort alleviate pain. Pain caused by increased intra-articular pressure can be relieved by intermittent aspiration or surgical drainage. Bilateral suspension of the lower extremities in abduction with traction may prevent subluxation or dislocation of a septic hip joint, especially in infants and children.

B. Specific Measures: Definitive treatment is based on surgery and effective drug therapy. The specific operation depends in part upon the infecting agent, the stage of the infection, and the response of the patient.

During the first 48–72 hours after onset, drainage of the joint may be replaced by intermittent aspiration to relieve intra-articular tension and to evacuate exudates. When the infection is due to *Staphylococcus aureus*, open or tube drainage is preferable because of the chondrolytic nature of the altered synovial secretions. If infection is not recognized or not treated effectively within the first 72 hours, immediate drainage by open or closed tube methods is advocated for most cases.

C. Drug Therapy: Antibiotics should be given based on smear and culture reports.

Course & Prognosis

If effective treatment can be instituted within the first 48–72 hours of onset, a prompt favorable response can be expected in an otherwise healthy patient. Defervescence, disappearance of pain, return of uninhibited joint motion, resorption of joint effusion, and a decreasing sedimentation rate are some of the factors that indicate a response to treatment.

Lloyd-Roberts GC: Suppurative arthritis in infancy. J Bone Joint Surg 42B:706–720, 1960.

Nelson JD, Koontz WC: Septic arthritis in infants and children. Review of 117 cases. Pediatrics 38:965–970, 1966.

Rimoin DL, Wennberg JE: Acute septic arthritis complicating chronic rheumatoid arthritis. JAMA 196:617–621, 1966.

Watkins MB, Samilson RL, Winters DM: Acute suppurative arthritis. J Bone Joint Surg 38A:1313–1320, 1956.

2. GONORRHEAL ARTHRITIS

Acute gonorrheal arthritis caused by *Neisseria gonorrhoeae*, is almost always secondary to infection of the genitourinary tract. At one time, joint involvement occurred in 2–5% of all gonococcal infections, but it is now seen more frequently in women who have occult genitourinary infections and sometimes in children. Joint symptoms are likely to appear during the third week of an active infection.

Joint infection is via the blood stream. Clinical evidence of involvement of multiple joints is often present at onset, but symptoms are usually transient in all joints except one. Large weight-bearing joints are affected most frequently. Systemic symptoms may accompany acute arthritis. The initial synovitis with effusion progresses to a purulent exudate with destruction of cartilage which may lead to fibrous or bony ankylosis.

The precise diagnosis is established by recovery of the causative microorganism from the involved joint by culture.

Gonorrheal arthritis must be differentiated from rheumatoid arthritis, pyogenic arthritis caused by other organisms, acute synovitis, Reiter's disease, and gout.

Nonspecific treatment includes immobilization of the joint, bed rest, and analgesics as necessary for pain. If the joint fluid is purulent and recurs rapidly, systemic antibiotic treatment can be supplemented by instillation into large joints of 25—50 thousand units of penicillin G in 5 ml saline, repeated once or twice at daily intervals.

The prognosis for preservation of joint function is good if the diagnosis is established promptly and treatment is vigorous.

Cooke CL & others: Gonococcal arthritis. JAMA 217:204—205, 1971.

Fink CW: Gonococcal arthritis in children. JAMA 194:123—124, 1965.

Hess EV, Hunter DK, Ziff M: Gonococcal antibodies in acute arthritis. JAMA 191:531—534, 1965.

3. CHRONIC PYOGENIC ARTHRITIS

Chronic pyogenic arthritis may follow acute primary or secondary pyogenic arthritis. Pyogenic cocci and enteric gram-negative rods are the most common organisms. Although a previously identified pathogen is likely to persist, superinfection can occur, especially after open surgical treatment and antibiotics. The original bacterial strain is sometimes supplanted by another during treatment, or a mixed infection may occur.

The infection can be continuously or intermittently active. Uninterrupted progress from the acute stage is characterized by continued local pain and swelling, restriction of joint motion, sinus formation, and increasing deformity. X-rays show progressive destruction of cartilage manifested by narrowing of the joint cleft, erosion of bone, and even infraction or cavitation. Even though the course is indolent, it is that of continued deterioration. Episodic abatement may follow treatment with antibiotics in the recurrent type. Occult infections may be unrecognized for long periods since they do not produce striking clinical findings. They may occur concomitantly with other joint diseases or may complicate surgical operations on joints, especially after surgical implants or antibiotic prophylaxis of postoperative infection.

Chronic pyogenic arthritis must be differentiated from chronic nonpyogenic microbial infections of joints, gout, rheumatoid arthritis, and symptomatic degenerative arthritis.

The goal of treatment is eradication of infection and restoration of maximum joint function. Bacterial sensitivity tests provide a basis for selection of antimicrobial drugs. Operative destruction of the joint by arthrodesis or resection is often necessary to eliminate chronic infection.

Jergesen F, Jawetz E: Pyogenic infections in orthopaedic surgery. Combined antibiotic and closed wound treatment. Am J Surgery 106:152—63, 1963.

TUMORS & TUMOR-LIKE LESIONS OF BONE

OSTEOMA

Osteoma is an uncommon benign tumor (or hamartoma) that arises from membranous bone. Symptoms usually appear during adulthood and are apt to be due to protrusion of the tumor mass superficially, where it becomes visible, or deeply, where it interferes with the function of adjacent structures.

Osteoma must be differentiated from osteochondroma, osteophytes occurring in tendons and ligaments, and reactive hyperostosis of the skull. It should not be confused with "parosteal osteoma," which may be locally invasive.

Surgical removal is curative.

OSTEOCHONDROMA
(Osteocartilaginous Exostosis, Osteochondromatosis, Hereditary Multiple Exostoses)

Osteochondroma can occur as a single lesion, but, because of the familial tendency, multifocal lesions are commonly referred to as hereditary multiple exostoses.

This common lesion characteristically arises from the surface of enchondral bone near an epiphyseal plate, but it also occurs in flat bones. It may have a sessile or pedunculated configuration and arises from cortically deficient cancellous bone.

Symptoms are likely to be caused by protrusion of the tumor, especially when a thick layer of soft tissue does not cover it. Initial subjective symptoms may be tenderness caused by pressure on adjacent structures. Occasionally, limitation of joint motion is present.

X-rays reveal a sessile lesion superimposed upon

the underlying bone. It may simulate nonosteogenic fibroma or chondromyxoid fibroma.

Thorough surgical removal with the enveloping periosteum is curative.

OSTEOID OSTEOMA

Osteoid osteoma, a lesion lacking certain characteristics of neoplasia, is a tumor-like nidus composed of osteoid and traveculas of newly formed bone deposited in a substratum of highly vascularized osteogenic connective tissue. It can occur in cancellous or compact bone. About half of cases involve the lower extremity.

Pain varies in severity and is frequently intensified at night. Where the lesion is superficial, localized tenderness and swelling may occur. Reactive sclerosis tends to be less intense about a lesion in spongy bone.

Osteoid osteoma must be differentiated from benign tumors of bone (eg, benign osteoblastoma) and localized infections.

Surgical removal of the nidus, which is rarely more than 1 cm in its greatest dimension, gives prompt relief of pain and is curative.

Kendrick JI, Evarts CM: Osteoid-osteoma: A critical analysis of 40 tumors. Clin Orthop 54:51–59, 1967.
Phelan JT: Osteoid osteoma. Surg Gynec Obst 121:112–116, 1965.

NONOSTEOGENIC FIBROMA
(Nonossifying Fibroma, Fibrous Cortical Defect, Metaphyseal Fibrous Defect)

This common lesion of bone is now considered to be nonneoplastic. Certain easily recognized examples—especially those encountered about the posteromedial aspect of the lower femoral metaphysis during infancy and childhood—which do not produce symptoms and tend to undergo spontaneous regression to the point of disappearance have been assigned a separate category, **subperiosteal cortical defect**. Grossly, the tissue is firm and may have a grayish-white, yellowish, or brownish color.

This lesion occurs most frequently in the metaphyses of major long bones—especially those of the lower extremity—during childhood and adolescence. It may be discovered fortuitously by x-ray examination because of injury, etc. In the metaphysis, it is likely to be located eccentrically, near the periosteum. An area of radiolucency involving compact bone of the cortex and adjacent spongiosa is oriented so that its greatest dimension parallels the long axis of the involved bone. In slender bones (eg, fibula and those of the forearm), larger lesions occupy a more central position and may

cause fusiform expansion. Superficially, a thin wall of compact bone may be preserved although elevated beyond the level of the surrounding normal cortex. Deeply, it is demarcated by a layer of sclerotic bone which separates the tumor mass from spongy bone.

Pain calls attention to the condition, and local tenderness or swelling may be noted. Occasionally, pathologic fracture is the first sign. Biopsy of lesions that simulate other conditions, eg, fibrous dysplasia, solitary cysts, histiocytosis X, bone infarct, chondromyxoid fibroma, and chronic osteomyelitis may be necessary to establish a precise diagnosis.

Treatment can be deferred because of the propensity of this lesion to heal spontaneously. Pain and signs of aggressiveness are indications for surgical treatment, which consists of removal of the focus either by curettement or excision.

Morton KS: Bone production in non-osteogenic fibroma. J Bone Joint Surg 46B:233–243, 1964.
Selby S: Metaphysial cortical defects in the tubular bones of growing children. J Bone Joint Surg 43A:395–400, 1961.

BENIGN OSTEOBLASTOMA
(Osteogenic Fibroma, Ossifying Fibroma, Osteofibroma, Fibrous Osteoma)

Benign osteoblastoma includes a group of benign osteoblastic neoplasms with varied histologic and clinical features which may simulate giant cell tumor or osteogenic sarcoma. It is encountered most frequently from childhood to early adulthood but may occur in later life. Although it is found in the skull and the vertebras, the long bones of the lower extremities are more common sites. Local pain calls attention to the lesion. X-rays demonstrate rarefying destruction of normal bone, cortical expansion, and focal osteosclerosis which gives an overall impression of mottling.

Surgical removal of the tumor by local resection followed by bone grafting, if necessary, is applicable to accessible lesions of the flat bones and those of the extremities. In the vertebras, complete removal by curettage or resection may not be feasible. In this circumstance, x-ray therapy has been recommended in addition to surgery.

Goldman RL: Periosteal counterpart of benign osteoblastoma. Am J Clin Path 56:73–78, 1971.
Lichtenstein L, Sawyer WB: Benign osteoblastoma. J Bone Joint Surg 46A:755–765, 1964.

CHONDROMYXOID FIBROMA

Chondromyxoid fibroma of bone is a rare tumor of varying aggressiveness that contains both chondroid and myxoid elements. The tumor may be encountered at any age. It involves the metaphyses of major long bones, bones of the hand and foot, and flat bones. Grossly, the tumor is firm and may contain grit-like foci of calcified cartilage.

Pain calls attention to the lesion, and swelling and tenderness may be apparent where its position is superficial. The x-ray appearance is not characteristic and may simulate that of nonosteogenic fibroma or indolent primary malignant tumors of bone. It may appear as an ovoid or elongated focus of rarefaction and cortical expansion with erosion, demarcated from cancellous bone by a thin zone of osteosclerosis.

Treatment is by surgical excision. Curettement has been followed by recurrence.

Feldman F & others: Chondromyxoid fibroma of bone. Radiology 94:249–260, 1970.

Schajowicz F, Gallardo H: Chondromyxoid fibroma (fibromyxoid chondroma) of bone: A clinico-pathologic study of thirty-two cases. J Bone Joint Surg 53B:198–215, 1971.

ENCHONDROMA

A solitary enchondroma is a mass of cartilage cells that lack the characteristics of neoplasia. The multifocal manifestation is now referred to as enchondromatosis and includes **dyschondroplasia** (Ollier's disease) and **Maffucci's syndrome**, the simultaneous occurrence of enchondromatosis and multiple cavernous hemangiomas.

Solitary enchondroma involves predominantly phalanges, metacarpals, and metatarsals but may be encountered in the metaphyses of major long bones and in flat bones. Although the lesion probably begins before skeletal maturation is complete, it may not be discovered until adulthood. Grossly, the lesion is a globoid mass of pale, firm tissue that may appear lobulated.

Minor trauma may cause pathologic fracture, or indolent progression may cause mild pain, tenderness, or swelling. The characteristic x-ray picture of lesions of the hand or foot is that of a discrete focus of radiolucency with mottling or compartmentalization caused by incomplete ridges of sclerotic bone. Cortical expansion occurs without extensive erosion.

Multiple lesions are likely to cause bizarre deformity because of their size and to disturb longitudinal growth of the involved skeletal segments. Malignant transformation of solitary lesions of the hand or foot is unlikely.

Treatment of a symptomatic solitary lesion of the hand or foot is by thorough curettement and supplemental bone grafting.

Cauble WG, Bowman HS: Dyschondroplasia and hemangiomas (Maffucci's syndrome). Arch Surg 97:678–681, 1968.

Mainzer F & others: The variable manifestations of multiple enchondromatosis. Radiology 99:377–392, 1971.

CHONDROBLASTOMA
(Epiphyseal Chondromatous Giant Cell Tumor, Codman's Tumor)

Chondroblastoma is an uncommon benign tumor that is encountered predominantly in the epiphyseal regions of adolescents, usually in the major tubular bones but also in flat bones. Although the tumor involves the epiphysis primarily, it may involve the metaphysis adjacent to the epiphyseal plate and may erode articular cartilage. Pain in the region of a major joint often calls attention to the tumor. An ovoid focus of radiolucency in the epiphysis or adjacent metaphysis with a demarcating wall of sclerotic bone and punctate areas of mottling caused by calcification within the tumor are significant x-ray findings.

Although this tumor is considered to be benign, instances of aggressiveness have been reported.

Surgical treatment by thorough curettement is usually adequate.

Kahn LB, Wood FM, Ackerman LV: Malignant chondroblastoma. Arch Path 88:371–376, 1969.

Schajowicz F, Gallardo H: Epiphysial chondroblastoma of bone: A clinico-pathological study of sixty-nine cases. J Bone Joint Surg 52B:205–226, 1970.

CHORDOMA

Chordoma, a rare skeletal tumor that apparently arises from notochordal elements, occurs predominantly at the base of the skull or in the sacrococcygeal region but occasionally involves other vertebral segments as well. Symptoms are related to the specific structures encroached upon since the tumor grows slowly, metastasizes late, and manifests local aggressiveness by destruction of adjacent bone and spread into contiguous soft tissues. Local pain and tenderness or peripheral neurologic deficits are the usual clinical features. X-ray findings are not characteristic but do demonstrate an osteolytic lesion with varying degrees of calcification. Biopsy establishes the diagnosis. This tumor may metastasize widely.

Surgical resection may be feasible for limited lesions in the coccyx or distal sacrum. Most lesions are surgically inaccessible but incomplete excision is palliative. The tumor is relatively radioresistant; for significant palliation, less than 4000 rads is likely to be ineffective.

Chalmers J, Heard BE: A metastasing chordoma: A further note. J Bone Joint Surg 54B:526–529, 1972.

Pearlman AW, Friedman M: Radical radiation therapy of chordoma. Am J Roentgenol 108:333–341, 1970.

GIANT CELL TUMOR
(Osteoclastoma)

Giant cell tumor of bone apparently arises from connective tissue of the marrow. Osteoid and new bone may be encountered. Giant cell tumor is observed most commonly from late adolescence to middle adulthood. The majority occur in the ends of major long bones, especially about the knee or in the lower radius, but they have also been observed in other bones of the extremities and in the spine. Pain and swelling are the principal symptoms. X-rays show an osteolytic focus with a foam-like appearance. Biopsy is necessary to differentiate this tumor from other lesions, especially unicameral bone cyst, aneurysmal cyst, chondromyxoid fibroma, osteoblastoma, chondroblastoma, and "brown tumor" of hyperparathyroidism.

The treatment is surgical. Whenever possible, excision is preferred to curettement. When the lesion is extensive and ominous, segmental resection is preferred and may require supplemental bone grafting. In surgically inaccessible areas, partial removal of the tumor supplemented by x-ray therapy is justified. This tumor tends to be locally aggressive but does metastasize.

Dahlin DC & others: Giant-cell tumor: A study of 195 cases. Cancer 25:1061–1070, 1970.
Goldenberg RR & others: Giant-cell tumor of bone: An analysis of 218 cases. J Bone Joint Surg 52A:619–664, 1970.

EWING'S SARCOMA

Ewing's sarcoma is a fairly common primary malignant neoplasm of bone that apparently arises from the marrow, but the nature of the parent cell remains in dispute. The propensity for this tumor to metastasize to the viscera and the common finding of multiple skeletal lesions has raised the question whether it is multicentric or merely tends to metastasize to other bones. Grossly, the tumor tissue is soft, frequently becomes necrotic to the point of liquidity, and destroys surrounding bone.

This tumor is encountered most frequently during adolescence and early adulthood. Initially, it is likely to be discovered in the shaft of a major tubular bone. Local pain is the outstanding symptom. Local tenderness and increase in skin temperature accompany swelling and induration. Mild anemia and leukocytosis are frequently observed.

In the long bones, the tumor is located in the diaphysis. X-rays show diffuse osteosclerosis of the cortex with a fusiform configuration, subperiosteal lamination ("onion peel"), and, occasionally, periosteal reaction resembling a "sunburst" pattern. Growth of the tumor causes medullary destruction which may be identified as diffuse rarefaction or nondescript mottling.

The differential diagnosis includes osteomyelitis, osteogenic sarcoma, adrenal neuroblastoma, Hodgkin's disease, and lymphosarcoma. The precise diagnosis must be established by biopsy. Metastases are frequently present when the lesion is first discovered.

Supervoltage radiation and chemotherapy provide the most effective palliation. Radical surgery, resection, or amputation has little to offer.

Boyer CE Jr & others: Ewing's sarcoma. Cancer 20:1602–1606, 1967.
Johnson R, Humphreys SR: Past failures and future possibilities in Ewing's sarcoma: Experimental and preliminary clinical results. Cancer 23:161–166, 1969.

PLASMA CELL MYELOMA
(Multiple Myeloma)

Plasma cell myeloma is a primary malignant tumor of bone that arises from the hematopoietic reticulum of marrow. It may be primary in the viscera or soft tissues. Although it may present as a solitary lesion, it usually demonstrates multifocal skeletal involvement. The tumor cell resembles a plasma cell, but its precise nature has not been established. Grossly, the tumor tissue is soft, dark red or grayish in color, and richly vascularized. This tumor is encountered predominantly after the age of 40 and is roughly twice as frequent in men as women. Pain is the most common symptom. Swelling and induration are local signs. Diffuse involvement of the spine is characterized by kyphosis and flattening of the lumbar curve with loss of body height. Pathologic fracture is common. When this condition is discovered early, laboratory tests may be normal. As the disease progresses, organ systems other than the bone marrow become involved and anemia, hypercalciuria, hypercalcemia, hyperglobulinemia, Bence Jones proteinuria, and hyperuricemia may be found. X-ray findings are variable, and, because of widespread involvement, diffuse osteoporosis may be the only significant manifestation. Collapse of vertebral bodies may occur. Myeloma is generally osteolytic, but rarely the lesions are sclerotic or mixed.

Although myeloma presents a fairly characteristic clinical picture, biopsy may be necessary to establish a precise diagnosis.

Complications arise from encroachment of the tumor on vital structures such as the spinal cord or cauda equina.

The rate of progress is variable, and periods of apparent remission are frequently observed. Palliative x-ray therapy is useful for the relief of intractable pain. Chemotherapy may ameliorate symptoms and prolong life in selected patients.

Surgical removal of a solitary focus may cure that lesion, but the disease is ultimately fatal.

Alexanian R & others: Treatment for multiple myeloma. JAMA 208:1680–1685, 1969.

Velez-Garcia E, Maldonado N: Long-term follow-up and therapy in multiple myeloma. Cancer 27:44–50, 1971.

OSTEOGENIC SARCOMA

With the exception of myeloma, osteogenic sarcoma is the most common primary malignant tumor of bone. It is encountered most commonly from preadolescence through early adulthood and is about twice as common in males as females. The primary tumor is almost always solitary. The metaphyses of major long bones are common locations, and about 50% involve the knee region.

Weight loss and anemia are common by the time the diagnosis is made. Pain occurs gradually and becomes progressively more severe. Local swelling due to tumor may be the initial complaint. Increase in local heat, venous engorgement, and tenderness are variable local manifestations.

Biopsy is the most useful diagnostic procedure. The features vary somewhat, but anaplastic connective tissue stroma and formation of tumor osteoid and bone are general histologic characteristics. The serum alkaline phosphatase level rises in relation to the degree of osteoblastic activity.

The x-ray findings vary depending upon the osteolytic or sclerosing nature of the tumor. Diffuse rarefaction may reflect the vascularity. Foci of osteolysis of spongy bone are caused by tumor destruction and incomplete replacement with less dense osteoid. Almost without exception, the cortex is eroded or replaced by disorderly formation of new bone. Bone spicules oriented perpendicularly to the normal cortical surface—the classic "sunburst" effect—are likely to appear in sclerosing lesions. X-ray of the chest may show metastases. Bone scans may demonstrate occult lesions and metastases. Arteriography may demonstrate soft tissue invasion not apparent with routine x-ray technics.

The differential diagnosis includes other primary malignant tumors of bone (chondrosarcoma, fibrosarcoma, and giant cell tumor), myositis ossificans, eosinophilic granuloma, and fibrous dysplasia.

Amputation offers the best hope of control when the lesion is accessible and metastasis has not occurred. Five-year survival rates in large series have varied from zero to about 20%. When a solitary pulmonary metastasis is present, its removal is justifiable because of sporadic reports of 5-year survival afterward.

Radiation therapy alone may relieve pain by decreasing the rate of tumor growth. It is a useful palliative step for tumors not amenable to operative treatment.

The more distant the lesion is from the trunk, the more favorable the outlook. In general, the prognosis is less favorable for large tumors. A greatly elevated preoperative serum alkaline phosphatase is a poor prognostic sign. The outlook for tumors involving the trunk which cannot be radically excised is extremely poor. When osteogenic sarcoma complicates Paget's disease, the outlook is hopeless.

Marcove RC & others: Osteogenic sarcoma under the age of 21: A review of 145 operative cases. J Bone Joint Surg 52A: 411–423, 1970.

Nonsanchuk JS & others: Osteogenic sarcoma: Prognosis related to epiphyseal closure. JAMA 208:2439–2441, 1969.

O'Hara JM & others: An analysis of 30 patients surviving longer than 10 years after treatment for osteogenic sarcoma. J Bone Joint Surg 50A:335–354, 1968.

Sweetnam R & others: Bone sarcoma: Treatment by irradiation, amputation, or combination of the two. Brit MJ 2:363–367, 1971.

PAROSTEAL SARCOMA
(Parosteal Osteoma, Parosteal Osteogenic Sarcoma, Juxtacortical Sarcoma, Desmoid of Bone)

Parosteal sarcoma is a primary tumor of extracortical origin which is seen most commonly in adolescents and young adults. The distal metaphysis of the femur, especially the popliteal aspect, is a common site; the tibia and humerus are other locations. The histologic picture is variable.

Because of the indolent nature of this tumor, a mass is commonly the initial feature. X-ray demonstrates a mass distorting adjacent soft tissues and, in some lesions, foci of nebulous calcification. Others may be so extensively ossified as to be radiopaque near the cortex while the more superficial zone demonstrates mottling. The diagnosis is dependent upon critical correlation of clinical, x-ray, and biopsy findings.

This tumor must be differentiated from the osteoblastic variety of osteogenic sarcoma, myositis ossificans, calcified hematoma, and osteochondroma.

Once the diagnosis has been established, segmental resection with reconstruction of the resulting defect by bone grafting or prosthetic replacement is preferred to local excision. Extensive involvement of soft tissues or a neurovascular bundle may make amputation necessary.

This tumor is slowly aggressive, and pulmonary metastases have been reported even after a prolonged interval following apparent eradication of the local lesion. The 5-year survival rate is about 70% following ablative surgery.

Farr GH, Huvos AG: Juxtacortical osteogenic sarcoma: An analysis of fourteen cases. J Bone Joint Surg 54A: 1205–1216, 1972.

Van der Heul, RO, von Ronnen JR: Juxtacortical osteosarcoma:
     Diagnosis, differential diagnosis, treatment, and an analy-
     sis of 80 cases. J Bone Joint Surg 49A:415–439, 1967.

FIBROSARCOMA

Fibrosarcoma of bone does not produce tumor osteoid or new bone. It is encountered predominantly during adult life in major long bones, especially those of the lower extremity. Since it tends to destroy compact bone of the cortex and to invade adjacent soft tissues, it must be differentiated from fibroblastic tumors (eg, periosteal fibrosarcoma and parosteal sarcoma) that arise extracortically and invade bone. Multicentric lesions have been reported.

The patient complains of pain and swelling. Precise diagnosis depends upon biopsy.

Fibrosarcoma may complicate Paget's disease or fibrous dysplasia, or may occur in bone irradiated many years previously.

Well-differentiated tumors may be treated by local resection. In most cases, however, amputation with or without preliminary irradiation is indicated.

The prognosis is poor, although perhaps better than with osteogenic sarcoma.

Eyre-Brook AL, Price CHG: Fibrosarcoma of bone: Review of
     50 consecutive cases from the Bristol Bone Tumour Regis-
     try. J Bone Joint Surg 51B:20–37, 1969.

CHONDROSARCOMA

Chondrosarcoma of bone is a primary malignant tumor that arises from cartilage. It comprises about 5–10% of all malignant primary bone tumors.

Difficulty occurs in making the histopathologic diagnosis. It requires experience and judgment on the part of the pathologist, especially when radical surgery is contemplated.

The initial symptom may be either pain or swelling, or a combination of both; neither is diagnostic. X-rays show destruction of bone, both the spongiosa and the cortex. Areas of mottled calcification in the osteolytic zone are common. Where the lesion involves the shaft of a tubular bone, the cortex may be thickened and expanded, giving a fusiform configuration. Peripheral chondrosarcoma presents as a mass. Calcification in the tumor mass may have a nebulous, mottled, or occasionally a streak-like appearance. The site of origin of the tumor from the cortex may show evidence of erosion.

Histologic diagnosis must precede radical surgery.

Angiography shows tumor vascularity and may be diagnostic of malignancy. Because of its selective concentration in cartilage, radioactive sulfur has been used for scintigraphy and may be useful in detecting occult metastatic deposits.

Complications include pathologic fracture, recurrence after incomplete surgical removal, and dissemination of viable tumor cells in the wound during biopsy.

Radical removal of the lesion by local excision, segmental resection, or amputation is the treatment of choice.

The tumor grows slowly, with long intervals between recurrence and the appearance of metastases In general, the prognosis of properly treated chondrosarcoma is much more favorable than that of osteogenic sarcoma.

Henderson ED, Dahlin DC: Chondrosarcoma of bone: A study
     of 288 cases. J Bone Joint Surg 45A:1450–1458, 1963.
Marcove RC & others: Chondrosarcoma of the pelvis and upper
     end of the femur: An analysis of factors influencing sur-
     vival time in one hundred and thirteen cases. J Bone Joint
     Surg 54A:561–572, 1972.

RETICULUM CELL SARCOMA

Reticulum cell sarcoma is a rare malignant tumor comprising less than 5% of primary bone tumors. It may originate either in the medullary cavity of tubular bones or from cancellous bone in any location but is encountered most frequently in the major long bones of the lower extremity.

Pain is frequently mild and may be of many months' duration; it may be referred to an adjacent joint, especially when the lesion is in the metaphysis of a long bone.

Special examinations which may be helpful are angiography to demonstrate soft tissue extension and the characteristic vascular pattern of malignant bone disease. Bone scans may be of diagnostic value.

Pathologic fracture is common and may be the initial manifestation of the disease.

Reticulum cell sarcoma must be differentiated from Ewing's sarcoma, which it mimics in many respects.

Since the tumor is highly radiosensitive, x-ray is usually the best treatment, especially for lesions of the pelvis and spine. Surgery is reserved for control of local disease of the extremities.

Important factors in the prognosis are the location of the primary tumor, the extent of the lesion, and the stage of development. Metastasis is likely to occur to adjacent lymph nodes before the lungs.

Shoji H, Miller TR: Reticulum cell sarcoma of bone. Cancer
     28:1234–1244, 1971.
Wang CC, Fleischli DJ: Primary reticulum cell sarcoma of bone.
     Cancer 22:994–998, 1968.

METASTATIC TUMORS TO BONE

Most malignant tumors of bone are metastases from an extraskeletal primary, usually an epithelial tumor. Occasionally, a primary bone tumor will metastasize to bone (eg, Ewing's sarcoma).

Pain and swelling are the initial complaints. Pathologic fracture may be the first manifestation in some cases. Elevation of the serum alkaline phosphatase may be associated with widespread metastatic lesions of bone, especially those that are osteoblastic. Biopsy and x-rays are the principal diagnostic tests. The early changes may be quite subtle and can be overlooked unless the x-rays are of superior quality. Laminagraphy, arteriography, and intraosseous phlebography (osteography) may demonstrate lesions inapparent by conventional technics. Radioisotope scanning may reveal metastatic foci in the skeleton before they can be demonstrated by x-ray.

If the osseous focus is amenable to irradiation, chemotherapy, or hormonal therapy, such treatment is indicated, especially when progressive enlargement of the lesion causes pain or predisposes to fracture. In general, if life expectancy is longer than a few weeks, definitive treatment should be undertaken for pathologic fractures.

Legge DA & others: Radioisotope scanning of metastatic lesions of bone. Mayo Clin Proc 45:755–761, 1970.
Parrish FF, Murray JA: Surgical treatment for secondary neoplastic fractures. J Bone Joint Surg 52A:665–686, 1970.

INJURIES TO THE SPINE

Traumatic injuries to the spine may vary from comparatively minor soft tissue injuries such as contusions, muscle strains, and sprains to severe fracture-dislocations with extensive neurologic impairment. Disease of the spine (eg, osteoarthritis) that existed before the traumatic injury may modify signs and symptoms and adversely affect the prognosis.

These injuries commonly result from indirect violence such as hyperextension or hyperflexion. They may also be caused by axial compression (eg, a blow on the top of the head) or by lateral flexion, torsion, or shearing, either singly or in combination. Blunt trauma is more likely to fracture a spinous process, rarely the lamina, and occasionally a transverse process in the lumbar region. Open fractures are usually due to penetrating injuries.

In most cases of injury to the spine, neither the spinal cord nor the nerve root is injured, but the possibility of such injury, especially in the cervical region, is always present. The greatest permanent disability caused by injury to the spine is due to associated injury to the spinal cord or the spinal nerves. Injury to the cord or nerves may result from displaced bone fragments, portions of the intervertebral disk, or segment of an intact but dislocated vertebra. Neurologic injury may be caused by the initial accident or may be the result of subsequent manipulation. Initial x-rays do not necessarily reflect the degree of displacement which may have occurred. Severe neurologic deficit may be present even though only minor fracture or minimal subluxation—or neither—can be demonstrated.

Concomitant injury at multiple levels of the spine may occur as the result of severe trauma. Because of its more dramatic clinical findings, a major injury, especially when it is proximal, may mask a lesser one even in the conscious patient. In addition to physical examination, survey x-rays of the entire spine may be warranted in the unconscious patient.

Careful inquiry should be made concerning any period of unconsciousness which may require interpretation of the mechanism of a spinal injury. A precise history of the time of onset of motor or sensory deficit can provide information of prognostic value.

The physical examination must be complete. Superficial soft tissue lesions such as abrasions, contusions, and lacerations may indicate the direction of applied force and its comparative magnitude. Tenderness may suggest the location of a deep lesion. Palpation may reveal an abnormal prominence suggesting a compression fracture of the body, or an abnormal separation of adjacent processes may indicate tearing of posterior ligaments with dislocation.

A record of the neurologic examination must be kept beginning as soon after injury as possible. A clear distinction must be drawn between damage to the spinal cord and to the nerve roots and the time of onset of paraplegia or quadriplegia—whether immediate or delayed—must be noted.

The comparative anatomic level in the spine of neurologic interruption may be determined by x-rays. Comparison of the x-ray findings with the physical findings—which establish the upper level of the total neurologic lesion—will indicate that part due to cord damage and that due to root damage. Retained muscle or sensory function below the level of the cord lesion during the first 24 hours after injury indicates that it is partial; the presence of reflex activity under similar circumstances indicates that function of the distal segment of the cord is not suppressed by spinal shock, which lasts no longer than 24 hours. The presence of reflex activity within 24 hours after injury or its subsequent return without recovery of any sensation or motor function distal to the level of the cord lesion within 24 hours after injury denotes complete and permanent damage to the cord.

The prevention of decubitus ulcers after spine injury with paraplegia or quadriplegia requires stabilization of the injured skeletal segment to permit turning the patient every 2 hours. This can be accomplished by a combination of padded plaster shells, half of which can be removed for proper skin care, and a turning frame. In this way, encircling plaster casts are

TABLE 46–1. Trauma to cervical spine.

Disorder and Mechanism	Common Symptoms	Common Signs	Neurologic Findings	Radiologic Findings
Sprain of cervical spine due to sudden movement of neck	Dull aching pain in neck radiating to adjacent areas. Stiffness. Relieved by immobility.	Stiffness with symmetric limitation of movement. Diffuse tenderness.	No objective findings.	None.
Dislocations				
Forward bilateral dislocation due to forced flexion with rotation	Localized tenderness posteriorly. Discomfort increased on extension if facets locked.	Head held in slight flexion without tilting.	Neurologic deficits most marked on complete dislocation and may be severe. Incomplete subluxation may have no cord symptoms.	Oblique views and stereoroentgenography needed to detect locked facets.
Unilateral dislocation due to forward flexion with marked rotation	May be only slight pain.	Head in slight flexion with head tilted toward lesion and chin rotated to opposite side. Tenderness over site of dislocation.	Asymmetric and noted on side of displacement.	Upper articular process displaced forward. Body of vertebra displaced forward less than half its depth. Spinous process rotated to side of dislocation.
Unilateral subluxation due to minimal injury; can occur in sleep	Slight discomfort on neck movements.	Head tilted away from side of subluxation and held immobile. Resistance to movements to affected side.	None.	Dislocation may show on lateral stereoroentgenograms.
Atlantoaxial dislocation (traumatic; after URI in children and in arthritis)	Pain is mild to severe. Tenderness is suboccipital.	Head rotated from affected side and tilted toward it in unilateral subluxation. In bilateral, head is flexed and chin down. Movements restricted.	Can be severe in traumatic type and may cause instant death. Variable in other forms.	Subluxation (incomplete dislocation) will show on lateral stereoroentgenograms.
Extension dislocation due to forced extension with rotation	Pain on head or neck movement.	Head held rigidly. Position depends on presence of dislocation.	Incomplete or extensive cord lesions.	Widening of space of involved disk. Dislocation may or may not be present.
Fractures				
Fracture of atlas due to severe blow to top of head	Pain in suboccipital region. Headache.	Restriction of neck movements.	Usually none.	Fracture clefts seen on special views.
Fracture of odontoid process due to complex stresses and shearing force	Suboccipital pain, headache. May have associated injuries of accident.	Severe restriction of movement.	No neurologic lesion in undisplaced fracture.	Fracture observed usually on standard films; laminagrams may be needed.
Compression fracture of vertebral body due to blow to head	Localized pain.	Restriction of movement.	Usually none unless dislocation occurs.	Wedge-shaped deformity seen in lateral x-rays. Dislocation may occur or may have reduced spontaneously.

TABLE 46–1 (cont'd). Trauma to cervical spine.

Disorder and Mechanism	Common Symptoms	Common Signs	Neurologic Findings	Radiologic Findings
Comminuted fracture of vertebral body due to severe blow on head	Localized pain and headache. Unconsciousness.	Severe restriction of movement.	High incidence of neurologic complications.	X-ray shows fragmented body of vertebra. Postero-inferior fragment may be driven into spinal canal.
Fracture of spinous process due to severe flexion (avulsion) or severe extension	Pain in back of neck; localized tenderness.	Restriction and guarding of movements.	None.	Lateral views usually show fracture, but oblique views may be needed.
Fracture of odontoid process of axis and dislocation of atlas due to severe complex forces	Suboccipital pain, headache. May be associated injuries.	Severe restriction of movement.	May have some neurologic findings.	Fracture usually observed in standard films. Special views or technics may be needed.
Fracture-dislocation of axis (rare)	Suboccipital pain.	Restriction of movement.	Usually none.	Dislocation of axis seen on roentgenograms.
Compression fracture of vertebral body with dislocation.	Localized pain.	Restriction of movement.	Neurologic complications may occur.	Standard x-rays usually show fracture and displacement.
Lateral flexion fracture-dislocation	Unilateral localized pain.	Restriction of motion with head tilted toward lesion.	Asymmetric lesions of cord or brachial plexus.	Oblique views needed to show facet subluxation. Other technics may be needed.

avoided.

Injuries of the spine are discussed here according to regional location because the extent of any neurologic deficit resulting from spinal cord or nerve injury depends in part upon the level at which injury occurs.

Holdsworth F: Fractures, dislocations, and fracture-dislocation of the spine. J Bone Joint Surg 45B:6–20, 1963.

SPRAIN OF THE CERVICAL SPINE

Indirect injury of the cervical spine that does not cause fracture or dislocation or objective neurologic disturbance may involve only the muscles and supporting soft tissues of joints; such injuries are considered here. When the extremes of the accustomed range of movements of the cervical spine are exceeded suddenly, the resulting sprain of joints or strain of neck muscles can be manifested predominantly by subjective symptoms. "Whiplash" is a term used to describe a mechanism of injury—sudden hyperflexion followed by extension recoil—that causes a variety of lesions of the cervical region. The term has been construed—especially by the laity—to denote a nonspecific post-traumatic cervical syndrome consequent to motor vehicle accidents. Accidents involving motor vehicles account for most of these injuries; a lesser number are due to sports mishaps.

The diagnosis of sprain of the cervical spine is based upon critical differentiation of this condition from structural lesions of bones and joints that can be demonstrated by x-ray and from lesions of the brain, spinal cord, and nerve roots that produce objective findings. A detailed history of the accident is necessary to assess the significance of certain symptoms. A period of unconsciousness or transitory amnesia immediately after the accident and the presence of other more serious injuries may cause temporary disregard of less dramatic complaints or findings related to the neck. When motor vehicles are involved, an indirect index of severity of injury to the neck region may be suggested by the extent of injury to other parts of the body and by an estimate of the degree of structural damage to the vehicle.

Clinical Findings

A. Symptoms and Signs: The onset of symptoms may be immediate or late. Delayed onset is more often associated with minor injury. The principal clinical feature is dull, aching pain vaguely distributed to the back of the neck and the trapezius regions; it may radiate into the occipital or interscapular region or down the arm. The pain is accentuated by neck movement, and a sensation of stiffness is common; both are relieved by immobility. Radiation of pain to a dermatome supplied by a cervical root should alert the examiner to the possible presence of a lesion involving the respective anatomic segment of the spine. Similar distribution of paresthesia, especially when accompanied by other sensory disturbances such as hypesthesia or hypalgesia, increases the likelihood that a focal lesion is present. Occipital or frontal headache is a frequent complaint. Persistent headache requires investigation of sources other than the neck. Difficulty in swallowing has been attributed to edema of the pharynx, but this indicates a more serious condition than a cervical spine. Continuing ocular symptoms such as blurring of vision or diplopia require investigation by an ophthalmologist. Dizziness and tinnitus suggesting vestibular and auditory dysfunction of the eighth cranial nerve are frequent complaints. Posttraumatic vertigo has been attributed to transient ischemia due to vertebral artery injury and to hemorrhage in the labyrinth. When these complaints persist, their assessment requires diagnostic technics such as electroencephalography and vestibular and auditory testing. Functional complaints such as anxiety, inability to concentrate, loss of memory, depression, sweating, and coldness of the extremities are likely to persist in the emotionally labile patient. There is a greater frequency of prolonged complaints following rear-end automobile collisions in comparison with those following front-end collisions.

Physical findings require critical evaluation. Restriction of active neck motion is likely to be symmetric and to involve all components. Persistent asymmetric limitation of motion suggests the possibility of fracture or dislocation. Symmetric limitation may be due to unconscious muscle guarding or conscious inhibition. Bizarrely performed active neck movements through a near-average range in all directions and accompanied by theatrical grimacing suggests malingering. Tenderness, like pain, is frequently diffuse, and the site is poorly defined during sequential examinations. Persistent, localized tenderness may identify the site of an occult fracture or joint derangement. Muscle spasm as determined by palpation is difficult to perceive and quantitate because it is commonly associated with diffuse deep tenderness.

B. X-Ray Examination: X-ray examination of the cervical spine must be thorough because differentiation of sprain from other lesions discussed below may depend entirely upon the reliability of this study. In addition to the routine projections, which include lateral views in flexion and extension, laminagraphy and cineradiography may help to differentiate sprain

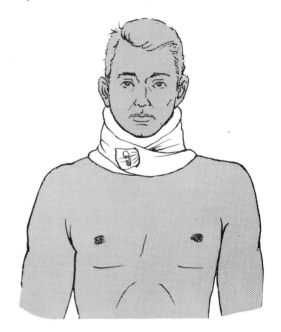

FIG 46–4. Cervical collar.

from fracture or dislocation. Myelography can demonstrate intervertebral disk derangements. Patients with osteoarthritis which antedated the injury may exhibit restriction of motion in the lower cervical segments when the involved joint is more proximal.

Treatment

Immobilization may be accomplished by external cervical support such as a felt collar (Fig 46–4) or by recumbency at bed rest; light cervical traction by means of a head halter can give further relief from discomfort. Analgesics and sedatives for apprehensive patients generally suffice for relief of mild pain. Some observers find that muscle relaxants are helpful. A persistent localized area of pain and tenderness may respond favorably to local anesthetic injections. The application of heat or cold may give temporary relief from pain.

Prognosis

Where litigation or emotional lability is not a factor, symptoms generally respond promptly to conservative measures. Younger patients can be expected to become asymptomatic more rapidly than older ones with osteoarthritis.

Breck LW & others: Medicolegal aspects of cervical spine sprains. Clin Orthop 74:124–128, 1971.

Burke DC: Hyperextension injuries of the spine. J Bone Joint Surg 53B:3–12, 1971.

Janes JM, Hooshmand H: Extension-flexion injury of the neck. Mayo Clin Proc 40:353–369, 1965.

Pang LQ: The otological aspects of whiplash injuries. Laryngoscope 81:1331–1387, 1971.

Williams JS & others: The nature of seat belt injuries. J Trauma 11:207–218, 1971.

DISLOCATIONS, FRACTURES, & FRACTURE-DISLOCATIONS OF THE CERVICAL REGION

Dislocations, fractures, and fracture-dislocations of the cervical spine comprise fewer than 1% of all cervical spine injuries and about 15% of all spine injuries. Concomitant injury to the cord and nerve roots can be expected in about 25% of severe injuries to the cervical spine. Injuries that reduce the diameter of the spinal canal account for most instances of lesions of the cord or nerve roots. Any neck injury severe enough to cause these lesions also involves the possibility of neurologic damage, and this hazard exists from the moment of the accident until any displacement of anatomic structures has been corrected and permanent stability provided. Extensive damage to the cord may be present without x-ray evidence of fracture or dislocation, and, conversely, dramatic skeletal injury may be present without neurologic deficit.

The diagnosis is suggested by the history and confirmed by physical examination and x-ray studies. Accurate diagnosis of the extent of skeletal and neurologic injury is essential to treatment, which should be started as soon as possible. In addition to the general examination, the patient with neurologic deficit must be evaluated within the first 24 hours to differentiate between complete and partial spinal cord injury.

The fourth cervical cord segment is situated at about the level of the body of the third cervical vertebra. Therefore, a complete lesion at this site or at a more proximal point causes death by respiratory paralysis. An incomplete lesion may be identified by spared perianal sensation and the presence of any voluntary action of the toe flexors. Permanent and complete division of the distal cord segment from the proximal segment can be assumed if these minimal findings are not present within 24 hours after injury. Some improvement of motor, sensory, and reflex function can be anticipated if findings of cord sparing are exhibited within 24 hours after injury. Spinal cord sparing must be distinguished from recovery of function temporarily lost because of root injury. Voluntary bowel and bladder control may be recovered in partial cord lesions when motor and sensory function of the sacral segments is retained. Reflex automatic bowel and bladder function may be recovered after complete cord lesions when anal and bulbocavernosus reflex activity is preserved.

Other mechanisms of injury and other lesions may also cause spinal cord disruption. Forced flexion can cause retropulsion of the nucleus pulposus even though compression fracture of the body or complete dislocation does not occur. This mechanism may cause serious cord damage when associated with minor wedge-shaped compression fracture of the body. Forced extension with or without dislocation may also cause cord damage.

Partial loss of cord function may occur as a result of contusion injuries to the cervical spine without apparent alteration of bony alignment. When this occurs, damage to the posterior columns and the lateral spinothalamic tracts may be either transient or permanent, and the resulting impairment of motor function is greater in the upper extremities than in the lower. Bladder dysfunction and varying degrees of sensory loss below the level of the lesion can also be present. Return of bladder function follows motor recovery in the lower extremities, and both precede return of muscle function in the upper extremities. Sensory deficit varies from minor to complete and immediate loss, and recovery does not follow any predictable pattern. Vascular insufficiency caused by compression of the vertebral arteries may be an indirect mechanism of damage to the cord which may account for the minimal or absent sensory impairment observed in some patients.

Radiologic Examination

The surgeon should supervise transfer of the patient to the x-ray table for the preliminary examination. Further injury may be avoided by temporary stabilization with an adjustable brace or by light traction applied manually with a head halter. Initial anteroposterior and lateral films of the entire cervical and upper thoracic spines should be taken to determine whether any extensive skeletal lesion is present. If so, the configuration of the fracture, the extent and direction of displacement of bone fragments, and the presence of dislocation will dictate whether to initiate skeletal traction before further manipulation to accomplish definitive x-ray studies. Routine studies should include films prepared in both oblique projections and open-mouth odontoid views. When these studies do not adequately demonstrate suspected lesions, special technics such as laminagraphy and cineradiography may be helpful. Myelography is useful to localize obstruction of the spinal canal and to differentiate complete from incomplete blockage. When evidence of neurologic deficit is lacking and dislocation is not apparent, films may be prepared in the lateral projection with actively assisted but limited flexion and extension to determine whether gross instability exists.

Treatment

A prime objective of treatment is to protect the spinal cord, spinal nerves, and vertebral arteries during transportation of the patient, during diagnostic and x-ray procedures, and throughout definitive treatment.

A. Emergency Treatment: Initially, the patient can be transported on a flat surface in the supine decubitus position with bolsters at the side of the head and neck to prevent rotation. When medical help becomes available, a head halter with 3–4 kg of force directed axially to the spine while maintaining the head in anatomic posture can be substituted for the bolsters.

B. Definitive Treatment: Although the head halter is useful for the application of heavy traction for short periods, it is not suitable for continuous traction because more than 3–4 kg of force causes pain in the regions of the chin and occiput. When halter traction is used continuously for prolonged periods, even with light loads, the submental region and the occiput should be carefully padded to prevent pressure necrosis of skin and ulceration. Skeletal traction applied to the cranial vault or the zygomatic arches will support as much as 30 kg of force over prolonged periods without causing significant discomfort. To effect closed reduction after application of a skeletal traction apparatus, the initial force of 5–8 kg is gradually increased by increments of 2.5 kg every 30 minutes with the patient awake and with periodic physical examination and x-ray control. Gentle and limited manipulation of the head during this critical period may be necessary to facilitate reduction. Once this has been accomplished, the force is gradually reduced to 4–5 kg, which is usually sufficient to maintain reduction.

Closed reduction by manipulation with concomitant skull traction under general anesthesia can be effective in the hands of experts. Heavy manual traction and forceful manipulation, with or without general anesthesia, are hazardous to the spinal cord and nerves.

Specific Treatment of Various Lesions

A. **Dislocations of the Cervical Spine:** Although the physical examination and understanding of the mechanism of injury are important in diagnosis, the x-ray examination is the most important part of the evaluation of injuries to the cervical spine. Only after an accurate x-ray diagnosis has been established can proper treatment be instituted.

1. **Forward dislocation of the cervical spine**–(Fig 46–5.)

a. **Bilateral complete dislocation**–Treatment of bilateral complete dislocation is directed toward reduction of the dislocation and stabilization of the injured vertebrae to prevent redislocation. Locked facets may be difficult to reduce even with the aid of skeletal traction, and reduction may be impossible even with the aid of general anesthesia. This is especially true when 2–4 weeks have elapsed since the injury. Immediate strong axial traction or traction in extension may firm the locking mechanism. When neurologic deficit is present–and especially when a spinal cord lesion is incomplete–reduction must be done promptly to prevent further damage. With the patient awake, reduction is attempted with skeletal traction and judicious manipulation. With the aid of frequent x-ray examination in the lateral projection, 2–2.5 kg of force are exerted in such a way as to cause slight flexion. When the locked facets are freed, visible lengthening of the neck may be apparent or unlocking may be observed on x-ray. The traction is then gradually increased by adding weights periodically until both facets are minimally distracted. Reduction can then be completed by extending the neck to the neutral position. Traction should then be gradually reduced to 2.5–3 kg.

If reduction by the foregoing technics is not successful, closed reduction under general anesthesia may be resorted to by the expert. Some authorities believe that open reduction is less hazardous.

Further treatment after closed reduction is controversial. Ligaments heal slowly and may not provide adequate stability because redislocation or subluxation can occur, especially when traction or external immobilization is discontinued early. Early arthrodesis by either the anterior or posterior approach has been advocated, especially when quadriplegia is present, because the period of traction is shortened, some problems of nursing care are made easier, and rehabilitation is expedited. A reasonable program for those patients who do not have extensive neurologic damage is a period of 6 weeks in skull traction followed by 6–10 weeks in a Minerva jacket (Fig 46–6) or a carefully fitted plastic collar. Dislocations of more than 4 weeks' duration should be treated by open reduction, recognizing that open reduction is hazardous to the spinal cord. If pain is a disabling factor in old unreduced dislocation, fusion in the position of deformity is safest.

b. **Bilateral incomplete dislocation (subluxation)**–Bilateral incomplete dislocation may accompany wedge-shaped compression fracture of a cervical vertebra or may occur alone. Neurologic damage is not likely, and, when it occurs, other accompanying lesions should be sought to explain the neurologic lesion. Uncomplicated bilateral subluxation can be treated by gentle manual traction with the patient awake, letting the head extend over the mattress so that its weight will provide the traction force, or by halter traction with 2.5–3 kg of force. The neck should be stabilized afterward with a felt collar for 2–3 weeks. Resubluxa-

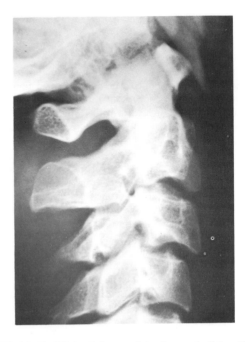

FIG 46–5. Bilateral incomplete forward dislocation of the third on the fourth cervical vertebra in a 19-year-old man. There were no neurologic symptoms.

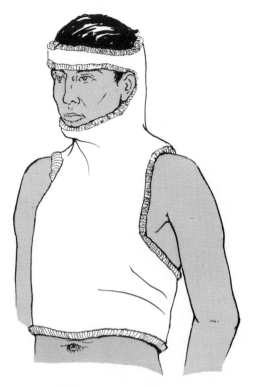

FIG 46—6. Minerva jacket.

tion may occur.

2. Unilateral dislocation of the cervical spine—
Reduction may be accomplished by skeletal traction with the patient awake as described for complete dislocation. While traction is applied, the head is tilted to the side opposite the dislocation. When unlocking has been accomplished, the head is rotated toward the side of the lesion. Open reduction is indicated early when closed reduction is unsuccessful and painful radicular symptoms exist or progressive cord deficit cannot be attributed to reasons other than dislocation. This lesion is mechanically stable and is not likely to displace further when unreduced.

Continued root symptoms associated with dislocation of more than 2—4 weeks' duration may respond to foraminotomy or fusion of the involved vertebras.

3. Unilateral subluxation of the cervical spine—
Reduction can usually be accomplished by gentle manual traction or by a head halter using 2.5—3 kg force for 12—24 hours. The neck should be stabilized and protected by a felt collar for 10—14 days afterward or until discomfort and restriction of movement disappear. Recurrence of subluxation must be ruled out if symptoms persist.

4. Atlantoaxial dislocation—

a. Pathologic atlantoaxial subluxation in children—Treatment consists of reduction of the displacement and stabilization of the cervical spine until healing is sound. Manipulative reduction by the Walton maneuver is hazardous except in experienced hands. Reduction may be accomplished in younger children by letting the head hang or by head halter traction with 1.5—3 kg of force in older children. In acute cases, reduction is likely to occur within 24—72 hours. The neck should then be supported by a felt collar, brace, or Minerva plaster jacket until flexion and extension x-rays in the lateral projection demonstrate that stability has been recovered. The period of protection may be a few weeks.

b. Pathologic atlantoaxial subluxation in arthritis—In the early stages, treatment can be by external cervical support. Subsequent observation may show that the condition has become stabilized. If signs of neurologic deficit are present or if x-rays show progressive displacement, treatment should be aggressive. It is directed toward maximal reduction of displacement and stabilization by spine fusion of the involved segments. The patient should be observed periodically after spine fusion because displacement may occur at the level distal to the arthrodesis.

5. Extension dislocation of the cervical spine—
This lesion is stable when the cervical spine is in slight flexion and can be treated effectively by external support and care of any neurologic complication.

B. Fractures of the Cervical Spine:

1. Fracture of the atlas—Treatment of isolated, undisplaced fracture can be by external cervical support by means of a surgical collar or bracing. Fractures complicated by displacement of the condyles or those associated with fracture of the axis require a preliminary period of traction to regain stability before resorting to external support.

2. Fracture of the axis—

a. Fracture of the odontoid process—For undisplaced fractures without neurologic complications, traction provides adequate stabilization and should be continued for 6 weeks. Subsequent support can be provided by a Minerva plaster jacket for an additional 10 weeks or more. Periodic x-rays are necessary to determine whether displacement has recurred. Some authorities believe that fibrous healing of the fracture or persisting pseudarthrosis is not acceptable in a patient who expects to lead an active life; this attitude becomes an indication for arthrodesis of the first and second cervical vertebrae. Fracture of the odontoid process with dislocation of the atlantoaxial articulation is discussed below.

3. Compression fracture of the vertebral body—
Deformity is not significant, and no attempt at reduction should be made. Treatment is nonoperative and depends initially upon the severity of pain. When pain is marked, bed rest with head halter traction and analgesics for a few days is apt to suffice. As soon as symptoms warrant, the patient can be mobilized with external cervical support in the form of a metal brace or surgical collar. Sound healing can be expected within 8—12 weeks. Overtreatment by prolonged external support is to be avoided.

4. Comminuted fracture of the cervical vertebral body—The most important aspect of treatment is that provided for complicating neurologic injury. Because the ligaments are intact, the fracture is essentially

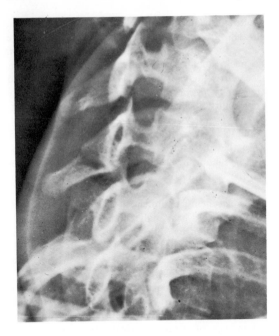

FIG 46—7. Avulsion fracture of the spinous process of the first thoracic vertebra in a 21-year-old woman caused by a rear-end automobile collision.

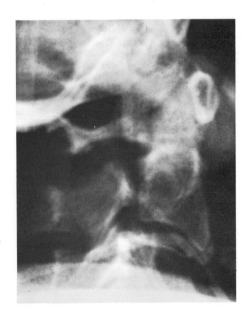

FIG 46—8. Bilateral fracture of the lateral masses of the axis with forward dislocation of the body section in a 61-year-old man.

stable and can be treated adequately by skull traction for 4—8 weeks while initial bone healing takes place. When neurologic damage does not occur, subsequent treatment can be by external support with a Minerva jacket or a plastic collar until healing is sound, which often takes more than 16 weeks.

5. Fracture of the spinous processes—(Fig 46—7.) Treatment is symptomatic. Failure of bony healing is not likely to cause persistent symptoms, and excision of the unhealed distal fragment is seldom warranted.

C. Fracture-Dislocations of the Cervical Spine:

1. Fracture of the odontoid process of the axis and dislocation of the atlas—Reduction can generally be accomplished by skull traction, which should be used for 6—8 weeks. Plaster immobilization afterward must be maintained for at least another 10 weeks because healing of the odontoid process is slow. Bony healing may not take place in spite of prolonged immobilization. Operative fusion of the atlas to the axis may be necessary to prevent redisplacement, with the hazard of injury to the spinal cord.

2. Fracture-dislocation of the axis—(Fig 46—8.) Bilateral fracture of the lateral mass of the axis in the coronal plane with dislocation of its body forward on the third cervical vertebra occurs rarely. A similar lesion has been observed elsewhere in the spine, notably at the lumbosacral level, and some authors prefer to use the designation traumatic spondylolisthesis. The advisability of traction in the treatment of this lesion has been questioned, and some surgeons have performed early operative fusion. Others have preferred closed treatment early and have reserved spine fusion

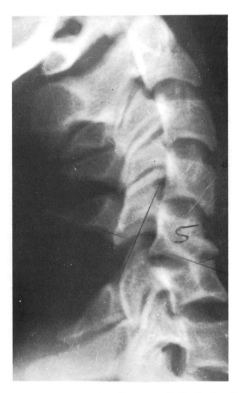

FIG 46—9. Compression fracture of the body of the sixth cervical vertebra with incomplete forward dislocation 4 months after injury in a 17-year-old girl. Neurologic symptoms in the left arm and leg were transient. Spontaneous fusion between the bodies is occurring.

for those cases where instability of the spine persists.

3. Compression fracture of the vertebral body with dislocation—(Fig 46—9.) Because of impaction of the bone fragments, fracture healing is not a problem. Treatment is directed to the accompanying dislocation (see above).

4. Lateral flexion fracture-dislocation—Injury to the brachial plexus may not be detected initially. Treatment by traction may be harmful, and external support by a cervical collar is recommended.

Dislocations of Cervical Spine

Barnes R: Paraplegia in cervical spine injuries. J Bone Joint Surg 30B:234—244, 1948.

Beatson TR: Fractures and dislocations of the cervical spine. J Bone Joint Surg 45B:21—35, 1963.

Braakman R, Vinken PJ: Unilateral facet interlocking in the lower cervical spine. J Bone Joint Surg 49B:249—257, 1967.

Burke DC: Hyperextension injuries of the spine. J Bone Joint Surg 53B:3—12, 1971.

Burke DC, Berryman D: The place of closed manipulation in the management of flexion-rotation dislocations of the cervical spine. J Bone Joint Surg 53B:165—182, 1972.

Evans DK: Reduction of cervical dislocations. J Bone Joint Surg 43B:552—555, 1961.

Holdsworth F: Fractures, dislocations, and fracture-dislocations of the spine. J Bone Joint Surg 52A:1534—1551, 1970.

Hollin SA & others: Management of cervical spine dislocations with locked facets. Surg Gynec Obst 124:521—524, 1967.

McKeever FM: Atlanto-axoid instability. S Clin North America 48:1375—1390, 1968.

Roaf R: A study of the mechanics of spinal injuries. J Bone Joint Surg 42B:810—823, 1960.

Rodgers WA: Fractures and dislocations of the cervical spine. An end-result study. J Bone Joint Surg 39A:341—376, 1957.

Schneider RC: Cervical traction, with evaluation of methods, and treatment of complications. Surg Gynec Obst 104:521—530, 1957.

Schneider RC, Schemm GW: Vertebral artery insufficiency in acute and chronic spinal trauma. J Neurosurg 18:348—360, 1961.

Stauffer ES & others: Diagnosis and prognosis of acute cervical spinal cord injury. J Bone Joint Surg 53A:1242, 1971.

Taylor AR: The mechanism of injury to the spinal cord in the neck without damage to the vertebral column. J Bone Joint Surg 33B:543—547, 1951.

Taylor AR, Blackwood W: Paraplegia in hyperextension cervical injuries with normal radiographic appearances. J Bone Joint Surg 30B:245—248, 1948.

Willard DeFP, Nicholson JT: Dislocation of the first cervical vertebra. Ann Surg 113:464—475, 1941.

Fractures of Cervical Spine

Ewald FC: Fracture of the odontoid process in a seventeen-month-old infant treated with a halo. J Bone Joint Surg 53A:1636—1640, 1971.

Holdsworth F: Fractures, dislocations, and fracture-dislocations of the spine. J Bone Joint Surg 52A:1534—1551, 1970.

Jefferson G: Fracture of the atlas vertebra. Brit J Surg 6:407—422, 1920.

Jefferson G: Remarks on fractures of first cervical vertebra. Brit MJ 2:153—157, 1927.

Schatzker J & others: Fractures of the dens (odontoid process). J Bone Joint Surg 53B:392—405, 1971.

Sherk HH, Nicholson JT: Fractures of the atlas. J Bone Joint Surg 52A:1017—1024, 1970.

Venable, JR & others: Stress fracture of the spinous process. JAMA 190:881—885, 1964.

Weston WJ: Clay shoveler's disease in adolescents (Schmitt's disease). Brit J Radiol 30:378, 1957.

Fracture-Dislocations of Cervical Spine

Blockey NJ, Purser DW: Fractures of the odontoid process of the axis. J Bone Joint Surg 38B:794—817, 1956.

Cornish BL: Traumatic spondylolisthesis of the axis. J Bone Joint Surg 50B:31—43, 1968.

Roaf R: Lateral flexion injuries of the cervical spine. J Bone Joint Surg 45B:36—38, 1963.

Rogers WA: Fractures and dislocations of the cervical spine. J Bone Joint Surg 39A:341—376, 1957.

Schneider RC, Kahn EA: Chronic neurological sequelae of acute trauma to the spine and spinal cord. J Bone Joint Surg 38A:985—997, 1956.

FRACTURES OF THE THORACIC SPINE

The thoracic spine is comparatively stable. Fracture results either from direct violence, which may involve only a spinous process; or indirect violence, which may result in compression of the body of the vertebra. Occasionally an avulsion fracture of the spinous process of the seventh cervical or first thoracic vertebra is caused by muscle activity ("clay shoveler's fracture").

Compression fractures of the thoracic vertebrae are rare in young children and are caused only by severe trauma in older children. In this age group, therefore, unless there is a positive history of severe trauma, a wedge-shaped deformity in the thoracic spine should suggest pathologic fracture. This must not be confused with Calvé's or Scheuermann's disease or deformity due to traumatic fracture.

Minimal (frequently unrecognized) trauma may cause compression fracture of the body of the thoracic vertebrae in adults with osteoporosis. Disability is not great, and reduction is not indicated. If rest in bed for 3—4 days does not relieve the pain, a surgical corset with shoulder restraints or brace (Taylor or Arnold type) may provide comfort and permit early ambulation.

Compression fractures of the thoracic spine caused by severe trauma are characterized by wedge-shaped deformity of the vertebral body. No adequate method has been devised for the reduction of these injuries. However, because of the inherent stability of the thoracic spine, prolonged immobilization is not necessary. In fracture of the upper thoracic region, if immobilization is required for relief of pain, a plaster Minerva jacket may be the only adequate method of external support that will provide relief from pain.

Rotational fracture-dislocations near the thoracolumbar junction and shear fractures of the thoracic spine are commonly associated with paraplegia. Rotational fracture-dislocation is inherently unstable because of extensive rupture of supporting ligaments, fracture of the vertebral body in the transverse plane, and disruption of the articular facet joints by fracture or dislocation. These fractures may or may not be stable, and fusion may be necessary to minimize injury to the cord.

Shear fracture is a term used to describe a fracture-dislocation of the thoracic spine whereby dislocation takes place at or near the intervertebral disk with fracture of the articular processes or the pedicles. Forward displacement takes place in the transverse plane.

Holdsworth F: Fracture, dislocations, and fracture-dislocations of the spine. J Bone Joint Surg 52A:1534–1551, 1970.

Roberts JB, Curtiss PH Jr: Stability of the thoracic and lumbar spine in traumatic paraplegia following fracture or fracture-dislocation. J Bone Joint Surg 52A:1115–1130, 1970.

FRACTURES OF THE LUMBAR SPINE

Uncomplicated Compression Fractures

Compression fractures of the vertebral bodies caused by hyperflexion injury are the most common fractures of the lumbar spine and occur most often near the thoracolumbar junction. The widespread use of seat belts in automobiles has been accompanied by an increasing incidence of fractures that occur near the lumbosacral level as the result of accidents. More than one vertebral body is often involved, but deformity may be greatest in one segment. Acute angulation of the spine caused by a compression deformity of the body of a vertebra may be associated with varying degrees of disruption of the facet joints, from sprain to complete dislocation.

Anteroposterior, lateral, and oblique x-rays are required to demonstrate the characteristic lesions such as wedge-shaped deformity of the body and the presence of dislocation of the facets, comminuted fracture of the body, and fracture of the pedicle. Laminagraphy is a useful adjunctive technic for disclosure of lesions that might not be demonstrated by routine x-ray studies.

Treatment depends upon the age of the patient, the presence of preexisting disease, and the severity of injury. In older patients with preexisting degenerative arthritis where there is mild deformity involving no more than one-fourth of the anterior height of the body of the vertebra, the surgeon may elect not to

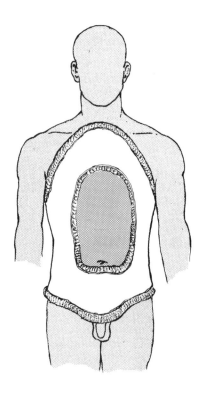
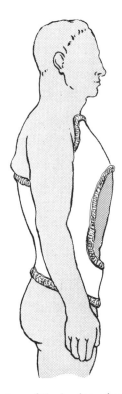

FIG 46–10. Hyperextension plaster for compression fracture of the lumbar spine.

reduce the deformity but merely to place the patient at bed rest for a few days. As soon as acute pain is relievd, the back should be braced and increasing physical activity encouraged within the tolerance of pain. In the more active age group when the compression deformity involves more than one-half of the anterior height of the body of the vertebra, reduction by hyperextension and immobilization in a plaster jacket (Fig 46–10) is the treatment preferred by some surgeons for these uncomplicated fractures.

Comminuted Fractures

Comminuted fracture of the vertebral body is characterized by disruption of the adjacent intervertebral disks and varying degrees of displacement of the fragments. The end plates of the body are forced into the centrum together with the disk. The extent of fragmentation (comminution) of the body depends upon the severity of the causative injury. A large fragment of the body may be displaced anteriorly. Posteriorly displaced fragments are apt to cause compression of the cord or cauda equina; and the facet joints may be fractured or dislocated. Therefore, careful physical and x-ray examinations are mandatory before treatment is instituted.

The method of treatment may be dictated by the extent of bone injury and the presence of neurologic complications. When neurologic involvement is absent and comminution is not manifest by extensive fragmentation, reduction may not be necessary. Under these circumstances, immobilization in a plaster jacket may be sufficient. It must be determined whether dislocation has occurred or is likely because of posterior element injury (see below). Mobilization of the patient from recumbency should be controlled by periodic physical and x-ray examinations to determine incipient displacement of fragments which may herald or accompany the onset of neurologic deficit. When the posterior elements are intact and compression of the body has been greater than one-fourth to one-third its former height, reduction by extension of the spine and immobilization in a plaster jacket should be considered in young adults. When cauda equina injury has occurred, laminectomy may be indicated, in which case spine fusion may also be performed. Bone healing is likely to be slow, and immobilization should be prolonged until stabilization has occurred. Cautiously executed biplane bending x-ray studies give helpful guidance in determining the soundness of healing and the extent to which mechanical stability is restored.

Fracture of the Transverse Processes

Fracture of the transverse processes may result from direct violence, such as a crushing injury, or may be incidental to a more serious fracture of the lumbar spine. It may result also from violent muscle contraction alone. One or more segments may be involved. If displacement is minimal, soft tissue injury is likely to be minor. Extensive displacement of the fragments indicates severe soft tissue tearing and hematoma formation.

Treatment depends upon the presence or absence of associated injuries. If fracture of the transverse process is the sole injury, and if pain is not severe upon guarded motions of the back, strapping and prompt ambulation may be sufficient. If displacement and soft tissue injury are extensive, bed rest for a few days followed by prolonged support in a corset or brace may be necessary and slow symptomatic recovery may be anticipated.

FRACTURE-DISLOCATION OF THE LUMBAR SPINE

Severe compression trauma may cause fracture-dislocation with rupture of one disk or, if comminution occurs, rupture of 2 disks. Varying degrees of injury to the posterior elements occur, including unilateral or bilateral dislocation of the facets or fracture of the pedicles or facets. Accompanying fractures of spinous and transverse processes, and tearing of the posterior ligaments and adjacent muscles can add to the complexity of this severe lesion. The dislocation of the upper segment may be solely in the anteroposterior plane, or it may be complex, with additional displacement in the coronal plane with torsion around the longitudinal axis of the spine.

Treatment depends upon the type of injury. If there is no neurologic involvement and dislocation was associated with fracture of the pedicles or facets, reduction may be attempted by cautious extension with traction on the lower extremities under x-ray control without anesthesia. When dislocation has been corrected, immobilization in a plaster body cast with a spica extension to incorporate at least one thigh may be necessary for adequate support. Mobilization of the patient from the recumbent position should be accomplished slowly because displacement of fragments can occur and neurologic complications may result. When reasonable doubt exists, it is preferred to continue recumbency for 8–12 weeks until initial healing has provided mechanical stability. If closed reduction is not successful, or if extension causes neurologic symptoms, the attempt should be abandoned at once in favor of open reduction.

In complete dislocation of one or both facets, reduction can be accomplished by open operation.

Fletcher BD, Brogden BG: Seat-belt fractures of the spine and sternum. JAMA 200:167–168, 1967.

Holdsworth F: Fractures, dislocations, and fracture-dislocations of the spine. J Bone Joint Surg 52A:1534–1551, 1970.

Peltier LF, Volz RG: Fractures of the dorsolumbar spine uncomplicated by injury of the spinal cord. Surg Gynec Obst 116:205–212, 1963.

Rennie W, Mitchell N: Flexion distraction fractures of the thoracolumbar spine. J Bone Joint Surg 55A:386–390, 1973.

FRACTURE OF THE SACRUM

Fracture of the sacrum may accompany fracture of the pelvis. It may also appear as an isolated lesion as a result of direct violence. Linear fracture of the sacrum without displacement should be treated symptomatically. Strapping of the buttocks of males and the wearing of a snug girdle by females can provide some comfort during the acutely painful stage. If the fracture extends through a sacral foramen and is associated with displacement, there may be injury to 1 of the sacral nerves and consequent neurologic deficit. If the sacral fragment is displaced anteriorly, reduction should be attempted by means of bimanual manipulation. Great care should be exercised to prevent injury to the rectal wall by pressure of the palpating finger against a sharp spicule of underlying bone.

FRACTURE OF THE COCCYX

Fracture of the coccyx is usually the result of a blow on the buttock. No specific treatment is required other than protection. Strapping the buttocks together for a few days may minimize pain. Pressure on the coccygeal region can be avoided by selecting a firm chair in which to sit or placing a support beneath the ghighs to relieve pressure. The patient should be warned that pain may persist for many weeks. Fracture-dislocation can be reduced by bimanual manipulation, but recurrence of the deformity is likely. Every effort toward conservative management should be made before coccygectomy is considered for treatment of the painful unhealed or malunited fracture.

FRACTURES OF THE PELVIS

AVULSION FRACTURES OF THE PELVIS

Avulsion fractures of the pelvis include those involving the anterior superior and anterior inferior iliac spines and the apophysis of the ischium. The ischial apophysis may be avulsed indirectly by violent contraction of the hamstring muscles in the older child or adolescent. If displacement is minimal, prompt healing without disability is to be expected. If displacement is marked (ie, more than 1 cm), reattachment by open operation is justifiable.

FRACTURE OF THE WING OF THE ILIUM

Isolated fracture of the wing of the ilium without involvement of the hip or sacroiliac joints most often occurs as a result of direct trauma. With minor displacement of the free fragment, soft tissue injury is usually minimal and treatment is symptomatic. Wide displacement of the free fragment may be associated with extensive soft tissue injury and hematoma formation. Healing may be accompanied by ossification of the hematoma with exuberant new bone formation.

ISOLATED FRACTURE OF THE OBTURATOR RING

Isolated fracture of the obturator ring, involving either the pubis or ischium with minimal displacement, is associated with little or no injury to the sacroiliac joints. This is also true of minor subluxation of the symphysis pubis. Initial treatment consists of bed rest for a few days followed by ambulation on crutches. A sacroiliac belt or pelvic binder may give additional comfort. As soon as discomfort disappears, unsupported weight-bearing may be permitted.

COMPLEX FRACTURES OF THE PELVIC RING

Complex fractures of the pelvic ring are due either to direct violence or to force transmitted indirectly through the lower extremities. They are characterized by disruption of the pelvic ring at 2 points: (1) anteriorly, near the symphysis pubis, manifested either by dislocation of that joint or by fracture through the body of the pubis, by unilateral or bilateral fracture through the obturator ring, or by fracture through the acetabulum; and (2) disruption of the pelvic ring through or in the vicinity of the sacroiliac joint. The disruption can extend partially through the sacroiliac joint as a dislocation and extend into the sacrum or into the adjacent ilium as a fracture. The magnitude of displacement of the fragments may indicate the severity of soft tissue injury. These complex injuries are often associated with extensive hemorrhage into the soft tissues or injury to the bladder, urethra, or intra-abdominal organs. When anterior and posterior disruptions are ipsilateral, the entire involved hemipelvis and extremity may be displaced proximally. Anterior disruption may occur on one side, and posterior disruption on the opposite side with wide opening of the pelvic ring.

When severe and complex fractures of the pelvic ring are suspected, the extent of associated injuries must be determined at once by physical and x-ray examination. Shock due to blood loss may be present. Treatment of the fracture by reduction should not be instituted until the extent of associated injuries has been determined. Treatment of some of those injuries may be more urgent than that of the fracture lesion. A careful search must be made for possible injury to bowel, bladder, ureters, and major blood vessels (see Chapter 44).

If displacement and soft tissue injury are minimal, a pelvic sling to facilitate nursing care may be all that is required. When the hemipelvis has been displaced proximally, skeletal traction on the distal end of the femur on the affected side with suspension of the extremity may permit reduction.

If the sacroiliac joint has been dislocated and the ilium is rotated posterior to the sacrum, with opening of the anterior fracture, closed reduction can be attempted. Postmanipulation maintenance of reduction is accomplished by a pelvic sling or a short bilateral thigh spica.

INJURIES OF THE SHOULDER GIRDLE

FRACTURE OF THE CLAVICLE

Fracture of the clavicle may occur as a result of direct trauma or indirect force transmitted through the shoulder. Most fractures of the clavicle are seen in the distal half, commonly at the junction of the middle and distal thirds. About two-thirds of clavicular fractures occur in children. Birth fractures of the clavicle vary from greenstick to complete displacement.

Because of the relative fixation of the medial fragment and the weight of the arm, the distal fragment is displaced downward and toward the midline. Anteroposterior x-rays should always be taken, but oblique projections are occasionally of more value. Although injury to the brachial plexus or subclavian vessels is not common, such complications can usually be demonstrated on physical examination.

Treatment

Fracture of the outer third of the clavicle distal to the coracoclavicular ligaments is comparable to dislocation of the acromioclavicular joint. If the coracoclavicular ligaments are intact and the fragments are not widely displaced, immobilization in a sling and swathe is adequate. If the coracoclavicular ligaments have been lacerated and extensive displacement of the main medial fragment is present, treatment is similar to that advocated for acromioclavicular dislocation.

A. Without Displacement: Immobilization of greenstick fractures is not required in children, and healing is rapid. Complete fractures should be immobilized for 10–21 days. A figure-of-eight dressing made of sheet cotton and an elastic bandage is adequate (Fig 46–11). In adolescents and adults, treatment is by immobilization in a sling and swathe for 4–6 weeks.

B. With Displacement: In infants and small children, apply a figure-of-eight dressing of sheet cotton and elastic bandage reinforced with adhesive tape. Healing usually takes 2–4 weeks. Older children and adolescents require reduction by closed manipulation and immobilization with a figure-of-eight dressing reinforced with plaster. Reduction need not be exact, since exuberant callus formation will be partially or completely obliterated by remodeling of bone architecture incidental to the late stage of the fracture reparative process.

C. With Displacement or Comminution (in Adults):

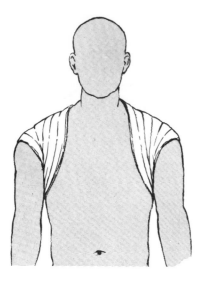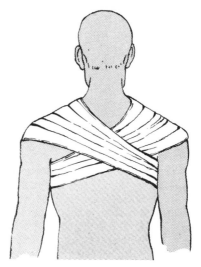

FIG 46–11. Figure-of-eight dressing.

1. Closed reduction—Comminuted fractures of the clavicle with displacement can usually be managed successfully by closed reduction, although in women greater effort must be made to secure accurate realignment without deformity. A plaster shoulder spica (Fig 46–12) gives more secure immobilization than the figure-of-eight dressing. Immobilization must be maintained for 6–12 weeks. The patient should remain ambulatory if possible, but in some cases the position of the fragments requires bed rest initially, with skin traction applied to the abducted upper arm and a sandbag between the shoulders to permit the distal fragment to fall into position and to aid in maintaining reduction. Recumbency in this position may be necessary for 5–6 weeks or even longer until stabilization has occurred.

2. Open reduction—Open reduction may be justifiable occasionally to prevent delay of healing where there is interposition of soft tissue.

ACROMIOCLAVICULAR DISLOCATION

Dislocation of the acromioclavicular joint may be incomplete or complete. A history of a blow or fall on the tip of the shoulder can often be obtained. The acromial end of the clavicle is displaced upward and backward; the shoulder falls downward and inward. Careful physical examination generally demonstrates this deformity. Anteroposterior x-rays should be taken of both shoulders with the patient erect. Displacement is more likely to be demonstrated when the patient holds a 5–8 kg weight in each hand. An axillary projection will demonstrate backward displacement of the acromial end of the clavicle.

Incomplete dislocation (subluxation) is associated with only minor tearing of the acromioclavicular ligaments, since complete dislocation requires rupture of the conoid and trapezoid components of the coracoclavicular ligament. These ligaments may be torn within their substance, or may be avulsed with adjacent periosteum from the acromial end of the clavicle.

Treatment

Unreduced acromioclavicular dislocations usually cause no disability; however, painful posttraumatic arthritis may require excision of the distal 4 cm of the clavicle. In general, reduction is indicated for both complete and incomplete dislocations.

A. Incomplete Dislocation: When displacement is minimal, initial treatment may be by sling until acute pain from movement and the weight of the upper extremity has been relieved. Stimson's dressing (Fig 46–13) can be used for injuries of intermediate severity, where displacement is greater but not complete. It is applied as follows: A strip of 3-inch adhesive tape is applied to the chest anteriorly and carried obliquely upward over the acromial end of the clavicle, which has been padded with felt. An assistant then presses downward on the acromial end of the clavicle and lifts the patient's arm upward and backward. The strip of adhesive is then continued posteriorly along the upper arm and over the elbow, where another felt pad is placed over the olecranon and proximal ulna. The strip is then continued along the anterior aspect of the upper arm, across the acromial end of the clavicle, and posteriorly over the scapula. The hand and forearm are supported by a sling. This dressing must be maintained for at least 4 weeks; frequent adjustment is necessary to maintain immobilization in the correct position. The patient is encouraged to sleep in a semireclining position.

B. Complete Dislocation: It is difficult to maintain reduction and adequate immobilization of complete acromioclavicular dislocations by closed methods. Stimson's dressing or its modifications may be

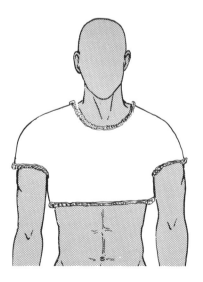
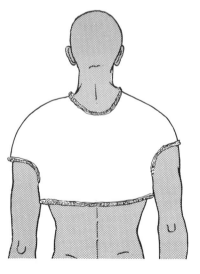

FIG 46–12. Plaster shoulder spica for fracture of clavicle.

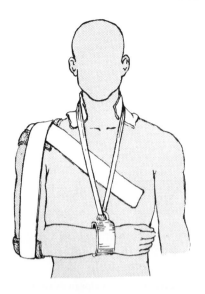

FIG 46–13. Stimson's dressing.

used successfully only if the patient can be kept under constant observation and frequent x-ray examinations made. Open reduction with temporary internal fixation offers the best possibility to restore anatomic alignment. Open reduction is most successful if it can be carried out within a few days after the injury. If it is deferred for 3 weeks or longer, the ligaments will have partially healed with elongation, so that the deformity can be expected to recur when immobilization is discontinued.

STERNOCLAVICULAR DISLOCATION

Displacement of the sternal end of the clavicle may occur superiorly, anteriorly, or, less commonly, inferiorly. Retrosternal displacement is rare. Complete dislocation can be diagnosed by physical examination. Anteroposterior and oblique x-rays confirm the diagnosis.

For incomplete dislocation, a plaster shoulder spica is adequate. Complete dislocations are not difficult to reduce, but external dressings are not adequate to maintain reduction. Open reduction with repair of torn sternoclavicular and costoclavicular ligaments with or without internal fixation are normally required to maintain adequate reduction of complete dislocations. Additional protection by external immobilization should be continued at least while the internal fixation apparatus is in situ.

Painful symptoms caused by posttraumatic degenerative arthritis from anatomically reduced or unreduced sternoclavicular dislocation may be persistent. Extraperiosteal resection of the medial two-thirds of the clavicle may be necessary for relief.

FRACTURE OF THE SCAPULA

Unless fracture of the scapula is complicated by dislocation of the shoulder joint, no treatment is usually required except as noted below.

Fracture of the neck of the scapula is most often caused by a blow on the shoulder or by a fall on the outstretched arm. The degree of fragmentation varies from a crack to extensive comminution. The main glenoid fragment may be impacted into the body fragment. The treatment of impacted or undisplaced fractures in patients 40 years of age or older should be directed toward the preservation of shoulder joint function, since stiffness may cause prolonged disability. In young adults especially, unstable fractures require arm traction with the arm at right angles to the trunk for about 4 weeks and protection in a sling and swathe for an additional 2–4 weeks. Open reduction is rarely required even for major displaced fragments except for those involving the articular surface when associated with dislocation of the humeral head. These fractures are likely to involve only a segment of the articular surface and may be impacted.

Fracture of the acromion or spine of the scapula requires reduction only when the displaced fragment is apt to cause interference with abduction of the shoulder. Persistence of an acromial epiphysis should not be confused with fracture.

Fracture of the coracoid process may result from violent muscular contraction or, rarely, may be associated with anterior dislocation of the shoulder joint.

When fracture of the body of the scapula is caused by direct violence, fractures of underlying ribs may be associated. Treatment of uncomplicated fracture should be directed toward the comfort of the patient and the preservation of shoulder joint function.

FRACTURE OF THE PROXIMAL HUMERUS

Fracture of the Surgical Neck of the Humerus

Fracture of the surgical neck is the most frequent fracture of the proximal humerus and occurs most often in elderly patients. It is commonly the result of indirect trauma such as a fall on the hand with the arm outstretched. Swelling of the shoulder region and restriction of motion due to pain are the prominent clinical features. The diagnosis is established by transthoracic and anteroposterior x-rays.

Undisplaced fractures require little treatment beyond the use of a sling and guarding of the shoulder until discomfort has disappeared. Restoration of bone continuity normally occurs in 8–12 weeks.

The head fragment may be impacted on the shaft in relative varus or valgus. An impacted fracture in marked varus may cause restriction of abduction, but the deformity is rarely sufficient in the elderly adult to warrant disruption of the impaction and reduction.

Impacted fractures of the surgical neck can be treated by means of a sling and swathe with early institution of active motion to preserve shoulder joint function.

Under anesthesia, attempted manipulation of unstable and displaced fractures of the surgical neck without complicating injury is justifiable, but in such instances the lesion must be stabilized by impacting or locking the fragments. When the shaft fragment has been displaced anteriorly and medially (in relation to the head fragment), prompt recurrence of the displacement may follow reduction if the fracture is not stable. Redisplacement is even more likely to occur with an unstable fracture which has been immobilized with the arm in abduction. Continuous traction, either by Buck's extension or by means of a Kirschner wire through the proximal ulna with the arm in abduction, and the elbow flexed, is advisable when the fracture cannot be stabilized (Fig 46–14). Traction must be continued for about 4 weeks before partial healing causes stability.

An unstable fracture in varus position may be reduced by traction and abduction of the arm in external rotation, so that the shaft is brought into alignment with the head fragment. In this position, the fracture may become stable and can then be immobilized in a spica. To avoid stiffness of the shoulder in abduction, the fracture can be stabilized with one or 2 stiff Kirschner wires. This will permit immobilization of the extremity at the side. The wires can be introduced percutaneously and obliquely in the deltoid region through the distal fragment into the head of the humerus with the fracture reduced. With the fragments stabilized, the arm is then brought to the side and immobilized either by a sling and swathe or by a plaster Velpeau dressing (Fig 46–15). Open reduction of fracture of the surgical neck to ensure an adequate functional result is not commonly required.

Fracture of the Greater Tuberosity of the Humerus

Fracture of the greater tuberosity of the humerus

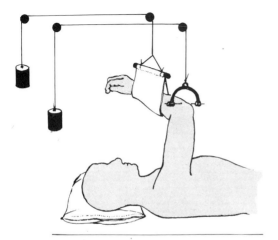

FIG 46–14. Method of suspension of upper extremity with skeletal traction on olecranon.

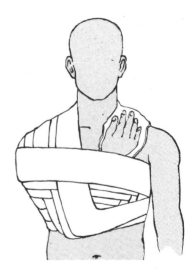

FIG 46–15. Velpeau dressing.

with no associated injury is apt to be undisplaced, and may require little treatment other than relief of pain and preservation of shoulder joint function. Fracture of the greater tuberosity with displacement is likely to be associated with anterior dislocation of the head of the humerus.

Comminuted Fracture of the Proximal Humerus

Comminuted fracture of the proximal humerus is not common, but its prognosis is unfavorable. The configuration of the fracture may vary, but 4 main fragments usually can be identified: 2 tuberosities, the head, and the shaft. Since little or no soft tissue attachment to the head fragment remains, avascular necrosis is apt to occur. The head fragment may be completely displaced anterior or posterior to the glenoid, or it may be impacted on the shaft. In elderly patients, if the fracture is impacted and the head fragment is not dislocated, reduction should not be attempted. Early mobilization is indicated to preserve as much shoulder joint function as possible. If the head fragment is dislocated from the glenoid fossa, open reduction offers the best chance of salvaging shoulder joint function. If the blood supply to the head fragment has been destroyed, the fragment may be removed and the upper end of the humerus placed in the glenoid or a prosthesis inserted. The prognosis for optimal functional recovery is poor in these cases.

Separation of the Epiphysis of the Head of the Humerus

When this injury occurs as a result of birth trauma, it is difficult to recognize because of the absence of a bony nucleus in the capital epiphysis. Even though x-ray examination is negative, the injury should be suspected when there is swelling of the shoulder region and limitation of active movements of the arm. Fracture through the epiphyseal plate may be encountered in older children. The principles of treatment are the same as for fracture of the surgical neck of the humerus. Open reduction is rarely desirable, and every effort should be made to obtain reduction by manipulation or traction.

DISLOCATION OF THE SHOULDER JOINT

Over 95% of all cases of shoulder joint dislocation are anterior or subcoracoid. Subglenoid and posterior dislocations comprise the remainder.

Anterior Dislocation of the Shoulder Joint

Anterior dislocation presents the clinical appearance of flattening of the deltoid region, anterior fullness, and restriction of motion due to pain. Both anteroposterior and axillary x-rays are necessary to determine the site of the head and the presence or absence of complicating fracture which may involve either the head of the humerus or the glenoid. Anterior dislocation may be complicated by (1) injury to major nerves arising from the brachial plexus; (2) fracture of the upper extremity of the humerus, especially the head or greater tuberosity; (3) compression or avulsion of the anterior glenoid; and (4) tears of the capsulotendinous rotator cuff. The most common sequel is recurrent dislocation. Before manipulation, careful examination is necessary to determine the presence or absence of complicating nerve or vascular injury. Under general anesthesia, reduction can usually be accomplished by simple traction on the arm for a few minutes or until the head has been disengaged from the coracoid. If reduction cannot be achieved in this way, the surgeon should apply lateral traction manually to the upper arm, close to the axilla, while the assistant continues to exert axial traction on the extremity. This is a modification of **Hippocrates' manipulation** in which the surgeon exerts traction on the arm while the heel of his unshod foot in the axilla provides countertraction and simultaneously forces the head of the humerus laterally from beneath the acromion.

If neither of the foregoing technics proves successful, **Kocher's method** may be useful. This maneuver, however, must be carried out gently or spiral fracture of the humerus may result. The elbow is flexed to a right angle and the surgeon applies traction and gentle external rotation to the forearm in the axis of the humerus. The surgeon continues traction to the arm while gentle external rotation about the longitudinal axis of the humerus is applied, using the forearm flexed to a right angle at the elbow as a lever. The maneuver can be completed by shifting the elbow across the anterior chest while traction is continuously exerted and, finally, slow internal rotation of the arm until the palm of the affected side rests on the opposite shoulder.

After closed reduction of an initial dislocation the extremity is immobilized in a sling and swathe for 3 weeks before active motion is begun. If a second epi-

sode is the result of minor trauma, the lesion is considered permanent and treated accordingly.

Subcoracoid Dislocation of the Shoulder Joint

Uncomplicated subcoracoid dislocation can almost always be reduced by closed manipulation. With associated fracture, or when the dislocation is old, open reduction may be necessary. Even when the dislocation is old, however, closed reduction by skeletal traction should be tried before open reduction is elected.

Posterior Dislocation of the Shoulder Joint

Posterior dislocation is characterized by fullness beneath the spine of the scapula and by restriction of motion in external rotation. An axillary x-ray view demonstrates the position of the head of the humerus in relationship to the glenoid. This uncommon lesion may be reduced by the same combination of coaxial and transverse traction as described for anterior dislocation. Immobilization following an initial episode should be accomplished by plaster spica, with the arm in approximately 30 degrees external rotation and the elbow flexed to a right angle.

Recurrent Dislocation of the Shoulder Joint

Recurrent dislocation of the shoulder is almost always anterior. Various factors can influence recurrent dislocation. Avulsion of the anterior and inferior glenoid labrum or tears in the anterior capsule remove the natural buttress that gives stability to the arm with abduction and external rotation. Other lesions which impair the stability of the shoulder joint are fractures of the posterior and superior surface of the head of the humerus (or of the greater tuberosity) and longitudinal tears of the rotator cuff between the supraspinatus and subscapularis. Reduction of the acute episodic dislocation is by closed manipulation. Immobilization does not prevent subsequent dislocation, and it should be discontinued as soon as acute symptoms subside, usually within a few days.

Adequate curative treatment of recurrent dislocation of the shoulder, so that unrestricted normal use of the joint is possible, almost always requires plastic repair of the anterior capsulotendinous cuff by operations such as those recommended by Bankhart, Putti and Platt, or Magnuson and Stack.

FRACTURES OF THE SHAFT OF THE HUMERUS

Fracture of the shaft of the humerus is more common in adults than in children. Direct violence is accountable for the majority of such fractures, although spiral fracture of the middle third of the shaft may result from violent muscular activity such as throwing a ball. The diagnosis is based upon the history and physical examination. Localized tenderness, swelling, and deformity are apparent. Palpation may elicit crepitus. Anteroposterior and transthoracic x-rays show the location and configuration of the fracture. Before initiating definitive treatment, a careful neurologic examination should be done (and recorded) to determine the status of the radial nerve. Injury to the brachial vessels is not common.

Fracture through the metaphysis proximal to the insertion of the pectoralis major is classified as fracture of the surgical neck of the humerus.

Fracture of the Upper Third of the Shaft of the Humerus

Fractures between the insertions of the pectoralis major and the deltoid commonly demonstrate adduction of the distal end of the proximal fragment, with lateral and proximal displacement of the distal fragment. Medial displacement occurs with fracture distal to the insertion of the deltoid.

Treatment depends upon the presence or absence of complicating neurovascular injury, the site and configuration of the fracture, and the magnitude of displacement.

In infants, skin traction for 1–2 weeks will permit sufficient callus to form so that immobilization can be maintained by a sling and swathe or a Velpeau dressing. Open reduction for the sole purpose of accurate positioning of the fragments is rarely justified in children and adolescents, since slight shortening and minor degrees of angulation will be compensated during growth. Torsional displacement, however, will not be compensated, and must be corrected initially.

In the adult, an effort should be made to reduce completely displaced transverse or slightly oblique fractures by manipulation. An injection of 10–15 ml of 2% procaine directly into the hematoma at the fracture site will provide adequate anesthesia for manipulation. If the ends of the fragments cannot be approximated by manipulative methods, traction on the skin or skeletal traction with a wire through the olecranon is indicated (Fig 46–34). In young patients, the olecranon wire should be placed opposite the coronoid process to avoid injury to the epiphysis. Traction should be continued for 3–4 weeks until stabilization occurs, after which time the patient can be ambulatory with an external immobilization device.

Fracture of the Middle & Lower Thirds of the Shaft of the Humerus

Spiral, oblique, and comminuted fractures of the shaft below the insertion of the pectoralis major may be treated by Caldwell's hanging cast, which consists of a plaster dressing from the axilla to the wrist with the elbow in 90 degrees of flexion and the forearm in midposition (Fig 46–16). The cast is suspended from a bandage around the neck by means of a ring at the wrist. Alignment should be verified on anteroposterior and transthoracic x-rays with the patient standing. Angulation may be corrected by lengthening or

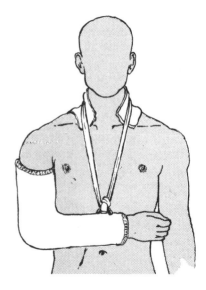

FIG 46–16. Caldwell's hanging cast.

shortening the suspension bandage. When lateral convex angulation cannot be corrected by adjustment of the bandage, moving the suspension ring closer to the elbow may be effective. Traction is afforded by the weight of the plaster. The patient is instructed to sleep in the semireclining position. As soon as clinical examination demonstrates stabilization (in about 6–8 weeks), the plaster may be discarded and a sling and swathe substituted.

If the configuration of the fracture approaches the transverse and is located between the insertions of the pectoralis major and the deltoid, the distal end of the proximal fragment may be in relative adduction. To prevent recurrence of medial convex angulation and maintain proper alignment, it may be necessary to bring the distal fragment into alignment with the proximal by bringing the arm across the chest and immobilizing it with a plaster Velpeau dressing (Fig 46–15).

When fracture of the shaft of the humerus is associated with other injuries which require confinement to bed, initial treatment may be by skin or skeletal traction (Fig 46–14).

Fractures of the shaft of the humerus—especially transverse fractures—may heal slowly. If stabilization has not taken place after 6–8 weeks of traction, more secure immobilization, such as with a plaster shoulder spica (Fig 46–17), must be considered. It may be necessary to continue immobilization for 6 months or more.

When complete loss of radial nerve function is apparent immediately after injury, open operation is indicated to determine the type of nerve lesion or to remove impinging bone fragments. If partial function of the radial nerve is retained, exploration can be deferred since spontaneous recovery sometimes occurs and may be complete by the time the fracture has healed. Open reduction of closed fractures is indicated also if arterial circulation has been interrupted or (in

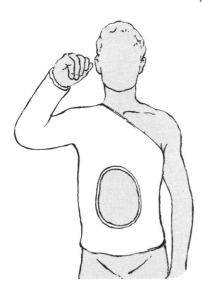

FIG 46-17. Plaster shoulder spica for fracture of humerus.

the adult) if adequate apposition of major fragments cannot be obtained by closed methods, as is likely to be the case with transverse fractures near the middle third of the shaft. When 4–5 months of treatment by closed methods have not resulted in clinical or x-ray evidence of healing, operative treatment should be considered.

INJURIES OF THE ELBOW REGION

FRACTURE OF THE DISTAL HUMERUS

Fracture of the distal humerus is most often caused by indirect violence. Therefore, the configuration of the fracture cleft and the direction of displacement of the fragments are likely to be typical. Injuries of major vessels and nerves and elbow joint dislocation are apt to be present.

Clinical findings consist of pain, swelling, and restriction of motion. Minor deformity may not be apparent because swelling usually obliterates landmarks. The type of fracture is determined by x-ray examination. Especially in children, it is advisable to obtain films of the opposite elbow for comparison.

Examination for peripheral nerve and vascular injury must be made and all findings carefully recorded before treatment is instituted.

Supracondylar Fracture of the Humerus

Supracondylar fracture of the humerus occurs

proximal to the olecranon fossa; transcondylar (diacondylar) fracture occurs more distally and extends into the olecranon fossa. Neither fracture extends to the articular surface of the humerus. Treatment is the same for both types.

Supracondylar fractures are observed more commonly in children and adolescents, and they may extend into the epiphyseal plates of the capitellum and trochlea. Transcondylar fracture is very rare in children.

The direction of displacement of the distal fragment from the midcoronal plane of the arm serves to differentiate the "extension" from the less common "flexion" type. This differentiation has important implications for treatment.

A. Extension-Type Fractures: The significant direction of displacement of the distal fragment in the "extension" type of fracture is posterior and proximal. The distal fragment may also be displaced laterally and, less frequently, medially. The direction of these displacements is identified easily on biplane x-ray films. Internal torsional displacement, however, is more difficult to recognize; and unless torsional displacement is reduced, relative cubitus varus with loss of carrying angle will persist.

Displaced supracondylar fractures are surgical emergencies. Immediate treatment is required to avoid occlusion of the brachial artery and to prevent or to avoid further peripheral nerve injury. If hemorrhage and edema prevent complete reduction of the fracture at the first attempt, a second manipulation will be required after swelling has regressed.

1. Manipulative reduction—Minor angular displacements (tilting) may be reduced by gentle forced flexion of the elbow under local or general anesthesia, followed by immobilization in a posterior plaster splint in 45 degrees of flexion (Fig 46–18). If displacement is marked but normal radial pulsation indicates that circulation is not impaired, closed manipulation under general anesthesia should be done as soon as possible. If radial pulses are absent or weak on initial examination and do not improve with manipulation, traction is indicated (see below). Capillary flush in the nail beds cannot be relied on as the sole indication of competency of deep circulation. After reduction and casting the patient should be placed at bed rest, preferably in a hospital, with his elbow elevated on a pillow and the dressing arranged so that the radial pulse is accessible for frequent observation. Swelling can be expected to increase for 24–72 hours. During this critical period continued observation is necessary so that any circulatory embarrassment which may lead to Volkmann's ischemic contracture can be identified at once. The circular bandage must be adjusted frequently to compensate for initial increase and subsequent decrease of swelling. If during manipulation it was necessary to extend the elbow beyond 45 degrees to restore radial pulses, the joint should be flexed to the optimal angle as swelling subsides to prevent loss of the reduction.

In children stabilization will take place in 4–5 weeks, after which time the plaster splint may be dis-

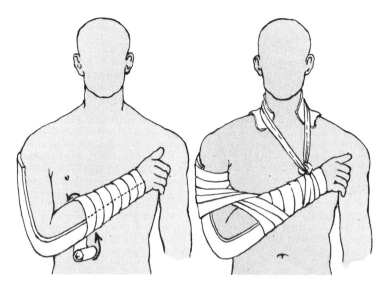

FIG 46—18. Posterior plaster splint for supracondylar fracture.

carded and a sling worn for another 2 weeks before active motion is permitted. In adults healing is less rapid and immobilization must be continued for 8—12 weeks or even longer before active exercise is permitted.

2. Traction and immobilization—In certain instances supracondylar fractures of the humerus with posterior displacement of the distal fragment should be treated by traction (Figs 46—19 and 46—20): (1) If comminution is marked and stability cannot be obtained by flexion of the elbow, traction is indicated until the fragments have stabilized. (2) If 2 or 3 attempts at manipulative reduction have been unsuccessful, continuous traction under x-ray control for 1—2 days is justifiable before further manipulation. (3) If the radial pulse is absent or weak when the patient is examined initially and does not improve with manipulation, traction may be necessary to prevent displacement of the fracture and further embarrassment of circulation. During the early phase of treatment by continuous traction, flexion of the elbow beyond 90 degrees should be avoided since this may jeopardize circulation.

B. Flexion-Type Fracture: Flexion-type fracture of the humerus is characterized by anterior and sometimes also torsional and lateral displacement of the main distal fragment. Treatment is by closed manipulation. A posterior plaster splint is then applied from the axillary fold to the level of the wrist, with the forearm in supination and the elbow in full extension. Elevation is advisable for at least 24 hours or until soft tissue swelling has reached the maximum, after which time the patient may be ambulatory. Immobilization is then continued for 4—6 weeks. When satisfactory reduction cannot be accomplished by closed manipulation, treatment should be by traction with the elbow in full extension until the fragments become stabilized.

Separation of the Distal Humeral Epiphyses

An uncommon variation of supracondylar fracture is separation of the distal humeral epiphyses with or without appreciable displacement. Sprains of the elbow do not commonly occur in children; injury more often involves the distal humeral epiphyses. X-ray comparison of the injured elbow with the uninjured elbow may show no deviation, but careful physical examination may demonstrate posterior tenderness over the lower epiphyses and also swelling. This combination of swelling and tenderness should suggest epiphyseal separation, and warrants protection from further injury by means of a sling worn for about 3 weeks.

The direction of displacement is determined by careful clinical and radiographic examinations. Depending upon the direction of angulation of the osseous nuclei of the capitellum and trochlea (as demonstrated in the lateral x-ray), immobilization is as described for supracondylar fractures.

Intercondylar Fracture of the Humerus

Intercondylar fracture of the humerus is classically described as being of the T or Y type (or both), according to the configuration of the fracture cleft observed on an anteroposterior x-ray. This fracture is usually seen in adults, commonly as the result of a blow over the posterior aspect of the flexed elbow. Open fracture and other injuries to the soft tissues are frequently present. The fracture often extends into the trochlear surface of the elbow joint, and unless the articular surfaces of the distal humerus can be accurately repositioned, restriction of joint motion, pain, instability, and deformity can be expected.

A. Closed Reduction: If the fragments are not widely displaced, closed reduction may be successful. Since comminution is always present, stabilization is difficult to achieve and maintain by manipulation and external immobilization.

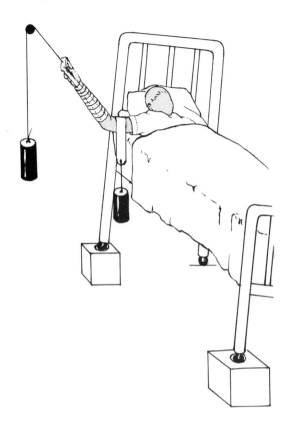

FIG 46–19. Dunlop's traction for supracondylar fracture.

1. Anterior displacement may be treated first by a combination of continuous skin traction with the elbow in full extension and closed manipulation of the main fragments. If adequate positioning can be achieved in this manner, traction is continued until stabilization occurs. The extremity may then be immobilized in a tubular plaster cast.

2. Significant posterior displacement requires overhead skeletal traction by means of a Kirschner wire inserted through the olecranon (Fig 46–20). It may be necessary to apply a swathe around the arm and body for simultaneous transverse traction.

B. Open Reduction: Open reduction may be indicated if adequate positioning cannot be obtained by closed methods. A requirement for acceptable results of open reduction and internal fixation is that the fragments be sufficiently large so that they can be fixed to one another. Comminution may be so extensive that satisfactory stabilization cannot be accomplished by current technics of internal fixation. Under such circumstances, it is better to abandon open operation and to accept the imperfect results of closed treatment.

Fracture of the Lateral Condyle of the Humerus

The 3 major varieties of fracture of the lateral condyle of the humerus are (1) fracture of a portion of the capitellum in the coronal plane of the humerus,

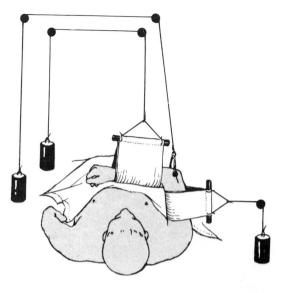

FIG 46–20. Skeletal traction for supracondylar fracture.

with or without extension into the trochlea (seen only in adults); (2) isolated fracture of the lateral condyle without extension into the trochlea; and (3) separation of the capitellar epiphysis (in children).

A. Fracture of the Capitellum: This is characterized by proximal displacement of the anterior detached fragment, and probably occurs as one component of a spontaneously reduced incomplete dislocation of the elbow joint. The lesion is most clearly demonstrated on lateral x-rays. Closed reduction should be attempted by forcing the elbow into acute flexion. After reduction the extremity is immobilized in a posterior plaster splint with the elbow in full flexion to prevent displacement of the small distal fragment.

When accurate reduction cannot be accomplished by closed technics, open operation may be desirable to avoid subsequent restriction of elbow movement. If the small distal fragment retains sufficient soft tissue attachment to assure adequate blood supply, it may be temporarily fixed to the main fragment in anatomic position by a Kirschner wire. If the articular fragment lacks significant soft tissue bonds, removal is recommended since avascular necrosis is likely to follow.

B. Isolated Complete Fracture: Isolated complete fracture of the lateral condyle without extension into the trochlea* is uncommon, and is not usually associated with major displacement of the detached fragment. The extremity should be supported by a sling. If tense hemarthrosis is present, aspiration may minimize

---

*Fracture which involves the entire capitellum and extends into the trochlea is associated with proximal and lateral displacement of the detached fragment and lateral subluxation of the elbow. This lesion is discussed below.

pain. Guarded active motions of the elbow should be initiated as soon as pain subsides.

C. Separation of the Capitellar Epiphysis: Fracture of the lateral condyle of the humerus in children is essentially separation of the capitellar epiphysis, even though the fracture may extend into the metaphysis and the trochlear epiphysis. If the center of ossification of the capitellum is small, minor displacement may be missed on initial examination; further displacement will then result from unguarded use. The fact that a part of the extensor muscles originates on the fragment is an important factor in displacement.

1. Closed reduction—Minor displacement may be treated by manipulative reduction and external immobilization in a posterior plaster splint which extends from the posterior axillary fold to the level of the heads of the metacarpals. X-rays are taken at least twice a week for the first 3 weeks to determine whether displacement has recurred.

2. Open reduction—When anatomic reduction cannot be achieved by one or 2 manipulations, open reduction is indicated.

Avulsion of the Medial Epicondylar Apophysis

Avulsion of the medial epicondylar apophysis in children may occur without dislocation of the elbow. Minor displacement causing localized tenderness and swelling over the medial aspect of the elbow can be treated by immobilization in a sling and swathe for a few days. More extensive injury should be suspected if tenderness and swelling are diffuse. When separation is greater than 1–2 mm, treatment is similar to that for dislocation of the elbow associated with separation of the apophysis (see below).

FRACTURE OF THE PROXIMAL ULNA

Common fractures of the proximal ulna include fracture of the olecranon and fracture of the coronoid process. Fracture of the coronoid process is a complication of posterior dislocation of the elbow joint, and is discussed below.

Fracture of the olecranon which occurs as the result of indirect violence (eg, forced flexion of the forearm against the actively contracted triceps muscle) is typically transverse or slightly oblique. Fracture due to direct violence is usually comminuted and associated with other fracture or anterior dislocation of the joint. Since the major fracture cleft extends into the elbow joint, treatment should be directed toward restoration of anatomic position to afford maximal recovery of range of motion and functional competency of the triceps.

Treatment

The method of treatment depends upon the degree of displacement and the extent of comminution.

A. Closed Reduction: Minimal displacement (1–2 mm) can be treated by closed manipulation with the elbow in full extension, assisted by digital pressure over the proximal fragment, and immobilization in a volar plaster splint which extends from the anterior axillary fold to the wrist. X-rays should be taken twice weekly for 2 weeks after reduction to determine whether reduction has been maintained. Immobilization must be continued for at least 6 weeks before active flexion exercises are begun.

B. Open Reduction and Internal Fixation: Open reduction and internal fixation are indicated if closed methods are not successful in approximating displaced fragments and restoring congruity to articular surfaces. The extremity is then immobilized in 90 degrees of flexion for at least 6–8 weeks before active flexion exercises are instituted.

FRACTURE OF THE PROXIMAL RADIUS

Fracture of the Head & Neck of the Radius

Fracture of the head and neck of the radius may occur in adults as an isolated injury uncomplicated by dislocation of the elbow or the superior radioulnar joint. This fracture is caused by indirect violence, such as a fall on the outstretched hand, when the radial head is driven against the capitellum. Care must be taken to obtain true anteroposterior and lateral x-rays of the proximal radius as well as of the elbow joint, since minor lesions may be obscured by a change in position from midposition to full spination during exposure of the films.

A. Conservative Measures: Fissure fractures and those with minimal displacement can be treated symptomatically, with evacuation of tense hemarthrosis by aspiration to minimize pain. The extremity may be supported by a sling or immobilized in a posterior plaster splint with the elbow in 90 degrees of flexion. Active exercises of the elbow are to be encouraged within a few days. Recovery of function is slow, and slight restriction of motion (especially extension) may persist.

B. Surgical Treatment: When the fracture involves the articular surface and is comminuted, or when displacement is greater than 1–2 mm, excision of the entire head of the radius is generally recommended. However, simple removal of a minor fragment of the head which comprises less than a quarter of the articular surface is compatible with recovery of satisfactory elbow function.

Fracture of the Upper Epiphysis of the Radius

Fracture of the upper radial epiphysis in a child is not a true epiphyseal separation since the fracture cleft commonly extends into the neck of the bone. Because the articular surface of the proximal fragment remains intact, the prominent features of displacement are angulation and impaction. Wide displacement of the minor proximal fragment may mean that the elbow joint was dislocated but has reduced spontaneously since the injury.

A. Closed Reduction: Every effort should be made to reduce these fractures by closed manipulation. Several x-rays taken with the forearm in various degrees of rotation should be examined so that the position can be selected which is best suited for digital pressure on the proximal fragment. Anteroposterior and lateral x-rays with the elbow in flexion are then taken; if angulation has been reduced to less than 45 degrees, the end result is likely to be satisfactory.

B. Open Reduction: If closed reduction is not successful, open reduction and repositioning under direct vision is indicated even in the child.

SUBLUXATION & DISLOCATION OF THE ELBOW JOINT

Subluxation of the Head of the Radius

This injury occurs most frequently in infants between the ages of 18 months and 3 years, usually when the child is suddenly lifted by his hands with the forearm in pronation. Because of comparative laxity of the interosseous membrane and other supporting ligamentous structures, the direction of displacement of the radial head is distal in the direction of the longitudinal axis of the shaft. It has been suggested that this permits the proximal part of the annular ligament to become infolded between the radial head and the capitellum. In unreduced subluxations, in addition to tenderness about the radial head and restriction of supination, swelling and tenderness may be present in the region of the ulnar head at the level of the inferior radioulnar joint. The infant holds the forearm semiflexed and pronated. If spontaneous reduction has occurred, diagnosis is dependent upon finding slightly restricted supination associated with discomfort. X-rays are not helpful at this stage.

Reduction by forced supination of the forearm can be accomplished easily without anesthesia. The arm should be protected in a sling for 1 week to prevent recurrence.

Dislocation of the Elbow Joint Without Fracture

Dislocation of the elbow joint without major fracture is almost always posterior. It may be encountered at any age but is most common in children. Complete backward dislocation of the ulna and radius implies extensive tearing of the capsuloligamentous structures and injury to the region of insertion of the brachialis muscle. The coronoid process of the ulna is usually displaced posteriorly and proximally into the olecranon fossa, but it may be displaced laterally or medially. Biplane x-rays of the highest quality are necessary to determine that no fracture is associated.

Peripheral nerve function must be carefully assessed before definitive treatment is instituted. The ulnar nerve is most likely to be injured.

In recent dislocations, closed reduction can be achieved (under general anesthesia) by axial traction on the forearm with the elbow in the position of deformity. Hyperextension is not necessary. Lateral or medial dislocation can be corrected during traction. As soon as proximal displacement is corrected, the elbow should be brought into 90 degrees of flexion and a posterior plaster splint applied which reaches from the posterior axillary fold to the wrist. Active motion is permitted after 3 weeks.

Closed reduction should be attempted even if unreduced dislocation has persisted for 2 months following the injury.

FRACTURE-DISLOCATION OF THE ELBOW JOINT

Dislocation of the elbow is frequently associated with fracture. Some fractures are insignificant and require no specific treatment; others demand specialized care.

Fracture of the Coronoid Process of the Ulna

Fracture of the coronoid process of the ulna is the most frequent complication of posterior dislocation of the elbow joint. Treatment is the same as for uncomplicated posterior dislocation of the elbow joint (see above).

Fracture of the Head of the Radius With Posterior Dislocation of the Elbow Joint

This injury is treated as 2 separate lesions. The severity of comminution and the magnitude of displacement of the radial head fragments are first determined by x-ray. If comminution has occurred or the fragments are widely displaced, the dislocation is reduced by closed manipulation; the head of the radius is then excised.

If fracture of the head of the radius is not comminuted and the fragments are not widely displaced, treatment is as for uncomplicated posterior dislocation of the elbow joint.

Fracture of the Olecranon With Anterior Dislocation of the Elbow Joint

This very unstable injury usually occurs from a blow on the dorsum of the flexed forearm. Fracture through the olecranon permits the distal fragment of the ulna and the proximal radius to be displaced anterior to the humerus, and may cause extensive tearing of the capsuloligamentous structures around the elbow joint. The dislocation can be reduced by bringing the elbow into full extension, but anatomic reduction of the olecranon fracture by closed manipulation is not likely to be successful and immediate open reduction is usually indicated. Recovery of function is likely to be delayed and incomplete.

Fracture of the Medial Epicondylar Apophysis With Dislocation of the Elbow Joint

Dislocation of the elbow joint in children may be complicated by avulsion of the medial epicondylar apophysis. The direction of dislocation may have been lateral, posterior, or posterolateral. Physical and x-ray examination may not demonstrate the extent of displacement at the time of injury since partial reduction may have occurred spontaneously. X-rays of the uninjured elbow in similar projections are desirable to compare the exact locations of the 2 apophyses. The free fragment is normally displaced downward by the action of the flexor muscles. If partial spontaneous reduction has occurred, the detached apophysis may be found incarcerated within the elbow joint between the articular surfaces of the trochlea and the olecranon. This may happen also during manual reduction. Ulnar nerve function must be evaluated before definitive treatment is given.

Dislocation of the elbow joint may be reduced by closed manipulation, but accurate repositioning of a widely separated apophysis cannot be achieved by closed methods. Opinion differs concerning the necessity for anatomic reduction of the apophysis if it is not incarcerated within the elbow joint. Some authorities maintain that fibrous healing of the apophysis causes no disability; others anticipate weakness of grasp or subsequent pain as the result of development of a pseudarthrosis between the apophysis and the medial condyle. Exuberant bone formation around the apophysis may cause tardy ulnar paralysis. If it is elected not to reduce displacement of an apophysis outside the elbow joint, the extremity should be immobilized at a right angle for 3 weeks in a tubular plaster cast before active motion is permitted.

If the ulnar nerve has been injured, or if the apophysis cannot be displaced from the elbow joint by closed manipulation, open reduction is advisable.

Fracture of the Lateral Condyle With Lateral Dislocation of the Elbow Joint

Fracture of the lateral condyle of the humerus with lateral dislocation of the elbow joint must be differentiated from fracture of the lateral condyle with or without posterior dislocation of the joint (see below). Neither lesion is common. A complicating feature of fracture of the lateral condyle with lateral dislocation is inclusion not only of the entire capitellum but also extension of the fracture cleft into the trochlea. This creates an unstable mechanism which cannot be reliably immobilized in either flexion or extension even though closed reduction has been successful. If closed methods of treatment are not adequate, open reduction is recommended.

Fracture of the Lateral Condyle With Posterior Dislocation of the Elbow Joint

Treatment should be divided into 2 phases. The dislocation should be reduced first by closed manipulation. This maneuver may also simultaneously accomplish adequate reduction of the condylar fracture. If the condylar fragment cannot be adequately repositioned by closed manipulation, open reduction and internal fixation are justifiable to assure anatomic restoration of the articular surfaces.

INJURIES OF THE SHAFTS OF THE RADIUS & ULNA

FRACTURES OF THE SHAFTS OF THE RADIUS & ULNA

General Considerations

A. Causative Injury: Spiral and oblique fractures are likely to be caused by indirect injury. Greenstick, transverse, and comminuted fractures are commonly the result of direct injury.

B. Radiography:

1. In addition to anteroposterior and lateral films of the entire forearm, including the elbow and wrist joints, oblique views are often desirable.

2. The lateral projection is usually taken with the forearm in midposition (between complete pronation and supination).

3. For the anteroposterior projection care must be taken to prevent any change in relative supination of the radius; if this happens, the distal radius will be the same in both views.

4. Especially in children, films of the uninjured forearm are desirable for comparison of epiphyses and for future reference if growth is impaired.

C. Anatomic Peculiarities: Both the radius and the ulna have biplane curves which permit 180 degrees of rotation in the forearm. If the curves are not preserved by reduction, full rotatory motion of the forearm may not be recovered or derangement of the radioulnar joints may follow.

Torsional displacement by muscle activity has important implications for manipulative treatment of certain fractures of the radial shaft. The direction of torsional displacement of the distal fragment following fracture of the shaft is influenced by the location of the lesion in reference to muscle insertion. If the fracture is in the upper third (above the insertion of the pronator teres), the proximal fragment will be drawn into relative supination by the biceps and supinator and the distal fragment into pronation by the pronator teres and pronator quadratus. The relative position in torsion of the proximal fragment may be determined by comparing the position of the bicipital tubercle on an anteroposterior film with similar projections of the uninjured arm taken in varying degrees of forearm rotation. In fractures below the middle of the radius (below the insertion of the pronator teres), the proximal fragment characteristically remains in midposition and the distal fragment is pronated; this is due to the antagonistic action of the pronator teres on the biceps and supinator.

D. Closed Reduction and Splinting: With fracture and displacement of the shaft of either the radius or the ulna, injury of the proximal or distal radioulnar joints should always be suspected. The presence of swelling and tenderness around the joint may aid in localization of an occult injury when x-rays are not helpful.

In both adults and children, closed reduction of uncomplicated fractures of the radius and ulna should be attempted. The type of manipulative maneuver depends upon the configuration and location of the fracture and the age of the patient. The position of immobilization of the elbow, forearm, and wrist depends upon the location of the fracture and its inherent stability.

Fracture of the Shaft of the Ulna

Isolated fracture of the shaft of the proximal third of the ulna (above the insertion of the pronator teres) with displacement is often associated with dislocation of the head of the radius. Reduction of an undislocated transverse fracture may be achieved by axial traction followed by digital pressure to correct displacement in the transverse plane. With the patient supine, the hand is suspended overhead and countertraction is provided by a sling around the arm above the flexed elbow. After the fragments are distracted, transverse displacement is corrected by digital pressure. With the elbow at a right angle and the forearm in midposition, the extremity is then immobilized in a tubular plaster cast extending from the axilla to the metacarpophalangeal joints. During the first month, weekly examination by x-ray is necessary to determine whether displacement has occurred. Immobilization must be maintained until bone continuity is restored (usually in 8–12 weeks).

Fracture of the shaft of the ulna distal to the insertion of the pronator teres is apt to be complicated by angulation. The proximal end of the distal fragment is displaced toward the radius by the pronator quadratus muscle. Reduction can be achieved by the maneuver described above. To prevent recurrent displacement of the distal fragment, the plaster cast must be carefully molded so as to force the mass of the forearm musculature between the radius and ulna in the anteroposterior plane. Care should be taken to avoid pressure over the subcutaneous surfaces of the radius and ulna around the wrist. Healing is slow, and frequent radiologic examination is necessary to make certain that displacement has not occurred. Stabilization by bone healing may require more than 4 months of immobilization.

An oblique fracture cleft creates an unstable mechanism with a tendency toward displacement, and immobilization in a tubular plaster is not reliable. Open reduction and rigid internal fixation with bone plates or an intramedullary rod are indicated.

Open reduction of uncomplicated fracture of the ulna in children is rarely justifiable because accurate

reduction is not imperative; in children under 12 years of age an angular deformity as great as 15 degrees may be corrected by growth. Torsional displacement of uncomplicated fractures of the shaft is not likely to occur. Deformity caused by transverse displacement will be corrected by growth and remodeling.

Fracture of the Shaft of the Radius

Isolated closed fracture of the shaft of the radius can be caused by direct or indirect violence; open fracture usually results from penetrating injury. Closed fracture with displacement is usually associated with other injury (eg, fracture of the ulna or dislocation of the distal radioulnar joint). X-rays may not reveal dislocation, but localized tenderness and swelling suggest injury to the distal radioulnar joint.

If the fracture is proximal to the insertion of the pronator teres, closed reduction is indicated. The extremity should then be immobilized in a tubular plaster cast which extends from the axilla to the metacarpophalangeal joints, with the elbow at a right angle and the forearm in full supination (Fig 46–21).

If the fracture is distal to the insertion of the pronator teres, manipulation and immobilization are as described above except that the forearm should be in midrotation rather than full supination. Since injury to the distal radioulnar joint is apt to be associated with fracture of the radial shaft below the insertion of the pronator teres, weekly anteroposterior and lateral x-ray projections should be taken during the first month to determine the exact status of reduction.

If the configuration of the fracture cleft is transverse rather than oblique, displacement is less apt to take place following anatomic reduction. In the adult, if stability cannot be achieved or if reduction does not approach the anatomic, open reduction and internal fixation are recommended since deformity as a result of displacement of fragments is likely to cause limitation of forearm and hand movements. Children under 12 years of age are likely to recover function provided that torsional displacement has been corrected and angulation does not exceed 15 degrees. Especially if it

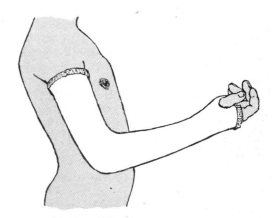

FIG 46–21. Full upper extremity plaster for fracture of both bones of the forearm.

is convex anteriorly, angulation greater than 15 degrees should be corrected in children even though open reduction is required.

In adults, a snug plaster should be maintained for 8–12 weeks or even longer, since healing may be slow. Healing is rapid in children even though reduction is not anatomic; open reduction to promote bone healing in children is not necessary.

Fracture of the Shafts of Both Bones

The management of fractures of the shafts of both bones of the forearm is essentially a combination of those technics which have been described for the individual bones. If both bones are fractured at the same time, dislocation of either radioulnar joint is not likely to occur. If the configuration of the fracture cleft is approximately transverse, stability can be attained by closed methods provided reduction is anatomic or nearly so. Oblique or comminuted fractures are unstable.

Treatment depends in part upon the degree of displacement, the severity of comminution, and the age of the patient.

A. Without Displacement: In adults, fracture of the shaft of the radius and ulna without displacement can be treated by immobilization in a tubular plaster cast extending from the axilla to the metacarpophalangeal joints with the elbow at a right angle and the forearm in supination (fractures of the upper third) or midposition (fractures of the mid and lower thirds). Immobilization for 8–12 weeks is generally sufficient for restoration of bone continuity in children; immobilization for a longer time is necessary for adults. To avoid late angulation or refracture, the elbow should be included in the plaster until the callus is well mineralized.

B. Greenstick Fractures: Greenstick fractures of both bones of the forearm are common in children. With fractures of the lower third in children under 12 years of age, if angulation is no more than 15 degrees and convex posteriorly, satisfactory correction of the deformity can be expected to occur spontaneously with growth. If angulation is greater than 15 degrees or if the apex is directed anteriorly, deformity should be corrected and the extremity immobilized in a tubular plaster cast extending from the axilla to the bases of the fingers, the elbow at a right angle, the forearm in pronation, and the wrist in the neutral position. Reduction is maintained by snug anteroposterior molding of the plaster over the distal third of the forearm rather than by placing the wrist in volar flexion.

Greenstick fracture of both bones proximal to the distal third of the shaft has a tendency toward increased angular deformity if angulation alone is corrected without completion of the fracture. It is recommended that the fracture be completed by sharply reversing the direction of angulation until a palpable "snap" indicates that intact fibers of bone and periosteum on the convex surface have ruptured. The extremity is then immobilized in a plaster cast similar to that used for lower third fractures, with the forearm in semisupination.

C. With Displacement: Although it is not always possible to correct displaced fractures of both bones of the forearm by closed methods, an attempt should be made to do so both in adults and in children if x-ray studies show a configuration whereby stabilization can be accomplished without operation. Manipulative reduction is recommended if the patient is treated soon after injury and overriding is less than 1 cm. It is essential that good apposition of the fragments of each bone be obtained. Once adequate reduction has been achieved, and while traction is maintained, a padded tubular plaster cast is applied from the bases of the fingers to the axilla.

If treatment is delayed until hemorrhage and swelling have caused induration by infiltration of the soft tissues, or if overriding is more than 1 cm, sustained traction for 2–3 hours will probably be necessary to overcome shortening. Traction on the skin with countertraction on soft tissues is hazardous in these circumstances because of the possibility of decubiti or vascular injury. Skeletal traction is indicated. When correction of the overriding is demonstrated by x-ray, the fragments are manipulated into position under local or general anesthesia. A plaster cast with wires incorporated is then applied and the tension bows maintained to keep the wires taut.

Persistent overriding without angulation in children is not a problem since 0.5 cm of shortening may be corrected by growth. If overriding of more than 0.5 cm is demonstrated, continuous skin traction upon the fingers with elastic bands attached to a banjo loop incorporated into the tubular plaster is indicated (Fig 46–22).

In adults, if accurate apposition of fragments or

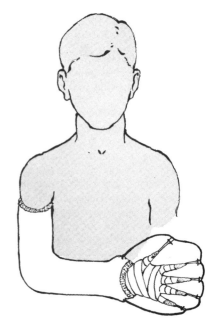

FIG 46–22. Banjo splint and skin traction for fracture of the forearm in children (Blount).

stability cannot be achieved in fractures of both bones, open reduction and internal fixation are recommended provided that experienced personnel and adequate equipment are available. Persistent displacement of the fragments of one or both bones may be associated with delay of healing, restriction of forearm movements, derangement of the radioulnar joints, and deformity. In those fractures in which open reduction is justifiable in the adult, rigid internal fixation is indicated; a technical pitfall to be avoided is the use of a single wire loop or transfixation screw, a short bone plate attached with unicortical screws, or small intramedullary wires. Even though excellent stability is achieved at operation with internal devices, the extremity should be protected by external fixation until bone healing is well under way.

FRACTURE-DISLOCATIONS OF THE RADIUS & ULNA

Fracture of the Ulna With Dislocation of the Radial Head (Monteggia's Fracture)

Fracture of the shaft of the ulna near the junction of the middle and upper thirds may be associated with anterior or posterior dislocation of the head of the radius. Lateral dislocation of the head of the radius with convex angulation of the shaft of the ulna in the same direction is not common.

A. Closed Reduction:

1. Anterior dislocation of the head of the radius— Although this lesion is usually caused by direct violence upon the dorsum of the forearm, it may also be caused by forced pronation. The annular ligament may be torn, or the head may be displaced distally from beneath the annular ligament without causing a significant tear. The injured ligament may be interposed between the articular surface of the head of the radius and the capitellum of the humerus or the adjacent ulna.

Closed reduction can be achieved under general anesthesia. Lateral and posteroanterior x-rays are then taken, and a posterior plaster splint is applied from the axillary fold to the head of the metacarpals with the elbow in 45 degrees of flexion (Fig 46−18) while the films are prepared. If reduction is anatomic, the arm is elevated and observed frequently for signs of circulatory embarrassment for at least 72 hours. Bandages must be adjusted at appropriate intervals to prevent displacement of the splint. As soon as the dressings have been applied, the x-ray examination should be repeated. Examination should be done again on the third day after reduction. Thereafter, for at least 1 month, biplane x-rays are taken once a week. Immobilization is maintained until bone continuity of the ulna is restored; this usually requires 10−12 weeks or even longer, since healing is likely to be slow. Acute flexion of the elbow in plaster should not be decreased before the eighth week.

2. Posterior dislocation of the head of the radius— This lesion is caused by direct violence to the volar surface of the forearm. Treatment is by closed reduction. Anteroposterior and lateral x-rays are then taken, and a tubular plaster cast or stout posterior plaster splint is applied from the metacarpal heads to the axilla with the elbow in full extension and the forearm in midposition. Careful postreduction observation as for anterior dislocation (see above) is essential.

B. Open Reduction: If accurate reduction of the fracture and the dislocation cannot be achieved by closed methods, open reduction by the technic of Boyd is indicated. Plaster immobilization is indicated until bone healing is well under way.

Fracture of the Shaft of the Radius With Dislocation of the Ulnar Head

In fracture of the shaft of the radius near the junction of the middle and lower thirds with dislocation of the head of the ulna (Dupuytren's fracture, Galeazzi's fracture), the apex of major angulation is usually directed anteriorly while the ulnar head lies volar to the distal end of the radius. (Convex dorsal angulation with the ulnar head posterior to the lower end of the radius is rare.)

A. Closed Reduction: Anatomic alignment is difficult to obtain by closed manipulation and difficult to maintain in plaster, but these technics should be tried before open reduction is used. After reduction, anteroposterior and lateral x-rays are taken and developed before application of the cast. If reduction is adequate, a tubular plaster cast is applied from the axilla to the knuckles with the elbow at a right angle, the forearm in pronation, and the wrist in neutral position. Weekly x-ray examination is indicated during the first month. Immobilization in a snug tubular plaster cast is continued until healing of the radius is complete.

Immobilization of the rare posterior type is with the forearm in supination.

B. Open Reduction: If anatomic reduction cannot be achieved by closed methods, open reduction of recent fracture of the radius is recommended.

INJURIES OF THE WRIST REGION

SPRAINS OF THE WRIST

Isolated severe sprain of the ligaments of the wrist joint is not common, and the diagnosis of wrist sprain should not be made until other lesions, eg, injury to the lower radial epiphysis (in children) and carpal fractures and dislocations (in adults), have been ruled out. If symptoms persist for more than 2 weeks, and especially if pain and swelling are present, x-ray examination should be repeated.

Treatment may be by immobilization with a volar splint extending from the palmar flexion crease to the elbow. The splint should be attached with elastic bandages so that it can be removed at least 3 times daily for gentle active exercise and warm soaks.

COLLES' FRACTURE

Abraham Colles described the fracture that bears his name as an impacted fracture of the radius 4 cm above the wrist joint. Modern usage has extended the term Colles' fracture to include a variety of complete fractures of the distal radius characterized by convex volar angulation and by varying degrees of dorsal displacement of the distal fragment.

The fracture is commonly caused by a fall with the hand outstretched, the wrist in dorsiflexion, and the forearm in pronation, so that the force is applied to the palmar surface of the hand. Colles' fracture is most common in middle life and old age.

The fracture cleft may be transverse or oblique, and extends across the distal radius. It may be comminuted, extending into the radiocarpal joint. Displacement is often minimal, with dorsal impaction caused by tilting of the distal fragment and volar convex angulation. As displacement becomes more marked, dorsal and radial tilt of the distal fragment causes increased angulation and torsional displacement in supination of the distal fragment. The normal volar and ulnar inclination of the carpal articular surface of the radius is reduced or reversed.

Avulsion of the styloid process is the usual injury to the distal ulna. Extension of the fracture cleft into the ulnar notch may injure the distal radioulnar articulation. The carpus is displaced with the distal fragment of the radius. Marked displacement at the fracture site causes dislocation of the distal radioulnar and ulnocarpal articulations, and tearing of the triangular fibrocartilage, both radioulnar ligaments, and the volar ulnocarpal ligament. If the ulnar styloid is not fractured, then the collateral ulnar ligament is torn. The head of the ulna lies anterior to the distal fragment of the radius.

Clinical Findings

Clinical findings vary according to the magnitude of injury, the degree of displacement of fragments, and the interval since injury. If the fragments are not displaced, examination soon after injury will demonstrate only slight tenderness and insignificant swelling; pain may be absent. Marked displacement produces the classic "silver fork" or "bayonet" deformity, in which a dorsal prominence caused by displacement of the distal fragment replaces the normal convex curve of the lower radius and the ulnar head is prominent on the anteromedial aspect of the wrist. Later, swelling may extend from the fingertips to the elbow.

Complications

Derangement of the distal radioulnar joint is the most common complicating injury. Direct injury to the median nerve by bone spicules is not common. Compression of the nerve by hemorrhage and edema or by displaced bone fragments is frequent and may cause all gradations of sensory and motor paralysis. Initial treatment of the fracture by immobilization of the wrist in acute flexion can be a significant factor in aggravation of compression. Persistent compression of the nerve creates classic symptoms of the carpal tunnel syndrome, which may require operative division of the volar carpal ligament for relief. Other complicating injuries are fractures involving the carpal navicular, the head of the radius, or the capitellum. Dislocation of the elbow and shoulder and tears of the capsulotendinous cuff of the shoulder may be associated.

Treatment

Complete recovery of function and a pleasing cosmetic result are goals of treatment which cannot always be achieved. The patient's age, sex, and occupation, the presence of complicating injury or disease, the severity of comminution, and the configuration of the fracture cleft govern the selection of treatment.

Open reduction of recent closed Colles' fracture is rarely the treatment of choice. Many technics of closed reduction and external immobilization have been advocated; the experience and preference of the surgeon determine the selection.

A. Minor Displacement: Colles' fracture with minimal displacement is characterized by absence of comminution and slight dorsal impaction. Deformity is barely perceptible, or may not be visible even to a trained observer. In the elderly patient, treatment is directed toward early recovery of function. In young patients, prevention of further displacement is the first consideration.

Reduction is not necessary. The wrist is immobilized for 3–5 days in a volar plaster splint extending from the distal palmar flexion crease to the elbow. Thereafter the splint may be removed periodically (4–5 times daily) to permit active exercise of the wrist. Soaking the hand and forearm for 15–20 minutes in warm water 2–3 times a day tends to relieve pain and stiffness. The splint can usually be discarded within 2 weeks.

B. Marked Displacement: Early reduction and immobilization are indicated. When reduction has been delayed until preliminary healing is advanced, open reduction may be elected or correction of the deformity can be deferred until healing is sound. The malunion can then be corrected by osteotomy and bone grafting.

In an old person with complicating arthritis, when impaction causes stability, the mild deformity may be accepted in favor of early restoration of function.

1. Stable fractures–Colles' fracture is characterized by comminution of the dorsal cortex. Correction of the deformity creates a wedge-shaped area of fragmented and impacted cancellous bone. The base of the wedge is directed dorsally, and there is no buttress to prevent recurrence of displacement. In part, stability is attained by bringing the volar cortices of the fragments into anatomic apposition.

Muscular relaxation of the extremity can usually be attained more readily under general anesthesia, but local anesthesia is commonly the better choice for the elderly patient.

Reduction is by manipulation. Success of manipulation is determined by clinical examination. Swelling is dissipated by massaging the volar and lateral aspects of the radius until the subcutaneous border can be palpated. Restoration of the normal convex curve of the distal radius implies that transverse displacement and angulation are absent. Proximal displacement has been reduced if the radial styloid process can be palpated 1 cm distal to the ulnar styloid.

A lightly padded tubular cast extending above the elbow or a "sugar tong" splint (Fig 46–23) is preferred. The plaster should extend distally only to the palmar flexion crease, with the forearm in midposition and the wrist in slight volar flexion and ulnar deviation. In obese patients, immobilization is more reliable if the elbow is included in the plaster. After the plaster has been applied, it is molded carefully around the wrist until it has set. X-rays are taken while anesthesia is continued. If x-rays show that reduction is not adequate, remanipulation is carried out immediately.

X-ray examination is repeated on the third day and thereafter at weekly intervals during the first 3 weeks. The plaster must remain snug; if loosening occurs after absorption of hemorrhagic exudate, a new cast should be applied.

2. Unstable fractures–If x-rays show extensive comminution with intra-articular extension and involvement of the volar cortex, the fracture is likely to be unstable and skeletal distraction is probably indicated by means of traction on Kirschner wires (Fig 46–24). Traction is continued while the plaster is applied. To ensure maximal external support, the extremity is immobilized in a tubular plaster cast extending from the axilla to the palmar flexion crease, with the elbow at a right angle, the forearm in midposition, and the wrist in slight ulnar deviation and volar flexion. The Kirschner wires are incorporated in the plaster, and the bows are maintained to hold the wires taut (Fig 46–25). The wires are left in place for 6 weeks. The fracture is protected for an additional 2 weeks following removal of the wires by a gauntlet or a "sugar tong" splint.

Postreduction Treatment

Frequent observation and careful management can prevent or minimize some of the disabling sequelae of Colles' fracture. The patient's full cooperation in the exercise program is essential. If comminution is marked, if swelling is severe, or if there is evidence of median nerve deficit, the patient should remain under close observation (preferably in a hospital) for at least 72 hours. The extremity should be elevated to minimize swelling, and the adequacy of circulation determined at frequent intervals. Active exercise of the fingers and shoulder is encouraged. In order that the extremity should be used as much as possible, the plaster should be trimmed in the palm to permit full finger flexion.

As soon as the plaster is removed, the patient is advised to use the extremity for customary daily care but to avoid strenuous activity that might cause refracture.

Complications & Sequelae

Joint stiffness is the most disabling sequel of Colles' fracture. Derangement of the distal radioulnar joint may be caused by the original injury and perpetuated by incomplete reduction; it is characterized by restriction of forearm movements and pain. Late rupture of the extensor pollicis longus tendon is relatively uncommon. Symptoms of median nerve injury due to compression caused by acute swelling alone usually do not persist more than 6 months. Prolonged symptoms can cause carpal tunnel syndrome. Failure to

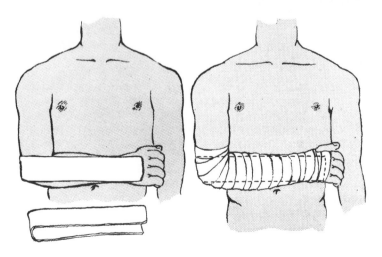

FIG 46–23. "Sugar tong" plaster splint.

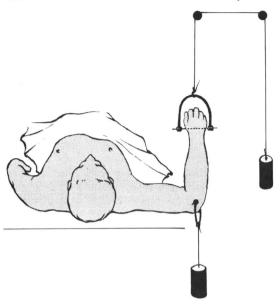

FIG 46—24. Skeletal distraction for closed manipulation of fracture of the forearm or wrist.

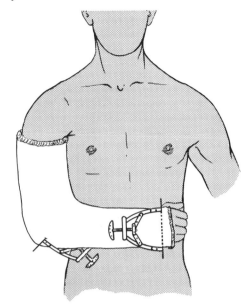

FIG 46—25. Full upper extremity plaster with Kirschner wires incorporated.

perform shoulder joint exercises several times daily can result in disabling stiffness.

SMITH'S FRACTURE
("REVERSED COLLES")

The distal fragment of the radius is displaced forward and the apex of angulation is directed dorsally so that the normal volar convexity of the lower radius is increased. The ulnar head may be displaced dorsally and there may be derangement of the inferior radioulnar joint.

The fracture can be reduced by closed manipulation, and immobilized with the wrist in dorsiflexion and ulnar deviation.

FRACTURE OF THE RADIAL STYLOID

Forced radial deviation of the hand at the wrist joint can fracture the radial styloid. A large fragment of the styloid is usually displaced by impingement against the carpal navicular. Avulsion of the tip of the styloid by the radial collateral ligament occurs less frequently, and may be associated with dislocation of the radiocarpal joint. If the fragment is large, it can be displaced farther by the brachioradialis muscle, which inserts into it.

Because the fracture is intra-articular, reduction of large fragments should be anatomic. If the styloid

fragment is not displaced, immobilization in a plaster gauntlet for 3 weeks is sufficient. If the fragment is displaced, manipulative reduction should be tried. If the distal, smaller fragment tends to displace but can be apposed by digital pressure, percutaneous fixation can be achieved by a medium Kirschner wire inserted through the proximal anatomic snuffbox so as to transfix both fragments. The wrist is then immobilized in a snugly molded plaster gauntlet for 6 weeks. X-ray examination is repeated every week for at least 3 weeks.

If closed methods fail, open reduction is indicated since persistent displacement is likely to cause posttraumatic degenerative arthritis relatively early.

FRACTURE OF THE DISTAL
RADIAL EPIPHYSIS

Fracture through the distal radial epiphyseal plate in children is the counterpart of Colles' fracture in the adult. Wrist sprain is rare in childhood and should be differentiated as early as possible from fracture of the distal epiphysis. Such an injury is usually caused by indirect violence due to a fall on the outstretched hand. The magnitude of displacement of the epiphyseal fragment varies.

In some cases, separation and displacement of the epiphysis cannot be demonstrated by radiologic examination and may be quite difficult to identify on clinical examination. The patient may complain of pain in the region of the wrist joint, and slight swelling may be present. Pressure with a blunt object, eg, the eraser of a lead pencil, may demonstrate maximal tenderness at the epiphyseal plate instead of at the wrist joint. Buckling of the adjacent metaphyseal cortex manifests greater displacement.

Displacement is posterior and to the radial side. Marked displacement may be accompanied by crushing of the epiphyseal plate, tear of the triangular fibrocartilage of the distal radioulnar articulation, displacement of the distal ulnar epiphysis, or avulsion of the ulnar styloid.

Both wrists should be examined by x-ray if injury to the distal radial epiphysis is suspected. Severe injury, crushing the epiphyseal cartilage and fracturing the epiphysis, is likely to impede growth and may even lead to early epiphyseal fusion; continued growth of the distal ulnar epiphysis produces derangement of the distal radioulnar joint.

If radial deviation of the hand becomes marked, symptomatic Madelung's deformity may result.

Open reduction is rarely necessary. The trauma of the operation superimposed on the injury is likely to cause early arrest of epiphyseal growth. Closed reduction by manipulation is usually successful if it can be done within the week following injury. Immobilization is with a plaster gauntlet or "sugar tong" splint. The plaster should be worn for 4–6 weeks. Permanent stiffness due to immobilization of the wrist is not to be feared.

The child should be examined yearly to determine whether there is any growth disturbance.

FRACTURE-DISLOCATIONS OF THE RADIOCARPAL JOINT

Dislocation of the radiocarpal joint without fracture is rare. Dislocation without injury to one of the carpal bones is usually associated with fracture of the anterior surface of the radius or the ulna. Comminuted fracture of the distal radius may involve either the anterior or posterior cortex and extends into the wrist joint. Subluxation of the carpus may occur at the same time. The most common fracture-dislocation of the wrist joint involves the posterior or anterior margin of the articular surface of the radius.

Anterior Fracture-Dislocation of the Radiocarpal Joint (Barton's Fracture)

Anterior fracture-dislocation of the wrist joint is characterized by fracture of the volar margin of the carpal articular surface of the radius. The fracture cleft extends proximally in the coronal plane in an oblique direction, so that the free fragment has a wedge-shaped configuration. The carpus is displaced volar and proximally with the articular fragment. This uncommon injury should be differentiated from Smith's fracture by x-ray examination.

Treatment by closed reduction may be successful, especially in cases in which the free fragment of the radius does not involve a large portion of the articular surface. Immobilization is with a tubular plaster cast extending from the palmar flexion crease to above the elbow with the wrist in volar flexion and the elbow at a right angle. Immediate x-rays are taken in 2 projections. If reduction is not anatomic and the fracture is unstable, skeletal distraction may be necessary. Weekly x-ray examination should be repeated during the first month. Skeletal distraction should be continued for 6 weeks or until preliminary bone healing has stabilized the fracture.

Posterior Fracture-Dislocation of the Radiocarpal Joint

Posterior fracture-dislocation of the wrist joint should be differentiated from Colles' fracture by x-ray. In most cases the marginal fragment is smaller than in anterior injury, and often involves the medial aspect where the extensor pollicis longus crosses the distal radius. If reduction is not anatomic, fraying of the tendon at this level may lead to late rupture.

Treatment is by manipulative reduction as for Colles' fracture and immobilization in a snug plaster gauntlet with the wrist in dorsiflexion.

DISLOCATION OF THE DISTAL RADIOULNAR JOINT

The triangular fibrocartilage is the most important structure in preventing dislocation of the distal radioulnar joint. The accessory ligaments and the pronator quadratus muscle play a secondary role. Complete anterior or posterior dislocation implies a tear of the triangular fibrocartilage and disruption of accessory joint ligaments. Tearing of the triangular fibrocartilage in the absence of major injury to the supporting capsular ligaments causes subluxation or abnormal laxity of the joint. Since the ulnar attachment of the triangular fibrocartilage is at the base of the styloid process, x-rays may demonstrate associated fracture. Widening of the cleft in comparison with the opposite radioulnar joint, which is apparent by x-ray examination, demonstrates diastasis of the radius and ulna if frank anterior or posterior displacement is not present.

Complete anterior or posterior dislocation of the distal radioulnar joint is rare. Medial dislocation is associated with fracture of the radius. The direction of dislocation is indicated by the location of the ulnar head in relation to the distal end of the radius.

FRACTURES & DISLOCATIONS OF THE CARPUS

Injury to the carpal bones occurs predominantly in men during the most active period of life. Because it is difficult to differentiate these injuries by clinical examination, it is imperative to obtain x-ray films of the best possible quality. The oblique film should be taken in midpronation, the anteroposterior film with the wrist in maximal ulnar deviation. Special views, such as midsupination to demonstrate the pisiform, and carpal tunnel views for the hamate, may be necessary.

Fracture of the Carpal Navicular

The most common injury to the carpus is fracture of the navicular. Fracture of the carpal navicular should be suspected in any injury to the wrist in an adult male unless a specific diagnosis of another type of injury is obvious. If tenderness on the radial aspect of the wrist is present and fracture cannot be demonstrated, initial treatment should be the same as if fracture were present (see below) and should be continued for at least 3 weeks. Further x-ray examination after 3 weeks may demonstrate an occult fracture.

Three types of fracture are distinguished:

(1) **Fracture of the tubercle:** This fracture usually is not widely displaced, and healing is generally prompt if immobilization in a plaster gauntlet is maintained for 2–3 weeks.

(2) **Fracture through the waist:** Fracture through the narrowest portion of the bone is the most common type. The blood supply to the proximal fragment is usually not disturbed, and healing will take place if reduction is adequate and treatment is instituted early. If the nutrient artery to the proximal third is injured, avascular necrosis of that portion of the bone may occur.

X-ray examination in multiple projections is necessary to determine the direction of the fracture cleft and displacement of the proximal fragment. If the proximal fragment is displaced, it can be reduced under local anesthesia by forced dorsiflexion and radial deviation of the wrist. Immobilization in a plaster gauntlet with the wrist in slight dorsiflexion is necessary. The plaster should extend distally to the palmar flexion crease in the hand and to the base of the thumbnail. If reduction has been anatomic and the blood supply to the proximal fragment has not been jeopardized, adequate bone healing can be expected within 10 weeks. However, such healing must be demonstrated by the disappearance of the fracture cleft and restoration of the trabecular pattern between the 2 main fragments. X-ray examination to verify healing should be repeated 3 weeks after removal of the cast.

(3) **Fracture through the proximal third:** Fracture through the proximal third of the navicular is likely to be associated with injury to the arterial supply of the minor fragment. This can be manifested by avascular necrosis of that fragment. If the lesion is observed soon after injury, reduction and immobilization in a plaster gauntlet will promote healing. The plaster gauntlet should be applied snugly, and must be changed if it becomes loose; it is usually necessary to renew the gauntlet every 4 weeks. X-rays should be taken once a month to determine the progress of bone healing; it

may be necessary to prolong immobilization for 4–6 months. The same criteria of radiographic examination as are used for healing of fractures through the waist are used in fractures of the proximal third. It is advisable to make an additional x-ray examination 3–4 weeks after removal of the cast.

If evidence of healing is not apparent after immobilization for 6 months or more, further immobilization will probably not be effective. This is especially true if x-rays show that the fracture cleft has widened and if sclerosis is noted adjacent to the cleft. If the interval between the time of injury and the establishment of a diagnosis is 3 months or more, a trial of immobilization for 2–3 months may be elected. If obliteration of the fracture cleft and evidence of restoration of bone continuity are not visible in x-rays taken after this trial period, some form of operative treatment will be necessary to initiate bone healing. Bone grafting is probably more successful. Prolonged immobilization in a plaster gauntlet is necessary before bony continuity is restored.

If avascular necrosis has occurred in the proximal fragment, bone grafting is less likely to be successful. Although excision of the avascular fragment may relieve painful symptoms for a time, the patient usually notes weakness of grasp and discomfort after prolonged use. Posttraumatic arthritis is apt to develop late.

Prolonged failure of bone healing predisposes to posttraumatic arthritis. Bone grafting operations or other procedures directed toward restoration of bone continuity may be successful, but arthritis causes continued disability. Arthrodesis of the wrist gives the best assurance of relief of pain and a functionally competent extremity.

Fracture of the Lunate

Fracture of the lunate may be manifested by minor avulsion fractures of the posterior or anterior horn. Careful multiplane x-ray examination is necessary to establish the diagnosis. Either of these lesions may be treated by the use of a volar splint for 3 weeks.

Fracture of the body may be manifested by a crack, by comminution, or by impaction. A fissure fracture can be treated by immobilization in plaster for 3 weeks.

One complication of this fracture is persistent pain in the wrist, slight restriction of motion, and tenderness over the lunate. X-ray examination can demonstrate areas of sclerosis and rarefaction. Impaction or collapse can be accompanied by arthritic changes surrounding the lunate. This x-ray appearance is referred to as Kienböck's disease, osteochondrosis of the lunate, or avascular necrosis.

Fracture of the Hamate

Fracture of the hamate may occur through the body and is shown on x-ray as a fissure or compression. Fracture of the base of the hamulus is less common and more difficult to diagnose; special projections are necessary to demonstrate the cleft. If the hamulus is displaced, closed manipulation will not be effective. Prolonged painful symptoms or evidence of irritation of the ulnar nerve may require excision of the loose fragment.

Fracture of the Triquetrum

Fracture of the triquetrum is caused commonly by direct violence and is often associated with fracture of other carpal bones. Treatment is by immobilization in a plaster gauntlet for 4 weeks.

Dislocation of the Lunate

Dislocation of the lunate is the second most common injury of the carpus. Dislocation is caused by forced dorsiflexion of the wrist, and the direction of dislocation is almost always anterior. The diagnosis is usually made by x-ray examination. Dislocation may be manifest by dorsal displacement of the capitate while the lunate retains contact with the radius. A further degree of injury is manifested by complete displacement of the lunate from the radius, so that it comes to lie anterior to the capitate and loses its relationship to the articular surface of the radius. If x-ray examination is adequate, the diagnosis can be established easily.

Reduction may be achieved by closed manipulation. X-rays are then taken to determine the success of treatment. If reduction is adequate, the extremity is immobilized in a plaster gauntlet with the wrist in full volar flexion for about 2 weeks. The plaster is then removed and another applied with the wrist in neutral position for an additional 2 weeks. If x-rays show that this manipulative maneuver has not caused reduction, skeletal distraction by means of Kirschner wires may separate the radiocarpal joint sufficiently to permit manipulative reduction (Fig 46–24). If closed methods are not successful, open reduction should be done promptly.

Dislocation of the Capitate

Dislocation of the capitate is most often associated with other lesions of the carpus and is commonly called transcarpal or midcarpal dislocation. The most frequent accompanying injury is fracture of the carpal navicular, in which case the lunate and the proximal fragment of the navicular retain their relationship to the articular surface of the radius whereas the distal fragment of the navicular, the capitate, and the remainder of the carpus are displaced dorsally. Thus the dislocation is retrolunar.

Subluxation of the navicular is less often associated with dislocation of the lunate. The direction of this dislocation is also retrolunar. Fracture of the radioulnar styloid processes is likely to be present also.

X-rays of poor technical quality may not demonstrate the lesion satisfactorily; anteroposterior and true lateral projections are necessary.

The comparatively uncommon midcarpal dislocation can be reduced by closed manipulation if the lesion is uncomplicated and recognized within 10–14 days after injury. Immobilization in a plaster gauntlet

with the wrist in slight dorsiflexion for 4 weeks is sufficient for stabilization by early ligamentous healing. If fracture complicates the dislocation, treatment is divided into 2 phases. Reduction of the fracture-dislocation is accomplished by closed manipulation. The navicular fracture is then treated as outlined above.

INJURIES OF THE HIP REGION

BIRTH FRACTURE OF THE UPPER FEMORAL EPIPHYSES

Birth injury to the upper femoral epiphyses is rare, and the diagnosis by physical examination alone is difficult because the skeletal structures involved are deeply situated. Swelling of the upper thigh and pseudoparalysis of the extremity following a difficult delivery suggest the injury. X-ray examination may demonstrate outward and proximal displacement of the shaft of the femur. Formation of new bone in the region of the metaphysis may be demonstrated in 7–10 days. If displacement has occurred, treatment for 2–3 weeks by Bryant's traction (Fig 46–31) is recommended. Otherwise, protection by a perineal pillow splint for the same length of time is adequate.

DISPLACEMENT & SEPARATION OF THE CAPITAL FEMORAL EPIPHYSIS

Displacement of the capital femoral epiphysis due to trauma in the normal child should be differentiated from idiopathic slipped epiphysis (epiphysiolysis, adolescent coxa vara) due possibly to endocrine or metabolic dysfunction. However, between the ages of 10 and 16 years, differentiation may be impossible. Mild injury may cause sudden separation and displacement because of weakening of the plate by antecedent idiopathic disturbance of cartilage growth.

Traumatic separation of the capital femoral epiphysis is rare in normal children, but it may occur as a result of a single episode of severe trauma which otherwise might cause fracture of the femoral neck. The direction of displacement is likely to be the same as in adolescent coxa vara. Although anatomic reduction can be obtained by closed manipulation, immobilization in a plaster spica should not be trusted since redisplacement is possible; internal fixation is more reliable. Traumatic separation of the capital epiphysis associated with dislocation of the hip joint (epiphysis and proximal femur) is a rare lesion with an unfavorable prognosis. Avascular necrosis of the epiphysis is almost certain.

FRACTURE OF THE FEMORAL NECK

Fracture of the femoral neck occurs most commonly in patients over the age of 50. If displacement has occurred, the extremity is in external rotation and adduction. Leg shortening is usually obvious. Motion of the hip joint causes pain. If the fracture is impacted in the valgus position, the injured extremity may be slightly longer than the opposite side and active external rotation may not be possible. If the fragments are not displaced and the fracture is stable, pain at the extremes of passive hip motion may be the only significant finding. The fact that the patient can actively move the extremity often interferes with prompt diagnosis.

Before treatment is instituted, anteroposterior and lateral films of excellent quality must be obtained; if adequate detail is not demonstrated in the initial films, repeated exposure should be made. Gentle traction and internal rotation of the extremity while the anteroposterior film is exposed may provide a more favorable relation of fragments to demonstrate the fracture cleft.

Fractures of the femoral neck may be classified as abduction or adduction fractures.

Abduction Fracture of the Femoral Neck

Abduction describes the relationship between the neck and shaft fragment and the head, which creates a coxa valga deformity. Abduction fractures occur most often in the proximal femoral neck adjacent to the head. Displacement is apt to be minimal, and impaction is often present. The direction of the fracture cleft approaches the transverse plane of the body, and the angle is 30 degrees or less (Fig 46−26). The anteroposterior x-ray may show a wedge-shaped area of increased density whose base is directed superiorly. A good lateral film will demonstrate both the anterior and posterior cortices of the femoral neck. In this plane the neck and shaft fragment may be angulated slightly, so that only the posterior cortex appears to be impacted and the anterior cortices of the fragments appear to be separated.

Impaction is precarious and undependable as a fixation mechanism; if internal fixation is not used, separation may occur before healing is sound. If firm impaction can be demonstrated in both the anterior

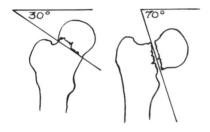

FIG 46−26. Pauwel's angles.

and posterior x-rays, some surgeons recommend conservative treatment, ie, bed rest with the extremity in balanced suspension for 4−8 weeks. The patient is then permitted to be ambulatory with crutches, but full weight-bearing is not permitted until complete healing can be demonstrated by x-rays (usually 4−12 months after injury). Other surgeons prefer internal fixation because it permits the patient to be out of bed soon after the operation even though unsupported weight-bearing is not permitted any sooner than after nonoperative treatment.

If examination in the lateral projection does not show firm impaction of both cortices at the fracture site, closed manipulation and internal fixation are indicated.

Adduction Fracture of the Femoral Neck

Adduction fracture is characterized by coxa vara deformity. The fracture may be at any level of the neck, and the direction of the fracture cleft approaches that of the sagittal plane of the body. Displacement is usually present. The relatively vertical configuration of the fracture cleft favors proximal displacement of the distal fragment by the force of any axial thrust transmitted through the extremity. The fracture should be considered unstable if the angle between the fracture cleft and the transverse plane of the body is greater than 30 degrees (Pauwels) (Fig 46−26). Internal fixation is necessary to prevent displacement after reduction since immobilization in a spica or treatment by traction is not reliable.

Adduction fracture of the femoral neck is a life-endangering injury; treatment is directed toward the preservation of life and restoration of function of the hip joint. Some surgeons believe that immediate operative treatment is required; others reply that 1−2 days of evaluation of the general health status of the patient while in traction is associated with a lowered mortality rate.

Preliminary treatment may be by skin or preferably by skeletal traction. X-rays are repeated in 12−24 hours to determine the adequacy of reduction. Comminution which was not evident on the initial examination will often be demonstrated on films taken with the fracture fragments in a more anatomic position.

Open operation is the treatment of choice. If internal fixation is adequate, postoperative immobilization is not necessary. The patient can be free in bed and can be mobilized at an early date; complications are minimized. If fixation is precarious, traction in balanced suspension for 1−4 months may be necessary until preliminary healing gives additional stability.

Weight-bearing should not be permitted until bone continuity is restored and avascular necrosis is not an immediate threat. The agile and cooperative patient may be ambulatory on crutches (but without weight-bearing) within a few days after operative treatment. Crutch walking is hazardous in elderly patients since inadvertent loading is likely to disrupt the fracture relationship.

The most common sequelae of cervical fracture of

the femur are redisplacement after reduction, failure of bone healing, and osteonecrosis (avascular or aseptic necrosis) of the head fragment. Posttraumatic arthritis appears relatively late.

Femoral Neck Fracture in Childhood

Traumatic cervical fracture of the femur in childhood (rare) must be differentiated from congenital coxa vara. Traumatic fracture is usually caused by severe injury. Anatomic reduction by closed manipulation and immobilization in a plaster spica are necessary to prevent deformity. Internal fixation with wires or screws may be necessary. Removal of the fixation apparatus after healing may prevent early fusion of the epiphysis.

Osteonecrosis of the capital epiphysis is a frequent sequel.

TROCHANTERIC FRACTURES

Fracture of the Lesser Trochanter

Isolated fracture of the lesser trochanter is quite rare but may develop as a result of the avulsion force of the iliopsoas muscle. It occurs commonly as a component of intertrochanteric fracture.

Fracture of the Greater Trochanter

Isolated fracture of the greater trochanter may be caused by direct injury, or may occur indirectly as a result of the activity of the gluteus medius and gluteus minimus muscles. It occurs most commonly as a component of intertrochanteric fracture.

If displacement is less than 1 cm and there is no tendency to further displacement (determined by repeated x-ray examinations), treatment may be by bed rest with the affected extremity in balanced suspension until acute pain subsides. As rapidly as symptoms permit, activity can increase gradually to protected weight-bearing with crutches. Full weight-bearing is permitted as soon as healing is apparent, usually in 6–8 weeks. If displacement is greater than 1 cm and increases on adduction of the thigh, extensive tearing of surrounding soft tissues may be assumed and open reduction is indicated, followed by internal fixation with 2–3 loops of stainless steel wire.

Intertrochanteric (Including Pertrochanteric) Fractures

These fractures occur most commonly among elderly persons. The cleft of an intertrochanteric fracture extends upward and outward from the medial region of the junction of the neck and lesser trochanter toward the summit of the greater trochanter. Pertrochanteric fracture includes both trochanters, and is likely to be comminuted.

It is important to determine whether comminution has occurred and the magnitude of displacement. These fractures may vary from fissure fracture without

significant separation to severe comminution into 4 major fragments: head-neck, greater trochanter, lesser trochanter, and shaft. Displacement may be so marked that the head-neck fragment forms a right angle with the shaft fragment and the distal fragment is rotated externally through an arc of 90 degrees.

Failure of restoration of bone continuity by healing of intertrochanteric fractures is unlikely and, when it occurs, the causes are usually apparent. Of the many factors that influence the rate of healing, those of particular significance are inadequate treatment as manifested by incomplete reduction with unsatisfactory apposition of fragments and unsustained immobilization; comminution; and osteopenia (osteoporosis and disuse atrophy). Healing in malposition (varus and external rotation) is abetted by the major stresses that cause displacement (gravity and muscle activity).

Initial treatment of the fracture in the hospital can be by balanced suspension and, when indicated, by the addition of traction. The selection of definitive treatment—closed or operative technics—depends in part upon the general condition of the patient. Because of the elderly age group in which intertrochanteric fracture is likely to occur, multiple system disease is a determinant of the mortality rate and for that reason the incidence of complications is diminished by the avoidance of prolonged recumbency in bed. Some surgeons are of the opinion that delay in open treatment is hazardous to the life of the patient, and they prefer to operate promptly. Others believe that an evaluation of the general health status of the patient should be made and that preliminary treatment of the fracture—reduction by closed technics—can proceed simultaneously.

Undisplaced fractures can be treated by balanced suspension of the lower extremity until the fragments are stabilized by preliminary bone healing. These fractures can also be treated initially by immobilization in a plaster spica. Sufficient healing generally occurs within 2–3 months to permit the patient to follow a bed and wheelchair existence until partial weight-bearing with crutches can be initiated. Unsupported weight-bearing should not be resumed until the fracture cleft has been obliterated by healing.

If comminution is present and displacement is significant, skin or (preferably) skeletal traction by a Kirschner wire through the tibial tubercle must be added to provide immobilization and to accomplish reduction. Definitive treatment of the fracture can be given in this way or it can be used as a preliminary to open operation.

Open operation may be done electively or may be mandatory for optimal treatment. Reduction of the fracture can be accomplished by closed technics, or it can be an integral part of the open operation. Some surgeons do not prefer to anatomically reduce unstable fractures caused by comminution of the medial femoral cortex. It is maintained that medial displacement of the upper end of the main distal fragment enhances mechanical stability (although it may cause concomitant varus deformity), and this advantageously permits

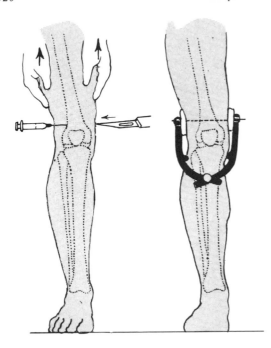

FIG 46–27. Technic of insertion of Kirschner wire in the supracondylar region of the femur.

earlier weight-bearing and more prompt healing. The chief intent of open operation is to provide sufficient fixation of the fragments by a metallic surgical implant so that the patient need not be confined to bed during the healing process.

Intertrochanteric fracture during childhood can be treated by skeletal traction with a Kirschner wire inserted through the lower femur above the epiphyseal line (Fig 46–27) or by closed reduction and internal fixation. Varus deformity should be avoided if possible. The incidence of avascular necrosis of the capital femoral epiphysis following this fracture is high.

SUBTROCHANTERIC FRACTURE

Subtrochanteric fracture due to severe trauma occurs below the level of the lesser trochanter at the junction of cancellous and cortical bone. It is most common in men during the active years of life. Soft tissue damage is extensive. The direction of the fracture cleft may be transverse or oblique. Comminution occurs and the fracture may extend proximally into the intertrochanteric region or distally into the shaft. Muscle is often interposed between the major fragments.

Closed reduction should be attempted by continuous traction to bring the distal fragment into alignment with the proximal fragment. If comminution is not extensive and the lesser trochanter is not detached, the proximal fragment is often drawn into relative

flexion, external rotation, and abduction by the predominant activity of the iliopsoas, gluteus medius, and gluteus minimus muscles.

Prolonged skeletal traction by means of a Kirschner wire inserted through the supracondylar region of the femur (with the hip and knee flexed to a right angle) is necessary (Fig 46–28). X-ray is repeated every 4–8 hours until reduction has been accomplished. If soft tissue interposition is not a factor, reduction can be achieved within 48 hours. Thereafter the extremity is left in this position with an appropriate amount of traction until stabilization occurs, usually in 8–12 weeks. The angle of flexion is then reduced by gradually bringing the hip and knee into extension. After 2–3 months of continuous traction, the extremity can be immobilized in a plaster spica provided stabilization of the fracture has occurred. Weight-bearing must not be resumed for 6 months or even longer, until bone healing obliterates the fracture cleft.

Interposition of soft tissue between the major fragments may prevent closed reduction. Open reduction of this fracture is difficult and should be undertaken early; if treatment is delayed until the third week following injury, extensive bleeding at the fracture site is likely to be encountered.

After open reduction has been performed, internal fixation is required to prevent redisplacement. If comminution is present, or if it is important to avoid prolonged immobilization, biplane fixation is recommended.

The activity status after operation depends upon the adequacy of internal fixation. If fixation is precarious, skeletal traction in balanced suspension should be continued until healing is well under way. Otherwise, if the patient is agile and cooperative, he may be ambulatory on crutches (but without weight-bearing) a few days after the operation.

DISLOCATION OF THE HIP JOINT

Dislocation of the hip joint may occur with or without fracture of the pelvis. It occurs most commonly during the most active years of life as a result of severe trauma. The femoral head can be completely dislocated from the acetabulum only if the ligamentum teres is ruptured.

Posterior Hip Dislocation

The head of the femur is usually dislocated posterior to the acetabulum while the thigh is flexed, eg, as may occur in a head-on automobile collision when the passenger's knee is driven violently against the dashboard.

The significant clinical findings are shortening, adduction, and internal rotation of the extremity. Anteroposterior, transpelvic, and, if fracture of the acetabulum is demonstrated, oblique projections are

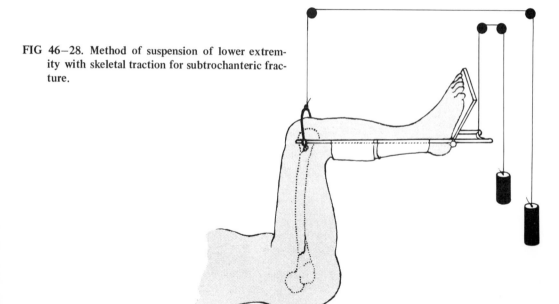

FIG 46–28. Method of suspension of lower extremity with skeletal traction for subtrochanteric fracture.

required. Common complications are fracture of the acetabulum, injury to the sciatic nerve, and fracture of the head or shaft of the femur. The head of the femur may be displaced through a rent in the posterior hip joint capsule, or the glenoid lip may be avulsed from the acetabulum. The short external rotator muscles of the hip joint are commonly lacerated. Fracture of the posterior margin of the acetabulum can create an unstable mechanism.

If the acetabulum is not fractured or if the fragment is small, reduction by closed manipulation either by Bigelow's or Stimson's method is indicated.

The success of reduction is determined immediately by anteroposterior and lateral x-rays. Interposition of capsule substance will be manifest by widening of the joint cleft. If reduction is adequate the hip will be stable with the extremity in extension and slight external rotation.

Postreduction treatment may be by immobilization in a plaster spica or by balanced suspension. Since this is primarily a soft tissue injury, sound healing should take place in 4 weeks. Active hip joint movements may be instituted then, but even partial weight-bearing should be deferred for at least 3 months and full weight-bearing for 6 months.

If the posterior or superior acetabulum is fractured, dislocation of the hip must be assumed to have occurred even though displacement is not present at the time of examination. Undisplaced fissure fractures may be treated by bed rest for 3 weeks and avoidance of weight-bearing for 2 months. Frequent examination is necessary to make certain that the head of the femur has not become displaced from the acetabulum.

Minor fragments of the posterior margin of the acetabulum may be disregarded unless they are in the hip joint cavity. Larger displaced fragments often cannot be reduced adequately by closed methods. If the fragment is large and the hip is unstable following closed manipulation, open operation is indicated. If the sciatic nerve has been injured it should be exposed and treated by appropriate neurosurgical technics when the posterior hip joint is exposed. The fragment is then placed in anatomic position and fixed with 1–2 bone screws.

After the operation the patient is placed in bed with the extremity in balanced suspension (Fig 46–29) under 5–8 kg of skeletal traction on the tibial tubercle for about 6 weeks or until healing of the acetabular fracture is sound. Full weight-bearing is not permitted for 6 months or more.

Anterior Hip Dislocation

In anterior hip dislocation the head of the femur may lie medially on the obturator membrane, beneath the obturator externus muscle (obturator or thyroid dislocation), or, in a somewhat more superior direction, beneath the iliopsoas muscle and in contact with the superior ramus of the pubis (pubic dislocation). The thigh is classically in flexion, abduction, and external rotation, and the head of the femur is palpable anteriorly and distal to the inguinal flexion crease. Anteroposterior and lateral films are required; films prepared by transpelvic projection are likely to be helpful.

Closed manipulation with general anesthesia is usually adequate. Postreduction treatment may be by balanced suspension or by immobilization in a plaster spica with the hip in extension and the extremity in neutral rotation. Active hip motion is permitted after 3 weeks.

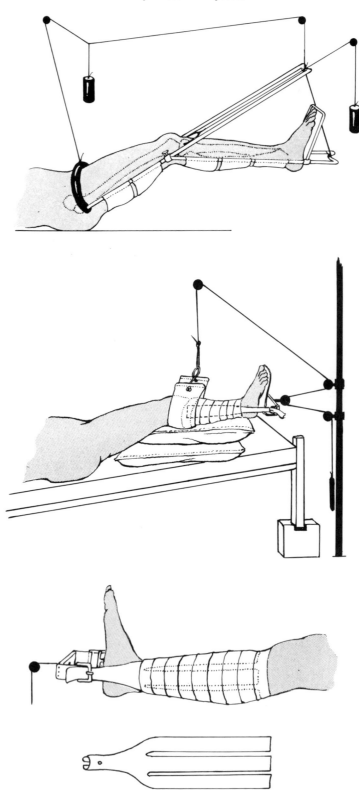

FIG 46–29. Methods of traction for lower extremity fractures. *Top:* Method of suspension of lower extremity with skeletal traction on tibial tubercle. *Center:* Russell's traction. *Bottom:* Method of application of skin traction.

Central Dislocation of the Hip
With Fracture of the Pelvis

Central dislocation of the head of the femur with fracture of the acetabulum may be caused by crushing injury or by an axial force transmitted through the abducted extremity to the acetabulum. Comminution is commonly present. There are usually 2 fragments: superiorly, the ilium with the roof of the acetabulum; inferiorly and medially, the remainder of the acetabulum and the obturator ring. Fracture occurs near the roof of the acetabulum, and the components of the obturator ring are displaced inward with the head of the femur. Extensive soft tissue injury and massive bleeding into the soft tissues are likely to be present. Intra-abdominal injury must not be overlooked. Initially, stereoanteroposterior and oblique x-rays are required.

In the absence of complicating injury or immediately after such an injury has received priority attention, closed treatment of the fracture-dislocation by skeletal traction is required. Open reduction is hazardous and technically difficult; it should not be attempted except by the expert. Bidirectional traction is likely to achieve the most satisfactory results in all but the exceptional case. For the average adult, approximately 10 kg of force are applied axially to the shaft of the femur, in neither abduction nor adduction, through a Kirschner wire placed preferably in the supracondylar region. A second Kirschner wire is inserted in the anteroposterior plane between the greater and lesser trochanters (in substantial cortical bone). Force is applied at a right angle to the direction of axial traction and the magnitude is the same. The extremity is placed in balanced suspension. Progress of reduction is observed by portable x-rays made 3 times a day until adequate positioning is manifested by relocation of the head of the femur beneath the roof of the acetabulum. Bidirectional traction is maintained for 4–6 weeks. Thereafter, the transverse traction component is gradually diminished under appropriate x-ray control until it can be discontinued. Axial traction is maintained until stabilization of the fracture fragments by early bone healing has occurred, usually about 8 weeks after injury. During the next 4–6 weeks, while balanced suspension is continued, gentle active exercises of the knee and hip are encouraged. After discontinuation of balanced suspension, more elaborate exercises designed to aid recovery of maximal hip function are performed frequently during the day. Full and unprotected weight-bearing should not be advised before 6 months.

Sequelae are common and the patient should be warned of their probable occurrence. Anatomic reduction is an unattainable goal in most severely comminuted and widely displaced fractures of this type. Scarring within and around the hip joint, with or without ectopic bone and exuberant callus formation, is incidental to the healing process and can be a significant factor in restriction of motion in varying degrees. Osteonecrosis of the femoral head and posttraumatic degenerative arthritis are common sequelae that appear somewhat later.

FRACTURE OF THE SHAFT
OF THE FEMUR

FRACTURE OF THE SHAFT OF THE FEMUR IN ADULTS

Fracture of the shaft of the femur usually occurs as a result of severe direct trauma. Indirect violence, especially torsional stress, is likely to cause spiral fractures that extend proximally or, more commonly, distally into the metaphyseal regions. These fractures are likely to be encountered in bone that has become atrophic as a result of disuse or senescence. Most are closed fractures; open fracture is often the result of compounding from within. Extensive soft tissue injury, bleeding, and shock are commonly present.

If the fracture is through the upper third of the shaft, the proximal fragment is apt to be in flexion, external rotation, and abduction, with proximal displacement or overriding of the distal fragment. In midshaft fracture the direction of displacement is not constant, but the distal fragment is almost always displaced proximally if the fracture is unstable; and angulation is commonly present with the apex directed anterolaterally. In complete fracture of the lower third of the shaft the distal fragment is often displaced proximally; the upper end of the distal fragment may be displaced posteriorly to the distal end of the upper fragment.

The most significant features are severe pain in the thigh and deformity of the lower extremity. Surgical shock is likely to be present. Careful x-ray examination in at least 2 planes is necessary to determine the exact site and configuration of the fracture cleft. Splints should be removed either by the surgeon or by a qualified assistant so that manipulation will not cause further damage. The hip and knee should be examined for associated injury.

Injuries to the sciatic nerve and to the superficial femoral artery and vein are not common but must be recognized promptly. Surgical shock and secondary anemia are the most important early complications. Later complications are essentially those of prolonged recumbency, eg, the formation of renal calculi.

Treatment

Treatment depends upon the age of the patient and the site and configuration of the fracture. Displaced, oblique, spiral, and comminuted fractures are unstable, and can rarely be treated successfully by closed manipulation and external plaster fixation. Traction followed by closed manipulation should be tried. Skeletal traction is generally the most effective form of closed treatment.

After preliminary traction, biplane x-rays are made to determine the progress of correction of overriding. If alignment and apposition of fragments are not satisfactory, closed manipulation, preferably under general anesthesia, should be carried out while traction is continued.

If soft tissue interposition prevents reduction by closed methods, open reduction may be required in the adult to avoid delay of bone healing.

A. Fracture of the Upper Third: The treatment of subtrochanteric fracture is discussed above. If a comminuted subtrochanteric fracture extends into the upper third of the femoral shaft, it may be necessary to use skeletal traction through the supracondylar region of the femur and suspend the extremity with the hip and knee at a right angle (Fig 46–28). Otherwise, skeletal traction can be through either the lower femur or the tibial tubercle with the extremity at a less acute angle in balanced suspension. Russell's traction can be used if the patient is small and muscular development is not great. External rotation and abduction of the extremity are usually required to bring the lower fragment into alignment with the proximal fragment.

B. Fracture of the Middle Third: The deformity caused by fracture at this level is not constant. Angulation is commonly present with the apex directed anterolaterally. Treatment may be by skeletal traction through the tibial tubercle or the lower end of the femur (Fig 46–29). Tr action in the transverse plane by a swathe around the thigh may be necessary to prevent recurrence of angulation.

C. Fracture of the Lower Third: In transverse and comminuted fractures, the proximal end of the distal fragment is likely to be displaced posterior to the distal end of the proximal fragment. The same displacement is likely to be encountered in supracondylar fracture. Russell's traction should not be used for comminuted or widely displaced fractures since it may injure the femoral or popliteal vessels. Simultaneous skeletal traction through the distal femur at right angles to the tibial tubercle can correct displacement of the distal fragment. The same mechanism of traction is used for supracondylar fracture (Fig 46–30).

After reduction has been accomplished by traction, biplane x-ray examination should be repeated at least weekly to determine maintenance of reduction and the progress of healing. When sufficient callus has formed to assure stabilization of the fragments, generally after 12 weeks or more, further immobilization can be given by a one and one half plaster spica. Prior to application of the spica, there should be a period of observation in balanced suspension without traction to determine whether displacement of the fracture fragments by overriding will occur. Angulation can generally be corrected in plaster by appropriate wedging.

Elective indications for open reduction and internal fixation may be based upon the desire to avoid prolonged recumbency in bed and hospitalization. Some mandatory indications include inability to obtain adequate reduction by closed technics and delay of bone healing. The purpose of open reduction is generally to provide anatomic reposition and clinically rigid fixation that will permit the patient to be ambulatory without such external supportive apparatus as casts, splints, or braces. Unprotected weightbearing without crutches until restoration of bone continuity should not be a goal of open operation of most fractures.

FRACTURE OF THE SHAFT OF THE FEMUR IN INFANTS & CHILDREN

Femoral fracture at birth occurs most often in the middle third. Comminution is usually not present.

Skin traction and plaster immobilization are adequate, although skeletal traction may be necessary in older children. Open reduction is rarely necessary.

Fracture of the proximal or middle third of the femur in a child under 5 years of age can be treated with Bryant's traction (Fig 46–31). Adhesive strips are

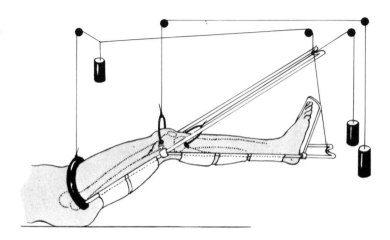

FIG 46–30. Method of suspension of lower extremity with biplane skeletal traction for supracondylar fracture.

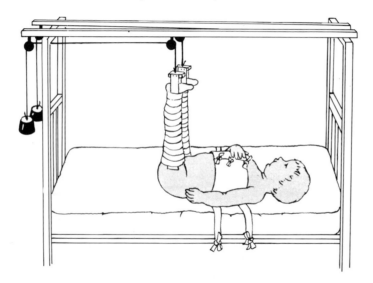

FIG 46–31. Bryant's traction.

applied to both extremities from the upper thirds of the thighs to the supramalleolar regions, and held firm by circular bandages. Both hips are flexed to a right angle, and the knees are maintained in full extension. Sufficient traction force is applied to raise the buttocks free of the bed. Circulatory adequacy must be observed carefully, and another method substituted if swelling, cyanosis or pallor of the foot, or obliteration of pedal pulsations cannot be managed by adjustment of dressings.

As a rule, sufficient callus is present at the fracture site after 3–4 weeks so that traction can be discontinued. If callus formation is adequate, infants who have not yet begun to walk need no further protection; walking infants may require a single plaster hip spica for an additional 4–6 weeks.

Preliminary treatment of unstable fracture of the femur in children over 5 years of age can be by Russell's traction (Fig 46–29). If the child is uncooperative, or if adequate correction cannot be obtained, it may also be necessary to place the sound extremity in traction. Traction should be continued until the fracture is stabilized; if traction is discontinued before the reparative callus is sufficiently mature, the deformity (especially angulation) may recur even though the extremity is protected by a plaster spica. Correction of angulation and torsional displacement around the long axis of the femur are mandatory. Slight shortening (1–2 cm) can be compensated by growth. Close apposition of fragments is not necessary, since healing will take place in spite of minimal soft tissue interposition.

It is usually necessary to continue traction for 6–8 weeks or until sufficient callus has formed to prevent recurrence of the deformity. Immobilization in a plaster spica should be maintained for another 2 months. Weight-bearing must not be resumed until x-rays show that healing is sound.

INJURIES OF THE KNEE REGION

FRACTURES OF THE DISTAL FEMUR

Supracondylar Fracture of the Femur

This comparatively uncommon fracture (at the junction of cortical and cancellous bone) may be transverse, oblique, or comminuted. The distal end of the proximal fragment is apt to perforate the overlying vastus intermedius, vastus medialis, or rectus femoris muscles, and may penetrate the suprapatellar pouch of the knee joint to cause hemarthrosis. The proximal end of the distal fragment is usually displaced posteriorly and slightly laterally.

Since the distal fragment may impinge upon the popliteal vessels, circulatory adequacy distal to the fracture site should be verified as soon as possible. Absence of pedal pulsations is an indication for immediate reduction. If pulsation does not return promptly after reduction, immediate exploration and appropriate treatment of the vascular lesion is indicated.

A less frequent complication is injury to the peroneal or tibial nerve.

If the fracture is transverse or nearly so, closed manipulation under general anesthesia will occasionally be successful. Stable fractures with minimal displacement can be immobilized in a single plaster hip spica with the hip and knee in about 30 degrees of flexion. Frequent x-ray examination is necessary to make certain that redisplacement has not occurred.

Stable or unstable uncomplicated supracondylar fracture is best treated with biplane skeletal traction if soft tissue interposition does not interfere with reduction (Fig 46–30). If adequate reduction cannot be obtained, it may be necessary to manipulate the fragments under general anesthesia, using skeletal traction to control the distal fragment.

Traction must be continued for about 6 weeks or until stabilization occurs. The wires can then be removed and the extremity immobilized in a single plaster spica for an additional 2–3 months.

An alternative method of treatment (applicable only to stable fractures) is to incorporate the wires into a plaster spica after reduction.

Supracondylar fracture is likely to be followed by restriction of knee motion due to scarring and adhesion formation in adjacent soft tissues.

Intercondylar Fracture of the Femur

This uncommon comminuted fracture, which occurs only in older patients, is classically described as T or Y according to the x-ray configuration of the fragments. Closed reduction is difficult when the proximal shaft fragment is interposed between the 2 main distal fragments. Maximal recovery of function of the knee joint requires anatomic reduction of the articular components. If alignment is satisfactory and displacement minimal, immobilization for about 4 months in a plaster spica will be sufficient. If displacement is marked, skeletal traction through the tibial tubercle (with the knee in flexion) is required. Manual molding of the distal fragments may be necessary. Open reduction and bolt fixation of the distal fragments may be indicated to restore articular congruity. Further treatment is as described for supracondylar fracture.

Condylar Fracture of the Femur

Isolated fracture of the lateral or medial condyle of the femur is a rare consequence of severe trauma. Occasionally only the posterior portion of the condyle is separated. The cruciate ligaments or the collateral ligament of the opposite side of the knee are often injured.

The objective of treatment is restoration of anatomic intra-articular relationships. If displacement is minimal, the knee can be manipulated into varus or valgus (opposite the position of deformity). If anatomic reduction cannot be obtained by closed manipulation, open reduction and fixation of the minor fragment with 2–3 bone screws is recommended. The ligaments must be explored, and repaired if found to be injured.

Separation of the Distal Femoral Epiphysis

Traumatic separation of the distal femoral epiphysis in children is the counterpart of supracondylar fracture in the adult. The direction of displacement of the epiphyseal fragment is most commonly anterior. Torsional displacement around the long axis of the femur may be associated.

Reduction of anterior displacement can be achieved by closed manipulation. After reduction is complete, the knee is flexed to a right angle and a tubular plaster cast is applied from the inguinal region to the toes. If the thigh is obese, the plaster should be extended proximally to include the pelvis in a single hip spica.

Peripheral circulation must be observed carefully. After 4 weeks the plaster is changed and flexion of the knee reduced to 135 degrees. At the end of the second month the patient may be permitted to be free in bed until he regains complete knee extension.

FRACTURES OF THE PROXIMAL TIBIA

Fracture of the Lateral Tibial Condyle

Fracture of the lateral condyle of the tibia is commonly caused by a blow on the lateral aspect of the knee with the foot in fixed position, producing an abduction strain. Hemarthrosis is always present, as the fracture cleft involves the knee joint. Soft tissue injuries are likely to be present also. The tibial collateral and anterior cruciate ligaments may be torn. A displaced free fragment may tear the overlying lateral meniscus. If displacement is marked, fracture of the proximal fibula may be present also.

The objective of treatment is to restore the articular surface and normal anatomic relationships, so that torn ligaments can heal without elongation. In cases of minimal displacement where ligaments have not been extensively damaged, treatment may be by immobilization for 6 weeks in a tubular plaster cast extending from the toes to the inguinal region with the knee in slight flexion. Reduction of marked displacement can be achieved by closed manipulation unless comminution is severe. After x-ray verification of reduction, the extremity can be immobilized in a tubular plaster cast extending from the inguinal region to the toes, preferably with the knee in full extension.

Many fractures of the lateral condyle of the tibia, especially comminuted fractures, cannot be reduced adequately by closed methods. Open reduction and stabilization with a bolt or multiple bone screws may be necessary.

Fracture of the Medial Tibial Condyle

Fracture of the medial condyle of the tibia is caused by the adduction strain produced by a blow against the medial aspect of the knee with the foot in fixed position. The medial meniscus and the fibular collateral ligament may be torn. Severe comminution is not usually present, and there is only one major free fragment.

Treatment is by closed reduction to restore the articular surface of the tibia so that ligamentous healing can occur without elongation. After reduction the extremity is immobilized for 10–12 weeks in a tubular plaster cast extending from the inguinal region to the toes with the knee in full extension. Weight-bearing is not permitted for 4 months at least.

Fracture of Both Tibial Condyles

Axial force, such as may result from falling on the

foot or sudden deceleration with the knee in full extension (during an automobile accident), can cause simultaneous fracture of both condyles of the tibia. Comminution is apt to be severe. Swelling of the knee due to hemarthrosis is marked. Deformity is either genu varum or genu valgum. X-ray examination should include oblique projections.

Severe comminution makes anatomic reduction difficult to achieve by any means and difficult to maintain following closed manipulation alone. Sustained skeletal traction is usually necessary. When stability has been achieved, the extremity can be immobilized for another 4–6 weeks in a tubular plaster cast extending from the toes to the inguinal region with the knee in full extension. Unassisted weight-bearing is not permitted before the end of the fourth month.

If closed methods are not effective, open reduction must be attempted.

Instability and restriction of motion of the knee are common sequelae. If reduction is not adequate, posttraumatic arthritis will appear early.

Fracture of the Tibial Tuberosity

Violent contraction of the quadriceps muscle may cause avulsion of the tibial tuberosity. Avulsion of the anterior portion of the upper tibial epiphysis, uncommon in childhood, must be differentiated from Osgood-Schlatter disease (osteochondrosis of the tibial tuberosity).

When avulsion of the tuberosity is complete, active extension of the knee is not possible.

If displacement is minimal, treatment is by immobilization in a tubular plaster cast extending from the inguinal to the supramalleolar region with the knee in full extension. Immobilization is maintained for 8 weeks or until stabilization occurs.

A loose fragment which has been displaced more than 0.5 cm can be treated either by closed reduction and percutaneous fixation, with plaster immobilization, or by open reduction.

Fracture of the Tibial Tubercle

This injury usually occurs in association with comminuted fracture of the condyles. The medial intercondyloid tubercle may be avulsed with adjacent bone attached to the anterior cruciate ligament, and injury to that structure is of greater importance. In addition to avulsion of the anterior cruciate ligament, there may also be injury to the tibial collateral ligament and the medial knee joint capsule. Hemarthrosis is always present.

Isolated and undisplaced fracture may be treated by immobilization of the extremity for 6 weeks in a tubular plaster cast extending from the inguinal region to the toes with the knee in slight flexion. The treatment of displaced fracture is the same as that of rupture of the anterior cruciate ligament (see below).

Separation of the Proximal Tibial Epiphysis

Complete displacement of the proximal tibial epiphysis is rare; partial separation due to forceful hyperextension of the knee is more common. The distal metaphyseal fragment is displaced posteriorly.

If no circulatory or neurologic deficit is present, immediate treatment by closed manipulation is indicated. Reduction can be accomplished by forced flexion of the knee. Anteroposterior films are then exposed by holding the plate against the anterior surface of the leg with the beam directed through the lower thigh. A lateral film is also prepared. If x-rays show that reduction is adequate, a heavy anterior plaster splint is applied from the inguinal region to the bases of the toes, with the knee in acute flexion. The splint is maintained in position with circular bandages around the foot, ankle, and upper thigh. The bandages are wrapped in figure-of-eight fashion around the thigh and leg (as is done for supracondylar fracture of the humerus). Peripheral circulation must be observed frequently for at least 72 hours. After 3 weeks the knee may be brought to a right angle and a tubular plaster cast applied from the inguinal region to the toes for another 3–4 weeks. Even guarded weight-bearing must be avoided until the end of the second month.

Injury to the proximal tibial epiphyseal plate as a result of a blow on the lateral aspect of the knee causes compression but only minor displacement. This lesion, analogous to fracture of the lateral condyle in the adult, is apt to retard or arrest the growth of the lateral aspect of the tibia and thus cause tibia valga, or knock-knee. Surgical arrest of the growth of the medial tibial epiphysis may be necessary to prevent this deformity.

FRACTURE OF THE PROXIMAL FIBULA

Isolated fracture of the proximal fibula is uncommon; this fracture is usually associated with fracture of the femur or of the tibia or fracture-dislocation of the ankle joint. The apex of the fibular head may be avulsed by the activity of the biceps femoris muscle or detached with the fibular collateral ligament by an adduction strain of the knee.

The fracture usually requires no treatment, but avulsion of the apex of the head may necessitate operative repair of the ligament or tendon.

Fracture in this region may be associated with paralysis of the common peroneal nerve.

DISLOCATION OF THE PROXIMAL TIBIOFIBULAR JOINT

This extremely rare lesion is caused by the activity of the biceps femoris muscle. Displacement is posterior, and can be reduced by digital pressure over the head of the fibula in the opposite direction.

FRACTURE OF THE PATELLA

Transverse Fracture of the Patella

Transverse fracture of the patella is the result of indirect violence, usually with the knee in semiflexion. Fracture may be due to sudden voluntary contraction of the quadriceps muscles or sudden forced flexion of the leg when these muscles are contracted. The level of fracture is most often in the middle. The extent of tearing of the patellar retinacula depends upon the degree of force of the initiating injury. The activity of the quadriceps muscles causes displacement of the proximal fragment; the magnitude of displacement is dependent upon the extent of the tear of the quadriceps expansion.

Swelling of the anterior knee region is caused by hemarthrosis and hemorrhage into the soft tissues overlying the joint. If displacement is present, the defect in the patella can be palpated and active extension of the knee is lost.

Open reduction is indicated if the fragments are separated more than 2–3 mm. The fragments must be accurately repositioned to prevent early posttraumatic arthritis of the patellofemoral joint. If the minor fragment is small (no more than 1 cm in height), it may be excised and the rectus or patellar tendon (depending upon which pole of the patella is involved) sutured directly to the major fragment. If the fragments are approximately the same size, repair by wire cerclage is preferred.

Removal of 50% of the patella causes incongruity of joint surfaces, and posttraumatic arthritis may occur early.

Comminuted Fracture of the Patella

Comminuted fracture of the patella is caused only by direct violence. Little or no separation of the fragments occurs because the quadriceps expansion is not extensively torn. Severe injury may cause extensive comminution of the articular cartilages of both the patella and the opposing femur. If comminution is not severe and displacement is insignificant, plaster immobilization for 8 weeks in a cylinder extending from the groin to the supramalleolar region is sufficient.

Severe comminution requires excision of the patella and repair of the defect by imbrication of the quadriceps expansion.

TEAR OF THE QUADRICEPS TENDON

Tear of the quadriceps tendon occurs most often in patients over 40 years of age. Preexisting attritional disease of the tendon is apt to be present, and the causative injury may be minor. The tear commonly results from sudden deceleration, such as stumbling, or slipping on a wet surface. A small flake of bone may be avulsed from the superior pole of the patella, or the tear may occur entirely through tendinous and muscle tissue.

Pain may be noted in the anterior knee region. Swelling is due to hemarthrosis and extravasation of blood into the soft tissues. The patient is unable to extend his knee completely. X-rays may show avulsion of a bit of bone from the superior patella.

Operative repair is required for complete tear. If treatment is delayed until partial healing has occurred, the suture line can be reinforced by transplantation of the iliotibial band from the upper extremity of the tibia.

TEAR OF THE PATELLAR LIGAMENT

The same mechanism which causes tears of the quadriceps tendon, transverse fracture of the patella, or avulsion of the tibial tuberosity may also cause tear of the patellar ligament. The characteristic clinical finding is proximal displacement of the patella. A bit of bone may be avulsed from the lower pole of the patella if the tear takes place in the proximal patellar tendon.

Operative treatment is necessary for complete tear. The ligament is resutured to the patella and any tear in the quadriceps expansion is repaired. The extremity should be immobilized for 8 weeks in a tubular plaster cast extending from the inguinal to the supramalleolar region. Guarded exercises may then be started.

DISLOCATION OF THE PATELLA

Traumatic dislocation of the patellofemoral joint may be associated with dislocation of the knee joint. When this injury occurs alone it may be due to direct violence or muscle activity of the quadriceps, and the direction of dislocation of the patella may be lateral. Spontaneous reduction is apt to occur if the knee joint is extended; if so, the clinical findings may consist merely of hemarthrosis and localized tenderness over the medial patellar retinaculum. Gross instability of the patella, which can be demonstrated by physical examination, indicates that injury to the soft tissues of the medial aspect of the knee has been extensive. Recurrent episodes require operative repair for effective treatment.

DISLOCATION OF THE KNEE JOINT

Traumatic dislocation of the knee joint is uncommon in adults and extremely rare in children. It is caused by severe trauma. Displacement may be transverse or torsional. Complete dislocation can occur only after extensive tearing of the supporting ligaments, and is apt to cause injury to the popliteal vessels or the tibial and peroneal nerves.

Signs of neurovascular injury below the site of dislocation are an absolute indication for prompt reduction under general anesthesia, since failure of circulation will undoubtedly result in gangrene of the leg and foot. Axial traction is applied to the leg and a shearing force is exerted over the fragments in the appropriate direction. If pedal pulses do not return promptly, the popliteal fossa should be explored at once for treatment of any vascular injury.

Anatomic reduction of uncomplicated dislocation should be attempted. If impinging soft tissues cannot be removed by closed manipulation, arthrotomy is indicated. After reduction the extremity is immobilized in a tubular plaster cast extending from the inguinal region to the toes with the knee in slight flexion. (In the obese patient, a single hip spica should be applied.) A window should be cut in the plaster over the dorsum of the foot to allow frequent determination of dorsalis pedis pulsation. After 8 weeks' immobilization the knee can be protected by a long leg brace. Intensive quadriceps exercises are necessary to minimize functional loss.

INTERNAL DERANGEMENTS OF THE KNEE JOINT

Internal derangements of the knee joint mechanism may be caused by trauma or attritional disease. Although ligamentous and cartilaginous injuries are discussed separately, they may occur as combined lesions.

Injury to the Menisci

Injury to the medial meniscus is the most frequent internal derangement of the knee joint. Any portion of the meniscus may be torn. A marginal tear permits displacement of the medial fragment into the intercondylar region ("bucket-handle tear"). A fragment of cartilage displaced between the articular surfaces of the femur and tibia prevents either complete extension or complete flexion.

The significant clinical findings after acute injury are swelling (due to hemarthrosis) and varying degrees of restriction of flexion or extension. Motion may cause pain over the anteromedial or posteromedial joint line. Tenderness can often be elicited at the point of pain. Forcible external rotation of the foot with the knee flexed to a right angle may cause pain over the medial joint line. If symptoms have persisted for 2–3 weeks, weakness and atrophy of the quadriceps femoris may be present.

Injury to the lateral meniscus less often causes mechanical blockage of joint motion. Pain and tenderness may be present over the lateral joint line. Pain can

be elicited by forcible rotation of the leg with the knee flexed to a right angle.

Initial treatment may be conservative. Swelling and pain caused by tense hemarthrosis can be relieved by aspiration. If pain is severe, the extremity should be immobilized in a posterior plaster splint with the knee in slight flexion. Younger patients usually prefer to be ambulatory on crutches, but immediate weight-bearing must not be permitted. As long as acute symptoms persist, isometric quadriceps exercises should be performed frequently throughout the day with the knee in maximum extension (as a "straight leg lift"). Unrestricted activity must not be resumed until complete motion is recovered and healing is complete.

Exploratory arthrotomy is advisable for recurrent "locking," recurrent effusion, or disabling pain. Isometric quadriceps exercises are instituted immediately after the operation and gradually increased in frequency. As soon as the patient is able to perform these exercises comfortably, graded resistance maneuvers should be started. Exercises must be continued until all motion has been recovered and the volume and competency of the quadriceps are equal on both sides.

Injury to the Collateral Ligaments

The collateral ligaments prevent excursion of the joint beyond normal limits. When the knee is in full extension, the collateral ligaments are taut; in flexion, only the anterior fibers of the tibial collateral ligament are taut.

A. Tibial Collateral Ligament: Forced abduction of the leg at the knee, which is frequently associated with torsional strain, causes injury varying from tear of a few fibers to complete rupture of the ligament. A bit of bone may be avulsed from its femoral or tibial attachment.

A history of a twisting injury at the knee with valgus strain can usually be obtained. Pain is present over the medial aspect of the knee joint. In severe injury joint effusion may be present. Tenderness can be elicited at the site of the lesion. When only an isolated ligamentous tear is present, x-ray examination may not be helpful unless it is made while valgus stress is applied to the extended knee. Under local or general anesthesia the extremities are bound together in full extension at the knee joint, and an anteroposterior film is made with the legs in forced abduction. Widening of the medial joint cleft suggests complete rupture.

Treatment of incomplete tear consists of protection from further injury while healing progresses. Painful hemarthrosis should be relieved by aspiration. The knee may be immobilized in a posterior plaster splint or a tubular cast extending from the inguinal to the supramalleolar region.

Complete rupture should be repaired immediately so that healing will take place without ligamentous elongation and subsequent instability of the knee joint. Tear of the medial collateral ligament is frequently associated with other lesions, such as tear of the medial meniscus, rupture of the anterior cruciate ligament, or fracture of the lateral condyle of the tibia.

B. Fibular Collateral Ligament: Tear of the fibular collateral ligament is often associated with injury to surrounding structures, eg, the popliteus muscle tendon and the iliotibial band. Avulsion of the apex of the fibular head may occur, and the peroneal nerve may be injured.

Pain and tenderness are present over the lateral aspect of the knee joint, and hemarthrosis may be present. X-rays may show a bit of bone avulsed from the fibular head. If severe injury is suspected, x-ray examination under stress, using local or general anesthesia, is required. A firm, padded nonopaque object about 20–30 cm in diameter is placed between the knees and the legs are forcibly adducted while an anteroposterior exposure is made. Widening of the lateral joint cleft indicates severe injury.

The treatment of partial tear is similar to that described for partial tear of the medial collateral ligament. If complete tear is suspected, and especially if the peroneal nerve has been injured, exploration is indicated. The extremity is protected for 8 weeks in a plaster cylinder extending from the inguinal region to above the ankle.

Injury to the Cruciate Ligaments

The function of the anterior and posterior cruciate ligaments is to restrict anterior and posterior gliding of the tibia when the knee is flexed. If the tibia is rotated internally on the femur, the ligaments twist around themselves and become taut; if the tibia is rotated externally, they become lax.

A. Anterior Cruciate Ligament: Injury to the anterior cruciate ligament is usually associated with injury to the medial meniscus or the tibial collateral ligament. The cruciate ligament may be avulsed with a part of the medial tibial tubercle or may rupture within the substance of its fibers.

The characteristic clinical sign of tear of either cruciate ligament is a positive "drawer" sign: the knee is flexed at a right angle and pulled forward; if excessive anterior excursion of the proximal tibia (in comparison with the opposite normal side) can be noted, a tear of the anterior ligament is likely.

Complete recent rupture of the anterior cruciate ligament within its substance can occasionally be repaired with stout sutures. When manifest by avulsed tibial bone that is displaced, attachment of the fragment in anatomic position by arthrotomy is necessary. When the fragment of bone is large, displaced, and not treated until 4 weeks or more after injury, excision of the fragment and reinsertion of the ligament may be necessary to eliminate the blocking effect of the bone fragment and to permit recovery of function. Old tears may require reconstructive procedures.

B. Posterior Cruciate Ligament: Tear of the posterior ligament may occur within its substance or may be manifest by avulsion of a fragment of bone of variable size at its tibial attachment. Tear of the posterior cruciate ligament can be diagnosed by the "drawer" sign: the knee is flexed at a right angle and the upper tibia is pushed backward; if excessive posterior excursion of

the proximal tibia can be noted, tear of the posterior ligament is likely.

Treatment is directed primarily at the associated injuries and maintenance of the competency of the quadriceps musculature. Primary repair of tears within the fibers is difficult and of dubious value. Open reduction and fixation of a fragment of tibia with the attached ligament is feasible and is likely to restore functional competency of the ligament.

FRACTURES OF THE SHAFTS OF THE TIBIA & FIBULA

Fracture of the shaft of the tibia or fibula occurs at any age but is most common during youth and active adulthood. In general, open, transverse, comminuted, and segmental fractures are caused by indirect violence. Fracture of the middle third of the shaft (especially if comminuted) is apt to be complicated by delay of bone healing.

If fracture is complete and displacement is present, clinical diagnosis is not difficult. However, critical local examination is of utmost importance in planning treatment. The nature of the skin wounds which may communicate with the fracture site often suggests the mechanism of compounding, whether it has occurred from within or from without. A small laceration without contused edges suggests that the point of a bone fragment has caused compounding from within. A large wound with contused edges, especially over the subcutaneous surface of the tibia, suggests compounding from without. The presence of abrasions more than 6 hours old, blebs, pyoderma, and preexisting ulcers precludes immediate open treatment of closed fracture. Extensive swelling due to hemorrhagic exudate in closed fascial compartments may prevent complete reduction immediately. Extensive hemorrhagic and edematous infiltration can complicate and make difficult satisfactory closure of the subcutaneous tissue and skin incidental to elective open reduction. Neurovascular integrity below the level of the fracture must be verified before definitive treatment is instituted.

X-rays in the anteroposterior and lateral projection of the entire leg, including both the knee and ankle joints, are always necessary, and oblique projections are often desirable. The surgeon must know the exact site and configuration of the fracture, the severity of comminution, and the direction of displacement of fragments. Inadequate x-ray examination can lead to an incomplete diagnosis.

FRACTURE OF THE SHAFT
OF THE FIBULA

Isolated fracture of the shaft of the fibula is uncommon and is usually caused by direct trauma. Fibular shaft fracture is usually associated with other injury of the leg, such as fracture of the tibia or fracture-dislocation of the ankle joint. If no other lesion is present, immobilization for 4 weeks in a plaster boot (equipped with a walking surface) extending from the knee to the toes is sufficient for displaced, painful fractures. Undisplaced fractures require no immobilization, but discomfort can be minimized during the early days after injury by the use of crutches or a cane. Complete healing of uncomplicated fracture can be expected.

FRACTURE OF THE SHAFT
OF THE TIBIA

Isolated fracture of the shaft of the tibia is likely to be caused by indirect injury, such as a torsional stress. Such a fracture is mechanically stable.

Fracture of the shaft of the tibia is comparatively stable unless the fibula is fractured also. Marked displacement does not usually occur, and overriding is not significant unless there is associated dislocation of either tibiofibular joint.

If the fragments are not displaced, treatment may be by immobilization in a tubular plaster cast extending from the inguinal region to the toes with the knee in about 30 degrees of flexion and the foot in neutral position. The plaster should be changed 2–4 weeks after the injury to correct the loosening which will occur as a result of absorption of hemorrhagic exudate and atrophy of the thigh and calf muscles. Immobilization should be continued for at least 10 weeks, or until early bone healing is demonstrated by x-ray.

If the fragments are displaced, manipulation under anesthesia may be necessary. Fractures with a comparative transverse cleft tend to be stable after reduction. Oblique and spiral fractures tend to become displaced unless the fragments are locked.

A tubular plaster cast is applied as for undisplaced fracture. If x-rays do not show satisfactory apposition of fragments, alternative methods of treatment should be used (see below).

FRACTURE OF THE SHAFTS OF
BOTH BONES IN ADULTS

Fracture of the shafts of the tibia and fibula are unstable lesions which tend to become displaced following reduction. Treatment is directed toward reduction and stabilization of the tibial fracture until healing takes place. For adequate reduction the fragments must be apposed almost completely, and angulation and torsional displacement of the tibial fracture must be corrected.

If reduction by closed manipulation is anatomic and angular and torsional displacement are corrected, transverse fractures tend to be stable. Repeated x-rays are necessary to determine whether displacement has recurred. The plaster must remain snug at all times. Recurrent angular displacement can be corrected by dividing the plaster circumferentially and inserting wedges in the appropriate direction. If apposition is disturbed, another type of treatment must be substituted.

If oblique and spiral fractures are unstable following manipulation and immobilization, internal fixation or skeletal traction is usually required (Fig 46–32). This can be accomplished by closed reduction and skeletal distraction. While traction is continued, a tubular plaster cast with pins or wires incorporated is applied.

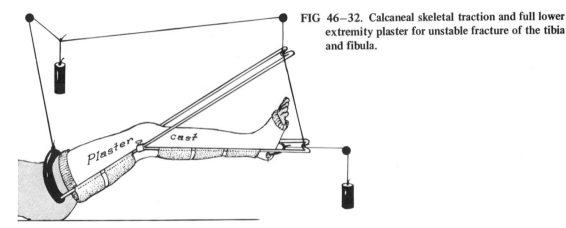

FIG 46–32. Calcaneal skeletal traction and full lower extremity plaster for unstable fracture of the tibia and fibula.

An alternative method is continuous skeletal traction. Traction must be continued for about 6 weeks until preliminary healing causes stabilization. The extremity is then immobilized in plaster for at least 12 weeks until bone continuity has been restored.

If adequate apposition and correction of the deformity cannot be achieved by closed methods, open reduction and internal fixation are required.

The blood supply to intermediate fragments is likely to be disturbed in comminuted and segmental fractures. These unstable fractures can usually be treated successfully only by closed reduction and external immobilization. If the patient wishes to remain ambulatory, percutaneous fixation of the major fragments with Steinmann pins or Kirschner wires will maintain reduction and alignment. However, continuous skeletal traction in plaster with a Kirschner wire inserted through the calcaneus is usually preferred until stabilization occurs (Fig 46–32).

FRACTURE OF THE SHAFTS OF THE TIBIA & FIBULA IN CHILDREN

Open reduction and internal fixation of closed fractures of the tibia or fibula in children are rarely necessary. If a tibial fracture is stable because of the configuration of the ends of the fragments, or if the fibular shaft is intact, closed reduction of axial displacement (overriding) is desirable; angular and torsional displacement must be corrected also. If proper alignment is secured, 1 cm of overriding is acceptable.

Comminuted or oblique tibial fractures with displacement or fractures of both bones require continuous skeletal traction by means of a Kirschner wire inserted through the calcaneus until early bone healing stabilizes the fragments. Further immobilization in a tubular plaster cast is necessary until bone healing is sufficiently well along to permit weight-bearing.

INJURIES OF THE ANKLE REGION

ANKLE SPRAIN

Sprain of the ankle joint during childhood is rare. In the adult, ankle sprain is most often caused by forced inversion of the foot, as may occur in stumbling on uneven ground. Pain is usually maximal over the anterolateral aspect of the joint; greatest tenderness is apt to be found in the region of the anterior talofibular and talocalcaneal ligaments. Eversion sprain is less common; maximal tenderness and swelling are usually found over the deltoid ligament.

Sprain is differentiated from major partial or complete ligamentous tears by anteroposterior, lateral, and 30 degrees internal oblique x-ray projections; if the joint cleft between either malleolus and the talus is greater than 4 mm, major ligamentous tear is probable. Occult lesions can be demonstrated by x-ray examination under inversion or eversion stress after infiltration of the area of maximal swelling and tenderness with 5 ml of 2% procaine.

If swelling is marked, elevation of the extremity and avoidance of weight-bearing for a few days is advisable. The ankle can be supported with a Gibney strapping (Fig 46–33). Adhesive support for another 2 weeks will relieve pain and swelling. Further treatment may be by warm foot baths and elastic bandages. Continue treatment until muscle strength and full joint motion are recovered. Tears of major ligaments of the ankle joint are discussed below.

FRACTURES & DISLOCATIONS OF THE ANKLE JOINT

Fractures and dislocations of the ankle joint may be caused by direct injury, in which case they are apt to be comminuted and open; or by indirect violence, which often causes typical lesions (see below).

Pain and swelling are the prominent clinical findings. Deformity may or may not be present. X-rays of excellent technical quality must be prepared in a sufficient variety of projections to demonstrate the extent and configuration of all major fragments. Special oblique projections may be required.

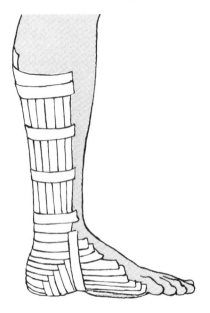

FIG 46–33. Gibney ankle strapping.

Fracture of the Medial Malleolus

Fracture of the medial malleolus may occur as an isolated lesion of any part of the malleolus (including the tip), or may be associated with (1) fracture of the lateral malleolus with medial or lateral dislocation of the talus, and (2) dislocation of the inferior tibiofibular joint with or without fracture of the fibula. Isolated fracture does not usually cause instability of the ankle joint.

Undisplaced isolated fracture of the medial malleolus should be treated by immobilization in a plaster boot extending from the knee to the toes with the ankle flexed to a right angle and the foot slightly inverted to relax the tension on the deltoid ligament (Fig 46–34). Immobilization must be continued for 6–8 weeks or until bone healing is sound.

Displaced isolated fracture of the medial malleolus may be treated by closed manipulation under general or local anesthesia. The essential maneuver consists of anatomic realignment by digital pressure over the distal fragment, followed by immobilization in a plaster boot (as for undisplaced fracture) until bone healing is sound (Fig 46–34). If anatomic reduction cannot be obtained by closed methods, open reduction and internal fixation with 1–2 bone screws are required.

Fracture of the Lateral Malleolus

Fracture of the lateral malleolus may occur as an isolated lesion, or may be associated with fracture of the medial malleolus, tear of the deltoid or posterior lateral malleolar ligament, or avulsion of the posterior tibial tubercle. If the medial aspect of the ankle is injured, lateral dislocation of the talus is apt to be present. The tip of the lateral malleolus may be avulsed by the calcaneofibular and anterior talofibular liga-

ments. Transverse or oblique fracture may occur. Oblique fractures commonly extend downward and anteriorly from the posterior and superior aspects.

If swelling and pain are not marked, isolated undisplaced fracture of the lateral malleolus may be treated by Gibney ankle strapping (Fig 46–33). Otherwise, a plaster boot should be applied for 6 weeks and an elastic bandage worn thereafter until full joint motion is recovered and the calf muscles are functioning normally.

Isolated displaced fracture of the lateral malleolus should be treated by closed manipulation. The foot should be immobilized in slight inversion, which tautens the ligaments over the lateral aspect of the ankle joint and tends to prevent displacement.

If anatomic reduction cannot be achieved by closed methods, open reduction is required.

Combined Fracture of the Medial & Lateral Malleoli

Bimalleolar fractures are commonly accompanied by displacement of the talus, usually in a medial or lateral direction. In conjunction with dislocation in the coronal plane, concurrent displacement may take place in the sagittal plane, either anteriorly or posteriorly, or in torsion about the longitudinal axis of the tibia.

Bimalleolar fracture may be treated by closed manipulation. A tubular plaster cast is then applied from the inguinal region to the toes with the knee in about 45 degrees of flexion and the foot in neutral position. Immediate open reduction must be resorted to if x-rays show that perfect anatomic reduction has not been achieved by closed manipulation.

Fractures of the Distal Tibia

Fracture of the distal tibia is usually associated with other lesions.

A. Fracture of the Posterior Margin: Fracture of the posterior articular margin may involve part or all of the entire posterior half and is apt to be accompanied by fracture of either malleolus and posterior dislocation of the talus. It must be differentiated from fracture of the posterior tibial tubercle, which is usually caused by avulsion with the attached posterior lateral malleolar ligament.

Anatomic reduction by closed manipulation is required if the fracture involves more than 25% of the articular surface. The extremity is immobilized in a plaster cast extending from the inguinal region to the toes with the knee in about 40 degrees of flexion, the ankle at a right angle, and the foot in neutral position.

Frequent x-ray examination is necessary to make certain that redisplacement does not occur. The plaster should be changed as soon as loosening becomes apparent. Immobilization must be maintained for at least 8 weeks. Weight-bearing must not be resumed until bone healing is sound, usually in about 12 weeks.

B. Fracture of the Anterior Margin: Fracture of the anterior articular margin of the tibia (rare) is likely to be caused by forced dorsiflexion of the foot. If displacement is marked and the talus is dislocated, tear

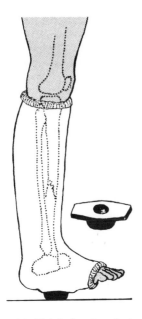

FIG 46–34. Weight-bearing plaster boot.

of the collateral ligaments or fractures of the malleoli are likely to be present.

Reduction is by closed manipulation. If comminution is present, the extremity should be immobilized for about 12 weeks. Healing is apt to be slow.

C. Comminuted Fractures: Extensive comminution of the distal tibia ("compression type" fracture) presents a difficult problem of management. The congruity of articular surfaces cannot be restored by closed manipulation, and satisfactory anatomic restoration is usually not possible even by open reduction. The best form of treatment for extensively comminuted and widely displaced fractures is closed manipulation and skeletal traction (Fig 46–32). After traction has been applied and impaction of fragments has been disrupted, displacement in the transverse plane is corrected by manual molding with compression. A tubular plaster cast is applied from the inguinal region to the toes with the knee in 10–15 degrees of flexion and the foot in neutral position. With the extremity immobilized in plaster, continuous skeletal traction can be maintained for 8–12 weeks or until stabilization by early bone healing occurs. An alternative is distraction with a wire or pin in the calcaneus and one or 2 wires or pins in the shaft of the tibia.

Healing is likely to be slow. If the articular surfaces of the ankle joint have not been properly realigned, disabling posttraumatic arthritis is likely to occur early. Early arthrodesis is indicated to shorten the period of disability.

Dislocation of the Ankle Joint

A. Complete Dislocation: The talus cannot be completely dislocated from the ankle joint unless all ligaments are torn. This lesion is rare.

B. Incomplete Dislocation: Major ligamentous injuries in the region of the ankle joint are usually associated with fracture.

1. Tear of the deltoid ligament—Complete tear of the talotibial portion of the deltoid ligament can permit interposition of the posterior tibial tendon between the medial malleolus and the talus. Associated injury is usually present, especially fracture of the lateral malleolus with lateral dislocation of the talus.

Pain, tenderness, swelling, and ecchymosis in the region of the medial malleolus without fracture suggest partial or complete tear of the deltoid ligament. If fracture of the lateral malleolus or dislocation of the distal tibiofibular joint is present, the cleft between the malleolus and talus is likely to be widened. If significant widening is not apparent, x-ray examination under stress is necessary.

Interposition of the deltoid ligament between the talus and the medial malleolus often cannot be corrected by closed manipulation. If widening persists after closed manipulation, surgical exploration is indicated so that the ligament can be removed and repaired by suture.

Associated fracture of the fibula can be treated by fixation with a coaxial intramedullary standard bone screw or a bone nail to assure maintenance of anatomic reduction.

2. Tear of the talofibular ligament—Isolated tear of the anterior talofibular ligament is caused by forced inversion of the foot. X-ray examination under stress may be necessary, using local or general anesthesia. Both feet are forcibly inverted and internally rotated about 20 degrees while an anteroposterior film is exposed. If the tear is complete, the talus will be seen to be axially displaced from the tibial articular surface.

Rupture of the anterior talofibular ligament may be associated with tear of the calcaneofibular ligament. Tear of both ligaments may be associated with fracture of the medial malleolus and medial dislocation of the talus.

Instability of the ankle joint, characterized by a history of recurrent sprains, may result from unrecognized tears of the anterior talofibular ligament.

Recent isolated tear of the anterior talofibular ligament or combined tear of the calcaneofibular ligament should be treated by immobilization for 4 weeks in a plaster boot. Associated fracture of the medial malleolus creates an unstable mechanism. Unless anatomic reduction can be achieved and maintained by closed methods, open reduction of the malleolar fragment is indicated, followed by internal fixation of the fracture and repair of the ligamentous injury.

Dislocation of the Distal Tibiofibular Joint

Both the anterior and posterior lateral malleolar ligaments must be torn before dislocation of the distal tibiofibular joint can occur. Lateral dislocation of the talus is also an essential feature, and this cannot occur unless the medial malleolus is fractured or the deltoid ligament is torn. The distal fibula is commonly fractured, but it may remain intact, and dislocation may be caused by a tear of the interosseous ligament.

Anatomic reduction by closed manipulation is difficult to achieve, but should be tried. Under general anesthesia, the foot is forced medially by a shearing maneuver and a snug plaster cast is applied from the inguinal region to the toes. If immediate and repeated x-ray examinations do not demonstrate that anatomic reduction has been achieved and maintained, open reduction and internal fixation should be performed as soon as possible.

Separation of the Distal Tibial & Fibular Epiphyses

The most common injury of the ankle region of children is traumatic separation of the distal tibial and fibular epiphyses. Sprain is rare in children. Separation of the distal fibular epiphysis may occur as an isolated injury, or may be associated with separation of the tibial epiphysis.

If displacement has occurred, treatment is by closed manipulation and plaster immobilization. Open reduction is seldom justifiable. If injury has been severe, disturbance of growth is likely to follow.

INJURIES OF THE FOOT

FRACTURE & DISLOCATION OF THE TALUS

Dislocation of the Subtalar & Talonavicular Joints

Dislocation of the subtalar and talonavicular joints without fracture occasionally occurs. The talocrural joint is not injured. Displacement of the foot can be either in varus or valgus. Reduction by closed manipulation is usually not difficult. Incarceration of the posterior tibial tendon in the talonavicular joint may prevent reduction by closed manipulation. After reduction, the extremity should be immobilized in a plaster boot for 4 weeks.

Fracture of the Talus

Major fracture of the talus commonly occurs either through the body or through the neck; the uncommon fracture of the head involves essentially a portion of the neck with extension into the head. Indirect injury is usually the cause of closed fracture as well as most open fractures; severe comminution is not commonly present. Compression fracture or infraction of the tibial articular surface may be caused by the initial injury or may occur later in association with complicating avascular necrosis. The proximal or distal fragments may be dislocated.

A. Fracture of the Neck: Forced dorsiflexion of the foot may cause this injury. Undisplaced fracture of the neck can be treated adequately by a non-weight-bearing plaster boot for 8–12 weeks. Dislocation of the body or the distal neck fragment with the foot may complicate this injury. Fracture of the neck with anterior and frequently medial dislocation of the distal fragment and foot can usually be reduced by closed manipulation. Subsequent treatment is the same as that of undisplaced fracture.

Dislocation of the proximal body fragment may occur separately or may be associated with dislocation of the distal fragment. If dislocation of the body fragment is complete, reduction by closed manipulation may not be possible. If reduction by closed manipulation is not successful, open reduction should be done as soon as possible to prevent or to minimize the extent of the avascular necrosis. Bone healing is likely to be retarded since some degree of avascular necrosis is probable.

Complete dislocation of the neck fragment from the talonavicular and subtalar joints is rare, but if it does happen avascular necrosis of the fragment is to be expected even though anatomic reduction is promptly accomplished. If satisfactory reduction by closed manipulation is not possible, immediate open operation with reduction of the fragment or its removal is advisable since delay may cause necrosis of overlying soft tissues.

B. Fracture of the Body: Closed uncomminuted fracture of the body of the talus with minimal displacement of fragments is not likely to cause disability if immobilization is continued until bone continuity is restored. If significant displacement occurs, the proximal fragment is apt to be dislocated from the subtalar and ankle joints. Reduction by closed manipulation can be achieved best by traction and forced plantar flexion of the foot. Immobilization in a plaster boot with the foot in equinus for about 8 weeks should be followed by further casting with the foot at a right angle until the fracture cleft has been obliterated by new bone formation as evidenced by x-ray examination. Even though prompt adequate reduction is obtained by either closed manipulation or by open operation, extensive displacement of the proximal body fragment is likely to be followed by avascular necrosis. If reduction is not anatomic, delayed healing of the fracture may follow and posttraumatic arthritis is a likely sequel. If this occurs, arthrodesis of the ankle and subtalar joints may be necessary to relieve painful symptoms.

C. Compression Fracture: Compression fracture or infraction of the dome of the talus from the initial injury (which is likely to have been violent) cannot be reduced. When this lesion occurs as a separate entity or in combination with other fractures of the body, prolonged protection from weight-bearing is the major means of preventing the further collapse that is so likely to occur in the area of healing.

FRACTURE OF THE CALCANEUS

Fracture of the calcaneus is commonly caused by direct trauma. Since this fracture is likely to occur as a result of a fall from a height, fracture of the spine may also be present. Comminution and impaction are general characteristics. Minor infractions or impactions and fissure fractures are easy to miss on clinical examination, and x-rays must be prepared in multiple projections to demonstrate adequately some fracture clefts. In some instances, minor impactions of articular surfaces will be evident only by tomography.

Various classifications have been advocated. Fractures that are generally comminuted and disrupt the subtalar and calcaneocuboid articulations should be distinguished from those that do not; this differentiation has important implications for treatment and prognosis.

Fracture of the Tuberosity

Isolated fracture of the tuberosity is not common. It may occur in a vertical or a horizontal direction.

A. Horizontal Fracture: Horizontal fracture may be limited to the superior portion of the region of the former apophysis and represents an avulsion by the Achilles tendon. Where the superior minor fragment is widely displaced proximally with the tendon, open reduction and fixation with a stout wire suture may be necessary to obtain the most satisfactory functional result.

Further extension of the fracture cleft toward the subtalar joint in the substance of the tuberosity creates the "beak" fracture. The minor fragment may be displaced proximally by the action of the triceps surae. If displacement is significant, reduction can be achieved by skeletal traction applied to the proximal fragment with the foot in equinus. Immobilization is obtained by incorporation of the traction pin or wire in a full extremity plaster with the knee flexed 30 degrees and the foot in plantar flexion. If adequate reduction cannot be accomplished in this way, open reduction is advised.

B. Vertical Fracture: Vertical fracture occurs near the sagittal plane somewhat medially through the tuberosity. Because the minor medial fragment normally is not widely displaced, plaster immobilization is not required. Comfort can be enhanced by limitation of weight-bearing with the aid of crutches.

Fracture of the Sustentaculum

Isolated fracture of the sustentaculum tali is a rare lesion which may be caused by forced eversion of the foot. Where displacement of the larger body fragment occurs, it is lateral. Incarceration of the tendon of the flexor hallucis longus in the fracture cleft has been reported. Generally this fracture occurs in association with comminution of the body.

Fracture of the Anterior Process

Fracture of the anterior process is caused by forced inversion of the foot. It must be differentiated from midtarsal and ankle joint sprains. The firmly attached bifurcate ligament (calcaneonavicular and calcaneocuboid components) avulses a bit of bone. Maximum tenderness and slight swelling occur midway between the tip of the lateral malleolus and the base of the fifth metatarsal. The lateral x-ray view projected obliquely is the most satisfactory to demonstrate the fracture cleft. Treatment is by a non-weight-bearing plaster boot with the foot in neutral position for 4 weeks.

Fracture of the Body

Fracture of the body may occur posterior to the articular surfaces, in a general vertical but somewhat oblique plane, without disruption of the subtalar joint. Most severe fractures of the calcaneal body are comminuted and extend into the subtalar and frequently the calcaneocuboid joints. Fissure fractures without significant displacement cause minor disability and can be treated simply by protection from weight-bearing, either by crutches alone or in combination with a plaster boot until bone healing is sufficiently sound to justify graded increments of loading.

A. Nonarticular Fracture: Where fracture of the body with comminution occurs posterior to the articular surface, the direction of significant displacement of the fragment attached to the tuberosity is proximal,

causing diminution of the tuber joint angle. Since the subtalar joint is not disrupted, symptomatic posttraumatic degenerative arthritis is not an important sequel even though some joint stiffness persists permanently. Marked displacement should be corrected by skeletal traction applied to the main posterior fragment to obtain an optimal cosmetic result, especially in women. Success of reduction can be judged by the adequacy of restoration of the tuber joint angle.

B. Articular Fracture: Articular fractures are of 3 general types:

1. Noncomminuted—Fracture of the body without comminution may involve the posterior articular facet. Where displacement of the posterior fragment of the tuberosity occurs, the direction is lateral. Fractures of this category with more than minimal displacement should be treated by the method advocated for nonarticular fracture of the body.

2. With minor comminution—In fractures with minor comminution, the main cleft occurs vertically, in a somewhat oblique lateral deviation from the sagittal plane. From emergence on the medial surface posterior to the sustentaculum it is directed forward and rather obliquely laterally through the posterior articular facet. The sustentaculum and the medial portion of the posterior articular facet remain undisplaced with relation to the talus. The body below the remaining lateral portion of the posterior articular facet with the tuberosity are impacted into the lateral portion of the posterior articular facet. Since anatomic reduction cannot be achieved by closed technics, Palmer has advocated open reduction and bone grafting. Lack of precise reduction, determined in part by restoration of the normal tuber joint angle, causes derangement of the subtalar joint, and symptomatic posttraumatic arthritis is a frequent sequel.

3. With extensive comminution—Fracture with extensive comminution extending into the subtalar joint may involve the calcaneocuboid joint as well as the tuberosity. The multiple fracture clefts involve the entire posterior articular surface, and the facet is impacted into the substance of the underlying body. There are many variants; the clefts may extend across the calcaneal groove into the medial and anterior articular surfaces, and detachment of the peroneal tubercle may be a feature. This serious injury may cause major disability in spite of the best treatment since the bursting nature of the injury defies anatomic restoration.

Some surgeons advise nonintervention. Displacement of fragments is disregarded. Initially, a compression dressing is applied and the extremity is elevated for a week or so. Warm soaks and active exercises are then started, but weight-bearing is avoided until early bone healing has taken place. In spite of residual deformity of the heel, varying degrees of weakness of the calf, and discomfort in the region of the subtalar joint (which may be intensified by weight-bearing), acceptable functional results can be obtained, especially among vigorous men who are willing to put up with the discomforts involved.

Other surgeons, notably Hermann and Böhler, advocate early closed manipulation which can partially restore the external anatomic configuration of the heel region, a cosmetic goal particularly desirable for women.

Persistent and disabling painful symptoms originating in the deranged subtalar joint may require arthrodesis for adequate relief. Concomitant involvement of the calcaneocuboid joint is an indication for the more extensive triple arthrodesis.

FRACTURE OF THE TARSAL NAVICULAR

Minor avulsion fractures of the tarsal navicular may occur as a feature of severe midtarsal sprain and require neither reduction nor elaborate treatment. Avulsion fracture of the tuberosity near the insertion of the posterior tibialis muscle is uncommon and must be differentiated from a persistent, ununited apophysis (accessory scaphoid) and from the supernumerary sesamoid bone, the os tibiale externum.

Major fracture occurs either through the middle in a horizontal or, more rarely, in the vertical plane, or is characterized by impaction of its substance. Only noncomminuted fractures with displacement of the dorsal fragment can be reduced. Closed manipulation by strong traction on the forefoot and simultaneous digital pressure over the displaced fragment can restore it to its normal position. If a tendency to redisplacement is apparent, this can be counteracted by temporary fixation with a percutaneously inserted Kirschner wire. Comminuted and impacted fractures cannot be anatomically reduced. Some authorities offer a pessimistic prognosis for comminuted or impacted fractures. It is their contention that even though partial reduction has been achieved, posttraumatic arthritis supervenes, and that arthrodesis of the talonavicular and cuneonavicular joints will be ultimately necessary to relieve painful symptoms.

FRACTURE OF THE CUNEIFORM & CUBOID BONES

Because of their relatively protected position in the midtarsus, isolated fracture of the cuboid and cuneiform bones is rarely encountered. Minor avulsion fractures occur as a component of severe midtarsal sprains. Extensive fracture usually occurs in association with other injuries of the foot and often is caused by severe crushing. Simple classification is impractical because of the complex character and the multiple combinations of the whole injury.

MIDTARSAL DISLOCATIONS

Midtarsal dislocation through the cuneonavicular and the calcaneocuboid joints or, more proximally, through the talocalcaneonavicular and the calcaneocuboid joints may occur as a result of twisting injury to the forefoot. Fractures of varying extent of adjacent bones are frequent complications. When treatment is given soon after the accident, closed reduction by traction on the forefoot and manipulation is generally effective. If reduction is unstable and displacement tends to recur upon release of traction, stabilization for 4 weeks by percutaneously inserted Kirschner wires is recommended.

FRACTURES & DISLOCATIONS OF THE METATARSALS

Fractures of metatarsals and tarsometatarsal dislocations are likely to be caused by direct crushing or indirect twisting injury to the forefoot. Besides osseous and articular injury, complicating soft tissue lesions are often present. Tense subfascial hematoma of the dorsum of the forefoot, if not relieved, may cause necrosis of overlying skin or may even lead to gangrene of the toes by interruption of the arterial supply.

Tarsometatarsal Dislocations

Possibly because of strong ligamentous support and relative size, dislocation of the first metatarsal at its base occurs less frequently than similar involvement of the lesser bones. If dislocation occurs, fracture of the first cuneiform is likely to be present also. More often, however, tarsometatarsal dislocation involves the lesser metatarsals, and associated fractures are to be expected. Dislocation is more commonly caused by direct injury but may be the result of stress applied indirectly through the forefoot. The direction of displacement is ordinarily dorsal, lateral, or a combination of both.

Attempted closed reduction should not be deferred. Skeletal traction applied to the involved bone by a Kirschner wire or a stout towel clamp can be a valuable aid to manipulation. Even though persistent dislocation may not cause significant disability, the resulting deformity can make shoe fitting difficult for men and the cosmetic effect undesirable to women. Open reduction with evacuation of dorsal subfascial hematoma and Kirschner wire stabilization is a preferred alternative to unsuccessful closed treatment. When effective treatment has been deferred 4 weeks or even longer, early healing will prevent satisfactory reduction of persisting displacement by closed technics. Under such circumstances, it. is better to defer open operation and to direct treatment toward recovery of function. Extensive operative procedures and continued immobilization can increase joint stiffness.

Reconstructive operation can be planned more suitably after residual disability becomes established.

Fractures of the Shafts

Undisplaced fractures of the metatarsal shafts cause no permanent disability unless failure of bone healing is encountered. Displacement is rarely significant where fracture of the middle metatarsals is oblique and the first and fifth are uninjured, since they act as splints. Even fissure fractures should be treated by a stiff-soled shoe (with partial weight-bearing) or, if pain is marked, by a plaster walking boot.

Great care should be taken in displaced fractures to correct angulation in the longitudinal axis of the shaft. Persistent convex dorsal angulation causes prominence of the head of the involved metatarsal on the plantar aspect with the implication of concentrated local pressure and production of painful skin callosities. Deformity of the shaft of the first metatarsal due to convex plantar angulation can transfer weight-bearing stress to the region of the head of the third metatarsal. After correction of angular displacement, the plaster casing should be molded well to the plantar aspect of the foot to minimize recurrence of deformity and to support the longitudinal and transverse arches.

If reduction is not reasonably accurate, fractures through the shafts near the heads (the "neck") may cause great discomfort from concentrated pressure beneath the head on the plantar surface and reactive skin callus formation. Every effort should be made to correct convex dorsal angulation by disrupting impaction and appropriate manipulation. Unstable fracture can be treated by sustained skeletal traction using a Kirschner wire inserted through the distal phalanx and traction supplied by an elastic band attached to a "banjo" bow. The efficacy of closed treatment should be determined without delay, and, where it is lacking, open operation should be substituted.

Fatigue Fracture of the Shafts

Fatigue fracture of the shafts of the metatarsals has been described by various terms, eg, march, stress, and insufficiency fracture, and by a variety of other terms in the French and German literature. Its protean clinical manifestations cause difficulty in precise recognition, even to the point of confusion with osteogenic sarcoma. Commonly, it occurs in active young adults, such as military recruits, who are unaccustomed to vigorous and excessive walking. A history of a single significant injury is lacking. Incipient pain of varying intensity in the forefoot which is accentuated by walking, swelling, and localized tenderness of the involved metatarsal are cardinal manifestations. Depending upon the stage of progress, x-rays may not demonstrate the fracture cleft and extracortical callus formation may ultimately be the only clue. More striking findings may vary from an incomplete fissure to an evident transverse cleft. Persistent unprotected weight-bearing may cause arrest of bone healing and even displacement of the distal fragment. The second and third metatarsals are most frequently involved near the junction of the middle and distal thirds. The lesion can occur more proximally and in other lesser metatarsals. Since weight-bearing is likely to prolong and aggravate symptoms, treatment is by protection in either a plaster walking boot or a heavy shoe with the sole reinforced by a steel strut. Weight-bearing should be restricted until painful symptoms subside and restoration of bone continuity has been demonstrated by x-ray examination.

Fracture of the Tuberosity of the Fifth Metatarsal

Forced adduction of the forefoot may cause avulsion fracture of the tuberosity of the fifth metatarsal, and, where supporting soft tissues have been torn, activity of the peroneus brevis muscle may increase displacement of the avulsed proximal fragment. If displacement of the minor fragment is minimal, adhesive strapping or a stiff-soled shoe is adequate treatment. If displacement is significant, treatment should be by a walking boot until bone healing occurs (Fig 46–34). Rarely does healing fail to occur. Fracture should be differentiated from a separate ossific center of the tuberosity in adolescence and the supernumerary os vesalianum pedis in adulthood.

FRACTURES & DISLOCATIONS OF THE PHALANGES OF THE TOES

Fractures of the phalanges of the toes are caused most commonly by direct violence such as crushing or stubbing. Spiral or oblique fractures of the shafts of the proximal phalanges of the lesser toes may occur as a result of indirect twisting injury.

Comminuted fracture of the proximal phalanx of the great toe, alone or in combination with fracture of the distal phalanx, is the most disabling injury. Since wide displacement of fragments is not likely, correction of angulation and support by an adhesive dressing and splint usually suffices. A weight-bearing plaster boot may be useful for relief of symptoms arising from associated soft tissue injury. Spiral or oblique fracture of the proximal phalanges of the lesser toes can be treated adequately by binding the involved toe to the adjacent uninjured member. Comminuted fracture of the distal phalanx is treated as a soft tissue injury.

Traumatic dislocation of the metatarsophalangeal joints and the uncommon dislocation of the proximal interphalangeal joint usually can be reduced by closed manipulation. These dislocations are rarely isolated and usually occur in combination with other injuries to the forefoot.

FRACTURE OF THE SESAMOIDS OF THE GREAT TOE

Fracture of the sesamoid bones of the great toe is rare, but may occur as a result of crushing injury. It must be differentiated from partite developmental lesions. Undisplaced fracture requires no treatment other than a foot support or a metatarsal bar. Displaced fracture may require immobilization in a walking plaster boot with the toe strapped in flexion. Persistent delay of bone healing may cause disabling pain arising from arthritis of the articulation between the sesamoid and the head of the first metatarsal. If a foot support and metatarsal bar do not provide adequate relief, excision of the sesamoid may be necessary.

. . .

ARTHROPLASTY OF THE HIP JOINT

Fracture of the head or neck of the femur or the acetabulum or traumatic dislocation of the hip joint is frequently followed by disability due to ischemic osteonecrosis of the femoral head, failure of bony healing of the fracture, or posttraumatic arthritis. The most disabling symptom is pain, which may require operative treatment for adequate relief. To minimize morbidity and invalidism and to avoid secondary operative procedures, there has been an increasing tendency to perform primary prosthetic replacement of the femoral head/neck segment for the treatment of certain cervical fractures. The general indications for primary replacement have been (1) debility due to poor general health, (2) preexisting disease of a major system, (3) preexisting arthritis of the affected joint, and (4) senility. In addition to the foregoing, displaced fractures at the cervicocapital junction are likely to be complicated by compromised vascularity of the head segment which can be correlated with osteonecrosis.

The overall results of primary hemiarthroplasty using an intramedullary femoral prosthesis have been variable. They have been more gratifying in elderly patients with limited functional demands. Failures have been attributed to postoperative infection, loosening of the implant from the femur, and acetabular deterioration secondary to wear.

Hemiarthroplasty has also been used for the treatment of sequelae of traumatic hip joint disabilities that are not complicated by infection. When infection is a factor, replacement arthroplasty is hazardous and should be reserved for the occasional treatment of a specific problem by an experienced surgeon. Otherwise, removal of the implant and treatment of the infection is safer, even though the patient will have residual disability which may or may not require subsequent operative treatment.

Increasing interest in total hip joint replacement has been generated during the past 10 years both abroad and in the USA. This technic implies substitution of at least the articular surfaces of both the acetabulum and the head of the femur by implants made of metal or plastic. In general, the femoral component is made of metal—either a chrome-cobalt alloy or stainless steel—and the acetabular constituent may be of the same metal or a plastic. Depending upon the specific design, the implants may be attached to the respective bone by their configuration or a cementing substance may be used as an intermediary. The Ring prosthesis is a practical example of an all-metal implant pair that is applied without a cementing substance. The Charnley type apparatus is composed of a metal femoral segment and a polyethylene acetabular component; both are stabilized in bone by self-curing polymethylmethacrylate.

The precise indications for total hip joint replacement in the primary treatment of fractures of the femoral head and neck have not been established. Total hip joint replacement has gained popularity in the treatment of cases of failure after hemiarthroplasty and sequelae of fracture and dislocation which have been mentioned previously but in which infection does not complicate. Total hip joint replacement is still considered a salvage operation. Because the long-term reliability has not been established, the operation should be reserved for patients over 50 years of age unless specific factors warrant its use in younger individuals.

Charnley J: The long-term results of low-friction arthroplasty of the hip performed as a primary intervention. J Bone Joint Surg 54B:61–76, 1972.

Dupont JA, Charnley J: Low-friction arthroplasty of the hip for the failures of previous operations. J Bone Joint Surg 54B:77–87, 1972.

Hinchey JJ, Day PL: Prostheses in femoral neck fractures. J Bone Joint Surg 46A:223–240, 334, 1964.

Patterson FP, Brown CS: The McKee-Farrar total hip replacement: Preliminary results and complications of 368 operations performed in five general hospitals. J Bone Joint Surg 54A:257, 1972.

Stinchfield FE & others: Low friction arthroplasty. Surg Gynec Obst 135:1–10, 1972.

Whittaker RP & others: Fifteen years' experience with metallic endoprosthetic replacement of the femoral head for femoral neck fractures. J Trauma 12:799–806, 1972.

. . .

General References

Abel MS: *Occult Traumatic Lesions of the Cervical Vertebrae.* Warren H. Green, 1971.

Aergerter E, Kirkpatrick JA: *Orthopedic Diseases,* 3rd ed. Saunders, 1968.

American Academy of Orthopedic Surgeons: *Symposium on Sports Medicine.* Mosby, 1969.

Bateman JE: *The Shoulder and Neck.* Saunders, 1972.

Compere EL: *Pictorial Handbook of Fracture Treatment,* 5th ed. Year Book, 1963.

Crenshaw AH (editor): *Campbell's Operative Orthopaedics,* 5th ed. Mosby, 1971.

Cruess RL, Mitchell NS (editors): *Surgery of Rheumatoid Arthritis.* Lippincott, 1971.

De Palma AF: *The Management of Fractures and Dislocations,* 2nd ed. Saunders, 1970.

Ferguson AB Jr: *Orthopaedic Surgery in Infancy and Childhood,* 3rd ed. Williams & Wilkins, 1968.

Gustilo RB & others: Analysis of 511 open fractures. Clin Orthop 66:148–154, 1969.

Holdsworth AA: Fractures, dislocations, and fracture-dislocations of the spine. J Bone Joint Surg 52A:1534–1551, 1970.

Hollander JL: *Arthritis and Allied Conditions,* 8th ed. Lea & Febiger, 1972.

Jackson RW, Abe I: The role of arthroscopy in the management of disorders of the knee: An analysis of 200 consecutive examinations. J Bone Joint Surg 54B:310–322, 1972.

Jaffee HL: *Metabolic, Degenerative, and Inflammatory Diseases of Bones and Joints.* Lea & Febiger, 1972.

Jawetz E, Melnick JL, Adelberg EA: *Review of Medical Microbiology,* 10th ed. Lange, 1972.

Jones R: An orthopaedic view of the treatment of fractures. Clin Orthop 75:4–16, 1971.

Lichtenstein L: *Bone Tumors,* 4th ed. Mosby, 1972.

Margolics MN & others: Arteriography to manage hemorrhage from pelvic fractures. New England J Med 287:317–320, 1972.

O'Donoghue DH: *Treatment of Injuries of Athletes,* 2nd ed. Saunders, 1970.

Paul LW, Juhl JH: *Essentials of Roentgen Interpretation,* 3rd ed. Harper & Row, 1972.

Raney RB Sr, Brashear HR: *Shands' Handbook of Orthopaedic Surgery,* 8th ed. Mosby, 1971.

Schmorl G: *The Human Spine in Health and Disease.* Grune & Stratton, 1971.

Schumacher HR Jr, Kulka JP: Needle biopsy of the synovial membrane: Experience with the Parker-Pearson technic. New England J Med 286:416–419, 1972.

Scharrard WJW: *Paediatric Orthopaedics and Fractures.* Davis, 1971.

Smith DR: *General Urology,* 7th ed. Lange, 1972.

Stauffer RN, Coventry MD: Anterior interbody lumbar spine fusion. J Bone Joint Surg 54A:256–268, 1972.

Tachdjian MO: *Pediatric Orthopedics.* Vols 1 and 2. Mosby, 1972.

Tullos HS & others: Unusual lesions of pitching arm. Clin Orthop 88:169, 1972.

Turek SL: *Orthopaedics: Principles and Their Application,* 2nd ed. Lippincott, 1967.

Waddel JP & others: Occult injuries in pedestrian accidents. J Trauma 11:844–852, 1971.

White AA III, Southwick WO, De Ponte RJ: Cervical spine fusions: Psychological and social considerations. Arch Surg 126:150–154, 1973.

Young HH: *Year Book of Orthopedics and Traumatic Surgery.* Year Book, 1972.

Zinn WM (editor): *Idiopathic Ischemic Necrosis of the Femoral Head in Adults.* University Park Press, 1972.

47 . . .

Plastic Surgery

William J. Morris, MD

In order to obtain the best possible result in plastic surgery—ranging from simple wound closure to complicated procedures such as tissue transplantation—strict attention must be paid to the principles of atraumatic surgery. Improper or rough handling of tissue may cause necrosis and hematoma formation, which provides a medium for bacterial growth and sepsis. This results in further necrosis and tissue loss, delayed healing, and excessive scar formation. As a consequence, the desired fine-line scar or the successful "take" of the tissue transplant may not be achieved.

Important factors in atraumatic technic are as follows:

(1) Use of hooks to handle skin edges during wound closure rather than forceps or clamps that crush tissue.

(2) Inclusion of the smallest amount of tissue possible in the ligation of blood vessels.

(3) Minimal use of electrocoagulating instruments.

(4) Absolute hemostasis.

(5) Use of sharp, fine instruments, fine needles, and fine sutures.

(6) Avoidance of hot wound packs.

WOUND CLOSURE

Primary Closure

The ideal type of wound closure is primary approximation of the skin and subcutaneous tissues immediately adjacent to the wound defect, producing a fine-line scar and the optimal cosmetic result in skin texture, thickness, and color match. Closure by adjacent rotational or transposed pedicle grafts usually produces the next best cosmetic result. Closure by free skin grafts or nonadjacent skin pedicle grafts is less satisfactory and should be considered only when sufficient adjacent tissues are not available.

Normal Skin Lines & Fine-Line Scars

In most cases, fine "hairline" scars can be achieved only if the line or lines of incision are placed in or parallel to the skin lines of minimal tension. These lines lie perpendicular to the underlying muscles. On the face, they are obvious as "wrinkle lines" or lines of facial expression which become more pro-

nounced with age since they are secondary to repeated muscle contraction. On the neck, trunk, and extremities, the lines of minimal tension are most noticeable as horizontal lines of skin relaxation on the anterior and posterior aspects of areas of flexion and extension.

So-called Langer's lines, which were determined by cadaver study, probably show the direction of fibrous tissue bundles in the skin and are no longer considered accurate guides for placing skin incisions.

If the lines of expression cannot be followed, the line of incision should (if possible) be placed at the junction of unlike tissues such as the hairline of the scalp and the forehead, the eyebrow and the forehead, the mucosal and skin junction of the lips, or the areolar and skin margins of the breast. Scars will be partially hidden if incisions are placed in inconspicuous areas such as the crease of the nasal ala and cheek, the auricular-mastoid sulcus, or the submandibular-neck junction. Lines of incision should never purposely cross flexor surfaces such as the neck, axilla, antecubital fossa, or popliteal space or the palmar surfaces of the fingers and hand.

Elliptical Excision (Fig 47–1.)

If a lesion is to be excised, an elliptical excision placed parallel to the skin lines of minimal tension will give the best result if the amount of tissue to be excised does not preclude primary closure.

If the ellipse is too broad or short, a protrusion of skin, commonly called a "dog-ear," will occur at each pole of the wound closure (Fig 47–2). This is most easily corrected by excising the dog-ear as a small ellipse.

A dog-ear may also be present if one side of the ellipse is longer than the other (Fig 47–3). In this case, it may be easier to excise a small triangle of skin and subcutaneous tissue from the longer side.

SKIN GRAFTS

Generally speaking, skin grafts may be classified as free grafts or pedicle grafts. The advantages and disadvantages and some specific indications for both types are summarized in Tables 47–1 and 47–2. Free

TABLE 47−1. Advantages and disadvantages of various types of skin grafts.

Type of Graft	Advantages	Disadvantages
Thin split thickness	Survive transplantation most easily. Donor sites heal most rapidly.	Fewest qualities of normal skin. Maximum contracture. Least resistance to trauma. Sensation poor. Cosmetically poor.
Thick split thickness	More qualities of normal skin. Less contracture. More resistant to trauma. Sensation fair. Cosmetically more acceptable.	Survive transplantation less well. Donor site heals slowly.
Full thickness	Nearly all qualities of normal skin. Minimal contracture. Very resistant to trauma. Sensation good to excellent. Cosmetically excellent.	Survive transplantation least well. Donor site must be closed surgically. Donor sites are limited.
Pedicle	Possess all qualities of normal skin. Minimal to no contracture. Greatest resistance to trauma. Sensation excellent to normal. Cosmetically may be excellent. Maximal padding over long bony surfaces. Will survive transplantation over avascular surfaces.	Transplantation requires highest degree of technical skill. Cosmetically may be poor. May be too bulky. Usually require multiple operative procedures.

grafts may be either partial or full thickness sheets or sections of skin which are completely separated from their donor sites, ie, their blood supply is completely interrupted. They are transferred to the recipient area and depend for their survival upon vascularization from the bed of the recipient area. Pedicle grafts always remain attached to the donor site or to an intermediate transfer site and therefore carry their own blood supply. Although they depend upon vascularization from the recipient site for healing, they do not depend upon it for survival. Pedicle grafts usually include the full thickness of skin plus all or a portion of the subcutaneous adipose tissue.

FREE GRAFTS

Types of Free Grafts

Free skin grafts are classified on the basis of their thickness as split thickness or full thickness (Fig 47–4).

A. Split Thickness Grafts: Split thickness grafts are further classified as thin, intermediate, and thick, depending upon the amount of dermis that is included with the graft. Since skin may vary in thickness from 0.09 inch to as much as 0.15 inch, an intermediate thickness graft from an area such as the eyelid would be much thinner than an intermediate thickness graft

TABLE 47−2. Indications for various types of skin grafts.

Type of Wound	Type of Graft	Reason for Choice
Infected wounds (including burns)	Thin split thickness	Difficulty in obtaining successful take of thicker grafts.
Wounds with poorly vascularized surfaces	Thin split thickness or pedicle	Difficulty in obtaining successful take of thicker grafts.
Small superficial facial wounds	Full thickness or local pedicle	Produces best cosmetic result.
Large superficial facial wounds	Thick split thickness or pedicle	Cannot use full thickness graft because of limited size of donor sites.
Noninfected wounds on a flexor surface	Thick split thickness, full thickness, or pedicle	Produces minimal contracture.
Full thickness eyelid loss	Local pedicle or composite	Repair requires more than one tissue element.
Deep loss of nasal tip	Local pedicle or composite	Repair requires thicker tissue than present in split or full thickness grafts.
Avulsive wounds with exposed tendons and nerves	Pedicle	Requires thick protective coverage without graft adherence to tendons and nerves.
Exposed avascular cortical bone or cartilage	Pedicle	Free grafts will not survive on avascular recipient site.
Wounds resulting from excision of deep x-ray "burn"	Pedicle	Free grafts will not survive on avascular recipient site.

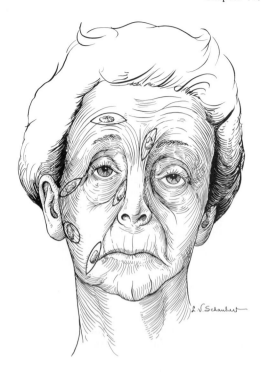

FIG 47—1. Sites of elliptical incisions corresponding to wrinkle lines on the face.

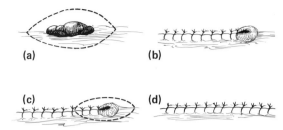

FIG 47—2. Correction of dog-ear.

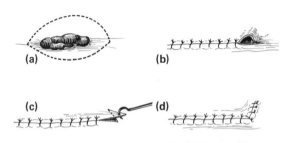

FIG 47—3. Alternative method of correction of dog-ear.

from the back. However, using the standard donor site areas such as the skin of the thigh or the lateral buttocks for reference, the average thin split thickness graft will measure 0.010–0.012 inch, the intermediate split thickness graft 0.016–0.018 inch, and the thick split thickness graft 0.022–0.024 inch.

Each type of split thickness graft has definite characteristics depending upon the thickness of dermis and the number of skin appendage elements that are present.

Each thickness presents certain advantages and disadvantages (Table 47—1). The major advantage of the thinner split thickness grafts is that they become vascularized more rapidly and thus survive transplantation more readily. This is of importance in grafting less than ideal recipient sites such as infected wounds, burn surfaces, and poorly vascularized surfaces. A second advantage in their use is that donor sites for these thinner grafts heal more rapidly, so that they can be reused within a relatively short period of time (7–10 days) in critical cases such as major burns.

In general, the disadvantages of the thin split thickness grafts outweigh the advantages. Thin grafts exhibit the highest degree of postgraft contracture, offer the least amount of resistance to surface trauma, and possess the least number of elements that are present in normal skin such as normal texture, suppleness, pore pattern, and hair growth. Hence, they are usually unacceptable from a cosmetic standpoint.

Conversely, the advantages of the thicker split thickness skin grafts are that they contract less, are more resistant to surface trauma, and possess to a greater degree the desirable elements of normal skin. They are cosmetically more acceptable than thin split thickness grafts, though they are not as acceptable as full thickness grafts.

The disadvantages of thick split thickness grafts are relatively few. They are less easily vascularized than

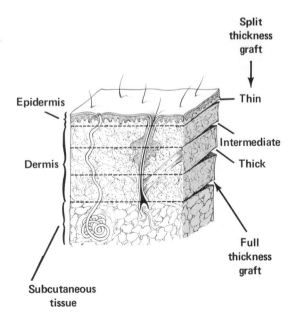

FIG 47—4. Depths of split thickness and full thickness grafts.

thin grafts and thus result in fewer successful "takes" when used on less than ideal surfaces. Their donor sites are slower to heal (requiring 10–18 days) and heal with more scarring than the donor sites for thin split thickness grafts, which may prevent their reuse.

Donor sites for split thickness grafts heal spontaneously by epithelization. This process depends upon the presence of sweat glands, sebaceous glands, or hair follicles whose epithelial cells proliferate and spread across the wound surface.

B. Full Thickness Grafts: Full thickness skin grafts include the epidermis and all of the dermis. They are the most cosmetically desirable of all free grafts since they include the highest number of skin appendage elements, undergo the least amount of contracture, and have a greater ability to withstand trauma.

There are several limiting factors in the use of full thickness grafts: the limited availability of donor sites, the necessity for closing the donor site since no epidermal elements remain to produce epithelization, and the difficulty in obtaining successful transplantation.

Only areas of thin skin can be utilized as donor sites for full thickness grafts because adequate vascularization of thick grafts will not occur before the graft dies. These areas of thin skin include the eyelids and the skin of the postauricular, supraclavicular, submammary, antecubital, inguinal, and genital areas. In grafts thicker than approximately 0.015 inch, the results of transplantation are consistently poor.

Borger AF: *Elective Incisions and Scar Revision.* Little, Brown, 1973.

Converse JM: Introduction to plastic surgery. Chap 1, pp 3–20, in: *Reconstructive Plastic Surgery.* Vol I. Converse JM (editor). Saunders, 1964.

Grabb WC, Smith JW: *Plastic Surgery: A Concise Guide to Clinical Practice,* 2nd ed. Little, Brown, 1973.

Kraissel CJ: The selection of appropriate lines for elective surgical incisions. Plast Reconstr Surg 8:1, 1951.

SKIN GRAFTING TECHNICS

OBTAINING THE GRAFT

Split Thickness

Various instruments are available for obtaining split thickness grafts. These include razor blades, skin grafting knives (Blair, Ferris Smith, Humby), manual dermatomes of either the suction (Barker) or drum variety (Padgett, Reese), and power-driven dermatomes of either the electric (Brown) or air variety (Hall).

The Blair and Ferris Smith knives are of limited value since successful use requires the special skill of the surgeon who uses them constantly. Even the tech-

nically improved Humby knife with its adjustable roller to control the thickness of the graft is not to be recommended for the occasional user. Except in the hands of a very skilled surgeon, skin grafting knives generally produce narrow, inferior grafts of uneven thickness with irregular scalloped edges.

The more precise drum type dermatomes are more reliable. Because their thickness gauges are the most dependable, they more consistently produce a graft of the desired thickness. However, their use requires skill and experience as well as time since their surfaces must first be coated with an adhesive or adhesive-bearing tape. Another disadvantage is that, since the maximum length of the drum is 20 cm (8 inches), longer grafts cannot be obtained without preparing the drum surface again between each cutting. They also require a fairly flat donor site if the surgeon desires a graft that measures the full 10 cm (4-inch) width of the drum.

Although the electric and air-powered dermatomes are not as precise as the drum type, they enjoy far wider popularity since the average surgeon, even without prior experience, is able to successfully obtain skin grafts with these instruments. They do not require the use of an adhesive, and the fact that they can be rapidly assembled and used to cut multiple grafts quickly without cleaning and reapplying an adhesive is an important advantage in treating a patient with extensive skin loss (such as a burn patient), when it is desirable limit the time of the surgical procedure. They also cut better than drum dermatomes on surfaces that are not perfectly flat, so that a wider choice of donor sites is available. The only major disadvantages are that they tend to produce grafts of uneven thickness and that the thickness tends to vary from the setting on the thickness gauge. The greatest width of graft that they will cut is 7.5 cm (3 inches), which is narrower than that obtained with the drum dermatome. However, grafts of any length can be obtained depending only upon the length of the donor site.

Full Thickness

Full thickness grafts are almost always cut to fit a small defect with an irregular outline. Because of this—and because they are cut precisely at the level of the junction of the dermis and the subcutaneous adipose layer—they are best obtained free-hand with a small scalpel blade, generally a No. 15. The plane of dissection is readily found if saline or lidocaine with epinephrine is injected into the subcuticular zone. A pattern is traced from the defect to be grafted by overlaying it with transparent plastic sheeting or exposed x-ray film and outlining the wound margins on the sheeting with marking ink. The pattern is then transferred to the donor area and precisely traced with marking ink. An incision is made along these margins into the dermis but not into the adipose layer. Using adequate countertension, the graft is cut along the desired plane and any fat that is inadvertently removed with the graft is trimmed away with a small curved plastic scissors.

Applying the Graft

After the graft has been applied directly to the prepared recipient surface, it may or may not be sutured in place and may or may not be dressed. Whenever the maximum cosmetic result is desired, the graft should be cut to fit the recipient area exactly and meticulously sutured into position without overlapping edges. Very large thick split thickness grafts and full thickness grafts will usually not survive without pressure. In areas such as the forehead, scalp, and extremities, adequate immobilization and pressure can be obtained by circular dressings. Tie-over pressure stent dressings are advisable for grafts in areas where pressure cannot be obtained by simple wraparound dressings (such as the cheek) or where movement is present (such as the anterior neck, where swallowing causes constant motion), and for grafts in areas of irregular contour (such as the axilla). This is accomplished by leaving the ends of the fixation sutures long and tying them over a bolus of gauze fluffs, cotton, sponge, or other suitable material (Fig 47–5).

When grafts are applied to freshly prepared or relatively clean surfaces, they are generally sutured into place and dressed with pressure. A single layer of fine mesh gauze impregnated with an ointment such as bismuth tribromophenate (Xeroform) to make it nonadherent is applied directly over the graft. Immediately over this are placed several thicknesses of flat gauze which have been cut by means of a pattern which exactly fits the graft. On top of this is placed a bulky dry dressing consisting of gauze fluffs, cotton, sponge, etc. Pressure is then obtained by wraparound dressings, adhesive tape, or the tie-over stent method.

In many cases it is permissible—and in some cases even preferable—to leave a skin graft site open with no dressing. This is particularly true in infected wounds, where the skin graft tends to "float off" in the purulent discharge that the wound produces. These wounds are better treated with exposed small sheets or stamp-size pieces of skin so that any liquid material that forms between the graft and wound bed can be evacuated by rolling the purulent drainage out from under the graft to the edge, where it can be wiped off. This same principle holds true in noninfected wounds that produce an unusual amount of serous or lymphatic drainage, as occurs following radical groin dissections.

In severely ill patients such as those with major burns, where it is essential to keep anesthetic time to a minimum, large sheets of split thickness skin grafts are rapidly applied without suturing, which is time-consuming. Grafts on these wounds may be left open if the area is small, but if the area is large or circumferential a pressure dressing should be applied.

ENSURING THE "TAKE"

In order to ensure survival of the graft, 4 conditions must be satisfied: (1) adequate vascularization of the recipient bed, (2) complete contact between the graft and the bed, (3) adequate immobilization, and (4) relative freedom from infection as far as the recipient area is concerned.

Since survival of the graft is dependent upon the ingrowth of capillary buds into its raw undersurface, vascularization of the recipient area is of prime importance. Conditions such as advanced radiation damage, chronic ulcers, bone or cartilage denuded of periosteum or perichondrium, and tendon without its paratenon are examples of avascular surfaces that will not generally accept free grafts. In these conditions, vascularity must be provided by excision down to healthy

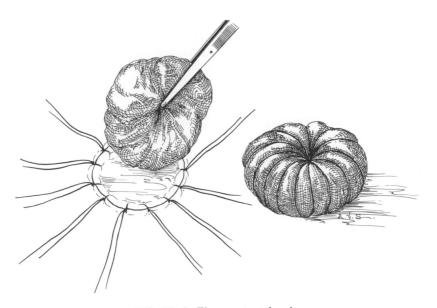

FIG 47–5. Tie-over stent dressing.

tissues, light scraping of unhealthy granulation tissue, or the production of granulation tissue by diligent wound care or by surgical means such as drilling holes through exposed cortical bone into healthy cancellous bone from which granulation tissue will form. If adequate vascularity cannot be provided, pedicle grafts (see below) are generally indicated.

Inadequate contact between the graft and the recipient bed can be caused by collection of blood, serum, lymph fluid, or purulent fluid between the graft and bed or by movement of the graft on the bed.

Thorough hemostasis is a cardinal rule in skin grafting and can be accomplished in most instances. In areas where adequate hemostasis with ligatures cannot be obtained, such as exposed cancellous bone from which the cortical surface has been removed, pressure must be relied upon for hemostasis. The standard tie-over pressure stent dressing is the best method of doing this.

The stent dressing is also useful in preventing serum or lymph collection under the graft and is essential in areas where movement cannot be controlled, such as in anterior neck wounds, where constant swallowing is present. In these areas, basting sutures through the graft to the underlying surface may be used.

If infection is present in the wound that is to be grafted, it is best controlled by diligent local wound care with saline compresses, conservative debridement, local antibiotics, and systemic antibiotics if indicated. Complete freedom from infection in open wounds is never obtained, but local care should be given until the wound is in optimum condition to receive the graft as demonstrated by the presence of clean, healthy granulation tissue.

Skin graft dressings may be left undisturbed for 5–7 days after grafting if the grafted wound was free of infection, if complete hemostasis was obtained, if fluid collection is not expected, and if immobilization is adequate. If any one of these conditions is not met, the dressing should be changed within 24–48 hours and the graft inspected. If blood, serum, or purulent fluid collection is present, evacuation of this collection should be accomplished—usually by making a small incision through the graft with a scalpel blade and applying pressure with cotton-tipped applicators. The pressure dressing is then reapplied and changed daily so that the graft can be examined and fluid expressed as it collects. Meticulous local care of the graft is essential, including debridement of any necrotic tissue that will allow colonization of bacteria beneath the graft surface, supporting infection that will further imperil the graft.

DONOR SITES

Factors to Consider in Choosing the Donor Site

The ideal donor site would provide a graft identical to the skin surrounding the area to be grafted.

Since skin varies greatly from one area to another as far as color, thickness, hair-bearing qualities, and texture are concerned, the ideal donor site (such as upper eyelid skin to replace skin loss from the opposite upper eyelid) is usually not found. However, there are definite principles that should be followed in choosing the donor area.

A. Color Match: In general, the best possible color match is obtained when the donor area is located close to the recipient area. Color and texture match in facial grafts will be much better if the grafts are obtained from above the region of the clavicles. However, the amount of skin obtainable from the supraclavicular areas is limited. If larger grafts for the face are required, the immediate subclavicular regions of the thorax will provide a better color match than areas on the lower trunk or the buttocks and thighs. When these more distant regions are used, the grafts will usually be lighter in color than the facial skin in Caucasians; in people with dark skin, hyperpigmentation occurs, producing a graft that is much darker than the surrounding facial skin.

B. Thickness of the Graft and Donor Site Healing: Donor sites heal by epithelization from the epithelial elements remaining in the donor bed. These include hair follicles, sweat glands, sebaceous glands, and their ducts. The ability of the donor area to heal and the speed with which it heals thus depend upon the number of these elements present. Donor areas for very thin grafts will heal in 7–10 days, whereas donor areas for intermediate thickness grafts may require 10–18 days and those for thick grafts 18–21 days or longer. This may be of critical importance in the treatment of severely burned patients, in whom sites may have to be reused within 7–10 days.

Since there is a normal anatomic variation in the thickness of skin, donor sites for thicker grafts must be chosen with the potential for healing in mind and should be limited to regions on the body where the skin is thick. Infants, debilitated adults, and elderly people have thinner skin than healthy younger adults. Grafts that would be split thickness in the normal adult may be full thickness in these patients, resulting in a donor site that has been deprived of the epithelial elements necessary for healing.

C. Hair-Bearing Qualities of the Graft: Since the hair follicles are usually present at the lowermost level of the dermis and the upper regions of the subcutaneous adipose layer, they are rarely transplanted with split thickness skin grafts. However, it is generally advisable to avoid hair-bearing donor sites in obtaining thick grafts that are to be used on hairless surfaces.

D. Cosmetic Appearance of the Donor Site: While donor sites for very thin grafts may heal with minimal or almost invisible scarring, donor areas for thicker grafts can heal with scarring that is quite conspicuous. In these cases it is more desirable to obtain grafts from areas such as the lateral hips and buttocks than from the thighs since these regions can more easily be hidden by clothing.

Care of the Donor Site

It has been common practice to cover the donor area with a sterile dressing and leave it unattended for 2–3 weeks. This practice is to be condemned since this type of dressing may provide ideal conditions for bacterial colonization with ensuing infection that destroys the epithelial elements that produce wound healing.

The care of the donor site must be as meticulous as the care of the grafted area. The method of care may vary, but the general principles are as follows: A layer of sterile, fine mesh, nonadherent gauze (such as 5% bismuth tribromophenate [Xeroform]) is placed directly over the wound. Several layers of sterile absorbent gauze bandages are placed over the nonadherent gauze. This dressing is then taped in place or held by a circumferential dressing. Oozing blood or serum will be absorbed by the dressing. This is removed in 24 hours, leaving in place the nonadherent gauze that is in direct contact with the wound. If a thin graft has been cut from this site, no further oozing will occur and the wound can be left open with the nonadherent gauze in place. If a thick graft has been cut, leaving a deep donor site, further oozing of serum can be expected. A fresh dressing of several layers of absorbent gauze is reapplied to collect this material, so that it will not form a crust over the wound under which bacteria will colonize. This is removed 24 hours later and the wound is left with only the nonadherent gauze covering. Heat lamps or warm air blowers may be used (with care) to facilitate drying of the wound. As epithelization occurs, the nonadherent gauze separates and is trimmed away. If isolated areas of superficial infection occur beneath the nonadherent gauze, the gauze is trimmed away over these areas so that saline compresses and local antibiotics can be applied. The entire gauze covering is not removed since at this time there is a temporary adherence to the wound and removing it will strip away the new epithelium that is being formed.

PEDICLE GRAFTS

A pedicle graft is a section of skin and subcutaneous tissue that is raised from one site and transferred to another. In contrast to free grafts, it always remains attached to its original donor site or to an intermediate transfer site.

The survival of free skin grafts depends upon the growth of vascular elements from the recipient bed into their undersurfaces. In the case of partial or full thickness skin grafts, this occurs readily. However, because pedicle skin grafts include a layer of subcutaneous adipose tissue beneath the skin, their thickness prevents this ingrowth at a rapid enough rate to maintain their survival. For this reason, they must always remain attached to a source of blood supply.

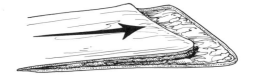
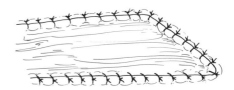

FIG 47–6. Advancement pedicle flap.

Types of Pedicle Grafts

Pedicle grafts may be classified into several general categories: They may be local or distant, depending upon whether they were obtained from tissues adjacent to or distant from the recipient wound. They may be single or double, depending upon the number of points of attachment. If an exposed raw area exists on the undersurface between the donor and recipient sites, they are called open pedicle flaps; if no exposed raw surface exists, they are called closed flaps. If they consist of more than skin and adipose tissue—such as skin with attached cartilage or bone—they are called composite pedicle grafts.

These grafts may also be classified as advancement flaps, transposed flaps, rotation flaps, jump flaps, and tube pedicle grafts.

A. Advancement Flaps: The simplest example of the advancement flap is one produced by undermining the skin edges of a tense wound to provide for adequate relaxation for closure (Fig 47–6). These are local pedicles that are advanced along a straight axis without transposition or rotation. Several methods have been devised to construct these grafts. They depend upon the skin being either loose enough or elastic enough to provide for the necessary relaxation.

The V-Y advancement (Fig 47–7) is a useful modification of this type of flap.

B. Transposed Flaps: Transposed flaps are local flaps that are advanced along an axis that forms an

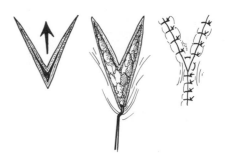

FIG 47–7. V-Y advancement flap.

Relaxing incision

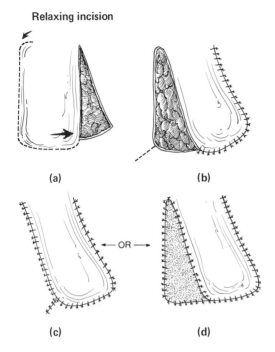

(a)   (b)

←— OR —→

(c)   (d)

FIG 47—8. Transposed flap.

angle to the original position of the flap (Fig 47—8a and b). They are usually rectangular and are generally transposed from an area where the skin is loose enough to provide for primary closure of the donor area (Fig 47—8c).

If this laxity is absent, the donor site must be closed with another graft, usually a split thickness free graft (Fig 47—8d).

On occasion, the pedicle flap cannot be transposed without tension on the flap. A short relaxing incision extending partially across the base may provide the needed relaxation if it does not interfere with the blood supply of the flap (Fig 47—8a).

At times the flap may be open, a portion of its exposed undersurface passing over intervening skin to reach the recipient area (Fig 47—9a and b). After a sufficient period of time has passed to allow for complete vascularization of the pedicle graft from the recipient site (usually 3 weeks), the pedicle is divided across its base and transfer is completed. The unused portion of the flap may be replaced to the donor site or sacrificed (Fig 47—9c).

C. Rotation Flaps: Rotation flaps are usually local closed flaps that are similar to transposed flaps but differ in that they are semicircular and rotate around a greater axis (Fig 47—10a). As with transposed flaps, they are generally rotated from areas where the skin is lax enough to allow for primary closure of the donor area (Fig 47—10b). A short relaxing incision may be necessary (Fig 47—10a) or, as with transposed flaps, a split skin graft may be used to close the donor site when it cannot be closed primarily.

D. Jump Flaps: Jump flap pedicle grafts are raised in the same fashion as the single based flaps illustrated above. Instead of being transferred immediately to their recipient areas, they are "jumped" or transferred to an intermediate carrying site. An example would be a rectangular flap raised from the abdomen and attached to the forearm to be later transferred to another region of the body. They may be open or closed, depending upon whether the undersurface is closed primarily or skin-grafted.

E. Tube Pedicle Flaps: Tube pedicles are bipedicled flaps that are formed by undermining the skin and the adjacent adipose layer between 2 parallel incisions and then rolling the skin edges under and suturing them together (Fig 47—11a, b, and c). Therefore, they are closed flaps that are especially suitable for transfer

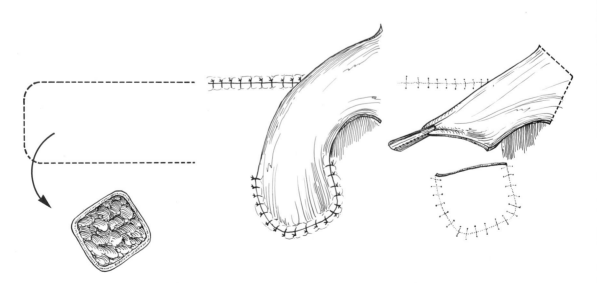

FIG 47—9. Flap passed over intervening skin to recipient area.

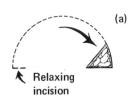

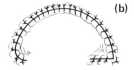

Relaxing incision

(a)

(b)

FIG 47–10. Rotation flap.

to a distant recipient site via a carrier such as the forearm or by migration by end-over-end transfer (Fig 47–12a and b).

Classic donor areas for tube pedicle flaps are the neck, the acromial-pectoral region of the anterior chest, the thoracoabdominal region of the trunk, the anterior abdominal wall, and the anteromedial aspect of the thigh. Any area on the body can be reached by a

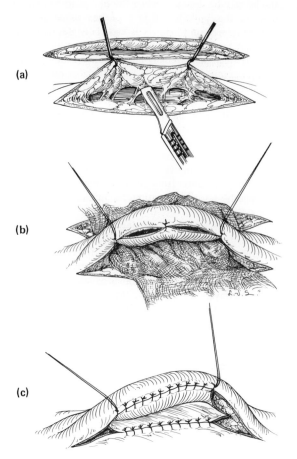

(a)

(b)

(c)

FIG 47–11. Construction of tube pedicle graft.

minimum number of transfer or migration procedures from one of these areas.

F. Island Pedicle Flaps: Island flaps consist of islands of skin and subcutaneous tissue which are transferred to new sites through a tunnel beneath the skin. The skin in the base of the island flap is removed, leaving only a neurovascular pedicle, so that skin will not be buried in the tunnel. The narrowness of this pedicle provides for great mobility, so that the flap may be transferred from one area to another in one stage, eg, from the forehead to the nose or cheek, or from one finger to another (Fig 47–13).

The intact nerve in the neurovascular pedicle provides the flap with normal sensation. Sensation can be restored to the anesthetic tip of an injured index finger by transferring an island flap from the tip and lateral aspect of the less important fourth finger.

G. Z-Plasty: (Fig 47–14). Z-plasty is actually a technic by which 2 triangular transposition pedicle flaps are elevated and transposed so that each flap occupies the other's original position. It has proved to be a very useful technic with 2 major applications: (1) lengthening a scar contracture line (flexion contractures across the neck, axilla, fingers, etc, congenital constriction bands, circular scars of body orifices); and (2) changing the direction of a scar (scars of the face that run across normal skin lines of minimal tension).

Characteristics of Pedicle Grafts

By definition, pedicle skin grafts remain attached to a donor site by a pedicle and possess their own blood supply through this pedicle. They also differ from free skin grafts in that they have a layer of sub-

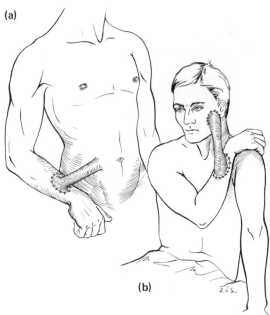

(a)

(b)

FIG 47–12. Transfer of pedicle graft via wrist carriers.

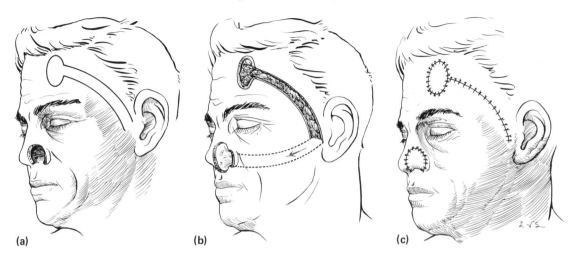

(a)   (b)   (c)

FIG 47—13. Island pedicle flap.

cutaneous adipose tissue lying beneath the full thickness of skin. These 2 factors make the use of pedicle grafts mandatory when the areas to be grafted are either avascular or require thick coverage to protect the underlying structures from trauma.

Examples of avascular surfaces are exposed bone, cartilage, or tendon without periosteum, perichondrium, or paratenon; exposed joint surfaces; wounds resulting from the excision of areas of radiation necrosis; and areas of extremely dense scar tissue.

Examples of structures or regions that require thick covering to protect them from trauma are bony surfaces and prominences; weight-bearing surfaces; densely scarred areas; and areas of decubitus ulcer formation.

There are numerous other characteristics of pedicle skin grafts that determine their use. Above all, they maintain all of the characteristics of normal skin. Their color and skin texture remain the same as before their transfer. For this reason, adjacent pedicle grafts usually provide for the best cosmetic appearance in reconstruction of facial defects if primary closure cannot be performed. By the same token, abdominal pedicles are not desirable for use on the face since they will continue to look like abdominal skin—different in color and with different skin texture, hair-bearing pattern, and thickness.

Hair growth, sebaceous secretion, and sometimes sweating are maintained by pedicle grafts. These factors—especially hair growth—make them undesirable for covering non-hair-bearing surfaces.

The bulkiness of pedicle grafts obtained from the abdomen and sometimes from the chest, buttocks, and thighs may be desirable when the defect to be grafted requires this bulk to fill in depressed tissue defects. This bulkiness or thickness is especially desirable for covering bony prominences and decubitus ulcer sites. Bulkiness can be extremely undesirable on the face and neck, where it obliterates normal facial contours and features; and in the hand, where it interferes with normal function.

Sensation is maintained in pedicle grafts. The degree of sensation is related directly to that of the donor site. Grafts of abdominal or chest skin will not provide adequate sensation to the fingertip, but grafts from adjacent fingers or the palmar surfaces will. Island pedicle grafts from adjacent fingers will provide for nearly normal sensation, including 2-point discrimination.

Whereas free grafts undergo varying degrees of contracture, pedicle grafts do not. This is an advantage in areas of scar contracture when free grafting has failed, and in relaxing circumferential scar constriction around orifices and within tubular passageways such as nasal airways, the pharynx, the esophagus, and the vagina. In these instances, Z-plasty should usually

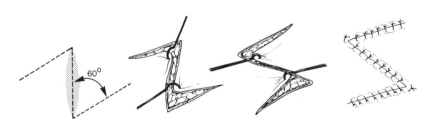

FIG 47—14. Z-plasty.

receive first consideration.

The layer of adipose tissue present in pedicle grafts makes them less adherent to underlying tissues than free skin grafts. Normally movable tissues such as tendons, joints, and muscles should be covered by pedicle grafts so that their movement will be restricted as little as possible.

In some cases, grafting over alloplastic materials is necessary. Examples are grafting over a vitallium or plastic cranioplasty and replacement of parietal pleura by a sheet of plastic mesh in wounds that extend completely through the chest wall. These materials can only be covered by grafts supplying their own blood supply.

Pedicle graft coverage is essential wherever secondary procedures such as tendon or nerve repairs or bone grafts are necessary. Because of their excellent blood supply, incisions can be made through pedicle flaps, and they can be raised by undermining to expose the structures that they cover. Split thickness skin grafts are not sufficiently vascularized to permit this.

Another desirable characteristic of pedicle grafts is that they maintain the same growth rate as the donor site, so that contracture does not occur when they are used as grafts in children.

Pedicle Grafting Technics

A. Construction: Although the technics for construction of pedicle flaps may vary with different types, there are certain basic principles that apply to the construction of all flaps.

Careful planning is essential to successful transfer. Following the principles that have been discussed, the type of graft and the donor site are selected. The size and shape of the flap are easiest to determine if an exact outline of the recipient area is made in thick pliable material such as gauze, leather, or felt. This pattern is then laid over the area to be grafted and the pattern transferred backward to the donor through exactly the same steps that will be taken during the actual transfer (Fig 47–15).

The ratio of the length of the pedicle flap to the width of the base is extremely important (Fig 47–16). Most flaps are of the single pedicle type that will be severed from the surrounding skin on 3 sides and will be completely separated from the donor bed. The entire blood supply must come from one base. The width of the base determines the number of blood vessels entering the graft. If the graft is too long in proportion to the width of the base, the distal portion of the flap will not survive due to lack of blood supply.

In general, single pedicle flaps require a 1:1 ratio between length and width and bipedicle flaps require a ratio of 2.5:1. However, there are several exceptions to this rule. If the pedicle flap possesses large arteries and veins within its base that traverse the length of the flap, the ratio of length to width can be greatly increased. Examples are the midline forehead flap, which includes in its base the frontalis artery and vein on each side of the midline; and the thoraco-epigastric tube pedicle based on the long thoracic artery

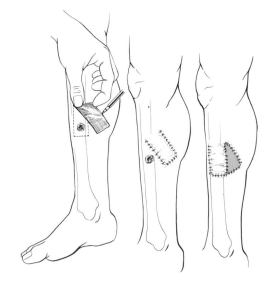

FIG 47–15. Use of pattern in construction of pedicle graft.

superiorly and the superficial epigastric artery inferiorly.

The ratio of length to width may also be increased (1) when the flap is to be constructed in areas with an abundant vascular supply, such as the head and neck, the hands, and the genital area; (2) in younger patients; and (3) when delay procedures on the pedicle flap are planned.

In areas of poor circulation, such as the lower regions of the legs and the back, and in older arteriosclerotic patients, greater caution must be observed.

B. Donor Sites: The ideal donor site would provide a graft identical to the skin that it is to replace. Important factors to consider are color match, thickness, sensation, hair-bearing qualities, and cosmetic appearance. These factors have been discussed above

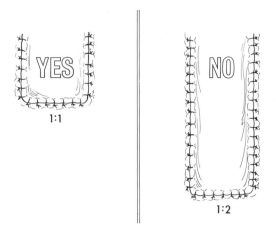

FIG 47–16. Ratio of length to width of base of pedicle graft.

(see p 946); however, there are 2 other important considerations.

(1) Pedicle grafts, like full thickness free skin grafts, leave a donor bed that is devoid of epithelial elements. Spontaneous healing therefore does not occur without contracture and undesirable scar tissue formation. Primary closure of the donor site is essential. This can be achieved by advancement and suturing of the wound edges if the pedicle is small. If the pedicle is large, the donor site must be closed by free split thickness skin grafts, or sometimes by another pedicle graft. Care should be taken to design pedicle grafts so that their grafted donor sites do not produce functional or cosmetic problems.

(2) Pedicle grafts should be constructed as close as possible to the recipient area so that multiple stages of surgical transfer can be avoided or minimized.

C. Delay of Pedicle Flaps: To delay a pedicle flap means to develop it in more than one stage by partially dividing it from its blood supply during each stage. This is done to enhance its vascularity and to condition it to respond less and less to hypoxia. Experimental and clinical studies have shown that after the sides of the pedicle flap have been incised in stages and after the flap has been undermined in stages, the vascular network within the flap becomes better aligned parallel to the long axis of the pedicle, with increase in both the number and size of the blood vessels. These changes occur in 1 week and reach their maximum in 18–21 days. For this reason, 21 days is the standard interval allowed between successive delays and transfers of pedicle flaps.

D. Transfer of Pedicle Flaps: All adjacent pedicle flaps are transferred directly to their recipient sites, either in one stage or after delay procedures depending upon their site of origin or their ratio of length to width.

Distant pedicles are transferred by migration from one intermediate site to another (tube pedicle flaps) or via a carrier such as the arm or wrist (jump flaps or tube pedicle flaps).

After the flap has been transferred, a period of 3 weeks is usually allowed to pass for full development of its blood supply. In regions of profuse vascularity, this period of time may be shortened.

To shorten the distance of transfer and the number of transfers, the graft is constructed as near as possible to the recipient area as long as the previously described requirements for the type of graft and the donor site are met.

Tube pedicles are usually transferred in stages. One end of the tube is first divided from its donor base. This will leave a circular open end of the pedicle (Fig 47–17). A flap that is shaped as a half-circle is then raised at the intermediate transfer site so that when it is reflected it will expose a circular recipient site to receive the end of the tube. After 21 days, the other end of the tube is severed from its base and transferred to a similarly created intermediate transfer area or to the final recipient site.

Jump flaps are usually rectangular, so that the

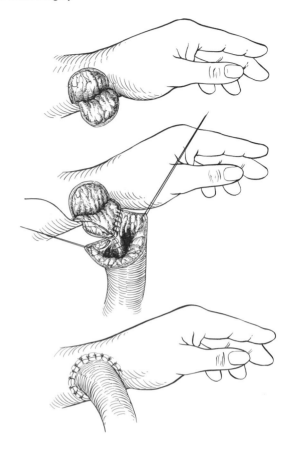

FIG 47–17. Method of transfer of tube pedicle flap.

flap that is raised on the carrier arm is similar in shape (Fig 47–15).

Whenever possible, all raw surfaces created by raising either the donor flap or the intermediate carrier flap should be closed by split thickness skin grafting to prevent infection.

Several adverse factors must be avoided to ensure successful transfer of pedicle flaps. Kinking of the base of the flap, undue tension on the flap, or excessive pressure by dressings may occlude the blood supply. Hematoma formation or infection at the recipient site may prevent successful transfer. These factors can be minimized by strict attention to details and adherence to the basic principles of plastic surgery.

Borger AF: *Elective Incisions and Scar Revision.* Little, Brown, 1973.

Brown JB, McDowell F: *Skin Grafting,* 3rd ed. Lippincott, 1958.

Converse JM, Brauer RO: Transplantation of the skin. Chap 2, pp 21–80, in: *Reconstructive Plastic Surgery.* Vol I. Converse JM (editor). Saunders, 1964.

Edgerton MT, Hanson FC: Matching facial color with split thickness skin grafts from adjacent areas. Plast Reconstr Surg 25:455, 1960.

Gillies HD, Millard DR Jr: *Principles and Art of Plastic Surgery.* 2 vols. Little, Brown, 1957.

SPECIFIC DISORDERS TREATED BY PLASTIC SURGERY

HYPERTROPHIC SCARS & KELOIDS

In response to any injury that is severe enough to break the continuity of the skin or produce necrosis, the skin heals by scar formation. Under ideal circumstances a fine, flat, "hairline" scar will result.

However, hypertrophy may occur, causing the scar to become raised and thickened, or a keloid may form. A keloid is a true tumor arising from the connective tissue elements of the dermis. By definition, keloids grow beyond the margins of the original injury or scar, and in some instances may grow to enormous size.

Healing and scar formation progress through 3 definite phases: exudative, proliferative, and maturation. During the exudative phase, blood and tissue fluids form an adhesive coagulum and a fibrinous network that serve to bind the wound surfaces.

Proliferation of endothelial and fibroblastic elements bridges the wound surfaces or fills in the spaces created by the loss of tissue. During this phase, the scar usually appears red and may be quite firm or hard. In the case of a fine incision, this phase may be short and the response minimal; in the case of a large open wound following avulsive injuries or burns, it may be prolonged and the response maximal.

The maturation phase begins as soon as the phase of fibroblastic proliferation has ceased. As the fibroblasts mature, the scar becomes less cellular and less vascular and begins to appear flat and white. Slow contracture also occurs.

Hypertrophic scars and keloids are produced during the second and third phases of scar formation. The tendency should be resisted to regard all thickened scars as keloids and to label as "keloid formers" all patients with unattractive scars. Hypertrophic scars and keloids are distinct entities, and the clinical course and prognosis are quite different in each case. The overreactive process that results in thickening of the hypertrophic scar ceases within a few weeks—before it extends beyond the limits of the original scar—and in most cases some degree of maturation occurs and gradual improvement take place. In the case of keloids, the overreactive proliferation of fibroblasts continues for weeks or months. By the time it ceases, an actual tumor is present that typically extends well beyond the limits of the original scar, involves the surrounding skin, and may become quite large. Maturation with spontaneous improvement does not usually occur.

Hypertrophic scars and keloids are difficult to differentiate by tissue staining methods. Tissue culture methods can be used for this purpose, but this is not practical. Clinical observation of the course of the scar is the only practical means of differentiation.

Treatment

Since nearly all hypertrophic scars will undergo some degree of spontaneous improvement, they do not require treatment in the early phases. If the scar is still hypertrophic after 6 months, surgical excision and primary closure of the wound are indicated. Improvement may be expected when the hypertrophic scar was originally produced by excessive endothelial and fibroblastic cell proliferation, as is present in open wounds, burns, and infected wounds. However, little or no improvement can be anticipated if the hypertrophic scar followed uncomplicated healing of a simple surgical incision. Hypertrophic scars across flexion surfaces such as the anterior elbow or the fingers cannot be improved unless a procedure such as a Z-plasty is performed to change the direction of the scar.

The treatment of choice for keloids is the injection of triamcinolone acetonide, 10 mg/ml (Kenalog-10 Injection), directly into the lesion. In the case of larger lesions, injection is made into more than one site. There is evidence that keloids may respond better to early than to late treatment.

Lesions are injected every 3–4 weeks, and treatment should not be carried out longer than 6 months. The following dosage schedule is used:

Size of Lesion	Dose per Injection
1–2 sq cm	20–40 mg
2–6 sq cm	40–80 mg
6–10 sq cm	80–110 mg

For larger lesions, the maximum dose should be 120 mg. The maximum doses for each treatment for children are as follows:

Age	Maximum Dose
1–2 years	20 mg
3–5 years	40 mg
6–10 years	80 mg

There is a tendency to inject the drug into the scar too often or in too high a dosage. Either may produce too vigorous a response, resulting in excessive atrophy of the skin and subcutaneous tissues surrounding the lesion and in depigmentation of darker skins. Both of these adverse responses will improve spontaneously in 6–12 months.

The response varies greatly; some lesions become flat after 2–3 injections, and some fail to respond at all.

Topical corticosteroid therapy is of no value.

Before the advent of corticosteroid injection therapy, surgical excision and radiation therapy were the only methods of treatment of keloids. Both methods are disappointing; surgical resection usually leads to recurrence of a larger lesion; with very few exceptions, radiation therapy produces no result. At present, surgical excision is used only in conjunction with intralesional corticosteroid therapy. Excision is usually confined to the larger lesions in which steroid therapy would exceed safe dosages. The wound is injected at the time of surgery and then postoperatively according to the schedule recommended above. Care should be taken to avoid extending surgical incisions out into the normal skin around the keloid since the growth of a new keloid may occur in these scars.

Conway H & others: Differential diagnosis of keloids and hypertrophic scars by tissue culture technique with notes on therapy of keloids by surgical excision and Decadron. Plast Reconstr Surg 25:117, 1960.

Crikelair GF: Surgical approach to facial scarring. JAMA 172:160, 1960.

Crikelair GF, Ju DMC, Cosman B: Scars and keloids. Chap 9, pp 161–186, in: *Reconstructive Plastic Surgery*. Vol 1. Saunders, 1964.

Ketchum LD, Robinson DW, Masters FW: Follow-up on treatment of hypertrophic scars and keloids with triamcinolone. Plast Reconstr Surg 48:256, 1971.

Maguire HC: Treatment of keloids with triamcinolone acetonide injected intralesionally. JAMA 192:325, 1965.

FACIAL INJURIES

Initial emergency care of severe facial injuries should be directed toward maintaining the airway and control of hemorrhage. Manual removal of blood clots and suctioning, if available, will usually free the oral airway. The unconscious patient should be positioned prone so that the tongue and the structures of the floor of the mouth do not occlude the oral pharynx. Tracheostomy is rarely necessary except in severe crushing injuries of the mid face.

Bleeding is best controlled by pressure until careful clamping of severed vessels under direct inspection can be done. Unless there has been massive bleeding from a major arterial laceration or other associated injury, shock is usually not present in the patient with maxillofacial injuries.

Extensive soft tissue injuries of the face should be repaired in the operating room under aseptic conditions as soon as possible. Treatment of concomitant injuries to the CNS, chest, or abdomen may take precedence. Because of the generous blood supply to the head and neck, repair of soft tissue lacerations may be safely delayed for up to 24 hours after injury. Soft tissue injuries should not be repaired until the possibility of injury to deeper structures has been ruled out by careful examination. This includes evaluation of facial nerve function, levator muscle function in the eyelid, and signs of injury to the parotid and lacrimal ducts. Delayed wound repair usually should be accompanied by antibiotic coverage. As in wounds elsewhere which may be contaminated, tetanus prophylaxis is indicated (see p 000). In immunized patients, a booster will suffice; tetanus-immune human globulin must be considered in nonimmunized patients with severely contaminated wounds.

Surgical Treatment

Local anesthesia is preferred to general anesthesia except in the case of very severe injuries when prolonged operating time and extensive skin grafting may be necessary. If intracranial injury is suspected, the type of anesthesia should be chosen after neurosurgical evaluation. With preliminary analgesic sedation, even small children and infants are usually cooperative when local anesthesia is used.

After local infiltration of the anesthetic, meticulous mechanical cleansing of the wound and adjacent skin is performed. Sterile drapes are then applied and the wound carefully explored using sterile saline irrigation to remove any imbedded foreign material. Suspected injuries to deeper structures can be verified at this time.

Debridement must include removal of all obviously devitalized tissues.

In special areas such as the eyelids, ears, nose, lips, and eyebrows, debridement must be very cautiously done since the tissue lost by debridement may be difficult to replace. Where tissues are more abundant, such as in the cheek, chin, and forehead areas, debridement may be more extensive. Small irregular or ragged wounds in these areas can be excised completely to produce clean, sharply cut wound edges which, when approximated, will produce the finest possible scar.

Because the blood supply in the face is plentiful, damaged tissues of questionable viability should be retained rather than debrided away. The chances for survival are good.

After debridement and wound irrigation, meticulous suture approximation will often obviate the need for secondary revision or reconstruction. A lacerated parotid or lacrimal duct should be repaired over a silicone or polyethylene catheter of appropriate size. Severed major branches of the facial nerves should be repaired by fine sutures when possible, or at least identified by small metal clips.

Closure of skin wounds should begin by approximation of key points. These include accurate rejoining of the borders of the lips, ears, and nose and reapproximation of such features as the vermilion border of the lip, the margins of the eyebrow, and the scalp hairline. Dead space, which can lead to hematoma formation and infection, is prevented by approximation of subcutaneous adipose and muscular tissues by buried absorbable sutures.

Undermining of the skin at the subdermal layer may be necessary to prevent wound tension where there has been significant skin loss. Either 4–0 or 5–0 sutures should be used, either nonabsorbable or absorbable. Where extensive contamination has occurred, absorbable material is preferable for buried sutures. Careful closure of the wound with subdermal sutures is followed by accurate approximation of the skin edges with fine nylon or silk sutures. Approximation without tension, using sutures that are not tied excessively tight, provides the most satisfactory cosmetic result.

Complicated lacerations such as complex stellate wounds or avulsion flaps often heal with excessive scarring. Because of the associated subcutaneous tissue injury, U-shaped or trap-door avulsion lacerations almost always become unsightly as a result of wound contracture. Small lacerations of this type are best excised and closed in a straight line initially; larger flaps that must be replaced usually require secondary revision. Extensive loss of skin is generally best treated by initial split thickness skin grafting followed later by secondary reconstruction. Primary attempts to reconstruct with local flaps may fail because of unsuspected injury to these adjacent tissues. The decision to convert avulsed tissues to free grafts which may not survive and thus delay healing requires sound surgical judgment.

Pressure dressings are useful in preventing hematoma formation and severe edema, which may result in poor wound healing. Dressings should be changed early and the wound inspected for hematoma or signs of infection. Hematoma evacuation, appropriate drainage, and antibiotic therapy based on culture and sensitivity studies may be required. Removal of sutures in 3–5 days, followed by splinting of the incision with paper tape or collodion gauze strips, will minimize scarring from the sutures themselves.

Prognosis

The final result of facial wound repair depends on the nature and location of the wounds, individual propensity to scar formation, and the passage of time. A year or more must often pass before resolution of scar contracture and erythema result in maximum improvement. Only after this time can a decision be made regarding the desirability of secondary scar revision.

Kazanjian VH, Converse JM: *The Surgical Treatment of Facial Injuries*, 3rd ed. Williams & Wilkins, 1963.

Plastic and Maxillofacial Trauma Symposium, Educational Foundation of the American Society of Plastic and Reconstructive Surgeons. Mosby, 1969.

FRACTURES OF THE FACIAL BONES

The bones of the nose are the most commonly fractured facial bones. Next in frequency are the mandible, the zygomatic-malar bones, and the maxilla. Multiple combined fractures are common as a result of automobile collisions at high speed.

Soft tissue edema may develop rapidly, making it difficult to palpate a displaced facial fracture. Radiologic examination, including the Waters view, basal view, and oblique views of the mandible, is imperative for accurate diagnosis.

Dingman RO, Natvig P: *Surgery of Facial Fractures*. Saunders, 1964.

Georgiade NG: *Plastic and Maxillofacial Trauma Symposium.* Vol 1. Mosby, 1969.

NASAL FRACTURES

Simple displaced fractures of the nasal bones may be treated immediately if the patient is seen before significant edema has developed. Local anesthesia is preferred, using either topical tetracaine or cocaine with epinephrine intranasally and lidocaine infiltration of the skin. The nasal bones may be disimpacted with an intranasal forceps or periosteal elevator, and aligned properly by means of external molding or pressure. Fractures of the nasal septum should be recognized and realigned in conjunction with manipulation of the external nasal bones.

If massive edema is already present when the patient is first seen, it is best to reduce the swelling with local cold compresses and proceed with closed reduction of the fractures when the edema has cleared enough so that the degree of displacement of the bones can be accurately evaluated. Compound fractures of the nose require prompt repair of the skin wound and either early or late reduction of the displaced nasal bones, depending upon the degree of local swelling.

External splinting, which is essentially a protective dressing, in conjunction with intranasal packing using nonadherent gauze, is appropriate following reduction of simple fractures of the nasal bones.

If there is extensive comminution of the bony nasal pyramid with posterior displacement into the piriform aperture, additional fixation may be required. After reduction and molding of the nasal bones, a fine stainless steel wire may be passed in a figure-of-eight fashion through the skin and across the base of the bony pyramid. Externally, the wire is passed through large buttons or soft lead plates to help mold the multiple comminuted fragments. Swelling of the soft tissues should be anticipated, and the wires should not be twisted so tight that external scarring will result. The fixation is maintained for 7–10 days.

MANDIBULAR FRACTURES

Mandibular fractures are most commonly bilateral, generally occurring in the region of the mid body at the mental foramen, the angle of the ramus, or at the neck of the condyle. A frequent combination is a fracture at the mental region of the body with a condylar fracture on the opposite side. Displacement of the fragments results from the force of the external blow as well as the pull of the muscles of the floor of the mouth and the muscles of mastication. The diagnosis is suggested by derangement of dental occlusion associated with local pain, swelling, and often crepitation upon palpation. Appropriate x-rays confirm the diagnosis. Special views of the condyle, including tomograms, may be required to evaluate fractures in this area.

Restoration of normal dental occlusion is the most important consideration in treating mandibular fractures. In patients with an adequate complement of teeth, arch bars or interdental wires can be placed. Local nerve block anesthesia is preferable for this procedure, though certain patients may require general anesthesia. Intermaxillary elastic traction will usually correct minor degrees of displacement and bring the teeth into normal occlusion. When the fracture involves the base of a tooth socket with suspected devitalization of the tooth, extraction of the tooth should be considered. Particularly in the incisor region, such devitalized teeth may be a source of infection, leading to the development of osteomyelitis and nonunion of the fracture.

If the patient is partially or completely edentulous, either his dentures or appropriate dental splints are used to maintain the mandible and maxilla in normal occlusion and provide a means of intermaxillary fixation. The dentures or splints may be wired directly by circumferential wires to the mandible and fixed to the maxilla either by pinning to the alveolar process or by suspensory wiring from above, entering the mouth through the upper buccal sulcus.

Intermaxillary fixation with wires immobilizes the mandible to the maxilla. This fixation should be maintained for 6 weeks in the case of fracture of the body and ramus. Earlier resumption of mandibular motion is indicated in cases of condylar fractures to prevent fibrotic ankylosis, which may accompany injury to the tempomandibular joint.

Open reduction of mandibular fractures is indicated where there is marked displacement that cannot be reduced or maintained by simple intermaxillary fixation. This may be the case in severely displaced fractures at the angle with muscle interposition that prevents reduction. Fractures of the body of the mandible in edentulous patients may require open reduction and wiring or plating the fragments together for adequate fixation. Open reduction is followed by intermaxillary fixation, using arch bars or splints, after normal occlusion is achieved.

Open reduction is not advised in condylar fractures except in the rare case where the condylar fragment may be so severely displaced as to prevent motion of the mandible because of impingement on the coronoid process or zygomatic arch. Even markedly displaced condylar fractures remodel after simple intermaxillary fixation to maintain normal occlusion. Early guided motion generally results in normal function.

ZYGOMATIC FRACTURES

Fractures of the zygomatic bones may involve just the arch of the zygomatic bone or the entire body of the zygoma (the malar eminence) and the lateral wall and floor of the orbit. The so-called tripod fracture characteristically occurs at the zygomatic frontal and zygomatic maxillary sutures as well as at the arch. Displacement of the body of the zygoma results in flattening of the cheek and depression of the orbital rim and floor.

Important diagnostic signs are subconjunctival hemorrhage, disturbances of extraocular muscle function (which may be accompanied by diplopia), and loss of sensation in the upper lip and alveoli on the involved side as a result of injury to the infraorbital nerve. Reduction of a displaced zygomatic fracture is seldom an emergency procedure and may be delayed until the patient's general condition is satisfactory for anesthesia. Local anesthesia will suffice only for reduction of fractures of the zygomatic arch. More extensively displaced fractures usually require general anesthesia.

Depressed fractures of the zygomatic arch only can best be elevated using the Gillies technic. Through a temporal incision above the hairline, an instrument is passed beneath the temporalis fascia and under the arch and body of the zygoma. The fracture can be elevated in conjunction with overlying palpation to achieve accurate reduction.

If extensive disruption of the orbital floor is suspected in conjunction with the zygomatic fracture, reduction of the fracture should be accompanied by direct visualization and repair of the orbital floor. Several approaches may be used for disimpaction and reduction of the displacement. These include the Gillies elevation and the transantral (Caldwell-Luc) approach directly through the antrum to the orbital floor. This latter technic is particularly helpful when there is extensive comminution of the antral portion of the zygoma and the adjacent maxilla. In complicated fractures, one or more of the approaches may be combined with direct visualization of the fracture sites and, if necessary, direct interosseous wiring to maintain reduction of unstable fragments. Elevation by grasping the zygoma with a towel clip is not recommended since it is difficult to control the reduction of comminuted fractures by this method and since unsatisfactory scarring may develop where the instrument pierces the skin.

"Blowout" fracture of the orbit refers to extensive disruption of the orbital floor which may occur as a result of blunt trauma directly to the orbit with no associated fracture of the body of the zygoma or the orbital rim. Such fractures may result in depression of the ocular globe due to prolapse of orbital fat into the antrum. The extraocular muscles may also be entrapped by the fragments of the disrupted floor. Diplopia occurs in either case. Careful x-ray examination, including orbital tomograms, is required to evaluate such an injury.

Repair of blowout fracture is effected after surgical exploration of the orbital floor. This may require the transantral (Caldwell-Luc) approach to elevate the depressed fragments of the floor, accompanied by packing of the antrum for support. In cases where there is extensive comminution and loss of bony fragments into the antrum, an implant to the orbital floor may be required to maintain support for the ocular structures. A thin sheet of alloplastic material such as silicone has been satisfactory for this purpose, although bone grafts have been recommended. Even with careful anatomic reduction of the disruption of the orbital floor, there may be late ocular problems due to resorption of the injured orbital fat. Follow-up evaluation by an ophthalmologist is mandatory.

MAXILLARY FRACTURES

Maxillary fractures range in complexity from partial fractures through the alveolar process to extensive displacement of the mid facial structures in conjunction with fractures of the frontonasal bones and orbital maxillary region. Hemorrhage and airway obstruction will require emergency care, and in severe cases tracheostomy is often indicated. Mobility of the maxilla can be elicited by palpation in extensive fractures. "Dish-face" deformity of the retruded displaced maxilla may be disguised by edema, and careful x-ray studies are necessary to determine the extent and complexity of the midfacial fracture. Treatment may have to be delayed because of other severe injuries. A delay of as long as 10–14 days may be safe before reduction and fixation, but the earliest possible restoration of maxillary position and dental occlusion is desirable to prevent late complications.

In the case of unilateral fractures or bilateral fractures with little or no displacement, splinting by intermaxillary fixation for 4 weeks will suffice. Fractures are usually displaced inferiorly or posteriorly and require direct surgical disimpaction and reduction. In certain severe cases, external traction may be necessary. Manipulation is directed toward restoring normal occlusion and maintaining the reduction with intermaxillary fixation to the mandible in association with direct fixation or supporting wires from other intact facial or cranial bones. Complicated fractures may require external fixation utilizing a head cap and intraoral splints in conjunction with multiple surgical incisions for direct wire fixation. Coexisting mandibular fractures usually necessitate open reduction and fixation at the same time.

CONGENITAL ANOMALIES

HEAD & NECK ANOMALIES

Cleft Lip & Cleft Palate

Cleft lip, cleft palate, or a combination of the 2 are the most common congenital anomalies of the head and neck. The incidence of facial clefts has been reported to be between 1 in every 650–750 live births, making it second only to clubfoot in frequency as a reported birth defect.

The cleft may involve the floor of the nostril and lip on one or both sides and may extend through the alveolus, the hard palate, and the entire soft palate. A useful classification based on embryologic and anatomic aspects divides the structures into primary and secondary palate. The dividing point between the primary and the secondary palate is the incisor foramen. Clefts can thus be classified as partial or complete clefts of the primary or secondary palate (or both) in various combinations. The most common clefts are left unilateral complete clefts of the primary and secondary palate and partial midline clefts of the secondary palate, involving the soft palate and part of the hard palate.

Most infants with cleft palate present some feeding difficulties, and breast feeding may be impossible. As a rule, enlarging the openings in an artificial nipple or using a syringe with a soft rubber feeding tube will solve difficulties in sucking. Feeding in the upright position helps prevent regurgitation or aspiration. Severe feeding problems and recurrent aspiration may complicate Pierre Robin syndrome, in which the palatal cleft is associated with a receding jaw and posterior displacement of the tongue, obstructing the oropharyngeal airway. A surgical procedure such as the tongue-lip adhesion operation may be necessary to prevent fatal aspiration in these patients.

Surgical repair of cleft lip is not considered an emergency. The optimal time for operation can be described as the widely accepted "rule of ten." This includes body weight of 5 kg (10 lb) or more and a hemoglobin of 10 g/100 ml or more. This is usually at some time after the 10th or 12th week of life. In most cases, closure of the lip will mold distortions of the cleft alveolus into a satisfactory contour. In occasional cases where there is marked distortion of the alveolus, such as in severe bilateral clefts with marked protrusion of the premaxilla, preliminary maxillary orthopedic treatment may be indicated.

General endotracheal anesthesia via an orally placed endotracheal tube is the anesthetic technic of choice. A variety of technics for repair of unilateral clefts have evolved over many years. Earlier procedures ignored anatomic landmarks and resulted in a characteristic "repaired harelip" look. The operation now employs an incision in the medial side of the cleft to allow the cupid's bow of the lip to be rotated down to a normal position. The resulting gap in the medial side of the cleft is filled by advancing a flap from the lateral side. This principle can be varied in placement of the incisions and results in most cases in a symmetric lip with normally placed landmarks. Bilateral clefts, because of greater deficiency of tissue, present more challenging technical problems. Maximum preservation of available tissue is the underlying principle, and most surgeons prefer simple approximation of the central and lateral lip elements in a straight line closure.

Secondary revisions are frequently necessary in the older child with a repaired cleft lip. A constant associated deformity in patients with cleft lip is distortion of the soft tissue and cartilage structures of the tip of the nose. Some correction of these deformities can be done at the time of initial surgery, but most cases require late revision after growth of the cartilagenous structure is complete. Many of the secondary procedures are minor in nature, including revisions of the scar and adjustments of local tissue deficiencies by either Z-plasties or V-Y advancement procedures. A tight upper lip due to severe tissue deficiency may be corrected in a 2-stage transfer of a pedicle flap from the lower lip—the Abbé flap operation.

Palatal clefts may involve the alveolus, the bony hard palate, or the soft palate, singly or in any combination. Clefts of the hard palate and alveolus may be either unilateral or bilateral, whereas the soft palate cleft is always midline, extending back through the uvula. The width of the cleft varies greatly, making the amount of tissue available for repair and reconstruction also variable. The bony palate, with its mucoperiosteal covering, forms the roof of the anterior mouth and the floor of the nose. The posteriorly attached soft palate is composed of 5 paired muscles of speech and swallowing.

Surgical closure of the cleft is the treatment of choice. However, in certain instances of severe tissue deficiency or in older patients with unrepaired clefts, closure of the defect with a dental prosthesis may be desirable. The consensus is that repair of the palate should be done between the first and second year since more tissue is available in the older baby. It is desirable to have the palate repaired and functioning as well as possible by the time the child undertakes serious speech, usually around age 2. If the soft palate seems to be long enough, simple approximation of the freshened edges of the cleft after freeing of the tissues through lateral relaxing incisions may suffice. If the soft palate is too short, a pushback type of operation is required. In this procedure, the short soft palate is retrodisplaced closer to the posterior pharyngeal wall, utilizing the mucoperiosteal flaps based on the posterior palatine artery.

Satisfactory speech following surgical repair of cleft palate is achieved in 70–90% of cases. Significant speech defects usually require secondary operations when the child is older. The most widely used technic is the pharyngeal flap operation, in which the palatopharyngeal space is reduced by attaching a flap of posterior pharyngeal muscle and mucosa to the soft palate. Various other kinds of pharyngoplasties have been useful in selected cases.

Blackfield HM & others: Cinefluorographic analysis of the surgical treatment of cleft palate speech. Plast Reconstr Surg 31:542, 1963.

Cronin TD: Surgery of the double lip and protruding premaxilla. Plast Reconstr Surg 19:389, 1957.

Grabb WC: *Cleft Lip and Palate: Surgical, Dental, and Speech Aspects.* Little, Brown, 1971.

Johansen B, Ohlsson A: Bone grafting and dental orthopedics in primary and secondary cases of cleft lip and palate. Acta chir scandinav 122:112, 1961.

Millard DR Jr: Wide and/or short cleft palate. Plast Reconstr Surg 29:40, 1962.

Nylen BO: Cleft palate and speech. Acta radiol Suppl 203, 1961.

Owsley JQ Jr & others: Experience with the high attached pharyngeal flap. Plast Reconstr Surg 38:232, 1966.

Pruzansky S: Presurgical orthopedics and bone grafting for infants with cleft lip and palate: A dissent. Cleft Palate J 1:164, 1964.

Randall P: A triangular flap operation for the primary repair of unilateral cleft of the lip. Plast Reconstr Surg 23:331, 1959.

Woolf CM, Woolf RR, Broadbent TR: Genetic and nongenetic variables related to cleft lip and palate. Plast Reconstr Surg 32:65, 1963.

Other Anomalies

The first and second branchial arch syndrome presents with deformities of variable severity. Deformities include absence of the external ear, partial or complete absence of the involved hemimandible, and lateral facial clefts.

Treacher-Collins syndrome presents a characteristic facies associated with mandibulofacial dysostosis.

Crouzon's syndrome, due to premature fusion of the facial sutures, is a rare anomaly. The major problems in these cases are related to the marked exophthalmos as well as the grotesque facies.

ANOMALIES OF THE HANDS & EXTREMITIES

The most common hand anomaly is syndactyly, or webbing of the digits. This may be associated with normal digits or with absence of portions of the fingers and occasionally with an extra digit. Surgical correction by division of the webbed cleft—and repair with appropriate local flaps and skin grafts—should be accomplished prior to school age.

Flexion contractures of the hands or digits may require surgical release and appropriate skin grafting. Congenital ring constriction of the extremities may be associated also with congenital amputation. The ring constrictions are best treated in stages by excision and Z-plasty.

GENITOURINARY ANOMALIES

Hypospadias and epispadias are the most commonly seen anomalies in the male and, depending on the severity, require one or more stages of surgical correction, usually starting when the child is 2–3 years of age. Epispadias may be associated with exstrophy of the bladder, which also occurs in females. This serious anomaly usually requires urinary diversion procedures and reconstructive surgery of the lower abdominal wall after excision of the bladder exstrophy.

Congenital absence of the vagina is quite uncommon. It is associated with an absent uterus, but the ovaries are usually normal. A satisfactory vaginal tract can usually be constructed with split thickness skin grafts using an inlay technic.

Converse JM: Vol II, Part 2, The Head and Neck, and Vol VI, Part 6, The Genitourinary System and Anorectal Malformations, in: *Reconstructive Plastic Surgery*. Saunders, 1964.

Grabb WC, Smith JW: *Plastic Surgery: A Concise Guide to Clinical Practice*, 2nd ed. Little, Brown, 1973.

Mustarde JC: *Plastic Surgery in Infancy and Childhood*. Saunders, 1971.

SKIN TUMORS

Tumors of the skin are by far the most common of all of the tumors that are seen in humans. They arise from each of the histologic structures that make up the skin—epidermis, connective tissue, gland, muscle, and nerve elements—and are correspondingly numerous in variety.

Skin tumors are conveniently classified as benign, premalignant, and malignant. Only those tumors that are commonly seen by the plastic surgeon will be discussed here.

Allen AC: *The Skin*, 2nd ed. Grune & Stratton, 1966.

Conway H: *Tumors of the Skin*. Thomas, 1956.

Fitzpatrick TB (editor): *Dermatology in General Medicine*. McGraw-Hill, 1971. [Chapters 10 and 11.]

Maddin S: *Current Dermatologic Management*. Mosby, 1970.

BENIGN SKIN TUMORS

The many benign tumors that arise from the skin rarely interfere with function. Since most are removed for cosmetic reasons, they are quite commonly treated by the plastic surgeon. The majority are small and can be simply excised under local anesthesia following the principles of elliptical excision and wound closure discussed above. General anesthesia may be necessary for larger lesions requiring excision and repair by skin grafts or those occurring in young children.

Most superficial lesions (seborrheic keratoses, verrucae, squamous cell papillomas) can be easily treated by simpler technics such as electrodesiccation, curettage and electrodesiccation, cryotherapy, and topical cytotoxic agents.

Seborrheic Keratosis

Seborrheic keratoses are superficial noninvasive tumors that originate in the epidermis. They appear in older people as multiple, slightly elevated, yellowish, brown, or brownish-black, irregularly rounded plaques with waxy or oily surfaces. They are most commonly present on the trunk and shoulders but are frequently seen on the scalp and face.

Curettage and electrodesiccation is usually the treatment of choice.

Verrucae Vulgaris

Verrucae vulgaris (common warts) are usually seen in children and young adults, commonly on the fingers and hands. They appear as round or oval elevated lesions with rough surfaces composed of multiple rounded or filiform keratinized projections. They may be skin-colored or gray to brown.

Verrucae are caused by a virus and are autoinoculable, which can result in multiple lesions around the original growth or frequent recurrences following treatment if the virus is not completely eradicated. They may disappear spontaneously.

Treatment by electrodesiccation is effective but is frequently followed by slow healing. Repeated applications of bichloroacetic acid, liquid nitrogen, or liquid CO_2 are also effective. Surgical excision is not recommended since the wound may become inoculated with the virus, leading to recurrences in and around the scar.

Because recurrences are common despite thorough treatment, it is reasonable to delay treatment of asymptomatic lesions for several months to determine if they will disappear spontaneously.

Cysts

A. Sebaceous Cyst: Although sebaceous cyst is the commonly used term, these lesions more properly should be called epidermal or keratinous cysts since they are composed of thin layers of epidermal cells filled with epithelial debris. (True cysts arising from sebaceous epithelial cells are uncommon.)

Sebaceous cysts are soft to firm, usually elevated, and are filled with an odorous cheesy material. Their most common sites of occurrence are the scalp, face, ears, neck, and back. They are usually covered by normal skin, which may show dimpling at the site of skin attachment.

Treatment consists of surgical excision.

B. Dermoid Cyst: Dermoid cysts are deeper than sebaceous cysts. They are not attached to the skin but frequently are attached to or extend through underlying bony structures. They may appear in many sites but are most common around the nose or the orbit, where they may extend to meningeal structures.

Treatment is by surgical excision, which may necessitate sectioning of adjacent bony structures.

Pigmented Nevi

A. Junction Nevi: Junction nevi are well-defined pigmented lesions appearing in infancy. They are usually flat or slightly elevated, light to dark brown in color, and contain no hair. They may appear on any part of the body, but most nevi seen on the palms, soles, and genitalia are of the junction type. Histologically, a proliferation of melanocytes is present in the epidermis at the epidermal-dermal junction. A varying amount of cellular activity in the form of cellular division with mitotic figures may be seen. Partly because of this, it has been widely accepted that junction nevi give rise to malignant melanoma and that all junction nevi should be excised for prophylactic reasons. However, most investigators now feel that junction nevi are not precancerous. If there is no change in their appearance, treatment is unnecessary. Any change such as inflammation, darkening in color, halo formation, increase in size, bleeding, or ulceration calls for immediate treatment.

Surgical excision is the only safe method of treatment.

B. Intradermal Nevi: Intradermal nevi are the typical dome-shaped, sometimes pedunculated, fleshy to brownish pigmented "moles" that are characteristically seen in adults. They frequently contain hairs and may occur anywhere on the body.

Microscopically, melanocytes are present entirely within the dermis and, in contrast to junction nevi, show little activity. They are rarely if ever malignant and require no treatment except for cosmetic reasons.

Surgical excision is nearly always the treatment of choice except in areas such as the nasal tip, where adverse scarring occurs. In such cases, more conservative dermatologic methods of treatment may be indicated, but pigmented nevi must never be treated without obtaining tissue for histologic examination.

C. Compound Nevi: Compound nevi exhibit the histologic features of both junction and intradermal nevi in that melanocytes lie both at the epidermal-dermal junction and within the dermis. They are usually elevated, dome-shaped, and light to dark brown in color.

Because of the presence of nevus cells at the epidermal-dermal junction, the indications for treatment are the same as for junction nevi. If treatment is indicated, surgical excision is the method of choice.

D. Benign Juvenile Melanoma: Benign juvenile melanomas are rapidly growing pigmented lesions that appear in children and exhibit some of the microscopic and clinical features of malignant melanoma. They usually appear on the face as distinctive small, pinkish or reddish, soft, nodular lesions. They increase in size rapidly, but the average lesion reaches only 6–8 mm in diameter, remaining entirely benign without invasion

or metastases. Microscopically, the lesion can be confused with malignant melanoma by the inexperienced pathologist.

The usual treatment is excisional biopsy.

E. Blue Nevi: Blue nevi are small, sharply defined, round, dark blue or gray-blue lesions that may occur anywhere on the body but are most commonly seen on the face, neck, hands, and arms. They usually appear in childhood as slowly growing, well-defined nodules covered by a smooth, intact epidermis. Microscopically, the melanocytes that make up this lesion are limited to (but may be found in all layers of) the dermis. An intimate association with the fibroblasts of the dermis is seen, giving the lesion a fibrotic appearance not seen in other nevi. This, together with extension of melanocytes deep into the dermis, may account for the blue rather than brown color.

Treatment is not necessary unless the patient desires removal for cosmetic reasons or fear of malignancy. Surgical excision is the treatment of choice.

F. Giant Hairy Nevi: Unlike most nevi arising from melanocytes, giant hairy nevi are congenital. They may occur anywhere on the body and cover large areas. They may be large enough to cover the entire trunk (bathing trunk nevi). They are of special significance for several reasons: (1) their large size is especially deforming from a cosmetic standpoint; (2) they show a definite predisposition for developing malignant melanoma; and (3) they may be associated with neurofibromas or melanocytic involvement of the leptomeninges and other neurologic abnormalities.

Microscopically, a varied picture is present. All of the characteristics of intradermal and compound nevi may be seen, along with those associated with juvenile melanoma. Neurofibromas may also be present within the lesion. Malignant melanoma may arise anywhere within the large lesion, the rate of occurrence being as high as 13.7% in one reported study. Malignant melanoma with metastases can arise in childhood and even in infancy.

The only treatment is complete excision and skin grafting. Large lesions may require excision and grafting in stages. Some lesions are so large that excision is not possible.

Hemangioma

It is confusing to attempt to classify hemangiomas on the basis of their histology. For example, the histologic term capillary hemangioma is used to designate both the common involuting hemangioma of childhood that disappears by 7 years of age and the port wine stain that persists into adulthood. The term cavernous is used to designate several types of hemangiomas that behave quite differently. Some hemangiomas are true neoplasms arising from endothelial cells and other vascular elements (such as involuting hemangiomas of childhood, endotheliomas, and pericytomas). Others are not true neoplasms but rather malformations of normal vascular structures (eg, port wine stains, cavernous hemangiomas, and arteriovenous fistulas).

A simple classification based upon whether or not the hemangioma undergoes spontaneous involution is proposed in Table 47–3.

A. Involuting Hemangioma: Involuting hemangiomas are the most common tumors that occur in childhood and comprise at least 95% of all the hemangiomas that are seen in infancy and childhood. They are true neoplasms of endothelial cells but are unique among neoplasms in that they undergo complete spontaneous involution.

Typically, they are present at birth or appear during the first 2–3 weeks of life. They grow at a rather rapid rate for 4–6 months, when growth ceases and spontaneous involution begins. Involution progresses slowly but is complete by 5–7 years of age.

Involuting hemangiomas appear on all body surfaces but are seen more often on the head and neck. They are seen twice as often in girls as in boys and show a predisposition for fair-skinned individuals.

Three forms of involuting hemangioma are seen—superficial, combined superficial and deep, and deep. Superficial involuting hemangiomas appear as sharply demarcated, bright red, slightly raised lesions with an irregular surface that has been described as resembling a strawberry. Combined superficial and deep involuting hemangiomas have the same surface characteristics, but beneath the surface a firm bluish tumor is present that may extend deeply into the subcutaneous tissues. Deep involuting hemangiomas present as deep blue tumors covered by normal-appearing skin.

The histologic findings in involuting hemangiomas are quite different from those seen in other types of hemangiomas. There is a constant correlation between the histologic picture and the clinical course. During the growth phase, the lesion is composed of solid fields of closely packed round or oval endothelial cells. As would be expected during the growth phase, cellular division with mitotic figures is seen, so that the lesion is sometimes called a hemangioendothelioma by the pathologist. This term must not be used, however, since it is commonly used to denote the highly malignant angiosarcoma that is seen in adults.

As the phase of involution progresses, the histologic picture changes, with the solid fields of endothelial cells breaking up into closely packed, capillary-sized, vessel-like structures composed of several layers of endothelial cells supported by a sparse fibrous stroma. These vascular structures gradually become fewer in number and spaced more widely apart in a loose, edematous fibrous stroma. The endothelial cells continue to disappear, so that by the time involution is complete the histologic picture is entirely normal with no trace of endothelial cells.

Treatment is not usually indicated since the cosmetic appearance following spontaneous regression is nearly always superior to the scars that follow surgical excision. Complete surgical excision of lesions that involve important structures such as the eyelids, nose, or lips results in the unnecessary destruction of these important structures that are difficult to repair.

Partial resection of a portion of a hemangioma of the brow or eyelid is indicated when the lesion is large enough to prevent light from entering the eye–a condition that will lead to blindness. The same type of treatment may be necessary for lesions of the mucosal surfaces of the lips when they project into the mouth and are traumatized by the teeth. In these cases, surgery should be very conservative–resecting only enough of the lesion to alleviate the problem and leaving the remaining portions to involute spontaneously.

In approximately 8% of cases, ulceration will occur. This may be accompanied by infection, which is treated by the use of compresses of warm saline or potassium permanganate and by the application of antibiotic powders and lotions. Bleeding from the ulcer is not common, and when it does occur it is easily controlled by the application of pressure.

After involution of large lesions, superficial scarring may be present or the involved skin may be thin, wrinkled, or redundant. These conditions may require conservative plastic surgery procedures. Telangiectasia may be present which may be improved by electrodesiccation of the involved capillaries, but the results of this type of treatment are usually disappointing.

The application of local agents such as dry ice to the surface of these lesions has been popular. This type of treatment has no effect on the deep portions of the hemangioma. It will destroy superficial lesions but results in severe scarring. Injections of sclerosing agents (eg, sodium morrhuate) have no effect. There is no place for radiation therapy in the treatment of these benign lesions.

B. Noninvoluting Hemangioma: Most noninvoluting hemangiomas are present at birth. In contrast to involuting hemangiomas, they do not undergo rapid growth during the first 4–6 months of life but grow in

TABLE 47–3. Proposed classification of hemangiomas based on appearance and clinical course of lesion.

Proposed Term	Terms in Common Use*
Involuting hemangioma	
Superficial	Strawberry nevus
	Nevus vasculosus
	Capillary hemangioma
Superficial and deep	Strawberry nevus
	Capillary hemangioma
	Capillary and cavernous hemangioma
Deep	Cavernous hemangioma
Noninvoluting hemangioma	
Port wine stain	Port wine stain
	Capillary hemangioma
	Nevus flammeüs
Cavernous hemangioma	Cavernous hemangioma
Venous racemose aneurysm	Cavernous hemangioma
Arteriovenous fistula	Arteriovenous fistula

*Confusing because different terms are used to denote the same lesion and because the same term is sometimes used to denote different lesions.

proportion to the growth of the child. They persist into adulthood, when they may cause severe cosmetic and functional problems. Some, such as arteriovenous fistulas, may cause death due to cardiac failure.

Unfortunately, treatment of noninvoluting hemangiomas is difficult and usually far from satisfactory.

Port wine stains are by far the most common of the noninvoluting hemangiomas. They may involve any portion of the body but most commonly appear on the face as flat patchy lesions that are reddish to purple in color. The light red lesions may fade to a varying degree but persist into adulthood. Some of the deep red or purplish lesions that have a stippled appearance show a propensity for growth later in life, in which case they become raised and thickened, with nodules appearing on the surface.

Microscopically, port wine stains are made up of thin-walled capillaries that are arranged throughout the dermis. The capillaries are lined with mature flat endothelial cells. In the lesions that produce surface growth, groups of round proliferating endothelial cells and large venous sinuses are seen.

Results following treatment of the port wine stain are uniformly disappointing. Since most lesions occur on the face or neck, patients seek treatment for the cosmetic problem they present. The simplest and still the most effective method of treatment is camouflaging. Unfortunately, this is difficult because the port wine stain is darker than the surrounding lighter skin.

Tattooing with skin-colored pigments may offer some measure of disguise in the lighter lesions but generally is unsatisfactory because the pigment deposited in the skin looks artificial and tends to be absorbed unevenly, producing a mottled appearance.

Superficial methods of treatment such as dry ice, liquid nitrogen, electrocoagulation, and dermabrasion are ineffective unless they destroy the upper layers of the skin, which produces severe scarring.

Radiation therapy, including the use of x-rays, radium, thorium-X, and grenz x-rays, is to be condemned. If it is administered in doses high enough to destroy the vessels involved, it also destroys the surrounding tissues and the overlying skin.

If the lesion is small, surgical excision with primary closure may be indicated. Unfortunately, most lesions are large, and surgical excision requires split thickness skin grafting. Because of the scar present around the edge of the graft and the loss of normal skin texture—along with the inability to obtain a good color match between the graft and the facial skin—the results of excision with skin grafting are far less than ideal.

Most port wine stains should be left alone.

C. Cavernous Hemangioma: Cavernous hemangiomas are bluish or purplish lesions that are usually elevated. They may occur anywhere on the body but, like other hemangiomas, are more common on the head and neck. They are composed of mature, fully formed venous structures that are present in tortuous masses which have been described as feeling like "a bag of worms."

Cavernous hemangiomas are usually present at birth but do not usually grow except to keep pace with normal body growth. In many cases, growth occurs later in life and may interfere with normal function.

Microscopically, cavernous hemangiomas are made up of large dilated, closely packed vascular sinuses that are engorged with blood. They are lined by flat endothelial cells and may have muscular walls like normal veins.

Treatment is difficult. In only a few cases is the lesion small enough or superficial enough to permit complete surgical excision. Most lesions involve deeper structures—including muscle and bone—so that complete excision is impossible without radical surgery. Since most lesions are cosmetic problems, radical surgery is rarely indicated.

Other forms of treatment such as x-ray and radium therapy are of no value since the mature vessels are not sensitive to radiation. Suture ligation of surrounding vessels, multiple intralesional ligations, and injections of sclerosing solutions usually have no effect upon the lesions and have been discarded.

Andrews GC, Domonkos AN: Cutaneous angiomas and their treatment. New York J Med 57:1436, 1957.
Blackfield HM & others: Management of visible hemangiomas. Am J Surg 94:313, 1957.

PREMALIGNANT SKIN LESIONS

Actinic Keratoses

Actinic keratoses are the most common of the precancerous skin lesions. They usually appear as small, single or multiple, slightly elevated, scaly or warty lesions ranging in color from red to yellow, brown, or black. Since they are related to sun exposure, they occur most frequently on the face and the backs of the hands in fair-skinned Caucasians whose skin shows evidence of actinic elastosis.

Microscopically, actinic keratoses consist of well-defined areas of abnormal epithelial cells limited to the epidermis. Approximately 15−20% of all lesions become malignant, in which case invasion of the dermis as squamous cell carcinoma occurs.

Since the lesions are limited to the epidermis, superficial treatment in the form of curettement and electrodesiccation or the application of chemical agents such as liquid nitrogen, phenol, bi- or trichloroacetic acid, or fluorouracil is curative. The application of fluorouracil (5-FU) cream is of particular benefit in preventive treatment in that it will destroy lesions of microscopic size—before they can be detected clinically—without causing damage to uninvolved skin.

Chronic Radiation Dermatitis

There are 2 distinct types of radiation dermatitis. The first and most common follows the acute administration of relatively high dosages of ionizing radiation over relatively short periods of time—almost always for the treatment of malignancy. It is characterized by an acute reaction that begins near the third week of therapy, when erythema, blistering, and sloughing of the epidermis start to occur. Burning and hyperesthesia are commonly present.

This initial reaction is followed by scarring characterized by atrophy of the epidermis and dermis along with loss of skin appendages (sweat glands, sebaceous glands, and hair follicles). Marked fibrosis of the dermis occurs, with gradual endarteritis and occlusion of the dermal and subdermal vessels. Telangiectasia of the surface vessels is seen, and areas of both hypo- and hyperpigmentation occur.

The second type of radiation dermatitis follows chronic exposure to low doses of ionizing radiation over prolonged periods of times. It is usually seen in professional personnel who handle radioactive materials or administer x-rays or in patients who have been treated for dermatologic conditions such as acne or excessive facial hair. Therefore, the face and hands are most commonly involved. The acute reaction described above does not usually occur, but the same process of atrophy, scarring, and loss of dermal elements occurs. Drying of the skin becomes more pronounced, and deepening of the skin furrows is typically present.

In both types of radiation dermatitis, late changes may occur such as the following: (1) the appearance of hyperkeratotic growths on the skin surface, (2) chronic ulceration, and (3) the development of either basal cell or squamous cell carcinoma. Ulceration and malignancy, however, are seen much less commonly in the first type of chronic radiation dermatitis than in the second. When malignant growths appear, basal cell carcinomas are seen more frequently on the face and neck and squamous cell carcinomas more frequently on the hands and body.

Treatment of chronic radiation dermatitis or the malignant lesions that develop is complicated by the marked scarring that is present and by the avascularity of the involved tissues secondary to endarteritis.

Surgical excision is the treatment of choice. Primary wound closure is feasible for only the smallest lesions. Free skin grafting can be performed only for the most superficial lesions, where damage to the vascular supply of the subcutaneous structures is not advanced. Lesions that involve the deeper subcutaneous tissues require surgical excision followed by pedicle skin grafting.

Bowen's Disease

Bowen's disease is characterized by single or multiple, brownish or reddish plaques that may appear anywhere on the skin surface but often on covered surfaces. The typical plaque is sharply defined, slightly raised, scaly, and slightly thickened. The surface is often keratotic, and crusting and fissuring may be present. Ulceration is not common, but when present suggests malignant degeneration with dermal invasion. Some authorities believe that all cases of Bowen's disease are secondary to the ingestion of arsenic. (A significant number of cases are related to arsenic-induced malignancies of internal organs.)

Histologically, hyperplasia of the epidermis is seen, with pleomorphic malpighian cells, giant cells, and atypical epithelial cells which are limited to the epidermis.

Treatment of small or superficial lesions consists of total destruction by curettement and electrodesiccation or by any of the other superficially destructive methods (cryotherapy, cytotoxic agents). Excision and skin grafting is preferred for larger lesions and for those that have undergone early malignant degeneration and invasion of the dermis.

Erythroplasia of Queyrat

Erythroplasia of Queyrat is almost identical to Bowen's disease both clinically and histologically but is confined to the glans penis and the vulva, where the lesions appear as red, velvety, irregular, slightly raised plaques.

Treatment is as described for Bowen's disease.

MALIGNANT SKIN TUMORS

1. BASAL CELL CARCINOMA

Basal cell carcinoma is the most common skin cancer. The lesions usually appear on the face and are more common in men than women. Since exposure to ultraviolet rays of the sun is a causative factor, basal cell carcinoma is most commonly seen in geographic areas where there is significant sun exposure and in people whose skins are most susceptible to damage from exposure, ie, fair-skinned individuals with blue eyes and blond hair. It may occur at any age but is not common before age 40.

The growth rate of basal cell carcinoma is usually slow but nearly always steady and insidious. Several months or years may pass before the patient becomes concerned. Without treatment, widespread invasion and destruction of adjacent tissues may occur, producing massive ulceration. Penetration into the bones of the facial skeleton and the skull is not uncommon. Basal cell carcinomas rarely metastasize, but death can occur because of direct intracranial extension or because of erosion of major blood vessels.

Typical individual lesions appear as small, translucent or shiny ("pearly") elevated nodules with central umbilication and rolled, pearly edges. Telangiectatic vessels are commonly present over the surface, and pigmentation is sometimes present. Superficial ulceration occurs early. When invasion of the dermis and subcutaneous tissues occurs along with deeper ulceration, the lesion is termed a rodent ulcer.

A less common type of basal cell carcinoma is the sclerosing or morphea carcinoma, consisting of elongated strands of basal cell cancer which infiltrate the dermis, with the intervening corium being unusually compact. These lesions are usually flat and whitish or waxy in appearance and firm to palpation—similar in appearance to localized scleroderma.

The superficial erythematous basal cell cancer ("body basal") occurs most frequently on the trunk. It appears as reddish plaques with atrophic centers and smooth, slightly raised borders. These lesions are capable of peripheral growth and wide extension but do not become invasive until late.

Pigmented basal cell carcinomas may be mistaken for melanomas because of the large number of melanocytes present within the tumor. They may also be confused with seborrheic keratoses.

Treatment

There are several methods of treating basal cell carcinoma. All may be curative in some lesions, but no one method is applicable to all. The special features of each basal cell cancer must be considered individually before proper treatment can be selected.

Since most lesions occur on the face, cosmetic and functional results of treatment are important. However, the most important consideration is whether or not therapy is curative. If the basal cell carcinoma is not eradicated by initial treatment, continued growth and invasion of adjacent tissues will occur. This will result not only in additional tissue destruction but also in invasion of the tumor into deeper structures, making cure impossible.

The principal methods of treatment are curettage and electrodesiccation, surgical excision, and radiation therapy. Chemosurgery, topical chemotherapy, and cryosurgery are not often used but may have value in selected cases.

A. Curettage and Electrodesiccation: Curettage and electrodesiccation is the most frequently used method of treatment. After infiltration with suitable local anesthetic, the lesion and a 2–3 mm margin of normal-appearing skin around it are thoroughly curetted with a small skin curet. The resultant wound is then completely desiccated with an electrosurgical unit to destroy any tumor cells that may not have been removed by the curet. The process is then repeated once or twice if necessary. The wound is left open and allowed to heal secondarily.

With experience, the soft and friable tumor cells in superficial lesions can be differentiated by the curet from the firm surrounding dermis. This permits the detection and removal of infiltrative strands of basal cells. However, in deeper lesions, as soon as these extensions of tumor invade beyond the dermis, they can no longer be accurately detected.

When used as treatment for superficial basal cell carcinoma, curettage and electrodesiccation is a simple, quick, and inexpensive procedure that will cure nearly all superficial lesions. However, this method of treatment should not be used in the deeper infiltrative and morphea type lesions. These should be treated by surgical excision, x-ray therapy, or chemosurgery.

B. Surgical Excision: Surgical excision, following the principles outlined earlier in this chapter, offers many advantages in the treatment of basal cell carcinoma: (1) Most lesions can be quickly excised in one procedure. (2) Following excision, the entire lesion can

be examined by the pathologist, who can determine if the tumor has been completely removed. (3) Deep infiltrative lesions can be completely excised, and cartilage or bone can be removed if they have been invaded. (4) Lesions that occur in dense scar tissue or in other poorly vascularized tissues cannot be treated by curettage and desiccation, radiation therapy, or chemosurgery since healing is poor. Excision with pedicle grafting may be the only method of treatment in these conditions. (5) Recurrent lesions in tissues that have been exposed to maximum safe amounts of radiation can be excised and grafted.

Small to moderate-sized lesions can be excised in one stage under local anesthesia. The visible and palpable margins of the tumor are marked on the skin with marking ink. The width of excision is then marked 3–5 mm beyond these margins. If the margins of the basal cell carcinoma are vague, the width of excision will have to be wider to ensure complete removal of the lesion. The lines of incision are drawn along these margins parallel to the normal skin creases in an elliptical shape. This ellipse of tissue is excised, taking care to leave a margin of normal-appearing subcutaneous tissue around the deep margins of the tumor. Frozen sections may be obtained at the time of excision to aid in determining whether or not tumor-free margins have been obtained.

Wounds resulting from the excision of some moderate-sized tumors and nearly all large tumors may necessitate closure by a free skin graft or a pedicle graft. Larger lesions may require excision and wound closure by free skin grafts or pedicle grafts. This can nearly always be performed in one stage.

The disadvantages of surgical excision are as follows: (1) Specialized training and experience are necessary to master the surgical technics. (2) Whereas curettage and desiccation may be performed in the office, surgical excision requires specialized facilities. (3) In lesions with vague margins, an excessive amount of normal tissue may have to be excised to ensure complete removal. (4) Structures that are difficult to reconstruct such as the eyelids, nasal tips, and lips have to be sacrificed when they are extensively infiltrated.

C. X-Ray Therapy: In the past, many radiologists and dermatologists tended to treat carcinoma of the skin by a single massive dose of ionizing radiation or by a few large individual doses over a short period of time. In addition, treatments were often administered with machines of low kilovoltage potential (kVp) that produces x-rays of poor quality. These factors led to excessive tissue damage and resulted in a high incidence of radiation dermatitis and radiation necrosis with associated undesirable cosmetic and functional results.

These problems have been almost completely eliminated by modern technics. The use of machines of higher kVp and application of the principle of treatment by fractionation are the 2 most important reasons for the excellent results now being obtained. Fractionation implies treatment with multiple relatively small doses (usually 4–6 per week) rather than the administration of higher individual doses every 3–7 days.

Many factors influence the quality of radiation used, the total dose to be given, the number of fractions, and the time period involved. Of the various types of radiation therapy, treatment with Roentgen rays generally is the most convenient and flexible with respect to adjusting the quality of the rays, the field size, and fractionation.

Carcinomas of the skin overlying cartilage, such as on the ear or nose, require special attention. Lesions in such locations require greater fractionation of dose and a higher quality of radiation in order to avoid painful chronic chondritis. Eyelid lesions are treated using a small cup-shaped lead shield to protect the eye.

The radiation therapist must estimate the extent of the lesion on a 3-dimensional basis, as the surgeon must, by inspection and palpation to determine adequate treatment. Fields of treatment should extend up to 1 cm or more beyond the evident borders of the lesion including both the lateral and deep margins. Larger, deeply invasive lesions require a wider margin of treatment.

Therefore, most small early lesions require fields of treatment at least 2 cm in diameter with a quality of radiation adequate to carry the desired dose to 1 cm in depth. For such lesions, Moss recommends using radiations produced at 110 kV with a filter of 0.25 mm copper and 1 mm aluminum. When lesions require treatment fields larger than 4 cm, he recommends radiations produced at 200 kV filtered with 0.5 mm copper and 1 mm aluminum.

Small lesions, except those of the eyelids or over cartilage, may be treated by administering a total of 4000 rads in 10 fractions over 10–12 days; but when the lids, ears, or nose are involved, he advises using 4200–5000 rads fractionated over a 3- to 4-week period. In treating large lesions (up to 8–10 cm in diameter) which infiltrate bone or cartilage, he advises using 6500–7500 rads over an 8-week period. In most cases, the dose is divided into 5 fractions per week.

The advantages of x-ray therapy are as follows: (1) Structures that are difficult to reconstruct such as the eyelids, tear ducts, and nasal tips can be preserved when they are invaded by but not destroyed by tumor. (2) A wide margin of tissue can be treated around lesions with poorly defined margins to ensure destruction of nondiscernible extensions of tumor. (3) It may be less traumatic than surgical excision to elderly patients with advanced lesions. (4) Hospitalization is not necessary.

The disadvantages are as follows: (1) Only well-trained, experienced physicians can obtain good results. (2) Expensive facilities are necessary. (3) Improperly administered radiation therapy may produce severe sequelae, including scarring, radiation dermatitis, ulceration, and malignant degeneration. (4) Baldness will result in hair-bearing areas. (5) It may be difficult to treat areas of irregular contour, ie, the ear and the auditory canal. (6) Repeated treatments over a period of 2–4 weeks may be necessary.

2. SQUAMOUS CELL CARCINOMA

Squamous cell carcinoma is the second most common cancer of the skin and is even more common than basal cell carcinoma in darkly pigmented racial groups. As with basal cell carcinoma, sunlight is the most common causative factor in Caucasians, and most lesions occur in fair-skinned individuals. The most common sites of occurrence are the ears, the cheeks, the lower lip, and the backs of the hands. Other causative factors are chemical and thermal burns, scars, chronic ulcers, chronic granulomas (tuberculosis of the skin, syphilis), draining sinuses, contact with tars and hydrocarbons, and exposure to ionizing radiation.

Since exposure to the sun is the greatest stimulus for the production of squamous cell carcinoma, most of these lesions are preceded by actinic keratosis on areas of the skin showing chronic solar damage. They may also arise from other premalignant skin lesions and from normal-appearing skin.

The natural history of squamous cell carcinoma may be quite variable. It may present as a slowly growing, locally invasive lesion without metastases or as a rapidly growing, widely invasive tumor with early metastatic spread. In general, squamous cell carcinomas that develop from actinic keratoses are of the slowly growing type, whereas those that develop from Bowen's disease, erythroplasia of Queyrat, chronic radiation dermatitis, scars, and chronic ulcers tend to be more aggressive in nature. Lesions that arise from normal-appearing skin and from the lip, genitalia, and anal regions also tend to be aggressive.

Early squamous cell carcinoma usually appears as a small, firm, erythematous plaque or nodule with indistinct margins. The surface may be flat and smooth or may be verrucous. As the tumor grows it becomes raised, and, because of progressive invasion, becomes fixed to surrounding tissues. Ulceration may occur early or late but tends to appear earlier in the more rapidly growing lesions.

Histologically, malignant epithelial cells are seen extending down into the dermis as broad, rounded masses or slender strands. In squamous cell carcinomas of low malignancy, the individual cells may be quite well differentiated, resembling uniform mature squamous cells having intracellular bridges. Keratinization may be present, and layers of keratinizing squamous cells may produce typical round "horn pearls." In highly malignant lesions the epithelial cells may be extremely atypical, abnormal mitotic figures are common, and intracellular bridges are not present and keratinization does not occur, so that "horn pearls" are absent.

As with basal cell carcinomas, the method of treatment that will eradicate squamous cell carcinomas and produce the best cosmetic and functional result varies with the characteristics of the individual lesion. Factors that determine the optimal method of treatment include the size, shape, and location of the tumor as well as the histologic pattern that determines its aggressiveness. The most common form of squamous cell carcinoma—that arising from actinic keratosis—is the least aggressive and requires less vigorous therapy than the more malignant types arising from Bowen's disease, scars, ulcers, chronic radiation dermatitis, and apparently normal skin.

The same methods of therapy that are discussed under treatment of basal cell carcinomas are used for the treatment of squamous cell carcinomas. The advantages and disadvantages of each type of therapy are discussed above. Since basal cell carcinomas are relatively nonaggressive lesions that very rarely metastasize, failure to eradicate the lesion will result only in local recurrence. Although this may result in extensive local tissue destruction, there is rarely a threat to life. Aggressive squamous cell carcinomas, on the other hand, may metastasize to any part of the body, and failure of treatment may have fatal consequences. For this reason, total eradication of each lesion is the imperative goal of treatment.

Because the overall incidence of lymph node metastasis is relatively low, most authorities agree that node resection is not indicated in the absence of palpable regional lymph nodes except in the case of very aggressive carcinomas of the genitalia and anal regions.

3. MALIGNANT MELANOMA

Malignant melanomas are not nearly as common as basal cell or squamous cell carcinomas, but they have a far greater potential for widespread invasion, metastasis, and subsequent mortality.

Clinical & Histologic Classification

Although all melanomas arise from the common melanocyte, 3 distinct clinical lesions are seen: (1) lentigo maligna melanoma, (2) superficial spreading melanoma, and (3) nodular melanoma. Each presents with different shapes, sizes, and shades of color and with different potentials for aggressive behavior.

A. Lentigo Maligna Melanoma: Lentigo maligna melanomas usually occur on exposed surfaces of the body in older individuals (65–70 years). They are usually large (3–5 cm), flat, freckle-like lesions with multicolored surfaces composed of light brown, dark brown, or black areas. Depigmented areas are sometimes present. Small black nodules are present on the surface, and the dark brown or black areas are sometimes raised. At times they are preceded by lentigo maligna.

The histologic morphology of the individual melanocytes that make up each lesion varies with the surface appearance. In the light brown areas, a proliferation of malignant melanocytes is present along the basal layer of the epithelium. These melanocytes vary in appearance from normal to very atypical. In the flat black areas, atypical malignant melanocytes are more numerous and replace the normal basal layer, with the adjacent papillary layer of the dermis being densely infiltrated by lymphocytes and macrophages filled with melanin pigment. In the areas where black surface nodules are present, nests of malignant melanocytes invade the underlying dermis.

B. Superficial Spreading Melanoma: Superficial spreading melanomas are usually smaller than lentigo maligna melanomas (2–3 cm) and occur in a slightly younger age group (50–60 years). The surface tends to be flat or slightly elevated and the edges irregular and indented. As with lentigo maligna melanomas, bizarre combinations of light brown, dark brown, black, red, or pink lesions may be seen. Numerous small nodules may also be present.

Histologically, the malignant melanocytes are rather uniform in appearance. These malignant cells usually involve both the epidermis and the dermis.

C. Nodular Melanoma: Nodular melanomas tend to occur in a younger age group (30–60 years). They are smaller than the other 2 types and are entirely elevated above the surface of the surrounding skin rather than flat. They are almost always uniformly dark brown or black, not showing the variations in color that are present in the other lesions. At times they exhibit a very rapid rate of growth and may become quite large.

Histologically, the malignant melanocytes arise from the epidermal-dermal junction and invade the underlying dermis. Whereas involvement of the epidermis is a prominent feature of lentigo maligna and superficial spreading melanomas, in nodular melanomas the epidermis remains free of invasion of melanocytes unless there is a direct extension of malignant cells from those invading the dermis. Complete invasion of the dermis and extension into the subcutaneous tissues is more commonly seen in this type of melanoma.

Treatment

The treatment of malignant melanoma consists of surgical excision. Nearly all lesions except small lentigo maligna melanomas must be excised widely enough so that skin grafting is required. Lymph node dissection is usually not necessary in lentigo maligna melanoma except in rare cases when palpable nodes are present. The same is true of superficial spreading melanoma unless invasion is present. There is considerable controversy regarding the value of prophylactic node dissection for melanoma. At present, most authorities feel it is not indicated for superficial spreading melanoma since excellent results follow wide excision alone. In nodular melanoma with invasion to level III or IV, the regional nodes are nearly always clinically involved and therapeutic dissection is indicated. Unfortunately, the prognosis with this lesion is so poor that genuine benefit from removal of clinically uninvolved nodes (prophylactic node dissection) is difficult to establish. Regional perfusion with antitumor drugs has been performed both by arterial and endolymphatic routes. Remarkable regressions have followed such therapy, but adequate clinical trials to establish its exact place are needed. Malignant melanoma sometimes regresses spontaneously. Moreover, dramatic regressions have followed a variety of immunologic treatments such as vaccination with smallpox vaccine, transfusion with blood from patients whose tumors have previously undergone spontaneous regression, and nonspecific stimulation of the immune system with BCG. A circulating tumor-specific antibody has been identified in cases of malignant melanoma, and there is some evidence for the existence of a common melanoma antigen shared by most, if not all, malignant melanomas. The prospect of controlling the disease in the near future by immunotherapy appears promising.

Prognosis

An accurate estimation of the prognosis of a patient with malignant melanoma can only be made by correlating the clinical appearance of the lesion with its histologic picture. In general, lentigo maligna melanomas are less aggressive and less apt to metastasize than superficial spreading melanomas, and both of these lesions tend to be less aggressive than nodular melanomas.

Clark has offered a helpful classification of malignant melanomas based on their clinical and pathologic features correlated with the level of histologic invasion of the lesion: level I, in situ melanoma, above the basement membrane; level II, through the basement membrane into the papillary level of the dermis but not into the reticular layer; level III, filling the papillary layer of the dermis and extending to the junction of the papillary and reticular layers but not into the reticular layer; level IV, into the reticular layer of the dermis; and level V, into the subcutaneous adipose tissue.

In Clark's opinion, lentigo maligna and superficial spreading melanomas that do not invade the dermis beyond level II do not cause death in more than 10% of cases. When nodular melanoma is first treated, it usually extends at least to level III and causes death in approximately 45% of cases. He feels that—regardless of the type of tumor—the mortality rate increases with the depth of invasion at the time of treatment.

Knutson CO, Hori JM, Spratt JS Jr: *Melanoma: Current Problems in Surgery.* Year Book, 1971.
Melanoma and Skin Cancer. Proceedings of the International Cancer Conference, Sydney, Australia, 1972. VCN Bright, Government Printer. Sydney, NSW Australia.

COSMETIC SURGERY

Cosmetic plastic surgery has an application in all age groups. Procedures include corrective otoplasty for the lop-eared child, rhinoplasty for the teen-age boy or girl, or a blepharoplasty or facelift for the aging man or woman.

Educational Foundation of the American Society of Plastic and Reconstructive Surgeons: *Symposium on Aesthetic Surgery of the Face, Eyelid, and Breast.* Mosby, 1972.
Masters FW, Lewis JR Jr (editors): *Symposium on Aesthetic Surgery of the Face, Eyelid, and Breast.* Vol 4. Mosby, 1972.
Symposium on cosmetic surgery. S Clin North America 51:261–531, 1971.

Otoplasty

Young children with protruding ears due to the absence of the conchoscaphal angle are frequently teased unmercifully by other children. The corrective surgical procedure which recreates the cartilage fold through a postauricular incision can be performed with a brief hospitalization and convalescence. Preschool age is probably the ideal time for operation, as the child's ears have reached nearly their full potential growth by age 6. The surgical technic is fairly standard with minor variations, and complications are rare.

Rhinoplasty

Variations in the appearance of the nose from aesthetically desirable standards may be a result of ethnic developmental deformities or secondary to an injury. Nasal fractures are frequently unrecognized in a young child, and the resulting deformity may only become manifest at a much later age. The large humped nose with bulbous or drooping tip is often a tragedy to the sensitive teen-age boy or girl with an emerging awareness of social competition. Cosmetic nasal reconstruction is usually recommended when the patient's nose shows evidence of maturity. This may be as early as age 13 in girls, but usually averages somewhere between 15 and 17 years. Boys are generally operated on at a slightly later age than girls. The operation is done through intranasal incisions, usually under local anesthesia, and requires only a brief period of hospitalization. Postoperative swelling and periorbital ecchymosis are associated with a convalescence of 10–14 days following operation.

Proper selection of the candidate for surgery is important both from a psychologic and anatomic point of view. Certain patients may present with other profile problems associated with a receding chin. In selected cases, a complementary chin augmentation with a silicone implant may enhance the surgical result. Rhinoplasty has proved to be a very satisfactory procedure, as attested by the fact that it is the most widely performed cosmetic surgical operation.

Mammoplasty

Cosmetic breast surgery, particularly the augmentation mammoplasty, has become a frequently requested operation. The general surgeon who operates for breast malignancy can attest to the tremendous psychologic significance of the breasts to the average woman. The development of the silicone breast prosthesis for augmentation mammoplasty in the past decade has made this procedure a safe operation with excellent long-term results. An appropriately sized implant containing silicone gel in a sealed silicone bag is placed in a prepared retromammary pocket through a small incision in the inferior submammary fold. The scars are usually quite inconspicuous after a few months. The improvement in contour is predictably good, and the breast is authentic to palpation unless too large an implant has been placed, resulting in overly tight skin coverage.

Direct injection of silicone fluid into the breast is

not only illegal at the present time but is strongly contra-indicated since it has been demonstrated experimentally that significant volumes of the injected fluid are gradually lost from the local site, and local reactions to the silicone fluid injection have been recorded. In addition, localized collections of fluid may simulate carcinoma.

Reduction mammoplasty, while it has significant cosmetic implications, is in fact a reconstructive surgical procedure. The chronic symptoms associated with carrying greatly enlarged breasts are well recognized, and the operation is indicated to relieve back and neck pain as well as posture problems.

The most common procedures used are those in which the nipple is displaced upward on a pedicle of breast tissue around which the reduced skin brassiere is tailored following excision of the excess breast tissue and skin. Nursing ability can be preserved with this technic, although nipple sensation may be lost. Small but ptotic breasts can be cosmetically improved utilizing this technic.

Another method of reduction mammoplasty which is suitable for the older patient with massively enlarged breasts employs the technic of transplantation of the nipple as a free graft. This is combined with a simpler plan of skin and breast tissue excision, and wound healing is usually free of complications.

Blepharoplasty

Removal of redundant drooping eyelid skin and eyelid "bags" can correct the evidence of aging around the eyes. The procedure is often performed at the same time as a facelift. The scars are placed so as to blend into normal skin creases. "Bags" of bulging orbital fat are removed after dissection from beneath the orbicularis oculi muscles.

Castanares S: Blepharoplasty for herniated intraorbital fat; anatomical basis for a new approach. Plast Reconstr Surg 8:46, 1951.

Facelift

The facelift, or rhytidectomy, is a very satisfactory operation in properly selected patients. The procedure is usually performed under local anesthesia combined with sedation and can be accomplished with a brief hospitalization and convalescence of 2–3 weeks. The operation is designed primarily to correct the sagging of redundant skin beneath the chin and along the neck and jawline that develops with advancing age. The lines of expression, such as the nasolabial folds and the so-called laugh lines around the lateral canthi of the eyes, are only minimally affected. The surgery is of value in the patient with sufficient laxity of the face and neck skin so that significant correction can be achieved. In such a patient, a worthwhile interval will pass before the sagging gradually occurs again. It is not uncommon for a patient to have a second facelift or even, occasionally, a third.

●   ●   ●

General References

Artz CP, Moncrief JA: *The Treatment of Burns,* 2nd ed. Saunders, 1969.

Barsky AJ: *Principles and Practice of Plastic Surgery,* 2nd ed. Williams & Wilkins, 1950.

Borger AF: *Elective Incisions and Scar Revision.* Little, Brown, 1973.

Brown JB, McDowell F: *Skin Grafting,* 3rd ed. Lippincott, 1958.

Clark WH Jr, Mihm MC: Chap 11 in: *Dermatology in General Medicine.* Fitzpatrick TB (editor). McGraw-Hill, 1971.

Converse JM: Introduction to plastic surgery. Chap 1, pp 3–20, in: *Reconstructive Plastic Surgery.* Vol I. Converse JM (editor). Saunders, 1964.

Converse JM (editor): *Reconstructive Plastic Surgery Principles and Procedures in Correction, Reconstruction, and Transplantation.* 5 vols. Saunders, 1964. Vol I: Part 1, *General Principles.* Vols II and III: Part 2, *The Head and Neck.* Vol IV: Part 3, *The Hand and Upper Extremity;* Part 4, *The Lower Extremity.* Vol V: Part 5, *The Trunk;* Part 6, *The Genitourinary System and Anorectal Malformations;* Part 7, *Tissue Transplantation and Burn Shock.*

Converse JM: *Surgical Treatment of Facial Injuries,* 3rd ed. Williams & Wilkins, 1973.

Converse JM (editor): Symposium on reconstructive plastic surgery. S Clin North America 47:259–549, 1967.

Dingman RO, Natvig P: *Surgery of Facial Fractures.* Saunders, 1964.

Edgerton MT, Hanson FC: Matching facial color with split thickness skin grafts from adjacent areas. Plast Reconstr Surg 25:455, 1960.

Educational Foundation of the American Society of Plastic and Reconstructive Surgeons: *Plastic and Maxillofacial Trauma Symposium.* Mosby, 1969.

Goldwyn RM (editor): *The Unfavorable Results in Plastic Surgery: Avoidance and Treatment.* Little, Brown, 1972.

Grabb WC, Smith JW: *Plastic Surgery: A Concise Guide to Clinical Practice,* 2nd ed. Little, Brown, 1973.

Longacre JJ: *Scar Tissue: Its Use and Abuse: The Surgical Correction of Deformities Due to Hypertrophic Scar and the Prevention of Its Formation.* Thomas, 1972.

Maddin S: *Current Dermatologic Management.* Mosby, 1970.

Murray JE: Annual discourse: Organ replacement, facial deformity, and plastic surgery. New England J Med 287:1069–1074, 1972.

Mustarde JC: *Plastic Surgery in Infancy and Childhood.* Saunders, 1971.

Pinckus H, Stoll HL, Van Scott EJ: Chap 10 in: *Dermatology in General Medicine.* Fitzpatrick TB (editor). McGraw-Hill, 1971.

Polk HC Jr, Stone HH: *Contemporary Burn Management.* Little, Brown, 1971.

Rees T, Wood-Smith D: *Cosmetic Facial Surgery.* Saunders, 1973.

48 . . .

Surgery of the Hand

Eugene S. Kilgore, MD, & William P. Graham III, MD

Both in industry and in the home, the hand is the most commonly injured part of the body. A disorder of the hand rarely jeopardizes life but often results in a handicap that may hamper vocational capacity.

assumed, without intention, after injury, paralysis, and the onset of painful states; it is also called the **position of injury**. Stiffening in this attitude jeopardizes function.

INTRODUCTION

The prime functions of the hand are feeling (sensibility) and grasping. **Sensibility** is important on the radial sides of the index, long, and ring fingers and on the opposing ulnar side of the thumb, where it is indispensable to be able to feel, pinch, pick up, and hold things. This sensibility is mediated by the median nerve. The ulnar side of the little finger and its metacarpal, upon which the hand usually rests, must register the sensations of contact and pain to avoid burns and other trauma.

Mobility is critical for grasping. The upper extremity is a cantilevered system extending from the shoulder to the fingertips. It must be adaptable to varying rates and kinds of movements with the maintenance of stability.

The specialization of the thumb ray has endowed man with superior aptitudes for defense, work, and dexterity. The thumb has exquisite sensibility and is a highly mobile structure of appropriate length, with a well-developed adductor and thenar (pronating) musculature. It is the most important digit of the hand, and every effort must be made to preserve its function.

The **position of function** of the upper extremity favors reaching the mouth and perineum as well as comfortable, forceful, and unfatiguing grip and pinch. The elbow is held at or near a right angle, the forearm neutral between pronation and supination, and the wrist extended 30 degrees with the fingers furled to almost meet the opposed (pronated) tip of the thumb (Fig 48–1A). This is the desired stance of the extremity if stiffness is likely to occur, and it should be adopted when joints are immobilized by splinting, arthrodesis, or tenodesis.

Opposite to the position of function is the **position of rest**, in which the flexed wrist extends the digits, making grip and pinch awkward, uncomfortable, weak, and fatiguing (Fig 48–1B). The forearm is usually pronated and the elbow extended. This habitus is

ANATOMY

All references to the forearm and hand should be made to the radial and ulnar sides (not lateral and medial), and to the volar (or palmar) and dorsal surfaces. The digits should be identified as the thumb, index finger, long finger, ring ringer, and little finger, or referred to as rays I, II, III, IV, and V.

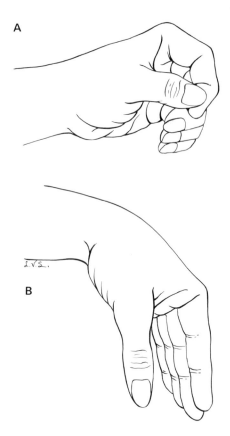

FIG 48–1. Positions of function (*A*) and rest (injury) (*B*).

*Nerve disorders of the hand are discussed in Chapter 41.

Skin

Skin is the elastic outer sleeve and glove of the arm and hand. Sacrifice of its surface area or elasticity by debridement and fibrosis can severely curtail range of motion and constrict circulation. In the adult hand, the dorsal skin stretches about 4 cm in the longitudinal and in the transverse planes when the fist closes, and the volar skin stretches a similar amount when the palm is flattened and spread. The long finger can easily have 48 sq cm of skin cover, and the whole hand (exclusive of digits) 210 sq cm.

For pinch and grasp to be stable, the volar skin is anchored to bone by a network of fascial bands. If swelling occurs, these bands prevent expansion and may convert the skin into a constrictive sleeve which can lead to fibrosis or necrosis if not treated adequately.

Dorsal skin does not need such stability. It is, therefore, loose and elastic and houses the majority of veins and lymphatics draining the hand. It covers the path of least resistance for sequestered fluid. Thus, swelling of the hand and flexion of the wrist stretch the dorsal skin. This destroys the position of function by extending the metacarpal joints and interferes with decongestion by compressing veins and lymphatics.

The tethered volar skin is more prone to cuts; the untethered dorsal skin is more apt to undergo avulsion. The thick, sweat-producing volar skin is less prone to third degree burns than the thin, dry, dorsal skin. Because the volar skin is far more sensitive than dorsal skin, palmar scars are more painful than dorsal scars.

Well-vascularized skin with or without fat padding is desired over any healing bone, tendon, nerve, or vessel and may be a prerequisite to adequate function later. Skin replacement is possible by split or full thickness or pedicle grafts. The choice is determined by the location and size of the deficit or the need for padding, stretch, resistance to wear and tear, and sensibility.

Fat

Fat performs an indispensable cushioning function and must not be surgically sacrificed or abused. Once lost, it does not regenerate. As a quilt under the skin and around healing structures, it absorbs shocks and prevents choking and restraint of motion due to unyielding scars. It may be transferred to a zone of injury by pedicle flaps but rarely by free graft. The need for it is greatest on the volar aspect of the hand.

Fascia

This tough, inelastic, and relatively avascular white tissue exists as sheets, fibers, bands, tendon sheaths and pulleys, and ligaments. It anchors volar skin to bone to make pinch and grip stable; the mid-lateral fibers of "Cleland's ligament" keep the skin sleeve from twisting about the digit (Fig 48–2). In the form of sheaths and pulleys, fascia holds tendons in the concavity of arched joints to convey mechanical efficiency and power. The fascial sleeve of the forearm, hand, and digits must sometimes be slit along with skin to relieve posttraumatic swelling. Any fascial compartment of the hand provides a space for infection or an avenue for its dissemination. Components critical to function should, however, be spared whenever possible, eg, vertical volar fibers anchoring distal digit skin and fat pad to the phalanx and flexor tendon pulleys. Components which are actually or potentially restrictive to joint motion or tendon glide or constrictive to neurovascular structures may be divided or resected.

Bones, Joints, & Ligaments

Intricate positioning and dexterity of the hand are facilitated by a diverse range of motion of the many joints of the upper extremity. One or more joints may be fused in a position favoring most functions, and their loss may be adequately compensated for by that of the remaining joints. For example, the shoulder compensates well for loss of forearm and wrist motion while the back, neck, and wrist compensate for the elbow. Each finger has 4 joints (MC, MP, PIP, and DIP—see accompanying box), any 2 of which may be fused and still leave adequate overall function. The thumb has only 3 joints (MC, MP, and IP), and every effort must be made to preserve at least two. The wrist is the master joint of the hand since its position governs the efficiency of extrinsic muscle contraction.

The stability of the digital joints and their planes of motion are governed by the length of the ligaments and the anatomy of their articulating surfaces. Circumduction occurs at all the MP joints, which are hinged off center. The IP joints move entirely in the AP plane. Tightness of the ligaments after injury jeopardizes joint motion and the functional arches of the hand.

The longitudinal and transverse arches of the hand are architectural prerequisites to gripping, pinching, and cupping and are maintained by the passive tone and active contraction of the intrinsic muscles. The arches create the "position of function" (Fig 48–3); when the arches are collapsed, the hand assumes the "position of rest" or "position of injury." The irretrievable loss of these arches is most often initiated by edema. They may be preserved by splinting in the position of function, elevation without constriction, and early restoration of active and vigorous joint motion.

Each MP and IP joint has a volar trap door called the volar plate (Fig 48–4) in addition to collateral ligaments stabilizing the joint on either side (Fig 48–5).

Abbreviations Used in This Chapter	
DIP	Distal interphalangeal
IC	Intercarpal
IP	Interphalangeal
MC	Metacarpocarpal
MP	Metacarpophalangeal
PIP	Proximal interphalangeal
RC	Radial-carpal
RU	Radial-ulnar

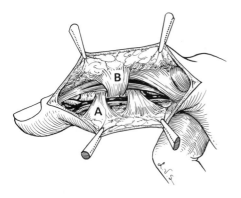

FIG 48–2. *A:* Cleland's ligament. *B:* Transverse retinacular ligament.

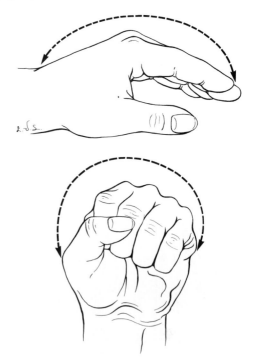

FIG 48–3. Longitudinal (top) and transverse arches.

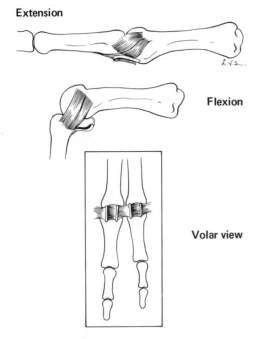

Extension

Flexion

Volar view

FIG 48–4. Volar plate.

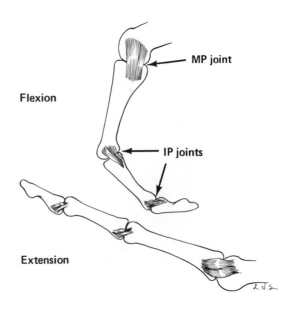

MP joint

Flexion

IP joints

Extension

FIG 48–5. Collateral ligaments.

Muscles, Tendons, Bursae, & Pulleys

The extrinsic flexor tendons are contained in fibrous **sheaths** to prevent bowstringing and preserve mechanical efficiency as the fingers furl into the palm. **Pulleys** (hypertrophied sections of the sheath) resist the points of greatest tendency to bowstring. Sheaths are inelastic and relatively avascular. Therefore, they crowd and congest any swollen, inflamed, or injured tendons and curtail glide by friction, constriction, and generation of inelastic adhesions. The term no-man's-land refers to the zone from the middle of the palm to the middle finger joint, wherein the superficialis and profundus lie ensheathed together and recovery of glide is so difficult after wounding (Fig 48–6).

Across the wrist, the dense volar carpal ligament closes the bony carpal canal **(carpal tunnel)** through which pass all 8 finger flexors as well as the flexor pollicis longus and median nerve (Fig 48–6). The **ulnar bursa** is the continuation of the synovial sheath of the little finger through the carpal tunnel, encompassing the other finger flexors which interrupted their separate sheaths at the midpalm level. The **radial bursa** is the flexor pollicis longus sheath continued through the carpal tunnel. These 2 bursae may intercommuni-

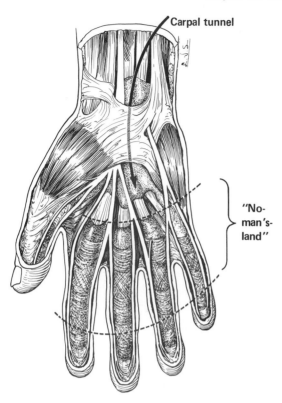

FIG 48—6. Carpal tunnel and no-man's-land.

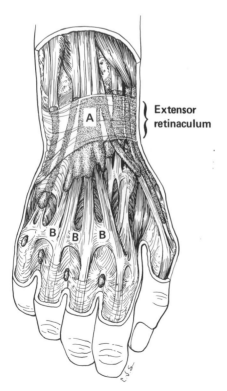

FIG 48—7. *A:* Extensor retinaculum. *B:* Juncturae tendinum (conexus intertendineus).

cate. **Parona's space** is that tissue plane of the distal forearm deep to the radial and ulnar bursae and on top of the pronator quadratus muscle.

The extensor tendons are ensheathed in 6 compartments at the wrist beneath the extensor retinaculum, which predisposes to adhesions (Fig 48—7).

The 20 intrinsic muscles provide digital dexterity, maintain the arches, and add power, particularly to the act of pinching. They govern the lateral movements of the digits as well as MP joint flexion and IP joint extension. The complex interaction of the intrinsic and extrinsic extensors is mediated by the triangular dorsal hood mechanism through the central slip and lateral bands (Fig 48—8).

Circulation

Veins and lymphatics are located predominantly on the dorsum of the hand and volar aspect of the elbow and are easily compressed.

Loss of either the radial or ulnar artery is in most instances compensated for through the collateral circulation of the deep and superficial palmar arches.

There are 4 arteries to each digit, but the 2 principal ones lie on the radial and ulnar sides of the volar aspect deep to the digital nerve.

Nerves

The nerves of greatest importance to hand function are the musculocutaneous, radial, ulnar, and median. The importance of the radial nerve is its innervation of the extensor muscles which stabilize the wrist and extend the digits. The ulnar nerve innervates 15 of the 20 intrinsic muscles. The median nerve, by its sensory innervation is "the eye of the hand"; through its motor innervation, it maintains the long flexors and

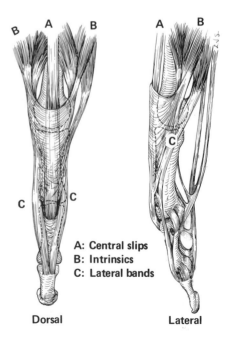

A: Central slips
B: Intrinsics
C: Lateral bands

Dorsal   Lateral

FIG 48—8. **Hood mechanism.**

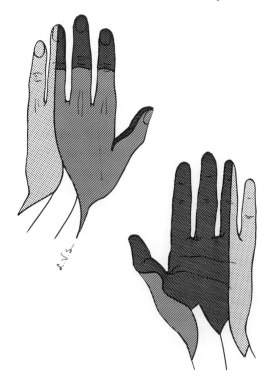

FIG 48−9. Sensory distribution in the hand. Dotted area, ulnar nerve; diagonal area, radial nerve; darker area, median nerve.

thenar muscles. Fig 48−9 shows the sensory distribution of the ulnar, radial, and median nerves.

Kaplan EB: *Functional and Surgical Anatomy of the Hand,* 2nd ed. Lippincott, 1965.
Lampe EW: *Surgical Anatomy of the Hand.* Ciba Clinical Symposia, vol 9, No. 1. Ciba Pharmaceutical Products, 1957.
Milford LW: *Retaining Ligaments of the Digits of the Hand.* Saunders, 1968.

starting with the head and neck and working down to the fingertips. Observe habitus, wasting, hypertrophy, deformities, skin changes, skin temperature, and scars. Feel the wrist pulses and the sweat of the finger pads, and test reflexes and the sensibility of the median, ulnar, and radial nerves.

The usual obstacles to diagnosis are inability to communicate (eg, those who speak a foreign language, a child, or psychologically handicapped patients); a fresh injury, causing withholding of movement due to pain or "protective" anesthesia which mimics loss of nerve function; incomplete x-ray, laboratory, or nerve conduction studies; or the willful withholding or distortion of information by the patient because of pain or anger or the hope of secondary gain. Two or more reassessments, hours, days, or weeks apart may be necessary to establish the diagnosis. The malingerer is usually exposed by the anatomic and functional inconsistencies of his complaints and performance. He usually becomes befuddled when asked to perform rapidly and repetitively.

Serial x-rays and laboratory procedures may clarify a problem with an indolent evolution (eg, Kienböck's aseptic necrosis of the lunate, causing unexplained wrist pain). Contralateral and multiple view x-rays in different planes (even tomograms) are often helpful. This is especially true in patients who have persistent perplexing bone and joint pain or limited motion or in patients who have not attained adult growth.

The diagnosis is often made by noting the response to therapy. This is particularly true in the case of local corticosteroids injected at the site of non-infectious inflammatory conditions (eg, carpal tunnel syndrome, trigger finger).

Committee On Rating of Mental and Physical Impairment: *Guides to the Evaluation of Permanent Impairment.* American Medical Association, 1971.
Lucas GL: *Examination of the Hand.* Thomas, 1972.
Swanson AB: Evaluation of impairment of function in the hand. S Clin North America 44:925, 1964.

CLINICAL EVALUATION OF HAND DISORDERS

The present complaint must be recorded explicitly and in complete detail with regard to its mechanism of onset, evolution, aggravating factors, and relieving factors. Age, sex, hand dominance, occupation, and relevant matters pertaining to the patient's general health and his emotional and socioeconomic status must be recorded also.

The examination should follow an orderly routine. Observe the neck, shoulders, and both upper extremities and the action and strength of all muscle groups, and be certain that all parts can pass painlessly and coordinately through a normal range of motion,

GENERAL OPERATIVE PRINCIPLES

Tidy, gentle, and effective surgery on the hand requires attention to certain principles. This precise surgery requires good light, adequate help, specialized instruments, and (invariably) an arterial tourniquet (a blood pressure cuff inflated to 250−300 mm Hg). Magnification with a loupe or microscope should also be available. The patient as well as the surgeon must be comfortable during the surgical procedure. Whatever anesthesia is used must effectively relax the musculature and prevent pain. Pain or the fear of pain unfavorably influences the course of recovery.

Preparation of the skin for surgery is reliably achieved with iodine and alcohol, which should be

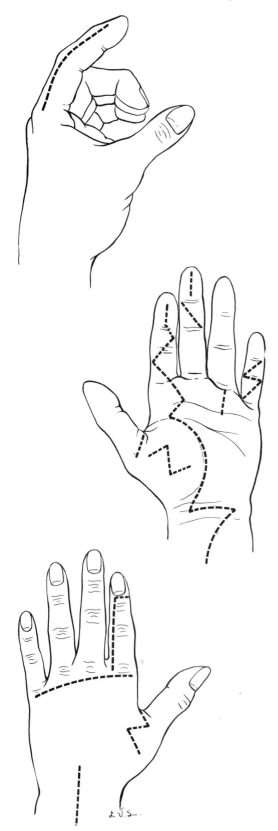

FIG 48–10. Proper placement of skin incisions.

kept away from the open wound. Preoperative shaving is not necessary; a waterproof draping is preferred.

Incisions, Dressings, Splints, & Immobilization

An incision must never compromise function; must give ideal access without a struggle for exposure; and must preserve vascular integrity (veins are just as important as arteries). Incisions must either be zigzagged across flexion and extension creases or run longitudinally in "neutral" zones (eg, between the lateral limits of the flexion and extension creases of the digits); and, whenever possible, must be designed so that a skin-fat flap is raised over the zone of a tendon or nerve suture.

Incisions made in accordance with these precepts are not painful once healed. Hence, a longitudinal midline incision of any flexor digital pad (sparing the crease) is the desired method for incision and drainage procedures or exposure for excision or incision of a great variety of digital and palmar lesions. This type of incision causes minimal trauma to neurovascular structures which enter the operative area from either side of the digit. A zigzag incision is preferable over the thenar area to avoid symptomatic hypertrophy. Fig 48–10 depicts some advisable choices for effective volar incisions. On the dorsum of the hand or digit, the surgeon must meticulously preserve the venous and lymphatic drainage.

Proper evaluation and treatment of a fresh injury often requires extension of the wound. This facilitates recognition of structures which can then be traced into the zone of injury, where blood and trauma so often make their identification difficult or impossible. The design of wound extension should be dictated by the foregoing guidelines and the surgeon's projected concepts of exploration and reconstruction. A complementary incision, rather than extension of an existing wound, is sometimes more useful.

Viable skin should not be sacrificed to make a wound look tidy when doing so will make the closure tight. The venous constriction that results may nullify the entire surgical effort. It is better to leave the wound open and to graft it primarily or secondarily rather than to close it under tension.

The entire success of operative and nonoperative management often depends upon the nature and adequacy of the dressings and immobilization—an art in itself. Constriction and tension must be avoided at all costs. The dressing should be applied evenly to the skin without wrinkles. The wound should be covered with a single layer of fine mesh gauze followed by a wet spongy medium (fluffs, mechanic's waste, Rest-On, Kling, or Kerlix). Wetness facilitates the drainage of blood into the dressing, which should be applied with gentle pressure to curtail dead space.

Splinting is paramount in controlling pain and favoring healing. In general, plaster (fast-setting) is preferred because of its adaptability to specific requirements. More often than not, the master joint (the wrist) requires immobilization along with any other part of the hand. Proper padding prevents any constriction and allows one the advantage of a boxing-glove type cast (Figs 48–11 and 48–12).

It must be appreciated that effective immobilization of a finger (even a fingertip) most often requires concomitant immobilization of one or more adjacent fingers, usually in the position of function. Forearm casts may be egg-shell thin as long as the wrist portion is properly keeled. Straight splints such as tongue blades involve a hazard of digital stiffness and distortion and should not be used.

Persistence of pain signifies inadequate immobilization and, if throbbing is present, congestion. Congestion must be promptly relieved by elevation and sectioning of the cast and dressing and, if necessary, the skin and fascia.

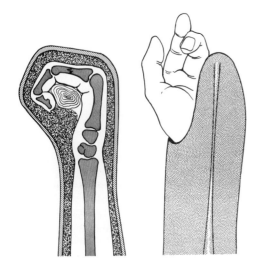

FIG 48–11. Casting.

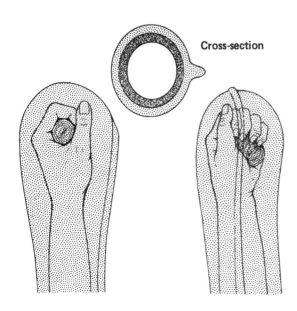

Cross-section

FIG 48–12. Casting.

TENDON DISORDERS

Tendon disorders are most commonly due to trauma or to inflammatory or degenerative conditions. These may be restricted to one or more tendons or may be part of a generalized disorder involving other tissues and structures. Neoplastic and congenital disorders of the tendons are rare.

The prerequisites to successful tendon surgery are (1) that the tendons be covered with healthy padded and pliable skin; (2) that the joints to be moved by the tendons have an adequate passive range of motion; (3) that the muscles to the tendons be elastic, and that they be innervated or capable of being so; (4) that the patient be motivated and capable of responsibility for the rehabilitative effort; (5) that the surgeon have the appropriate training, skill, and technical facilities; and (6) usually, that the musculotendinous units involved not be spastic and the digits involved not irrevocably anesthetic.

Adhesions invariably form wherever tendons are even slightly inflamed or injured and can completely nullify tendon function; even so, adhesions are indispensable to repair. No divided tendon will reestablish its continuity and no tendon graft will develop its own blood supply without the ingrowth of capillaries and fibroblasts from the tendon bed. Thus, it is not only the quantity of adhesions but also their pliability that determines whether or not the tendon will glide. With much active and passive effort over many months, tendon glide can be increased as a consequence of maturation and molding of the collagen in the adhesions. If this does not take place and the adhesions remain thick and hard, tendon excursion fails.

The experience of the surgeon influences the functional results of tenorrhaphy. Preoperative treatment of fresh lacerations consists of immobilization and prophylactic antibiotics. Such cases can be deferred for definitive primary repair for 24 hours or more. The timing of delayed secondary procedures depends upon the resolution of wound edema and callus (ie, how soft and pliable it is). After 6–8 weeks, tendons that retract over 2.5 cm may defy full excursion because the muscle elasticity has been lost.

Tendon Repair

All tendon surgery should be performed with adequate facilities. Using fine forceps, the tendon is held only on its cut surface at the very ends. By suitable positioning of the wrist, tension may be relieved so that the ends approximate easily. Needles should be very sharp and mounted atraumatically on the suture material, which should be smooth, nonreactive, nonabsorbable, and size 4–0 or, occasionally, 5–0 or 6–0. Needle punctures of the tendon should be minimal. Sutures should have sufficient purchase on the tendon to avoid slippage.

Tendon Grafting

The palmaris longus, plantaris, or one of the

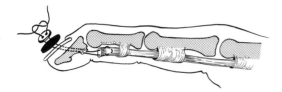

FIG 48–13. Tenodesis.

superficialis or long toe extensors are the most common sources of a graft. In removing the graft, make sure that its surface is smooth and glistening, which will be the case if the paratenon is left behind. It must not be allowed to dry and should be threaded into the recipient bed promptly and with minimal handling. After the graft has been attached at one end, length and tension are set with a preliminary suture and tested by motion of the wrist. Immobilization is necessary for 3–4 weeks.

Tenodesis (See Fig 48–13.)

Tenodesis will occur if the surface of the tendon and the surface where adherence is desired are roughened. The best anchoring surface is either bone, ligament, or a tendon pulley. Immobilization is necessary for 3–4 weeks and may require a Kirschner wire or plaster cast (or both).

Tenolysis

The access to tenolysis should be through a wound offering effective exposure and placed where the immediate active and passive joint motion that must follow will not jeopardize healing of the wound by undue stretching or direct pressure. The most common causes of failure are immobilization of the tendon for longer than 24 hours after lysis; failure in the tendon's work of repeated active contraction of the musculotendinous unit; carrying out a concomitant procedure requiring immobilization (ie, neurorrhaphy); or separation of the tendon.

Tendon Lengthening

Tendon lengthening is used to advance a tenorrhaphy beyond a point of constriction (eg, pulley) or to elongate a contracted musculotendinous unit.

Immobilization

The position of immobilization needed to relieve tension on the tendon sutures is ideally determined when the wound is still open and the tendon juncture is in view. Avoiding extreme flexion or extension, the wrist joint is generally positioned for the control of tension. This allows the digital joints to be more relaxed and more nearly in the position of function.

Mobilization

The patient must understand that the subsequent musculotendinous and joint mobilization is a time-consuming process, often taking many weeks or months. **Work** is the key to progress, and this should

be regular and disciplined with regard to duration, frequency, and vigor. Exercise should be sufficient to make progress but not so much as to cause lingering pain and swelling. A sensible program of exercise is 15 minutes 3 times a day, advancing over a period of 2–4 weeks to 15 minutes every hour. All of this is new and worrisome to the patient. He needs guidance, and should be seen at least twice a week for 2–4 weeks when his cast is removed.

"Ball-squeezing" has no place in getting tendons to glide early since it blocks the movement of digital joints. Once glide has been achieved, however, ball-squeezing may strengthen the muscles.

Diagnosis & Treatment of Tendon Injuries

Tendon injury may be single or multiple and may be complicated by injury to nerve or bone. Diagnosis, treatment, and prognosis may be difficult. One must know the terminal joint that a given tendon moves, where overlap of function may mask the loss of action of a specific tendon, and how to block the action of tendons that conflict with functional testing of their fellow travelers.

Repeated testing will serve to confirm a tendon injury and differentiate unconscious or willful withholding of pertinent clinical information. The history, the habitus of the joints, and the results of specific tendon testing are the 3 crucial elements in the diagnosis of tendon deficits. The normal musculotendinous unit moves its target joints with force and through a full range of motion. When active joint motion is weak and when active range of motion is less than the passive range, one must suspect derangement of the unit. Identification of structures during surgical exploration is facilitated by experience, a dry operative field, and a methodical dissection which is begun with normal, identifiable structures and proceeds into the diseased or damaged ones. Normal tendons are whiter and firmer than nerves, which have a pearly luster and an epineural vessel running along on the surface.

The state of the wound and the complexity of the injury are the principal issues the hand surgeon must weigh in choosing a **primary** or **secondary** tenorrhaphy and its type. Clean wounds generally favor primary tenorrhaphy. Primary tenorrhaphy is defined as one that is done within 24–48 hours after injury. If a wound has been surgically prepped and closed and the hand immobilized within a few hours of injury, tenorrhaphy can then be scheduled for a time when facilities are ideal rather than as an emergency under unfavorable conditions.

When wounds are untidy, contaminated, or complicated by fracture or ischemia, formal tenorrhaphy is usually delayed for weeks or months until the tendon bed is more favorable to healing and glide. This does not preclude tacking 2 easily accessible tendon ends together when the wound receives initial care.

The retrieval of a proximal tendon stump which has recoiled must be accomplished without trauma to the tunnel (see Kilgore & others reference on p 978.)

"Mallet" finger ("baseball" or "drop" finger) (Fig 48−14) is due to division or attenuation of the extensor to the distal phalanx. A distal joint which can be passively but not actively extended is diagnostic. The injury most commonly results from sudden forceful flexion of the digit when it is held in rigid extension. Either the extensor is partially or completely ruptured, or the dorsal lip of the bone is avulsed. Less frequently, the injury is due to direct trauma such as a laceration or a crush force. An x-ray should be taken to determine the presence and extent of any fracture.

Treatment may not be necessary if the loss of active extension is less than 15 degrees and any existing fracture is only a chip. More severe injury requires 6 weeks of continuous splinting in full distal joint extension (**not** hyperextension) with or without 40 degrees of PIP joint flexion. Skillful joint fixation with fine Kirschner wire, padded aluminum, plastic, or even plaster splints is equally effective. A lacerated tendon should be delicately reapproximated. When a fracture fragment represents one-third or more of the surface of the joint, it should be carefully reduced and held by wiring or pinning. In selected cases, smaller fracture fragments may be removed. If there is sufficient articular disruption, one may consider joint fusion. Tendon grafting is difficult and easily leads to a poor cosmetic and functional result. It should be done only rarely.

Swan-neck deformity (Fig 48−14) is a frequent complication of mallet finger, but it may also be the result of disparity of pull between the extrinsic flexors and extensor hood with or without attenuation of the DIP joint extensor. It is seen in congenitally hypermobile joints, spastic and rheumatoid states, and following resection of the superficialis tendon. The dorsal hood acts to extend the distal joint but is held back by its insertion at the base of the middle phalanx, which it therefore hyperextends ("PIP joint recurvatum"). This in turn increases the tension on the profundus, which hyperflexes the DIP joint. If the mallet deformity is 25 degrees or less and there is some active distal joint extension, it may be treated by severing the middle phalangeal insertion of the dorsal hood.

The **"buttonhole"** or **"boutonniere" deformity** (Fig 48−15) appears as the opposite of the swan-neck deformity: hyperextension of the DIP joint and flexion of the PIP joint. There is attenuation or separation of the dorsal hood, so that the lateral bands shift volar to the PIP joint axis and the joint buckles dorsalward. Active extension of the PIP joint becomes impossible, and the entire extrinsic-intrinsic force on the hood passes onto the lateral bands which flex the PIP joint and hyperextend the DIP joint. This deformity may develop suddenly or, more often, insidiously after trauma over the dorsum of the PIP joint.

To avoid this complication, fresh extensor tendon lacerations and severe contusions over the PIP joint should be sutured if necessary but should always have the PIP joint alone splinted in extension for 3−4 weeks. A small, oblique Kirschner wire provides good immobilization. Established deformities can be treated by such immobilization or by operative correction.

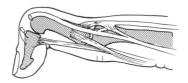

FIG 48−14. Mallet finger with swan-neck deformity.

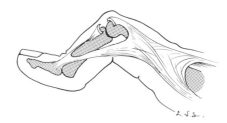

FIG 48−15. Buttonhole deformity.

Tendon rupture, subluxation, and drift: The most frequent rupture of a healthy tendon is that of the distal joint extensor of one of the fingers as a result of sudden, forceful flexion (see mallet finger, above). Other tendons rupture where they have been weakened by division and repair, partial transection, crushing, or attritional fraying over roughened bone. The synovial thickening, tendon nodularity, and roughening of articular bone seen in the rheumatoid hand easily dispose to rupture by mechanical abrasion and circulatory depletion of tendons. Much can be done prophylactically by synovectomy, sectioning of constricting tendon sheaths, and resection of sharp bony spurs and tendon nodules. If correction of a rupture is indicated, the methods of doing so include repair, tendon graft, tendon transfer, or tenodesis.

The most common subluxations and drifts of tendons are 2-fold: (1) volar drift of the intrinsic tendons as they pass the PIP joint of the fingers, causing the "buttonhole" deformity (see above); and (2) ulnar drift of the extrinsic extensors (central slips) as they pass the MP joints. The latter may result from trauma that divides or attenuates the lateral expansion of the extensor hood on the radial side of the central slip. It more commonly results from attenuation of the entire extensor hood over the MP joint as a consequence of marked distention of the joint space and thickening of the synovium in rheumatoid arthritis. Treatment of ulnar drift involves repositioning of the extensor tendon to a point central to the MP joint and holding it by appropriate reefing of the lateral fibers of the hood on the radial side.

Evaluation of Results

The excursion and force of centripetal pull of the operated tendon should be compared with the normal one in the opposite hand and objective measurements recorded at least once a month. It then becomes readily apparent whether or not progress is being made. If the conscientious patient makes no progress in 2–3 months, his disability is probably static and he should be considered for further surgical treatment or released from care. Often, however, 6–12 months are required before maximal function is restored.

Two types of measurements of mobility and one of strength are needed. With the back of the hand on a flat surface, the distance between the nail and the table should be measured to gauge digital extension. Flexion should be gauged by having the patient touch the proximal palm (MP and PIP joints flexed), mid palm (MP and both IP joints flexed), and distal palm (IP joints flexed) and the distance from fingertip to palm recorded. Thumb motion is gauged by the distance between its tip and the base of the little finger in flexion and by the angle it makes with the index finger in abduction. Significant differences between active and passive motion should be noted.

In addition, the angles made by digital joints in full extension and full flexion should be compared with the same joints of the opposite hand. This is usually recorded as a fraction: injured side/uninjured side. The range of motion (ROM) and the difference in range of motion between injured and uninjured sides can be readily calculated and serves as a guide to progress. An excellent result is achieved in a flexor tenorrhaphy if the fingertip can be actively flexed to within 12 mm of the mid palm and extended to within 12 mm of a straight line.

Strength can be gauged on one of the commercially available grip dynamometers. This should be compared to the opposite hand.

Boyes JH, Stark HH: Flexor-tendon grafts in the fingers and thumb. J Bone Joint Surg 53A:1332–1342, 1971.

Hunter J: Artificial tendons. Am J Surg 109:325–338, 1965.

Kilgore ES & others: Atraumatic flexor tendon retrieval. Am J Surg 122:430–431, 1971.

Littler JW: The severed flexor tendon. S Clin North America 39:435–447, 1959.

Potenza AD: Prevention of adhesions to healing digital flexor tendons. JAMA 187:187–191, 1964.

Verdan C: Primary repair of the flexor tendons. J Bone Joint Surg 42A:647–657, 1960.

Verdan C: Half a century of flexor-tendon surgery: Current status and changing philosophies. J Bone Joint Surg 54A: 472–491, 1972.

FRACTURES, DISLOCATIONS, & LIGAMENTOUS INJURIES

Stiffness and pain are the 2 most common disabling effects of these injuries. In some cases they are compounded by (1) excessive efforts to restore "absolutely normal" anatomy, and (2) by excessive immobilization. The posttraumatic sequestration of serum and blood invites initial stiffness from swelling and secondary stiffness from contractures and adhesions. Experience and judgment must be exercised in the management of these problems. Above all, the treatment of injury to one bone or one joint must not cause stiffness and pain in many joints. The older and tougher the hand, the more readily it swells and stays swollen and stiff after injury and surgery. Active joint motion milks away sequestered fluid and must be initiated at the proper time and to the proper extent according to the needs of a given case. Bone deformity per se is not bad as long as the overall painless function of the hand and its digits is preserved.

Diagnosis

A detailed account of the mechanism of injury greatly facilitates diagnosis. Of particular significance is the direction, speed, and magnitude of the force causing the injury. The prior existence of deformity, stiffness, or pain must also be ascertained. Examine the entire upper extremity and often the whole patient before focusing on the affected part. The injured bone or joint must be compared with its counterpart in the other hand. Carefully inspect any acquired deformity, noting crepitation and pain on motion or stress, or associated abnormal motion. Pressing, impacting, or percussing a fractured bone or stretching an incompletely torn ligament usually elicits diagnostic pain.

Fractures should be determined by routine x-ray studies and often by comparative views of injured and uninjured hands, multiple views in different planes, tomograms, and serial views at 1–2 week intervals. In the case of ligamentous injuries, joint views with and without stress on the ligament may contribute to the diagnosis and evaluation of treatment.

Treatment

Whenever reduction and alignment are necessary, manipulation should be painless and done without force. After suitable anesthesia with good relaxation is achieved, closed reduction is preferred over open reduction unless the estimate of difficulty favors an open procedure.

The wrist and digits should be generally maintained in the position of function after reduction. Unstable alignment may require internal fixation to hold reduction. At all costs, avoid extremes of joint position and forceful pressure of external splints and plaster. Constant digital traction is hazardous because it leads to joint stiffness. To minimize stiffness, immobilization should be maintained for the shortest time consistent with adequate control of pain and tissue repair.

Elevation of the forearm and removal of all jewelry and snug sleeves are essential to control edema. The patient's responsibilities in this regard must be carefully explained to him. When swelling is excessive, it must be reduced and the soft tissues rendered pliable as soon as possible. Reduction of the displaced fracture or dislocated joint sometimes makes the soft tissues pliable again. A releasing incision of skin and fascia may be needed to overcome brawny induration. It can be closed later with a split thickness skin graft.

Open injuries involving bones and joints should be

treated prophylactically with antibiotics administered systemically and often in the wound or joint as well (see Chapter 10). Active or passive tetanus immunization must be administered if needed.

SPECIFIC FRACTURES

Wrist Fractures

No injured wrist with joint pain lasting a week or more can be considered only sprained until serial x-rays rule out fracture or aseptic necrosis. Hence, a cast should be applied which provides sufficient immobilization to relieve pain; if an imperceptible fracture is present, this will be adequate treatment until later x-rays demonstrate the break.

The distal **radius** and **ulna** are the most frequently fractured wrist bones. Distortion may range from minimal soft tissue swelling with no bone displacement to marked bone displacement and so much swelling that median and sometimes ulnar nerves are paralyzed. The mode of injury is usually a fall on the palm forcing the wrist into extreme extension. The ensuing typical **Colles' fracture** presents a "silver fork" or hunchback deformity by the dorsal and recessed displacement of the distal radius. There is an associated fracture of the ulnar styloid.

The reverse deformity occurs if the fall is carried on the back of the hand, forcing the wrist into extreme flexion with volar displacement of the distal radius (**Smith's fracture**).

When reduction is necessary, adequate centrifugal traction on the thumb and index finger against countertraction at the level of the axilla or the flexed elbow should precede manipulation to make it minimally traumatic to the soft tissues. Comminuted and displaced fractures require a long arm cast for 4 weeks and a forearm cast for an additional 2 weeks.

A **fractured navicular** should be immobilized in the same way. The MP joint of the thumb should be included in the cast. If at 6 weeks there is no x-ray evidence of union, immobilization should be continued for an additional 6 weeks. Failing any improvement by x-ray, one must then decide whether to continue with much prolonged immobilization (eg, 6–12 months), or to resect the proximal pole or bone-graft the ununited waist fracture with or without radial styloidectomy. Surgical alternatives in late cases of intractable pain due to nonunion are replacement of the navicular by a Silastic prosthesis or fusion of the wrist.

Chip fracture of the dorsum of the **triquetrum** is a common carpal fracture requiring immobilization more for relief of pain than for consideration of bone repair. Fracture of the hook of the **greater multangular** or **hamate** should be suspected by the location of palmar tenderness following direct violence. Splinting is not necessary, but pain may be prolonged. The x-ray diagnosis is made by a carpal tunnel view. The hamate fracture may paralyze the deep motor branch of the ulnar nerve. Other carpal fractures occur but are rare.

Metacarpals & Phalanges

Immobilization of fractures of these bones is generally for 3–4 weeks.

Fractures of **metacarpals** and **proximal** and **middle phalanges** tend to bow and to rotate. Rotation of a finger causes it to cross over an adjacent finger during flexion, thus blocking digital excursion, fistmaking, and grasp. Rotation is avoided by having the injured finger flexed alongside an adjacent finger.

Dorsal and volar bowing is caused by the pull of intrinsic and extrinsic flexor and extensor forces. These forces can be most effectively neutralized by immobilizing the wrist and the digits in the position of function. The risk of reduction of bowing is the added predisposition to joint stiffness and tenodesis incident to the iatrogenic manipulation or surgery. Therefore, if the bowing is less than 20–30 degrees, this risk must be weighed carefully, for such deformity may not be functionally significant. Greater angles of bowing of the phalanges must, however, be corrected by either closed or open methods. Angulation of up to 40 degrees can be tolerated in some metacarpal fractures.

In immobilizing the fingers, the MP joints must be maintained in functional flexion. In the case of the ring and little fingers, this function means between 60–80 degrees of flexion. Malleable and rigid readymade volar splints cannot be applied without a threat to this important angle of MP joint flexion or (equally harmful) a threat of too much compression of the soft tissue of the palm.

After closed or open reduction, a preferred method of immobilization is to furl the digits over a volar roll of soft gauze which allows the position of function to be maintained (Figs 48–11 and 48–12). The forearm and pertinent digits are then wrapped in loosely applied cast padding followed by a light circumferential plaster cast, keeled for strength across the extended wrist. This immobilization is usually maintained for 3 weeks.

Two basal metacarpal fractures deserve special mention:

(1) Bennett's intra-articular fracture is an impaction of the thumb metacarpal, causing an oblique separation of the volar base from the dorsal base. The latter usually subluxates dorsally. The ideal treatment is reduction by centrifugal pulling on the thumb and pressure volarward on the base of the metacarpal followed by fixation with a Kirschner wire. If satisfactory realignment is not achieved, open reduction is advocated.

(2) A spiral or displaced fracture of the **base of the fifth metacarpal** always deserves an immediate and repeated check on the function of the first dorsal interosseus muscle to establish the integrity of the deep motor branch of the ulnar nerve, which is easily injured by this fracture.

Distal phalangeal fractures are located at the tuft, shaft, or base. Pain is the prime reason for treatment, and may be compounded if subungual hematoma is also present. The simplest way to treat the latter problem is to burn a hole through the nail with the tip of a paper clip heated to a red glow over a candle or alcohol lamp. This is quite painless if done gently. Marked pain and swelling can be best controlled by applying a well-padded circumferential cast to the forearm and, if the fracture involves a finger, incorporating the injured digit and at least one adjacent digit in the cast. After 1—2 weeks, a digital guard can take the place of the cast.

Digital Joint Fracture

Minute marginal joint fractures usually need no more than 1—2 days of immobilization. Stiffness and pain will best be avoided by early mobilization. Fractures with involvement of one-fourth to one-third of the joint surface require careful reduction and immobilization for 3 weeks. In some cases, the fragment should be resected. Mangled joints should be set at a functional angle for fusion or, in select circumstances, replaced by a Silastic joint if tendons are functioning. If the distal joint has been injured, an arthrodesis is often the best treatment.

In closed or open **crushing fractures** with a lot of swelling, the prime consideration should be preservation of the circulation, particularly venous return. Anatomic reduction of the bone is of secondary importance. Leaving a wound open or even slitting skin and fascia to loosen the tissues may be the best way to aid the circulation and may also make it possible to secure alignment and the position of function. Reduction is often well maintained by molding a roll of very wet, loose gauze to the injured digits or whole hand and then applying a well-cushioned boxing-glove type of cast to the appropriate digits or all of the hand. Internal fixation is advisable in selected cases.

Open reduction is the technic of choice in injuries which present a gaping wound with exposed fractures. It is also the preferred technic in the following circumstances: (1) when perfect reduction is important for subsequent function, as in intra-articular fractures, or when indicated for the removal of a potentially troublesome displaced small fragment; (2) if it allows reduction with less soft tissue trauma than closed reduction; or (3) to facilitate internal fixation in difficult reductions. The technic of open reduction must not jeopardize the circulation. Excessive periosteal stripping must be avoided.

Internal fixation can be achieved in many ways, including unthreaded or threaded rods, screws with or without plates, or malleable wire loops and sutures. Unthreaded Kirschner wires are most often used. Their insertion is not always easy. Threading the medullary cavity in open reductions may be facilitated by first skewering the distal segment through the fracture site, pushing the wire through the skin until its proximal end is flush with the fracture line, and then, after reduction, reversing the thrust of the wire. It will then easily engage the medullary cavity of the proximal segment, and, at the same time, impact distal and proximal segments together. If one pin does not adequately immobilize the fracture, another one parallel or oblique to it will give stability.

Fractures with loss of substance and shortening, particularly of a metacarpal, should be bone-grafted as soon as the risk of infection has passed. Pending this repair, length can be maintained by a longitudinal threaded Kirschner wire or transverse Kirschner wires holding the distal segment to the adjacent metacarpal.

DISLOCATIONS

Dislocations of the wrist and fingers are far less frequent than fractures. Swelling may completely mask the bone displacement, but motion is usually limited and painful. X-rays may be indispensable to the diagnosis. In the case of the wrist, multiple views and comparison of right and left may be necessary.

Dislocations are most easily reduced by accentuating the position that produced the deformity with simultaneous centrifugal traction on the distal segment followed by firmly pressing the displaced bone into its anatomic position. A reduction snap may be heard and is often promptly followed by excellent range of motion. A postreduction x-ray should usually be taken.

Limited progressive mobilization is usually advisable to avoid stiffness. It should start within 3—4 weeks for the wrist and a week for the digits. A concomitant fracture or an open dislocation would interdict mobilization so early. Compound dislocations require prophylactic treatment with antibiotics.

Open reduction is indicated whenever closed reduction requires much force. A chronic dislocation may defy even an open reduction.

Dislocations About the Wrist

These most often involve the lunate or the navicular. The **lunate** usually tears its dorsal ligament and flips volarward. In fresh cases, forthright reduction is often easy with wrist hyperextension, centrifugal traction on the hand, and a bit of thumb pressure on the lunate from the volar aspect. Late cases may be quite difficult to reduce and require open reduction from a volar approach to simultaneously decompress the median nerve. If there is avascular necrosis, the lunate should be resected and replaced with a Silastic prosthesis, or the proximal row of carpals should be removed.

In **perilunate dislocation of the carpus,** the volar ligaments are ruptured and the hand shifts dorsalward with the shear being between the lunate and navicular proximally and the remaining carpal bones distally. The navicular rotates in relation to the radius and the lunate, or it fractures through its waist with the distal half going dorsally with the hand—so-called **trans-navicular perilunate fracture-dislocation.** Although reduction may be easy, there is extensive ligamentous injury. The fractured navicular is likely to require bone grafting if its reduction is poor and the nonunion is painful.

Dislocation of the wrist develops insidiously in

chronic **rheumatoid arthritis**. Here the ulnar styloid shifts dorsally and often needs resection (Darrach operation). Wrist fusion is often the only or the most expeditious answer to intractable arthritic pain.

Dislocations About the Digits

The most common dislocation is a dorsal displacement of the distal segment on the proximal one. When ligaments are intact, reduction may be difficult. The most difficult is the dislocated MP joint of one of the fingers, which normally requires open reduction. It traps the head of the metacarpal in a noose formed by the lumbrical radially, the flexor tendons and pretendinous palmar fascia band ulnarly, the volar plate and transverse palmar fascia in the web distally, and the transverse palmar fascia proximally. Volar exposure and section of the fascia proximally and distally makes reduction quite easy, although section of the ulnar collateral ligament must sometimes be added.

Dislocation of an interphalangeal joint is most often reduced by the patient himself or a bystander at the time it occurs and requires little or no immobilization. Failure of reduction can mean that the displaced phalangeal head has escaped sideways from under the hood of the extensor mechanism, which then closes in between the head and the base of the more distal phalanx and locks the deformity. Failure of flexion after reduction usually means that the volar plate has come to lie like a wedge inside the joint. Recurrence of the dislocation usually means that the volar plate has been torn off at its origin distally. All 3 of these difficulties require open procedures to restore normal anatomic relationships. Repair of the volar plate requires 3–4 weeks of immobility. One obliquely placed Kirschner wire is sufficient fixation of the joint.

Chronic dislocations with erosion of the joint should be handled by replacing the joint with a Silastic prosthesis if the surrounding tendons are functionally intact; otherwise, the joints should be fused in the position of function. **Rheumatoid arthritis** causes a variety of insidious dislocations. The most common is at the MP joint. This consists of volar and **ulnar drifting** of the proximal phalanx in relation to the metacarpal as a result of the mean force of intrinsic-extrinsic tendon pull in association with pathologically attenuated joint capsules and ligaments. When intrinsic muscles atrophy and fibrose, these distortions may be irreducible without soft tissue surgery. At the PIP and DIP joint levels, the distortion may be of the **swan-neck** (PIP hyperextension and DIP flexion) or **button-hole** type (PIP flexion and DIP hyperextension).

LIGAMENTOUS INJURIES

Ligamentous Injuries of the Wrist

Pure ligamentous injuries of the wrist do occur, but the diagnostic pitfall is mistaking an unrecognized fracture or dislocation for a sprain. Accordingly, in the presence of pain and x-rays which show no fracture after violence, always apply a cast sufficient to totally relieve pain. The cast should remain in place for at least 1–2 weeks or until follow-up x-rays with multiple views rule out the presence of fracture. Fracture of the navicular is especially apt to present in this way.

Ligamentous Injuries of the Fingers

The ligaments of the **MP and PIP joints** are the most commonly injured. These vary from total ruptures to tears without any loss of stability. Either the ligament tears, or its bony attachment is avulsed, or both ligament and bone are torn. Those of the MP joint are usually due to violent abduction, whereas PIP ligaments rupture with equal proclivity on the radial or ulnar sides. Diagnosis may depend on stress x-ray views showing abnormal joint widening.

Except for the thumb, treatment of purely ligamentous injuries is rarely surgical. Splinting should often be brief to avoid excessive stiffness and pain which may result. As long as there is intact intrinsic and extrinsic tendon function and the patient is careful to avoid further injury, early motion within 2–3 days of injury is often desirable. One finger can be splinted by loosely strapping to an adjacent digit for 2–4 weeks. The pain of these injuries is notoriously slow to resolve irrespective of treatment.

Twisting injuries and falls may rupture the radial collateral ligament of the thumb by an adduction force; most commonly, however, the injury is an abduction force which tears the ulnar collateral ligament. Partial tears with limited instability may be treated by immobilization for 4–6 weeks. Total tears should be repaired or reconstructed surgically.

If there is a sizeable avulsed bone fragment in any of these injuries, it must be accurately reduced or, if it involves less than one-fourth of the surface area of the PIP or MP joint, removed. One may try local injections of small amounts of corticosteroid and lidocaine for chronic pain, or resection of scarred intrinsic muscle and the leading edge of the intermetacarpal ligament for intractable pain in the finger webs.

HAND INFECTIONS

Pyogenic infections of the hand often develop and spread as a result of failure to preserve or restore good venous and lymphatic drainage following trauma. In order to prevent as well as to treat infection, it is necessary to control swelling and congestion of tissues and to avoid any dead space filled with stagnant blood or serum. Inflammation causes tissue tension by sequestration of edema fluid. This in turn impairs tissue oxygenation by compressing the blood vessels, and a vicious cycle may develop which can lead to necrosis within the constrictive sleeves of fascia and skin.

Any circumstance that leads to acute swelling predisposes to infection, especially if there has been contamination through a puncture or open wound. Tissues and structures with a limited blood supply—or a blood supply that is easily choked off—are most susceptible to infection. Tissues around the nails, joints, tendon sheaths, and bones have the least natural resistance to infection.

Prevention & Treatment of Pyogenic Infections

A detailed history and careful physical examination are the basis of proper management. Tissue oxygenation depends upon adequate circulating blood volume. Constrictive clothing, jewelry, dressings, casts, and even a tightly closed wound can impair oxygenation. Comfortable immobilization and elevation of the hand above the level of the heart will help to control swelling. Throbbing pain is a symptom of excessive swelling that demands prompt mechanical relief and not analgesics. If pain, swelling, and induration progress despite other mechanical measures, immediate slitting of skin and fascia in one or more areas is mandatory and must be done in the operating room. This is usually done either along the dorsoradial or the dorsoulnar side of the digits, the hand, and the forearm, with care to avoid injury to nerves, major vessels, and tendons. A dorsal transverse skin incision over the heads of the metacarpals (sparing the veins) allows the MP joints of the swollen hand to flex and assume the functional position. Prophylactic local and systemic antibiotics are indicated for all contaminated wounds or whenever the circulation has been compromised. Clearly definable and easily recovered foreign bodies and nonviable tissue should be removed without endangering residual function. The evacuation of blood, serum, and foreign fluids can be facilitated by loosely fitting drains and wet dressings. Tetanus immunization should be given as indicated.

Immobilization

Adequate immobilization usually requires a splint of the wrist. In serious cases or uncooperative patients, the elbow should be splinted also and the patient kept flat in bed with his hand propped up on pillows. Without immobilization, the infection may be "milked" into uninvolved areas and progress farther.

Antibiotics

The need for antibiotics is determined by the extent of the infection. If the process is already well localized, simple drainage may be all that is needed. Since 80% of pyogenic infections are due to *Staphylococcus aureus* or beta-hemolytic streptococci, begin with antibiotics empirically while waiting for cultures. Methicillin and lincomycin are the most commonly effective agents. Bacitracin (50,000 units in 500 ml of saline) is an effective antibiotic for wound irrigation, which may be maintained for several days by means of inflow and outflow catheters. Specific antibiotics should be given when the results of cultures and sensitivity tests become available.

Incisions (Done in Operating Room)

When incision and drainage of an abscess is necessary, it should always be done at the point of maximum tenderness or the point of maximum fluctuation, where the overlying tissues are thinnest. The drainage wound should run parallel to and not across the paths of nerves, arteries, and veins. Wounds should be made long enough—and should be zigzagged, when necessary—to avoid secondary contractures. (See General Operative Principles, above, and Fig 48–10.)

Tourniquet

A bloodless field should be achieved for the purpose of incision and drainage by simple elevation of the extremity and then compression of the upper arm by tourniquet. Avoid centripetal wrapping to exsanguinate the part since this will spread the infection.

Carter SJ, Merscheimer WL: Infections of the hand. Orthop Clin North America 1:455, 1970.

Eaton RG, Butsch DP: Antibiotic guidelines for hand infections. Surg Gynec Obst 130:119–122, 1970.

Stone HH & others: Empirical selection of antibiotics for hand infections. J Bone Joint Surg 51A:899–903, 1969.

SPECIFIC INFECTIONS OF THE HAND

Furuncle & Carbuncle

These most commonly arise in a hair follicle. An incipient furuncle may be aborted by immobilization and elevation and antibiotics specific for *Staphylococcus aureus.* Once central necrosis has developed, adequate surgical decompression and drainage followed by moist or zinc oxide dressings allows sequestration of the "core."

Abrasions, Burns, & Granulating Wounds

These are best "cleaned up" with continuous 0.5% silver nitrate-soaked dressings; with ointment containing 25 mg hydrocortisone acetate and 5 mg neomycin sulfate per gram (eg, Neo-Cortef); or by means of surgical debridement. Staphylococci, streptococci, and pseudomonas are the predominant pathogens. The wound should be rendered suitable for split thickness skin grafting as promptly as possible, using postage stamp or mesh grafts. A take of the skin graft eradicates surface infection. Wet dressings aid sequestration of exudate and facilitate the skin take in its first 24–48 hours.

Cellulitis, Lymphangitis, & Adenitis

Cellulitis is manifested by local swelling, warmth, redness, and tenderness. It usually demands immobilization and elevation, and sometimes fasciotomy, in addition to antibiotics.

Lymphangitis and adenitis are most often due to streptococci and require elevation and immobilization as well as antibiotics.

Pyogenic Granuloma

Pyogenic granuloma is a mound of granulation tissue 3–20 mm (or more) in diameter. It most often develops under a chronically moist dressing, and may form around a suture knot. It should be scraped flush with the skin under local anesthesia. A small granuloma (less than 6–7 mm in diameter) exposed to the air will soon dry up and epithelize, whereas larger ones should be covered with a split thickness skin graft. If the granuloma is adjacent to the nail, one must be certain that the nail is not acting as a foreign body aggravating the reaction.

Pyoderma

Pyoderma (subepithelial abscess) is the forerunner of **collar-button abscess.** These infections develop within the skin in a hair follicle or infected blister. Failure to treat a blister or puncture wound deep to a callus commonly leads to this abscess, which becomes collar-button in configuration when it points into the subdermal fat, the path of least resistance. Treatment by means of incision, debridement of a blister or callus, drainage, water-soaked or zinc oxide dressings, rest, and elevation is usually sufficient.

Infections Around the Nail (Paronychia)

The rigidity of the fingernail causes it to press upon and aggravate any inflammation of the soft tissues surrounding it. The nail fold is often traumatized and becomes secondarily inflamed, leading to a paronychia on the radial or ulnar side. The lesion is called an eponychia if it involves the base of the nail; a "run-around" if the entire fold is involved; and a subungual abscess if pus develops and extends under the nail. Subonychia is inflammation between the nail bed and the bony phalanx. Because of the early and unrelenting tissue tension that develops, these entities are quite painful. Abscess formation often results, occasionally at some distance proximal to the nail fold (para-eponychial abscess). Early treatment is by means of water-soaked or zinc oxide dressings, elevation, immobilization, and antibiotics. Most abscesses can be drained painlessly with a needlepoint scalpel, cutting through the insensible necrotic skin cap where it points (Fig 48–16). Sagittal incisions forming a "trap door" of the eponychium should be reserved for the longstanding case in which a dense fibrous callus of the nail fold must be excised. Occasionally, the nail must be basally excised or totally avulsed, after which the eponychial fold should be separated from the nail matrix by a loose pack. Chronically wet nails of dishwashers may develop tissue changes and nail deformities which defy treatment. Fungal infections should be diagnosed and treated, and the fingers should be protected from water or excessive sweating.

Space Infections

The skin and fascia compartmentalize certain areas of the hand and forearm, predisposing these spaces to increased tissue tension and the progression of infection to abscess formation. The treatment of

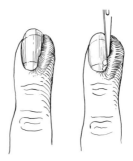

FIG 48–16. Incision and drainage of paronychia.

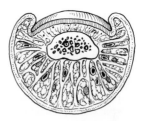

FIG 48–17. Cross-section of distal phalanx.

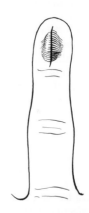

FIG 48–18. Incision of felon.

early space infection involves elevation, immobilization, and antibiotics administered systemically. If this does not arrest the progression of symptoms and signs within a few hours—or if the space is already tense when first examined—incision and drainage are required. Recovery is expedited by an antibiotic drip into the space administered through a fine catheter.

The proper technic of drainage of specific spaces is as follows:

A. Volar Digital Pulp (Fat Pad) Spaces of the Fingers: (Fig 48–17.) Whether in the proximal, middle, or distal pad, any abscess that points to the center of the pad should be drained by an incision which is precisely central and runs longitudinally but does not cross the flexion crease **(felon).** This preserves the important digital arteries and nerves. In the case of a felon (distal pad infection), a central longitudinal incision should also be used (Fig 48–18). Fishmouth, lateral, and transverse incisions have made far too many fingertips gangrenous or anesthetic. Division of the vertical fascial fibers of the pulp was recommended in the past but can irretrievably deprive the pad of the tethering it needs for stable pinching.

B. Web Spaces: The web spaces are the path of least resistance for pus from infected distal palm calluses, puncture wounds, and infections of the lumbrical canals. In the case of the thenar space, the thumb web often represents its watershed. A dorsal sagittal incision is usually most desirable between the fingers. A dorsal incision in the web of the thumb may be zigzagged to prevent contracture (Fig 48–10).

C. Midpalmar Space: The midpalmar space becomes infected by direct puncture or by extension of infections from the flexor sheaths of rays II, III, or IV. Only the skin should be incised over the point of fluctuation. The rest of the dissection should be carried out by gentle spreading with a blunt clamp to avoid injury to arteries, nerves, and tendons. Infection spreads easily from this space along the lumbrical canals and to the thenar space.

D. Hypothenar and Thenar Spaces: A hypothenar space abscess is usually a product of a penetrating wound and should be drained where it points. The same is true for a thenar space abscess, which may point in the palm rather than the thumb web.

E. Space of Parona: This space lies over the pronator quadratus beneath the flexor muscles in the distal forearm. Infection here is usually due to extension of pus from the flexor sheaths of the thumb (radial bursa) or little finger (ulnar bursa). Drainage should be along the ulnar side of the forearm deep to the flexor tendons and the ulnar nerve and artery.

F. Dorsal Subaponeurotic and Subcutaneous Spaces: The subaponeurotic space lies deep to the extensor tendons on the back of the hand, and the subcutaneous space is superficial to it. Either or both may become infected by puncture, by open injury, or by extension of infection from the digits and web spaces. Drainage is best done through the dorsoradial side of ray II or the ulnar side of ray V. A superficial transverse incision, sparing the veins, may be made over the metacarpal heads for additional drainage and to allow flexion of the MP joints into the position of function.

Septic Tenosynovitis

The flexor and extensor synovial tendon sheaths (bursae) are avenues for the spread of infection. The ulnar bursa extends from the level of the distal joint of the little finger to incorporate all flexors of the other fingers as they pass through the carpal tunnel. Here it often communicates with the radial bursa coming from the thumb. The bursae of the index, long, and ring fingers usually terminate at the mid palm. Intercommunication of bursae is variable. The 6 dorsal tendon compartments under the extensor retinaculum of the wrist have separate synovial bursae.

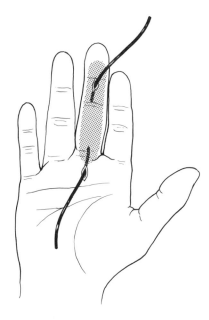

FIG 48–19. Drainage and irrigation for septic tenosynovitis.

The cardinal sign of tenosynovitis is moderate to severe pain along a given synovial sheath when the tendon therein is made to glide a short distance actively and passively. Passive motion must be performed by touching no more than the patient's fingernail, thus avoiding misdiagnosis by limiting the stimulus to motion of the synovial sheath.

Only unresponsive, tense, and toxic cases need incision and drainage. With rest, elevation, and antibiotics, it is safe to observe most cases for several hours. The preferred method of incision and drainage (Fig 48–19) is to make a short sagittal distal wound immediately over the tendon and introduce a small plastic catheter for irrigating with solutions of antibiotics. Another catheter should be inserted for drainage through a counterincision in the palm. These incisions do not cross flexion creases. The hand should then be elevated and immobilized in the position of function and covered by continuous wet or zinc oxide dressings. Phlegmonous tenosynovitis usually requires opening of the entire synovial sheath (often through a lateral midaxial incision) and, frequently, excision of necrotic tendon and sometimes amputation of a digit.

Bone & Joint Infections

The limited circulation of these structures makes them very susceptible to infection. Any open wound of bone or joint deserves immediate treatment as though infection were already established. Penetrating tooth wound infections (eg, human bite infections) are among the most virulent. They often involve the dorsum of the MP and PIP joints as a result of striking a blow with a closed fist. Osteomyelitis responds well to antibiotics and sequestrectomy where indicated.

Miscellaneous Infections

A. Streptococcal Gangrene: This is a very toxic process which causes rapid necrosis of tissues and requires emergency fasciectomy and excision of necrotic tissue, continuous compresses with 0.5% silver nitrate, and massive antibiotic therapy. Microaerophilic streptococcal infection (Meleney's phagedenic ulcer, sloughing ulcer) is a similar process that must be treated promptly in the same way.

B. Tuberculosis: Tuberculous infection of the hand is usually chronic and may be relatively painless. Some cultures take months to become positive. Tuberculosis commonly involves only one hand, which may be the only focus of infection in the body. Bones and joints may be infected, but the infection more commonly involves the tendon sheaths, which become fused to the tendons. Treatment is by means of synovectomy and antituberculosis drug therapy for 6–12 months.

C. Leprosy: Leprous neuritis of the median and ulnar nerves causes sensory and motor loss to the hand. Crippling claw deformities develop due to intrinsic muscle palsy. Open sores appear on the hands as a result of trauma to anesthetic digits. Reconstructive surgery and occupational training are required as part of the rehabilitation program.

D. Fungal Infections: Fungal infections involve primarily the nails. Tinea unguium (onychomycosis) may be caused by many organisms, including *Epidermophyton floccosum,* trichophyton, and *Candida albicans.* Prolonged treatment with antifungal drugs— griseofulvin systemically or nystatin topically—may be necessary, along with daily applications of fungicidal agents such as tolnaftate.

E. Herpes Simplex: This should be suspected if there is a history or observation of multiple tiny vesicles, usually about the distal phalanx. It is usually self-limiting in about 3 weeks. Idoxuridine ointment (a specific antiviral drug) applied directly on the opened vesicles may accelerate the resolution.

F. Rare Infections: Gas gangrene, syphilis, deep fungal infections (eg, coccidioidomyocosis, actinomycosis, blastomycosis, sporotrichosis), tularemia, anthrax, yaws, and glanders are unusual infections which can only be diagnosed by means of a pertinent history of exposure, chronicity, and laboratory studies to identify the pathogen.

NONINFECTIOUS INFLAMMATORY DISORDERS OF THE HAND

The entities in this group have little in common except a greater or lesser degree of inflammatory or collagen reaction and change. They include wear-and-tear conditions, degenerative states, rheumatic and collagen diseases, and gout. Pain is often the presenting complaint, and there may be a coexisting abnormality of appearance or mechanical function.

DESMITIS, TENDINITIS, & MYOSITIS

Desmitis (inflammation of a ligament) is often impossible to distinguish from inflammation of juxtaposed tendon (tendinitis) or muscle (myositis), and in any case the distinction is somewhat academic. The diagnosis is made by finding the trigger point of tenderness. The disorder may be idiopathic, secondary to direct trauma, or due to acute or chronic repetitive strain. The first spring day of gardening often precipitates acute **myositis crepitans** of muscle groups—most commonly the abductor pollicis longus and the extensor pollicis brevis. Even more common is **lateral epicondylitis** ("tennis elbow") or **medial epicondylitis.** Pain and tenderness are also very common around the dorsal and volar radial and ulnar ligaments and tendons of the wrist, or the collateral ligaments of any of the digital joints. If the area is swollen and inflamed, as many of the joints should be splinted as necessary to relieve the pain. In the absence of heat and swelling, splinting is not usually necessary, and relief can be rendered by the local injection of lidocaine mixed with triamcinolone (10–40 mg/ml). This should be done slowly, avoiding vessels and nerves, and without aggravating pain. Patients should be warned of the possibility of a postinjection flare-up of misery for 6–12 hours (when the lidocaine wears off) and should be given a systemic analgesic to cover it. Prolonged splinting is undesirable because it leads to muscle atrophy, which compounds the disability. Effective systemic treatment may be given with phenylbutazone, 100–200 mg 3 times daily with meals or with antacids. Radiation therapy is occasionally successful for epicondylitis. Failing relief from this and all other therapy, surgical stripping of the muscle wad from its epicondylar origin may be of benefit. The patient must sometimes develop a compensatory technic of using his extremity or relinquish certain types of activity (eg, gardening) to forestall exacerbations.

CONSTRICTIVE CONDITIONS

In stenosing tenosynovitis there is a disproportion between the clearance inside a tendon pulley or tunnel and the diameter of the tendon or tendons that must glide through it. Any pulley or tunnel may be incriminated. The more common sites are as follows:

(1) The proximal digital pulleys in the distal palm, causing **trigger finger** (stenosing flexor tenosynovitis). The manifestations are local tenderness of the pulley; pain, which may be referred to the PIP joint:

and (usually but not always) locking of the digit in flexion with a painful jog as it goes into extension (ie, as the bulge in the tendon passes through the tight pulley).

(2) The pulley over the radial styloid housing the abductor pollicis longus and extensor pollicis brevis, causing **DeQuervain's tenosynovitis.** Local tenderness and pain occur if these tendons are actively or passively stretched.

(3) The volar carpal ligament, causing **carpal tunnel syndrome.** The "soft" median nerve is compressed against the ligament by the 9 "hard" tendons in the tunnel with it. Mild compression causes pathognomonic mid-sleep aching and numbness over the distribution of the nerve, but always sparing the little finger. Severe constriction causes constant hypesthesia and thenar paralysis.

(4) **Ulnar nerve compression** (less common) occurs as the nerve passes behind the medial epicondyle (the cubital tunnel) or along Guyon's canal from the pisiform bone to the hook of the hamate. The differential diagnosis is based on a knowledge of the anatomy of innervation. Electromyography and nerve conduction studies may be helpful in evaluating these nerve compressions.

These disorders are usually due to chronic adaptive hypertrophy of tendon and pulley alike in response to work or repetitive activity, coupled with factors of aging, but they can occur at any age. Other factors are distortion caused by trauma, tumor, rheumatoid synovitis, tendinitis, or rheumatoid nodules.

Relief can be achieved by local injections of triamcinolone or dexamethasone mixed with lidocaine or by means of surgical section of the constricting pulley or tunnel. Local injections may be tried 3–4 times at weekly intervals before resorting to surgery, which involves a hazard of nerve trauma or prolonged weakness. A disabling complication of surgery for DeQuervain's tenosynovitis is a very painful neuroma of the radial nerve. Immediate surgery is justified if the constriction is so tight that no tendon glide is possible, and in cases of unrelenting motor or sensory nerve impairment, irreversible rheumatoid or nonspecific synovial thickening, or other space-consuming lesions.

Surgery must never be done without a tourniquet or blindly. If nerves are involved, a loupe should be used for magnification. Adequate proximal and distal decompression is essential. If the epineurial sheath is also thickened or a nerve has an hourglass constriction, endoneurolysis is in order.

DUPUYTREN'S CONTRACTURE
(Palmar Fasciitis)

The cause of this common disorder among Caucasian populations is not known. It occurs predominantly in males over 50 who have been in sedentary occupations, and is bilateral in about half of cases.

There is a hereditary influence, and the incidence is higher among alcoholics and patients with chronic illnesses. The contracture may develop in women who do not work and (in laborers) in the hand that does the least work, so that it is not considered work-related.

Dupuytren's contracture manifests itself most commonly in the palm by thickening, which may be nodular, and therefore mistaken for a callosity; or cord-like, and therefore mistaken for a tendon abnormality because it passes into the digits and restricts their extension. This process typically involves the longitudinal and vertical components of the fascia but at times seems to exist apart from anatomically distinct fascia. The skin may fuse with it and become raised and rock-hard, or it may be greatly shrunken and sometimes drawn into a deeply puckered crevasse. It "invades" the palm but is never adherent to vessels, nerves, or musculotendinous structures. It has an unpredictable rate of progression, but the earlier it starts in life the more destructive and recurrent it is apt to be.

Dupuytren's contracture may involve the fascia of any digit or web space, but it affects predominantly the ring and little fingers. In long-standing cases the fingers may be drawn tightly into the palm, resulting in secondary cicatrization of joint ligaments and capsules or atrophic fibrosis of muscles.

Surgery is indicated when the disorder has progressed sufficiently to provoke a request for relief from the patient, who must be warned about the potential for recurrence and the increasing technical difficulty with progressive flexion and adduction contractures. These hands stiffen easily, and expert surgical technic is essential to good results. Use of a tourniquet, magnification, and meticulous hemostasis are mandatory for fasciectomy, which is the surgical procedure that gives the best long-term results. In selected cases where only the longitudinal pretendinous fascial band is involved and the skin moves freely over it, subcutaneous fasciotomy done carefully through a small longitudinal incision may release a contracture quite well with only a few days of postoperative disability. In the occasional case with acute and rapid onset of a tender nodule, local triamcinolone may be used for not only subjective but even objective relief.

Depending upon the amount of cutaneous shrinkage, skin grafts may be required for wound closure after fasciectomy. The hopelessly contracted little finger must sometimes be amputated.

Motion should be started within 3–5 days after surgery. Dynamic splints and postoperative injection of corticosteroids into joints and the zone of surgery may help the well-motivated patient.

The complications of surgery are digital infarction and ischemic skin flaps, hematoma formation, fibrosis and stiffness, anesthesia or neuromatous pain, and recurrence of fasciitis and contracture. In general, the functional reward to the patient is great and lasting at any age.

Davis JE: On surgery of Dupuytren's contracture. Plast Reconstr Surg 36:277, 1965.

DEGENERATIVE OSTEOARTHRITIS

This is a common condition in people over age 40. It affects women more often than men, and is first manifested about the distal finger joints. Heberden's nodes of hypertrophic cartilage and bone cause typical dorsal bossing with occasional associated synovial cyst (mucous cyst) formation. Such cysts (really ganglions) may press on the nail matrix and cause longitudinal grooving of the fingernail. If they are excised, magnification should be used. Methylene blue diluted and injected volarly into the distal joint helps to define the limits of these cysts and to trace their stalks into the joint. The subjacent bony spur which is often present should be excised to prevent recurrence. Joint deformity, pain, and stiffness may be treated by replacement of the joint with a prosthetic silicone rubber joint spacer or hinge (see below) or by joint fusion.

RHEUMATOID DISEASE

This disease of unknown cause affects all the tissues of mesenchymal origin in the hand, especially the synovial tissues. The x-ray changes vary from early marginal joint erosion with associated osteoporosis to advanced destructive changes and subluxation, particularly of the wrist and the MP and PIP joints. The disease often starts in the hands and involves the synovia of joints and tendons. Initially there is vague pain of insidious (sometimes acute) onset, swelling, stiffness, and local hyperthermia. In time, thickening of synovial tissues about the joints and tendons causes destruction and distortion. Tendons may rupture. Rheumatoid granulomatous nodules develop in the substance of tendons and tendon sheaths and subcutaneously over bony prominences. Stretched ligaments and retinacular tissues can no longer maintain the alignment of joints and tendons against the mean pulling forces, and a host of deformities may develop (swan-neck or boutonniere deformity, ulnar drift, and "intrinsic plus" deformity). With intrinsic muscle fibrosis and advanced joint destruction, many of these deformities become fixed.

The ideal management of these cases consists of combined medical and surgical supervision and guidance. It is always hoped that physical and emotional rest, heat, analgesia, therapeutic exercise, and anti-inflammatory agents (eg, corticosteroids, gold salts) will check the progression of disease. When these measures are not successful, the surgeon should offer surgical procedures (synovectomy, arthroplasty, tenoplasty, resection of nodules, arthrodesis, ulnar styloidectomy, etc) which may forestall further destruction and preserve function and cosmetic appearance.

The problems amenable to surgical correction are the following:

(1) Boggy synovitis about flexor and extensor tendons. (2) Boggy synovitis of wrist or digital joints. (3) Rheumatoid nodules. (4) Tendon rupture (mainly of extensors of the ring and little fingers and the thumb). (5) Constrictive conditions (stenosing tenosynovitis and median and ulnar nerve compression syndromes). (6) Joint erosions, subluxations, and fixed deformities.

• • •

Silicone Rubber Implants

Made of heat-vulcanized, medical grade silicone elastomer stock, these implants ("joint spacers") were developed for arthritic joint and carpal bone replacement. They have been effectively time-tested for replacement of the MP and PIP joints, the greater multangular, navicular, and lunate bones. If there has been much soft tissue reconstruction, immobilization is continued for 4–6 weeks; if not, motion may be guardedly initiated in 3 or 4 days with partial daytime and complete nighttime splinting for 4–6 weeks. The removal of carpal bones can be very difficult and hazardous. Piecemeal removal may prevent a disastrous surgical experience. Postoperative immobilization should be maintained for 4–6 weeks.

Flatt AE: *The Care of the Rheumatoid Hand*. Mosby, 1963.

Nalebuff EA: Symposium on surgical management of rheumatoid arthritis. S Clin North America 49:787–846, 1969.

Swanson AB: Flexible implant arthroplasty for arthritic finger joints: Rationale, technic, and results of treatment. J Bone Joint Surg 54A:435–455, 1972.

Swanson AB: Silicone rubber implants for replacement of arthritic or destroyed joints in the hand. S Clin North America 48:1113, 1968.

SCLERODERMA, LUPUS ERYTHEMATOSUS, & SARCOIDOSIS

These systemic diseases of unknown cause have distinctive—though not necessarily pathognomonic—manifestations in the hands.

Scleroderma initially produces joint stiffness, hyperhidrosis, and Raynaud's phenomenon. Unchecked, it leads to marked tautness of skin and rigidity of joints with associated osteoporosis (even absolution of the distal phalanges) and soft tissue calcifications.

Lupus erythematosus, which may be initiated or aggravated by certain drugs, foreign proteins, or psychic states, often causes polyarthritis indistinguishable from that of rheumatoid arthritis. It does not usually lead to similar joint destruction.

Sarcoidosis may produce digital nodules and articular swellings, and x-rays may show small punched-out lesions, particularly of the phalanges.

GOUT

Gout is a metabolic disorder of uric acid metabolism which affects about 1% of the population; approximately 50% of patients with gout have cheiragra (gouty hands).

The diagnosis is suggested by a sudden onset of severe pain and inflammatory signs about the joints and musculotendinous structures. The usual duration of an attack is 5–10 days. The serum uric acid is elevated in 75% of cases. Gout may coexist with rheumatoid disease.

In time, typical tophi form, consisting of toothpaste-like infiltrates of urate crystals. These arise in multilobulated form about the soft tissue structures that have been invaded. X-rays show characteristic punched-out lesions at the margins of articular cartilage.

The prophylactic medical treatment of gout consists of diet, uricosuric agents (eg, allopurinol), and avoidance of stress. Colchicine, 0.6 mg/hour with a glass of water for 6–8 doses or to the point of gastrointestinal distress, is the time-honored means of interrupting an attack, but phenylbutazone, corticotropin gel, and corticosteroids are also of value.

Surgical measures consist of drainage of abscessed tophi and tophectomy. The latter procedure is more often of cosmetic than functional value. Tophectomy is not technically tidy or absolute but consists of removal of as much tophaceous material as can be fairly easily recovered, being sure not to destroy ligaments, tenoretinacular structures, nerves, and vessels in the process.

BURNS OF THE HAND

The hands are a common site of thermal (including frictional), electrical, chemical, and radiation burns. Function is imperiled in all instances by swelling and scar formation. Prompt measures to preserve existing function are often urgently required. Delay may lead to irreversible impairment and deformity.

THERMAL BURNS

These are the most common types of hand burns. Thermal burns occur as a result of scalding, branding by contact with hot surfaces and sparks, and by contact with flames or friction. The thick keratinized palmar skin protects the palm from the deep second and third degree burns that commonly occur on the thin dorsal skin. Flame burns usually cause second and

third degree burns on the dorsal surfaces because of the protective reflex to shield the face with the hands by supinating the forearms. Hot liquids often burn both the dorsal and the volar surfaces. Hot tar cools fast and does not usually cause third degree burns, whereas hot grease often causes whitish, waxy-looking deep second or third degree burns. Hot water burns are often only first or second degree. Branding is apt to be no more than second degree because of protective withdrawal, whereas friction burns due to moving machinery and rope are often deep second or third degree.

The depth of the burn is indicated by the presence or absence of blisters, response to pinprick, and charring: first degree burn causes no blister; second degree burn is blistered; third degree burn is anesthetic to pinprick; and fourth degree burn is charred. Early, the burn interferes with function by distortion and stiffness due to swelling (congestion), infection, pain, and loss of substance. Cicatrix formation, shrinkage, and adhesions are later problems.

Treatment

A. Objective of Treatment: The urgent objective of treatment is to restore mobility as soon as possible (within 1–3 weeks) by the following measures: (1) Control of swelling (by elevation, fasciotomy, and escharotomy). (2) Control of pain (by cold compresses, elevation, analgesics, and grafting). (3) Prevention of infection (by topical anti-infective agents), immediate or early grafting, and control of congestion. (4) Prompt (even primary) debridement followed by grafting as soon as oozing has stopped and the wound appears ready.

B. Emergency Treatment: Immediate immersion in cold water prevents further heat damage. No ointments or home remedies (butter, etc) should be applied to burned surfaces at the scene. The burned hand should be covered with a clean (if possible, sterile), dry dressing and the patient transported as soon as possible to the hospital emergency department.

C. Definitive Treatment:

1. First degree burns—No treatment is required for first degree hand burns. Symptomatic relief may be achieved by the application of ice water compresses.

2. Second degree burns—Second degree burns should be debrided if blisters are bulky or already broken. Burns involving 2.5 sq cm or more may then be covered with a biologic dressing, if available, such as allograft (homograft) or xenograft (which are bacteriostatic) or amniotic membrane. All of these effectively control pain. Pigskin is an ideal xenograft (heterograft). If grafts are not available, an ideal emollient is a thick coating of zinc oxide ointment or an ointment made up of silver nitrate, 1 part; balsam of Peru, 5 parts; hydrous lanolin, 30 parts; and amber petrolatum, 30 parts. Motion is encouraged from the beginning, whereas dependency and the "position of injury" are discouraged. Splinting at night may be useful. When the epithelium no longer weeps, lanolin may be applied.

3. Deep second degree burns and third degree burns—A deep second degree burn or third degree burn which involves one-third to one-half or more of the surface area of a digit, hand, or forearm usually causes enough swelling to threaten loss of function. Hand swelling is greatest on the dorsum, where the skin is loose and the space beneath will accommodate a lot of water. This forces MP joint extension and thumb adduction, creating "a claw hand in disguise." The burned part must be constantly and carefully watched. If elevation alone is not effective and the patient becomes less able than formerly to close his fist and touch his thumb to his little finger—or if throbbing pain progresses followed by numbness—then immediate bedside escharotomy with biologic dressing and prompt operating room debridement and grafting must be considered. Brawny induration throughout the tissues must be prevented. The following releasing incisions are often necessary:

(1) Transversely over the metacarpal heads of rays II–V to allow the MP joints which are trapped in extension to fall into flexion. (*Note:* In doing this, cut only the skin—avoid veins and tendons.) At the same time, one should consider the insertion of Kirschner wires through the metacarpal heads across these joints until grafting is complete in 2–4 weeks, thus preventing an ultimate claw deformity.

(2) Longitudinal dorsoradial or dorso-ulnar incisions of the digits, the body of the hand, or forearm (often slitting the forearm fascia as well). Again, it is essential to spare veins and nerves.

(3) A zigzag dorsal incision from the crest to the base of the thumb web, followed by Kirschner wire fixation of the thumb metacarpal spread in pronation from the index metacarpal to prevent adduction contracture.

Early closure of the burn wound and early mobilization of joints and tendons is the essence of good care of these deep burns.

When motion is being lost or is already lost, it is far better to debride skin primarily or within the first week and have the hand grafted and mobilized within 10 days than to anxiously await for 3–4 weeks the possible survival of the burned skin at the expense of cicatrix formation and immobility.

Debridement incisions should be serrated on the radial and ulnar margins of the digits and in the webs to curtail hypertrophic scar formation and contracture. After debridement with a dermatome or scalpel, the ooze usually precludes immediate grafting. This, therefore, should be deferred for 24 hours. Thin (0.2–0.25 mm) postage stamp, mesh, or sheet grafts are most apt to take and should be used over beds of equivocal graft-sustaining quality. Few or no sutures need be used unless the bed is ideal. "Onlay" grafts will adhere to the bed in 8–24 hours if the bed is kept immobile. Meticulously applied dressings protected by plastic and a padded boxing glove cast for 1 or 2 days serve the purpose well. (The dressings are preferably moistened with bacteria-resistant fluid or ointment. If these are not available, use water to aid the sequestration of serum.) If open treatment is used, a conscientious attendant must daily remove any serum collections from beneath the graft.

Prolonged splinting should be avoided as much as possible except when the patient is resting or sleeping. At these times the hand should be propped up comfortably on pillows to keep it higher than the level of the heart. Isoprene splinting material is ideal for this purpose because it can be sterilized and heat-molded to fit the patient. The position of function must be maintained in modeling any splint, and constrictive wrappings must never be used. Hanging the extremity by a noose is to be condemned unless a long arm cast is applied with the elbow at 90 degrees. Elastic bandages are also dangerously constrictive.

4. Fourth degree burns—Fourth degree burns are usually associated with extensive second and third degree burns. The charred elements should be excised as soon as the general condition of the patient allows and the wounds closed as soon as possible.

Reconstructive Procedures

The proper initial care can prevent or limit many but not all of the functional disabilities caused by burns. The hand surgeon can do much by individualized procedures to reduce the extent of some of these disabilities. Resurfacing is accomplished with split thickness grafts for appearance, with full thickness grafts for release of flexion and web contractures, and with pedicle grafts when better padding is needed. Joints may be freed by capsulotomies and tenotomies, or they may be arthrodesed in a functional attitude.

Cosmesis and function can be well served by amputation. A ray resection of a useless index finger may greatly compensate for a thumb web contracture.

Restoration of movement. The patient with a burned hand must be helped and encouraged to move every joint of the upper extremity as soon and as often after injury as possible. It is tragic to have saved the life of the patient and neglected the function of his upper extremities. A claw hand is bad enough; add to that a frozen shoulder, fixed extension of the elbow, and fixed pronation of the forearm and the patient becomes an economically and psychologically destitute human being. The critically burned patient needs daily passive motion with encouragement for active motion. The patient must be disciplined to initiate frequent maximal movement and be educated concerning the greater value of his active effort than any passive movements by his medical attendants. Pain must be relieved by skin cover, analgesics, and emollients if mobilization is to be successful. Dependency must be avoided, and the selection of devices to assist the patient must be mechanically appropriate (eg, squeeze a sponge, **not** a ball) and psychologically challenging and stimulating rather than boring.

ELECTRICAL BURNS

High-voltage injuries to the extremity may be of great but hidden magnitude. Beneath the skin sleeve, extensive coagulation necrosis of vessels, nerves, and musculotendinous structures may be present, and its extent may not become manifest for several days. Electrical contact points usually have third degree skin burns. The treatment parallels that described for injection injuries (see p 995). It is not uncommon to have to amputate a hand or arm that has been damaged by an electrical burn. Early decompression by incisions of the skin and underlying fascia may limit progressive injury secondary to congestion.

CHEMICAL BURNS

Prolonged contact with certain chemicals (eg, picric acid) may saturate the skin enough to cause neuritis and vasculitis. By the time symptoms develop, the damage has already been done and one must wait for spontaneous recovery and regeneration. The skin itself may show no change.

Other caustic chemicals (acids or alkalies) may cause an immediate superficial burn. Treatment consists of immediate dilution by immersion in water and appropriate topical neutralization by alkaline (eg, sodium bicarbonate) or acid (eg, vinegar) solutions. The long-range treatment parallels that of thermal burns. Occasionally, the neutralizing agent can be injected in small amounts at the site of the burn (eg, 10% calcium gluconate at the site of a hydrofluoric acid burn).

RADIATION BURNS

These burns are not recognized at the moment of exposure and usually take many years (10–20 or more) to become manifest. Typical atrophic and telangiectatic changes of the skin develop which may lead to ulceration and malignant degeneration. Bone necrosis is common.

This type of injury was at one time common among dentists holding dental films in place for roentgenography.

If malignant change occurs, wide skin excision and resurfacing or even amputation may be necessary.

TUMORS & PSEUDOTUMORS OF THE HAND

Except for squamous cell carcinoma of the dorsal skin, malignancy in the hand is rare.

All tumors or pseudotumors do not need to be removed surgically, and removal can almost always be done electively. "Urgent" tumor surgery of the hand is usually unwarranted and may be harmful to hand function if the requisite skill is lacking.

Hand tumor surgery requires proper lighting, instruments, loupe magnification, and assistance and tourniquet-controlled ischemia. The incision must be carefully planned; should usually be made directly over the lesion; and must be long enough to make visualization atraumatic and the resection total.

A variety of lesions are found in the hand, including hematomas, scars, calluses, warts, nevi, cysts, xanthomas, enchondromas, giant cell tumors, fibromas, hemangiomas, carcinomas, and sarcomas. The most important ones are discussed on the following pages.

Hematoma & Foreign Body

There is usually a history of injury. Transillumination may reveal a dark area, and an x-ray with proper projection to exclude bone may show a radiopaque foreign body, including glass if it contains lead. Surgical evacuation of blood is often an unwarranted surgical insult when the blood infiltrates the interstitial fibers of tissues. Two to 3 weeks later, a hematoma, if present, may be easily removed through a small incision or, if liquefied, aspirated. Foreign bodies are generally no threat to the immobilized and elevated hand if antibiotics are given. Waiting 2–4 weeks for blood to clear will immensely aid the search when it is done. Obtaining x-ray views in several planes is a far better way to localize the foreign body than to use the traditional needles and x-ray technic.

Warts

Warts are caused by a DNA virus and are usually autoinoculated. Treatment consists either of local application of a 40% salicylic acid pad securely held over the wart with tape for 1 week or more or needle-tip electrocoagulation under lidocaine block anesthesia. In either case, after treatment the wart is curetted off flush with the skin. "Dry ice," liquid nitrogen, and 20% podophyllin in tincture of benzoin (must be thoroughly washed off in a few hours) are also effective but less favored by hand surgeons because they are more prone to cause nerve damage or ulceration if treatment is too deep and wide.

Ganglion & Mucous Cyst

Where there is a synovial lining, a protrusion may develop followed by later isolation of a closed pouch or cul-de-sac to form a cyst filled with the physiologic lubricant fluid of joints and tendons. The old concept of "mucoid degeneration" and development from embryologic cell rests has now been abandoned. If absorption of water occurs, the cyst will have a jelly-like consistency. Sudden, forceful bending of a joint may cause extrusion of the cyst between ligamentous fibers and the sudden appearance of a lump. More often, the cyst appears insidiously. Pain may be caused by tension within the cyst and pressure on adjacent tissues.

Most ganglions arise from the joints of the wrist, but any joint and tendon sheath can give rise to one. The path followed is along the tissue planes of least resistance. The length and pathway of a stalk are unpredictable. When there is protrusion through more than one fibrous tissue plane, the cyst may have an hourglass configuration.

A volar wrist ganglion always deserves a careful preoperative test of collateral arterial competency (Allen's test) to ensure good digital circulation if one artery must be divided in removing the ganglion. A flexor sheath ganglion is usually like a "pebble in the shoe." It may be mistaken for a sesamoid.

Treatment of a ganglion is not indicated unless the patient insists. Aspiration through a large-bore needle under lidocaine anesthesia followed by injection of triamcinolone may sustain many in remission. Some claim "cure" by this procedure. Midline flexor sheath ganglions that are off center should not be so treated, for in such cases the nerve and artery may be injured by the needle.

If surgery is required, the essence of skill is removal of the cyst unruptured until the joint or tendon sheath is entered and resection is completed without trauma to surrounding nerves or tendons. Recurrence and complications are usually caused by failure to use magnification, to explore adequately, and to visualize "satellite cysts" as one enters the joint. A rim of joint capsule or tendon sheath should be removed with the stalk. Injection of a small amount of methylene blue into the cyst with a fine needle helps to trace the cyst during the dissection. An exsanguinating Esmarch bandage, if used at all, must be wrapped on very carefully before inflation of the tourniquet or the ganglion may rupture. There is no need to close the joint capsule after ganglionectomy.

Inclusion Cyst

Injury can carry viable epidermal cells deep to the dermis, into fat, or even into bone. With growth of these cells, keratinized cells accumulate into a ball or cyst which compresses the tissue in which it lies. Bone may become eroded. At surgery, an inclusion cyst looks like a pearl and has a soft thin wall that surrounds its cheesy contents. If—with care—it is totally enucleated from its bed, it will not recur.

Posttraumatic Neuroma

This common lump only presents for treatment when it is painful. Such will be the case if it lies on a hard surface (eg, tendon or bone) at a point of pressure, or when it is trapped in scar tissue and subjected to stretching. (The treatment of neuromas is described in Chapter 41.)

Xanthoma (Giant Cell Tumor of Soft Tissue)

This is a hard, often multinodular tumor which arises from the fibrous flexor sheath or collateral ligaments. Even though benign, it extends under tendons and collateral ligaments and through joints. Unless all of the brownish-yellow tumor is removed, the tumor may recur.

Enchondroma, Giant Cell Tumor of Bone, & Aneurysmal Bone Cyst

Enchondromas constitute 90% of true bone tumors of the hand. The classic finding is calcific stippling of the lytic bone defect, most common in the proximal phalanges and distal half of the metacarpals. The carpal bones are spared. Aneurysmal bone cysts and giant cell tumors of bone are practically identical except for their vascularity. Pathologic fracture may be the presenting finding.

Treatment consists of curettement of the contents and wall of the lesion followed by packing of the hole with tiny cortical chips from the proximal third of the ulna.

Lipoma

This tumor usually occurs on the volar aspect of the digit or palm. If the proper plane is followed in the dissection, the lesion can be easily enucleated. Caution must be taken when these "invade" the carpal tunnel or extend about the major nerves.

Neurofibroma

Most of these tumors are multiple (Recklinghausen's disease) and consist of thickened nerve sheath elements. There is a rare tendency to malignant degeneration. The usual indication for resection of this tumor is cosmetic. It should be enucleated under magnification so as to spare the nerve. If growth is rapid, malignancy should be suspected and a long segment of the nerve resected or amputation contemplated.

Hemangioma

Hemangiomas in infants should never be treated by irradiation. The common strawberry angiomas will involute after their initial growth period. If the angioma is rapidly enlarging, it may be induced to involute by a course of corticosteroid therapy. In the older patient (and a few infants), surgical removal is the only means of treatment. Angiography may be helpful in determining the nature and extent of this group of tumors. They may be located primarily in skin, fat, or muscle—or, in the case of a cavernous hemangioma—may extend throughout all tissues and be impossible to totally remove without amputation or destroying digital or hand function.

Squamous Cell & Basal Cell Carcinoma

These tumors comprise 90% of malignancies of the hand. Squamous cell tumors are far more common than basal cell. Both types are seen primarily on the dorsum of the hand in fair-skinned patients with a long history of exposure to sunlight. Squamous cell tumors have also occurred in dentists who have held their hands in the path of radiation while taking dental x-rays. The preferred treatment is excision and closure with a skin graft or sliding or rotating flap. When lesions are multiple, total dorsal resurfacing may be necessary. If the tumor is clinically invasive or microscopically extends beyond the deep plane of the resected specimen, an appropriate amputation (partial or complete) must be considered. When an invasive squamous cell carcinoma exceeds 2 cm in diameter, axillary dissection should be considered.

Actinic Keratosis & Bowen's Disease

These lesions respond well to topical fluorouracil (5-FU), 1% solution in propylene glycol. Bowen's lesions are usually found on the dorsum of the hands in persons exposed chronically to sunlight, and present as blotchy, scaling, reddened areas.

Malignant Melanoma

Malignant melanoma is rare but must be suspected in any growing lesion—pigmented or unpigmented—of the skin or nail bed (melanotic whitlow). Digital melanoma should be treated with ray resection and axillary node dissection. Superficial melanomas of the hand and forearm (penetrating less than the upper third of the dermis) need only wide local excision and skin grafting to give a cure rate of almost 100%. Lesions more invasive than this should be treated by wide excision of skin and underlying fascia and regional lymph node dissection or proximal amputation if underlying periosteum is involved. Early radical treatment may result in a 5-year survival rate as high as 50% for invasive melanoma. Adjunctive chemotherapeutic limb perfusion has not influenced survival.

Glomus Tumor

This rare tumor, comprised of blood vessels and unmyelinated nerves of a heat-regulating arteriovenous shunt, causes extremely severe pain. It can develop anywhere but is most dramatic under the fingernail, where "pinpoint" pressure initiates the pain. Half of patients may have no symptoms except the visible or palpable lesion. Treatment consists of meticulous dissection and total excision under magnification.

COMPLEX INJURIES OF THE HAND

GENERAL PLAN OF MANAGEMENT

The Impact on the Patient

Sudden physical or functional loss of part or all

of the hand or arm is a shocking experience that deserves special recognition and attention on the part of the surgeon. Psychologic and physical comfort should be given, and the patient must be spared alarming comments as well as any false hopes of reimplantation or salvage. A surgeon who is confident of his experience in these matters is best qualified to discuss them with the patient and his family.

Amputation may be physical or functional. Injury and disease may functionally (though not physically) amputate by crushing, mangling, paralyzing, stiffening, causing pain, or otherwise destroying all or part of the hand beyond hope of useful recovery. In such cases, salvage may be impossible and surgical amputation is justified to improve the overall physical and psychologic effectiveness of the patient.

Referral

In referring cases, the injured part should be comfortably aligned and splinted without constriction. Bleeding should be controlled by compression or by ligation of the bleeder provided it is adequately exposed under tourniquet ischemia and loupe magnification to avoid injuring adjacent nerves. Wet dressings should be applied to open wounds to facilitate sequestration of blood and serum, and the extremity should be comfortably elevated. In the case of open injuries, prophylactic antibiotics should be given. An amputated part may be irrigated and, if possible, placed in a container or plastic bag with ice. Even if reimplantation is not feasible, tissue (eg, skin or bone) from the ablated part is sometimes of value in primary or secondary reconstructive procedures.

In Vivo Tissue Bank

A "nearly amputated," badly crushed, or mangled digit, hand, or arm may present a great challenge to good judgment and to the surgeon's technical skill in acting on a decision to attempt salvage. Viable structures and tissues can often be reimplanted or transferred to give maximal restoration of function, ie, the patient can serve as his own "in vivo tissue bank" if the surgeon keeps a functionally irretrievable digit or other forearm or hand structure alive for use elsewhere in reconstruction.

Areas requiring padded skin are shown in Fig 48–20.

Foreign Bodies

Foreign bodies should be removed only if they interfere with function, cause symptoms, or result in dead space or infection. If removal is necessary, it is often facilitated by a period of observation and waiting (eg, 2–3 weeks) until congestion and bloody extravasation have cleared. In the meantime, the hand should be splinted, elevated, and, in some cases, drained. Prophylactic antibiotics should be given.

Assessment of Problem

These injuries notoriously cause multilevel and multitissue involvement ("common wound"). All

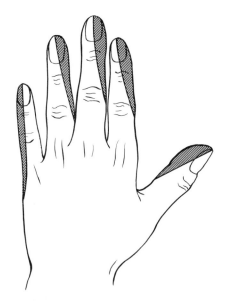

FIG 48–20. Areas requiring padded skin.

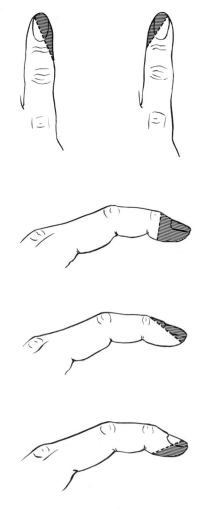

FIG 48–21. Distal digit amputation.

structures are congealed in the reactive process, culminating in a common scar (callus) with loss of structural independence.

The surgeon must individualize the treatment of complex hand injuries by considering such factors as age, occupation, hand dominance, economic status, cosmesis, emotional makeup, and general health. In other words, adequate salvage and maximal salvage are relative to the patient's needs, desires, and capacities. An extensive reconstructive effort is justified if, without it, there will be little or no function; but one must be careful not to destroy existing function and to spare the patient unwarranted disability and expense by heroic efforts that might fail. It is sometimes best to remove part or all of the hand in the interest of the patient's overall psychologic and functional competence and productivity.

AMPUTATION

Management of the Stump

The surgical objective in amputating a part is to create a painless stump with soft tissue cover which will meet the functional needs of the patient and will have good sensibility and adequate stability and pliability. Digital amputation will either be transverse or will face obliquely to the dorsal, volar, radial, or ulnar aspects of the digit (Fig 48–21). It may involve more than one phalanx.

If stump closure is by a local flap, it must be without any tension whatsoever. If it is tight, leave it open and graft it or resect bone to close it. If the flap is redundant, beware of trimming excessively – the slack may be needed to accommodate swelling.

When sufficient stump cover is not available locally, it must be obtained from grafts and flaps. The most predictable take is achieved by a thin (0.01–0.015 inch) split thickness graft; this should always be the first choice if there is any doubt about blood supply, infection, or joint stiffness. Sutures are not needed except in large grafts.

Primary and secondary advancement or pedicle grafts should be considered when it is necessary to give better skin cover over volar-oblique surfaces of all digits, the radial-oblique surface of the fingers, and the ulnar-oblique surface of the thumb; when one does not want to shorten digital bone on a transverse amputation surface; or when it is necessary to cover the body of the hand. Transverse digital stumps of infants will close by secondary intention with a result equal to or better than can be achieved by surgery.

In amputations through joints, cartilage should be left if possible. Chondritis will not develop even when the wound is left exposed to granulate in. Removing the cartilage may cause the skin to stick to the bone so much that it is forever abraded. When stumps need revision, what must be removed are all remnants of tough white tissue around the joint, ie, collateral ligaments, the volar plate, and flexor and extensor tendon stumps. For cosmetic reasons, condylar flares may be selectively reduced in size by rongeuring.

Amputations through bone should be tailored with the osteotome and rongeur to conform to function and to remove protruding sharp edges, fragments, and spicules.

Indications for Amputation

Irreversible ischemia is the only absolute indication for amputation. The other major indication is where salvage of the digit or part of it will threaten the overall function of the hand, the extremity, or the patient. Such may be the case with an overwhelmingly injured or infected finger which is hopelessly stiff or painful and may jeopardize the function of the other good fingers, or with malignant tumor (eg, malignant melanoma).

Degloving Injuries

These injuries are usually caused by having a ring torn violently from a digit, eg, in falling from a fence and simultaneously hooking the ring on a prong. The skin, fat, and neurovascular bundles are ripped off, flexor tendons may be avulsed, and middle and distal phalanges may be amputated. The other digits are usually not injured. The best treatment is usually to amputate. One has a choice of primary ray amputation or amputation through the proximal phalanx. Salvage and reconstruction are possible only rarely and involve a great deal of time, with several major surgical procedures and some jeopardy to the function of adjacent normal digits.

Amputation of Rays III & IV

Amputation of the long and ring fingers causes a gap through which material and liquid matter (eg, rice, nails, water) in the cupped hand will escape. This gap can be closed by removing the metacarpal at its proximal third (ray resection) and allowing the adjacent metacarpal heads to be approximated; or by the central transplantation of the adjacent osteotomized metacarpals onto the metacarpal stump of ray III or IV, or both (ray transfer). When the index, long, and ring fingers are gone, rotation osteotomy of the fifth metacarpal may be needed so that the little fingertip can comfortably oppose the thumb.

Thumb Amputation

Because most skills of man are hampered by loss of part or all of the thumb, preservation, reconstruction, or replacement of a thumb has great functional merit. The prime objectives are the preservation of length, the proper placement for opposition, and provision of a stable strut against which the fingers can flex with force. Ideally, there should be sensibility where the thumb and fingers meet in pinch, and this can be provided with a neurovascular island pedicle transfer. Not so urgent (but desirable) are motion and power,

particularly to control all the planes of movement of the metacarpal-carpal joint. If this exists, bone-strutted tube pedicle thumb reconstruction—or a digital transfer (pollicization) on a neurovascular pedicle—can compensate remarkably for a loss.

WRINGER, CRUSH, & COMPRESSION INJURIES

In wringer injury, part or all of the extremity is dragged into and compressed by one or more machine-driven rollers. It is common in industries where rolls or sheets of material are drawn between rollers for threading, printing, or compressing purposes or where conveyor belts are used; and in homes where washing machine wringers are still used.

The extremity is advanced until anatomic obstruction is met. As the rollers continue to turn, avulsion of skin and fat or a friction burn of the tissues (or both) may result. The thumb web is the first common obstruction, and the dorsal hand skin then becomes avulsed or burned. The next obstruction is the elbow, and the last the axilla.

Vessels, nerves, and muscles may be avulsed, and bones may be dislocated or broken. The most common unrecognized complication is secondary congestion, which can lead to paralysis and severe muscle fibrosis (eg, Volkmann's contracture) and joint stiffness if not arrested.

Most of these patients should be hospitalized, kept flat in bed with the extremity comfortably elevated, and observed hourly. One should consider the use of low molecular weight dextran, corticosteroids, and prophylactic antibiotics. Progressive throbbing pain leading to anesthesia and tightness of the skin and fascia sleeve of the finger, hand, or arm requires longitudinal slitting of skin and fascia for decompression. More than one muscle compartment may need decompression, and the pronator teres muscle and transverse carpal ligament must sometimes be sectioned to liberate the median nerve.

Skin avulsed by the wringer is usually in the form of a retrograde flap with imperiled circulation to it. One must judge the color by capillary filling of the flap; if this is poor or absent, debride all the fat from the flap and apply it as a full thickness graft, or discard it completely in favor of a primary or delayed split thickness skin graft. In most cases, fractures and dislocations should be reduced and aligned, but the overall circulation of the extremity is of more initial concern than definitive management of specific tissue and structural injuries. Abrasion burns are often third degree and, if so, require debridement and grafting when the integrity of the circulation is restored.

INJECTION INJURIES

These injuries are caused by the sudden introduction of substances under high pressure (ie, hundreds or thousands of pounds per square inch). The substances include air or other gases; liquids such as water, paint, oil, and a host of chemicals in various solutions; and solids and semisolids such as grease and molten plastic. Accordingly, these accidents occur principally in industry. Air pressure hoses in gasoline service stations, aerosol bombs, and sandblast hoses are typical sources of gas-driven injuries. Paint guns, oil and grease guns, and nozzles that inject molten plastic at high temperatures (eg, 260 C [500 F]) are among the most common other sources of these injuries.

The history is the most important clue to the severity of the injury and the need for immediate treatment. While operating a high-pressure device, the patient suddenly feels a strange sensation which ranges from very painful to not painful at all. He may present a totally normal-appearing hand with perhaps an almost undetectable pinpoint injection site; or the hand may be discolored or pale and cold, and tensely swollen due to the injected material.

Sometimes the injection is limited to a single digit, but often the great pressure forces the material to spread widely throughout the hand and even into the forearm. The greatest problems stem from the following: (1) The chemical irritant effect on all tissues, causing vascular thrombosis and toxic inflammation and necrosis. (2) The primary congestion effect of the material, leading within minutes or hours to secondary congestion due to the inflammatory response, all of which first interrupts venous flow and then leads to arterial arrest and gangrene. (3) Thermal burns (eg, from hot plastic). (4) Inability to remove enough of the offending material to forestall a short-term or long-term foreign body response, which ultimately leads to fibrosis that is so extensive that it destroys the functions of sensation and mobility of the part.

The examination should include an immediate x-ray to demonstrate, if possible, the distribution of material or gas in the hand; and a careful evaluation of sensibility, tenderness, induration, crepitation, color, temperature, and mobility. All such cases require immediate and continued unrelenting scrutiny, even if the part seems completely normal. With evidence of retained foreign material causing swelling, ischemia, or progressive throbbing pain, the hand must be explored if for no other reason than to release the tourniquet effect of the skin and fascia induced by the congestion. It is impossible to remove all of the foreign material when it is widespread and invasive. As much should be removed as can be done by gentle scraping and teasing —and that which lies in bloodless tissue—as long as one does not further damage the tissues to the point of greater congestion or ischemia and interfere with the normal process of demarcation and sequestration.

In addition to appropriate decompression and debridement, the hand must be drained and covered with compresses of zinc oxide, saline, or 0.5% silver nitrate solution. The hand must be held in the position of function and elevated, with the patient kept supine. Prophylactic antisludging agents (dextran 40), corticosteroids, antibiotics, and antitetanus medication must be administered. In most instances, hospitalization is urgent.

The objective of treatment is to minimize loss of function, and the most important initial effort must be to preserve circulation and avoid infection. If only one digit is involved and its functional fate is hopeless, amputation may be the most expeditious means of treatment.

GUNSHOT INJURIES OF THE HAND

Gunshot injuries of the hand may cause insignificant grazing or through-and-through injuries, or may severely maim the part. The damage depends upon the character and velocity of the missile, proximity to the muzzle, the concussion effect, and the amount of contamination of the wound by bacteria and foreign material (eg, clothing).

The essence of treatment is maintenance of circulation and the avoidance of infection by adequate drainage, antibiotics (systemically and often locally), discreet debridement of ischemic tissue and macrocontaminants (not stained, living tissues), immobilization and elevation, and, if necessary, decompression of skin and fascia. Primary reparative surgery must never be done if it will in any way compromise these prime objectives. Gentle reduction of gross bony distortions may complement them.

Progressive numbness and motor paralysis may demand emergency decompression of a nerve. Immediate paralysis can await nerve exploration until the tissues soften and circulation is ideal.

MANGLING INJURIES OF THE HAND

These injuries commonly cause various degrees of distortion of tissue and interruption of the circulation. The principles outlined at the beginning of this chapter must be followed in the treatment of these catastrophes. As always, initial emphasis must be on restoring circulation and preventing infection (ie, appropriate drainage, local and systemic antibiotics, and wound closure as soon as the circulation is adequate).

• • •

General References

Beasley RW: Principles and techniques of resurfacing operations for hand surgery. S Clin North America 47:389–413, 1967.

Beasley RW: Symposium on the hand. Orthop Clin North America 1:2, 1970.

Boyes JH: *Bunnell's Surgery of the Hand*, 5th ed. Lippincott, 1972.

Chase RA: Surgery of the hand. Medical Progress articles in 2 parts. New England J Med 287:1174–1181, 1227–1234, 1972.

Chase RA, Laub D: The hand: Therapeutic strategy for acute problems. Curr Probl Surg, June, 1966.

Correa LG: Cirugia de la Mano, IMSS. Seguridad Para Todos. Mexico, 1971.

Converse JM: Symposium on reconstructive surgery. S Clin North America 47:2, 1967.

Cramer LM, Chase RA: *Symposium on the Hand*. III. Educational Foundation of the American Society of Plastic and Reconstructive Surgeons. Mosby, 1971.

Dunphy JE, Van Winkle HW Jr: *Repair and Regeneration*. McGraw-Hill, 1969.

Eaton RG: *Joint Injuries of the Hand*. Thomas, 1971.

Entin MA: Symposium on practical surgery of the hand. S Clin North America 44:4, 1964.

Entin MA: Symposium on practical surgery of the hand. S Clin North America 48:5, 1968.

Flatt AE: *The Care of Minor Hand Injuries*, 3rd ed. Mosby, 1972.

Flynn JE: *Hand Surgery*. Williams & Wilkins, 1966.

Grabb WC, Smith JW: Hand and upper extremity, plastic surgery. Part IV, in: *Plastic Surgery: A Concise Guide to Clinical Practice*, 2nd ed. Little, Brown, 1973.

Littler JW: The hand and upper extremity. Vol IV, Part 3, in: *Reconstructive Plastic Surgery*. Converse JM (editor). Saunders, 1964.

Marble HC: *The Hand: A Manual and Atlas for the General Surgeon*. Saunders, 1960.

Milford L: The hand. Chap 4 in: *Campbell's Operative Orthopaedics*. Vol 1. Crenshaw AH (editor). Mosby, 1971.

Nichols HM: *Manual of Hand Injuries*, 2nd ed. Year Book, 1960.

Peacock EE, Van Winkle W: *Surgery and Biology of Wound Repair*. Saunders, 1970.

Rank BK, Wakefield AR: *Surgery of Repair as Applied to Hand Injuries*, 2nd ed. Williams & Wilkins, 1960.

Schneewind JH: Surgical emergencies of the hand. S Clin North America 52:203–218, 1972.

Seddon H: *Surgical Disorders of the Peripheral Nerves*. Williams & Wilkins, 1972.

Verdan C: Basic principles in surgery of the hand. S Clin North America 47:355–377, 1967.

White WL: Symposium on surgery of the hand. S Clin North America 40:2, 1960.

49...

Pediatric Surgery

Alfred A. deLorimier, MD

The surgical treatment of infants and children has advanced in recent years because of refinements in both surgical technic and in pre- and postoperative care. Physiologic norms in the young are now better understood than formerly. The newborn infant with a surgical lesion often has other disorders that are a threat to survival. Problems such as the difference between the small premature baby and the intrauterine deprived baby, the significance and treatment of hypoglycemia or hypocalcemia, and the metabolic and cardiopulmonary consequences of respiratory insufficiency are now better recognized. The vital functions of the critically ill infant can now be monitored, and the same intensive care can be applied that has been provided for adult patients.

CARE OF THE NEWBORN

Transportation of Newborn Surgical Patients

When transporting newborn infants for surgery, the following precautions must be observed: (1) Support normal body temperature by using an incubator maintained at 34 C (93.2 F). (2) Keep the airway clear by supplying a bulb syringe to aspirate mucus and vomitus. (3) Keep the stomach empty by giving nothing by mouth. Infants with intestinal obstruction should have a nasogastric tube placed in the stomach and aspirated at frequent intervals. (4) Provide proper identification and pertinent medical information if the infant is to be transported to a pediatric surgical center.

Determination of Gestational Age

Infants with surgically treatable lesions frequently weigh less than 2500 g. It is important to distinguish premature infants from "intrauterine growth-retarded infants." Premature infants have a high incidence of hyaline membrane disease, whereas growth-retarded infants are subject to intrauterine asphyxia with meconium aspiration, pneumothorax, and hypoglycemia and frequently have major congenital anomalies. The gestational age of the infant is calculated from the date of the last normal menstrual period. The weight of the baby can be correlated with the gestational age, and intrauterine growth retardation is defined as birth weight below the 25th percentile for the gestational age (Fig 49–1).

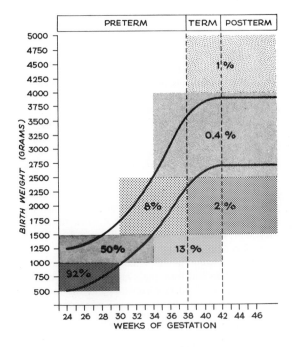

FIG 49–1. Neonatal mortality risk (in percent) related to weight and gestational age. Heavy curved lines outline the 10th and 90th percentiles. (Colorado data, 1958–1968. Reproduced, with permission, from Kempe CH, Silver HK, O'Brien D: *Current Pediatric Diagnosis & Treatment,* 2nd ed. Lange, 1972.)

Five physical signs may be useful in assessing gestational age. Infants of 36 weeks' gestational age or less have (1) fine fuzzy hair, (2) ears that lack cartilaginous support, (3) a breast nodule less than 3 mm in diameter, (4) testicles in the inguinal canal and a small scrotum with few rugae, and (5) skin on the feet with few transverse creases confined to the balls of the feet anteriorly.

Battaglia FC, Lubchenco LO: A practical classification of newborn infants by weight and gestational age. J Pediat 71:159, 1967.

Usher R, McLean F, Scott KE: Judgement of fetal age. II: Clinical significance of gestational age and an objective method for its assessment. P Clin North America 13:835–848, 1966.

Temperature Loss & Regulation

A. Simple Heat Loss: Infants and children have a relatively greater body surface area and thinner subcutaneous fat than adults. Therefore, heat loss by conduction and radiation may be 4 times that of the adult. Infants respond to hypothermia by norepinephrine secretion that increases the metabolic rate in most tissues, particularly the myocardium, and produces vasoconstriction with impaired tissue perfusion and increased lactic acid production which may result in shock and cardiac arrest. The neutral thermal environmental temperature occurs when the oxygen consumption of the infant is minimal, ie, when the gradient between the skin surface (particularly the face) and the environmental temperature is less than 1.5 C (2.7 F). The optimal environmental temperature should be 34 C (93.2 F) (slightly higher environmental temperatures are required for premature infants). Although the environmental temperature can be servo-controlled from skin or rectal temperature, it is difficult to detect fever or hypothermia due to sepsis by this technic.

B. Effect of Drugs: Depressant and anesthetic drugs abolish the thermoregulatory response of the patient, and oxygen consumption will decrease during hypothermia. Although the metabolic rate is decreased at this time, hypothermia also produces cardiac and respiratory depression. Following anesthesia, high oxygen consumption—during an interval when the respiratory and cardiac responses are depressed—results in severe hypoxia, acidosis, and cardiorespiratory failure.

C. Prevention of Heat Loss: Infants should be transported to and from the x-ray department or operating room in a warm incubator, and the incubator temperature should be maintained when the baby is removed. In the operating room, the temperature of the infant must be continuously recorded by placing a thermistor in the rectum or esophagus. Conservation of body heat may be accomplished by wrapping the extremities with sheet wadding and by using a circulating heating pad and an infrared lamp, but these measures are not sufficient in small infants. The operating room should be prewarmed and the temperature kept at about 20–27 C (68–80.6 F). Wet sponges and drapes exaggerate evaporative heat losses. Plastic drapes against the skin help contain body heat and keep the skin dry. When large volumes of blood are required, the blood should be warmed by circulating it through tubing immersed in warm water (37 C [98.6 F]) or prewarmed in the container before being transfused.

Adamsons K: The role of thermal factors in fetal and neonatal life. P Clin North America 13:599–619, 1966.

Roe CF, Santulli TV, Blair CS: Heat loss in infants during general anesthesia and operations. J Pediat Surg 1:266–274, 1966.

Cardiorespiratory Control

A. Postoperative Position: Although the pain threshold of a young infant is quite high, the protective response to pain is to remain immobilized. The young infant breathes primarily with his diaphragm, and his respiratory excursion becomes limited following the pain of an operative incision in the chest or abdomen. Therefore, it is important to rotate the young infant from side to side at least every hour to prevent atelectasis. It is usually necessary to restrain the arms to prevent dislodgement of the nasogastric and intravenous tubes. When the arms are restrained, it must be done with the baby on his side and the 2 arms together—the arms must never be restrained on the opposite sides of the crib because the baby might aspirate vomitus.

B. Cardiorespiratory Resuscitation: Newborn infants with surgically treatable diseases frequently are asphyxiated during birth. Causes of asphyxia include antepartal hemorrhage, prolonged labor, respiratory insufficiency due to aspiration pneumonitis, and congenital diaphragmatic hernia. The resulting hypoxia, hypercapnia, and acidosis produce generalized vasoconstriction. In particular, increased pulmonary vascular resistance occurs when the P_{O_2} falls below 50 mm Hg and the pH is less than 7.3. Normally, a right-to-left shunt of 20% of the cardiac output is present in newborn infants. During asphyxia, this shunt will be increased, and the existing hypoxia and acidosis may become exaggerated. Cyanosis is an inadequate sign of hypoxia in the newborn because fetal hemoglobin will be 85% saturated at P_{O_2} levels of 42 mm Hg, whereas in the adult, hemoglobin is 85% saturated at P_{O_2} levels of 52 mm Hg. Therefore, in circumstances which produce asphyxia in the newborn, resuscitation should be established promptly before obvious clinical signs are present.

At birth, the pharynx should be aspirated of mucus, amniotic fluid, or meconium. Respirations should be assisted or controlled with bag and mask, and prolonged respiratory support may require endotracheal intubation. A small air leak between the endotracheal tube and the airway is necessary to minimize laryngeal trauma. The required tube diameter may be 2.5–5 mm. The trachea from the glottis to the carina in the newborn is 5–7.5 cm long, and placement of the tube into the right or left bronchus must be avoided. An oral-tracheal tube is preferred to a nasotracheal tube in order to minimize trauma and subsequent infection in the nasal passages. The ventilatory pressure must be carefully monitored to prevent rupture of the lung.

Infants who have had asphyxia but who are ventilating well without assistance should be placed in an incubator with a humidified oxygen atmosphere. In the absence of abnormal diffusion or shunting, an inspired oxygen concentration of 40% will result in an arterial P_{O_2} of 110–116 mm Hg. The inspired oxygen concentration must be frequently monitored with an oxygen analyzer. Prolonged hyperoxia (arterial P_{O_2} of 160 mm Hg) may cause retrolental fibroplasia in premature infants and pulmonary oxygen toxicity. When an infant has pulmonary insufficiency and requires greater oxygen concentrations, with or without assisted ventilation, it is essential to repeatedly measure the arterial P_{O_2} and regulate the inspired oxygen concentration to keep the blood P_{O_2} between 60 and 80 mm Hg.

The frequent monitoring of these infants is most easily accomplished by inserting a polyvinyl catheter into the umbilical artery and threading it 10 cm into the distal aorta. Blood pressure may be recorded by connecting the catheter to a strain gauge and recorder. A blood pH of < 7.3 should be corrected with sodium bicarbonate or tromethamine with electrolytes (THAM-E). Sodium bicarbonate (44.4 mEq in 50 ml) may be given intravenously in amounts of 3–8 ml at a rate of 1 ml/kg/minute. After an equilibration period of 5–10 minutes, the pH and base deficit measurements should be repeated and the requisite amount of additional sodium bicarbonate or tromethamine calculated (see below). When asphyxia has been present for prolonged periods, the resulting vasoconstriction may produce a decreased blood volume. Correction of hypoxia and acidosis, however, can sometimes result in vasodilatation and hypovolemic shock. The blood volume will have to be replenished by transfusing 5% albumin solution or whole blood. The requirements for assisted respiration, high oxygen concentration, buffering, and volume replacement can be determined only by repeated evaluation of the patient, the blood pressure, and the P_{O_2}, P_{CO_2} and pH status of the blood.

C. Assisted Ventilation: Following certain operations—particularly after thoracotomy or tight abdominal wall closure—lung volume is diminished and diaphragmatic motion is greatly impaired. Assisted ventilation may be required for 24 hours or more. This is best accomplished by firmly fixing an endotracheal tube in place and connecting it to a Norman elbow and Sommers T-piece with attached "elephant" tubing and a 500 ml reservoir bag (Fig 49–2). The gas mixture flowing into the Norman elbow should be carefully controlled by an air and oxygen mixing device, and the oxygen concentration should be regulated according to analysis of blood oxygen tensions. The gas should be humidified by using a heated or ultrasonic nebulizer. Water absorption in the lung may be very great, and parenteral fluid may have to be restricted. The side-arm of the Sommers T-piece is connected to an aneroid manometer, and the end of the tubing is immersed in a graduate tube filled with water 25–30 cm in depth. This serves as a pop-off valve should excessive airway pressure develop. Manual positive pressure should be applied to the bag hourly to open up areas of atelectatic lung.

When alveolar collapse tends to develop, such as in hyaline membrane disease or with persistent atelectasis, the terminal airways can be kept open by continuous positive airway pressure breathing. This is accomplished by closing the reservoir bag with a screw clamp on the tailpiece and by observing the end-expiratory pressure on the aneroid manometer. End-expiratory pressures as high as 12 mm Hg may be required initially. The infant can be allowed to breathe on his own effort with this system. During continuous positive pressure breathing, an inspired oxygen mixture is

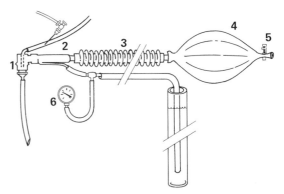

FIG 49–2. System for continuous positive pressure breathing. The system consists of endotracheal tube with a Norman elbow (1) and Sommers T-piece (2). The inhaled gases are conveyed to the airway via the Norman elbow. Elephant tubing (3) and a 500 ml reservoir bag (4) provide a means of applying positive pressure. The screw clamp on the tailpiece (5) regulates the amount of continuous positive pressure in the airway. The side-arm of the Sommers T-piece is connected to an aneroid manometer (6) to monitor the airway pressure. One end of this side-arm is placed in a column of water at the desired depth (usually 30 cm) for a pop-off if the intratracheal pressure exceeds the desired level. (Redrawn and reproduced, with permission, from Gregory GA & others: New England J Med 284:1333–1340, 1971.)

selected which will maintain a blood oxygen tension of 50–70 mm Hg. When the P_{aO_2} exceeds 70 mm Hg, the inspired oxygen concentration is gradually lowered 5–10% at a time. When a 40% oxygen mixture is reached, the continuous positive airway pressure is lowered in 1 mm Hg decrements, while keeping the P_{aO_2} above 50 mm Hg. When the end-expired airway pressure is atmospheric, the endotracheal tube is removed. At this time the inspired oxygen concentration should be increased to 10% greater than during the period of positive pressure. The inspired oxygen concentration may then be lowered toward that of room air, as indicated by the blood gas changes.

Chest percussion, endotracheal suctioning by careful sterile technic, and rocking from side to side are necessary while the endotracheal tube is in place.

The continuous positive pressure does not impair venous return, and its primary effect is to keep open airways that tend to collapse at atmospheric pressure. This is very important in the care of infants who are not ventilating adequately.

Gluck L (editor): Symposium on respiratory disorders of the newborn. P Clin North America 20:273–505, 1973.

Gregory GA & others: Treatment of the idiopathic respiratory-distress syndrome with continuous positive airway pressure. New England J Med 284:1333–1340, 1971.

Stern L: The use and misuse of oxygen in the newborn infant. P Clin North America 20:447–464, 1973.

Tunstall ME: Neonatal resuscitation. Brit J Anaesth 36:591–599, 1964.

Blood Loss & Replacement

A. Determination of Blood Loss: Defects in the coagulating mechanism may occur in newborn infants as a result of vitamin K deficiency, thrombocytopenia, and temporary hepatic insufficiency due to immaturity, asphyxia, or infection. Prior to operation, newborn infants should receive phytonadione (vitamin K_1; AquaMephyton, Konakion), 1–2 mg IV or IM. If an extensive surgical procedure is anticipated, freshly drawn blood should be typed and cross-matched.

The blood volume of a newborn infant ranges from 50–100 ml/kg body weight (average, 85 ml/kg). This wide variation is due principally to the timing and technic of clamping the umbilical cord. By 1 month of age, the blood volume in premature and full-term infants is approximately 75 ml/kg.

The blood lost during operation varies greatly according to the extent of the operative procedure, the disease being treated, and the effectiveness of hemostasis. Mild blood loss, amounting to less than 10% of the blood volume, usually does not require transfusion. In a 3.5 kg infant, mild blood loss would be a volume up to 30 ml. Since blood loss greater than 10% should be corrected—and since these volumes are quite small—it is imperative to develop methods for closely monitoring the amount of blood lost during operation. Dry sponges should be used and weighed shortly after use to minimize error from evaporation. The suction line, connected to a calibrated trap on the operating table, should be short to diminish the dead space of the tubing and to provide immediate quantitation of accumulated blood loss. Visual observation of blood loss may be used as a rough guide but tends to be underestimated.

B. Replacement of Blood Loss: Whenever an operation results in a blood loss greater than 10% of blood volume, a cutdown should be performed. Procedures associated with blood loss > 20% of blood volume should be preceded by a jugular vein cutdown with the catheter tip directed into the right atrium. This catheter should be connected to a manometer for measuring central venous pressure and a 3-way stopcock for taking samples for blood gas and pH measurements.

In infants with hematocrits greater than 50%, blood loss may be replaced by transfusion with 5% albumin solution to compensate for losses of up to 25% of total blood volume. Greater blood losses should be replaced with freshly drawn whole blood. Transfusion of old blood may result in cardiac arrest and death as a result of hyperkalemia, hypocalcemia, acidosis, hypothermia, and air embolism. The transfused blood should be prewarmed to body temperature by running it through coiled tubing immersed in water at 37 C (98.6 F). ACD (acid-citrate-dextrose) blood that is older than 3 days may have a pH of less than 6.1, a P_{CO_2} greater than 80 mm Hg, a base deficit greater than 15, a potassium content greater than 10 mEq/liter, citrate which binds serum magnesium and calcium, and deficient clotting factors and platelets. The acidosis that results from the transfusion of ACD blood may be partially corrected by adding 30 ml of 0.3 M tromethamine, but the pH should be checked to prevent overcorrection and alkalosis. Citrate-phosphate-dextrose (CPD) is a better blood preservative because it maintains the carrying capacity and release of oxygen for a longer period than ACD preservative. After transfusion, subsequent metabolism of the citrate to bicarbonate may produce a metabolic alkalosis. Heparinized blood diminishes the metabolic complications of ACD blood, but protamine sulfate may be required to correct a prolonged clotting time. Hypocalcemia, produced by complexing calcium with citrate, may be treated by giving 2 ml of 10% calcium gluconate for each 100 ml of ACD blood transfused.

Oski FA, Naiman JL: *Hematologic Problems in the Newborn.* Saunders, 1966.

Humidity

A high environmental humidity may be desired for liquefaction of viscid pulmonary secretions or for treatment of croup. An ultrasonically generated mist is the only effective means of getting water droplets as far as the larynx or upper trachea. The mist should be delivered through a face mask, hood, or incubator. Infants can absorb a significant volume of ultrasonic mist water, and they may develop pulmonary edema if not carefully monitored.

Infants with an endotracheal tube or a tracheostomy must be given humidified gases to breathe. Ultrasonic humidification should not be used, in these cases, because of excessive water absorption. These babies should have the mist generated by a heated nebulizer.

Overgrowth of bacteria, such as pseudomonas, will occur in the mist generator and incubator within a short time. Therefore, the incubator and generator will have to be changed and cleaned at least every 2 days. The fluid requirements of these babies are greatly decreased when high humidification is used. Body temperature may be elevated as a result of heat retention in an environment with high humidity.

FLUID & ELECTROLYTE CONTROL

Fluid & Electrolyte Management; Caloric Intake

Fluid and electrolyte therapy requires a knowledge of normal basic requirements, preexisting deficits, and continuing losses. This subject is covered in Chapter 12. Special considerations of pediatric interest are as follows.

A. Newborn Requirements: Fluid administration in the first 3 days of life is usually restricted. Normally, a newborn infant loses 5–10% of his birth weight in the first 3 days. Part of the weight lost is meconium, vernix, and urine; however, the major component is excess total body water. During the first 4 days on oral feedings, a normal newborn infant will have a urine volume of 20–30 ml/kg/day and an insensible water loss of 20–25 ml/kg/day. The total urinary excretion of sodium, potassium, and chloride is less than 0.9 mEq/kg. Oliguria and shift in the potassium/nitrogen ratio due to increased aldosterone secretion do not occur following stress in the first few weeks of life. A sodium-excreting factor following stress has been postulated since urinary sodium and chloride retention do not occur when there are large extrarenal losses of these ions. The usual amount of water given during the first 4 days after birth is 80 ml/kg/day. The maximum tolerance for sodium and chloride is 1.5 mEq/kg/day; for potassium, 1 mEq/kg/day. Therefore, the postoperative maintenance fluid in the first 4 days after birth should consist of dextrose, 10%, in 0.2% saline, given at a rate of 50–80 ml/kg/day. Potassium chloride or bicarbonate, 15 mEq/liter, and calcium gluconate, 150 mg/kg/day, are usually added to the solution. Additional potassium, calcium, bicarbonate, and glucose may be added according to the blood chemistry analysis and the clinical status of the patient.

Many stressed newborn infants develop low blood levels of potassium, calcium, magnesium, and glucose. A deficiency of any one of the substances will produce such signs as vomiting, abdominal distention, poor feeding, apneic spells, cyanosis, limpness, eye rolling, high-pitched cry, tremors, or convulsions. Convulsions and tetany due to hypocalcemia should be treated with intravenous 10% calcium solution (chloride, lactate, or gluconate) given at a rate of 1 ml/minute while carefully monitoring the heart sounds. Hypocalcemia can be largely eliminated by routinely adding calcium salts to intravenous solutions. Subcutaneous infiltration of calcium solutions may produce severe vasoconstriction and skin necrosis.

Hypoglycemia frequently occurs in infants with low birth weight for gestational age, respiratory distress, asphyxia, or CNS abnormalities. Hypoglycemia is defined as a blood glucose less than 20 mg/100 ml in the premature or low birth weight infant; less than 30 mg/100 ml in full-sized infants within the first 72 hours after birth; and less than 40 mg/100 ml thereafter in full-term infants. The treatment of hypoglycemia consists of giving 50% glucose, 1–2 ml/kg IV, followed by a continuous infusion of 10–15% glucose solutions at a rate equivalent to that needed for maintenance water requirements.

B. Fluid & Electrolyte Requirements for Older Infants and Children: Three methods are available for determining the physiologic limits for water, based upon (1) total body weight, (2) body surface area, and (3) calculated basal caloric expenditure related to body weight.

The **average** water requirements are as follows: 130 ml/kg up to 10 kg; 110 ml/kg up to 20 kg; 100 ml/kg to 30 kg; 90 ml/kg up to 40 kg; and 80 ml/kg above 40 kg. The physiologic limits are 35 ml/kg above or below the mean daily requirement (Fig 49–3).

The surface area can be determined from nomograms by knowing the height and weight of the patient or the weight alone (see p 1084). The physiologic range of fluid tolerance is 1200–3500 mg/sq m/day (Fig 49–3). With this method, 1500 mg/sq m should be considered the usual minimum water requirement.

In the caloric system, the **minimum** water requirement is 100 ml/100 Cal expended. The basic caloric requirements related to weight are as follows: up to 10 kg, 100 Cal/kg; 10–20 kg, 1000 Cal for the first 10 kg plus 50 Cal for each kg above 10; over 20 kg, 1500 Cal for the first 20 kg plus 20 Cal/kg over 20 kg. Additional water should be given according to the state of hydration, body temperature, and estimated caloric expenditure above basal activity.

The normal daily sodium requirement is usually 30–35 mEq/sq m (1–2.5 mEq/kg), but it may vary from 10–250 mEq/sq m in extreme cases. The usual range of potassium required is the same as that of sodium. The large reserve of calcium and magnesium in the skeleton makes short-term intravenous replacement unnecessary, especially for older children.

Continuing losses such as gastric juice, ileostomy output, pleural fluid, and "third space" fluid must be replaced as rapidly as they occur, preferably within 4–8 hours. Gastric juices should be replaced by 5% dextrose in 0.45% saline plus KCl, 20 mEq/liter. Small bowel, bile, or pancreatic losses may be replaced with lactated Ringer's injection to which potassium chloride, 10 mEq/liter, has been added. During operative procedures, "third space" losses in the injured serosal surfaces, bowel wall, and lumen should be replaced by giving lactated Ringer's injection, 5–15 ml/kg/hour; the amount to be given depends upon the magnitude of the operative procedure. Eight to 24 hours postoperatively, 5% dextrose in Ringer's lactate is continued at a rate calculated for greater than average maintenance.

The status of hydration, intake and output, and weight of infants and small children should be assessed at frequent intervals. The orders for intravenous fluids should be rewritten at least every 8 hours.

By knowing the ranges of tolerance for fluid and electrolytes, polyionic solutions can be made using concentrated electrolyte solutions. The volume of a repair solution is usually given at a rate close to maximal tolerance, and, therefore, the glucose content should be 5% to prevent osmotic diuresis. Maintenance solutions can be made with 10% glucose.

Existing deficits may occur from external losses, such as hemorrhage, vomiting, diarrhea, or starvation, or from internal "third space" losses such as in the bowel lumen, peritoneal space, or burned tissues.

Patients with dehydration or shock will require rapid volume expansion. A catheter should be placed in the right atrium via the jugular or subclavian vein. The central venous pressure, blood pH, and blood gases may be constantly monitored from this catheter. Rapid volume replacement may be accomplished by

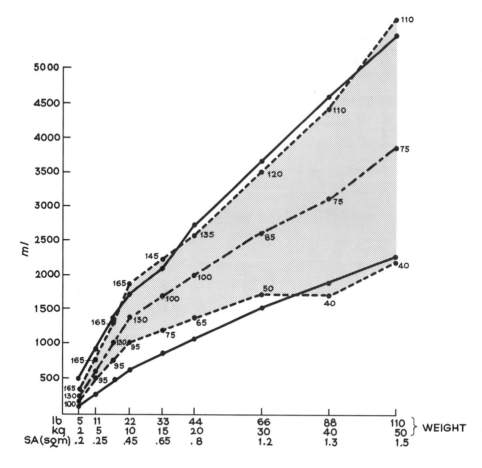

FIG 49–3. Comparison of 2 methods of calculating intravenous fluid requirements. Solid lines show the maximum (3000 ml/sq m) and minimum (1200 ml/sq m) fluid requirements by surface area. The broken lines show the mean (ml/kg) and the range (±35 ml/kg) from the mean total fluid requirements. The surface area system underestimates the requirements in infants weighing less than 10 kg, probably because of errors in the nomograms.

using normal saline, lactated Ringer's injection, or 5% albumin solution in amounts of 10–20 ml/kg given as rapidly as possible but not exceeding a right atrial pressure of 15 cm water. If anemia exists, whole blood is substituted for these solutions as soon as the type and cross-match are done. Following this initial expansion of the blood volume, rehydration is continued with 5% dextrose in lactated Ringer's injection at the maximum physiologically tolerated rate until a rise in central venous pressure occurs or urine flow has been established. A repair solution is then continued at close to physiologic maximal rates until the existing deficits have been restored. This is determined by clinical examination of the status of central venous pressure, hydration, pulse, urine output and specific gravity or osmolarity, hemoglobin, hematocrit, electrolyte changes, and, when possible, measurement of right atrial pressure.

Replacements of sodium deficits may also be calculated as follows:

$$\frac{\text{mEq sodium}}{\text{needed}} = \frac{(140-\text{patient's serum}}{\text{sodium in mEq})} \times \frac{(60\% \text{ body}}{\text{weight in kg})}$$

If dehydration is also present, sodium should be replaced by using normal saline. Hyponatremia associated with abnormal retention of water should be treated by restriction of water intake.

Significant acidosis (serum HCO_3^- less than 15 mEq/liter or base deficit greater than 8) should be corrected with sodium bicarbonate. When the base deficit is determined from the Siggaard-Andersen nomogram, the replacement requirement is calculated by multiplying the base deficit (mEq/liter) by the estimated extracellular volume (30% total body weight in kg). The result is the required number of mEq of $NaHCO_3$ that must be given intravenously. If the magnitude of acidosis is known only by the serum bicarbonate level, a rule of thumb for $NaHCO_3$ (in a concentration of 44.5 mEq/50 ml) replacement is 4 ml/kg, to raise the serum HCO_3^- by 5 mEq/liter.

For patients with severe acidosis and excessive

total body sodium (eg, congestive heart failure), tromethamine with electrolytes (THAM-E) may be preferred to $NaHCO_3$ as a buffer. A 0.3 M solution is isotonic, and the amount of 0.3 M tromethamine to be given (in ml) = (body weight in kg) X (base deficit in mEq/liter). When the fluid volume must also be restricted, tromethamine can be made up as an 0.6 or 0.9 M solution. Tromethamine is usually given over a 1-hour period. It diffuses freely both intracellularly and extracellularly, is rapidly excreted in the urine (50—70% in the first 24-hour period), and produces an osmotic and potassium diuresis. The hazards of tromethamine include hypercalcemia, hypoglycemia, hypoventilation, local irritation, and vasospasm.

When oliguria occurs, a frequent concern is whether it is due to dehydration and hypovolemia or acute renal shutdown. An effective method of establishing diuresis when oliguria is due to prerenal causes is to give 25% mannitol, 3.5 ml/kg IV, in 20—30 minutes, or furosemide, 0.5—1 mg/kg IV.

Comblath M, Schwartz R: *Disorders of Carbohydrate Metabolism in Infancy,* Saunders, 1966.

Holliday MA: Fluid and electrolyte disturbances in pediatrics. Chap 13 in: *Clinical Disorders of Fluid and Electrolyte Metabolism.* Maxwell MH, Kleeman CR (editors). McGraw-Hill, 1962.

Mizrahi A, London R, Gribetz D: Neonatal hypocalcemia: Its causes and treatment. New England J Med 278:1163—1165, 1968.

Moore FD: Tris buffer, mannitol and low viscous dextran. S Clin North America 43:577—596, 1963.

Suzuki H & others: Water and electrolyte metabolism of newborn infants after surgical operations. Tohoku J Exp Med 94:187—202, 1968.

Talbot NB, Richie RH, Crawford JD: *Metabolic Homeostasis.* Harvard Univ Press, 1969.

Parenteral Alimentation (See also Chapter 13.)

The indications for parenteral alimentation include the following: (1) expected period of prolonged ileus, eg, following repair of gastroschisis or jejunal atresia; (2) intestinal fistulas; (3) supplementation of oral feedings, as in intractable diarrhea, short bowel syndrome, or various malabsorption syndromes; (4) intrauterine growth retarded infants; and (5) catabolic wasting states such as infections or tumors when gastric feedings are inadequate. Total parenteral alimentation was usually limited in the past because the concentrated solutions and polyethylene catheters produced thrombophlebitis. Nonreactive polyvinyl or Silastic catheters can now be placed into the right atrium via the jugular or subclavian veins, avoiding this complication. When this technic is used, a constant infusion pump should be employed to regulate a steady rate of infusion and to prevent blood from backing into the catheter during straining or crying. If a fibrin clot develops in the tube lining, bacterial growth is enhanced and sepsis will occur. A bacterial filter between the infusion pump and the atrial catheter may help protect against sepsis. Careful placement of the catheter under ideal sterile conditions is best accomplished with general anesthesia in an operating room.

A solution for parenteral alimentation may be prepared with protein hydrolysate or crystalline amino acids, dextrose, balanced electrolytes, vitamins, iron, and trace metals. With the exception of the crystalline amino acid solutions, approximately half of the nitrogen content is in the form of polypeptides which are not utilizable and are excreted in the urine. Each of the available solutions has a different electrolyte content. The relatively high titratable acidity and ammonia level must be appreciated in anticipation of complications (Table 49—1).

The concentration of the various electrolytes can be altered according to the individual patient, recognizing the electrolyte content of the basic amino acid solutions. A standard solution which is suitable for infants and young children must contain a sufficient amount of calcium, magnesium, and phosphate to allow for bone growth.

Trace metals are also added to the basic solution, and this solution is infused in volumes calculated to be slightly above the usual maintenance water requirements for a 24-hour period at a constant rate with an infusion pump. If it is necessary to restrict the volume of infusion, more concentrated glucose solutions of 25% and 30% can be made by using anhydrous dextrose.

Complications of prolonged intravenous alimentation are numerous. The most frequent problem is sepsis, particularly due to candida, and immediate discontinuation of the catheter usually results in prompt clinical improvement. Accidental dislodgment

TABLE 49—1. Composition of parenteral amino acid solutions.

	Hyprotogen 10%	Amigen 5%	Aminosol 5%	FreAmine 8.5%
Sodium	50 mEq/liter	25 mEq/liter	10 mEq/liter	10 mEq/liter
Potassium	36 mEq/liter	20 mEq/liter	17 mEq/liter	. . .
Calcium	10 mEq/liter	5 mEq/liter	2 mEq/liter	. . .
Magnesium	40 mEq/liter	20 mEq/liter	2 mEq/liter	. . .
Chloride	36 mEq/liter	18 mEq/liter	10 mEq/liter	45 mEq/liter
Phosphate	50 mEq/liter	25 mEq/liter	. . .	. . .
Ammonia	10^3-30^3 μg/100 ml	10^3-30^3 μg/100 ml	10^3-30^3 μg/100 ml	10^2-10^3
Titratable acidity	. . .	26 mEq/liter	. . .	. . .

of the catheter is a frequent problem which can be prevented by careful fixation by use of skin sutures and taping. Thrombosis of the superior vena cava and right atrium is usually controlled by adding 1 unit of heparin per ml of solution. Emphasis on a constant rate of infusion will minimize hyper- or hypoglycemia. Small newborn infants usually do not tolerate concentrations greater than 10% glucose during the first week of life, but the glucose concentrations can be increased beyond the first week. Repeated blood chemistries must be performed to anticipate electrolyte imbalances and metabolic acidosis due to the high titratable acidity of the solution, and these patients should be observed for ammonia intoxication and for vitamin or trace mineral deficiency. Until intravenous fat solutions become available in the USA, these solutions are deficient in linoleic acid, an essential fatty acid. Deficiency in linoleic acid is characterized by thrombocytopenia, thin, scaly, flushed skin, and a peculiarly firm subcutaneous fat. The latter can be corrected with intravenous Intralipid or with orally administered fats such as Lipomul. Hepatitis with hepatic necrosis of uncertain origin occurs after prolonged alimentation and is characterized by a progressive hepatomegaly and jaundice. This syndrome subsides with cessation of the intravenous alimentation solution. Severely starved patients may develop a syndrome characterized by progressive coma with or without convulsions, hypophosphatemia, and death. This is probably a consequence of using solutions which contain a phosphate.

Cowan GSM Jr, Scheetz WL (editors): *Intravenous Hyperalimentation.* Lea & Febiger, 1972.

Shaw JCL: Parenteral nutrition in the management of sick low birthweight infants. P Clin North America 20:333–358, 1973.

Shils ME: Guidelines for total parenteral nutrition. (AMA Council on Foods and Nutrition.) JAMA 220:1721–1729, 1972.

Van Way CW: Parenteral alimentation in surgery. Ann Surg 117:103–111, 1973.

LESIONS OF THE HEAD & NECK

DERMOID CYSTS

Dermoid cysts are congenital inclusions of skin and appendages which are commonly found on the scalp and eyebrows and in the midline of the nose, neck, and upper chest. They present as painless swellings which may be completely mobile or fixed to the skin and deeper structures. Dermoid cysts of the eyebrows and scalp may produce a depression in the underlying bone which will appear as a smooth, punched-out defect on radiographs of the skull. These cysts contain a cheesy material which is produced by

desquamation of the cells of the epithelial lining. Dermoid cysts of the neck may be confused with thyroglossal duct cysts, but they usually do not move with swallowing or protrusion of the tongue as thyroglossal cysts do. Dermoid cysts may produce cosmetic deformities and tend to become infected. Those of the nose may extend into the nasal passages and the cribriform plate of the skull. These cysts should be excised intact, since incomplete removal will result in recurrence. Those arising on the eyebrows should be excised through an incision within the hairline. The eyebrows should not be shaved.

BRANCHIOGENIC ANOMALIES

Branchiogenic anomalies include sinuses, cysts, cartilaginous rests, cervical fistulas (Fig 49–4), and cervical cysts. These lesions are probably remnants of the branchial apparatus present during the first month of fetal life. The primitive neck develops 4 external clefts and 4 pharyngeal pouches which are separated by a membrane. Between the clefts and pouches are branchial arches.

Preauricular sinuses, cysts, and cartilaginous rests probably arise from anomalous development of the auricle. Fistulas which arise above the hyoid bone and communicate with the external auditory canal represent persistence of the first branchial cleft. Fistulas which communicate between the anterior border of the sternocleidomastoid muscle and the tonsillar fossa are of second branchial origin, and those that extend into the piriform sinus are derived from the third bran-

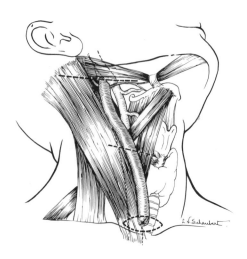

FIG 49–4. Branchiogenic fistula from second branchial cleft origin. The fistula extends along the anterior border of the sternocleidomastoid muscle and courses between the internal and external carotid arteries and cephalad to the hypoglossal nerve to enter the tonsillar fossa.

chial pouch. Fourth branchial fistulas have not been described.

A tract of branchial origin may form a complete fistula, or one end may be obliterated to form an external or internal sinus, or both ends may resorb, leaving an aggregate of cells forming a cyst. First branchial cleft tracts are always lined by squamous epithelium based on thick connective tissue. Cysts and sinuses of second or third branchial origin are lined by squamous, cuboidal, or ciliated columnar epithelium. Cervical fistulas and cysts have a prominent lymphoid stroma beneath the epithelial lining which may contain germinal centers and Hassall's corpuscles.

Clinical Findings

In the preauricular area, the anomalies may take the form of cysts, sinuses, skin tabs, or cartilaginous nubbins. A sinus or fistulous opening along the anterior border of the sternocleidomastoid muscle is readily seen at birth and usually discharges a mucoid or purulent material. The patient may complain of a foultasting discharge in the mouth upon massaging the tract, but the internal orifice is rarely recognized. Lateral cervical cysts, without an external sinus, are usually not recognized in childhood but become evident in young adulthood. The cysts are characteristically found anterior and deep to the upper third of the sternocleidomastoid muscle, or they may be located within the parotid gland, pharyngeal wall, over the manubrium, or in the mediastinum. Branchiogenic anomalies occur with equal frequency on each side of the neck, and 10% are bilateral.

Differential Diagnosis

Granulomatous lymphadenitis due to mycobacterial infections may produce cystic lymph nodes and draining sinuses, but these are usually distinguishable by the chronic inflammatory reaction which preceded the purulent discharge. Hemangiomas, cystic hygromas, and lymphangiomas are soft, spongy tumor masses which might be confused with cervical cysts, but the latter have a firmer consistency. Cystic hygromas and lymphangiomas transilluminate, and cervical cysts do not. Carotid body tumors are quite firm, are located at the carotid bifurcation, and occur in older patients. Lymphomas produce firm masses in the area where branchial remnants occur, but multiple, matted nodes rather than a solitary cystic tumor distinguish these lesions. Mucoid material may be expressed from the openings of branchial sinuses or fistulas, and a firm cord-like tract may be palpable along its course.

Complications

The sinuses and cysts are prone to become repeatedly infected, producing cellulitis and abscesses. Very rarely, carcinoma may occur.

Treatment & Prognosis

Superficial skin tabs and cartilaginous rests can be easily excised under sedation and local anesthesia.

Preauricular sinus tracts may be very deceptive in their extent, and the surgeon should be prepared for an extensive dissection under general anesthesia to completely excise these lesions. General anesthesia is required for proper excision of branchial fistulas and cysts. Cervical cysts are excised through transverse incisions directly over the mass.

Infected sinuses and cysts will require initial incision and drainage. Excision of these tracts should be attempted only after the acute inflammatory reaction has subsided.

Albert GD: Branchial anomalies. JAMA 183:399–409, 1963.

Henzel JH, Pories WJ, DeWeese MS: Etiology of lateral cervical cysts. Surg Gynec Obst 125:1–8, 1967.

THYROGLOSSAL DUCT REMNANTS

The thyroid gland develops from an evagination in the floor of the primitive pharynx, between the first pair of pharyngeal pouches, during the fourth week of gestation. If the anlage of the thyroid does not descend normally, the thyroid gland may form in the tongue or remain as a mass anywhere in the midline of the neck from the submandibular fossa to the pretracheal area. If the thyroglossal duct persists, the tract forms a cyst which usually communicates with the foramen cecum of the tongue. The thyroglossal duct descends through the second branchial arch anlage, the hyoid bone, prior to its fusion in the midline. Because of this, the tract of a persistent thyroglossal duct usually extends through the hyoid bone (Fig 49–5).

Thyroid follicles may be found in 30–40% of the specimens. Three or more tracts between the thyroglossal cyst and the base of the tongue are present in more than 75% of cases.

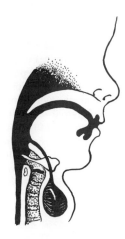

FIG 49–5. Thyroglossal cyst and duct courses through the hyoid bone to the foramen cecum of the tongue.

Clinical Findings

The most common finding is a rounded, cystic mass of varying size in the midline of the neck just below the hyoid bone. When infected, the acute inflammatory reaction may herald the presence of a cyst. The fluid content of the cyst is usually under pressure and may give the impression of a solid tumor. Cysts and aberrant midline thyroid glands move with swallowing and with protrusion of the tongue. When a solid midline mass is detected, evidence of athyreosis should be sought such as hypothyroidism and absence of the palpable lateral lobes of the normal thyroid.

Differential Diagnosis

Only lymph nodes, dermoid cysts, and enlarged Delphian nodes containing metastases are confused with thyroglossal remnants in the midline of the neck. Dermoid cysts do not move with swallowing. Lingual thyroids may be confused with hypertrophied lingual tonsil or with a dermoid cyst, fibroma, angioma, sarcoma, or carcinoma of the tongue. These lesions and thyroglossal cysts may be distinguished from aberrantly located thyroid glands by needle aspiration or by radioiodine scintiscan.

Complications

Lingual thyroid glands may produce dysphagia, dysphonia, dyspnea, hemorrhage, or pain. Carcinoma develops more frequently in ectopic thyroid tissue than in normal thyroid glands. Thyroglossal cysts are prone to become infected, and spontaneous drainage or incision and drainage of an abscess will result in a chronically draining fistula. Excision of an ectopic thyroid usually removes all remaining thyroid tissue, producing subsequent hypothyroidism.

Treatment

Acute infection in thyroglossal tracts should be treated with local heat and antibiotics. Abscesses should be incised and drained. After complete subsidence of the inflammatory reaction, thyroglossal cysts and ducts should be excised.

Ectopic thyroid glands are usually associated with athyreosis of the 2 lobes. These remnants of thyroid may produce sufficient hormones until early childhood and adolescence, at which time hypothyroidism develops. Because of increased stimulation by thyrotropic hormone, the aberrant thyroid tissue enlarges. The residual hypertrophic thyroid remnants usually recede in response to administration of thyroid hormone, and in many instances surgical excision is not necessary. If an ectopic thyroid is excised and is the only remnant of thyroid gland, allotransplantation of the duct gland into the rectus or sternocleidomastoid muscle may be successful.

Brown PM, Judd ES: Thyroglossal duct cysts and sinuses: Results of radical (Sistrunk) operation. Am J Surg 102:494–501, 1961.

Choy FJ, Ward RK, Richardson R: Carcinoma of the thyroglossal duct. Am J Surg 108:361–369, 1964.

MUSCULAR TORTICOLLIS

Infants with congenital muscular torticollis may initially develop a nontender, hard, fusiform swelling diffusely involving the sternocleidomastoid muscle. The muscle tumor may be present at birth but is usually not noticed until the second to sixth weeks of life. The tumor appears with equal frequency in both sexes and on each side of the neck. Rarely, there is more than one tumor in the muscle or both sternocleidomastoid muscles are involved. The tumor resolves in 6–7 months, and in about half of cases the sternocleidomastoid muscle becomes fibrotic. A history of breech delivery is present in 20–30% of these children. Older children (2–15 years of age) may develop sternocleidomastoid fibrosis and torticollis without an initial history of tumor formation.

Clinical Findings

The sternocleidomastoid tumor or fibrosis may be present with or without torticollis. When torticollis occurs, the sternocleidomastoid muscle is shortened, the mastoid process on the involved side is pulled down toward the clavicle and sternum, and the head is tilted and directed toward the opposite shoulder. The shoulder on the affected side is raised, and there may be cervical and thoracic scoliosis. The fusiform mass may be palpable in the affected sternocleidomastoid muscle, or the muscle may feel like a tight, hard band. Passive rotation of the head to the ipsilateral side of the involved muscle will be resisted and limited to varying degree, and the muscle will appear as a protuberant band. Because of persistent pressure when the patient is recumbent, the ipsilateral face and contralateral occiput will be flattened or hypoplastic.

Complications

If the torticollis is corrected late in the course, the adjacent neck structures may also become shortened and division of the sternocleidomastoid muscle will not be sufficient to correct the deformity.

Treatment & Prognosis

The infant with a sternocleidomastoid tumor or fibrosis should be treated by forcefully rotating in a full range of motion. This procedure should be performed at least 4 times a day even though it may be quite uncomfortable for the child. If the muscle continues to become progressively shortened, with facial and occipital skull deformity, both heads of the sternocleidomastoid muscle should be divided through a small transverse incision just above the clavicle. After the muscle is divided, the head should be turned to the ipsilateral side and any surrounding muscle or fascial contracture should also be divided. It is unnecessary to excise the tumor, which involves a risk of injuring the spinal accessory nerve. Only the platysma muscle and skin layers are closed. When postoperative pain has subsided, exercises to provide a full range of neck motion must be carried out. The use of a neck brace is rarely indicated.

If surgical division of the muscle is performed early, the cosmetic deformity is greatly improved or corrected within several months.

Jones PG: *Torticollis in Infancy and Childhood.* Thomas, 1968.

CERVICAL LYMPHADENOPATHY

1. PYOGENIC LYMPHADENITIS

Infections in the upper respiratory passages, scalp, ear, or neck produce varying degrees of secondary lymphadenitis. Most of the causative organisms are streptococci and staphylococci. In infants and young children, the clinical course of the suppurative lymphadenitis may greatly overshadow a seemingly insignificant or inapparent primary infection. Scalp or ear infections produce pre- or postauricular and suboccipital lymph node involvement; submental, oral, tonsillar, and pharyngeal infections affect the submandibular and deep jugular nodes.

Clinical Findings

With significant lymphadenitis, the regional lymph nodes become greatly enlarged and produce local pain and tenderness. Fever is high initially and then becomes intermittent and may persist for days or weeks. The regional nodes may remain enlarged and firm for prolonged periods, or they may suppurate and produce surrounding cellulitis and edema. Subsequently, the nodes may involute or a fluctuant abscess may form, resulting in redness and thinning of the overlying skin.

Differential Diagnosis

A smoldering lymphadenitis which neither resolves nor forms an abscess can be confused with granulomatous lymphadenitis, lymphoma, or metastatic tumor. After several weeks, there will usually be a reduction in the size and firmness of pyogenic adenitis. Excisional biopsy is occasionally required to differentiate these lesions. Suppurative lymphadenitis can be distinguished from granulomatous lymphadenitis by the signs of acute inflammation and a short history of fever, pain, and exquisite tenderness over the lymph nodes.

Complications

The complications are principally those of bacterial infection, including sepsis, abscess formation, and sensitivity reactions such as glomerulonephritis.

Treatment

In the acute phase, the patient should be treated with appropriate antibiotics. In the subacute or chronic phase, the presence of pus in the node may be confirmed by needle aspiration of the mass. When an abscess is present, a general anesthetic should be given and the abscess should be incised and drained. An incision is made in the skin and the tract is bluntly dissected to avoid transecting an adjacent nerve. The loculated areas should be broken down and a gauze wick placed to keep the tract open. Packing an abscess with gauze is necessary only for excessive hemorrhage; it should be removed within several days to allow free drainage of the pus and obliteration of the abscess cavity.

2. GRANULOMATOUS LYMPHADENITIS

Although typical tuberculous cervical adenitis is very rare in the USA, "atypical" or "anonymous" mycobacteria frequently cause chronic suppuration in the cervical, axillary, and inguinal lymph nodes.

Granulomatous lymphadenitis and caseation may occur in the regional nodes draining the inoculation site of BCG.

Cat-scratch disease causes a caseating lymphadenitis in regional lymph nodes.

Clinical Findings

Children under 6 years of age are most frequently affected. The initial manifestation is a painless, progressive enlargement of the lymph nodes in the deep cervical chain and the parotid, suboccipital, submandibular, and supraclavicular nodes. The duration of lymphadenopathy is usually 1–3 months or longer. The nodes may be large and mobile or, with progressive disease, may become matted, fixed, and finally caseate to form a cold abscess. Incision or spontaneous breakthrough of the skin will result in a chronically draining sinus. In tuberculosis, both sides of the neck or multiple groups of nodes are infected and the chest x-ray indicates pulmonary involvement. In atypical mycobacterial lymphadenitis, pulmonary disease is rare and the cervical adenitis is unilateral. The tuberculin skin test is weakly positive in over 80% of patients with atypical infection. Skin test antigens from the various strains of atypical mycobacteria are available.

Cat-scratch fever is usually acquired by a bite or scratch from a kitten. It is an acute illness characterized by fever, malaise, and occasionally a pustular lesion at the site of the scratch. Two to 4 weeks later, regional lymphadenitis produces painless, fixed suppurative nodes which may produce a chronically draining sinus.

Differential Diagnosis

The firm, rubbery, or fixed nodes resemble lymphoma or metastatic tumor (neuroblastoma or thyroid carcinoma) and may be distinguished only by excisional biopsy. A positive skin test helps differentiate granulomatous adenitis from malignant lymphadenopathy. A fluctuant node can be confused with branchial cleft or thyroglossal cysts.

Complications

Granulomatous lymphadenitis progresses to caseation and breakdown of the overlying skin in the great majority of affected children.

Treatment & Prognosis

Chemotherapeutic agents for pyogenic infections and tuberculosis may be effective, but they have been ineffective against atypical mycobacteria. Tetracyclines may shorten the course of cat-scratch disease and prevent suppuration.

The procedure of choice is surgical excision of involved nodes before caseation occurs. Once the nodes become fluctuant or a draining sinus forms, a wedge of involved skin should be excised and the underlying necrotic nodes should be curetted out, taking care not to injure the neighboring branches of the nerve. The wound edges and skin should be closed primarily. The value of continuing chemotherapy is influenced by sensitivity tests on the cultured material. Excision and primary closure usually result in excellent healing with good cosmetic results.

Carithers HA, Carithers CM, Edwards RO Jr: Cat-scratch disease: Its natural history. JAMA 207:312–316, 1969.

Salyer KE, Votteler TP, Dorman GW: Surgical management of cervical adenitis due to atypical mycobacteria in children. JAMA 204:1037–1040, 1968.

LYMPHOID TUMORS

Primary tumors of lymphatic origin in children and their incidence are as follows: lymphosarcoma, 50%; Hodgkin's disease, 40%; reticulum cell sarcoma, 8%; and giant follicular lymphoma, 2%. The lymphoma group of tumors accounts for 10% of childhood neoplasms. They are considered in this section because 70% of these tumors are first recognized by lymph node enlargement. Although there are cases with features that do not readily distinguish each of these types of lymphoma, most of the tumors conform to a fairly typical histologic pattern and clinical course.

The most common initial manifestation is asymptomatic unilateral enlargement of the cervical, inguinal, or axillary lymph nodes. Intra-abdominal, nasopharyngeal, skin, and bone sites of origin occur in one-third of cases. Systemic symptoms of malaise, fever, weight loss, sweating, pruritus, and local pain may occur initially. In most patients, these symptoms become evident within several months after the original asymptomatic tumor mass is treated.

The role of the surgeon in the management of patients with lymphoid tumors is largely to obtain suitable tissue specimens for the diagnosis and staging of tumors. Exploratory abdominal operations for diag-nostic purposes, treatment of complicating acute surgical emergencies, or even radical lymphadenectomy may be necessary.

Megavoltage radiation therapy may be extremely effective or even curative for certain lymphoid tumors, especially if the tumor is confined to a single node or one anatomic area. Chemotherapy with antineoplastic agents, with or without x-ray therapy, may be of value in widespread systemic disease.

X-ray therapy is "curative" for stages I, II, and perhaps III of Hodgkin's disease. Giant follicular lymphoma tends to remain localized and has a 30% cure rate. The 5-year cure rate for lymphosarcoma is 10%. The prognosis for reticulum cell sarcoma is even poorer.

Hoogstraten B & others: Combined chemotherapy in lymphosarcoma and reticulum cell sarcoma. Blood 33:370–378, 1969.

Jenkins RDT & others: Primary gastrointestinal tract lymphoma in childhood. Radiology 92:763–767, 1969.

Jones B, Klingberg WG: Lymphosarcoma in children. J Pediat 63:11–20, 1963.

Kaplan HS: Clinical evaluation and radiotherapeutic management of Hodgkin's disease and the malignant lymphomas. New England J Med 278:892–899, 1968.

Lukes RJ, Butler JJ, Hicks EB: Natural history of Hodgkin's disease as related to its pathologic picture. Cancer 19:317–344, 1966.

•   •   •

SURGICAL RESPIRATORY EMERGENCIES IN THE NEWBORN

Respiratory distress may be produced by airway obstruction, displacement of lung volume, or pulmonary parenchymal insufficiency.

Certain aspects of respiration peculiar to the infant must be appreciated. The newborn baby is an obligate nasal breather except when he is crying. The ability to breathe through the mouth may take weeks or months to learn. Inspiration is primarily accomplished by diaphragmatic excursion, and the intercostal and accessory muscles contribute little to ventilation. Impaired inspiration results in retraction of the sternum, costal margin, and neck fossae; the resulting paradoxic motion may contribute to respiratory insufficiency. The airway is small and flaccid, so that it is readily occluded by mucus or edema, and it collapses readily under slight pressure. Dyspneic infants swallow large volumes of air, and the distended stomach and bowel may further impair diaphragmatic excursion.

Classification

   A. **Upper Airway:**

      1. Micrognathia—Pierre Robin syndrome.

      2. Macroglossia—Muscular hypertrophy, hypothyroidism, lymphangioma.

      3. Choanal atresia.

      4. Tumors, cysts, or enlarged thyroid remnants

in the pharynx or neck.

    5. Laryngeal or tracheal stenosis, webs, cysts, tumors, or vocal cord paralysis.

B. Intrathoracic:

    1. Atelectasis.

    2. Pneumothorax and pneumomediastinum.

    3. Pleural effusion or chylothorax.

    4. Pulmonary cysts, sequestration, and tumors.

    5. Tracheomalacia or bronchomalacia.

    6. Congenital lobar emphysema.

    7. Diaphragmatic hernia or eventration.

    8. Esophageal atresia or tracheo-esophageal fistula.

    9. Vascular rings.

    10. Mediastinal tumors and cysts.

1. PIERRE ROBIN SYNDROME

Pierre Robin syndrome is a congenital defect characterized by micrognathia and glossoptosis, often associated with a cleft palate. The small lower jaw and strong sucking action of the infant allow the tongue to be sucked back and occlude the laryngeal airway and may be life-threatening.

Most infants (mild cases) should be kept in the prone position during care and feeding. A nasogastric or gastrostomy tube may be necessary. Nasohypopharyngeal intubation is effective in preventing occlusion of the larynx. If conservative measures fail, prompt attention to maintaining an open airway by tracheostomy is indicated. The tongue may be sutured forward to the lower jaw, but this frequently breaks down. In time, the lower jaw develops normally. These infants eventually learn how to keep the tongue from occluding the airway.

Dennison WM: The Pierre Robin syndrome. Pediatrics 36: 336–341, 1965.

2. CHOANAL ATRESIA

Complete obstruction at the posterior nares due to choanal atresia may be unilateral and relatively asymptomatic. It may be membranous (10%) or bony (90%). When it is bilateral, severe respiratory distress is manifest by marked chest wall retraction on inspiration and a normal cry.

There is arching of the head and neck in an effort to breathe, and the baby is unable to eat. The diagnosis is confirmed by inability to pass a tube through the nares to the pharynx. With the baby in a supine position, radiopaque material may be instilled into the nares and lateral x-rays of the head taken to outline the obstruction.

Emergency treatment consists of maintaining an oral airway by placing a nipple, with the tip cut off, in the mouth. The membranous or bony occlusion may then be perforated by direct transpalatal excision, or it may be punctured and enlarged by using a Hegar dilator. The newly created opening must be stented with plastic tubing for 5 weeks to prevent stricture.

3. CONGENITAL PHARYNGEAL OR LARYNGEAL TUMORS, CYSTS, & STENOSES

Tumors affecting the airway of the pharynx include lingual thyroid and teratoma. The pharynx and larynx may be obstructed by hemangioma, lymphangioma, neurofibroma, and fibrosarcoma. Thyroglossal cysts, pharyngeal inclusion cysts, and laryngeal cysts may compromise breathing. Stenoses of the larynx result from fibrous webs, which are remnants of epithelial ingrowths during embryonic formation of the larynx. They may be located at the true cords or may be supraglottic.

Clinical Findings

Retractions of the chest occur on inspiration, and a prolonged expiratory wheeze may be noted. A hoarse, weak, or completely absent cry indicates involvement of the larynx. In the absence of other obvious causes of airway obstruction such as tumors of the neck, direct laryngoscopy and bronchoscopy should be performed.

Treatment

The paramount concern of treatment is to provide an adequate airway; treatment of the obstructing lesion is of secondary importance. An endotracheal tube should be placed in the trachea and anchored with tape to the lips. Emergency tracheostomy may be required. A lingual thyroid can be made smaller by the administration of thyroid hormone. Some hemangioendotheliomas may respond to adrenocorticosteroids; or they may involute spontaneously. Cavernous hemangiomas are extremely difficult to excise intact when adjacent normal structures are involved. Cysts of the pharynx may be aspirated or marsupialized until excision can be accomplished. Laryngeal webs may be excised by cup forceps. Thicker webs may require repeated laryngeal dilatations.

Holinger PH: Clinical aspects of congenital anomalies of the larynx, trachea, bronchi, and esophagus. J Laryng 75: 1–44, 1961.

4. ATELECTASIS

The airway of the unborn infant is normally filled with fluid which is formed in the lungs. This fluid flows out of the trachea to contribute to amniotic fluid. During asphyxia, the unborn baby may attempt to breathe, resulting in inhalation of amniotic fluid, meconium, or blood. When the airways are filled with this debris, they may become plugged at birth and prevent aeration of the lungs. Mucous secretions may cause atelectasis when an endotracheal tube or tracheostomy tube has been used without humidified air, or in infants with cystic fibrosis.

Clinical Findings

Prenatal asphyxia should be suspected when there is prolonged and difficult labor and when bradycardia occurs in the infant. Babies who are small for gestational age and depressed infants with low Apgar scores are particularly prone to aspiration. Meconium will be noted in the amniotic fluid and pharynx. With the onset of breathing, respirations will be labored, but chest wall retractions are not usually prominent. Chest x-rays will indicate lack of aeration in some areas or hyperaeration in areas where partial obstruction of the bronchus occurs. Bacterial pneumonia and sepsis frequently follow prolonged atelectasis.

Treatment

An asphyxiated, meconium-stained, or depressed newborn infant should be treated by pharyngeal aspiration and immediate insertion of an endotracheal tube into the trachea. The trachea should also be aspirated of debris before ventilatory resuscitation is attempted. Bronchoscopy and direct aspiration of the plugged bronchus may be necessary. Increased concentrations of inspired oxygen with ultrasonic humidification should be given to maintain the peripheral arterial P_{O_2} at about 60–80 mm Hg. Intensive physical therapy with postural drainage and chest cupping will be needed. Because of the risk of pneumothorax, positive pressure ventilation should be avoided unless it is required to maintain adequate oxygenation.

Schaffer AJ: Massive aspiration syndrome. Chapter 7, pp 76–85, in: *Diseases of the Newborn,* 2nd ed. Saunders, 1965.

5. CONGENITAL DIAPHRAGMATIC HERNIA & EVENTRATION OF THE DIAPHRAGM

Fusion of the transverse septum and pleuroperitoneal folds normally occurs during the eighth week of embryonic development. If diaphragmatic formation is incomplete, the pleuroperitoneal hiatus (foramen of Bochdalek) persists. The intestine normally returns from the umbilicus for rotation and fixation within the abdomen at the tenth week of gestation. If the bowel should herniate into the chest at this early stage, nonfixation of the mesentery and colon will occur. Since the transition from the glandular to the bronchial phase of pulmonary development occurs at about the 15th week of gestation, severe impairment of pulmonary development may occur when the bowel compresses the lung (Fig 49–6). Experimental studies have shown that pulmonary hypoplasia is due to the herniation of bowel and not just an association of anomalies. The earlier in gestation the hernia occurs, the more severe the pulmonary hypoplasia.

Eventration of the diaphragm may be congenital or acquired. Congenital eventration may consist of only pleural and peritoneal membranes, with attenuation of muscular and fibrous layers. The diaphragmatic serosal membranes may protrude slightly into the pleural space or may line it completely. When intact pleural membranes exist, the distinction between eventration and Bochdalek's hernia may be quite arbitrary. Varying degrees of pulmonary hypoplasia also occur with diaphragmatic eventration.

Acquired diaphragmatic eventration may occur as a result of direct injury to the phrenic nerve associated with brachial or cervical plexus trauma during birth or during thoracotomy.

Clinical Findings

Symptoms may appear immediately after birth or not until the infant is several months old. Severe respi-

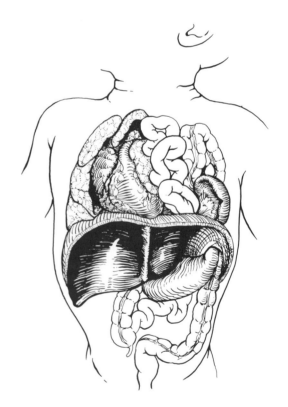

FIG 49–6. Congenital posterolateral (Bochdalek) diaphragmatic hernia. Bowel, spleen, and liver herniate into the chest and severely compromise lung development in utero and ventilation after birth. (Reproduced, with permission, from Wilson JL: *Handbook of Surgery,* 4th ed. Lange, 1969.)

ratory distress may be characterized by gasping respirations with cyanosis. Pulmonary hypoplasia is the most frequent cause of death. The left diaphragm is affected 4–5 times as frequently as the right. The abdomen is usually scaphoid. The chest on the side of the hernia may be dull to percussion, but bowel sounds are not usually appreciated. When the hernia is on the left, the heart sounds may be heard best on the right side of the chest. A chest x-ray will show bowel in the thorax with a shift of the mediastinal structures to the opposite side.

Treatment

An endotracheal tube should be placed in the trachea and assisted ventilation controlled to prevent a positive pressure greater than 30–35 cm water. A nasogastric tube should be placed in the stomach to aspirate swallowed air and to prevent distention of the herniated bowel, which further compresses the lungs. An umbilical artery catheter should be inserted to the level of the lower aorta, and metabolic acidosis must be corrected.

A rectus or transverse abdominal incision should be made and the herniated bowel reduced from the pleural space. The negative pressure between the bowel and the chest wall may make reduction difficult. This negative pressure may be broken by inserting a tube along the pleura and injecting air through it. A hernia sac should be searched for and excised. Following reduction of the bowel, a chest tube should be placed in the pleural space and connected to a water seal and not to vacuum. No attempt should be made to expand the collapsed and hypoplastic lung by positive pressure. The diaphragmatic defect should be closed by nonabsorbable sutures. In rare instances, a synthetic material, fascia, or muscle flap from the abdominal wall is required to close the defect. A gastrostomy tube should be placed in the stomach so that the nasogastric tube can be withdrawn. The abdominal cavity is often too small and undeveloped to accommodate the intestine and permit closure of the abdominal wall muscle and fascial layers. In such cases, abdominal wall skin flaps should be mobilized and closed over the protruding bowel. The resulting ventral hernia can be repaired later when the infant is thriving. Continued respiratory support and treatment of hypoxia, hypercapnia, and acidosis are required postoperatively. Localized eventration may be approached better by means of a posterolateral thoracotomy.

Prognosis

The mortality rate depends upon the severity of pulmonary hypoplasia, associated anomalies, and the quality of care provided for these critically ill infants. Surgical units which are immediately adjacent to obstetric services have mortality rates as high as 80% because infants with severe pulmonary hypoplasia will be recognized and treated immediately. Infants that survive transfer to surgical centers remote from the delivery area usually have less pulmonary insufficiency, and the mortality rate will be less than 50%.

Bonham Carter RE, Waterston DS, Aberdeen E: Hernia and eventration of the diaphragm in childhood. Lancet 1:656–659, 1962.

deLorimier AA, Tierney DF, Parker HR: Hypoplastic lungs in fetal lambs with surgically produced congenital diaphragmatic hernia. Surgery 62:12–17, 1967. ·

Snyder WH, Greaney EM: Congenital diaphragmatic hernia: Seventy-seven consecutive cases. Surgery 57:576–588, 1965.

Thomas TV: Non-paralytic eventration of the diaphragm. J Thoracic Cardiovas Surg 55:586–593, 1968.

6. CONGENITAL LOBAR EMPHYSEMA

Lobar emphysema consists of massive hyperinflation of a single lobe; rarely, more than one lobe is affected. The upper and middle lobes are most frequently involved. The cause of lobar emphysema is usually unknown but has been related to deficient bronchial cartilage support, redundant mucosa, bronchial stenosis, mucous plug, and bronchial compression by anomalous vessels or other mediastinal structures.

Clinical Findings

In one-third of patients, respiratory distress is noted at birth; in only 5% of cases do symptoms develop after 6 months. Males are affected twice as frequently as females. The signs include progressive and severe dyspnea, wheezing, grunting, coughing, cyanosis, and difficulty with feedings. Increased dimensions of the chest and retractions may be seen. The chest is hyperresonant, and decreased breath sounds may be noted over the affected lobe. Chest x-rays show radiolucency of the emphysematous lobe with bronchovascular markings extending to the lung periphery. Compression atelectasis of the adjacent lung, shift of the mediastinum, depression of the diaphragm, and anterior bowing of the sternum are usually seen. The emphysematous lobe, if untreated, will continue to expand, compressing adjacent lung and airways and asphyxiating the infant.

Treatment & Prognosis

Occasionally, the emphysema may be due to a mucous plug in the bronchus which may be aspirated by bronchoscopy. Compression of the bronchus by mediastinal masses may be relieved by removal of the tumor or repair of anomalous vessels. Treatment of mildly symptomatic cases may not be necessary.

Most patients with lobar emphysema are severely symptomatic, and pulmonary lobectomy is necessary. Anesthesia should not be started until all personnel are ready for emergency thoracotomy. Excessive positive pressure ventilation should be avoided. Following surgical relief of the lobar emphysema, the prognosis is excellent. Some patients may show residual disease in the remaining lung.

DeMuth GR, Sloan H: Congenital lobar emphysema: Long-term effects and sequelae in treated cases. Surgery 59:601–607, 1966.

Hendren WH, McKee DM: Lobar emphysema of infancy. J Pediat Surg 1:24–39, 1966.

ESOPHAGEAL ANOMALIES

Classification (See Fig 49–7.)
  A. With Esophageal Atresia:
    1. With a blind proximal pouch and a fistula between the distal end of the esophagus and the trachea (85% of cases).
    2. With a blind proximal esophageal pouch, no tracheo-esophageal fistula, and a rudimentary distal esophagus (10% of cases).
    3. With fistulas between both proximal and distal esophageal segments and the trachea (0.5% of cases).

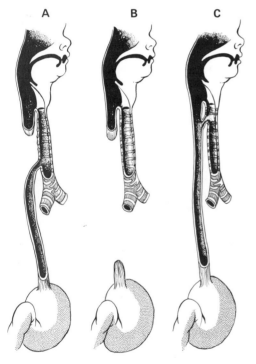

FIG 49–7. Congenital esophageal anomalies. The most common is esophageal atresia with a tracheo-esophageal fistula to the distal segment (A). The second most common is esophageal atresia without a tracheo-esophageal fistula (B). Tracheo-esophageal fistula without esophageal atresia (C) is the third most common anomaly, and two-thirds of these fistulas are located above the first thoracic vertebra. (Reproduced, with permission, from Wilson JL: *Handbook of Surgery,* 4th ed. Lange, 1969.)

4. With a fistula between the proximal esophagus and the trachea (0.3% of cases).
  B. Without Esophageal Atresia:
    1. With an H-type tracheo-esophageal fistula (4–5% of cases).
    2. With esophageal stenosis consisting of a membranous occlusion between the mid and distal thirds of the esophagus (rare).
    3. With a laryngotracheo-esophageal cleft consisting of a linear communication between these structures (very rare).

Clinical Findings

Shortly after birth, the infant with esophageal atresia is noted to have excessive salivation and repeated episodes of coughing, choking, and cyanosis. Attempts at feeding result in choking, gagging, and regurgitation. Infants with tracheo-esophageal fistula in addition to esophageal atresia will have reflux of gastric secretions into the tracheobronchial tree which produces severe chemical bronchitis and pneumonia. Pneumonic infiltrates are usually noted first in the right upper lobe.

A size 12F catheter should be passed into the esophagus, either by way of the nose or mouth; if esophageal atresia is present, the tube will not go down the expected distance to the stomach. Smaller tubes will coil in the upper esophageal pouch or may pass from the tracheo-esophageal fistula to the stomach, giving a false impression of normal esophagus. With the tube in the upper pouch, saliva should be aspirated and no more than 2 ml of barium in saline solution should be instilled into the tube and pushed into the blind pouch by injecting air after it. Too much contrast material will result in aspiration. A lateral chest x-ray will show the contrast medium in the blind pouch and its relationship to the vertebrae. If a tracheo-esophageal fistula connects to the lower esophageal segment, air will be present in the stomach and bowel. Absence of air below the diaphragm usually means that distal tracheo-esophageal fistula is not present. Injection of contrast medium through a gastrostomy with reflux into the distal esophagus will determine the distance between the 2 esophageal ends.

Tracheo-esophageal fistula without esophageal atresia will produce repeated coughing, cyanosis, and pneumonia. These episodes are more apt to occur with swallowing liquids than with solid foods. Abdominal distention is a prominent finding because the Valsalva effect of coughing and crying forces air through the fistula into the stomach and bowel. The diagnosis may be difficult. A cine-esophagogram taken from a lateral position is required. The swallowed material should be a thin barium mixture or diatrizoate (Hypaque). Diatrizoate is hyperosmolar and irritating to the tracheal mucosa but may shrink the mucosa of the fistula to allow its visualization. In rare cases it is necessary to verify the presence and position of the fistula by esophagoscopy. A general anesthetic is used, and dilute methylene blue is instilled into the endotracheal tube. During positive pressure ventilation, the blue color and gas bubbles can be seen through the esophagus at the level of the fistula. Two-thirds of the fistulas are located in the neck; the remainder are within the thorax.

Laryngotracheo-esophageal cleft produces symptoms similar to tracheo-esophageal fistula but of much greater severity. Laryngoscopy shows the cleft between the arytenoids and larynx.

Differential Diagnosis

Newborn infants may have transient dysphagia with aspiration of feedings due to an uncoordinated swallowing mechanism. This usually subsides within the first 2 days after birth. Prolonged swallowing dysfunction may occur with brain anomaly or injury.

Treatment

Aspiration pneumonia must be treated before surgical treatment is begun. A sump suction catheter should be placed in the infant's upper esophageal pouch and connected to continuous suction. The head of the bed should be elevated. The infant should be placed in a humidified incubator, turned from side to side every hour, and stimulated to cry and cough. Ampicillin, 100 mg/kg, and kanamycin, 7 mg/kg, should be given every 12 hours IM. Infants that are fully mature and without severe anomalies should have a gastrostomy and an extrapleural thoracotomy for division of tracheo-esophageal fistula and primary esophageal anastomosis. The operation should be staged for premature babies, for infants with associated severe anomalies, or for babies with a short upper esophageal segment. The first stage consists of a gastrostomy and transpleural division of the tracheo-esophageal fistula. A sump suction catheter is maintained in the upper esophageal pouch, and the baby is fed by gastrostomy until he has become strong enough to tolerate the second stage procedure. A short upper pouch can be elongated with a 22–24F Hurst bougie over a period of 2–3 weeks. The second stage procedure consists of an extrapleural thoracotomy followed by anastomosis of the 2 esophageal segments.

The infant with esophageal atresia and no tracheo-esophageal fistula requires cervical esophagostomy and gastrostomy. He is fed through the gastrostomy tube until he weighs 9–11 kg, at which time a colon interposition is used to establish continuity between the cervical esophagus and the stomach.

In infants with an H-type tracheo-esophageal fistula, the fistula is located above the thoracic inlet in two-thirds of cases. These fistulas may be divided through a left transverse cervical incision. Intrathoracic fistulas may be divided by an extrapleural right thoracotomy. A gastrostomy is commonly employed for feeding until the esophageal closure is healed.

Esophageal webs respond readily to esophageal dilatation. This is usually accomplished with Hurst or Maloney mercury-weighted bougies. Dilatations are repeated until healing occurs without recurrence. Esophagoscopy and excision of portions of a tough or thick web, using biopsy forceps, may be required in addition to dilatation.

Prognosis

The survival rate for a full-term infant without associated anomalies is excellent. Deaths do occur, however, as a result of pulmonary complications, severe associated anomalies, prematurity, and sepsis due to anastomotic disruption. Anastomotic leaks occur either as a result of technical problems or because the distal esophageal wall is very weak. In performing the anastomosis, the extrapleural approach prevents the development of empyema and maintains infection to a small localized area. Swallowing is a reflex response that must be reinforced early in infancy. If establishment of esophageal continuity is delayed for more than 4–6 weeks, it may take many months to teach the infant to swallow. Babies with cervical esophagostomy should be encouraged to suck, eat, and swallow during gastrostomy feedings.

Dysphagia may occur weeks or months following successful repair of esophageal atresia. Stricture of the anastomosis may require one or more dilatations, with a filiform and follower, or by using antegrade or retrograde dilators. Another cause of dysphagia may be neuromuscular incoordination, usually associated with esophageal anomalies. This frequent problem improves with age.

Most of these infants have an alarming, barking cough and rattling sound with respiration, probably due to a reed-like protrusion of the membranous portion of the trachea at the site of tracheo-esophageal fistula. A whispering, soft voice may also be noted. These findings improve with increasing age.

Swallowed foreign bodies will lodge at the site of anastomosis and require removal with esophagoscopy. Hiatus hernia with reflux esophagitis occasionally follows successful repair, which requires surgical treatment.

Blackburn WR, Amoury RA: Congenital esophago-pulmonary fistulas without esophageal atresia: An analysis of 260 fistulas in infants, children, and adults. Rev Surg 23:153–175, 1966.

deLorimier AA: Treatment of esophageal atresia with a short proximal esophageal segment. JAMA 195:697–698, 1966.

Holder TM & others: Esophageal atresia and tracheo-esophageal fistula: A survey of its members by the Surgical Section of the Academy of Pediatrics. Pediatrics 34:542–549, 1964.

VASCULAR RINGS

Tracheobronchial and esophageal compression by the great vessels may occur as a result of anomalies of the aortic arch or of abnormally located or enlarged pulmonary arteries. The genesis of aortic vascular rings may be understood if the embryo is considered to have

2 aortic arches, each with a carotid and subclavian artery and a ductus arteriosus (Fig 49−8). In the normal development of the aortic arch, the distal portion of the right arch is obliterated. There are 5 main types of vascular rings: (1) persistence of both arches gives rise to double aortic arch (Fig 49−9); (2) obliteration of the left distal arch generates right aortic arch and persistent left ligamentum arteriosum; (3) obliteration of the right arch between the right carotid and subclavian arteries results in anomalous origin of the right subclavian artery; (4) incorporation of the right proximal arch into the left arch produces anomalous origin of the innominate artery; and (5) incorporation of the left proximal arch into the right arch gives rise to an anomalous origin of the right common carotid artery.

When the left pulmonary artery arises from the right pulmonary artery, it encircles the right side of the trachea and courses between the trachea and esophagus to the left lung. This sling effect produces significant compression of the lower trachea and proximal main bronchi. Aneurysmal dilatation of the pulmonary artery usually occurs in association with ventricular septal defect and infundibular stenosis. Other forms of congenital heart defects are frequent. Each of these anomalies may compress and encircle the trachea and esophagus, producing respiratory distress and symptoms of obstruction on swallowing.

Clinical Findings

These infants have a characteristic inspiratory and expiratory wheeze, stridor, or croup. The head is held in an opisthotonic position to prevent compression of the trachea. If the head is forcibly flexed, the stridor is increased and apnea may be produced. There may be hesitation on swallowing, with episodes of choking−so-called dysphagia lusoria. Chest x-rays may show compression of the trachea. Anteroposterior and lateral esophagograms show indentation of the esophagus at the level of T3 and T4. When there is no esophageal indentation, a tracheogram may be necessary to demonstrate tracheal compression due to anomalous origin of the innominate or left common carotid artery. An angiocardiogram is not necessary for isolated aortic arch anomalies but is required for assessing congenital heart lesions associated with anomalies of the pulmonary artery. Esophagoscopy and bronchoscopy may be helpful in assessing the degree and level of compression.

Treatment

The aortic arch anomaly must be completely dissected and visualized through a left thoracotomy. The smallest component of a double aortic arch must be divided. An anomalous right subclavian artery is divided at its origin. The anomalous innominate or left carotid arteries are pulled forward by placing sutures between their adventitia and the sternum. The accompanying fibrous bands and sheaths constricting the trachea and esophagus must also be divided. Pulmonary artery slings are corrected by dividing the origin of the left pulmonary artery and anastomosing it to the main pulmonary artery anterior to the trachea. Aneurysmal dilatation of the pulmonary artery is relieved by correcting the congenital heart defect; occasionally, the pulmonary artery requires reduction in size by direct surgical resection.

Occasionally, symptoms persist postoperatively because of deformed tracheocartilaginous rings. This may require tracheostomy and endotracheal intubation for a prolonged period of time. If tracheomalacia is present, sleeve resection of the abnormal portion of the trachea and bronchi with anastomosis should be accomplished.

Lincoln JCR & others: Vascular anomalies compressing the esophagus and trachea. Thorax 24:295−306, 1969.

Mahoney EB, Manning JA: Congenital abnormalities of the aortic arch. Surgery 55:1−14, 1964.

Park CD & others: Tracheal compression by the great arteries in the mediastinum. Arch Surg 103:623−632, 1971.

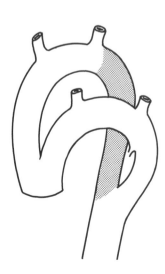

FIG 49−8. Normal embryonic aortic arch.

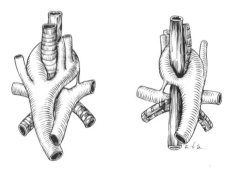

FIG 49−9. Anterior (left) and posterior views of double aortic arch constricting the trachea and esophagus.

CHALASIA OF THE ESOPHAGUS

Chalasia of the esophagus refers to an incompetent cardioesophageal sphincter mechanism. Studies of esophageal motility and manometric measurements of the cardioesophageal junction show disordered peristalsis and absence of a high-pressure zone in the lower esophagus in most newborn infants. Change to the normal adult pattern of peristalsis and the development of a competent cardioesophageal sphincter develops after several months. Until this occurs, many infants suffer varying degrees of regurgitation after feeding. Repeated gastric reflux may produce peptic esophagitis and interfere with subsequent development of a competent sphincter mechanism.

Symptoms consist of repeated, effortless regurgitation of feedings, particularly when the baby is placed in a recumbent position. The baby will be hungry and will readily feed after vomiting. Persistent regurgitation may result in poor weight gain, peptic esophagitis with appearance of blood in the vomitus, or occult bleeding, producing anemia. Aspiration of vomitus, particularly during sleep, produces recurrent pneumonia.

The symptoms are the same as those occurring with esophageal hiatus hernia and incompetent cardioesophageal sphincter. The diagnosis is established by esophagography under fluoroscopic vision or with cineradiography.

Conservative treatment is successful in most cases. The feedings should be thickened with rice cereal, and the baby should be maintained upright at all times in an "infant seat." If a prolonged trial of this conservative approach fails and significant complications of growth failure, anemia, or pneumonia persist, an antireflux procedure such as the Nissen gastric fundoplication is indicated.

Bettex M, Kuffer F: Long-term results of fundoplication in hiatus hernia and cardioesophageal chalasia in infants and children. J Pediat Surg 4:526, 1969.

Strawczynski H & others: The behavior of the lower esophageal sphincter in infants and its relationship in gastroesophageal regurgitation. J Pediat 64:17–23, 1964.

HYPERTROPHIC PYLORIC STENOSIS

Pyloric stenosis results from hypertrophy of the circular and longitudinal muscularis of the pylorus and distal antrum of the stomach (Fig 49–10). The cause is not known. The male/female sex incidence is 4:1. The disorder is more common in first-born infants and occurs 4 times more often in the offspring of mothers who had the disease as infants than in those whose fathers had the disease. If one monozygotic twin is affected, the other will have the disorder also in two-thirds of cases. A seasonal variation is noted in the occurrence of symptoms, with peaks in spring and fall.

Clinical Findings

A. Symptoms and Signs: The "typical" affected infant was full-term when born and had been feeding and growing well until he was 2 weeks old. Occasional regurgitation of some of the feedings occurred initally. Several days later, however, the vomiting became more frequent and projectile. The vomitus contained the previous feeding and no bile. Blood may be seen in the vomitus in 5% of cases, and coffee-ground or occult blood is frequently present. Shortly after vomiting, the infant acts starved and will feed again. The stools become infrequent and firm in consistency as dehydration occurs. The premature and weak, chronically starved infant does not have the strength to have projectile vomiting.

Less frequently, symptoms occur earlier—even shortly after birth—or as much as 4 months later.

Weight loss follows progressive starvation. Jaundice with indirect hyperbilirubinemia occurs in fewer than 10% of cases. Gastric peristaltic waves can usually be seen moving from the left costal margin to the area of the pylorus. The pyloric "tumor" or "olive" can be palpated when the infant is relaxed in over 95% of cases. Abdominal relaxation may be accomplished by sedation or by feeding clear fluids and simultaneously aspirating the stomach contents with a nasogastric tube.

B. X-Ray Findings: A gastrointestinal series is indicated in those cases in which a pyloric tumor cannot be palpated. Radiographic diagnostic signs, preferably using small amounts of meglumine diatrizoate (Gastrografin), include (1) outlining of the narrow pyloric channel by a single "string sign" or "double track" due to folds of mucosa; (2) a pyloric "beak" where the pyloric entrance from the antrum occurs; (3) the "shoulder" sign, in which the pyloric mass bulges into the antrum; (4) the pyloric "tit," where the contrast bulges on the lesser curvature between peristaltic waves; and (5) complete obstruction of the pylorus.

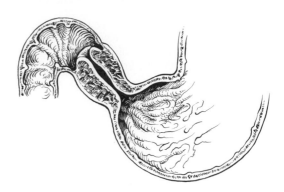

FIG 49–10. Hypertrophic pyloric stenosis. Note that the distal end of the hypertrophic muscle protrudes into the duodenum (arrow), accounting for the ease of perforation into the duodenum during pyloromyotomy.

Differential Diagnosis

Repeated nonbilious vomiting in early infancy may be due to feeding problems, intracranial lesions, incompetence of the cardio-esophageal sphincter (chalasia) with or without hiatus hernia, pylorospasm, duodenal stenosis, malrotation of the bowel, or adrenal insufficiency.

Complications

Repeated vomiting with inadequate intake of formula results in hypochloremic, hypokalemic alkalosis, dehydration, and starvation. Gastritis and reflux esophagitis occur frequently and may contribute to an incompetent cardio-esophageal sphincter. Aspiration of vomitus may produce pneumonia or suffocation.

Treatment & Prognosis

Conservative treatment with antispasmodics has been advocated by some, but this requires prolonged, constant vigilance and care to maintain nutrition and prevent aspiration of vomitus. After many months, the pyloric hypertrophy may subside with relief of obstructive symptoms.

The preferred operative treatment is the Fredet-Ramstedt pyloromyotomy, which should be undertaken only after dehydration and hypokalemic hypochloremic alkalosis have been corrected. A nasogastric tube should be placed preoperatively to empty the stomach.

Postoperatively, nasogastric suction is continued for 8–12 hours. Following this, the infant is fed 10% dextrose solution, 30 ml for 3 feedings; the regular formula is then resumed, giving 45 ml every 3 hours for 3 feedings and then increasing the volume 15 ml at a time until the normal intake is being given. The hospital stay averages 3 days. Occasionally, an infant will vomit persistently, and prolonged nasogastric suction may be required for several days until normal motility returns. Careful management should result in no mortality and prompt recovery.

Carter CO, Evans KA: Inheritance of congenital pyloric stenosis. J Med Genet 6:233–254, 1969.

Kwok RH, Avery G: Seasonal variation of congenital hypertrophic pyloric stenosis. J Pediat 70:963–965, 1967.

Shuman FI, Darling DB, Fisher JH: The radiographic diagnosis of congenital hypertrophic pyloric stenosis. J Pediat 71:70–74, 1967.

INTESTINAL OBSTRUCTION IN THE NEWBORN

The cardinal signs and symptoms of intestinal obstruction are (1) polyhydramnios in the mother, (2) vomiting, (3) abdominal distention, and (4) failure to pass meconium. Polyhydramnios is related to the level of obstruction, occurring in approximately 45% of women who have infants with duodenal atresia and 15% of those who have infants with ileal atresia. When a tube is routinely passed into the stomach of a newborn, a residual greater than 40 ml is diagnostic of obstruction. Vomiting occurs early in upper intestinal obstruction, and it is bile-stained if the obstruction is distal to the ampulla of Vater. Abdominal distention is related to the level of obstruction, being most marked for distal obstructions. Meconium is passed in 30–50% of newborn infants with intestinal obstruction, but failure to pass meconium within the first 24 hours is distinctly abnormal.

Causes of neonatal intestinal obstruction include intestinal atresia or stenosis, annular pancreas, malrotation with peritoneal bands or volvulus, meconium ileus, Hirschsprung's disease, and meconium plug syndrome. Atresia of the bowel occurs in the duodenum in 40%, in the jejunum in 20%, in the ileum in 20%, and in the colon in 10% of cases.

1. CONGENITAL DUODENAL OBSTRUCTION

Duodenal atresia and stenosis produce obstruction at the level of the ampulla of Vater. In 75% of cases, the bile is diverted to the proximal duodenum. Annular pancreas is almost always associated with hypoplasia of the duodenum at the level of the ampulla. In about half of cases, multiple congenital anomalies are present, including Down's syndrome in 30% and congenital heart disease in 20%. Birth weight is less than 2500 g in half of these infants.

Clinical Findings

Vomiting, usually with bile, occurs shortly after birth and during attempted feedings. Distention of the upper abdomen may be noted. Meconium is passed in over 50% of cases. Abdominal x-rays show a distended stomach and duodenum ("double bubble" sign). Gas in the small and large intestine indicates incomplete obstruction. Barium (in saline) enema identifies the presence or absence of malrotation, and the colon may be noted to be unused (microcolon).

Treatment & Prognosis

The abdomen is explored through a right upper transverse abdominal incision. The hepatic flexure may have to be mobilized to expose the duodenum. Although it is tempting to perform a Heineke-Mikulicz duodenoplasty for stenosis and webs, there is a risk of injuring the ampulla of Vater. A retrocolic, side-to-side duodenojejunostomy is the procedure of choice. A gastrostomy should also be performed for decompression of the stomach and duodenum and to check gastric residual during graded feedings. Persistent functional obstruction may be obviated by performing a long side-to-side duodenojejunostomy from the pylorus to the point of obstruction. A fine Silastic catheter may be passed alongside the gastrostomy tube and through the anastomosis into the jejunum for purposes of feeding until duodenal peristalsis becomes functional. Gastrojejunostomy should not be done because the blind duodenal pouch may cause repeated vomiting. The mortality rate is high because of prematurity and associated anomalies.

Fonkalsrud EW, deLorimier AA, Hays DM: Congenital atresia and stenosis of the duodenum. Pediatrics 43:79–83, 1969.

2. ATRESIA & STENOSIS OF THE JEJUNUM, ILEUM, & COLON

Atresia and stenosis of the jejunum, ileum, and colon are caused by a mesenteric vascular accident in utero such as may result from hernia, volvulus, or intussusception, producing aseptic necrosis and resorption of the necrotic bowel. Although atresia may occur in any portion of the intestine, most cases occur in the proximal jejunum or distal ileum. A short area of necrosis may produce only stenosis or a membranous web occluding the lumen. A more extensive infarct may leave a fibrous cord between the 2 bowel loops, or the proximal and distal bowel may be completely separated with a V-shaped defect in the mesentery (Fig 49–11). Multiple atresias occur in 10% of cases.

Clinical Findings

Vomiting of bile, abdominal distention, and failure to pass meconium indicate intestinal obstruction. Plain abdominal x-rays will give an estimate of how far along the intestine the obstruction exists; small bowel, however, cannot be distinguished from colon in the newborn. No contrast material should be given by mouth to newborn babies with complete intestinal obstruction. A barium (in saline) enema may be indicated to detect the level of obstruction and the coexistence of anomalous rotation. In obstructions which occur in the distal bowel and which appear relatively early in gestation, the colon will be empty of meconium and will appear abnormally narrow. When the obstruction is proximal, or when it occurs late in pregnancy, meconium will be passed into the colon. Barium enema will then outline a more generous-sized colon with its contents. Rarely, a microcolon is not just unused bowel but is due to Hirschsprung's disease. In older children with evidence of partial intestinal obstruction, a small bowel series may be indicated to identify intestinal stenosis.

Treatment

A transverse upper abdominal incision is preferred. Infants with jejunal atresia usually have greatly dilated bowel from the stomach to the point of obstruction. This overly distended jejunum should be resected—to the ligament of Treitz, if necessary—since it is a source of persistent functional obstruction if it is retained. This same principle applies for membranous

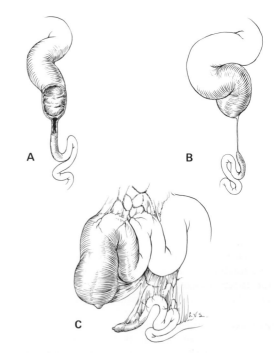

FIG 49–11. Types of intestinal atresia: *A:* A membranous web. *B:* Fibrous band connecting 2 blind ends. *C:* Complete separation of the 2 ends with V-shaped defect in the mesentery.

atresia, and the temptation to resect the web and perform a Heineke-Mikulicz resection should be resisted.

In patients with ileal atresia, only the most distal blind end is bulbously dilated, and this should be excised. More proximal resection of ileum should not be performed to prevent the complication of malabsorption. A great discrepancy between the diameter of the segments of intestine proximal and distal to the atresia is the rule. Therefore, the preferred anastomosis will be end-to-oblique or end-to-side.

A gastrostomy is preferred to help in postoperative decompression and to provide graded feedings.

Atresia of the proximal colon should be treated by resection of the dilated bowel and ileocolostomy. Atresia of the distal colon may be treated by proximal end colostomy or by a Mikulicz side-to-side colostomy. Later, the continuity of the distal colon may be established by end-to-end anastomosis.

Prognosis

The high mortality rate is related to sepsis, malfunctioning proximal bowel and anastomosis, prematurity, and coexisting meconium peritonitis. In contrast to duodenal atresia, associated anomalies are unusual in small bowel and colon atresia.

Coran AG, Eraklis AJ: Atresia of the colon. Surgery 65:828–831, 1969.

deLorimier AA, Fonkalsrud EW, Hays DM: Congenital atresia and stenosis of the jejunum and ileum. Surgery 65:819–827, 1969.

Louw JH: Resection and end-to-end anastomosis in the management of atresia and stenosis of the small bowel. Surgery 62:940–950, 1967.

DISORDERS OF INTESTINAL ROTATION

The midgut of the 10-week-old fetus normally returns from the umbilicus to the abdominal cavity and undergoes counterclockwise rotation about the superior mesenteric artery axis. The duodenojejunal portion of gut rotates posterior to the superior mesenteric vessels for 270 degrees. The duodenojejunal junction becomes fixed at the ligament of Treitz and located to the left of and cephalad to the superior mesenteric artery. The cecocolic portion of the midgut also rotates 270 degrees counterclockwise, anterior to the superior mesenteric artery; and the cecum normally becomes fixed in the right lower abdomen.

Pathogenesis & Classification

Anomalies of rotation and fixation (twice as common in males as in females) include (1) nonrotation, (2) incomplete rotation, (3) reversed rotation, and (4) anomalous fixation of the mesentery.

A. Nonrotation: When rotation does not occur, the midgut is suspended from the superior mesenteric vessels, with the small bowel located on the right side of the abdomen and the large bowel in the left abdomen. No fixation occurs, and adhesive bands are not present. This anomaly is usually found in patients with omphalocele, gastroschisis, and congenital diaphragmatic hernia.

B. Incomplete Rotation: Incomplete rotation may affect the duodenojejunal segment, the cecocolic portion of the bowel, or both. Adhesive bands are usually present. In the most common form of incomplete rotation, the cecum is adjacent to the root of the superior mesenteric vessels and dense peritoneal bands extend from the right abdomen to the cecum, obstructing the duodenum (Fig 49–12). Because the base of the mesentery is quite short and does not extend (as normally) from the ligament of Treitz in the left upper abdomen to the cecum in the right lower abdomen, volvulus frequently occurs, with clockwise twisting of the bowel about the superior mesenteric vessels.

C. Reversed Rotation: In reversed rotation, the bowel rotates varying degrees in a clockwise direction about the superior mesenteric axis. The duodenojejunal loop is anterior to the superior mesenteric artery. The cecocolic loop may be prearterial or may be rotated clockwise or counterclockwise in a retroarterial position. In either case, the cecum may be right-sided or left-sided. The most frequent anomaly is retroarterial clockwise rotation, which produces obstruction of the right colon.

D. Anomalous Fixation of Mesentery: Anomalies of mesenteric fixation account for internal mesenteric and paraduodenal hernias, mobile cecum, or obstructing adhesive bands in the absence of anomalous bowel rotation.

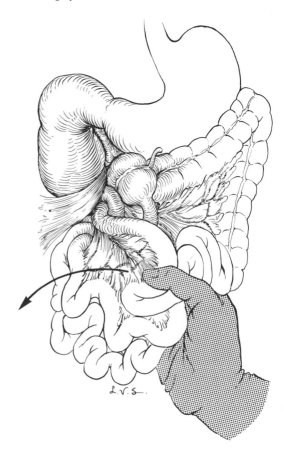

FIG 49–12. Malrotation of the midgut with volvulus. Note cecum at the origin of the superior mesenteric vessels. Fibrous bands cross and obstruct the duodenum as they adhere to the cecum. Volvulus is derotated in a counterclockwise direction.

Clinical Findings

Anomalies of intestinal rotation may cause symptoms related to intestinal obstruction, peptic ulceration, or malabsorption. Three-fourths of patients develop intestinal obstruction in infancy. Older patients may develop intermittent obstruction. The obstruction occurs in the duodenum or upper jejunum as a result of adhesive bands or midgut volvulus. Vomiting of bile occurs initially. Older patients may appear thin and wasted, presumably because of early satiety due to chronic partial obstruction or malabsorption. When the obstruction is due to bands, abdominal distention is not prominent. When volvulus occurs, abdominal distention may be very great. Bloody stools and signs of peritonitis indicate infarction of the bowel. Plain abdominal x-rays may show a "double bubble" sign which mimics duodenal stenosis. Distribution of gas throughout the intestines may be normal. When volvulus with gangrene occurs—the most disastrous complication—the bowel will be distended with gas and the intestinal walls will be thickened. Barium enema will show abnormal position of the cecum. With chronic intermittent symptoms of obstruction and a normal position of the cecum noted on barium enema, an upper gastrointestinal and small bowel series will show distention of the duodenum and narrowing at the point of obstruction.

Duodenal and antral stasis presumably account for the presence of peptic ulcer in 20% of patients. Malabsorption with steatorrhea occurs as a result of partial venous and lymphatic obstruction, and coarse rugal folds of the small bowel may be noted.

Treatment

Through a transverse upper abdominal incision, the entire bowel should be delivered from the abdominal cavity to assess the anomalous arrangement of the intestinal loops. Volvulus should be untwisted in a counterclockwise direction (Fig 49—12). The Ladd procedure consists of division of adhesive bands between the duodenum and proximal colon and the lateral abdominal wall. The appendix is removed. The cecum is then placed in the left lower quadrant and the duodenum moved to the right lateral abdomen. When duodenal obstruction exists without evident anomalous rotation of the colon, the right colon should be mobilized to expose the duodenum and the duodenum is moved to the right lateral abdomen. A Kocher maneuver should be accomplished, with complete mobilization of the third and fourth portions of the duodenum. Upon completion of the above procedures, a gastrostomy should be performed and a Foley catheter threaded through it down the duodenum and jejunum. The balloon should then be inflated and withdrawn to the stomach. This maneuver will detect an intrinsic web partially obstructing the bowel, which may coexist with the anomalies of rotation and fixation.

Prognosis

Once correction of the anomaly has been accomplished, the long-term results are excellent. Some patients tend to form adhesions that cause recurrent intestinal obstruction. Recurrent volvulus is rare after the Ladd procedure.

Amir-Jahed AK: Classification of reversed intestinal rotation. Surgery 64:1071—1074, 1968.

Bill AH, Grauman D: Rationale and technic for stabilization of the mesentery in cases of nonrotation of the midgut. J Pediat Surg 1:127—136, 1966.

Louw JH: Intestinal malrotation and duodenal ileus. J Roy Coll Surg Edinb 5:101—126, 1960.

Rees JR, Redo SF: Anomalies of intestinal rotation and fixation. Am J Surg 116:834—840, 1968.

MECONIUM ILEUS

In 20% of infants born with cystic fibrosis, the thick mucous secretions of the small bowel produce obturant obstruction due to inspissated meconium. This usually occurs in the mid ileum but may develop in the jejunum or colon. Although there is no clear correlation between pancreatic insufficiency and the development of inspissated meconium, meconium ileus also occurs in patients with pancreatic duct obstruction and pancreatic aplasia. Meconium obstruction without any apparent cause has also been described in newborn infants.

Meconium ileus may be complicated by volvulus of the heavy, distended loops of bowel. Depending upon how early in fetal life this occurs, the volvulus may progress to gangrene of the bowel, perforation with meconium peritonitis, or atresia of the ileum—singly or in combination (Fig 49—13).

Meconium ileus equivalent is obturant intestinal obstruction from viscid mucous secretions occurring after the newborn period. All of these patients have cystic fibrosis. The age at onset varies from several days after birth to early adulthood, but most cases occur within the first year. A respiratory infection and fever with dehydration usually precede the obstruction. Paradoxically, these patients usually have symptoms of pancreatic insufficiency with steatorrhea prior to the onset of intestinal obstruction.

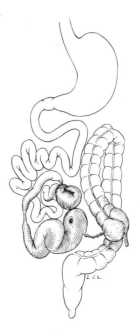

FIG 49—13. Complicated meconium ileus. Includes malrotation, volvulus of the heavy, meconium-filled bowel, and ischemic necrosis of the bowel, producing stenosis, atresia, or perforation with meconium peritonitis.

Clinical Findings

The infant typically has a normal birth weight. The abdomen is usually distended, and may be large enough to cause dystocia. In most cases, no meconium is passed. Vomiting of bile occurs early. Loops of thick, distended bowel may be seen and palpated. Plain abdominal x-rays show loops of bowel which vary greatly in diameter; the thick meconium gives a ground-glass appearance. When air mixes with the meconium, the so-called "soap bubble" sign is produced, usually in the right lower quadrant. X-rays taken shortly after the infant has been placed in an upright position may fail to show air-fluid levels because the thick, viscid meconium fails to layer out rapidly. An x-ray contrast enema will show microcolon with some meconium flecks. Reflux of contrast medium into the terminal ileum will outline a small terminal ileum with inspissated mucus; more proximally, the bowel is progressively distended with packed meconium. In complicated meconium ileus, perforation may be detected by the presence of calcification or extraluminal air. The sweat chloride test is usually impractical in the newborn because very little sweat can be collected. The albumin content of meconium in babies with cystic fibrosis is high, whereas no protein is found normally. Histologic sections of resected bowel will show an increase in number and size of the goblet cells, and the intestinal glands will be engorged with inspissated mucus.

Complications

The most common complication of meconium ileus is repeated pulmonary infection with chronic bronchopneumonia, bronchiectasis, atelectasis, and lung abscess. Malabsorption due to pancreatic insufficiency will require enzyme replacement with feedings. Rectal prolapse and intussusception are related to the inspissated stools of these patients.

Treatment

A nasogastric tube should be inserted into the stomach and connected to suction. Under fluoroscopic control, enemas containing full-strength meglumine diatrizoate (Gastrografin), which is hygroscopic, or acetylcysteine (Mucomyst), which is mucolytic, may effectively unplug the meconium in uncomplicated cases. The enema must be given to a well-hydrated infant, and intravenous infusions must be continued to prevent hypovolemia following the enema. Most patients, however, have bowel gangrene, atresia, or perforation due to volvulus, and require a right lower quadrant transverse incision and Mikulicz resection of the most dilated portion of the ileum. The proximal and distal bowel loops may then be irrigated with acetylcysteine. Subsequently, the Mikulicz enterostomy is closed.

These patients must be placed in an environment with high humidity to keep the tracheobronchial secretions fluid. Ultrasonic mist is preferable. Postural drainage with cupping of the chest should be taught to the parents so that they will continue to maintain tracheobronchial toilet indefinitely. Long-term prophylactic antibiotics are not indicated since infection with antibiotic-resistant pseudomonas and klebsiella organisms usually develop.

Pancreatic enzyme replacement in the form of pancreatin (Viokase) or pancrelipase (Cotazym) may be required. A low-fat formula in the newborn may produce better absorption and growth than standard formulas.

Meconium ileus equivalent should be treated conservatively by nasogastric suction, meglumine diatrizoate or 4% acetylcysteine enemas, and 4% acetylcysteine instilled into the stomach. Many patients develop mucous impaction of the bowel because of failure to take pancreatic enzymes orally. Respiratory infection and fever with dehydration usually precipitate meconium ileus equivalent.

Prognosis

The most frequent cause of death is progressive respiratory insufficiency due to plugging of bronchi with mucus, producing chronic bronchitis, atelectasis, pneumonia, and lung abscess. About 50% of these children die by age 10. Chronic malabsorption develops as a result of pancreatic insufficiency and because the viscid mucus produces a barrier between the bowel lumen and the intestinal mucosa. Progressive cirrhosis with portal hypertension also occurs in many long-term survivors.

Cordonnier JK, Izant RJ: Meconium ileus equivalent. Surgery 54:667–672, 1963.

Graham WP, Jaffee BF, deLorimier AA: Late intestinal obstruction in patients surviving neonatal meconium ileus. California Med 103:171–174, 1965.

Holsclaw DS, Eckstein HB, Nixon HH: Meconium ileus. Am J Dis Child 109:101–112, 1965.

Noblett HR: Treatment of uncomplicated meconium ileus by Gastrografin enema: A preliminary report. J Pediat Surg 4:190–197, 1969.

Thomaidis TS, Arey JB: The intestinal lesion in cystic fibrosis of the pancreas. J Pediat 63:444–453, 1963.

HIRSCHSPRUNG'S DISEASE

Hirschsprung's disease (aganglionic megacolon) is due to absence of the parasympathetic myenteric nervous plexuses in the lower portion of the colon or sometimes even in the entire organ. The aganglionic rectum and colon produce a functional obstruction because the bowel does not have normal propulsive waves and contracts en masse in response to distention. Short segment aganglionosis involving only the terminal rectum occurs in about 10% of instances. The disease extends to the sigmoid colon in 65% of cases. In 10%, more proximal colon is involved, and in 10–15% of cases the entire colon lacks ganglion cells. Extensive involvement of the small bowel is rare.

Males are affected 5 times more frequently than

females in cases where the involvement is of the usual length. Females tend to have longer aganglionic segments. A familial association occurs in 5–10% of cases—more frequently when females are affected. The length of involvement tends to be consistent in familial cases. Other anomalies are present also in 10–15% of patients.

Clinical Findings

A. Symptoms and Signs: The symptoms vary widely in severity but almost always occur shortly after birth. The infant passes little or no meconium within 24 hours. Thereafter, chronic or intermittent constipation usually occurs. Progressive abdominal distention, vomiting, reluctance to feed, listlessness, irritability, and poor growth and development follow. A rectal examination in the infant may be followed by expulsion of stool and flatus with remarkable decompression of abdominal distention. However, foul-smelling diarrhea and abdominal distention should be considered Hirschsprung's disease until proved otherwise. In older children, chronic constipation and abdominal distention are characteristic. Passage of flatus and stool requires great effort, and the stools are small in caliber. These children are sluggish, with wasted extremities and flared costal margins. Rectal examination in older children usually reveals a normal or contracted anus and a rectum without feces. Impacted stools can be palpated across the lower abdomen because of the greatly dilated and distended sigmoid colon.

B. Laboratory Findings: Definitive diagnosis is made by rectal biopsy. This requires removing a 1 × 2 cm full thickness strip of rectum from the posterior rectum proximal to the dentate line. A sample of this size is sufficient for the pathologist to determine whether ganglion cells are or are not present in Meissner's plexus or Auerbach's plexus.

C. X-Ray Findings: Plain abdominal x-rays in infants show dilated loops of bowel, but it is difficult to distinguish small and large bowel in infancy. A barium (in saline) enema x-ray should be performed. There should be no attempt to clean out the stool before barium enema, for this will obscure the change in caliber between aganglionic and ganglionic bowel. The barium enema may not show a transition zone in the first 6 weeks after birth since the liquid stool can pass the aganglionic bowel and the proximal intestine may not be dilated. The aganglionic segment appears relatively narrowed compared to the dilated proximal bowel. The proximal aganglionic intestine can be dilated by impacted stool or enema, giving a false impression of the level of the normal colon. Irregular, bizarre contractions which do not encircle the aganglionic portion of the bowel may also be recognized. The dilated proximal bowel may have circumferential, smooth, parallel contractions, similar in appearance to jejunum, which are exaggerated contraction waves. Contrast medium should not be refluxed much beyond the transition zone, for marked distention of the aganglionic area may conceal the diagnostic signs. Lateral x-rays should be taken of the pelvis to demonstrate the rectum, the transition zone, and the irregular contractions which may otherwise be obscured by the redundant sigmoid colon on anteroposterior views. X-ray examinations of the abdomen and lateral pelvis should be repeated after evacuation and 24–48 hours later. The barium will be retained for prolonged periods, and saline enemas may be required to evacuate it. The delayed film may show the transition zone and the bizarre irregular contractions more clearly than the initial study.

Differential Diagnosis

Low intestinal obstruction in the newborn infant may be due to rectal or colonic atresia, meconium plug syndrome, or meconium ileus. Hirschsprung's disease in patients who develop enterocolitis and diarrhea may mimic other causes of diarrhea. Chronic constipation due to functional causes may suggest Hirschsprung's disease. Although functional constipation may occur early in infancy, the stools are normal in caliber, soiling is frequent, and enterocolitis is not usually a problem. In functional constipation, stool is palpable in the lower rectum and a barium enema shows uniformly dilated bowel to the level of the anus. However, short segment Hirschsprung's disease may be difficult to differentiate, and rectal biopsy may be necessary. Segmental dilatation of the colon is a rare cause of constipation which may appear similar to Hirschsprung's disease.

Complications

The mortality rate of untreated aganglionic megacolon in infancy may be as high as 80%. Nonbacterial, nonviral enterocolitis is the principal cause of death. This putrefactive diarrhea tends to occur more frequently in infants but may appear at any age. The cause is not known but seems to be related to the high-grade partial obstruction. There is no correlation between the length of aganglionosis and the occurrence of enterocolitis. Perforation of the colon and appendix may result from the distal bowel obstruction. Atresia of the distal small bowel or colon also develops secondary to bowel obstruction due to Hirschsprung's disease in utero.

Following definitive surgical treatment (see below), anastomotic leak with perirectal and pelvic abscess is the most serious problem. This should be treated immediately by proximal colostomy until the anastomosis has healed. Necrosis of the pulled-through colon may occur if the bowel has not been mobilized sufficiently to prevent tension on the mesenteric blood supply. It is occasionally necessary to divide the inferior mesenteric artery. For this reason, a left transverse colostomy should be avoided (unless it is the position of the transition zone) because the collateral blood supply between the middle and left colic arteries may be divided.

Treatment

The large bowel obstruction and enterocolitis may be relieved initially by placing a large tube in the

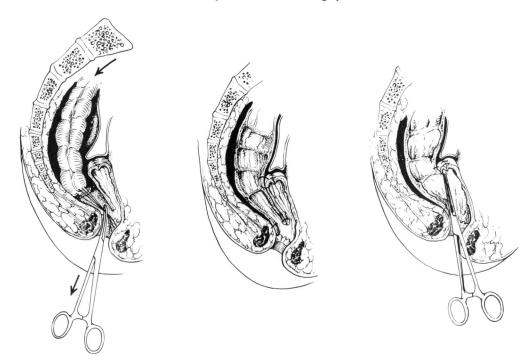

Duhamel abdominoperineal pull-through

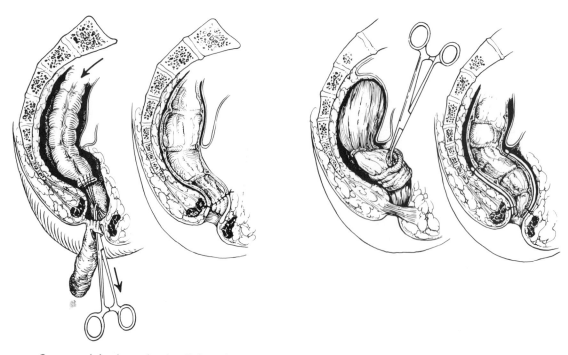

Swenson abdominoperineal pull-through

Soave endorectal pull-through

FIG 49–14. Three methods of surgical treatment of Hirschsprung's disease. (Reproduced, with permission, from Wilson JL: *Handbook of Surgery,* 4th ed. Lange, 1969.)

rectum and repeatedly washing out the colon contents with saline solution. Infants less than 1 year of age should have a preliminary colostomy. Conservative measures with enemas may not prevent further obstruction and enterocolitis. The colostomy should be placed at the transition zone, and the presence of ganglion cells at the colostomy site must be confirmed by frozen section biopsy. In total aganglionic colon, an ileostomy is necessary. Because loop colostomies tend to prolapse in infants, it is preferable to divide the bowel, close the distal end, and bring the proximal colon through by suturing the seromuscular portion of the bowel wall to all abdominal wall layers.

The definitive surgical procedure should be performed when the patient weighs about 9 kg. Long-term follow-up studies have documented the effectiveness of 4 operative procedures. Three are illustrated in Fig 49–14.

A. Swenson Operation: In the Swenson procedure, the overly dilated and aganglionic colon and rectum are excised to the mucocutaneous junction of the anus posteriorly and laterally, and to a more proximal level anteriorly. The transected end of the normally ganglionated bowel is sutured end-to-end with the distal anorectal segment.

B. Duhamel Operation: Both in the Duhamel and the Soave (see below) procedures, the overly dilated and aganglionic bowel is removed down to the rectum at the level of the pelvic peritoneal reflection. In the Duhamel operation, the proximal bowel is brought between the sacrum and the rectum and sutured end-to-side to the rectum above the dentate line. The intervening spur of rectum and bowel is crushed to form a side-to-side anastomosis.

C. Soave Operation: The Soave operation consists of dissecting the mucosa out of the residual rectal stump, pulling the proximal bowel through, and suturing it to the rectum just above the dentate line.

Prognosis

Although in the neonatal period the mortality rate is high in untreated infants, most patients who are properly treated for Hirschsprung's disease do very well. Problems with occasional incontinence and soiling may occur in a few cases. Episodic constipation and abdominal distention is more common since the aganglionic internal anal sphincter is intact. These patients respond to anal dilatation. Occasionally, an internal sphincterotomy may be necessary. Smaller children may still develop enterocolitis after definitive treatment, and they should be vigorously treated with a large rectal tube and enemas.

Asch MJ & others: Total colon aganglionosis: Report of nine cases. Arch Surg 105:74–78, 1972.

Boley SJ & others: Endorectal pull-through procedure for Hirschsprung's disease with and without primary anastomosis. J Pediat Surg 3:258–262, 1968.

deLorimier AA, Benzian SA, Gooding CA: Segmental dilatation of the colon. Am J Roentgenol 152:100–104, 1971.

Hyde GA, deLorimier AA: Colon atresia and Hirschsprung's disease. Surgery 64:976–978, 1968.

Lynn HB: Rectal myomectomy for aganglionic megacolon. Mayo Clin Proc 41:289–295, 1966.

Martin LW: Surgical management of Hirschsprung's disease involving the small intestine. Arch Surg 97:183–189, 1968.

INTUSSUSCEPTION

Telescoping of a segment of bowel (intussusceptum) into the adjacent segment (intussuscipiens) is the most common cause of intestinal obstruction in children under 2 years of age (Fig 49–15). The process of intussusception may result in gangrene of the intussusceptum. The terminal ileum is usually telescoped into the right colon, producing ileocolic intussusception, but ileoileal, ileoileocolic, jejunojejunal, and colocolic intussusceptions also occur. In 95% of infants and children, an obvious cause is not found. The most frequent occurrence is in midsummer and midwinter, and there is a positive correlation with adenovirus infections. In most cases, hypertrophied Peyer's patches are noted to be a leading edge. Causes such as Meckel's diverticulum, polyps, intramural hematoma (Henoch-Schönlein purpura), and intestinal lymphoma are identified with increasing frequency in patients over age 1. The ratio of males to females is 3:1. The peak age is in infants 5–9 months old; 80% of patients are less than 2 years old.

Clinical Findings

A. Symptoms and Signs: The typical patient is a healthy child who has a sudden onset of crying and doubles his knees up because of abdominal pain. The pain is intermittent, lasts for about 1 minute, and is followed by intervals of apparent well-being. Reflex

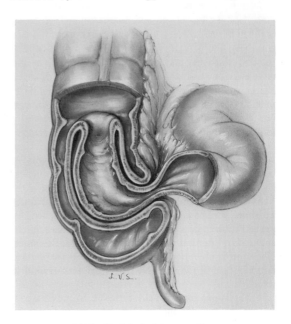

FIG 49–15. Intussusception.

vomiting is a frequent early sign, but vomiting due to bowel obstruction occurs later in the course. Blood and mucus produce a "currant jelly" stool. In small infants—and in postoperative patients—the colicky pain may not be apparent; these babies become withdrawn, and the most prominent symptom is vomiting. Pallor and sweating are common signs during colic. A mass is usually palpable along the distribution of the colon. A hollow right lower quadrant may be noted. Occasionally, the intussusception is palpable on rectal examination.

B. Laboratory Findings: The blood count usually shows polymorphonuclear leukocytosis and hemoconcentration.

C. X-Ray Findings: Intravenous administration of sodium pertechnetate Tc 99m and abdominal scanning may outline an intussusception. Plain films of the abdomen may demonstrate evidence of mechanical intestinal obstruction or a soft tissue mass. The diagnosis is usually established by barium enema.

Complications

Repeated vomiting and bowel obstruction will produce progressive dehydration. Prolonged intussusception produces edema and hemorrhagic or ischemic infarction of the intussusceptum. Delayed treatment of infarcted bowel may result in cardiovascular collapse and death.

Treatment

Initial efforts are concerned with correction of hypovolemia and dehydration. A cutdown or right atrial catheter is indicated for very sick patients. Expansion of blood volume with whole blood or albumin solution may be required. Barium enema should not be attempted until the patient has been resuscitated sufficiently so that he can tolerate an operative procedure. The baby should be sedated with meperidine, 1–2 mg/kg subcut, and secobarbital, 1–2 mg/kg orally. The enema bag must not be raised more than 75 cm above the patient, and under fluoroscopic control the barium enema may distend the intussuscipiens and reduce the intussusceptum in more than 50% of cases. If the initial enema is unsuccessful, it should be repeated 2 or 3 times following evacuation of the barium before reduction by enema can be considered a failure. Barium enema will not reduce gangrenous bowel.

Operation is required when there are signs of bowel perforation and peritonitis. If enema reduction has failed, the patient is explored through the right transverse lower abdominal incision. When no obvious gangrene is present, reduction is accomplished by gentle, retrograde compression of the intussuscipiens and not by traction on the proximal bowel. Resection of the intussusception is indicated if the bowel cannot be reduced or if the intestine is gangrenous. A Mikulicz resection may be necessary in critically ill patients.

The appendix is usually removed to prevent confusion about abdominal pain in later years when the patient has an abdominal incision.

Prognosis

Intussusception recurs in 2–4% of barium enema reductions and 1–2% of operative reductions. In the hands of an experienced surgeon, the mortality rate should approach zero. Deaths do occur if treatment of gangrenous bowel is delayed.

Frye RR, Howard WHR: The handling of ileocolic intussusception in a pediatric medical center. Radiology 97:187–191, 1970.

Levy JL Jr, Linder LH: Etiology of "idiopathic" intussusception in infants. South MJ 63:642–646, 1970.

Ravitch MM: *Intussusception.* Chap 56, pp 914–931, in: *Pediatric Surgery.* Mustard WT & others (editors). Year Book, 1969.

Stevenson EOS, Hays DM, Snyder WH: Post-operative intussusception in infants and children. Am J Surg 113:562–566, 1967.

DUPLICATIONS OF THE GASTROINTESTINAL TRACT

Duplications may occur at any point along the gastrointestinal tract from the mouth to the anus. Duplications occur (in order of decreasing frequency) in the ileum (50% of cases), mediastinum, colon, rectum, stomach, and neck. Intrathoracic and small bowel duplications are usually spherical. Colonic duplications are commonly long and tubular (Fig 49–16). Characteristically, the intra-abdominal duplications are within the mesentery and have a common wall with the intestine. Combined thoracoabdominal duplications also occur in which the thoracic saccular component extends through the esophageal hiatus or a separate diaphragmatic opening to empty into the duodenum or jejunum. Associated cardiovascular, neurologic, urologic, and gastrointestinal anomalies recur in more than a third of cases. A tract of the duplication may extend through the anomalous vertebrae into the spinal canal.

Clinical Findings

A. Symptoms and Signs: Two-thirds of patients with duplications are symptomatic in the first year of life. Duplications of the neck and mediastinum produce respiratory distress by compression of the airway. Thoracic duplications may also ulcerate into the lung and lead to pneumonia or hemoptysis. Intestinal duplications usually produce abdominal pain due to spastic contraction of the bowel, excessive distention of the duplication, or peptic ulceration resulting from ectopic gastric mucosa. Intestinal obstruction due to intussusception, volvulus, or encroachment on the lumen by an intramural cyst also occurs. An isolated asymptomatic mass may be the only finding. Peptic ulceration caused by ectopic gastric mucosa may produce massive gastrointestinal bleeding.

B. X-Ray Findings: X-ray studies include films of the chest and thoracolumbar spine, barium enema,

Bishop HC, Koop CE: Surgical management of duplications of the alimentary tract. Am J Surg 107:434–442, 1964.

Favara BE, Franchiosi RA, Akers DR: Enteric duplications. Thirty-seven cases: A vascular theory of pathogenesis. Am J Dis Child 122:501–506, 1971.

Forshall I: Duplication of the intestinal tract. Postgrad MJ 37:570–589, 1961.

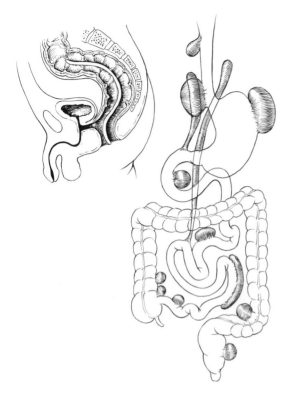

FIG 49–16. Duplications of the gastrointestinal tract. Duplications may be saccular or tubular. They usually arise within the mesentery, having a common wall with the intestine. Thoracoabdominal duplications arise from the duodenum or jejunum and extend through the diaphragm into the mediastinum.

esophagography, and gastrointestinal series. If an intraspinal extension of a duplication is suspected, a myelogram may be indicated.

Treatment

Duplications not intimately adherent to adjacent organs should be excised. Isolated spherical duplications can be excised with the adjacent segment of bowel and an end-to-end anastomosis of the bowel performed. Long tubular duplications can be decompressed by establishing an anastomosis between the proximal and distal ends of the adjacent bowel. Noncommunicating duplications, which would require radical resection of surrounding structures, should be drained by a Roux-en-Y technic. Duplications which cannot be removed completely and which contain gastric mucosa should be opened (without jeopardizing the blood supply of the normal bowel) and the mucosal lining excised. During resection of a mediastinal duplication, extension of the lesion into the spine and abdomen must be recognized and removed. An intra-abdominal extension is closed at the level of the diaphragm, and complete excision by laparotomy is accomplished at a later date.

OMPHALOMESENTERIC DUCT ANOMALIES

Omphalomesenteric or vitelline duct anomalies are remnants of the embryonic yolk sac. When the entire duct remains intact, it is recognized as an **omphalomesenteric fistula.** When the duct is obliterated at the intestinal end but communicates with the umbilicus at the distal end, it is called an **umbilical sinus.** When the epithelial tract persists but both ends are occluded, an umbilical cyst or intra-abdominal **enterocystoma** may develop. The entire tract may be obliterated, but a fibrous band may persist between the ileum and the umbilicus (Fig 49–17).

The most common remnant of the omphalomesenteric duct is Meckel's diverticulum, which is present in 1–3% of the population. Meckel's diverticulum may be lined wholly (or in part) by small intestinal, colonic, or gastric mucosa, and it may contain aberrant pancreatic tissue. Heterotopic tissue is found in 5% of asymptomatic and 60% of symptomatic cases. In contrast to duplications and pseudodiverticula, Meckel's diverticulum is located on the antimesenteric border of the ileum, 10–90 cm from the ileocecal valve.

Clinical Findings

Meckel's diverticulum is often asymptomatic and occurs as an incidental finding during operation for some other disease. Symptomatic omphalomesenteric remnants (male/female incidence 3:1) produce rectal bleeding in 40%, intussusception in 20%, diverticulitis or peptic perforation in 15%, umbilical fistula in 15%, intestinal obstruction in 7%, and abscess in 3%. Tumors such as carcinoids, leiomyomas, or leiomyosarcomas are very rare.

Rectal bleeding associated with Meckel's diverticulum is due to peptic ulceration of ectopic gastric mucosa. Over 50% of these patients are under 2 years of age. The blood is mixed with stool and is most often dark red or bright red; tarry stools are unusual. A history of a previous episode of bleeding may be elicited in 40% of cases. Occult bleeding from Meckel's diverticulum is very rare. Younger patients tend to bleed very briskly and may exsanguinate rapidly.

Diverticulitis or free perforation will present with abdominal pain and peritonitis identical to acute appendicitis. The pain and tenderness occur in the lower abdomen, most commonly near the umbilicus. An almost pathognomic sign is cellulitis of the umbilicus.

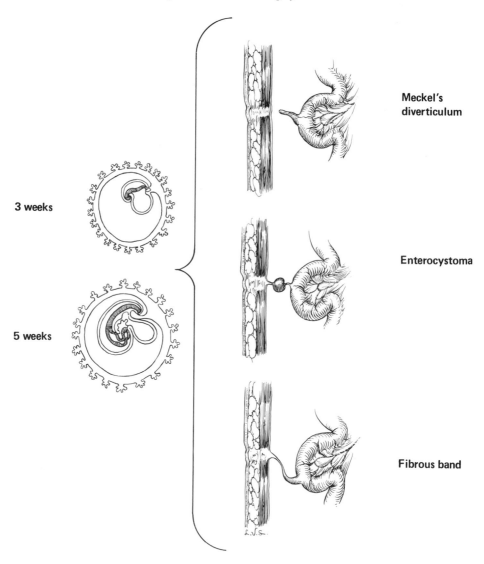

3 weeks

5 weeks

Meckel's
diverticulum

Enterocystoma

Fibrous band

FIG 49–17. Omphalomesenteric duct anomalies arise from the primitive yolk. Remnants include Meckel's diverticulum, enterocystoma, or a fibrous band or fistulous tract between the ileum and the umbilicus.

A mucoid, purulent, or enteric discharge and excoriation about the umbilicus characterizes an umbilical sinus or omphalomesenteric fistula. Recurrent cellulitis or deep abdominal wall abscess about the umbilicus also occurs.

Intestinal obstruction may develop as a result of volvulus of the bowel about a persistent band between the umbilicus and the ileum or as a result of herniation of bowel between the mesentery and a persistent vitelline or mesodiverticular vessel. Infarction of the incarcerated hernia not uncommonly occurs, disturbing the blood supply to a Meckel's diverticulum.

Treatment & Prognosis

After depleted blood volume has been restored and fluid and electrolyte disturbances have been corrected, the patient should be explored through a transverse abdominal incision. An omphalomesenteric remnant with a narrow base may be treated by amputation and closure of the bowel defect. In cases where the anomaly has a wide mouth with ectopic tissue or where an inflammatory or ischemic process involves the adjacent ileum, intestinal resection with the diverticulum and anastomosis may be necessary. Involvement of Meckel's diverticulum by tumor would require intestinal resection with the lymphatic pathways of the mesentery. Morbidity and mortality may increase if operation is delayed.

Rutherford RB, Akers DR: Meckel's diverticulum: A review of 148 pediatric patients, with special reference to the pattern of bleeding and to meso-diverticular bands. Surgery 59:618–626, 1966.

Weinstein EC, Cain JC, ReMine WH: Meckel's diverticulum: Fifty-five years of clinical and surgical experience. JAMA 182:251–253, 1962.

ANORECTAL ANOMALIES

Anomalies of the anus result from abnormal growth and fusion of the embryonic anal hillocks. The rectum has usually developed normally, and the sphincter mechanism, consisting of the internal anal muscle, the puborectalis muscle, and the external sphincter, is usually intact. With proper treatment, the sphincter will function normally. Anal agenesis is an exception to this because the internal sphincter may be deficient.

Anomalies of the rectum develop as a result of faulty division of the cloaca into the urogenital sinus and rectum by the urorectal septum. In anomalies of the high type, the internal sphincter has not formed and the external sphincter is hypoplastic and does not serve as a functional sphincter following surgical repair.

Classification

A. Low Anomalies: In the low (translevator) anomalies, the rectum has traversed the puborectalis portion of the levator ani muscle (Fig 49–18). The anus may be in the normal position, with a narrow outlet due to stenosis or an anal membrane. There may be no opening in the perineum, but the skin at the anal area is heaped up and may extend as a band in the perineal raphe completely covering and occluding the anal opening. More commonly, the covering of the anus is incomplete because of a small fistula that extends from the anus anteriorly to open in the raphe of the perineum, scrotum, or penis in the male or the vulva in the female. Finally, the anus may be ectopically placed anterior to the normal position.

B. Intermediate Anomalies: In the intermediate anomaly the bowel extends to the puborectalis muscle but either ends blindly or has a fistula between the rectum and the bulbous urethra in the male or the low vagina in the female. Another form consists of stenosis of the anorectal junction.

C. High Anomalies: In the high (supralevator) anomalies, the bowel ends above the puborectalis muscle, which is contracted against the urethra in the male and the vagina in the female (Fig 49–l8). The bowel may end blindly, but more commonly there is a fistula to the urethra or bladder in the male or the upper vagina in the female. Communication may be directly to the bladder in the female, and the fistula extends between the 2 halves of a bicornuate uterus. In females, the cloaca is an anomaly consisting of a short urethra with a urethrovaginal fistula and a rectovaginal fistula.

Clinical Findings

A. Signs: The most important means of establishing the type of anorectal anomaly is by physical examination. In low anomalies, an ectopic opening from the rectum can be detected in the perineal raphe in males or in the lower vagina, vestibule, or fourchette in females. An intermediate or high anomaly exists when meconium is found at the urethral meatus, in the urine, or in the upper vagina.

B. X-Ray Findings: X-rays are useful when the clinical impression is unclear. After the infant has had enough time to swallow an adequate amount of air (at least 8–10 hours), he should be placed upside down for more than 5 minutes to allow the air to displace the meconium in the distalmost rectum. A lateral x-ray is then centered over the greater trochanter with the baby upside down and his legs straight. A lead marker may be placed in the anal dimple, but measurement between this and the level of the rectum is not sufficient to demonstrate the type of anomaly. When a line is drawn on the x-ray film from a point just below the superior pubic ramus to the last sacral vertebra (the pubococcygeal line), the highest level of the puborectalis portion of the levator ani is outlined. A line through the lowest level of the ischial bone and parallel to the pubococcygeal line describes the lower level of the puborectalis muscle. When air in the rectum ends above the lower line, the anomaly may be the high type; when it ends below the line, it is probably a low anomaly. This method is inaccurate because the air may not have completely displaced the meconium, giving a falsely high impression; or the infant may cry or strain, so that the puborectalis muscle and rectum may actually descend below the ischium, giving a falsely low diagnosis. Gas in the bladder clearly indicates a rectourinary fistula. Anomalies of the vertebrae and the urinary tract occur in two-thirds of patients with high (rectal) atresia and in one-third of male patients with low (anal) atresia. Vertebral anomalies in females invariably indicate a high or intermediate anomaly.

Complications

Delay in the diagnosis of imperforate anus may result in excessive large bowel distention and perforation of the cecum.

Associated anomalies are frequent and include the following: esophageal atresia, anomalies of the gastrointestinal tract, agenesis of one or more sacral vertebrae (agenesis of S1, S2, or S3 is associated with comparable neurologic deficit, resulting in neurogenic bladder and greatly impaired continence), genitourinary anomalies, and anomalies of the heart and lungs.

The presence of a rectourinary fistula allows reflux of urine into the rectum and colon, and absorption of ammonium chloride may cause acidosis. Colon contents will reflux into the urethra, bladder, and upper tracts, producing recurrent pyelonephritis. A divided right transverse colostomy rather than a loop colostomy will prevent this until the fistula can be closed at a later date.

Treatment

A. Low Anomalies: Low anomalies are usually repaired from the perineal approach in the newborn. The anteriorly placed anal opening is mobilized to the level of the levator ani and transferred to the normal position. After healing, the anal opening must be

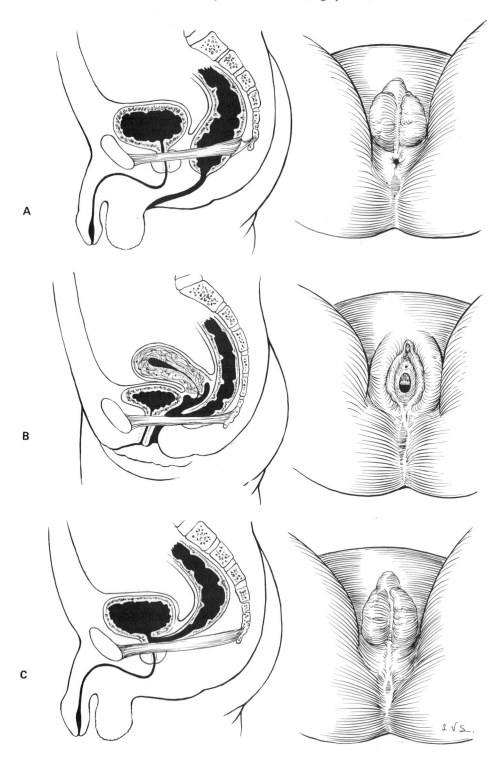

FIG 49–18. Three types of anorectal anomalies. *A:* Translevator anal atresia with anoperineal fistula. *B:* Supra-levator anorectal atresia with rectovaginal fistula. *C:* Supralevator anorectal atresia with rectourethral fistula.

dilated daily for 6−8 months to prevent stricture and to allow for growth.

B. Intermediate and High Anomalies: These should be treated by preliminary right transverse colostomy. If there is doubt about the diagnosis of a high or low anomaly, it is better to perform a colostomy than to attempt a perineal repair and have the anomaly prove to be a high one. The colostomy should be divided to prevent movement of stool into the distal loop, producing recurrent urinary tract infection. After the baby gains to approximately 9 kg, the definitive abdominoperineal pull-through procedure, in which the distal colon is brought anterior to the puborectalis muscle and sutured to the perineum, can be performed. It is important to preserve the afferent and efferent portion of the defecation reflex arc as well as the existing sphincter muscles.

In the high and intermediate anomalies, the external anal sphincter is inadequate and the internal sphincter is absent. Therefore, continence is dependent upon a functioning puborectalis muscle.

Surgical complications include damage to the nervi erigentes with poor bladder and bowel control and failure of erection. Division of rectourethral fistula some distance from the fistula may serve as a pocket for recurrent infection and stone formation, and cutting the fistula too short may result in urethral stricture. Erroneously attempting to repair a high anomaly from the perineal approach will leave a persistent rectourinary fistula. An abdominoperineal pull-through procedure performed for a low type of anomaly will invariably produce an incontinent patient who might otherwise have had an excellent prognosis.

Prognosis

Most patients with imperforate anus also have constipation as an inherent part of the disease. This is fortunate for individuals who have defective sphincter control but requires considerable attention to prevent obturant obstruction. Patients with low anomalies usually have good fecal control. Children with high anomalies do not have an internal sphincter which provides continuous, unconscious, and unfatiguing control against soiling. However, in the absence of a lower spine anomaly, perception of rectal fullness, ability to distinguish between flatus and stool, and conscious voluntary control of rectal discharge by contraction of the puborectalis muscle can be accomplished. When the stools become liquid, sphincter control is usually impaired in patients with high and intermediate anomalies.

Berdon WE & others: The radiologic evaluation of imperforate anus. Radiology 90:466−471, 1968.

Stephens FD, Smith ED: *Ano-Rectal Malformations in Children.* Year Book, 1971.

NEONATAL JAUNDICE, BILIARY ATRESIA, & HEPATITIS

Jaundice in the first week of infancy is usually due to indirect (unconjugated) hyperbilirubinemia. The causes include (1) "physiologic jaundice" due to immaturity of hepatic function; (2) Rh, ABO, and rarer blood group incompatibilities, producing hemolysis; and (3) infections.

Jaundice that persists beyond the first week is due to elevated indirect and conjugated bilirubin levels and presents difficult problems in diagnosis and treatment. The most frequent cause (60%) of prolonged jaundice in infancy is biliary atresia; various forms of hepatitis occur in 35%; and choledochal cyst is found in 5% of cases of obstructive jaundice.

Extrahepatic biliary atresia is the absence of patent bile ducts draining the liver. Biliary atresia is probably not congenital but acquired after birth because no cases have been described in autopsies of newborn infants. Furthermore, conjugated bilirubin is not cleared by the placenta as unconjugated bilirubin is, and jaundice due to conjugated hyperbilirubinemia with biliary obstruction has not been recognized in newborn infants. The atretic ducts consist of solid fibrous cords which may contain occasional islands of biliary epithelium. The extent of duct involvement varies greatly.

In the only surgically correctable form of biliary atresia, the common bile duct or the gallbladder (or both) is obliterated but the common hepatic duct and intrahepatic ducts are patent (5%).

In infants with extrahepatic biliary atresia, the liver develops progressive periportal fibrosis and the liver cords eventually become disrupted by the cirrhotic process. Proliferation of the bile canaliculae, containing inspissated bile, and lakes of extravasated bile may also be noted.

Intrahepatic biliary atresia is very rare. The extrahepatic bile ducts are patent, but repeated liver biopsy shows progressive disappearance of the intrahepatic portal ducts. Cirrhosis is not a prominent finding, and these patients may live for 3−5 years with persistent or intermittent jaundice.

Biliary hypoplasia has been described as a distinct entity causing jaundice in which the bile ducts are very small. A more likely explanation is that these cases represent hepatitis or intrahepatic biliary atresia in which the bile ducts are unused and therefore do not distend to normal size. In some cases, the bile ducts are very thickened and the lumen is very narrow. These patients were probably affected by the same process producing biliary atresia, but the lumen was not completely obliterated.

The infant who develops jaundice is usually full-term with an uneventful neonatal course. Jaundice is first noted in 2 or 3 weeks. He may have normal or clay-colored stools and dark urine. The stools contain an increased quantity of fat but are of normal consistency and not frothy. The liver may be of normal size early, but it becomes enlarged with time. The infant with surgical obstructive jaundice develops a hard liver as a consequence of progressive cirrhosis; patients with hepatitis have an enlarged liver of softer consistency. Splenomegaly usually develops in all forms of prolonged jaundice in infancy.

Liver function tests are of no help in distinguishing obstructive jaundice from medical jaundice in infants. The bilirubin levels may vary considerably from day to day. Serum transaminase levels are often high in all forms of jaundice, and the serum albumin decreases and serum globulin increases after 4 months in medical or surgical jaundice. Stool excretion of rose bengal sodium I 131 greater than 10% of an intravenous dose indicates patent bile ducts but does not rule out choledochal cyst; excretion of less than 10% occurs in patients with hepatitis as well as those with biliary atresia.

Needle biopsy of the liver may be safely performed at any age if the bleeding and clotting tests are normal. A diagnosis based on needle biopsy is accurate in 60%, equivocal in 16%, and erroneous in 24%. A diagnosis based on the combined results of abdominal exploration, cholangiography, and open liver biopsy is accurate in 98% of cases.

Differential Diagnosis

Other causes of obstructive jaundice are choledochal cyst, inspissated bile syndrome, and hepatitis. A choledochal cyst is identified by the presence of a palpable mass in the right upper quadrant and a gastrointestinal series showing indentation of the duodenum. Inspissated bile syndrome follows a hemolytic process in which a large bilirubin load is excreted into the bile ducts, where it becomes coalesced and impacted. This is recognized by cholangiography.

Hepatitis is most commonly of unknown cause but may be due to a variety of infections, often of maternal origin.

Complications

Delayed treatment of patients with correctable forms of biliary atresia will result in progressive cirrhosis. However, operative exploration may increase the risk of progressive cirrhosis in patients with neonatal hepatitis. As a general rule, severe grades of hepatic fibrosis take 3 months to develop in infants with biliary atresia, whereas the jaundice usually clears during this interval in some infants with hepatitis. Therefore, surgical exploration for neonatal jaundice is usually delayed until the age of 6 weeks. If the liver of a jaundiced infant becomes hard, some form of mechanical obstructive jaundice is probably present and operative exploration should not be further delayed.

Treatment

Preoperative care includes correction of anemia and administration of intravenous glucose and K vitamins. The operation should be scheduled in the morning so that the infant will be on a "nothing by mouth" regimen no longer than 6 hours. X-ray facilities should be made ready in the operating room, and the anesthetic period is made as short as possible. Through a transverse abdominal incision, the gallbladder should be located and cannulated. Diatrizoate (Hypaque) diluted to 25% should be gently instilled into the biliary tree, taking care to prevent pressure which might disrupt the bile ducts. If x-rays show a patent common duct but no reflux into the liver, a rubber-shod bulldog clamp may be placed on the distal common duct and the cholangiogram repeated. During development of the x-ray films, a wedge of liver is obtained for biopsy. If atresia of the bile duct is found, the hilus of the liver must be carefully explored with the hope of finding a patent common hepatic duct which communicates with normal intrahepatic ducts. When this is found, a Roux-en-Y choledocho- or hepaticojejunostomy is performed and a tube stent is inserted through the anastomosis. Excision of fibrous cords and hilar tissue anterior to the portal vessels, followed by Roux-en-Y jejunostomy to the perihilar liver capsule, has been curative (portojejunostomy).

Patients with uncorrectable atresia will develop progressive ascites, making their care difficult; they eat poorly and become rapidly wasted. Palliation of ascites can be achieved by diuretics or by a peritoneal to right atrial shunt via the saphenofemoral vein and inferior vena cava, using Silastic tubing and a valve. The only hope for patients with uncorrectable biliary atresia is liver transplantation.

Choledochal cysts are best handled by cystduodenostomy or -jejunostomy.

Prognosis

Patients with correctable forms of atresia may do very well. Cholangitis occurs frequently, related to anastomotic stricture or bile duct fibrosis with peripheral bile duct abscesses. Reexploration and revision of the anastomosis should be performed in these instances. Preliminary jejunal diversion by an isolated skin jejunostomy loop may prevent cholangitis and sepsis in young infants with significant cirrhosis. The average life span for infants with uncorrectable biliary atresia is 19 months. Death is due to progressive liver failure, bleeding from esophageal varices, or sepsis.

Bennett DE: Problems in neonatal obstructive jaundice. Pediatrics 33:735–748, 1964.

deLorimier AA: Current concepts: Surgical treatment of neonatal jaundice. New England J Med 288:1284–1286, 1973.

Hays DM & others: Diagnosis of biliary atresia: Relative accuracy of percutaneous liver biopsy, open liver biopsy and operative cholangiography. J Pediat 71:598–607, 1967.

Kasai M & others: Surgical treatment of biliary atresia. J Pediat Surg 3:665–675, 1965.

Schweitzer IL & others: Hepatitis and hepatitis-associated antigen in 56 mother-infant pairs. JAMA 220:1092–1095, 1972.

Smetana HF, Edlow JB, Glunz PR: Neonatal jaundice: A critical review of persistent obstructive jaundice in infancy. Arch Path 80:553–574, 1965.

ABDOMINAL WALL DEFECTS

1. INGUINAL HERNIA & HYDROCELE

The processus vaginalis remains patent in over 80% of newborn infants. With increasing age, the incidence of patent processus vaginalis diminishes. At 2 years, 40–50% are open, and in adults 25% are persistently patent. Actual herniation of bowel into a widely patent processus vaginalis develops in 1–4% of children; 45% occur within the first year of life. Indirect inguinal hernia occurs 8 times more frequently in males. Direct and femoral hernias occur in children but are very rare.

Clinical Findings

The diagnosis of hernia in infants and children can be made only by the demonstration of an inguinal bulge originating from the internal ring. The bulge often cannot be elicited at will, and signs such as a large external ring, the "silk glove" sign, and thickening of the cord are not dependable. Under these circumstances, a reliable history alone may be sufficient. Hernias are found on the right side in 60% of cases, on the left side in 25%, and bilaterally in 15%. Bilateral hernias are more frequent in premature infants. The processus vaginalis may be obliterated at any location proximal to the testis or labium. When the bowel herniates into the scrotum, it is called complete indirect inguinal hernia; when it extends to a level proximal to the testis in the male or the external ring in the female, it is an incomplete inguinal hernia.

Incarcerated inguinal hernia accounts for approximately 10% of childhood hernias, and the incidence is highest in infants. In 45% of females with incarcerated hernia, the contents of the sac consist of various combinations of ovary, tube, and uterus. These structures are usually a sliding component of the sac.

Hydroceles almost always represent peritoneal fluid trapped in a patent processus vaginalis; hence, they are commonly called communicating hydroceles. A hydrocele is characteristically an oblong, nontender, soft mass that transilluminates with light.

Differential Diagnosis

A hydrocele under tension is often confused with incarcerated inguinal hernia. Transillumination of the scrotum or groin with a flashlight distinguishes fluid from bowel. The sudden appearance of fluid confined to the testicular area may represent a noncommunicating hydrocele secondary to torsion of the testis or testicular appendage, or to epididymo-orchitis. Rectal examination and palpation of the peritoneal side of the inguinal ring may distinguish an incarcerated hernia from a hydrocele or other inguinoscrotal mass.

Complications

Failure to treat an inguinal hernia in infancy shortly after the diagnosis has been made may allow the hernia to become incarcerated and subsequently strangulated. About a third of incarcerated inguinal hernias in infancy show evidence of strangulation, and in 5% of cases the bowel is gangrenous. Compression of the spermatic vessels by an incarcerated hernia may produce hemorrhagic infarction of a testicle.

Treatment

Inguinal hernia in infancy and childhood should be repaired soon after diagnosis. In premature infants under constant surveillance in the hospital, hernia repair may be deferred until the baby is strong enough to be discharged home. Ordinarily, high ligation and excision of the hernia sac at the internal ring is all that is required. When there is a large internal ring, it may be necessary to narrow the internal ring with sutures placed in the transversalis fascia, but use of abdominal muscle for repair is unnecessary.

An incarcerated hernia in an infant can usually be reduced initially before operation. This is accomplished by sedation with meperidine, 2 mg/kg IM, and secobarbital, 2 mg/kg IM, and by elevating the foot of the bed to keep intra-abdominal pressure from being exerted against the inguinal area. When the infant is well sedated, the hernia may be reduced by gentle pressure over the internal ring in a manner that milks the bowel into the abdominal cavity. During this time, nasogastric suction and intravenous fluid replacement should be started. If the bowel is not reduced after a few hours, operation is required. If the hernia is reduced, operative repair may be delayed for 24 hours to allow edema in the tissues to subside. It is not necessary to delay repair in females, in whom there is no risk of injuring the vas deferens or spermatic vessels. Bloody stools and edema and red discoloration of the skin around the groin suggest strangulated hernia, and reduction of the bowel should not be attempted. Emergency repair of incarcerated inguinal hernia is technically difficult because the edematous tissues are friable and tear readily. When gangrenous intestine is encountered, the hemorrhagic fluid in the sac should be prevented from entering the abdominal cavity. The gangrenous bowel should be resected and an end-to-end intestinal anastomosis performed. Black, hemorrhagic discoloration of the testis or ovary does not require excision of the gonad.

Fonkalsrud EW, deLorimier AA, Clatworthy HW: Femoral and direct inguinal hernias in infants and children. JAMA 192:597–599, 1965.

Holcomb GW: Routine bilateral inguinal hernia repair. Am J Dis Child 109:114–120, 1965.

Nyhus LM, Harkins HN: *Hernia.* Lippincott, 1964.

Rowe MI, Clatworthy HW: Incarcerated and strangulated hernias in children. Arch Surg 101:136–139, 1970.

2. UMBILICAL HERNIA

A fascial defect at the umbilicus is frequently present in the newborn, particularly in premature infants. The incidence is higher in blacks. In most children, the umbilical ring progressively diminishes in size and eventually closes. Fascial defects less than 1 cm in diameter spontaneously close by the age of 6 years in 95% of cases. When the fascial defect is greater than 1 cm in diameter, only 40% close spontaneously. Protrusion of bowel through the umbilical defect rarely results in incarceration. Surgical repair is not indicated unless the intestine becomes incarcerated or unless the fascial defect persists after the age of 4 or 5 years

Walker SH: The natural history of umbilical hernia. Clin Pediat 6:29–32, 1967.

3. OMPHALOCELE

Omphalocele is a very rare defect of the periumbilical abdominal wall in which the coelomic cavity is covered only by peritonium and amnion. More than half of these babies are born prematurely. The omphalocele may contain small and large bowel, liver, spleen, stomach, pancreas, and bladder. The abdominal musculature is usually well developed, but the "prune belly" syndrome, with absence of abdominal muscles, occurs occasionally.

Treatment

Omphaloceles with small abdominal defects can be treated by excising the omphalocele sac and by reapproximating the abdominal wall muscles and skin edges. Because of the high mortality rate with the surgical treatment of omphaloceles greater than 8 cm in diameter, nonoperative management is advised. The membrane becomes vascularized beneath the eschar, and over a period of time contraction of the wound and skin growth will occur over the granulating portion of the omphalocele.

Prognosis

The survival rate for infants with the fetal type of omphalocele is excellent since the lesion is easily repaired. The mortality rate following surgical correction of large omphaloceles is over 50%. When the conservative approach is used, the mortality rate is less than 10%.

Firor HV: Omphalocele—and appraisal of therapeutic approaches. Surgery 69:208–214, 1971.
Schuster SR: A new method for the staged repair of large omphaloceles. Surg Gynec Obst 125:837–850, 1967.

4. GASTROSCHISIS

Gastroschisis is a rare defect in the abdominal wall which usually is to the right of a normal insertion of the umbilical cord. It is probably produced by rupture of the embryonic umbilical sac in utero. The remnants of the amnion are usually reabsorbed. The skin may continue to grow over the remnants of the amnion, and there may be a bridge of skin between the defect and the cord. The small and large bowel herniate through the abdominal wall defect. Having been bathed in the amnionic fluid, the bowel wall has a very thick, shaggy membrane covering it. The loops of intestine are usually matted together, and the intestine appears to be abnormally short.

Complications

Since the bowel has not been contained intraabdominally, the abdominal cavity fails to enlarge and cannot accommodate the protuberant bowel. Over 70% of the infants are premature, and associated anomalies are frequent. Nonrotation of the midgut is present. Intestinal atresia occurs frequently because segments of intestine which have herniated through the defect become infarcted in utero.

Treatment & Prognosis

Initially, the bowel should be covered by forming a tube from silicone-coated fabric and incorporating the protuberant bowel into the tube. The end of the tube is tied off and suspended from an incubator top. As edema and shaggy membrane of the protuberant intestine are absorbed, the bowel will spontaneously reduce into the abdominal cavity. Reduction is aided by tying the protuberant end of the tube adjacent to the bowel each day. When the bowel has completely returned within the abdomen, the silicone-coated tube is removed and the abdominal wall is closed in layers. A gastrostomy is valuable in the postoperative care of the baby.

The mortality rate for infants with gastroschisis has been greatly reduced by this technic.

Allen RG, Wrenn EL: Silon as a sac in the treatment of omphalocele and gastroschisis. J Pediat Surg 4:3–8, 1969.

TUMORS IN CHILDHOOD

1. NEUROBLASTOMA

Of all childhood neoplasms, neuroblastoma is exceeded only by leukemia and brain tumors in frequency. Two-thirds of cases occur within the first 5 years of life. This tumor is of neural crest origin and may originate anywhere along the distribution of the sympathetic chain. Neuroblastomas originate in the retroperitoneal area in 65% of cases; 40% arise from the adrenal gland. The biologic behavior varies with the age of the patient, the site of primary origin, and the extent of the disease.

Clinical Findings

The most common finding is the presence of a mass, which may be primary or metastatic. Nonspecific symptoms include vomiting, diarrhea, constipation, weight loss, and fever. In infants, metastases confined to the liver or subcutaneous fat are very frequent and bone metastases are unusual. In older children, metastases to lymph nodes and bone are found in over 70% of cases at diagnosis. Pain in areas of bony involvement and joints with associated myalgia and fever suggest rheumatic fever. Hypertension may occur. Abdominal neuroblastoma may be distinguished from other tumors by the hard, irregular surface of the tumor and the tendency to cross the midline. X-ray films show a soft tissue mass displacing surrounding structures, and calcification is present in 45% of tumors. For retroperitoneal tumors, an intravenous urogram shows displacement or compression of the adjacent kidney without distortion of the renal calyces. Chest x-ray, complete bone survey, and bone marrow aspiration for histologic examination are indicated because of the frequency of bony metastases. About 70% of neuroblastomas produce norepinephrine and its metabolites. The breakdown products of excess norepinephrine production, vanilmandelic acid (VMA), and homovanillic acid (HVA) should be measured in urine specimens at intervals so that the clinical course of the patient can be followed.

Treatment

A localized neuroblastoma should be excised and the local area of the tumor should be irradiated. Unresectable neuroblastomas should be treated initially by radiation therapy and surgical resection performed for residual tumor. Most neuroblastomas are radiosensitive and respond to 3000 rads or less of radiation. Patients with disseminated disease should be treated with chemotherapeutic agents such as cyclophosphamide (Cytoxan), 5–10 mg/kg/day IV for 10 days, repeated every 6 weeks, or 2–5 mg/kg/day orally. Vincristine (Oncovin), 0.03–0.05 mg/kg IV once a week, may be given simultaneously or alternately with cyclophosphamide. Excessive x-ray therapy and chemotherapy must be avoided.

Prognosis

Of the patients that die from neuroblastoma, 92% do so within 14 months after diagnosis. The overall 2-year survival rate for infants less than 1 year old is almost 60%; for children older than 2 years, it is less than 10%. For infants with tumor confined to the site of primary origin or with adjacent regional spread, the cure rate is greater than 80%; the 2-year survival rate with distant metastases to the liver and subcutaneous fat is close to 100%. Cure of neuroblastoma in older children is frequent for localized disease and rare if regional or distant metastasis has occurred.

Spontaneous regression of neuroblastoma probably occurs more frequently (5%) in patients with neuroblastoma than with any other neoplasm. However, spontaneous regression occurs only in patients under 2 years of age.

D'Angio GJ, Evans AE, Koop CE: Special pattern of widespread neuroblastoma with a favorable prognosis. Lancet 1: 1046–1049, 1971.

deLorimier AA, Bragg KU, Linden G: Neuroblastoma in childhood. Am J Dis Child 118:441–450, 1969.

2. NEPHROBLASTOMA (WILMS'S TUMOR)

With rare exceptions, this tumor arises within the capsule of the kidney and consists of a variety of epithelial and sarcomatous cell types such as abortive tubules and glomeruli, smooth and skeletal muscle fibers, spindle cells, cartilage, and bone. Hence, the tumor is also called embryoma, carcinosarcoma, and mixed tumor of the kidney. Eighty percent of patients are under 4 years of age. Bilateral tumors occur in 5–10% of cases. Metastases occur most commonly in the liver and lungs, and rarely in the brain and bones. Nephroblastoma accounts for 8% of childhood malignancies.

Clinical Findings

Symptoms consist of abdominal enlargement in 60% of cases, pain in 20%, hematuria in 15%, malaise, weakness, anorexia, and weight loss in 10%, and fever in 3% of patients. An abdominal mass is palpable in almost all cases. The mass is usually very large, firm, and smooth and does not ordinarily extend across the midline. Hypertension is noted in more than 50% of patients and may be sufficient to produce congestive heart failure. Aniridia, hemihypertrophy, hypospadias, cryptorchidism, and urinary anomalies are frequently associated. An intravenous urogram shows distortion of the calyces and kidney. Nonvisualization on the urogram indicates tumor extension into the ureter or renal vessels. Cystoscopy and retrograde urograms are not necessary. Renal arteriograms are helpful in differentiating retroperitoneal tumors and in detecting small or bilateral nephroblastomas. An inferior venacavagram may show obstruction of the vena cava, but it does not differentiate compression from tumor invasion.

Differential Diagnosis

Abdominal masses may be caused by hydronephrotic, multicystic, or duplicated kidneys, neuroblastoma, teratoma, hepatoma, and rhabdomyosarcoma as well as nephroblastoma. An intravenous urogram distinguishes nephroblastoma from these other tumors because calyceal distortion indicates intrarenal origin of the tumor. Calcification occurs in 10% of cases of nephroblastoma and tends to be more cres-cent-shaped, discrete, and peripherally located, whereas the calcification of neuroblastoma is finely stippled.

Complications

The tumor can extend into the renal vein and inferior vena cava. These vessels should be carefully palpated during abdominal exploration, and the tumor should be removed in such a way that tumor embolus will not occur.

Treatment

The preferred treatment is immediate nephrec-tomy and excision of all the surrounding tissues within Gerota's fascia, followed by radiation therapy to the tumor bed. Very large tumors should be treated with radiation therapy preoperatively to reduce the size of the tumor. A significant reduction in size usually occurs in 7–10 days, after which nephrectomy is read-ily performed. Nephrectomy is accomplished through an abdominal or thoracoabdominal incision, and the renal artery and vein are divided before any other dis-section is performed. Dactinomycin (Cosmegen) should be given with preoperative x-ray treatment or intraoperatively if x-ray therapy does not precede nephrectomy. The course of dactinomycin should be repeated in 6 weeks and every 3 months thereafter for 2 years. Vincristine (Oncovin) is also effective and less toxic, but it does not have the radiomimetic effect of dactinomycin.

Metastases develop in 30% of patients who had none at diagnosis. Solitary metastases in the lung should be resected. Hepatic metastases and multiple pulmonary metastases should be irradiated. Any resid-ual tumor following radiation therapy—including mul-tiple lesions—should be resected.

Bilateral nephroblastoma occurs in 3–10% of cases. X-ray therapy followed by radical nephrectomy on one side and partial nephrectomy, if possible, on the contralateral side is preferred. Radioresistant tumors which diffusely involve both kidneys require bilateral radical nephrectomy and kidney transplanta-tion.

Prognosis

Of those patients that die of nephroblastoma, 98% die within 2 years following treatment. Nephrec-tomy and x-ray therapy alone or with one course of dactinomycin provide a cure rate of 50% at best. When sequential dactinomycin is used, the survival rate is greater than 80%. When pulmonary or hepatic metas-tases are present at diagnosis, the survival rate follow-ing combined treatment with surgery, x-ray therapy, and chemotherapy is 50%.

deLorimier AA & others: Treatment of bilateral Wilms' tumor. Am J Surg 122:275–280, 1971.
Wolff JA & others: Single versus multiple dose dactinomycin therapy of Wilms' tumor. New England J Med 279: 290–294, 1968.

3. TERATOMA

Teratomas are congenital neoplasms derived from all 3 basic germ cells of the early embryo. Sites of origin (in order of frequency) are the ovaries, testes, anterior mediastinum, presacral and coccygeal regions, and the retroperitoneum.

These tumors should be excised because of their malignant potential and the symptoms produced by their size. Some of the malignant tumors respond to x-ray therapy, and some metastatic lesions have regressed with combined cyclophosphamide, vin-cristine, and dactinomycin therapy.

Donnellan WA, Swenson O: Benign and malignant sacrococ-cygeal teratomas. Surgery 64:834–846, 1968.
Willis RA: *The Borderland of Embryology and Pathology.* Butterworths, 1962.

RHABDOMYOSARCOMA

Rhabdomyosarcomas are the third most common solid malignant tumor in children, exceeded only by neuroblastoma and Wilms's tumor. Embryonal rhabdo-myosarcoma occurs in infants and young children, and, when it develops in submucosal areas such as the blad-der, vagina, or nose, it develops multiple fleshy, grape-like excrescences called sarcoma botryoides.

Localized tumors should be resected with wide surgical margins. Rhabdomyosarcomas tend to recur locally and metastasize to regional lymph nodes. Pul-monary metastases frequently occur early in the course of the disease. Rhabdomyosarcomas arising in the head and neck are treated primarily by radiation therapy with good response.

Tumors developing in the genitourinary tract and extremities tend to be radioresistant and require radi-cal resection with or without postoperative radio-therapy. Because of the early and frequent occurrence of distant metastases, repeated courses of chemo-therapy may improve the survival rate. Cure rates of sarcoma botryoides may be as high as 60%; survival from orbital tumor is approximately 75%; tumors in other areas of the head, neck, and extremities have a cure rate of 20%. Genitourinary rhabdomyosarcoma in males has a poorer prognosis than in females. The prog-nosis for infants and young children is better than for older patients.

Grosfeld JL, Clatworthy HW, Newton WA: Combined therapy in childhood rhabdomyosarcoma: An analysis of 42 cases. J Pediat Surg 4:637–645, 1969.
Sutow WW & others: Prognosis in childhood rhabdomyosar-coma. Cancer 25:1384–1390, 1970.

CONGENITAL DEFORMITIES
OF THE CHEST WALL
(Pectus Excavatum, Pectus Carinatum)

Anomalous development of the costal cartilages and sternum produces a variety of chest wall deformities. Failure of fusion of the 2 sternal bands during embryonic development produces congenital sternal cleft, which may involve the upper, lower, or entire sternum. This defect is usually associated with protrusion of the pericardium and heart (ectopia cordis) and congenital heart lesions.

Clinical Findings

Most children are noted to have the deformity at birth. In some cases, the defect does not occur until late childhood. Paradoxic motion in the area of the pectus excavatum is commonly seen in infants. The deformity may stabilize, but most progress in severity with age. The incidence in girls and boys is probably equal, but surgical consultation is requested 3–4 times more frequently in boys.

In pectus excavatum, the xiphoid is the deepest portion of the depression. The sternum curves posteriorly from the manubriosternal junction, although the manubrium may also be posteriorly directed. The costal cartilages, curving posteriorly to insert on the sternum, are deformed and fused. The third, fourth, and fifth ribs are usually affected, although the second through the eighth costal cartilages and ribs may be involved. The severity of the defect varies greatly from a mild, insignificant depression to an extreme where the xiphoid bone is adjacent to the vertebrae. Chest x-ray shows the posterior depression and displacement of the heart to the left. Angiocardiograms may show impingement of the sternum on the right atrium or ventricle.

These patients are typically round-shouldered, with stooped posture, potbelly, and an asthenic appearance. They tend to be withdrawn and refuse to participate in sports activities, particularly if their deformity might be exposed. Many patients complain of easy fatigability or inability to compete in exertional activities. Cardiopulmonary function studies show impaired stroke volume and cardiac output during upright exercise. Following repair, parents and children comment upon the great improvement in their well-being and exercise tolerance.

Treatment & Prognosis

The operation is performed both for cosmetic reasons and to improve cardiopulmonary function. Mild deformities should be left alone and the patient followed to observe for progression. Moderate to severe defects should be repaired, particularly when the patient or parent indicates a desire for improvement. The ideal age is 4–5 years. Operation in older children requires greater operative time, and a good result is easier to achieve in young children. Blood for transfusion should be available. Preoperatively, older children should be taught how to use a mechanical ventilator to assist in treating and preventing atelectasis postoperatively.

A stainless steel strut or Kirschner wire may be passed beneath the sternum and anchored by sutures to the fourth or fifth rib laterally on each side. This serves to ensure ideal position of the sternum and minimizes postoperative paradoxic motion and pain. The strut may be removed 6 or more months later.

The round-shouldered, slouched posture will persist postoperatively. A new acquired habit of maintaining an erect posture is established by using a T-brace fitted for the patient, which must be worn during waking hours for a minimum of 6 months. Exercises such as pull-ups and push-ups are initiated 3 weeks postoperatively.

Another technic, purely for improving cosmetic depression deformities, is to fill the space with a Silastic subcutaneous implant.

Removal of the defect improves vigor, endurance, and well-being.

Bieser GD & others: Impairment of cardiac function in patients with pectus excavatum, with improvement after operative correction. New England J Med 287:267–272, 1972.

Mason JK, Payne WS, Gonzales JB: Pectus excavatum: Use of preformed prosthesis for correction in the adult. Plast Reconstr Surg 46:399–402, 1970.

Polgar F, Koop CE: Pulmonary function in pectus excavatum. Pediatrics 32:209–215, 1963.

Ravitch MM: Congenital deformities of the chest wall. Pages 317–338 in: *Pediatric Surgery*, 2nd ed. Vol I. Mustard WT & others (editors). Year Book, 1969.

• • •

General References

Brown JJM: *Surgery of Childhood*. Williams & Wilkins, 1963.

Gans SL (editor): *Surgical Pediatrics*. Grune & Stratton, 1972.

Gans SL (editor): Symposium on surgical pediatrics. P Clin North America 16:529–766, 1969.

Gray SW, Skandalakis JE: *Embryology for Surgeons: The Embryological Basis for Treatment of Congenital Defects.* Saunders, 1972.

Gross RE: *The Surgery of Infancy and Childhood*. Saunders, 1953.

Mustard WT & others (editors): *Pediatric Surgery*, 2nd ed. Vol I and II. Year Book, 1969.

Norman AP (editor): *Congenital Abnormalities in Infancy.* Davis, 1971.

Rickham PP, Johnston JH: *Neonatal Surgery*. Appleton-Century-Crofts, 1969.

Swenson O: *Pediatric Surgery*. Appleton-Century-Crofts, 1969.

White JJ, Haller JA: Symposium on pediatric surgery. S Clin North America 50:753–952, 1970.

50 . . .

Oncology & Cancer Chemotherapy

Samuel D. Spivak, MD

In any given year, nearly 1 million Americans are under medical care for neoplastic disease and over 600,000 new cases are diagnosed. Cancer is responsible for about 17% of all deaths and (next to heart disease) is the second leading cause of death. The incidence of neoplasia by site and sex is shown in Table 50–1.

TABLE 50–1. Cancer incidence (in %) by site and sex.

	Male	Female
Skin	23%	13%
Oral	3	2
Lung	18	3
Breast	. . .	23
Colon and rectum	11	13
Other digestive	10	8
Prostate	10	. . .
Uterus	. . .	15
Urinary tract	7	3
Leukemia and lymphomas	7	6
All other	11	14

CLASSIFICATION OF TUMORS

Although the term tumor originally denoted any mass or swelling, the present meaning is now generally synonymous with neoplasm (a new pathologic growth of tissue). A neoplasm may be characterized as benign or malignant depending upon its histologic, gross, and clinical features. Malignant neoplasms usually show imperfect differentiation and structure atypical of the tissue of origin, an infiltrative growth pattern not contained by a true capsule, and relatively frequent and abnormal mitotic figures. Growth rarely ceases, although the rate of growth may be irregular, and many malignant tumors have a propensity for metastasis. Benign tumors generally lack these features, although they may be fatal as a result of impingement on other structures and impairment of function.

Neoplasms are classified according to their tissue of origin. Those from mesenchyme (muscle, bone, tendon, cartilage, fat, vessels, lymphoid, and connective tissue) are called sarcomas. Malignant tumors of epithelial origin are carcinomas and may be further classified, according to their histologic appearance, as adenocarcinomas (glandular), squamous (epidermoid), transitional, or undifferentiated. Tumors may be composed of one neoplastic cell type (although also containing nonneoplastic stromal elements such as blood vessels); may contain several neoplastic cell types of common derivation from the same germ cell layer (mixed tumors); or may derive from more than one embryonic germ cell layer (teratomas).

ETIOLOGIC FACTORS IN TUMOR FORMATION

Immunologic Disease & Cancer

Malignancy as a sequel to immunologic derangements has long been observed and is thought to represent a failure of immunity surveillance or ineffective immunity control. Neoplasms are more common when cell-mediated immunity is impaired, and some tumors have a distinctly better prognosis when lymphocytic infiltration of the tumor or regional nodes is noted histologically. Tumor-specific antigens are present in experimental animal tumors induced by chemicals and viruses. Human colon cancer contains carcinoembryonic antigens capable of eliciting an immunologic response. Recently, similar evidence has also been forthcoming for Burkitt's lymphoma, malignant melanoma, neuroblastoma, and osteosarcoma. Serum "blocking factors" which impair lymphocyte-mediated tumor inhibition have been demonstrated in patients with progressive, uncontrolled neuroblastoma and are absent in patients whose disease is controlled. Immunologic manipulations aimed at reconstituting host immune defenses are now being investigated, although no specific form of "immunotherapy" has yet been established as effective in the prevention or treatment of human neoplasms.

Smith RT: Possibilities and problems of immunologic intervention in cancer. New England J Med 287:439–450, 1972.

Zamcheck N & others: Immunologic evaluation of human digestive tract cancer: Carcinoembryonic antigens. New England J Med 286:83, 1972.

Chemical Oncogenesis

Chemical carcinogenesis induced by coal tars, aromatic amines, azo dyes, aflatoxins, or alkylators is a 2-stage phenomenon consisting of tumor initiation and subsequent neoplastic growth with a variable but distinct latent period between these 2 stages. Carcinogenesis requires cell proliferation once the malignant initiation phase has occurred. Carcinogens are dose-dependent, additive, and irreversible. According to the Huebner hypothesis of oncogenesis, carcinogens may activate the "oncogene" or may modify host RNA in such a way that faulty "reverse transcription" occurs in the Temin model (see below).

Ryser HJP: Chemical carcinogenesis. New England J Med 285:721, 1971.

Radiation Oncogenesis

Radiation oncogenesis is a complex process that appears to involve irreversible injury to chromosomes. The incidence of the spontaneous human neoplasms is increased by radiation, probably in proportion to its spontaneous incidence in the population at risk. The list includes chronic myelocytic leukemia, all forms of acute leukemia, malignant lymphomas, osteosarcoma, breast and lung carcinoma, and pancreatic, pharyngeal, thyroid, and colon carcinomas—ie, those neoplasia which account for 85% of human cancer morbidity and mortality are increased in populations exposed to radiation above background levels.

Gofman JW & others: Radiation, cancer, and environmental health. Hosp Practice 5:91, 1970.

Viral Oncogenesis

The contention that viruses may cause cancer in man rests mainly on analogous reasoning from observations in other species, particularly laboratory animals. Of the oncogenic DNA viruses, a human herpesvirus of major interest is the Epstein-Barr (EB) virus which was discovered by electron microscopy in cultured Burkitt's lymphoma cells and subsequently found in many isolates of Burkitt's lymphoma. Nasopharyngeal carcinoma has also been associated with EB virus, but the causal role in that illness is far from certain. A herpesvirus has also been associated with cancer of the uterine cervix, since more women so affected have viral antibodies than control populations.

Oncogenic RNA viruses (oncornaviruses) have recently been thought to cause some human cancers. An RNA tumor virus might produce a stable genetic trait if viral RNA served as the template for DNA synthesis and the latter became integrated into the host genome, resulting in neoplastic transformation. This revolutionary concept challenged the classic Watson-Crick hypothesis that information flow was unidirectional from DNA → RNA → protein. This hypothesis became more tenable with the demonstration that "reverse transcriptase" existed in nearly all RNA viruses with oncogenic potential, in human lymphoblastic leukemia cells, in virus-like C particles

from human milk in patients with breast cancer, and to a lesser extent in their seemingly normal relatives.

Two interesting theories of oncogenesis have recently been proposed on the basis of these data:

(1) Huebner's oncogene theory states that many (if not all) vertebrates contain the genetic information for producing C-type RNA viruses. This information (virogene) is transmitted vertically from one generation to the next and from one cell to the daughter cells. A portion of the virogene is responsible for neoplastic transformation (oncogene) and is expressed in undifferentiated fetal cells but not in normal, mature nonproliferative cells. Exposure to a carcinogenic stimulus (x-ray, chemical, or tumor virus) and the host genotype itself determine whether activation of the oncogenome will occur. This theory is based on the idea that a regulatory switch mechanism controls a stable alteration in genotype.

(2) Temin's protovirus theory proposes the origin of C particles from cellular genes which have incorporated a "protovirus" as a product of action of reverse transcriptase upon a cellular RNA template. Alterations or abnormal integrations of protovirus (due to changes in RNA, DNA, or the transcriptase) lead to oncogenesis.

The available evidence does not permit a clear choice between these 2 theories. Both have already broadened the conceptual role of viruses in oncogenesis and may have more general biologic import.

Allen DW & others: Viruses and human cancer. New England J Med 286:70, 1972.
Gallo RC: RNA-dependent DNA polymerase in viruses and cells. Blood 39:117, 1972.

VALUE OF GRADING & STAGING IN MALIGNANT DISEASE

For most curable neoplasms, the first therapeutic attempt must be definitive if cure is to be achieved; this means that initial therapy must be radical enough to encompass and extirpate or sterilize all existing foci of disease. An accurate delineation of the stage and extent of disease is thus an important initial step in consideration of the most appropriate treatment for the patient.

Grading and staging of neoplasms are attempts to describe the degree of malignancy and the dissemination of the malignancy. Histologic grading determines the degree of anaplasia of tumor cells, varying from grade I (very well differentiated) to grade IV (undifferentiated). Grading has prognostic value in some tumors (transitional cell carcinoma of bladder, astrocytoma, and chondrosarcoma) but is of little predictive value in others (melanoma or osteosarcoma). Staging of cancer is based upon the extent of its spread rather than on histologic appearance and has been standardized for many cancers by use of the TNM system. T refs to the degree of local extension at the primary site, N to the clinical findings in regional nodes, and M to the presence of distant metastases. Some cancers are staged by clinical examination alone (eg, squamous cell carcinoma of the cervix), whereas for others (eg, transitional cell carcinoma of the bladder and adenocarcinoma of the colon) the stage is determined on the basis of findings in the resected surgical specimen. In both instances, there is an excellent correlation of stage with prognosis.

For many neoplasms, both the histologic grading and the clinical staging have relevance to the choice of treatment and prognosis.

Glatstein E & others: Surgical staging of abdominal involvement in unselected patients with Hodgkin's disease. Radiology 97:425–432, 1970.

Feinstein AR: A new staging system for cancer and reappraisal of "early" treatment and "cure" by radical surgery. New England J Med 279:747–753, 1968.

THERAPY OF MALIGNANT DISEASE

1. SURGERY

Surgery is the most effective curative method for many malignancies and may also serve to palliate obstructive or compressive complications of unresectable or disseminated disease. Specific surgical approaches are discussed in other chapters.

2. IRRADIATION

Radiation therapy may also serve as definitive treatment of certain malignant diseases, alone or in conjunction with surgery or chemotherapy. Local obstructions and inoperable masses are frequently and effectively controlled by radiation therapy as discussed in Chapter 7.

3. CHEMOTHERAPY

Scientific Basis of Chemotherapy

A. Selective Toxicity; the Qualitative Approach: A basic goal of cancer chemotherapy is the development of agents with "selective toxicity" against replicating tumor cells which at the same time spare replicating host tissues. Such an ideal drug has not yet been found, and only the hormones and L-asparaginase (and, to a lesser extent, mitotane [o,p'DDD; Lysodren] and streptozotocin) approach this goal. Al-

though these drugs have important side-effects, their toxicity is not primarily directed against normal replicating cells.

B. The Quantitative Kinetic Approach: Since in most instances qualitative metabolic differences between normal and neoplastic cells have not been discovered, the chemotherapist must base his attack upon quantitative differences in the proliferative kinetics of normal and neoplastic cell growth if he is to achieve tumor regression without major host toxicity. Early bacteriologists, in their study of germicidal agents, formulated the concept of "the logarithmic order of cell kill." According to this theory, any particular treatment will kill a certain fraction of cells *independently* of the total number of cells present (provided the growth rate is constant). Thus, "cure," in the sense of killing the last remaining tumor cells, is more readily achieved by drugs when the total tumor cell burden is small. For example, a drug that is 99% efficient kills 2 logs of cells regardless of the total number of cells present and will reduce a tumor cell population of 100 to a single remaining cell, whereas it will leave 10,000 remaining cells of an initial tumor cell number of 1 million.

The quantitative evaluation of drug effects on normal and neoplastic tissues was furthered by the development of an in vivo assay system to allow measurement of the dose-response relationship of a variety of agents against both neoplastic and normal hematopoietic stem cells. As a result of these experiments, at least 3 cell survival curves are generated (Fig 50–1). The first (left) curve shows decimation of both normal and neoplastic cells to almost the same degree, whereas the other 2 curves (middle and right) show a much greater decimation of tumor cells than of normal stem cells. The selectivity of the agents in the last 2 classes was attributed to a differential effect of the agents on proliferating cells in the mitotic cycle while sparing resting cells not in mitotic division. Thus arose the classification of forms of therapy into (1) cell cycle specific (CCS) agents, which attack only actively proliferating cells engaged in DNA synthesis, and the mitotic cycle; and (2) cell cycle nonspecific (CCNS) agents, which kill both normal and tumor cells regardless of their proliferative state.

The important implications of these data are borne out by evidence in experimental tumor systems and to some extent in man: (1) Differences in sensitivity of normal hematopoietic precursors and neoplastic cells are a function of the difference in their proliferative states and not a result of any inherent qualitative biochemical differences between the 2 cell types. (2) An injured or "stimulated" marrow or normal tissue which is proliferating as rapidly as neoplastic tissue will be affected to the same extent as neoplastic tissue.

As a general rule, any tissue, normal or neoplastic, manifests an early logarithmic phase of exponential growth during which most cells are in active mitosis. When a certain bulk is achieved there is a transition to a later "steady state" plateau phase of growth during

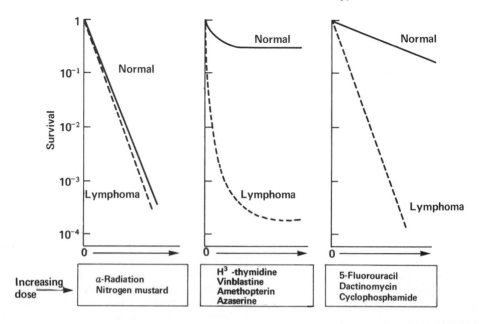

FIG 50–1. The form of the dose-survival curves for normal hematopoietic and lymphoma colony-forming cells exposed to 9 different anticancer agents for 24 hours in vivo. Three classes of dose-survival curves are evident. (Reproduced, with permission, from Bruce WR & others: Comparison of the sensitivity of normal hematopoietic and transplanted lymphoma colony-forming cells to chemotherapeutic agents administered in vivo. J Nat Cancer Inst 37:233, 1966.)

which a lesser fraction of cells is in the proliferative cycle. To maximize the therapeutic effects of CCS antineoplastic agents, resting cells must be induced to enter the proliferative cycle without at the same time increasing normal tissue vulnerability. This implies a reduction of tumor bulk with a reentry from the plateau phase into the log phase of exponential growth. Methods for reducing tumor bulk presently include treatment by CCNS agents such as x-ray or mechlorethamine and removal of gross tumor masses at surgery, but these stratagems all too often have attendant toxicities.

Utilizing these concepts, Schabel has proposed an approach to "curative" sequential chemotherapy of advanced tumors using a CCNS agent followed by a CCS agent in repeated courses.

While this is an idealized approach to curative therapy, similar principles have resulted in cure of laboratory-induced neoplasms, and such concepts form the basis for several successful new antileukemic regimens—particularly for childhood leukemia. Clearly, this approach will be furthered by a better understanding of human tumor cell kinetics in individual patients, by new knowledge about the dose, duration, and site of action of antitumor agents, by the development of new "marrow-sparing" agents, and by appropriately synergistic combinations of drugs as well as better means of measuring their effects on grossly unmeasurable tumors.

Bergevin PR, Tormey DC, Blom J: Guide to the use of cancer chemotherapeutic agents. Mod Treat 9:185–273, 1972.

Bruce WR & others: Comparison of the sensitivity of normal hematopoietic and transplanted lymphoma colony-forming cells to chemotherapeutic agents administered in vivo. J Nat Cancer Inst 37:233, 1966.

DeVita VT: Cell kinetics and the chemotherapy of cancer. Cancer Chemother Rep 2:23, 1971.

DeVita VT, Schein PS: The use of drugs in combination for the treatment of cancer. New England J Med 288:998–1006, 1973.

Greenwald ES: *Cancer Chemotherapy: Medical Outline Series.* 2nd ed. Med Exam Pub, 1973.

Schabel FM: The use of tumor growth kinetics in planning "curative" chemotherapy of advanced solid tumors. Cancer Res 29:2384, 1969.

Skipper HE & others: Implications of biochemical, cytokinetic, pharmacologic, and toxicologic relationships in the design of optimal therapeutic schedules. Cancer Chemother Rep 54:431, 1970.

The choice of therapy in the treatment of malignancy. Med Lett Drugs Ther 15:9–16, 1973.

GUIDELINES FOR THE INSTITUTION OF CANCER CHEMOTHERAPY

Establish the Diagnosis

A firm diagnosis of neoplastic disease must be made before treatment is started. This will usually (and

Synonyms of Anticancer Drugs

Adriamycin*
Allopurinol (Zyloprim)
Asparaginase* (L-asparaginase, Elspar)
BCNU* (see Carmustine)
Bleomycin
Busulfan (Myleran)
CCNU* (see Lomustine)
Carmustine* (bischloroethylnitrosourea, BCNU)
Chlorambucil (Leukeran)
Cyclophosphamide (Cytoxan)
Cytarabine (cytosine arabinoside, arabinosylcytosine, Ara-C, Cytosar)
Dactinomycin (actinomycin D, Cosmegen)
Daunomycin*
Dimethyltriazenoimidazole carboxamide (imidazole carboxamide)
Fluorouracil (5-FU, Efudex)
Hydroxyurea (Hydrea)
Imidazole carboxamide (dimethyltriazenoimidazole carboxamide)
Lomustine* (cyclohexylchloroethylnitrosourea, CCNU)
Mechlorethamine (nitrogen mustard, HN2, Mustargen)
Mercaptopurine (6-MP, Purinethol)
Methotrexate (amethopterin)
Methyl-CCNU (methylcyclohexylchloroethylnitrosourea)
Mithramycin (Mithracin)
Mitotane (o,p'DDD, Lysodren)
Phenylalanine mustard (melphalan, Alkeran, L-sarcolysin)
Procarbazine (Matulane)
Streptozotocin*
Thioguanine (6-TG)
Thiotepa (triethylenethiophosphoramide)
Vinblastine sulfate (Velban)
Vincristine sulfate (Oncovin)

*See Note to Reader, below.

preferably) include a histologic diagnosis, but in some instances the diagnosis may be based solely on analysis of exfoliative cytology. In rare instances, a biochemical parameter (eg, chorionic gonadotropin) in a consistent clinical setting may constitute a rationale for institution of therapy, although tissue diagnosis is always preferable. In emergency situations (eg, superior vena cava syndrome), it may be necessary to institute appropriate therapy without histologic or biochemical documentation; in such cases, appropriate diagnostic procedures are required after stabilization has been achieved.

Note to reader: Agents designated with an asterisk in the following discussion and in Tables 50–3 and 50–4 are investigational and not generally available to the practicing physician. Further information concerning these agents may be obtained from the various regional or national cooperative cancer chemotherapy study groups or the National Cancer Institute.

Delineate the Stage & Extent of Disease

This can frequently be achieved by correlating symptoms and the known natural history of the neoplasm with appropriate radiologic, chemical, and surgical staging data. The lymphomas are staged according to the modified Rye classification; many solid tumors are best staged by the TNM system.

Establish Goal of Therapy

The histologic diagnosis and extent of the disease frequently define the goal of therapy as either curative or palliative with or without hope for prolongation of survival, and frequently determine the most appropriate treatment—surgery, radiotherapy, chemotherapy, or a combination of these.

Measure Antitumor Response

After treatment is started, serial observations of objectively measured parameters are essential to judge antitumor response (measurable mass, tumor product, or remote effect) and to monitor the toxicity of the treatment. For example, in the treatment of gestational trophoblastic disease, assay of chorionic gonadotropin measures a tumor product which correlates directly with the numbers of neoplastic cells and will reveal subclinical amounts (10^6 cells or less) of tumor which must continue to receive chemotherapy. The sensitivity of this assay is largely responsible for the 90% cure rate of trophoblastic disease. In contrast, a "complete clinical remission" of acute leukemia (a normal bone marrow) occurs with a tumor cell mass of 10^9; most solid tumors contain $10^{10}-10^{11}$ (10–100 g) of tumor cells before the mass can be detected clinically.

Acceptable Drug Toxicity

The degree of toxicity that is acceptable depends on the probability and risks of achieving the therapeutic goal, other clinical characteristics of the individual patient, and the availability of supportive facilities to manage the anticipated toxicity.

Status of Patient

The patient's subjective and functional status must always be considered in formulating and instituting a therapeutic program. Subjective symptoms of disease usually parallel objective parameters of progression or regression of the neoplasm. When this is not so, other factors such as unrecognized drug toxicity, unreliable parameters of tumor response, and the masking of disease progression by certain forms of therapy (eg, corticosteroids) must be considered. The Karnofsky performance index (Table 50–2) is useful for following the functional status of the patient and must be accorded at least equal importance as objectively measurable parameters, especially when the goal of treatment is palliation.

The above considerations apply generally to cancer chemotherapy. Experimental drugs or treatment protocols may be considered if all of the following criteria are met:

TABLE 50–2. Karnofsky performance index.

	%	
Able to carry on normal activity. No special care is needed.	100	Normal. No complaints. No evidence of disease.
	90	Able to carry on normal activity. Minor signs or symptoms of disease.
	80	Normal activity with effort. Some signs or symptoms of disease.
Unable to work. Able to live at home and care for most personal needs. A varying amount of assistance is needed.	70	Cares for self. Unable to carry on normal activity or to do active work.
	60	Requires occasional assistance but is able to care for most of his needs.
	50	Requires considerable assistance and frequent medical care.
Unable to care for self. Requires equivalent of institutional or hospital care. Disease may be progressing rapidly.	40	Disabled. Requires special care and assistance.
	30	Severely disabled. Hospitalization is indicated, although death is not imminent.
	20	Very sick. Hospitalization necessary.
	10	Moribund. Fatal processes progressing rapidly.
	0	Dead.

(1) Proved methods of effective therapy have been exhausted.

(2) Data collection and dissemination of the information obtained will contribute toward answering the question asked in the protocol.

(3) The patient's human rights are fully protected, and informed consent has been obtained.

(4) There is a reasonable expectation that the treatment will do more good than harm.

CHEMOTHERAPEUTIC AGENTS
(See Tables 50–3 and 50–4.)

Chemotherapeutic Agents With Selective Toxicity

Only the adrenocortical hormones, sex hormones, and L-asparaginase* have demonstrated a predictable

*See Note to Reader on p 1040.

selective killing power of tumor cells based on metabolically exploitable differences between neoplastic and normal tissue.

A. Glucocorticoids: The glucocorticoids exert a "lympholytic" effect which can repeatedly induce remission of acute lymphoblastic leukemia, especially in combination with vincristine. This lympholytic effect, which does not depend on the mitotic activity of the tumor, is also useful in chronic lymphocytic leukemia, lymphomas, and myeloma.

The adrenal corticosteroids are also beneficial for certain hormonally sensitive tumors such as breast and prostatic cancer. They improve cerebral edema accompanying brain tumors; palliate hemolytic anemias associated with chronic lymphocytic leukemia and the lymphomas; and correct hypercalcemia due to various neoplasms. Their antineoplastic effects are less if given on an intermittent schedule; large daily doses for the shortest time necessary to produce the desired effect are preferred. Toxicity may be metabolic (hyperglycemia, sodium retention, potassium wasting), gastrointestinal (peptic ulceration), or immunosuppressive (increased susceptibility to infection). Myopathies, psychosis, hypertension, and osteoporosis are important side-effects of long-term administration.

B. Estrogens: The estrogenic steroids were used in the early 1940s for prostatic carcinoma and represented one of the first successful attempts at rational cancer chemotherapy. Shortly thereafter, estrogens were found useful in postmenopausal patients with breast cancer. Diethylstilbestrol, the most widely used estrogen, is potent, inexpensive, and effective when given orally but may cause gastrointestinal disturbance, fluid retention, feminization in males, and uterine bleeding. Its administration may cause hypercalcemia and "tumor flare" of disseminated breast carcinoma.

C. Synthetic Progestational Agents: These drugs are useful in pharmacologic doses for disseminated or uncontrolled carcinoma of the endometrium and occasionally for hypernephroma.

D. Androgens: The androgens are used principally in the treatment of disseminated breast cancer, especially in pre- and perimenopausal (1–4 years) women. They also have a role in the stimulation of erythropoiesis in anemic patients with several neoplastic and myelophthisic diseases. The toxic effects of androgens include excessive virilization of females, prostatism in males, and fluid retention; tumor flare and hypercalcemia occur occasionally. The halogenated androgens, which are effective when given orally, can produce cholestatic jaundice, although the parenteral nonhalogenated compounds do not do so.

The Alkylators

The alkylators, whose prototype is mechlorethamine, react with nucleophilic substances within the cell to form cross-links at the guanine residues of parallel double DNA strands. With the possible exception of cyclophosphamide, the alkylators are cell cycle nonspecific and affect both resting and dividing cells; both normal and malignant cells are injured.

TABLE 50–3. Solid tumors responsive to chemotherapy.

Neoplasm	Current Drugs of Choice	Other Useful Agents
Hodgkin's disease	MOPP (mechlorethamine, Oncovin [vincristine], prednisone, procarbazine)	Vinblastine (Velban), adriamycin,* bleomycin, BCNU*
Non-Hodgkin's lymphoma	CVP (cyclophosphamide, vincristine [Oncovin], prednisone)	Bleomycin, adriamycin,* BCNU*
Multiple myeloma	Melphalan and prednisone	Cyclophosphamide, procarbazine, vincristine
Squamous carcinoma of head and neck	Methotrexate	Bleomycin, (?) alkylators
Squamous carcinoma of lung	Cyclophosphamide and other alkylators	Methotrexate, imidazole carboxamide,* adriamycin*
Squamous carcinoma of cervix	Alkylators	
Transitional carcinoma of bladder	Adriamycin*	
Malignant melanoma	Imidazole carboxamide*	BCNU,* hydroxyurea (Hydrea), adriamycin,* vincristine (Oncovin)
Adenocarcinoma of gastrointestinal origin	Fluorouracil	(?) Methyl-CCNU*
Adenocarcinoma of breast	Hormone manipulation (estrogens for postmenopausal, androgens for premenopausal), fluorouracil	Alkylators, adriamycin*; various combinations of prednisone, fluorouracil, alkylator, methotrexate, vincristine
Adenocarcinoma of ovary	Alkylators	Fluorouracil, methotrexate, vincristine, (?) mercaptopurine, adriamycin*
Renal cell carcinoma	Progestagens	Androgens, glucocorticoids
Testicular carcinoma	Combination: Cyclophosphamide, vincristine, dactinomycin (and mithramycin for embryonal cell type)	Bleomycin, methotrexate, vinblastine (Velban), adriamycin*
Endometrial carcinoma	Progestagens	(?) Adriamycin*
Prostatic carcinoma	Estrogen	Prednisone, fluorouracil, (?) adriamycin*
Various soft tissue sarcomas	Combination: Cyclophosphamide, vincristine, dactinomycin	Combination: Adriamycin* plus imidazole carboxamide*; methotrexate
Insulinoma	Streptozotocin*	
Adrenocortical	Mitotane (o,p'DDD)	
Carcinoid	Cyclophosphamide	Fluorouracil, (?) dactinomycin
Wilms's tumor	Dactinomycin, with surgery and radiotherapy	
Neuroblastoma	Cyclophosphamide, vincristine	Dactinomycin, adriamycin*
Choriocarcinoma	Methotrexate, or vincristine plus dactinomycin	Vinblastine, mercaptopurine, alkylators

*See Note to Reader on p 1040.

Mechlorethamine (nitrogen mustard, HN2, Mustargen) is the alkylator of choice in the treatment of Hodgkin's disease, either singly or in combination with other drugs. For Burkitt's lymphoma, cyclophosphamide may be curative, and it is also the agent of choice for undifferentiated small cell carcinoma of the lung. Cyclophosphamide has a unique role in childhood acute leukemia, in which other alkylators are ineffective. For most purposes, however, equivalent doses of the various alkylators produce equivalent responses, and there is cross-resistance among the various alkylators except for the nitrosoureas (see below). The choice of alkylators thus rests upon the desired route and mode of administration and variations in toxicity.

Chlorambucil (Leukeran) has had its major use in chronic lymphocytic leukemia, Hodgkin's disease, and Waldenström's macroglobulinemia. Its major advantage is its narrow spectrum of toxicity (hematopoietic only) and ease of administration (oral). **Phenylalanine mustard (melphalan)** is usually given for multiple myeloma, but this may be merely traditional; **busulfan (Myleran)** is customarily used in chronic myelocytic leukemia and in polycythemia vera; all alkylators are equally effective against ovarian carcinoma.

Mechlorethamine is a vesicant if extravasated. **Cyclophosphamide (Cytoxan)** and **thiotepa** are much less irritating if applied directly to tissues because they must first be metabolized to the active form. The immediate effects of intravenous alkylator administration are nausea and vomiting beginning within 30 minutes and persisting for 8–10 hours; premedication with phenothiazine is preventative. The important delayed effects of alkylators are principally on rapidly proliferating tissues (hematopoietic, gonadal, skin, and gastrointestinal), with bone marrow suppression being the most prominent. In the marrow, cell necrosis begins at 12 hours; the nadir of blood count depression is at 7–10 days, and marrow regeneration time limits the administration of mechlorethamine to intervals of 4–6 weeks.

Several of the alkylators cause relatively characteristic adverse reactions. Examples are alopecia and hemorrhagic cystitis (cyclophosphamide), and melanosis and pulmonary fibrosis (busulfan). All alkylators have the potential to cause hypospermia, menstrual irregularities, and fetal anomalies.

Thiotepa is discussed in Table 50–4.

The Nitrosoureas

BCNU,* CCNU,* and methyl-CCNU* are cell cycle nonspecific synthetic chemicals which act much like the classic alkylators but have several unique and exploitable properties, including lipid solubility, and delayed onset of marrow suppression compared to the alkylators (see above). Moreover, there appears to be no cross-resistance with other alkylators. These drugs are effective in Hodgkin's disease, but less effective in non-Hodgkin's lymphomas; they appear promising for metastatic and primary CNS neoplasms because of their lipid solubility. BCNU* is administered intravenously; CCNU* and methyl-CCNU* are given orally.

Structural Analogues (Antimetabolites)

The antimetabolites are specific cytotoxic agents closely related to substrates normally utilized by cells for metabolism and growth. The structural analogues interfere with nucleic acid synthesis to impair proliferation of normal and neoplastic cells. They are generally cell cycle specific, with proliferating cells being more vulnerable to their effects than are resting cells.

A. Methotrexate: Methotrexate competitively inhibits dihydrofolate reductase; acquired resistance to methotrexate results from increased dihydrofolate reductase activity since the rate of enzyme synthesis exceeds the rate of methotrexate uptake by resistant cells.

Methotrexate toxicity may be hematologic, gastrointestinal, hepatic, and dermatologic. These effects may be alleviated or prevented by the prompt (preferably within 1 hour, but no longer than several hours) administration of folinic acid (citrovorum factor). One treatment regimen has used folinic acid to "rescue" the marrow after administration of toxic doses, although it is not yet certain that the antitumor effect is more pronounced. Methotrexate may be administered orally, intramuscularly, intravenously, or intrathecally, and is bound to plasma protein, metabo-

*See Note to Reader on p 1040.

lized by the liver, and excreted in the urine. Hepatic or renal failure are contraindications; leukopenia, thrombocytopenia, stomatitis, or gastroenteritis with diarrhea are the toxic side-effects which may require a reduction in dosage.

Although methotrexate has been used for over 20 years, critical questions regarding dosage and scheduling have not been fully answered. Intermittent (twice-weekly) administration is superior to daily administration for maintenance of remission in childhood acute leukemia. In acute leukemia, "resistance" to methotrexate is relative and may be overcome by revising the schedule of administration and dosage. Intrathecal methotrexate is effective for CNS leukemia deposits even when marrow disease has become "resistant." Methotrexate can cure most cases of gestational choriocarcinoma. It has been used extensively in the treatment of epithelial neoplasia of the head and neck and is useful in breast cancer, testicular tumors, lung cancer, medulloblastomas, and other brain tumors.

B. Mercaptopurine and Thioguanine: Mercaptopurine (6-MP) and thioguanine (6-TG) are purine antagonists; mercaptopurine is the analogue of adenine and thioguanine the analogue of guanine (with both having a mercapto substitution of the 6-amino group). Although the actions of these 2 drugs are quite similar and they share cross-resistance, they are probably not identical. Thioguanine (but not mercaptopurine) is synergistic in combination with cytarabine for induction of remission in acute myelocytic leukemia. Mercaptopurine is metabolized via the xanthine oxidase pathway, which is blocked by allopurinol. Therefore, the dose of mercaptopurine must be reduced to 25% of the usual dose if allopurinol is administered concomitantly. Full doses of thioguanine may be given in conjunction with allopurinol.

The purine analogues suppress purine synthesis through "pseudofeedback" inhibitory mechanisms which inhibit formation and interconversion of the intermediary compounds. The major toxicity is marrow suppression, which may be delayed in onset for several weeks. Its major clinical role is in induction and maintenance of remission in the acute leukemias and in blastic transformation of chronic myelocytic leukemia. It may be of some benefit in lymphomas and ovarian carcinoma.

C. Fluorouracil: Fluorouracil (5-FU) is a thymidine analogue which in vivo interferes with thymidylate synthetase, an enzyme involved in the formation of thymidylic acid, a DNA precursor. The agent is first metabolized to FUDR. FUDR itself is now available for use by perfusion but has not been shown to have a clear advantage over the parent compound. Fluorouracil is principally metabolized in the liver. Its major toxicities include stomatitis, enteritis, and marrow suppression; significant atrophic dermatitis is occasionally reported; neurotoxicity is rare.

Fluorouracil has been most useful in breast and colonic adenocarcinoma, but it is also beneficial against pancreatic, gastric, ovarian, and prostatic cancer. The preferred schedule of administration is

TABLE 50–4. Cancer chemotherapeutic drugs useful against solid tumors.*

Agent	Response > 50%	Response in 30–50%	Response in 20–30%	Route	Toxicity	Usual Adult Dose†	Specificity‡
Hormones							
Glucocorticoids	Hypercalcemia, Hodgkin's disease and other lymphomas (in combination), tumor edema of brain.	Breast carcinoma, multiple myeloma.	Hypernephroma.	Orally. (IV and IM preparations also available.)	Sodium retention, potassium wasting, hyperglycemia, peptic ulcer, immunosuppression, hypertension, osteoporosis.	Prednisone: 1–2 mg/kg/day for brief intervals (< 6 weeks if possible); then maintain at minimal required daily dosage.	Not known
Estrogens	Prostatic carcinoma.	Breast carcinoma.		Orally	Sodium retention, feminization, uterine bleeding, nausea and vomiting.	Diethylstilbestrol: 5–25 mg/day for breast; 2.5–5 mg/day for prostate. Ethinyl estradiol: 3 mg/day for breast.	Not known
Progestagens		Endometrial carcinoma.	Hypernephroma.	Orally, IM	Sodium retention.	Hydroxyprogesterone: 1 g 2–3 times weekly IM. Medroxyprogesterone: 200–600 mg orally twice weekly.	Not known
Androgens		Myelophthisic and refractory anemias; breast carcinoma.	Hypernephroma.	Orally, IM	Sodium retention, masculinization; cholestatic jaundice with oral preparations.	Testosterone propionate: 100 mg 2–3 times weekly. Fluoxymesterone: 10–40 mg/day orally. Calusterone: 200 mg/day orally.	Not known
Alkylators							
Mechlorethamine (nitrogen mustard, HN2, Mustargen)	Hodgkin's disease, neoplastic effusions.	Non-Hodgkin's lymphomas.	Melanoma, cervical carcinoma, head and neck carcinoma, bronchogenic carcinoma.	IV, intracavitary	Nausea and vomiting, marrow depression, ulcer if extravasated, hypogonadism, fetal anomalies, alopecia.	0.4 mg/kg IV as single dose every 4–6 weeks; 0.4 mg/kg by intracavitary injection.	CCNS
Cyclophosphamide (Cytoxan)	Burkitt's lymphoma, Hodgkin's disease, other lymphomas.	Multiple myeloma, neuroblastoma, breast carcinoma, ovarian carcinoma.	Oat cell carcinoma of lung, cervical carcinoma, Ewing's sarcoma.	IV, orally	Nausea and vomiting, marrow depression, alopecia, hemorrhagic cystitis.	40–60 mg/kg IV every 3–5 weeks; 5 gm/kg/day orally for 10 days, then 1–3 mg/kg/day as maintenance.	(?) CCNS
Chlorambucil (Leukeran)	Hodgkin's disease.	Non-Hodgkin's lymphomas, breast carcinoma, ovarian carcinoma.	(?) Cervical carcinoma.	Orally	Marrow depression, gastroenteritis.	0.1–0.2 mg/kg/day.	CCNS
Phenylalanine mustard (melphalan, Alkeran)		Myeloma, ovarian carcinoma.		Orally	Marrow depression (occasionally prolonged), gastroenteritis.	0.25 mg/kg/day orally for 4 days every 6 weeks; 2–4 mg/day as maintenance.	CCNS
Thiotepa		Ovarian carcinoma, neoplastic effusions.		IV, intracavitary	Marrow depression.	0.8 mg/kg IV as single dose every 4–6 weeks; 0.8 mg/kg by intracavitary injection.	CCNS
Nitrosoureas*							
Carmustine (BCNU), lomustine (CCNU), methyl-CCNU		Primary and metastatic brain tumors, meningeal carcinomatosis, Hodgkin's disease and other lymphomas.	Melanoma.	BCNU, IV; CCNU and methyl-CCNU, orally	Nausea and vomiting, prolonged marrow depression, local phlebitis.	BCNU: 75–100 mg/sq m IV daily for 2 days every 4–6 weeks. CCNU: 130 mg/sq m orally every 6 weeks.	CCNS

Drug				Route	Toxicity	Dosage†	
Structural analogues							
Methotrexate (amethopterin)*	Choriocarcinoma, Burkitt's lymphoma.	Squamous carcinoma of head and neck, testicular, breast carcinoma.	Various brain tumors, squamous cell carcinoma of lung.	Orally, IV, intrathecally	Ulcerative mucositis, gastroenteritis, dermatitis, marrow depression, hepatitis, abortion.	20–40 mg IV twice weekly; 5–15 mg intrathecally weekly; 2.5–5 mg/day orally.	CCS
Fluorouracil (5-FU, Efudex)		Breast carcinoma, colon and rectal carcinoma.	Other carcinomas of gastrointestinal origin, ovarian, prostatic carcinoma.	Orally, IV, intra-arterial infusion	Atrophic dermatitis, gastroenteritis, mucositis, marrow depression, neuritis.	15–20 mg/kg IV weekly for at least 6 weeks; 15 mg/kg orally weekly.	CCS
Dimethyltriazeno-imidazole carboxamide*			Melanoma, (?) lung carcinoma.	IV	Gastroenteritis, marrow depression, hepatitis, phlebitis.	150 mg/sq m/day IV for 5 days every 4–6 weeks.	Not known
Cytotoxic antibiotics							
Dactinomycin (actinomycin D, Cosmegen)	Wilms's tumor, choriocarcinoma.	Testicular carcinoma.	Soft tissue sarcomas.	IV	Nausea and vomiting, stomatitis, gastroenteritis, proctitis, marrow depression, ulcer if extravasated, alopecia; radiation potentiator.	0.01 mg/kg/day for 5 days every 4–6 weeks.	CCS
Adriamycin*		Lymphomas, transitional cell carcinoma of bladder, breast carcinoma.	Various sarcomas.	IV	Alopecia, marrow depression, myocardiopathies, ulcer if extravasated.	1 mg/kg/week; total cumulative dose should not exceed 550 mg/sq m.	CCNS
Mithramycin (Mithracin)	Hypercalcemia of malignancies.	Testicular embryonal carcinoma.		IV	Marrow depression, nausea and vomiting, complex coagulopathies, hepatotoxicity.	0.05 mg/kg IV every other day to toxicity or 8 doses per course.	Not known
Bleomycin (Blenoxane)	Lymphomas, testicular carcinoma.	Squamous cell carcinoma of head and neck.		IV, IM, subcut	Allergic dermatitis, pulmonary fibrosis, fever, mucositis.	15 mg twice weekly; total cumulative dosage should not exceed 300 mg.	Not known
Vinca alkaloids							
Vinblastine (Velban)	Hodgkin's disease.	Choriocarcinoma.	Breast, testicular carcinoma, non-Hodgkin's lymphomas.	IV	Marrow depression, alopecia, ulcer if extravasated, nausea and vomiting, neuropathy.	0.1–0.2 mg/kg IV weekly.	CCS
Vincristine (Oncovin)	Hodgkin's disease, other lymphomas, Wilms's tumor, neuroblastoma, medulloblastoma, choriocarcinoma.		Ewing's sarcoma, testicular, breast carcinoma, brain tumors, (?) multiple myeloma.	IV	Alopecia, neuropathy (peripheral and autonomic), ulcer if extravasated; rarely, marrow depression.	1.5 mg/sq m weekly or less. No individual dosage should exceed 2 mg.	CCS
Miscellaneous agents							
Mitotane (Lysodren, o,p'DDD)	Hypersecretion in adrenocortical carcinoma.		Reduction of tumor mass in adrenocortical carcinoma.	Orally	Gastroenteritis, dermatitis, CNS abnormalities.	5–12 g daily orally.	Not known
Streptozotocin*	Insulinoma.			IV	Nephrotoxicity, gastroenteritis.	1 g/sq m.	Not known
Procarbazine (Matulane)	Hodgkin's disease.		Lymphomas, oat cell carcinoma.	Orally	Marrow depression, gastroenteritis, dermatitis, CNS abnormalities.	50–150 mg/sq m/day to toxicity or response; maintain with 50–100 mg/day orally.	Not known

*See Note to Reader on p 1040.

†Modifications of drug dosages: If white count is > 4500 and platelet count > 150,000, give full dose; if white count is 3500–4500 and platelet count is 100–150 thousand, give 75% of full dose; if white count is 3000–3500 and platelet count is 75–100 thousand, give 50–75% of full dose; if white count is < 3000 and platelet count is < 75,000, give 0–25% of full dose.

‡CCS = cell cycle specific.   CCNS = cell cycle nonspecific.

once weekly rather than the 4-day loading dose schedule initially advocated, since the latter is more toxic without being more effective. The dosage should be in the range of 15–20 mg/kg IV, weekly as tolerated.

D. Cytarabine, Allopurinol, and Hydroxyurea: These agents are currently under study.

E. Imidazole Carboxamide*: This drug probably functions as an antimetabolite and has significant activity against malignant melanoma.

Cytotoxic Antibiotics

These agents, the first of which was dactinomycin, were isolated in the 1940s by Waksman from soil strains of bacteria of the Streptomyces class.

A. Dactinomycin: Dactinomycin (actinomycin D, Cosmegen) is an inhibitor of DNA-dependent synthesis of RNA by ribosomes. Its toxicities include hematopoietic suppression, ulcerative stomatitis, and gastroenteritis. It causes intense local tissue necrosis if extravasated. The drug is retained for a considerable time intracellularily, and acquired resistance is thought to correlate with poor cellular uptake or poor retention of the drug. The major use for dactinomycin is in sequential combination with radiation therapy for Wilms's tumor; "maintenance" long-term administration of the drug adds significantly to the salvage obtained with combinations of surgery, radiation therapy, and "adjuvant" short-term courses of the drug. Dactinomycin is of proved value in trophoblastic malignancy, soft tissue sarcomas, and testicular carcinoma, especially in combination with alkylators and antimetabolites. The optimal scheduling and combination of drugs with dactinomycin is not known, but the most customary has been in courses of several days at dosages of 15 μg/kg/day IV repeated after 2–4 weeks as toxicity allows.

B. Daunomycin* and Adriamycin*. Daunomycin* and its related compound, adriamycin,* are tumoricidal antibiotics whose major toxicity is severe marrow suppression, although myocardial necrosis is also an important side-effect of both drugs. Both agents have established activity against acute leukemia, and adriamycin* appears to be effective against a variety of solid tumors, including bladder carcinoma and Ewing's sarcoma.

C. Mithramycin: Mithramycin (Mithracin) is useful in the treatment of hypercalcemia resistant to hydration and steroids, and the dosage may be less than that required for tumoricidal activity although still within the toxic range. Its major usefulness is in embryonal cell carcinoma and other testicular tumors, and its toxicity includes marrow suppression, hepatic and gastrointestinal injury, and complex coagulopathies.

D. Bleomycin: Bleomycin (Blenoxane) is a new agent which is important because it is effective against squamous cell carcinomas and lymphomas without

causing myelosuppression. Toxicity appears to be related to its squamous tropism and includes skin rash and pulmonary fibrosis.

The Plant Alkaloids

The plant alkaloids include the periwinkle (*Vinca rosea*) derivatives, vincristine and vinblastine, 2 closely related compounds with widely different toxicities and somewhat different spectra of activity. Both Vinca alkaloids are bound to cytoplasmic precursors of the mitotic spindle in S phase, with polymerization of the microtubular proteins which comprise the mitotic spindle.

A. Vinblastine: Vinblastine sulfate (Velban) is a major agent against Hodgkin's disease and has lesser efficacy in the non-Hodgkin's lymphomas. The toxicity of vinblastine is primarily marrow suppression, but gastroenteritis, neurotoxicity, and alopecia also occur—the latter much less commonly than with vincristine. The drug is usually given once a week. Severe local ulceration may occur if the drug is extravasated.

B. Vincristine: Vincristine sulfate (Oncovin) is primarily neurotoxic and may induce peripheral, autonomic, and, less commonly, cranial neuropathies. Alopecia occurs in 20% of patients, but hematologic suppression is unusual. The drug is extremely effective in inducing remissions in acute lymphoblastic leukemia, especially in combination with prednisone, and is quite active in all forms of lymphoma. It is one of the most effective agents against childhood tumors, choriocarcinoma, and various sarcomas. Because of its lack of significant overlapping toxicity with most other chemotherapeutic agents, vincristine is receiving wide use in combination with other agents. The optimal dosage and scheduling for this agent remain to be elucidated; weekly administration is customary but may not be the best regimen.

Miscellaneous Compounds

Mitotane* (o,p'DDD) is a DDT congener which may cause adrenocortical necrosis and plays a useful role in reducing excessive steroid output in 70% of patients with adrenocortical carcinoma; in a lesser number (about 35%), an objective decrease in tumor mass is also recorded. Toxicities include dermatitis, gastroenteritis, and CNS abnormalities.

Streptozotocin,* an antibiotic derived from Streptomyces, has been useful in the treatment of metastatic insulinoma; 16 of 23 treated patients in a recent series experienced a reduction of hyperinsulinism, and several had objective decrease in tumor mass. Toxicities are primarily renal and gastrointestinal. Marrow function is not significantly impaired by the drug.

Procarbazine (Matulane) is a monoamine oxidase inhibitor whose exact mechanism of action is uncertain. It may cause both oxidation and alkylation of cellular constituents. Procarbazine is effective in Hodgkin's disease and may have some effect in various solid tumors, including oat cell carcinoma of the lung and melanoma. It finds wide use in combination chemo-

---

*See Note to Reader on p 1040.

therapy as part of the MOPP regimen for Hodgkin's disease, and higher dose regimens are also being evaluated in the treatment of other solid tumors. The dose-limiting toxicity is hematologic, CNS, or gastrointestinal, although tolerance to the gastrointestinal side-effects may develop. Occasional drug dermatitis is also reported.

Asparaginase* is an enzyme which has been partially purified and derived from several sources, including guinea pig serum and cultures of *Escherichia coli*. It catalyzes the hydrolysis of L-asparagine to L-aspartic acid and ammonia. Certain tumor cells, especially lymphoblasts, require exogenous asparagine for protein synthesis and optimal growth, while most normal mammalian cells are able to synthesize sufficient endogenous asparagine. Asparaginase has proved efficacy only in acute lymphoblastic leukemia, but it has stimulated great interest because it exploits a rarely found biochemical difference between normal and neoplastic tissue. Toxicity has proved to be severe, and includes the expected allergic effects of intravenous administration of a foreign protein as well as pancreatitis and hepatic dysfunction.

Livingston RB, Carter SK: *Single Agents in Cancer Chemotherapy*. Plenum Press, 1970.

SURGICAL ADJUVANT CHEMOTHERAPY

It has been suggested that surgical or radiotherapeutic (cell cycle nonspecific) measures which reduce tumor bulk and increase the growth fraction of a tumor might increase tumor sensitivity to chemotherapy agents (cell cycle specific) without increasing marrow sensitivity. Thus, chemotherapeutic agents given after operation might improve results when there is no clinical evidence of residual disease but recurrence is statistically likely. In 1957, in order to test the validity of this reasoning, the National Surgical Adjuvant Breast Project began trials in which patients with clinically curable breast cancer were randomly given thiotepa for 2 days after radical mastectomy; controls received no chemotherapy. As yet there is no noticeable benefit to the treated group, and adjuvant chemotherapy for breast cancer is still reserved for controlled clinical trials.

Adjuvant chemotherapy with fluorouracil is also undergoing evaluation for colorectal neoplasms. In Duke's stage B and C carcinoma (nodal involvement), fluorouracil therapy was administered after "curative" resection for at least 4 courses, and a "second look" operative procedure was performed later.

Adjuvant chemotherapy has been of documented worth in Wilms's tumor and neuroblastoma and may be of benefit in stages II–IIIB Hodgkin's disease in conjunction with radiation therapy. Among other promising tumors for controlled studies of adjuvant chemotherapy are ovarian carcinoma, testicular tumors, and certain sarcomas.

Rhabdomyosarcoma in children can now be treated effectively by wide local excision (avoiding amputation) followed by irradiation and repeated cyclic therapy with dactinomycin and vincristine.

Fisher F & others: Surgical adjuvant chemotherapy in cancer of the breast: Results of a decade of cooperative investigation. Ann Surg 168:337, 1968.

Kelman JW & others: Reasonable surgery for rhabdomyosarcoma: A study of 67 cases. Ann Surg [in press].

Mackman S, Curreri AR, Ansfield FS: Second look operation for colon carcinoma after fluorouracil therapy. Arch Surg 100:527, 1970.

Rousselot CM & others: A 5-year progress report on the effectiveness of intraluminal chemotherapy (5-fluorouracil) adjuvant to surgery for colon rectal cancer. Am J Surg 115:140, 1968.

SOLITARY METASTASIS

Even though more than 80% of apparently solitary metastases are eventually found to be multiple, an occasional cure results from their excision. In patients with a solitary lung metastasis, lobectomy gives 5-year survival rates of 15–60% depending upon the tissue of origin, the histologic characteristics of the tumor, and the time of appearance of the metastasis. The best results have been achieved when the metastasis was discovered more than 2 years after treatment of the primary. Surgery is much less successful for solitary brain metastases from lung tumors. The prognosis for solitary bony and liver metastases is poor, but occasional cures have followed removal of metastases from hypernephroma, testicular, and gynecologic neoplasms, various sarcomas, and occasional intestinal tumors.

Long-term palliation sometimes follows radiation therapy for metastases from certain radiosensitive tumors such as Wilms's tumor, seminoma, neuroblastoma, and some sarcomas.

Radiotherapy has also produced long-term survival in patients with metastases in neck nodes from an occult primary, presumably in the oro- or nasopharynx.

Adkins PC & others: Thoracotomy on the patient with previous malignancy: Metastasis or new primary? J Thoracic Cardiovas Surg 56:351, 1968.

Rubin P, Green J: *Solitary Metastases*. Thomas, 1968.

INFUSION & PERFUSION THERAPY

Selective arterial infusion has been used to deliver higher concentrations of drugs to the tumor than could

*See Note to Reader on p 1040.

be tolerated by systemic administration. One worker gave fluorouracil by hepatic arterial infusion to 200 patients with hepatic metastases, most of whom had failed to respond to intravenous fluorouracil. About 60% of the patients objectively improved and survived an average of 8.7 months; nonresponders lived an average of 2.5 months.

Regional perfusion is an experimental technic that has given promising results in the following situations: (1) melanoma of an extremity perfused with mechlorethamine, phenylalanine mustard, or imidazole carboxamide* and (2) head and neck tumors performed through the carotid artery with alkylators, fluorouracil, or methotrexate.

Ansfield FJ & others: Intrahepatic arterial infusion with 5-fluorouracil. Cancer 28:1147, 1971.

Freckman HA: Chemotherapy for metastatic colorectal liver carcinoma by intra-aortic infusion. Cancer 28:1152, 1971.

Krementz ET, Creech O Jr, Ryan RF: Evaluation of chemotherapy of cancer by regional perfusion. Cancer 20:834, 1967.

COMBINATION CHEMOTHERAPY

Combinations of drugs which block multiple biosynthetic pathways are given in an attempt to obtain a synergistic effect on the tumor. The drugs of a combination are selected to avoid overlapping toxicity. This approach has been of greatest value where no single agent is highly effective. Thus, vincristine plus prednisone or cytarabine plus thioguanine produce more complete remissions of acute leukemia than either agent alone, and toxicity is not enhanced. Survival is prolonged proportionate to the length of remission, which documents the importance of achieving a complete remission.

The cyclic administration of mechlorethamine, vincristine (Oncovin), prednisone, and procarbazine ("MOPP") produces 81% complete remissions of Hodgkin's disease in untreated stage III and stage IV; 76% complete remissions after radiotherapy alone; and 50% complete remissions after prior radiotherapy and chemotherapy. Seventy percent of complete responders were alive after 5 years, and 50% were continuously free of disease during that period. Single agent therapy with these drugs is much less successful. Improved—but less striking—results have also followed chemotherapy of non-Hodgkin's lymphoma. The combination of cyclophosphamide, vincristine, and prednisone ("CVP"), produces about 60% complete remissions with a median duration of 5 months.

In breast cancer, the combination of an alkylator (usually thiotepa) with methotrexate or fluorouracil and varying combinations of testosterone and prednisone, have given a 50–60% response rate. Approximately 80% of patients with visceral and skin metasta-

ses have responded to a 5-drug program: daily oral cyclophosphamide and prednisone; weekly intravenous fluorouracil after a 4-day loading dose program; and methotrexate and vincristine for 8 weeks (if possible) with maintenance at more widely spaced intervals and with varying dosages.

Nearly 50% of patients with testicular carcinoma improved on a triple regimen consisting of an alkylator (chlorambucil), an antimetabolite (methotrexate), and dactinomycin.

The lack of adequate controls makes interpretation of these combination studies difficult, but a controlled investigation of the MOPP regimen in conjunction with radiation therapy is currently in progress. In addition, it will be necessary to study the dosage schedule of each proved combination to determine the optimal regimen.

DeVita VT, Serpick AA, Carbone PP: Combination chemotherapy in the treatment of advanced Hodgkin's disease. Ann Int Med 73:881, 1970.

Greenspan EM: Combination cytotoxic chemotherapy in advanced disseminated breast carcinoma. J Mt Sinai Hosp 33:1, 1966.

Li MC & others: Effects of combined drug therapy on metastatic cancer of the testis. JAMA 174:1291, 1960.

Luce JK: Chemotherapy for lymphomas: Current status. Page 295 in: *Leukemia-Lymphoma.* Year Book, 1969.

PALLIATION OF LOCAL COMPLICATIONS OF NEOPLASIA*

Effusions

At least half of all patients with lung and breast cancer will develop a pleural effusion at some time during their illness. Ascites is a common complication of ovarian carcinoma. Lymphomas may be associated with chylous or nonchylous pleural effusion of either or both sites. One-fourth of all effusions are neoplastic in origin, and where pulmonary infarction is unlikely, most bloody effusions are from neoplasm. The diagnosis in malignant pleural effusions can be established by cytologic study of the fluid and pleural biopsy with the Cope needle.

Diuretics may be sufficient to control neoplastic effusions. However, when recurrent accumulations of fluid cause dyspnea, abdominal distention, or pericardial tamponade, palliative control should be attempted.

A. Pleural Effusions: Control of pleural effusions is best achieved by obliteration of the pleural space with sclerosing agents such as mechlorethamine. The lung must be fully expanded, and negative intrathoracic pressure must be applied to oppose the pleural surfaces for several days with a large thoracostomy

---

*See Note to Reader on p 1040.

*Spinal cord compression and cerebral edema are discussed in Chapter 41.

tube connected to water-sealed drainage. If the lung is not expandable—because of endobronchial obstruction with massive atelectasis, fibrothorax with "trapped lung," or massive intraparenchymal replacement by tumor—obliteration of the pleural space is contraindicated. When the pleural surfaces are opposed, freshly prepared mechlorethamine, 0.4 mg/kg in 50 ml of saline, is instilled intrapleurally through the clamped chest tube and the patient is positioned for 1 minute each in the prone, left decubitus, supine, right decubitus, and knee-chest positions to distribute the drug. After 1 hour, the tube is unclamped and drainage reestablished for 24–48 hours or until no further fluid is forthcoming. Lower dosages of mechlorethamine are used in the face of marrow depression. The procedure may be repeated in 3–4 weeks if the first attempt is unsuccessful.

Using this technic up to 90% of pleural effusions can be palliated. If the attempt fails or if the bone marrow is too compromised to permit the use of mechlorethamine, quinacrine can be used.

B. Ascitic Effusions: Ascites is generally best treated by attempting to control the underlying disease, which is usually ovarian carcinoma or malignant lymphoma. Mechlorethamine frequently induces a chemical peritonitis. Thiotepa does not have a vesicant action on tissues and is thus more gentle.

C. Pericardial Effusions: Most pericardial effusions are best treated by irradiation except (1) those due to radioresistent tumors or (2) when previous radiotherapy has included the proposed field. Impending tamponade must always be anticipated and treated by pericardiocentesis, creation of a pericardial window, or pericardiectomy. If needle pericardiocentesis is performed for a malignant effusion, thiotepa may be instilled into the pericardial cavity (in systemic doses) at the termination of the procedure. Mechlorethamine should not be used since it induces a too severe inflammatory response.

Obstructions & Lytic Lesions of Bone

A. Caval Obstruction: Superior vena caval obstruction is a medical emergency which should be treated by a combination of chemotherapy and radiotherapy. It is characterized by venous congestion and distention of tributaries of the superior vena cava, and thus presents clinically as edema of the face and arms—frequently associated with dyspnea and the hazard of cerebral venous thrombosis or cerebral edema. The syndrome may occur with various diseases affecting the mediastinum, but neoplastic disease—especially bronchogenic carcinoma and the malignant lymphomas—is by far the most common cause. Although a biopsy should be obtained whenever possible, this should not delay the start of therapy. Surgery or endoscopy should not be performed, since such intervention produces increased morbidity and mortality. Treatment should be started as soon as the clinical syndrome is recognized and consists of diuretics, corticosteroids, and maintenance of the upright posture. An intravenous alkylator should be given through an uninvolved vein (eg, femoral vein) and radiotherapy begun immediately. Cyclophosphamide or thiotepa is preferable to mechlorethamine since the former agents induce less vomiting. Venography determines the extent and location of the tumor and the propagating thrombus which is frequently present.

B. Bony Lytic Lesions: Palliation of metastases to weight-bearing bones is best achieved by irradiation. If pathologic fracture is impending, prophylactic fixation can minimize morbidity, especially in areas such as the femoral neck that are susceptible to considerable stress. Prolonged bed rest should be avoided whenever possible, for, in addition to the usual complications, patients with bony disease are prone to develop hypercalcemia, and this tendency is accentuated by immobilization. Supportive bracing is often a useful adjunct for vertebral involvement.

Metabolic Complications of Neoplasia

A. Hypercalcemia Associated With Neoplastic Disease: Hypercalcemia occurs most commonly with myeloma, breast carcinoma, and lung carcinoma and is occasionally seen in patients with prostatic carcinoma, lymphomas, and leukemia. It has also been reported with a wide variety of metastatic or disseminated neoplasms. Symptoms include confusion, somnolence, nausea and vomiting, constipation, dehydration with polyuria, and general clinical deterioration which can easily be mistaken for progressive disease or direct neurologic involvement by tumor. The true nature of this metabolic complication may easily be overlooked, resulting in hypercalcemic death secondary to cardiac, neurologic, and renal toxicity. Hypercalcemia may be due to elaboration of a parathormone-like substance by tumor (lung carcinoma), to osteolytic sterols (as secreted by breast tumors), or to increased bone resorption by invasion and neoplastic destruction of bone (as in myeloma).

The mainstay of therapy to reduce calcium is hydration with isotonic saline (to promote a diuresis of 2–3 liters per 24 hours) in addition to appropriate tumoricidal therapy, mobilization of the bedridden, institution of a low-calcium diet devoid of dairy products, and appropriate treatment of bacterial infections. If the patient was receiving androgens or estrogens for breast carcinoma, they should be withdrawn. Chelating agents such as sodium citrate promote renal excretion of calcium, and potent diuretics such as furosemide or ethacrynic acid also inhibit calcium resorption by the renal tubule. These measures, however, may not be appropriate in patients with impaired renal failure or congestive heart failure or may not be sufficient of themselves, and other measures such as glucocorticoids (prednisone, 60–100 mg daily) may be required. The corticosteroids appear to act by reducing calcium resorption from bone. Oral phosphate is often rapidly effective, but intravenous phosphates are too hazardous to recommend their use. Mithramycin, 25 µg/kg IV, is also a prompt and effective agent to be considered if the above measures fail to control hypercalcemia. It is not known whether it acts by exerting a direct toxic effect on the osteoclast or by some other mechanism.

B. Hyperuricemia in Neoplastic Disease: Hyperuricemia is a potentially lethal result of high nucleic acid turnover associated with some malignancies—especially after effective cytotoxic therapy. Uric acid nephropathy is related to intraluminal precipitation of uric acid in the distal renal tubule and collecting duct, with progressive intrarenal obstruction and failure. This sequence of events can often be avoided by maintaining satisfactory hydration and alkalinization of the urine to pH 7.0 by oral sodium bicarbonate (10–15 g/day) or by giving acetazolamide (Diamox) (0.5–1 g/day). Although allopurinol does not replace these measures, the preventive use of this drug (300–800 mg/day) should be considered in patients with leukemia, lymphomas, and myeloproliferative disorders, especially if radiotherapy is instituted. If mercapto-purine is being given, the dose must be reduced to one-fourth to one-third of usual when allopurinol is started.

Lambert CJ: Treatment of malignant pleural effusions by closed trochar tube drainage. Ann Thoracic Surg 3:1, 1967.

Lenhard RE Jr (editor): Clinical case records in chemotherapy: The management of hypercalcemia complicating cancer. Cancer Chemother Rep 55:509, 1971.

Levitt SH & others: Treatment of malignant superior vena caval obstruction. Cancer 24:447, 1969.

Millburn L, Hibbs GG, Hendrickson FR: Treatment of spinal cord compression from metastatic carcinoma. Cancer 21:447, 1968.

Perez CA, Bradfield JS, Morgan HC: Management of pathologic fractures. Cancer 29:684, 1972.

Rubin P & others: Superior vena caval syndrome: Slow low dose versus rapid high dose schedule. Radiology 81:388, 1963.

•   •   •

General References

Brodsky I, Kahn SB, Moyer JH: *Cancer Chemotherapy,* 2nd symposium. Grune & Stratton, 1972.

Cline MJ: *Cancer Chemotherapy.* Saunders, 1971.

National Cancer Institute Chemotherapy Program: *First Joint Working Conference.* Cancer Chemother Rep, vol 2, 1971.

Symposium: A critical evaluation of cancer chemotherapy. Cancer Res, vol 29, Dec 1969.

Symposium: Medical aspects of cancer. M Clin North America, vol 55, May 1971.

Veidenheimer MC (editor): Symposium on the care and treatment of the cancer patient. S Clin North America 47:557–802, 1967.

51 . . .

Organ Transplantation

Samuel L. Kountz, MD, & Folkert O. Belzer, MD

There are 3 types of tissue and organ transplantation: **(1) autotransplantation (autograft)**, in which tissue is moved from one location to another within the same individual; **(2) homotransplantation (allograft)**, in which an organ or tissue is moved from one individual to another of the same species; and **(3) heterotransplantation (xenograft)**, in which an organ or tissue is transplanted from a member of one species to a member of another, eg, from ape to man. Autotransplantation elicits no immune response and is widely used in clinical practice. Heterotransplantation (xenografting) elicits a severe immune response except when the organ or tissue has been specifically treated, as in transplantation of lyophilized pigskin to a severely burned patient. This is used solely as a temporary procedure. Heterotransplants must presently be regarded as purely experimental because there is as yet no way to control the vigorous rejection phenomenon that characteristically occurs.

At present, the major emphasis in clinical transplantation is on homotransplantation in which the immune process can be partially controlled so as to allow retention of the transplanted organ for long periods.

The success of tissue grafts between individuals of the same species depends upon the degree of histoincompatibility between donor and recipient. Rejection occurs because antigens present on the donor cells are absent on the cells of the recipient tissue. These so-called histocompatibility antigens are genetically determined and are present mainly on the surfaces of the cells. The major cell for testing is the leukocyte, and the major antigenic system is called HL-A. Rejection is minimized to the extent that HL-A antigens between donor and recipient are compatible. Related donors are more likely to have compatible HL-A antigens. Identical antigens are found in the cells of identical twins; cells of other siblings and parents are less compatible; and cells of unrelated donors are least compatible (Fig 51–1).

In addition to HL-A antigens, the ABO blood group antigens also determine transplant compatibility. These must also be tested and used as a basis for prediction of success in homograft transplantation.

Two crucial observations led to investigation of the role of the HL-A antigen system in organ transplantation. The first was the finding that rabbits preimmunized by injection of allogeneic leukocytes developed a second set rejection of a subsequent skin graft from the immunizing donor. The second was the discovery that human leukocytes could be serologically classified by a unique series of genetic markers—ie, the HL-A antigens. The construction of this system coincided with the evolution of clinical kidney transplantation in man, and it was logical that attempts would be made to correlate the HL-A system with graft survival. At present, the HL-A antigens appear to be related to histocompatibility because when kidneys are transplanted from HL-A identical siblings the postoperative course is smooth and graft survival is prolonged. Where kidney pairs are mismatched for one or more HL-A specificities, both in related and in unrelated groups, the results are not as good.

The following clinical guidelines have proved useful in the selection of donors based on tissue typing:

(1) Verification of ABO compatibility and a negative leukocyte cross-match to avoid hyperacute rejections during surgery must be the first step. If a more sensitive technic were available, it might be possible to prevent some losses that occur in the first 3 weeks after operation.

(2) If the donor is a sibling, the best choice is an identical genotype based on a family study. Lacking a family study, the second choice is an identical phenotype.

(3) In parent-child combinations, matching (other than ABO) is not mandatory, but the information derived from matching may be useful in determining which antigens (if any) are most active in rejection.

(4) In transplants from unrelated donors, an identical phenotype seems to give the best results. It should be emphasized, however, that a clinically acceptable frequency of graft survival follows the transplant of a kidney mismatched for 4 HL-A antigens.

To determine the precise role of the HL-A system in organ transplantation, there is urgent need for (1) regional exchange of organs based on a large recipient pool, (2) long-term follow-up of transplanted patients, and (3) a very cautious analysis made jointly by all investigators of the worldwide data.

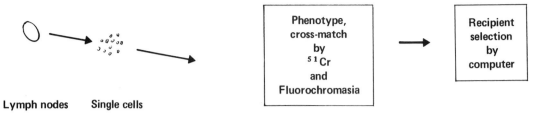

FIG 51−1. Recipient selection by kidney and lymphocyte phenotyping.

AUTOTRANSPLANTATION

Skin

Autotransplantation of skin to cover burned areas and reconstruct traumatic and congenital defects.

Teeth

Autotransplantation of the third molar in young people to replace the first molar.

Vascular System

Where trauma or disease requires replacement of an artery, autografts using another artery may be used. Vein autografts may be used to replace smaller arteries, and they withstand the increased pressures in the arterial system quite well. Autologous vessels must be used instead of prostheses in a contaminated field.

Gastrointestinal Tract

The stomach and the large and small intestines have been used to bypass or reconstruct the esophagus. Loops of ileum are used to replace a bladder which has been removed or severely diseased. Small intestine is often interposed between esophagus and duodenum after total gastrectomy.

Genitourinary Tract

Ureters are commonly transplanted into the bladder because of abnormal ureterovesical connections or into ileal loops when these are used to replace the bladder. Ureters are also connected to the colon as well as directly to outside skin under certain circumstances.

The kidney may be transplanted to the pelvis to compensate for loss of ureteral length.

Musculoskeletal Tissues

Cartilage, bone, fascia, tendons, and nerves may be used as autografts in the repair of traumatic and congenital defects. Whole hands, arms, and legs have been replanted following traumatic amputation.

Malt RA, McKhann CF: Replantation of severed arms. JAMA 189:716, 1964.

Bone Marrow

Bone marrow may be removed from the sternum or iliac crest and stored under sterile conditions prior to drug administration. Once the chemotherapeutic agent has been fixed to the body tissues, the cells are reinfused to repopulate the marrow.

Endocrine Tissues

Autotransplantation of the parathyroids, adrenals, ovaries, and testes are performed under specific circumstances.

Hardy JD, Laugford HG: Surgical management of Cushing's syndrome: Including studies of adrenal autotransplants, body composition and pseudotumor cerebri. Ann Surg 159:711, 1964.

Kearns WM: Testicular transplantation: Successful autoplastic graft following accidental castration. Ann Surg 114:886, 1941.

HOMOTRANSPLANTATION

Homotransplantation is performed for endstage organ diseases. Three major problems limit widespread use of this procedure: (1) inability to completely control the immune response, (2) the paucity of donor organs offered for transplantation, and (3) lack of technics for resuscitation and storage of cadaver organs after death. Homotransplant organs include kidney, heart, liver, pancreas, and lung. There are other transplants such as bone and cornea.

The Rejection Reaction

The length of survival of homografts in the absence of immunosuppressive therapy depends upon the genetic disparity between donor and recipient. Most of our earlier knowledge about this immune reaction was obtained from investigations with skin grafts. However, the basic immunologic process may be similar for each organ or tissue, and the pathophysiologic expression depends upon the specific organ undergoing rejection. Antigens in the donor tissue that are lacking in the recipient are responsible for initiation of the rejection process. These antigens, believed to be glycoproteins or lipoproteins, are processed by the macrophages. Lymphocytes and plasma cells then infiltrate the graft and destroy the endothelium of the blood vessels. The reaction of host cells and specific cytotoxic antibodies against the grafted tissue continues until ultimate destruction occurs.

In spite of many attempts to elucidate the various steps in the rejection process, our knowledge remains incomplete. It was first observed by Medawar that the application of a second skin graft from the same donor results in a more rapid rejection than the first—this due to cytotoxic antibodies preformed in response to sensitization from the first skin graft. Dempster demonstrated cross-reaction between antigens of the skin and the kidneys. It is now known that sensitization to skin, kidney, and other organs can be achieved by injections of lymphocytes and cross-reaction with bacterial antigens.

In the kidney, the rejection process begins immediately after transplantation. Electronmicroscopic studies by Williams & others (see reference, below) demonstrated changes as early as 24 hours after grafting which were distinct from those observed in autotransplants (Fig 51−1). Lymphocytes from the host initially attack the endothelial cells of the peritubular capillaries. Evidence that the cells that infiltrate homotransplanted kidneys are from the host is of 2 types: (1) If the host is given total body irradiation to destroy the lymphocytes, cells are not seen in the graft several days after transplantation. (2) In the labeling studies of Porter & Calne and Williams & others (see references), lymphocytes of the host were labeled with tritiated thymidine and the kidneys were then transplanted. The lymphocytes that infiltrated the graft were labeled. Recently, it has been shown that lymphocytes from the donor ("passenger lymphocytes") can be transferred with the donor organ and play an important role in immunizing the host. In animals, if the lymphocytes of the donor are destroyed by x-ray radiation or antilymphocyte serum before transplantation, skin, kidneys, and hearts survive longer. This technic has not been used in clinical organ transplantation, but the potential clinical applications are obvious.

The initial area of attack of host lymphocytes on the grafted tissue is the peritubular capillaries. In this area, blood flow is slower and the endothelial cells are more widely separated. This causes early swelling of the organ. Host lymphocytes are observed to attack the vascular endothelial cells in the peritubular capillaries, and cytoplasmic discontinuity has been observed. In the early phase of the rejection process, the major cell population consists of lymphocytes; later, immature plasma cells are observed in increasing numbers. A number of mediators are released during the interaction of host and graft cells, but their role is incompletely understood. It is well established that humoral antibodies play an important role in the destruction of homografts. Specific cytotoxic antibody has been shown to produce rejection in passive transfer experiments. In addition, cytotoxic antibody eluted from rejected grafts has been shown to destroy donor cells in vitro. Both the cellular and humoral arms of the immune response are greatest during the final phase, when the blood vessels of the graft are progressively destroyed and blocked by cells and cell debris,

and death of the graft is due to the resulting ischemia. In the case of renal allografts, glomerular and tubular function is anatomically intact until this final phase.

Cochrum KC & others: Renal autograft rejection initiated by passive transfer of immune plasma. Transplant Proc 1:301, 1969.

Dempster WJ: Kidney homotransplantation. Brit J Surg 40:447, 1953.

Egdahl RH, Hume DM: Immunologic studies in renal homotransplantation. Surg Gynec Obst 102:450, 1956.

Gowans JL, McGregor DD, Cowen DM: Initiation of immune responses by small lymphocytes. Nature 196:651, 1962.

Hume DM: Homotransplantation of kidneys and of fetal liver and spleen after total body irradiation. Ann Surg 152:354, 1960.

Knudsen DM & others: Serial angiograms in canine renal allografts. Transplantation 5:257, 1967.

Kountz SL & others: Mechanism of rejection of homotransplanted kidneys. Nature 199:257, 1963.

Medawar P: Second study of behavior and fate of skin homografts in rabbits: Report to War Wounds Committee of Medical Research Council. J Anat 79:157, 1945.

Porter KA, Calne RY: Origin of the infiltrating cells in skin and kidney homografts. Transplant Bull 26:458, 1960.

Williams PL & others: Ultrastructural and hemodynamic studies in canine renal transplants. J Anat 98:545, 1964.

KIDNEY TRANSPLANTATION

Renal homotransplantation is indicated for patients with end stage renal failure. It is estimated that 20−40 patients per million are candidates each year for treatment by transplantation. This means that in the USA an estimated 8−10 thousand patients could benefit from this procedure each year. Chronic hemodialysis has been an important factor in making renal homotransplantation possible, especially for recipients of cadaver kidneys.

SOURCES OF DONOR KIDNEYS

There are 3 sources of kidneys for renal homotransplantation: (1) living related donors, (2) living unrelated donors, and (3) cadaver donors. Of all the patients who are acceptable candidates for transplantation, only about 15−20% have an acceptable volunteer living related donor. The donor must be ABO compatible with the recipient. Living donors should be in good health both physically and psychologically. Above all, the donor should be a volunteer and must clearly understand the nature of the procedure so that he can give his informed consent to the operation. The law requires that donors be adults.

Living Donors

Over the last decade, about 5000 individuals have donated one kidney. The life of a healthy donor is not shortened by the loss of one kidney. There are no diseases that affect the kidneys in which the donor will be better off with 2 kidneys than with only one. In young donors, the remaining kidney hypertrophies and in a few months provides 75–80% of the original renal function. Women with one kidney do not have an increased incidence of urinary infections during pregnancy. Some transplant surgeons have advocated removal of the right kidney in women of childbearing age because of the increased chance of the uterus partially obstructing the only ureter during pregnancy.

The main risk to a donor is the anesthesia and the operation itself. The mortality rate is estimated to be 0.1%–about the same risk as in driving 8–10 thousand miles a year in an automobile.

The most common complication following nephrectomy is wound infection, which occurs in about 2–3% of cases and is usually superficial. Renal failure occurred postoperatively in one of our donors but cleared spontaneously. Superficial pain and hernias may occur, but rarely.

After the donor has been judged to be a true volunteer and the risks and complications have been explained to him, he is admitted to the hospital for special studies. A detailed history is taken, and a physical examination is performed. The routine work-up includes chest x-ray, ECG, urinalysis, complete blood count, fasting blood sugar, serum bilirubin, creatinine clearance, and BUN. If these are normal, an intravenous urogram is performed; if that is normal, a renal arteriogram is performed. Kidneys with multiple renal arteries may be transplanted, but if the vessel is too small the chance of thrombosis is increased. When there are multiple renal veins, the smaller veins may be ligated since there is free communication of the veins within the kidney. If the arteriogram is normal, the patient is an acceptable donor.

In the early days of transplantation, many centers included psychiatric evaluation as part of the preoperative assessment of living donors. In a study by Sadler & others of living unrelated and related donors over a 5-year period, true altruism was exhibited in many donors, including the living unrelated donor. Sibling donors appear to show the most anxiety, especially when the donor has just married and has young children. Follow-up studies on donors show that they have good renal function and suffer no ill effects from the procedure either physically or psychologically. Many donors–especially living unrelated donors–have a desire to identify with the transplant team.

Psychiatric evaluation of donors is not a requirement. Adequate evaluation by the donor's own physician is all that is needed.

Cadaver Kidneys

Since only 20% of recipients have a suitable volunteer living donor, the only way to offer transplantation to the vast majority of patients is to use cadaver kidneys, and there is a shortage of available cadaver organs. It is essential to the success of the procedure that the transplanted organ be of good quality. This means that the organ must be removed before or immediately after cardiac arrest. This requirement has made it difficult to obtain enough donor organs, and the advent of heart and liver homotransplantation has raised moral and ethical questions that have perhaps been overstated. A Harvard Committee has established criteria of death in which the diagnosis of death may be determined neurologically when the donor is on the respirator. Such donors are usually patients with irreversible loss of cerebral circulation who have received no drugs and show the following: (1) lack of spontaneous respiration, (2) areflexia, (3) no response to pain or other stimuli, and (4) a flat EEG. This definition of death is no different from that used by physicians for centuries–ie, the patient is considered dead when the organism as a whole is dead and not when the whole organism is dead. The kidneys may be removed for transplantation up to 1 hour after cardiac arrest provided the donor has relatively normal renal function at the time of death and phenoxybenzamine or another vasodilator is given to prevent renal vasospasm during the agonal phase. To obtain more organs for transplantation, more physicians will have to base the diagnosis of death on neurologic criteria so that the transplantation teams will have time to obtain the organs. To ease the logistics, a special method has been devised for removing kidneys after cardiac arrest.

There are 2 technics for short-term preservation of kidneys: (1) surface cooling with Ringer's solution and (2) perfusion with cryoprecipitated plasma. Kidneys can be preserved by surface cooling for 12–18 hours and for 50 hours or more by perfusion. Short-term preservation eases the logistics of transplantation because patients awaiting kidneys may be a long distance from the transplant center in their homes on dialysis. In addition, smaller transplant teams are required and more time is available for preoperative preparation of the recipient.

Our experience with procuring cadaver kidneys indicates that enough kidneys and other organs will not be available to meet transplant demands until the public accepts and supports organ donation. Many individuals are now carrying Uniform Donor Cards which comply with the Uniform Anatomical Act adopted by all 50 states of the USA. Further research in resuscitative technics may make more cadaver organs available. The age limit for donors has been from birth to age 65, but kidneys from young donors appear to fare better. The donor should be free of cancer (except for primary brain cancer) and systemic fungal infections such as histoplasmosis and coccidioidomycosis.

A preservation apparatus has been developed which can be transported in a specially designed truck. This apparatus has the advantage of being able to differentiate kidneys severely damaged with little chance of survival in the recipient from those with minimal damage with a good chance of survival. Empirical observations indicate that kidneys removed from donors with serum creatinines below 2 mg/100 ml have a good chance of adequate initial function. In addition, if such donors are treated with phenoxybenzamine, posttransplant dialysis is required in fewer than 10% of cases.

Belzer FO, Kountz SL: Preservation and transplantation of human cadaver kidneys: A two-year experience. Ann Surg 172:395, 1970.

Blaufox DM & others: Physiologic responses of the transplanted human kidney. New England J Med 280:62, 1969.

Bricker NS & others: Studies on the functional capacity of a denervated homotransplanted kidney in an identical twin with parallel observations in the donor. J Clin Invest 35:1364, 1956.

Collins GM, Bravo-Shugarman M, Terasaki PI: Kidney preservation for transplantation. Lancet 1:620, 1970.

Dempster WJ, Kountz SL: Recent concepts of the causes of functional arrest of homotransplanted kidneys. Rev Surg 23:5, 1966.

Dempster WJ, Kountz SL, Jovanovic M: Simple kidney storage technique. Brit MJ 1:407, 1964.

Kountz SL & others: Kidney transplants using living unrelated donors. Transplant Proc 2:427, 1970.

Kron AG, Ogden DA, Holmes JH: Renal function in 29 healthy adults before and after nephrectomy. JAMA 196:110, 1966.

Shorter RG: Renal function in donors and recipients of renal allotransplantation: Radioisotopic measurements. Ann Int Med 66:105, 1967.

SELECTION OF RECIPIENTS

During the developmental days of renal homotransplantation, most of the patients accepted for transplantation were in the younger age group from 15–45 years. In recent years, the age range has been extended in both directions—children below age 1 and adults up to age 83. It was noted earlier that children between ages 1–15 do as well as adults below the age of 50. Although transplantation is not contraindicated in older people, the success rate is lower because associated diseases are more frequent, resistance to infection is less, and the surgical risk is greater. If older patients are accepted for transplantation and enough cadaver kidneys are not available, the donor problems will reverse, ie, many patients will be candidates to receive kidneys from their children at the most crucial time of their children's lives.

The ideal recipient is a young person who has no serious infections or lower urinary tract disease, with minimal and reversible systemic disease secondary to renal failure. Recipients with the following primary renal diseases have been successfully transplanted: glomerulonephritis, pyelonephritis, polycystic kidney disease, malignant hypertension, congenital bladder neck obstruction with reflux pyelonephritis, Goodpasture's syndrome, congenital renal hypoplasia, renal cortical necrosis, Fabry's syndrome, and Alport's syndrome. Patients with certain systemic diseases in which the kidney is one of the end organs have been successfully transplanted: cystinosis, systemic lupus erythematosus, and Kimmelstiel-Wilson disease. Oxalosis is one disease in which transplantation is contraindicated at present because the disease immediately reappears in the transplant.

Transplants have been performed successfully in patients with Wilms's tumors of both kidneys, in patients with bilateral hypernephromas, and in patients with bilateral renal tuberculosis. When there is absence (congenital or atrophic) of the bladder, a Bricker or a cutaneous ureterostomy has been used to obtain urinary drainage. Patients with peptic ulcer disease have been successfully transplanted and have shown no increased hazard due to corticosteroid therapy. Some patients have required vagotomy and pyeloplasty for treatment of peptic ulcer after transplantation.

Emotional instability or psychosis has been thought to be a contraindication to transplantation, but successful transplantation has been observed to cure these patients if their emotional difficulties were due to uremia or poor response to dialysis. Unfortunately, there is no way to tell if the psychiatric symptoms are a reflection of the physical problems of the patients.

Advanced retinopathy and peripheral neuropathy due to uncontrolled hypertension frequently improve after transplantation. One patient had been successfully transplanted after therapy for pulmonary cryptococcosis, but she died of the disease after 2½ years even though the transplant was successful.

Transplantation should not be performed in patients with generalized septicemia due to viral, fungal, or bacterial infection.

The decision to accept patients in the poorer risk groups is usually based on the available dialysis facilities and the number of cadaver kidneys offered for transplantation.

Once a patient has been selected as a transplant recipient, he is usually started on hemodialysis. If he is to receive a kidney from a living related donor, only 2 or 3 dialyses are required before transplantation or bilateral nephrectomy. Recipients awaiting a cadaver kidney will require longer hemodialysis; if possible, they should be trained to dialyze themselves at home. Bilateral nephrectomy should be performed if required to control the blood pressure or if there is infection in the kidneys.

There is no evidence that splenectomy is of value before transplantation.

Hamburger J, Crognier J, Durmont J: Experience with 45 renal homotransplantations in man. Lancet 1:985, 1965.

Murray JE, Wilson RE, O'Connor NE: Evaluation of long-functioning human kidney transplants. Surg Gynec Obst 124:509, 1967.

Russel PS: Kidney transplantation. Am J Med 44:776, 1968.

CONTROLLING THE REJECTION REACTION

The first successful renal allografts were done before the advent of immunosuppressive drugs and were between identical twins. These transplants, known as isografts, did not undergo a rejection process. Homografts always involve the problem of rejection. Two procedures have been developed to predict acceptance of the graft by the host: close histocompatibility matching and immunosuppressive drug preparation. At present, there are 2 methods of histocompatibility testing: (1) HL-A phenotyping, and (2) mixed leukocyte culture (MLC).

Mixed Leukocyte Culture (MLC) & Matching

Histocompatibility antigens are shared by all tissue cells, but the lymphocyte is the only cell capable of responding to a foreign antigen by blast-like formation and increased DNA synthesis. This response can be measured in vitro by culturing the cells of 2 individuals together for 5 days. On the fifth day, the mixed cell cultures and appropriate control cultures (containing each cell population alone) are labeled with tritiated thymidine. This isotope is incorporated into any new DNA being produced so that the level of cellular radioactivity becomes an indicator of the degree of cellular response. The amount of DNA produced in mixed culture above the base level of DNA produced by the same cells cultured alone represents the degree of antigenic disparity between the cells being tested.

Mixed leukocyte culture (MLC) done in this way measures the response of both populations of cells to one another (ie, a "2-way" reaction). Since the response of the donor to the recipient is not really pertinent to transplantation, several modifications of the test have been developed which measure only the response of the recipient's cells to his donor's antigens (ie, a "one-way" reaction). Donor cells may be rendered nonresponsive by treatment with mitomycin C or x-irradiation, yet they still maintain their antigenicity. Work has also been done using donor cells of different types such as skin, kidney, or buccal mucosa, which are not able to respond to antigenic stimulation themselves but still display the donor's antigenic makeup. These mixed culture technics have proved useful in the selection of donor-recipient pairs for related transplantation.

They are particularly helpful in selection of the best related donor within a family in combination with HL-A typing. The value of MLC matching in addition to HL-A typing is that the matching technic measures the total immune response. Hamburger reported a positive correlation between MLC results and related transplant survival. Cochrum & others have shown the same positive correlation in relation grafts and, more importantly, have shown a high positive correlation in cadaver grafts. This is important since the correlation between HL-A typing and cadaver graft survival is low. The importance of mixed cell culture for transplantation has been sufficiently well established so that it is now a primary goal to shorten the test from the existing 5 days in order that it may benefit the recipients of cadaver organs as well.

HL-A Typing

It has now been established that the HL-A system is composed of 2 segregant series. Many of the antigens in each series have been identified, but new antigens are continually being described. An individual can be considered to be well typed if both antigens for each segregant series have been found. When this has not been accomplished, the remaining antigen or antigens were not detected, or homozygosity exists for one or more antigens.

Immunosuppression

As a working hypothesis, it is assumed that the closer the histocompatibility match, the less immunosuppression by drugs will be required to achieve graft acceptance. The use of immunosuppressive agents imposes an increased risk of death and complications due to viral, fungal, and bacterial infections.

The first immunosuppressive agent used was total body sublethal x-ray radiation, but this was rapidly abandoned because it could not be controlled and because the mortality rate was exceedingly high. Because the spleen and thymus in lower animals have been shown to mediate the immune response, they have been removed in man, but there is no clinical evidence that splenectomy or thymectomy in man alters the immune response. Some centers have observed an increased incidence of thromboembolic disease after splenectomy; others have not. It is believed that splenectomy corrects some of the bleeding abnormalities in uremia and permits the administration of larger doses of immunosuppressive agents, but this is an area of controversy. Very few thymectomies have been performed, and the value of this procedure in transplantation is unsettled.

The major drugs used in immunosuppressive therapy are azathioprine (Imuran) and the adrenal corticosteroids. Azathioprine is one of the mercaptopurine class of drugs and inhibits nucleic acid synthesis. It is given daily in doses of 2–3 mg/kg. In the case of living donors, the drug is started 2–3 days before transplantation. In the case of recipients of cadaver transplantation, 4–5 mg/kg are given just before the transplant. The patients are maintained on approximately 2 mg/kg indefinitely, and the dosage is reduced only if there are complications. The drug may cause depression of the bone marrow elements (leukocytes and platelets) and may cause jaundice. Some patients develop a polycythemia-like syndrome after transplantation, and this can be controlled by increasing the dose of azathioprine. This drug is never given in increased doses during an acute rejection episode, and the dosage may have to be reduced during rejection when renal function is poor.

Prednisone is almost always used with azathioprine. The dosage must be regulated carefully so as to prevent complications such as aseptic necrosis of the hips, cataracts, the development of cushingoid features and hypertension, increased bruisability, and acne. At the University of California Medical Center in San Francisco, prednisone is started 2 days before transplantation for recipients of living related kidneys and on the day of transplantation for recipients of cadaver kidneys. The oral dosage is 120 mg for 3 days. The dose is reduced by 20 mg every 3 days until a maintenance dosage of 30 mg/day is achieved. After 2 years of normal function, the dosage may be further reduced. In addition to oral prednisone, large initial doses (1–2 g) of methylprednisone may be given intra-arterially or intravenously. This may be repeated 1–3 times to treat rejection crises.

The exact site of action of corticosteroids on the immune response is not known, but it is believed that they inhibit the inflammatory aspect of rejection.

High doses of prednisone in children inhibit growth and distort the features of young women to the point that severe emotional problems may arise. This may be circumvented by alternate day treatment, administering the drug once in the morning. The exact dosage has not been precisely defined, but 2 mg/kg in children on alternate days has permitted growth. When a rejection crisis occurs, the corticosteroids are increased to their initial level and the same schedule repeated. If this is required more than 3 times during the first 3 months, it is better to remove the graft and return the patient to chronic hemodialysis or perform another transplant.

Dactinomycin (actinomycin D; Cosmegen) is frequently used as an adjunct immediately after transplantation in doses of 250–500 µg/day for 3–5 days; the same doses are given as treatment for a rejection crisis. Five hundred micrograms of dactinomycin may be added to 1–2 g of methylprednisolone and administered intravenously as a push.

X-Ray Radiation

X-ray radiation in doses of 450–600 rads may be given immediately after transplantation or for treatment of a rejection crisis. It is frequently given by the method of Hume, which consists of delivering 150 rads to the area of the graft every other day for 3 or 4 doses.

Thoracic Duct Drainage

Most patients have undergone renal transplants without thoracic duct drainage because of the complications and difficulty of maintaining the patient's drainage system. Nevertheless, removal of lymphocytes via the thoracic duct has reduced the rejection rate in recipients.

Antilymphocyte Globulin

An adjunct of proved value is antilymphocyte globulin (ALG). This material may be made in the horse, rabbit, or sheep, but the main source at present is the horse. Lymphocytes from human peripheral blood, spleen, lymph nodes, or thymus are injected into the animal. After immunization, the serum is harvested and the active globulin fraction isolated. Another source has been cultured lymphoblast. These can be phenotyped to contain all HL-A antigens, whereas donors of other cells must be selected from a large pool if all HL-A antigens are to be represented in the injection mixture. Once the IgG fraction is obtained, it is administered intramuscularly or intravenously. To be effective, it should have a high cytotoxicity titer and should have been shown to prolong skin grafts in subhuman primates. This biologic test system has made it difficult to evaluate ALG preparations, as each batch may be of a different titer and produce different clinical results. Much effort is being directed toward developing standardization procedures and a standardized product.

Because the material is made in horses, it has the potential of producing glomerulonephritis. ALG manufactured from cultured lymphoblasts does not produce antigen-antibody complexes in the kidney, but ALG manufactured from spleen cells and lymphocytes—because of their stroma—does produce complexes. However, clinical glomerulonephritis has not developed in any of the patients receiving ALG.

Bach FH: Transplantation: Pairing of donor and recipient. Science 168:1170, 1970.

Dempster WJ, Harrison CV, Shackman RM: Rejection processes in human homotransplanted kidneys. Brit MJ 2:969, 1964.

Hume DM & others: The comparative results of cadaver and related donor renal homografts in man, and the immunological implications of the outcome of second and paired transplants. Ann Surg 164:352, 1966.

Kountz SL, Cohn R: Initial treatment of human renal allografts with large doses of intrarenally administered immunosuppressive drugs. Lancet 1:338, 1969.

Kountz SL & others: Selection of allograft recipients by leukocyte and kidney cell phenotyping. Surgery 68:69, 1970.

Murray JE & others: Study on transplantation immunity after total body irradiation and clinical and experimental investigation. Surgery 48:272, 1960.

Murray JE & others: Prolonged survival of human kidney homografts by immunosuppressive drug therapy. New England J Med 268:1315, 1963.

Patel R, Terasaki PI: Significance of the positive cross-match test in kidney transplantation. New England J Med 280:735, 1969.

Rapaport FT, Dausset J: Ranks of donor-recipient histocompatibility for human transplantation. Science 167:1260, 1970.

Starzl TE & others: Heterologous antilymphocyte globulin, histoincompatibility matching, and human renal homotransplantation. Surg Gynec Obst 126:1023, 1968.

OPERATIVE TECHNICS

The left kidney of a living donor is preferred because it has the longest renal vein and the renal artery does not run in close proximity to the inferior vena cava. The kidney may be removed through a transabdominal approach, but a subcostal retroperitoneal approach is preferred. The major difference between nephrectomy for transplantation and nephrectomy for disease is that the quality of the donor kidney should be preserved. This means that every attempt should be made to minimize renal ischemia and damage to the ureters. Renal ischemia may be minimized by hydrating the donor and administering an osmotic diuretic to promote a urine flow rate of 3–4 ml/minute at the time of nephrectomy. Since the blood supply for the ureter arises from the renal artery, the ureter should not be skeletized and dissected high in the renal pedicle. Great care should be taken in removal of the kidney.

Recipient Operation

There is no good evidence that splenectomy is of value in renal homotransplantation. Removal of the recipient's kidneys is necessary when they are infected or responsible for uncontrolled hypertension. These procedures should be performed 1 week or more before allotransplantation.

A donor left kidney is transplanted to the right iliac fossa (Fig 51–2), turned over so that the pelvis is dependent. The renal artery is usually anastomosed end-to-end to the hypogastric artery and the renal vein end-to-side to the common iliac vein. Meticulous attention should be paid to hemostasis and ligation of the lymphatics, since inadequate attention to this may result in a postoperative seroma or lymphocele. The

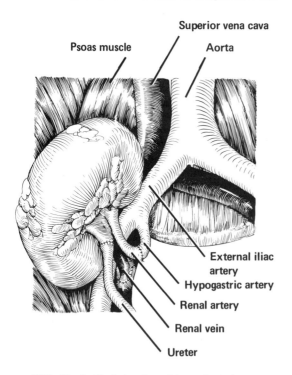

Psoas muscle

Superior vena cava

Aorta

External iliac artery

Hypogastric artery

Renal artery

Renal vein

Ureter

FIG 51–2. Technic of renal transplantation.

ureter is implanted into the bladder. A uretero-ureteral anastomosis or ureteropyelostomy may be performed under special conditions. It is better that these be reserved for complications of the transplanted ureter.

POSTOPERATIVE MANAGEMENT

Recipients who have received transplants from living donors usually undergo immediate diuresis and natriuresis. The magnitude is related to how overhydrated the patient was before transplantation. In the absence of a rejection crisis, the process may continue for 3–4 days, and the patient may develop postural hypotension and require added salt or blood transfusion. The diuresis and natriuresis occur because the transplanted kidney is vasodilated, but the glomerular filtration rate as measured by inulin clearance is rarely above that expected for a single kidney. The kidney has been found to have a low PAH extraction ratio and a low filtration fraction but a normal T_mPAH. How long vasodilatation persists after transplantation is not known.

Once this phase has passed, the patient maintains a relatively stable weight, although the weight may rapidly increase because of increased appetite and food intake. The urethral catheter may be removed after 4 days, although some recommend that it be left in place for as long as 7 days to ensure healing of the bladder incision. Most recipients may be started on a solid food diet with no added salt on the first to third postoperative days.

GRAFT REJECTION

The major hazard for the postoperative allograft recipient is rejection. Most rejections occur within the first 6–8 weeks. Four types of rejections have been clinically recognized: **(1) Hyperacute rejection** is due to preformed cytotoxic antibodies against donor lymphocytes or renal cells. This reaction occurs immediately after completion of the anastomosis, and complete graft destruction occurs in 24–48 hours. Initially, the graft is pink and firm, but it then becomes blue and soft with evidence of diminished blood flow. There is no effective method of treating this reaction, and patients who have preformed antibodies against donor cells should not be transplanted with a kidney from that donor. **(2) Accelerated rejection** has been described recently. This appears within 5–9 days after a period of good function. It is believed to be related to subliminal preformed cytotoxic antibodies against donor cells not detected by the usual cytotoxicity technics. It has also been suggested that sensitized cells could bring about this reaction. Skillful use of immunosuppressive therapy may overcome some of these reactions. **(3) The classic rejection reaction** usually occurs within 1–6 weeks. **(4) Chronic rejection** may take place any time after transplantation.

Although these 4 types of rejection reactions are recognized, they are only important as a guide. Rejection is a summation of numerous events many of which are still not understood.

DETECTING A REJECTION CRISIS

Since a rejection may occur at any time after transplantation, it may at times be difficult to differentiate from other conditions. In the immediate postoperative period, graft rejection must be differentiated from technical and urologic problems and acute tubular necrosis. Its clinical manifestations are frequently a change in mood of the patient and a sudden fever of 39–40 C (102.2–104 F). Many recipients are apprehensive, with increased anxiety, and may have tachycardia. There are 2 important physical findings: (1) the transplanted kidney is enlarged and tender on palpation. The tenderness is due to stretching of the peritoneum overlying the kidney. (2) As the process proceeds, the patient will gain weight and become hypertensive, and will have a falling urine output.

Laboratory Studies (Fig 51–3)

There is no single study that will pinpoint a rejection crisis. The BUN and serum creatinine rise. There will be a decline in the clearances of inulin, PAH, and ^{131}I-hippuran. A fall in the effective renal plasma flow (ERPF) as measured by the single injection of ^{131}I-hippuran also occurs. The GFR as measured by creatinine clearance also declines. The urine shows an increase in protein and lymphocytes, and urinary

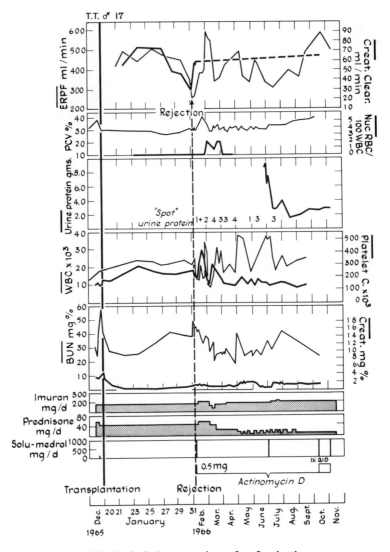

FIG 51–3. Laboratory signs of graft rejection.

sodium is low. If the kidney does not function well initially, as may occur with cadaver kidneys, a ^{131}I-hippuran renogram may be used to detect graft viability. The vasculature of the graft may be visualized by the use of techneticum 99m pertectnetate.

Perhaps the best way to accurately diagnose a rejection reaction is by renal biopsy, but this is impractical.

The diagnosis is made by analysis of the total clinical and laboratory findings. Although most patients will experience a rejection crisis (HL-A identical siblings tend to have very few), most can be successfully treated and the patient may survive with normal renal function. After the first rejection, others are less frequent. This has led to the belief that some sort of "adaptation" has taken place between the host and the graft. There is some evidence that the endothelium of the blood vessels of the graft is replaced by cells of the host. Also, there is evidence that a "blocking" antibody is formed which prevents host cells from attacking the graft's vascular endothelium. Whatever the mechanism, most grafts that are lost are rejected within the first 3 months; very few grafts are lost after 2 years.

Since most rejection reactions occur within the first 3 months, the mortality rate from immunosuppressive drugs is highest during this period.

Chronic rejection has a different manifestation. It may present as chronic and increasing proteinuria followed by edema and the nephrotic syndrome. This frequently responds to intensive immunosuppressive therapy. However, very few patients reject their grafts after 2 years.

Blaufox MD, Merrill JP: Evaluation of renal transplant function by iodohippurate sodium-I^{131}. JAMA 202:575, 1967.

Cochrum KC & others: The correlation of MLC with graft survival. Transplant Proc 5:391–395, 1973.

Kissmeyer-Nielsen F & others: Hyperacute rejection of kidney allografts associated with pre-existing humoral antibodies against donor cells. Lancet 2:662, 1966.

Kountz SL, Laub DR, Cohn R: Detecting and treating early renal homotransplant rejection. JAMA 191:997, 1965.

Slapak M, Lee HM, Hume DM: Transplant lung and lung complications in renal transplantation. Page 769 in: *Advances in Transplantation.* Dausset J, Hamburger, Mathe G (editors). Williams & Wilkins, 1968.

Starzl TE: *Experience in Renal Transplantation.* Saunders, 1964.

HEART TRANSPLANTATION

The immunologic barriers to clinical heart allotransplantation are probably no greater than those for the kidney. The logistical problems, however, are far greater. Unlike the donor kidney, the donor heart must be of excellent quality at the time of transplantation, because it must immediately take over the total circu-

latory system. Cardiopulmonary bypass to support the host circulatory system during removal of the heart at transplantation is essential, but this cannot be maintained for a long period of time.

The heart was first transplanted heterotopically (ie, to the necks of recipient dogs) by Alexis Carrel in 1905. Between 1905 and 1967, when the first human heart was successfully transplanted orthotopically, a number of experimental observations had shown that the acutely denervated heart could adequately support the circulation. The clinical technic which made orthotopic cardiac homotransplantation possible was first described in 1959 by Lower, Stofer, and Shumway in dogs. Autotransplantation of the heart in dogs was pursued at length by Hurley and his associates at Stanford, who achieved long-term survivals, documenting that the nerves do regenerate.

Operative Technics

The technic in use by the Stanford group is shown in Fig 51–4. Central cannulations of the aorta and vena cava are performed to place the recipient on cardiopulmonary bypass. The recipient's diseased heart is removed by severing the atrium in a plane just posterior to the base of both atrial appendages and the great vessels just above the semilunar valves. The entrances of the 2 vena cavas and the pulmonary veins are left in situ at the end of the posterior walls of both atria. The donor heart is removed by severing the inferior and superior vena cavas and the great vessels at the pericardial reflections, and the pulmonary veins at their entrance into the left atrium. The left atrium is opened by interconnecting the pulmonary vein orifices. The superior vena cava is ligated. The right atrium is opened with a lateral incision extending from the inferior vena cava to the base of the atrial appendages.

Immunosuppression & Histocompatibility Testing

The immunosuppressive regimen used in cardiac homotransplantation is the same as that used in renal homotransplantation. The only notable exception is that most patients who receive cardiac transplants have received intravenous or intramuscular antilymphocyte globulin. A second difference is that selection of donor-recipient pairs on the basis of matching is not possible at present for clinical cardiac homotransplantation because the donor heart cannot be preserved for a long period and recipients cannot be maintained until a phenotypically HL-A identical heart becomes available. Therefore, maximum immunosuppression that is safe for survival is used during the months following transplantation.

Selection of Recipients

Cardiac homotransplantation, although it has a great future, must be regarded as experimental and developmental at present. As of this writing, 173 cardiac homotransplantations have been performed, with a total survival of 23 patients, several of whom are past 2 years. Stanford University has accumulated the largest series, with a total 1-year survival rate of 38%.

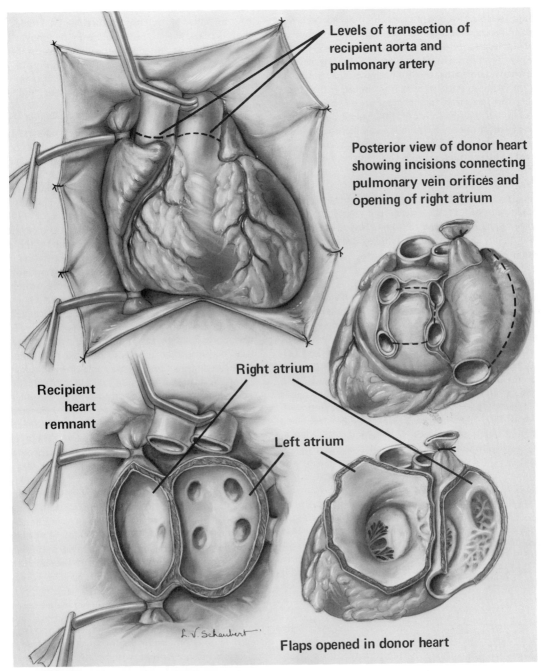

Levels of transection of recipient aorta and pulmonary artery

Posterior view of donor heart showing incisions connecting pulmonary vein orifices and opening of right atrium

Recipient heart remnant

Right atrium

Left atrium

Flaps opened in donor heart

L.V. Schaubert

FIG 51–4. *Top left:* Recipient heart showing levels of transection across aorta and pulmonary artery. *Lower left:* Implantation site with recipient heart removed. *Top right:* Posterior view of donor heart showing lines of incision connecting pulmonary vein orifices and opening the right atrium in preparation for implantation. *Lower right:* Flaps opened in donor heart in preparation for implantation.

The patient selected for cardiac homotransplantation must be in end stage cardiac failure for which no other medical or surgical therapy can be of benefit. However, patients with severely elevated pulmonary vascular resistance have an extremely poor prognosis following cardiac transplantation. This is because the normal right ventricle of the grafted heart is unable to work at the near-systemic pressures which are present in the lesser circulation. Progressive graft failure and patient death are the results of such transplants. It is currently felt that any patient whose pulmonary vascular resistance is less than 5 units and whose mean pulmonary artery pressure is less than 40 mm Hg does not face an increased risk of right ventricular failure postoperatively, as do those patients who have a very high pulmonary vascular resistance. Patients with a pulmonary vascular resistance greater than 10 units or a pulmonary artery pressure greater than 50 mm Hg have an extremely poor prognosis following cardiac transplantation. Younger patients appear to do better than older ones; this is related to the duration of their disease. Infection at the time of cardiac transplantation renders the patient a poor risk. Infection and increased pulmonary vascular resistance in the same patient are believed to be contraindications to the procedure.

Selection of Donors

Donors for cardiac transplantation must be young people who satisfy the criteria for neurologic death. This is essential because the donor heart must be of good quality, and immediate autopsy must be permissible on the basis of neurologic death.

Postoperative Course

The postoperative course following cardiac homotransplantation may vary depending upon whether or not the heart undergoes a rejection crisis. The diagnosis of rejection in heart transplants is a summary of all of the findings, the major one being changes in the ECG. This is noted by changes in the height of the R wave. The rhythm of these patients is frequently sinus, with a rate of 70–150 beats per minute. The rate increases with exercise, but the rate of increase is much slower. Several dogs demonstrated Stokes-Adams syncopal attacks, which are believed to be due to conduction defects. To prevent this, most patients have had a pacemaker inserted for a short time following transplantation.

Bieber CP & others: Cardiac transplantation in man. VII: Cardiac allograft pathology. Circulation 41:753, 1970.

Hurley EJ, Lower RR, Shumway NE: Stokes-Adams attacks in transplanted hearts. Surg Forum 16:218–219, 1965.

Lower RR: Pages 259–269 in: *Cardiovascular Transplantation: Present and Future in Human Transplantation.* Rapaport F, Dusset J (editors). Grune & Stratton, 1968.

LIVER TRANSPLANTATION

Liver transplantation has been studied extensively in the past 15 years, clinically as well as experimentally. Two surgical approaches have been used. The first approach is to transplant the liver as an extra organ in an animal or in a human (auxiliary transplants), a method first described by Welch in 1955. This procedure has been performed in 36 clinical cases. The second (much more common) approach is to replace the liver in its normal anatomic location after recipient hepatectomy (orthotopic transplantation). Although technically more difficult, orthotopic transplantation has been more successful, and some patients are still alive more than 3 years after transplantation.

In spite of extensive experimental studies and clinical trials, liver transplantation in man must still be considered an experimental procedure. Liver transplantation presents many problems. First, it is probably the most difficult transplant to perform since it requires an arterial anastomosis, 3 venous anastomoses, and a biliary anastomosis.

The donor organ obviously must come from a cadaver, and a major problem in early clinical transplantation was to obtain well-preserved cadaver organs capable of immediate and sustained function from the time of transplantation. The recognition and acceptance of brain death, in which the liver can be removed from the so-called heart-beating cadaver, has alleviated some of these problems.

Operative complications such as vascular thrombosis or biliary leaks are still common in the early postoperative period, and in many patients the cause of death has been technical rather than immunologic. In addition to the usual rejection episodes, which can occur at any time in the postoperative period, a separate type of rejection, called "septic infarction of the liver," is common in clinical cases. Septic infarction is probably caused by severe rejection involving the vascular supply of the liver with secondary infection by enteric organisms normally traveling through the portal system, resulting in infection and abscess formation in the ischemic infarcts. Rejection is best prevented by adequate immunosuppression. Starzl has recently introduced cyclophosphamide (Cytoxan) in place of azathioprine (Imuran). Its equal immunosuppressive but lesser hepatotoxic effects have given encouraging results. In Starzl's recent experience with 10 liver transplants, 8 patients are still alive in a follow-up period ranging from 1 month to 1 year. Although liver transplantation should only be performed by transplant centers with extensive experience in clinical and experimental transplantation, the slow but definite improvement in technics and survival suggests that patients with terminal nonmalignant liver disease can be considered for liver transplantation.

Calne RY, Williams R: Survival after orthotopic liver transplantation: A follow-up report of two patients. Brit MJ 3:436–437, 1970.

Starzl TE & others: Indications for orthopic liver transplantation: With particular reference to hepatomas, biliary atresia, cirrhosis, Wilson's disease and serum hepatitis. Transplant Proc 3:308–312, 1971.

PANCREATIC TRANSPLANTATION

Although pancreatic transplantation involves transplantation of a nonessential organ as compared to liver, heart, or kidney, it has an enormous potential in the management of patients with juvenile diabetes. In the juvenile diabetic, even though insulin and diet are carefully controlled, vascular injury to small arteries relentlessly continues. Many patients develop severe retinopathy at an early age, leading to blindness, renal disease and uremia, and peripheral vascular disease with severe neuropathy or limb loss.

Although pancreatic transplantation in animals has been extensively studied, animals (unfortunately) do not spontaneously develop diabetes mellitus, which would allow an investigation of the vascular change.

Transplantation of isolated and viable islet cells may become the procedure of choice in future. At present, pancreatic transplantation by vascular anastomoses has been more successful, and animals have lived for long periods with normal blood sugars after total pancreatectomy and pancreatic allotransplantation. In man, 2 technics have been used: (1) transplantation of the pancreas and a portion of duodenum with its vascular supply, and (2) transplantation of the pancreas only. Gliedman recently reported 3 patients in whom the pancreas was transplanted by anastomosing the pancreatic vessels to the iliac vessels and the ureter of the recipient to the pancreatic duct of the donor organ. Two of the 3 patients survived for at least 3 months with normal pancreatic function. In most clinical transplants, a portion of donor duodenum was attached to the pancreas. Complications in the postoperative period were often directly due to the transplanted duodenum rather than to the pancreas, indicating that this is probably not the best procedure. Although clinical survival of patients with pancreatic transplants is still far from encouraging, clinical pancreatic transplantation should be continued in centers with a particular interest in this problem and in which all patients can be extensively studied in the postoperative period. If a normally functioning transplanted pancreas could reverse or influence the vascular lesions of diabetes mellitus—and if, by technical and immunologic improvements, the operation could be made more successful—pancreatic allografting could become one of the most frequent organ transplants in man. Especially for the juvenile diabetic, it might provide a more favorable prognosis than does the use of insulin.

Lillehei RC & others: Pancreatico-duodenal allotransplantation: Experimental and clinical experience. Ann Surg 172:405–436, 1970.

Lillehei RC & others: Current state of pancreatic allotransplantation. Transplant Proc 3:318–324, 1971.

LUNG TRANSPLANTATION

Thirty-two patients have received all or a part of a lung from an unrelated donor, but only one has survived for more than 1 month. Infection, hemorrhagic consolidation, and rejection are the major causes of failure. Because lungs ventilate air, which may contain microorganisms, lung transplants are more susceptible to infection than are transplants of other organs. Furthermore, denervation of the lung abolishes the cough reflex and temporarily alters the amount and character of mucus in the airways. These factors and the problem of obtaining uncontaminated donor lungs make infection a major barrier to successful lung transplantation.

Many patients and experimental animals develop hemorrhagic consolidation of the lung after transplantation. Although this complication may result from imperfect vascular anastomoses, pressure-flow studies show that pulmonary blood flow can increase to more than 3 times resting flows with only a slight increase in pulmonary vascular resistance. Hemorrhagic consolidation is not caused by changes in vascular resistance in the transplanted lung. It is probably caused by edema and congestion after division of lymphatics and an inflammatory process which accompanied rejection.

Rejection is the most serious barrier to successful lung transplantation. The process attacks pulmonary microvessels initially and is extremely difficult to control in unrelated animals or man. Physiologic alterations and problems in procurement and preservation can be controlled or solved, but, since the lung is primarily a vascular organ, successful lung transplants require improved methods for controlling rejection or improved technics of donor-recipient matching. At present, lung transplants cannot be considered to be of therapeutic value to the thousands of patients suffering from severe chronic respiratory insufficiency.

Derom F: Current state of lung transplantation. Transplant Proc 3:313–317, 1971.

Veith FJ, Blumenstock DA: Lung transplantation. J Surg Res 11:33, 1971.

•   •   •

General References

Birtch AG, Moore FD: Organ transplantation in New England: An anniversary note. New England J Med 287:129–131, 1972.

Caine RY (editor): *Clinical Organ Transplantation.* Davis, 1971.

Hamburger J & others (editors): *Renal Transplantation: Theory and Practice.* Williams & Wilkins, 1972.

Hardy JD (editor): *Human Organ Support and Replacement: Transplantation and Artificial Prostheses.* Thomas, 1971.

Lowrie EQ & others: Chronic hemodialysis and renal transplantation: Survival rates. New England J Med 288:863–867, 1973.

Moore FD: *Transplant: The Give and Take of Tissue Transplantation.* Simon & Schuster, 1972.

Najarian JS, Simmons RL (editors): *Transplantation.* Lea & Febiger, 1972.

Veith FJ & others: Experience in clinical lung transplantation. JAMA 222:779–782, 1972.

Weiss W & others: Risk of lung cancer according to histologic type and cigarette dosage. JAMA 222:799–801, 1972.

52...

Surgical Diagnostic & Therapeutic Procedures

Robert C. Lim, Jr, MD

The purpose of this chapter is to describe some of the more common procedures encountered in the practice of surgery. Descriptions of operating room equipment, instruments, and the emergency resuscitative setup are beyond the scope of this chapter and will not be presented.

LOCAL ANESTHESIA

Surgical procedures on ambulatory patients usually require only local anesthesia. On rare occasions, regional block anesthesia may be necessary, and these patients will usually need a period of observation. Mild premedication may be indicated for agitated or apprehensive patients. Precautions must be taken against hypersensitivity. Transportation home should be arranged as a further safety measure.

For descriptions of the technics of local anesthesia and the management of toxicity, see Chapter 14.

LACERATIONS

The healing of lacerations is dependent upon a number of factors, including the patient's age and nutritional and endocrine status, local temperature, blood supply, mechanical stresses, infections, and the presence of foreign bodies. Wound healing is discussed in Chapter 9.

The first step in the care of a simple laceration of the skin and subcutaneous tissues is cleansing and debridement of devitalized tissue. Irregular skin edges should be trimmed to allow accurate approximation of the wound. It is vital that hemostasis be achieved before wound closure is attempted. In closing, subcutaneous tissues are approximated with fine catgut sutures and the skin is closed with interrupted sutures of fine nylon or other nonabsorbable material. Good cosmetic results demand accurate approximation of subcutaneous and epithelial layers. If the wound is grossly contaminated or first seen more than 6–8 hours after the actual injury, it should be debrided, irrigated clean, and left open to allow healing by second or third inten-

tion. It is customarily dressed with iodoform gauze (to maintain the skin edge separation) and then covered with sterile dressings. Caution must be taken not to close a contaminated wound (or one that contains a foreign body) since the end result of doing so is nearly always infection and abscess formation.

Wounds created by human or animal bites are heavily contaminated and therefore are usually left open. After adequate debridement of devitalized and necrotic tissue, the patient should be treated with prophylactic antibiotics. If treated promptly, wounds about the head and neck may be closed because the blood supply to these areas is copious. Such procedures must be followed closely so that skin sutures can be removed and the wound opened at the first sign of infection. A culture should be taken immediately. In addition, further debridement may be necessary.

Management of Lacerations

Three things should be kept in mind in the management of lacerations: (1) prevention of infection, (2) the cosmetic result, and (3) preservation of function. The wound should be meticulously prepared by thorough mechanical cleansing, irrigation with isotonic saline, and surgical debridement of all necrotic tissue and foreign bodies. Areas around the laceration are prepared by painting them with appropriate antiseptic agents. Inject 0.5% or 1% lidocaine into the wound edges to obtain anesthesia before debridement of the contused tissues (Fig 52–1). Hemostasis is usually obtained by gentle pressure on the edges of the wound or by the use of fine absorbable ligatures. Raised flaps of skin should be thoroughly cleansed and

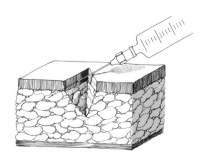

FIG 52–1. Injection of local anesthetic for wound closure.

assessed for viability. Irregular skin edges should be trimmed to allow accurate approximation.

Minor lacerations can be repaired by simple interrupted fine nylon skin sutures. In facial lacerations, the most commonly used sutures are 6–0 or 5–0 monofilament nylon. In other areas of the body, 5–0 or 4–0 sutures are used. In deeper wounds, the fascia and subcutaneous tissue is approximated in layers with interrupted 4–0 or 3–0 plain catgut sutures. The skin is then approximated with interrupted fine nylon sutures. A dry, sterile dressing is usually placed over the wound for protection.

In facial lacerations, where cosmetic result is of greatest importance, the finest suture material possible yields the best results. If the wound is clean and dry and no more than 3–4 mm wide, it can be closed with Steri-Strips instead of suture. This technic is especially useful in children and is performed as follows (Fig 52–2): (1) The skin is cleaned and dried. (2) Tincture of benzoin is applied to the skin and allowed to dry until tacky. (3) Half of each strip is placed on one side of the skin edge. (4) Gentle traction is applied to bring the 2 edges together. (5) The unattached half of each Steri-Strip is firmly placed on the opposite side of the wound.

In principle, if lacerations are deep, subcutaneous tissue must be approximated to eliminate dead space and to relieve the tension from the skin sutures.

Skin sutures should be left in place for approximately 7–10 days. Where cosmetic results are important, skin sutures can be removed in 2 or 3 days and the wound edges supported with Steri-Strips or collodion strips. Care of the wound after repair of the laceration should include keeping the area clean and dry. Undue stress on the wound edges should be kept

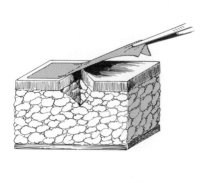

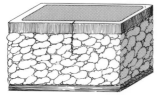

FIG 52–2. *Top:* Gentle traction is applied on the Steri-Strip to approximate the edges. *Bottom:* Closure of wound.

to a minimum. In some cases, immobilization with a splint may be necessary.

ABSCESSES

An abscess is a walled-off collection of pus. The terms boil, furuncle, and carbuncle refer to abscesses in the skin and subcutaneous tissue. A boil refers to a collection of pus which lies within the subcutaneous tissue. A furuncle is an abscess which originates in the sweat glands or hair follicles. A carbuncle refers to an abscess which has extended into the subcutaneous tissue and is multiloculated, with individual compartments formed by anatomic fascial attachments of the skin to the deep fascia. Common sites for a carbuncle include the nape of the neck and the pulp of the digits. Abscesses of the integument are usually caused by staphylococci; however, they may become secondarily infected by gram-negative organisms. They may also be the result of contamination from penetrating wounds (eg, those seen with drug abuse).

Management of Abscesses

Adequate incision and drainage are important in the management of abscess. Local or regional anesthesia may be used. A skin incision is made over the fluctuant area, and a closed hemostat is then inserted through the subcutaneous tissue into the center of the abscess. Care should be taken not to penetrate too deeply. Once the abscess cavity is entered, the blades of the hemostat are spread apart to break up loculations. If the abscess cavity is large, digital examination should be performed to confirm complete drainage. The skin incision should extend the entire length of the abscess cavity to afford adequate drainage. Cruciate incisions should be used only rarely.

Carbuncles are best managed by total excision with the electrocautery. Care should be taken that the advancing edge of the infection in the multiloculated compartments has been excised. The wound is packed open. Rapid closure by wound contraction without the need for skin grafting is the rule.

After evacuation of the abscess cavity, the wound should be drained by loosely inserting a strip of plain or iodoform fine-mesh gauze. Excessive oozing may be controlled by packing the cavity more firmly. Firm packing must be removed after 6–12 hours and replaced by loose gauze so that drainage is not impeded. Antibiotics are usually not used except when there are systemic manifestations of infection or persistent localized cellulitis in the region. The indications for antibiotics may be liberalized in treating wounds in special areas (eg, the hands) because the consequences of uncontrolled infection may be more severe.

Management of Other Pyogenic Infections

The treatment of cellulitis and lymphangitis due to nonsuppurative infection of the subcutaneous tissues consists of rest, heat, elevation, immobilization, and antibiotics (see Chapter 10). If the inflammatory process does not respond after 48 hours of therapy, suppuration and abscess formation should be suspected and drainage of any recognized collection is indicated.

When there is infection of the face, especially in the nasolabial area (the area with its border extending from the nasolabial fold to the outer canthus of each eye), aggressive antibiotic therapy is indicated because infection in this location carries a hazard of intra-cranial septic thrombophlebitis by spread from the nasal veins into the cavernous sinus. Morbidity and mortality are high when this occurs. Areas that are in close proximity to the occipital, mastoid, and frontal emissary veins should be of similar concern.

Management of Dental Abscess

Alveolar or apical abscess is usually related to poor oral hygiene and carious teeth. With necrosis of the dental pulp, periapical abscess causes severe pain and localized osteomyelitis around the root of the tooth. With further extension, the abscess will rupture through the buccal mucosa. If the abscess is pointing in the buccal mucosa and submucosal fluctuation is demonstrated, the abscess should be drained through an incision parallel to the gum margin. The patient should be given systemic antibiotics, and the tooth should be removed or a root canal should be done by a dentist. Occasionally, a periapical alveolar abscess will erode through the mandible to the outside of the face. Treatment in such cases is directed toward removal of the abscessed tooth, which is usually decayed and slightly loose.

SUPERFICIAL LESIONS

Excisional biopsy of subcutaneous tumors or skin lesions in an ambulatory patient is easily performed under local anesthesia. Infiltration of the skin and sub-cutaneous tissue around the lesion with 1% or 0.5% lidocaine will provide adequate anesthesia. The general principle in excisional biopsy is to make a skin incision which allows removal of the entire lesion with a margin of normal tissue. Hemostasis must be maintained to prevent seroma or hematoma formation, which will lead to wound complications. An elliptical incision should be made around the lesion parallel to the lines of skin tension. The incision should include a margin of 1–2 mm of normal skin. The length of the incision should be at least twice the width. Following removal of the lesion, the edges of the skin should be under-mined to facilitate approximation without tension or puckering. The subcutaneous layer may be closed with interrupted fine catgut sutures if necessary to eliminate the dead space. The skin should be closed with fine monofilament sutures. If the lesion is in the subcutane-ous tissue, a linear skin incision is placed over the center along the lines of skin tension. Skin flaps are

created and the lesion is completely excised with a margin of normal subcutaneous tissue. Following exci-sion of such a lesion, subcutaneous tissue layers may be sutured or not depending upon the size and extent of the wound. For small wounds, a few skin stitches may be all that is necessary. A dry sterile dressing should then be applied.

INTRAVENOUS CANNULATIONS

The indications for catheterization of a major vein are to establish an avenue for administration of blood and fluid during resuscitation, to measure cen-tral venous pressure in monitoring patients, and to administer intravenous hyperalimentation in malnutri-tional states. The sites most commonly used are the subclavian, internal and external jugular, basilic, and saphenous veins. The surgeon must be thoroughly familiar with the anatomy of these vessels before the procedures are attempted.

Standard Leg Cutdown

The origin of the long saphenous vein can be used for intravenous cannulation for the administration of fluids and blood, but cutdowns in this location in adults are complicated by a high rate of thrombo-phlebitis. The vein always lies anterior to the medial malleolus. A small transverse skin incision is made as illustrated (Fig 52–3). Blunt dissection is done with a small curved hemostat to identify the saphenous vein, which usually lies just superficial to the deep fascia and periosteum. The saphenous nerve must be separated from the vein. Plain catgut (3–0 in adults and 4–0 or 5–0 in children) is used to encircle the vein on both sides of the site of cannulation. The distal ligature is tied and gentle traction is applied to put the vein on stretch. The surgeon is best positioned at the foot of the bed, facing the patient. A transverse or lon-gitudinal venotomy is made depending on personal preference.

The transverse venotomy is quickly accomplished by inserting a No. 11 Bard-Parker scalpel blade through the midportion of the vein with its cutting edge directed distally (Fig 52–3). The blade is then turned 90 degrees, directing the cutting edge upward and incising the upper half of the vein. This maneuver creates a small lip to grasp in exposing the lumen.

A small mosquito clamp is used to dilate the vein. An appropriate-sized plastic cannula is inserted into the lumen and secured in place with the proximal liga-ture. The skin is closed with 4–0 or 5–0 nylon sutures, allowing the cannula to exit through the skin incision. Antibiotic ointment and a sterile dressing are applied at the cannula exit site.

Cannulation of the Basilic Vein

Central venous cannulation through the basilic vein is best done by a surgical cutdown unless the

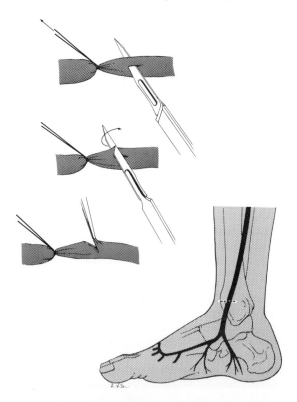

FIG 52–3. Leg cutdown with transverse venotomy.

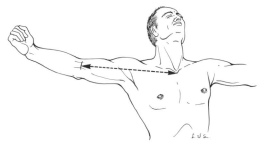

FIG 52–4. Length of catheter for basilic vein cannulation.

patient has large, prominent arm veins which permit the percutaneous approach. In hypovolemic shock, the peripheral veins are usually collapsed, and time is often wasted in multiple attempts to cannulate them percutaneously. Surgical cutdown is preferred under these conditions. The patient is placed in the supine position with his right arm abducted 90 degrees. The antecubital area is prepared and draped aseptically. After infiltration of local anesthetic, a small transverse skin incision is placed anteromedially proximal to the antecubital crease over a demonstrable vein. A venous tourniquet may be helpful to delineate the vein. After the vein is isolated, the tourniquet should be removed. A ligature is placed around the vein distally, and gentle traction is maintained. A small venotomy is made with a pointed scalpel blade. The lumen of the vein is gently dilated by the insertion of a mosquito clamp. A premeasured catheter whose length equals the distance from the cutdown site to the suprasternal notch is inserted (Fig 52–4). This distance corresponds to the distance from the venotomy to the superior vena cava. When positioned, the tip of the catheter will be in the right location to measure central venous pressure. If there is any question, portable x-rays can be done with radiopaque dye in the catheter to confirm its location. The catheter is then secured with a ligature around the proximal segment of the basilic vein. The wound is closed with several skin sutures. Antibiotic ointment is placed around the catheter exit site.

One of the complications of this type of cutdown

is inadvertently opening the brachial artery. One should always feel for a pulse before incising the vessel, but the pulse may be difficult to detect in shock. If an opening is made in the brachial artery, it should be repaired immediately with several sutures of fine cardiovascular silk. Care must also be exercised in identifying peripheral nerves in this region which may, at times, be mistaken for veins.

Cutdown of the Saphenofemoral Junction

The saphenous vein can be surgically approached at its junction with the femoral vein. The groin area is aseptically prepared and draped. After infiltration with local anesthetic, a small transverse incision is made over the saphenofemoral junction approximately 3–4 cm lateral and inferior to the pubic spine. Dissection is carried through the subcutaneous tissue, isolating the saphenous vein and identifying the saphenofemoral junction. A ligature is placed distally around the saphenous vein, a small venotomy is made, and a catheter is passed through the saphenous vein into the femoral vein as far as the inferior vena cava. The appropriate length of the catheter may be estimated by measuring it from the cutdown site to the umbilicus. The catheter is secured with a ligature at the saphenofemoral junction. The wound is closed with interrupted catgut sutures in the subcutaneous tissue and nylon sutures to the skin. Antibiotic ointment is applied to the catheter wound site.

VENOUS CATHETERIZATION

Percutaneous Subclavian Catheterization

The patient should be supine and in a slight Trendelenburg position to avoid air embolism during this procedure. This is especially important in hypovolemic shock since the veins are usually collapsed. The head is placed in a neutral position or turned to the opposite side. The infraclavicular area is widely prepared aseptically. A small skin wheal is made with 1% lidocaine solution approximately 1 cm below the midportion of the clavicle. A large-bore needle attached to a 2 or 5 ml syringe is introduced through

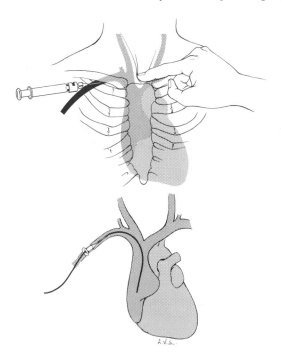

FIG 52–5. Percutaneous subclavian catheterization.

the skin wheal and directed toward the suprasternal notch (Fig 52–5). As the needle is advanced, slight negative pressure is applied to the syringe by pulling back on the plunger; when the vein is entered, blood will flow back freely. At this point, the syringe is removed and a catheter of appropriate size is inserted through the needle and advanced gently. After the catheter is advanced the desired length, the needle is withdrawn slowly and manual pressure is applied over the puncture site. The catheter is then secured in place with a small skin stitch to prevent it from slipping into the vein or being pulled out inadvertently. Antibiotic ointment is placed over the puncture site to minimize ascending bacterial contamination.

The major complications resulting from subclavian catheterization are air embolism, embolization of the catheter, pneumothorax, and hematoma formation.

To avoid catheter embolization, the catheter should never be withdrawn through the needle because a segment of the soft plastic may be sheared off by the beveled point inside the lumen of the vein, allowing it to float freely to the heart. Both catheter and needle must be withdrawn at the same time. Moreover, once the catheter is advanced, it must not be manipulated back and forth in an attempt to advance it further. If the catheter cannot be advanced to the desired length with ease, both the catheter and the needle should be removed and a different site used for cannulation.

To prevent hematoma formation after the needle is withdrawn, gentle pressure should be applied over the puncture site. Pressure should be maintained while the patient is taken out of the Trendelenburg position.

Gentle compression maintained for several minutes will allow the puncture site to seal around the catheter.

If the subclavian artery is entered, the needle is withdrawn immediately and manual pressure is maintained over the puncture for 10–15 minutes or longer.

Pneumothorax, due to inadvertent puncture of the cupula of the lung, occurs less often with the infraclavicular approach than with the supraclavicular approach. With the infraclavicular approach, the position of the first rib prevents advancement of the needle into the pleural cavity. Auscultation of the chest should be done after completion of the procedure. If there is any suspicion of pneumothorax, a portable chest x-ray should be obtained.

Percutaneous Catheterization of the Internal Jugular Vein

The patient should be supine and in a slight Trendelenburg position. The head is extended and turned acutely to the opposite side. A small skin wheal is made with local anesthesia at the midportion of the sternocleidomastoid muscle at its posterior border. A needle with a syringe attached is introduced through the skin wheal and passed behind the muscle. As the needle is advanced toward the suprasternal notch, gentle negative pressure is applied on the syringe (Fig 52–6). Once the needle enters the jugular vein, blood will be drawn back. The syringe is then removed and a catheter of appropriate size is passed through the needle into the internal jugular vein for the desired distance. The needle is then withdrawn while the catheter is held in place. As the needle is withdrawn from the vein, gentle pressure is placed over the punc-

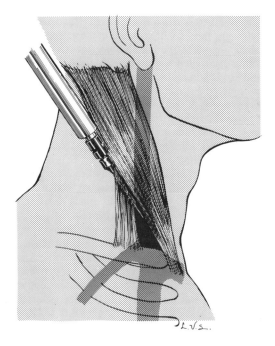

FIG 52–6. Internal jugular vein catheterization (posterior approach).

ture site for several minutes to allow a hemostatic seal to form around the catheter. The patient is taken out of the Trendelenburg position, and the catheter is secured with a simple skin stitch.

Another approach to the internal jugular vein is anteriorly. The patient is prepared as above except that the head is extended and turned to the opposite side. The needle is introduced overlying the juncture of the sternal and clavicular heads of the sternocleidomastoid muscle (Fig 52–7) and is directed inferiorly toward the clavicle at an angle of about 45 degrees from the coronal plane. The internal jugular vein usually lies deep to this area. If the internal jugular is not entered, the needle is withdrawn and then redirected several degrees laterally. The common carotid artery is avoided because it is medial and posterior to the internal jugular vein. Once the vein is entered, blood will be aspirated freely into the syringe. The syringe is removed and a 15–20 cm (6–8 inch) catheter is advanced. The needle is then withdrawn and the catheter is secured to the skin with a simple skin stitch. Antibiotic ointment is placed at the puncture site as with the subclavian cannulation.

The major complications of internal jugular puncture are a large hematoma (secondary to carotid arterial puncture), catheter embolization, and, rarely, pneumothorax. If the common carotid artery is entered, the needle should be withdrawn and gentle pressure maintained over the puncture site for 10–15

minutes or longer. Precautions in avoiding catheter embolization are the same as described for the subclavian cannulation. Pneumothorax can be avoided if the manipulation of the needle is confined to the neck and the needle is not advanced too far into the inlet of the thoracic cavity.

Percutaneous Approach to the External Jugular Vein

The external jugular vein is a subcutaneous structure that runs vertically across the sternocleidomastoid muscle from the inferior tip of the parotid gland to the posterior triangle of the neck. The patient is positioned in a slight Trendelenburg position with his head extended and turned acutely to the opposite side. The external jugular vein should be visible, but it can be accentuated if the patient performs a Valsalva maneuver. Cannulation of this vessel is done as described above for cannulation of the subclavian or internal jugular vein.

INSERTION OF CHEST TUBE
(Tube Thoracostomy)

Tubes for drainage are inserted into the thoracic cavity to evacuate a pneumothorax, hemothorax, or empyema (pyothorax). Experience has shown that attempts to remove intrathoracic collections with needle aspiration are usually unsatisfactory, and this technic is rarely employed except occasionally for a small pneumothorax.

Pneumothorax. If a tension pneumothorax exists, it should be immediately decompressed by a needle introduced through the second anterior intercostal space. A tube thoracostomy can then be performed unhurriedly.

For pneumothorax, a chest tube is usually inserted through the second or third anterior intercostal space in the midclavicular line and directed toward the apex of the thorax. The tube is attached to the suction device, and the rate of escape of air is indicated by the appearance of bubbles in the second of the 3 bottles. When bubbling ceases, this suggests that the pulmonary air leak has become sealed. Chest x-rays should be taken at intervals to verify full expansion of the lung. The tube is usually left in place for about 24 hours after the leak has sealed and full expansion has been achieved and is then removed.

Hemothorax. To evacuate a hemothorax, a tube is usually inserted through the fifth or sixth intercostal space slightly posterior to the anterior axillary line. This level is preferable to a lower one immediately over the center of the collection because it avoids the hazard of penetrating the diaphragm during insertion of the tube. Drainage is just as satisfactory in this location because, as the hemothorax becomes smaller, the residual blood takes a more lateral position and rises to the tube as a result of capillary forces along the pleural surfaces.

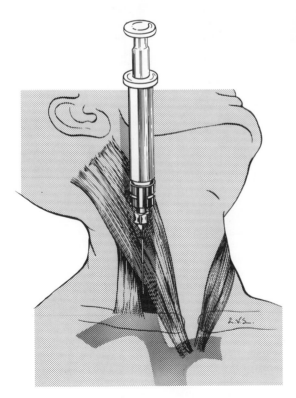

FIG 52–7. Internal jugular vein catheterization (anterior approach).

Empyema. The tube is usually inserted over the center of the collection as determined by x-ray. With small collections, fluoroscopy is sometimes desirable to accurately pinpoint the site. After a stab wound is made, a large (40–45F) Malecot catheter is inserted to drain the pus. Loculations are often present and must be broken down with a finger in order to accomplish thorough drainage. If the pus is especially thick and contains fibrin or necrotic tissue fragments, it should be lavaged vigorously by injecting saline through the thora-

costomy tube. In some cases, proteolytic enzymes may be used to decrease the viscosity of the exudate. Strepto-kinase-streptodornase (Varidase) diluted in 100 ml of saline can be instilled into the cavity; the tube is clamped for several hours and then reopened. The technic can be repeated as necessary if the secretions remain thick.

Technic of Tube Thoracostomy

The patient is positioned supine with his arm abducted at a 90 degree angle. The skin is prepared and

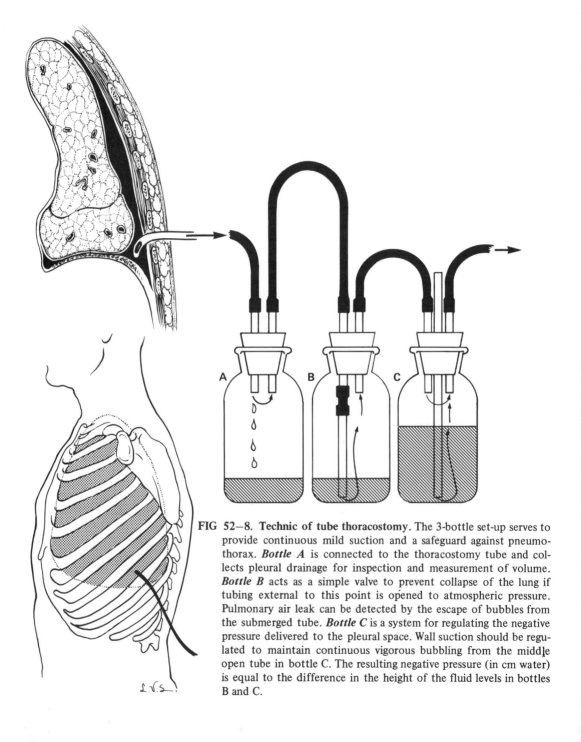

FIG 52–8. **Technic of tube thoracostomy.** The 3-bottle set-up serves to provide continuous mild suction and a safeguard against pneumothorax. ***Bottle A*** is connected to the thoracostomy tube and collects pleural drainage for inspection and measurement of volume. ***Bottle B*** acts as a simple valve to prevent collapse of the lung if tubing external to this point is opened to atmospheric pressure. Pulmonary air leak can be detected by the escape of bubbles from the submerged tube. ***Bottle C*** is a system for regulating the negative pressure delivered to the pleural space. Wall suction should be regulated to maintain continuous vigorous bubbling from the middle open tube in bottle C. The resulting negative pressure (in cm water) is equal to the difference in the height of the fluid levels in bottles B and C.

draped aseptically. The skin and subcutaneous tissues are anesthetized with 1% lidocaine, and a 2.5 cm (1 inch) transverse skin incision is made over the superior border of the rib at the site selected for the tube. The pleural space is entered by blunt dissection over the edge of the rib with a curved clamp. The jaws of the clamp are spread, enlarging the opening enough to permit the introduction of a finger into the pleural cavity. Digital examination should be performed to confirm the absence of pleural adhesions; this will prevent inadvertent insertion of the tube into adherent lung parenchyma. If the lung is adherent, it can easily be separated by gentle blunt dissection with the finger. The chest tube is grasped with a clamp and inserted into the thorax and positioned for optimal drainage. During insertion, the tube may slide into a subcutaneous space, and the malposition may go unrecognized unless tube function is tested. After the position is checked, the tube is connected to sealed underwater suction regulated to 10–20 cm water negative pressure (Fig 52–8). The tube should be fixed to the chest wall with No. 0 silk suture placed so that it can be used to close the wound site after the tube is removed. A sterile dressing is then applied.

THORACENTESIS

The optimal site for aspiration is selected by correlation of x-ray (or fluoroscopic) localization with the chest wall area of maximal flatness to percussion. Thoracentesis is rarely productive when performed below the eighth interspace in the midaxillary line even if a large volume of fluid is present. The most common mistake is to choose a location which is too low, which results in an unsuccessful tap because the diaphragm is sucked up against the needle. Shoulder and neck discomfort due to phrenic nerve pain referral may suggest this early in the procedure.

The easiest position for the patient is straddling an armless straight-backed chair, facing the back with his forearms resting on the top. The operator can sit on another chair behind him or to one side. If the patient becomes faint or dizzy, he can rest his head on his folded arms without altering the position of his thorax.

The chest wall is prepared widely, using sterile precautions. A small skin wheal is raised with 1% lidocaine or comparable local anesthetic at the appropriate site. A 25-gauge needle is used, and the local anesthetic is injected as the needle is slowly advanced. Care should be taken to proceed slowly with this phase of the procedure and to fully anesthetize the chest wall. When the parietal pleura is reached, minimal resistance will be perceived and more anesthetic is injected. A slight "popping" sensation is felt as the needle tip passes through the parietal membrane and enters the pleural space. The infiltration needle is withdrawn, and a small nick is made with a pointed scalpel. A short-beveled, blunt-tipped 13-guage aspirating needle

attached to a 50 ml glass (not plastic) Luer-Lok syringe by means of a 3-way stopcock which has both a female and a male Luer-Lok attachment at the proximal and distal ends, respectively, is gently advanced into either the mid or lower portion of the pleural space. One hand pushes on the syringe as the other hand acts as a "brake" or control on the needle at the skin surface so that the introduction is accomplished smoothly. Aspiration is facilitated by lubricating the syringe barrel and plunger with lidocaine solution throughout its full length at the beginning of the procedure. Steady, gentle withdrawal of the syringe barrel prevents the visceral pleura from being sucked up against the needle orifice and permits a free flow of even very thick, fibrin-containing exudate. The stopcock handle is turned to allow discharge of the material through the sidearm (with a short length of tubing attached) into a large sterile flask containing heparin. During collection, it is important for the nurse assistant to agitate the container gently to prevent clotting of the fluid, which otherwise will occur when the effusion is high in fibrin and protein content. When most of the fluid has been removed from the pleural space, it will flow freely only during the inspiratory phase of the respiratory cycle; at this point, the patient is asked to take slow, gradual, deep breaths and to lean backward toward the side of involvement, holding onto the back of the chair much as one holds onto the tow bar when water-skiing.

When a known malignant effusion is being evacuated, it is best to stop just short of complete withdrawal of all obtainable fluid so that 20 mg of mechlorethamine or another antitumor agent dissolved in 50 ml of normal saline can be instilled into the pleural space. The needle is then withdrawn and the patient is placed for 1 hour supine, for 1 hour with the involved side down, and for 1 hour prone to distribute the medication over all serous surfaces. A chest x-ray should be taken 6–12 hours later because there is usually a reaccumulation of fluid as a result of the chemical pleuritis caused by the irritant effect of mechlorethamine. Repeat thoracentesis is then performed in an effort to tap the chest "dry" and give the pleural surfaces the best opportunity for adhesive fusion. Successful obliteration of the pleural space is the usual result and prevents further accumulation of fluid.

LUMBAR PUNCTURE

Lumbar puncture is an easily performed but frequently misused and potentially lethal diagnostic tool. It should be done only in an effort to answer a specific clinical question—never "routinely" and never (unless essential to diagnosis) when signs of increased intracranial pressure are present.

Technic

The patient should be placed on his side in the fetal position (Fig 52–9). The lumbosacral area is pre-

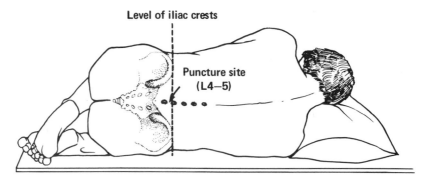

FIG 52—9. Lying position for lumbar puncture. (Reproduced, with permission, from Krupp MA & others: *Physician's Handbook,* 17th ed. Lange, 1973.)

pared with an antiseptic solution; the skin over the L3—4 or L4—5 interspace is infiltrated with local anesthetic; and a 19- or 20-gauge needle is introduced with its bevel parallel to the spinal axis. (Since the spinal cord does not terminate before reaching approximately the level of L2, punctures at or above this level could damage the cord. Cisterna magna and lateral cervical punctures can be done, but only in special situations by experienced personnel.) The needle is connected to a manometer; if the opening pressure is elevated, only the CSF in the manometer should be withdrawn.

Indications

A. Diagnosis of Hemorrhage: When subarachnoid hemorrhage is suspected, red cells in the CSF will be diagnostic. Truly bloody CSF can be differentiated from the bloody CSF due to a traumatic tap because, with the latter, the CSF will become progressively clearer with each successive specimen. One should centrifuge bloody CSF and examine the supernatant for xanthochromia. The degree of xanthochromia will provide some index of the length of time the red cells have been in the CSF. Crenation of red blood cells is a meaningless sign. The presence of red cells in the CSF may be associated with a lowered CSF glucose, but the length of time the cells have been present does not affect the level of glucose.

B. Diagnosis of Infection: In the patient with purulent meningitis, lumbar puncture is usually diagnostic: the pressure will be increased; white cells will be present, the number and type depending on the etiologic agent; the protein will be increased; and the glucose will be decreased. CSF should be obtained for routine culture as well as for cultures for anaerobic bacteria, fungi, and tubercle bacilli.

A traumatic lumbar puncture may produce confusing CSF findings.

The CSF may be normal in cases of brain abscess, subdural empyema, or epidural abscess, although the pressure is frequently elevated. CSF findings in meningeal metastatic carcinoma may simulate those of meningitis but can frequently be differentiated by cytologic studies. Active neurosyphilis produces CSF abnormalities, the exact findings depending on the type of involvement: serologic tests on blood and CSF may be positive; the pressure may be increased; the protein and cell count (lymphocytes) may be increased; and the colloidal gold curve may be abnormal.

C. Evaluation of Spinal Trauma: In cases of spinal trauma, lumbar puncture is frequently done to determine if a block is present in the spinal CSF pathway. After the needle is inserted, the jugular veins are compressed while the examiner notes the rise and fall of CSF pressure (Queckenstedt's test). When this test is performed, one should be prepared to proceed with contrast medium myelography if indicated.

Lumbar puncture is seldom useful following acute head injuries, but it may be useful in more chronic situations to determine the presence of blood or elevated CSF pressure.

Contraindications & Side-Effects

Lumbar puncture should not be done in the presence of papilledema or other manifestations of increased intracranial pressure unless essential for diagnosis. *Note:* In such situations, lumbar puncture may be fatal.

At least 20% of patients will complain of headache and stiff neck after diagnostic lumbar puncture. This will be self-limiting but may persist for days. It is absent when the patient lies flat, and can usually be prevented if the patient remains flat for 12 hours after the procedure. It is presumably related to persistent leakage of CSF at the site of needle puncture. The headache is occasionally associated with fever and is essentially an aseptic meningitis. Rarely, a septic process will result. Local structures in the area of the lumbar puncture, including the intervertebral disk, may be traumatized by the procedure, but this rarely happens.

CATHETERIZATION OF THE BLADDER

Urinary catheters are introduced into the bladder both for diagnostic purposes, as in blunt trauma with

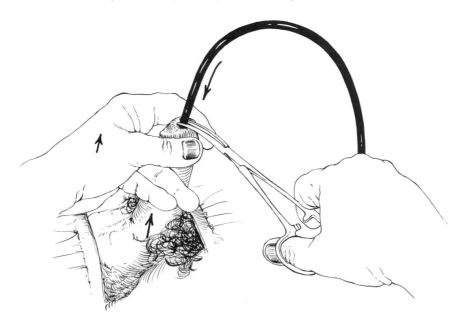

FIG 52–10. Technic of catheterization. A sterile water-soluble lubricant is first instilled into the urethra by means of a bulb syringe. The penis is drawn taut with one hand. The catheter, held near its tip with a sterile clamp, is introduced into the urethra; the other end of the catheter is held between the fourth and fifth fingers of the hand holding the clamp. The clamp is then moved up on the catheter and the catheter introduced farther into the urethra. (Reproduced, with permission, from Smith DR: *General Urology,* 7th ed. Lange, 1972.)

renal injuries or pelvic fractures, and for the relief of urinary retention, as in prostatic obstruction. Indwelling catheters (Foley) are inserted to allow for continuous monitoring of urine output.

The size of the catheter will depend upon the size of the patient. In men, catheters that are too small tend to bend and coil within the urethra. Size 18–22F catheters may be used in adults with very little trauma. In children, size 8–12F may be used.

Catheterization in Males

The genital area is draped and the penis is held taut with one hand. The meatus and glans are prepped aseptically. The catheter can be introduced with a sterile gloved hand or with a sterile clamp. The catheter should be well lubricated with water-soluble lubricant. In some patients with bladder neck obstruction, the lubricant should be instilled into the urethra with a syringe before the catheter is introduced. As the catheter is advanced, there will be a momentary obstruction at the external sphincter. By maintaining gentle pressure on the catheter and keeping the penis perpendicular and taut, the catheter tip will usually overcome the sphincteric spasm and enter the bladder (Fig 52–10).

Before inserting a Foley catheter, the balloon is blown up to check its integrity. It is then deflated and the catheter introduced into the bladder as described above. The balloon is reinflated to the appropriate volume with sterile saline and the catheter connected to a closed drainage system.

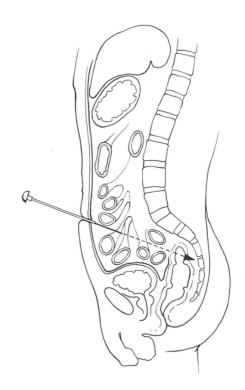

FIG 52–11. Direction of insertion of stylet for abdominal paracentesis.

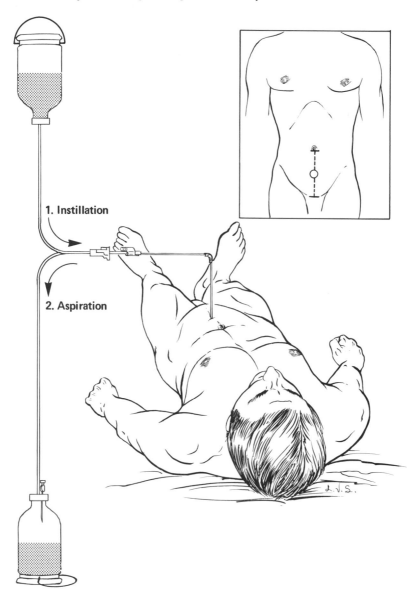

FIG 52–12. Technic of peritoneal lavage.

If there is a tight urethral stricture, it will be necessary to use sounds or filiforms and followers to dilate the area of obstruction.

Catheterization in Females

The genital area is draped and the labia held apart with one hand. The labia and meatus are cleansed with antiseptic solution. With a sterile gloved hand or a clamp, the catheter is introduced and passed into the bladder.

PERITONEAL LAVAGE

Peritoneal lavage is a useful diagnostic test for intra-abdominal bleeding after blunt trauma. It is more accurate than the 2- or 4-quadrant needle aspiration maneuver. The indication for peritoneal lavage is the same as for diagnostic needle aspiration, ie, suspected intra-abdominal bleeding when the physical findings are equivocal. This test is reserved for patients who are conscious and able to cooperate. It is contraindicated in those who are stuporous or unconscious and in patients with previous abdominal surgery, in whom the intestine may be fixed by adhesions. The incidence of false-positive results due to iatrogenic injury to the mesenteric vessels or the bowel is high in these types of patients.

The patient is positioned supine and the lower abdomen prepared aseptically by applying tincture of iodine followed by 70% alcohol. The skin and subcutaneous tissues are infiltrated with local anesthetic at the site of introduction of the dialysis catheter. The most commonly used site is in the lower midline, halfway between the umbilicus and the pubis. The bladder must be empty. The patient is instructed to slightly flex his head and to tighten his anterior abdominal muscles as the catheter with a stylet in place is passed into the peritoneal cavity. A small stab wound in the skin will often facilitate the introduction of the catheter (Fig 52–11). Once the catheter pops through the peritoneum, the stylet is withdrawn and the catheter is advanced gently with caution, aiming it toward the hollow of the sacrum. If blood wells up through the catheter as it is advanced, a positive interpretation for intra-abdominal bleeding is made. The catheter is then withdrawn and the patient prepared for immediate operation.

For the usual test, after positioning the catheter, 1000 ml of normal saline or lactated Ringer's solution is instilled into the peritoneal cavity over a period of 10–15 minutes. Gravity aspiration of the fluid is accomplished by placing the empty infusion bottle on the floor. An air vent is created by inserting a large-bore needle through the top of the empty bottle (Fig 52–12).

A negative test is one in which the fluid returning into the bottle is clear or very slightly tinged with blood. Anything that resembles rosé wine or has a deeper color indicates intra-abdominal bleeding. One should familiarize oneself with the color of the different shades of red as 1, 2, 5, and 10 ml of whole blood are mixed with 1 liter of saline.

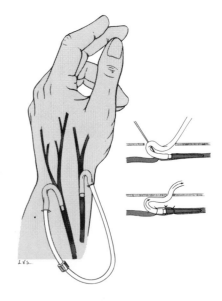

FIG 52–13. Scribner shunt.

INSERTION OF SCRIBNER SHUNT

Scribner shunts are used for hemodialysis in acute renal failure and for administering hyperosmotic nutrient solutions (hyperalimentation). The sites most readily used are at the ankle, where the long saphenous vein and the posterior tibial or anterior tibial arteries can be cannulated, and in the forearm, where the cephalic vein and radial artery can be cannulated.

The patient is placed in the supine position. The operative area is prepared and draped aseptically. Local anesthesia is achieved by infiltration with 1% lidocaine. Longitudinal skin incisions are made over the artery and vein. The vessels are dissected and isolated with 3–0 nonabsorbable sutures. The largest size Teflon cannula tip that will fit into the vessel with ease is selected and connected to a Silastic tube with a reverse U curve at the end. Heparin-saline solution is injected into the tubing and cannula to evacuate the air, and the free end of the Silastic tube is clamped. Through a longitudinal venotomy and arteriotomy, the cannulas are introduced into the vein and artery, respectively. They are secured in place with several ligatures around the vessel and tubing in the manner illustrated (Fig 52–13). The loop of the Silastic tubing is positioned under the skin, avoiding angulation or axial twisting of the vessel. The free ends of the tubing are brought out through separate small skin incisions and are reconnected to each other. A rapid flow should be noted in the arteriovenous connection when the occluding clamps are removed. The operative site is closed with interrupted catgut sutures to the subcutaneous tissue and fine nylon sutures to the skin. Antibiotic ointment is applied around the tubing at its exit sites.

Appendix

CHEMICAL CONSTITUENTS OF BLOOD & BODY FLUIDS

Aldolase, Serum: Normal: 3–8 units/ml (Bruns). Males, < 33 units; females, < 19 units (Warburg and Christian). 0–8 IU/liter.

A. Precautions: Serum should be separated promptly. If there is to be any delay in the determination, the serum should be frozen.

B. Physiologic Basis: Aldolase, also known as zymohexase, splits fructose-1,6-diphosphate to yield dihydroxyacetone phosphate and glyceraldehyde-3-phosphate. Because it is present in higher concentration in tissue cells than in serum, destruction of tissue results in elevation of serum concentration.

C. Interpretation: Elevated levels in serum occur in myocardial infarction, muscular dystrophies, hemolytic anemia, metastatic prostatic carcinoma, leukemia, acute pancreatitis, and acute hepatitis. In obstructive jaundice or cirrhosis of the liver, serum aldolase is normal or only slightly elevated.

Ammonia, Blood: Normal (Conway): 40–70 μg/100 ml whole blood.

A. Precautions: Do not use anticoagulants containing ammonia. Suitable anticoagulants include potassium oxalate, EDTA, and heparin that is ammonia-free. The determination should be done immediately after drawing blood. If the blood is kept in an ice-water bath it may be held for up to 1 hour.

B. Physiologic Basis: Ammonia present in the blood is derived from 2 principal sources: (1) In the large intestine, putrefactive action of bacteria on nitrogenous materials releases significant quantities of ammonia. (2) In the process of protein metabolism, ammonia is liberated. Ammonia entering the portal vein or the systemic circulation is rapidly converted to urea in the liver. Liver insufficiency may result in an increase in blood ammonia concentration, especially if protein consumption is high or if there is bleeding into the bowel.

C. Interpretation: Blood ammonia is elevated in hepatic insufficiency or with liver by-pass in the form of a portacaval shunt, particularly if protein intake is high or if there is bleeding into the bowel.

D. Drug Effects on Laboratory Results: Elevated by methicillin, ammonia cycle resins, chlorthalidone, spironolactone. Decreased by monoamine oxidase inhibitors, oral antimicrobial agents.

Amylase, Serum: Normal: 80–180 Somogyi units/100 ml serum. (One Somogyi unit equals amount of enzyme which will produce 1 mg of reducing sugar from starch at pH 7.2.) 0.8–3.2 IU/liter.

A. Precautions: If storage for more than 1 hour is necessary, blood or serum must be refrigerated.

B. Physiologic Basis: Normally, small amounts of amylase (diastase) originating in the pancreas and salivary glands are present in the blood. Inflammatory disease of these glands or obstruction of their ducts results in regurgitation of large amounts of enzyme into the blood.

C. Interpretation:

1. Elevated in acute pancreatitis, obstruction of pancreatic ducts (carcinoma, stone, stricture, duct sphincter spasm after morphine), mumps, occasionally in the presence of renal insufficiency, occasionally in diabetic acidosis, and occasionally with inflammation of the pancreas from a perforating peptic ulcer. Rarely, combination of amylase with an immunoglobulin produces elevated amylase activity (macroamylasemia).

2. Decreased in hepatitis, acute and chronic; pancreatic insufficiency, and occasionally in toxemia of pregnancy.

D. Drug Effects on Laboratory Results: Elevated by morphine, codeine, meperidine, methacholine, pancreozymin, sodium diatrizoate, cyproheptadine, perhaps by pentazocine, thiazide diuretics. Pancreatitis may be induced by indomethacin, furosemide, chlorthalidone, ethacrynic acid, corticosteroids, histamine, salicylates, and tetracyclines. Decreased by barbiturate poisoning.

Amylase, Urine: Normal: Varies with method. 40–250 Somogyi units/hour.

A. Precautions: If the determination is delayed more than 1 hour after collecting the specimen, urine must be refrigerated.

B. Physiologic Basis: See Amylase, Serum. If renal function is adequate, amylase is rapidly excreted in the urine. A timed urine specimen (ie, 2, 6, or 24 hours) should be collected and the rate of excretion determined.

C. Interpretation: Elevation of the concentration of amylase in the urine occurs in the same situations in which serum amylase concentration is elevated. Urinary amylase concentration remains elevated for up to 7 days after serum amylase levels have returned to normal following an attack of pancreatitis. Thus the determination of urinary amylase may be useful if the patient is seen late in the course of an attack of pancreatitis. An elevated serum amylase with normal or low urine amylase excretory rate may be seen in the presence of renal insufficiency.

Bicarbonate, Serum or Plasma (measured as CO_2 content): Normal: 24—28 mEq/liter or 55—65 vol %.

A. Precautions: Plasma or serum is preferably drawn under oil and handled anaerobically.

B. Physiologic Basis: Bicarbonate-carbonic acid buffer is one of the most important buffer systems in maintaining normal pH of body fluids. Bicarbonate and pH determinations on plasma serve as a basis for assessing "acid-base balance."

C. Interpretation:

1. Elevated in—

(a) Metabolic alkalosis (arterial blood pH increased) due to ingestion of large quantities of sodium bicarbonate, protracted vomiting of acid gastric juice, accompanying potassium deficit.

(b) Respiratory acidosis (arterial blood pH decreased) due to inadequate elimination of CO_2 because of pulmonary emphysema, poor diffusion in alveolar membrane disease, heart failure with pulmonary congestion or edema, ventilatory failure due to any cause, including oversedation, narcotics, or inadequate artificial respiration (elevated P_{CO_2}).

2. Decreased in—

(a) Metabolic acidosis (arterial blood pH decreased) due to diabetic ketosis, starvation, persistent diarrhea, renal insufficiency, ingestion of excess acidifying salts, or salicylate intoxication.

(b) Respiratory alkalosis (arterial blood pH increased) due to hyperventilation (decreased P_{CO_2}).

Bilirubin, Serum: Normal: Direct (glucuronide), 0.1—0.4 mg/100 ml. Indirect (unconjugated), 0.2—0.7 mg/100 ml.

A. Precautions: The fasting state is preferred to avoid turbidity of serum. For optimal stability of stored serum, samples should be frozen and stored in the dark.

B. Physiologic Basis: Destruction of hemoglobin yields bilirubin, which is conjugated in the liver to the diglucuronide and excreted in the bile. Bilirubin accumulates in the plasma when liver insufficiency exists, biliary obstruction is present, or the rate of hemolysis increases. Rarely, abnormalities of enzyme systems involved in bilirubin metabolism in the liver (eg, absence of glucuronyl transferase) result in abnormal bilirubin concentrations.

C. Interpretation:

1. Direct and indirect forms of serum bilirubin are elevated in acute or chronic hepatitis, biliary tract obstruction (cholangiolar, hepatic, or common ducts), toxic reactions to many drugs, chemicals, and toxins, and Dubin-Johnson and Rotor's syndromes.

2. Indirect serum bilirubin is elevated in hemolytic diseases or reactions and absence or deficiency of glucuronyl transferase, as in Gilbert's disease and Crigler-Najjar syndrome.

D. Drug Effects on Laboratory Results: Elevated by acetaminophen, chlordiazepoxide, novobiocin, acetohexamide. Many drugs produce impairment of liver function.

Calcium, Serum: Normal: 9—10.6 mg/100 ml or 4.5—5.3 mEq/liter.

A. Precautions: Glassware must be free of calcium. The patient should be fasting. Serum should be promptly separated from the clot.

B. Physiologic Basis: Endocrine, renal, gastrointestinal, and nutritional factors normally provide for precise regulation of calcium concentration in plasma and other body fluids. Since some calcium is bound to plasma protein, especially albumin, determination of the plasma albumin concentration is necessary before the clinical significance of abnormal serum calcium levels can be interpreted accurately.

C. Interpretation:

1. Elevated in hyperparathyroidism, secretion of parathyroid-like hormone by malignant tumors, vitamin D excess, milk-alkali syndrome, osteolytic disease such as multiple myeloma, invasion of bone by metastatic cancer; Paget's disease of bone, Boeck's sarcoid, and immobilization. Occasionally elevated with hyperthyroidism and with ingestion of thiazide drugs.

2. Decreased in hypoparathyroidism, vitamin D deficiency (rickets, osteomalacia), renal insufficiency, hypoproteinemia, malabsorption syndrome (sprue, ileitis, celiac disease, pancreatic insufficiency), severe pancreatitis with pancreatic necrosis, and pseudohypoparathyroidism.

Calcium, Urine, Daily Excretion: Ordinarily there is a moderate continuous urinary calcium excretion of 50—150 mg/24 hours, depending upon the intake.

A. Procedure: The patient should remain upon a diet free of milk or cheese for 3 days prior to testing; for quantitative testing a neutral ash diet containing about 150 mg calcium per day is given for 3 days. Quantitative calcium excretion studies may be made on a carefully timed 24-hour urine specimen. The screening procedure with the Sulkowitch reagent is simple and useful.

B. Interpretation: On the quantitative diet a normal person secretes 125± 50 mg of calcium per 24 hours. Normally, a slight (1+) cloud reaction (Sulkowitch) occurs if milk and cheese are not present in the diet. In hyperparathyroidism, the urinary calcium excretion usually exceeds 200 mg/24 hours. Urinary calcium excretion is elevated in almost all situations in which serum calcium is high.

Carbon Dioxide Combining Power, Serum or Plasma: Normal: 24—29 mEq/liter or 55—75 vol/100 ml.

Plasma or serum CO_2 combining power is elevated or decreased in the same clinical circumstances as plasma or serum bicarbonate. Anaerobic handling of the specimen is not necessary. The method is the same as for bicarbonate determination except that the serum or plasma is exposed to an "alveolar" air concentration of CO_2 (ie, 40—50 mm Hg partial pressure or 5—6% CO_2) prior to the determination.

See Bicarbonate, above, for interpretation.

Chloride, Serum or Plasma: Normal: 100–106 mEq/ liter or 350–375 mg/100 ml.

A. Precautions: Determination on whole blood yields lower results than those obtained using serum or plasma as the specimen. Always use serum or plasma.

B. Physiologic Basis: Chloride is the principal inorganic anion of the extracellular fluid. It is important in maintenance of acid-base balance even though it exerts no buffer action. When chloride as HCl or NH_4Cl is lost, alkalosis follows; when chloride is retained or ingested, acidosis follows. Chloride (with sodium) plays an important role in control of osmolarity of body fluids.

C. Interpretation:

1. Elevated in renal insufficiency (when Cl intake exceeds excretion), nephrosis (occasionally), renal tubular acidosis, ureterosigmoid anastomosis (reabsorption from urine in gut), dehydration (water deficit), and overtreatment with saline solution.

2. Decreased in gastrointestinal disease with loss of gastric and intestinal fluids (vomiting of acid gastric juice, diarrhea, gastrointestinal suction), renal insufficiency (with salt deprivation), overtreatment with diuretics, chronic respiratory acidosis (emphysema), diabetic acidosis, excessive sweating, adrenal insufficiency (NaCl loss), hyperadrenocorticism (chronic K^+ loss), and metabolic alkalosis ($NaHCO_3$ ingestion; K^+ deficit).

Chloride, Urine:

Urine chloride content varies with dietary intake, acid-base balance, endocrine "balance," body stores of other electrolytes, and water balance. Relationships and responses are so variable and complex that there is little clinical value in urine chloride determinations other than in balance studies.

Cholesterol, Plasma or Serum: Normal: 150–280 mg/100 ml.

A. Precautions: The fasting state is preferred.

B. Physiologic Basis: Cholesterol concentrations are determined by metabolic functions which are influenced by heredity, nutrition, endocrine function, and integrity of vital organs. Cholesterol metabolism is intimately associated with lipid metabolism.

C. Interpretation:

1. Elevated in familial hypercholesterolemia (xanthomatosis), hypothyroidism, poorly controlled diabetes mellitus, nephrotic syndrome, chronic hepatitis, biliary cirrhosis, obstructive jaundice, hypoproteinemia (idiopathic, with nephrosis or chronic hepatitis), and lipemia (idiopathic, familial).

2. Decreased in acute hepatitis and Gaucher's disease, occasionally in hyperthyroidism, acute infections, anemia, malnutrition.

D. Drug Effects on Laboratory Results: Elevated by bromides, anabolic agents, trimethadione, oral contraceptives. Decreased by cholestyramine resin, haloperidol, nicotinic acid, salicylates, thyroid hormone, estrogens, clofibrate, chlorpropamide, phenformin, kanamycin, neomycin, phenyramidol.

Creatine Phosphokinase (CPK), Serum: Normal: Varies with method. 10–50 IU/liter.

A. Precautions: The enzyme is unstable, and the red cell content inhibits enzyme activity. Serum must be removed from the clot promptly. If assay cannot be done soon after drawing blood, serum must be frozen.

B. Physiologic Basis: CPK splits creatine phosphate in the presence of ADP to yield creatine + ATP. Skeletal and heart muscle and brain are rich in the enzyme.

C. Interpretation: Normal values vary with the method.

1. Elevated in the presence of muscle damage such as with myocardial infarction, trauma to muscle, muscular dystrophies, polymyositis, severe muscular exertion, hypothyroidism, and cerebral infarction (necrosis). Following myocardial infarction, serum CPK concentration increases rapidly (within 3–5 hours), and remains elevated for a shorter time after the episode (2 or 3 days) than does GOT or LDH.

2. Not elevated in pulmonary infarction or parenchymal liver disease.

Creatinine, Plasma or Serum: Normal 0.7–1.5 mg/100 ml.

A. Precautions: Other materials than creatinine may react to give falsely high results.

B. Physiologic Basis: Creatinine, which is derived from creatine, is excreted by filtration through the glomeruli of the kidney. Endogenous creatinine is apparently not excreted by renal tubules. Retention of creatinine is thus an index of glomerular insufficiency. Creatinine clearance closely approximates the inulin clearance and is an acceptable measure of filtration rate.

C. Interpretation: Creatinine is elevated in acute or chronic renal insufficiency, urinary tract obstruction, and impairment of renal function induced by some drugs. Values of less than 0.7 mg/100 ml are of no known significance.

D. Drug Effects on Laboratory Results: Elevated by ascorbic acid, barbiturates, sulfobromophthalein, methyldopa, and phenolsulfonphthalein, all of which interfere with the determination of the alkaline picrate method (Jaffe reaction).

Glucose, Plasma, Serum: Normal: Fasting "true" glucose, 65–110 mg/100 ml. Because of the difference in glucose concentration in erythrocytes and plasma, whole blood concentrations will vary depending on the hematocrit.

A. Precautions: If determination is delayed beyond 1 hour, sodium fluoride, about 3 mg/ml blood, should be added to the specimen. The filtrates may be refrigerated for up to 24 hours. Errors in interpretation may occur if the patient has eaten sugar or received glucose solution parenterally just prior to the collection of what is thought to be a "fasting" specimen. Determination of serum or plasma concentration is preferred over whole blood.

B. Physiologic Basis: The glucose concentration in

extracellular fluid is normally closely regulated, with the result that a source of energy is available to tissues and no glucose is excreted in the urine. Hyperglycemia and hypoglycemia are nonspecific signs of abnormal glucose metabolism.

C. Interpretation:

1. Elevated in diabetes mellitus, hyperthyroidism, adrenocortical hyperactivity (cortical excess), hyperpituitarism, and hepatic disease (occasionally).

2. Decreased in hyperinsulinism, adrenal insufficiency, hypopituitarism, hepatic insufficiency (occasionally), functional hypoglycemia, and by hypoglycemic agents.

D. Drug Effects on Laboratory Results: Elevated by corticosteroids, chlorthalidone, thiazide diuretics, furosemide, ethacrynic acid, triamterene, indomethacin, oral contraceptives (estrogen-progestin combinations), isoniazid, nicotinic acid (large doses), phenothiazines, and paraldehyde. Decreased by acetaminophen, phenacetin, cyproheptadine, pargyline, and propranolol.

Iodine, Protein-bound (PBI), Thyroxine (T_4), Serum: Normal: PBI, 4–8 μg/100 ml; T_4 (by column), 2.9–6.4 μg/100 ml; T_4 (by competitive protein binding), 3–7 μg/100 ml.

A. Precautions: Avoid iodine contamination of glassware and the use of iodine on the skin prior to venipuncture. The patient need not be fasting.

B. Physiologic Basis: Thyroid hormone is normally the only organic iodine compound present in blood in significant concentration. The protein-bound iodine is, therefore, a measure of circulating thyroxine. Newer methods of determining thyroxine (by column or by competitive protein binding) eliminates much or all of the interference from other iodine-containing compounds. Free T_4 (that not bound to thyroid-binding globulin) is the metabolically active moiety. The concentration of free T_4 normally is in the range of 0.0016 μg/100 ml serum.

C. Interpretation:

1. Elevated in hyperthyroidism, thyroiditis (during active stage), and pregnancy. Factitiously high levels may result from (1) administration of large doses of thyroid hormone (desiccated thyroid, thyroxine), (2) ingestion of inorganic and organic iodides, and (3) administration of organic iodides used in x-ray diagnostic tests (cholecystograms, urograms, myelograms, bronchograms, uterosalpingograms). These diagnostic compounds may produce elevated iodine levels for 1 year or more.

2. Decreased in hypothyroidism, after use of mercurial diuretics (effect is only of few days' duration), during administration of reserpine, or during administration of triiodothyronine (which suppresses thyroxine production by the thyroid gland).

D. Drug Effects on Laboratory Results: Elevated by sulfobromophthalein, oral contraceptives (estrogen-progestin combinations), estrogens, pyrazinamide, chlormadinone, and Metrecal. Decreased by salicylates, anabolic steroids, progestogens, bishydroxycoumarin,

diphenylhydantoin, para-aminobenzoic acid, tolbutamide, tolazamide, and thiocyanate.

Lactate Dehydrogenase, Serum, Serous Fluids, Spinal Fluid, Urine: Normal: Serum, 200–450 units (Wrobleski), 60–100 units (Wacker), 90–200 IU/liter. Serous fluids, lower than serum. Spinal fluid, 15–75 units (Wrobleski); 6.3–30 IU/liter. Urine, less than 8300 units/8 hours (Wrobleski).

A. Precautions: Any degree of hemolysis must be avoided because the concentration of LDH within red blood cells is 100 times that in normal serum. Heparin and oxalate may inhibit enzyme activity.

B. Physiologic Basis: LDH catalyzes the interconversion of lactate and pyruvate in the presence of NADH or $NADH_2$. It is distributed generally in body cells and fluids.

C. Interpretation: Elevated in all conditions accompanied by tissue necrosis, particularly those involving acute injury of the heart, red cells, kidney, skeletal muscle, liver, lung, and skin. Marked elevations accompany hemolytic anemias, and the anemias of vitamin B_{12} and folate deficiency, and polycythemia rubra vera. The course of rise in concentration over 3–4 days followed by a slow decline during the following 5–7 days may be helpful in confirming the presence of a myocardial infarction; however, pulmonary infarction, neoplastic disease, and megaloblastic anemia must be excluded. Although elevated during the acute phase of infectious hepatitis, enzyme activity is seldom increased in chronic liver disease.

Lipase, Serum: Normal: 0.2–1.5 units.

A. Precautions: None. The specimen may be refrigerated up to 24 hours prior to the determination.

B. Physiologic Basis: A low concentration of fat splitting enzyme is present in circulating blood. In the presence of pancreatitis, pancreatic lipase is released into the circulation in higher concentrations, which persist, as a rule, for a longer period than does the elevated concentration of amylase.

C. Interpretation: Serum lipase is elevated in acute or exacerbated pancreatitis and in obstruction of pancreatic ducts by stone or neoplasm.

Nonprotein Nitrogen (NPN), Blood, Plasma, or Serum: Normal: 15–35 mg/100 ml.

A. Precautions: See Urea, below.

B. Physiologic Basis and Interpretation: See Urea, below, and Creatinine, above.

Phosphatase, Acid, Serum: Normal: Bodansky units, 0.5–2; King-Armstrong, 1–5; Gutman, 0.5–2; Shinowara, 0–1.1; Bessey-Lowry, 0.1–0.63. Females: 0.2–9.5 IU/liter. Males: 0.5–11 IU/liter.

A. Precautions: Avoid hemolysis of the specimen, which releases erythrocyte phosphatase to give factitiously high results. Serum may be refrigerated 24–48 hours prior to determination.

B. Physiologic Basis: Phosphatase active at pH 4.9 is present in high concentrations in the prostate gland and in erythrocytes. In the presence of carcinoma of the prostate which has gone beyond the capsule of the gland or has metastasized, serum acid phosphatase concentration is increased.

C. Interpretation: Increased in carcinoma of the prostate, metastatic or invasive beyond the capsule of the gland, and occasionally in acute myelocytic leukemia.

Phosphatase, Alkaline, Serum: Normal: Bodansky, 2–5 units; King-Armstrong, 5–13 units; Gutman, 3–10 units; Shinowara, 2.2–8.6 units; Bessey-Lowry, children, 2.8–6.7 units; Bessey-Lowry, adults, 0.8–2.3 units. 30–85 IU/liter.

A. Precautions: Serum may be kept in refrigerator 24–48 hours, but values may increase slightly (10%). The specimen will deteriorate if not refrigerated. Do not use fluoride or oxalate.

B. Physiologic Basis: Alkaline phosphatase is present in high concentration in growing bone, in bile, and in the placenta. The phosphatase in serum consists of a mixture of isoenzymes not yet clearly defined. It appears that the enzyme of hepatic origin is resistant to heat; that of osseous origin is sensitive to heat.

C. Interpretation:

1. Elevated in—

a. Children (normal growth of bone).

b. Osteoblastic bone disease—Hyperparathyroidism, rickets and osteomalacia, neoplastic bone disease (osteosarcoma, metastatic neoplasms), ossification as in myositis ossificans, Paget's disease (osteitis deformans), and Boeck's sarcoid.

c. Hepatic duct or cholangiolar obstruction due to stone, stricture, or neoplasm.

d. Hepatic disease resulting from drugs such as chlorpromazine, methyltestosterone.

e. With no clinical correlate to account for an elevated enzyme level in the serum, an indication of the source of the increased concentration may be obtained by measuring activity before and after heating the serum at 56 C for 10 minutes.

Bone: residual activity < 25% of control.

Hepatic: residual activity > 35% of control.

"Normal" or "mixed": residual activity 25–30% of control.

2. Decreased in hypothyroidism and in growth retardation in children.

D. Drug Effects on Laboratory Results: Elevated by acetohexamide, tolazamide, tolbutamide, chlorpropamide, allopurinol, sulfobromophthalein, carbamazepine, cephaloridine, furosemide, methyldopa, phenothiazine, and oral contraceptives (estrogen-progestin combinations).

Phosphorus, Inorganic, Serum: Normal: Children, 4–7 mg/100 ml. Adults, 3–4.5 mg/100 ml or 0.9–1.5 mM/liter.

A. Precautions: Glassware cleaned with phosphate cleaners must be thoroughly rinsed. The fasting state is necessary to avoid postprandial depression of phosphate associated with glucose transport and metabolism.

B. Physiologic Basis: The concentration of inorganic phosphate in circulating plasma is influenced by parathyroid gland function, intestinal absorption, renal function, bone metabolism, and nutrition.

C. Interpretation:

1. Increased in renal insufficiency, hypoparathyroidism, and hypervitaminosis D.

2. Decreased in hyperparathyroidism, hypovitaminosis D (rickets, osteomalacia), malabsorption syndrome (steatorrhea), some forms of renal tubular insufficiency, postprandial state, and after insulin.

Potassium, Serum or Plasma: Normal: 3.5–5 mEq/liter; 14–20 mg/100 ml.

A. Precautions: Avoid hemolysis, which releases erythrocyte potassium. Serum must be separated promptly from the clot or plasma from the red cell mass to prevent diffusion of potassium out of erythrocytes.

B. Physiologic Basis: Potassium concentration in plasma determines the state of neuromuscular and muscular irritability. Elevated or decreased concentrations of potassium impair the capability of muscle to contract.

C. Interpretation:

1. Increased in renal insufficiency (especially in the presence of increased rate of protein or tissue breakdown); adrenal insufficiency; and too rapid administration of potassium salts, especially intravenously and with spironolactone (Aldactone) administration.

2. Decreased in—

a. Inadequate intake (starvation).

b. Inadequate absorption or unusual enteric losses—Vomiting, diarrhea, or malabsorption syndrome.

c. Unusual renal loss—Secondary to hyperadrenocorticism (especially hyperaldosteronism) and to adrenocorticosteroid therapy, metabolic alkalosis, use of diuretics such as chlorothiazide and its derivatives and the mercurials, and renal tubular defects such as the De Toni-Fanconi syndrome and renal tubular acidosis.

d. Abnormal redistribution between extracellular and intracellular fluids—Familial periodic paralysis, testosterone administration.

D. Drug Effects on Laboratory Results: Elevated by triamterene, phenformin. Decreased by degraded tetracycline, phenothiazines, and sodium polystyrenesulfonate resin.

Proteins, Serum or Plasma (Includes Fibrinogen): Normal: See Interpretation, below.

A. Precautions: Serum or plasma must be free of hemolysis. Since fibrinogen is removed in the process of coagulation of the blood, fibrinogen determinations cannot be done on serum.

B. Physiologic Basis: Concentration of protein determines colloidal osmotic pressure of plasma. The concentration of protein in plasma is influenced by the nutritional state, hepatic function, renal function,

TABLE 1. Protein fractions as determined by electrophoresis.

	Percentage of Total Protein
Albumin	52–68
α_1 globulin	2.4–4.4
α_2 globulin	6.1–10.1
β globulin	8.5–14.5
γ globulin	10–21

occurrence of disease such as multiple myeloma, and metabolic errors. Variations in the several fractions of plasma proteins may signify the presence of specific disease.

C. Interpretation:

1. **Total protein, serum**–Normal: 6–8 g/100 ml. See albumin and globulin fractions, below.

2. **Albumin, serum or plasma**–Normal: 3.5–5.5 g/100 ml.

a. **Elevated** in dehydration, shock, hemoconcentration, administration of large quantities of concentrated albumin "solution" intravenously.

b. **Decreased** in malnutrition, malabsorption syndrome, acute or chronic glomerulonephritis, nephrosis, acute or chronic hepatic insufficiency, neoplastic diseases, and leukemia.

3. **Globulin, serum or plasma**–Normal: 1.5–3 g/100 ml.

a. **Elevated** in hepatic disease, infectious hepatitis, cirrhosis of the liver, biliary cirrhosis, and hemochromatosis; disseminated lupus erythematosus; acute or chronic infectious diseases, particularly lymphopathia venereum, typhus fever, leishmaniasis, schistosomiasis, and malaria; multiple myeloma; and Boeck's sarcoid.

b. **Decreased** in malnutrition, congenital agammaglobulinemia, acquired hypogammaglobulinemia, and lymphatic leukemia.

4. **Fibrinogen, plasma**–Normal: 0.2–0.6 g/100 ml.

a. **Elevated** in glomerulonephritis, nephrosis (occasionally), and infectious diseases.

b. **Decreased** in disseminated intravascular coagulation (accidents of pregnancy including placental ablation, amniotic fluid embolism, violent labor, meningococcal meningitis, metastatic carcinoma of the prostate and occasionally of other organs, and leukemia), acute and chronic hepatic insufficiency, and congenital fibrinogenopenia.

Sodium, Serum or Plasma: Normal: 136–145 mEq/ liter.

A. Precautions: Glassware must be completely clean.

B. Physiologic Basis: Sodium constitutes 140 of the 155 mEq of cation in plasma. With its associated anions it provides the bulk of osmotically active solute in the plasma, thus affecting the distribution of body water significantly. A shift of sodium into cells or a

loss of sodium from the body results in a decrease of extracellular fluid volume with consequent effect on circulation, renal function, and nervous system function.

C. Interpretation:

1. **Increased** in dehydration (water deficit), CNS trauma or disease, and hyperadrenocorticism due to hyperaldosteronism or to corticosterone or corticosteroid excess.

2. **Decreased** in adrenal insufficiency; renal insufficiency, especially with inadequate sodium intake; renal tubular acidosis; as a physiologic response to trauma or burns (sodium shift into cells); unusual losses via the gastrointestinal tract, as in acute or chronic diarrhea, intestinal obstruction or fistula, and in unusual sweating with inadequate sodium replacement. In some patients with edema associated with cardiac or renal disease, serum sodium concentration is low even though total body sodium content is greater than normal; water retention and abnormal distribution of sodium between intracellular and extracellular fluid contribute to this paradoxical situation. Hyperglycemia occasionally results in shift of intracellular water to the extracellular space, producing a dilutional hyponatremia.

Transaminase Enzyme Tests, Serum or Serous Fluid: Normal: Glutamic-oxaloacetic transaminase (SGOT), 5–40 units (6–25 IU/liter). Glutamic-pyruvic transaminase (SGPT), 5–35 units (3–26 IU/liter).

A. Precautions: None.

B. Physiologic Basis: Glutamic oxaloacetic transaminase, glutamic pyruvic transaminase, and lactic dehydrogenase are all intracellular enzymes involved in amino acid or carbohydrate metabolism. The enzymes are present in high concentrations in muscle, liver, and brain. Elevations of concentrations of these enzymes in the blood indicate necrosis or disease, especially of these tissues.

C. Interpretation: Elevated in myocardial infarction; acute infections or toxic hepatitis; cirrhosis of the liver; liver neoplasm, metastatic or primary; and in transudates associated with neoplastic involvement of serous cavities. SGOT is elevated in muscular dystrophy, dermatomyositis, and paroxysmal myoglobinuria.

D. Drug Effects on Laboratory Results: Elevated by a host of drugs, including anabolic steroids, androgens, clofibrate, erythromycin (especially estolate) and other antibiotics, isoniazid, methotrexate, methyldopa, phenothiazines, oral contraceptives, salicylates, acetaminophen, phenacetin, indomethacin, acetohexamide, allopurinol, bishydroxycoumarin, carbamazepine, chlordiazepoxide, desimipramine, codeine, morphine, meperidine, tolazamide, propranolol, and guanethidine.

Triglycerides, Serum: Normal: < 165 mg/100 ml.

A. Precautions: Subject must be in a fasting state (preferably for at least 16 hours). The determination may be delayed if the serum is promptly separated from the clot and refrigerated.

B. Physiologic Basis: Dietary fat is hydrolyzed in the small intestine, absorbed and resynthesized by the mucosal cells, and secreted into lacteals in the form of chylomicrons. Triglycerides in the chylomicrons are cleared from the blood by tissue lipoprotein lipase (mainly adipose tissue) and the split products absorbed and stored. Free fatty acids derived mainly from adipose tissue are precursors of the endogenous triglycerides produced by the liver. Transport of endogenous triglycerides is in association with β lipoproteins, the very low density lipoproteins. In order to assure measurement of endogenous triglycerides, blood must be drawn in the postabsorptive state.

C. Interpretation: The concentrations of triglycerides, cholesterol, and the lipoprotein fractions (very low density, low density, and high density) are interpreted collectively. Disturbances in normal relationships of these lipid moieties may be primary or secondary.

1. Elevated (hyperlipoproteinemia)—

a. Primary—Type II hyperbetalipoproteinemia, type III broad beta hyperlipoproteinemia, type I hyperlipoproteinemia (exogenous hyperlipidemia), type IV hyperlipoproteinemia (endogenous hyperlipidemia), and type V hyperlipoproteinemia (mixed hyperlipidemia).

b. Secondary—Hypothyroidism, diabetes mellitus, nephrotic syndrome, chronic alcoholism with fatty liver, ingestion of contraceptive steroids, biliary obstruction, stress.

2. Decreased (hypolipoproteinemia)—

a. Primary—Tangier disease (a-lipoprotein deficiency), abetalipoproteinemia, and a few rare, poorly defined syndromes.

b. Secondary—Malnutrition, malabsorption, and occasionally with parenchymal liver disease.

Urea & Urea Nitrogen, Blood, Plasma, or Serum: Normal: BUN, 8–20 mg/100 ml.

A. Precautions: *Do not use* ammonium oxalate or "double oxalate" as anticoagulant, for the ammonia will be measured as urea (see Method). Do not use too much oxalate, for it will impair urease activity.

B. Physiologic Basis: Urea, an end-product of protein metabolism, is excreted by the kidney. In the glomerular filtrate the urea concentration is the same as in the plasma. Tubular reabsorption of urea varies inversely with rate of urine flow. Thus urea is a less useful measure of glomerular filtration than is creati-

nine, which is not reabsorbed. BUN varies directly with protein intake and inversely with the rate of excretion of urea.

C. Interpretation:

1. Elevated in—

a. Renal insufficiency—Nephritis, acute and chronic; acute renal failure (tubular necrosis), urinary tract obstruction.

b. Increased nitrogen metabolism associated with diminished renal blood flow or impaired renal function—Dehydration from any cause, gastrointestinal bleeding (combination of increased protein absorption from digestion of blood, plus decreased renal blood flow).

c. Decreased renal blood flow—Shock, adrenal insufficiency, occasionally congestive heart failure.

2. Decreased in hepatic failure, nephrosis not complicated by renal insufficiency, and cachexia.

D. Drug Effects on Laboratory Results: Elevated by many antibiotics that impair renal function, guanethidine, methyldopa, indomethacin, isoniazid, propranolol, and potent diuretics (decreased blood volume and renal blood flow).

Uric Acid, Serum or Plasma: Normal: 3–7.5 mg/100 ml.

A. Precautions: If plasma is used, lithium oxalate should be used as the anticoagulant; potassium oxalate may interfere with the determination.

B. Physiologic Basis: Uric acid, an end-product of nucleoprotein metabolism, is excreted by the kidney. Gout, a genetically transmitted metabolic error, is characterized by an increased plasma or serum uric acid concentration, an increase in total body uric acid, and deposition of uric acid in tissues. An increase in uric acid concentration in plasma and serum may accompany increased nucleoprotein catabolism (blood dyscrasias, therapy with antileukemic drugs), thiazide diuretics, or decreased renal excretion.

C. Interpretation:

1. Elevated in gout, toxemia of pregnancy (eclampsia), leukemia, polycythemia, therapy with antileukemic agents, and renal insufficiency.

2. Decreased in acute hepatitis (occasionally), treatment with allopurinol, probenecid.

D. Drug Effects on Laboratory Results: Elevated by thiazide diuretics, ethacrynic acid, spironolactone, furosemide, and triamterene. Decreased by salicylates (small doses), methyldopa, ascorbic acid, clofibrate, phenylbutazone, cinchophen, sulfinpyrazone, and phenothiazines.

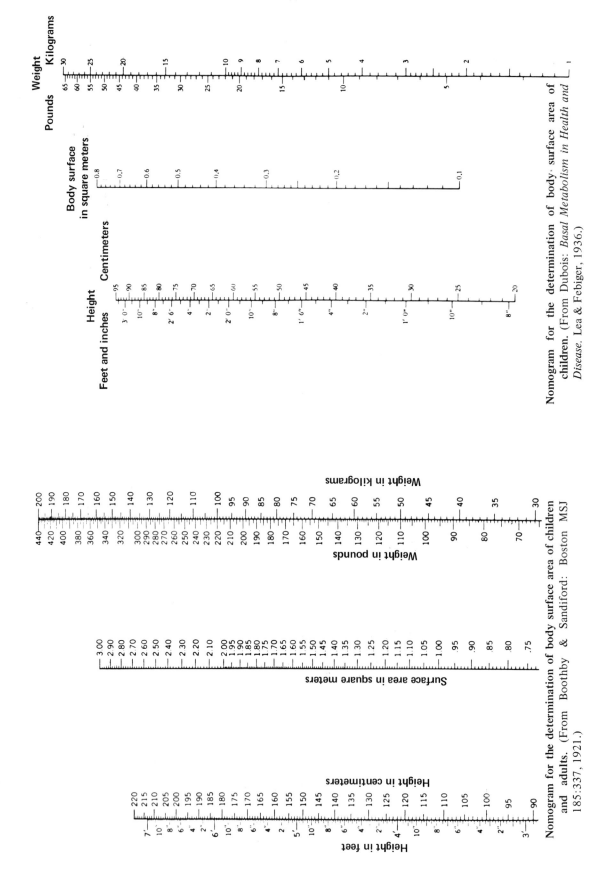

Nomogram for the determination of body surface area of children. (From Dubois: *Basal Metabolism in Health and Disease.* Lea & Febiger, 1936.)

Nomogram for the determination of body surface area of children and adults. (From Boothby & Sandiford: Boston MSJ 185:337, 1921.)

Index